Athletic Injuries and Rehabilitation

Athletic Injuries and Rehabilitation

James E. Zachazewski, MS, PT, SCS, ATC

Supervisor, Outpatient Services
　　Department of Physical Therapy
　　Newton-Wellesley Hospital
　　Newton, Massachusetts
Adjunct, Clinical Assistant Professor,
　　Graduate Programs in Physical Therapy
　　MGH Institute of Health Professions
　　Boston, Massachusetts
Academic Faculty
　　Orthopedic Physical Therapy Program &
　　　　Clinical Residency
　　Kaiser Permanente Medical Center
　　Hayward, California

David J. Magee, PhD, BPT, CAT(C), SPDIII

Professor, Department of Physical Therapy
　　Faculty of Rehabilitation Medicine
　　University of Alberta
　　Edmonton, Alberta, Canada
Consulting Physical Therapist
　　Edmonton Oilers Hockey Club
　　Edmonton Eskimos Football Club
　　Edmonton, Alberta, Canada
Consulting Physical Therapist
　　Glen Sather Sports Medicine Clinic &
　　　　Strathcona Physiotherapy Inc.
　　Edmonton, Alberta, Canada
Team Physical Therapist
　　Canadian Synchronized Swimming Team
　　Synchro Canada
　　Gloucester, Ontario, Canada

William S. Quillen, PhD, PT, SCS

Associate Professor and Chair
　　Department of Physical Therapy
　　College of Mount St. Joseph
　　Cincinnati, Ohio
Physical Therapist
　　Sports Medicine Clinic
　　Children's Hospital Medical Center
　　Cincinnati, Ohio

W.B. SAUNDERS COMPANY
A Division of Harcourt Brace & Company
Philadelphia　London　Toronto　Montreal　Sydney　Tokyo

W.B. SAUNDERS COMPANY
A Division of Harcourt Brace & Company

The Curtis Center
Independence Square West
Philadelphia, Pennsylvania 19106

Library of Congress Cataloging-in-Publication Data

Athletic injuries and rehabilitation / [edited by] James E. Zachazewski, David J. Magee, William S. Quillen.

p. cm.

ISBN 0-7216-4946-7

1. Sports injuries. 2. Sports injuries—Patients—Rehabilitation. 3. Sports physical therapy. I. Zachazewski, James E. II. Magee, David J. III. Quillen, William S.

RD97.A86 1996   617.1'027—dc20
DNLM/DLC   95-23428

Athletic Injuries and Rehabilitation   ISBN 0-7216-4946-7

Printed in the United States of America.

Last digit is the print number: 9 8 7 6 5 4

DEDICATION

To our mentors—our wise and trusted counselors
To you we dedicate this volume with appreciation and thanks

To our students
who gave us purpose and, in reality,
have taught us more
than we have taught them

ACKNOWLEDGMENTS

We would like to gratefully acknowledge the assistance of the following individuals without whom we would have not been able to complete this project.

Margaret M. Biblis–Senior Acquisitions Editor, W.B. Saunders Co.
Scott W. Weaver–Developmental Editor, W.B. Saunders Co.
Bev Aindow–Editorial Assistant to David Magee
Larry Ward–Artist

PREFACE

As society's emphasis on continued physical activity and athletics throughout the lifespan has increased, so have the knowledge and skill required by the community of health care providers involved in managing the related injuries. Our purpose in developing this text was to bring together noted members of the Sports Medicine community (basic scientists, exercise physiologists, physicians, surgeons, nutritionists, psychologists, athletic trainers, and physical therapists) to share their knowledge, expertise, and clinical insight. We believe that by combining the talents of the individuals in each of these disciplines, *ATHLETIC INJURIES AND REHABILITATION* will offer practicing clinicians, as well as students in the advanced stages of their training, a well-referenced resource, written by acknowledged experts who are respected by their peers for both their scientific knowledge and their ability to apply this knowledge in the practice environment.

Contributors to the book hail from the United States, Canada, and Australia. Where possible, we have tried to have chapters written by interdisciplinary teams. Each discipline involved in the Sports Medicine continuum brings a valuable and unique interpretation of the body of knowledge and perspective to working with injured athletes. The basic scientist and exercise physiologist contribute knowledge and insight into the most recent research available concerning the anatomic, physiologic, and pathologic consequences attributable to exercise and athletic injuries. Physician and surgeon contributors provide information on the disease and injury process as well as the diagnostic, medical, and surgical management of injuries associated with this unique population. The physical therapists and athletic trainers who have contributed to this text provide the reader with current information on rehabilitative concerns, methodology, and techniques enabling the athlete to return to participation in the shortest possible time. We hope that our approach of fusing international, interdisciplinary, collegial teams will assist in breaking down the professional "territorial" barriers that all too often exist. We can, and must, share and learn from each other to provide the injured athlete with the most effective, cost-efficient care possible.

All health care providers associated with the care and rehabilitative management of athletic injuries will find valuable in-depth information in this liberally illustrated text. The text is divided into five sections: *Arthrology and Tissue Physiology, Physiology of Rehabilitation, Applied Sport Biomechanics in Rehabilitation, Clinical Considerations and Management,* and *Special Topic Areas.* These divisions were chosen so that information presented occurs in a logical sequence and the reader does not encounter repetition in subsequent sections.

Beginning with the sections *Arthrology and Tissue Physiology* and *Physiology of Rehabilitation,* the framework and scientific basis for the body's normal and pathologic response to injury, exercise, and rehabilitation are presented. The contributing authors effectively show on a conceptual basis how to apply the information contained in the chapters to the clinical environment. Subsequent chapters in the section *Applied Sport Biomechanics in Rehabilitation* present the biomechanical basis of selected sports activities. Normal mechanics of these activities are presented to give the reader further insight into how to avoid injury commonly associated with these activities and how to most appropriately utilize the mechanics in the rehabilitative process. The section entitled *Clinical Considerations and Management* presents state of the art information on the medical, surgical, and rehabilitative management of athletic injuries. This section discusses not only the clinical management of these injuries but also the emergency medical/on-the-field management. The final section, *Special Topic Areas,* focuses on topic areas that enhance the health care providers' knowledge of the care and prevention of athletic injuries associated with special athletic populations.

We believe that *ATHLETIC INJURIES AND REHABILITATION* will prove a valuable resource for students and practicing clinicians from all disciplines because of its comprehensive makeup, topic areas, and interdisciplinary author panel. This text will serve as a valuable resource to assist clinicians in preparing for specialty examinations within their respective fields. It can also provide the basis for formal course work in athletic health care.

We hope that readers will find this text a valuable source of information relevant to their clinical practice and interests. We look forward to feedback from clinicians, teachers, and students from the many disciplines that contribute to Sports Medicine so that we may further develop and improve *ATHLETIC INJURIES AND REHABILITATION*.

James E. Zachazewski
David J. Magee
William S. Quillen

FOREWORD

The Physician's Perspective

The editors of *ATHLETIC INJURIES AND REHABILITATION* have undertaken and completed a very important and much needed project, namely, compiling in one work the pertinent available scientific and clinical information necessary for the education of physical therapists, athletic trainers, and physicians committed to a career in Sports Medicine. This text brings together in one resource valuable information that until now was scattered throughout the medical literature in a variety of subspecialty publications. The editors have assembled a group of superb contributors, representing the disciplines involved in the diagnosis, management, and rehabilitation of athletic injuries. These contributing authors have extensive experience in their respective fields and include well-known experts from the United States, Canada, and Australia.

One of the most helpful features of this text is the large number of photographs, drawings, diagrams, and graphs. In a hands-on field such as Sports Medicine, a picture is indeed worth a thousand words, especially for the busy practitioner. The content of this text is effectively combined to present both the orthopaedist and the primary care provider interested in Sports Medicine with a single resource that includes detailed medical science, practical information regarding the care and rehabilitation of athletic injuries, and medical problems that commonly occur in athletes and other physically active individuals.

In the first section, the editors present the basic scientific material necessary to understand the normal and pathophysiologic changes that occur in bone, ligament, tendon, articular cartilage, muscle, and nerve as a response to trauma. The next section presents the physiologic principles that govern exercise, conditioning, training, and rehabilitation. The third section details the normal and abnormal biomechanics of the most common sports activities (swimming, throwing, running, and cycling) that are often associated with overuse type injuries but are also commonly used for general fitness, conditioning, and rehabilitation. We believe that these sections are important aspects of this text, giving the reader the foundation to understand the underlying nature of athletic injuries and the rationale for the use of specific therapeutic exercise techniques and modalities in the management and rehabilitation of these injuries.

The final two sections of the text contain the clinical material necessary to make an accurate diagnosis of injuries involving specific anatomic areas. What makes this text unique is that the contributing authors take an interdisciplinary approach. The physician authors are indeed among the leaders in their specialties, as are the physical therapists and athletic trainers who have contributed to these sections. The interdisciplinary authorship adds a dimension that is not demonstrated in other texts on athletic injuries. There is useful overlap of material presented in the basic science and clinical chapters that serves to reinforce the basic scientific principles and effectively illustrate the treatment protocols available for a variety of acute and chronic athletic injuries. While the primary focus is on the musculoskeletal injuries commonly associated with athletics, the text goes beyond its title and includes practical chapters on emergency care, dermatology, general medicine, the female athlete, the youthful athlete, nutrition, drugs, and problems due to heat, cold, and altitude.

We would like to congratulate the editors and authors on their accomplishment. We believe that this book will be of great value to all those involved in the care of athletes and that it clearly emphasizes and addresses the need for an interdisciplinary approach in the management of these challenging problems.

Arthur L. Boland, MD
Assistant Clinical Professor of Orthopaedic Surgery
Harvard Medical School

Chief of Orthopaedics
Harvard University Health Services

Head Surgeon
Department of Athletics
Harvard University

Department of Orthopaedic Surgery
Massachusetts General Hospital

Richard H. Strauss, MD
Professor of Preventive and Internal Medicine
The Ohio State University

Editor in Chief
The Physician and Sports Medicine

FOREWORD

Physical Therapist's and Athletic Trainer's Perspective

I'm a physical therapist—you're an athletic trainer—she's a physical therapist and an athletic trainer—he used to be an athletic trainer but now he's a physician's assistant. Sometimes we get way too hung up on credentials, degrees, titles, or how many letters we can tack on after our name. In doing this we tend to forget what our primary focus should be—providing competent, quality health care to the injured athlete.

Sports Medicine is an umbrella term that encompasses many different areas of professional specialization, all of which are in some way related to either enhancing athletic performance or caring for the injured athlete. Exercise physiologists, biomechanists, nutritionists, sport psychologists, strength and conditioning coaches, nurses, physicians, physician's assistants, athletic trainers, and physical therapists can all legitimately claim to be "specialists" in Sports Medicine. Certainly, each of these areas of specialization can make a significant contribution to getting athletes fit for competition, helping them perform to their maximal potential, and guiding them back to competitive levels following injury.

It is essential for all Sports Medicine professionals to realize that a **team approach,** which takes maximal advantage of the collective knowledge, talent, and expertise of all these specialists in a collaborative effort, affords the athlete the optimal conditions for successful performance. The problem that currently seems to exist is that many practitioners in these areas of specialization are still trying to determine exactly how and where they can best fit into the system of health care provision for the athletic population. Unfortunately, in the past there has been far too much effort expended in "turf protection" and "profession bashing" related to areas of common ground, rather than in seeking ways of combining efforts toward a common goal.

The field of Sports Medicine is still in its infancy relative to many other well-established fields in health care. As those of us who call ourselves Sports Medicine professionals struggle to define our position within the scope of our health care system, we must make every effort to expand our knowledge base by engaging in both experimental and clinical research that documents and substantiates the efficacy of various techniques and procedures used when caring for the injured athlete. This collective body of research-based information must be synthesized into scholarly textbooks that serve to define and establish standards by which we choose to practice our specialty.

ATHLETIC INJURIES AND REHABILITATION represents a long-term effort on the part of the three editors to assemble an advanced text, written by professionals from various specializations within the field of Sports Medicine. The contributors to this text are clinicians, educators, and researchers, all of whom have earned respect from their peers and colleagues for their expertise and knowledge. As the body of information pertaining to Sports Medicine continues to grow and expand rapidly, the need arises to integrate this new research-based information into a text that can be used as a reference source. A number of well-done, comprehensive textbooks in Sports Medicine already exist. This particular text is unique, however, in that it is directed at the advanced student or clinician who wishes to gain a more in-depth understanding of the science and theory underlying Sports Medicine practice. The text addresses all aspects of Sports Medicine, including getting the athlete fit and ready to compete and correcting biomechanical faults in performance technique (both of which are essential in injury prevention). Most importantly, it emphasizes techniques for rehabilitation of various injuries sustained by the athlete.

We commend and congratulate the editors, Jim Zachazewski, David Magee, and Sandy Quillen, for their effort in producing a text that can be used as a reference by all of us in the Sports Medicine community regardless of our particular areas of specialization.

Jack Rockwell, MS, PT, ATC
Consultant
HEALTHSOUTH Rehabilitation Corporation
Birmingham, Alabama

Bill Prentice, PhD, PT, ATC
Professor, Coordinator of the Sports Medicine Program
Department of Physical Education, Exercise and Sport Science
Clinical Professor, Division of Physical Therapy
Department of Medical Allied Professions
Associate Professor of Orthopedics
School of Medicine
The University of North Carolina
Chapel Hill, North Carolina

Director of Sports Medicine Education and Fellowship Programs
HEALTHSOUTH Rehabilitation Corporation
Birmingham, Alabama

Ron Peyton, MS, PT, ATC
President
Dogwood Institute
Atlanta, Georgia

CONTRIBUTORS

Richard T. Abadie, Jr., BA, EMC
Equipment Manager, Certified
　Department of Athletics
　University of Virginia
　Charlottesville, Virginia
Protective Equipment Considerations

Jeffrey M. Anderson, MD
Director of Sports Medicine
　University of Connecticut
　Storrs, Connecticut
Emergency Care of the Injured Athlete

Mark A. Anderson, PhD, PT, ATC
Associate Professor and Director of Graduate Studies
　Department of Physical Therapy
　College of Allied Health
　University of Oklahoma Health Sciences Center
　Oklahoma City, Oklahoma
Return to Competition: Functional Rehabilitation

James R. Andrews, MD
Medical Director
　American Sports Medicine Institute

Orthopaedic Surgeon
　Alabama Sports Medicine and Orthopaedic Center
　Birmingham, Alabama

Clinical Professor, Orthopaedics and Sports Medicine
　University of Virginia
　Charlottesville, Virginia
Biomechanics of Throwing

Elizabeth A. Arendt, MD
Assistant Professor of Orthopaedics
　Director, Sports Medicine Institute
　Department of Orthopaedic Surgery
　University of Minnesota Medical School

Medical Director and Orthopaedic Consultant
　Varsity Athletic Teams
　University of Minnesota
　Minneapolis, Minnesota
The Female Athlete

William D. Bandy, PhD, PT, SCS, ATC
Associate Professor
　Department of Physical Therapy

University of Central Arkansas
　Conway, Arkansas
Adaptability of Skeletal Muscle: Response to Increased and Decreased Use

Arnold T. Bell, PhD, PT, SCS, ATC
Associate Professor of Physical Therapy
　Division of Physical Therapy
　Florida A & M University

Rehabilitation Specialist
　Department of Intercollegiate Athletics
　Florida A & M University
　Tallahassee, Florida
The Use of Ergogenic Aids in Athletics

T. A. Blackburn, MEd, PT, ATC
Adjunct Assistant Professor
　University of Miami School of Medicine
　Physical Therapy Program
　Miami, Florida

Co-Founder and Director
　Berkshire Institute of Orthopaedic and Sports
　　Physical Therapy, Inc.
　Wyomissing, Pennsylvania
Preparticipation Sports Physicals

Cal Botterill, PhD
Professor
　Department of Physical Activity and Sport Studies
　University of Winnipeg
　Winnipeg, Manitoba, Canada
Psychology of the Injured Athlete

David Butler, BPHTY, GDAMT
Lecturer
　School of Physiotherapy
　University of South Australia
　South Australia, Australia
Nerve: Structure, Function, and Physiology

Daniel J. Cipriani, MEd, PT
Associate Professor
　The Medical College of Ohio School of Allied Health
　Department of Physical Therapy
　Toledo, Ohio
Physiologic Principles of Resistance Training and Rehabilitation

Mark W. Cornwall, PhD, PT

Associate Professor
Department of Physical Therapy
Northern Arizona University
Flagstaff, Arizona

Applied Sports Biomechanics in Rehabilitation: Running

Ron Courson, PT, ATC, NREMT

Instructor
School of Exercise Science
University of Georgia

Director of Sports Medicine
University of Georgia Athletic Association
Athens, Georgia

Pharmacology and Drugs in Sports: Common Use, Abuse, and Testing

Susan Cummings, MS, RD

Assistant Professor
MGH Institute of Health Professions

Clinical Dietitian
Massachusetts General Hospital
Boston, Massachusetts

Nutritional Concerns in Athletes

Kathleen A. Curtis, PhD, PT

Associate Professor
Department of Physical Therapy
California State University
Fresno, California

The Athlete With a Disability

Sandra L. Curwin, BSc(Physio), MSc, PhD

Director and Associate Professor
Husson College
Bangor, Maine

Tendon Injuries: Pathophysiology and Treatment

Bruce H. Dick, MD, FACSM

Associate Professor of Family Medicine
Albany Medical College
Albany, New York

Head Physician, US Field Hockey Association
Colorado Springs, Colorado

Director of Sports Medicine
Siena College
Loudonville, New York

Emergency Care of the Injured Athlete

Caroline D. Drye, MS, PT

Clinical Instructor
PT Residency Program in Advanced Orthopaedic
Manual Therapy
Kaiser Hospital

Hayward, California

Peripheral Nerve Injuries

Kim Dunleavy, MS, PT, OCS

Assistant Professor
Department of Physical Therapy
Wayne State University
Detroit, Michigan

Adaptability of Skeletal Muscle: Response to Increased and Decreased Use

Daniel A. Dyrek, MS, PT

Assistant Professor
Graduate Programs in Physical Therapy
MGH Institute of Health Professions
Boston, Massachusetts

President
Orthopaedic Physical Therapy Services
Wellesley, Massachusetts

Injuries to the Thoracolumbar Spine and Pelvis

Rafael F. Escamilla, PhD

Biomechanist
American Sports Medicine Institute
Birmingham, Alabama

Biomechanics of Throwing

Jeffrey E. Falkel, PhD, PT, CSCS

Golfcordz, Inc.
Highlands Ranch, Colorado

Physiologic Principles of Resistance Training and Rehabilitation

Glenn S. Fleisig, PhD

Director of Research
American Sports Medicine Institute
Birmingham, Alabama

Biomechanics of Throwing

Frances A. Flint, PhD, ATC

Coordinator
Sport Therapy Certificate Program
York University School of Physical Education
North York, Ontario, Canada

Psychology of the Injured Athlete

Susan Foreman, MEd, MPT, ATC

Instructor
Curry School of Education

Instructor of Orthopaedic Surgery
University of Virginia

Associate Athletic Trainer
Department of Athletics
University of Virginia
Charlottesville, Virginia

Protective Equipment Considerations

Terri L. Foreman, MS, PT, SCS

Adjunct Assistant Professor
  Department of Physical Therapy
  College of Allied Health
  University of Oklahoma Health Sciences Center
  Oklahoma City, Oklahoma

Clinical Manager, START Center
  South Tulsa Advanced Rehabilitation Therapy
  Tulsa Regional Medical Center
  Tulsa, Oklahoma

Return to Competition: Functional Rehabilitation

Eileen Fowler, PhD, PT

Adjunct Assistant Professor
  Department of Orthopedic Surgery
  School of Medicine
  University of California, Los Angeles
  Los Angeles, California

Biomechanics of Cycling

C. B. Frank, MD, FRCS(C)

Professor and Alberta Heritage Scientist
  Department of Surgery
  University of Calgary

Research and Clinical Director
  Sports Medicine Center
  University of Calgary
  Calgary, Alberta, Canada

Ligament Injuries: Pathophysiology and Healing

Beau J. Freund, PhD

Research Physiologist
  U.S. Army Research Institute of Environmental
    Medicine
  Natick, Massachusetts

Environmental Considerations for Exercise

Freddie H. Fu, MD

Blue Cross Professor of Orthopaedic Surgery

Executive Vice Chairman and Professor
  Department of Orthopaedic Surgery
  University of Pittsburgh School of Medicine

Medical Director, Center for Sports Medicine
  University of Pittsburgh Medical Center
  Pittsburgh, Pennsylvania

The Knee: Ligamentous and Meniscal Injuries

John Fulkerson, MD

Clinical Professor of Orthopaedic Surgery
  University of Connecticut Medical School
  Farmington, Connecticut

Staff Physician
  University of Connecticut Health Center
  Hartford Hospital

Hartford, Connecticut

The Knee: Patellofemoral and Soft Tissue Injuries

Robert S. Gailey, Jr., MSEd, PT

Instructor, Division of Physical Therapy
  Department of Orthopedics
  University of Miami School of Medicine
  Coral Gables, Florida

The Athlete With a Disability

William E. Garrett, Jr., MD, PhD

Professor of Surgery
  Division of Orthopaedic Surgery
  Duke University
  Durham, North Carolina

Muscle: Deformation, Injury, Repair

Gary Geissler, MS, PT ATC, SCS

Adjunct Faculty
  Sargent College, Boston University, and Graduate
    Programs of Physical Therapy
  MGH Institute of Health Professions
  Boston, Massachusetts

Clinical Director of Rehabilitation
  Department of Intercollegiate Athletics
  Harvard University
  Cambridge, Massachusetts

Traumatic Injuries to the Cervical Spine

Joe H. Gieck, EdD, PT, ATC

Professor of Clinical Orthopaedics
  Curry School of Education
  Head Athletic Trainer, Department of Athletics
  University of Virginia
  Charlottesville, Virginia

Hand and Wrist Injuries

Robert J. Gregor, PhD

Professor
  Department of Health and Performance Science
  Georgia Institute of Technology
  Emory University
  Atlanta, Georgia

Biomechanics of Cycling

Peter Grigg, PhD

Professor of Physiology
  University of Massachusetts Medical School
  Worcester, Massachusetts

Articular Neurophysiology

Don Groot, MD, FRCP(C), FACP

Associate Clinical Professor of Medicine
  University of Alberta

Active Staff, Royal Alexandra Hospital

Team Physician and Dermatologist
Edmonton Oilers Hockey Club
Edmonton, Alberta, Canada
Dermatologic Considerations in Athletics

Brian Halpern, MD

Clinical Assistant Professor of Sports Medicine

Fellowship Director, Sports Medicine
Robert Wood Johnson School of Medicine
University of Medicine & Dentistry of New Jersey
New Brunswick, New Jersey

Assistant Attending Physician
Hospital for Special Surgery
New York Hospital
Cornell Medical Center
New York, New York
Preparticipation Sports Physicals

Donald H. Hangen, MD

Instructor in Orthopaedic Surgery
Harvard Medical School
Boston, Massachusetts

Associate
Orthopaedic Associates of Marlborough
Marlborough, Massachusetts
Traumatic Injuries to the Cervical Spine

Omar D. Hussamy, MB, BChir, MD

Division of Sports Medicine and Hand Surgery
University of Virginia School of Medicine
Charlottesville, Virginia
Hand and Wrist Injuries

Lydia Ievleva, PhD

Lecturer in Sport Psychology
Department of Sport Studies
University of Western Sydney, Macarthur
Bankstown Campus
Australia
Psychology of the Injured Athlete

Brian Incremona, MD

Clinical Instructor
University of Medicine & Dentistry of New Jersey
Piscataway, New Jersey

Director of Sports Medicine
Rutgers, The State University of New Jersey
New Brunswick, New Jersey
Preparticipation Sports Physicals

James J. Irrgang, MS, PT, ATC

Assistant Professor and Vice Chair
Clinical Department of Physical Therapy
University of Pittsburgh School of Health
and Rehabilitation Sciences

Director of Physical Therapy
University of Pittsburgh Medical Center
Pittsburgh, Pennsylvania
The Knee: Ligamentous and Meniscal Injuries

Frank W. Jobe, MD

Clinical Professor, Department of Orthopaedics
University of Southern California
School of Medicine
Los Angeles, California

Associate
Kerlan-Jobe Orthopaedic Clinic
Inglewood, California
Biomechanics of Swimming

Patricia Johnston, MClSc, MBA

President
InForum
Edmonton, Alberta, Canada
Dermatologic Considerations in Athletics

John P. Kelly, DMD, MD, FACS

Chairman and Associate Professor
Oral and Maxillofacial Surgery
State University of New York at Stony Brook
Stony Brook, New York

Chief of Oral and Maxillofacial Surgery
Long Island Jewish Medical Center
New Hyde Park, New York
Maxillofacial Injuries

James J. Kinderknecht, MD

Clinical Assistant Professor
Family and Community Medicine

Assistant Team Physician
Department of Intercollegiate Athletics
University of Missouri
Columbia, Missouri
Head Injuries

Barbara J. Loitz-Ramage, PhD, PT

Assistant Professor
Department of Kinesiology
University of Wisconsin
Madison, Wisconsin
Bone Biology and Mechanics

David J. Magee, PhD, BPT, MS, SPDIII, CAT(C)

Professor
Department of Physical Therapy
Faculty of Rehabilitation Medicine
University of Alberta
Edmonton, Alberta, Canada

The Process of Athletic Injury and Rehabilitation
Injuries to the Thoracolumbar Spine and Pelvis
Shoulder Injuries
Leg, Foot, and Ankle Injuries

Terry R. Malone, EdD, PT, ATC

Associate Professor and Director of Physical Therapy
University of Kentucky
Lexington, Kentucky

Muscle: Deformation, Injury, Repair

Jenny McConnell, B App Sci, GDMT, M Biomed Eng

Director
McConnell Institute
Mossman, NSW
Australia

The Knee: Patellofemoral and Soft Tissue Injuries

Frank C. McCue, III, MD

Alfred R. Shands Professor of Orthopaedic Surgery
and Plastic Surgery of the Hand

Professor of Plastic Surgery

Director, Division of Sports Medicine & Hand
Surgery
School of Medicine

Professor of Education
Curry School of Education

Team Physician
Department of Intercollegiate Athletics
University of Virginia
Charlottesville, Virginia

Hand and Wrist Injuries

William H. McDonald, BS, MA

Head Athletic Trainer
The University of Alabama
Tuscaloosa, Alabama

Pharmacology and Drugs in Sports: Common Use, Abuse,
and Testing

Paula F. McFadyen, MSc

Senior Laboratory Instructor
Department of Physical Education
University of Victoria
Victoria, British Columbia, Canada

Physiologic Principles of Conditioning

Ross McFadyen, BSc

Director
Yates Orthopedic and Sports Physiotherapy Clinic
Victoria, British Columbia, Canada

Physiologic Principles of Conditioning

Thomas G. McPoil, PhD, PT, ATC

Professor
Department of Physical Therapy
Northern Arizona University
Flagstaff, Arizona

Applied Sports Biomechanics in Rehabilitation: Running

Lyle J. Micheli, MD

Associate Clinical Professor of Orthopaedic Surgery
Harvard Medical School

Director, Division of Sports Medicine
Children's Hospital
Boston, Massachusetts

Injuries to the Thoracolumbar Spine and Pelvis

Scott J. Montain, PhD

Research Physiologist
U.S. Army Research Institute of Environmental
Medicine
Natick, Massachusetts

Environmental Considerations for Exercise

Aurelia Nattiv, MD

Assistant Clinical Professor
Division of Family Medicine
Department of Orthopaedic Surgery
School of Medicine
University of California, Los Angeles

Assistant Team Physician
UCLA Department of Intercollegiate Athletics
Los Angeles, California

The Female Athlete

William C. Nemeth, MD

Clinical Associate Professor
Southwest Texas State University
Hill Country Sports Medicine
San Marcos, Texas

Hip and Thigh Injuries

Andrew W. Nichols, MD

Associate Professor
Family Practice and Community Health
John A. Burns School of Medicine

Head Team Physician
Department of Intercollegiate Athletics
University of Hawaii at Manoa
Honolulu, Hawaii

Abdominal and Thoracic Injuries

Robert P. Nirschl, MD, MS

Associate Clinical Professor of Orthopedic Surgery
    Georgetown University Medical Center
    Washington, D.C.

Fellowship Director, Nirschl Orthopedic Fellowship
    Program
    Nirschl Orthopedic Sports Medicine Clinic
    Arlington, Virginia

Elbow Injuries

Marilyn M. Pink, PhD, PT

Director
    Biomechanics Laboratory
    Centinela Hospital Medical Center
    Inglewood, California

Biomechanics of Swimming

James C. Puffer, MD

Professor and Chief
    Division of Family Medicine
    University of California, Los Angeles,
        School of Medicine

Chief of Service
    Family Medicine
    UCLA Medical Center
    Los Angeles, California

Medical Problems in Athletes

William S. Quillen, PhD, PT, SCS

Associate Professor and Chair
    Department of Physical Therapy
    College of Mount St. Joseph
    Cincinnati, Ohio

The Process of Athletic Injury and Rehabilitation

**David C. Reid, MD, BPT, MCh(Orth), MCSP,
MCPA, FRCS(C)**

Professor
    Department of Surgery
    Faculty of Medicine

Director
    Glen Sather Sports Medicine Clinic
    University of Alberta
    Edmonton, Alberta, Canada

Shoulder Injuries

Mary Jane Rewinski, RD, BS

Clinical Dietitian
    Massachusetts General Hospital
    Boston, Massachusetts

Nutritional Concerns in Athletes

Rich Riehl, ATC

Head Athletic Trainer
    Pepperdine University
    Malibu, California

The Female Athlete

James B. Robinson, MD

Associate Clinical Professor
    Family Practice and Sports Medicine
    College of Community Health Sciences

Medical Director
    DCH Sports Medicine

Team Physician
    Department of Athletics
    The University of Alabama
    Tuscaloosa, Alabama

*Pharmacology and Drugs in Sports: Common Use, Abuse,
and Testing*

Marc R. Safran, MD

Assistant Clinical Professor
    Department of Orthopaedic Surgery
    University of California, San Diego

Associate
    Alvarado Orthopaedic Medical Group
    San Diego, California

The Knee: Ligamentous and Meniscal Injuries

Ethan Saliba, PhD, ATC, PT, SCS

Assistant Professor
    Curry School of Education

Assistant Professor
    Orthopedic Surgery
    University of Virginia

Senior Associate Athletic Trainer
    Department of Intercollegiate Athletics
    University of Virginia
    Charlottesville, Virginia

Protective Equipment Considerations

Barbara Sanders, PhD, PT, SCS

Associate Professor
    Department of Physical Therapy
    Southwest Texas State University

Consultant
    Institute for Sports Medicine and Human
        Performance
    Southwest Texas State University
    San Marcos, Texas

Hip and Thigh Injuries

Clyde Smith, BSc, DPT, SPDIII

Clinical Instructor
  Department of Family Practice
  University of British Columbia

Senior Physiotherapist
  Allan McGavin Sports Medicine Centre
  Physiotherapy Division
  University of British Columbia
  Vancouver, British Columbia, Canada

Leg, Foot, and Ankle Injuries

Janet Sobel, BS, PT

Clinical Coordinator
  Suburban Physical Medicine Center
    at Chevy Chase
  Chevy Chase, Maryland

Elbow Injuries

William T. Stauber, PhD

Professor
  Departments of Physiology and Neurology
  Division of Physiotherapy
  West Virginia University
  Morgantown, West Virginia

Delayed-Onset Muscle Soreness and Muscle Pain

Jack Taunton, BSc(Kin), MSc, MD

Professor
  Department of Family Practice
  School of Human Kinetics
  University of British Columbia

Co-Director
  Allan McGavin Sports Medicine Centre
  Vancouver, British Columbia, Canada

Leg, Foot, and Ankle Injuries

Lori A. Thein, MS, PT, SCS, ATC

Associate Lecturer
  Department of Kinesiology
  Program in Physical Therapy

Clinical Specialist
  University of Wisconsin Clinics, Research Parks
  Madison, Wisconsin

The Young and Adolescent Athlete

Joan M. Walker, PhD

Professor
  School of Physiotherapy
  Dalhousie University
  Halifax
  Nova Scotia, Canada

Cartilage of Human Joints and Related Structures

Steve Weintraub, DO, BS

Clinical Instructor
  Primary Care Sports Medicine Fellowship
  Robert Wood Johnson University Hospital
  New York College of Osteopathic Medicine

Attending Physician, Family Practice
  Helene Full Medical Center

Consulting Physician, Orthopaedics
  Medical Center of Ocean County
  Bricktown, New Jersey

Preparticipation Sports Physicals

Howard A. Wenger, PhD

Professor
  University of Victoria
  Victoria
  British Columbia, Canada

Physiologic Principles of Conditioning

Kenneth E. Wright, DA, ATC

Associate Professor and Director
  Athletic Training Education
  The University of Alabama
  Tuscaloosa, Alabama

Pharmacology and Drugs in Sports: Common Use, Abuse, and Testing

James E. Zachazewski, MS, PT, SCS, ATC

Adjunct, Assistant Clinical Professor
  Graduate Programs of Physical Therapy
  MGH Institute of Health Professions
  Boston, Massachusetts

Academic Faculty
  Orthopaedic Physical Therapy Program and
    Clinical Residency
  Kaiser Permanente Medical Center
  Hayward, California

Supervisor, Outpatient Services
  Department of Physical Therapy
  Newton-Wellesley Hospital
  Newton, Massachusetts

The Process of Athletic Injury and Rehabilitation
Muscle: Deformation, Injury, Repair
Traumatic Injuries to the Cervical Spine
Peripheral Nerve Injuries

Ronald F. Zernicke, PhD

Professor and Heritage Medical Scholar
  Department of Surgery
  Faculties of Medicine, Engineering, and Kinesiology
  University of Calgary
  Calgary, Alberta, Canada

Bone Biology and Mechanics

CONTENTS

SECTION II

Physiology of Rehabilitation

CHAPTER 11

Physiological Principles of Conditioning 189

Howard A. Wenger PhD
Paula F. McFadyen MSc
Ross McFadyen BSc, PT

CHAPTER 12

Physiologic Principles of Resistance
Training and Rehabilitation 206

Jeffrey E. Falkel PhD, PT, CSCS
Daniel J. Cipriani MEd, PT

CHAPTER 13

Return to Competition:
Functional Rehabilitation 229

Mark A. Anderson PhD, PT, ATC
Terri L. Foreman MS, PT, SCS

CHAPTER 14

Environmental Considerations for Exercise 262

Scott J. Montain PhD
Beau J. Freund PhD

SECTION III

Applied Sport Biomechanics in Rehabilitation

CHAPTER 16

CHAPTER 17

CHAPTER 24

Daniel A. Dyrek MS, PT
Lyle J. Micheli MD, FAAOS, FACSM
David J. Magee BPT, PhD, MS

CHAPTER 25

Andrew W. Nichols MD

CHAPTER 26

David J. Magee PhD, BPT, MSc, SPD III, CAT (C)
David C. Reid MD, MCh (Ortho)

CHAPTER 27

Janet Sobel PT
Robert P. Nirschl MD, MS

CHAPTER 28

Hand and Wrist Injuries 585

Frank C. McCue III MD
Omar D. Hussamy MB, B Chir, MD
Joe H. Gieck EdD, PT, ATC

CHAPTER 29

Hip and Thigh Injuries 599

Barbara Sanders PhD, PT, SCS
William C. Nemeth MD

CHAPTER 30

The Knee: Ligamentous and Meniscal Injuries 623

James J. Irrgang MS, PT, ATC
Marc R. Safran MD
Freddie H. Fu MD

CHAPTER 38

Brian Halpern MD
T. A. Blackburn MEd, PT, ATC
Brian Incremona MD
Steve Weintraub DO, BS

CHAPTER 39

Susan Cummings MS, RD
Mary Jane Rewinski BS, RD

CHAPTER 40

Ethan Saliba PhD, ATC, PT, SCS
Susan Foreman MEd, MPT, ATC
Richard T. Abadie, Jr. BA, EMC

CHAPTER 41

Lori A. Thein MS, PT, SCS, ATC

CHAPTER 42

The Athlete With a Disability 959

Kathleen A. Curtis PhD, PT
Robert S. Gailey, Jr. MSEd, PT

CHAPTER 43

Pharmacology and Drugs in Sports:
Common Use, Abuse, and Testing 981

Ron Courson ATC, PT, NREMT
William H. McDonald MA, ATC
James B. Robinson MD
Kenneth E. Wright DA, ATC

Arthrology and Tissue Physiology

CHAPTER 1

The Process of Athletic Injury and Rehabilitation

WILLIAM S. QUILLEN *PhD, PT, SCS*
DAVID J. MAGEE *PhD, PT, CAT(C), SPD III*
JAMES E. ZACHAZEWSKI *MS, PT, ATC, SCS*

Sports and recreational pursuits constitute a major element of the structure of most societies. Individuals have competed athletically both against themselves and against others throughout recorded history and, as a result, have sustained injuries during preparatory practice or actual competition. The study, diagnosis, and management of these injuries have evolved into the multidisciplinary field of sports medicine, involving physicians, therapists (both physical and athletic), sports scientists, and other health care professionals who have an interest in the area of sports injury prevention and care. Thus, a multitude of health care professionals, researchers, and educators devote all or part of their respective professional careers and practices toward the prevention, treatment, and rehabilitation of athletic injuries and the return of the individual to the highest level of activity possible.[1-15]

Prevention can often be the key to lessening the chance of injury. Proper progression, intensity, timing, and loading can lead to a decrease in injuries, especially those resulting from overuse. Although prevention has long been a topic for discussion, little has been done in this area. This attitude is gradually changing as prevention is being accepted as one of the essentials of the care continuum.

The goal of treatment of athletic injury has been the restoration of athletic function, to the greatest degree possible, in the shortest time possible.[3-5,8,14,16-20] The safe and successful return of an athlete to his or her preinjury level of performance remains the desired outcome for any sports medicine practitioner. Scientifically based practice, focused on managing the time course of initial inflammatory reaction and subsequent healing processes, recognizing the healing constraints of neuromusculoskeletal soft tissues, and based on an appreciation of joint mechanics, performance physiology, and psychology of the athlete regarding the injury, has hastened the resolution of many injuries.[8,21]

EPIDEMIOLOGY OF INJURY

The incidence of athletic injury continues to rise in competitive athletics and among the general population because of the continued emphasis upon fitness as a preventive medicine measure.[22-25] Specific sports activity as well as age, sex, and physical condition of the participant may contribute to the incidence and severity of injuries. Broadly defined, an athletic injury is (1) any injury that is sports or physical activity related and results in keeping the individual out of practice, activity, or competition on the day following the injury; or (2) any injury requiring medical attention.[24]

Injuries may be considered either acute or chronic, resulting from macrotraumatic or microtraumatic forces. Macrotraumatic injuries are those involving sudden direct or indirect trauma causing immediately noticeable injury, including sprains, strains, dislocations, and fractures, to various structures of the body. The microtraumatic category of injury is often collectively referred to as overuse syndromes and today may be as common in

TABLE 1–1
Ten Most Common Sites of Athletic Injuries in Adults

Women		Men	
Injury Site	%	*Injury Site*	%
Knee	29	Knee	27
Ankle	10	Ankle	10
Lower back	9	Lower back	9
Lower leg	6	Lower leg	7
Metatarsal region	3	Achilles tendon	7
Toes	3	Lower leg	4
Calf	3	Hip	3
Achilles tendon	3	Elbow	3
Sole	2	Heel	3
Hip	2	Calf	3

From Kannus P, Niitymakis S, Jarvinen M: Sports injuries in women. Br J Sports Med 1987; 21:37–39.

TABLE 1–2
Common Athletic Injuries Involving Neuromusculoskeletal Tissues

Osseous	Soft Tissue	Nerve
Fractures	Contusion	Neurapraxia
Closed	Hemorrhage	Axonotmesis
Open	Hematoma	
Comminuted	Strain	
Avulsion	Sprain	
Incomplete	Myositis ossificans	
Torus	Tenosynovitis	
Greenstick	Bursitis	
Bow	Osteochondritis	
Physical		
Stress		
Pathologic		
Dislocation		
Subluxation		

children as in adults.[25] By definition, an overuse injury is defined as a "long-standing or recurrent musculoskeletal problem that was not initiated by an acute (macrotraumatic) injury."[25] Continued use or overuse, often in an incorrect manner or as a compensatory mechanism because of macrotrauma in another area, will lead to injury if not corrected soon enough.

Athletic injuries most often involve the musculoskeletal system.[26] In children, many acute injuries result in fractures of the growth plate or avulsion at the physis, as these areas are weaker than the bone itself. Injuries experienced by adults are clustered in the joints of the lower extremity, with the knee being the anatomic region most commonly involved (Table 1–1).[23] In sports involving the upper limb, the shoulder, because of its extensive mobility and minimal inherent stability, is the primary focus of injuries.

Certain types of injuries are more prevalent in different populations as lifetime sports and fitness activity increases. For example, Matheson et al.[22] reviewed sports-related injuries in a large series of both young and older patients presenting to a sports medicine clinic. They found that the older population suffered from certain types of injuries more frequently (for example, metatarsalgia, plantar fasciitis, and degenerative meniscal lesions). However, they found no clear relationship between the injury and the given sport, fitness, or activity type.

CATEGORIES OF ATHLETIC INJURIES

As previously stated, the majority of athletic injuries involve the neuromusculoskeletal system. Common osseous, soft tissue, and nerve injuries are summarized in Table 1–2.[22] Fractures are simply a complete or incomplete loss of continuity of bone or cartilage, or both. A variety of descriptions have been applied to further delineate the degree of discontinuity or specific structure involved.[26,27] Joint injuries primarily involve dislocations and subluxations. Soft tissue injuries include trauma to skin (e.g., laceration, abrasion), underlying tissue (e.g., contusion), fascia (e.g., fasciitis),

musculotendinous units (e.g., strains, tendinitis), and ligaments (e.g., sprains). Most often, they are clinically assessed as mild, moderate, or severe (grades I to III) based upon severity and extent of loss of structural integrity.[1,12,26] These injuries primarily result from macrotraumatic forces imposed upon the body. They are among the most frequent injuries experienced by sports participants and are the classic "lumps, bumps, and bruises" whose morbidity is frequently disproportionate to the injury severity.[21,28] Microtraumatic injuries involve osseous and musculotendinous structures and result from the repetitive overloading of the body associated with continuous training or competition.[22,23,25] Injuries to the peripheral or central nervous system usually result from macrotraumatic forces and those involving the central nervous system and are potentially catastrophic or life-threatening.

A complete taxonomy of athletic injury descriptions may be found in the American Medical Association's *Standard Nomenclature of Athletic Injuries*.[29] As Rachun has stated:

> fundamental to an increasingly sophisticated health supervision of sports . . . is a common language that permits the sharing of accurate and complete information.

Uniformity of the terminology applied to injuries and those structures most frequently injured through athletic participation ensures an accurate and timely diagnosis, provides an appropriate index of injury grading, and forms the basis for timely and appropriate intervention.

RESPONSE TO ATHLETIC INJURY

INFLAMMATORY PHASE

The body's response to trauma follows a predictable sequence and time course of events[8,16,21,30] relative to the severity, extent, and type of tissue disruption. Although appropriate postinjury management and timely surgical and rehabilitative intervention, in addition to the athlete's health and psychologic and nutritional status, may optimize conditions for healing and recovery, in reality, there is no absolute factor that will accelerate this phenomenon.[10]

The initial response to trauma is inflammation. Without the inflammation response, normal healing could not proceed.[21] Inflammation triggers local and systemic responses to initiate the repair process. Figure 1–1 summarizes the cycle of athletic injury and related events. Interventions are directed at optimizing conditions for tissue regeneration and repair.

Inflammation is the body's response to trauma and ultimately results in healing and replacement of damaged tissue with an associated restoration of function. Primary injury results from the disruptive traumatic force that affects the physical integrity and matrix of the tissue. The inflammatory response, accompanying the primary injury, is sometimes referred to as the secondary injury, or hypoxia. It is initiated by the release of chemical mediators that alter vascular tone and capillary permeability.[8,16,21] All cell death from local hypoxia initiates the further release of chemical mediators. Among these are histamine and bradykinin, which alter capillary permeability, allowing blood plasma and proteins to escape into tissues surrounding the injury to produce characteristic edema.[8,14,21,28]

The postinjury response of the body is to concentrate its defensive elements, usually found in the circulation, at the injury site. Blood flow is reduced, allowing margination of white blood cells around the vessels intimate to the injury site. Phagocytosis is initiated by macrophages, which scavenge cellular debris that may impede the repair process. Once inflammatory debris has been removed, the repair process can begin.[14,21] It is important to note that inflammation is necessary for repair but true tissue repair and regeneration will not occur until the inflammatory process subsides. If the inflammatory process does not subside, a chronic condition, often with low-grade inflammation that can be resistant to treatment, results. Attempts to significantly alter the time course of this acute inflammatory phase via pharmacologic or physical means have been problematic.[8,10,21] Contradictory in vitro and in vivo findings have been reported in the literature for both pharmacologic and physical agents.

The "vicious circle" (Fig. 1–2) described by Stokes and Young[31] and demonstrated by Fahere et al.[32] demonstrates the absolute necessity for the sports medicine professional to moderate inflammatory response symptoms and keep the period of immobilization to an absolute minimum.[17,20]

REPARATIVE PHASE

Repair proceeds with resolution of the inflammatory response. Nonviable tissues are replaced through the process of fibroblastic proliferation. A dense network of capillaries and connective tissue bridges the defect. Subsequently, significant amounts of collagen are laid down such that a loose matrix of fibrous connective tissue occupies the injured area.[8,16,21] This fragile tissue remains highly vascularized. As the quantity of collagen at the injury site increases, the number of fibroblasts diminishes. This is the process of tissue repair, in which the original tissue is replaced by scar tissue. In any healing process there is a "race" between repair, which is the replacement of the original tissue by scar tissue, and regeneration, which is replacement by the original type of tissue. Both processes occur with healing, but, invariably, repair wins, with more scar tissue than the original type of tissue being formed. Proper care, however, may enhance the regenerative process, although it seldom "wins the race" over the reparative phase. The end of fibroblastic

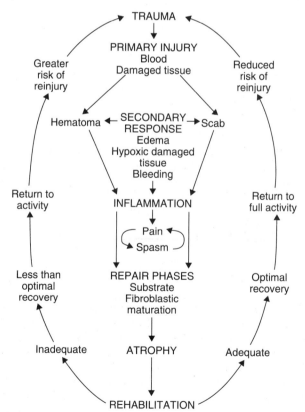

FIGURE 1–1. Cycle of athletic injury. (From Booher JM, Thibodeau GA: Athletic Injury Assessment, 3rd ed. St. Louis, Times Mirror/Mosby College Publishing, 1994.)

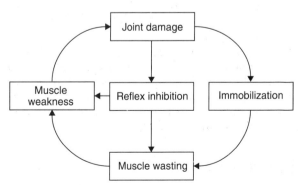

FIGURE 1–2. Vicious circle. (From Stokes M, Young A: The contribution of reflex inhibition to arthrogenous muscle weakness. Clin Sci 1984; 67: 7–14.)

proliferation marks the beginning of the maturation phase of healing.[8,21]

MATURATION PHASE

During the maturation phase, pronounced changes occur in the newly formed fibrous connective tissue. The initial random arrangement of collagen fibers aligns along lines of imposed physical stress, resulting in a more organized pattern with increasing tensile strength. This repaired tissue, however, is seldom as strong as the original tissue that it replaces. Tissue repair, remodeling, and maturation follow a similar continuum in all vascularized connective tissues. Detailed and tissue-specific sequences can be found in the chapters on ligament (Chapter 2), tendon (Chapter 3), muscle (Chapters 5 and 6), bone (Chapter 7), cartilage (Chapter 8), and nerve (Chapter 10). Restoration of tissue integrity to preinjury status is highly variable in timing and outcome and remains one of the major areas of sports medicine research.

IMMOBILIZATION EFFECTS

With limb and joint injuries, immobilization is often indicated as part of an initial treatment regimen to decrease pain and to provide a suitable healing environment.[7,11] Immobilization, while contributing to the resolution of inflammation and supporting/protecting injured structures during the early reparative phase, is not without its own morbidity. Muscular inhibition and atrophy and joint hypomobility, as observed clinically, are the most obvious consequences of immobilization.[18,31] Joints may also be adversely affected by immobilization. In addition to the adaptive shortening that occurs in capsular and other connective tissue structures supporting the joint, lack of motion leads to loss of lubrication between joint surfaces,[14,16] and lack of alternating compression deprives articular cartilage of nutrition, hastening degeneration of the cartilage matrix.[16]

Ligament and tendon size and strength are a function of speed and direction of joint, limb, and muscle loading. With immobilization, stress is eliminated and collagen structures weaken and become more compliant, thus losing their ability to stabilize, guide joint motion, and transmit muscular force.[8,16]

Dehne[33] (Fig. 1–3) summarized the clinical dilemma faced by those who treat neuromusculoskeletal injuries with his classic "spinal adaptation syndrome" model. Competitive states of health and repair (injury), with attendant symptoms, necessitate timely intervention to moderate acute symptoms and the secondary sequelae of prolonged immobilization.

ATHLETIC REHABILITATION

Unlike conventional rehabilitation, athletic rehabilitation requires not only the complete restoration of

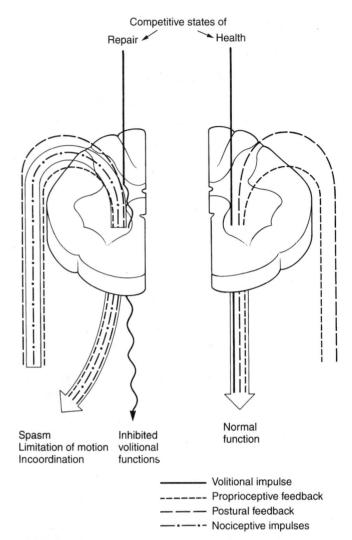

FIGURE 1–3. The spinal adaptation syndrome. (From Dehne E: The spinal adaptation syndrome. Clin Orthop Rel Res 1995; 5: 211–220.)

preinjury performance of the injured limb or joint but also maintenance of peak cardiovascular conditioning of the body as a whole.[3–5,7,9,10,17] Athletic injury rehabilitation is founded in the science of tissue healing constraints, knowledge of joint biomechanics, physiology of muscular strength and endurance, and the neurophysiological basis of skill retraining. Physical change, i.e., hypertrophy, trails functional performance improvements by many weeks. Each sports activity imposes unique demands on the body. Successful athletic rehabilitation programs are constructed on an understanding of tissue healing constraints, which, when properly applied, permit the progressive stressing of joints and muscles. Muscular strength, endurance, and power can be redeveloped while the necessary structural flexibility and general cardiovascular fitness are maintained.[3–5,9,12,17,19,20]

Goals for rehabilitation of an athletic injury should be structured in an ordered sequence that builds on the successful attainment of each preceding stage[20]; each step should contribute to the larger goal of return to sport (Fig. 1–4).[5,9,17] A close athlete-provider relationship, built upon mutual goal setting and attainment, can facilitate the necessary attention to the athlete's "emotional rehabilitation."[11]

An athlete's injury may result in a profound loss of self-worth and identity (Chapter 34). Providing emotional support during the early days of rehabilitation helps the athlete regain a sense of competency, achievement, and acceptance. Although the source of self-worth differs from that of athletic competition, the injured athlete does have a lifeline to initiate his or her rehabilitation efforts. The sports medicine professional must convey a genuine sense of care and concern during this period.[11]

Restoring proprioceptive control and balance as a prelude to motor skill reacquisition precedes the completion of a planned sequence of sport-specific skills—a functional activities progression.[34] Progressing from general to specific, simple to complex, easy to difficult with ever-increasing repetition and intensity, the athlete's injured limb or joint is reintroduced to the performance demands of the sport's environment. Determining when the end point has been reached in the rehabilitation of an athletic injury can be a difficult task.

Clinical tests and measurements, however sophisticated, cannot predict the complex interactions of a rehabilitated joint or limb in response to the specific imposed demands of a sport's environment.[12,20] Careful observation of the athlete's bodily control, maintenance of carriage or form, and confidence in the performance of the activity can be critical in determining readiness for return to competition.[20]

CONCLUSION

The demand to return to former levels of performance drives athletes to expect a full recovery following even the most severe injuries. The pressure to enhance healing or to speed recovery may lead the athlete or provider to embrace unconventional treatment regimens. Proper rehabilitation of athletic injuries requires (1) immediate and accurate initial diagnosis of the nature and severity of the injury with specific tissues involved; (2) immediate initiation of appropriate treatments directed toward moderating the secondary effects of the inflammatory reaction; (3) an ordered sequence of rehabilitation, including exercises, progressive in nature, to enhance the healing of soft tissue structures; (4) integration of functional activities to assist in the restoration of coordinated movement patterns; and (5) the successful completion of sport-specific activities with confidence and bodily control.[12,20]

Goals should be jointly established by the athlete, physician, and therapist-trainer, keeping in mind the athlete's psychological status.[11] Successful rehabilitation is an active, participative process in which the athlete is motivated to meet successive criteria, thereby progressing through a rehabilitation continuum that is highly structured yet truly individualized.[9,12] Contemporary athletic rehabilitation is a process shared by physicians, surgeons, physical therapists, athletic trainers, sport scientists, conditioning specialists, and coaches.[2] To be effective, the process must be scien-

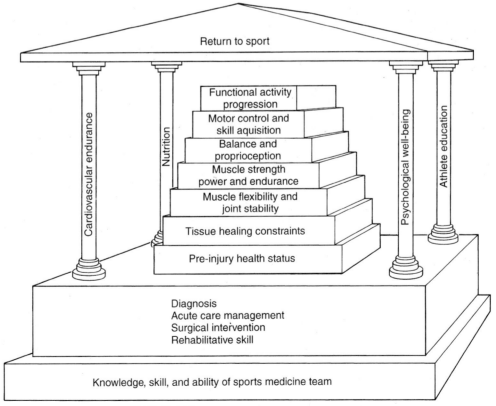

FIGURE 1–4. The athletic rehabilitation pyramid.

tifically founded in anatomy, biomechanics, applied and performance physiology, and rehabilitative therapeutics.

This introduction has provided the reader with a brief overview of the process of injury and rehabilitation. Subsequent chapters on the basic and applied science and clinical topics cover contemporary management of athletic injuries. In presenting this overview, the editors' intent is to firmly support athletic injury treatment and rehabilitation on a scientific rather than an anecdotal foundation.

REFERENCES

1. Garrick J, Webb D: Sports Injuries: Diagnosis and Management. Philadelphia, WB Saunders, 1990.
2. Mellion M, Walsh W, Shelton G (eds): The Team Physician's Handbook. Philadelphia, Hanley & Belfus, 1990.
3. Torg J, Vegso J, Torg E (eds): Rehabilitation of Athletic Injuries. Chicago, Year Book Medical Publishers, 1987.
4. Bernhardt D (ed): Sports Physical Therapy. New York, Churchill Livingstone, 1986.
5. Prentice W (ed): Rehabilitation Techniques in Sports Medicine. St Louis, CV Mosby, 1990.
6. Cantu RC, Micheli L (eds): ACSM's Guidelines for the Team Physician. Philadelphia, Lea & Febiger, 1991.
7. Peterson L, Renstrom P: Sports Injuries: Their Prevention and Treatment. Chicago, Year Book Medical Publishers, 1986.
8. Hubbel S, Buschbacher R: Tissue injury and healing: Using medications, modalities and exercise to maximize recovery. In Buschbacher R, Branddom R (eds): Sports Medicine and Rehabilitation: A Sports Specific Approach. Philadelphia, Hanley & Belfus, 1994, pp 19–30.
9. Gould J, Davis G: Orthopaedic and sports rehabilitation. In Gould J, Davies G (eds): Orthopaedic and Sports Physical Therapy. St. Louis, CV Mosby, 1985, pp 181–198.
10. Reid DC: Sports Medicine and Therapy: Sports Injury Assessment and Rehabilitation. New York, Churchill Livingstone, 1992.
11. Kuland D: The athletic trainer and rehabilitation. In Gieck J (ed): The Injured Athlete. Philadelphia, JB Lippincott, 1982, pp 177–205.
12. Roy S, Irvin R: Injury Rehabilitation. Sports Medicine. Englewood Cliffs, NJ, Prentice-Hall, 1983.
13. Booher JM, Thibodeau GA: Athletic Injury Assessment, 3rd ed. St. Louis, Times Mirror/Mosby College Publishing, 1994.
14. Harrelson G: Physiologic factors of rehabilitation. Introduction to rehabilitation. In Andrews J, Harrelson G (eds): Physical Rehabilitation of the Injured Athlete. Philadelphia, WB Saunders, 1991, pp 13–39, 165–195.
15. Marino M: Current concepts of rehabilitation in sports medicine. In Nicholas J, Hershman E (eds): The Lower Extremity in Sports Medicine. St. Louis, CV Mosby, 1988, pp 126–128.
16. Buckley P, Grana WA, Pascale M: The biomechanical and physiological basis of rehabilitation. In Grana WA, Kalenak A (eds): Clinical Sports Medicine. Philadelphia, WB Saunders, 1991, pp 233–250.
17. Ryan EJ, Stone J: Specific approaches to rehabilitation of athletic injury. In Grana WA, Kalenak A (eds): Clinical Sports Medicine. Philadelphia, WB Saunders, 1991, pp 255–263.
18. Erriksson E: Rehabilitation of muscle function after sports injury—major problem in sports medicine. Int J Sports Med 1981; 2:1–6.
19. Cooper DL, Fair J: Reconditioning following athletic injuries. Phys Sports Med 1976; 4(9):125.
20. Knight K: Guidelines for rehabilitation of sports injuries. Clin Sports Med 1985; 4:405–416.
21. Leadbetter WB, Buckwalter JA, Gordon SL (eds): Sports Induced Inflammation. Rosemont, IL, American Academy of Orthopaedic Surgeons, 1990.
22. Matheson GO, MacIntyre JG, Taunton JE, et al: Musculoskeletal injuries associated with physical activity in older adults. Med Sci Sports Exerc 1989; 21:379–385.
23. Kannus P, Niitymakis S, Jarvinen M: Sports injuries in women: A one year prospective follow up study at an outpatient sports clinic. Br J Sports Med 1987; 21:37–39.
24. Noyes FR, Lindenfeld TN, Marshall MT, et al: What determines an athletic injury? Am J Sports Med 1988; 16:(S1) 365–368.
25. McKeag DB: The concept of overuse: The primary care aspect of overuse syndromes in sports medicine. Prim Care 1984; 1:43–59.
26. Berquist TH: Epidemiology and Categories of Sports Injuries. Imaging of Sports Injuries. Gaithersburg, MD, Aspen Publishers, 1992, pp 1–10.
27. Muckle DS: An Outline of Fractures and Dislocations. Bristol, John Wright and Sons, 1985.
28. Puffer JC, Jachazewski JE: Management of overuse injuries. Pract Ther 1988; 38(3): 225–232.
29. Rachun A, Allman FL, Blazina M, et al: Standard Nomenclature of Athletic Injuries. Chicago, American Medical Association, 1968; pp vii–viii.
30. Bucci LR: Nutrition Applied to Injury Rehabilitation and Sports Medicine. Boca Raton, CRC Press, 1995, pp 1–20.
31. Stokes M, Young A: The contribution of reflex inhibition to arthrogenous muscle weakness. Clin Sci 1984; 67: 7–14.
32. Fahere H, Rentsch HU, Gerber NJ, et al: Knee effusion and reflex inhibition of the quadriceps. J Bone Joint Surg 1988; 70B: 635–638.
33. Dehne E: The spinal adaptation syndrome. Clin Orthop 1995; 5:211–220.
34. Tippet SR, Voight ML: Functional Progressions for Sport Rehabilitation. Champaign, IL, Human Kinetics, 1995.

CHAPTER 2

Ligament Injuries: Pathophysiology and Healing

C. B. FRANK MD, FRCS(C)

NORMAL LIGAMENTS

DEFINITION AND ANATOMY

The word "ligament" is derived from the Latin "ligare," meaning "to tie" or "to bind."[1] Skeletal ligaments have thus been defined historically as bands of grossly parallel fibrous dense connective tissue that "tie" or "bind" bones together at or near the margins of bony articulation.[2] Since well over 120 movable bones make up the major diarthrodial joints of the human body, with a number of ligaments connecting each articulation between these bones, it can be estimated that there are several hundred ligaments.[3]

The majority of the ligaments that have been defined in this way have been named for the bones into which they insert (e.g., glenohumeral, scapholunate, coracoacromial). However, other features, such as their shape (deltoid), relationships to a joint (collateral, on either side), and relationships to each other (cruciate, crossed), also have been used. These well-characterized ligaments are, by definition, anatomically quite distinct and are therefore often portrayed schematically as typical ligaments (Fig. 2–1). Such descriptions imply that ligaments are rather simple structures both anatomically and, by implication, functionally. This is almost certainly not the case.

The first evidence that ligaments are not simple is that each of the above-noted "anatomically distinct," "simple" ligaments, upon more careful inspection, can be seen to insert into very specific and geometrically complex areas on the bones.[4] These insertion sites and the movements of insertions relative to each other in three-dimensional space during typical joint function have a great deal of influence on ligament parts, different parts appearing to tighten or loosen during movement. With such observation during joint movement it becomes clear that ligaments contain "functional subunits," components that tighten or loosen in different joint positions (Fig. 2–2). These functional subunits have been described best in the ligaments of the knee joint, including the anterior cruciate ligament (ACL) and the medial collateral ligament (MCL).[5–9] There is every reason to believe that functional subdivisions are likely to be found in all ligamentous structures. Therefore, each apparently "simple" ligament is designed to function effectively in numerous positions of its parent joint. This fact by itself has profound functional, diagnostic, and therapeutic significance.

The second piece of evidence in support of ligament complexity is that many ligaments are parts of anatomically inseparable structures known as joint capsules.[3] These sheetlike capsules have been so named because they clearly "encapsulate" a major diarthrodial joint. Some of these capsules contain relatively discrete

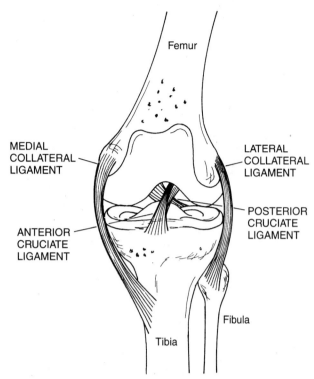

FIGURE 2–1. Typical schematic showing the four "anatomically distinct" ligaments of the knee joint.

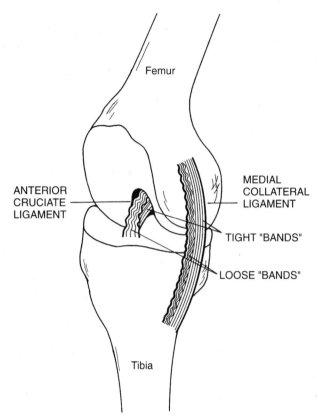

FIGURE 2–2. Schematic of the functional subunits of the anterior cruciate ligament (ACL) and the medial collateral ligament (MCL). At approximately 15 degrees of flexion, the anterior portion of both the ACL and the MCL is relatively "loose" in comparison with the "tight" posterior parts.

fibrous bands with functionally distinguishable roles (e.g., the insertion of the semimembranosus tendon into the posteromedial aspect of the knee joint capsule contributes to the so-called posterior oblique ligament).[10] Owing to the complex interdigitation of fibers in other parts of these capsules, however, no attempt has been made to distinguish individual ligaments. Rather, it has been more convenient to consider the capsule as the functional unit. Since capsules clearly tighten or loosen in different joint positions, this too is a gross oversimplification. Many of the "ligaments" within joint capsules have, at least thus far, probably escaped specific anatomic definition while no doubt sharing in some of the functions of their more anatomically obvious neighbors.

The third piece of evidence supporting ligament complexity comes from a variety of sources showing that many ligaments share functions.[11–13] The ACL, for example, is the primary restraint to anterior translation of the tibia relative to the femur (it prevents the tibia from sliding forward).[14–16] To a lesser extent, the collateral ligaments of the knee and the posterior capsule of the knee also share this function.[15,17,18] In other words, since the anatomic subunits of a variety of ligamentous structures around a joint are likely to be oriented in functionally similar ways, ligaments work together to stabilize joints and control their movements. Thus, in a functional sense, ligaments are not the discrete units that one perceives during anatomic dissection. This perspective has a profound effect on one's understanding of ligament functions, injuries, and therapies.

LIGAMENT FUNCTIONS

Ligaments have long been thought to have two primary roles: the passive guidance of bone position during normal joint function, and joint stabilization (i.e., prevention of abnormal bony displacements) during the application of extrinsic load. There is little doubt that these functions are served by ligaments, since when ligaments are torn or cut, bones no longer maintain normal kinematic relationships[15,18] and can be shown to displace in abnormal directions during the application of external forces.[15,16] This fact is a main feature in the clinical diagnosis of ligament injuries.

A different function that has recently been brought back into consideration[19] is the ligament's potential role as a proprioceptor (position sensor). Nerves within ligaments are speculated to be sensory end-organs that are thought to feed back information through the central nervous system to the periarticular muscles, potentially affecting the quality or quantity of muscular function. There is some appealing contemporary evidence to support this speculation, including the documented presence of proprioceptive type nerve endings in some ligaments[20–22] and the evidence that joint motion can cause periarticular nerve signals.[22] Further, the denervation of joints that are ligament deficient appears to increase the incidence of arthritis.[23] Despite the evidence, the actual magnitude and relative importance of proprioception in ligaments remain unknown.

GROSS APPEARANCES

The anatomically well-defined ligaments are dense white bands or cords of connective tissue that run between specific sites on bones (Fig. 2–3). From a gross perspective, they look like juxta-articular tendons, which are also dense and white but are more often cordlike. Tendons, of course, connect muscle to bone, while ligaments connect bone to bone. Their anatomic locations and orientations are subsequently almost always clearly different.

Upon closer inspection, even with the naked eye, many ligaments can be seen to be composed of roughly parallel fibers of material that tighten or loosen in different joint positions or as different forces are applied to the joint. Not all ligaments, however, have easily distinguishable fibers, at least not without considerable fine dissection. The removal of surrounding tissues or surface layers of ligaments during their anatomic dissection has never been thought to have any particular significance, since these tissues are believed to be nonligamentous. However, these obscuring surface

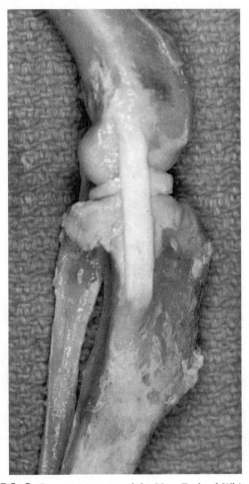

FIGURE 2–3. Gross appearance of the New Zealand White rabbit MCL.

layers may, in fact, be a very important component of the ligament. For example, the MCL has, in some models, been shown to have a very thin superficial layer of tissue attached to it that obscures the view of its fibrous architecture.[24] This layer is analogous to the synovial layer on the surface of the ACL, which is similarly attached to its outer surface and often obscures the gross view of the ACL structure in the joint. The main concept that must be appreciated is that, even at a gross level, ligaments are not homogeneous tissues.

As alluded to earlier, there are many ligaments that are much less distinct than those commonly described. These capsular ligaments are worthy of note, since despite their relative lack of definition, they clearly have major functional roles.[10,25–27]

BLOOD SUPPLY AND INNERVATION

Ligaments are not as richly endowed with blood vessels or nerves as many other tissues. This does not mean that their vascularity or innervation is not important. Ligaments have a ligament-specific blood and nerve supply. Details are only beginning to be defined, since it has only been within the last few years that ligaments have been recognized as being "alive."

The ACL receives its arterial supply from a branch of the middle geniculate artery.[28–30] As with the blood supply to other ligaments, it appears that this vessel branches and ramifies quickly at the surface of the ligament, entering its substance after coursing into and through the superficial layers in specific locations along the length of the soft tissue component of the ligament.[31] Blood vessels do not appear to enter the ligament through its bony interfaces. Nerves in the ACL appear to include C-type pain fibers as well as certain proprioceptive nerve endings.[32] The distribution and type of these nerves remain the subject of many investigations in a variety of models.[31]

The MCL receives its blood supply from a branch of the superior medial geniculate artery. Its microvasculature, like that of the ACL, appears to enter the substance of the ligament through the epiligamentous (surface) layer, ramifying deeper within the substance of the ligament into smaller neurovascular bundles that run parallel to the dominant fibrous structure.[33] The surface of the MCL, including its epiligamentous layer (like the synovium of the ACL), is thus highly vascular (Fig. 2–4). Deeper levels of the ligament are less vascular but still appear to contain neurovascular elements at regular intervals (see Fig. 2–4). The longitudinal distribution of vessels in the MCL is somewhat similar to that in the ACL. No vessels cross the bony interface in the mature ligament. In the soft tissue part of the ligament, near the bony insertions, vessels enter the surface of the ligament substance, making these areas relatively richly vascularized. Vessels enter the remaining length of the MCL at various locations.[33] Like the blood supply, MCL innervation is greatest at its surface, particularly in the epiligament.[24] Some C-type pain fibers and some myelin-encapsulated, specialized

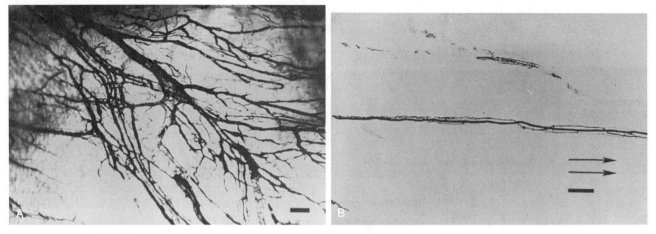

FIGURE 2—4. Vascular perfusion of the New Zealand White rabbit lateral collateral ligament with an ink/gelatin solution. Collagen and matrix are unstained and therefore not visible. Bar = 50 μm. *A*, The surface (epiligamentous) layer. Note the high number of branching blood vessels. *B*, Deep substance. Double arrows = long axis of ligament, bar = 50 μm. Note the large area that is devoid of vessels. (From Bray RC, Fisher AWF, Frank CB: Fine vascular anatomy of adult rabbit knee ligaments. J Anat 1990; 172: 69–79. Reprinted with the permission of Cambridge University Press.)

nerve end-organs have also been seen on the surfaces of the MCL.

From a functional view, ligaments therefore have the innervation to perceive pain and, as noted above, are likely to possess nerves to assist with position sense and feedback. Complete ligament tears probably disrupt the pattern of innervation completely. Ligaments also have a sufficient number of blood vessels both in their substance and on their surface to cause local bleeding (seen as bruising or as a hemarthrosis, depending upon whether bleeding tracks outward toward the skin or inward into the adjacent joint).

MICROSCOPIC AND ULTRASTRUCTURAL ORGANIZATION

At a microscopic level, a ligament is defined as extending from insertional bone at one end, through its major soft tissue portion, to the bone at the other end. Ligaments are heterogeneous from surface to deep both in their substance and along their length. Further, it is clear that there are differences in the microscopic organization of different ligaments.[34–36] The main organizational features of ligaments are described below.

The main soft tissue portion of ligaments is made up of relatively densely packed, relatively parallel fibered material (compared with loose connective tissues, such as skin) with a few interspersed cells (Fig. 2–5A). The relative paucity of cells in ligaments, compared with other connective tissues, has led to the impression that ligaments are inert. This is not the case. Ligament fibroblasts are metabolically active[37] and participate in the turnover of the ligament substance at a rate that is likely to extend from months to years.

Using polarizing filters, it can be seen that the fibers within the substance of the ligament are kinked or

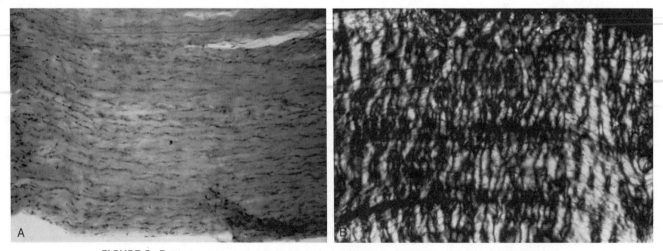

FIGURE 2—5. Photomicrographs of the New Zealand White rabbit MCL showing densely packed parallel fibrous material interspersed with a small number of cells (*A*) and the wavy "crimped" appearance of the fibers (*B*). Hematoxylin and eosin stain.

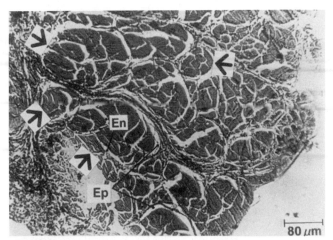

FIGURE 2–6. Microphotograph of a canine ACL cut transversely at the tibial level. Arrows indicate fascicles of different sizes covered by epitenon (Ep) and with nearly elliptical outlines. Each fascicle is subdivided into subfascicles by the endotenon (En). Hemalinpholoxin-Safran Stain, × 40. (From Yahia LH, Drouin G: Microscopical investigation of canine anterior cruciate ligament and patellar tendon: Collagen fascicle morphology and architecture. J Orthop Res 1989; 7: 243–251.)

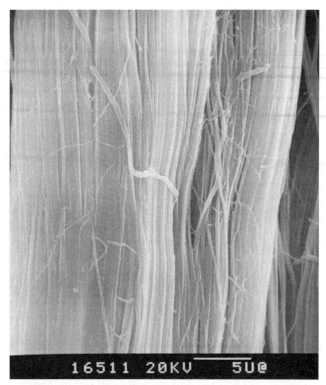

FIGURE 2–7. Scanning electron micrograph of midsubstance New Zealand White rabbit MCL showing a small number of collagen fibers that appear to cross-connect roughly perpendicular to the predominant fiber direction.

crimped (Fig. 2–5B).[2] The main material present is fibrillar collagen.[38,39] Several types of collagen as well as a number of other substances exist in ligaments. The fibrous nature of the ligament midsubstance cannot therefore be attributed to collagen alone.

Ligament midsubstance is not homogeneous. Bundles of fibrous material can be seen to be separated by other bundles of loose connective tissue in the ACL (Fig. 2–6) that provide a clear microscopic separation into functionally distinct subunits. These bundles are less clear in the MCL owing to the relative lack of the loose endoligamentous spacers in that structure.[35] However, functional subdivisions can still be distinguished. These subdivisions allow different parts of the ligament to tighten at different positions of the joint by enabling interbundle shearing to occur. There are, in addition, some cross-connecting fibrils in the ligament substance that help bind the ligament together, particularly within the bundles themselves (Fig. 2–7). Cells appear to differ between the dense and loose connective tissue areas of the same ligament, demonstrating that there is probably more than one cell type present, even within a fairly small region of the ligament. The predominant cell present is the fibroblast or fibrocyte. There appears, however, to be a significant morphologic variation even in this relatively homogeneous cell type.

Different ligaments have different cellular appearances (Fig. 2–8) and, as noted above, different matrix architecture. Cruciate ligaments appear to contain more chondroid (round) nuclei than collateral ligaments,[34] for reasons that are not at all clear. As will be discussed later, this may help explain interligamentous differences in appearance, function, and healing.

As ligaments approach bones, their matrix architecture and cellular appearance change. This appears to be somewhat age and ligament specific,[40,41] but certain features of insertional changes can be emphasized. Collagen fibers that make up the ligament appear to be

cemented into the bone during ligament growth and development,[42] forming so-called Sharpey's fibers at the ligament insertions. The cells at the bone–soft tissue interface in ligaments are different from those in the midsubstance.[40,41,43] It appears that the ligament cells undergo a transition from fibroblasts (cells that produce and maintain the ligament midsubstance), through fibrocartilaginous cells (producing fibrocartilaginous material within 100 μm of the bone interface), to an area where fibrocartilage calcifies (at the surface of the bone) into an area with bone (Fig. 2–9). From a functional point of view, this transition permits a progressive stiffening of the ligament as it approaches bone, decreasing the likelihood of the concentration of stresses at a relatively sharp material interface and thus minimizing the chance of failure at that site.

As noted above, ligaments are also heterogeneous at their surfaces. The MCL of the rabbit, for example, has been shown to have a very thin superficial layer named the epiligament,[24] which is only a few cell layers thick and contains many of the neurovascular elements discussed earlier. Polarized light shows that the organization of this layer is completely different from that of the ligament proper, having smaller diameter collagen fibrils that appear to encircle the main mass of the ligament rather than running parallel to it.[43] Although its function is currently unknown, we have speculated that this layer may be a very active participant in the healing process, probably contributing cells and blood vessels to the scar that forms. Further, we speculate that its vascularity, innervation, and superficial location on

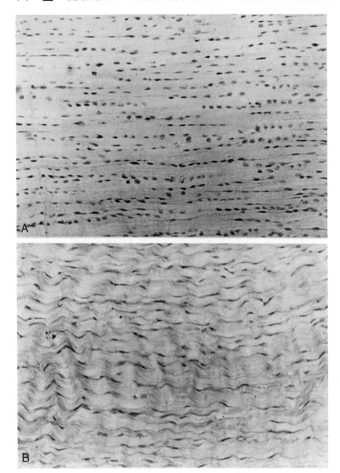

FIGURE 2—8. Differing appearances of cells in the New Zealand White rabbit ACL (*A*) and the New Zealand White rabbit MCL (*B*). Note the more rounded appearance of the ACL nuclei in contrast to the elongated MCL nuclei.

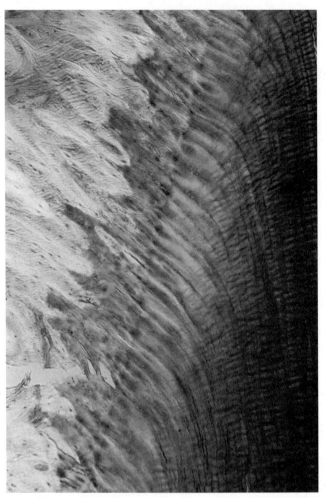

FIGURE 2—9. The femoral insertion of a canine ACL. The femur is on the left, the calcified zone in the center, and the ACL proper on the right. The characteristic elongated midsubstance fibroblast nuclei are the black areas between the parallel-appearing collagen fibers on the bottom right. These fibroblast nuclei become chondroid (rounded) in the calcified zone. (Courtesy of Dr. John Matyas.)

the ligament make this epiligament an important potential source of water regulation in the underlying ligament. As with the synovium on the surface of the ACL,[36] that it is a volumetrically small part of the ligament does not mean that it may not be functionally very important.

BIOCHEMICAL COMPOSITION

Ligaments are roughly two-thirds water and one-third solid (Fig. 2–10). Water is therefore a critical component, contributing to cellular function (the distribution of nutrients, removal of wastes, and other potential movement-related influences) and viscoelastic behavior.[44] The amazing ability of normal ligaments to adapt to loads and load histories within seconds is due in part to this water content.

Of the solid components of ligaments, the major family of proteinaceous constituents is the collagens. Collagen makes up roughly 75 percent of the dry component. The structures and definitions of the collagens can be found in a number of reviews.[45–47] In summary, approximately 15 different types of collagen have been characterized biochemically, with specialized structures and functions. Ligaments have been shown to contain approximately 85 percent type I collagen (the major fibrillar component), less than 10 percent type III collagen (an embryonic, vascular, more microfibrillar type), and a very small percentage of type VI collagen (also microfibrillar and found in the pericellular and interfibrillar spaces).

The second family of solid components, as found in other connective tissues, is the proteoglycans. These protein-sugars have major water-binding properties and appear to be at least partially responsible for controlling water composition and water distribution in ligaments. The most common proteoglycan that has been found in ligaments thus far is a small dermatan sulfate.[48] These make up a very small proportion of the ligament by weight (<1 percent).

The third solid component of ligaments, present in very small proportions, is elastin. Elastin makes up less than 1 to 2 percent of most ligaments but may be an important contributor to their low load recovery.

Other proteins and glycoproteins have been described in ligaments, including actin, laminin, and the integrins, although their quantities, qualities, and relationships to the other components of the matrix remain subjects of ongoing investigation. As of this writing, roughly 20 percent of the dry weight of ligaments remains uncharacterized.

BIOMECHANICAL BEHAVIOR

Ligaments are typical of all connective tissues in the body in having very complex but functionally very important biomechanical behaviors. The interested reader is referred to other sources for a detailed discussion of these behaviors.[49–52] In this section, only those attributes that have clinical significance will be discussed. The reader will be familiarized with some of the engineering terminology commonly used in the literature to describe connective tissue properties in order to demystify the language to some extent. It is hoped that those familiar with engineering terminology will forgive the simplification.

There are three fundamentally different biomechanical attributes of connective tissues that have clinical significance. These are structural (load-deformation) behavior, material (stress-strain) behavior, and viscoelastic (relaxation and creep) behavior.

STRUCTURAL (LOAD-DEFORMATION) BEHAVIOR

Structural behavior refers to how a ligament behaves in its entirety, regardless of its composition or its geometry, when it is mechanically tested in a particular way. For example, if one ligament is isolated between two bones and the two bones are pulled apart, that ligament will exhibit specific structural properties. It will resist the displacement with an increasing stiffness until some part of that ligament complex fails. The ligament itself may fail, as could its insertions into bone, or the bones themselves. The structural strength of the ligament complex does not take into consideration which part of the complex was the weak link but refers only to the load and deformation at the point where the ligament did fail. This load is usually the number quoted by many authors as the strength of that tissue.[53,54]

The structural behavior of a ligament is, therefore, entirely dependent upon the "boundary conditions" of the test. The direction of load (relative to the ligament or bone axis) is a particularly important determinant of apparent ligament complex strength. In other words,

the direction in which a ligament is pulled can change its apparent strength by as much as 50 to 100 percent![53] This has obvious clinical significance in that ligament complex strengths depend, to a certain extent, on the direction in which the joint (and its ligaments) are loaded. This also has significance for the interpretation of any experimental comparisons of ligament strength. Results must be normalized, or at least qualified, to the boundary conditions of the test, with joint angle being a particularly important factor. Quoting "ligament strengths" in absolute terms is therefore a risky business!

The increasing tensile resistance (stiffness) of ligaments as they are distracted is known as nonlinear structural behavior. The farther the ligament is pulled, the more force it takes to continue the displacement (up to the point of yield and failure). This increasing stiffness is due to the recruitment of parts of the ligament (fibers in it becoming tight) as the ligament ends are pulled apart (Fig. 2–11). Exactly how and when the parts of the ligament become tight depends on how the ligament is pulled. If different parts of each ligament are tight in different joint angles, then it is clear that those parts will be the first to be loaded if the ligament ends are distracted suddenly with the joint fixed at that angle of flexion or rotation. The relatively loose parts of the ligament will then become tight as the displacement continues. The parts of the ligament that were tightest at first (when the load began) are likely to be the first to fail.

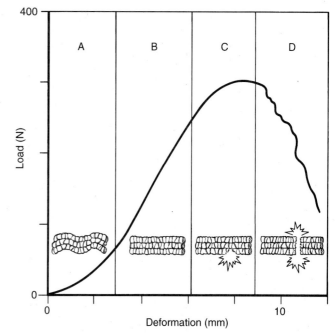

FIGURE 2–11. Graph illustrating the structural behavior of ligaments subject to tensile deformation. As the ligament complex is distracted, fibers become progressively recruited into tension (*A*) until all the fibers are tight (*B*). The parts of the ligament that tightened first are likely to be the first to fail (*C*) as the ligament reaches its "yield point." Progressive fiber failure quickly results in catastrophic ligament rupture (*D*). (Adapted from Curwin S, Stanish WD: Tendinitis: Its Etiology and Treatment. Lexington, MA, The Collamore Press, 1984.)

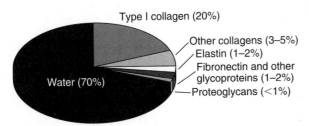

FIGURE 2–10. Pie chart illustrating the biochemical constituents of a typical ligament. Note the predominance of water.

Until recently, the reasons for differing tightness or looseness of ligament parts were not entirely clear. It is now apparent that there are probably several reasons for this to occur. The first reason for relative looseness of part of a ligament is the presence of crimp, as noted earlier. Straightening of collagen fiber crimp occurs at relatively low strains with low amounts of force. Thus, there is effectively a small amount of relative slack built into the fibrillar system that allows some elongation to occur with low amounts of energy and without any damage to the fibrils themselves. At higher loads, there are greater displacements and fibrils themselves begin to carry increasing loads. As the distraction of ligament ends continues beyond this crimp region, an increasing number of ligament fibers are recruited into tension. As the number of fibers increases, the stiffness of the ligament also increases. At the point of maximal ligament stiffness, the maximum number of fibers in the ligament (for that joint position) have been recruited. Yield and failure of the ligament then result from progressive fibril failure in the ligament. If loads are sustained, or if distraction continues to increase, the amount of stress (force per unit area) on the remaining ligament increases dramatically as the number of fibrils present that can carry load drops. Catastrophic rupture then occurs very quickly.

Most clinical tests of joints are really structural tests. The joint is gripped and displaced in some direction, and the examiner feels the stiffness of the joint (its resistance to load) under those conditions. The ligaments of the joint will be recruited to resist the force being applied, depending on the position of the joint. The feeling of stiffness that the examiner perceives is clearly an aggregate of whichever ligaments (or parts thereof) resist force in that direction (plus, of course, the contributions to resistance of all nonligamentous tissues, which may be considerable in some joints and some joint positions). The examiner simulates forces that the joint would encounter during function, hoping to reveal an abnormally low stiffness of the joint in that plane of displacement. Forces during a clinical examination are, of course, very much lower than forces that the joint would encounter during an injury (probably in the range of about 10 percent of their failure loads). Clinical examinations are therefore being conducted in what is known as the toe region of a load-deformation curve for the joint (see below).

To summarize, both joints and isolated ligaments exhibit nonlinear load-deformation behavior. In the case of isolated ligament tests, as the ligament ends move apart the ligament begins to take up a load. With increasing distraction, the load increases slowly. At some point, the amount of load increase in the ligament is linearly proportional to the amount of displacement. With further distraction, however, the ligament begins to yield. Catastrophic rupture of the ligament then occurs. The amount of force and the amount of displacement that it takes to rupture any ligament are dependent on the size of the ligament (usually related to the size of the individual), the age

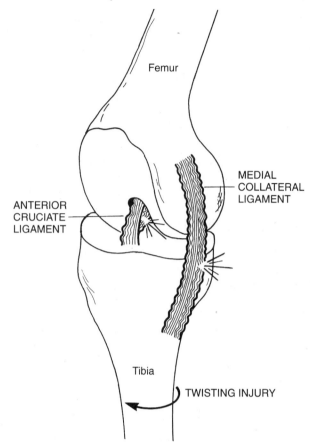

FIGURE 2–12. Changes in knee ligament load-sharing patterns following a typical injury with the knee at approximately 15 degrees of flexion. The portions of the ligaments that are taut at the time of injury (see Figs. 2–2 and 2–11) are likely to be the first to rupture. Once rupture has occurred, neighboring portions of affected ligaments must assume load-bearing responsibilities. Compare with Figure 2–2.

of the host (ligaments reach peak energy-absorbing ability at the time of skeletal maturity), and the position of the joint when loads are applied (which determines how and when fibers within the ligament will be recruited).[11,53,55–57] When entire joints are being loaded, the "load-sharing pattern" of ligaments under the conditions in which the load is applied (direction, magnitude, and rate) will determine which ligaments, or parts thereof, will be damaged. Thus, the nonlinear load-deformation behavior of ligaments explains why the majority of joint injuries are actually combined injuries, involving parts of a number of ligaments (Fig. 2–12).

MATERIAL PROPERTIES

The material properties of a ligament are those load-deformation behaviors that have been normalized for the size of the ligament and for local changes in its length known as its stress-strain behavior. Stress is the amount of force per unit area in the ligament and is thus derived by measuring cross-sectional areas and calculating force (load being carried) per unit area of the ligament. Strain is the change in length divided by the original length of the part of the ligament being measured and is thus a very localized measure. Like the load-deformation behavior, the stress-strain behavior of ligaments is nonlinear, with increasing material stiffness (known as the modulus of elasticity of the material) as stress and strain increase.

Material measures allow ligament tissue to be compared with other biologic materials (e.g., tendons) or artificial materials and are generally of more interest to researchers (who are trying to duplicate normal ligament material behaviors) than to clinicians (who are more interested in reproducing structural properties). A large amount of an inferior material can produce a structure with reasonable structural stiffness and strength. The duplication of normal ligament material behaviors,[17,58] however, would allow replacement of the structural behaviors with something that is the same size as the original.

VISCOELASTIC BEHAVIOR

Ligaments exhibit a combination of viscous and elastic behaviors, besides having an interesting ability to change the proportions of each behavior as conditions demand it. Being viscous means that the ligament behaves as though it contains a thick fluid that is being squeezed through a porous medium. Being elastic means that the ligament has complete recoverability to its resting length after being stretched (like an elastic band or a spring). The combination produces behaviors that are somewhere in between.[59] The ligament absorbs energy as it stretches and recovers in a nonlinear way; at lower loads the viscous behaviors dominate, whereas at the higher loads, elastic behaviors dominate. At all levels of load, both behaviors can be measured, but during clinical tests, viscous behaviors are so subtle that they are usually not appreciated. As will be discussed below, however, they are likely to influence some clinical impressions of joint laxity, particularly those due to changes in ligament lengths or loads after different load histories.

When a ligament is pulled to a fixed length, a certain amount of force is required. If the ligament is held at that length, the amount of load in it decreases. This decrease is due to the load-relaxation of the viscous component of that ligament. The ligament behaves as if some component of the ligament adjusts to the new length by flowing to a new location. This relaxation behavior minimizes the amount of force in the ligament within seconds to minutes (although the phenomenon can continue for hours to days to a lesser extent); it has clinical significance in that it is likely to be one means by which the joint can adjust loads within a tissue to decrease its chances of injury. The same behavior occurs with the cycling of a ligament to a fixed deformation. The load in the ligament decreases with successive cycles until the load in the whole structure achieves a new equilibrium.

When a ligament experiences a fixed load, the ligament length continues to increase, up to either a new equilibrium or the point of ligament failure (depending on the magnitude of the load), a behavior known as ligament creep. Cyclic loading to a fixed level similarly increases the ligament length. From a clinical point of view, it can be seen that cyclic loading of a joint during exercise will effectively alter the lengths of the ligaments that were experiencing loads and will effectively alter subsequent clinical impressions of their length (e.g., joint laxities). Fortunately, from a clinical point of view, these adjustments in length are likely to be only fractions of millimeters in normal cases and probably do not influence clinical impressions too much.

Nonetheless, the functional significance of viscoelastic behavior is that ligaments demonstrate an amazing ability to adjust their length (or intrinsic load) according to actual loads or loading history. Adjusting the balance between viscous and elastic behavior allows ligaments to function within a fairly wide range of loads without being damaged and probably contributes considerably to the homeostatic balance of loads within all the joint tissue.

EFFECTS OF AGING

Like all connective tissues, all the aforementioned structural, material, and viscoelastic properties of ligaments change as a function of age. In general, ligaments reach their peak performance, in a mechanical sense, shortly after the time of skeletal maturity (i.e., age 18 to 20 years), owing to an optimization of their cellular and matrix behaviors.[56]

Prior to skeletal maturation, ligaments are slightly more viscous.[60–62] These ligaments have smaller cross-sectional areas and are thus relatively compliant (low stiffness). Joints thus appear to be relatively loose upon clinical manipulation. At higher loads, insertions are common sites of weakness, since ligaments are not yet firmly cemented into bones.[42,63,64] Insertions are thus common injury sites in children.

After skeletal maturation, ligament cells begin to slow down their metabolic functions, probably performing a less efficient replacement of ligament substance over time. Ligaments reach their maximum size and structural stiffness and are less viscous (more elastic) than their immature counterparts. In middle age, both ligament and ligament insertional bone begin to weaken, resulting in progressive losses in structural strength. Ligament viscosity decreases further, and the collagen in ligaments becomes more highly cross-linked.[65] Ligaments thus become even less compliant, and joints appear to become tighter over time.

In old age, bones are usually more fragile than ligaments and become clinically significant sites of weakness in joint injuries. Ligaments lose mass, stiffness, strength, and viscosity in the elderly. Probably because of decreasing loads on the ligaments and decreasing activity levels in the elderly, these changes in the ligaments are usually are not part of any obvious clinical problem. If joints deform as a result of changes in bone shapes, however, and ligaments experience excessive loads as a result, ligaments may creep excessively and contribute to pathologic joint laxities.

For a more detailed description of the effects of growth, maturation, and aging on ligament properties, the reader is referred to specific references on this topic.[65,66]

EFFECTS OF IMMOBILIZATION AND EXERCISE

IMMOBILIZATION

Although the mechanisms are not clear, ligament complexes are extremely sensitive to load and load history. Load deprivation (joint immobilization) causes a rapid deterioration in ligament biochemical and mechanical properties, partially due to atrophy (a decrease in ligament mass), which causes a net loss in ligament strength and stiffness.[2,67–69] Experimental evidence suggests that immobility causes a net shift in ligament cell metabolism from a balanced (homeostatic) state or a net anabolic (building) state to a more catabolic (destructive) state.[37] A few weeks of immobilization causes the ligament matrix to decrease in quantity. Ligament cells also apparently produce inferior quality ligament material, which contributes to the structural weakening of the ligament complex. Bone begins to resorb, causing a focal weakness at the sites of insertion. The loss of ligament complex strength with immobilization appears to be exponential over time.[68,70,71] While there is only slight weakening in the first few weeks, ligament complexes that have been completely immobilized for periods of 6 to 9 weeks are only about 50 percent as strong and stiff as normal controls.[67,72] From a functional therapeutic view, this implies that periods of joint immobilization should ideally, for the sake of the ligaments at least, be minimized.

Joint stiffness following immobilization is probably not caused by ligament deterioration. Rather, ligaments are less stiff after periods of immobilization. Joint stiffness is probably caused by the binding together (cross-linking) of the nonligamentous periarticular tissues. Joint stiffness is not, therefore, a good index of ligament function following immobilization, since nonligamentous structures contribute to this impression. In fact, true ligament function cannot be tested for a long period of time in intact joints following the remodeling of this nonligamentous tissue.

PREVENTION OF ATROPHY CAUSED BY IMMOBILIZATION

To date, it is not clear how much movement is required to maintain normal ligament behavior. If ligaments were analogous to bone, only a minimal number of cyclic loads (e.g., only a few cycles of a joint per day) would be required to maintain baseline ligament behaviors.[73–75]

RECOVERY FROM IMMOBILIZATION

Experimental evidence suggests that different parts of the ligament complex recover at different rates

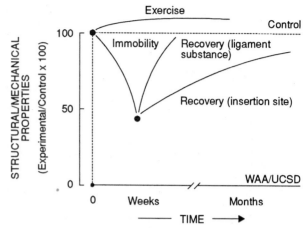

FIGURE 2–13. Schematic diagram illustrating ligament responses to immobilization and exercise. (From Woo SL-Y, Gomez MA, Sites TJ, et al: The biomechanical and morphological changes in the medial collateral ligament of the rabbit after immobilization and remobilization. J Bone Joint Surg 1987; 69A: 1200–1211.)

following a significant period of immobilization.[67,76,77] The bony insertions appear to recover more quickly than the substance of the ligament itself. The former occurs in a period of weeks following the removal of immobilization. The recovery of the latter occurs over many months (Fig. 2–13).

It is not clear what dose-response relationship may exist between the recovery of ligament behavior following immobilization and the exercise protocol used. Presumably there is some, as yet undefined, optimal amount of load or optimal number of loading cycles that would, in turn, optimize the metabolic recovery of ligament cells in each ligament. Until this information is available, the protocols for joint recovery must remain empirical.

EFFECTS OF EXERCISE

Ligaments respond to joint exercise by becoming slightly stronger and stiffer.[78] In most cases, however, ligaments receive the minimum amount of mechanical stimulation necessary for them to maintain a substantial baseline (which appears to be roughly 80 to 90 percent of their mechanical potential). Exercise, therefore, appears to have the potential to increase ligament strength and stiffness by probably no more than that additional 10 to 20 percent (see Fig. 2–13). As with immobilization, the effects of exercise may be ligament specific. A certain "window of loading" is likely to be positive for each ligament, whereas loads outside that window (too much or not enough) probably result in ligament deterioration.

LIGAMENT INJURY

MECHANISMS OF INJURY

Based on the above-noted understanding of ligament structures and functions, it is now possible to provide a clearer understanding of how ligaments are injured and how clinical diagnostic methods work (or fail to work).

In any particular position of any joint, it should be clear that parts of several ligaments around that joint are likely to be in a taut state. In other words, a certain proportion of specific ligament fiber bundles will have been recruited and will be somewhere within the relatively linear portion of their load-deformation curve (see under Biomechanical Behavior). Since ligaments share loads around the joint in order to maintain a mechanical equilibrium, it is unlikely that only one ligament will be loaded at any point in time. If an extrinsic load is then applied to the joint (e.g., a twisting injury to a knee joint), the tight (loaded) portions of those restraining ligaments will absorb the greatest amount of energy. They will deform past their elastic (recovery) limit and will fail. Other fibers in those structures will simultaneously become recruited into tension. Depending upon how far the bones are allowed to displace (from the forces being applied and resistance of other periarticular structures, e.g., muscles), a certain proportion of several ligaments will be damaged. The ligament, the primary restraint to the force being applied (e.g., the MCL is the main restraint to a valgus knee force), will be the primary structure damaged. Secondary ligamentous restraints will be damaged to a lesser degree. It is therefore unlikely for a truly "isolated" ligament injury to ever occur. There will often be some (possibly minor and subclinical) damage to other ligaments around a damaged joint, which should be sought in a careful history and physical examination. More than one ligament may be partially torn while the functional part of one anatomic structure is completely torn.

Ligament "sprains" must therefore be re-evaluated in this context. Ligament injuries have historically been graded according to the severity of a tear, grade I being an incomplete tear (no joint instability noted), grade II being a more significant tear that is not complete (some instability), and grade III being a complete tear (complete instability). The grade III case, almost by definition, involves the tearing of multiple ligaments, making joint instability obvious upon clinical examination. Some structures are likely to be partially torn in these types of instabilities (structures that were secondary restraints to the injury forces). Grade II injuries, which also have some obvious clinical instability, may be due to complete tearing of one structure (e.g., the MCL) plus incomplete tears of other structures (e.g., capsular ligaments or ACL). Alternatively, instability could be due to only partial tears of several structures, which may have a different clinical prognosis than the previous scenario. Grade I injuries are the most difficult for the clinician to detect. It is possible that ligaments have been damaged so minimally that the joint is not clinically unstable. On the other hand, it seems possible that some of these injuries are simply not being examined in the right way with respect to joint position or direction of force, causing a latent instability to be missed. It is possible that these types of injury become the chronic instabilities that are so often seen clinically. A high index of suspicion and a very careful examination will probably lead to further refinements in defining ligament injuries in all joints.

The fact that partial ligament injuries are likely to be very common has one extremely important clinical consequence—clinicians must be aware that partial injuries will be common and that they must be extremely careful in examining a joint in order to discover them. The most important principle in this regard is that the joint will be unstable only in the position in which it was injured. A knee that was injured with the knee flexed at 20 degrees will therefore be likely to be unstable (i.e., the ligaments will not provide normal resistance to forces) only in that degree of flexion and in the direction in which the injury forces were applied. This is the basis on which the Lachman test[79] has proved to be a much more sensitive test for torn ACLs than the anterior drawer test. The former tests the knee at the degree of flexion in which most knees are injured (slight flexion). Few knees are ever injured at 90 degrees of flexion (the anterior drawer position). In fact, the portion of the ACL that is taut at 90 degrees of flexion[80,81] is often uninjured in most first-time knee injuries, and knees will still be stable in that position when tested clinically. The clinician should also be aware that a second injury will often "finish off" a ligament (such as the remaining part of the ACL) if it has become the main restraint in the direction needed to pathologic bony displacement. Prevention of second injuries should therefore become the focus of treatment by attempting to protect the joint within its range of instability during, and subsequent to, its healing.

This principle is almost certainly true of all joint injuries and is based on the knowledge that individual ligaments (as perceived anatomically) do not have single, simple functions.

PHASES OF HEALING

BLEEDING AND INFLAMMATION

When ligaments tear, there is immediate local pain (due to pain fibers within the ligament) and bleeding (due to tearing of vessels in and around the ligament). As with bleeding anywhere, an immediate inflammatory response is initiated. With extra-articular ligaments, bleeding occurs into a subcutaneous space, where tamponade can ensue. With intra-articular ligaments (e.g., cruciate ligaments), bleeding proceeds unchecked into the joint space until either clotting occurs spontaneously or pressure builds to the point that ligament vascular pressure is exceeded and tamponade also occurs. The next steps are, to some extent, ligament and environment specific.

In all cases, platelets promote clotting. A fibrin clot is deposited and substances (growth factors) are released that promote an inflammatory cascade. Local vessels dilate, acute inflammatory cells infiltrate, and fibroblastic scar cells begin to appear. The first phase of ligament healing, lasting for hours to days, comprises this acute cascade of events.

PROLIFERATION OF BRIDGING MATERIAL

The second phase of ligament healing involves the production of scar matrix.[2] Unfortunately, there is no evidence that normal ligament matrix can be produced during this phase of healing, for any ligament. Different quantities (and *possibly* qualities) of scar matrix can be produced (which can be altered by different therapies, as discussed below), but there appears to be some fundamental inability for completely disrupted ligaments to regenerate normal ligament matrix. Thus the proliferating scar fibroblasts (whose source remains unknown but probably involves some combination of local fibroblasts and the differentiation of circulating cells, e.g., macrophages) become the local workers, attempting to produce a new bridging matrix for the torn ligament. Inflammatory cells simultaneously remove damaged ligament and clot debris and attempt to leave only a dense scar matrix in place of the gap in the ligament.

The gap in extra-articular ligaments (e.g., the MCL) probably becomes filled with a very viscous scar matrix within days. The scar progressively becomes less viscous and more elastic over several weeks as inflammation decreases.

Contrary to popular belief, which seems to hold that the ACL is incapable of any healing response, scar tissue is apparently produced in many ACL injuries. Based on clinical observations, bridging scar appears to occur frequently between the torn ACL and the PCL, or between the torn ACL and some other location in the intercondylar notch in the joint.[82] Unfortunately, the scar tissue appears to occur in functionally useless locations and probably often involves the same inferior-quality scar that is found in extra-articular ligament healing. The combination of inferior quality material in the wrong position in the joint is likely to explain the high incidence of failure to heal in the ACL. The principle, however, is that in this phase of healing, healing material must connect torn ligament ends to the correct anatomic locations. The failure to reconnect appropriate locations on bones (i.e., between the anatomic insertions that were presumably optimized by nature for that ligament) is one cause of healing failure. The failure to produce enough scar is a second cause of failure (i.e., the scar tissue is structurally inadequate). The third cause is the failure to produce the correct material (probably the cause of failure in ligaments that have been surgically repaired).

MATRIX REMODELING

The third phase of ligament healing is matrix remodeling. Once bridging has occurred, the scar matrix contracts, becomes less viscous, and becomes both denser and more highly ordered. Defects in the scar (such as debris, fat cells, loose matrix, hypercellular inflammatory areas, and areas without matrix) become filled in.[83,84] Although ligament scar matrix becomes more ligament-like with time, it still has some very major differences in composition and architecture.[84-86] Improvement in scar quality occurs over time, depend-

ing on a variety of factors, including, for example, joint motion.

For those interested in more detailed reviews of the morphologic, biochemical, metabolic, and biomechanical events that occur during ligament healing in experimental models of healing, some specific articles are recommended.[2,87-90]

EFFECTS OF VARIOUS TREATMENTS ON LIGAMENT HEALING

From a clinical point of view, to be effective, treatments must both improve joint function and decrease secondary disability caused by ligament injuries. Unfortunately, the quantitative proof that any treatment results in true improvement of either of these areas is plagued by the lack of quantitative assessment tools, the myriad of clinical variables that can influence the natural history of healing in any individual case, and the unknown contributions of other structures (which can compensate to variable degrees) in the healing process. The reader should therefore not have any false illusions. As of 1995, there is not yet a clear picture of what any treatment truly does in a clinical setting. At best, there are general ideas about what some commonly used clinical modalities do to alter the healing processes of ligamentous tissues in some circumstances. These have been derived using animal models under certain boundary conditions and with some very specific markers as indices of improvement. Based on the foregoing discussions of ligament structure and function, it should be appreciated that ligaments have many structural elements, a complex composition and organization, and a complicated biomechanical behavior. Further, they never act in isolation in a joint. Only a few of these features can be studied in any experiment, and none should be portrayed as being the most important characteristic of the ligament. In other words, the reader should be cautioned that any parameter, such as ligament strength, for example, while important, may not be the most important outcome measure. Similarly, collagen content, or types of collagen present, may not have any functional meaning. Because one cannot say which behaviors are most important, discussions usually revolve around how "healing is different from normal."

The current understanding of experimental effects of various therapies on ligament healing will be summarized below, but the reader is cautioned to be critical of this interpretation and should refer to other sources for a more in-depth appreciation of this very complex subject.[90,91]

IMMOBILIZATION

The immobilization of an injured joint almost certainly decreases the loads and load history of injured ligaments in that joint. As noted above, immobilization will have detrimental mechanical effects on noninjured ligaments, making them weaker and less stiff. This is a

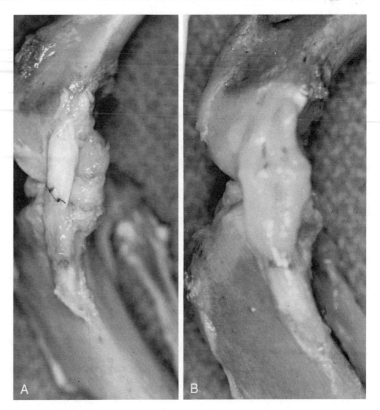

FIGURE 2–14. New Zealand White rabbit MCL scars subject to immobilization (*A*) and exercise (*B*). Note that the scar from the immobilized ligament is small compared with the scar of the exercised ligament.

long-lasting effect that takes months to reverse after remobilization.

The effects of immobilization on the other tissues in the injured joint should also be considered. Long-term, rigid immobility has been shown to have detrimental effects on diarthrodial joints.[92] Cartilage surfaces become damaged, bones atrophy, and the joint becomes fibrosed (stiffened). A joint that has been destabilized owing to a significant ligament injury appears to undergo other types of damage. Bones form osteophytes; cartilage fibrillates, then erodes; and the joint becomes inflamed. These changes are known as osteoarthritis.[93] In fact, certain ligament deficiencies, for example, ACL deficiency, have been used to produce osteoarthritis in animal models.[94] In these cases, joint immobilization has some beneficial effects. Short-term periods of immobilization decrease these osteoarthritic changes.[95] If the joint does not move, it appears to be kinematically stable and is thereby relatively protected. Presumably the detrimental effects of immobilization are present, but they do not appear to be as rapid or as destructive as those seen with instability in the same models. It is not known whether there are any long-term protective effects of such immobilization on the joint surfaces once these unstable joints are remobilized, since these experiments, to the author's knowledge, have not yet been performed. It can be assumed, however, that if the period of immobility does not facilitate increased stability of the joint (e.g., allow the damaged structure to heal, or produce some compensatory net stiffening of other structures), the instability will subsequently cause osteoarthritis as well.

The immobilization of ligament scar tissue appears to inhibit scar mass and scar quality.[84,96] Scars in legs that have been immobilized are thus smaller, structurally weaker, and less stiff than are larger scars from knee joints that have been allowed to move (Fig. 2–14). Immobilized scars are also less viscous (relax less) and are materially weaker than their nonimmobilized counterparts. At equal points in time, these scars are therefore less able to resist stresses without straining. They would, presumably, be more subject to subsequent reinjury at comparable levels of load or deformation on the joint.

The biggest unknown regarding ligament immobilization (or exercise) is the effect upon ligament length. Ligament length refers to the amount of bone deformation that must occur in the normal plane of the ligament in question before that ligament takes up any load. This would correspond to the clinical term "laxity." It is clear that in certain joint instabilities, healing ligaments are effectively much "longer" than their normal counterparts. In the combined MCL/ACL–deficient rabbit knee, for example, the healing MCL is initially much more lax.[95] Immobilizing the joint during the early phase of healing prevents this laxity and may thus confer some degree of low-load stability to the knee. On the other hand, it simultaneously prevents scar mass and inhibits scar qualities that would allow that MCL scar to resist higher loads. On balance, it would appear that this short-term benefit does not compensate for the resultant disability. This appears to be borne out by clinical studies, which have thus far failed to show that immobilizing MCL/ACL–injured joints provides any long-term benefit to the outcome.[97]

This clearly remains controversial, however, and is still worthy of further investigation.

EXERCISE

As with normal ligaments, exercise has some powerful influences on ligament scars. Joint movement during ligament healing definitely has some beneficial effects on the joint tissues, the noninjured ligaments, and the healing ligament so long as forces on the healing tissues are not too great. What force is too great, however, is unknown at present. Further, it is not clear, in most cases, how loads on healing ligaments can be modified, since it is not even clear how much load a normal ligament carries in a joint, let alone when it or some of its load-sharing partners have been damaged.

The current concept is that very low cyclic loads on a ligament scar will promote scar proliferation and material remodeling, thus making the scar stronger and stiffer structurally[98] and, possibly, materially. As far as is known, the definitive experiment demonstrating that the loading of a ligament scar can accelerate either the rate of its material improvement or its material end point has not yet been carried out. It has been shown, however, that animals that are presumably more active during healing (dogs) form better quality scars in collateral ligaments than do less active animals (rabbits).[17] Canine MCL scars apparently can reach 75 percent of normal material strength, whereas those in rabbits appear to reach their peak at 30 to 40 percent of normal. If these differences are real and if they are due to joint movement, there is experimental support for controlled motion during ligament repair. Loads can presumably be increased slowly as the stiffness of ligament scars increases, in terms of load-resisting ability, for several months after injury.

Until the limits of load are defined, and until loads on the ligaments of interest in the clinic can be determined under both normal and pathologic (injured) conditions, the current empirical forms of controlled motion should probably still be employed.

ICE AND HEAT

Based more on clinical than on experimental evidence, it appears that the use of ice immediately following a ligament injury decreases bleeding, swelling, and inflammation. This is certainly helpful in minimizing the masking signs of pain and swelling. The inhibition of inflammation may also limit secondary damage to the other joint structures, which may decrease secondary stiffness of the joint, if periarticular scar formation is inhibited.

The effects of ice on scar formation are unknown. If scar mass is dependent upon inflammatory mediators, ice-mediated scar inhibition may also inhibit the structural maturation of a ligament scar. Bleeding and inflammation may be important to the healing process itself. As with many aspects of therapeutic intervention, this requires further study.

The anecdotal and experimental results suggesting that ice can be used to manipulate blood flow to a tissue[99] could be invoked to suggest that ligament healing may be influenced through that mechanism, even during the chronic phases of healing. This has not been studied in ligaments, and it remains unknown whether blood flow is a limiting factor in their healing at all.

The same holds true for heat. In the short term, heat increases inflammation, swelling, and blood flow. It is not known what the consequences are of these changes to the quality or the quantity of ligament healing. Similarly, the effects of ultrasound on scar tissue are, to the author's knowledge, unknown.

SURGICAL REPAIR

The surgical apposition of torn ligament ends has been noted in the past to induce faster and stronger healing through a process that was likened to regeneration rather than scar formation.[100,101] Subsequent work, however, has shown that even in cases in which ligament ends are surgically apposed immediately, scar tissue still forms between the ends and may or may not withstand subsequent loads. In the case of the ACL, such reapposition usually fails, both in the clinic and experimentally.[87,101–103] In the case of the MCL, apposition of ends makes the MCL complex slightly stronger and stiffer at comparable points in time,[58] but it does not cause true regeneration. Even in this best-case scenario (immediate overlapping repair of a Z-plasty cut in an extra-articular rabbit ligament), the complex recovers only to about 80 to 90 percent of normal structural strength. Larger gaps in the rabbit model cause a relative weakness of the MCL complex owing to the increased prevalence and size of defects in the scars.[83] These defects (see under Phases of Healing) are removed over time but cause bigger scar gaps to be weaker than smaller ones for the first few months of healing.[58]

If repair could be shown to restore immediate normal joint kinematics while the scar forms and remodels, it would probably be an advantage. However, since repairs are unlikely to provide enough initial tensile resistance, this is seldom the case. Further, since it appears that in most cases (at least for most extra-articular ligaments) ligament ends are likely to be in reasonable apposition, repair is probably not justifiable for the small degree of structural improvement that gap minimization would create.

In situations in which gaps are known to be large (e.g., if ends are seen to be far apart on a magnetic resonance imaging [MRI] scan), in which large forces may maintain a ligament gap (e.g., arm weight distracting ends of coracoclavicular ligaments), or in which a large anatomic gap may exist (e.g., the ACL), the surgical repair of ligament ends may be justified. Since it appears that, in at least some cases, scars are capable of contracting to minimize joint laxity[88] and most of the foregoing conditions occur only rarely, the operative approach to repair of ligaments should probably remain restricted.

SURGICAL REPLACEMENT (GRAFTING)

There has been a great deal of work on the surgical replacement of ligament complexes with both nonbiologic (i.e., artificial) and biologic (i.e., tendons, fascia) substances. It is far beyond the purpose of this chapter to review all these results. A few points, however, are worth making.

No ligament replacement has ever been shown to restore normal function totally. Most replacements have been aimed primarily at restoring ligament complex strength or stiffness and secondarily at restoring low-load behaviors such as joint laxity. None has been aimed at restoring viscoelastic behaviors, and none has even begun to look at the possibility of restoring proprioceptive functions (if they exist). Even the most successful ligament replacements have achieved only 80 to 90 percent of normal ligament strength and stiffness under optimal circumstances.[104–107] The best replacements of the ACL in animals have achieved only about 50 percent of normal ACL strength, even after many months of healing.[108,109]

Ligament grafts, if performed acutely and if fixed with adequate means to ensure immediate joint motion, offer a distinct advantage in facilitating healing of the joint according to the principles espoused above. If the graft controls joint kinematics in the same way as its damaged predecessor did, and if the joint can be cyclically loaded within the window of acceptable forces after the replacement, joint healing will presumably be facilitated. The potential advantages and disadvantages of this approach are, of course, the subject of many ongoing investigations.[50,110–112]

SUMMARY

Ligaments are biologically complex connective tissues that are only beginning to be understood. They are heterogeneous both structurally and functionally, and many share functions with other ligaments within any given joint.

Ligaments are metabolically active and are constantly changing over time. Normal ligaments respond to their environment, including the therapeutic modalities of immobilization and exercise.

Ligaments are rarely injured in isolation, and it is common for different parts of ligaments to be damaged in a joint injury. Ligaments do not regenerate when injured. They appear to heal, when able, with variations in scar tissue.

Ligament scars respond to therapeutic modalities. Exercise and immobilization are powerful modifiers of scar quantity and probably scar quality. Controlled joint motion, within a (yet to be defined) "window" of stress on the healing tissues, appears to be the optimal way to enhance ligament healing. Other modalities have more speculative effects.

A great deal of clinical and experimental work remains to be done before a scientifically rational approach to therapy for all ligament injuries will be possible.

ACKNOWLEDGMENTS

The author wishes to acknowledge the financial support of the Medical Research Council of Canada, the Canadian Arthritis Society, and the Alberta Heritage Foundation for Medical Research as well as the editorial assistance of Ms. Jackie Wilson.

REFERENCES

1. Webster AM: Webster's Seventh New Collegiate Dictionary. Springfield, MA, G & C Merriam Company, 1970.
2. Akeson WH, Woo SL-Y, Amiel D, Frank CB: The chemical basis of tissue repair. The biology of ligaments. *In* Hunter LY, Funk FJ (eds): Rehabilitation of the Injured Knee. St. Louis, CV Mosby, 1984, pp 93–148.
3. Basmajian JV, Slonecker CE: Grant's Method of Anatomy. A Clinical Problem-Solving Approach, 11th ed. Baltimore, Williams & Wilkins, 1989.
4. Girgis FG, Marshall JL, Al Monajem ARS: The cruciate ligaments of the knee joint. Clin Orthop 1975; 106: 216–231.
5. Furman W, Marshall JL, Girgis FG: The anterior cruciate ligament. A functional analysis based on post-mortem studies. J Bone Joint Surg 1976; 58A: 179–185.
6. Girgis FG, Marshall JL, Monajem ARS: The cruciate ligaments of the knee joint. Anatomical, functional and experimental analysis. Clin Orthop 1975; 106: 216–231.
7. Warren LF, Marshall JL, Girgis FG: The prime static stabilizer of the medial side of the knee. J Bone Joint Surg 1974; 56A: 665–674.
8. Kennedy JC, Fowler PJ: Medial and anterior instability of the knee. An anatomical and clinical study using stress machines. J Bone Joint Surg 1971; 53A: 1257–1260.
9. Grood ES, Noyes FR, Butler DL, Suntay WT: Ligamentous and capsular restraints preventing straight medial and lateral laxity in intact human cadaver knees. J Bone Joint Surg 1981; 63A: 1257–1269.
10. Hughston JC, Eilers AF: The role of the posterior oblique ligament in repairs of acute medial (collateral) ligament tears of the knee. J Bone Joint Surg 1973; 55A: 923–940.
11. Ahmed AM, Burke DL, Duncan NA, Chan KH: Ligament tension pattern in the flexed knee in combined passive anterior translation and axial rotation. J Orthop Res 1992; 10:854–867.
12. Chao TT, Lew WD, Lewis JL, et al: Biomechanical effect of a two-segment anterior cruciate ligament graft with separate femoral attachments and differing levels of prescribed load sharing. J Orthop Res 1992; 10:868–877.
13. Hanley P, Lew WD, Lewis JL, et al: Load sharing and graft forces in anterior cruciate ligament reconstructions with the Ligament Augmentation Device. Am J Sports Med 1989; 17: 414–422.
14. Butler DL: Anterior cruciate ligament: its normal response and replacement. J Orthop Res 1989; 7: 910–921.
15. Wroble RR, Grood ES, Cummings JS, et al: The role of the lateral extraarticular restraints in the anterior cruciate ligament–deficient knee. Am J Sports Med 1993; 21: 257–262.
16. Noyes FR, Grood ES, Suntay WJ: Three-dimensional motion analysis of clinical stress tests for anterior knee subluxations. Acta Orthop Scand 1989; 60: 308–318.
17. Woo SL-Y, Inoue M, McGurk-Burleson E, Gomez MA: Treatment of the medial collateral ligament injury. II. Structure and function of canine knees in response to different treatment regimens. Am J Sports Med 1987; 15: 22–29.
18. Grood ES, Stowers SF, Noyes FR: Limits of movement in the human knee. Effect of sectioning the posterior cruciate ligament and posterolateral structures. J Bone Joint Surg 1988; 70A: 88–97.
19. Brand RA: A neurosensory hypothesis of ligament function. Med Hypotheses 1989; 29: 245–250.
20. Bray RC, Fisher AW, Salo P, et al: Neurovascular anatomy of collateral knee ligaments as revealed by vascular injection and metallic impregnation techniques. Orthop Trans 1989; 13(3): 670.
21. Brand RA: Knee ligaments: A new view. J Biomech Eng 1986; 108: 106–110.

22. Marshall KW, Tatton WG: Joint receptors modulate short and long latency muscle responses in the awake cat. Exp Brain Res 1990; 83: 137–150.

23. O'Connor BL, Visco DM, Brandt KD, et al: Neurogenic acceleration of osteoarthrosis. The effects of previous neurectomy of the articular nerves on the development of osteoarthrosis after transection of the anterior cruciate ligament in dogs. J Bone Joint Surg 1992; 74A: 367–376.

24. Chowdhury P, Matyas JR, Frank CB: The "epiligament" of the rabbit MCL: A quantitative morphological study. Connect Tissue Res 1991; 27(1): 33–50.

25. Warren LF, Marshall JL: The supporting structures and layers on the medial side of the knee. J Bone Joint Surg 1979; 61A: 56–62.

26. Hughston JC, Andrews JR, Cross MI, Moschi A: Classification of knee ligament instabilities. 1. Medial compartment and cruciate ligaments. J Bone Joint Surg 1976; 58(2)A: 159–172.

27. Hughston JC, Andrews JR, Cross MJ, Moschi A: Classification of knee ligament instabilities. 2. Lateral compartment. J Bone Joint Surg 1976; 58(2)A: 173–179.

28. Arnoczky SP: Blood supply to the anterior cruciate ligament and supporting structures. Orthop Clin North Am 1985; 16(1): 15–28.

29. Marshall JL, Arnoczky SP, Rubin RM, Wickiewicz TL: Microvasculature of the cruciate ligaments. Phys Sports Med 1979; 7: 87–91.

30. Scapinelli R, Little K: Observations on the mechanically induced differentiation of cartilage from fibrous connective tissue. J Pathol 1970; 101: 85–91.

31. Bray RC, Fisher AWF, Frank CB: Fine vascular anatomy of adult rabbit knee ligaments. J Anat 1990; 172: 69–79.

32. Bray RC, Frank CB, Miniaci A: Structure and function of diathrodial joints. In McGinty JB (ed): Operative Arthroscopy. New York, Raven Press, 1991, pp 79–123.

33. Bray RC, Rangayyan RM, Eng K, Frank CB: A study of vascular behaviour in normal and healing medial collateral ligaments. Trans Orthop Res Soc 1993; 18: 57(Abstract).

34. Amiel D, Frank CB, Harwood FL, et al: Tendons and ligaments—A morphological and biochemical comparison. J Orthop Res 1983; 1: 257–265.

35. Yahia L-H, Drouin G: Microscopical investigation of canine anterior cruciate ligament and patellar tendon: Collagen fascicle morphology and architecture. J Orthop Res 1989; 7: 243–251.

36. Kennedy JC, Weinberg HW, Wilson AS: Anatomy and function of the anterior cruciate ligament—as determined by clinical and morphologic studies. J Bone Joint Surg 1974; 56(2)A: 223–235.

37. Frank CB, Hart DA: The biology of tendons and ligaments. In Mow VC, Ratcliffe A, Woo SL-Y (eds): Biomechanics of Diarthrodial Joints. New York, Springer-Verlag, 1990, pp 39–62.

38. Frank CB, Woo SL-Y, Andriacchi TP, et al: Normal ligament: Structure, function and composition. In Woo SL-Y, Buckwalter JA (eds): Injury and Repair of the Musculoskeletal Soft Tissues. Rosemont, IL, American Academy of Orthopaedic Surgeons, 1988, pp 45–101.

39. Chaudhuri S, Nguyen H, Rangayyan RM, et al: A Fourier domain directional filtering method for analysis of collagen alignment in ligaments. IEEE Trans Biomed Eng 1987; 34(7): 509–518.

40. Cooper RR, Misol S: Tendon and ligament insertion. A light and electron microscope study. J Bone Joint Surg 1970; 52A: 1–20.

41. Woo SL-Y, Maynard J, Butler DL, et al: Ligament, tendon and joint capsule insertions into bone. In Woo SL-Y, Buckwalter JA (eds): Injury and Repair of the Musculoskeletal Soft Tissues. Rosemont, IL, American Academy of Orthopaedic Surgeons, 1988, pp 133–166.

42. Matyas JR, Bodie D, Andersen M, Frank CB: The developmental morphology of a "periosteal" ligament insertion: Growth and maturation of the tibial insertion of the rabbit medial collateral ligament. J Orthop Res 1990; 8(3): 412–424.

43. Matyas JR: The Structure and Function of the Insertions of the Rabbit Medial Collateral Ligament. University of Calgary, PhD thesis, 1990.

44. Woo SL-Y, Gomez MA, Woo YK, Akeson WH: Mechanical properties of tendons and ligaments. I. Quasi-static and nonlinear viscoelastic properties. Biorheology 1982; 19:385–396.

45. Nimni ME: Collagen. Volume II. Biochemistry and Biomechanics. Boca Raton, CRC Press, 1988.

46. Miller EJ, Gay S: Collagen structure and function. In Cohen IK,

Diegelmann RF, Lindblad WJ (eds): Wound Healing. Biochemical and Clinical Aspects. Philadelphia, WB Saunders, 1992, pp 130–151.

47. Parry DAD, Craig AS: Collagen fibrils during development and maturation and their contribution to the mechanical attributes of connective tissue. In Nimni ME (ed): Collagen, Vol II. Biochemistry and Biomechanics. Boca Raton, CRC Press, 1988, pp 1–23.

48. Vogel KG, Ordog A, Pogany G, Olah J: Proteoglycans in the compressed region of human tibialis posterior tendon and in ligaments. J Orthop Res 1993; 11: 68–77.

49. Woo SL-Y, Young EP: Structure and function of tendons and ligaments. In Mow VC, Hayes WC (eds): Basic Orthopaedic Biomechanics. New York, Raven Press, 1991, pp 199–243.

50. Woo SL-Y, Adams DJ: The tensile properties of human anterior cruciate ligament (ACL) and ACL graft tissues. In Daniel DM, Akeson WH, O'Connor JJ (eds): Knee Ligaments. Structure, Function, Injury and Repair. New York, Raven Press, 1990, pp 279–289.

51. Butler DL, Grood ES, Noyes FR, Zernicke RF: Biomechanics of ligaments and tendons. Exerc Sports Sci Rev 1978; 6:125–182.

52. Woo SL-Y, Weiss JA, MacKenna DA: Biomechanics and morphology of the medial collateral and anterior cruciate ligaments. In Mow VC, Ratcliffe A, Woo SL-Y (eds): Biomechanics of Diarthrodial Joints. New York, Springer-Verlag, 1990, pp 63–104.

53. Woo SL-Y, Hollis JM, Adams DJ, et al: Tensile properties of the human femur–anterior cruciate ligament–tibia complex. The effects of specimen age and orientation. Am J Sports Med 1991; 19(3): 217–225.

54. Noyes FR, Butler DL, Grood ES, et al: Biomechanical analysis of human ligament grafts used in knee-ligament repairs and reconstructions. J Bone Joint Surg 1984; 66A: 344–352.

55. Grood ES, Butler DL, Noyes FR: Comment on "Effects of knee flexion angle on the structural properties of the rabbit femur-anterior cruciate ligament-tibia complex." J Biomech 1988; 21: 688–691 (Letter).

56. Woo SL-Y, Orlando CA, Gomez MA, et al: Tensile properties of the medial collateral ligament as a function of age. J Orthop Res 1986; 4: 133–141.

57. Lewis JL, Lew WD, Hill JA, et al: Knee joint motion and ligament forces before and after ACL reconstruction. J Biomech Eng 1989; 111:97–106.

58. Chimich DD, Frank CB, Shrive NG, et al: The effects of initial end contact on medial collateral ligament healing—A morphological and biomechanical study in the rabbit model. J Orthop Res 1991; 9:37–47.

59. Woo SL-Y, Gomez MA, Akeson WH: The time- and history-dependent viscoelastic properties of the canine medial collateral ligaments. J Biomech Eng 1981; 103: 293–298.

60. Lam TC, Frank CB, Shrive NG: Changes in the cyclic and static relaxations of the rabbit medial collateral ligament complex during maturation. J Biomech 1993; 26(1): 9–17.

61. Chimich DD, Shrive NG, Frank CB, et al: Water content alters viscoelastic behaviour of the normal adolescent rabbit medial collateral ligament. J Biomech 1992; 25(8): 831–837.

62. Lam TC: The Mechanical Properties of the Maturing Medial Collateral Ligament. University of Calgary, PhD thesis, 1988.

63. Hurov JR: Soft tissue interface: How do attachments of muscles, tendons and ligaments change during growth? A light microscopic study. J Morphol 1986; 189: 313–325.

64. Videman T: An experimental study of the effects of growth on the relationship of tendons and ligaments to bone at the site of diaphyseal insertion. Part II. Determination of growth patterns and inhibitions of displacement using metal markers. Ann Chir Gynaecol Fenn 1970; 59: 22–34.

65. Amiel D, Kuiper SD, Wallace CD, et al: Age-related properties of medial collateral ligament and anterior cruciate ligament: A morphologic and collagen maturation study in the rabbit. J Gerontol 1991; 46(4): B159–B165.

66. Frank CB, Matyas JR, Hart DA: Aging of the medial collateral ligament (MCL): Interdisciplinary studies. In Buckwalter JA, Goldberg VM, Woo SL-Y (eds): Musculoskeletal Soft-Tissue Aging: Impact on Mobility. Rosemont, IL, American Academy of Orthopaedic Surgeons, 1994, pp 305–322.

67. Woo SL-Y, Gomez MA, Sites TJ, et al: The biomechanical and morphological changes in the medial collateral ligament of the

rabbit after immobilization and remobilization. J Bone Joint Surg 1987; 69A: 1200–1211.

68. Woo SL-Y, Matthews V, Akeson WH, et al: Connective tissue response to immobility. Correlative study of biomechanical and biochemical measurements of normal and immobilized rabbit knees. Arthritis Rheum 1974; 18(3): 257–264.

69. Tipton CM, Matthes RD, Maynard JA, Carey RA: The influence of physical activity on ligaments and tendons. Med Sci Sports 1975; 7(3): 165–175.

70. Amiel D, Woo SL-Y, Harwood FL, Akeson WH: The effect of immobilization on collagen turnover in connective tissue: A biochemical-biomechanical correlation. Acta Orthop Scand 1982; 53(3): 325–332.

71. Woo SL-Y, Wang CW, Newton PO, Lyon RM: The response of ligaments to stress deprivation and stress enhancement. Biomechanical studies. In Daniel DM, Akeson WH, O'Connor JJ (eds): Knee Ligaments: Structure, Function, Injury and Repair. New York, Raven Press, 1990, pp 337–350.

72. Noyes FR: Functional properties of knee ligaments and alterations induced by immobilization. A correlative biomechanical and histological study in primates. Clin Orthop 1977; 123: 210–242.

73. Akeson WH, Amiel D, Woo SL-Y: Immobility effects on synovial joints. The pathomechanics of joint contracture. Biorheology 1980; 17:95.

74. Akeson WH: An experimental study of joint stiffness. J Bone Joint Surg 1961; 43A: 1022–1034.

75. Rubin CT, Lanyon LE: Regulation of bone formation by applied dynamic loads. J Bone Joint Surg 1984; 66A: 397–402.

76. Weir TMB: Recovery of the MCL After Immobilization. University of Calgary, MSc thesis, 1992.

77. Larsen NP, Forwood MR, Parker AW: Immobilization and retraining of cruciate ligaments in the rat. Acta Orthop Scand 1987; 58: 260–264.

78. Woo SL-Y, Gomez MA, Woo YK, Akeson WH: Mechanical properties of tendons and ligaments. II. The relationships of immobilization and exercise on tissue remodeling. Biorheology 1982; 19: 397–408.

79. Torg J, Conrad W, Kalen V: Clinical diagnosis of anterior cruciate ligament instability in the athlete. Am J Sports Med 1976; 4: 84–93.

80. Jackson DW, Campbell AJ: Diagnosis of partial ruptures of the anterior cruciate ligament. Orthop Trans 1981; 5: 441 (Abstract).

81. Jackson RW: The torn ACL: Natural history of untreated lesions and rationale for selective treatment. In Feagin JA (ed): The Cruciate Ligaments. New York, Churchill Livingstone, 1988, pp 341–348.

82. LeBlanc PE: A descriptive anatomic study of the anterior cruciate ligament in patients with failed non-operative therapy. Annual Surgeons' Day, University of Calgary 1992; 10 (Abstract).

83. Shrive NG, Chimich DD, Marchuk L, et al: "Flaws" in scar matrix correlate with material properties of ligament scars. J Orthop Res (in press).

84. Padgett LR, Dahners LE: Rigid immobilization alters matrix organization in the injured rat medial collateral ligament. J Orthop Res 1992; 10: 895–900.

85. Frank CB, Schachar NS, Dittrich D: Natural history of healing in the repaired medial collateral ligament. J Orthop Res 1983; 1: 179–188.

86. Frank CB, Amiel D, Woo SL-Y, Akeson WH: Normal ligament properties and ligament healing. Clin Orthop 1985; 196: 15–25.

87. O'Donoghue DH, Frank GR, Jeter GL, et al: Repair and reconstruction of the anterior cruciate ligament in dogs. Factors influencing long term results. J Bone Joint Surg 1971; 53A: 710–718.

88. Frank CB, Woo SL-Y, Amiel D, et al: Medial collateral ligament healing. A multidisciplinary assessment in rabbits. Am J Sports Med 1983; 11(6): 379–389.

89. Woo SL-Y, Tkach LV: The cellular and matrix response of ligaments and tendons to mechanical injury. In Leadbetter WB, Buckwalter JA, Gordon SL (eds): Sports-Induced Inflammation. Rosemont, IL, American Academy of Orthopaedic Surgeons, 1990, pp 189–204.

90. Tipton CM, Vailas AC, Matthes RD: Experimental studies on the influences of physical activity on ligaments, tendons and joints: a brief review. Acta Med Scand (Suppl) 1986; 711:157–168.

91. Woo SL-Y, Young EP, Kwan MK: Fundamental studies in knee ligament mechanics. In Daniel DD, Akeson WH, O'Connor JJ (eds): Knee Ligaments. Structure, Function, Injury and Repair. New York, Raven Press, 1990, pp 115–134.

92. Salter RB: The biologic concept of continuous passive motion of synovial joints. The first 18 years of basic research and its clinical application. Clin Orthop 1989; 242: 12–25.

93. Mankin HJ: The response of articular cartilage to mechanical injury. J Bone Joint Surg 1982; 64A: 460–466.

94. Adams ME: Target tissue models: cartilage changes in experimental osteoarthritis in the dog. J Rheumatol(Suppl)1983; 11: 111–113.

95. Bray RC, Shrive NG, Frank CB, Chimich DD: The early effects of joint immobilization on medial collateral ligament healing in an ACL-deficient knee: A gross anatomic and biomechanical investigation in the adult rabbit model. J Orthop Res 1992; 10(2): 157–166.

96. Gomez MA, Woo SL-Y, Inoue M, et al: Medial collateral ligament healing subsequent to different treatment regimens. J Appl Physiol 1989; 66(1): 245–252.

97. Anderson AF, Lipscomb AB: Analysis of rehabilitation techniques after anterior cruciate reconstruction. Am J Sports Med 1988; 17(2): 154–160.

98. Frank CB, Akeson WH, Woo SL-Y, et al: Physiology and therapeutic value of passive joint motion. Clin Orthop 1984; 185: 113–125.

99. Leadbetter WB, Buckwalter JA, Gordon SL (eds): Sports-Induced Inflammation. Rosemont, IL, American Academy of Orthopaedic Surgeons, 1990.

100. O'Donoghue DH, Rockwood CA, Zaricznyj B, Kenyon R: Repair of knee ligaments in dogs. I. The lateral collateral ligament. J Bone Joint Surg 1961; 43A: 1167–1178.

101. O'Donoghue DH, Rockwood CA, Frank GR, et al: Repair of the anterior cruciate ligament in dogs. J Bone Joint Surg 1966; 48A: 503–519.

102. Feagin JAJ, Cabaud HE, Curl WW: The anterior cruciate ligament: radiographic and clinical signs of successful and unsuccessful repairs. Clin Orthop 1982; 164: 54–58.

103. Feagin JAJ, Blake WP: Postoperative evaluation and result recording in the anterior cruciate ligament reconstructed knee. Clin Orthop 1983; 172: 143–147.

104. Sabiston CP, Frank CB, Lam TC, Shrive NG: Transplantation of the rabbit medial collateral ligament. 1. Biomechanical evaluation of fresh autografts. J Orthop Res 1990; 8(1): 35–45.

105. Sabiston CP, Frank CB, Lam TC, Shrive NG: Allograft ligament transplantation. A morphological and biochemical evaluation of a medial collateral ligament complex in a rabbit model. Am J Sports Med 1990; 18(2): 160–168.

106. Sabiston CP, Frank CB, Lam TC, Shrive NG: Transplantation of the rabbit medial collateral ligament. 2. Biomechanical evaluation of frozen-thawed allografts. J Orthop Res 1990; 8(1): 46–56.

107. King GJW: A Biomechanical Evaluation of Orthoptic Ligament Transplantation in a Rabbit Model. University of Calgary, MSc thesis, 1991.

108. Grood ES, Butler DL, Noyes FR: Models of ligament repairs and grafts. In Finnerman G (ed): American Academy of Orthopaedic Surgeons: Symposium on Sports Medicine: The Knee. St. Louis, CV Mosby, 1985, pp 169–181.

109. Noyes FR, Butler DL, Paulos LE, Grood ES: Intra-articular cruciate reconstruction. I: Perspectives on graft strength, vascularization, and immediate motion after replacement. Clin Orthop 1983; 172: 71–77.

110. Shino K, Inoue M, Horibe S, et al: Reconstruction of the anterior cruciate ligament using allogenic tendon. Long term follow-up. Am J Sports Med 1990; 18(5): 457–465.

111. Horibe S, Shino K, Nakamura H, et al: Replacing the medial collateral ligament with an allogenic tendon graft. An experimental canine study. J Bone Joint Surg 1990; 72B(6): 1044–1049.

112. Noyes FR, Barber SD, Mangine RE: Bone-patellar ligament-bone and fascia lata allografts for reconstruction of the anterior cruciate ligament. J Bone Joint Surg 1990; 72A(8): 1125–1136.

CHAPTER 3

Tendon Injuries: Pathophysiology and Treatment

S A N D R A L. C U R W I N   *BSc (Physio), MSc, PhD*

Tendons are important structures in the musculoskeletal system. They transmit the forces generated by muscles to bony attachments, thus moving these skeletal levers. They are relatively small but are tremendously strong—perhaps half as strong as steel. Yet, tendons do become injured. Some injuries are unavoidable, the result of accidents such as the severing of flexor tendons in the hand. More commonly, the gradual onset of pain and tenderness alerts the athlete to a lesser tendon injury—tendinitis. This "simple" overuse injury can cause prolonged disability for the competitive athlete and a dilemma for both athletes and care providers. How can mobility and strength be best maintained while healing occurs? Should tendons be exercised while healing? Can tendons respond to changes in loading? If so, how rapidly? What type, and how much, exercise is beneficial? When should it be started? Does tendinitis follow the same healing process as ruptured or severed tendons? Can exercise prevent injury to tendons? These and many other questions about tendon behavior remain unanswered. Experts cannot even agree if the problem should be called tendinitis!

The purpose of this chapter is to describe the structure, physiology, and mechanics of tendon, to describe what happens to an injured tendon, and to speculate on how one can manipulate the tendon's environment. A successful treatment strategy will both treat the injured tendon and prevent it from becoming reinjured or perhaps prevent an injury from ever occurring. The design of such a strategy requires knowledge and understanding of tendon structure and function and their alteration in pathologic conditions such as tendinitis. One can then use this knowledge to successfully treat tendon injuries.

STRUCTURE AND FUNCTION

STRUCTURE OF THE TENDON AND ITS COMPONENTS

Tendons and ligaments are often called "dense, parallel-fibered connective tissues" and are considered similar in structure. They are both composed of cells and matrix, and both tissues are unique because their behavior is determined not by their cell content but by their extracellular components. Many differences exist, however, between ligaments and tendons; indeed, the details of fine structure of tendons themselves may vary

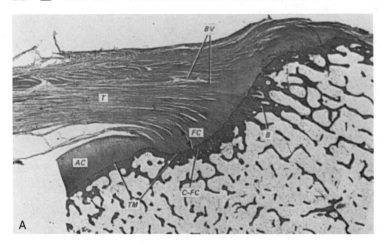

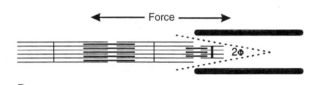

FIGURE 3–1. *A,* The bone-tendon junction. The bony insertion of the supraspinatus tendon, showing the four distinct zones Tendon (T), unmineralized fibrocartilage (FC), mineralized fibrocartilage (C-FC), and bone (B). There are no blood vessels (BV) in the fibrocartilage zones. There is a prominent line, the tidemark (TM), between the mineralized and unmineralized zones; this is analogous to that seen in articular cartilage. (From Benjamin M, Evans EJ, Copp L: J Anat 1986; 149:89. Reprinted with the permission of Cambridge University Press.) *B,* The structures of the muscle-tendon junction. Muscle cells and collagen fibers interact directly and are connected via adhesions crossing the muscle cell membrane. The strength of the junction is largely due to frictional forces between the overlapping surfaces. (Adapted from Tidball JG: Cell Motil 1983; 3:439. Copyright 1983. Reprinted by permission of John Wiley & Sons, Inc.)

among species and even between different tendons in the same animal.[1–3] Despite these variations, all tendons are alike in attaching muscle to bone at each end of the muscle. The distal tendon is often larger and better developed and is ropelike in structure, whereas the proximal end is composed of much shorter, smaller fibers and has a fleshy attachment into the bone. At most tendon-bone interfaces the collagen fibers insert directly, at a 90 degree angle, into the bone.[4] There is a gradual transition in material composition, over a distance of about 1 mm, through four zones: tendon, fibrocartilage, mineralized fibrocartilage, and bone.[4] Some fibers join the bone at an acute angle, blending gradually into the periosteum.[5] The ultrastructure of most bone-tendon junctions is similar, even though they may vary widely in gross anatomic appearance, from a flat aponeurosis to a rounded cord. The structure of the bone-tendon junction is illustrated in Figure 3–1A.

Each myotendinous junction is a layered region of infoldings connecting the terminal actin filaments of the sarcomeres to tendon collagen fibers via transmembrane proteins.[6–8] The infoldings increase the surface contact area so that stress is reduced, ensure that junctions are loaded in shear rather than tension, and minimize areas of stress concentration.[6] Muscle cells are surrounded by collagenous tissue, so the entire surface of the muscle fiber, not just the end, is capable of transferring tension across the cell membrane to the tendon.[6,7] The geometry of these attachments is illustrated in Figure 3–1B.

Tendons are complexes composed primarily of collagen and other proteins, glycosaminoglycans, elastin, glycolipids, cells, and water.[9–11] Collagen is a family of molecules divided into two major groups (Table 3–1). At least 13 collagens, the products of 20 distinct genes, have so far been identified.[12] These collagen molecules can be divided into two classes, the fiber-forming collagen types (I, II, III, V, XI), and other types that do not form regular fibers (IV, VI, VII, VIII, IX, X, XII, XIII).[12] Types II and XI collagen are found only in cartilage. The collagen in tendons is mainly type I; it composes 70 to 80 percent

TABLE 3–1
Types of Collagen

Type	Tissue	Form
Type I	Skin bone, tendon	Fibrillar
Type II	Cartilage, disc	Fibrillar
Type III	Skin, blood vessels, tendon, healing tissues	Fibrillar
Type V	With Type I	Fibrillar
Type XI	With Type I	Fibrillar
Type IV	Basal lamina (around cell)	Three-dimensional network
Type VII	Epithelial basement membrane	Anchoring fibril
Type VIII	Endothelial basement membrane	Unknown
Type VI	Widespread	Microfilaments
Type IX	Cartilage	Cross-linked to type II
Type X	Hypertrophic cartilage	Unknown
Type XII	Tendon, other?	Unknown
Type XIII	Endothelial cells	Unknown

Adapted from Eyre DR: The collagens of musculoskeletal soft tissues. *In* Leadbetter WB, Buckwalter JA, Gordon SL (eds): Sports-Induced Inflammation. Rosemont, IL, American Academy of Orthopaedic Surgeons, 1990, p 162.

of the dry weight of the tissue after all water is removed. There is also some type V collagen in tendon, about 3 percent of the amount of type I, and a variable amount of type III collagen depending on the maturity of the tissue. Type III collagen is found in fairly large amounts in immature or healing tendon but usually constitutes less than 5 percent of the total collagen found in mature tendons.[13] Type IV collagen is also found in tendons, but it does not contribute to the mechanical properties of the tissue. Because type I collagen is the major load-bearing component in dense connective tissues,[12] tendons and ligaments provide an excellent opportunity to explore the mechanical properties of this collagen. All the extracellular elements of the tendon are synthesized inside cells called fibroblasts, where a variety of influences can alter the amount and type of each component.[14]

The tendon also contains *ground substance,* a mixture of water and glycosaminoglycan (GAGs) compounds. The ground substance provides the friction that causes collagen fibrils to adhere to one another, yet also provides lubrication and spacing so that fibrils can slide past one another.[9,15] The GAGs form only about 1 percent of the tissue dry weight but are important because they bind water, which forms 65 to 75 percent of the total weight of the tendon. The GAGs are bimolecular sugar type molecules. They may combine with other GAGs to form long chains or with a protein core to form proteoglycans.[9,10] Tendon proteoglycans (PGs) are organized like those found in cartilage but are much smaller. They also have a different GAG composition, containing mostly dermatan sulfate, whereas cartilage contains large amounts of chondroitin sulfate.[10,16] PGs associate with the surface of the collagen molecule,[15] probably in the gap zone near where the collagen molecules overlap in a head-to-tail fashion (see Fig. 3–2). PGs play a role, as yet undefined, in the organization of collagen into fibrils, both directing and limiting this organization.[9,15,17]

PROCESSING INSIDE AND OUTSIDE THE CELL

Most proteins are "processed" inside the cells that produce them and remain largely unchanged after leaving the cell. Processing may include such things as hydroxylation or glycosylation of amino acids, cleaving of terminal peptides, folding into a tertiary formation, and covalent bonding.[14] Collagen undergoes many of these same intracellular processes but also undergoes a number of extracellular modifications that contribute to its function. In fact, it is the extracellular processing of collagen that gives rise to the unique mechanical properties of connective tissues such as skin, ligaments, and tendons.[12] Extracellular events include cross-linking between molecules and the organization into a fibrillar structure that gives collagen its unique load-bearing properties.[18–21] This is an extremely important feature of dense connective tissues such as tendon, for the *amount* of tissue depends largely on intracellular events, whereas the *quality* of the final

tissue is determined outside the cell. These processes are summarized in Figure 3–2.

Cross-linking between and within collagen molecules prevents their enzymatic, mechanical, or chemical breakdown and helps direct the organization of collagen molecules into fibrillar structures.[12,18] Some cross-links have a short-lived function, such as the disulfide bonds that form intracellularly between cysteine residues in the amino- and carboxy-terminals of the procollagen chain that facilitate the triple helix arrangement of the molecule.[14] These termini are later cleaved from the molecule by peptidase enzymes outside the cell, leaving the tropocollagen molecule. Other cross-links are formed after the molecules leave the cell. These cross-links, called immature or reducible, form between modified lysine and/or hydroxylysine amino acid residues in adjacent amino acid chains. The chains may be from the same or neighboring molecules. These cross-links are basically enzyme-facilitated chemical rearrangements of adjacent amino acids, the enzyme being lysyl oxidase. Lysine-derived cross-links predominate in some tissues, while hydroxylysine-derived cross-links predominate in other tissues such as tendon that are subjected to higher tensile loads.[12] It has been shown that the amount of hydroxylysine-based cross-links can be directly affected by increasing the load on a tendon, suggesting a feedback mechanism to the cell or its environment.[22] After the bimolecular cross-links form, they gradually rearrange to make up trimolecular cross-links such as hydroxypyridinium. These cross-links, derived from hydroxylysine-based immature cross-links, are thought to take weeks or months to form under normal circumstances.[22] Their presence is a reflection of the mature load-bearing ability of the tendon, giving the tendon its ability to withstand high levels of tensile force.[12,21]

DEFECTS IN COLLAGEN PROCESSING AND ORGANIZATION

There are a number of defects in collagen metabolism that can lead to clinical disorders (Table 3–2). Some are genetic disorders, such as the various forms of Ehler-Danlos syndrome,[24] osteogenesis imperfecta (OI), chondrodysplasias, some forms of epidermolysis nervosa, Marfan syndrome, and others.[25] Some gene mutations cause decreased cross-linking, resulting in weaker tissues that elongate readily when force is applied. Others cause defects in collagen molecular structure or organization. There is a wide spectrum of severity of these disorders, depending on the location of the gene mutation.[25] Milder phenotypes may appear as the more common disorders of osteoarthritis, osteoporosis, and some disorders of vascular integrity. Increased cross-linking is more likely to occur in diabetic patients, resulting in stiffer tissues that require more force to stretch, which may explain why adhesive capsulitis is up to ten times more prevalent in diabetic patients compared with age-matched control subjects.[26] This is environmental, rather than genetic, and appears to be due to an increase in nonenzymatic cross-linking

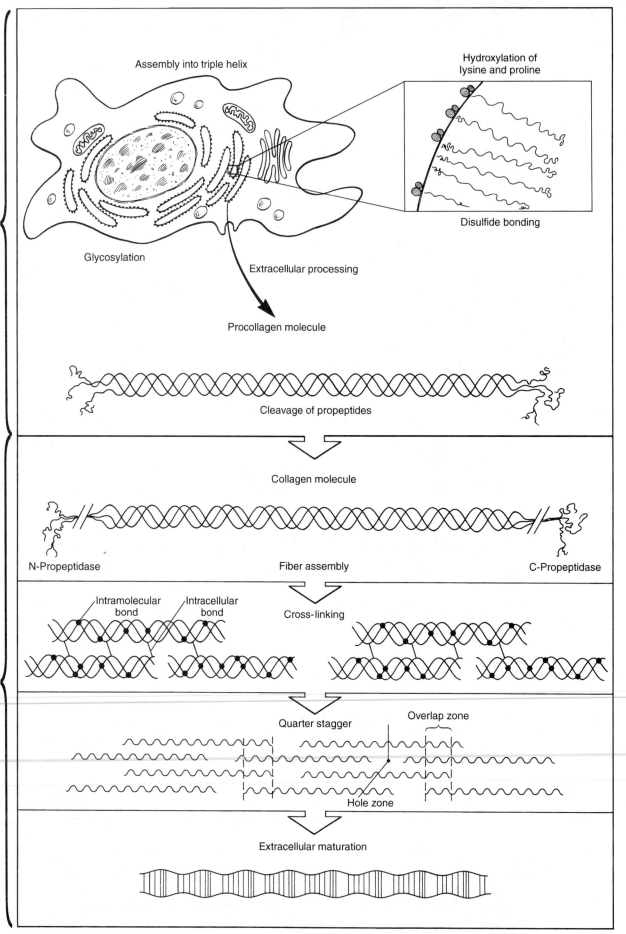

FIGURE 3–2. Extracellular modifications of collagen. Collagen is synthesized in ribosomes; the triple helix forms in the rough endoplasmic reticulum. Several modifications occur here as well, such as hydroxylation and glycosylation. After secretion into the extracellular space, in the confines of cellular infoldings, further modifications take place that allow the collagen to assemble into a fibrillar structure. Mature cross-links form later. (Adapted from Prockop D, Guzman NA: Hosp Pract 1977; 12:61. Reprinted with permission.)

TABLE 3–2
Some Disorders of Collagen Metabolism

Level of Defect	Collagen Defect	Reason	Clinical Manifestations	Clinical Name
Regulation of synthesis	Decreased or abnormal type I collagen	Lack of gene, or mutation	Fragile bones and soft tissues, multiple fractures, blue sclera; variable in severity depending on genetic pattern	Osteogenesis imperfecta (OI) (several types exist)
	Decreased or abnormal type III collagen	Lack of gene, or mutation	Weak arteries, skin, intestine, uterus (organs may rupture); easy bruising	Ehler-Danlos syndrome type IV
	Decreased type I collagen	Severe vitamin C deficiency, fasting	Growth suppression, poor wound healing, fragile skin	Scurvy
Structural defects	Decreased collagen fibril formation, failure to remove amino-terminal propeptide	Structural mutation in one procollagen chain	Skin fragility and hyperextensibility, easy bruising, bilateral hip dislocation	Ehler-Danlos syndrome type VI
	Decreased hydroxyproline	Vitamin C deficiency (cofactor for prolylhydroxylase enzyme)	Same as above	Scurvy
Enzyme defects	Decreased cross-linking	Decreased lysyl oxidase enzyme	Loose skin, hypermobility in joints of digits	Ehler-Danlos syndrome type V
	Decreased cross-linking	Decreased lysyl hydroxylase enzyme	Skin hyperextensibility, poor wound healing, musculoskeletal deformities	Ehler-Danlos syndrome type VI
Lysyl oxidase inhibition	Decreased cross-linking	Copper deficiency, decreased lysyl oxidase activity	As for Ehler-Danlos type V	
	Decreased cross-linking	Poisoning due to β-aminopropionitrile ingestion	As for Ehler-Danlos type V	Lathyrism

related to glycosylation of hydroxylysine residues while in the rough endoplasmic reticulum or Golgi complex of the cell. Immature cross-links are also increased in capsular tissues after joint immobilization, whereas they are decreased in tendons and ligaments around the same joint.[27–29] This leads to decreased joint range of motion and increased friction with joint movement, thus requiring a greater muscle effort to produce the same range of motion.[27–29]

ASSEMBLY INTO A FIBRILLAR STRUCTURE

Collagen molecules aggregate linearly in an overlapping head-to-tail fashion after leaving the fibroblast,[3,14] but the exact nature of their supramolecular organization is not certain, probably because it varies among tissues. For example, both the cornea and the tendon contain mostly type I collagen; however, that of the cornea is organized randomly to produce a transparent sheet, while that of tendon is organized into bundles.[12] The reasons for this difference are not known. Once the procollagen chains have been secreted from the cell, but while they are still contained within infoldings of the cell membrane, the ends of the triple helix molecules are enzymatically removed, leaving collagen (tropocollagen). This step is essential for subsequent assembly into fibrils; linear and lateral aggregation of the molecules then begins. The molecules assemble laterally in groups of five (microfibrils), overlapped linearly in a head-to-tail fashion that is dictated by cross-linking ability and by the type and amount of GAGs already present.[3,9] Each microfibril is about 4 nm wide. A variable number of microfibrils associate to form col-

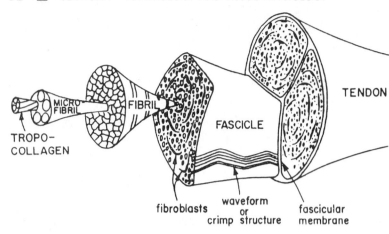

FIGURE 3–3. The hierarchical structure of tendon. (Redrawn with permission from Kastelic J, Galseki A, Baer E: Connect Tissue Res 1978; 6:11.)

lagen fibrils ranging from 30 to 400 nm in diameter. It is at the subfibrillar levels that intermolecular cross-linking normally occurs.[9,12,29] The space between fibrils is usually too large to allow cross-linking between adjacent fibrils, although this may sometimes occur during immobilization.[27,29] The interfibrillar matrix probably plays its greatest role in adhesion between collagen fibrils.[15,17]

Collagen fibrils are the smallest tendon units capable of resisting load under laboratory conditions. Tissue strength, especially during healing, is closely correlated with collagen content, but this collagen must be organized and cross-linked before it can function as a load-bearing unit.[30] Masses of nonorganized collagen molecules are incapable of resisting tensile force application.[13] The ground substance modifies the organization of collagen in the tissue, both directing and somehow limiting fibril organization.[9,11,15,17] New microfibrils may be added to existing nearby fibrils, increasing their size, or they may associate to form new fibrils, which are typically much smaller in diameter than the older fibrils.[31,32] Fibroblasts become squeezed between the growing fibrils and end up as columns of flattened, spindle-shaped cells with thin cytoplasmic processes extending among the fibrils. The strongest tendons contain large numbers of large-diameter fibrils. These are generally the oldest fibrils, which also contain the largest numbers of mature cross-links.[12,31,32] Immature and healing tissues contain larger amounts of type III collagen, which forms smaller diameter fibrils than does type I.

Collagen fibrils group together to form successively larger primary bundles, which are also known as fibers (see Fig. 3–3). They are the smallest units visible in light microscopy, with a diameter of 1 to 10 μm. Groups of fibers are surrounded by a loose connective tissue sheath called the *endotenon,* which also encloses the nerves, lymphatics, and blood vessels supplying the tendon, to form a *fascicle* (secondary bundle).[3,33] The fascicles are considered the smallest functional, i.e., "real-life," load-bearing units within the tendon. Individual fascicles are associated with discrete groups of muscle fibers (or motor units) at muscle-tendon junctions. Several fascicles may form a larger group (tertiary bundle) also surrounded by endotenon; enveloping all the secondary bundles and their endotenon coverings is

another sheath, the *epitenon.* The sheaths may be differentiated by their location and also by their collagen type content. The endotenon contains more type III collagen, organized as small-diameter fibrils, while the epitenon, which contains more type I, has larger diameter fibrils. An additional double-layered sheath of areolar tissue, the *peritenon* or *paratenon,* is loosely attached to the outer surface of the epitenon. The peritenon may become a synovial fluid–filled sheath, the *tenosynovium,* in tendons that are subjected to friction. A simplified version of the hierarchical organization of the tendon is illustrated in Figure 3–3.[3] There is some evidence to suggest that the organization may vary from place to place within the tendon, which may explain why there is no universally accepted model of tendon organization.[34]

MECHANICAL BEHAVIOR OF THE TENDON

The organization of the tendon determines its mechanical behavior. The ground substance "shrinks" the resting tendon, causing it to have a slightly crimped, or wavelike, appearance.[1,2] The crimp can be straightened by application of a load, but the tendon will immediately recover its original resting length if the load is removed. This results in a "toe" region in the force-elongation curve (Fig. 3–4). The tendon is very elastic at low loads, with small increases in force resulting in large changes in length. It is the straightening of the crimped fibrils that is responsible for mechanical behavior in this region of the curve; little or no physical deformation of the collagen fibrils themselves takes place.[1,3] The force-elongation curve can be transformed into a stress-strain curve by dividing the force by the tissue cross-sectional area, and the change in length by the original tissue length (Fig. 3–5).[1]

STRUCTURAL PROPERTIES

Many factors can affect the force-elongation curve. The total amount of force the tendon can resist, and the absolute change in length during loading, will depend on the size (cross-sectional area) and length of the tendon, as shown in Figure 3–6. Larger tendons will be

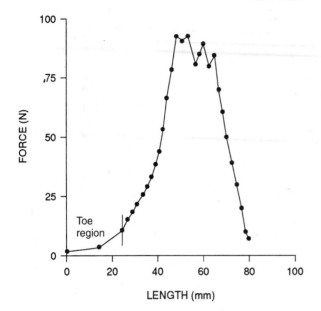

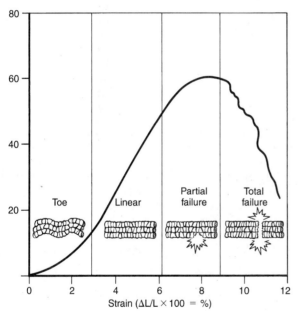

FIGURE 3—4. A force-length curve for a tendon loaded until failure. The tendon lengthens as force is increased, and the collagen fibrils straighten, then stretch under the applied force. First, a few fibers fail and the load drops, rising as remaining fibers "take up" the load. Finally, more fibers rupture, tissue failure occurs, and force drops rapidly.

FIGURE 3—5. A stress-strain curve for a tendon loaded until failure. In this case, the force is divided by the size (cross-sectional area) of the tendon to give the stress, while the increase in length is divided by original length to give the strain ([ΔL/L] × 100). In the toe region of the curve, the crimped collagen fibrils straighten, which requires little force. In the linear region, the straightened collagen fibrils resist the load, and ever-increasing amounts of force are required to produce the same percentage elongation. The slope of this part of the curve represents the stiffness of the tissue. It is in this region of the curve that changes in material properties, such as increased cross-links or larger diameter fibrils, will have the most influence. Less physical deformation (increased tissue stiffness) should reduce the likelihood of injury. After the linear region, the stress-strain curve becomes less predictable as fibers fail sequentially.

able to tolerate larger forces, and longer tendons will undergo greater absolute (but not percentage) changes in length before fibril disruption than will shorter tendons. These size-dependent features are referred to as the structural properties of the tendon.[1] They depend on the physical dimensions of the tendon.

MATERIAL PROPERTIES

Variability in tendon composition, such as differences in collagen concentration or cross-link number, can also cause differences in the force-elongation curve. The inability to distinguish whether size or composition is responsible for changes makes comparison of the mechanical behavior of different tendons difficult, unless the influence of one factor is somehow removed.[1] The effect of size can be removed by calculating the force relative to the cross-sectional area of the tendon,

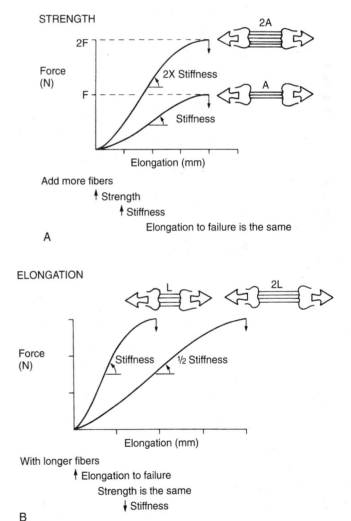

FIGURE 3—6. Structural properties of tendon (those determined by size and length). Generally, a larger tendon will withstand greater forces at the same percentage elongation, while a longer tendon will undergo a greater overall length change in response to the same magnitude of applied load. (Redrawn from Butler DL, Grood ES, Noyes FR, Zernicke RF: Biomechanics of ligaments and tendons. Exerc Sports Sci Rev 1978; 6:144.)

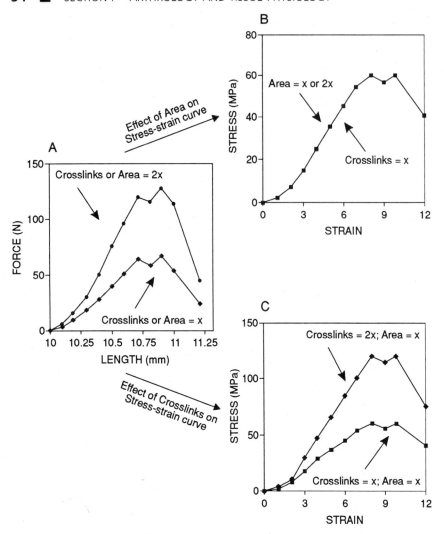

FIGURE 3–7. The effects of changing size and/or composition on tendon behavior. Changes in structural properties (size-related) or material properties (composition-related) can have the same, or very different, mechanical effects. *A*, Both increased cross-links and increased size can increase the force that can be applied to the tendon during tensile loading. *B*, When force is divided by area to yield stress, the different-sized tendons are revealed to have the same material properties, i.e., the same stress-strain curve. *C*, When cross-linking differs between tendons, this will always be reflected in a different stress-strain curve. This would apply whether the area was the same or different.

i.e., stress, and by expressing length changes as a percentage of the original length, i.e., strain. Thus, the force-elongation curve becomes the stress-strain curve (see Fig. 3–5), a representation that is independent of area or length. Differences in the stress-strain curves of different tendons are said to reflect the material properties of the tendons.[1,29,34] These properties are due to such factors as differing collagen fibril organization, differences in cross-linking, varying ground substance concentration, and perhaps different collagen types. They are dependent on the material of which the tendon is made, not how much material the tendon contains.

An increase in cross-linking would be expected to alter the material properties of a tendon and make it stronger than a tendon of the same size containing fewer cross-links. Similarly, an overall increase in area but no change in cross-linking or collagen concentration could result in a tendon able to withstand larger loads. Both these adaptations take place in tendons exposed to altered physiologic conditions. The effects of changes in composition and size are illustrated in Figure 3–7.

Differences in collagen type also may affect tissue mechanical behavior. Tissues with large amounts of type III collagen usually are less stiff and have lower tensile strength than those composed of mostly type I collagen[12,19,32]; however, it is unknown whether there is actually any difference in the tensile strength of type I vs. type III collagen, or whether tissue strength differences are more closely related to fibril architecture and cross-link number.[12] Type I and type III collagen have been found in the same fibrils, but the effect of this commingling on tensile strength is unknown.[12]

PHYSICAL CHANGES DURING LOADING

Force application beyond the toe region (2 to 4 percent elongation) causes progressive deformation of the tendon's components and structure.[34] There is a linear relationship between applied force and resulting tissue deformation beyond the toe region, with stress applied directly to the now-straightened collagen fibrils.[35,36] It is in this region of the curve that cross-linking and adhesion between fibrils play the most important role, and differences in the slope of the linear region of the stress-strain curve may be interpreted to reflect differences in collagen concentration (or type), cross-linking, or ground substance concentration. X-ray diffraction techniques show that as loading is increased, the first structural damage is intrafibrillar slippage (between molecules), then interfibrillar slipping (between fibrils), and finally gross disruption of the collagen fibrils/fibers themselves.[35-37] Intrafibrillar slippage is probably governed by cross-linking, interfibrillar slippage by ground substance, and gross disruption by these factors plus fibril size. After the first fibrils rupture, the force curve plateaus, then drops off rapidly as the remaining fibrils fail in sequence. Total mechanical failure usually occurs at about 8 to 10 percent elongation from the starting length.[34]

Most tendon injuries, except frank ruptures or cuts, probably result from loading that extends into the linear region. Increasing severity of injury may be due to a progressive collapse of lateral cohesion between components that begins at the fibrillar level, a collapse that can result in an even greater reduction in tensile strength than is suggested by the number of torn fibrils or fibers observed on tissue examination.[34] In other words, the tissue is more severely damaged than it appears. Such damage can occur not only during tissue loading but also during rapid unloading, perhaps as a result of shearing within the tendon.[35] This may explain why both sudden or unexpected force application and release are often associated with tendinitis.

The breaking strength of the tendon, i.e., the magnitude of the force being applied at the point of tendon rupture, has historically been used to assess the tensile strength of the tendon.[1] Ensuring proper gripping of tendon specimens for tensile testing is difficult, which can lead to large errors in the measurement of deformation and force at the end points of mechanical testing. These data are useful for comparing different tendons or ligaments or for assessing the effects of experimental interventions on a tendon. Most tendons, however, probably function in the toe and early linear regions under physiologic loading conditions, leading some authors to suggest that the slope of the linear portion of the curve ($\Delta F/\Delta L$), the stiffness, may be a better indicator of the tendon's in vivo mechanical behavior.[29,34] Tendons rarely rupture under normal loading conditions unless previously injured or diseased,[38] so one can probably assume that they are seldom loaded in vivo to the maximum levels used to rupture tendons in laboratory testing.[2] Understanding the physical changes occurring in the linear region of the stress-strain curve may be more important in explaining the tissue damage that occurs during tendinitis than is a knowledge of the maximum load that the tendon can tolerate before breaking.[39] Maximum tensile load is probably more representative of tendon rupture, which is far less common than tendinitis.

RESULTS OF TESTING AND INDIRECT CALCULATIONS

There is a strong relationship between the size of a tendon and the maximum force that its attached muscle can produce.[40] Tendons of fusiform muscles tend to have smaller cross-sectional areas relative to muscle strength than do tendons of penniform muscles, suggesting that the former have higher tensile strengths than the latter. It has been estimated that the tensile strength of a tendon is about four times the maximum force produced by its attached muscle, and that tendons in vivo are rarely stressed to more than one-quarter their maximum physiologic strength,[2] probably into the toe region of the stress-strain curve. Such loads should not damage a normal tendon.

Estimates of in vivo tendon strength have been extrapolated from in vitro testing, but it is difficult to obtain direct measures of in vivo stress-strain behavior. Studies using transducers implanted on animal tendons support the theory that tendons are strained only within the toe region of the stress-strain curve during normal daily activities such as walking and trotting.[41,42] It is difficult to see why tendons would be injured during activities, given such a large margin between physiologic and maximum loading. Perhaps physiologic animal loads are not representative of the loads to which humans are willing to subject their tendons during athletic activities?

Human data have usually been acquired through indirect calculations based on biomechanical models and kinematic and kinetic data. Barfred estimated maximum forces of about 4340 N in a person who, while running, suddenly changed direction and ruptured his Achilles tendon; ordinary push-offs were calculated to be about 2000 N.[43] This represents an increase of over 100 percent between normal and maximal loading. The larger value was similar to data obtained from in vitro testing of human tendons, which found maximum tensile strength of about 4000 N, and suggests that tendons may be loaded maximally during activities.[21] This author has estimated Achilles tendon forces from 2000 to 5000 N in various activities such as running and jumping (Fig. 3–8).[44] Other examples of estimated tendon forces in various tendons during different activities suggest that tendons may often be loaded to more than 4000 N during athletic activities.[44] However, these are still only estimates of tendon force. Gregor and Komi placed buckle transducers on the Achilles tendon of volunteers (including themselves!) and recorded forces in the range of 5000 to 6000 N during cycling and running.[45] Forces of up to 4000 N were recorded during hopping on one foot; these forces were higher than those observed during countermovement jumps for maximal height.[46]

The data from estimates and direct measurement of human tendon forces suggest that tendons can indeed be subjected to large loads under daily conditions. The confusion may arise from the definition of "physiologic loading," which can vary between individuals. Forces during walking and light exercise may be only 20 to 30 percent of those observed during vigorous exercise. It thus appears that athletes' tendons are frequently subjected to potentially damaging loads, though they are rarely injured. The reasons for this paradox remain unknown. Perhaps all athletes have structural defects at the submicroscopic level in their tendons, and it is only when some threshold is reached that symptoms and dysfunction occur.

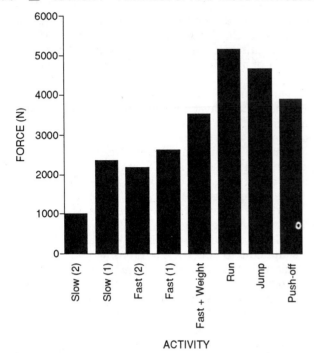

FIGURE 3–8. Increasing Achilles tendon forces during toe-raising exercises over the edge of a step and three sports-related activities. Slow 1, Fast 1 = weight on one foot; slow or fast speed. Slow 2, Fast 2 = weight on both feet, slow or fast speed. Fast + Weight = extra weight added to body. Run = sprint running. Jump = landing from 50 cm. Push-off = a change in direction from backward to forward running. The slow and fast movements represent progressive steps in the clinical exercise program to treat Achilles tendinitis.

EFFECTS OF EXERCISE AND DISUSE ON TENDONS

The effects of disuse and immobilization on tissues such as muscle, ligament, joint capsule, and tendon have been well established.[27–29,47–53] All musculoskeletal tissues atrophy under conditions of decreased load. Protein degradation exceeds synthesis such that a net decrease in collagen develops.[29] Both collagen and cross-link concentration decline, and the tissues become weaker both structurally and materially.[28] These findings have led to the concept of using early motion and gradual stress application to treat many hard and soft tissue injuries.[55–58]

Both healing and normal tendons adapt to increased loads either by becoming larger and hypertrophying, as muscle does, or by changing their material properties to become stronger per unit area.[1,35,59,60] Almost all musculoskeletal tissues seem to respond to increased load with an increase in tensile strength.[1,61,62] Muscle rapidly hypertrophies under increased load conditions and may also increase its connective tissue content.[60] Ligament and tendon have been shown to behave in a similar fashion.[39,61,63,64]

Increased loading is usually associated with exercise such as running and jumping. It is now well documented that some sports-related activities can stress tendons to large percentages of the theoretical maximum for mammalian tendon (Table 3–3).[44,65] The association of tendinitis or tendon rupture with par-

ticular sports (such as badminton with Achilles tendon rupture) implies that the high demands placed on these tissues during many movements in sports and dance may cause injury.[44,65–71] The incidence of tendon injuries after sudden increases in the amount of training, or when training is resumed at a high level after a period of inactivity, suggests that the tendon is being subjected to loads that exceed its tensile strength and thus cause damage.

Some athletes may develop tendinitis for no apparent reason while training at the same level of intensity. It is hard to imagine why loads previously well tolerated by the tendon should now produce an injury. Such occurrences suggest that the relationship between training intensity, load, and tendon physiology is more complex than previously thought. Different types of exercise may not have the same influence on tendon.[72,73] There is evidence to suggest that cross-linking in the Achilles tendon may be increased with chronically increased loads but decreased by an intermittent strenuous running program (even though the latter would be expected to load the Achilles tendon and indeed is often used as a model of increased tendon loading).[73] Other factors may also be capable of inducing changes in the tendon such that previously safe levels of loading are now capable of damaging the tendon. Recent animal studies suggest that the duration of loading is also important, with physiologic loads capable of inducing tendinitis if repeated over a prolonged period.[74,75]

TENDON INJURY

THE INJURED TENDON

Armed with a thorough understanding of normal tendon structure and function, one can predict changes that would make the tendon susceptible to injury (Table 3–4). The most basic principle in the etiology of tendinitis seems to be that the tendon is exposed to forces that cause it to be damaged.[51,66,69,74] The key to treating the problem lies in determining whether the cause is external to an otherwise healthy tendon or whether the tendon itself is "sick."[76] The nature of the actual damage probably varies with the *type* of force (compressive vs. tensile) as well as its *magnitude* and *pattern* of application.[38,51]

EXTRINSIC VS. INTRINSIC TENDINITIS

Tendinitis resulting from forces outside the tendon is often called "extrinsic" tendinitis.[51,77] Some examples are shown in Figure 3–9. The cause is usually excessive compressive force applied to the tendon. The compression may come from an article worn by the athlete; for example, tight laces in a hightop sneaker or skate may cause tenosynovitis of the extensor tendons at the ankle joint.[78] Pressure from the athlete's own anatomic structures may also be responsible.[77] A large acromion process may cause pressure on the supraspinatus

TABLE 3–3
Tendon Forces During Activities

Activity	Tendon	Force (N)	Reference
Running	Achilles	5000	Curwin, 1984[44]
	Patellar	7500–9000	Alexander and Vernon, 1975[65]
Jumping	Achilles	4000–5000	Curwin, 1984[44]
	Patellar	8000	Alexander and Vernon, 1975[65]
Cycling	Achilles	5500	Gregor et al, 1987[45]
Kicking	Patellar	5000	Curwin and Stanish, 1984[54]
Rupture	Patellar	14,000	Zernicke et al, 1977[86]
Mechanical testing	Various	5000–10,000	Harkness, 1968[21]

tendon, leading to shoulder impingement syndrome. Similarly, retinacula at the wrist can cause various forms of tenosynovitis, usually in combination with repeated use during occupational or recreational activities.[67] These cases of tendinitis are best treated by early removal of the external cause.

Tendinitis may also result from changes or inadequacies within the tendon, the so-called intrinsic forms of tendinitis. In such cases, there are no obvious external causes, and tendinitis is attributed to a change in tendon structure.[68] It should be recognized, however, that factors outside the tendon almost always induce the change, except in rare cases involving genetic abnormalities or diseases affecting connective tissue structure.[14,23,25] The tendon is simply not strong enough to tolerate the tensile loads to which it is subjected. There are basically two long-term solutions to this problem: (1) remove or reduce the tensile forces, or (2) cause the tendon to become stronger. Frequently the loading pattern is within normal limits for the athlete, and force reduction is not a viable long-term solution, although it may be necessary for short periods.[51,78] There are many athletes and dancers who suffer from chronic tendon pain because they are unable or unwilling to reduce the forces applied to their injured tendons.[66,70] Inability to modify loading

creates a situation whereby the tendon must be modified to match its environment. Many forms of intrinsic tendinitis fall into this category, most of which are referred to as overuse injuries.

THE OVERUSE INJURY

Overuse injury is probably the term most commonly used to describe chronic tendinitis. An otherwise normal tendon is chronically subjected to relatively large loads, perhaps extending into the linear region of the stress-strain curve.[38] The overuse theory holds that this chronic loading causes partial rupture (microscopic failure) of some of the fibrils within the tendon or slippage between fibrils, which leads to tendon injury.[78,79] Such injuries have been likened to the stress fractures that occur in bones subjected to chronic load.[66] The injury is thought to be the result of fatigue of the loaded structure, just as metal beams will fatigue with repeated loading. Individual loads may be within the physiologic range but are repeated so often that recovery cannot occur and the structure fatigues. This concept is supported by animal studies.[34,36,74,75] Since tendon structure recovers with rest, even after loading into the linear region, time is probably an important

TABLE 3–4
Potential Causes of Tendon Dysfunction

Stimulus	Response	Possible Effects
Immobilization	Atrophy at myotendinous junction	Partial rupture, microtears
	Increased cross-linking in joint capsule	Increased resistance to joint movement, increased muscle work
Prolonged endurance exercise	Hormonal changes leading to increased collagen turnover	Weaker tendon, microtears
Intense exercise	Rupture of cross-links or collagen fibrils; release of collagen components into circulation	Inability to withstand forces during daily activities, inflammatory response
Prolonged increased mechanical loading	Increased cross-links, decreased collagen	Effect on tendon function unknown
Injection	Mechanical disruption of fibrils, decreased collagen synthesis	Weaker tendon, possible rupture
Nonsteroidal medication	Decreased inflammation	Effect on tendon function unknown
Intermittent resistance exercise	Unknown	Effect on tendon function unknown

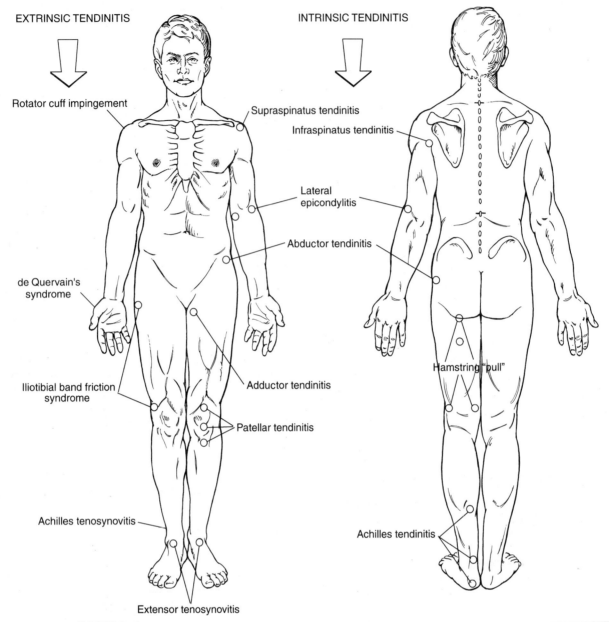

FIGURE 3–9. Some examples of extrinsic and intrinsic tendinitis that are commonly seen in clinical practice. It is to cases of intrinsic tendinitis that the information in this chapter applies most closely.

element in producing these injuries. This is the type of tendinitis that seems to develop very gradually and is often related to high training levels, such as distance running.[51,68,78–80] It may be appropriate to consider this another form of overtraining, and the analogy can be helpful when explaining this disorder to athletes, since most are familiar with situations in which high intensities of training result in no improvement, or even a decline, in performance.[81–83]

It is not only high-level athletes who are afflicted with this type of tendinitis, although this group does account for most of the eponyms, such as tennis elbow and jumper's knee, that are used for many cases of chronic tendinitis. Many older individuals involved in recreational sports also suffer, as well as nonathletes[80] involved in repetitive loading activities.

SUDDEN LOADING/EXCESSIVE FORCE

The tendon may be damaged by loading patterns other than the chronic submaximal variety. Sudden force application, particularly involving lengthening (eccentric) muscle contractions, may lead to muscle or tendon injury.[68,84,85] A sudden maximum muscle activation results in a larger than normal force being very rapidly applied to the tendon, perhaps causing partial or complete rupture. The filming of a competitive weightlifter during a lift in which his patellar tendon ruptured (Fig. 3–10) revealed that the disruption occurred as the lifter changed from downward to upward motion, i.e., the end of the eccentric phase.[86] The force on the patellar tendon was estimated at about 14.5 kN, over 17 times body weight!

Sudden force application can cause more damage than a gradual force increase to the same level of loading, and the sudden removal of a given force level is also more likely to cause disruption than a gradual reduction of the same force. The reasons for this are not entirely known, although a disruption of the relationship between the collagen fibrils and their surrounding matrix appears to be involved.[34,35] The distribution of stress within the tendon also remains largely unknown, although it is generally assumed to be symmetric across the tendon cross-sectional area. However, not every motor unit within a muscle fires during each activation of the muscle. Slow movements, low force levels, and the maintenance of posture require the use of small motor units composed of slow muscle fibers. The tendon fascicles associated with these motor units are therefore regularly loaded during daily activities. Very rapid loading may cause the firing of fast motor units that are seldom used at lower force levels. Presumably, the tendon fascicles associated with these seldom used motor units have not been exposed to the same loading history as other fascicles within the tendon. This suggests possible asymmetries in the pattern of loading and fascicle strength within the tendon.[7,87] It may be possible that some tendon fascicles are actually weakened as a result of little or no loading during daily activities and that they are thus more easily injured when a sudden demand is made on the muscle for rapid force production.

ROLE OF ECCENTRIC MUSCLE ACTIVATION

Muscle physiology experiments on both isolated and in vivo human muscle have shown that force increases as the velocity of active muscle lengthening increases, while the opposite is true during concentric (shortening) muscle activations (Fig. 3–11).[88–90] This may explain the frequent connection between eccentric loading and tendon injury.[54,78,84] The tendon is exposed to larger loads during eccentric loading, especially if the movement occurs rapidly.[41,46,54,84,85] This is exactly the situation that occurs in landing from or preparing for a jump (patellar tendinitis),[66,69] midstance during run-

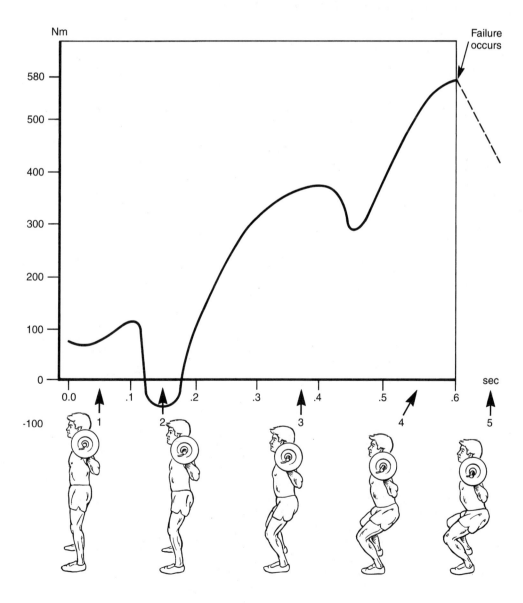

FIGURE 3–10. Rupture of the patellar tendon during weight lifting. Knee joint moments are shown from the beginning of the jerk movement until 0.04 sec after tendon rupture. Dividing by a moment arm of 4 cm (.04 m) reveals a load of approximately 14,500 N, more than 17 times body weight, at the time of rupture. Such loads are much greater than the 5000–7000 N during most daily activities. (Redrawn with permission from Zernicke RF, Garhammer J, Jobe FW: J Bone Joint Surg 1977; 59A:179.)

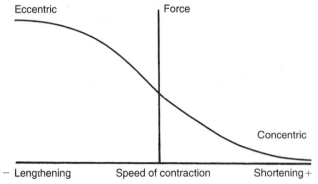

FIGURE 3–11. The force-velocity relationship for eccentric and concentric muscle contractions. As shortening velocity increases, force decreases; as lengthening velocity increases, force also increases. (From Curwin SL, Stanish WD: Tendinitis: Its Etiology and Treatment. Lexington, MA, DC Heath, 1984.)

ning[46] or during a demi-plié in ballet[70] (Achilles tendinitis), and when hitting a backhand in tennis (lateral epicondylitis).[91]

Almost all shortening activations of muscle-tendon units are preceded by lengthening while the muscle is active. This activation pattern stretches the muscle-tendon unit (MTU), creating a passive force in the muscle due to the elongation of its elastic elements and providing elastic energy *if* the muscle is allowed to immediately shorten after being lengthened.[88–90] This storage of elastic energy allows the muscle to produce more force at less metabolic cost. Unfortunately, it also results in maximum force and maximum elongation being simultaneously applied to the tendon, which may cause damage. Figure 3–12 shows the loading patterns on the Achilles tendon associated with some different activities and exercises. It is well known that muscle damage after unaccustomed exercise is closely associated with eccentric muscle contraction, presumably because of higher load levels, and this appears to be true for tendon as well.[85,91,92]

OTHER FACTORS IN TENDON INJURY

ENDOCRINE

It is often difficult to explain to athletes why they have developed tendinitis, when no apparent change in loading or training has occurred and there have been no examples of sudden, unexpected force application (although this may have happened but gone unnoticed by the athlete). This suggests that there may sometimes be other reasons why tendons, previously pain free, become symptomatic. Emphasis is placed on the word apparent, since only after all external influences have been eliminated as potential causes should other factors be considered as possible primary causes. Endocrine responses to stress, such as increased glucocorticoid and catecholamine release,[93,94] may have negative effects on connective tissue,[95,96] increasing turnover and resulting in decreased cross-linking.[12,73] Hormones can influence connective tissues such as tendon, but no relationship has yet been demonstrated in athletic cases of tendinitis.

Nevertheless, tendon injury is closely linked with other clinical disorders such as renal transplantation, and it has even been suggested that the ABO blood group may be associated with a higher incidence of tendinitis.[98–100] It is interesting to speculate that an endocrine response to chronic levels of overtraining[82,93,94,97] may be at least a partial explanation for cases of tendinitis that develop spontaneously. Similar influences have been suggested

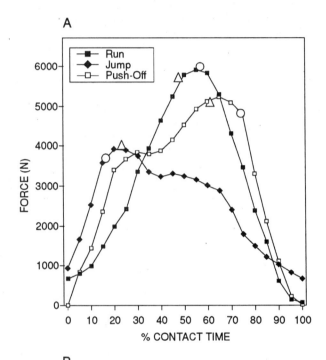

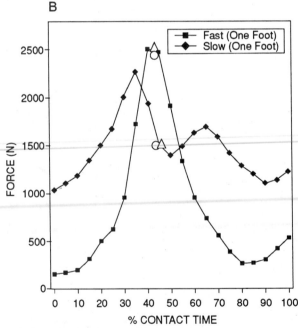

FIGURE 3–12. Achilles tendon forces during three sports-related activities (A) and a slow and rapid heel drop over the edge of a step. B, Forces were indirectly estimated using force platform and film data; muscle lengths for the soleus and gastrocnemius were also estimated from the film records. Maximum muscle lengths (soleus maximum = Δ, gastrocnemius maximum = ○) usually occur at or near the peak force observed during the activity.

for lateral epicondylitis (lack of estrogen),[91] and the relationship between chronic steroid administration and tendon rupture is well known.[95,96,99]

COMPRESSIVE LOADING

The tensile strength of the tendon may gradually decline over time if it is subjected to chronic compressive loads or if turnover is increased markedly, resulting in less mature cross-linking.[101] Less collagen, fewer collagen cross-links, and more ground substance all result in decreased tissue tensile strength.[9,10,12] This could be a factor in rotator cuff tendinitis and may suggest a role for loading the supraspinatus tendon with tensile forces during rehabilitation.[102] Such loading would be expected to induce a change in tendon composition if applied gradually, such that collagen content and cross-linking actually were increased.[101] Compressive loading may also result in a decrease in blood flow through the tendon, as has been demonstrated for supraspinatus tendinitis.[102]

NUTRITIONAL

Adequate amounts of amino acids supplied by a normal healthy diet are required for all protein synthesis, including collagen. Cofactors such as vitamin A, vitamin C, and copper are known to be important in collagen synthesis and cross-linking.[14] Iron deficiency can also have a negative influence on healing.[103] The tensile strength of the myotendinous junction has recently been shown to be partially dependent on calcium, suggesting that a dietary deficiency in calcium could somehow influence junctional injuries.[104] There is some evidence to suggest that collagen synthesis is more severely affected than some other proteins during fasting, which may have some implications for athletes involved in sports that emphasize a slender build, such as gymnastics and ballet.[96] The nutritional influences on chronic tendinitis, however, remain largely unexplored.

REFERRED PAIN

This is a largely unrecognized cause of tendinitis-like pain and is due to peripherally produced (somatic referred) pain from irritation of spinal structures such as joint capsule and ligament. It is probably most common in cases of tennis elbow, in which degenerative changes in the cervical spine cause symptoms that exactly mimic those of tennis elbow.[91] These cases are probably not common in the athletic population, but the clinician should be very suspicious if a "tendinitis" fails to respond to treatment, and one should always conduct a spine examination in parallel with peripheral examination, especially if the athlete falls in the appropriate age category for degenerative spinal changes.

TENDON HEALING

Much is known about the healing of severed tendons. This work comes from models in which the tendon has been divided, surgically or accidentally, and the severed ends reopposed and held in place via immobilization or suture.[30,105-109] These models have told us a tremendous amount about tendon healing under these conditions, particularly the timing of the biochemical and mechanical changes that take place in the healing tendon. The initial inflammatory stage triggers an increase in GAG synthesis within days; this is rapidly followed by collagen synthesis, such that the healing wound can be subjected to low levels of force within a matter of days.[55,109,110] It is known that the application of some force (but not too much!) is ideal in encouraging the new collagen fibrils to align with the direction of force application. Furthermore, healing tissues that are subjected to loading are almost always stronger than unloaded tissues, whether the example be skin, ligament, or tendon.[51,53,55,56,61,109] The application of these principles in plastic surgery has led to the design of early motion programs after tendon repair as well as rehabilitation programs based on scientific principles.

Unfortunately, there remains a great deal of confusion when it comes to applying information about tendon healing to tendinitis. Just what is tendinitis? Does tendinitis follow the same healing pattern described for complete lacerations? Little is known about the inflammatory response to the type of mechanical trauma that produces chronic tendinitis. Any injury that involves the tendon or its associated sheaths may be referred to as tendinitis, but a plethora of other terms also exists: tendinosis (degeneration of the tendon without inflammation), tenosynovitis (inflammation of the sheath surrounding the tendon), paratenonitis, peritendinitis. Some authors argue that, with cases of chronic tendinitis that developed very gradually and never appeared to have an acute stage, there is no associated inflammation of the tendon or the tendon sheath, and so the condition should be called tendinosis.[68,74,76,111,112] This conclusion is based primarily on observations of human tissue obtained during surgical procedures aimed at relieving chronic tendinitis. These observations probably represent the late, fibrotic stage of tendinitis and do not eliminate the possibility of the earlier presence of inflammation.

One of the major difficulties in evaluating chronic tendinitis has been the lack of a suitable animal model for chronic tendinitis. Racehorses frequently develop chronic tendinitis and, indeed, are responsible for much of what is now known about chronic tendinitis.[113,114] They cannot be used by most researchers because of expense, and the amount (time and/or magnitude) of loading responsible for the tendinitis is unknown. Recently, the first animal model was designed to simulate the type of overloading that often leads to human tendon dysfunction.[74,75] The ankle joints of anesthetized rabbits were repeatedly flexed and extended for 2 hours daily while the triceps surae muscle was electrically stimulated. After 4 weeks of exercise, palpation of the exercised tendons showed that all had irregular thickening, with nodules a short distance from the tendon's insertion into the calcaneus. Light microscopy showed degenerative changes in the tendon and thickening of the tendon sheath (paratenon).[74] Blood flow was increased (about twofold) to both the paratenon and the tendon.[75] Most cellular changes suggestive of an inflammatory response were found in the tendon sheath, with degenerative changes in the central portion of the tendon. This model is the first to produce tendon dysfunction through reproducible loading and suggests that inflammation is an integral part of the injury response. Other animal models used to evaluate submaximal tendon injuries have caused damage by partial laceration or chemical injection and may not be as closely representative of naturally occurring injuries.[79,114,115]

The findings from human surgical and post-mortem specimens and from animal studies suggest that most of the inflammatory changes take place in the paratenon and are accompanied (preceded? followed?) by areas of focal degeneration within the tendon.[68,111] These findings also suggest that injury to the tendon structure does not occur in isolation and that it would be uncommon for tendon degeneration to occur without accompanying inflammatory changes. In other words, it should be possible to have paratenonitis without tendinosis (as can occur with extrinsic tendinitis) but not tendinosis without some inflammation of the tendon sheath. A scenario for the progression of tendon injury is presented in Figure 3–13.

It is unlikely, then, that tendon damage takes place without symptoms being present at some point. Athletes may not complain of pain serious enough to prevent them from participating in activities that they consider enjoyable (or unavoidable). Careful questioning, however, will often reveal that symptoms were and may continue to be present during activities that load the tendon or that a more acute episode took place at an earlier time. The clinical signs of tenderness with palpation and pain on loading may be interpreted to reflect the presence of an inflammatory response.[115] The response, while mostly in the tendon sheath, reflects and accompanies the structural damage to the tendon, but the exact relationship is not yet known.[74,75] The sheath inflammation may resolve while the degenerative changes in the tendon itself remain or even progress.

In most clinical cases it is impossible to determine which portion of the tendon is the source of pain. Palpation involves both the tendon and its sheath, and muscle contraction will apply force to an inflamed sheath and its damaged tendon. One can perhaps define tendinitis as "a syndrome of pain and tenderness localized over an area of tendon, aggravated by activities that apply tensile force to the tendon, and either caused or followed by degenerative changes in tendon structure." The syndrome can include inflammation of the tendon sheath, as in tenosynovitis and tenovaginitis, as well as actual inflammation of the tendon substance itself. The degree of degenerative change can vary from microscopic to complete rupture. It is unlikely that pathologic changes can be determined for most athletes, since such analysis would require a sample of tendon tissue. This means that any classification system for chronic tendon injury based on pathology alone probably does not apply to the vast majority of clinical

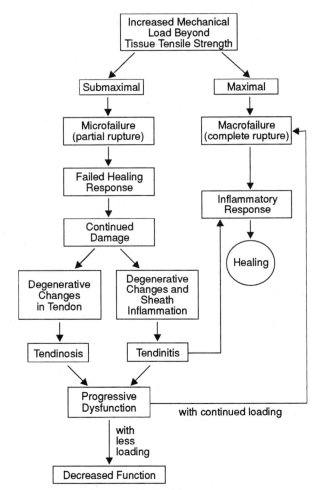

FIGURE 3–13. The possible progression of tendon injury. The inflammatory response may be very limited, and thus barely noticed by the athlete, while degenerative changes continue. As the remaining collagen fibers are overloaded and more are damaged, the inflammatory response will reappear. This may be weeks or months after the initial injury. Once the tendon is in the inflammatory stage, it can be treated as an acute injury and should heal normally. In rare cases, the tendon may rupture because applied forces exceed the tensile strength of the now-weakened tendon.

cases of tendinitis. It may be more helpful to use a classification system based on pain and function, which can be determined clinically, even though the exact relationship between symptoms and pathology remains unknown. Such a system is presented in Table 3–5.[54]

TREATING THE INJURED TENDON

ACUTE TENDON INJURIES

Most of what we know about healing tendons comes from work on severed or ruptured tendons. Little or nothing is known about the healing process of injuries such as the chronic tendon injuries that most athletes suffer. If the exact time of injury is known, as it may be after a sudden loading incident, the principles of soft tissue healing can be used to guide treatment (Table 3–6). The principal aims are to avoid reinjuring the tendon early in the healing process while tensile strength is low, while simultaneously preventing the ill

TABLE 3–5
Classification of Tendon Disorder Based on Pain and Disability

Intensity	Level	Pain	Disability
Mild	1*	No pain	No effect on activities
	2	Pain with extreme exertion; stops when activity ceases	No effect on activities
Moderate	3	Pain with extreme exertion; lasts 1–2 hours afterward	Little effect on activities; may limit more intense physical activities
	4	Pain with any moderate exertion; increases with activity; lasts 4–6 hours afterward	Performance level decreased; unable to perform some necessary tasks
Severe	5	Pain with any exertion; rapidly increases in intensity; lasts 8–24 hours	Causes immediate withdrawal from activity
	6	Pain during daily activities	Unable to participate in any sports; daily activities may also be restricted

*Level 1 is almost the same as normal tendon but can be reached only from one of the higher levels. There may be some residual strength or functional deficits, as explained in the text, which should be ruled out before calling the tendon "normal."
Adapted from Curwin SL, Stanish WD: Tendinitis: Its Etiology and Treatment. Lexington, MA, DC Heath, 1984.

effects of disuse on other, unaffected tissues in the same limb. Later, the emphasis shifts to the healing tissue itself.

CHRONIC TENDON INJURIES

The main difficulty with treating chronic injuries is that the exact placement of the tissue in the healing process is unknown. Can one assume that the tissue is in the remodeling phase if a considerable length of time, say 6 months, has elapsed since the onset of symptoms? This would call for exercise and tissue loading in treatment. Or should it be assumed that the tissue is "stuck" in an earlier stage of healing, continually reinjured by the athlete's activities so that no true healing has taken place? In this case, PRICEMM is the treatment of choice—Protection, Rest, Ice, Compression, Modalities, Medication—as it is in any acute injury.[116] There are several promising diagnostic techniques on the horizon, such as magnetic resonance imaging (MRI), but none is yet able to resolve lesser tendon injuries such as tendinosis/tendinitis.[117] Serum and urine markers of collagen metabolism may eventually be useful.[118–120]

SOME ASSUMPTIONS ABOUT CHRONIC TENDINITIS

Because the current understanding of chronic tendinitis remains inadequate, the development of a rational treatment strategy requires making some assumptions. These assumptions may or may not be true, but they allow the development of a logical, and successful, approach to the treatment of tendinitis.

TABLE 3–6
Tendon Healing and Suggested Therapies

	Stage of Healing		
	Inflammatory	Fibroblastic/Proliferation	Remodeling/Maturation
Time (days)	0–6	5–21	20 days and onward Progressive stress on tissue
Suggested Therapy	Rest, ice Anti-inflammatory modalities Decreased tension	Gradual introduction of stress Modalities to increase collagen synthesis	
Physiologic Rationale	Prevent prolonged inflammation Prevent disruption of new blood vessels and collagen fibrils Promote ground substance synthesis	Increase collagen Increase collagen cross-linking Increase fibril size and alignment	Increase cross-linking (tendons and ligaments) Decrease cross-linking (joint capsule) Increase fibril size
Main Goals	Avoid new tissue disruption	Prevent excessive muscle and joint atrophy	Optimize tissue healing

ASSUMPTION ONE—ALL CASES OF TENDINITIS CAN BE TREATED APPROPRIATELY IF THEY ARE IN THE ACUTE STAGE. Acute tendon injuries by definition will pass through the stages of healing as defined in Table 3–6 and so can be treated appropriately. Almost all cases of tendinitis will be fully resolved in 6 weeks or less if the time of injury is known. Chronic tendinitis has presumably already passed through the acute stage but, if returned to it, can also be treated appropriately. There is probably no harm in assuming that all cases of tendinitis are in the acute stage, if treatment is adjusted accordingly! Treatment would begin at a low level of intensity and progress according to the patient's symptoms. This approach ensures that chronic injuries in the inflammatory or proliferative phases are treated correctly and minimizes the chance that the athlete's condition will be made worse. Chronic injuries are often made worse because they are assumed to be in the remodeling phase of healing and thus deserving of vigorous treatment. Time alone does not define the stage of healing.

The flare-up that occurs after too vigorous treatment usually convinces the clinician that a more conservative approach is required. The advantage is that the time of injury is now known—it was the last treatment!

ASSUMPTION TWO—THE CHRONICALLY INJURED TENDON WILL HEAL THE SAME WAY AS THE SEVERED OR RUPTURED TENDON. Because we have no information on the sequence of steps in the healing of tendinitis, it is difficult to form a framework for the physiologic progression of the tendon during treatment. This assumption allows us to visualize the changes taking place in the tendon during the treatment process. The appropriate use of modalities and the progression of tensile loading is matched with the stage of healing, producing an evolving treatment strategy (see Table 3–6). If the tendon injury has inadvertently been returned to the acute stage, the treatment progression becomes easier to visualize.

ASSUMPTION THREE—INFLAMMATION OF THE TENDON SHEATH REFLECTS THE DEGREE OF DAMAGE TO THE TENDON. If this relationship holds, the signs of inflammation (pain, tenderness, dysfunction) can be monitored to assess the progression of tendon damage or recovery. This assumption is very important, because the successful treatment of chronic tendinitis is based on the theory that pain is a reflection of the inflammatory response occurring in the tendon. This means monitoring pain and function to determine whether improvement is occurring and modifying treatment as the pain or inflammation changes. There are drawbacks to this approach because pain is a very subjective perception, but it appears to be the most clinically useful way to monitor patient progress (see Table 3–5). While it can be argued that many patients have degenerative changes without inflammation, the fact remains that affected athletes have pain. This suggests the presence of an inflammatory response somewhere in the tendon "complex."

ASSUMPTION FOUR—THE EFFECTS OF EXERCISE AND DISUSE WILL BE THE SAME FOR CHRONICALLY INJURED TENDONS AS FOR OTHER CONNECTIVE TISSUE STRUCTURES. If the effects of exercise and disuse are the same for chronic tendinitis as for normal and healing tendons and ligaments, exercise should have a positive influence on the healing tendon and should therefore be beneficial in the treatment of chronic tendinitis.

There is no way of knowing at present whether these assumptions are correct. They are theories that have not been tested. Much research remains to be done in determining the sequence of events in tendon healing in tendinitis and in examining the correlation between clinical symptoms of soft tissue injury and serum or urine markers of connective tissue metabolism.[118–120] These markers have been used successfully to monitor bone healing, osteoporosis, and osteogenesis imperfecta, and it is reasonable to speculate that they may have a place in monitoring other collagen disorders, such as chronic tendinitis.

GENERAL PRINCIPLES FOR TREATING TENDINITIS

There are many principles, physiologic and mechanical, that should be considered when treating chronic tendinitis. Many were touched upon earlier. It is helpful to develop an approach that can be applied to all forms of chronic tendon injury, whether extrinsic or intrinsic. This helps reduce the possibility that the clinician will miss something that may be a factor in an individual athlete's case. The following guidelines, also shown in Figure 3–14, can be used for treating all forms of tendinitis.

1. *Identify and remove all negative external forces/factors.*
   With extrinsic tendinitis, the outside force is usually pressure on the tendon. Treatment involves identification and removal of the source of pressure; this is essential if further tendon damage is to

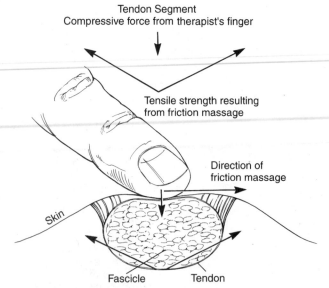

FIGURE 3–14. Transverse friction massage may create tensile forces on the tendon through a "bowstring" effect. (Reprinted from Gross MT: J Orthop Sports Phys Ther 1992; 16:248 with the permission of the American Physical Therapy Association.)

be avoided.[54] A simple example is tenosynovitis of the extensor tendons at the ankle joint caused by pressure from tight laces in a skate or shoe. The pressure may be removed by loosening the laces or designing a device to redistribute the force.[78] A more complicated example is the classic shoulder impingement syndrome, in which the appropriate treatment is removal of the cause of impingement. In cases in which glenohumeral motion is restricted, impingement occurs when the head of the humerus fails to glide downward on the glenoid as the humerus rolls upward during abduction. Treatment involves physical therapy, usually joint mobilization techniques, to restore normal elasticity to the tight joint capsule.[121] In long-standing cases of degenerative cuff changes that require repair, or faulty configuration of the acromion, surgery may be necessary.[122] There are also cases of impingement syndrome in which the glenohumeral joint is hypermobile, and the head of the humerus glides upward during abduction because of lack of adequate stabilization by the shoulder girdle and/or rotator cuff muscles.[123] This type of impingement, usually found in younger athletes, requires a very different treatment strategy and highlights the need for individual patient assessment rather than treatment by diagnosis. Other forms of treatment, such as modalities, however helpful in relieving the symptoms of extrinsic tendinitis, can be considered only temporary or adjunctive. Eliminating the cause is the fundamental treatment.

In some cases, external factors may be contributing to or causing intrinsic tendinitis. Excessive foot pronation can cause the medial side of the Achilles tendon, or the tibialis posterior muscle-tendon unit, to be overstretched. Under these circumstances, the medial side of the Achilles tendon is forced to elongate more than the lateral side.[124,125] Excessive lateral shoe wear, or a varus hindfoot, may lead to iliotibial band syndrome as the lateral aspect of the lower limb is subjected to increased stress. Many of these problems are easily corrected with a shoe orthotic or simply by buying new shoes.[124,125]

Probably the single most common contributing factor in almost all cases of chronic tendinitis is a lack of flexibility of the involved muscle-tendon unit. For this reason, a thorough and specific stretching program is nearly always an essential part of the rehabilitation strategy. Despite the fact that there is little scientific evidence to show that stretching prevents injuries or reduces the rate of reinjury, extending the physiologic joint range of motion seems logical when treating athletes in whom it is restricted.[125]

2. *Estimate the phase of healing (stage of tendinitis).*

This is a very imprecise process, requiring judgment based on the examiner's clinical experience to be truly successful. Generally, the more severe the patient's symptoms, the more closely the choice and timing of treatment should resemble that used for an acute tendon injury. Treatment should progress as it would for an acute injury. Those who have worked with large numbers of athletes will better recognize the appropriate starting point for loading; however, there is no harm in underestimating the load and "catching up" over a few days to a week. If the condition is made worse, remember assumption one and treat the injury as if it were in the acute phase.

3. *Determine the appropriate focus for initial treatment.*

This involves matching treatment with the stage of healing. Most cases of chronic tendinitis should be in the remodeling phase of healing, when force application is the most effective treatment. Time alone, however, does not define the stage of healing, as noted above. More severe cases should be assumed to be acute injuries and should be treated with judicious rest, ice, and modalities for a short period, followed by gradual stress increase, as would be the case for any acute tendon injury or repair.

4. *Institute an appropriate tensile loading program.*

The healing tendon must be loaded if collagen synthesis, alignment, and maturation via cross-linking are to be ideal.[110] The more acute or severe the injury, the lower the force.[55] Passive movement produces very little tensile force, is safe immediately after injury, and is known to have beneficial mechanical effects on tendon.[127] Gentle stretching would be the next step, followed by increased stretching force and then active exercise.

5. *Control pain and inflammation.*

The appropriate use of loading during healing should ensure that inflammation is not provoked by mechanical disruption and reinjury. There may be cases in which additional help is needed to reduce a prolonged inflammatory response. In such cases, drugs, ice, and modalities can be used as adjuncts to treatment.[54,78,116]

SPECIFIC FORMS OF TREATMENT

MODALITIES

Physical therapists employ a wide variety of modalities in treating soft tissue disorders, including ultrasound, laser, ice, heat, pulsed electromagnetic current, electromagnetic field therapy, high-voltage galvanic stimulation, acupuncture, and interferential current. Most are proposed to "decrease inflammation and promote healing." There is only limited evidence to date to support these claims.

Ultrasound is one of the most commonly used modalities. Generally, pulsed ultrasound is recommended for acute injuries in order to avoid a thermal effect, and continuous ultrasound is used for more long-standing injuries.[128,129] Although there have been reports of no influence on healing tendon,[130] studies have shown that ultrasound increases collagen synthesis by fibroblasts,[131] speeds wound healing,[128] and results in increased tensile strength in healing tendons.[132,133] Ultrasound has little or no effect on inflammation.[134] None of the models used in the laboratory simulates the clinical situation of chronic tendinitis, forcing reliance upon the second assumption, that the chronically injured tendon will heal like the severed tendon. Given that one of the explanations for chronic tendinitis is "failed healing response,"[112] it is uncertain whether this assumption will always be true. Ultrasound probably has its most important effect when the synthetic activity of the fibroblasts is maximal, i.e., in the proliferative stage of healing. However, because of the nature of chronic injuries, it is probably most widely used clinically during the remodeling stage. It would be interesting to see whether ultrasound increases the synthesis of collagen during all stages of healing, especially during remodeling, when the synthesis rate of collagen has declined. This would, in effect, prolong or renew the proliferative phase of healing. There would seem to be little indication for using ultrasound for prolonged periods of time.

Another modality widely used in Europe and Canada is laser.[135] Like ultrasound, laser has been shown to increase fibroblasts' synthesis of GAGs and collagen and to speed superficial wound healing; unlike ultrasound, however, it has also been shown to decrease inflammation.[136] The use of lasers in nonsuperficial cases, such as chronic tendinitis, remains speculative, however; there is as yet no clinical or scientific evidence to support its use for treating deeper tissues such as tendon or to suggest its superiority to ultrasound. Given the wide variety of laser types and dosages, much more research is needed on the effects of this modality.

Electrical stimulation is a modality that has also been demonstrated to have a positive influence on tendon healing.[137–140] Like most studies on modalities, results were obtained using an acute tendon healing model and so may not represent chronic tendon injuries. Both direct electrical stimulation[138,139] and indirect current via electromagnetic field induction[137,140] seem to augment tendon healing. Pulsed electromagnetic fields can treat both deep and superficial tissues and cover larger areas than ultrasound or laser.[137] Questions about timing and dosage remain, but it appears that treatment needs to be prolonged to several hours daily to have an influence on tissue, since clinical use for shorter periods has not shown the same positive effects.[140]

One of the most widely used modalities for all soft tissue injuries is ice. Its use is recommended immediately after injury to prevent excessive soft tissue swelling. It is thought to act mainly by decreasing the activity of inflammatory mediators and decreasing the overall metabolic rate of the injured tissue.[141] Another important effect is analgesia, which allows the use of appropriate forms of exercise, such as passive motion, that otherwise might be uncomfortable for the patient. The rationale for the use of ice with chronic injuries is less clear, although it can be used for its analgesic effect, and it may help offset inflammatory changes induced by mechanical injury to the tendon during exercise.[54]

The use of modalities, although widespread, remains largely speculative in the treatment of chronic soft tissue injuries. Scientific studies suggest that increased synthetic activity by fibroblasts is the major effect of most modalities except ice. Clinicians should keep in mind that this synthetic activity occurs mainly during the proliferative phase of healing, and this is probably the phase in which modalities will have the greatest effect on healing tissues. The effects of modalities on chronic injuries remain largely unexplored, and more well-designed clinical trials are needed to determine their efficacy in the clinical setting.

Mechanical forces are required during remodeling as soon as the newly synthesized collagen begins to assemble into a fibrillar structure. Loading causes the fibrils to align themselves parallel to the direction of the tensile load, thus reducing the likelihood of restricted movement due to cross-linking between disorganized "haystack" fibrils.[27] In a structure such as skin or ligament, in which forces occur in different directions, a less uniform fibril arrangement may be desirable. However, since only the fibrils aligned with a load can resist it, in tendon it is far better to have all fibrils parallel. As cross-links form between the aligned fibrils, the healing tendon will develop into a structure capable of withstanding even greater tensile loads.

TRANSVERSE FRICTION MASSAGE

This technique was recommended by Cyriax as a treatment for chronic tendinitis and is widely used by physical therapists.[142] It is thought that adhesions between tendon and surrounding tissue may cause continuous tissue irritation and inflammation and that transverse friction massage will release these adhesions. An increase in local blood flow from the hyperemic response to finger pressure is also thought to occur. Transverse friction massage may also create a tensile force as the downward pressure on the tendon creates a "bowstring" effect (Fig. 3–14).[78] The exact effects of friction massages are not known, and although both positive and "no effects" have been claimed, the technique is widely recommended by experienced clinicians.[142–145]

DRUGS

The most potent anti-inflammatory drugs are the corticosteroids, which are sometimes used, via local injection, to treat chronic tendinitis. The negative effects of systemic corticosteroid use are well known,[96,99] but the effects of local injection are less clear. Both negative and "no effects" have been reported.[146,147] There now seems to be general agreement that injection into the tendon substance should be avoided.[147,148] This is due to the effects of the drug (which decreases collagen synthesis), the mechanical disruption caused by the needle and the volume of fluid injected, and the irritant effect of the solvent in which the drug is dissolved.[148] Since most inflammatory changes occur in the paratenon, injection into the tendon sheath may be useful when inflammation is marked or prolonged.[148] If the tendon proper has been injected, tensile force should be reduced for 10 to 14 days, and the tendon should be treated as if it had suffered an acute injury, i.e., ice, rest, and modalities, followed by progressive loading starting at about 2 weeks. Repeated steroid injections into a tendon are almost certain to result in substantial mechanical disruption and should be avoided.[147]

Nonsteroidal anti-inflammatory agents (NSAIDs) are also widely used in the treatment of acute soft tissue injuries but less so for chronic injuries such as tendinitis.[149,150] They limit inflammation by inhibiting prostaglandin synthesis or release, depending on the drug. Unlike corticosteroids, they do not inhibit fibroblast or macrophage activity.[150] Although there is some evidence to show that preventive use of indomethacin may reduce subsequent muscle injury in cases of delayed-onset muscle soreness (DOMS),[149] most clinical studies have not been well enough designed to firmly conclude whether the use of NSAIDs has a beneficial effect on postinjury recovery.[150]

Some athletes may be self-administering another class of drugs known to affect connective tissues, anabolic steroids.[151] Although the exact effects of these agents are unknown owing to difficulties in determining use and dosage, there is both scientific and anecdotal evidence to suggest that anabolic steroid users are more likely to develop a tendon injury.[152] Users of these substances claim that recovery time after injuries is reduced, but the effect of anabolic steroids on the healing of acute and chronic tendon injuries remains largely unexplored. Clinicians should be alert to the possibility of anabolic steroids, since their use by young males has become widespread.[151]

SURGERY

There is very little place for surgery in the treatment of chronic tendinitis unless the tendon ruptures and the ends need to be approximated.[153] Some authors advocate the removal of scar tissue and repair of the injured tendon,[154] but it is just as likely that the postoperative healing response and carefully progressed treatment, rather than the surgery itself, cause the improvement in the patient's condition. There have been no controlled studies to examine this possibility. Some forms of surgical treatment for chronic tendinitis are not far removed from methods previously used, but now discarded, in treating chronic tendon injuries in racehorses. Almost all cases of chronic tendinitis can be successfully treated without surgery.[54]

THE ROLE OF EXERCISE IN TREATING CHRONIC TENDINITIS

Many forms of treatment are used for chronic tendinitis. One man with tennis elbow recently brought a "progress note" from his physical therapist with him to clinic. The list of treatments given included ultrasound, interferential current, laser, ice, TENS, acupuncture, deep friction massage, muscle stimulation, pulsed magnetic field, and an exercise program! After 2 months of this treatment, the patient's condition remained unimproved. The note also contained the information that weakness was noted on eccentric testing and that the patient's symptoms were worse after maximal testing on an isokinetic device. Strength tests involve maximal eccentric loading and are almost certain to reproduce the injury if used before full recovery has occurred. It is therefore inappropriate to carry out such tests before complete functional recovery has occurred, although less demanding tests, such as grip strength, may be useful to monitor progress.

Cases like the one described above, and a growing appreciation for tendon physiology and mechanics, suggest that a modality-based approach to the treatment of chronic tendinitis is inadequate. This does not mean that modalities and drugs should be abandoned but rather that they should not form the basis of a treatment strategy for chronic tendinitis. An understanding of tendon's ability to adapt to increased loads, and the belief that chronic tendon injuries are the result of tensile loads exceeding the tendon's mechanical strength, suggest that exercise should be the cornerstone of treatment. Mechanical problems demand mechanical solutions!

BASIC PRINCIPLES OF EXERCISE

Basic exercise principles must be followed for any exercise program to succeed. In the treatment of chronic tendinitis, the following are most important.

SPECIFICITY OF TRAINING. Training must be anatomically specific to the affected muscle-tendon unit (MTU) and must also be activity-specific in terms of the type of loading (tensile, eccentric) and the magnitude and speed of loading. Activity specificity is achieved by simulating the movement pattern associated with maximal tendon forces, i.e., a lengthening of the active MTU followed by shortening contraction. The initial magnitude and speed of loading are based on the estimated stage of healing. The more acute the injury, the lower the magnitude of the force, and the lower the speed of eccentric loading. The affected tendon must be subjected to isolated tensile loading without systemic influences. For example, the Achilles tendon is loaded by having the patient stand at the edge of a step and drop his or her heels downward, rather than running. This specific exercise is aimed at countering the potentially negative effects associated with stressful training (e.g., hormonal) with the positive effects of exercise on the MTU (increased strength). Functional activities are also gradually progressed as symptoms abate.

MAXIMAL LOADING. Maximal loading is essential to induce adaptation in musculoskeletal tissues.[31] Clinically, the maximum load is determined by the tendon's tolerance, which is judged by the athlete's pain level during exercise. It has been determined empirically that the patient should experience some pain and fatigue between the twentieth and thirtieth repetition of the movement.[54] Pain felt before this point generally is accompanied by worsening of symptoms. No pain by 30 repetitions usually results in no change in symptoms, suggesting that the stimulus is inadequate to induce a change in the tendon.

PROGRESSION OF LOADING. As the tendon adapts to the loads being applied by increasing its tensile

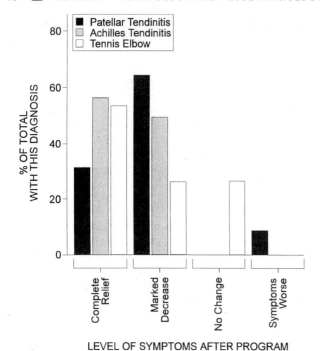

FIGURE 3–15. Response to the eccentric exercise program. (Data from Curwin SL, Stanish WD: Tendinitis: Its Etiology and Treatment. Lexington, MA, DC Heath, 1984.)

strength, the magnitude of loading must be progressed. This ensures that maximal loads are applied, creating a stimulus for adaptation. Progress can be made by increasing the speed of movement (eccentric muscle activation) or increasing the magnitude of the tensile force by changing the external resistance (isometric, concentric, and eccentric muscle activation). The progression is determined by the patient's symptoms (Fig. 3–15).

ECCENTRIC EXERCISE PROGRAM

The principles outlined above have been incorporated into an "eccentric exercise program" for treating chronic tendinitis.[54] The principles can be applied to any injured tendon, following the guidelines in Figure 3–16. The overall program has five steps, which are performed in the order listed:

1. *Warm-up*

A generalized exercise such as cycling or light jogging is used to increase body temperature and increase circulation. This exercise is not intended to load the tendon and should not cause local pain or discomfort. It is possible that local heating modalities, such as hot packs or ultrasound, may be useful.

2. *Flexibility*

As noted earlier, lack of flexibility is a common finding in chronic tendinitis. It is recommended that the athlete perform at least two 30-second static stretches of the involved MTU and its antagonist(s). More stretching may be done if lack of flexibility is felt to be a major factor in causing the patient's symptoms, i.e., if functional range of motion is far from normal.

3. *Specific exercise*

This is done following the guidelines in Figure 3–16, based on the principles outlined above. It is suggested that the athlete perform three sets of ten repetitions, with a brief rest or a stretch between each set. Symptoms should appear after 20 repetitions. The level of discomfort should be similar to that felt during activities and should not be severe or steeply increasing in intensity. If pain is felt earlier than 20 repetitions, reduce the speed of movement, or decrease the load; if no pain is experienced by 30 repetitions, increase speed *or* load (not both). If this is the first exercise session and the initial level of loading is being determined, the intensity of exercise may be increased until symptoms are reproduced. A less intense level of exercise can then be chosen as a starting point and the 30 repetitions carried out. The response to this treatment will determine whether subsequent treatment should be more or less vigorous. Since it is much easier to increase exercise intensity incrementally than to recover from overzealous loading, it is recommended that clinicians err on the side of underloading during initial treatment sessions.

4. *Repeat flexibility exercises*
5. *Apply ice*

Ice is applied for 10 to 15 minutes to the affected (painful to palpation) area. It is hoped that this will help prevent any inflammatory response provoked by microscopic damage to the tendon that might occur during the exercise. It will also decrease pain.

Many athletes with chronic tendinitis are able to participate in athletic activity but find their participation

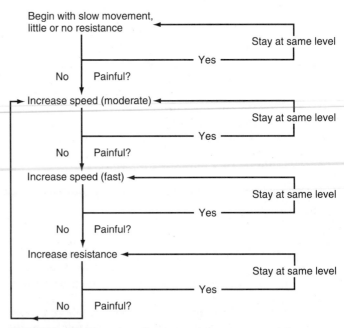

FIGURE 3–16. Flow chart illustrating the progression of the eccentric exercise program according to the athlete's symptoms. (From Curwin SL, Stanish WD: Tendinitis: Its Etiology and Treatment. Lexington, MA, DC Heath, 1984.)

painful (level 2/3) or their performance impaired (level 4/5). *It is not essential for these athletes to cease participating in sports while carrying out the eccentric exercise program, unless they are unable to perform their activity satisfactorily or their symptoms are becoming worse.* In fact, the ideal scenario is that nothing changes, except for the addition of the exercise program. This means that only one variable has changed, allowing the effect of treatment to be more accurately assessed. A decrease in physical activity, a second variable, usually causes a parallel decrease in symptoms. This makes it difficult to distinguish whether it is reduced activity or the clinical intervention that is responsible for improvement. It is recommended, however, that athletes not participate in sports immediately before or after the therapeutic exercise program (especially before), as this may alter their pain response during exercise or activity.

Athletes can often be successfully treated with a home program and periodic rechecks, since the exercise is easily done independently, and most people become asymptomatic within 6 to 8 weeks. Athletic involvement can be increased gradually as symptoms abate; the progression will generally be slower when full withdrawal from sports was necessary. It is recommended that close supervision be given in the early stages of the program until the level of loading, rate of progression, compliance with instructions, and response to treatment are well established.

The exercise program is performed daily, with continuous progression, until symptoms are no longer present during activity. Strength testing should not be performed until treatment is complete and the athlete is asymptomatic and has returned to activity, since the maximum force levels generated during testing may damage the healing tendon. After this point, testing is helpful to detect residual deficits or left-right asymmetries. Strength deficits may persist even after the symptoms of tendinitis have been reduced, suggesting that testing may be beneficial in some cases to determine whether strength training (progressive loading) should be continued.[155]

Modification of activity may be necessary if symptoms are more severe or are continually present. Professional attention is seldom deemed necessary until function is affected, so many athletes will have already been forced to curtail their activity. Level 5/6 symptoms, especially, are interpreted as reflecting a process of acute tendinitis, even though symptoms may be longstanding. Treatment is commenced at a very low level: ice, gentle stretching, passive movement, modalities to stimulate collagen synthesis, medication if deemed necessary. Treatment is progressed as healing progresses, so that by 2 weeks more vigorous exercise can usually be introduced, as the symptoms will have subsided. Continued progression as described in Figure 3–16 is then possible.

The stage between ending a rehabilitation program and resuming full activity is the biggest challenge for both the injured athlete and the clinician, because so little is known about the best way to return to activities. This is especially true if athletes have had to cease all sports activities during treatment. When athletes have been able to continue activity in parallel with treatment, this is not so great a problem.

Guidelines are available,[156] but there are no strict rules to guide reintroduction to activity after tendinitis. In tendinitis cases, it is recommended that there be no symptoms during nonathletic activities and that the athlete be performing the appropriate eccentric exercise rapidly. It is safer and more satisfying for the athlete and clinician to start at a low level and progress, rather than try to resume participating at the preinjury level and find this impossible to achieve. A too rapid return to preinjury levels of involvement is probably the most common cause of recurrence of tendon injuries. Athletic participation can be started at about 25 percent of the preinjury level (duration or intensity, depending on the sport and movement) and should initially be done on alternate days to avoid muscle soreness and to evaluate the tendon's response to training. Assuming that few or no symptoms are produced, progression can be made in approximately 10 percent increments until full training has been resumed. This should take about 8 weeks. The entire treatment period for tendinitis therefore ranges from about 2 weeks for very mild cases with no interruption of activity, to 12 to 16 weeks for severe cases in which no activity was possible until 4 to 6 weeks of treatment had been carried out.

SUCCESS OR FAILURE OF THE PROGRAM. Curwin and Stanish monitored more than 200 chronic tendinitis patients who were treated using the eccentric exercise program (including many who had been unsuccessfully treated with several alternative therapies) and found that most had minimal or no symptoms after 6 weeks (see Figure 3–15)[54]. Similar improvements have been noted by others using eccentric training programs.[78,155] At least 6 weeks of treatment are usually required, although a few people will experience complete resolution in 2 to 3 weeks, and a very few others will need to continue for 12 to 16 weeks. Modalities can be employed if desired, especially if symptoms are acute or prolonged and the clinician suspects that the collagen-synthesizing ability of the tendon is decreased. A similar rationale can be used by the physician to decide whether to use NSAIDs in patients in whom the inflammatory phase is thought to be prolonged.

If eccentric exercise is not successful in treating an athlete's tendinitis, several explanations are possible:

1. *Incorrect diagnosis*

   The athlete does not have tendinitis. Joint pathology is causing the problem, or symptoms are being referred from another musculoskeletal location, usually the spine. More rarely, there is a nonmusculoskeletal reason for the patient's pain and dysfunction. Careful history taking and the clearing of all joint signs before starting exercise treatment will help reduce the possibility of errors.

2. *Unrecognized external factors*

   The clinician has failed to identify an external cause for the athlete's symptoms. This may be footwear, training errors, or other factors of which the clinician is unaware. For eccentric exercise treatment to be successful, symptoms must be caused by tensile loading, and all outside factors must first be removed. Be sure that joint range of motion, both physiologic and accessory, is normal and pain free. Pain should be elicited during eccentric muscle work even if other muscle tests are negative, but large forces may be required to provoke symptoms with some athletes. Eccentric exercise should *not* be used for all cases of tendinitis; it is best suited to cases in which the history suggests an overuse type injury due to tensile loading.

3. *Noncompliance*

The athlete is not complying with the exercise program. In many cases, the clinician will discover that the athlete is performing 300, rather than 30, repetitions of the exercise program. More rarely, the athlete is not performing the exercises. It is recommended that athletes be monitored closely for the first 2 weeks, after which supervision can be reduced.

4. *Incorrect program progression*

In cases in which the clinician is confident of the diagnosis of tendinitis, the most common reason for lack of success is incorrect program progression. Either the injured athlete was started at too high a level (increased symptoms), or he or she has not progressed to the next level of training intensity (no change in symptoms). A slight increase in symptoms during activity may be noted in the first 2 to 3 weeks of carrying out the exercise, but the pain should not be severe and should *not* be progressively increasing. Exercise programs require time to be successful, since tissue adaptation is needed, but under no circumstances should treatment be continued without modification if no improvement in symptoms takes place after 2 to 3 weeks (about 10 to 15 daily exercise sessions). The physician and physical therapist may need to consider other causes of the athlete's symptoms, and a thorough re-examination should be performed. All joint signs should be cleared, and metabolic considerations, such as diet and hormonal status, may need to be investigated. Ask another clinician to assess the athlete if you arrive at the same diagnosis, but treatment remains unsuccessful.

SUMMARY

Chronic tendinitis remains a dilemma for many clinicians, and the best treatment is not always possible or recognized. Ideally, treatment should combine both resolution and prevention of symptoms and should be based on good science and common sense. The use of exercise to treat chronic tendinitis relies on both—the science of tendon adaptation to increased stress and the common sense of participation based on ability to perform. In order to be successful, exercise cannot be used in isolation if other factors are also involved, but a knowledge of the beneficial effects of tensile loading on tendon can be used to treat almost all tendon injuries.

REFERENCES

1. Butler DL, Grood ES, Noyes FR, Zernicke RF: Biomechanics of ligaments and tendons. Exerc Sports Sci Rev 1978; 6:125–182.
2. Elliott DH: Structure and function of mammalian tendon. Biol Rev 1965; 40:392–421.
3. Kastelic J, Galseki A, Baer E: The multicomposite structure of tendon. Connect Tissue Res 1978; 6:11–23.
4. Cooper RR, Misol S: Tendon and ligament insertion: A light and electron microscopic study. J Bone Joint Surg 1970; 52A:1–21.
5. Benjamin M, Evans EJ, Copp L: The histology of tendon attachments to bone in man. J Anat 1986; 149:89–100.
6. Trotter JA, Hsi K, Samora A, et al: A morphometric analysis of the muscle-tendon junction. Anat Rec 1985; 213:26–32.
7. Trotter JA: Functional morphology of force transmission in skeletal muscle. Acta Anat 1993; 146:205–222.
8. Tidball JG: The geometry of actin filament-membrane associations can modify adhesive strength of the myotendinous junction. Cell Motil 1983; 3:439–447.
9. Flint MH: Interrelationships of muco-polysaccharides and collagen in connective tissue remodelling. J Embryol Exp Morphol 1972; 27:481–495.
10. Gillard GC, Reilly HC, Bell-Booth PG, et al: A comparison of the glycosaminoglycans of weight-bearing and nonweight-bearing human dermis. J Invest Dermatol 1977; 69:257–261.
11. Scott JE, Hughes EW: Proteoglycan-collagen relationships in developing chick and bovine tendons: influence of the physiological environment. Connect Tissue Res 1986; 14:267–278.
12. Eyre DR: The collagens of the musculoskeletal soft tissues. *In* Leadbetter WB, Buckwalter JA, Gordon SL (eds): Sports-Induced Inflammation. Rosemont, IL, American Academy of Orthopaedic Surgeons, 1990; pp 161–170.
13. Evans JH, Barbenel JC: Structure and mechanical properties of tendon related to function. Equine Vet J 7:1-8, 1975.
14. Prockop D, Guzman NA: Collagen diseases and the biosynthesis of collagen. Hosp Pract 1977; 12:61–68.
15. Scott JE: The periphery of the developing collagen fibril: Quantitative relationships with dermatan sulphate and other surface-associated species. Biochem J 1984; 218:229–233.
16. Koob TJ, Vogel KG: Proteoglycan synthesis in organ cultures from different regions of bovine tendon subjected to different mechanical forces. Biochem J 1987; 246:589–598.
17. Vogel KG, Trotter JA: The effect of proteoglycans on the morphology of collagen fibrils formed in vitro. Collagen Relat Res 1987; 7:105–114.
18. Bailey AJ, Robins SP, Balian G: Biological significance of the intermolecular crosslinks of collagen. Nature 1974; 251:105–109.
19. Hardy MA: The biology of scar formation. Phys Ther 1989; 69:1014–1024.
20. Viidik A: Tensile properties of achilles tendon systems in trained and untrained rabbits. Acta Orthop Scand 1969; 40:261–272.
21. Harkness RD: Mechanical properties of collagenous tissues. *In* Gold BS (ed): Treatise on Collagen, vol 2. Biology of Collagen Part A. London, Academic Press, 1968, pp 247–310.
22. Gerriets JE, Curwin SL, Last JA: Tendon hypertrophy is associated with increased hydroxylation of nonhelical lysine residues at two specific cross-linking sites in Type I collagen. J Biochem 1993; 268:25553–25560.
23. Schultz RM: Proteins II: physiological proteins. *In* Devlin TM (ed): Textbook of Biochemistry with Clinical Correlations. New York, John Wiley & Sons, 1982.
24. Ihme A, Krieg T, Nerlich A, et al: Ehler-Danlos syndrome type VI: Collagen type specificity of defective lysyl hydroxylation in various tissues. J Invest Dermatol 1984; 83:161–165.
25. Byers PH, Pyeritz RE, Uitto J: Research perspectives in heritable disorders of connective tissues. Matrix 1992; 12:333–342.
26. Monnier VM, Vishwanth V, Frank KE, et al: Relation between complications of type I diabetes mellitus and collagen-linked fluorescence. N Engl J Med 1986; 314:403–408.
27. Akeson WH, Amiel D, Abel MF, et al: Effects of immobilization on joints. Clin Orthop 1987; 219:28–37.
28. Amiel D, Akeson WH, Harwood FL, et al: The effect of immobilization on the types of collagen synthesized in periarticular connective tissue. Connect Tissue Res 1980; 8:27–35.
29. Amiel D, Woo SL-Y, Harwood FL, Akeson WH: The effect of

immobilization on collagen turnover in connective tissue: a biochemical-biomechanical correlation. Acta Orthop Scand 1982; 53:325.

30. Postacchini F, DeMartino C: Regeneration of rabbit calcaneal tendon: maturation of collagen and elastic fibers following partial tenotomy. Connect Tissue Res 1980; 8:41–47.

31. Michna H: Morphometric analysis of loading-induced changes in collagen-fibril populations in young tendons. Cell Tissue Res 1984; 236:465–470.

32. Doillon CJ, Dunn MG, Bender E, et al: Collagen fiber formation in repair tissue: development of strength and toughness. Coll Relat Res 1985; 5:481–492.

33. Edwards DAW: The blood supply and lymphatic drainage of tendons. Anatomy 1946; 80:147–152.

34. Butler DL, Grood ES, Noyes FR, et al: Effects of structure and strain measurement technique on the material properties of young human tendons and fascia. J Biomech 1984; 17:579–596.

35. Knorzer E, Folkhard W, Geercken W, et al: New aspects of the etiology of tendon rupture: An analysis of time-resolved dynamic-mechanical measurements using synchrotron radiation. Arch Orthop Trauma Surg 1986; 105:113–120.

36. Mosler E, Folkhard W, Knorzer E, et al: Stress-induced molecular rearrangement in tendon collagen. J Mol Biol 1985; 182:589–596.

37. Steven FS, Minns RJ, Finlay JB: Evidence for the local denaturation of collagen fibrils during the mechanical rupture of human tendons. Injury 1975; 6:317–319.

38. Barfred T: Experimental rupture of the Achilles tendon: comparison of various types of experimental rupture in rats. Acta Orthop Scand 1971; 42:528–543.

39. Woo SL-Y, Rittel MA, Amiel D, et al: The biomechanical and biochemical properties of swine tendons—long-term effects of exercise on the digital extensors. Connect Tissue Res 1980; 7:177–183.

40. Elliott DH, Crawford GNC: The thickness and collagen content of tendon relative to the strength and cross-sectional area of muscle. Proc R Soc Med 1965; 162:137–146.

41. Barnes GRG, Pinder DN: In vivo tendon tension and bone strain measurement and correlation. J Biomech 1974; 7:35–42.

42. Silver IA, Rossdale PD: A clinical and experimental study of tendon injury, healing and treatment in the horse. Equine Vet J 1983; (Suppl 1):1–43.

43. Barfred T: Kinesiological comments on subcutaneous ruptures of the achilles tendon. Acta Orthop Scand 1971; 42:397–405.

44. Curwin SL: Force and length changes of the gastrocnemius and soleus muscle-tendon units during a therapeutic exercise program and three selected activities. Dalhousie University, MSc Thesis, 1984.

45. Gregor RJ, Komi PV, Jarvinen M: Achilles tendon forces during cycling. Int J Sports Med 1987; 8(Suppl):9–14.

46. Komi PV, Fukashiro S, Jarvinen M: Biomechanical loading of Achilles tendon during normal locomotion. Clin Sports Med 1992; 11:521–531.

47. Booth FW: Effect of limb immobilization on skeletal muscle. J Appl Physiol 1982; 52:1113–1118.

48. Booth FW, Gould EW: Effects of training and disuse on connective tissue. Exerc Sports Sci Rev 1975; 3:83–107.

49. Jozsa L, Kannus P, Thoring J, et al: The effect of tenotomy and immobilization on intramuscular connective tissue. A morphometric and microscopic study in rat calf muscles. J Bone Joint Surg 1990; 72B:293–297.

50. Klein L, Sawson MH, Heiple KG: Turnover of collagen in the adult rat after denervation. J Bone Joint Surg 1977; 59A:1065–1067.

51. Noyes FR, Torvik PJ, Hyde WB, DeLucas JL: Biomechanics of ligament failure II. An analysis of immobilization, exercise, and reconditioning effects in primates. J Bone Joint Surg 1974; 56A:1406–1418.

52. Vailas AC, Deluna DM, Lewis LL, et al: Adaptation of bone and tendon to prolonged hindlimb suspension in rats. J Appl Physiol 1988; 65:373–378.

53. Zuckerman J, Stull GA: Ligamentous separation force in rats as influenced by training, detraining and cage restriction. Med Sci Sports Exerc 1973; 5:44–49.

54. Curwin SL, Stanish WD: Tendinitis: Its Etiology and Treatment. Lexington, MA, DC Heath, 1984.

55. Hitchcock TF, Light TR, Bunch WH, et al: The effect of immediate constrained motion on the strength of flexor tendon repairs in chickens. J Hand Surg 1987; 12A:590–595.

56. Karpakka J, Vaananen K, Virtanen P, et al: The effects of remobilization and exercise on collagen biosynthesis in rat tendon. Acta Physiol Scand 1990; 139:139–145.

57. Loitz B, Zernicke R, Vailas A., et al: Effects of short-term immobilization versus continuous passive motion on the biomechanical and biochemical properties of the rabbit tendon. Clin Orthop Rel Res 1989; 244:265–271.

58. Matsuda JJ, Zernicke RF, Vailas AC, et al: Structural and mechanical adaptation of immature bone to strenuous exercise. J Appl Physiol 1986; 60:2028–2034.

59. Becker H, Diegelman RF: The influence of tension on intrinsic tendon fibroplasia. Orthop Rev 1984; 13:65–71.

60. Blanchard O, Cohen-Solal L, Tardieu C, et al: Tendon adaptation to different long-term stresses and collagen reticulation in soleus muscle. Connect Tissue Res 1985; 13:261–267.

61. Tipton CM, Matthes RD, Maynard JA, Carey RA: The influence of physical activity on ligaments and tendons. Med Sci Sports Exerc 1975; 7:165–175.

62. Vailas AC, Zernicke RF, Curwin SL, et al: Adaptation of rat knee meniscus to prolonged exercise. J Appl Physiol 1986; 60:1031–1034.

63. Heikkinen E, Vuori I: Effect of physical activity on the connective tissue metabolism in mice. Scand J Clin Lab Invest (Suppl) 1979; 113:36–41.

64. Kiiskinen A: Physical training and connective tissues in young mice: physical properties of Achilles tendons and long bones. Growth 1977; 41:123–137.

65. Alexander R McN, Vernon A: The dimensions of knee and ankle muscles and the forces they exert. J Hum Movement Stud 1975; 1:115–123.

66. Blazina M: Jumper's knee. Orthop Clin North Am 1973; 2:665–678.

67. Casanova J, Casanova J: "Nintendinitis." J Hand Surg 1991; 16:181 (Letter).

68. Clancy WG: Tendon trauma and overuse injuries. In Leadbetter WB, Buckwalter JA, Gordon SL (eds): Sports-Induced Inflammation. Rosemont, IL, American Academy of Orthopaedic Surgeons, 1990, pp 609–618.

69. Colosimo AJ, Bassett FH: Jumper's knee. Diagnosis and treatment. Orthop Rev 1990; 19:139–149.

70. Fernandez-Palazzi F, Rivas S, Mujica P: Achilles tendinitis in ballet dancers. Clin Orthop 1990; 257:257–261.

71. Jorgensen U, Winge S: Injuries in badminton. Sports Med 1990; 10:59–64.

72. Vailas AC, Pedrini VA, Pedrini-Mille A, et al: Patellar matrix changes associated with aging and voluntary exercise. J Appl Physiol 1985; 58:1572–1576.

73. Curwin SL, Vailas AC, Wood J: Immature tendon adaptation to strenuous exercise. J Appl Physiol 1988; 65:2297–2301.

74. Backman C, Boquist L, Friden J, et al: Chronic Achilles paratenonitis with tendinosis: an experimental model in the rabbit. J Orthop Res 1990; 8:541–547.

75. Backman C, Friden J, Widmark A: Blood flow in chronic Achilles tendinosis. Radioactive microsphere study in rabbits. Acta Orthop Scand 1991; 62:386–387.

76. Puddu G, Ippolito E, Postacchini F: A classification of Achilles tendon disease. Am J Sports Med 1976; 4:145–150.

77. Fredenburg M, Tilley G, Yagoubian E: Spontaneous rupture of posterior tibial tendon secondary to chronic non-specific tenosynovitis. Foot Surg 1983; 22:198.

78. Gross MT: Chronic tendinitis: Pathomechanics of injury, factors affecting the healing response, and treatment. J Orthop Sports Phys Ther 1992; 16:248–261.

79. Fackleman BE: The nature of tendon damage and its repair. Equine Vet J 1973; 5:141–149.

80. Matheson GO, Macintyre JG, Taunton JE, et al: Musculoskeletal injuries associated with physical activity in older adults. Med Sci Sports Exerc 1989; 21:379–385.

81. Bonen A, Keizer HA: Pituitary, ovarian and adrenal hormone responses to marathon running. Int J Sports Med 1987; 8(Suppl 3):161–167.

82. Bosenberg AT, Brock-Utne JG, Gaffin SL, et al: Strenuous exercise causes systemic endotoxemia. J Appl Physiol 1988; 65:106–108.

83. Vailas AC, Morgan WP, Vailas JC: Physiologic and cellular basis of overtraining. *In* Leadbetter WB, Buckwalter JA, Gordon SL (eds): Sports-Induced Inflammation. Rosemont, IL, American Academy of Orthopaedic Surgeons, 1990, pp 677–686.

84. Stanish WD, Rubinovich RM, Curwin SL: Eccentric exercise in chronic tendinitis. Clin Orthop Rel Res 1986; 208:65–68.

85. Stauber WT: Eccentric action of muscles: Physiology, injury and adaptation. Exerc Sports Sci Rev 1989; 17:157–185.

86. Zernicke RF, Garhammer J, Jobe FW: Human patellar tendon rupture. J Bone Joint Surg 1977; 59A:179–183.

87. Tidball JG: Myotendinous junction: Morphological changes and mechanical failure associated with muscle cell atrophy. Exp Mol Pathol 1984; 40:1–12.

88. Komi PV: Measurement of the force-velocity relationship in human muscle under concentric and eccentric contractions. Med Sport 1973; 8:224–229.

89. Komi PV: Neuromuscular performance: factors influencing force and speed production. Scand J Sports Sci 1979; 1:2–15.

90. Bosco C, Komi PV: Potentiation of the mechanical behaviour of the human skeletal muscle through pre-stretching. Acta Physiol Scand 1982; 14:543–550.

91. Nirschl RP: The etiology and treatment of tennis elbow. J Sports Med 1974; 2:308–319.

92. Horswill CA, Layman DK, Boileau RA, et al: Excretion of 3-methyl-histidine and hydroxyproline following acute weight-training exercise. Int J Sports Med 1988; 9:245–248.

93. Alen M, Pakarinen A, Hakkinen K, et al: Responses of serum androgenic-anabolic and catabolic hormones to prolonged strength training. Int J Sports Med 1988; 9:229–233.

94. Kjaer M: Epinephrine and some other hormonal responses to exercise in man: with special reference to physical training. Int J Sports Med 1989; 10:2–15.

95. Newman RA, Cutroneo KR: Glucocorticoids selectively decrease the synthesis of hydroxylated collagen peptides. Mol Pharmacol 1978; 14:185–198.

96. Oxlund H, Manthorpe R: The bio-mechanical properties of tendon and skin as influenced by long-term glucocorticoid treatment and food restriction. Biorheology 1982; 19:631–646.

97. Davis JM, Pate RR, Burgess WA, et al: Stress hormone response to exercise in elite female distance runners. Int J Sports Med 1987; 8(Suppl 2):132–135.

98. Agarwal S, Owen R: Tendinitis and tendon ruptures in successful renal transplant recipients. Clin Orthop 1990; 252:270–275.

99. Murison MS, Eardley J, Slapak M: Tendinitis—a common complication after renal transplantation. Transplantation 1990; 48:587–589.

100. Gillard GC, Reilly HC, Bell-Booth PG, Flint MH: The influence of mechanical forces on the glycosaminoglycan content of the rabbit flexor digitorum profundus tendon. Connect Tissue Res 1979; 7:37–47.

101. Kukjula UM, Jarvinen M, Natri A, et al: ABO blood groups and musculoskeletal injuries. Injury 1992; 23:131–133.

102. Rathbun JB, MacNab I: The microvascular pattern of the rotator cuff. J Bone Joint Surg 1970; 52B:540–553.

103. Andrews FJ, Morris CJ, Lewis EJ, et al: Effect of nutritional iron deficiency on acute and chronic inflammation. Ann Rheum Dis 1987; 46:859–865.

104. Law DJ, Lightner VA: Divalent cation-dependent adhesion at the myotendinous junction: ultrastructure and mechanics of failure. J Muscle Res Cell Motil 1993; 14:173–185.

105. Abrahamsson S-O, Lundborg G, Lohmander LS: Tendon healing in vivo. An experimental model. Scand J Reconstr Surg 1989; 23:199–205.

106. Morcos MB, Aswad A: Histological studies of the effects of ultrasonic therapy on surgically split flexor tendons. Equine Vet J 1978; 10:267.

107. Nistor L: Surgical and non-surgical treatment of Achilles tendon rupture. J Bone Joint Surg 1981; 63A:394–399.

108. Steiner M: Biomechanics of tendon healing. J Biomech 1982; 15:951–958.

109. Enwemeka CS, Spielholz NI, Nelson AJ: The effect of early functional activities on experimentally tenotomized Achilles tendons in rats. Am J Phys Med Rehabil 1988; 67:264–269.

110. Enwemeka CS: Inflammation, cellularity and fibrillogenesis in regenerating tendon: implications for tendon rehabilitation. Phys Ther 1989; 69:816–825.

111. Kannus P, Jozsa L: Histopathological changes preceding spontaneous rupture of a tendon. A controlled study of 891 patients. J Bone Joint Surg 1991; 73A:1507–1525.

112. Leadbetter WB: Cell-matrix response in tendon injury. Clin Sports Med 1992; 11:533–578.

113. Watkins P, Auer JA, Gay S, et al: Healing of surgically created defects in the equine superficial digital flexor tendon: collagen-type transformation and tissue morphologic reorganization. Am J Vet Res 1985; 46:2091–2096.

114. Watkins P, Auer JA, Morgan SJ, et al: Healing of surgically created defects in the equine superficial digital flexor tendon: effects of pulsing electromagnetic field therapy on collagen-type transformation and tissue morphologic reorganization. Am J Vet Res 1985; 46:2097–2103.

115. Hargreaves KM: Mechanisms of pain sensation resulting from inflammation. *In* Leadbetter WB, Buckwalter JA, Gordon SL (eds): Sports-Induced Inflammation. Rosemont, IL, American Academy of Orthopaedic Surgeons, 1990, pp 383–392.

116. Nirschl RP: Elbow tendinosis: tennis elbow. Clin Sports Med 1992; 11:851–870.

117. Pope CF: Radiologic evaluation of tendon injuries. Clin Sports Med 1992; 11:579–600.

118. Gertz BJ, Shao P, Hanson DA, et al: Monitoring bone resorption in early postmenopausal women by an immunoassay for cross-linked collagen peptides in urine. J Bone Mineral Res 1994; 9:135–141.

119. Seibel MJ, Robins SP, Bilezikian JP: Urinary pyridinium cross-links of collagen. Trends Endocrinol Metab 1992; 3:263–270.

120. Seibel MJ, Duncan A, Robins SP: Urinary hydroxy-pyridinium crosslinks provide indices of cartilage, bone involvement in arthritic diseases. J Rheumatol 1989; 16:964–970.

121. Nicholson GG: The effects of passive joint mobilization on pain and hypomobility associated with adhesive capsulitis of the shoulder. J Orthop Sports Phys Ther 1985; 6:238–251.

122. Tibone J, Jobe F, Kerland R, et al: Shoulder impingement syndrome in athletes treated by an anterior acromioplasty. Clin Orthop Rel Res 1985; 198:134.

123. Boissonault WG, Janos SC: Dysfunction, evaluation and treatment of the shoulder. *In* Donatelli R, Wooden MJ (eds): Orthopaedic Physical Therapy. New York, Churchill Livingstone, 1989, pp 151–172.

124. Clement DB, Taunton JE, Smart GW: Achilles tendinitis and peritendinitis: Etiology and treatment. Am J Sports Med 1984; 12:179–184.

125. Galloway MT, Jokl P, Dayton OW: Achilles tendon overuse injuries. Clin Sports Med 1992; 11:771–781.

126. Stanish WD, Curwin SL, Bryson G: The use of flexibility exercises in preventing and treating sports injuries. *In* Leadbetter WB, Buckwalter JA, Gordon SL (eds): Sports-Induced Inflammation. Park Ridge, IL, American Academy of Orthopaedic Surgeons, 1990, pp 731–746.

127. Loitz B, Zernicke R, Salem G, et al: Influence of continuous passive motion on the mechanical properties of tendon in rabbit. Phys Ther 1988; 68:265–271.

128. Dyson M, Pond JB, Joseph J, et al: The stimulation of tissue regeneration by means of ultrasound. Clin Sci 1968; 35:273–285.

129. Gieck JH, Saliba E: Therapeutic ultrasound: influence on inflammation and healing. *In* Leadbetter WB, Buckwalter JA, Gordon SL (eds): Sports-Induced Inflammation. Park Ridge, IL, American Academy of Orthopaedic Surgeons, 1990, pp 479–492.

130. Morcos MB, Aswad A: Histological studies of the effects of ultrasonic therapy on surgically split flexor tendons. Equine Vet J 1978; 10:267.

131. Harvey W, Dyson M, Pond JB, Grahame R: The stimulation of protein synthesis in human fibroblasts by therapeutic ultrasound. Rheumatol Rehabil 1975; 14:237.

132. Enwemeka CS: The effects of therapeutic ultrasound on tendon healing. A biomechanical study. Am J Phys Med Rehabil 1989; 68:283–287.

133. Frieder S, Weisberg J, Fleming B, et al: A pilot study: The therapeutic effect of ultrasound following partial rupture of Achilles tendons in male rats. J Orthop Sports Phys Ther 1988; 10:39–46.

134. Snow CJ, Johnson KA: Effect of therapeutic ultrasound on acute inflammation. Physiotherapy Can 1988; 40:162–167.

135. Basford JR: Low-energy laser therapy. *In* Leadbetter WB,

Buckwalter JA, Gordon SL (eds): Sports-Induced Inflammation. Park Ridge, IL, American Academy of Orthopaedic Surgeons, 1990, pp 499–508.

136. Enwemeka CS: Laser biostimulation of healing wounds: specific effects and mechanisms of action. J Orthop Sports Phys Ther 1988; 9:333–338.

137. Frank C, Schachar N, Dittrich D, et al: Electromagnetic stimulation of ligament healing in rabbits. Clin Orthop 1983; 175:263–272.

138. Nessler JP, Mass DP: Direct-current electrical stimulation of tendon healing in vitro. Clin Orthop 1987; 217:303–312.

139. Stanish WD, Rubinovich M, Kozey J, et al: The use of electricity in ligament and tendon repair. Phys Sports Med 1985; 13:109–116.

140. Watkins JP, Auer JA, Morgan SJ, et al: Healing of surgically created defects in the equine superficial digital flexor tendon: effects of pulsing electromagnetic field therapy on collagen-type transformation and tissue morphologic reorganization. Am J Vet Res 1985; 46:2097–2103.

141. Knight KL: Cold as a modifier of sports-induced inflammation. In Leadbetter WB, Buckwalter JA, Gordon SL (eds): Sports-Induced Inflammation. Park Ridge, IL, American Academy of Orthopaedic Surgeons, 1990, pp 463–477.

142. Cyriax J: Textbook of Orthopaedic Medicine, vol. II. Treatment by Manipulation, Massage and Injection, 11th Ed. London, Bailliere Tindall, 1984.

143. Vasseljen D: Low-level laser versus traditional physiotherapy in the treatment of tennis elbow. Physiotherapy 1992; 78:329–334.

144. Stratford PW, Levy DR, Gauldie S, et al: The evaluation of phonophoresis and friction massage as treatments for extensor carpi radialis tendinitis: a randomised controlled trial. Physiother Can 1989; 41:93–99.

145. Chamberlain GJ: Cyriax's friction massage: a review. J Orthop Sports Phys Ther 1982; 4:16–22.

146. Kennedy JC, Willis RB: The effects of local steroid injections on tendons: A biomechanical and microscopic correlative study. Am J Sports Med 1976; 4:11–21.

147. Nirschl RP: The etiology and treatment of tennis elbow. J Sports Med 1974; 2:308–319.

148. Leadbetter WB: Corticosteroid injection therapy in sports injuries. In Leadbetter WB, Buckwalter JA, Gordon SL (eds): Sports-Induced Inflammation. Park Ridge, IL, American Academy of Orthopaedic Surgeons, 1990, pp 527–545.

149. Salminen A, Kihlstrom M: Protective effect of indomethacin against exercise-induced injuries in mouse skeletal muscle fibers. Int J Sports Med 1987; 8:46–49.

150. Abramson SB: Nonsteroidal anti-inflammatory drugs: mechanisms of action and therapeutic considerations. In Leadbetter WB, Buckwalter JA, Gordon SL (eds): Sports-Induced Inflammation. Park Ridge, IL, American Academy of Orthopaedic Surgeons, 1990, pp 421–430.

151. Haupt HA: The role of anabolic steroids as modifiers of sports-induced inflammation. In Leadbetter WB, Buckwalter JA, Gordon SL (eds): Sports-Induced Inflammation. Park Ridge, IL, American Academy of Orthopaedic Surgeons, 1990, pp 449–454.

152. Michna H: Tendon injuries induced by exercise and anabolic steroids in experimental mice. Int Orthop 1987; 11:157–162.

153. Nistor L: Surgical and non-surgical treatment of Achilles tendon rupture. J Bone Joint Surg 1981; 63A:394–399.

154. Clancy WG, Neidhart D, Brand RL: Achilles tendinitis in runners: a report of five cases. Am J Sports Med 1976; 4:46–56.

155. Reid DC: Sports Injury Assessment and Rehabilitation. New York, Churchill Livingstone, 1992.

156. Jensen K, DiFabio RP: Evaluation of eccentric exercise in treatment of patellar tendinitis. Phys Ther 1989; 69:211–216.

CHAPTER 4

Adaptability of Skeletal Muscle: Response to Increased and Decreased Use

WILLIAM D. BANDY *PhD, PT, SCS, ATC*
KIM DUNLEAVY *MS, PT, OCS*

The controlled contraction of muscle allows individuals to move their limbs, maintain posture, and perform a variety of tasks with great precision.[1] In order for the clinician to adequately plan and conduct programs to increase the efficiency of muscle, a knowledge of the muscular system is imperative. In the text that follows, the anatomic structure and function of skeletal muscle, as well as its embryonic development, are briefly reviewed. Once the microscopic "building blocks" of muscle and the process by which these various structures contribute to muscle function are presented, the mechanisms associated with the adaptation, or mutability, of muscle in response to increased demand (such as resistance training) and decreased use (such as immobilization) are discussed. In addition, special consideration is given to muscle adaptation that occurs as a result of increased use across the age span, as well as changes that occur due to gender differences.

The intent of this chapter is to provide information that will serve as a scientific foundation for training and rehabilitation. As noted by previous authors, "an understanding of muscle biology applied by practitioners in any area of physical therapy can only serve to increase the effectiveness of treatment."[2]

STRUCTURE AND FUNCTION OF MUSCLE

TYPES OF MUSCLE

Contractility, a fundamental property of all animal cells, attains its greatest expression in muscle tissue. Muscle tissue is composed of long and narrow cells, called muscle fibers, that are specialized to contract and pull two ends of the cell closer together.[3] Given the various kinds of contractions required for the different functions of the body, three types of muscle tissues exist, each with its own characteristic fiber: cardiac muscle, specific to the heart[4]; smooth muscle, found particularly in thin sheets forming part of the wall of hollow organs, such as the digestive tract and blood vessels[5]; and voluntary skeletal muscle.[3]

Cardiac muscle, which comprises the heart walls and the large veins entering the heart, possesses an intrinsic ability to contract, doing so in the absence of impulses from the central nervous system. Cardiac muscle is a network of striated muscle fibers that differs from the other two types of tissue mainly by the presence of interweaving, anastomosing fibers forming a continuous network, called a syncytium. Whereas each fiber in skeletal muscle is a discrete entity and can contract individually, tissue innervation in cardiac muscle results in a wavelike contraction that passes through this entire network of muscle fibers of the heart. The function of the cardiac muscles is the rhythmic contraction of the heart organ.[4]

Smooth muscle, the simplest of the three types of muscle, lacks cross striations when viewed through a microscope, hence its name. The fibers of smooth muscle are commonly arranged in sheets and constitute one or more layers of the walls of tubes and certain hollow structures of the body, examples being blood vessels, tubes conducting air into and out of the lungs, the urinary bladder and gallbladder, and all regions of the digestive tract. The chief role of the smooth muscle in the walls of such tubular or bladder-like structures is to regulate the size of their lumina or cavities by the degree of contraction. In some cases, smooth muscle also propels the contents of these tubes along with waves of contraction.[5]

Skeletal muscle, which in this chapter is referred to simply as "muscle," is the only type of muscle in which the specialized function of generating force and producing movement is directly responsive to volitional control. Most of these muscles are attached by at least one end to some part of the skeleton, and contraction of these muscles causes its movement.[3,6]

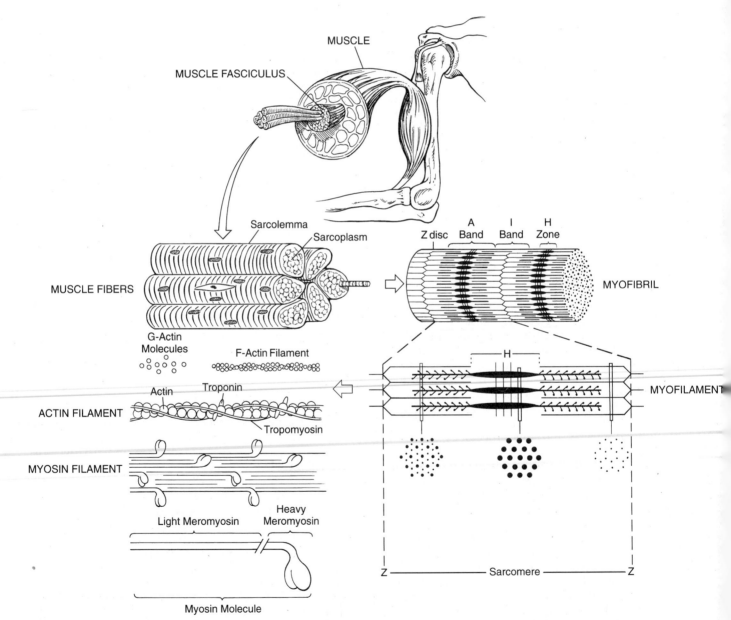

FIGURE 4–1. Organization of skeletal muscle. (Adapted from Bloom W, Fawcett DW: A Textbook of Histology, 10th ed. Philadelphia, WB Saunders, 1975.)

STRUCTURE OF SKELETAL MUSCLE

The size, shape, and gross structure of skeletal muscle (Fig. 4–1) vary greatly in accordance with their particular function and workload, ranging from the 1.4 cm length of the dorsal interossei to the 30 cm length of the sartorius muscle. The basic cellular structure that is common to all muscle is the cylindrically shaped individual muscle fiber, the diameter ranging from 10 to 100 μm (1 meter = 10^2 cm, 10^3 mm, 10^6 μm, 10^9 nm) and length ranging up to 70 mm. The muscle and muscle fiber are surrounded and supported by connective tissue components, which serve as a medium for a rich nerve and blood supply, as well as providing a noncontractile framework through which the contraction of muscle is transmitted to the bone.[3,6]

Each individual muscle fiber is surrounded by a thin sheathlike covering of connective tissue containing extensive capillaries and nerve fibers, called the endomysium. Up to 150 muscle fibers are collected into bundles, called fascicles (see Fig. 4–1), and covered with a thicker layer of connective tissue called the perimysium, which allows lymphatic vessels, nerve fibers, and blood vessels to enter or leave the interior of the muscle. The endomysium and perimysium are continuous with the outer, tough sheath of connective tissue enclosing the entire muscle, the epimysium. Continuations of the tissue of the epimysium merge with the connective tissue of the tendon, which then attaches the muscle to the bony components.[3,6–9]

Evidence exists that the connective tissue matrix forms a passive elastic component of muscle that plays a vital role in force transmission, serving in more than a merely supportive role to the muscle fiber.[7–10] Because each single muscle fiber does not run the entire length of the muscle, or even the length of a fasciculus, these connective tissue sheaths—endomysium, perimysium, and epimysium—are necessary to transmit the force of muscle contraction from the muscle fiber to the tendons, which act on the bones. Since all connective tissue in muscle is interconnected and surrounds the muscle fibers in parallel, lengthening or shortening of the muscle also leads to lengthening or shortening of the connective tissue. Therefore, the potential for increase or decrease in passive tension available in the connective tissue of muscle can substantially affect the total force available for muscle contraction.[7,10]

STRUCTURE OF THE MUSCLE FIBER

Each individual muscle fiber is enclosed in a special membrane, the sarcolemma, which lies just inside and attaches to the endomysium and surrounds the cytoplasm of the muscle cell, the sarcoplasm (see Fig. 4–1). The sarcolemma plays an important role in conducting contraction-eliciting impulses along and into the muscle fiber, as well as acting as a diffusion medium for oxygen and nutrients from nearby capillaries outside the cell into the sarcoplasm. The sarcoplasm is a semifluid substance containing structures that are of vital importance to cell metabolism and muscle contraction, including the eccentrically placed cell nuclei, about 40 for each millimeter length of fiber; the mitochondria, containing the respiratory enzymes that are so important for the active metabolism of muscle fibers; sarcoplasmic reticulum, which is composed of anastomosing membranous channels within the myofibrils, containing a large calcium-storage capacity; ribosomes, performing the tremendously important task of protein synthesis; deposits of glycogen, which can quickly take up, store, or give up oxygen to the muscle on a short-term basis as needed; and longitudinal bundles of myofibrils, the contractile structural units of a muscle fiber.[1,3,9,11]

Under the light microscope, the myofibrils appear as continuous bands of alternating light (isotropic or I) and dark (anisotropic or A) bands, giving the structure a striated appearance. Hence, skeletal muscle is also known as striated muscle. When examined with electron microscopy, the myofibrils are found to consist of repeated cylindrical units 2 to 3 μm in length and 1 μm in diameter separated by thin Z discs, forming units called sarcomeres, the ultimate contractile structure of striated muscle (see Fig. 4–1). The sarcomere is composed of two distinct myofibrillar proteins, generally called myofilaments; more specifically, it is divided into thin and thick filaments.[3,6–9,11]

Electron microscopy reveals that in relaxed muscle fiber, the darker A bands are the result of the presence of thick filaments (about 1 μm long and 10 nm in diameter), and the lesser density of the I band is the result of its containing only thin filaments (about 1 μm long and 5 nm in diameter). The thin filaments lying at each end of the relaxed sarcomere project into the A band approximately one-quarter of its length, leaving a less dense middle section in the A band where no overlap of the thin and thick filaments occurs, corresponding to the lighter H zone seen with the light microscope (see Fig. 4–1).[3,6–9,11]

Estimates based on electron microscopy are that each muscle fiber contains thousands of sarcomeres (a muscle fiber 5 mm long contains about 20,000 such divisions). Each sarcomere, in turn, contains about 3 million myofilaments (actin and myosin). As an example, a single muscle fiber 100 μm in diameter and 1 cm long contains about 8000 myofibrils, and each myofibril consists of 4500 sarcomeres, resulting in a total of 16 billion thick and 64 billion thin filaments.[8]

The main constituents of the thin filaments are pairs of chainlike strings of polymerized actin molecules (G actin and F actin) wound around each other in a helix formation. Within the groove formed by the paired strands of actin is a long filamentous protein called tropomyosin, with a small molecular complex called troponin attached to the tropomyosin filament at regular intervals (Fig. 4–1). The troponin and tropomyosin molecules control the binding of actin and myosin.[3,7–9,11]

The thick filaments are composed of about 250 myosin molecules bundled together, forming long filaments. Each of the myosin filaments resembles a golf club, consisting of a globular enlargement, called the head group (the heavy meromyosin), and a long tail (the light meromyosin) (see Fig. 4–1). The myosin

TABLE 4–1
Hierarchy of Skeletal Muscle Structure

Structure	Length*	Diameter*
Whole skeletal muscle and muscle fascicle	1–30 cm	Varies
Muscle fiber	1–70 mm	10–100 μm
Myofibril		
Sarcomere	2–3 μm	1 μm
Myofilament	1 μm	5–10 nm

*1 meter = 10^2 cm, 10^3 mm, 10^6 μm, 10^9 nm.

molecule is flexible at the junction of the heavy and light meromyosin portions, allowing the globular heads to swivel and attach to the actin molecule, thereby playing a vital role in muscle contraction and relaxation.[7–9]

The myosin-containing (thick) and actin-containing (thin) filaments interdigitate to form a hexagonal lattice (see Fig. 4–1). Together, these microscopic myofilaments produce muscle shortening.[7–9]

In summary, the structure of muscle is arranged in what Lieber[1] termed an "elegant hierarchy" (Table 4–1). From the gross whole skeletal muscle to the smallest myofilament, "structural hierarchy organization is the rule, not the exception."[1]

SLIDING FILAMENT THEORY

Muscle contraction occurs because the sarcomeres shorten to as little as half their resting length, a phenomenon described by Huxley[3] as the sliding filament theory. Upon stimulation of the muscle by the arrival of the nerve impulse, chemical changes occur in the sarcomere, causing the thin filaments to move further between the thick filaments, with their free ends almost meeting at the middle of the sarcomere during full muscle contraction. Since the length of the myofilaments remains unchanged, the only way that the thin filaments can move between the thick filaments is by pulling the Z lines to which they are attached, thereby pulling the ends of all sarcomeres closer together. During relaxation, the thin myofilaments slide out again from between the thick filaments and the sarcomere lengthens, as does the entire muscle fiber.[3,6–9,12]

Electron microscopy indicates that the H zone (see Fig. 4–1) virtually disappears in fully contracted sarcomeres because, as the thin filaments move, the A band becomes uniformly dense, revealing no H band; this occurs because the sarcomere now contains both thick and thin myofilaments from end to end. During relaxation, the sarcomere lengthens and the lighter H band returns.[3,6–9]

The muscle contraction occurs because, at the molecular level, the globular heads of the myosin molecules attach themselves to receptor sites on the actin molecules, forming cross-bridges between the thick and thin filaments. The myosin heads' access to the attachment sites on the actin molecules is regulated by troponin, which repositions the tropomyosin molecules so that receptor sites on the actin molecules are free and binding can occur. After some cross-bridges are formed, the myosin heads undergo a conformational change, causing the heads to swivel in an arc, resulting in the actin molecule being pulled along the myosin molecule. Finally, the myosin heads detach themselves from the actin and the cycle starts over.[3,7–9,12]

The formation, breaking, and re-formation of cross-bridges can continue until a maximum overlap of the filaments has occurred. At this point, all possible sites for cross-bridge formation have been filled in the shortened muscle, and further cross-bridge formation cannot occur. When the sarcomere is considerably shortened, the myosin molecules are completely overlapped with the actin molecules, but not, as indicated previously, because either filament has changed in length.[3,6–9,12]

In order for the mechanical linkages between actin and myosin filaments to form, break, and re-form cross-bridges, resulting in shortened sarcomeres, two major intermolecular processes are necessary: (1) an electrical impulse and depolarization must trigger the coupling (via the action potential, myoneural junction, endoplasmic reticulum, and so on), and (2) chemical reactions must provide for the development of tension (via excitation coupling, adenosine triphosphate [ATP], and so on).[7–9] A description of the processes of electrical depolarization and energy provision is beyond the scope of this chapter. For a more thorough description of chemical and mechanical events that control muscle contraction, the reader is referred to texts on histology and the physiology of muscle.[1,7–9]

MOTOR UNIT

The ability of the central nervous system to control the amount of force with which a contraction occurs is largely dependent on the final pathway of the nervous system, the motor unit.[13,14] The motor unit—defined as a single motor cell in the anterior horn of the spinal cord, its axon and terminal branches, and all the individual muscle fibers supplied by the axon—is considered the basic functional unit of skeletal muscle. The innervation ratio, defined as the total number of motor axons divided by the total number of muscle fibers in a muscle, varies according to the primary function of each muscle. Muscles involved in delicate movements of the eye have a very small innervation ratio (1:4), whereas large postural muscles not requiring a fine degree of control have an innervation ratio that is significantly larger (1:1000).[13,14]

Motor units control muscle tension through two primary mechanisms: the number of motor units recruited and the rate of firing of each motor unit. First, force generated by a muscle is accomplished by simultaneous contraction of increased numbers of motor units (spatial summation). Since all the fibers composing a motor unit contract in unison and maximally, variations in the strength of contractions are partly the result of the number of motor units employed. Only a few motor units contract during a weak contraction, whereas a greater number of motor units contract simultaneously for a strong contraction. Should all the motor units contract at the same time, the contraction would be maximal.[15]

Second, the force of a muscle contraction is affected by the frequency of stimulation of each motor unit (temporal summation). If a muscle fiber is stimulated several times in succession, a new contraction begins before the previous one is completed. Each succeeding contraction then adds to the force of the preceding one, and the overall strength of the contraction is increased. A weak contraction occurs when the muscle fiber is stimulated only a few times per second, and a strong contraction occurs when the fiber is stimulated many times per second into a smooth, continuous contraction.[16,17]

In summary, the force of a muscle contraction is attained by utilizing a combination of recruitment and rate of firing. During a weak contraction, only one or two motor units contract at only two or three times per second, but the contractions are spread one after another among the different motor units. Relatively smooth performances are achieved by low discharge rates of motor units firing asynchronously, or out of phase, so that when one group of fibers is contracting another group is resting.[14,15] When a stronger contraction is desired, a greater number of motor units are recruited simultaneously and fire more frequently. If the majority of the motor units are discharging together at maximal frequency, the force of the muscle will be greatest, and the motor units are said to be synchronous or in phase.[17,18]

Obviously, the ability of the muscle to maximally generate force as a result of all motor units firing synchronously cannot be sustained indefinitely, and eventually muscular fatigue occurs. During maximal muscle contraction, fatigue is accompanied by a decrease in motor unit activity (as measured by electromyography [EMG]), which may be partially caused by a failure in the neural system or impaired myoneural transmission. Although several factors have been suggested as being related to muscle fatigue during all-out activity, the precise mechanism for this "neural fatigue" is not yet known and remains under study.[19]

MUSCLE FIBER TYPES

Although it contains the same architectural organization and microscopic structure, skeletal muscle is not simply a homogeneous group of fibers with similar metabolic and functional properties. Human muscle is composed of various types of muscle fibers. Many classification systems for muscle fiber types have been proposed (Table 4–2), based on physiological, histochemical, and biochemical properties.[20–22] A review of literature by Rose and Rothstein[2] combined classification schemes of previous studies and described three muscle fiber types as follows:*

1) Type I (Slow oxidative, slow twitch) fibers have large amounts of oxidative enzymes and small amounts of glycolytic enzymes. These fibers primarily use aerobic metabolism, are associated with extensive capillary density, have a high number of mitochondria. . . . These muscles generate a relatively small amount of tension, have a slow contraction time, and are resistant to fatigue.

2) Type IIB (Fast glycolytic, fast twitch–fast fatiguable) fibers are well supplied with glycolytic enzymes and are poorly endowed with oxidative enzymes, which indicate a high capacity for anaerobic metabolism. These fibers are associated with relatively sparse capillary density, have few mitochondria. . . . These muscle units generate a large amount of tension in a short time, but they fatigue rapidly.

3) Type IIA (Fast oxidative glycolytic, fast twitch–fatigue resistant) fibers possess intermediate amounts of oxidative and glycolytic enzymes, which indicates the use of both anaerobic and aerobic metabolism. These fibers have cytological properties that fall between the type I and type IIB fibers.

*Reprinted from Rose SJ, Rothstein JM: Muscle mutability. Phys Ther 1982; 62:1773–1787. With permission of the APTA.

TABLE 4–2
Characteristics of Different Muscle Fiber Types

Property	Muscle Fiber Type		
	Slow-Twitch	*Intermediate*	*Fast-Twitch*
Muscle fiber diameter	Small	Intermediate	Large
Color	Red	Red	White
Myoglobin content	High	High	Low
Mitochondria	Numerous	Numerous	Few
Oxidative enzymes	High	Intermediate	Low
Glycolytic enzymes	Low	Intermediate	High
Glycogen content	Low	Intermediate	High
Myosin ATPase activity	Low	High	High
Major source of ATP	Oxidative phosphorylation	Oxidative phosphorylation	Glycolysis
Speed of contraction	Slow	Intermediate	Fast
Rate of fatigue	Slow	Intermediate	Fast
Other names used	Type I	Type IIB	Type IIA
	SO (slow oxidative)	FOG (fast oxidative glycolytic)	FG (fast glycolytic)

Adapted from Burke RE, Edgerton VR: Motor unit properties and selective involvement in movement. Exerc Sport Sci Rev 1975; 3:31–35. © American College of Sports Medicine.

The size principle described by Henneman and colleagues[23,24] implies that motor units are recruited in order, according to their fiber type. Slow-twitch muscle fibers (type I), which are used for submaximal contractions, are recruited first, followed by intermediate fibers (type IIB). Finally, fast-twitch fibers (type IIA) fire when a force of maximal contraction is needed.[14] During long-lasting endurance activities, all motor units fire at moderate rates, but as soon as the activity is less than maximal, the neurons with the highest threshold (fast-twitch) drop out. In contrast, during short-lasting maximal performance, such as resistance training, all motor units fire.[14]

The percentage distribution of muscle fiber type varies broadly among individuals, as well as among different muscle groups within the same individual.[25–27] Although some investigations indicate a possibility of transformation of fiber type under conditions of prolonged and specific training,[28–30] most researchers agree that the predominant muscle fiber distribution is established before birth or early in life and is largely determined by genetic factors.[31–34] Through appropriate endurance or resistance training, fiber types can be significantly improved in metabolic capacity, but the transformation of one fiber type to another is uncommon.[31]

Some researchers believe that the possibility of muscle fiber transformation is overrated and is not as important as performance. According to Lieber,[1] "even if transformation does occur, its influence on performance is relatively small compared to intrinsic architectural and kinematic musculoskeletal properties. Muscle fiber types are clearly related to performance, but are not the cause for performance at a particular level."

EMBRYONIC DEVELOPMENT OF MUSCLE: MYOGENESIS

The specialized structure and function that allow a muscle to contract are a culmination of an intricate embryologic developmental sequence referred to as myogenesis (Fig. 4–2).[1,35] Embryologically, skeletal muscle cells are derived from the mesodermal germ layer in the limb buds (limb musculature), somites (trunk muscles), and branchial segments (neck and cranial muscles). Early in myogenesis (at about the fourth or fifth week of fetal development), certain closely packed mesodermal cells accumulate at certain sites to form elongated, spindle-shaped cells called presumptive myoblasts, which are later differentiated to form clusters of small mononucleated cells called myoblasts. A primary activity of both the presumptive myoblasts and the myoblasts, which intense proliferation in number by mitosis; these structures do not synthesize myofibrillar protein.[1,35–37]

During the seventh to ninth week of fetal development, these myoblastic cells (stimulated by conditions not yet fully understood) cease dividing and fuse with one another to form multinucleated cylindrical structures known as myotubes. Once the myoblasts have

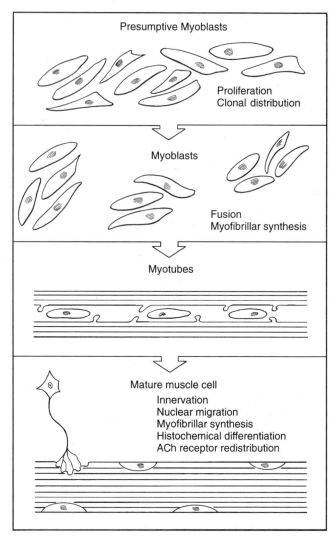

FIGURE 4–2. Embryonic development of skeletal muscle. (Redrawn from Cruess RL: The Musculoskeletal System: Embryology, Biochemistry, and Physiology. New York, Churchill Livingstone, 1982.)

fused, the resulting myotubes no longer have the capacity for cell division, and synthesis of the myofibrillar components—actin and myosin—begins.[1,35–37]

As development progresses, myotubes increase in size and number as more and more myoblasts leave the proliferation cycle and fuse at the ends of the myotubes. Between the tenth and fifteenth week of fetal development, the myotube begins to look more like a mature muscle fiber, with the nuclei being forced from the fiber center to the periphery because of the progressive filling with contractile protein. The myotube diameter continues to increase as a result of ongoing synthesis and the coordinated assembly of myofibrils, giving the muscle a striated appearance. Formation of the sacrotuberous system, proliferation of the mitochondria, deposition of glycogen, and, lastly, innervation follow.[1,35]

The differentiation and fusion that occur with myogenesis take place without neurologic influence. However, the maintenance of the differentiated state of the mature muscle cell and the continued functional growth of muscle in the postnatal period require innervation. In addition, the physiological properties, ultrastructural and histochemical characteristics, and myofibrillar ATPase activity of muscle are all influenced by the specific nerve that contacts the myotube. Following formation of the myotube, the motor neurons begin to send axon processes into the muscle, forming myoneural junctions and bringing the muscle under the control of the central nervous system. From this point on, the muscle fiber depends on its motor neuron not only to provide a means of initiating a contraction but also for the continued survival and development of the muscle fiber. If the nerve fibers to the muscle are severed or the motor neurons destroyed, the denervated muscle fibers become progressively smaller, their actin and myosin content decreases, and proliferation of connective tissue around the muscle fibers occurs. It appears that action potentials in the nerve fibers release chemical substances to the embryonic muscle that are necessary for the functional state of the muscle.[1,35]

The predominant muscle fiber type in the early fetus is a primitive, undifferentiated fast-twitch fiber. As the neurologic and muscular systems mature and as limb, diaphragm, and trunk muscles begin to function in the womb, fiber differentiation occurs so that the histochemically identifiable fiber types become distinguishable (types I, IIA, and IIB).[38]

Although muscle development is not complete at birth, the number of muscle fibers available is probably established at birth, and continued muscle growth is the result of an increase in fiber size (hypertrophy), in both width and length.[39] As growing myofibrils approach their maximum diameter, increase in the width of the muscle occurs as the fibrils split longitudinally and create more myofibrils. Muscle fibers also increase in length as the muscle elongates by the addition of sarcomeres to the ends of fibers.[39]

Although wide variation exists in the number of fast-twitch and slow-twitch fibers present at birth, as in adults, the majority of muscle fibers during the first year of life are slow twitch. The increased proportion of slow-twitch fibers may be explained by the infant's need for these postural muscles to maintain spinal position and initiate locomotion. After the first year of life, however, the fiber types are established in an equal percentage within muscle (about 50 percent fast twitch and 50 percent slow twitch), and the greatest change is not in the distribution but in the increase in diameter of each fiber type.[38] The developmental addition of sarcomeres and the hypertrophy of muscle fibers continue until growth ceases and adult fiber size is attained, usually at about the age of 15 years.[40]

MUSCLE ADAPTATION TO INCREASED USE

HYPERTROPHY

The maximal force that can be generated by a muscle is closely related to the cross-sectional area of the muscle, with a large muscle generating greater force than a small muscle.[41–45] Muscle growth in response to overload training occurs primarily from the enlargement of individual fibers, called hypertrophy.[41,43,44,46–51] Investigations into the occurrence of hypertrophy in humans have used primarily two designs: cross-sectional research designs, in which muscles of "normal" subjects were compared with those of subjects engaged in extensive resistance training programs, and longitudinal research designs, in which the change in cross-sectional area was measured across time in subjects beginning a resistance training program.

Cross-sectional studies in humans indicate that weight lifters have similar percentages of fast-twitch and slow-twitch fibers as nonexercising subjects but exhibit preferential hypertrophy of fast-twitch fibers.[41,43,46,47] Evaluating the cross-sectional area of the muscles of weight lifters and sedentary individuals, Haggmark and colleagues[41] reported that weight lifters had greater muscle cross-sectional area than sedentary subjects. These results were supported in a later study by MacDougall and coworkers,[43] who reported that the average cross-sectional area for both elite and intermediate bodybuilder groups was significantly greater than that for sedentary groups.

Using longitudinal designs, Ikai and Fukunaga[49] reported a 23 percent increase in the cross-sectional area of the elbow flexors after 100 days of isometric training; Luithi and associates[42] reported an 8.4 percent increase in cross-sectional area of the vastus lateralis muscle after 6 months of training using dynamic, concentric training; MacDougall and colleagues[44] demonstrated an 11 percent increase in arm circumference after a 5-month training study; and Moritani and deVries[50] reported a 7 percent increase in cross-sectional area following 8 weeks of training the elbow flexors. More recently, Frontera and coworkers[51] reported a 9.3 percent increase in the cross-sectional areas of the quadriceps muscles in older men following 12 weeks of resistance training.

The authors of each of these investigations, irrespective of whether a cross-sectional or a longitudinal design was used, concluded that the increase in cross-sectional area following resistance training was the result of the enlargement of the skeletal muscle fiber, not the result of increased fiber numbers.[41–44,49–51]

The process of hypertrophy is directly related to the synthesis of cellular material, particularly the thickening of myofibrils and the increase in their number. In addition, as muscle activity is increased during resistance training, more sarcomeres are formed as protein synthesis accelerates and protein breakdown decreases.[46,52,53] In fact, Goldberg and associates[52] emphasized that "there is little question that the enhancement of protein synthesis is largely responsible for the increased protein content" that occurs during hypertrophy following resistance training. They also suggested that the primary requirement for initiating work-induced hypertrophy is the increased tension or force that the muscle is called on to generate during exercise, which is independent of the variety of hormonal influences required for growth of muscle during postnatal development.[52]

HYPERPLASIA

Previous researchers theorized that an increase in the number of muscle fibers in muscle, called hyperplasia or fiber splitting, occurs when intense resistance training creates maximal hypertrophy of the muscle cells, making further increases in muscle size impossible. These researchers suggested that after maximal hypertrophy is obtained, additional strength gains can be made only through a process of longitudinal fiber splitting in which the split fibers form two individual daughter cells through a process of lateral budding.[54-56]

Early evidence supporting the process of longitudinal fiber splitting following extensive resistance training was reported by Edgerton[57] in the muscle fibers of rats. Since Edgerton's work, additional studies have reported hyperplasia following resistance training in other animals, such as chickens[58] and cats.[54,55,59] Although fiber splitting has been reported in several different animals, conclusive evidence supporting an increase in the numbers of muscle fibers via hyperplasia in human muscle following resistance training does not exist.[59]

One of the problems often encountered with animal research is generalizing the findings to humans. For example, most animals do not undergo the extensive hypertrophy that is possible in humans following resistance training. Therefore, fiber splitting may be the only compensatory adjustment to progressive overload for animals. In addition, research supporting hyperplasia in animals has been criticized because of methodologic problems associated with the estimation of fiber numbers from histologic sections.[46] Gollnick and coworkers[46] warned that the biopsy techniques used in the studies supporting hyperplasia in animals lacked reliability, and conclusions based on such biopsy techniques provided no evidence of whether the total number of fibers in a muscle increased, decreased, or remained constant as a result of resistance training.

Therefore, most researchers agree that increased cross-sectional area of muscles following resistance training is primarily the result of hypertrophy.[43,44,46,60] In fact, McArdle and colleagues[61] suggest that even if findings of hyperplasia in animals are replicated in humans, "the greatest contribution to muscular strength with overload training is made by the increase in size (hypertrophy) of existing individual muscle cells."

NEUROLOGIC FACTORS

Information collected using longitudinal studies with humans following resistance training indicates that the percentage increase in muscle force is often greater than the percentage increase in cross-sectional area, with some studies reporting changes in muscle force without any measurable change in cross-sectional area.[30,32,42,49] These changes in the force of the muscle that occur with little or no change in cross-sectional area are the result of the influence of the nervous system and are referred to as neural adaptation.[62]

Neural adaptation of muscle is commonly measured by a surface electrode over the active muscle (EMG) to record the motor unit activity during a maximal contraction before and after resistance training.[62] Motor unit activation during maximal contraction has been documented to increase after various types of resistance training.[50,63-65] Moritani and deVries[50] reported that both isometric muscle force and motor unit activation (as measured by EMG) increased following 8 weeks of isotonic elbow flexion exercise. The authors concluded that the increased force production following resistance training was the result of a combination of increased neural input and hypertrophy of contractile tissue.

Hakkinen, in cooperation with various co-investigators,[63-65] examined the concept of neural adaptation in three studies. Evaluating the adaptation of the knee extensor muscles following 24 weeks of a dynamic squat-lift exercise program, two studies reported marked improvement in muscle force and significant increases in neural activation of the motor units of knee extensor muscles (as measured by EMG).[63,64] A third study[65] supported previous findings of increased force and enhanced motor unit activation after 24 weeks of resistance training using explosive jumping activities. In each of these three investigations, the conclusion was that the increased EMG activity noted during maximal contraction following resistance training resulted from a combination of recruitment of an increased number of motor units and an increased firing rate of each unit.

SPECIAL CONSIDERATION: MUSCLE ADAPTATION TO INCREASED USE ACROSS GENDER AND AGE

MUSCLE ADAPTATION IN CHILDREN

Although resistance training has been well documented to cause hypertrophy in adults, only a few studies have examined the effect of resistance training on muscle size in children. Information concerning possible changes in muscle size and function following resistance training indicates that gains in strength are possible in prepubescent children, but these changes occur independent of muscle hypertrophy.[66-68] McGovern,[66] examining the effect of 12 weeks of circuit weight training, and Weltman and colleagues,[67] studying the effect of 14 weeks of hydraulic training of the elbow flexors and knee extensors, reported significant increases in limb strength but no hypertrophy. More recently, Ramsay and coworkers[68] examined the response of 13 boys, aged 9 to 11 years, to 20 weeks of progressive resistance training. Again, the results of the study indicated significant increases in strength, but even after intense exercise for 20 weeks, there was no change in cross-sectional area of the muscle.

Therefore, progressive resistance training in prepubescent boys has been shown to increase strength without any change in cross-sectional area. The authors of each of these studies suggest that the increased strength is the result of neural adaptation or improved coordination of muscle groups involved in the exercise rather than altered fiber size.[66–68]

MUSCLE ADAPTATION IN WOMEN

ABSOLUTE STRENGTH

Research investigating the differences between men and women in absolute strength (strength without regard for muscle or body size) indicates that general muscle strength in women is approximately two-thirds that of men, but it varies according to muscle group.[69] For example, in comparison with men, women are weaker in the chest, arms, and shoulders but as strong in the lower extremities.[69,70] One reason for the difference in absolute strength in the upper and lower extremities may be the fact that both men and women use their legs to a similar degree (standing, walking, running, climbing stairs), but females have traditionally had less opportunity to use their upper limb muscles in a way that would increase strength.

Greater absolute strength in men as compared with women is the result of women typically averaging 60 to 85 percent of the total cross-sectional area of muscle found in men.[71–73] The difference in cross-sectional area between untrained men and women is the result of differences in both the number of muscle fibers and the muscle fiber size. It has been suggested that the increased number of fibers in men is an intrinsic, genetically based gender difference.[74] The difference in the size of each individual muscle fiber may reflect both a genetic gender difference and a behavior difference in the physical activity of men and women.[74] Therefore, the greater number of fibers and larger initial fiber size allow for larger absolute strength gains in men as compared with women following resistance training.

RELATIVE STRENGTH

The relative muscle strength of men and women has been studied by measuring the strength of an individual and dividing this strength by the cross-sectional area of the muscle. Research indicates that when relative muscle strength is taken into consideration, the strength differences between men and women are reduced.[75] Early studies by Ikai and Fukunaga[75] plotted the strength of the elbow flexors in men and women against their muscle size and found that there is little or no difference in the relative strength of men and women. The authors suggested that although men have larger muscle size than women, the force exerted by equal-sized muscle is the same.[75] In other words, the quality of the muscle fiber in exerting force is independent of gender.

EFFECTS OF RESISTANCE TRAINING

Research indicates that women are capable of achieving increased levels of strength following resistance training.[69,74,76–79] A controversy exists, however, when measuring changes in muscle hypertrophy. An early study by Brown and Wilmore[76] reported "substantial" strength gains in female athletes following 6 months of training but only "minimal evidence" of muscular hypertrophy. The authors suggested that the female athletes' previous levels of activity may have already caused muscle hypertrophy and therefore minimized any changes in muscle size that might have occurred through further resistance training.

Wilmore[77] reported that even though the absolute increase in strength was greater in men than in women, significant increases in strength occurred in women following 10 weeks of resistance training. In contrast to the study by Brown and Wilmore,[76] significant increases in several circumferential measurements were reported in both men and women following 16 weeks of heavy resistance training, and the percentage change in muscle hypertrophy was similar for both men and women. Wilmore[77] concluded that "relative changes in strength and muscle hypertrophy consequent to weight training are similar in men and women." In addition, he reported percentage increases in strength that were greater than the percentage change in muscle cross-sectional area in both men and women, further supporting the theory that improvement in strength is the result of a combination of hypertrophy and neural adaptation, regardless of gender.[77]

In summary, research indicates that men and women can increase strength to a similar degree following resistance training. Although some previous investigations indicated that men and women can hypertrophy to the same level following resistance training, the majority of research indicates that muscle hypertrophy is much less pronounced in women.[76,77,79]

Some researchers have speculated that less hypertrophy in women may result from differences in hormonal levels between genders. Specifically, men have 20 to 30 times higher production levels of the androgen testosterone, which has been shown to have a strong anabolic function in tissue building in muscle.[78,79] However, other researchers have suggested that no relation exists between naturally occurring blood testosterone levels and the extent of hypertrophy consequent to resistance training in men or women.[80,81] More research is required before a definitive statement can be made concerning the role of circulating androgens in the response of men and women to resistance training. In addition, when evaluating the similarities and differences between men's and women's ability to hypertrophy following resistance training, other factors to consider are the smaller cross-sectional area of muscles in females (60 to 85 percent that of men) and the greater subcutaneous fat stores, which tend to "soften" the muscular definition in women.[82]

AGING AND MUSCLE ADAPTATION

Maximum strength in men and women is generally achieved between the ages of 20 and 30 years, when the cross-sectional area is usually the largest. This is followed by a plateau through the age of 50, followed by a loss of strength by age 65 and a progressive decline

TABLE 4–3
Size of Fast-Twitch Muscle Fibers With Age

Age Group (Years)	N	Mean Age (Years)	Fiber Type Distribution %, Type II	Fiber Areas (μm²)	
				Type I	Type II
20–29	11	26.1 (0.8)	59.5 (3.9)	2944 (249)	3663 (224)
30–39	10	35.3 (1.0)	63.2 (1.5)	2854 (178)	3509 (282)
40–49	8	42.6 (0.8)	51.8 (5.1)	3133 (230)	3361 (296)
50–59	12	54.5 (0.6)	48.3 (3.0)	2877 (160)	2802 (125)
60–65	10	61.6 (0.6)	45.0 (4.5)	2264 (245)	2120 (174)

From Larsson L, Grimby G, Karlsson J: Muscle strength and speed of movement in relation to age and muscle morphology. J Appl Physiol 1979; 46:451–456.

as age increases beyond 65 years.[83–85] The progressive decline in strength that occurs with aging is the result of a reduced muscle mass that reflects a loss of total muscle protein and a change in fiber type brought about by aging itself and by lower levels of physical activity, which produce a decline in function.[86] Although somewhat controversial, recent evidence suggests that resistance training in the elderly may delay the strength decrement that occurs with aging.[84]

FACTORS UNDERLYING LOSS OF MUSCLE

The loss of strength that occurs with aging is the result, in part, of a loss of muscle mass caused by a decrease in the number of muscle fibers. More specifically, several studies have reported that loss of muscle mass is the result of reduced size in the fast-twitch (type II) fibers,[87–89] as indicated in Table 4–3. Research by Lexall and associates[90] and Grimby and Saltin[89] suggests that "quantitative" rather than "qualitative" changes within muscle account for most of the loss of strength. In other words, reduction in the total number of fast-twitch muscle fibers causes strength loss as aging progresses.

The theory of a decreased number of fast-twitch fibers is supported by EMG studies indicating loss of functioning fast-twitch motor neurons in the elderly.[91,92] One possible explanation for the selective loss of fast-twitch motor neurons in the elderly is that fast-twitch motor neurons may be susceptible to damage arising from local ischemia as a result of atherosclerotic lesions in the peripheral circulation, which is common in the aging population.[93]

In addition, Bemben and colleagues[83] reported that although maximal force production by muscle decreases with age, changes in lean body mass do not decrease to the same degree. Based on these findings, the authors suggested that the decline in strength is related to neural factors, "possibly in terms of the ability to coordinate motor unit firing." Changes at the neuromuscular junction that slow synaptic transmissions needed for muscle contraction may also occur,[94,95] and this may explain the decreased ability to "coordinate motor unit firing" in the elderly. More research concerning the mechanisms of change that lead to decreased muscle strength as a result of aging is required.

Other changes in muscle that occur with aging and lead to a decrease in muscle strength include alteration in the balance between protein synthesis and protein degradation, as well as changes in the connective tissue in the muscle.[96,97] As indicated previously, protein synthesis plays an important role in muscle growth and maintenance of strength. Evaluating the changes that occur with aging, Markrides[96] reported that synthesis of protein is reduced and degradation of protein is increased, resulting in the loss of total muscle protein and a further decrease in the efficiency of muscle. Aging has also been reported to cause changes in connective tissue within the muscle belly, specifically, an increase in the concentration of endomysium and perimysium.[97] Alnaqeeb and associates[97] suggested that this increase in connective tissue in muscle is correlated to an increase in muscle stiffness experienced as aging progresses, which may have a deleterious effect on the muscle's ability to develop appropriate passive connective tissue tension and ultimately affect the total force output of muscle.

EFFECTS OF RESISTANCE TRAINING

The extent to which reduction in muscle mass with aging may be overcome by resistance training is somewhat uncertain. However, recent studies suggest that older individuals may retain the potential for significant increases in strength performance and hypertrophy in response to overload.

Investigating the effects of resistance training on cross-sectional area in the elderly, previous authors have reported inconsistent results. Moritani and deVries[98] reported no change in upper arm girth after 8 weeks of training in elderly men, but the weight-lifting capacity of the trained elbow flexors increased 23 percent. Similarly, Aniansson and Gustafsson[99] reported no change in cross-sectional area in the quadriceps muscle following 12 weeks of training in older adults, even though significant increases in torque of the knee extensors occurred. The authors of these two studies suggested that, although resistance training can result in increased strength in older persons, the muscle adaptation mode may differ from that observed in younger individuals. More specifically, the increased ability to recruit motor units was the primary mechanism for improved strength in the elderly; hypertrophy of muscle was not believed to contribute to enhanced strength.[98,99]

In contrast, more recent studies by Frontera and coworkers[51] and Brown and colleagues[100] indicate that older muscle responds to resistance training with increases not only in weight-lifting performance but also in muscle mass and muscle fiber size, specifically, increases in type II fiber area. Frontera and associates[51] reported increases of greater than 100 percent in the strength of the knee flexors and extensors, an 11.9 percent increase in muscle cross-sectional area, and a 27.6 percent increase in type II fiber area after 12 weeks of training in subjects ranging in age from 60 to 70 years. In addition, they reported that the muscle hypertrophy was accompanied by an increased rate of myofibrillar turnover, indicating the possibility of an increase in protein synthesis that had not been reported in previous literature. In comparison, Brown and coworkers[100] reported a smaller increase in weight-lifting performance (48 percent), a greater increase in muscle cross-sectional area (17.4 percent), and a similar increase in type II fiber area (30 percent) following 12 weeks of resistance training of the elbow flexors in 60- to 70-year-old volunteers. Both of these studies demonstrate the ability of older individuals to respond to progressive resistance training by increasing strength through hypertrophy of muscle. They do not support previous reports of strength gains occurring exclusively as a result of neural function.[51,100]

Despite the fact that muscle strength has been reported to progressively decrease after the age of 50,[83–85] and despite the fact that previous research indicates that muscles' ability to adapt to resistance training may change with age,[98,99] recent studies indicate that exercise training can reverse this trend of negative effects due to aging.[51,100] Observations from researchers reporting hypertrophy of muscle in the elderly comparable to responses seen in younger individuals "raise the encouraging prospect that the rate of decline in strength and muscle mass in old age and the accompanying loss of independent functional capacity can be reduced or even reversed by appropriate resistance training programs."[100]

MUSCLE ADAPTATION TO DECREASED USE: ATROPHY

Just as muscle adapts to increased use by changes in physical characteristics (hypertrophy) and neurologic function, muscle also adapts to decreased use, as has been observed by clinicians noting "disuse atrophy" following forced or voluntary reduction in muscle utilization. Clinical signs of atrophy include decreases in circumferential size, muscle strength, and endurance, with the decrease in strength and endurance becoming a primary concern during rehabilitation after injury or when resuming training.[101] Diminished muscular support may lead to increased stress on joint structures, abnormal movement patterns, and the increased risk of injury. Understanding the adaptations involved with decreased use can assist in the planning of effective rehabilitation programs.

Muscular atrophy is a decrease in the size of muscle tissue that may result from muscle pathologies,[102] malnutrition, denervation,[1,98] or disuse.[1,101,103] The emphasis of this section is on the changes that occur when muscle use is limited after trauma—by immobilization or bed rest—or following voluntary decrease in exercise intensity.

Changes that occur with atrophy are decreases in the gross circumferential size and volume of muscle as well as in the microscopic cross-sectional diameter of muscle fibers.[101,103,104] Sargeant and colleagues[104] reported a 12 percent decrease in leg volume measured anthropometrically after limb immobilization in healthy male subjects after fractures. This small change in volume was in contrast to a large decrease in cross-sectional diameter of fibers (42 percent) measured from the vastus lateralis muscle. The authors suggested that the different degree of change in limb volume and cross-sectional area in the same subjects could have been the result of extracellular fluid accumulation, connective tissue changes, or differing amounts of atrophy in the muscles constituting the upper thigh compartment, none of which could be assessed with anthropometric measurement of humans.[104]

HISTOLOGIC AND HISTOCHEMICAL CHANGES

Animal studies have been used extensively to differentiate the cellular changes that may occur during the decrease in muscle cross-sectional area as a result of muscle atrophy. The advantages of animal studies include the ease of weighing animal tissue as well as the relative ease with which microscopic muscle fiber diameter can be measured in animals as compared with humans.[103] Two of the most frequently used methods of inducing atrophy in animals are cast immobilization and suspension.

Using cast fixation, the muscle is maintained at a fixed length (an important determinant of the amount of atrophy that takes place), promoting a state of hypokinesia in which the muscle is limited from full excursion through range of motion. The suspension method (suspending animals in a horizontal position by a sling or by the tail, with the hind limbs in the air; Fig. 4–3) involves a state of hypodynamia that describes a reduction in mechanical loading and incorporates differences in circulatory response as well as altered biomechanical forces. The suspension method differs from cast immobilization in that the limbs are free to move, although muscles are obviously not required to produce the forces necessary for ambulation. In addition, the suspension method allows the muscles to maintain full range of motion, thereby avoiding the changes associated with limited length positioning found with the cast immobilization method.[101,103,105]

Changes in fiber size that occur with atrophy result from a decreased rate of protein synthesis[106–108] and an increased rate of protein catabolism or degradation,

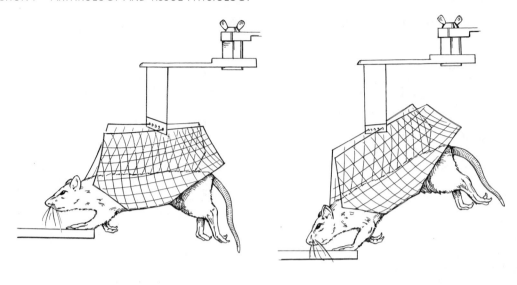

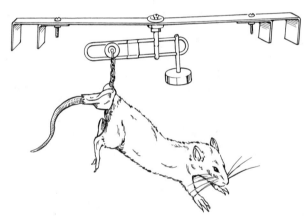

FIGURE 4–3. Suspension methods in which animal is suspended in horizontal position by sling or by the tail. (Adapted from Musacchia XJ: A model for hypokinesia: effects of muscle atrophy in the rat. J Appl Physiol 1980; 48:479–486; and from Jaspers SR, et al: Atrophy and growth failure of rat hindlimb muscle in tail-cast suspension. J Appl Physiol 1984; 57:1472–1479.)

with the latter being the major mechanism whereby protein content in muscle decreases in immobilized muscle.[109] Using casts to prevent the movement of rat hind limbs, Booth and Seider[110] reported a significant decline in the rate of protein synthesis starting as early as 6 hours after immobilization. These findings were later supported by Thomason and associates,[111] who determined that protein synthesis rates in the soleus muscle were decreased from 5.9 percent a day to 4.6 percent a day after 5 hours of hind limb suspension, decreasing to 2.4 percent by day 7.

Total protein content diminishes with a specific reduction in the myofibrillar protein, not only as a result of decreased protein synthesis but also as a result of protein degradation.[112] Templeton and colleagues[113] reported that activity of lysosomal protease, an important enzyme involved with the degradation of protein, is increased during the time of maximal loss of muscle weight. Furthermore, the authors reported that type I (slow-twitch) myosin was shown to be affected most; type II (fast-twitch) myosin levels remained relatively constant after suspension for 3 weeks.[113]

In addition to the decreased rate of protein synthesis and increased rate of protein degradation that occur with immobilization, research indicates that actual weight loss occurs in the muscle as early as 2 days after immobilization, with a steady decline until day 10 to 14, when the rate of atrophy decreases.[110,114] Maximal muscle atrophy has been reported to occur in 14 to 30 days in animal models.[104]

EFFECT OF IMMOBILIZATION ON FIBER TYPE

In contrast to the preferential type II (fast-twitch) atrophy that is associated with muscular diseases such as myopathies and muscular dystrophy,[102] disuse atrophy that occurs with hypodynamia or hypokinesia is more likely to demonstrate greater atrophy of type I slow-twitch fibers (although some atrophy of fast-twitch fibers does occur).[113,115–117] Templeton and associates[113] reported that following 4 weeks of suspension, the soleus muscle of rats consisted of 50 percent slow-twitch fibers, in contrast to control values of 70 to 90 percent slow-twitch fibers. Examining differences in atrophy in the quadriceps muscle in dogs, Lieber and colleagues[118] reported that the slow-twitch fibers of the vastus medialis muscle atrophied more than the slow-twitch fibers of the vastus lateralis and rectus femoris muscles, with the rectus femoris demonstrating the least atrophy. Since all muscles were immobilized in the same position, the differences could not be accounted for by length-associated preferential atrophy. One explanation proposed was that the vastus medialis muscle has an important postural function in stabilizing the patella during knee movement, which necessitates a higher percentage of slow-twitch fibers to sustain low-intensity prolonged contractions.[118] In addition, Herbison and coworkers[119] reported that the primarily slow-twitch soleus muscle was affected more than the primarily fast-twitch gastrocnemius and plantar muscles when exposed to immobilization, supporting the claim of Lieber and colleagues[118] that selective atrophy of slow-twitch muscle occurs following immobilization.

Results of these studies suggest that the extent of atrophy depends on the primary function of the muscle that is immobilized. It could be suggested that during normal everyday activity, slow-twitch fibers constantly fire to sustain postural control, and when this stimulus for contraction is removed by immobilization, these fibers undergo less than the normal daily contraction levels. Conversely, fast-twitch fibers are recruited for maximal contractions of short durations and are not recruited as often as slow-twitch fibers. Therefore, the muscles that are most susceptible to atrophy may be the more frequently used slow-twitch fibers, which play an important part in maintaining posture.

OTHER FACTORS AFFECTED BY IMMOBILIZATION

EFFECT ON NEURAL TISSUE

As previously described, utilization of motor units has been reported to improve with repetition and to account for changes in force output without hypertrophy.[62] Changes that have been documented to occur following limb immobilization include decreased motor unit activity (as measured by EMG)[120] and motor end-plate degeneration.[121] Sale and associates[122] recorded decreased EMG reflex potentiation after immobilization of human thenar muscles, which the authors interpreted as indicating impaired activation of motor units during maximum voluntary contractions. The impaired activation may then lead to decreased neural efficiency, which might contribute to observed loss of voluntary strength.[122] Although documentation exists that neural tissue is adversely affected by muscle atrophy, the cause and effect of these neural changes occurring with immobilization have yet to be established.[115]

EFFECT ON MUSCLE LENGTH

In addition to decreased cross-sectional diameter of individual muscle fibers, changes in the length of individual sarcomeres and muscle fibers occur if the muscle is immobilized in a fixed position other than the resting length. Tabary and associates[123] immobilized cats in full plantar flexion (shortened muscle) and full dorsiflexion (lengthened muscle) for 4 weeks. The researchers noted a decrease in the length of individual sarcomeres and a 19 percent increase in the number of sarcomeres in series when the muscle was immobilized in the fully lengthened position. When the muscle was immobilized in the fully shortened position, there was a 40 percent decrease in the number of sarcomeres in series, with little or no change in sarcomere length. In addition, the amount of atrophy was far greater when the muscle was immobilized in the shortened position than in the lengthened position. The authors concluded that adjustments in the number of sarcomeres functioned to place the muscle filaments in a position to maximize the sliding and cross-bridging potential.[123] Jaspers and colleagues[124] also investigated the effect of immobilization on muscle tissue in varying lengths, reporting similar results. They suggested that the change in sarcomere number was necessary to enable development of maximum tension when muscle excursion was limited.[124]

EFFECT OF PAIN

Pain, which inhibits motor activity, has been noted clinically to be associated with specific muscle atrophy. The concept of a facilitated segment has been theorized by Korr,[125,126] in which incoming noxious stimuli produce sustained guarding of postural muscles supplied by the same spinal reflex level. Korr[125,126] hypothesized that this protective mechanism is intended to prevent further damage to injured structures. If the painful stimulus continues over an extended period, constant contraction of the affected muscle could decrease circulation to the muscle, causing depletion of oxygen and nutrients. Inability to restore circulation to the area leads to a buildup of waste products and, over time, can become the stimulus for eventual protein depletion and, finally, muscle atrophy.[125,126] Further research in this area of chronic pain eventually leading to muscle atrophy is needed to confirm Korr's hypothesis.

RECOVERY OF FUNCTION

Once activity is resumed following atrophy, function at the cellular level returns to normal. Protein synthesis of previously immobilized muscle increases to normal levels during the first 6 hours of renewed activity, remains at normal levels for 2 days, and then exceeds (about doubling) control levels by the fourth recovery day in animal experiments.[106,127,128] Aerobic or anaerobic activity at the cellular level following resumed activity results in additional increases in enzyme activity.[106] In addition, adaptations in sarcomere number that occur with immobilization have been shown to be temporary, and the number and length of sarcomeres return to normal once activity is resumed, irrespective of whether the muscle was immobilized in a lengthened or shortened position.[123]

SUMMARY

Almost 15 years have passed since Rose and Rothstein[2] defined muscle as "the biological element therapists have worked with since the inception of the profession." This chapter has summarized the existing knowledge of muscle structure, function, and development and presented concepts involved in the adaptations of muscle that occur with increased (hypertrophy and neural adaptation) and decreased (atrophy) use. As more is learned about the anatomic and physical properties of muscles, including the dynamics of muscle hypertrophy and atrophy, better methods of treating patients with musculoskeletal pathology will follow.

REFERENCES

1. Lieber RL: Skeletal Muscle Structure and Function. Baltimore, Williams & Wilkins, 1992.
2. Rose SJ, Rothstein JM: Muscle mutability. Part 1. General concepts and adaptations to altered patterns of use. Phys Ther 1982; 62:1773–1787.
3. Huxley H: The structural basis of muscular contraction. Proc R Soc Med 1971; 178:131–149.
4. Stinger RJ, Spiro D: The ultrastructure of mammalian cardiac muscle. J Biophys Biochem Cytol 1961; 9:325–351.
5. Bois RM: The organization of the contractile apparatus of vertebrate smooth muscle. Anat Rec 1973; 177:61–72.
6. Lehmkuhl D: Local factors in muscle performance. Phys Ther 1966; 46:473–484.
7. Williams PL, Warwick R, Dyson M, et al (eds): Gray's Anatomy, 37th ed. London, Churchill Livingstone, 1989.
8. Vander AJ, Sherman JH, Luciano DS: Human Physiology: The Mechanism of Body Function. New York, McGraw-Hill, 1990.
9. Berne RM, Levy MN: Physiology. St. Louis, CV Mosby, 1988.
10. Ounjian M, Roy RR, Eldred E, et al: Physiological and developmental implications of motor unit anatomy. J Neurobiol 1991; 22:547–599.
11. Garrett WE, Mumma M, Lucavecke CL: Ultrastructural differences in human skeletal muscle fiber types. Orthop Clin North Am 1983; 14:413–425.
12. Pollack GH: The cross-bridge theory. Physiol Rev 1983; 63:1049–1113.
13. Buchthal F, Schmallruch H: Motor unit of mammalian muscle. Physiol Rev 1980; 60:90–142.
14. English A, Wolf SL: The motor unit: anatomy and physiology. Phys Ther 1982; 62:1763–1772.
15. Milner-Brown HS, Stein RB, Yemm R: The orderly recruitment of human motor units during voluntary isometric contractions. J Physiol 1973; 230:359–370.
16. Hoffer JA, O'Donovan MJ, Pratt CA, et al: Discharge patterns of hindlimb motoneurons during normal cat locomotion. Science 1981; 213:466–468.
17. Kukula CG, Clamann HP: Comparison of the recruitment and discharge properties of motor units in human brachial biceps and adductor pollices during isometric contractions. Brain Res 1981; 219:45–55.
18. Monster AW: Firing rate behavior of human motor units during isometric voluntary contractions; relations to unit size. Brain Res 1979; 171:349–354.
19. Hermansen L, Osnes JB: Human Muscle Fatigue: Physiological Mechanisms. London, Pitman Medical, 1981.
20. Peter JB, Barnard RJ, Edgerton VR, et al: Metabolic profiles of three fiber types of skeletal muscle. Biochemistry 1972; 11:2627–2633.
21. Burke RE, Levine DN, Tsairis P, et al: Physiological types and histochemical profiles in motor units of the cat gastrocnemius. J Physiol 1973; 234:723–748.
22. Brooke MH, Kaiser KK: Muscle fiber types: how many and what kind? Arch Neurol 1970; 23:369–379.
23. Henneman E, Somjen G, Carpenter DO: Functional significance of cell size in spinal motoneurons. J Neurophysiol 1965; 28:560–580.
24. Henneman E, Somjen G, Carpenter DO: Excitability and inhibitability of motoneurons of different sizes. J Neurophysiol 1965; 28:599–620.
25. Saltin B, Henriksson J, Nygaard E, et al: Fiber types and metabolic potentials of skeletal muscles in sedentary man and endurance runners. Ann N Y Acad Sci 1977; 301:3.
26. Elder GC, Bradbury K, Roberts R: Variability of fiber type distributions within human muscles. J Appl Physiol: Respir Environ Exerc Physiol 1982; 53:1473–1480.
27. Gollnick PD, Matoba H: The muscle fiber composition of skeletal muscle as a predictor of athletic success. Am J Sports Med 1984; 12:212–217.
28. Baldwin KM, et al: Biochemical properties of overloaded fast-twitch skeletal muscle. J Appl Physiol 1982; 52:457.
29. Gollnick PD, Saltin B: Significance of skeletal muscle oxidative enzyme enhancement with endurance training. Clin Physiol 1982; 2:1.
30. Jansson E, Sjodin B, Tesch P: Changes in muscle fiber type distribution in man after physical training. Acta Physiol Scand 1978; 104:235.
31. Jansson E, Kaijser L: Muscle adaptation to extreme endurance training in man. Acta Physiol Scand 1977; 100:315.
32. Dons B, Bollerup K, Bonde-Peterson F, et al: The effects of weight-lifting exercise related to muscle fiber composition and muscle cross-sectional area in humans. Eur J Appl Physiol 1979; 40:95–106.
33. Thorstensson A, Hultin B, von Dobeln W, et al: Effect of strength training on enzyme activities and fibre characteristics in human skeletal muscle. Acta Physiol Scand 1976; 96:392–398.
34. Costill DL, Coyle EF, Fink WF, et al: Adaptations in skeletal muscle following strength training. J Appl Physiol 1979; 46:96–99.
35. Karpati G: Muscle: structure, organization, and healing. In Cruess RL (ed): The Musculoskeletal System: Embryology, Biochemistry, and Physiology. New York, Churchill Livingstone, 1982, p 323.
36. Konigsberg IR: Clonal analysis of myogenesis. Science 1963; 140:1273–1284.
37. Konigsberg IR: The embryological origin of muscle. Sci Am 1964; 211:61–66.
38. Vogler C, Bove KE: Morphology of skeletal muscle in children. Arch Pathol Lab Med 1985; 109:238–242.
39. Williams PE, Goldspink G: Longitudinal growth of striated muscle. J Cell Sci 1981; 9:751–767.
40. Bell RD, et al: Muscle fiber types and morphometric analysis of skeletal muscle in six-year-old children. Med Sci Sports 1980; 12:28–33.
41. Haggmark T, Jansson E, Svane B: Cross-sectional area of the thigh muscle in man measured by computed tomography. Scand J Clin Lab Invest 1978;38:355–360.
42. Luithi JM, Howald H, Claasen H, et al: Structural changes in skeletal muscle tissue with heavy resistance exercise. Int J Sports Med 1986; 7:123–127.
43. MacDougall JD, Sale DG, Alway SE, et al: Muscle fiber number in biceps brachii in body builders and control subjects. J Appl Physiol 1984; 57:1399–1403.
44. MacDougall JD, Sale DG, Elder G, et al: Ultrastructural properties of human skeletal muscle following heavy resistance training and immobilization. Med Sci Sports 1976; 8:72–73.
45. Young A, Stokes M, Tound JM: The effect of high-resistance training on the strength and cross sectional area of the human quadriceps. Eur J Clin Invest 1983; 13:411–417.
46. Gollnick PD, Timson BF, Moore RL, et al: Muscular enlargement

and number of fibers in skeletal muscle of rats. J Appl Physiol 1981; 50:936–943.

47. Alway SE, MacDoughall ID, Sale DG, et al: Functional and structural adaptations in skeletal muscle of trained athletes. J Appl Physiol 1988; 64:1114–1120.

48. Yarasheski KE, Lemon PWR, Gilloteaux J: Effect of heavy resistance exercise training on muscle fiber composition in young rats. J Appl Physiol 1990; 69:434–437.

49. Ikai M, Fukunaga T: A study of training effect of strength per unit cross-sectional area of muscle by means of ultrasonic measurement. Int Z Angew Physiol 1970; 28:173–180.

50. Moritani T, deVries HA: Neural factors vs hypertrophy in time course of muscle strength gain. Am J Phys Med Rehabil 1979; 58:115–130.

51. Frontera WR, Meredith CN, O'Reilly KP, et al: Strength conditioning in older men: skeletal muscle hypertrophy and improved function. J Appl Physiol 1988; 64:1038–1044.

52. Goldberg AL, Etlinger JD, Goldspink DF, et al: Mechanism of work-induced hypertrophy of skeletal muscle. Med Sci Sports 1975; 7:185–198.

53. Ashnore CR, Summers PJ: Stretch-induced growth of chicken wing muscles: myofibrillar proliferation. Am J Physiol 1981; 240(Cell Physiol 10):93.

54. Gonyea WF, Erickson GC: Experimental model for study of exercise induced skeletal muscle hypertrophy. J Appl Physiol 1976; 40:630–633.

55. Gonyea WJ: Role of exercise in inducing increases in skeletal muscle fiber number. J Appl Physiol 1980; 48:421–426.

56. Ho KW: Skeletal muscle fiber splitting with weight-lifting exercises in rats. Am J Anat 1980; 157:433.

57. Edgerton BR: Morphology and histochemistry of the soleus muscle from normal and exercised rats. Am J Anat 1970; 127:81–86.

58. Sole O, Christensen DL, Marten AW: Hypertrophy and hyperplasia of adult chicken anterior latissimus dorsi muscle following stretch with and without denervation. Exp Neurol 1973; 41:76–100.

59. Gonyea WF, Sale DG, Gonyea FB, et al: Exercise induced increases in muscle fiber number. Eur J Appl Physiol 1983; 54:1292–1297.

60. Tesch PA: Skeletal muscle adaptations consequent to long-term heavy resistance exercises. Med Sci Sports Exerc 1988; 20:S132–S134.

61. McArdle WD, Katch FI, Katch VL: Exercise Physiology: Energy, Nutrition, and Human Performance, 2nd ed. Philadelphia, Lea & Febiger, 1986, p 388.

62. Sale DG: Neural adaptation to resistance training. Med Sci Sports Exerc 1988; 20(suppl):S135–S145.

63. Hakkinen K, Alén M, Komi PV: Changes in isometric force- and relaxation-time, electromyographic and muscle fiber characteristics of human skeletal muscle during strength training and detraining. Acta Physiol Scand 1985; 125:573–585.

64. Hakkinen K, Komi PV: Electromyographic changes during strength training and detraining. Med Sci Sports Exerc 1983; 15:455–460.

65. Hakkinen K, Komi PV, Alén M: Effect of explosive type strength training on isometric force- and relaxation-time, electromyographic, and muscle fibre characteristics of leg extensor muscles. Acta Physiol Scand 1985; 125:587–600.

66. McGovern MB: Effects of circuit weight training on the physical fitness of prepubescent children. Diss Abstr Int 1984; 45:452-A.

67. Weltman A, Janney C, Rians B, et al: The effects of hydraulic resistance strength training in pre-pubertal males. Med Sci Sports Exerc 1986; 18:629–638.

68. Ramsay JA, Blimkie CJR, Smith K, et al: Strength training effects in prepubescent boys. Med Sci Sports Exerc 1990; 22:605–614.

69. Wilmore J: Body composition and strength development. J Phys Educ Rec 1975; 46:38–40.

70. Laubach L: Comparative muscular strength of men and women: a review of the literature. Aviat Space Environ Med 1976; 47:534–542.

71. Sale DG, MacDougall JD, Alway SE, et al: Voluntary strength and muscle characteristics in untrained men and women and male bodybuilders. J Appl Physiol 1987; 62:1786–1793.

72. Schantz P, Randall-Fox E, Norgren P, et al: The relationship between mean muscle fiber area and the muscle cross-sectional

area of the thigh in subjects with large differences in thigh girth. Acta Physiol Scand 1981; 113:537–539.

73. Schantz P, Randall-Fox E, Hutchison W, et al: Muscle fibre type distribution, muscle cross-sectional area and maximal voluntary strength in humans. Acta Physiol Scand 1983; 117:219–226.

74. Cureton KJ, Collins MA, Hill DW, et al: Muscle hypertrophy in men and women. Med Sci Sports Exerc 1988; 20:338–344.

75. Ikai M, Fukunaga T: Calculation of muscle strength per unit cross-sectional area of human muscle by means of ultrasonic measurements. Int Z Angew Physiol 1968; 26:26–32.

76. Brown C, Wilmore JH: The effects of maximal resistance training on the strength and body composition of women athletes. Med Sci Sports 1974; 6:174–177.

77. Wilmore JH: Alterations in strength, body composition and anthropometric measurements consequent of a 10-week weight training program. Med Sci Sports 1974; 6:133–138.

78. Hetrick GA, Wilmore JH: Androgen levels and muscle hypertrophy during an eight week weight training program for men/ women. Med Sci Sports 1979; 11:102.

79. Mayhew J, Gross P: Body composition changes in young women with high resistance weight training. Res Q 1974;45:433–440.

80. Fahey TD, Rolph R, Mongmee R, et al: Serum testosterone, body composition, and strength of young adults. Med Sci Sports 1976; 8:31–34.

81. Westerlind KC, Byrnes WC, Freedson PS, et al: Exercise and serum androgens in women. Phys Sports Med 1987; 15:87–94.

82. Fox E, Bartels R, Billings C, et al: Frequency and duration of interval training programs and changes in aerobic power. J Appl Physiol 1975; 38:481–484.

83. Bemben MG, Massey BH, Bemben DA, et al: Isometric muscle force production as a function of age in healthy 20- to 74-yr-old men. Med Sci Sports Exerc 1991; 23:1302–1310.

84. Kroll W, Clarkson PM: Aged isometric knee extension strength, and fractionated resisted response time. Exp Aging Res 1978; 4:389–409.

85. Larsson L, Viitasalo JH, Komi PV: Changes in reflex time and EMG signal characteristics in aging quadriceps muscle. Acta Physiol Scand 1978; 457(suppl):1–17.

86. Haskell WL: Physical activity and health: need to define the required stimulus. Am J Cardiol 1985; 55:4D–9D.

87. Aniansson A, Hedberg M, Henning GB, et al: Muscle morphology enzymatic activity, and muscle strength in elderly men: a follow-up study. Muscle Nerve 1986; 9:585–591.

88. Grimby G, Sanneskiold-Samsoe B, Hvid K, et al: Morphology and enzymatic capacity in arm and leg muscles in 78–81 year old men and women. Acta Physiol Scand 1982; 179:513–523.

89. Grimby G, Saltin B. The ageing muscle. Clin Physiol 1983;3:209–218.

90. Lexall J, Henriksson-Larsson K, Wimblad B, et al: Distribution of different fiber types in human skeletal muscle. 3. Effects of aging in m. vastus lateralis studies in whole muscle cross-sections. Muscle Nerve 1983; 6:588–595.

91. Campbell MJ, McComas AJ, Petito F: Physiological changes in aging muscles. J Neurol Neurosurg Psychiatry 1973; 36:174–182.

92. Carlsson KE, Alston W, Feldman DJ: Electromyographic study of aging in skeletal muscle. Am J Phys Med 1964; 43:141–145.

93. Sjostrom M, Neglen P, Friden J, et al: Human skeletal muscle metabolism and morphology after temporary incomplete ischaemia. Eur J Clin Invest 1982; 12:69–79.

94. Frolkis VV, Martynenko OA, Zamostyan VP: Ageing of the neuromuscular apparatus. Gerontology 1976; 22:244–279.

95. Gutmann E, Hanzlikova V: Basic mechanisms of aging in the neuromuscular system. Mech Ageing Dev 1972; 1:327–349.

96. Markrides SC: Protein synthesis and degradation during ageing and senescence. Biol Rev 1983; 58:343–422.

97. Alnaqeeb MA, Alzaid NS, Goldspink G: Connective tissue changes and physical properties of developing and aging skeletal muscle. J Anat 1984; 139:677–689.

98. Moritani T, deVries HA: Potential for gross muscle hypertrophy in older men. J Gerontol 1980; 35:672–682.

99. Aniansson A, Gustafsson E: Physical training in elderly men with special reference to quadriceps muscle strength and morphology. Clin Physiol 1981; 1:87–98.

100. Brown AB, McCartney N, Sale DG: Positive adaptations to weight-lifting training in the elderly. J Appl Physiol 1990; 69:1725–1733.

101. Booth FW, Gollnick PD: Effects of disuse on the structure and function of skeletal muscle. Med Sci Sports Exerc 1983; 15: 415–420.

102. Wheeler SD: Pathology of muscle and motor units. Phys Ther 1982; 62:1809–1822.

103. Musacchia XJ, Steffen JM, Fell RD: Disuse atrophy of skeletal muscle: animal models. Exerc Sport Sci Rev 1988; 16:61–87.

104. Sargeant AJ, Davies CTM, Edwards RHT, et al: Functional and structural changes after disuse of human muscle. Clin Sci Mol Med 1977; 52:337–342.

105. LeBlanc A, Marsh C, Evans H, et al: Bone and muscle atrophy with suspension of the rat. J Appl Physiol 1985; 58:1669–1675.

106. Tucker KR, Seider MJ, Booth FW: Protein synthesis rates in atrophied gastrocnemius muscles after limb immobilization. J Appl Physiol: Respir Environ Exerc Physiol 1981; 51:73–77.

107. Goldspink DF, Garlick PJ, McNurlan MA: Protein turnover measured in vivo and in vitro in muscles undergoing compensatory growth and subsequent denervation atrophy. Biochem J 1983; 210:89–98.

108. Watson PA, Stein JP, Booth FW: Changes in actin synthesis and A-Actin-mRNA content in rat muscle during immobilization. Am J Appl Physiol 1984; 247(Cell Physiol 16):C39–C44.

109. Goldspink DF: The influence of immobilization and stretch on protein turnover of rat skeletal muscle. J Physiol 1977; 264: 267–282.

110. Booth FW, Seider MJ: Early change in skeletal muscle protein synthesis after limb immobilization of rats. J Appl Physiol: Respir Environ Exerc Physiol 1979; 47:974–977.

111. Thomason DB, Biggs RB, Booth FW: Protein metabolism and B-myosin heavy-chain mRNA in unweighted soleus muscle. Am J Physiol 1989; 257(Regulatory Integrative Comp Physiol 26): R300–R305.

112. Witzmann FA, Kim DH, Fitts RH: Effect of hindlimb immobilization on the fatigability of skeletal muscle. J Appl Physiol: Respir Environ Exerc Physiol 1983; 54:1242–1248.

113. Templeton GH, Padalino M, Manton J, et al: Influence of suspension hypokinesia on rat soleus muscle. J Appl Physiol: Respir Environ Exerc Physiol 1984; 56:278–286.

114. Booth FW: Time course of muscular atrophy during immobilization of hindlimbs in rats. J Appl Physiol: Respir Environ Exerc Physiol 1977; 43:656–661.

115. Thomason DB, Booth FW: Atrophy of the soleus muscle by hindlimb unweighting. J Appl Physiol 1990; 68:1–12.

116. Fitts RH, Metzger JM, Riley DA, et al: Models of disuse: a comparison of hindlimb suspension and immobilization. J Appl Physiol 1986; 60:1946–1953.

117. Witzmann FA, Kim DH, Fitts RH: Hindlimb immobilization: length-tension and contractile properties of skeletal muscle. J Appl Physiol: Respir Environ Exerc Physiol 1982; 53:335–345.

118. Lieber RL, Friden JO, Hargens AR, et al: Differential response of the dog quadriceps muscle to external skeletal fixation of the knee. Muscle Nerve 1988; 11:193–201.

119. Herbison GJ, Jaweed MM, Ditunno JF: Muscle atrophy in rats following denervation, casting inflammation, and tenotomy. Arch Phys Med Rehabil 1979; 60:401–404.

120. Fuglsang-Fredrickson A, Scheel U: Transient decrease in number of motor units after immobilization in man. J Neurol Neurosurg Psychiatry 1978; 41:924–929.

121. Pachter BR, Eberstein A: Neuromuscular plasticity following limb immobilization. J Neurocytol 1984; 13:1013–1025.

122. Sale DG, McComas AJ, MacDougall JD, et al: Neuromuscular adaptation in human thenar muscles following strength training and immobilization. J Appl Physiol: Respir Environ Exerc Physiol 1982; 53:419–424.

123. Tabary JC, Tabary C, Tardieu C, et al: Physiological and structural changes in the cat's soleus muscle due to immobilization at different lengths by plaster casts. J Physiol 1972; 224:231–244.

124. Jaspers SR, Fagan JM, Tischler ME: Biochemical response to chronic shortening in unloaded soleus muscles. J Appl Physiol 1985; 59:1159–1163.

125. Korr I: The facilitated segment. Proc IFOMT 1977:81–92.

126. Korr I (ed): The Neurobiological Mechanisms in Manipulative Therapy. New York, Plenum Press, 1978.

127. Booth FW, Thomason DB: Molecular and cellular adaptation of muscle in response to exercise: perspectives of various models. Physiol Rev 1991; 71:541–585.

128. Morrison PR, Muller GW, Booth FW: Actin synthesis rate and mRNA level increase during early recovery of atrophied muscle. Am J Physiol 1987; 253:C205–C209.

CHAPTER 5

Muscle: Deformation, Injury, Repair

T E R R Y   R .   M A L O N E   *EdD, PT, ATC*
W I L L I A M   E .   G A R R E T T ,   J R .   *MD, PhD*
J A M E S   E .   Z A C H A Z E W S K I   *MS, PT, ATC, SCS*

Athletics requires varying degrees of neuromuscular coordination, cardiovascular and muscular endurance, speed, strength, and flexibility. Acute traumatic injuries to the musculotendinous unit are all too common in athletes, accounting for up to 50 percent of all injuries.[1–8] One of the most common injuries is muscle strain. Overall, the following quote from the U.S. Department of Health and Human Services Evaluation of the Musculoskeletal Disease Program in 1984 summarizes this problem well: "Little is known of the factors that predispose muscle to strain or the mechanisms of production of symptoms. . . . Scientific knowledge in this area is scanty and new investigative methods must be developed to elucidate the functional, physiological and biochemical events associated with muscle strain and soreness."

Although it is evident from the wealth of literature published on this subject that new scientific knowledge has been gained since that time, many areas remain to be explored, and questions need to be answered by basic science and applied clinical research. The majority of basic science studies that have explored muscle strain injury associated with athletics have used passive stretch or lengthening of an electrically stimulated and contracting muscle to induce these injuries. Clinically, muscle strain injuries are most often associated with muscle stretching with a simultaneous forceful eccentric muscle action. Injury and damage predominantly in the region of the musculotendinous junction are the result.

The purpose of this chapter is to describe the anatomy and normal physiology associated with muscle deformation, the pathophysiology associated with muscle strain injury, the repair process, and the associated clinical considerations.

ANATOMY

Muscle is a unique structure with contractile proteins (actin and myosin) and noncontractile viscoelastic collagenous elements. Muscle must be able to not only shorten and lengthen but also recover or return from shortened and lengthened positions. Muscle must be able to be lengthened to allow a single joint or a series of joints to move through their full available range of motion. This characteristic of muscle is often termed flexibility and is specific to the individual, the activity in which he or she is involved, and the joint or joints involved in that particular activity.[9,10] The inability of muscle to be deformed and lengthen readily may be described as stiffness, or resistance to elongation.

Historically, Stolov and Weilepp[11] identified the following anatomic elements as possible contributors to muscle stiffness: adhesion of one fibril to another, adhesion between muscle and overlying subcutaneous tissue, the epimysium, the perimysium and endomysium, and contractile elements within the muscle fiber. More recently, Garrett and various colleagues[12–16] have also identified the myotendinous junction as an anatomic area that is intimately involved with muscle deformation and pathophysiologic change due to injury.

MUSCLE FIBERS

Anatomically, muscle is a complex arrangement of contractile and noncontractile protein filaments. Muscles' ability to deform and recover from deformation is dependent on this complex arrangement.[17,18] The limitation of muscles' ability to stretch is predominantly dependent on its noncontractile components. These noncontractile protein elements are integrated into a viscoelastic network of connective tissue. These collagenous elements, which make up the series and parallel elastic components of muscle, provide functional stiffness to enhance the transmission of tension. (A description of the anatomic composition and makeup of the contractile elements may be found in Chapter 4.)

A large quantity of connective tissue is associated with muscle (Fig. 5–1). The majority of this connective tissue is composed of type I collagen. Types III and IV collagen make up the rest of the connective tissue element. The arrangement of the connective tissue allows muscle to be divided into three different layers — the endomysium, perimysium, and epimysium.

The endomysium is a delicate connective tissue sheath that invests and separates each individual muscle fiber. The endomysium provides for myocyte-to-myocyte connectives, myocyte-to-capillary connectives, and a collagenous weave associated with the basal laminae of the myocytes.[17] External to the basal lamina and the sarcolemma, the endomysium is composed primarily of two different-sized collagenous filaments. Neither of these filaments penetrate the basal lamina of the sarcolemma (Fig. 5–2A and B).[19] Collagen fibers of the thicker filament (50 μm in diameter) are arranged in a predominantly longitudinal direction. This orientation may reflect the endomysium's role in providing mechanical support for the fibers' surface and acting as an elastic device for contraction-relaxation cycles. The thinner filaments represent immature forms of collagen and intermingle with the thicker filaments. Figure 5–2C and D depict the collagenous fibrils that make up the endomysium. Although oriented predominantly parallel to the muscle fiber, these collagen fibrils also run in a variety of directions, over and between the different muscle fibers. The course and distance between the fibrils vary, depending on the degree of stretch or contraction of the muscle. When the muscle is contracted, the fibrils are close together and at right angles to one another, and when the muscle is stretched, they are parallel to the fibers. This arrangement of the connective tissue permits easy displacement of the muscle fibrils and offers increasing resistance to deformation at extreme lengthened ranges.[19,20] Arranged as a weave network

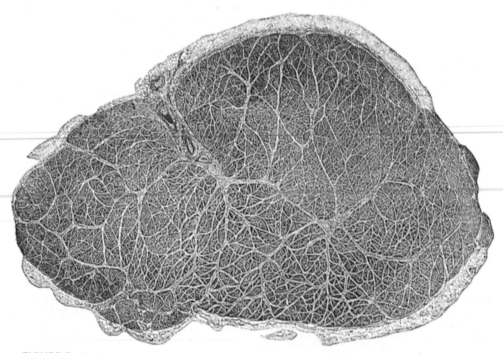

FIGURE 5–1. Connective tissue of muscle. Cross section through human sartorius muscle showing the connective tissue of the epimysium surrounding the entire muscle and the perimysium enclosing muscle fiber bundles of various sizes. (From Fawcett DW: Bloom and Fawcett: Textbook of Histology. New York, Chapman & Hall, 1986.)

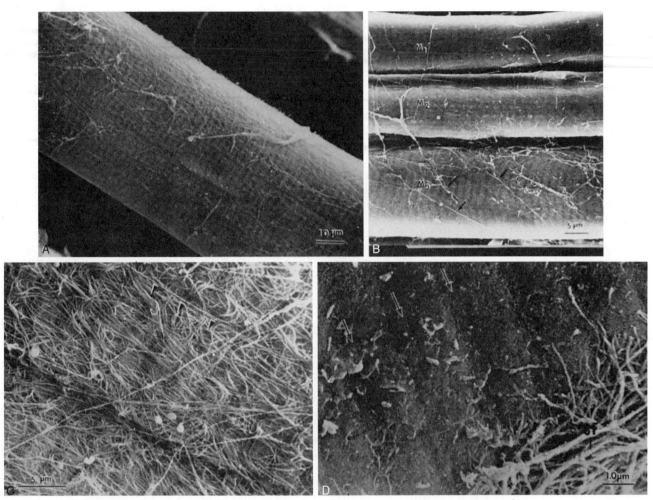

FIGURE 5–2. *A,* Fibrous endomysium. Frog sartorius muscle fiber. Fiber surface is covered by a fibrous layer, through which cross striations are visible. *B,* Teased preparation. Frog sartorius muscle (fixed with tannic acid–OsO$_4$). Skeletal muscle fibers (M1, M2, M3) appear as cylindrical units aligned in parallel bundles. Faint cross striations are visible along individual fibers. Coarse collagenous fibers of the endomysium run in various directions over and between muscle fibers *(arrows). C,* Fibrous connective tissue of muscle. Fibrous layer on surface of frog sartorius muscle fiber. Collagenous fibrils cover muscle fiber and take a predominantly longitudinal course. Cross striations can be seen through fibrous layer *(arrowheads). D,* Outer aspect of basal lamina of frog sartorius muscle fiber by use of low-power SEM. Basal lamina is exposed where fibrous layer (CF) is stripped off. Cross striations *(arrows)* can be seen more clearly through the lamina than through the fibrous layer. (From Ishikawa H, Sawada H, Yamada E: Surface and internal morphology of skeletal muscle. *In* Peachey LD, Adrian RH, Geiger SR (eds): Skeletal Muscle, Baltimore, American Physiological Society, 1983, pp 1–22.)

intimately associated with the basal lamina, the endomysium is an important factor in the passive series elastic component of muscle.

Each group of 10 to 20 muscle fibrils, which collectively form a fascicle, is surrounded by a thicker coating of connective tissue, the perimysium. The perimysium may be oriented in either a parallel or a circumferential direction to the fascicle. The perimysium is composed of varying amounts of collagenous, elastic, and reticular fibers and fat cells.[20] The collagen of the perimysium consists of tightly woven bundles of fibers, 600 to 1800 μm in diameter, that interconnect with the fascicles. During passive stretch, the amount and arrangement of the connective tissue in the perimysium may be more important than those in the endomysium. Nagel, as summarized by Borg

and Caulfield,[17] found that the perimysium, which is arranged in a spiral fashion during relaxation of the muscle, is wavy during muscle contraction, indicating little tension. This report allowed Borg and Caulfield to conclude that the perimysium could be a major component of the parallel elastic component of muscle, demonstrating importance in maintaining the proper position of the muscle bundles and distributing the stress associated with passive stretch. The fascicles of individual muscle are then grouped together and surrounded by the epimysium.

The percentage of elastin and collagen in the connective tissue associated with muscle varies with the function of the muscle. In the extremities, the elastic fibrils are more exclusively limited to the septa between fasciculi in the perimysium.

CONTRACTILE ELEMENTS AND MUSCLE STIFFNESS

Muscle fibers can exist in three states: relaxed, activated, and rigor.[21] Each of these states is characterized by tension (of the contractile elements) and stiffness (the change in force or tension produced by change in length). In a relaxed state, muscle does not generate active force and therefore does not possess a high degree of stiffness in the range of muscle length where most physiologic actions occur. With enough stretch, even relaxed muscle is stiffer than activated muscle. However, in the physiologic range, where the passive tension is not high, activation can significantly increase stiffness.

Opinion varies as to the exact contribution of each of these elements to passive tension. A large portion of the passive resting tension of a muscle may be due to the connective tissue that lies parallel to the muscle fibers, although some tension may be attributable to a small proportion of cross-bridges between actin and myosin filaments. These cross-bridges have been demonstrated to resist deformation in skinned muscle fiber (muscle fibers in which all connective tissue has been removed). The amount of stiffness or resistance to deformation provided by the cross-bridges increases as the velocity of the deforming force increases.[22,23] According to Hill,[24] these cross-bridges are very stable and may have a "long life."

The exact contribution of each of the anatomic elements to muscle stiffness, or the resistance to deformation, is unknown. The contribution of the contractile elements appears to be related to the velocity of deformation. As muscle is deformed or stretched, the contribution to stiffness from the noncontractile elements increases.

MYOTENDINOUS JUNCTION

A working knowledge of the anatomy of the myotendinous junction is important, as clinical and laboratory investigations of the morphology of muscle injury due to deformation or strain indicate that injury occurs at the myotendinous junction. This information has been well summarized by Garrett and Lohnes[25] and Garrett and Tidball.[26]

The musculotendinous junction occurs at the end of each long cylindrical muscle fiber. The location of this junction, where myofibrils attach to the cell membrane, supports its proposed function as the site of force transmission between the contractile elements and noncontractile collagenous tissue (although no direct physiologic evidence is available to demonstrate this). Each muscle cell originates and terminates with direct connections to the myotendinous junction on which it acts (Fig. 5–3A and B).

The cell membrane at the myotendinous junction is a continuous interface between the intracellular and extracellular compartments, possessing extensive folding so that the cell and extracellular connective tissue appear to interdigitate (Fig. 5–3C). The external surface of the myotendinous junction is covered by a basement membrane, which is continuous and morphologically identical to basement membrane elsewhere on the cell. The external region of the basement membrane, the reticular lamina, provides structural connections to tendon collagen fibers (Fig. 5–3D). For successful transmission of force across the muscle cell–tendon interface, the cell and tendon must form an adhesive junction at these sites. The load placed on the interface must not exceed the strength of the interface under these loading conditions, and the mechanical properties of the elastic and viscous elements must permit some mechanical energy to be transmitted at the junction. The role of the myotendinous junction as a force-transmitting structure therefore appears to be supported by its morphologic features.

The extensive folding at the myotendinous junction is an important structural correlate to the magnitude of the stress placed on the junction. This folding increases the membrane surface contact area, thereby reducing stress on the membrane when the junction is stressed by either contraction or deformation. Since muscle and the myotendinous junction are viscoelastic structures, their behavior under loading varies with the magnitude, frequency, duration, and rate of loading. Because of the effects of these forces on viscoelastic structures, junction failure may occur at different stresses during long-term loading and during rapidly applied, short-duration loading.

Folding at the myotendinous junction places the membrane at low angles relative to the force vectors generated by muscle contraction or deformation. If the membrane were not folded, load would occur in a tensile manner at right angles. Because of the angle of the folds, shear forces occur at the membrane. These folds and shear forces allow the myotendinous junction to behave like an adhesive joint. The strength of an adhesive joint varies with the angle of the interface. The closer the angle of the interface to zero, which is the case at the myotendinous junction, the stronger the junction. Tidball[27] noted that disuse atrophy of muscle results in an increase in the angle at the interface and failure at the myotendinous junction (Fig. 5–4). This increase in angulation may result in a decrease in strength or changes in the adhering surface at the myotendinous junction, but further research is needed to demonstrate any causal relationship.

Sarcomeres near the myotendinous junction tend to be shorter than other sarcomeres within skeletal muscle. Although these sarcomeres are not anatomically different, they must function in a different "environment." When functioning in this environment—the myotendinous junction—their biomechanical properties may be different from those of sarcomeres that are not adjacent to the myotendinous junction. Shorter sarcomeres at the myotendinous junction have a decreased force-generating capacity, an increased rate of contraction, and a decreased ability to change length (deform) compared with other sarcomeres within the same muscle fiber. It has also recently been demonstrated that fibers nearest the distal myotendinous junction may undergo the greatest strain during elongation.[28] These

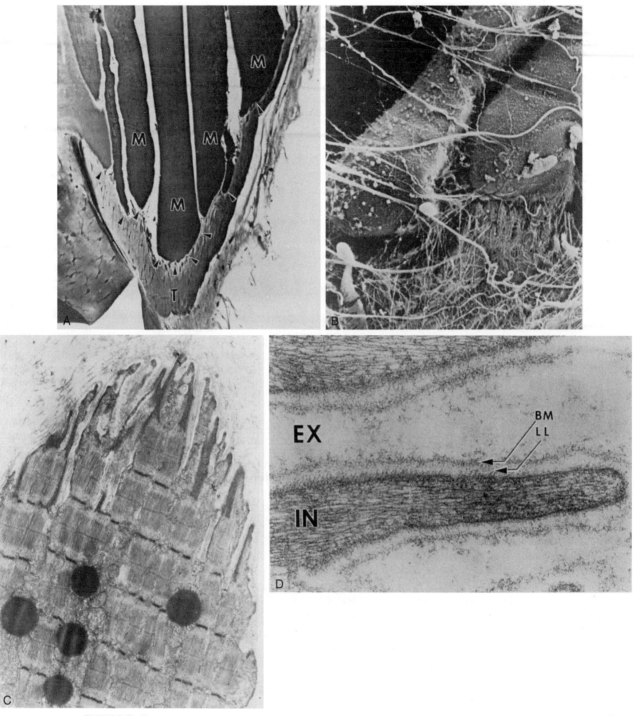

FIGURE 5–3. *A*, Light micrograph of longitudinal section through several frog semitendinosus muscle cells (M) attached to their tendon of insertion (T) at myotendinous junctions *(arrowheads)* (× 250). *B*, Two frog semitendinosus muscle cells terminating on tendon. Both bundles of collagen fibers pass from tendon to ends of the cylindrical cells (SEM, × 600). *C*, Longitudinal section through myotendinous junction of frog semitendinosus muscle cell. Note that the cell and surrounding connective tissue appear to interdigitate at the end of the cell. Also, note that the dense, fibrillar material extends from the terminal Z disc to the junctional plasma membrane (TEM, × 12,500). *D*, Single, digit-like process of skeletal muscle at myotendinous junction in longitudinal section. Note that thin filaments run along the length of the process (IN). External to the process (EX) the basement membrane (BM) is separated from the junctional membrane by the basal lucida (LL) (TEM, × 60,000). (*A* from Garrett WE, Tidball J: Myotendinous junction: Structure, function and failure. *In* Woo SL-Y, Buckwalter JA (eds): Injury and Repair of the Musculoskeletal Soft Tissues. Park Ridge, IL, American Academy of Orthopaedic Surgeons, 1988, pp 171–207. *B–D* from Tidball JG: Myotendinous junction: Morphological changes and mechanical failure associated with muscle cell atrophy. Exp Mol Pathol 1984; 40:1–12.)

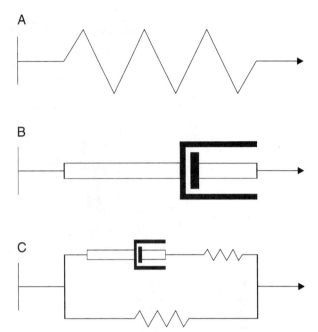

FIGURE 5–4. Diagram of a myotendinous junction. Muscle force is applied parallel to the longitudinal axis of the myofilaments and the collagen fibers. The junctional membrane lies at an angle relative to the myofilaments. (From Tidball JG: The geometry of actin filaments–membrane associations can modify the adhesive strength of the myotendinous junction. Cell Motil 1983; 3:439–447. © 1983 John Wiley & Sons, Inc. Reprinted by permission.)

physiologic correlates suggest that the myotendinous junction is first preloaded by forces generated by the terminal sarcomeres and then subjected to further increases in tension as other sarcomeres reach peak tension.[26]

ABILITY TO DEFORM AND RECOVER

TISSUE PROPERTIES

Like any collagenous tissue, the musculotendinous unit exhibits both physical and mechanical properties when undergoing deformation. These properties give the tissue high tensile stress, allowing it to respond to load and deformation appropriately.

Mechanically, the muscle-tendon unit functions as a composite viscoelastic structure.[10,29,30] The viscoelastic behavior of muscle is more complex because of the contractile components found within muscle; however, several of the noncontractile collagenous components exhibit typical viscoelastic properties. The elastic property implies that deformation of a change in length is directly proportional to the load or the force applied. When that load is removed, the change in length is completely recovered (Fig. 5–5A). Viscous properties are characterized by time and rate change dependency. The rate of deformation is directly proportional to the applied force when considering the viscous property of connective tissue (Fig. 5–5B). The muscle-tendon unit combines both of these patterns, functioning as a viscoelastic structure (Fig. 5–5C).[31–33] Viscoelastic behaviors explain many of the observed characteristics of the muscle-tendon unit.[29,30]

Intimately related to the viscoelastic properties of collagenous tissues are the physical properties of stress-relaxation, creep, and hysteresis. Stress-relaxation is exhibited by a tissue if a decrease in force is required to maintain the tissue, which has been stretched or deformed, at a constant length over time; creep is characterized by a continuance in deformation in response to a maintained load.[30,31,33] The hysteresis response is the amount of relaxation, or variation in the load-deformation relationship, that takes place within a single cycle of loading and unloading. During hysteresis, a greater amount of energy is absorbed by the tissue during loading than is dissipated during unloading, resulting in an increase in tissue temperature. Viscoelastic materials and tissues also exhibit strain rate dependence, exhibiting higher tensile stress at faster strain rates (Fig. 5–6).[30,34,35]

FIGURE 5–5. A, The hookean body. The perfect spring provides a model for elastic behavior. Deformation is proportional to force. B, The newtonian body. A model for viscous behavior is provided by a dashpot or hydraulic cylinder containing viscous fluid. Velocity of dashpot displacement is directly proportional to force. C, The viscoelastic model. A spring and dashpot are combined in parallel or series to exhibit viscoelastic behavior.

The effect of each of these properties on muscle has been illustrated by Taylor and colleagues[30] using an animal model. Controlled stretching of the muscle-tendon units of the long extensor muscle of the toes and the anterior tibial muscle was used in the rabbit model. Figure 5–7A presents the data from ten controlled stretches of the long extensor muscle. Each stretch was to 10 percent beyond resting length. The generated maximal tension (resistance to deformation) was recorded and is presented as a percentage of the initial stretch. The first four curves or stretches show significant difference, but no significant changes are seen beyond the fourth measure. Figure 5–7B presents the stress-relaxation sequence and shows significant changes only through the initial stretches. Figure 5–7C demonstrates that 80 percent of the total change in

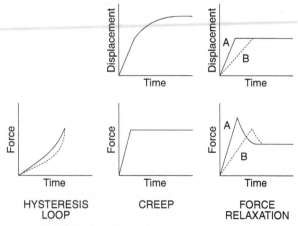

FIGURE 5–6. Physical properties of collagen.

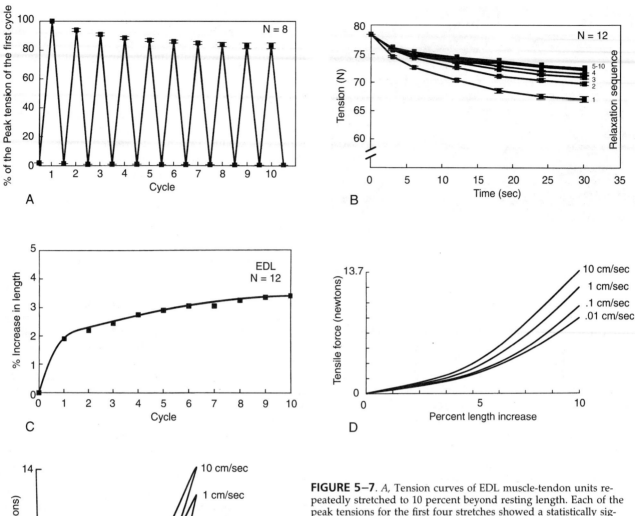

FIGURE 5–7. *A,* Tension curves of EDL muscle-tendon units repeatedly stretched to 10 percent beyond resting length. Each of the peak tensions for the first four stretches showed a statistically significant (p < .05) difference from the other peak tensions. The overall tension decrease was 16.6 percent. *B,* Relaxation curves for EDL muscle-tendon units stretched repeatedly to 78.4 N. The relaxation curves of the first two stretches demonstrated statistically significant differences from the other curves. There were no significant differences in curves 4–10. *C,* Graphic representation of EDL lengthening with repeated stretching to the same tension. Eighty percent of the length increase occurred during the first four stretches. *D,* Representative force-length relationships demonstrating the effect of stretch rate on a single TA muscle-tendon unit. *E,* Hysteresis loops observed in TA muscle during loading and unloading at constant rates of 0.01, 0.1, 1, and 10 cm/sec. (From Taylor DC, Dalton JD, Seaber AV, et al: Viscoelastic properties of muscle-tendon units: The biomechanical effects of stretching. Am J Sports Med 1990; 18:300–309.)

length is accomplished in the first four stretches of the long extensor muscle-tendon unit when ten repeated stretches were applied at the same level of tension; Figure 5–7D shows the hysteresis loops generated via loading-unloading at specific speeds. During each stretch, different amounts of energy are absorbed (during loading) and dissipated (during unloading), with the difference resulting in ultrastructural change or heat transfer. This process may also play a role in tissue temperature response to exercise.[36] Finally, a muscle strain rate dependency and a viscoelastic response with greater force (stiffer response) at higher velocity are demonstrated in Figure 5–7E. Throughout the data presented by Taylor and associates,[30] it is

apparent that the initial cycles of cyclic stretching and deformation are the most critical for causing change.

TYPES OF MUSCLE FLEXIBILITY

Static and dynamic flexibility is required in athletics and characterizes a healthy athlete. Although we believe that good flexibility is vital to athletic performance, the attributes of good flexibility have been difficult to demonstrate in clinical studies if these studies are subjected to rigid research criteria.

According to the literature, there are a number of benefits to good flexibility. Multiple reports in the

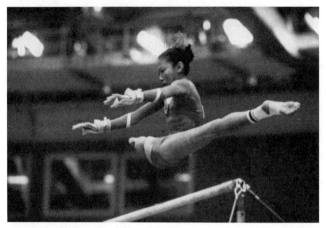

FIGURE 5–8. Demonstration of dynamic flexibility. (Courtesy of Tony Duffy/*Sports Illustrated*.)

literature have stated that having good flexibility assists in preventing or decreasing the incidence of injury.[37–43] This may happen because of the tissue's improved ability to accommodate the stress placed on it. However, a true cause-effect relationship between flexibility and the incidence of injury is difficult to establish if rigorous research criteria are applied.[44] The results of studies attempting to demonstrate that good flexibility influences movement efficiency and enhances athletic performance are conflicting or inconclusive.[45–49] More sensitive methods of assessing movement efficiency and change in athletic performance may be required to prove this commonly held hypothesis. Good flexibility and stretching after strenuous exercise have also been stated to decrease delayed-onset muscle soreness (DOMS).[9,50]

deVries has defined static flexibility as the measured range of motion available in a joint or a series of joints and dynamic flexibility as a measure of the resistance to active motion about a joint or a series of joints.[9] Resistance to tissue deformation (stiffness) decreases as dynamic flexibility increases. As a rule, good static flexibility is a prerequisite for good dynamic flexibility. Good static flexibility, however, does not ensure good dynamic flexibility. Dynamic flexibility may be critical for maximizing human performance and efficiency as well as minimizing the risk of injury, especially in high-velocity activities such as gymnastics (Fig. 5–8), hurdling, and sprinting, but further research is required before a definitive statement can be made. Periarticular connective tissue and muscle must be able to easily deform in the time required to perform specific activities. Dynamic flexibility is limited by the ability of the connective tissue to deform quickly and easily and by the integration of the neuromuscular system (contractile elements of muscle and its innervation).[10]

INFLUENTIAL FACTORS

AGE

During the normal aging process, increased stability of the collagen fibrils occurs as a result of changes within the ground substance; an increase in the collagen fibril diameter and the total collagen content of tendon, capsule, and muscle; and the maturation and development of complex intermolecular cross-links between tropocollagen molecules.[51–57] These changes can translate into decreased joint range of motion and muscle flexibility with aging. Clinically, this decrease has been reported in the young as part of the maturation process,[58,59] as well as throughout the life span.[60–64] Muscle flexibility that has decreased due to the aging process may be regained from participation in exercise programs that include stretching and range of motion exercises.[64–66]

IMMOBILIZATION

The length of time and position of immobilization are significant factors related to a muscle's response and its ability to recover its contractile characteristics and flexibility. The effect of rigid immobilization on muscle has been well detailed.[67–72] The results of restricted motion, where a joint and associated muscles are not allowed to move through their complete range, have not been well studied.

Stress-induced changes caused by immobilization tend to occur at the myotendinous junction.[26] An adjustment in the number and length of sarcomeres occurs at the myotendinous junction whether the imposed immobilization takes place in a shortened or a lengthened position. Sarcomeres are added when muscle is immobilized in a lengthened position and lost when immobilized in a shortened position.[67–71] A change in sarcomere number begins within 12 to 24 hours and continues until a normalization of tension occurs through regaining motion. Changes also occur in the connective tissue.

Biological adaptation to muscle growth or muscle immobilization in a stretch position occurs near the myotendinous junction. When muscle is immobilized in a shortened position, atrophy results in a loss of both contractile and noncontractile elements. Noncontractile elements are lost at a slower rate than contractile elements, resulting in a relative increase in connective tissue and a reduction in the extensibility of muscle. The thickness of the endomysium and perimysium may also increase.[57] These changes may result in an increase in the stiffness of the muscle. Similar changes have also been demonstrated in respiratory muscles that must function in chronically shortened positions.[73]

Biomechanically, muscle immobilized in a shortened position develops less force and stretches to a shorter length before tearing than does nonimmobilized muscle. Muscle immobilized in a lengthened position responds differently; greater force and a greater change in length are required to cause a tear than in nonimmobilized muscle. In both cases, the tear occurs at the myotendinous junction, indicating an alteration in the mechanical properties at the junction. Clearly, a key factor in determining the nature of the change at the myotendinous junction is the position of immobilization.[26]

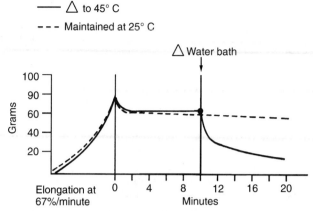

FIGURE 5—9. Effect of temperature on force relaxation response. (From Lehmann JF, Masock AJ, Warren CG, et al: Effect of therapeutic temperatures on tendon extensibility. Arch Phys Med Rehab 1970; 51:481–487.)

TEMPERATURE

Temperature has a profound effect on the physical and mechanical properties of collagen (Fig. 5–9). Collagenous tissues have an inverse temperature–elastic modulus relationship, especially at higher temperatures.[74–79] Historically, numerous investigators have explored the effects of therapeutic temperatures (which have an upper limit of 45° C) and load on the extensibility of collagen, using tendon as a model. All have demonstrated that temperature elevation results in increased elasticity and decreased stiffness when attempting to deform connective tissue.[80–84]

Recent studies on muscle demonstrate a similar relationship using the anterior tibial muscle and long extensor muscle of the toe in a rabbit model.[85,86] Although each study used a different testing temperature (39° C vs. 35° C[85]; 25° C vs. 40° C[86]), a significant increase in length or deformation was attained prior to failure by the warmer muscles in both of these studies. The thermal effects in the study completed by Noonan and co-workers[86] were dependent on the loading rate and contractile state of the muscle. Stiffness and energy absorbed to failure were significantly higher in the colder muscles, suggesting that warming a muscle may confer a protective effect against muscle strain injury. Warm muscles must undergo greater deformation prior to failure, which is advantageous in the prevention of injury. A warm muscle is less stiff than a cold muscle, developing less force for a given deformation. Some protection may be acquired by a warm muscle, assuming that a critical force needs to be attained for injury to occur (Fig. 5–10). It is still unclear, however, if the critical factor in the cause of injury is strain or load. If the critical factor is strain, a warm muscle might be prone to injury, since it undergoes greater deformation to attain a given load. Further research is needed in this area.

An increase in intramuscular temperature may be produced either by various means of external warming (environment, therapeutic modalities)[87] or through muscular contraction. Not only has exercise been demonstrated to increase intramuscular temperature,[88–90] but a single isometric contraction has been induced through muscle stimulation. Safran and colleagues[36] demonstrated that a single muscle contraction is able to warm a muscle by 1° C and alter the amount of stretch a muscle can withstand prior to failure.

CONTRACTION

The strength of muscle is defined as the maximum ability to produce contractive force. Muscle strength per se does not limit flexibility or the ability of muscle to lengthen. Strong muscle may provide a protective mechanism by which to minimize the chance of muscle strain injury. An appropriate balance of strength and flexibility must be attained by an athlete for maximal protection.

Garrett and associates[91] examined the biomechanical properties of passive (relaxed) and active (stimulated) muscle rapidly lengthened to failure in an animal model. The parameters of force to failure, change in length to failure, site of failure, and energy absorbed prior to failure were examined. With a rabbit model, the long extensor muscle of the toe was pulled to failure either while being stimulated electrically (tetanically or by wave summation [submaximally]) or while in a relaxed or passive state. Stimulated muscle required a significantly greater force to cause failure and absorbed more energy prior to failure than did nonstimulated, passive muscle. All muscles were injured at the distal myotendinous junction and demonstrated no difference in the length to failure (Fig. 5–11). Maximally stimulated muscle absorbed more energy prior to failure than did submaximally stimulated muscle. A muscle that can contract strongly and effectively is well equipped to absorb energy. A muscle that is developing more force is absorbing more energy while stretching the same degree. It is apparent that this could be a factor in preventing muscle strain injury.[91]

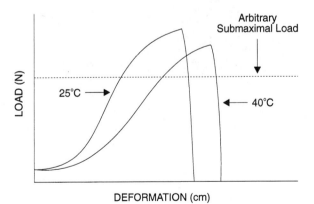

FIGURE 5—10. The biomechanical effects of warming a muscle. Warm muscle reaches an arbitrary submaximal load at a greater length than cold muscle. (From Noonan TJ, Best TM, Seaber AV, et al: Thermal effects on skeletal muscle tensile behavior. Am J Sports Med 1993; 21:517–522.)

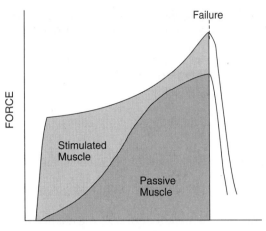

FIGURE 5–11. Differences in relative energy absorbed to failure in stimulated versus passive muscle shown schematically as the area under each length-tension curve. (From Garrett WE, Safran MR, Seaber AV, et al: Biomechanical comparison of stimulated and nonstimulated skeletal muscle pulled to failure. Am J Sports Med 1987; 15:448–454.)

INJURY

LOCATION AND PATHOPHYSIOLOGY

When a muscle strain injury occurs, it is because the tension generated exceeds the tensile capacity of the weakest structural element.[92] These indirect muscle injuries, caused by either stretching or a combination of muscle activation and stretching, have been demonstrated to occur near the region of the myotendinous junction[13–16,92] and, more recently, within random areas of the muscle belly.[93]

Although these in vitro studies used animal models, subsequent computed tomography (CT) and magnetic resonance imaging (MRI) studies demonstrated similar results on over 50 patients (Fig. 5–12).[94] MRI demonstrated that high-signal-intensity fluid collected at the site of the disruption (the myotendinous junction) and then dissected along the epimysium, at times breaking through to the epimysium or subcuticular tissues. Muscle tissue somewhat remote from the myotendinous junction also demonstrated signal changes consistent with edema and inflammation. These injuries may result in a complete or incomplete tear.

Disruption of fibers occurs near the myotendinous junction, not necessarily at the junction itself (Fig. 5–13). The disruption usually occurs a short distance from the tendon, ranging from 0.1 mm to several millimeters.[25,26] The response to injury at the myotendinous junction is limited to the area of injury and is usually extremely focal in nature. The basic early structural defect in this type of injury is thought to be a localized disruption of the sarcolemma of the muscle fiber, created by the force of stretching.[95] Some current research also suggests that following an acute muscle strain, an intracellular barrier may effectively restrict the injury response to less than 500 μm away from the initial site of rupture.[96]

After failure, muscle fibers may still be attached to the tendon. It is not presently known how this may relate

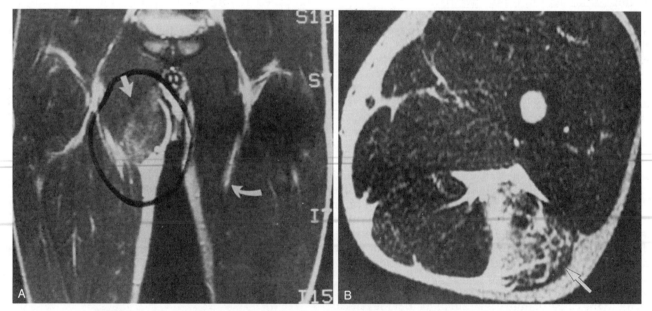

FIGURE 5–12. *A*, A T2 weighted coronal MR image (repetition time, 2000 msec; echo time, 70 msec) of a grade III distal adductor longus muscle strain with proximal retraction (*straight arrow*). The normal contour of the adductor longus is shown by the curved arrow. Note the high signal within the retracted muscle. *B*, A T2 weighted axial MR image (repetition time, 2200 msec; echo time 70 msec) of a biceps femoris muscle strain (*arrow*). Whole muscle involvement with edema and inflammation is present. The high-signal fluid has escaped the epimysium to abut adjacent structures. The biceps femoris and semitendinous muscles share a common tendon of origin situated between the two muscle bellies. The most intense changes in the biceps femoris can be seen to occur near the tendon. (From Speer KP, Lohnes J, Garrett WE: Radiographic imaging of muscle strain injury. Am J Sports Med 1993; 21:89–96.)

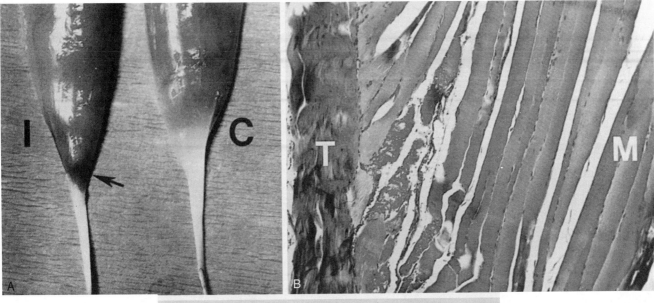

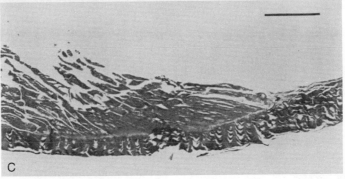

FIGURE 5–13. *A,* Gross appearance of tibialis anterior of rabbit following controlled strain injury. A small hemorrhage *(arrow)* is visible at the distal tip of injured muscle at 24 hours. I, injured; C, control. *B,* Histologic appearance of tibialis anterior immediately following strain injury showing limited rupture of the most distal fibers near the musculotendinous junction along with hemorrhage. T, tendon; M, intact muscle fibers. Masson stain (100 ×). *C,* Complete avulsion of muscle fibers from myotendinous junction. The tendon is at the lower margin. Approximately 2 mm of muscle fiber remains attached to the tendon (bar gauge = 1 mm). (*A* and *B* from Nikolaou PK, MacDonald BL, Glisson RR, et al: Biomechanics and histological evaluation of muscle after controlled strain. Am J Sports Med 1987; 5:9–14. C from Garrett WE, Tidball J: Myotendinous junction: Structure, function and failure. *In* Woo SL-Y, Buckwalter JA [eds]: Injury and Repair of the Musculoskeletal Soft Tissues. Park Ridge, IL., American Academy of Orthopaedic Surgeons, 1988, pp 171–207.)

to the membranous folding, angle of junctional loading, or increase in terminal sarcomere stiffness at the myotendinous junction. Although injury occurs within this region of limited extensibility, and structural differences are noted, full detailed studies of this anatomic area are lacking.

THRESHOLD AND CONTINUUM

Hassleman and colleagues[93] recently demonstrated that a threshold and continuum for injury induced by active stretch (lengthening of stimulated and contracting muscle) in the animal model exist, with fiber disruption occurring initially and connective tissue disruption resulting only with larger muscle deformation. In rabbits, anterior tibial muscles and long muscles of the toe were actively stretched at 10 cm per second

to 60, 70, 80, or 90 percent of the force required for passive failure. The effects on maximal isometric contractile force, tensile properties, and histologic changes are summarized in Table 5–1 and Figures 5–14, 5–15, and 5–16. This study, which induced partial injury, provides evidence that injury with active stretch is selective, with muscle fiber disruption occurring prior to connective tissue damage. Injury occurs not only at the myotendinous junction but also within the muscle belly. A threshold for injury with active stretch was demonstrated, and perhaps more importantly, injury was produced within the physiologic range of the muscles tested (EDL). Injury was initially demonstrated at the distal myotendinous junction and in distal fibers near the junction. Muscle fiber damage progressed in severity as force increased in the 70, 80, and 90 percent groups. Muscle belly injury was associated with higher-force injuries and also progressed in severity as the force

TABLE 5–1
Continuum of Injury

Injury Parameter	Force for Passive Failure			
	60%	70%	80%	90%
Maximal isometric contractile force	Unchanged	Decreased 20%	Decreased 50%	Decreased 80%
Failure properties	Unchanged	Unchanged	Unchanged	Altered
Histologic changes	Normal	Edema and bleeding Inflammatory cells Focal myotendinous junction fiber disruption Normal muscle belly	Edema and bleeding Inflammatory cells Moderate myotendinous junction fiber disruption Random fiber disruption in muscle belly	Edema and bleeding Inflammatory cells Major myotendinous junction fiber disruption Scattered fiber disruption in muscle belly Connective tissue disruption

From Hassleman CT, Best TM, Seaber AV, et al: A threshold and continuum of injury during active stretch of rabbit skeletal muscle. Am J Sports Med 1995; 23:65–73.

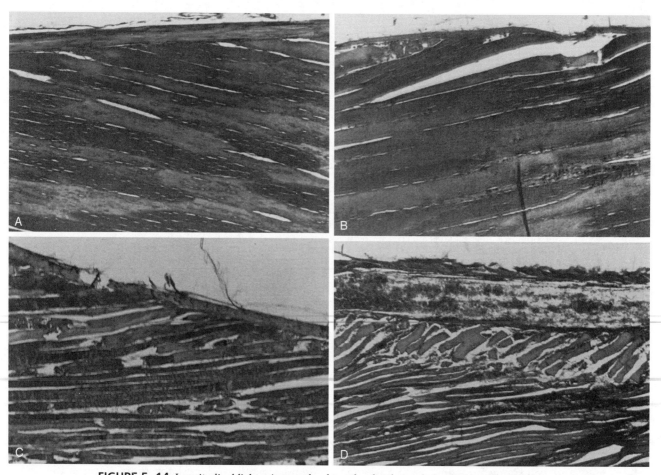

FIGURE 5–14. Longitudinal light micrographs show the distal muscle-tendon junction for the different strain groups using trichrome stain. Both tibialis anterior and extensor digitorum longus muscles had similar morphologic features in each group. *A,* The 60 percent group showed normal findings. *B,* The 70 percent group showed hemorrhage, edema, inflammatory cells, and focal fiber disruption. *C,* The 80 percent group showed findings similar to the 70 percent group, but damage was more widespread. *D,* The 90 percent group revealed connective tissue damage as well as significant muscle fiber disruption. (From Hassleman CT, Best TM, Seaber AV, et al: A threshold and continuum of injury during active stretch of rabbit skeletal muscle. Am J Sports Med 1995; 23:65–73.)

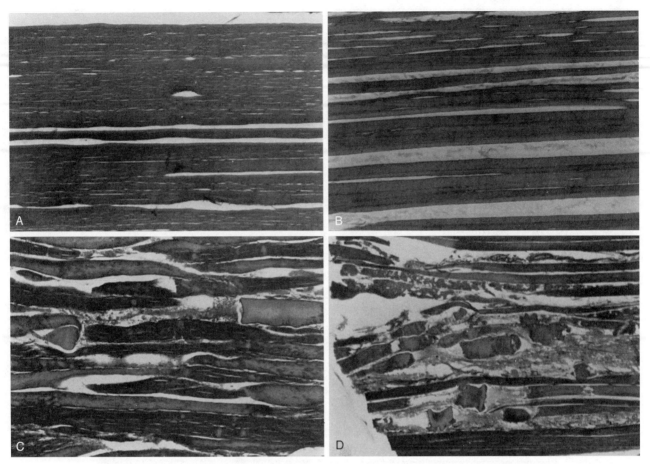

FIGURE 5–15. Longitudinal light micrographs show the distal muscle belly for the different strain groups using trichrome stain. The extensor digitorum longus and tibialis anterior tendons were similar in morphology for the different groups. *A,* The 60 percent group showed normal findings. *B,* The 70 percent group showed edema separating the muscle fibers. *C,* The 80 percent group showed random fiber disruption, edema inflammatory cells, and hemorrhage. *D,* The 90 percent group revealed connective tissue damage along with muscle fiber damage, edema, inflammatory cells, and hemorrhage. (From Hassleman CT, Best TM, Seaber AV, et al: A threshold and continuum of injury during active stretch of rabbit skeletal muscle. Am J Sports Med 1995; 23:65–73.)

increased. Connective tissue disruption was demonstrated only at the highest force (90 percent).

The mechanism of injury used in this study simulated the most common mechanism seen clinically, the active stretch, which does not usually result in complete rupture of the muscle. The histologic change seen at the distal muscle fibers and the mid muscle belly may explain why some athletes complain of diffuse muscle pain after a muscle strain injury. The fact that the contractile elements were initially involved and injured, and that injury to the connective tissue elements did not occur until the highest forces were imposed on the muscles, may assist in focusing prevention and rehabilitation efforts on the appropriate structures.[93]

REPAIR AND REGENERATION

Incomplete muscle tears are more common than complete tears.[26] The process of injury and repair is similar to that found in other collagenous tissues, with the exception of the activation of satellite cells.[16,97–102]

With complete tears, the healing process sets up two competitive events, the regeneration of muscle fibers and the production of fibrous scar tissue.[98,99] Initially, hemorrhage and edema occur. Soon after, degenerative change and necrosis are noted, but these are confined to the site of the injury.[96] Phagocytosis is then initiated to clear debris from the area. Satellite cells become activated and are subsequently transformed into myoblastic cells, myotubes, and new muscle fibers. A decrease in inflammation, with an increase in scarring and fibrosis, is evident a few days after injury. These events are summarized in Table 5–2.

The inflammatory process described above is a vital part of initiating tissue repair. Clinicians often seek to control the inflammatory process by limiting the amount of hemorrhage and edema. This is usually accomplished by the use of rest, ice, compression, and early mobilization. Nonsteroidal anti-inflammatory drugs (NSAIDs) are often given in an attempt to control pain and inflammation. The effect of the NSAID piroxicam (Feldene, Pfizer Inc., Groton, CT) on the histologic, biomechanical, tensile, and contractile char-

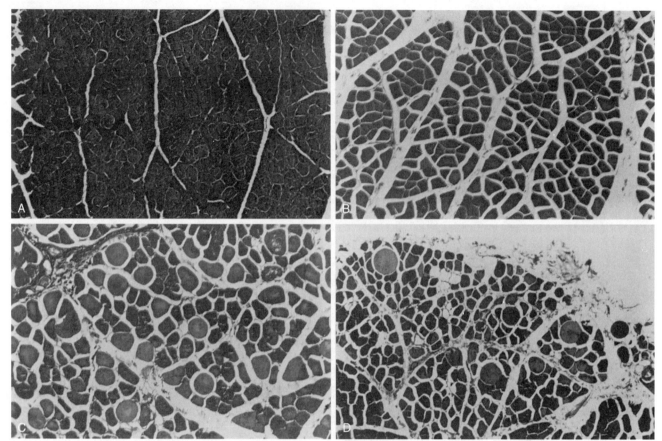

FIGURE 5–16. Cross-section light micrographs show the tibialis anterior middle muscle belly for the different strain groups using trichrome stain. *A,* Normal anatomy was noted in the 60 percent group. *B,* Edema was noted in the 70 percent group. *C,* The 80 percent group showed hemorrhage, edema, and a number of rounded, lightly staining cells that were two to three times the normal size. *D,* The 90 percent group was similar to the 80 percent group, except that connective tissue damage was noted as well. (From Hassleman CT, Best TM, Seaber AV, et al: A threshold and continuum of injury during active stretch of rabbit skeletal muscle. Am J Sports Med 1995; 23:65–73.)

acteristics of rat and rabbit muscle strained to failure has been investigated by Almekinders and Gilbert[104] and Obremsky and colleagues[105] from 1 to 7 days and 1 to 11 days after injury, respectively. In the study by Almekinders and Gilbert, the animal's test limb was immobilized following injury, whereas the animals in the study by Obremsky and associates were allowed free cage activity. The inflammatory response in the animal group receiving piroxicam was delayed in both studies. Tensile strength of the muscle was not significantly different in either study, but there was a trend toward decreased tensile strength. The contractile force able to be generated by electrical stimulation in the rabbit model used by the Obremsky group was increased on day 1 only and at no other time. Contractile force was not assessed by Almekinders and Gilbert. Although there appear to be no significant deleterious effects on tensile strength of muscle or contractile ability, dose response studies are lacking. An interesting note is that muscles of the sham control animals in the study by Almekinders and Gilbert demonstrated a progressive decrease in tensile strength with immobilization alone over an 11-day period. Although the effect of corticosteroid injections has not been specifically studied and reported in the literature, these injections are being used in major college and professional athletics in an effort to return injured players to competition sooner. The drugs may block pain, but the muscle may be more easily subjected to tensile forces above the threshold for complete rupture or rerupture, resulting in reinjury.[103,106]

Tensile strength of the healing tissue increases over time. Normal intramuscular collagenous tissue has a greater proportion of type I collagen than type III collagen.[97–99] Following injury, type III collagen demonstrates a significant increase over type I collagen in the area of repair as a function of the granulation response. As the tissue matures, collagen cross-links stabilize and gain strength, and the proportion of type I to type III collagen returns to normal. The response to healing and tissue maturation takes time. Although the active contractile tension that an injured muscle is able to generate from the remaining intact muscle fibers increases rapidly following muscle strain injury, the tissue maturation and collagenous strength do not increase as rapidly. The process by which collagenous strength is regained may take weeks.

TABLE 5–2
Muscle Repair and Regeneration

Finding*	Time From Injury						
	15 Minutes	3 Hours	8 Hours	16–24 Hours	48 Hours	3–6 Days	7 Days
Hemorrhage[100–103]	+	+	+	+			
Pyknosis[100–103]		+	+				
Sarcolemma breakup[100–103]		+	+				
Mitochondria disruption[100–103]		+	+				
Sarcoplasmic reticulum disruption[100–103]		+	+				
Interrupted sarcolemma[100–103]		+	+				
Phagocytosis[100–103]				+		+	
Satellite cell activation[100–103]				+	+	+	
Myotubes evident[100–103]						+	
Scarring and fibrosis[16]							+
Contractile ability (% of control)[16,106]	67–80			51.1	74.5		92.5
Peak load (% of control)[106]	63						
Elongation to rupture (% of control)[106]	79						

*Data compiled from the cited references.

CONTRACTILE AND TENSILE STRENGTH FOLLOWING INJURY

Nikolaou and associates[16] and Taylor and colleagues[106] examined the structural and functional strength of muscle immediately after an experimentally created strain injury using the long extensor muscles of the toe and the anterior tibial muscles in a rabbit model. A nondisruptive strain injury was created by stretching the experimental muscle just short of complete rupture. All failures occurred in the area of the myotendinous junction. Immediately following injury, the contractile ability of the muscles was 20 to 33 percent of control in the experiment conducted by Taylor and 70.5 percent of control in the data presented by Nikolaou. Nikolaou continued to test contractile ability up to 7 days following injury, demonstrating a further decrease to 51.1 percent at 24 hours, followed by a progressive return to 74.5 percent at 48 hours and 92.5 percent 7 days following injury (see Table 5–2). Immediately following injury, the peak load was 63 percent of control and elongation to rupture was 79 percent of control in the experiment conducted by Taylor.

Although contractile strength may demonstrate fairly rapid increases in a short period of time following injury in the animal model, tissue maturation and integrity do not occur in this short time span. Controlled mobility and stress are key considerations in the postinjury period. Scar formation, muscle regeneration, orientation of new muscle fibers, and tensile properties of muscle have been demonstrated to be enhanced in an animal model when subjected to controlled mobilization or movement compared with immobilization.[107] This fact must be considered relative to the results of the immobilized sham group from the study by Almekinders and Gilbert discussed above.[104]

Clinically, scarring and fibrosis, with their inability to tolerate the tension that uninjured contractile elements may generate, may explain the frequent recurrence of injury to strained muscles if excessive load or deformation is placed on the healing tissues too early.[16,103] The findings presented imply that, even in severely injured muscle, enough structural strength remains so that muscle may undergo functional rehabilitation in the form of low-force exercise designed to prevent muscle atrophy and to maintain muscle tone. Range of motion and muscle flexibility are able to be maintained with gentle stretching. A treatment regimen of complete rest and immobilization may be too conservative, prolonging recovery.[106,107]

MECHANISM OF INJURY

Muscle strain injury is an indirect injury caused by excessive intrinsic force production, excessive extrinsic stretch, or both. Muscle undergoing an extrinsic stretch with a simultaneous eccentric contraction (intrinsic force) may fail due to excessive load being applied while at a point of extreme deformation.

Factors that contribute to muscle strain injury—inadequate flexibility, inadequate strength or endurance, dys-synergistic muscle contraction, insufficient warm-up, or inadequate rehabilitation from previous injury—have been well reviewed and summarized.[44,108,109] Based on these factors, Worrell and Perrin[44] proposed a multiple-factor hamstring injury model (Fig. 5–17). This model appears to be supported

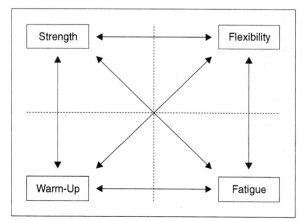

FIGURE 5–17. Multiple factor hamstring injury model. (From Worrell TW, Perrin DH: Hamstring muscle injury: The influence of strength, flexibility, warm-up and fatigue. J Orthop Sports Phys Ther 1992; 16:12–18.)

by the studies and information presented earlier. A compromise of one or more of these factors could predispose an athlete to injury or increase the chance of injury.

CLINICAL IMPLICATIONS

Clinically, muscle strain injury occurs often in athletics. Symptoms are pain on contraction and stretch, as well as ecchymosis and swelling with large or complete tears. Sometimes a palpable defect may be perceived by the clinician when swelling has resolved in the presence of large or complete tears or if the injury is palpated soon after occurring. The anatomic, physiologic, and biomechanical factors presented from the animal model studies discussed earlier in this chapter, as well as each of the causative factors presented by Worrell and Perrin, must be addressed in any flexibility program. These considerations hold true if the program is prophylactic in nature, intended to improve flexibility and prevent injury, or if an injury has occurred and the program is designed to return the athlete to function. If injury has occurred, the clinician must also take into consideration the time frame required for tissue repair and regeneration.

MUSCLE STRENGTH AND FATIGUE

A strong muscle is able to absorb greater energy and requires greater force to be imposed on it prior to failure. Although a muscle that is stimulated submaximally requires a greater force to failure and absorbs greater energy than a relaxed muscle, its injury resistance capacity is not as great as a tetanically stimulated muscle.[91] Therefore, the greater the strength and the fatigue resistance capacity of the muscle, the less likely it is to be injured. Extrapolating from the work of Hassleman and associates,[93] one might also hypothesize that the ability of muscle to undergo eccentric loading is a critical factor in the ability to prevent partial muscle strain injury that occurs within the available physiologic

range. Based on this hypothesis, incorporation of eccentric exercise and strength training appears to be integral in the prevention and treatment of muscle strain injuries.

Muscular strength does not limit muscle flexibility, provided the athlete pursues an active flexibility program. Changes in connective tissue strength due to hypertrophy of collagen fibers do not decrease the tissue's ability to deform but do increase its stiffness and resistance to deformation.[110]

If injury has occurred, the clinician must remember the physiologic and functional factors outlined in Table 5–2. Low-resistance exercise designed to prevent muscle atrophy and a loss of muscular endurance and gentle stretching exercises should be started 3 to 4 days following injury. The clinician must remember that following injury, less force and shorter stretch lengths are required to cause reinjury or complete rupture.[106] Forces must be controlled and progressively increased prior to the return to competition. Controlled exercise and mobilization, after a minimal time of rest and relative immobilization, have demonstrated positive results in an animal model.[107]

WARM-UP

The term "warm-up" must be further defined in athletics. The pregame warm-up, as traditionally defined, includes stretching and flexibility exercises. Also included are activities and drills. These activities are usually progressive in nature and relate to the velocity of the activity and its difficulty, the objective being to begin to simulate game or practice conditions.

Intramuscular temperature should be increased prior to stretching. An increase in tissue temperature has a beneficial effect on the ability of collagen and the myotendinous junction to deform, as described earlier. The critical temperature threshold for beneficial effects appears to be approximately 39° C or 103° F.[77,78,82–84] The effect of temperature must also be considered in relation to the innervation of the muscle-tendon unit. There are reports in the literature that the sensitivity of the Golgi tendon organ (GTO) to sustained stretch is increased with increasing temperature and that the GTO's sensitivity to tension is inversely correlated with the mechanical stiffness of the musculotendinous unit in which it lies.[111] The stiffer or less flexible the musculotendinous unit, the less sensitive the GTO is to firing and inhibiting the contractile element's ability to limit flexibility. An increase in tissue temperature may be achieved through the use of either therapeutic modalities or therapeutic exercise.

Henrickson and coworkers[112] and Lentell and associates[113] conducted clinical experiments using superficial heat (hot packs) and cold (ice) to enhance muscle flexibility when used in conjunction with stretching. Heat alone had no effect on flexibility.[112] Heat plus stretching produced a greater, though nonsignificant, increase in flexibility than stretching alone in the study by Henrickson using the hamstring muscles. Lentell assessed shoulder external rotation utilizing low-load prolonged stretching (LLPS) in conjunction with heat and cold or alone. Although gains were noted with all combinations in which LLPS was involved, the only significant gains demonstrated were when heat was combined with LLPS.[113] Little evidence exists, however, for any temperature elevation beyond 36° to 37° C in the depth of large muscle groups during external conductive heating, which could have affected Henrickson's results. Lentell and associates postulated that the increase in range of shoulder rotation exhibited by their subjects was from a reflexive decrease in muscle tone associated with the application of heat, not necessarily from changes at the tissue level. The change in muscle tone would allow the subjects to stretch farther and develop greater gains. This is supported by a clinical study by Cummings,[114] who demonstrated a significant increase in elbow extension in a group of nine subjects before and after they were paralyzed by succinylcholine chloride at the time of surgery.

The use of a cryostretching technique has been advocated by Knight.[115] Cryostretching is used whenever there is a need to reduce low-grade muscle spasm, which is often associated with muscle strain injury and postexercise soreness. Cold and cryostretching are more effective than heat and static stretching in reducing muscle pain and electrical activity in injured muscle within 24 hours of injury.[116] Clinical researchers using vapocoolants have reported mixed results.[117–119]

Physiologically, the most appropriate and easiest way to increase intramuscular temperature and warm up a muscle is by performing active exercise. Submaximal exercise, emphasizing those muscle groups to be stretched, should be performed. Temperature increases to approximately 39° C, close to the critical temperature for collagen deformation, are possible after 10 to 15 minutes of general exercise (Fig. 5–18). The increase in intramuscular temperature allows the muscle and the myotendinous junction to deform with greater ease and minimizes the chance of microtrauma.

An initial cyclic phase or building process of deformation may also occur at this time, stretching or deforming the muscle within its tolerable limits. This cyclic deformation may be very efficient prior to the addition of any stationary stretching. This cyclic process may influence the hysteresis response and the readily available elastic and viscoelastic deformation available within the muscle and myotendinous junction, as demonstrated by Taylor and colleagues[106] using muscle and by Viidik[120] using isolated tissue preparation. A further increase in tissue deformation may then be gained by static deformation, attempting to further influence the creep response of the tissue.

Upon completion of this "intramuscular warm-up," stretching exercises may be initiated. Stretching should also be considered upon completion of exercise, when muscles are at their highest intramuscular temperature, to avoid postexercise soreness (DOMS).[9,50]

Following the completion of a stretching program, a "neuromuscular warm-up" should be done.[10] During this type of warm-up, the activities performed by the athlete simulate the sport or activity for which he or she is preparing. The velocity of the activities chosen and

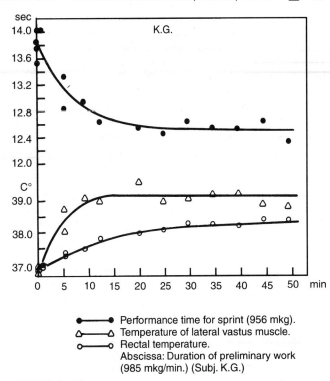

FIGURE 5–18. Effect of exercise on intramuscular temperature. (From Asmussen E, Boje OVE: Body temperature and capacity for work. Acta Phys Scand 1945; 10:1–22.)

the range through which they are carried out progressively increase over a series of repetitions, influencing the viscoelastic responses of the tissues and conditioning them to tolerate the stress to be imposed on them. Muscles are able to undergo progressive velocity transitions from agonist to antagonist, helping to avoid dys-synergistic contractions, which have been implicated as one of the causes of muscle strain injury.[108,109]

FLEXIBILITY

Following intramuscular warm-up, other stretching exercises should be initiated. The clinical literature presents three basic forms of muscle-tendon stretching: static stretching, ballistic stretching, and proprioceptive neuromuscular facilitory techniques. Although many authors have investigated the efficacy of these patterns and their influence on short-term or acute changes and long-term or chronic changes, no absolute answer has evolved as to the most appropriate form for increasing the flexibility of the muscle-tendon unit.[42,113,121–139] All of them improve muscle flexibility.

Static stretching involves the maintenance of a stationary position of muscle-tissue deformation over a period of time, usually at the end of the range of motion or the muscle's ability to deform. The duration of the stretch and the amount of force involved influence the effectiveness. Low-load prolonged deformation techniques have proved to be the best to facilitate long-lasting change for isolated tissue preparations.[80,81,83] Clinically, static stretching offers the advantages of being less likely to exceed the limits of tissue extensibility, requiring less energy, and not causing muscle soreness. The clinical literature states that each static stretch should be held a minimum of 15 to 30 seconds. There does not appear to be any distinct advantage to holding a stretch longer.[113,136,139] The concept of low load is extremely important, as the concepts of viscoelasticity state that high tensile resistance results in opposition to a rapidly applied force. Gentle elongation is demonstrated under slowly applied loads. Thus, static stretching provides less opportunity to cause injury as well as allowing effective treatment with lower levels of load.

Ballistic stretching is a dynamic, rapid action characterized by bobbing or jerky motions imposed on the muscle to be stretched. Motion is initiated by the antagonistic muscle group of the muscles to be stretched. Although these actions have been used effectively in athletics, they have fallen out of favor because of possible injury from uncontrolled force and proposed neurologic inhibitory influences associated with the rapid stretch.[9,10,129,134,140] Ballistic stretching has been demonstrated to be effective for increasing flexibility in athletes, but there is a greater chance of experiencing muscle soreness and injury.[42,121] If ballistic stretching is used, it should be preceded by an intramuscular warm-up and static stretching and confined to a small range of motion at the end of the available range of muscle flexibility. Care should be taken to make sure that the athlete understands the technique and that the amount of motion and force is well controlled. Ballistic stretching techniques should not be used by nonathletes.

The foregoing information seems to point to the application of static stretching in lieu of ballistic stretching. But it is reasonable to ask whether static stretching has been overemphasized in athletics at the expense of ballistic stretching.[10] The dynamic actions and interactions required of high-performance athletic movements imply the need for ballistic stretching maneuvers in athletes who participate in high-velocity ballistic activities such as karate, sprinting, or hurdling. Static stretching should be used predominantly early in the season. As the athlete's level of fitness and conditioning rises, ballistic stretching should be integrated into the program.

Zachazewski has proposed the use of a progressive velocity flexibility program (PVFP) whenever ballistic stretching is considered.[10] The PVFP takes the athlete through a series of stretching exercises in which the velocity and range of lengthening are combined and controlled on a progressive basis (Fig. 5–19). The athlete is progressed from slow, controlled, methodical stretching to high-velocity ballistic stretching. Control and range are the responsibility of the athlete. No outside force is exerted by anyone else. This program should be closely monitored initially to make sure that the athlete is not being overly aggressive in its incorporation. The time required to get to fast, full-range stretching may be days to weeks, depending on the athlete, his or her level of fitness and conditioning, and injury history. The PVFP may be incorporated as a part of an athlete's neuromuscular warm-up.

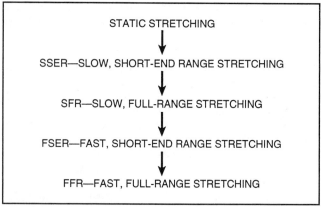

FIGURE 5–19. Progressive velocity flexibility program. (From Zachazewski JE: Flexibility for sports. *In* Sanders B (ed): Sports Physical Therapy. Norwalk, CT, Appleton and Lange, 1990, pp 201–238.)

Proprioceptive neuromuscular facilitation (PNF) techniques have been popularized based on the general neurologic concepts of stretch activation. These stretching activities involve the activation of either agonist or antagonistic muscle prior to the application of stretch. These sequences are designed to utilize the activation of the GTO, by inhibiting the stretched muscle, or the principles of reciprocal inhibition, as originally described by Sherrington.[141]

PNF stretching is accomplished by a contract relax (CR) sequence, a hold relax (HR) sequence, or a contract relax agonist contraction (CRAC) pattern.[123] These techniques are more time-consuming than static or ballistic stretching and frequently require extensive periods of athlete education.

Although various authors have concluded that PNF stretching techniques are effective in increasing flexibility, there is no consensus about which of the three techniques is the best.[122,124–131] PNF techniques have provided acute, short-term improvements in range of motion that are equal to or better than those achieved with static or ballistic stretching.[134,135] During each of these techniques, a contraction of the muscle being stretched occurs just prior to the stretch. This contraction may cause an increase in intramuscular temperature, similar to that reported by Safran and associates[36] using an animal model. This rise in temperature allows a greater relaxation and elongation at the myotendinous junction during the stretch that immediately follows. Contraction of antagonistic muscles while performing CRAC has demonstrated a reciprocal inhibition of the muscle being stretched, which would also allow for greater flexibility on an acute, short-term basis.[133,135]

Muscle flexibility can be increased regardless of which type of stretching technique is used—static, ballistic, or PNF. Studies are lacking on how long it takes to cause a lasting change in muscle flexibility once a stretching program has begun. However, the retention of gained range of motion was evaluated by Zebas and Rivera,[122] and Wallin and colleagues[124] examined how often a stretching program must be performed. Zebas and Rivera examined the changes demonstrated in a group of healthy subjects following a 6-week training program using ballistic, static, or PNF stretching. Significant gains were demonstrated in multiple muscle groups using all three stretching techniques. Two weeks after cessation of the program, a significant loss was also demonstrated for all stretching techniques. Further decreases were demonstrated at 4 weeks, but not to the initial level; thus, some improvement in flexibility remained. Wallin and coworkers[124] presented data that completion of a muscle flexibility program one time per week may be sufficient to maintain any flexibility gained. Engaging in a program three to five times per week results in an increase in muscle flexibility.

In summary, programs designed to improve muscle flexibility should include a minimum of a general warm-up to increase tissue temperature, specific stretching exercises, and controlled postparticipation stretching. The use of a PVFP or some other type of ballistic stretching program should be considered with specific athlete populations as part of a neuromuscular warm-up prior to activity. Postparticipation stretching should be performed as part of a cool-down to further enhance muscle flexibility and decrease exercise-induced muscle soreness.

SUMMARY

This chapter provides the basic science background of muscle deformation, injury, and repair and the possible clinical application of this information. It appears that most muscle strain injuries occur in the area of the muscle-tendon junction and involve a strong eccentric muscle activation with stretching. Less severe partial strain injuries may involve predominantly the contractile elements; more severe injuries and complete muscle tears also cause injury to the associated connective tissue structures. Significant alterations in extensibility of the musculotendinous unit can be provided through changes in temperature and the level of activation (contraction) as well as speed of applied load or force. Resistance to stretch is multifactorial, coming from the neural mechanisms, contractile elements, and connective tissue resistance. Strength, fatigue, warm-up, and flexibility are all critical factors associated with muscle strain injury. Clinicians should focus not only on injury prevention through the increase in flexibility but also on increases in strength, particularly emphasizing the eccentric pattern of muscle utilization. It is imperative to recognize that muscle typically functions as an energy absorption system in which the highest tensile loads and demands are greatest. Clinical studies have documented the usefulness of specific interventions, but further basic and applied clinical research is needed.

REFERENCES

1. Garrick JG, Requa RK: Epidemiology of women's gymnastic injuries. Am J Sports Med 1980; 8:261–264.
2. Garrick JG, Requa RK: Girls' sports injuries in high school athletics. JAMA 1978; 239:2245–2248.
3. Garrick JG: Characterization of a patient population in a sports medicine facility. Phys Sports Med 1985; 13:73–75.
4. Bass AL: Injuries of the leg in football and ballet. Proc R Soc Med 1967; 60:527–532.
5. Pritchett JW: High cost of highschool football injuries. Am J Sports Med 1980; 8:197–199.
6. Apple DV, O'Toole J, Annis C: Professional basketball injuries. Phys Sports Med 1982; 10:81–88.
7. Glick JM: Muscle strains: prevention and treatment. Phys Sports Med 1980; 8:73–77.
8. O'Donoghue DH: Treatment of Athletic Injuries. Philadelphia, WB Saunders, 1984.
9. deVries HA: Flexibility. In Physiology of Exercise for Physical Education and Athletics, 3rd ed. Dubuque, IA, Wm. C. Brown, 1980, pp 462–472.
10. Zachazewski JE. Flexibility for sports. In Sanders B (ed): Sports Physical Therapy. Norwalk, CT, Appleton & Lange, 1990, pp 201–238.
11. Stolov WC, Weilepp TG: Passive length tension relationship of intact muscle, epimysium, and tendon in normal and denervated gastrocnemius of the rat. Arch Phys Med Rehabil 1966; 47:612–620.
12. Garrett WE, Almekinders LC, Seaber AV: Biomechanics of muscle tears in stretching injuries. Trans Orthop Res Soc 1984; 9:384.
13. Almekinders LC, Garrett WE, Seaber AV: Pathophysiologic response to muscle tears in stretching injuries. Trans Orthop Res Soc 1984; 9:307.
14. Almekinders LC, Garrett WE, Seaber AV: Histopathology of muscle tears in stretching injuries. Trans Orthop Res Soc 1984; 9:306.
15. Garrett WE, Nikolaou PK, Ribbeck BM, et al: The effect of muscle architecture on the biomechanical failure properties of skeletal muscle under passive extension. Am J Sports Med 1988; 16:7–12.
16. Nikolaou PK, Macdonald BL, Glisson RR, et al: Biomechanical and histological evaluation of muscle after controlled strain injury. Am J Sports Med 1987; 15:9–14.
17. Borg TK, Caulfield JB: Morphology of connective tissue in skeletal muscle. Tissue Cell 1980; 12:197–207.
18. Mawghan DW, Godt RE: A quantitative analysis of elastic, entropic, electrostatic and osmotic forces within relaxed skinned muscle fibers. Biophys Struct Mech 1980; 7:17–40.
19. Ishikawa H, Sawada H, Yamada E: Surface and internal morphology of skeletal muscle. In Perchey LD, Adrian RH, Geiger SR, et al (eds): Skeletal Muscle. Baltimore, American Physiological Society, 1983, pp 1–22.
20. Kakulas BA, Adams RD: Diseases of Muscle: Pathophysiological Foundations of Clinical Myology, 4th ed. Philadelphia, Harper & Row, 1985, pp 3–60.
21. Podalsky JR, Schenbreg M: Force generation and shortening in skeletal muscle. In Perchey LD, Adrian RH, Geiger SR, et al (eds): Skeletal Muscle. Baltimore, American Physiological Society, 1983, pp 173–174.
22. Schoenberg M, Brenner B, Chalovich JM, et al: Cross bridge attachment in relaxed muscle. Adv Exp Med Biol 1984; 170:269–284.
23. Cecchi G, Griffiths PJ, Taylor S: The kinetics of crossbridge attachment and detachment studied by high frequency stiffness measurements. Adv Exp Med Biol 1984; 170:641–655.
24. Hill DK: Tension due to interaction between the sliding filaments in resting striated muscle: the effects of stimulation. J Physiol 1968; 199:637–684.
25. Garrett WE, Lohnes J: Cellular and matrix response to mechanical injury at the myotendinous junction. In Leadbetter WB, Buckwalter JA, Gordon SL (eds): Sports Induced Inflammation. Park Ridge, IL, American Academy of Orthopaedic Surgeons, 1990, pp 215–224.
26. Garrett WE, Tidball J: Myotendinous junction: structure, function and failure. In Woo SLY, Buckwalter JA (eds): Injury and Repair of the Musculoskeletal Soft Tissues. Park Ridge, IL, American Academy of Orthopaedic Surgeons, 1988, pp 171–207.
27. Tidball J: The geometry of actin filament-membrane associations can modify adhesive strength of the myotendinous junction. Cell Motil 1983; 3:439–447.
28. Best TM, McElhaney J, Garrett WE, et al: Axial strain measurements in skeletal muscle at various rates. J Biomech Eng, in press.
29. McHugh MT, Magnusson SP, Gleim GW, Nicholas JA: Viscoelastic

stress relaxation in human skeletal muscle. Med Sci Sports Exerc 1992; 24:1375–1382.

30. Taylor DC, Dalton JD, Seaber AV, Garrett WE: Viscoelastic properties of muscle-tendon units. Am J Sports Med 1990; 18:300–309.

31. Frankel VH, Burstein AH: Orthopaedic Biomechanics. Philadelphia, Lea & Febiger, 1970.

32. Wainwright SA, Biggs WD, Currey JD, et al: Mechanical Design in Organisms. Princeton, NJ, Princeton University Press, 1976.

33. Fung YCB: Biomechanics: Mechanical Properties of Living Tissues. New York, Springer-Verlag, 1981.

34. Garrett WE Jr: Muscle strain injuries: clinical and basic aspects. Med Sci Sports Exerc 1990; 22:436–443.

35. Malone TR, Garrett WE: Muscle strains: histology, cause, trauma and treatment. Surg Rounds Orthop 1989; 3:43–46.

36. Safran MR, Garrett WE, Seaber AV, et al: The role of warmup in muscular injury prevention. Am J Sports Med 1988; 16:123–129.

37. Ekstrand J, Gillquist J: The avoidability of soccer injuries. Int J Sports Med 1983; 4:1124–1128.

38. Ekstrand J, Gillquist J: The frequency of muscle tightness and injury in soccer players. Am J Sports Med 1982; 10:75–78.

39. Ekstrand J, Gillquist J, Lilzedahl S: Prevention of soccer injuries: supervision by doctor and physiotherapist. Am J Sports Med 1983; 11:116–120.

40. Corbin CB, Noble L: Flexibility: a major component of physical fitness. J Phys Educ 1980; 51:23–60.

41. Glick JM: Muscle strains: prevention and treatment. Phys Sports Med 1980; 8:73–77.

42. Schultz P: Flexibility: day of the static stretch. Phys Sports Med 1979; 7:109–117.

43. Hubley CL, Kozey JW, Stanish WD: Can stretching prevent athletic injuries? J Musculoskel Med 1984; 1:25–32.

44. Worrell TW, Perrin DH: Hamstring muscle injury: the influence of strength, flexibility, warm-up and fatigue. J Orthop Sports Phys Ther 1992; 16:12–18.

45. deVries HA: The "looseness" factor in speed and oxygen consumption of an anaerobic 100 yard dash. Res Q Exerc Sport 1963; 34:305–313.

46. Godges JJ, MacRae H, Longdon C, et al: The effects of two stretching procedures on hip range of motion and gait economy. J Orthop Sports Phys Ther 1989; 10:350–357.

47. Gleim GW, Stanchenfeld NS, Nicholas JA: The influence of flexibility on the economy of walking and jogging. J Orthop Res 1990; 8:814–823.

48. Wilson GJ, Elliott BC, Wood GA: Stretch shorten cycle performance enhancement through flexibility training. Med Sci Sports Exerc 1992; 24:116–123.

49. Godges JJ, MacRae H, Engelke KA: Effect of exercise on hip range of motion, trunk muscle performance and gait economy. Phys Ther 1993; 73:468–477.

50. deVries HA: Prevention of muscular distress after exercise. Res Q Exerc Sport 1961; 32:177–185.

51. Ippolito I, Natoli PH, Postacchini F: Morphological, immunological and biochemical study of rabbit Achilles tendon at various ages. J Bone Joint Surg 1980; 62A:583–598.

52. Hana H, Yamauro T, Takeda T: Experimental studies on connective tissue of capsular ligament. Acta Orthop Scand 1976; 47:473–479.

53. Mohan S, Radha E: Age related changes in muscle connective tissue: acid mucopolysaccharides and structural glycoproteins. Exp Gerontol 1981; 16:385–392.

54. Viidik A: Connective tissues: possible implications of the temporal changes for the aging process. Mech Age Dev 1979; 9:267–285.

55. Danielson CC: Thermal shrinkage of reconstituted collagen fibrils: Shrinkage characteristics upon in vitro maturation. Mech Aging Dev 1981; 15:269–278.

56. Balzas EA: Intracellular matrix of connective tissue. In Finch C, Hayflick L (eds): Handbook of the Biology of Aging. New York, Van Nostrand Reinhold, 1977, pp 222–240.

57. Alnaqeeb MA, Al Zaid NS, Goldspink G: Connective tissue changes and physical properties of developing and ageing skeletal muscle. J Anat 1984; 139(pt4):677–689.

58. Hunter SC, Etchison WC, Halpern BC: Standards and norms of fitness and flexibility in the high school athlete. J Ath Training 1985; 16:210–212.

59. Kendall HO, Kendall FP: Normal flexibility according to age groups. J Bone Joint Surg 1948; 30A:690–694.

60. Leighton JR: Flexibility characteristics of males ten to eighteen. Arch Phys Med Rehabil 1956; 37:494–499.

61. Tucker JE: Measurement of joint range of motion of older individuals. Master's thesis, Stanford University, Palo Alto, CA, 1964.

62. Smith JR, Walker JM: Knee and elbow range of motion in healthy older individuals. Phys Occup Ther Geriatr 1983; 2:31–38.

63. Walker JM, Sue D, Miles-Elkousy N, et al: Active mobility of the extremities in older subjects. Phys Ther 1984; 64:919–923.

64. Boone DC, Azen SP, Lin CM, et al: Reliability of goniometric measurements. Phys Ther 1978; 58:1355–1360.

65. Misner JE, Bassey BH, Bemben M, et al: Long term effects of exercise on the range of motion of aging women. J Orthop Sports Phys Ther 1992; 16:37–42.

66. Raab DM, Agre JC, McAdam J, et al: Light resistance and stretching exercise in elderly women: effect upon flexibility. Arch Phys Med Rehabil 1988; 69:268–272.

67. Williams PE, Goldspink G: The effect of immobilization on the longitudinal growth of striated muscle fibers. J Anat 1973; 116:45–55.

68. Williams PE, Goldspink G: Connective tissue changes in immobilized muscle. J Anat 1984; 138:343–350.

69. Griffin GE, Williams PE, Goldspink G: Region of longitudinal growth in striated muscle fibers. Nature 1971; 232:28–29.

70. Tabary JC, Tardieu C, Tardieu G, et al: Experimental rapid sarcomere loss with concomitant hypoextensibility. Muscle Nerve 1981; 4:198.

71. Tardieu C, Tabary JC, Tabary C, et al: Adaptation of connective tissue length to immobilization in the lengthened and shortened position in cat soleus muscle. J Physiol (Paris) 1982; 78:214.

72. Tabary JC, Tabary C, Tardieu C, et al: Physiological and structural changes in the cat's soleus muscle due to immobilization at different lengths by plaster casts. J Physiol 1972; 224:231–244.

73. Kelsen SG, Wolanski T, Supinski GS, Roessmann U: The effect of elastase-induced emphysema on diaphragmatic muscle structure in hamsters. Am Rev Respir Dis 1983; 127(3):330–334.

74. Aptar JT: Influence of composition on thermal properties of tissues. In Fung YC, Perrone N, Akliker M (eds): Biomechanics: Its Foundations and Objectives. Englewood Cliffs, NJ, Prentice-Hall, 1970, pp 217–235.

75. Walker PS, Amstutz HC, Rubinfeld M: Canine tendon studies II: biomechanical evaluation of normal and regrown canine tendons. J Biomed Mater Res 1976; 10:61–76.

76. Woo SLY, Lee TQ, Gomez MA, et al: Temperature dependent behavior of the canine medial collateral ligament. J Biomech Eng 1987; 109:68–71.

77. Rigby JB, Hirai N, Spikes JD, et al: The mechanical properties of rat tail tendon. J Gen Physiol 1959; 43:265–283.

78. Rigby JB: The effect of mechanical extension upon the thermal stability of collagen. Biochim Biophys Acta 1964; 79:334–363.

79. Mason T, Rigby BJ: Thermal transitions in collagen. Biochim Biophys Acta 1963; 66:448–450.

80. Kottke FJ, Pauley DL, Ptak RA: The rationale for prolonged stretching for correction of the shortening of connective tissue. Arch Phys Med Rehabil 1966; 47:345–352.

81. LaBan MM: Collagen tissue: implications of its response to stress in vitro. Arch Phys Med Rehabil 1962; 43:461–466.

82. Lehmann JF, Masock AJ, Warren CG, et al: Effect of therapeutic temperatures on tendon extensibility. Arch Phys Med Rehabil 1970; 51:481–487.

83. Warren CG, Lehmann JF, Koblanski JN, et al: Elongation of rat tail tendon: effect of load and temperature. Arch Phys Med Rehabil 1971; 52:465–474.

84. Warren CG, Lehmann JF, Koblanski JN: Heat and stretch procedures: an evaluation using rat tail tendon. Arch Phys Med Rehabil 1976; 57:122–126.

85. Strickler T, Malone T, Garrett WE: The effects of passive warming on muscle injury. Am J Sports Med 1990; 18:141–145.

86. Noonan TJ, Best TM, Seaber AV, et al: Thermal effects on skeletal muscle tensile behavior. Am J Sports Med 1993; 21:517–522.

87. Lehmann JF, DeLateur BJ: Therapeutic heat. In Lehmann JF (ed): Therapeutic Heat and Cold. Baltimore, Williams & Wilkins, 1982, pp 404–563.

88. Asmussen E, Boje OVE: Body temperature and capacity for work. Acta Phys Scand 1945; 10:1–22.

89. Saltin B, Hermansen L: Esophageal, rectal and muscle temperature during exercise. J Appl Physiol 1966; 21:1757–1762.

90. Saltin B, Gragge AP, Bergh U, et al: Body temperatures and sweating during exhaustive exercise. J Appl Physiol 1972; 32:635–643.

91. Garrett WE, Safran MR, Seaber AV, et al: Biomechanical comparison of stimulated and non-stimulated skeletal muscle pulled to failure. Am J Sports Med 1987; 15:448–454.

92. Garrett WE, Califf JE, Bassett HF: Histochemical correlates of hamstring injuries. Am J Sports Med 1984; 12:98–103.

93. Hassleman CT, Best TM, Seaber AV, et al: A threshold and continuum of injury during active stretch of rabbit skeletal muscle. Am J Sports Med 1995; 23:65–73.

94. Speer KP, Lohnes J, Garrett WE: Radiographic imaging of the muscle strain injury. Am J Sports Med 1993; 21:89–96.

95. LeCroy CM, Reedy MK, Seaber AV, et al: Limited sarcomere extensibility and strain injury in rabbit skeletal muscle. Trans Orthop Res Soc 1989; 14:316.

96. Reddy AS, Reddy MK, Seaber AV, et al: Restriction of the injury response following an acute muscle strain. Med Sci Sports Exerc 1992; 25:321–327.

97. Lehto M, Jarvinen M, Nelmarkka O: Scar formation after muscle injury: a histological and autoradiographical study in rats. Arch Orthop Trauma Scand 1986; 104:366–370.

98. Lehto M, Jarvinen M: Collagen and glycosaminoglycan synthesis of injured gastrocnemius muscle in rat. Eur Surg Res 1985; 17:179–185.

99. Lehto M, Duance VC, Restall D: Collagen and fibronecin in a healing skeletal muscle injury. J Bone Joint Surg 1985; 65B:820–828.

100. Carlson BM, Faulkner JA: The regeneration of skeletal muscle fibers following injury: a review. Med Sci Sports Exerc 1983; 15:187–198.

101. Snow M: Myogenic cell formation in regenerating rat skeletal muscle injured by mincing. Anat Rec 1977; 188:181–200.

102. Hurme T, Kalimo H: Activation of myogenic precursor cells after muscle injury. Med Sci Sports Exerc 1992; 24:197–205.

103. Hurme T, Kalimo H, Lehto M, et al: Healing of skeletal muscle injury: an ultrastructural and immunohistochemical study. Med Sci Sports Exerc 1991; 23:801–810.

104. Almekinders LC, Gilbert JA: Healing of experimental muscle strains and the effects of non-steroidal anti-inflammatory medications. Am J Sports Med 1986; 14:303–308.

105. Obremsky WT, Seaber AV, Ribbeck BM, et al: Biomechanical and histologic assessment of a controlled muscle strain injury treated with piroxicam. Am J Sports Med 1994; 22:558–561.

106. Taylor DC, Dalton JD, Seaber AV, et al: Experimental muscle strain injury: early functional and structural deficits and the increased risk for reinjury. Am J Sports Med 1993; 21:190–194.

107. Kvist M, Jarvinen M: Clinical, histochemical and biomechanical features in repair of muscle and tendon injuries. Int J Sports Med 1982; 3:12–14.

108. Agre JC: Hamstring injuries: proposed etiological factors, prevention and treatment. Sports Med 1985; 2:21–33.

109. Burkett LN: Causative factors in hamstring strains. Med Sci Sports Exerc 1970; 2:39–42.

110. Butler DL, Grood ES, Noyes FR, et al: Biomechanics of ligaments and tendons. Exerc Sport Sci Rev 1979; 6:126–282.

111. Fukami Y, Wilkinson RS: Responses on isolated Golgi tendon organs of the cat. J Physiol 1977; 265:673–689.

112. Henrickson AS, Fredricksson K, Persson I: The effect of heat and stretching on the range of hip motion. J Orthop Sports Phys Ther 1984; 6:110–115.

113. Lentell G, Hetherington T, Eagan J, et al: The use of thermal agents to influence the effectiveness of a low-load prolonged stretch. J Orthop Sports Phys Ther 1992; 5:200–207.

114. Cummings G: Comparison of muscle to other soft tissue in limiting elbow extension. J Orthop Sports Phys Ther 1983; 5:170–174.

115. Knight KL: Cryotherapy: Theory, Technique, and Physiology. Chattanooga, TN, Chattanooga Corp., 1986.

116. Prentice WE: An electromyographic analysis of the effectiveness of heat or cold and stretching for inducing relaxation in an injured muscle. J Orthop Sports Phys Ther 1982; 3:133–140.

117. Halkovich LR, Personius WJ, Clamann HP, et al: Effect of Flouri-Methane spray on passive hip flexion. Phys Ther 1981; 61:185–189.

118. Newton R: Effects of vapocoolants on passive hip flexion in healthy subjects. Phys Ther 1985; 65:1034–1036.

119. Koury S, Mamary M, Kagan R, et al: Effect of Fluori-Methane spray on hamstring extensibility during "contract-relax" and active stretching. Phys Ther 1986; 66:806.

120. Viidik A: Functional properties of connective tissue. Rev Connec Tissue Res 1973; 6:127–215.

121. deVries HA: Evaluation of static stretching procedures for improvement of flexibility. Res Q 1962; 3:222–229.

122. Zebas CJ, Rivera ML: Retention of flexibility in selected joints after cessation of a stretching exercise program. In Dotson CO, Humphrey JH (eds): Exercise Physiology: Current Selected Research Topics. New York, AMS Press, 1985.

123. Voss DE, Ionta MK, Myers GJ: Proprioceptive Neuromuscular Facilitation: Patterns and Techniques, 3rd ed. Philadelphia, J. B. Lippincott 1985.

124. Wallin D, Ekblom B, Grahn R, et al: Improvement of muscle flexibility, a comparison between two techniques. Am J Sports Med 1985; 13:263–268.

125. Cornelius W, Jackson A: The effects of cryotherapy and PNF on hip extensor flexibility. J Ath Training 1984; 19:183–184.

126. Prentice WE: A comparison of static stretching and PNF stretching for improving hip joint flexibility. J Ath Training 1983; 18:56–59.

127. Louden KL, Bolier CE, Allison KA, et al: Effects of two stretching methods on the flexibility and retention of flexibility at the ankle joint in runners. Phys Ther 1985; 65:698.

128. Markos PD: Ipsilateral and contralateral effects of proprioceptive neuromuscular facilitation techniques on hip motion and electromyographic activity. Phys Ther 1979; 59:1366–1373.

129. Moore M, Hutton R: Electromyographic investigation of muscle stretching techniques. Med Sci Sports Exerc 1980; 12:322–329.

130. Sady SP, Wortman M, Blanke D: Flexibility training: ballistic, static, or proprioceptive neuromuscular facilitation? Arch Phys Med Rehabil 1982; 63:261–263.

131. Tanigawa MC: Comparison of the hold relax procedure and passive mobilization of increasing muscle length. Phys Ther 1972; 52:725–735.

132. Condon SA, Hutton RS: Soleus muscle EMG activity and ankle dorsiflexion range of motion from stretching procedures. Phys Ther 1987; 67:24–30.

133. Entyre BR, Abraham LD: Antagonist muscle activity during stretching: a paradox reassessed. Med Sci Sports Exerc 1988; 20:285–289.

134. Entyre BR, Abraham LD: Ache-reflex changes during static stretching and two variations of proprioceptive neuromuscular facilitation techniques. Electroencephalogr Clin Neurophysiol 1986; 63:174–179.

135. Entyre BR, Lee EJ: Chronic and acute flexibility of men and women using three different stretching techniques. Res Q Exerc Sport 1988; 59:222–228.

136. Madding SW, Wong JG, Hallum A, et al: Effects of duration of passive stretching on hip abduction range of motion. J Orthop Sports Phys Ther 1987; 8:409–416.

137. Wiktorsson-Moeller M, Oberg B, Ekstrand J, et al: Effects of warming-up, massage, and stretching on range of motion and muscle strength in the lower extremity. Am J Sports Med 1983; 11:249–252.

138. Hubley CL, Kozey JW, Stanish WD: The effects of static stretching exercises and stationary cycling on range of motion at the hip joint. J Orthop Sports Phys Ther 1984; 6:104–109.

139. Bandy WD, Irion JM: The effect of time of static stretch on the flexibility of the hamstring muscles. Phys Ther 1994; 74:845–852.

140. Shindo M, Harayama H, Kondo K, et al: Changes in reciprocal Ia inhibition during voluntary contraction in man. Exp Brain Res 1984; 53:400–408.

141. Sherrington CS: The Integrative Action of the Nervous System. New Haven, CT, Yale University Press, 1906.

CHAPTER 6

Delayed-Onset Muscle Soreness and Muscle Pain

W I L L I A M   T.   S T A U B E R   *PhD*

Performance Deficit
Muscle Soreness and Muscle
   Damage
Location of the Soreness

Residual Muscular Swelling
Inflammation
Perception of Pain
Treatment for DOMS

Physical Modalities
Prevention

The pain or discomfort in muscles that have undergone unaccustomed exercise, particularly exercise involving eccentric muscle actions, is commonly called delayed-onset muscle soreness (DOMS). DOMS is characterized by the time course of pain that follows cessation of the activity. The soreness continues for several days regardless of whether there is further activity. Since eccentric muscle actions (lengthening contractions) are most often associated with DOMS, and since eccentric muscle actions (strains) produce tissue damage (Table 6–1),[1] tissue damage is important in the development of soreness (Fig. 6–1).[2]

Although the terms "pain" and "soreness" will be interchanged throughout this discussion, some comments should be made concerning the subjective experience of pain and soreness associated with muscle tissues. A wide variety of conditions, including exercise, can produce muscle pain (Table 6–2).[3,4] The common "burning" experienced during and immediately after a maximal exercise bout is similar in experience to the pain resulting from defective energy supply (e.g., intermittent claudication).[5] In both cases, the pain results from metabolic processes that produce noxious substances (e.g., low pH, potassium ion). Local ionic disturbances following alterations in pH and ion homeostasis can stimulate free nerve endings. In healthy individuals, the burning pain subsides within a couple of minutes of cessation of the activity. This reduction in pain experience is due to the removal of lactate, the return of high-energy phosphagens, and the restoration of ionic gradients.

Another type of pain, closely related to "burning," results from muscle cramps. The reason for the similarity in experience stems from the physiologic outcome of

a muscle cramp. A muscle cramp or spasm is the result of an uncontrolled muscle activation caused by high stimulation frequencies and muscles working in shortened positions.[6] Stretching the muscle relieves a cramp but exacerbates DOMS.

A muscle cramp is similar to a voluntary isometric muscle action held at the same tension level for the same amount of time. During any high-tension isometric muscle action, blood flow to active muscles decreases due to the high compressive forces generated by the muscle. Thus, it is useful to generalize and say that muscle pain results from metabolic factors common to ischemic conditions and fatiguing exercise; the intensity of the pain is proportional to the concentration of noxious stimuli.

Soreness is a curious type of muscle discomfort, since its intensity changes with movement or pressure. Active contraction, passive stretching, and manual palpation of the muscle increases the pain. In fact, one of the accepted methods for documenting this type of pain is to apply manual pressure to the muscle and note whether pain is experienced by the subject.[7] The experience of pain on palpation is called "tenderness."[8]

DOMS is a temporary condition that occurs after unaccustomed activity involving eccentric muscle actions that require muscles to absorb energy or perform negative work.[2] At the turn of the century, Hough[9] first hypothesized that the muscle damage that occurred following unaccustomed exercise was the result of mechanical stress to the muscles. Working with simple equipment and using himself as the subject, Hough described the experience and functional outcome of this type of exercise-induced muscle damage as well as accurately hypothesizing the mechanism of injury.

TABLE 6–1
Muscle Strain Continuum

Damage	Failure	Disruption
Subcellular	Sarcomere, sarcolemma, cytoskeleton, extracellular matrix	Disruption in structures smaller than the myofiber
Cellular	Myofiber	Rupture and retraction of one or more muscle cells
Organ	Muscle	Rupture of a fascicle or the entire muscle, involving myofiber fascia, and blood vessels (e.g., hamstring tears)

TABLE 6–2
Muscle Pain Experience

Finding	Presence (+) or Absence (−) of Pain
Degeneration/regeneration	−
Ischemia at rest	−
Inflammation	+ or −
Ischemic exercise	+
Defective energy metabolism	+
Acute fiber necrosis	+
Connective tissue damage	+
Eccentric muscle action (delayed onset)	+
Intramuscular injection (delayed onset)	+

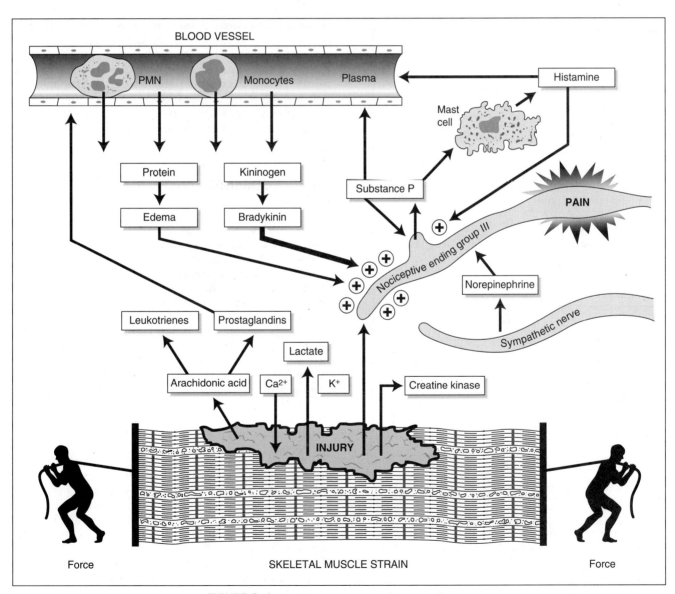

FIGURE 6–1. Muscle strain injury and pain production.

PERFORMANCE DEFICIT

The functional outcome of DOMS, as demonstrated by Hough,[9] was a reduction in muscular force output (weakness) immediately after the exercise and lasting several days. The performance deficit preceded the onset of muscle soreness, which began the day after the exercise session. The decrease in muscle performance is

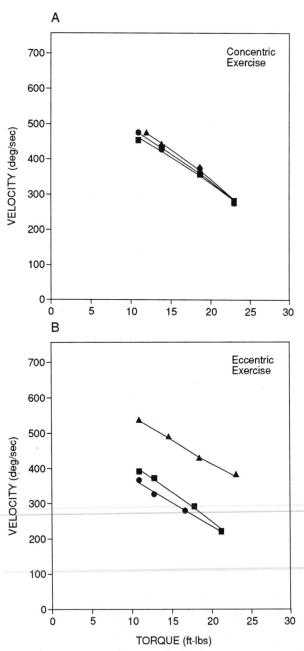

FIGURE 6–2. Torque-velocity tests of elbow flexors using a Dynatrac dynamometer before and following a fatiguing exercise protocol consisting of three bouts of 10 repetitions of concentric or eccentric muscle actions in college-age males. The load was approximately equal to the load calculated for the maximal power output of that subject. ▲ = values before the exercise bout; ● = values 5 minutes after the exercise bout; ■ = values 30 minutes after the exercise bout. Symbols represent mean ± standard deviation for three trials. The r^2 for all the linear regressions of the subjects was 0.96 ± 0.06 (n = 12).

due to a reduction in the muscle's intrinsic ability to produce force. Figure 6–2 illustrates the difference in loss of performance following three sessions of ten repetitions of isolated eccentric or concentric muscle actions of the elbow flexors. The reduction in maximal power output by more than 40 percent following eccentric muscle actions persisted even after 30 minutes of rest. Other researchers have shown that performance deficits can last for more than 5 days following such an exercise bout.[10,11]

It is well documented that pain and soreness reduce the voluntary muscle output of muscles,[12] including following exercise-induced injury.[13] However, normal force output can be restored in many painful musculoskeletal conditions by blocking the nociceptor system,[12] indicating that the intrinsic output of the muscle was normal. In individuals with DOMS, direct electrical stimulation of muscles revealed that the intrinsic force capability of the muscle was reduced.[13] In addition, in Hough's original description,[9] the force deficit remained reduced even though the pain often disappeared within a few minutes of renewed exercise. Subsequently, many different experimental models using human volunteers have demonstrated that the restoration of force and the sensation of soreness follow different time courses after exercise-induced muscle injury.[10] Thus, reduced performance occurs as a result of muscle tissue damage; it involves the intrinsic force-generating system independent of any pain-induced inhibition of muscle activation.

MUSCLE SORENESS AND MUSCLE DAMAGE

The theory of intrinsic muscle damage associated with muscle strains (eccentric muscle actions) has been supported by many studies using muscle biopsy to document both myofiber damage[14] and connective tissue damage.[15] The myofiber damage consisted of hypercontracted sarcomeres, Z line streaming, and refractory fibers that could be observed immediately after exercise,[16,17] when no pain was present. The connective tissue damage involved endomysial separations.[15] Although disruptions in the noncontractile tissue have been observed 2 days following eccentric muscle actions,[15] it is reasonable to assume that they too occur during exercise. Both types of structural disruptions could result in a functional impairment (strength deficit) requiring several days of tissue repair for recovery.

Recently, Zerba and colleagues[18] provided physiologic evidence of a force deficit immediately after exercise in rat hind limb muscles, which was followed by a secondary decline in strength 2 days later. The secondary decline in tension output of the muscles seemed to be related to free radical production by the injured tissue. Whether this free radical production is due to an inflammatory process or is a secondary response of injured muscle is unknown. However, there is evidence for a secondary response in humans following an exercise session that included eccentric muscle actions.[19] Many characteristics of this response resemble that associated with the stereotyped reactions following injury and infection known as the acute phase response. In particular, the mobilization of neutrophils and the production of cytokines may be an important part of this secondary strength deficit.

LOCATION OF THE SORENESS

Although much research has been devoted to understanding the nature of muscle damage and the time course of its recovery,[10] the cause of the soreness is less well understood. Since the location of soreness can be quantified using pressure algometers,[20] manual palpation techniques have been useful to document the distribution of pain following exercise-induced muscle injury. Newham and colleagues[21] reported that the discomfort was most intense in the region of the myotendinous junction after stepping exercise. This observation has led some researchers to believe that the myotendinous junction is more susceptible to damage.[22] However, most morphologic studies, both in humans and in animals, have revealed myofiber damage along the entire length of the muscle. To reconcile the difference between soreness localization and actual myofiber and connective tissue damage requires more definitive anatomic and physiologic knowledge of the location and properties of the nociceptive system of muscle. For example, if more nociceptors, sensitive to mechanical stimuli, are located in the area of the myotendinous junction, then more pain would be experienced in that region when it was palpated or moved. Alternatively, the enzymes responsible for the production of pain mediators might be localized in the region of the myotendinous junction. Recent reports of the localization of prostaglandin-synthesizing enzymes to the myotendinous junction in the rat soleus muscle provide evidence for the myotendinous junction as a prostaglandin synthesis site.[23] Prostaglandins are compounds that can sensitize the nociceptive system (see Fig. 6–1). However, evidence to support this finding is lacking for human muscles.

RESIDUAL MUSCULAR SWELLING

Muscle stiffness and swelling are commonly observed with DOMS. Increased muscle stiffness refers to an increase in the amount of force required to extend a limb (Hooke's law) and can result from muscular swelling. If the region of the myotendinous junction was a semirigid compartment, as in some muscles such as the tibialis anterior, then this region could respond to tissue damage and swelling as a whole muscle does, for example, during a compartment syndrome,[24] producing pain and increased stiffness.

The residual swelling would increase the tissue pressure,[25] causing a decreased blood flow and increased metabolite buildup, producing pain. Although

specific knowledge of the microcompartmentation of the myotendinous junction has not been published, arguments have been presented against the "compartment syndrome" resulting from fluid accumulation as a major participant in the development of DOMS.[8] However, blood flow to skeletal muscle is decreased following exercise that produces DOMS and remains subnormal for several days after the exercise session, but the decrease is not sufficient to cause ischemia.[26] It is not known whether this decline in blood flow could result in secondary responses similar to those seen following ischemia and reperfusion.[27] Exercises can be performed by these muscles even though the performance deficit remains.

INFLAMMATION

The classic inflammation response does not seem to be present following muscle overload injuries that lead to DOMS, although arguments have been presented to the contrary.[28] From the author's own experience,[29,30] the difference between exercise-induced muscle damage and trauma resides in the absence of bleeding following exercise-induced muscle damage. In contrast, contusions or muscle ruptures that are accompanied by bleeding manifest all the characteristics of inflammation. With injury to both muscle and vasculature, all the clotting factors (proteases) are present in the injured tissue, along with a unique class of injury factors.[19] In addition, the clot must be removed by phagocytic cell action, and restoration of an adequate blood supply (angiogenesis) must occur before the muscle regeneration begins. Since an inadequate blood supply would produce an anoxic environment, metabolites from cell activity would accumulate to produce constant pain. Pain, not soreness, is reported by people with muscle trauma.

If the classic scheme of inflammation is not operational, then what mediators of inflammation are present in DOMS? Heat, swelling, pain, and loss of function are characteristics of inflammation.[31] It is common experience that DOMS is characterized by warm, swollen muscles[32] that demonstrate loss of range of motion (stiffness) and weakness. However, when the tissue characteristics are monitored by morphologic techniques, not all the inflammation mediators are present. For example, vascular permeability, kinin production, mast cell degranulation, and macrophage infiltration are primary cellular responses during inflammation. With the exception of extensive macrophage infiltration, all the other characteristics have been shown to be present after exercise injury.[30] In contrast, when blood vessel rupture is present following muscle trauma, abundant macrophage infiltration is observed.

If "true" inflammation is not present in exercise-damaged muscle, then agents and modalities that are proved to assist in the process of pain reduction or tissue healing in inflammatory conditions might not be effective in the treatment or prevention of DOMS. Some evidence exists to support this hypothesis.[33]

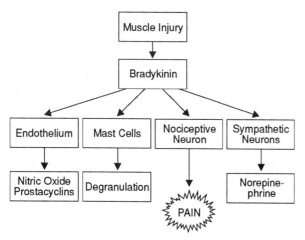

FIGURE 6–3. Schematic of bradykinin actions following muscle injury.

PERCEPTION OF PAIN

In muscle, as in many tissues, there are pain receptors or nociceptors that respond to mechanical or chemical stimuli or both. Substances such as bradykinin, serotonin, histamine, potassium, and prostaglandins may activate the nociceptive system during the inflammatory response of muscle.[34] Of these, bradykinin seems to be the most potent and important (Fig. 6–3).[34] Bradykinin and the other substances are produced by muscle tissues after muscle strains and exercise-induced damage and may require some time to accumulate before exerting a response. This time might account for the delayed onset of the muscle soreness.[2]

Bradykinin reduces the threshold of mechanoceptors so that normal tissue pressures such as those produced by movement are perceived as painful.[34] These nociceptive sensors transmit the sensation of dull, diffuse pain by the unmyelinated group IV afferent fibers. Therefore, bradykinin is an important mediator of hyperalgesia following tissue injury.[35]

Both pain and tenderness are common symptoms in some, but not all, patients with myositis (e.g., polymyositis)[36] or inflammatory diseases of muscle (see Table 6–2). Neurophysiologic assessments of the discharge properties of muscle receptors in inflamed human muscle are lacking. However, in an experimentally induced myositis, the properties of group III and IV muscle receptors have been measured.[37] Both group III and IV receptors showed an increased proportion of units having increased activity, although only the group III fibers were significantly different. In addition, the stimulation threshold for mechanical stimulation of the receptors was lower. Thus, bradykinin acts by increasing the sensitivity of pressure receptors to produce pain on movement. This change in sensitivity is probably the neurophysiologic basis for tenderness (hyperalgesia) in an injured muscle.

TREATMENT FOR DOMS

There have been many attempts to provide relief for DOMS, but few successful results have been reported.

In general, the soreness is accepted as a part of life, especially for active individuals. Again, if inflammation were the cause of pain, then common anti-inflammatory or analgesic drugs would be beneficial. To date, no drug has been reported to decrease the soreness in muscles, with the exception of calcium blockers given to patients with exertional pain syndromes[38,39] and protease inhibitors given to patients with intermittent claudication.[5] Although calcium blockers would be expected to influence a number of different physiologic responses—from variations in blood flow to mast cell granule release—calcium appears to be the most likely candidate for producing cellular damage[38,40,41] and the resulting muscle stiffness.[11] In addition, calcium can activate phospholipase A_2, leading to changes in membrane phospholipid metabolism and prostaglandin production.[42] It is interesting to note that tricyclic antidepressants, which depress calcium's inward movement,[43] have been successful in the treatment of myofascial pain and fibromyalgia, even at doses below an antidepressant action.[16,44]

The wide use of anti-inflammatory drugs may actually have an adverse effect on muscle[45] and skin[46] healing. Although prostaglandins have been documented to be involved in tissue degradation following injury, they are also involved in tissue growth. The important role of prostaglandins in muscle remodeling and repair may dominate over their catabolic actions. Thus, the action of drugs that act on the cyclo-oxygenase pathway of prostaglandin synthesis may give mixed results.

PHYSICAL MODALITIES

If swelling is a contributing factor to the activation of nociceptors, then specific modalities that promote fluid movement through the lymphatic system away from the muscle would be expected to result in decreased soreness. There is little documentation of pain reduction by physical modalities with the exception of exercise.[25] However, stretching, massage, and other physical manipulations would be expected to move fluid out of the muscle and reduce swelling.

PREVENTION

No known prevention technique or drug exists, even though DOMS was present even before Hough's first description. However, some types of exercise produce less damage, and they should be emphasized early in any training or rehabilitation program. Also, it is known that more muscle damage occurs when muscles are stretched at longer muscle lengths.[47] A clever exercise program could be developed that used specific muscles in their shortened positions under mild loads and gradually increased the range of movement with each training session, until the muscle was active throughout the entire range. The problem of exercising at short muscle lengths is the development of cramps.

It should be emphasized that the best prevention for DOMS is regular exercise. Although specificity of use prevents the protective effect from crossing over to all types of exercise, it is well recognized that repetition of an activity that contains eccentric muscle actions leads to protection from repeated injury.[48,49] Secondary muscle damage caused by free radical production can be prevented in part by dietary supplementation with antioxidants[18] such as vitamins C and E and beta carotene, but with varying degrees of effectiveness.[19]

In summary, there appears to be a continuum (see Table 6–1) of muscle damage in response to strain (eccentric muscle actions). Some types of muscle damage result in the production of substances that sensitize the muscle receptors so that movement and pressure become painful. The muscle pain is delayed in onset but lasts for several days after the injury event. At present, there is no known treatment or prevention. So if a once-a-year volleyball game is part of your annual picnic, perhaps a warning label should appear on the announcement: "Unaccustomed exercises may produce a temporary condition of muscular pain known as delayed-onset muscle soreness; this soreness will disappear after a few days without any intervention."

ACKNOWLEDGMENTS

The author wishes to thank Erin Barill, BS, ATC, a senior physical therapy student at West Virginia University, for the data on muscle performance deficits following fatigue. This work was supported in part by a grant from the National Institute for Occupational Safety and Health of the Centers for Disease Control (RO1 OHAR02918).

REFERENCES

1. Stauber WT: Eccentric action of muscles: physiology, injury, and adaptation. *In* Pandolf KB (ed): Exercise and Sport Sciences Reviews, vol 17. Baltimore, Williams & Wilkins, 1989, pp 157–185.
2. Armstrong RB: Mechanisms of exercise-induced delayed-onset muscle soreness: a brief review. Med Sci Sports Exerc 1984; 16:529–538.
3. Edwards RHT: Muscle fatigue and pain. Acta Med Scand Suppl 1987; 711:179–188.
4. Mills KR, Edwards RHT: Investigative strategies for muscle pain. J Neurol Sci 1983; 58:73–88.
5. Digiesi V, Bartoli V, Dorigo B: Effect of a proteinase inhibitor on intermittent claudication or on pain at rest in patients with peripheral arterial disease. Pain 1975; 1:385–389.
6. Bertolasi L, De Grandis D, Bongiovanni LG, et al: The influence of muscular lengthening on cramps. Ann Neurol 1993; 33:176–180.
7. Hasson SM, Daniels JC, Divine JG, et al: Effect of ibuprofen use on muscle soreness, damage, and performance: a preliminary investigation. Med Sci Sports Exerc 1993; 25:9–17.
8. Newham DJ: The consequences of eccentric contractions and their relationship to delayed-onset muscle pain. Eur J Appl Physiol 1988; 57:353–359.
9. Hough T: Ergographic studies in muscular soreness. Am J Physiol 1902; 7:76–92.
10. Ebbeling CB, Clarkson PM: Exercise-induced muscle damage and adaptation. Sports Med 1989; 7:207–234.
11. Howell JN, Chleboun G, Conaster R: Muscle stiffness, strength loss, swelling and soreness following exercise-induced injury in humans. J Physiol 1993; 464:183–196.
12. Stokes M, Young A: The contribution of reflex inhibition to arthrogenous muscle weakness. Clin Sci 1984; 67:7–14.
13. Davies CTM, White MJ: Muscle weakness following eccentric work in man. Pflugers Arch 1981; 392:168–171.
14. Friden J, Sjostrom M, Ekblom B: Myofibrillar damage following intense eccentric exercise in man. Int J Sports Med 1983; 4:170–176.
15. Stauber WT, Clarkson PM, Fritz VK, Evans WJ: Extracellular matrix disruption and pain after eccentric muscle action. J Appl Physiol 1990; 69:868–874.
16. Goldenberg DL, Felson DT, Dinerman H: A randomized, controlled trial of amitriptyline and naproxen in the treatment of patients with fibromyalgia. Arthritis Rheum 1986; 29:1371–1377.
17. Newham DJ, McPhail G, Mills KR, Edwards RHT: Ultrastructural changes after concentric and eccentric contractions of human muscle. J Neurol Sci 1983; 61:109–122.
18. Zerba E, Komorowski TE, Faulkner JA: Free radical injury to skeletal muscles of young, adult, and old mice. Am J Physiol 1990; 258:C429–C435.
19. Cannon JG, Meydani SN, Fieling RA, et al: Acute phase response in exercise. II. Associations between vitamin E, cytokines and muscle proteolysis. Am J Physiol 1991; 260:R1235–R1240.
20. Jaeger B, Reeves JL: Quantification of changes in myofascial trigger point sensitivity with the pressure algometer following passive stretch. Pain 1986; 27:203–210.
21. Newham DJ, Mills KR, Quigley BM, Edwards RHT: Pain and fatigue after concentric and eccentric muscle contractions. Clin Sci 1983; 64:55–62.
22. Garrett WE, Nikolaou PK, Ribbeck BM, et al: The effect of muscle architecture on the biomechanical failure properties of skeletal muscle under passive extension. Am J Sports Med 1988; 16:7–12.
23. McLennan IS, Macdonald RE: Prostaglandin synthetase in mature rat skeletal muscles: immunohistochemical localization to arterioles, tendons and connective tissues. J Anat 1991; 178:243–253.
24. Friden J, Sfakianos PN, Hargens AR: Muscle soreness and intramuscular fluid pressure: comparison between eccentric and concentric load. J Appl Physiol 1986; 61:2175–2179.
25. Friden J, Sfakianos PN, Hargens AR, Akeson WH: Residual muscular swelling after repetitive eccentric contractions. J Orthop Res 1988; 6:493–498.
26. Howell JN, Falkel J, Chleboun G: Blood flow to skeletal muscle during postexercise muscle soreness in humans. *In* Sperelakis N, Wood JD (eds): Frontiers in Smooth Muscle Research. New York, Alan R. Liss, 1990, pp 789–793.
27. Smith JK, Grisham MB, Granger DN, Korthuis RJ: Free radical defense mechanisms and neutrophil infiltration in postischemic skeletal muscle. Am J Physiol 1989; 256:H789–H793.
28. Smith LL: Acute inflammation: the underlying mechanism in delayed-onset muscle soreness? Med Sci Sports Exerc 1991; 23:542–551.
29. Stauber WT, Fritz VK, Dahlmann B: Extracellular matrix changes following blunt trauma to rat skeletal muscles. Exp Mol Pathol 1990; 52:69–86.
30. Stauber WT, Fritz VK, Vogelbach DW, Dahlmann B: Characterization of muscles injured by forced lengthening. I. Cellular infiltrates. Med Sci Sports Exerc 1988; 20:345–353.
31. Hargreaves KM: Mechanisms of pain sensation resulting from inflammation. *In* Leadbetter WB, Buckwalter JA, Gordon SL (eds): Sports-Induced Inflammation: Clinical and Basic Science Concepts. Park Ridge, IL, American Academy of Orthopaedic Surgeons, 1990, pp 383–398.
32. Howell JN, Chila AG, Ford G, et al: An electromyographic study of elbow motion during postexercise soreness. J Appl Physiol 1985; 58:1713–1718.
33. Kuipers H, Keizer HA, Verstappen FTJ, Costill DL: Influence of a prostaglandin-inhibiting drug on muscle soreness after eccentric work. Int J Sports Med 1985; 6:336–339.
34. Mense S: Physiology of nociception in muscles. *In* Fricton JR, Awad E (eds): Advances in Pain Research and Therapy, vol 17. New York, Raven Press, 1990, pp 67–85.
35. Raja SN, Campbell JN, Meyer RA, Colman RW: Role of kinins in pain and hyperalgesia: psychophysical studies in a patient with kininogen deficiency. Clin Sci 1992; 83:337–341.
36. DeVere R, Bradley WG: Polymyositis: its presentation, morbidity and mortality. Brain 1975; 98:637–666.
37. Berberich P, Hoheisel U, Mense S: Effects of a carrageenan-induced myositis on the discharge properties of group III and IV muscle receptors in the cat. J Neurophysiol 1988; 59:1395–1409.
38. Haverkort-Poels PJE, Joosten EMG, Ruitenbeek W: Prevention of

recurrent exertional rhabdomyolysis by dantrolene sodium. Muscle Nerve 1987; 10:45–47.

39. Sufit RL, Peters HA: Nifedipine relieves exercise-exacerbated myalgias. Muscle Nerve 1984; 7:647–649.

40. Duarte JAR, Soares JMC, Appell HJ: Nifedipine diminishes exercise-induced muscle damage in mouse. Int J Sports Med 1992; 13:274–277.

41. Jones DA, Jackson MJ, McPhail G, Edwards RHT: Experimental muscle damage: the importance of external calcium. Clin Sci 1984; 66:317–322.

42. Jackson MJ, Jones DA, Edwards RHT: Experimental skeletal muscle damage: the nature of the calcium-activated degenerative processes. Eur J Clin Invest 1984; 14:369–374.

43. Kamatchi GL, Ticku MK: Tricyclic antidepressants inhibit Ca^{2+}-activated K^+-efflux in cultured spinal cord neurons. Brain Res 1991; 545:59–65.

44. Carette S, McCain GA, Bell DA, Fam AG: Evaluation of amitriptyline in primary fibrositis. Arthritis Rheum 1986; 29:655–659.

45. Almekinders LC, Gilbert JA: Healing of experimental muscle strains and the effects of nonsteroidal antiinflammatory medication. Am J Sports Med 1986; 14:303–308.

46. Proper SA, Fenske NA, Burnett SM, Luria LW: Compromised wound repair caused by perioperative use of ibuprofen. J Am Acad Dermatol 1988; 18:1173–1179.

47. Newham DJ, Jones DA, Ghosh G, Aurora P: Muscle fatigue and pain after eccentric contractions at long and short length. Clin Sci 1988; 74:553–557.

48. Ebbling CB, Clarkson PM: Muscle adaptation prior to recovery following eccentric exercise. Eur J Appl Physiol 1990; 60:26–31.

49. Sacco P, Jones DA: The protective effect of damaging eccentric exercise against repeated bouts of exercise in the mouse tibialis anterior muscle. Exp Physiol 1988; 77:757–760.

CHAPTER 7

Bone Biology and Mechanics

BARBARA J. LOITZ-RAMAGE *PhD, PT*
RONALD F. ZERNICKE *PhD*

Although apparently inert macroscopically, bone is a dynamic structure that perpetually remodels in response to alterations in mechanical loads, systemic hormones, and serum calcium levels. Bone's dynamic structure-function relation—Wolff's law—makes it a prime focus for exercise and rehabilitation specialists interested in physically active individuals who place heightened mechanical and systemic demands on their skeleton. Maintaining a positive balance between adaptive and maladaptive skeletal responses is vital if participation and performance are to be optimized.

Here, after providing an overview of bone structure, the authors emphasize bone structure-function relations as well as what exercise- and disuse-related changes in bone dynamics reveal about underlying mechanisms of bone remodeling. The truncated discussion of bone's other functions reflects only the need to focus this chapter and does not connote a hierarchy of functional importance.

The skeleton provides levers from which muscles control movements, protects vital organs, serves as a mineral storehouse, and houses bone marrow hematopoietic cells.[1] Each of these functions is synergistically interrelated; that is, the specific anatomy of a bone reflects the specific function of that bone. For example, in the slender trabeculae of cancellous bone, osteocytes are located close to vascular channels, suggesting that cancellous bone contributes effectively to mineral mobilization.

SKELETAL ORGANIZATION

Bone is described as an organ, as a tissue, or in terms of its cells, and it is important to appreciate that bone is a functional entity at each of these organizational levels. As an organ, bone encompasses a substantial percentage of total body mass. A distinction is not made here regarding bone size, shape, or developmental origin, but it is as an organ that bone metabolic processes (e.g., hematopoiesis) can be described. Bone tissue can be classified as either cortical or cancellous. Although cortical and cancellous bone comprise the same cells, the mechanical behavior and adaptive responses differ. Many types of cells are native to bone tissue, and these cells function interactively to maintain bone as a tissue and as an organ.

DEVELOPMENT OF BONE

Skeletal development is an intricate, highly refined process, the full details of which are beyond the scope of this chapter. Nonetheless, in a clinically relevant context, the general milestones and terminology associated with bony development are introduced, with examples of the developmental phases that, if modified, can produce skeletal dysplasia. Particular note is made of the role of mechanical stress in the development of the skeleton. For an in-depth discourse on skeletal development, several excellent reviews are available.[2,3]

Skeletal development begins when mesenchymal cells derived from the primary germ layers (mesodermal cells) condense. In a few bones (cranium and facial bones and, in part, the ribs, clavicle, and mandible), the cellular condensations form fibrous matrices that subsequently ossify directly (intramembranous ossification). In this process, mesenchymal cells differentiate and begin producing the enzyme alkaline phosphatase. Soon thereafter, calcification and ossification of the fibrous matrix occur, forming individual bony trabeculae that, together, constitute a primary ossific center. Bone deposition continues in a centrifugal direction from the primary center until a bony island is formed. As centrifugal expansion slows, the periosteum thickens and develops mature osteoblasts on its deepest layer. The deep periosteal layer then becomes the primary site of continued bone growth.

In appendicular and axial bones, mesenchymal condensations form a cartilaginous model (anlage) of the bones rather than proceeding directly to calcification and ossification. The cartilage cells within the anlage are organized in five distinct zones that correspond histologically to the cartilage layers of the growth plate.[2] At the ends of the cartilage model, the cells of zone 1 are tightly packed with little extracellular matrix. Cells of zone 2 are flattened with their cellular axes oriented transverse to the anlage longitudinal axis. This orientation reflects the diametric growth that occurs in the cartilage anlage, in contrast to the longitudinal growth that predominates in the growing bone. Zone 3 cells are cuboidal in shape and begin to show vacuoles, indicative of active synthesis of matrix components. The neighboring cells of zone 4 are the largest of the chondrocytes. These cells actively produce extracellular matrix components. At the central, midshaft level of the anlage, the cells of zone 5 are rapidly involuting or dying, leaving large empty spaces, or lacunae. It is in this region where the initial deposition of osteoid tissue occurs. Circumferentially, the perichondrium surrounding zone 5 thickens and lays down a thin layer of osteoid tissue, which subsequently mineralizes and forms a bony collar at the midshaft level. Vascular channels penetrate the central region and bony collar, ultimately forming the primary ossific center. Ossification proceeds quickly toward the ends to form the bone diaphysis and metaphysis.

In the epiphyseal regions, the vascular channels directly invade the cartilage, which subsequently ossifies and forms secondary ossific centers. Vascular ingrowth is a mandatory step in the formation of the primary and secondary centers because the blood supply ensures the arrival and subsequent differentiation of osteogenic precursor cells.[4]

Between the bone formed by the primary and secondary ossific centers, the cartilage anlage persists as the epiphyseal (growth) plates between the shaft and ends of the long bone. The growth plate results from a compaction of the cellular zones of the cartilage anlage and thus contains analogous layers of chondrocytes. An important anatomic region within the developing long bone is the zone of Ranvier, found at the cortical margins of the growth plate toward the primary ossific center.[2] The zone of Ranvier contains the periosteal collar of bone that is advancing from the bony shaft toward the epiphysis, a region of undifferentiated mesenchymal cells that gives rise to chondrocytes along its deepest surface, as well as the junction between the periosteum, which covers the bony shaft, and the perichondrium, which covers the epiphyseal cartilage. This complex zone is important because it is here that the increase in metaphyseal diameter occurs during growth. Therefore, trauma that damages the zone of Ranvier may disrupt the normal circumferential growth of the long bone metaphysis.

Longitudinal bone growth occurs through activity of the chondrocytes within three functionally distinct regions of the growth plate: the regions of growth, maturation, and transformation (Fig. 7–1A). The region of growth contains two subpopulations of chondrocytes. Resting cells lie close to the secondary ossific center. These cells are associated with the small arterioles and capillaries from the epiphyseal vessels. The vessels are important in transporting undifferentiated cells to add to the pool of resting cells. Away from the resting cells is an area of active cell division. In this area, the cells are organized in longitudinal columns, and during a period of rapid growth, the columns may account for over half the height of the growth plate.[3]

The region of maturation is composed of chondrocytes that actively synthesize and secrete cartilaginous extracellular matrix. Adjacent to the region of growth, the cells are large and actively produce matrix components, whereas the cells near the ossific front become trapped in the rapidly calcifying matrix and, therefore, are not as active in matrix production.

The third zone is characterized as an area of transformation where the cartilage matrix becomes increasingly calcified and is invaded by metaphyseal blood vessels. The encroaching vessels bring the osteoblasts necessary for the formation of bone osteoid. The osteoid is rapidly mineralized to form true bony tissue.

Eventually, chondrocyte differentiation and proliferation slow in the regions of growth and maturation, allowing the bone mineralization—encroaching from the diaphyseal edge of the plate—to catch up. This brings together the bone formed initially by the primary and secondary centers and marks the culmination of long bone growth.

Both intramembranous and endochondral ossification can occur in the same bone. The shaft of the clavicle, for example, is formed by intramembranous ossification, but a secondary ossific center develops within a cartilaginous epiphysis to form the sternal end of the bone. The primary ossific center is present in most bones at birth, but the secondary ossific center of the distal femur is the only secondary center present at birth and is often used as a landmark to identify a full-term fetus. Both endochondral and intramembranous ossification persist postnatally during fracture repair (endochondral) and periosteal bone deposition (intramembranous), which occurs during an increase in the midshaft diameter of a long bone.

The initial condensation of mesodermal cells appears to be directed by a genetic message. Epigenetic factors,

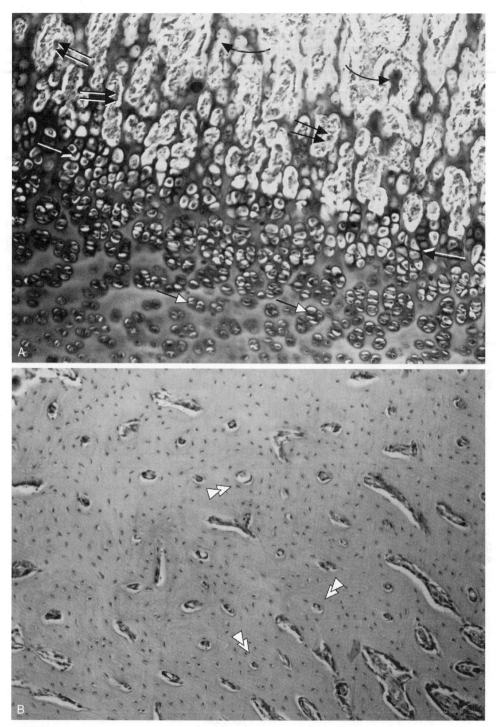

FIGURE 7–1. *A*, Histologic section of the growth plate of a rabbit acetabulum. Note the areas of proliferating *(open arrow)* and hypertrophied *(solid arrow)* chondrocytes. Trabeculae of the newly deposited woven bone *(double arrow)* surround small areas of cartilage matrix *(curved arrow)*. Paraffin-embedded section, stained with safranin O and light green; original magnification = 10×. *B*, Primary osteons *(double arrowheads)* are replacing woven bone. Osteocytes are embedded in the bony matrix that is deposited by osteoblasts within the vascular channels. Paraffin-embedded section, stained with safranin O and light green; original magnification = 25×.

such as mechanical stress, are unable to influence the developing structure until after the fundamental three-dimensional form is complete. After the initial form is present, however, specific changes occur, such as enlarged tuberosities or muscle insertion sites. The distinction between these processes is relevant in a discussion of the origins of skeletal abnormalities. If a genomic disturbance is present, the fundamental form of the bone may be altered, and a specific skeletal dysplasia may result. In contrast, although the fundamental form of the bone may be intact because of a competent genetic message, epigenetic factors can influence the functional, mature form. Achondroplasia is a good example of both processes. The decreased bone length seen in this condition reflects a genetic defect that influences the fundamental form of the developing cartilage anlage. A varus deformity—often present in an achondroplastic adult—results from the forces acting on the bone after the genetic defect is expressed. Thus, the bony deformity present in the adult reflects combined genetic and epigenetic influences.

Movement and its related forces during skeletal development have been investigated extensively to elucidate the stimuli that can influence the final skeletal form. Carter and colleagues[5] propose that the regulation of skeletal biology by mechanical forces is accomplished by the transfer of strain energy. To this end, these researchers believe that cyclic shear stresses generated during movement accelerate the rate of chondrocytic proliferation, maturation, degeneration, and ossification that occurs during endochondral ossification, whereas compressive stresses tend to retard the same sequence. Carter and colleagues propose that some of the energy imparted to the skeletal structures during movement is stored within the tissue and later released during unloading. The remaining energy is transferred to the tissue in the form of heat or a change in internal energy. This latter form of energy transfer may be an important factor in a bone's ability to recognize and respond to mechanical cues.

Extrinsic factors, such as hormones, influence the rate and extent of long bone growth. The growth cartilage is stimulated by thyroxine, growth hormone, and testosterone. Estrogen exerts a greater stimulatory influence on the bony tissue while suppressing cartilage growth. Such distinct influences of testosterone versus estrogen may account for the differences in the timing of physeal closure between boys and girls.[6]

Normal skeletal growth can be interrupted by trauma or fracture. Physeal injuries account for approximately 15 percent of all fractures in children.[6] Girls are more prone to physeal injury from 9 to 12 years of age, and boys are more prone between the ages of 12 and 15 years.[6] The periods of increased incidence parallel the times of rapid growth during which hormone-mediated changes in the growth plate cartilage may alter its response to mechanical stress.[7] Most pediatric fractures are classified according to a system developed by Salter.[8] The classification system considers, generally, the location of the fracture, whether the fracture disrupts the growth plate, and, if present, the extent of growth plate damage. Growth disturbances may result if the fracture and subsequent callus formation stimulate the premature closure of the growth plate, thereby preventing the normal longitudinal growth of the bone. Angular deformities may result if only one portion of the growth plate sustains damage, with normal growth occurring in the remaining portion of the growth plate.

Development of the muscular, vascular, neural, and articular anatomy happens at the same time as skeletal development and growth. Although understanding the development specifics of these other systems is not vital in the present context, recognizing the complexity of the interactive musculoskeletal development is important.

ANATOMY OF OSSEOUS TISSUE

MICROSCOPIC

CELLULAR COMPONENTS

Osteoblasts and osteocytes are responsible for bone formation. These two cell types are distinguished primarily by their location and only secondarily by their structure or function.[9] The osteoblast is the primary bone-forming cell located on the bony surface. It becomes an osteocyte when it has produced sufficient mineralized matrix to completely surround itself. Cells intermediate in the changeover from osteoblast to osteocyte have been identified (osteoid osteocyte, osteocytic osteoblast),[10] but demonstrable differences in function are yet to be found. The distinctions, then, among osteoblast, osteocyte, and the intermediate cells are related more to their differing developmental stages rather than to differing cell phenotypes.

Scanning electron micrographs of growing bone reveal active osteoblasts covering most of the bony surface. The more active the cells, the more closely packed they are. Osteoblasts assemble along surfaces created by active resorption of existing bone, thus creating a spatial and temporal coupling between resorption and deposition. Although osteoblasts identified in the growing, immature skeleton have a different origin from those identified in the remodeling, adult skeleton, in the present context, subtle differences between these can be blurred, without a loss of basic understanding. Active osteoblasts are plump, rounded cells with abundant cytoplasm filled with rough endoplasmic reticulum, mitochondria, and Golgi membranes, indicative of the active protein and polysaccharide synthesis being undertaken by the cell. The cells stain intensely with a basic stain, indicating the presence of large quantities of RNA.[9] When osteoblasts are not actively producing matrix (resting osteoblasts), their size decreases and there are spaces between adjacent cells. Most of the decreased size can be attributed to a decrease in cytoplasmic volume, with a concomitant decrease in the number of cellular organelles. When the active osteoblast begins the transition to osteocyte, cell volume decreases by 30 percent initially, and as the metabolic activity of the osteocyte gradually decreases, cell volume continues to decrease. The osteocyte slowly fills in its surrounding lacuna with matrix, and thus both cell and lacunar size decrease.

Neighboring osteocytes communicate with one another, and the deeper osteocytes communicate with the surface-covering osteoblasts by interconnecting processes housed within channels (canaliculi) in the extracellular matrix. Connections between adjacent processes are gap junctions, which allow for cell-cell communication by permitting ions and small molecules to move between the cells. The presence of gap junctions between bone cells suggests that the osteoblasts, osteocytes, and bone-lining cells form a functional syncytium that may play an integral role in many physiological functions, including the conversion of mechanical signals into remodeling activity and mineral movement into and out of the bone.[11]

Osteoclasts are easily identified using light microscopy because they are large (two to three times larger than osteoblasts), multinucleated cells with many cytoplasmic extensions that hint of cell mobility. Indeed, time-lapse microscopy reveals that the cells move along the surface and leave behind a trail of resorbed bone that has the appearance of an etched surface. The multiple nuclei reflect the osteoclast's origin as a union of several mononuclear cells. Osteoclast cytoplasm appears "foamy" because of multiple intracellular vacuoles and the lysing function of the cell. The most distinguishing feature of the osteoclast is the extensive infoldings of the cell plasma membrane that give rise to a "ruffled border." This border has important functional significance, because it greatly increases the surface area along which the cell can interact with the surrounding bony matrix. Adjacent to the ruffled border is an area of cytoplasm with a smooth plasma membrane and no cellular organelles. This "clear zone" always accompanies osteoclasts and may be an area where the cell attaches to the bone surface undergoing resorption. In this way, the cell can adhere to the surface while the highly motile ruffled border resorbs the targeted bone. Without the clear zone, the cell could not remain anchored to the surface long enough for resorption to occur.[9]

Because bone resorption and deposition are, typically, tightly coupled, osteoclasts and osteoblasts are often found in close proximity to one another. It is theorized that, during remodeling, osteoblasts initiate the signal to the osteoclasts to begin resorption.[11] In contrast, during modeling, one cortical surface undergoes resorption while the opposing surface is deposited (cortical drift, medullary expansion), and osteoclasts and osteoblasts are not in close proximity.

EXTRACELLULAR MATRIX

Bone matrix comprises three elements (Fig. 7–2): organic, mineral, and fluid. Organic components con-

stitute 39 percent of the total bone volume, containing 95 percent type I collagen and 5 percent proteoglycans. Minerals include primarily calcium hydroxyapatite crystals and contribute about half of total bone volume. Fluid-filled vascular channels and cellular spaces constitute the remaining volume.[12] Bone mechanical behavior reflects a balance between the mineral and organic phases, with mineral contributing stiffness and the organic matrix adding to bone strength.

Collagen deserves special attention not only because it provides the major structural support of all connective tissues but also because, in a clinical context, collagen abnormalities can have far-reaching effects on the skeleton's ability to resist mechanical stresses. Collagen derives its tensile strength from polypeptides arranged in α chains. Each α chain is composed of amino acids, with glycine, proline, and lysine being prominent. Three α chains coil together to form a triple helix called procollagen. Osteoblasts secrete procollagen into the surrounding matrix, where the terminal peptide of each α chain is cleaved, allowing procollagen bundles to link together. The linked procollagen bundles form tropocollagen. The tensile strength of collagen relies on cross-links between the hydroxylysine molecules of the procollagen. The degree of cross-linking changes with age and between types of collagen, with more cross-links producing a stiffer tissue.

Collagen orientation in immature (growing) and mature bone has been linked to the mechanical behavior of individual layers of bone (lamellae), individual osteons, and cortical sections of whole bone.[13,14] The question that should, perhaps, be addressed first is, how does the collagen become organized initially during bone development? Stopak and colleagues[15] injected collagen into the limb buds of developing chicks and saw collagen orientation change within 24 hours and persist for up to 9 days following the injection. They concluded that, even in this early developmental phase, traction forces exerted by the proliferating cells were sufficient to "organize" collagen fibrils in a systematic pattern. The relevance of this work to the present context is to illustrate that, although mechanical influences are predominantly generated by loads applied *to* the structure, forces *within* the structure may also affect the final form of the tissue.

More than 200 noncollagenous proteins are also found within bone's extracellular matrix,[16] although in terms of concentration, collagen occupies the greatest portion of the matrix. Among the noncollagen proteins are osteonectin, osteocalcin, and bone sialoproteins I and II. The noncollagen proteins may facilitate cell differentiation and growth, cell adhesion, and organization of the matrix and may also modulate resorptive processes related to maintaining calcium homeostasis. Therefore, the abundance of these proteins may be important diagnostically in metabolic bone dysfunctions and disease.[16]

Mineral content distinguishes bone from other connective tissues and provides bone with its characteristic stiffness, as well as providing a mineral storehouse. The mechanism responsible for calcification of the extracellular matrix of bone and not of other connective tissues

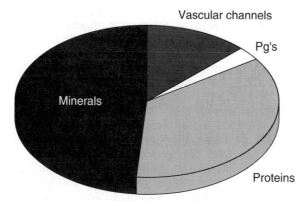

FIGURE 7–2. Relative amounts of the constituents of bone extracellular matrix (pg's = proteoglycans; proteins include collagen and noncollagenous proteins).

is not completely understood, but apparently, the ability to bind mineral crystallites is unique to type I collagen. Neither type II nor type III collagen can bind to minerals. This is a significant and active area of basic research, because if the process of calcification is revealed, clinical interventions to enhance or slow mineral deposition may be useful in the management of certain skeletal dysplasias.

BLOOD SUPPLY

All elements of bone, including the marrow, periosteum, metaphysis, diaphysis, and epiphysis, are richly supplied with blood. Gross and associates[17] estimated that, in dogs at rest, 11 percent of the cardiac output is sent to the skeleton. Blood reaches each area of the bone via extensive arterial anastomoses that feed a network of sinusoids. The sinusoids, in turn, empty into central venous channels deep within the medullary canal in long bones or a central canal in flat bones. The primary nutrient vessel enters the medullary canal via an obliquely oriented nutrient foramen. Once within the bone endosteum, the artery divides into longitudinal branches that course along the bone's length and then re-enter the cortical bone. This vascular distribution is consistent with reports by Singh and coworkers[18] that most of the blood flow in long bone is in a centrifugal (from endosteum to periosteum) rather than centripetal direction. In the epiphyses, the longitudinal vessels branch into extensive arcades that supply the bony ends. Medullary vessels pierce through the cortex and anastomose with periosteal vessels to supply the outer surfaces of the cortex.

Within the compact bone, primary arteries and veins travel parallel to the osteonal longitudinal axes within the haversian canals. Transversely oriented vessels are contained within the Volkmann canals, but apparently no branches are distributed from the arteries at this point.

MACROSTRUCTURE

Despite differences in size and mechanical properties, bone tissue is similar in all bones. Macrostructural differences, therefore, account in part for the functional differences between bones. At a tissue level, bone may be divided into woven, primary, and secondary bone. Woven bone is laid down rapidly as a disorganized arrangement of collagen fibers and osteocytes. Although the mineral content of woven bone may be similar to that of lamellar bone, the disorganized pattern and generally lower proportions of noncollagenous proteins (osteonectin and osteocalcin)[16] decrease the mechanical strength of woven bone compared with that of primary or secondary bone.[19] Developmentally, woven bone is unique because it can be deposited de novo, without a previous hard or cartilaginous model.[1] The cell-to-bone volume ratio is high in woven bone, confirming its role in providing temporary, rapid mechanical support, such as following traumatic injury. In the healthy adult skeleton, woven bone is not typically present but can be found in a fracture callus, areas undergoing active endochondral ossification, and some skeletal pathologies. During maturation, primary bone systematically replaces woven bone, providing the mature skeleton with the appropriate functional stiffness.[12]

Primary bone comprises several types of bone, each with unique morphology and function. A common factor among the types of primary bone, however, is that, unlike woven bone, primary bone must replace a pre-existing structure, either a cartilaginous model or previously deposited woven bone. Primary lamellar bone is composed of layers of bone matrix and cells organized circumferentially around the endosteal or periosteal surface of a whole bone. Vascular channels are infrequent in primary lamellar bone, so it can be very dense. Cancellous bone found in the vertebral bodies and in long bone epiphyses is primary lamellar bone. In this case, although vascular channels are not enclosed within the lamellar structure, the individual struts or trabeculae of cancellous bone are in intimate contact with a rich vascular supply. Because of this close proximity, cancellous bone assumes an important role in mineral homeostasis; calcium stores can be mobilized quickly in response to decreased serum calcium. Primary lamellae formed around individual vascular channels (rather than around the whole bone circumference) are called concentric lamellae (see Fig. 7–1B). The concentric lamellae that surround a common vascular channel, or haversian canal, constitute a primary osteon. In this case, individual lamellae are arranged in concentric rings that are 5 μm thick.[20] Developmentally, primary osteons are considered modified vascular channels, where sequential layers were deposited within existing vascular channels.

Secondary bone is deposited only during remodeling and replaces primary bone. Differences between the developmental process of primary and secondary bone imply that a different controlling mechanism may be responsible for the endosteal or periosteal deposition of primary bone versus the intracortical deposition of secondary bone during remodeling. Toward this end, the deposition of secondary osteons must be linked temporally and spatially to the resorption of existing bone by active osteoclasts. Histologically, secondary osteons can be distinguished from primary osteons because the secondary units are larger, with larger haversian canals, and secondary osteons are surrounded by a cement line between the osteon and the surrounding interosteonal bone matrix (Fig. 7–3). The cement line marks the reversal phase of osteonal remodeling, as resorption ceases and deposition begins.[21]

Each primary or secondary lamella contains osteocytes housed in lacunae and surrounded by extracellular matrix. Collagen orientation within each lamella is controversial, with some investigators suggesting that all fibrils within a lamella assume the same orientation.[13] Others suggest that although parallel-fibered bundles do exist, the bundles themselves do not necessarily lie in parallel.[22] Similarly, collagen orientation within the interlamellar spaces may differ between adjacent lamel-

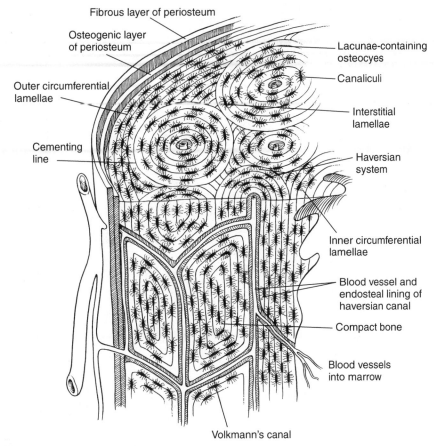

FIGURE 7–3. A longitudinal and transverse section through secondary haversian bone. Note the orientation of the vascular channels (haversian and Volkmann canals) relative to the secondary osteons. Cement lines demarcate the boundary of each secondary osteon. (From Ham AW: Bone. *In* Ham AW [ed]: Histology, 7th ed. Philadelphia, JB Lippincott, 1974.)

lae and adjacent osteons. These disparate views may reflect sampling artifacts that occur during tissue processing.[23] Collagen orientation is measured as the brightness of polarized images of the structure, with collagen fibers that lie orthogonal to the direction of the polarized light appearing dark, and fibers oriented longitudinally appearing light. Sampling artifacts may result if the sections being compared were not oriented similarly when cut or if the orientation of individual osteons differs between samples. From a functional perspective, this controversy is not trivial, because collagen orientation can influence the ability of the lamellae and osteons to resist mechanical loads.

Recently, Riggs and colleagues[14,24] examined the relationship among interosteonal collagen orientation, mechanical behavior, and in vivo strain patterns. Strain gauge data collected on the equine radius during walking revealed that the cranial cortex sustained tensile loads, whereas the caudal cortex was loaded in compression. Samples from each cortex were tested mechanically in compression and tension, and collagen orientation was measured from circularly polarized light (CPL) images of each sample. Their results revealed a high positive correlation between collagen orientation (as measured by CPL) and the radius cortical strength and stiffness. Collagen within the caudal cortex, loaded in compression in vivo, oriented more

obliquely or transversely (relative to the longitudinal axis of the bone), whereas the collagen within the cranial cortex oriented more nearly parallel to the bone's long axis. Samples from the cranial cortex were stiffer but absorbed less energy during loading than did the caudal samples. These findings provide important support for a strong relation between the functional loads sustained by a bone and its architecture. These data also strengthen a structure-function argument that microscopic architecture reflects the mechanical environment present during skeletal growth or remodeling.

FRACTURE HEALING

Fracture healing can be divided into three phases: inflammation, initial union of the bony ends, and remodeling of the callus. Of clinical importance are the findings that the timing and strength of the initial union can be influenced by the mechanical stability across the fracture site, thus giving the impetus for internal fracture fixation. The advantage of an internal fixator is that less external splintage is necessary, thereby decreasing the morbidity related to immobilization (e.g., joint contracture and loss of strength). Internal fixation with compression across the fracture line results in an insignificant external callus, but when the fracture is

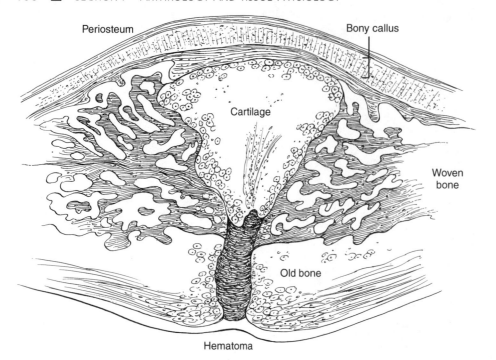

Periosteum

Bony callus

Cartilage

Woven bone

Old bone

Hematoma

FIGURE 7–4. Fracture callus of a rabbit rib 14 days after fracture. The bony callus has bridged the fracture. Osteoblasts covering the surfaces of the spicules of woven bone are depositing new bone. In addition, bone is replacing cartilage via endochondral ossification. A hematoma persists between the bone ends. (Adapted from Ham AW, Harris WR: *In* Bourne GH [ed]: The Biochemistry and Physiology of Bone, 2nd ed. vol III. New York, Academic Press, 1971.)

mechanically unstable, micromotion across the gap results in the formation of a large external callus.

Immediately following injury, a hematoma develops around the fracture site. Within 3 days, mesenchymal cells arrive in the area and produce a fibrous tissue that envelops the fractured bone ends. The outer layer of the fibrous material begins to form the new periosteum. Until this point, stable and unstable fractures react similarly, but between days 3 and 5 after a fracture, the degree of stability influences subsequent healing steps. Microscopic examination of the fibrous tissue reveals that in a stable fracture, the tissue is well vascularized, but in an unstable fracture, the fibrous tissue contains no vessels. Where the fibrous tissue meets the original bony cortex—in both stable and unstable fractures—new bony trabeculae are formed by osteoblasts lying on the old bone surface. In a stable fracture, new bone forms along the periosteal surface of the fibrous layer and bridges the fracture site. In an unstable fracture, new bone also forms along the periosteal surface of the fibrous material but does not bridge the fracture line. In rabbits, this union occurs 9 days after injury, but in humans, minimal periosteal bone formation is present at this point in healing, and periosteal union is further delayed. This difference, however, may be a consequence of damage to the periosteum and the resulting stimulation of osteoblasts in the rabbit fracture model, rather than resulting from damage to only the bone.[25] As bony trabeculae continue to form, the bony collar becomes more compact, and the periosteum increases in thickness.

In the gap between the bony ends (rather than along the periosteal surface), the first cells to invade after injury (approximately day 9) are macrophages, followed by fibroblasts and capillaries. Macrophages scavenge cell and matrix debris, and fibroblasts produce the structural foundation for cells and vessels. Osteoblasts

begin bone deposition by 2 weeks after a fracture, and bony union across the fractured ends is established (ideally) by 3 weeks. If bone adjacent to the fracture site dies secondary to disruption of its blood supply at the time of fracture, osteoclasts may be present to resorb the dead material. Otherwise, contrary to previous reports, osteoclasts are not routinely present in all fractures.[26] In small gaps (< 10 μm) or where fracture ends contact, healing is via direct haversian remodeling: osteoclasts resorb a cone of bone, osteoblasts deposit new haversian bone, and osteocytes maintain the new bone after mineralization. In 10 to 30 μm gaps (too large for haversian remodeling, but too small for cells to move), osteoclasts may resorb the bone to increase the gap width. Osteoblasts subsequently arrive to lay down disorganized lamellae across the gap. The disorganized bone is then remodeled.

In an unstable fracture, periosteal bone formation continues from the old bone ends toward the fracture line, but across the fracture line (where the fibrous material is avascular), chondrocytes proliferate and lay down a cartilage matrix. At the intersection of the cartilage-bone layers, a matrix forms with types I and II collagen. In 10 days (in rabbit), cartilage formation is completed and forms a *V* over the fracture site (Fig. 7–4). In a sequence identical to that which occurs during endochondral ossification of long bones, the cartilage bridging the fracture ends is gradually replaced by bone. In the rabbit, by 3 to 4 weeks after a fracture, bone has replaced most of the cartilage, and the bony callus offers good stability across the fracture site. In humans, this process takes slightly longer, with good stability generally achieved by 6 weeks. With the improved stability, blood vessels and fibroblasts proliferate in the fracture gap. The important milestones of fracture healing are summarized in Figure 7–5.

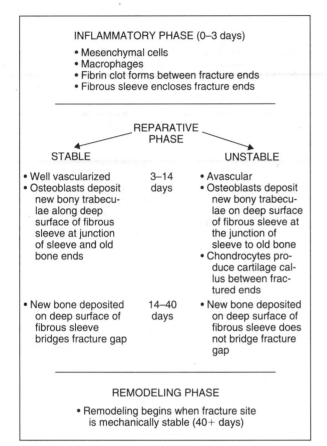

INFLAMMATORY PHASE (0–3 days)
• Mesenchymal cells
• Macrophages
• Fibrin clot forms between fracture ends
• Fibrous sleeve encloses fracture ends

REPARATIVE PHASE

STABLE — UNSTABLE

STABLE		UNSTABLE
• Well vascularized	3–14 days	• Avascular
• Osteoblasts deposit new bony trabeculae along deep surface of fibrous sleeve at junction of sleeve and old bone ends		• Osteoblasts deposit new bony trabeculae on deep surface of fibrous sleeve at the junction of sleeve to old bone
		• Chondrocytes produce cartilage callus between fractured ends
• New bone deposited on deep surface of fibrous sleeve bridges fracture gap	14–40 days	• New bone deposited on deep surface of fibrous sleeve does not bridge fracture gap

REMODELING PHASE
• Remodeling begins when fracture site is mechanically stable (40+ days)

FIGURE 7–5. Milestones of fracture healing, distinguishing how the process differs between stable and unstable fractures.

The formation of cartilage in an unstable fracture may arise because the mobility across the fracture site inhibits angiogenesis (blood vessel formation). Mathematical models predict where stresses will be high in fracture calluses, and such areas correspond with the regions where cartilage develops.[27] This association suggests that high stresses limit vascularization and subsequent bone deposition.

Remodeling of the fracture callus begins as soon as the fracture site regains stability. The dynamics of this remodeling are similar to those that occur in haversian remodeling, in that the old bone is resorbed by osteoclasts, and new bone is deposited by osteoblasts. The process is vigorous in the area where the periosteal callus meets the surface of the old bone. Prior to remodeling, this line is clearly visible, but after remodeling, the junction between the old bone and the callus is indistinguishable.

Factors contributing to fracture nonunion are poorly understood, but instability is thought to result in persistence of the fibrous material and type III collagen, both of which suggest that the fracture healing sequence has been altered. Type III collagen is typically present only during early healing and is indicative of immature callus. Its persistence suggests that the subsequent steps to replace the early tissue are altered. Also, type III collagen may be unable to bind minerals; thus, by persisting, type III collagen may block the mineralization of a newly formed matrix.

MECHANICAL BEHAVIOR OF BONE

CORTICAL BONE

The mechanical behavior of any structure can be assessed in a variety of ways, with each method yielding useful details about bone as a structure. Ostensibly, the method of testing is chosen to assess most closely the loading situation that the structure encounters in vivo. Because bone experiences multiaxial loads, however, it is difficult to test each direction in which a bone is loaded. Cortical bone is frequently treated as an elastic beam of uniform dimension and tested in three- or four-point bending, or a piece of bone of known dimension is machined out of a larger piece and tested in uniaxial tension or compression.

In three-point bending tests, a long bone shaft or a cortical strip of bone rests on two supporting points, while a load from above is applied at the midpoint, thus creating three points of contact (Fig. 7–6). Alternatively, the load from above can be applied at two contact points to produce four-point bending. As the load is applied, the bone sample bends with a compressive strain in the superior surface (concave) and a tension strain in the inferior surface (convex). During bending tests, the distance between the contact points should be maximized so that the loads bend the bone sample rather than crush it. In a typical bending test (see Fig. 7–6), when the bone is first loaded, the load-deformation curve is concave toward the load axis. As load application continues, load and deformation increase linearly (obeying Hooke's law). The slope of this linear region represents the bone's flexural rigidity (a measure of stiffness). The proportional limit indicates the end of the linear region, beyond which small increases in the applied load easily deform the sample. After this area of nonlinear deformation, the sample either reaches its maximum load and fails abruptly or reaches its maximum load and then decreases slightly before catastrophic failure. The area under the load-deformation curve quantifies the energy absorbed by the sample during loading. Each of these measures (stiffness, loads and energy at the proportional limit, and maximum and failure points) constitutes a structural property of the bone. If the geometry of the tested bone sample is known, the structural properties can be "normalized" (e.g., force per unit area) to better understand the

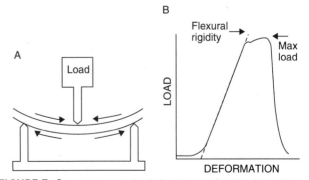

FIGURE 7–6. A structure is loaded in three-point bending (A), generating the load-deformation curve (B).

TABLE 7–1
Elastic Modulus and Stress at the Proportional Limit for Various Bones and Other Materials

Material Tested	Elastic Modulus (GPa)	Stress at Proportional Limit (MPa)	Author
20-yr-old human femur*	17.0	120	Burstein et al[112]
70-yr-old human femur*	16.3	111	Burstein et al[112]
20-yr-old human tibia*	18.9	126	Burstein et al[112]
70-yr-old human tibia*	19.9	120	Burstein et al[112]
8-wk-old chick TMT	–	113	Matsuda et al[49]
Adult rooster TMT	12.8	153	Loitz and Zernicke[56]
16-wk-old canine femur	7.1	60	Torzilli et al[113]
Adult canine femur	15.6	123	Torzilli et al[113]
18-wk-old rat tibia	11.4	146	Li et al[114]
Stainless steel	190.0	500	Beer and Johnston[115]
Wood	12.5	–	Beer and Johnston[115]

*Machined samples, tested in tension.
TMT = tarso metatarsus

behavior of the bone material itself. Elastic moduli and stresses at the proportional limit and at maximum and failure points are examples of a bone's material properties. For comparative purposes, stresses at the proportional limits and elastic moduli of different materials and bones from a variety of species are presented in Table 7–1.

Data recorded from isolated mechanical tests can be "translated" into terms that are relevant to the clinician. During normal, daily activities, bones sustain loads well within the linear region of the load-deformation curve, with the odd event placing high (but not catastrophic) loads on the bone. When loaded within the linear region, the bone bends but does not sustain permanent deformation. However, even within this region, if low loads are sustained repetitively over a short period of time, such as during long-distance running, fatigue-related damage to the bone may result. That is, although each loading cycle alone is not sufficient to cause damage, the cumulative effect of the loading events may result in failure, such as a stress fracture. When loads or stresses exceed the proportional limit, the bone sustains permanent deformation because of substantial microarchitectural damage. The bone elastic modulus is a measure of the resistance of the bone material to being deformed; a more highly mineralized matrix possesses a higher elastic modulus. There is an optimal mechanical balance created by varying the relative amounts of the various matrix components. Bone with a low elastic modulus deforms easily at relatively low loads and may result in permanent skeletal deformity, such as occurs with rickets. Conversely, bone that possesses a high elastic modulus may be too stiff to "give" with the daily loads placed on the skeleton, thereby increasing the risk of fracture.

Bone geometry influences its mechanical behavior. During bending, for example, the distribution of bone about the bending axis (second moment of area equals I) and the distance from the centroid to the tensile surface are pertinent. For example, assume that two bone samples with identical cortical cross-sectional areas are tested (Fig. 7–7). One is a perfect circle (hollow,

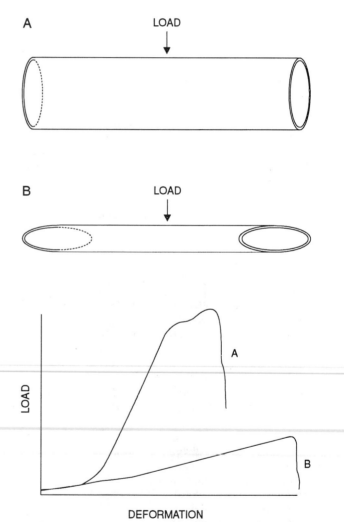

FIGURE 7–7. The hypothetical load-deformation curves that might result from loading a cylinder with uniform mass distribution (A) and a cylinder of nonuniform mass distribution bending about its major axis (B). Note the differences in maximum load and flexural rigidity between the two structures. Second moment of area (I), a mathematical expression of the distribution of cortical mass relative to the bending axis, is significantly greater in A because the distance between the bending axis and the cortical surface is much greater in A.

thick-walled cylinder) with its mass distributed uniformly around a constant radius. The other is an oval-shaped sample of the same total mass but with its mass distributed around a major axis that is twice as long as the minor axis. Even though the masses of the two samples are the same, their structural behavior will be different. But how do the data collected from each test differ? When the oval-shaped sample is tested with the bending occurring about the major axis (smaller I), the bone sample is less stiff and carries less load than the circular sample, or even the oval-shaped sample when tested in bending about the minor axis (larger I) (see Figure 7–7). To illustrate further how mass distribution (I) affects a structure's response during bending, consider the following. Imagine that you are standing, midlength, on a wooden plank (2 meters long by 4 cm thick by 30 cm wide) that is supported only at its two ends; the plank will be much stiffer and carry greater load when you stand (albeit precariously) on the plank's edge (4 cm surface down) than if the 30 cm side is placed down. In a comparable fashion, the redistribution of cortical bone following remodeling is significant because of the influence that geometry has on the bone's mechanical behavior.

Tensile tests of machined cortical samples also produce data for the same mechanical variables as the bending test. The advantage of working with machined samples is that the structural variables can be compared directly between samples because the geometry of each sample is identical. The disadvantage of machined samples is that, although great effort may be made to ensure that the machining does not damage the sample, any change or surface crack that happens as a result of heating of the sample or from a dull or imperfect cutting edge will affect the outcome.

CANCELLOUS BONE

The mechanical behavior of trabecular bone and how its behavior changes during aging and disease are of paramount importance to health care practitioners. In the United States, for example, there are more than 500,000 vertebral fractures, 250,000 hip fractures, and 200,000 distal radius fractures annually. Hip fractures can be fatal in up to 20 percent of these cases.[28] These statistics add an urgent tone to the efforts directed toward understanding trabecular bone mechanics and physiology.

Cancellous bone samples are generally tested in compression. Usually, a sample of trabecular bone is cored from a larger sample and then compressed. The variables measured are similar to those measured in cortical bone tests. The challenge in testing cancellous bone comes in identifying the effects of the trabecular pattern on the mechanical behaviors. The greatest problem comes from the anisotropic nature of cancellous bone; the mechanical behavior of an anisotropic structure differs among various parts of the structure. Trabecular pattern reflects the in vivo loading pattern sustained by the tissue and results in anisotropic mechanical behaviors. For example, if trabeculae are oriented predominantly parallel to the bone's longitudinal axis, a sample tested by loading in a transverse direction will have a very different mechanical response from a sample tested longitudinally.

Cancellous bone can also be tested in a whole bone preparation, such as may be performed on vertebrae or on the femoral neck. In these cases, the contribution of the cortical shell versus the cancellous bone can be quantified by digitizing photographic images of each bone cross section. This approach may be more relevant clinically, because the behavior of the integrated cortical and cancellous structure can be assessed. This approach is of limited utility, however, if the contribution of the cancellous bone alone is of interest.

Recently, Goldstein and associates[29] constructed a miniature system to test single trabeculae in three-point bending. The objective of this testing was to understand the contribution of individual trabeculae to the mechanical behavior of the entire structure. Because of the unique nature of this custom technique, however, its use is not widespread.

REMODELING OF BONE

Adaptation prompted by changes in the mechanical stress state, such as prolonged bed rest, spaceflight, or exercise, forms the basis for much of the research being done in bone physiology and mechanics, with the premise being that if function is altered, the resulting change in structure can be examined. As with most connective tissues, bone possesses strong structure-function interactions.

CELLULAR EVENTS

The remodeling process, by definition, is the resorption and replacement of existing bone. The sequence of events can be remembered as ARF — activation, resorption, formation (Table 7–2). The first step in remodeling is activation of osteoclasts to resorb existing bone. A line of osteoclasts (osteoclastic front) cuts a longitudinal cone through the bone by secreting acid phosphatase, collagenase, and other proteolytic enzymes.[30] The "cutting cone" resorbs approximately three times its volume and, when completed, leaves a resorptive channel 1 to 10 mm deep.[19]

New bone is deposited by osteoblasts that follow the resorptive front. Mineralized matrix is first laid down around the walls of the resorptive channel, forming the cement line. Osteoblasts then fill the remaining volume that was eroded by the osteoclasts. Deposition of new bone is a much slower process than resorption, taking three times longer, despite the fact that osteoblasts can outnumber osteoclasts by more than 200 to 1.[31] The distance between the osteoclasts and osteoblasts translates into the time lapse between resorption and formation. Generally, this latent period is about 1 week.[19] Initially, osteoblasts deposit a nonmineralized matrix that calcifies 8 to 10 days later. In so doing, the

TABLE 7–2
Summary of Modeling-Remodeling Differences

Factor	Modeling	Remodeling
Timing	Continuous	Cyclical (ARF)
Resorption and formation surfaces	Different	Same
Surfaces affected	100%	20%
Activation	Not required	Required
Balance	Net gain	Net loss
Coupling of formation and resorption	Systemic? (no ARF)	Loss

ARF = activation-resorption-formation.
Adapted from Parfitt AM: The cellular basis of bone remodeling: the quantum concept reexamined in light of recent advances in the cell biology of bone. Calcif Tissue Int 1984; 36:S37.

osteoblasts trap themselves within the matrix and become osteocytes.

Generally, skeletal remodeling is triggered in three circumstances: to release mineral stored in the bone in response to a low serum calcium level, to repair skeletal microdamage, and to balance the mechanical and mass needs of the skeleton.[32] Although each circumstance can explain the remodeling stimulus, experimental evidence describing the actual controlling mechanism in each case is lacking. It is difficult to conceive how the body's need for calcium, for example, could result in the site-specific, reproducible pattern of bone resorption that is seen.

Most commonly, in true remodeling, bone resorption and deposition are sequential events, and the responsible cells (osteoclasts and osteoblasts) are located within the same functional framework—the basic multicellular unit (BMU).[33] This "functional unit" reinforces the concept of the tightly coupled interaction between resorption and deposition, and current theory suggests that resting osteoblasts (bone-lining cells) are responsible for initiating the remodeling process and recruiting the osteoclasts to begin resorption.[21] In another example of coupled osteoclast-osteoblast activity, the respective cells are not active along the same surface. In modeling (change in bone architecture when bone deposition does not follow bone resorption), resorption occurs along one cortex, and deposition occurs along another (see Table 7–2). Because osteoclasts and osteoblasts do not populate the same bony areas, the stimulus that initiates this process is unclear.

Several observations support the role of mechanical stimuli in bone remodeling, including: (1) bone is always lost when mechanical stimuli are greatly reduced or eliminated (i.e., stress magnitude is decreased); (2) a change in the distribution of stresses on the bone stimulates adaptive remodeling; and (3) although the quantity of bone at various sites may be altered by varying mechanical stimuli, the quality of the bone matrix being deposited generally remains similar for all sites. That is, in response to mechanical stimuli, the body changes the quantity of bone but not its composition.

One of the prevailing theories of bone remodeling is the "mechanostat theory" postulated by Frost.[34] Frost suggests that a sensor exists within bone to monitor the mechanical usage of the bone and to adjust any imbalance between the mechanical usage and bone mass. The sensor establishes a "set point" or threshold, called the "minimum effective strain" (MES), that dictates the resorption-deposition balance. There are basically two ways to initiate remodeling. The first occurs when an imbalance exists between the MES and the daily mechanical use of the skeleton. Increased strains, such as those occurring during exercise, can slow bone remodeling and increase bone deposition. Second, the MES can be readjusted by various systemic factors, including serum concentrations of various hormones, or by disease or genetic factors. When any of these factors alters the set point, bone remodeling adjusts so that the mechanical behavior of the bone agrees with the new MES. For example, in the absence of estrogens, the MES may be raised, such that the mechanostat recognizes an excess of bone mass (i.e., strain is too low). In response, bone resorption exceeds deposition, resulting in a net loss of bone mass, an increase in strain close to the MES threshold, and the re-establishment of a new mechanostat set point. The mechanostat theory predicts that remodeling is stimulated by decreased mechanical usage (with a net loss of bone mass) and is inhibited by increased mechanical usage (with a net increase in bone mass).

In a similar vein, Lanyon[35] described functional remodeling as an "interpretation and purposeful reaction" to a bone's strain state, allowing for adaptation to both increased and decreased strains. "Functional strains are both the objective and the stimulus for the process of adaptive modeling and remodeling."[35] Rubin and Lanyon[36] hypothesized that if functional strains were too high, the incidence of damage and probability of failure increased. If strains were too low, the metabolic cost of maintaining unnecessary bone mass was too high. Thus, functional strain appeared to be a relevant parameter to control. The question remains, however, which attribute of strain (magnitude, rate of application, distribution, or gradient) has the greatest sensitivity.

Another remodeling theory related to mechanical use of the bone suggests that remodeling is stimulated by fatigue damage that occurs during physical activity. In an engineering sense, "fatigue" is the loss of strength and stiffness that occurs in materials subjected to repeated cyclic loads. In bone, fatigue has been attributed to the microscopic cracks that develop within and between the osteons.[1] In healthy bone, if damage is not excessive, remodeling resorbs the material around the crack, and new bone is deposited. If the damage is excessive and the normal remodeling process cannot keep up with the repair, macroscopic failure and fracture may result. Clinically, the accumulation of fatigue microdamage may result in a stress fracture, an injury common to athletes participating in activities that place highly repetitive, cyclic loads on the weight-bearing bones, such as ballet dancers, gymnasts, and long-distance runners.

The mechanism linking microcracks to cellular activation and remodeling remains controversial. Martin and Burr[1] suggest that when a crack propagates along a cement line, the osteon surrounded by the cement line becomes isolated from mechanical stresses. The resulting lack of mechanical stimuli may be likened to that which occurs during bed rest, immobilization, or spaceflight. A cutting cone would be initiated within the osteon, and new bone would be deposited. In contrast, Frost[37] argues that cracks disrupt the canalicular network and trigger a cellular membrane response. The osteocytes then initiate the signal to begin remodeling of the damaged matrix. Evidence exists in support of both postulates, and research is proceeding toward resolving this question.

Clinical evidence suggests that electrical phenomena alter remodeling and fracture repair and supports the premise that electrical effects may be important in the information transfer between mechanical deformation and cellular response. Although the mechanisms responsible for the production of electrical potentials are unknown, two possible sources of electrical phenomena exist—piezoelectricity and streaming potentials.

During deformation, crystals with a lattice structure and no central symmetry develop a net charge between the anions and cations. This charge separation causes a potential difference (piezoelectric potential) to develop between opposite ends of the crystal. Wet collagen within bone can act like a crystalline lattice when deformed, thus generating piezoelectric potentials in bone. The marked directionality of the piezoelectric potential is consistent with the different potentials generated in bone during compression versus tension.

Streaming potentials are generated when an ionized fluid flows through channels in a solid that carries a surface charge. As the fluid flows, ions from the fluid are attracted to the oppositely charged surface and form a charged layer along the surface. The remaining ions in the fluid create a charge of opposite polarity, and as the fluid flows, a current is generated. For example, if the surface charge along the walls of a channel is negative, positive ions will be attracted from the fluid and create a slow-moving, positively charged layer along the outer edges of the channel. The negative ions remaining in the fluid will accumulate in the middle of the channel, thereby creating a negatively charged current in the channel. Extracellular fluid in bone is charged and tends to move during deformation, thus developing streaming potentials.

Lanyon and Hartman[38] noted that when bending a sample of wet bone, the tensile surface developed a net positive charge, and the compressive surface carried a negative charge. The difference between the surface charges was dependent on both the rate and the magnitude of deformation. When the same magnitude load was applied statically rather than cyclically, the potential decayed to zero within a few seconds.[39] Eriksson[40] postulated that the polarization created during bending was a result of the decrease in fluid channel diameters on the compressive side, forcing the charged extracellular fluid to flow toward the open, tensile surface channels. This explanation is consistent with earlier data that static bending does not generate potentials and with the differential sensitivities to strain rate and magnitude.

Rubin and colleagues[41] examined the effectiveness of pulsed electromagnetic fields in preventing disuse osteoporosis. When the midshaft of a turkey ulna was stress-shielded by isolating it from the bony ends, cortical mass decreased 13 percent in 8 weeks. However, if the experimental stress-shielded limb was exposed to a daily 1-hour dose of electromagnetic current, the ulna mass increased 23 percent over the same time interval. The investigators suggested that electrical potentials generated by the electromagnetic current may have influenced cell activity, similar to the influences created by strain-related potentials generated during bending. This was the first published study of a dose-response relationship describing electrically induced osteogenesis.

Following fracture, the developing callus becomes electronegative with respect to the ends, suggesting that electrical currents may be used to enhance fracture healing.[42] The first reported use of electrical current in the management of nonunion was reported by Brighton and colleagues in 1977.[43] In this study, they reported an 84 percent success rate among 164 patients with 171 fractures. Since this early report, several studies have been conducted with reported success rates of greater than 50 percent.[44,45] In each study, the osteogenic range for stimulation has consistently been 1 to 10 mV/cm and 10 to 20 μA/cm^2. Currently, ongoing studies focus not only on the mechanism responsible for enhanced healing but also on whether electromagnetic fields can be used to enhance healing in fresh fractures as well as in those in which healing is delayed.[44]

EXERCISE-INDUCED CHANGES IN BONE

Exercise-related increases in cortical thickness[46,47] and bone mineral content[48] suggest that exercise can be a potent stimulus for bone remodeling. Over the past several years, exercise models have become a more common means for studying the influence of mechanical overload on bone remodeling. Interestingly, many studies suggest that the responses to similar exercise protocols differ between mature and immature (open physes) animals.

In growing chicks, 9 weeks of moderately strenuous exercise increased the cortical cross-sectional area of a weight-bearing bone (the tarsometatarsus, or TMT) but did not increase maximum bone strength.[49] In addition, the exercise apparently delayed longitudinal bone growth, as the TMTs of the exercised chicks were significantly shorter than those of the age-matched, sedentary controls. Forwood and Parker[50] described similar findings in growing rats. After a 1-month training program, tibial and femoral lengths were significantly less for the exercised animals compared with the sedentary controls. Also, the proximal epiphyseal cartilage in the tibia was thinner in the exercised rats, and the bones absorbed less energy to failure. These studies suggest that in growing animals, "competition" between exercise- and growth-related stimuli may alter the normal rate of calcification and longitudinal growth; in these animal models, growing bone did not benefit from strenuous exercise.

In cancellous bone, Hou and associates[51] examined the effects of strenuous exercise on the femoral neck and L-6 vertebral body in rats. After 10 weeks of training at 75 to 80 percent of maximum aerobic capacity, the material properties of the femoral neck were significantly diminished compared with sedentary controls. An increase in the percentage of trabecular bone, with a concomitant decrease in the cortical shell in the exercised femoral necks, apparently contributed to the detrimental changes. In contrast, no exercise-related changes in the lumbar vertebrae were noted.

Thus, *strenuous* endurance exercise can adversely affect the mechanical integrity of immature bone, but it is unclear whether a more moderate exercise regimen would have a positive effect. To investigate the response of immature trabecular bone to *moderate* exercise, Salem and coworkers[52] randomly assigned young female Sprague-Dawley rats (8 weeks old) to a basal-control, exercise, or age-matched control group. The basal-control rats were euthanized at 8 weeks of age, and the other two groups were euthanized at 18 weeks of age. Between 8 and 18 weeks, one group remained sedentary and the other group was trained progressively on a motor-driven treadmill at a moderate level of intensity. The femoral necks (FN) and the sixth lumbar vertebral bodies (L-6) were mechanically tested, and the bones were analyzed for calcium, hydroxyproline (to indicate collagen concentration), collagen cross-linking concentrations, and changes in geometry. L-6 calcium content, compressional stress, and elastic modulus were significantly less in the exercise group as compared with the age-matched sedentary group. Nonreducible collagen cross-links (hydroxylysylpyridinoline [HP] and lysylpyridinoline [LP] were significantly greater in the L-6 and FN of the older exercise and age-matched control groups. In the weight-bearing FN—but not L-6—the LP concentration in the exercise group was significantly greater than in the age-matched controls. FN mechanical properties were not affected significantly by the exercise regimen. Figure 7–8 illustrates the trend seen in the maximal load of the FN versus the L-6 vertebra between the age-matched control animals and the exercised group.

In discussing their results, Salem and colleagues[52] note that although both FN and L-6 are loaded during running in the rat, the FN must adjust to repetitive weight-bearing loads. During moderate exercise, the FN may be more influenced by mechanical loading than by

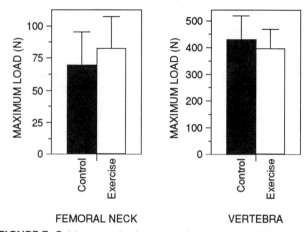

FIGURE 7–8. Maximum load, measured in newtons, of the rat femoral neck *(left)* and L_6 vertebrae *(right)* from age-matched, sedentary control animals and exercised animals. Note that exercise effects differ between the weight-bearing femoral neck and the vertebrae that has a less important weight-bearing role. Values are means ±SD. (Adapted from Salem GJ, Zernicke RF, Martinez DA, et al: Adaptations of immature trabecular bone to moderate exercise: geometrical, biochemical, and biomechanical correlates. Bone 1993; 14:647.)

systemic effects, to produce little net effect on FN mechanical properties. In contrast, L-6 may be more sensitive to systemic influences than to mechanical loading influences, with a resulting decrease in calcium concentration and L-6 material properties. These suggestions agree with the results of Seeman and colleagues[53] who found that glucocorticoids preferentially affected the axial skeleton rather than the appendicular skeleton, and with McDonald and coworkers,[54] who found that immature weight-bearing bones were sensitive to increased loading and immature non-weight-bearing bones were less sensitive to increased loads. Thus, endurance training of moderate intensity can have a mixed effect on the mechanical properties and matrix composition of immature L-6 and FN. These responses to exercise in growing bone suggest an intricate interplay between local mechanical effects and systemic factors that drive the adaptations in the bone.

Generalization of animal-based research to humans must be done cautiously because of differences in, for example, life span, basic physiology, and movement mechanics. These limitations notwithstanding, findings from the above-cited studies agree, generally, with human studies examining activity and skeletal mass in children, although such studies are limited in scope because of ethical restrictions on the types of data that can be collected from humans. As part of a longitudinal study, Slemenda and associates[55] enrolled 59 pairs of twins (5.3 to 14 years of age) and obtained self-reports and reports from the mothers regarding the youngsters' activity patterns. Bone mineral densities of the distal radius, proximal femur, and lumbar spine were assessed with single- and dual-photon absorptiometry. These authors reported a high positive correlation between the hours spent in weight-bearing activities and the density of the femur and radius. Vertebral density also correlated to activity, but the relationship was not as strong. Slemenda and coworkers concluded "that more active children may emerge from adolescence with

5–10% greater bone mass, depending on skeletal site. This may represent an important advantage in terms of peak skeletal mass, and this advantage may persist throughout adult life."[55]

The effects of strenuous exercise on mature bone (ceased longitudinal growth) are different from those on growing bone. In a follow-up to an earlier study that examined the effects of strenuous exercise on growing chick bone,[47] the authors examined the effects of a similar strenuous training program on the tarsometatarsus (TMT) of mature roosters.[56] The exercised birds ran a total of more than 150 km over the 9-week training program. When compared with those of age-matched, sedentary control birds, the exercised TMTs had similar cortical areas, but the medial and anterior cortices were thicker than those of the controls. None of the mechanical properties differed significantly between the exercise and sedentary groups. During treadmill walking, however, the in vivo strains recorded along the TMT anterior cortex were significantly greater (13 percent) in the exercised birds than in the sedentary roosters, suggesting that strain may not be the primary objective for bone remodeling. Although remodeling may have been driven by the need to maintain strain within an optimal range, the maximum amount of bone tissue that could be deposited to accomplish that goal may have been tempered by the need to minimize metabolic cost. Because exercise was the remodeling stimulus in this study, energy expenditure during running was a relevant parameter for the bird to minimize. If there was no limit on the mass of the bone, the exercised birds may have developed thick-walled, heavy bones in an effort to decrease strain. Metabolically, this solution would not be optimal. Therefore, the resulting adaptation may have represented a compromise between the desire to maintain optimal strains and the need to minimize energy expenditure.

Jee and colleagues[57] recently undertook a comprehensive study examining the effects of overload on the rat tibia. One hind limb of each rat (9 months old) was taped to the animal's abdomen so that the limb could not be used for weight bearing, and the contralateral hind limb was forced to sustain all the loads normally shared between the hind limbs. The geometry, mass distribution, and remodeling dynamics of the overloaded tibia were assessed after 2, 10, 18, or 26 weeks. Over these intervals, cortical area increased gradually in the overloaded bones, with a significant increase (10 percent) after 26 weeks. In the sedentary controls, endosteal resorption resulted in a significant increase in the bone endosteal diameter at each interval. This normal, age-related remodeling was altered in the overloaded bones, with the endosteal diameter remaining similar to the baseline throughout the entire 26 weeks. By comparing the relative positions and amount of fluorochrome labels incorporated into the bone, the degree of subperiosteal remodeling was also quantified. Their analysis revealed that the overload stimulus slowed the remodeling of existing bone and increased the rate of new bone deposition, resulting in a net increase in subperiosteal bone. The authors suggested that their data supported the mechanostat theory of Frost[34]—the increased mechanical use of the limb slowed age-related bone loss and increased the deposition of new bone around the periosteal surface.

STRESS FRACTURES

Although bone requires mechanical loads in order to maintain its mineral mass and strength, repetitive loading may result in structural failure, despite the magnitude of each loading cycle being within the physiological range. Historically, "march fracture" has been used to describe bone failure resulting from repetitive loading cycles.[58] This term identifies the high incidence of fracture among military recruits who spend many hours marching on hard surfaces without resilient footwear.[59,60] More recently, two terms have been used to describe distinct phases of this overuse injury. "Stress reaction" describes the series of pathophysiologic changes that occur with repetitive loading, and "stress fracture" is the structural failure of bone that may follow a stress reaction and results in a radiographically evident fracture line.[61]

Stress fracture risk was assessed recently by the authors in a multidisciplinary study in California. During the 1989–90 academic year at the University of California, Los Angeles (UCLA), 4.7 percent of the male and female intercollegiate athletes reported having had a stress fracture during that year or the prior year. However, among the runners on the women's cross-country and track teams, the incidence was 25 percent. These data provided the impetus for a larger ongoing study to examine the risk factors among women runners and to develop a risk profile that may assist the athletes, coaches, and medical personnel in identifying athletes who are prone to fracture.

Although the UCLA study is ongoing, the preliminary findings suggest that stress fracture etiology is a complex interaction among several factors, including mechanical (e.g., kinetic variables during running),[58] systemic (e.g., menstrual function),[62] dietary (calcium intake),[63] and psychosocial behaviors (e.g., eating disorders). The lack of a single causative factor makes it difficult to identify athletes at risk of sustaining stress fractures. Additionally, many of the individuals prone to fracture are highly trained elite athletes or highly motivated military personnel who may tend to "run through the pain," thereby preventing the medical team from managing the symptoms of a stress reaction before a frank stress fracture develops.

Jones and coworkers[61] proposed a grading system to assist in the accurate diagnosis of stress reaction and stress fracture. By standardizing the terminology, they also sought to facilitate identification of the actual incidence of such injuries among athletes. In this schema (Table 7–3), several clinical tools are used in forming a diagnosis: bone scan, plane x-ray, clinical symptoms (pain and tenderness, palpable mass), and history of recent increase in activity intensity or duration.

Treatment of a stress fracture generally follows two phases. Phase I consists primarily of therapeutic modalities aimed at pain reduction (ice, nonsteroidal anti-inflammatory medications) and reduced weight-bearing aerobic activities, such as swimming and run-

TABLE 7–3
Classification Scheme for Diagnosis of Stress Reaction and Stress Fracture

Grade 0	Grade 1	Grade 2	Grade 3	Grade 4
Normal remodeling	Mild stress reaction	Moderate stress reaction	Severe stress reaction	Stress fracture
Detectable by bone scan	Positive bone scan; undetectable on plane x-ray	Positive bone scan; minimal change on plane x-ray	Positive bone scan; positive plane x-ray	Positive bone scan; positive plane x-ray
	No structural compromise	No structural compromise	Structural changes evident	Structural failure
Asymptomatic	Local pain during activity; no pain at rest	Local pain during activity; tender to palpation	Significant pain does not abate after cessation of activity; palpable mass	Extreme pain with weight bearing

Adapted from Jones BH, Harris JM, Vinh TN, et al: Exercise-induced stress fractures and stress reactions of bone: epidemiology, etiology, and classifications. Exerc Sport Sci Rev 1989; 17:379; and Grimston SK, Zernicke RF: Exercise-related stress responses in bone. J Appl Biomech 1993; 9:2.

ning in water. After 3 weeks of pain-free participation in phase I activities, the individual begins phase II by gradually increasing weight-bearing activities and continues the modalities for pain management. Matheson and associates[64] reported that among 320 athletes with stress fractures, average rehabilitation time was 13 weeks from diagnosis to resumption of full activities. A recent report by Whitelaw and colleagues[65] suggests that the rehabilitation time can be reduced significantly to 3.6 weeks with the use of pneumatic leg braces during weight-bearing activities. The brace appears to act as a dynamic splint that provides enough support to the injured extremity to allow healing without substantial curtailment of weight-bearing activities. Multicenter studies examining the use of pneumatic braces are currently ongoing.

DISUSE-RELATED CHANGES IN BONE

Disuse-related changes in bone are commonly associated with bed rest, immobilization, or spaceflight. Animal studies examining disuse changes in bone suggest that lack of regular load bearing prompts remodeling in a variety of ways. Loads can be diminished through neurectomy, tenotomy, or cast or pinned-joint immobilization. Regardless of the specific methodology, however, the effects of disuse are profound. Disuse results in a substantially increased resorption and decreased deposition. Weinreb and colleagues[66] reported that bone resorption in a rat model increased dramatically within 30 hours after tenotomy or neurectomy because of a significant increase in the number of osteoclasts per millimeter of bone surface. A sustained decrease in the rates of both bone formation and mineral apposition contributed to a marked decrease in trabecular bone volume and bone mineral content at the end of the 42-day experiment.

Because disuse changes are comparatively clear-cut and immobilization may be unavoidable in certain circumstances, of greater clinical relevance is whether disuse-related changes can be reversed by remobiliza-

tion. Using a rat tibia and femur, Tuukkanen and colleagues[67] examined the effects of 1 or 3 weeks of immobilization followed by 3 weeks of remobilization. After 3 weeks of immobilization, tibial and femoral ash weights decreased (9 to 12 percent) compared with nonimmobilized controls, with the tibia and femur demonstrating similar losses. After remobilization, the tibia recovered 62 percent of its mineral mass, and the femur regained only 38 percent. The shorter immobilization period resulted in an improved recovery of mineral mass, although full return was not demonstrated. These data suggest that mineral loss prompted by immobilization can be reversed to some extent, although recovery does not occur rapidly. The degree of recovery is related to the duration of the immobilization. Clinically, the impact of these data is reflected, to some degree, in the recent surge in the use of fracture braces and early mobilization in the management of orthopaedic trauma.

Spaceflight induces similar dramatic changes in both cortical and trabecular bone. Interesting, as well, are the suggestions that weight-bearing bones may be more sensitive to decreased mechanical usage than non-weight-bearing or axial bones. Three-point bending tests of the tibia and humerus from rats after a 1-week spaceflight revealed a decrease in bone stiffness and strength, with the tibial changes more dramatic than those of the humerus.[68] In addition, the animals used in this study were rapidly growing, and the absence of mechanical loads appeared to delay the maturation of the humerus but not the tibia. These findings support the theory that the mechanical threshold that triggers remodeling may be bone specific, a premise supported by the extensive work of Biewener and colleagues,[69] who demonstrated site-specific optimal strains in growing chicks.

Trabecular bone appears to react to spaceflight with decreased stiffness and strength, as noted in rat lumbar vertebrae after 12.5 days in space.[70] The concentration of mature collagen cross-links was also diminished in the spaceflight rats compared with the earth-reared controls, indicating that bone maturation may have slowed during the flight. Similar to the above-noted relevance of remobilization, the pertinent question is whether these marked detrimental changes can be minimized during flight. This question continues to be investigated.

DISEASE-RELATED CHANGES IN BONE

DIABETES

In clinical studies with humans[71–76] and experimental studies with animals,[77–82] diabetic osteopathy has been reported, with diabetes-related effects being more pronounced in insulin-dependent (type I) diabetic patients. Non-insulin-dependent (type II) diabetic patients have more variable results.[73,83] Mechanical deterioration of diabetic bone has been reported for the femoral shaft[78,84] and femoral neck,[78] but the specific relationship between severity of diabetes and extent of osteopathy remains equivocal. McNair and colleagues[85] found a correlation between osteopenia and blood glucose level, but other clinical studies did not find such a relationship.[86,87] Schwartz and coworkers[88] indicated that bone growth, formation, and calcification decreased with glucose concentrations higher than 200 mg/dL, but the changes gradually reached a steady state. These mixed findings may, in part, be a consequence of the different severities and durations used in studies and the difficulties in establishing an adequate clinical control group, as diabetic patients vary widely in diets, treatment regimens, environment, and physical activity levels.

Animal studies indicate that severe diabetes can retard bone growth and development,[89] and the serum from diabetic rats with high glucose levels can retard the growth of rat fetuses in culture.[90] In one study,[79] it was shown that moderate type I diabetes can deleteriously affect rat femoral neck mechanical properties. Insulinopenia may account for these growth retardation effects,[84,91,92] as recent studies have shown that the potent effects of growth factors in bone (e.g., insulin-like growth factors I and II) are highly similar to insulin.[93,94] Indeed, with moderately diabetic rats, insulin therapy ameliorated growth-retardation effects on bone.[79]

More recently, the authors investigated the relation between the severity of diabetes and degree of osteopenia in rats.[80] The interactive effects of diabetes and insulin therapy on the geometric, biomechanical, and histomorphologic characteristics of the femoral neck in streptozotocin-induced insulin-dependent (type I) diabetic rats were studied. Female Sprague-Dawley rats (8 weeks old) were randomly assigned to one of three groups: control (C), severe diabetes (SDM), and severe diabetes with insulin treatment (SDI). Rats with severe insulin-dependent diabetes had significantly lower total body mass than controls, as well as significantly less femur mass, femur length, total bone cross-sectional area, and cortical shell cross-sectional area. Insulin therapy ameliorated some, but not all, of the detrimental effects of diabetes on femoral neck geometry. Compared with C and SDI rats, SDM rats had lower

femoral neck structural properties. SDM rats had significantly greater porosity in the femoral neck cortex than control rats.

Decrements in material properties of the rat femoral neck were linearly correlated with diabetic severity (blood glucose level), and insulin therapy mitigated diabetic osteopathy (Fig. 7–9). The data suggest that there are clear severity-related changes in diabetic bone—with the material properties being the most directly and adversely affected.[79,80]

OSTEOPOROSIS

Aging alone causes changes in the intracortical bones of people.[1] Most of these changes are associated with the BMU remodeling system, and their effects are found in the age-dependent alterations in bone geometry, size, and number of osteons.[1] As indicated earlier, bone at the tissue level undergoes remodeling; bone is continually resorbed and re-formed.[95] A negative balance between bone resorption and formation (in many cases related to excessive resorption) is the basic mechanism associated with many bone diseases.[95] Generally, increased age is associated with increased bone porosity. Increased porosity can be associated with increased numbers of haversian canals, more resorption spaces and incomplete refilling of osteons, and larger haversian canals.[1] Furthermore, cortical bone typically becomes weaker and slightly more brittle with increasing age.[1]

Osteoporosis is a disease characterized by reduced bone mineral mass and changes in bone's structural geometry. It is strongly associated with an increased probability of fractures, primarily of the hip, spine, and wrist.[96] Although it is recognized that osteoporosis is widely prevalent, the incidence of the disease is not well documented.[97] Praemer and colleagues[96] indicate that part of the difficulty associated with determining the prevalence of osteoporosis is that (1) some progressive loss of bone mass is a function of the normal aging process, (2) loss of bone can be caused by other disease processes, and (3) the amount of bone mass at one site is

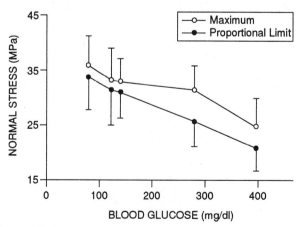

FIGURE 7–9. Relationship between the normal stress of the femoral neck at the proportional limit and maximum, and blood glucose levels. Values are means ±SD. (From Hou JC-H, Zernicke RF, Barnard J: Effects of severe diabetes and insulin on the femoral neck of the immature rat. J Orthop Res 1993; 11:263.)

not necessarily correlated with bone mass at other sites in the body. Currently, there are no internationally recognized survey data using objective diagnostic criteria for osteoporosis. Nevertheless, a recent longitudinal study on aging from the National Center for Health Statistics (United States) reported the prevalence of osteoporosis and hip fractures in individuals 70 years of age and older (Table 7–4). These data are probably an underestimate because they come from "self-reports" and lack radiologic detection. Many individuals are unaware of the existence of osteoporosis, particularly in the early stages.

Although standard radiographic techniques can be used to assess the degree of osteoporotic bone loss qualitatively, quantification of bone mineral content and the subsequent prediction of fracture risk due to osteoporosis require the use of quantitative computed tomography (QCT).[98] QCT provides a measure of the trabecular bone mass of the vertebrae or other sites with predominantly trabecular bone.

The mean normal vertebral mineral mass for young males and females is 175 mg/cm^3. By age 75, men have lost an average of 40 percent of that mineral mass (110 mg/cm^3); at the same age, women have lost 50 percent (approximately 90 mg/cm^3).[98] The fracture threshold has been estimated to be 110 mg/cm^3, with the fracture risk being low for individuals with mineral mass greater than the threshold. Although this is only an estimation and there is considerable overlap in vertebral mineral mass between normal women and those who have sustained atraumatic (non-accident-related) fracture, it can be used as a general guideline to assess fracture risk. QCT has also been useful in studies comparing vertebral mineral mass between amenorrheic elite athletes and cohorts with normal menstrual function.[99] The amenorrheic athletes were found to have 20 to 25 percent less mineral mass than the normal women, suggesting that estrogen deprivation has a powerful effect on trabecular mineral mass.

Hip fractures resulting from osteoporosis have significant social impact in terms of disability, medical costs, and mortality.[96–100] An estimated 250,000 hip fractures occur each year in the United States alone.[96,100] Because the frequency of hip fractures is rapidly increasing among the population, it is becoming a greater public health concern.[96] In addition to contributing substantially to morbidity and disability within the older population, hip fractures are associated with increased mortality for years after the fracture.[97] Based on census projections in the United States, there will be an estimated 340,000 hip fractures by the year 2000 and more than 650,000 hip fractures by the year 2050; half of these will be in individuals 85 years of age and older.[101,102] After the age of 50, there is an almost exponential increase in the incidence of hip fractures, with an approximate doubling of the incidence of fracture for every 5- to 6-year increase in age.[96,101] Of those who survive hip fractures, up to 50 percent may spend time in a long-term care setting.[96,97] Of those individuals who were living at home and independently prior to the fracture, approximately 20 percent remained in long-term institutions for at least a year after the fracture. Those people who sustained hip fractures had approximately a 15 percent higher mortality rate in the first year after the fracture compared with people of comparable ages, and most of those deaths occurred within the first 4 months after the fracture.[96,97]

Both men and women experience some loss of bone mass during normal aging, but osteoporosis progresses much more rapidly in postmenopausal women.[103] After 30 years of age, men typically lose bone mass at approximately the same rate for the remainder of their lives. In women, however, the loss of bone increases significantly for about 5 years after menopause and then slows to a more gradual loss.[103] Just after menopause, the rate of bone mass loss is up to 10 times faster in women than in men of the same age.[103] To retard the rapid loss of bone in postmenopausal women, therapeutic interventions and exercise have been proposed. In premenopausal adult women, the rates of bone formation and bone resorption are approximately equal, calcium balance is maintained, and there is no effective loss of bone mass.[104] After menopause, however, bone formation and resorption rates increase, but the rate of bone resorption increases more rapidly and produces a calcium imbalance and a net loss of bone.[103] One of the goals of osteoporosis prevention is to restore bone resorption and formation rates to premenopausal levels.

TABLE 7–4
Prevalence of Self-Reported Osteoporosis and Hip Fracture in Persons 70 Years of Age and Older: United States, 1984

Age and Gender	Type of Impairment (per 100 Persons)		
	Osteoporosis	Hip Fracture	Either Condition
Total (70 yr and older)	3.7	4.5	7.7
70–79 yr	3.5	3.2	6.2
80 yr and older	4.3	8.0	11.6
Male	0.6	2.7	3.3
70–79 yr	0.7	1.9	2.5
80 yr and older	0.4	5.5	5.9
Female	5.7	5.6	10.5
70–79 yr	5.5	4.0	8.8
80 yr and older	6.2	9.2	14.4

Source: U.S. National Center for Health Statistics, Longitudinal Study on Aging. Adapted from Praemer A, Furner S, Rice D: Musculoskeletal Conditions in the United States. Park Ridge, IL, American Academy of Orthopaedic Surgeons, 1992.

Various preventive and therapeutic agents are currently being used and investigated in the treatment of osteoporosis. Most researchers now agree that hormone replacement therapy, using estrogen alone or estrogen plus progesterone, may prevent osteoporosis in postmenopausal women.[104,105] In addition, Nilas and Christiansen[104] indicate that other treatments, including fluoride, calcitonin, bisphosphonates, and vitamin D metabolites, may exert a positive influence by decreasing the age-related loss of bone. Rodan[95] indicates that, among those therapeutic agents that inhibit bone resorption, only calcitonin and bisphosphonates have been shown to act directly on osteoclasts. Other hormones and agents influence bone turnover by acting on osteoblasts or cells of the osteoblast lineage. A significant amount of ongoing research continues in the area of bone metabolism, as bone is responsive to a host of influences, including parathyroid hormones, glucocorticoids, vitamin D, sex steroids, insulin, prostaglandins, growth factors, and many cytokines.

Frost[106] recently discussed the pathogenesis of osteoporosis in terms of mechanical usage. He indicates that decreased mechanical usage stops the deposition of bone by modeling and increases the removal of bone next to the marrow by remodeling. More data are becoming available that indicate that regular exercise may have a positive impact on bone mass and that there may be increased trabecular bone density as a result of exercise that specifically loads the affected bones in postmenopausal women.[107]

Recently, Snow-Harter and Marcus[108] wrote an extensive paper reviewing the relations among exercise, bone mineral density, and osteoporosis. Among the numerous issues presented, they summarized information about physical activity and bone mass from cross-sectional and interventional studies. Cross-sectional studies usually involve an assessment of an active versus a sedentary group of people at a single point in time. Generally, cross-sectional data reveal a positive correlation between activity level and bone mineral density,[109,110] although the duration, frequency, and intensity of the exercise regimen are often not detailed, and there are many confounding factors associated with the differences that are reported.

Interventional studies are prospective studies that assess the effect of an exercise program on bone mineral density. Snow-Harter and Marcus,[108] after reviewing a wide range of studies, concluded that, generally, there is a good indication that bone mineral density is enhanced as a result of an exercise program, but the effects are "site specific." Furthermore, it is still unknown which exercise *best* promotes bone density.[108] Running, jogging, and walking are usually the types of exercise prescribed to ameliorate bone loss related to menopause, but Snow-Harder and Marcus[108] suggest that exercise with higher loads at specific sites may provide a greater osteogenic response.

With physical training, it is well known that muscle mass and strength can increase. Discovering the interrelation between muscle strength and bone mineral density has become a target of more recent research.[109,111] Although there generally appears to be a site specificity between muscle strength and bone

mineral density, in some cases, postural and axial muscles apparently exert beneficial forces on bones.[108]

Snow-Harter and Marcus[108] state that the efficacy of exercise in preventing and treating osteoporosis is unknown. They summarize the known information, however, by answering the following questions: (1) Can exercise maximize peak bone mass? (2) Can exercise forestall or reduce age-related bone losses? (3) Does exercise enhance bone mineral density in those people with existing osteoporosis? (4) Can exercise replace estrogen replacement therapy during the postmenopausal years? Given reasonable caveats, the answer is positive to the first three questions. The answer to the fourth question, however, is no. To date, there is no basis to state that exercise alone is superior to estrogen replacement for maintaining bone mass and reducing the fracture risk for postmenopausal women.[108]

SUMMARY

Skeletal biology is the focus of substantial ongoing research, and it is impossible to summarize the essence of the field in a single chapter. However, within the context of sports medicine and rehabilitation, the authors have selected specific topics that are both pertinent and of interest to clinicians and sports medicine specialists. In a few words, the material presented here can be summarized as follows: Bone is a dynamic and highly complex organ that plays an integral role in many of the normal metabolic processes of the body. The close coupling that exists between bone and the external mechanical environment dictates that change in one will influence the other: a bone fracture changes the response of the tissue to mechanical load, and, conversely, change in the mechanical environment stimulates adaptation. Such interaction is particularly relevant clinically, because it is toward this that many therapeutic interventions are directed.

The goal of this chapter is to provide the clinician with a basic tool to which he or she can refer when reviewing research studies that describe bone adaptation or healing. In addition, the material is intended to help the clinician tie his or her clinical knowledge and skills to the ongoing basic research being done in this area. The materials referenced in the chapter are current and provide a good reference base to which the reader can turn if additional, in-depth study is desired.

REFERENCES

1. Martin RB, Burr DB: Structure, Function, and Adaptation of Compact Bone. New York, Raven Press, 1989.
2. Ogden JA, Grogan DP: Prenatal development and growth of the musculoskeletal system. *In* Albright JA, Brand RA (eds): The Scientific Basis of Orthopaedics, 2nd ed. Norwalk, CT, Appleton-Lange, 1987, p 47.
3. Ogden JA, Grogan DP, Light TR: Postnatal development and growth of the musculoskeletal system. *In* Albright JA, Brand RA (eds): The Scientific Basis of Orthopaedics, 2nd ed. Norwalk, CT, Appleton-Lange, 1987, p 91.
4. Caplan AI: Bone development. *In* Wiley J (ed): Cell and

Molecular Biology of Vertebrate Hard Tissues. Chichester, CIBA Foundation Symposium, 1988, p 3.

5. Carter DR, Fyhrie DP, Whalen R, et al: Control of chondro-osseous skeletal biology by mechanical energy. *In* Biomechanics: Principles and Applications, Proceedings of the European Society of Biomechanics. Amsterdam, Martinus Nijhoff, 1986, p 88.

6. Ogden JA: Anatomy and physiology of skeletal development. *In* Ogden JA (ed): Skeletal Injury in the Child, 2nd ed. Toronto, WB Saunders, 1990, p 42.

7. Muscher E, Desaulles PA, Schenk R: Experimental studies on tensile strength of and morphology of the epiphyseal cartilage at puberty. Ann Pediatr 1965; 205:112.

8. Ogden JA: Injury to the growth mechanisms. *In* Ogden JA (ed): Skeletal Injury in the Child, 2nd ed. Toronto, WB Saunders, 1990, p 97.

9. Holtrop ME: Light and electron microscopic structure of bone-forming cells. *In* Hall BK (ed): Bone, vol 1. Boca Raton, CRC Press, 1992, p 1.

10. Vernon-Roberts B: Morphological and functional interrelationships of bone cells and matrix. Aust N Z J Med 1979; 9:1.

11. Miller SC, Jee WSS: Bone lining cells. *In* Hall BK (ed): Bone, vol 4. Boca Raton, CRC Press, 1992, p 1.

12. Frost HM: Mechanical determinants of skeletal architecture. *In* Albright JA, Brand RA (eds): The Scientific Basis of Orthopaedics, 2nd ed. Norwalk, CT, Appleton-Lange, 1987, p 241.

13. Ascenzi A, Bonucci E, Ripamonti A, et al: X-ray diffraction and electron microscope study of osteons. Calcif Tissue Res 1978; 25:133.

14. Riggs CM, Vaughan LC, Evans GP, et al: Mechanical implications of collagen fibre orientation in cortical bone of the equine radius. Anat Embryol 1993; 187:239.

15. Stopak D, Wessells NK, Harris AK: Morphogenetic rearrangement of injected collagen in developing chicken limb buds. Proc Natl Acad Sci U S A 1985; 82:2804.

16. Termine JD: Non-collagen proteins in bone. *In* Wiley J (ed): Cell and Molecular Biology of Vertebrate Hard Tissues. Chichester, CIBA Foundation Symposium, 1988, p 178.

17. Gross PM, Heistad DD, Marcus ML: Neurohumeral regulation of blood flow to bones and marrow. Am J Physiol 1979; 237:H440.

18. Singh IJ, Sandhu HS, Herskovits MS: Bone vascularity. *In* Hall BK (ed): Bone, vol 3. Boca Raton, CRC Press, 1992, p 141.

19. Albright JA, Skinner HC: Bone: structural organization and remodeling dynamics. *In* Albright JA, Brand RA (eds): The Scientific Basis of Orthopaedics, 2nd ed. Norwalk, CT, Appleton-Lange, 1987, p 161.

20. Currey JD: The Mechanical Adaptations of Bones. Princeton, NJ, Princeton University Press, 1985.

21. Parfitt AM: The cellular basis of bone remodeling: the quantum concept reexamined in light of recent advances in the cell biology of bone. Calcif Tissue Int 1984; 36:S37.

22. Frasca P, Harper R, Katz JL: Collagen fiber orientations of human secondary osteons. Acta Anat 1977; 98:1.

23. Black J, Mattson R, Korostoff E: Haversian osteons: longitudinal variation of internal structure. J Biomed Mater Res 1974; 8:299.

24. Riggs CM, Lanyon LE, Boyde A: Functional associations between collagen fibre orientation and locomotor strain direction in cortical bone of the equine radius. Anat Embryol 1993; 187:231.

25. Ashhurst DE: Macromolecular synthesis and mechanical stability during fracture repair. *In* Hall BK (ed): Bone, vol 5. Boca Raton, CRC Press, 1992, p 61.

26. McKibbon B: The biology of fracture healing in long bones. J Bone Joint Surg 1978; 60B:150.

27. Carter DR, Blenman PR, Beaupre GS: Correlations between mechanical stress history and tissue differentiation in initial fracture healing. J Orthop Res 1988; 6:736.

28. Snyder BD, Hayes WC: Multiaxial structure-property relations in trabecular bone. *In* Mow VC, Ratcliffe A, Woo SL-Y (eds): Biomechanics of Diarthrodial Joints, vol 2. New York, Springer-Verlag, 1990, p 31.

29. Goldstein SA, Matthews LS, Kuhn JL, et al: Trabecular bone remodeling: an experimental model. J Biomech 1991; 24(S):135.

30. Buckwalter JA, Cooper RR: The cells and matrices of skeletal connective tissue. *In* Albright JA, Brand RA (eds): The Scientific Basis of Orthopaedics, 2nd ed. Norwalk, CT, Appleton-Lange, 1987, p 1.

31. Jaworski ZFG: Lamellar bone turnover system and its effector organs. Calcif Tissue Int 1984; 36:S46.

32. Kahn AJ, Partridge NC: Bone resorption in vivo. *In* Hall BK (ed): Bone, vol 2. Boca Raton, CRC Press, 1992, p 119.

33. Frost HM: The Laws of Bone Structure. Springfield, IL, Charles C. Thomas, 1964.

34. Frost HM: Bone "mass" and the "mechanostat": a proposal. Anat Rec 1987; 219:1.

35. Lanyon LE: Functional strain in bone tissue as an objective and controlling stimulus for adaptive bone remodeling. J Biomech 1987; 20:1083.

36. Rubin CT, Lanyon LE: Regulation of bone mass by mechanical strain magnitude. Calcif Tissue Int 1985; 37:411.

37. Frost HM: Bone Remodeling and Its Relation to Metabolic Bone Disease. Springfield, IL, Charles C. Thomas, 1973.

38. Lanyon LE, Hartman W: Strain related electrical potentials recorded in vitro and in vivo. Calcif Tissue Res 1977; 22:315.

39. Cochran GV, Pawluk RJ, Bassett CA: Electromechanical characteristics of bone under physiologic moisture conditions. Clin Orthop Rel Res 1968; 58:249.

40. Eriksson C: Electrical properties of bone. *In* Bourne GH (ed): The Biochemistry and Physiology of Bone, 2nd ed. vol 4. New York, Academic Press, 1976, p 329.

41. Rubin CT, McLeod KJ, Lanyon LE: Prevention of osteoporosis by pulsed electromagnetic fields. J Bone Joint Surg 1989; 71A:411.

42. Yasuda I: Fundamental aspects of fracture treatment. Clin Orthop Rel Res 1977; 124:5.

43. Brighton CT, Friedenberg ZB, Mitchell EI, et al: Treatment of nonunion with constant direct current. Clin Orthop Rel Res 1977; 124:106.

44. Aaron RK, Ciombor DM: Therapeutic effects of electromagnetic fields in the stimulation of connective tissue repair. J Cell Biochem 1993; 52:42.

45. Sharrard W: A double blind trial of pulsed electromagnetic fields for delayed union of tibial fractures. J Bone Joint Surg B 1990; 72:347.

46. Jones HH, Priest HB, Hayes WC, et al: Humeral hypertrophy in response to exercise. J Bone Joint Surg 1977; 59A:204.

47. Woo SLY, Kuei SC, Amiel D, et al: The effect of physical training on the properties of long bone: a study of Wolff's law. J Bone Joint Surg 1981; 63A:780.

48. Krolner B, Toft B, Nielsen SP, et al: Physical exercise as prophylaxis against involutional bone loss: a controlled trial. Clin Sci 1983; 64:541.

49. Matsuda JJ, Zernicke RF, Vailas AC, et al: Structural and mechanical adaptation of immature bone to strenuous exercise. J Appl Physiol 1986; 60:2028.

50. Forwood MR, Parker AW: Effects of exercise on bone growth: mechanical and physical properties studied in the rat. Clin Biomech 1987; 2:185.

51. Hou JC-H, Salem GJ, Zernicke RF, et al: Structural and mechanical adaptations of immature trabecular bone to strenuous exercise. J Appl Physiol 1990; 69:1309.

52. Salem GJ, Zernicke RF, Martinez DA, et al: Adaptations of immature trabecular bone to moderate exercise: geometrical, biochemical, and biomechanical correlates. Bone 1993; 14:647.

53. Seeman E, Wahner HW, Offord KP, et al: Differential effects of endocrine dysfunction on the axial and appendicular skeleton. J Clin Invest 1982; 69:1302.

54. McDonald R, Hegenauer J, Saltman P: Age-related differences in the bone mineralization pattern of rats following exercise. J Gerontol 1986; 41:445.

55. Slemenda CW, Miller JZ, Hui SL, et al: Role of physical activity in the development of skeletal mass in children. J Bone Miner Res 1991; 6:1227.

56. Loitz BJ, Zernicke RF: Strenuous exercise-induced remodelling of mature bone: relationships between in vivo strains and bone mechanics. J Exp Biol 1992; 170:1.

57. Jee WSS, Li XJ, Schaffler MB: Adaptation of diaphyseal structure with aging and increased mechanical usage in the adult rat: a histomorphometrical and biomechanical study. Anat Rec 1991; 230:332.

58. Grimston SK, Zernicke RF: Exercise-related stress responses in bone. J Appl Biomech 1993; 9:2.

59. Giladi M, Milgrom C, Simkin A, et al: Stress fractures: identifiable risk factors. Am J Sports Med 1991; 19:647.

60. Milgrom C, Giladi M, Stein H, et al: Stress fractures in military recruits: a prospective study showing an unusually high incidence. J Bone Joint Surg 1985; 67B:732.

61. Jones BH, Harris JM, Vinh TN, et al: Exercise-induced stress fractures and stress reactions of bone: epidemiology, etiology, and classifications. Exerc Sport Sci Rev 1989; 17:379.

62. Drinkwater BL, Nilson K, Chestnut CH, et al: Bone mineral content of amenorrheic and eumenorrheic athletes. N Engl J Med 1984; 311:277.

63. Myburgh KH, Hutchins J, Fataar AB, et al: Low bone density is an etiologic factor for stress fractures in athletes. Ann Intern Med 1990; 113:754.

64. Matheson GO, McKenzie DC, Taunton JE, et al: Stress fractures among athletes: a study of 320 cases. Am J Sports Med 1987; 15:46.

65. Whitelaw GP, Wetzler MJ, Levy AS, et al: A pneumatic leg brace for the treatment of tibial stress fractures. Clin Orthop Rel Res 1991; 270:301.

66. Weinreb M, Rodan GA, Thompson DD: Osteopenia in the immobilized rat hind limb is associated with increased bone resorption and decreased bone formation. Bone 1989; 10:187.

67. Tuukkanen J, Wallmark B, Jalovaara P, et al: Changes induced in growing rat bone by immobilization and remobilization. Bone 1991; 12:113.

68. Shaw SR, Vailas AC, Grindeland RE, et al: Effects of a 1-wk spaceflight on morphological and mechanical properties of growing bone. Am J Physiol 1988; 254:R78.

69. Biewener AA, Swartz SM, Bertram JE: Bone modeling during growth: dynamic strain equilibrium in the chick tibiotarsus. Calcif Tissue Int 1986; 39:390.

70. Zernicke RF, Vailas AC, Grindeland RE, et al: Spaceflight effects on biomechanical and biochemical properties of rat vertebrae. Am J Physiol 1990; 258:R1327.

71. Griffiths HJ: Diabetic osteopathy. Orthopedics 1985; 8:401.

72. Hough FS: Alterations of bone and mineral metabolism in diabetes mellitus. Part I. An overview. S Afr Med J 1987; 72:116.

73. Hough FS: Alterations of bone and mineral metabolism in diabetes mellitus. Part II. Clinical studies in 206 patients with type I diabetes mellitus. S Afr Med J 1987; 72:120.

74. Rosenbloom AL, Lezotte DC, Weber T, et al: Diminution of bone mass in childhood diabetes. Diabetes 1977; 26:1052.

75. Shore RM, Chesney RW, Mazess RB, et al: Osteopenia in juvenile diabetes. Calcif Tissue Int 1981; 33:455.

76. Soejima K, Landing BH: Osteoporosis in juvenile-onset diabetes mellitus: morphometric and comparative studies. Pediatr Pathol 1986; 6:289.

77. Dixit PK, Ekstrom RA: Decreased breaking strength of diabetic rat bone and its improvement by insulin treatment. Calcif Tissue Int 1980; 32:195.

78. Einhorn TA, Boskey AL, Gundberg CM, et al: The mineral and mechanical properties of bone in chronic experimental diabetes. J Orthop Res 1988; 6:317.

79. Hou JC-H, Zernicke RF, Barnard J: Effects of diabetes and insulin therapy on femoral neck geometry and biomechanics. Clin Orthop Rel Res 1991; 264:278.

80. Hou JC-H, Zernicke RF, Barnard J: Effects of severe diabetes and insulin on the femoral neck of the immature rat. J Orthop Res 1993; 11:263.

81. Hough S, Avioli LV, Bergfeld MA, et al: Correction of abnormal bone and mineral metabolism in chronic streptozotocin-induced diabetes mellitus in the rat by insulin therapy. Endocrinology 1981; 108:2228.

82. Shires R, Teitelbaum SL, Bergfeld MA, et al: The effect of streptozotocin-induced chronic diabetes mellitus on bone and mineral homeostasis in the rat. J Lab Clin Med 1981; 97:231.

83. McNair P: Bone mineral metabolism in human type I (insulin-dependent) diabetes mellitus. Dan Med Bull 1988; 35:109.

84. Dixit PK, Stern AMK: Effect of insulin on the incorporation of citrate and calcium into the bones of alloxan-diabetic rats. Calcif Tissue Int 1979; 27:227.

85. McNair P, Madsbad S, Christiansen MS, et al: Bone mineral loss in insulin-treated diabetes mellitus: studies on pathogenesis. Acta Endocrinol 1979; 90:463.

86. Frazer TE, White NH, Hough S, et al: Alterations in circulation vitamin D metabolites in the young insulin-dependent diabetic. J Clin Endocrinol Metab 1981; 53:1154.

87. Wiske PS, Wentworth SM, Norton JA, et al: Evaluation of bone mass and growth in young diabetics. Metabolism 1982; 31:848.

88. Schwartz Z, Ornoy A, Soskoline WA: The effects of insulin and glucose on bone modeling in vitro. Diabetes Res 1986; 3:321.

89. Tattersall RB, Pyke DA: Growth in diabetic children. Lancet 1973; 17:1105.

90. Ornoy A, Zusman I, Cohen M, et al: Effect of sera from Cohen genetically determined diabetic rats, streptozotocin diabetic rats and sucrose fed rats on the in vitro development of early somite rat embryos. Diabetes Res 1986; 3:43.

91. Sloan GM, Norton JA, Brennan MF: Influence of diabetes mellitus and insulin treatment on protein turnover in the rat. J Surg Res 1980; 28:442.

92. Weiss RE, Gorn AH, Nimni ME: Abnormalities in the biosynthesis of cartilage and bone proteoglycans in experimental diabetes. Diabetes 1981; 30:670.

93. Frolik CA, Ellis LF, Williams DC: Isolation and characterization of insulin-like growth factor-II from human bone. Biochem Biophys Res Commun 1988; 151:1011.

94. Hock JM, Centrella M, Canalis E: Insulin-like growth factor I has independent effects on bone matrix formation and cell replication. Endocrinology 1988; 122:254.

95. Rodan GA: Introduction to bone biology. Bone 1992; 13:S3.

96. Praemer A, Furner S, Rice DP: Musculoskeletal Conditions in the United States. Park Ridge, IL, American Academy of Orthopaedic Surgeons, 1992.

97. Cummings SR, Kelsey JL, Nevitt MC, et al: Epidemiology of osteoporosis and osteoporotic fractures. Epidemiol Rev 1985; 7:178.

98. Genant HK, Ettinger B, Harris ST, et al: Quantitative computed tomography in assessment of osteoporosis. In Riggs BL, Melton LJ (eds): Osteoporosis: Etiology, Diagnosis, and Management. New York, Raven Press, 1988, p 221.

99. Marcus R, Cann CE, Madvig P, et al: Menstrual function and bone mass in elite women distance runners. Ann Intern Med 1985; 102:158.

100. Lawrence RC, Hochberg MC, Kelsey JL, et al: Estimates of the prevalence of selected arthritic and musculoskeletal disease in the United States. J Rheumatol 1982; 16:427.

101. Brody JA: Aging in the 20th and 21st centuries. In Proceedings of the National Center for Health Statistics Conference "Data for an Aging Population: Issues in Health Research and Public Policy, Now and into the 21st Century." DHHS Pub PHS:88, 1987.

102. Brody JA: Prospects for an aging population. Nature 1985; 315:463.

103. Christiansen C: Prevention and treatment of osteoporosis: a review of current modalities. Bone 1992; 13:S35.

104. Nilas L, Christiansen C: Bone mass and its relationship to age and the menopause. J Clin Endocrinol Metab 1987; 65:697.

105. Christiansen C, Lindsay R: Estrogens, bone loss and preservation. Osteoporosis Int 1990; 1:7.

106. Frost HM: The role of changes in mechanical usage set points in the pathogenesis of osteoporosis. J Bone Miner Res 1992; 7:253.

107. Simkin A, Ayalon J, Leichter I: Increased trabecular bone density due to bone loading exercises in postmenopausal women. Calcif Tissue Int 1986; 40:59.

108. Snow-Harter C, Marcus R: Exercise, bone mineral density, and osteoporosis. Exerc Sport Sci Rev 1991; 19:351.

109. Nilsson BE, Westlin NE: Bone density in athletes. Clin Orthop Rel Res 1971; 77:179.

110. Pirnay F, Bodeux M, Crielaard JM, et al: Bone mineral content and physical activity. Int J Sports Med 1987; 8:331.

111. Sinaki M, Offord K: Physical activity in post menopausal women: effect on back muscle strength and bone mineral density of the spine. Arch Phys Med Rehabil 1988; 69:277.

112. Burstein AH, Reilly DT, Martens M: Aging of bone tissue: mechanical properties. J Bone Joint Surg 1976; 58A:82.

113. Torzilli PA, Takebe K, Burstein AH, et al: The material properties of immature bone. Trans ASME 1982; 104:12.

114. Li K-C, Zernicke RF, Barnard AF-Y, et al: Effects of a high fat-sucrose diet on cortical bone morphology and biomechanics. Calcif Tissue Int 1990; 47:308.

115. Beer FP, Johnston ER. Mechanics of Materials. Toronto, McGraw-Hill, 1981, p 585.

CHAPTER 8

Cartilage of Human Joints and Related Structures

J O A N M. W A L K E R *PhD*

Excellence in physical performance is dependent on the integration of the different components of the musculoskeletal system, all of which must perform effectively to attain this goal. This chapter describes the morphology and physiology of the articular cartilage, fibrocartilage, and synovial tissues and fluid. It considers innervation, nutrition, lubrication, loading, breakdown, repair, and the implications for rehabilitation. The hyaline articular cartilage (HAC) that covers synovial joint surfaces cannot be considered by itself. HAC is part of the load-bearing unit that consists of the HAC layer and the subchondral bone; it has important interactions with synovial fluid. The joint's static and dynamic stability is heavily dependent on the contour of the joint surfaces and the supporting structures—capsule, tendons, ligaments, and muscles—that surround the joint; these structures are detailed in other chapters.

The specialized HAC has many functions: to distribute and transmit loads and shear forces to the underlying bone, to protect the underlying bone, and to permit diarthrodial (synovial) joints to have a wide range of almost frictionless movement. HAC is aneural, largely avascular and acellular, and has a water content of up to 80 percent.[1]

CELLS AND MATRIX

The cells found in articular tissues are chondroblasts, chondrocytes, fibroblasts, and fibrocytes (chondrocyte-like cells). Chondrocytes are responsible for the synthesis of proteoglycans and collagen fibers, which principally constitute the cartilage matrix. Cartilage cells are embedded in a finely textured matrix, in small zones that conform to the cell shape. The "lacunae" described from light microscopy studies are believed to be shrinkage artifacts.[2] The thin pericellular matrix that surrounds the chondrocytes is up to 2 μm thick and contains a few well-defined collagen fibers. The chondrocyte and its pericellular matrix have been termed a "chondron." In contrast, cartilage cells in fibrocartilage are squashed between the thick bands of collagen fibers and thus appear elongated without any significant pericellular matrix surrounding them, except close to the osseous junction. The young cell or chondroblast is small and often flattened, with a regular contour and many surface projections. The mature cell, or chondrocyte, increases in size with age but still has small, rounded surface projections. Nuclei are round or oval. Multinucleated cells are common. The cell cytoplasm contains Golgi apparatus, mitochondria, granular endoplastic reticulum, a few fat goblets, pigment granules, and glycogen deposits. In immature cartilage, both the Golgi apparatus and the granular reticulum are particularly prominent.[3] Wilsman[4] described a monocilium on every chondrocyte and postulated that these may have a microtransductory function, detecting changes due to mechanical effects in the cell's environment and enabling it to respond.

Chondrocytes in the superficial layers are flattened, whereas those in the deeper layers are more rounded. "Cell density is at its highest at the articular surface and is progressively reduced in the mid- and deep zones to about one-half to one-third that of the superficial layer."[5] Cell density is also at its highest in fetal and newborn cartilages and decreases with increasing age. Cell density is low in HAC, and the decreased number of cells due to aging and to the move from superficial to deep greatly reduces the repair capacity of HAC. Cartilage cells, however, are capable of changing their shape. The isolated living chondrocyte constantly changes its shape, putting out and withdrawing pseudopodic processes. If in vitro, cells from the superficial layer are transplanted to a deeper layer; they change their shape and become more rounded.[6] Such findings contradict the traditional view that mature cells are effete, with minimal capacity to respond to injury or disease.

In the developing embryo, chondroblasts and mature chondrocytes are derived from progenitor mesenchymal cells. After the embryonic period, prechondrogenic mesenchyme forms cartilage even when transplanted to other sites.[7] The chondroblasts that will mature into the chondrocytes of HAC are similar in origin to the chondroblasts of fracture callus and growth plates. The latter develop into hypertrophic chondrocytes and have the capacity to form calcified cartilage, which acts as a scaffold for osteoblasts to deposit an osteoid.[8] Differences in chondrocyte function according to location may be related to the presence or absence of a receptor for the basic fibroblastic growth vector (bFGF), which all chondroblasts possess.[5] Whereas the chondrocyte of HAC retains a receptor for bFGF, the hypertrophic chondrocyte found in the growth plate or in fracture callus has no bFGF receptor. The factors that regulate the commitment of chondroblasts to develop into hypertrophic chondrocytes or chondrocytes of HAC are not yet fully established.[5] A further distinction between chondrocytes in the epiphyseal growth plate and those in HAC is that blood vessels are usually found in close proximity to the growth plate and fracture callus. Poole[5] commented that "for cartilage to calcify during endochondral ossification [and in fracture repair], angiogenesis appears to be required, which can be induced by chondrocytes." Since HAC is avascular even in development, angiogenesis apparently is not induced by HAC chondrocytes. Obviously, calcification of HAC is detrimental to its normal function. This is evident in aging cartilage, in which there is expansion of the deep calcified layer.

Angiogenesis is always present in developing growth plates and fracture sites, and hypertrophy of chondro-cytes precedes this vessel ingrowth in those situations. In contrast, although the deepest zone of HAC contains hypertrophic chondrocytes, vascular invasion of the calcified zone is limited or not present at all. The absence of vascularity is a critical factor in HAC's inability to respond to injury with the typical stages of inflammation and seriously impairs its repair capacity.

Cells of fibrocartilaginous structures, such as menisci and the anulus fibrosus of the intervertebral disc, are a chondrocytic type of cell (mature cells are termed fibrocytes) that synthesizes and secretes type I rather than type II collagen, which is synthesized and secreted by HAC cells. Where these structures carry significant loads, the cells synthesize proteoglycan aggrecan, which increases the stiffness of the fibrocartilage.[5]

EXTRACELLULAR MATRIX

Both the articular cartilage and the nucleus pulposus of the disc are specialized connective tissues in which cells are relatively sparsely distributed. There is abundant extracellular matrix associated with these tissues. It is this matrix that confers to the tissue its specialized loading and mechanical properties, such as the ability to withstand both static and dynamic loading stresses. The extracellular matrix is composed of collagens, proteoglycans, noncollagen protein proteoglycans (NCPs), and water. Between 65 and 80 percent of the extracellular matrix is water. The water content, greater in the superficial layers, is reduced in the deeper layers to between 65 and 70 percent.[9] The extracellular matrix of articular cartilage is largely composed of large protein aggregates (LPAs) and type II collagen (50 to 90 percent).

PROTEOGLYCANS

The proteoglycans and glycosaminoglycans (GAGs) in connective tissue, such as in articular cartilage ground substance, account for less than 100 g per person (between 22 and 38 percent dry weight in HAC; compare with 0.5 to 55 percent dry weight of NCP). These hydrophilic (water-loving) polyaminos play an important role in regulating the movement of water in the matrix and thereby greatly influence the mechanical and lubrication properties of cartilage.[10] By binding with water, the high proteoglycan content gives cartilage a low hydraulic permeability, which limits fluid loss when it is loaded in compression. Cartilage deforms reversibly, loses water to the joint space when loaded, and imbibes water when the load is released. Contributing to this mechanism is the LPA, an elastic molecule that can expand in solution and resist compression in a small volume.[11] It is this constraint of the proteoglycan aggregates and the dense network of collagen fibers that gives some remarkable mechanical properties (compressibility, elasticity, self-lubrication) to articular cartilage.

LPAs form a "noncovalent" association of collagen protein monomers (termed an "aggrecan"). Aggrecan is

CARTILAGE PROTEOGLYCAN AGGREGATE

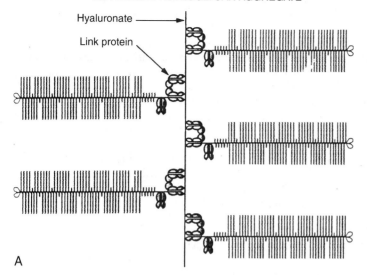

A

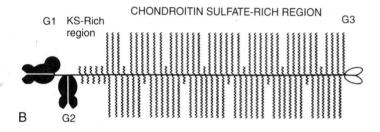

B

FIGURE 8–1. *A*, Diagrammatic model of the cartilage proteoglycan aggregate. The filamentous backbone of the aggregate is hyaluronate. Proteoglycan monomers (aggrecan molecules) of variable length arise at regular intervals from the opposite sides of the hyaluronate chain. Proteoglycan monomer core protein contains three globular domains designated G1, G2, and G3. G1 is located at the NH_2-terminus and contains the hyaluronate acid binding region. Link protein binds simultaneously to hyaluronate and G1 and stabilizes the aggregate against association. *B*, Diagrammatic model of the structure of the cartilage proteoglycan monomer (aggrecan). (*B* from Rosenberg L: Structure and function of cartilage proteoglycans. *In* McCarty DJ, Koopman WJ [eds]: Arthritis and Allied Conditions, 12th ed, vol 1. Philadelphia, Lea & Febiger, 1993, p 230.)

bound at intervals with a single central filament of hyaluronate and is stabilized with link proteins (Fig. 8–1). Aggrecans have three globular domains known as G1, G2, and G3. The major component of proteoglycans consists of chains of chondroitin sulfate (CS-6 and CS-4). Regions that are rich in keratan sulfate (KS) lie between domains G2 and G3.[11] CS and KS are linear polymers consisting of sugar residues, members of a group of polysaccharides called GAGs or mucopolyaminoglycans; they are found in the ground substance of several connective tissues. An entire aggrecan molecule has a molecular weight of 2 to 3 million (an aggrecan molecular protein core is about 220,000; CS chains about 20,000 to 30,000; and KS chains about 5000 to 10,000.[11] An important feature of CS and KS is that the repeating units of GAGs contain closely packed, negatively charged groups, so that when these chains are linked to the aggrecan core protein (ACP), they stand out like bristles on a brush.

The strongly repelling forces of the thousands of negatively charged groups mean that the protein aggregate (PA) would occupy a greater volume of solution in vitro, but in vivo, the PAs are constrained by the collagen network. It is this feature that gives articular cartilage its elastic properties. The elastic forces of PAs are balanced by the tensile forces of the collagen network. When cartilage is compressed, water (interstitial fluid) is extruded from the cartilage, and the aggregate is confined to a smaller area. With relief of pressure, the aggregate expands until limited by the

collagen fiber network; simultaneously, cartilage imbibes water and the volume of cartilage increases. This characteristic is vital to cartilage's ability to deform on loading yet withstand loading and thus protect the underlying subchondral bone from damage. (The reader is referred to Rosenberg[11] for a detailed account of the structure and function of proteoglycans.) The link protein (see Figure 8–1) stabilizes the aggregate against dissociation by binding with hyaluronate and to the G1 globular domain of the ACP. This arrangement is unstable at low pHs and will dissociate at pH 4.[11] Therefore, a greater amount of aggregate is present when the pH is about 7.

The other two proteoglycans are small interstitial dermatan sulfate proteoglycans (DSPGs). DSPG-1 is biglycan and DSPG-2 is decorin. Both the DSPGs have a core protein with a molecular weight of about 37,000; GAG chains have a molecular weight of about 30,000. These are "multifunctional macromolecules that bind to the extra-cellular matrix macromolecules and regulate or modulate their biological properties."[11] DSPGs inhibit the processes involved in tissue development and repair. They have been shown to bind to the surface of collagen fibers, inhibiting collagen fibrillogenesis, and to bind to fibronectin, thus inhibiting cell adhesion and thrombin activity in clot formation. Their activity could explain why lesions of articular cartilage do not heal well or repair spontaneously.[11] Mature articular cartilage contains biglycan and decorin in roughly equal amounts,"and they tend to be most concentrated near the articular surface and least in the deep zone."[5] The significance of this distribution is yet to be determined. There is no apparent difference in repair capacity of different levels of HAC; only defects involving the subchondral plate may show repair with HAC-like tissue.

COLLAGEN

The collagen family is now recognized to have at least 15 types, which are labeled from I to XV (Table 8-1).[12] The various types of collagen are strands of α chains that are composed of amino acids. Each collagen is composed of three polypeptides forming a triple-helical structure. Collagen constitutes approximately one third of the total body protein.[10]

The major type of collagen in the extracellular matrix of articular cartilage is type II, the fibrillar type. Fibrils, several thousand molecules in diameter, are packed in bundles to form large fibers. Articular cartilage also contains fiber-associated type IX (5 to 20 percent) and two types of short-chained type VI collagen, which are also found in ligaments. Some type X collagen, which is principally found in the hypertrophic cartilage of the growth plate, is also present. In articular cartilage, collagen forms about 55 g per 100 g dry weight, whereas proteoglycans form about 25 g per 100 g dry weight.[15] The collagen meshwork gives tensile strength to HAC and resists the swelling pressure of the proteoglycans, enabling HAC to withstand compressive loads.

The metabolic turnover of collagen is continuous through growth to maturity, when the collagen fibers become more metabolically stable and have half-lives of weeks or months.[15] Collagen turnover increases in conditions of malnutrition, starvation, Paget's disease, hypoparathyroidism, and metastatic diseases of bone.[15] The degradation of collagen under these conditions or diseases provides the body with a source of amino acids.

TABLE 8-1
Collagens of Joint Tissue[5,13-15]

Type	Distribution
I	Bone, ligament, tendon, fibrocartilage, capsule, synovial lining tissues, skin
II	Cartilage, fibrocartilage
III	Blood vessels, synovial lining tissues, skin
IV	Basement membranes
V	Pericellular region of articular cartilage when present,* bone, blood vessels
VI	Nucleus pulposus
VII	Anchoring fibers of various tissues
VIII	Endothelial cells
IX	Cartilage matrix*
X	Hypertrophic and ossified cartilage only
XI	Cartilage matrix*
XII	Tendon, ligament, perichondrium, periosteum
XIII	Skin, tendon

*Small amounts (<20%).

TABLE 8-2
Multistep Process in Collagen Synthesis

Intracellular Events

- Synthesis of mRNA specific for collagen
- Formation of polyribosomal clusters
- Association of polyribosomal and endoplasmic reticulum
- Formation of an alignment segment of the polypeptide chains
- Hydroxylation of specific proline and lysine residues
- Glycosylation of selected hydroxylysine residues
- Conversion of procollagen to collagen by procollagen peptidase and extrusion of tropocollagen into the extracellular milieu

Extracellular Events

- Formation of peptide-bound aldehydes as specific lysine and hydroxylysine
- Formation of intramolecular cross-links by an aldol condensation reaction
- Formation of intermolecular cross-links, peptide-bound aldehydes, and unmodified amino groups of lysine or hydroxylysine residues as Schiff bases
- Aggregation of collagen fibers in the extracellular matrix to reflect the specific structural characteristics of a given tissue[17]

From Castor CW: Regulation of connective tissue metabolism. *In* McCarty DJ, Koopman WJ (eds): Arthritis and Allied Conditions, 12th ed, vol 1. Philadelphia, Lea & Febiger, 1993, p 246.

It is hypothesized that, in these conditions, HAC is more vulnerable and should not be subjected to heavy loading stresses. It is suspected that mechanical forces, or enzymes, may degrade the "glue" that binds the collagen fibers into a network and be a contributing factor in the pathogenesis of osteoarthritis.[16]

Table 8-2 summarizes the intracellular and extracellular events in the synthesis of collagen. Collagen maturity is achieved in the extracellular matrix. Many factors are important in the multistep process of collagen formation (Fig. 8-2).[5] Among these factors is increased glucose transport, which is essential to all growth-related processes. Glucose transport is mediated by a group of glucose-transport proteins that have distinct tissue distributions in cartilage and in synovial cells; a connective tissue active protein (CTAP-III) is involved.[10] Amino acids are also transported into the cells. Other factors are insulin-like growth factors (IGF-I and IGF-II), which stimulate connective tissue cell replication and extracellular matrix synthesis—that is, the synthesis of proteoglycans. Osteogenin, a type of bone morphogenic protein (BMP), is present and is known to induce formation of both bone and cartilage; it is theorized that BMPs may be involved in bone and cartilage repair. The preceding account indicates the growing complexity of processes involved in cartilage metabolism—whether during growth or in repair. Such processes are dependent on a number of factors, including normal cartilage nutrition, in which motion and loading play a vital role.

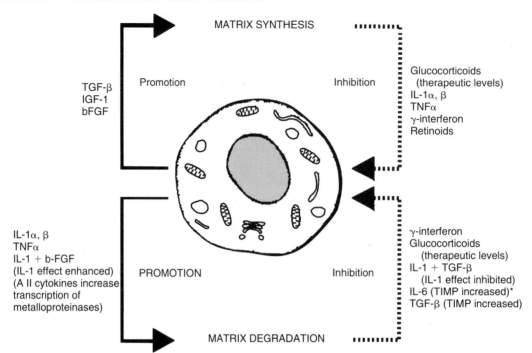

MATRIX SYNTHESIS

TGF-β
IGF-1
bFGF

Promotion

Inhibition

Glucocorticoids
(therapeutic levels)
IL-1α, β
TNFα
γ-interferon
Retinoids

IL-1α, β
TNFα
IL-1 + b-FGF
(IL-1 effect enhanced)
(A II cytokines increase
transcription of
metalloproteinases)

PROMOTION

Inhibition

γ-interferon
Glucocorticoids
(therapeutic levels)
IL-1 + TGF-β
(IL-1 effect inhibited)
IL-6 (TIMP increased)*
TGF-β (TIMP increased)

MATRIX DEGRADATION

FIGURE 8–2. Effects of cytokines that favor either cartilage matrix synthesis or degradation. (From Poole AR: Cartilage in health and disease. *In* McCarty DJ, Koopman WJ [eds]: Arthritis and Allied Conditions. 12th ed, vol 1. Philadelphia, Lea & Febiger, 1993, p 301.)

ELASTIN FIBERS

In contrast to the collagen fibers of HAC, fibroblasts are thought to be responsible for formation of the protein elastin, of which elastin fibers are chiefly composed. Elastin fibers are yellowish in color, tend to branch freely, and are usually thinner than collagen fibers. They stretch easily, although they may show some calcification and reduced elasticity with advancing age.[3] Although Buckwalter and associates[18] demonstrated elastin fibers in human intervertebral discs, to date, there is still controversy whether elastin fibers are found in HAC. Elastin fibers are found in the fibrous layer of the perichondrium. Cotta-Pereira and colleagues[19] used ultrastructural studies to demonstrate the presence of elaunin and oxytalan fibers in rat HAC, but not elastin fibers. Location of these elastic-related fibers suggests a modulation of elasticity from the perichondrium to HAC and may reflect resistance requirements of these tissues to mechanical stress. Surrounding soft tissues (capsule, ligaments, aponeurosis) also blend with the perichondrium and periosteum. The presence of elastic-like fibers should facilitate stretching at the extremes of range, recoil on return to neutral range, and enlargement of the joint space in the effused joint.

THE TISSUES

In this account dealing with human joints, only the two major subtypes of cartilage in synovial joints—hyaline cartilage and fibrocartilage—and the synovial lining tissues are considered.

HYALINE ARTICULAR CARTILAGE

HAC is a specialized type of hyaline cartilage that covers the joint surfaces, except for those of the sternoclavicular and temporomandibular joints, which ossify in membrane. These joints, along with the sacroiliac joint, have at least one fibrocartilaginous surface.[3,20,21] Figure 8–3 shows the typical two-layered arrangement of HAC. The superficial layer is uncalcified cartilage, and the deeper calcified cartilage layer is integrally bound to and merges with the subchondral bone. The tidemark forms the boundary between these two layers. Three zones are distinguished within the uncalcified cartilage: a superficial (tangential or gliding)

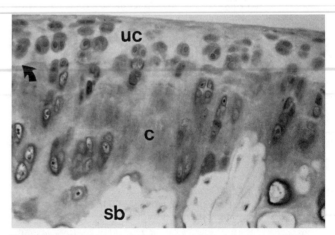

FIGURE 8–3. Light microscopy view of the articular cartilage. uc = uncalcified layer; c = calcified layer; sb = subchondral bone; arrow indicates the tidemark.

zone, a mid or transitional zone, and a deep or radial zone (Fig. 8–4). Each zone is unique with regard to cell number, cell shape, orientation, collagenous fiber arrangement, and nutrition. Cartilage is classified for convenience by the type of matrix. Three varieties are described—hyaline, fibro-, and elastic.[3]

TIDEMARK

The tidemark is a boundary in a metabolically active zone between the noncalcified and calcified articular cartilage (Figs. 8–4 and 8–5).[22,23] Oettmeier and coworkers[23] demonstrated in noncalcified preparations of human femoral heads that there were three structural components to the tidemark: (1) a PAS-positive, proteoglycan-containing tidemark line adjacent to the basal cartilage; (2) a subliminal light-colored zone; and (3) a demarcation line to the calcified cartilage. In life, there is calcifying activity in the tidemark region, so that the tidemark slowly advances in the direction of the noncalcified cartilage.[22] Variations in the subchondral bone volume are thought to influence the tidemark region and the changes in cartilage that lead to osteoarthrosis.[23] Lane and Bullough[24] demonstrated that the number of tidemarks increases significantly after the age of 60. This increase relates to the continuous remodeling that appears to occur with age and to changes that are related to endocartilaginous ossification affecting the calcified zone. The latter becomes thinner with age.

HAC ORGANIZATION

In light microscopy studies, some investigators have described HAC as having four zones or strata, whereas others described the two layers (as above) with three zones within the uncalcified cartilage (see Fig. 8–5). Hamerman and associates[25] and Lane and Weiss[26] described a superficial layer called "lamina splendens" on the surface of the superficial layer. This is a layer of fine fibers (4 to 10 mm) that can be peeled off with forceps and shear types of trauma. Other investigators did not distinguish the "lamina splendens" from the superficial zone. Cells in the superficial zone are oriented with their long axes parallel to the surface.[27] In the transitional zone, the cells are either rounded or oval.[27,28] In the radial zone, the cells are larger and rounded and may be paired in irregular columns numbering four to eight. Variation in descriptions of the cell shapes in HAC may be related to methods of tissue preparation and the plane of sectioning. Cell density decreases from the superficial to the deep layer.[29] Cells in the calcified zone are heavily encrusted with hydroxyapatite (crystals of calcium salts) and are surrounded with calcified matrix in mature cartilage. These cells are considered to be relatively metabolically inactive.[30]

Ultrastructural studies show that a thin layer of pericellular matrix immediately surrounding the cell can be distinguished. Surrounding the pericellular matrix is a wider layer of lighter-staining interterritorial matrix. The electron-dense zone between the two

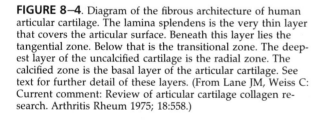

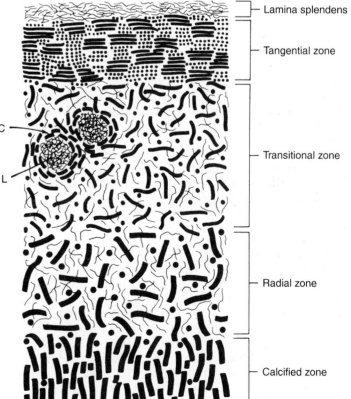

FIGURE 8–4. Diagram of the fibrous architecture of human articular cartilage. The lamina splendens is the very thin layer that covers the articular surface. Beneath this layer lies the tangential zone. Below that is the transitional zone. The deepest layer of the uncalcified cartilage is the radial zone. The calcified zone is the basal layer of the articular cartilage. See text for further detail of these layers. (From Lane JM, Weiss C: Current comment: Review of articular cartilage collagen research. Arthritis Rheum 1975; 18:558.)

Lamina splendens

Tangential zone

Transitional zone

Radial zone

Calcified zone

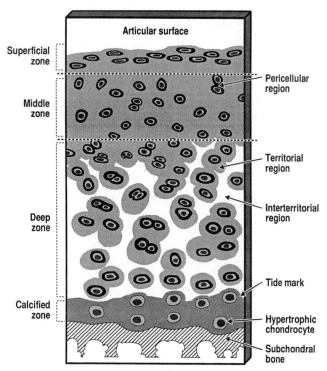

FIGURE 8–5. Regional organization of articular cartilage based on studies in adult cattle and humans. The pericellular region contains a high concentration of aggrecan, the proteoglycan decorin, and type VI collagen. The superficial zone contains thin collagen fibrils arranged parallel with the articular surfaces. The partially calcified cartilage of the calcified zone is indicated. The interterritorial zone is first recognizable at about 17 years of age in humans, based on changes in distribution of aggrecan and link protein. (From Poole AR: Cartilage in health and disease. *In* McCarty DJ, Koopman WJ [eds]: Arthritis and Allied Conditions, 12th ed, vol 1. Philadelphia, Lea & Febiger, 1993, p 282.)

probably reflects the pericellular capsule. Adjacent to and outside the interterritorial matrix is the territorial matrix (see Fig. 8–5).[28] The pericellular capsule is composed of fine fibrillar material. The interterritorial matrix has larger-diameter, more closely packed collagen fibers. It is also stiffer owing to a high concentration of keratan sulfate.[31] The KS concentration may enable the interterritorial matrix to better resist compressive deformation.[28] Abnormal KS concentration (decreased with immobilization, increased with aging) may contribute to cartilage pathology, because changes in matrix stiffness impact load bearing and dissipation of forces through cartilage.

The superficial zone of the uncalcified cartilage has been described as fibrillar,[2] hyaline-like,[32] and membrane-like;[33] as a dense, unfibrillated layer;[34] as a random fibrillated layer;[35] and as a biomechanical protecting membrane.[36] There is agreement that the bundles of fibers in the superficial zone lie in layers parallel to the joint cavity (see Fig. 8–4). In the transitional zone, the fibers are more randomly dispersed. Fibers in the superficial zone have a diameter of about 35 nm; the fibers in the transitional zone are slightly bigger (about 60 nm). In the radial zone, the fibers have an arcade-type pattern, with radial rows in the deepest regions. These fibers are coarser, about 80 nm in diameter.[36] The fibers in the calcified zone are greater than 100 nm in diameter and are oriented perpendicular to the surface.[26] The collagen fiber pattern in the deeper zones is similar to that described by Benninghoff.[37] The implications of the variation in fiber size are not fully known. Size appears to be related to structural stability, the ability to withstand horizontal stresses, providing a tight framework to contain matrix components, and, in the deep layers, to give a tight bonding to subchondral bone. Thicker fibers may be more stable, with a slow rate of turnover.

Muir and coworkers[38] suggested that the closely packed fibrils in the superficial zone make a less permeable layer than is present in the underlying zones and that this may function as a "skin" for the hydrated cartilage. Recently, Moses and colleagues[39] demonstrated that the calcified layer possesses antiangiogenic molecules. These molecules appear to confer an ability to inhibit the vascular invasion that would bring about ossification, similar to that in the growth plate. Thus, calcified cartilage can persist and be a buffer zone between the uncalcified articular cartilage and subchondral bone.[5]

AGING CHANGES OF HAC

Gross changes in HAC with aging include increased congruity of the articular surfaces and a variable fibrillation or fraying of the surfaces. However, Goodfellow and Bullough[40] related the latter more to joint type (multiaxial or uniaxial) and to joint mechanics than to aging. There is a change in HAC appearance from a transparent bluish to an opaque yellow. The functional significance of the pigment change is not known.

With light microscopy and histochemical staining, a number of changes have been revealed in HAC. There is an increased grainy or fibrillar appearance, thought to be due to the unmasking of collagen fibers. The number of tidemarks increases,[24] and there is a decrease in overall thickness,[41] but there is no change in the total amount of HAC. Blood vessels may penetrate from subchondral bone to the calcified cartilage layer, and this layer thickens. These changes make articular cartilage susceptible to osteoclastic resorption and eventual ossification, with consequential effects on cartilage resilience and compliance. Knets[36] commented that the "intensity of this process decreased with age," which is fortunate, since these changes not only impair normal load bearing but also may contribute to the development of osteoarthritis.

Intercellular components may display more aging changes.[42] Although the total content of collagen may not change,[43] older collagen remains in the extended state longer than younger collagen as it loses its ability to return to the resting state. Verzar[44] demonstrated an increased formation of cross-bridges, which give altered solubility to collagen. The increased cross-bridges involved both inter- and intramolecular cross-linking[45] and resulted in increased stiffness. With thicker and less resilient collagen fibers, and the calcification in the deeper zones, load-bearing properties of cartilage are affected. Theoretically, there is impairment to the chondrocytes' nutrition, which contributes to further deterioration.

With histochemistry, the loss of proteoglycans is demonstrated with a decrease in the articular cartilage's reaction to alcian blue staining and an increased reaction to Schiff reagent.[20] Several studies of aging have reported a decrease in GAGs,[46,47] a decrease in CS-4, an increase in CS-6, and an increase in the small molecular KS. However, there is variability in the reports as to whether these components, as well as cell frequencies, lipids,[48] and water content, actually increase or decrease.[29,41,49–52] Livne and associates[53] demonstrated in mice that the number of cells decreased and that the interstitial growth was very limited. Poole[5] summarized aging changes of the matrix proteoglycan aggrecan as an increase in KS molecules and the HAC binding region and a reduction in link protein molecular size, with accumulation of degradation products in the deep zone. Ziv and coworkers[54] demonstrated in aging human facet cartilage that there was a very high hydration, which increased from the fourth decade and was indicative of collagen damage and cartilage degeneration. With inference microscopy, Longmore and Gardner[43] revealed increased irregularities in the surface of the lateral femoral condyle cartilage, which appeared normal by naked eye examination (the oldest specimen examined was only 47 years). These investigators theorized that the changes were related to a loss of surface ground substance and exposure of fiber bundles.

The impact of these changes, indicating imbalance between synthesis and degradation of matrix components, is a decreased ability of cartilage to withstand shear forces and impulsive loading, and increased susceptibility to trauma. Cartilage is both softer and, in its deeper layers, stiffer; microfractures of subchondral bone may occur due to reduced dispersion of loads.

Although some investigators consider degenerative changes to typify the aging process,[53] it should be noted that it is difficult to distinguish among natural aging changes, functional adaptive changes, and degenerative changes that result from micro or macro trauma or disease.[51]

FIBROCARTILAGE

INTRA-ARTICULAR DISCS, MENISCI, AND LABRA

Intra-articular discs, menisci, and labra are found in certain joints in all species. In humans, these may take the form of the complete disc that subdivides the cavity into two separate compartments, as in the temporomandibular and sternoclavicular joints, or they may be incomplete structures, such as the menisci in the knee. These structures function to increase the congruity of the articulating surfaces. They may assist in joint lubrication and protect the edges of the joints; in the knee joint, menisci function as shock absorbers[55] and bear loads.[56] Whereas articular discs tend to be overall circular structures, possibly with a central perforation,[57] the menisci are semilunar or C-shaped structures with

an inferior flat surface and a superior concave surface. The degree of fixation of articular discs and menisci varies between species and joints (see Van Sickle and Kincaid[58] for a comparative arthrology review). Although menisci, labra, and articular discs are often termed "fibrocartilages," many have little or no fibrocartilage present, being principally composed of collagenous connective tissue.[58] The histologic appearance of these structures is a dominance of circumferential collagenous fibers.

Poole[5] defined fibrocartilage as being "characterized by the presence of chondrocytic cells that synthesize and secrete Type I rather than Type II collagen." On gross and light microscopic examination, the matrix of HAC appears translucent, homogeneous, and apparently structureless. White fibrocartilage, however, is characterized by collagen fibers arranged in abundant bundles of dense, white, fibrous tissue.[3] Scattered groups of cells with ovoid-shaped nuclei lie between the fiber bundles. The amount of visible matrix varies considerably between different structures and with age. Detail of the so-called fibrocartilaginous structures follows.

The fusiform cells of fibrocartilages that are visible with light microscopy may be "mistaken" for fibroblasts.[59] These are revealed by electron microscopy to be more like the cells in articular cartilage—zone 1 chondrocytes. These cells show a well-developed Golgi apparatus and rough endoplastic reticulum.

"Fibrocartilaginous" structures exhibit both territorial (former "lacunae" zone around the cells) and interterritorial (general) matrix. The latter is composed of sheets of collagen fibrils and fibers in a sparse interfibrillary matrix. Some radial and oblique fibers are seen, and these are thought to bind the dominant circumferential fibers. Bullough and associates[60] believed that the primary circumferential orientation of the meniscal collagenous fibers functioned to counteract the tensile forces to which the meniscus is exposed. Both meniscal and articular discs have tensile strength that is similar to that of HAC.[60] In comparison with HAC, the collagen is predominantly type I ($2\alpha_1$, $1\alpha_2$), which forms some 60 to 90 percent of organic solids in the menisci.[27] Water composes some 70 to 78 percent of menisci, and proteoglycans are less than 10 percent of the dry weight and are mainly chondroitin sulfates and dermatan sulfate, with very little keratan sulfate.[27] Differences between the structure and composition of discs and cartilage probably reflect the primary functions to resist tensile stresses and act as efficient shock absorbers. Variation in fiber thickness and orientation allows these structures to respond to a wide range of vibrations created by compressive forces.

Articular discs and menisci are largely aneural and devoid of lymphatics, but they do have a vascular supply, which tends to be rich at the periphery, where there is a bony attachment. Although the inner portion of menisci is avascular, vessels may penetrate the distal one third.[58,61,62] Nerves appear to be associated in the meniscus only with the vessels at the periphery.[2]

Labra, which Van Sickle and Kincaid[58] termed "marginal fibrocartilages," are located in the glenohumeral and hip joints. These structures serve to deepen the socket and assist in joint lubrication, and they may protect the joint edges. In the developing hip, the histologic structure resembles that of a ligament with no apparent matrix. The cells in the substance of the fetal hip labra resemble fibrocytes, being elongated and flattened between the collagenous bundles.[63] Labra are covered on both surfaces by synovial lining tissues.[3] In contrast, the load-bearing surfaces of the menisci are not covered with synovial lining tissues. A vascular synovial fringe, however, is adherent to the surfaces and extends 1 to 3 mm over the superior and inferior margins.[64]

Mikic[65] showed in human radioulnar discs that central perforations increased with age. The discs between the sternum and first costal cartilage and between the manubrium and the sternal body (manubriosternum joint [MSJ]) have been observed to ossify with age. The central portion of the MSJ disc in some 30 percent of people may be absorbed, converting the symphysis into more of a synovial-type joint.[3] A similar change may occur in the symphysis pubis, where the fibrocartilaginous disc is covered with a hyaline cartilage layer and is firmly united to the bone. A cavity is not seen before the tenth year, and it is not lined by synovial lining tissues.[3]

The thickness of articular discs varies among joints and is related to the joint contour. For example, the disc of the temporomandibular joint is thickest near the center, where it lies in the deepest part of the mandibular fossa.[3] In contrast, both labra and knee menisci are thicker on the periphery. Regeneration of menisci can occur, provided the whole breadth of the menisci is removed.[3] This regeneration occurs from the vascular fibroareolar tissue around the meniscal periphery and is thought to be of a fibrous variety. After injury, the vascular periphery permits healing within this zone, which is similar to that of other tissues and involves formation of a fibrin clot. Fibrous scar tissue forms within 10 weeks, but modulation into fibrocartilage may take several months.[64,66,67] These time periods for regeneration of tissues should be considered in planning rehabilitation programs and return to participation in serious training and sports activities (see also "Repair of Articular Cartilage"). Trauma to the inner two thirds, however, does not heal.[68] The periphery is probably chondrocytic "in origin and type."[27]

INTERVERTEBRAL DISCS

With the exception of the first two cervical levels, the opposing surfaces of free vertebra are separated by intervertebral discs, which form between one fifth and one third of the total length of the spine. Intervertebral discs, often described as fibrocartilaginous structures,[3] are composed of an inner nucleus pulposus (NP) and an outer anulus fibrosus (AF). Discs lie between and are adherent to the hyaline plates, which cover the inferior and superior surfaces of the vertebral end plates, forming symphyses. Discs occupy a greater proportion of the length of the cervical and lumbar regions in comparison with the thoracic region; thus, they confer

greater motion to the cervical and lumbar regions. The intervertebral discs are very firmly attached by connections with the anterior and posterior longitudinal ligaments and, in the thoracic region, by the intraarticular ligaments. The shape dimensions of the discs reflect the region in which they are situated. Discs are thicker in the cervical and lumbar regions than in the thoracic region and contribute to the convex forward alignment of those regions; they are thinnest in the upper thoracic region and thickest in the lumbar region.[3] For further details, the reader is referred to Holm and Urban[69] and Happey.[70] The functions of the disc are to transmit loads, act as impact or shock absorbers, sustain shearing forces, and resist wear. The AF, in particular, serves to absorb natural forces by resisting and modifying pressures through the stretching of its collagenous framework.

ANULUS FIBROSUS. The AF is the outer laminated layer that contains the inner NP. It consists of a series of concentric laminae that are visible to the naked eye in horizontal sections. The outer zone is chiefly collagenous fibers, and the wider inner zone is fibrocartilaginous. Laminar bundles form collars within which most of the collagen fibers lie in parallel. Laminae are convex from superior to inferior and pass obliquely between two adjacent vertebrae, subscribing an angle of between 40 and 70 degrees with the vertebrae.[70,71] Strong fibrous bands connect the concentric laminae. Between the contiguous bundles, fibers lie at obtuse angles and pass in different directions.[3,71] Inoue and Takeda,[71] in electron microscopy studies, examined the highly specialized organization of these collagenous fibers. There are 15 to 20 concentric laminae in the parallel bundles that average 10 to 50 μm in size. Each bundle has fine fibrils that vary between 0.1 and 0.2 mm in diameter. Laminae can vary between 200 and 400 mm in width, with the outer laminae being the thickest. In comparison, the collagenous fibers in the inner NP are finer (20 to 50 mm in diameter) and have a loose, irregular network.[71] The AF is anchored firmly to the cartilaginous end plates, with the fibers in the medial half anchored more deeply than those in the lateral half.[72] Johnson and colleagues[73] reported that up to 10 percent of fibers in the AF of human lumbar discs were of the elastic variety.

NUCLEUS PULPOSUS. The NP is encased by the AF and lies slightly more posteriorly within the disc. This structure demonstrates significant developmental and aging changes. The young nucleus is described as being semifluid, soft, and gelatinous. It consists of mucoid material with a few notochordal cells present; the latter disappear by the end of the first decade.[3] Gradually, the mucoid material is replaced by fibrocartilage, which appears to be derived from the cells in the AF or the contiguous vertebral end plates. The NP is united to the AF by fibers that connect to the AF inner zone; this transition zone is gradual. Compared with articular cartilage, the NP is soft, more compressible and deformable, and capable of considerable changes in its volume and shape with spinal motion. Aging changes, possibly as early as the fourth decade, gradually reduce this capacity. The consequence of these changes is decreased dissipation of forces from the nucleus to the AF, thereby concentrating forces transmitted to the vertebrae, with potential for microfractures of vertebral trabeculae.

With the exception of the inner NP, the cell elements of the disc and vertebral end plates are formed from embryonic mesoderm in early prenatal life, and the central portion of the NP is derived from the notochord. As in articular cartilage, the disc matrix is produced and maintained by cells of the disc. These cells are described as either chondrocytes or chondrocyte-like cells. They are rounded in the NP and more elongated in the AF. Maroudas and coworkers[74] described little variation in cell density between human AF and NP (4.3 cells/mm^2 in NP; 5.0 in AF). The discs, therefore, are relatively acellular. Investigators have reported that in both humans and animals, the young anulus does not contain cartilage cells; only fibroblasts are observed.[75,76] Chondroid-like cells, however, are frequently seen in the older AF.

VERTEBRAL END PLATE. The vertebral end plate, although not part of the intervertebral disc, is an integral part of the disc's structure and contributes to disc function (Fig. 8–6). The vertebral bony end plates are covered with a hyaline cartilage layer that is identical to HAC, except that it lacks "a discrete superficial surface."[27,77] The cartilage end plate serves as an anchor for the finer NP fibers and the coarser AF fibers. It also plays an important role in the nutrition of the NP. Although the outer portion of the plate appears impermeable, diffusion of nutrients occurs in the central portion, where blood vessels lie close to the plate. The NP may be solely nourished via the end plate.

DISC COMPOSITION. Water constitutes about 90 percent of the total disc content. Although water content decreases with age, it still remains high.[69] The AF is about 65 to 70 percent water, whereas the NP is between 88 and 65 percent water (from younger to older). The collagen content is higher in the AF, being 50 to 55 percent dry weight; in the NP, it is between 20 and 30 percent dry weight.[78,79] The collagen in the AF is predominately of type I; that in the NP is almost all type II. The proportion of type I collagen fibers decreases from the outer part of the AF, and the proportion of type II increases toward the center of the NP. In the calf disc, as in human articular cartilage, minor collagens of types V, VI, and IX are found.[69] Collagen and proteoglycans are the major structural macromolecules in the disc. There are some minor amounts of other glycoproteins, elastin, and some serum proteins.[79] The major GAGs (part of proteoglycans) are CS and KS. Compared with HAC, proteoglycans of the disc are smaller and richer in KS.[69] With aging or degeneration, there is a greater loss of the small proteoglycans, so that the larger ones remain. In the intracellular matrix, collagen content is higher in the outer anulus, and it decreases inward to the nucleus, whereas the values for proteoglycans are the reverse.[69]

NUTRITION. The level of hydration confers the mechanical properties to the disc, and changes in the

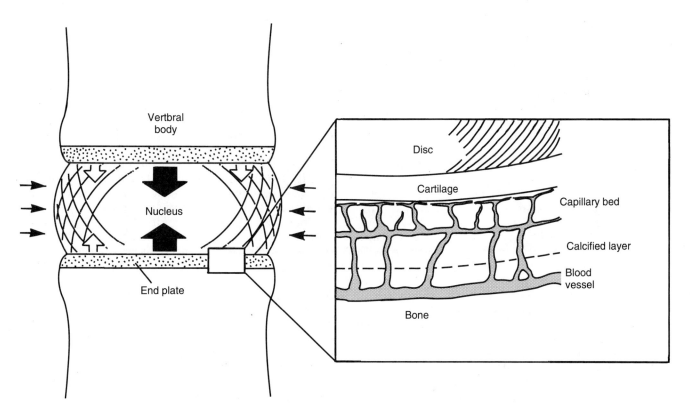

FIGURE 8–6. Schematic diagram of the nutritional routes into the intervertebral disc and an enlarged view of the area underneath the hyaline cartilage. (From Holm S, et al: Nutrition of the individual disc: Solute transport and metabolism. Connect Tissue Res 1981; 8:117.)

fluid content affect these properties. The creep or loss of disc height (1 to 2 cm between morning and night) is related to fluid loss. Changes in the microcirculation affect fluid flow patterns in the disc and its nutrition.[69] Since the cellularity of the disc is low, much of the water is interfibrillar and freely exchangeable. Proteoglycans maintain disc hydration by controlling osmotic pressure and the resistance of the tissue to fluid loss. The proteoglycan concentration in the collagen network determines the pore size of the matrix and thus the rate of fluid flow. Because of the avascularity of the disc, nutrients are derived by transport of solutes through the disc from the surrounding blood vessels, including, for the nucleus, vessels close to the central portion of the vertebral end plate.

The main mechanism for metabolite transport is diffusion, and the main route for supply of nutrients into the nucleus is via the end plate (see Fig. 8–6).[81] Holm and associates[81] demonstrated that the periphery of the vertebral end plate is practically impermeable. In the region of the NP, however, numerous blood vessels are in contact with the bony end plate. Only a small amount of glucose is predicted to be supplied by convection transport. It appears that most solutes are transported by diffusion. However, as Holm and Urban[69] noted, diffusion distances in humans can be large, and for about 16 hours of the day, the overall direction of fluid flow is outward. Oxygen retention is consistent through the AF but is much higher in the central portion of the NP.[81] This finding supports the theory of impermeability of the outer end plate and implies that the AF must derive its nutrition almost solely from the surrounding vasculature and not through the vertebral end plate.

INNERVATION. In a disc, only the AF is innervated. Bogduk and colleagues[82] found that nerves penetrated up to one-third of the total thickness of the AF of lumbar discs. Most of these nerves were remote from blood vessels; were of large diameter; and were derived from the lumbar sinuvertebral nerves, the ventral primary rami, and the gray rami communicans to innervate the posterior, posterolateral, and lateral aspects of the discs. Although most investigators have reported finding only free nerve endings,[83–86] Malinsky[87] described the presence of both encapsulated and nonencapsulated nerve endings on the lateral surface of the AF.

AGE CHANGES. With aging, the NP is less distinguished from the anulus. It becomes amorphous, with decreased elasticity and water-binding ability. Although Peacock[88] considered that the AF underwent comparatively few changes with age, Bernick and Cailliet[75] used light microscopy to demonstrate a progressive degeneration of the laminae from middle age onward. Chondroid material was deposited, and the collagen fibers became frayed and split and decreased in number. In the anuli of persons more than 70 years old, few laminae remained intact and discernible.[75] Clefts and fissures are visible after the third decade.[69] Additionally, with aging, cartilage end plates become calcified, which leads to resorption and replacement by bone.[75,89] There is also an apparent weakening

of the anchoring of the AF to the bony end plate, since the collagenous fibers are embedded only superficially into the end plate.[75]

Aging changes are largely detrimental to the intervertebral disc's function. This suggests that heavy impact loading and abrupt application of torques should be reduced as an individual ages.

FIBROUS CAPSULE

The joint cavity is lined by synovial tissues that cover all but the articulating surfaces of the joint and the contact surfaces of any intra-articular structure, such as menisci. Synovial tissues are intimately bound externally with the fibrous capsule, which is mostly type I collagen ($2\alpha_1$, $1\alpha_2$).[27] This type I collagen is similar but not identical to that in the dermis. It is hyperhydrated, with a water content estimated at about 70 percent. There is variability in the thickness and attachment of the capsule.[3] It may be thin and redundant, as in the shoulder joint, or thick and dense, as in the hip and the knee. Fiber diameter varies between 150 and 1500 nm, and fibers are organized in chiefly parallel bundles. Articular ligaments reinforce and may form the majority of the capsule. It is unique compared with other connective tissues involved in human articulations.

The extent of redundancy in the fibrous capsule, or lack thereof, has important consequences to the mobility of the joint (compare that of the hip and glenohumeral joints). Following injury, the unique characteristics of the specific joint must be restored. An inflamed capsule has a high potential for adhesion formation between redundant folds, indicating a need for early mobilization to prevent this occurrence.

It should be remembered that joint pathology and trauma invariably involve inflammation of synovial lining tissues. The fibrous phase may convert the proliferative fibro-fatty connective tissue formed in inflammation into adhesions, which, particularly when the part is immobilized, mature into strong scars. In small joints, where soft tissues are in close proximity, and in joints such as the shoulder, where redundant capsular folds may be present, this process can have profound effects on mobility and function.

When a joint is deprived of mechanical stimuli, there is decreased concentration of GAG and water.[90] The loss of the gel structure compromises connective tissue. Fiber-fiber distances and the lubrication between fibers that facilitates normal gliding are decreased, and adhesion formation and cross-linking between fibers are enhanced. The collagen arrangement is more random; fibers may be thicker as new fibers are laid down without regard to mechanical requirements. It is vital to control the inflammatory process. Therapy should avoid further aggravation until this is achieved, but there is considerable evidence that early motion should be encouraged. Continuous or intermittent passive motion has been demonstrated to be effective in the maintenance of mobility and the restoration of more normal tissue structure and function.[91,92]

INNERVATION

Articular cartilage is aneural. It is unknown how chondrocytes detect or transduce themselves into a biochemical response.[6] Chondrocyte shape is altered by mechanical stress. The chondrocytes can respond quickly and sensitively to small mechanical forces. It has been demonstrated that cultured chondrocytes and cartilage segments respond to both hydrostatic forces and deforming stress (stretch, directional), even when these are briefly applied.[93] Because most mechanical receptors (e.g., hair cell of the ear) possess monocilia of a nonmotile variety, Wilsman,[4] observing that one monocilium was present on every chondrocyte, hypothesized that this may provide a mechanotransductional function.

Stockwell[6] questioned whether the many cell processes that extend into the matrix pericellular zone may have connections with the collagen matrix framework via chondronectin or anchorin II, to give a sense of directionality when articular cartilage is loaded. Alternatively, it has been hypothesized that mechanical stress may provide a type of "pressure wave" to perturb the cell membrane and transform the mechanical stimulus into a chemical one, producing "receptor/catalytic" unit interaction or "greater activity of key enzymes." This process may involve cAMP, Ca²⁺, and adenyl cyclase, the inositol system in voltage-dependent channels.[94] The mechanoreceptor mechanism in articular cartilage remains to be found. The mechanisms causing the sensation of pain common to articular injuries are probably not derived from cartilage damage itself but are derived from increased pressure resulting from abnormal motion (as in chondromalacia patella)[95] and distention of the synovial lining tissues and fibrous capsule, periosteum, and other soft tissue structures related to the joint. A prime objective of injury management, therefore, must be reduction of inflammation to achieve pain relief.

Although cartilage is aneural, joint connective tissue structures (ligament, capsule, disc, fat pad) are well innervated with myelinated and unmyelinated fibers. Pain and vasomotor afferent fibers (about 45 percent) are small.[83,96] Most nerve endings are located in the fibrous portion of the capsule and not in the synovial lining tissues, with the exception of those accompanying vessels.[97-99] There is variability in location within and between joints and among species.[83] Space does not permit further consideration of the innervation of joints as a unit or arthrokinetic reflexes. The reader is referred to reviews by Wyke,[100,101] Dee,[83] Zimny,[102] and Johansson and Per Sjölander[103] for further information.

SYNOVIAL LINING TISSUES

The synovial lining tissue (synovium) is the soft connective tissue that borders the joint cavity and covers all intra-articular structures except for the central load-bearing portions of menisci and articular cartilage. The term "synovial membrane" is inappropriate be-cause there is no clearly defined membrane.[104,105] Synovial intima is the layer of lining cells that is immediately adjacent to the joint space. Beneath this inner layer, there is a supporting layer of subintimal tissue that merges on its external surface with the fibrous capsule of the joint or the fibrous outer coating of the tendon sheath or bursa. Synovium is a type of mesothelium, being derived from the original skeletoblastoma.[106]

There are two main types of cells in the synovium—type A and type B (the term "synoviocyte" is an alternative name for a synovial lining cell, but it is a general term and does not distinguish between the two main types of cell).[104] Synovial lining tissues have been described in a number of papers.[107,108] The synovial intima layer consists of a layer of cells 1 to 3 deep and set in a matrix (Fig. 8–7). Since this is not a continuous layer, both the synoviocytes and the matrix can come in contact with the joint fluid. Between the cells in the intimal layer, there are collagen fibers and some electron-dense, amorphous material that includes hyaluronate. A basement membrane is lacking, and cell processes—thin branching filaments—appear to provide a supportive membrane for the cells.

The subsynovial layer is a vascular connective tissue framework composed of fibrous, areolar, and fatty tissues (predominance of these tissues varies by site and within the joint), with some elements of the endothelial system and lymphatic.[108] Where fibrous tissue predominates, there is little difference between the amount of collagen fibers in the intima and that in the subsynovial tissues. In fatty or areolar varieties, however, few collagen fibers are seen in the intima.[104] Reticular fibers may be seen between the lining cells, and elastin fibers are found in the deep layer associated with capillaries. Synovial lining tissues are endowed with a rich plexus of blood vessels and lymphatics in the subsynovial layer; the latter are believed to be responsible for the transfer of nutrients into the synovial cavity and the formation of synovial fluid (Fig. 8–8).

Capillaries are located both in the subsynovial tissues and in the intima close to the surface. In the intima, capillaries are of the fenestrated variety, which is believed to facilitate movement of water and solutes into the tissues (Fig. 8–9). In the subsynovial tissues, the capillaries are of the continuous variety.[59] Vascularity varies both between joints and within a joint. Fibrous synovial surfaces are the least vascular.[62,109] Lymphatic vessels occur in groups, with arterioles and venules deep to the intima, and drain into regional lymph nodes. Blood sacs from the deeper lymphatic plexus penetrate the intima but do not reach the surface, as do capillaries.[110]

Although there are no free nerve endings in the subsynovial tissues, there are many autonomic fibers in the adventitia of blood vessels. Pacinian corpuscles have been noted at the border of the capsule and the synovial lining tissues.[111] Rodosky and Fu[112] noted that although the precise way in which pain is sensed from synovial lining tissues has not yet been elucidated, the surrounding tissues that are affected in synovitis are well innervated by pain fibers. The sensation of pain

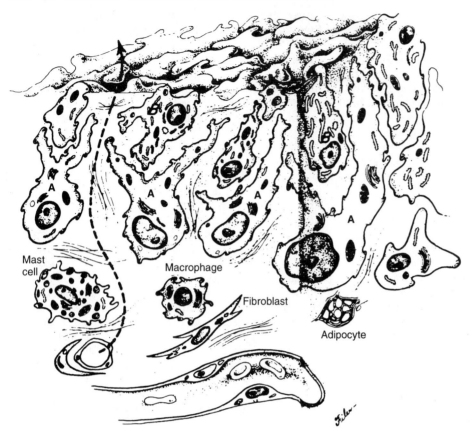

FIGURE 8–7. Normal synovium. The intimal layer consists of types A and B cells. The subintimal layer shows the vascular structures and various cell types seen normally. The arrow indicates the path taken by synovial fluid as it filters through the subintimal capillary and extracellular matrix on its way to the interior of the joint. (From Rodosky MW, Fu FH: Induction of synovial inflammation by matrix molecules, implant particles and chemical agents. *In* Leadbetter WB, Buckwalter JA, Gordon SL [eds]: Sports-Induced Inflammation. Park Ridge, IL, American Academy of Orthopaedic Surgeons. 1990, p 359.)

may be derived from pressure transmitted by the myelinated and nonmyelinated fibers and free nerve endings that have been observed close to blood vessels within the subsynovial fluid.[112,113] The functions of normal synovium are listed in Table 8–3.

SYNOVIAL LINING CELLS

Synovial lining cells, otherwise termed "synoviocytes," constitute the synovial intimal layer. These cells are distinguished by electron microscopic examination

to be composed of two major types: type A and type B (see Fig. 8–7). Cells with the features of both are quite common and are termed AB lining cells. The two major types of cells are not believed to represent two distinct lines but are functional variants of a single cell line.[108,114] Type A cells have prominent Golgi complexes, many vacuoles and vesicles, small amounts of rough endoplastic reticula, and many filopodia. Type B cells are essentially the converse of type A cells, with prominent nucleoli and long cytoplasmic processes. The type A cells appear to be equipped for phagocytosis and may

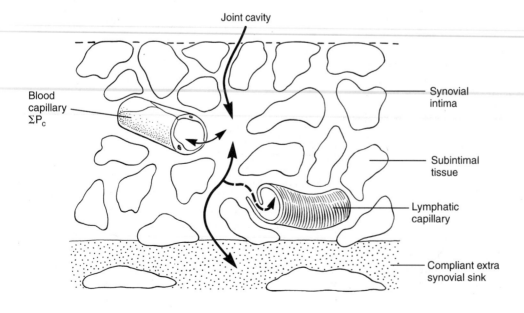

FIGURE 8–8. Diagram showing pathways for fluid exchange across the synovium. (From Levick JR: Synovial fluid dynamics. *In* Maroudes A, Holborow GJ [eds]: Studies in Joint Disease, vol 2. London, Pitman, 1983, p 165.)

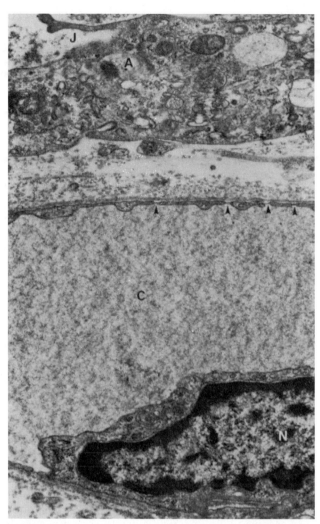

FIGURE 8–9. Synovial membrane of rabbit showing a large capillary (C) lying under a type A (A) synovial cell. An endothelial cell nucleus (N) is seen on the deep aspect of the capillary. Fenestra *(arrowheads)* are evident in the endothelial lining. Joint space (J) (× 28,000). (From Ghadially FN: Fine structure of joints. *In* Sokoloff L [ed]: The Joints and Synovial Fluid. London, Academic Press. 1978, p 148.)

be termed surface macrophages.[104] The type A cells have a capacity for endocytosis; they are thought to synthesize and may secrete hyaluronate into the joint fluid. Type B cells are equipped for protein secretion and are hypothesized to be responsible for polypeptide secretion due to their abundant rough endoplastic reticulum. They also have the capacity to secrete enzymes that can degrade cartilage. Type A cells can remove debris from the synovial fluid–cell interface and thus can clear the joint cavity.[112] This function has been shown in the retention of gold deposits in rheumatoid arthritis patients and the retention of artificial ligament wear fragments; both may be taken up by the synovial cells and persist indefinitely.[112] Retention of these substances reflects the slow turnover under physiologic conditions. However, the synovial lining cells do retain an ability for rapid cell division.[115]

Synovial lining cells also synthesize and release neutrophils or neutral proteinases that can degrade cartilage. In this function, type B cells may be primarily

involved. Collagenase can digest the collagenous lattice within the articular matrix. Other types produced are gelatinase and stromelysin.[116] Particularly, type A cells are believed to release cytokines such as interleukin-1 and prostaglandin E_2. Interleukin-1 is an inflammatory mediator that can cause chondrocytes to decrease matrix synthesis and resorb their surrounding matrix. The cytokines may play a major role in the perpetuation of synovitis.[115] Synovial cells are also activated by proteoglycans released from enzymatically digested cartilage. Synoviocytes may influence the immune response by presenting other targets for immune leukocytes or influence immune lymphocytes by expressing cell membrane molecules that affect the immune responses.[115]

ORIGIN OF SYNOVIAL LINING CELLS. Mitotic cells have not been reported in the intima of the synovium. Intimal cell replacement or regeneration appears to be derived from cells in the subintimal layer.[108,114,117] Henderson and Edwards[104] debated the origin of the synovial lining cells. Are they derived from a single cell line, and do they divide in situ? Or are they a mixture of connective tissue cells that arrive at a surface and whose behavior is distinguished from that of other connective tissue cells by the surface environment? The latter view is supported by evidence of regenerative tissue around artificial joints and the formation of adventitious bursa at sites of friction from sporting or occupational activities. These authors concluded that the synovial lining cells are probably a mixture of cells that in other sites would be described as macrophages and fibroblasts. Once at the surface, the cells undergo functional changes that may vary in different areas of the synovial lining. They are thus not a distinct population in terms of their origin and are more distinguished by position and arrangement. This is particularly true when viewed by light microscopy.

The intimal cells commonly have more long cytoplasmic processes than do the cells in the deep layers. Newer histologic techniques are constantly revealing new functional subpopulations.[104] Henderson and associates,[118] using the rat as an experimental model, induced a cavity with lining that resembled synovium. Their results suggested that tissue cavitation may stimulate fibroblasts and macrophages to differentiate into synovial lining cells. Fox and Kang[115] concluded

---

TABLE 8–3
Functions of the Synovial Lining Tissues[104,123]

- Provide low adherence of the surfaces
- Provide low friction lining
- Provide biological lubricants
- Provide deformable packing
- Provide blood supply for chondrocytes
- Control volume and composition of synovial fluid
- Transport nutrients into the joint space and remove metabolic wastes
- Play an important role in joint stability and joint health
- May have an antimicrobial effect

that the environment (synovial fluid, cells, and matrix) is necessary to maintain the differentiated state of these cells.

SYNOVIAL FLUID

Synovial fluid (SF) has a concentration of electrolytes and small molecules roughly the same as that of plasma.[119] However, it is not a dialysate of blood plasma, since synoviocytes secrete various substances in the SF, such as hyaluronate and glycoproteins. It is important to realize that there are only small amounts (a few drops) of free fluid in human joints and only a film of fluid covers the articulating structures within the joint. There are still no good methods to measure SF volume in healthy human joints, and values are reported only for the knee (0.5 to 4 mL).[120] Larger volumes than those found in the knee are reported in the shoulder or ankle, depending on the species studied. The joint cavity is a potential space, not a real space, as is often depicted diagrammatically. It has been shown that the thickness of SF between opposing articular surfaces is about 26 μm.[121] A gross analysis of normal joint fluid is given in Table 8–4. SF has no tensile force. The solute pressure (that exerted by dissolved substances, e.g., crystalloids) is balanced by extrinsic forces—that is, plasma hydrostatic and osmotic forces (exerted by proteins that are normally higher in plasma than in SF). Equilibrium between these forces is important in the control of fluid exchange between the joint space and synovial vessels; effusion is a result of imbalance.

SF volume is dependent on conditions in the lining interstitium, the forces acting upon it, and the permeability of the tissue surface to water and solutes. SF contains hyaluronic acid, a nonsulfated GAG, in higher concentration than that found in other connective tissue interstitial fluids. Hyaluronic acid is present in fluid as a complex with protein. There is no evidence that hyaluronic acid is actively exported by the synovial lining fluid cells,[104] but there is evidence that the cells synthesize hyaluronic acid.

SF is low in protein and has a high viscosity. It has a number of molecules with lubricating properties,

mainly glycoproteins, and its clearance rates are dependent on the molecular size. The glycoprotein-1 (termed "lubricin") is believed to be responsible for the lubricating ability of SF.[122] Although normal SF is mainly acellular,[120] differential white blood cell analysis shows, in decreasing values, monocytes, lymphocytes, plasmacytes, and polynuclear and synovial lining cells.[105] Protein is composed of approximately 60 percent of the small molecule albumin and 40 percent of the larger molecule globulin.[105] The albumin concentration is responsible for SF's colloid osmotic pressure. As SF does not contain fibrinogen or any clotting factors, it does not clot. Hyaluronate is responsible for the viscosity. Small molecules such as lactose, carbon dioxide, and inorganic pyrophosphate are produced by the joint tissues and diffused into the SF; glucose enters the SF by a facilitated diffusion. Despite the large amount of fat in synovium, little lipid is present in SF.[105] All plasma proteins can cross the vascular endothelium, traverse the synovial interstitium, and enter SF (see Figure 8–7). The major mechanism is a size-selective process of passive diffusion; small molecules such as albumin enter easily, whereas larger molecules such as fibrinogen are largely excluded.[123] The interstitium or tissue space of the synovial lining appears to be an important factor in the trans-synovial exchange of small molecules into SF.

Joints exist to provide motion within the constraints of the surrounding soft tissues. The synovial lining must adapt to a wide range of positions without being pinched. An effective lubrication system is vital. The synovial lining must be able to expand and contract with joint motion, a process of folding, unfolding, and elastic stretching of the tissue. Geborek and Wollheim[120] hypothesized that hyaluronate may assist in the adherence of joint surfaces, which, given the subatmospheric intracavity pressure, plays a role in maintaining surface alignment during distractive forces.

JOINT PRESSURES

Discrepancy between the colloid osmotic pressure of the synovium and SF may explain the negative subatmospheric intracavity pressure. The intra-articular pressure (IAP) helps keep the joint surfaces in contact, achieve congruency, and lessen strain on joint stabilizing structures such as ligaments.[123] Subatmospheric intracavity pressure of −8 to −12 cm of water in three noninfused human knees was reported by Müller[124] (Fig. 8–10). In the presence of an effusion, the IAP may be positive. The mechanism by which this pressure is maintained is unclear, but it is not thought to be due to the contraction of muscles or the pumping action of the lymphatics.[123] However, some authors believe that the latter plays a major role.[120] In active exercise, the mean IAP is increased, and it is reported to be between −25 and −102 mg Hg in human knees with simple isometric exercise.[125] However, the IAP is unchanged during passive joint motion.[126] If the pressure is driven sufficiently low, dissolved gases may come out of solution and give rise to the "knuckle crack" on sudden distraction of joint surfaces.[127]

TABLE 8–4
Gross Analysis of Joint Fluid[105]

Parameter	Normal Finding	
Volume (human knee)	<4 ml	
Color	Clear to pale yellow	
Clarity	Transparent	
Viscosity	High	
Mucin clot	Good	
Spontaneous clot	None	

Parameter	Range	Mean
pH	7.2–7.43	7.38
White blood cells/mm²	13–180	63
Total protein (g/dL)	1.2–3.0	1.8
Hyaluronate (g/dL)	–	0.3

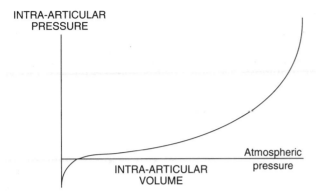

FIGURE 8–10. Pressure-volume relation in a diarthrodial joint when increasing the interarticular volume (modified after Levick, 1983[128]. (From Geborek P, Wollheim FA: Synovial fluid: *In* Wright V, Radin E [eds]: Mechanics of Human Joints. New York, Marcel Dekker, 1993, p 118. Reprinted by courtesy of Marcel Dekker, Inc.)

Clinicians should be aware that, in the presence of effusion, joint stability is compromised because the pressure becomes positive. Strain on supporting structures such as ligaments, already compromised by the inflammatory process, is increased.[120]

CARTILAGE NUTRITION

Cartilage nutrition is believed to be derived from three sources: from the vascular net in the perichondrium and the synovial tissue near its periphery, from the synovial fluid, and from blood vessels in the underlying marrow cavity. The importance of these sources is disputed.[3] Hunter, in 1743, first observed that the articular cartilage was devoid of blood vessels.[37] Since that time, there have been a number of studies that further elucidated cartilage nutrition, notably by Ekholm in 1951, who concluded, from studies using radioactive gold on rabbit joint cartilage, that nutrition was probably partly from synovial fluid and partly from direct contacts between the epiphyseal marrow spaces and basal layers of cartilage.[129] Later studies substantiated that immature articular cartilage received some nutrition via the subchondral route.[50,130,131]

Mow and colleagues[132] noted that even though HAC is very hydrated, being about 75 percent water, its pores are of a molecular size. This indicates that macromolecules that constitute the solid matrix, collagens, proteoglycans, and other glycoproteins are highly dispersed in the interstitial fluid. These authors proposed that the motion and deformation behavior of the tissues must be described by a genuinely valid and "finite deformation non-linearly permeable biphasic theory."[132] The rate of loading on this porous, free-draining surface or tissue causes a variable rate of fluid efflux at the loading surface or, at least, at the edges of the contact zones. Although fluid flow in cartilage and intervertebral discs is influenced by loading, the bulk of fluid flow in these tissues is largely passive.

The pore size is dependent on proteoglycan concentration. Pore size controls the rate at which water can flow through articular cartilage or the intervertebral disc, and it also controls the distribution of large solutes in the tissues. Small solutes, such as simple ions, can fit through all pores, but as the molecular size of the solutes increases, the ability to fit through the pores decreases. If there is a loss of proteoglycan in hyaline cartilage, the larger proteins can enter with increasing concentrations. The proteoglycan content is responsible for the osmotic pressure. The hydraulic permeability coefficient is also sensitive to the proteoglycan content. More notable in intervertebral discs, there is a higher load during day activities than at night, when the body is at rest. There is a net outflow of fluid from the intervertebral disc during the day and a net influx of fluid during the night that is sufficient to produce a discernible change in body height of about 1 to 2 cm between morning and evening.[133,134] Osmotic pressure depends more on the charge concentration than on the proteoglycan size or degree of aggregation. Fixed negative charges exclude anions such as Cl^- and SO_4, and cations such as Na^+, Ca^{2+}, Mg^{2+}, and K^+ have a higher concentration.

The subsynovial microvasculature and lymphatics obviously play a large role in cartilage nutrition, being the source of nutrients and the normal clearance mechanism, respectively. Imbalance between microvascular permeability, especially to proteins, and the normal clearance mechanism of the lymphatic outflow occurs in effusions. It is reflected by an increased protein concentration in synovial fluid. Regular motion may adequately clear the leaking protein, but rest, sleep, or immobilization allows the synovial lining tissues to become edematous; the individual experiences pain and stiffness. This indicates the importance of even once-daily movement through available range in effused joints.

Clinicians should be aware of the positive correlation between effective synovial plasma flow and intra-articular temperature.[135] Cooler, low-flow effusions are more likely to have metabolic evidence of ischemia and of low glucose, pH, and lactate.[136] This finding suggests that moderate heat modalities should be more effective in promoting clearance than cold therapy. In effused joints—either hot or cold—clinicians should be concerned not only with pain relief but also with achieving the primary goal of inflammation control and effusion reduction.

Production of the matrix is the responsibility of chondrocytes, and cell health is dependent on an adequate supply of nutrients and the efficient removal of metabolic waste products; solute diffusivity is important to this process. Holm and associates[81] showed that there is a negative correlation between oxygen concentration in the NP as a function of distance from the vertebral end plate. Since the end plate is almost totally impermeable, any solutes entering the NP must enter the blood vessels that surround the anulus on the periphery.[81] Thus, oxygen concentrations vary with the position in the intervertebral disc and are highest at the periphery and lowest at the center of the nucleus. This is similar in HAC, where the oxygen concentrations are highest at the surface closest to the synovial fluid, the source of diffusing oxygen from the blood supply within the synovial lining tissues, and lowest in the calcified zone of the cartilage adjacent to the subchondral plate. The latter is impervious in mature, healthy cartilage.

JOINT LUBRICATION

Healthy human synovial joints have a remarkable ability to permit reciprocal movements within a wide range of loads and speeds while maintaining stability. Their low frictional resistance makes human joints remarkably slippery. Our understanding of joint lubrication has evolved slowly over the last 3 decades. Models of human joint lubrication are theoretical, derived from engineering man-made bearings, and involve complex mathematics. There has been a lack of biological data to test the theoretical models, but those data are slowly growing. Experiments have been largely in vitro, which vastly simplifies the actual joint properties and physiologic conditions. Recently, computer modeling has been employed. Space does not permit an extensive account of the work that has led to the current opinions on how human joints are lubricated.

The reader is referred to papers by Unsworth,[137,138] McCutchen,[139] and Dintenfass.[140] In this section, the current theories are briefly reviewed.

Like engineering bearings, human joints should function with very low friction and wear, regardless of the loading conditions. The type of loading is an important factor in the mechanism of human joint lubrication. Human joints are subjected to steady (static or constant) loading (as in standing still) and dynamic (cyclic) loading (as in jumping or in gait). Loading can vary from very light loads, such as in the swing phase of gait (< 500 N), to three to five times body weight, such as at heel contact in the stance phase of gait when hip and knee forces are about 1500 N (40 lbs = 177 N).[137] High loads tend to occur for only brief periods (0.01 to 0.15 second), whereas low loads occur for longer periods (> 5 seconds). Table 8–5 gives the different mechanisms that are believed to play a role in lubrication of human joints (Fig. 8–11). Critical variables in the proposed mechanisms for joint lubrication are given in Table 8–6. Surface compliance is an important variable because the harder the surface, the higher the friction. Under loading, if the surface is compliant, more of the

TABLE 8–5
Proposed Mechanisms for Human Joint Lubrication

Mechanism	Author	Year	Definition
Hydrodynamic	MacConnaill[141]	1932	UL, wedgelike fluid film present to separate surfaces in unidirectional motion
Mixed (fluid film and boundary)	Jones[147,148] Linn[149]	1934, 1936 1968	H/C, rough points in contact but fluid present in "dips" to provide fluid film at those sites
Hydrostatic	McCutchen[142] Mow & Mansour[143]	1959 1977	High loads, cartilage compression, fluid extruded ahead of the loaded areas and in dips in rough surface
Boundary	Charnley[146]	1959	Low loads, thin layer of large molecules adsorbed on the surface, forming a gel to protect rough points in contact; inadequate compression for fluid extrusion from HAC
Weeping	McCutchen[142]	1959	H/C, surfaces kept apart owing to impervious subchondral bone, which causes fluid outflow during the creep phase of cartilage deformation
Elastohydrodynamic	Dintenfass[140]	1963	UL-L, wedge-film, model recognizes pliability of HAC to reduce friction
Squeeze film	Fein[145]	1966–67	L, pliability deformability of HAC reduces peak pressures and spreads load when loads are maintained after motion ceases
Boosted	Walker et al[150]	1968	H/C porosity of cartilage allows fluid efflux to augment fluid film between surfaces
Micro-elastohydrodynamic	Dowson & Jin[144]	1986	L, local pressures on high spots, given HAC deformability smooths surface, allows fluid film to exist

H/C = high and/or constant loading; L = brief loading, no motion; UL = unloaded; Ul-L = unloaded, free swinging (swing phase gait).

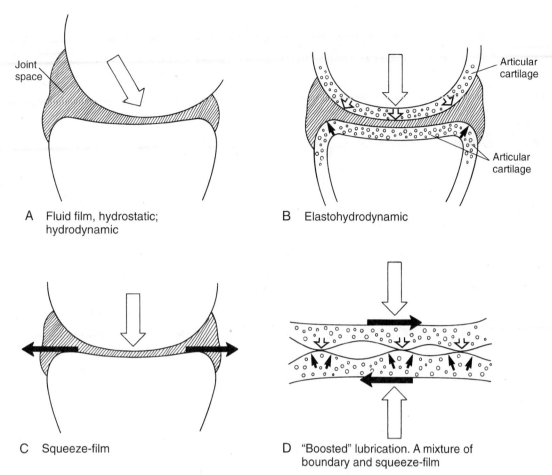

FIGURE 8–11. Theoretical models of lubrication (see text for details).

joint surface is brought into contact. In actual fact, under a no-load or light-load condition, joint surfaces are incongruent. With higher loads, because of the surface compliance, the joint surfaces become more congruent, increasing joint stability.

Surface roughness has been shown in all types of microscopy (Fig. 8–12).[59] It is considered that the surface roughness produces contact areas that may result in pools of fluid being trapped when the joint is loaded. Some investigators, however, consider the surface roughness detected by electron microscopy to represent only artifacts.[151]

The remarkable slipperiness of human joints is measured by the coefficient of friction (COF). The COF is the shear force needed to make one surface slide on another, divided by the normal force pressing them together. The lower the COF, the lower the resistance to sliding. For example, a skate on ice has a COF of 0.03, whereas the theorized COF for cartilage on cartilage is between 0.02 and 0.001.[152,153] The higher the coefficient, the greater the force that is required to move the bearing or joint under load. Where a fluid film is predicted to exist between the surfaces of a joint, the COF is approximately 0.01. In the fluid film model, rough points of the surfaces are always separated by a thin film of pressurized fluid. Where the boundary lubrication mechanism is proposed, the COF is 0.1 to 0.5 and is independent of the speed of sliding or load.[137] In the latter model, the surfaces are separated only by a thin layer of molecules adsorbed onto the surface (molecules too large to enter cartilage). In disease states in which the surfaces are fibrillated, the ability to have boundary lubrication is reduced, since larger molecules may enter HAC.

Synovial joints are characterized by a very low COF. Linn and Radin[154] disproved that hyaluronic acid was responsible for the lubrication by demonstrating that the boundary lubrication ability of synovial fluid was destroyed by trypsin but was unchanged by hyaluronidase treatment. These results suggested that the lubrication ability lay in some form of protein. Swann and coworkers[122] showed that the lubrication ability resided in glycoprotein-1 and suggested that the term "lubricin" be used for this glycoprotein. Questions concerning its synthesis and the rate and control of synthesis remain unanswered.

Synovial fluid has "thixotropic" flow characteristics, which means the slower the flow, the more viscous it becomes. The viscosity of synovial fluid is important for fluid film mechanisms.[27] The previously described synovial fluid protein lubricant plays an important role in the mechanism of boundary lubrication by adhering to the surfaces of the joint. Boundary lubrication is considered most effective at low loads.[155] Under low loading conditions, fluid replenishment cannot be relied on, because the cartilage is inadequately com-

TABLE 8–6
Critical Variables in Joint Lubrication Mechanisms

Variable	Effect of Change from Normal Values*
Surface compliance (elasticity)	When ↓ dispersion load, focal concentration of forces leading to microfracture of SCB, ↓ adjustment of surface to loads; therefore, EHD or M-EHD less effective, vulnerable to long-term, high-stress, cyclic loading
Surface roughness	When ↑ there is ↑ contact stresses and friction, ↓ potential for fluid film
Low coefficient of friction	↑ force required to move joint under load; boundary lubrication more likely to exist than fluid film
Rolling and sliding velocities	Normally sustain HDL and fluid film; absence ↑ contact, therefore, boundary lubrication, ↑ friction and wear
Synovial fluid viscosity	Owing to hyaluronate, NB lubricant of synovium, not cartilage, gives thixotrophy to SF (slower the flow, more viscous it becomes); inadequate lubrication of SLT where contact occurs
Synovial fluid protein lubricants	If ↓ loss of boundary lubricants, ↓ defense against distraction and ↓ joint stability, ↑ friction, ↑ slippage under load; inadequate lubrication in low-load states
Surface permeability	If ↑ larger molecules can penetrate, ↓ ability to have boundary lubrication conditions, therefore, ↑ wear; if ↓ impairs cartilage nutrition and removal of waste products, ↓ stiffness, inadequate protection of SCB from peak forces
Joint surface contour	Incongruity of unloaded joint permits deformation of SCB under loads; loss of normal variability in HAC across surfaces means > area in initial contact, ↓ load dispersion, more boundary lubrication conditions, ↑ wear

EHD = elastohydrodynamic lubrication; HAC = hyaline articular cartilage; HDL = hydrodynamic lubrication; M-EHD = micro-EHD; SCB = subchondral bone; SF = synovial fluid; SLT = synovial lining tissue.
*Variables are not acting alone to determine lubrication type and ease of motion.

pressed. In these instances, boundary lubrication, from macromolecules that adhere to the surface, is considered best. The hydrostatic mechanism is best at generating a fluid film under high loads when there is cartilage compression and fluid is extruded from the cartilage, especially on surfaces ahead of the load.[143] It is now believed that fluid film mechanisms can operate in healthy human joints under most conditions.

Figure 8–13 shows the theorized loading-lubricating mechanisms for the hip joint during the gait cycle.[137,156,157] In the swing phase, there is a light load and a fluid film exists, separating the two surfaces. At heel contact, the load is very high, with a low entraining velocity, and the fluid film, though reduced, still separates the joint surfaces. In mid-stance, the load is decreased, the entraining velocity is increased, and there is elastic deformation of the surface; the mechanism is one of elastohydrodynamic (EHD) lubrication (a rolling or sliding motion that pressurizes the viscous joint fluid and squashes cartilage, which changes the pressures generated in the fluid), which maintains a small fluid film. At toe-off, once again there is a very high load and a very low entraining velocity. It is theorized, however, that with high loads, the squeeze film mechanism (compliant, deformable surface and incompressible fluid) can maintain a small fluid film between the two surfaces for a few seconds. Therefore, because there are transient applications of variable loads, a fluid film mechanism can operate in a healthy human joint throughout the gait cycle.

When an individual stands for long periods, such as on guard duty, a condition is created in which the fluid film is not maintained. The cartilage, however, weeps in the noncontact areas just ahead of the load. Boundary lubrication is theorized to operate where surface-to-surface contact occurs, with pools in the roughened dips of the cartilage that are not in full contact. The larger molecule of the hyaluronic acid protein complex is unable to penetrate the cartilage and remains on the surface. This mechanism is termed "boosted lubrication," as fluid is extruded owing to pressure in the noncontact areas (see Fig. 8–11). Friction increases as more of the surface cartilage is in contact. The lubricant glycoprotein in the synovial fluid can reduce the friction

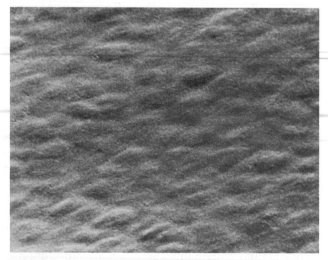

FIGURE 8–12. Normal adult rabbit articular cartilage showing numerous pits on the surface (× 400). (From Ghadially FN, Oryschak AF, Yong NK: Experimental production of ridges on rabbit articular cartilage: A scanning electron microscope study. J Anat 1976; 121:121.)

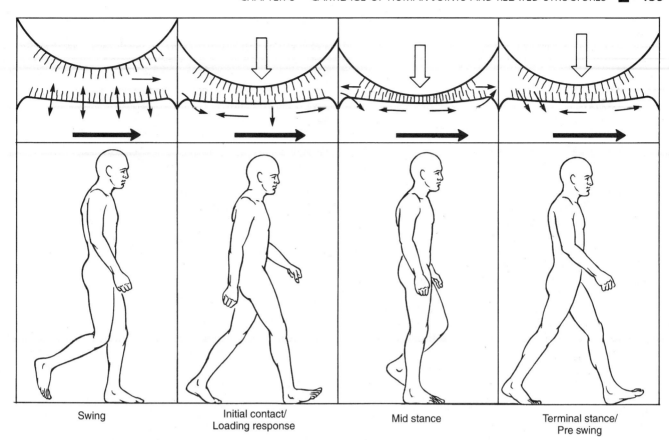

Swing   Initial contact/   Mid stance   Terminal stance/
                     Loading response   Pre swing

FIGURE 8–13. Lubrication mechanisms for the right hip joint. (From Unsworth A: Lubrication of human joints. *In* Wright V, Radin E [eds]: Mechanics of Human Joints. New York, Marcel Dekker, 1993, p 158. Reprinted by courtesy of Marcel Dekker, Inc.)

and wear when motion recommences, and the fluid film would be restored.[137] The boundary lubricating ability of synovial fluid becomes more important when it loses its viscosity because of injury or disease. Loss of cartilage compliance or deformability under loading, as occurs in aging, reduces the ability to maintain fluid film by the squeeze film or EHD mechanisms.

Clinicians need to be aware of the potential for synovial cells to release substances that soften and degrade cartilage matrix, as well as how cartilage is nourished (see the previous section). Lubrication mechanisms should be considered in planning rehabilitation and return to training. Modes of exercise that theoretically provide fluid film conditions rather than boundary conditions appear to be preferable. Studies of damaged cartilage (osteoarthrosis) and lubrication mechanisms suggest that clinicians should be particularly attuned to the theories that (1) the manner (type) of loading is more important than the actual load, (2) the potential for wear increases when the joint goes from static loading to high loads, (3) synovial fluid volume and lymphatic clearance increase with exercise, (4) friction is inversely related to the predicted thickness of the fluid film, (5) cartilage deteriorates in the unloaded state, and (6) repetitive impulsive loading (RIL), e.g., typing, using a pneumatic drill, skipping is detrimental to both articular cartilage and subchondral bone.

Insufficient data exist to scientifically prescribe ideal exercise programs to ensure a fluid film mechanism and avoid cartilage damage. However, prudence suggests that, in the presence of joint pathology, trauma, or effusion, passive motion should be accompanied by gentle traction to avoid compression of softened cartilage and overstretching of vulnerable, inflamed soft tissues such as ligaments and tendons. Pendular-type movements provide a fluid film and minimal or no wear. Static loading and isometric exercise, if used, should be very brief (a few seconds), as these conditions favor a mixed model of lubrication, with boundary friction predominating. High loading should be either very brief or avoided. High loading is possibly least harmful following low-load, high-velocity motion, since the latter encourages the presence of a fluid film region. If high loads are sustained for less than 0.5 second, a squeeze film mechanism should ensure that a fluid film exists. If resistance is applied in any form, the individual should work through the range, and holding periods at the end range (e.g., knee extension) should be *very* brief. Controlled eccentric loading creates large compressive (loading) forces; these should be avoided where cartilage damage may exist.

Research suggests that cartilage has such a low permeability that any fluid flow out of cartilage to contribute to lubrication of joint surfaces is negligible. Therefore, clinicians cannot predict that load-bearing exercises will provide an adequate fluid film by promoting fluid efflux from cartilage. However, load bearing will promote fluid influx into cartilage and facilitate cartilage nutrition. It is hoped that further research will elucidate this area for which minimal "hard" evidence currently exists.

MECHANISMS OF CARTILAGE BREAKDOWN

Since cartilage is avascular, it cannot demonstrate an inflammatory process, a normal response to injury and an important component of repair. Conditions in which breakdown of cartilage occurs are generally classified as inflammatory (e.g., rheumatoid arthritis) or noninflammatory (e.g., chondromalacia [nonprogressive], osteoarthrosis [progressive, leading to osteoarthritis]). Multiple factors are involved in cartilage breakdown, the imbalance between extracellular matrix synthesis, and degradation. Repetitive impulsive loading may be the major factor in cartilage breakdown leading to osteoarthrosis and osteoarthritis.[158] Other factors are stress deprivation (immobilization, bed rest, weightlessness), excessive loading (body weight), developmental etiologies leading to abnormal force transmission (e.g., developmental hip dysplasia, coxa valga, genu valgum), joint surface incongruity, and joint instability (generalized ligamentous laxity and cruciate ligament damage). In rheumatoid arthritis (RA), free radicals, cytokines, neutral proteinases, and catabolic enzymes (which may be derived from synoviocytes, chondrocytes, or polymorphonuclear leukocytes) play a primary role; they are also a factor in osteoarthritic cartilage breakdown.[5,41,57,159–167] Regardless of the cause of exudation, proliferation, or infiltration, the highly vascular synovial lining tissues can respond with an inflammatory process. This produces variable joint effusion and potentially eventual fibrosis and thickening, which may adversely affect synovial fluid production, cartilage nutrition, and joint space clearance.

The inflamed synovial lining tissues secrete enzymes and neutral proteinases, such as cholinase, as well as release neutral proteoglycans, which decrease cartilage matrix synthesis, break down and absorb matrix, degrade the collagenous matrix, and may play a role in maintenance of synovitis.[5,16,123]

The chondrocyte is at particular risk because of its location in avascular cartilage and the long transit route of its nutrition from subsynovial capillaries through synovial lining tissues, synovial fluid, and cartilage matrix. Chondrocytes also secrete degrading (catabolic) enzymes and protease inhibitors (see Fig. 8–2). Imbalance between anabolism and catabolism of cartilage matrix results in matrix destruction. The reader is referred to Poole[5] for a detailed review of factors affecting cartilage degradation.

The belief that repetitive impulsive loading is the principal mechanism of cartilage breakdown in osteoarthrosis has been proposed by Radin.[158] It is theorized that repetitive impulse loading leads to microfractures of subchondral bone and activation of the secondary center of ossification, which causes the tidemark to advance and duplicate, and the noncalcified cartilage layer to thin, perhaps totally. This process increases shear forces in the deeper layers, decreases dispersion of stresses within HAC, and leads to deep horizontal and vertical splitting, with surface fibrillation, as cartilage deteriorates. Proteoglycan loss occurs. Articular detritus is present in synovial fluid. This may act to perpetuate synovial effusion, leading to synovial tissues producing and releasing more cartilage-degrading substances into synovial fluid.

Osteoarthritic cartilage is characterized by hypertrophic chondrocytes and clustering of cells. This reflects an attempt by the cells to increase matrix synthesis.

With the loss of proteoglycans, there is an unmasking of collagen fibers within the cartilage matrix. In osteoarthritis, extensive damage to type II collagen fibers occurs, with eventual unwinding of the triple helix and the appearance of crimping of collagen fibrils. This process commences in the superficial layers and progresses to involve deeper layers.[5,15] As collagen fibers become exposed on the surface, normal joint motion gradually produces a roughened surface, encouraging splitting, cartilage detachment, and potentially complete cartilage abrasion. Since cartilage cannot regenerate, its destruction causes a reaction by subchondral bone consisting of osteosclerosis and osteophytes. Bone itself may be abraded and eburnated. Joint fluid detritus may lodge in the exposed medullary spaces, producing cysts. This end process is similar in both osteo- and rheumatoid arthritis. All phagocytosed structural elements, including bone calcium apatite crystals, contribute to joint space detritus, which provokes synovitis (secondary in osteoarthritis) or perpetuates it in RA-like conditions. Fassbender,[168] however, emphasized that the synovial tissue in secondary synovitis of osteoarthrosis or osteoarthritis does not destroy HAC as it does in RA. Exposure of subchondral bone provides blood vessels to the area as well as collagen fibers, enabling a scar pannus to form to provide a measure of repair.

In RA, there is proliferation of the synovial lining tissues. Mesenchymal cells migrate over the joint surface—a process thought to be facilitated by fibronectin—and eventually form a fibrous pannus.[115] This may lead to fibrous ankylosis.

Obviously and fortunately, not all individuals demonstrate the total degradation of cartilage described above.

REPAIR OF ARTICULAR CARTILAGE

POTENTIAL

It is well established that articular cartilage has a low potential for repair, for both the cellular and the matrix components.[5,41,169,179] When trauma or disease occurs, a tissue must have regenerative capacity for the repair process to result in the presence of tissue that is identical to the original tissue. This repair process is well known and involves an inflammatory reaction and formation of a fibrin clot, which provides the scaffold for new cells to come in and reconstitute the tissue. Sledge[170] noted that repair of articular cartilage is not intrinsically well programmed; the emphasis is on protection from damage. Many investigators have been unable to observe mitosis or any evidence of cell division in normal adult cartilage.[41]

The constraints on repair of articular cartilage are low cellularity, lack of a primitive cell population with chondrogenic potential, avascularity of the tissue, and great distance of cells from their nutritional sources.[168] Healing of articular cartilage appears to be dependent on whether the defect penetrates the subchondral plate. When subchondral plate penetration occurs, as in deeper injuries, there is extensive fibroblastic proliferation from cells in the adjacent bone, but "seldom is true hyaline cartilage produced."[170] Landells[172] noted that essentially no repair was evident by surviving or remaining cells when the cleft involved only the articular cartilage.

A few authors have reported the existence of mitotic activity. Havdrup and Telhag[169] demonstrated mitosis in unoperated and sham operated rabbits with traumatized cartilage. It was unknown whether the mitotic activity was due to a decrease in cell inhibitors or an increase in stimulation factors. Evidence of mitotic activity was also reported in rabbits that had been subjected to sustained pressure by clamping the limb in an abnormal position of full extension.[173]

Several investigators noted that in the presence of degeneration, as is characteristic in osteoarthritis, the HAC chondrocytes appear to recover their ability to undergo division.[174] The ability of chondrocytes in osteoarthritis to replicate their DNA appears to be an ability that cells of healthy HAC either suppress or lose.[175] It was also demonstrated that cartilage can undergo mitosis when grown in culture.[176] Poole noted that in both in vivo and in vitro studies of adult periosteum, it was demonstrated that the bone morphogenic molecules, such as osteogenin, can result in cartilage formation; adult periosteum appears to remain chondrogenic.[5,177,178] The latter is reflected in osteophyte formation at the periosteal-cartilage junction in osteoarthrosis. Cultured articular cartilage appears to have properties more like those of fibrocartilage than of articular cartilage.[176] There are species differences in the growth and behavior of mammalian chondrocytes. Articular cartilage, when repaired, has been reported in a number of studies to be similar to hyaline cartilage, particularly when examined with light microscopy. Biochemical and biomechanical studies, however, have clearly demonstrated that the cartilage formed in the repair process has characteristics that are more like those of fibrocartilage. There is a higher portion of type I collagen in repaired articular cartilage than in HAC.

Repair is controlled by numerous factors, mainly hormonal, synovial, and cartilage-derived chemical mediators, as well as mechanical stimuli. For a fuller discussion of these influences, the reader is directed to Sledge,[170] Buckwalter and Mow,[179] and Brandt and Mankin.[16] Knowledge of the factors governing the anabolic and catabolic processes that are crucial to the repair potential of cartilage is critical to understanding HAC's responsiveness to injury. Akeson and colleagues[92] stressed that a number of studies over the years—first by Convery and associates[180] and later by Salter and colleagues[91]—have amply demonstrated that healing by HAC occurs only in small defects (about one eighth of an inch in diameter) and does not occur in large or full-thickness defects, with or without motion. This finding has been demonstrated by histologic, biochemical, and biomechanical studies of the replacement tissue. It demonstrates that physical stimuli, such as motion and load, are critical to the repair of HAC and may either stimulate or inhibit the repair capacity. The collagen network may provide the substratum used by mesenchymal cells to migrate over the surface of cartilage defects.[11] The reader is referred to Buckwalter and coworkers,[165] Caterson and Buckwalter,[181] Byers and Brown,[182] Akeson and associates,[92] Buckwalter and Mow,[179] and Salter[91] for descriptions and discussions of current research involving studies of articular cartilage injury and methods of facilitating repair of articular cartilage. A brief description of these approaches is given below.

APPROACHES TO FACILITATE REPAIR

Current practice in severe joint damage is the surgical replacement of the joint by an artificial prosthesis. Joint replacement devices have a limited tolerance for heavy loading and vigorous wear. Particularly in younger patients, in whom implanted devices may work loose with growth, arthroplasties and arthrodeses do not provide satisfactory simulations of natural joints. Investigators continue to search for methods to stimulate repair of damaged cartilage and provide a near normal articulating surface. If techniques can be employed to simulate the coverage of load-bearing surfaces with tissue that has loading characteristics that permit functioning similar to that of natural HAC, in younger patients, joint replacement procedures can be deferred until after maturity. Methods explored to improve repair are biomechanical, biophysical, subchondral bone, grafting, surgical implantation, and various combinations of these methods.

BIOMECHANICAL

Biomechanical approaches that have shown variable success involve

1. Using osteotomies to alter the distribution of the load and improve the congruity or alignment of the joint surfaces.
2. Performing tendon transplants or muscle releases,[183] which alter the forces acting over the joint.
3. Decreasing the load through the weight-bearing surfaces by the use of different ambulatory aids (e.g., canes, crutches).
4. Using continuous or intermittent passive motion (CPM or IPM).

The biomechanical approach of CPM has shown a degree of success, as reported mainly by Salter and associates.[184] CPM may be delivered either continuously or cyclically. In adolescent rabbits, Salter and coworkers[185] demonstrated the healing of full-thickness drill hole defects by hyaline cartilage within 4 weeks, with a significant difference in the animals that had been treated by CPM. The percentage of HAC in the three experimental groups of rabbits was as follows: immobilized, 8 percent; free motion, 9 percent; CPM, 52 percent. O'Driscoll and Salter[186] had similar results using free intra-articular periosteal grafts. These results were less impressive in mature rabbits. It was not established how the newly synthesized HAC responded to normal loading over time. Both of these studies showed a combination of approaches—CPM and involvement of the subchondral bone with the use of full-thickness drill holes or periosteal grafts. The reader is referred to Salter[91] and Akeson and colleagues[92] for more detailed descriptions and discussions of the use of passive motion to promote healing of cartilage.

Recently, Coutts and associates[187] demonstrated in the mediofemoral condyles of adult rabbits with full-thickness defects and rib perichondrial grafts that nearly normal HAC was present in 55 percent of animals at 6 weeks; at 1 year, 82 percent demonstrated type II collagen. The shear moduli did not differ between the two groups (those exposed to cage activity alone and those having passive motion followed by cage activity). This study showed that HAC with biomechanical properties would develop and not degrade within 1 year after the full-thickness defects had been created. Also, the percentage of type II collagen may increase over time.[188] Moran and colleagues,[189] using rabbits with full-thickness defects and autogenous periosteal grafts, utilized either CPM or IPM. The tissue was examined with a variety of microscopy approaches and histochemistry, but no biomechanical tests were done. They demonstrated healing by hyaline cartilage that contained type II collagen, but with an irregular organization. This result was better in the animals that had been grafted and better in animals that had CPM rather than IPM.

It is important that either in vitro or in vivo methods to simulate, induce, or improve repair of articular cartilage be examined biomechanically to test the functional behavior of the tissues. Several studies using microscopy have shown that the repair tissue may have the appearance of hyaline cartilage, but it fails to perform like articular cartilage, especially over time. This suggests that a return to sports with repetitive impulsive loading (e.g., hurdling, running, ice skating with jumps) is probably ill-advised. Since it is shown in animals that type II collagen takes a year or more to develop, a very gradual return to high loading conditions would be prudent.

BIOPHYSICAL

Variable effects of electromagnetic fields on cartilage and chondrocytes have been demonstrated. No effect of pulsed electromagnetic fields on extracellular matrix synthesis of chondrocytes in high-density cultures has been observed.[190] However, increased proteoglycan and DNA synthesis occurred with chondrocytes grown in cultures with constant direct current.[191] Other studies revealed a stimulating effect of electromagnetic fields on chondrocyte activity.[192–194] Two studies demonstrated enhanced healing of osteochondral defects in rabbits, with the animals showing repair tissue resembling hyaline cartilage.[195,196] The long-term results and biomechanical characteristics of the repair tissue are not known, but it is reasonable that electromagnetic fields should have a biological effect. Current intensity may be a critical factor. On growth plate chondrocytes grown in electrical fields, Armstrong and coworkers[197] showed inhibited growth with strong electrical fields but enhancement of proliferation with weaker electrical fields.

Increased synthesis of proteoglycans and collagen was shown following exposure to carbon dioxide and Nd:YAG-laser irradiation in organ bovine cultures and chondrocyte cultures.[198] Better repair of superficial defects in guinea pig knee occurred with low-dose laser energy (25 J) compared with high-dose (125 J) and controls.[199] Long-term results were not reported, and although the mechanism is unknown, the authors theorized stimulation of cell replication mechanisms. For both electromagnetic and laser therapy, more research is needed.

SUBCHONDRAL BONE

Approaches that involve the subchondral bone are designed to disrupt the vascularity and promote fibrin clot formation, as well as provide a source of new cells from the bone marrow. Use of isolated drill holes has disadvantages, as these sites may not be loaded and thus may inadequately test the involvement of the subchondral bone.[179] Mitchell and Shepard[200] used multiple drill holes and obtained repair with HAC-like tissue, but it deteriorated within 1 year. Subchondral bone may be involved by some form of penetration, such as drill holes, or by resection of the cartilage through to the cancellous bone, a procedure called spongilization.[201] The latter procedure involves excising the damaged cartilage to below the subchondral plate to promote the growth of fibrocartilage. This technique can provide a biological resurfacing, particularly where the joint congruence is good and the load is well distributed over a large area.[202] When the entire surface of the patella is removed, the reduction in thickness has a decompressive effect, and only embryologic cells produced cartilage-like tissue.[202]

GRAFTING

Approaches employing grafting have used periosteal,[189] perichondrial,[187] or osteochondral[203] grafts. Grafts provide cells that have the potential to synthesize matrix, but osteochondral grafts (allo- and autogenic) tend to produce a severe immunologic rejection reaction.[203] Buckwalter and Mow[179] summarized the literature of graft studies in rabbits, dogs, and sheep. Generally, the graft tends to degenerate within 1 to 2 years, resulting in fibrillation and breakdown of the surfaces.

SURGICAL IMPLANTATION

Surgical implantation is designed to provide a new cell population and may involve the use of cultured or harvested chondrocytes,[203] mesenchymal cells,[204] a fibrin clot,[205] or an artificial synthetic matrix.[206] The latter involves using carbon fiber with a collagen and/or fibrin gel.[207,208] Implantation of cells may be used in conjunction with cartilage growth factors, such as osteogenin, fibroblast growth factors, platelet-derived growth factors, or the transforming growth factor β. Surgeons believe that these approaches should stimulate migration, proliferation, and matrix synthesis by mesenchymal cells. Surgeons have also utilized irrigation of defects with a saline solution or a solution containing the enzyme pepsin or Ringer's lactate. These solutions are hypothesized to degrade the proteoglycans and promote the formation of a fibrin clot.[179]

A number of investigators have used a combination of different approaches, such as Coutts and colleagues,[187] who used drill holes and CPM. Others have used joint resection plus motion or periosteal grafts and CPM. Buckwalter and Mow[179] noted several limitations of experimental studies. For example, if osteoarthritic joints are used, it should be remembered that the changes in osteoarthritis are not restricted to HAC. Animal models are often rabbits, guinea pigs, or rats, and their small joints do not permit extrapolation directly to the larger joints of humans. Additionally, HAC varies in thickness, cell density, composition, material properties, and function among joints and species. Also, when animal models are used, there is difficulty in assessing the long-term functional outcome. Most investigators have not studied the animals for an adequate period following the experimental procedure. Pain relief, often the primary objective of the intervention, is difficult to assess. Clinicians should be aware that "the available evidence indicates that, at a minimum, repair tissue must have initial protection from loading, followed by a regime of loading and motion that promotes remodelling,[209] but thus far experimental studies have not defined this optimal sequence of changes in the mechanical environment."[179] Clearly, it is not yet possible to give definitive direction to clinicians regarding progression of a rehabilitative program. However, repetitive high loads, as in long-distance running, should be avoided for perhaps a year, and when they are used, they should be applied briefly.

RESPONSE TO MECHANICAL STIMULI

In the last 3 decades, there have been a number of histologic, biochemical, and biomechanical studies, as well as analytic models, that have documented the response of articular cartilage and/or chondrocytes, both in vitro and in vivo, to mechanical stimuli. Frank and Hart[210] theorized that loads may influence cells "indirectly" (systemic, regional, and pericellular) and "directly" (cell related). Pericellular pH values and membrane ionic permeabilities are mechanisms that respond to loading. Cartilage tissue heterogeneity may influence the cells' regulation of anabolic and catabolic activities, which has been suggested by studies on bovine cartilage implants from different areas within the joint and similar areas from other joints.[211,212]

REDUCED LOADING

The suggestion that chondrocytes are sensitive to mechanical stimuli is supported by studies of denervated and immobilized joints.[6] In disuse atrophy (paraplegia, poliomyelitis)[213,214] and denervation,[215] it was observed that chondrocytes increased their synthetic activity with mechanical stress, whereas their activity was lowered with decreased compression on the loading surfaces. The decrease in the thickness of articular cartilage (atrophy) and in CS observed in these conditions was also observed in studies using animal models and hind paw amputations.[216,217] The latter studies also demonstrated a decrease in the synthesis of GAG. Compared with disuse atrophy conditions, partial amputation of a limb decreases compression but still allows motion in the remaining joints. Under these conditions, adult rabbits may show changes within 1 week. In dogs, similar changes may take 11 weeks to be detectable.[218,219] Some of the problems in the use of animal models for these studies are related to different ages and species. Another problem is variability in methods, such as the position of immobilization, the degree of compression of the joint surfaces, and the extent to which motion is limited. Reduced loading studies support the view that maintenance of healthy joint surfaces requires a regular program of loading. Encouraging seniors to walk regularly should be beneficial.

IMMOBILIZATION

Immobilization prevents motion, and, depending on the position, it may or may not provide an increase or decrease in loading to the contact area of the joint surfaces. This limitation in motion results in degenerative changes that are similar to those seen in osteoarthritis and may result in cell necrosis.[217,219–223] A number of investigators used clamps to produce immobilization, mostly of the knee joint in small animals, and intentionally or unintentionally, may have produced compression of the articular cartilage.[173,224–228] Cell death occurs with such rigid sustained pressure at focal points of the articular cartilage. This is presumably because of interference with nutrition to cells, which is dependent on the cyclic compression and expansion of articular cartilage that occurs with normal intermittent loading.[6] Tomlinson and Maroudas[229] considered that simple diffusion of small solutes was unaffected by cyclic loading. They suggested that changes, such as decreased articular cartilage amount, were due to the absence of mechanical stimuli to be sensed by the chondrocytes. Permeability of the cartilage did decrease with compression.[132] Maroudas[230] indirectly demonstrated that permeability of cartilage correlated inversely with hydration. Large deformation of cartilage regulates the manner and rate of fluid transport; the more rapid the applied load, the more rapid the efflux at the loading surface.

Simple immobilization without compression also causes atrophy and thinning of the articular cartilage.[231,232] In this condition, there is no report of change in cell density. Other changes include a decrease in GAGs and CS compared with the nonoperated or nonimmobilized side,[233] whereas intermittent compression of articular cartilage causes the reverse.[93,234,235] With the atrophy of articular cartilage that has been observed in immobilization, there is also an enhancement in collagen synthesis but not in the total amount of collagen. Tammi and coworkers[236] used splints to immobilize dogs and showed a 53 percent increase in collagen production. In comparison, there was only an 11 to 13 percent increase in the dogs that ran on a treadmill for 15 weeks. Cultured chondrocytes reportedly respond to mechanical stress in a comparable manner to articular cartilage in vivo.[93]

When immobilization is an essential component of, for example, fracture management or following surgery, clinicians should devise exercises that provide loading to immobilized joint surfaces.

EXCESSIVE LOADING

There have been a number of experiments in which the joint surfaces have been abnormally loaded. This may be done by having one non-weight-bearing limb, thereby creating an increased and altered load on the weight-bearing side. Alternatively, it could be done by putting backpacks on the animal or simulating weight gain as in the experiments performed by Simon and associates.[237] Severe excessive loading experiments have employed the "drop tower" procedure to subject articular cartilage to high stress levels. These studies have shown that chondrocytes can survive up to a 30 percent compressive strain, but if the stress exceeds 25 MN/m^2 and produces a strain that is greater than 40 percent, tissue death results.[238] This type of impact loading results in a loss of proteoglycans, fibrillation of the surfaces, and cell death.[166] Stockwell[6] noted that when loaded tissue extrudes interstitial fluid, it becomes less hydrated, which causes an increase in proteoglycan concentration. That, in itself, inhibits synthesis of proteoglycans. Parkkinen and colleagues,[239] in in vitro studies, observed that "static compressive pressures consistently inhibit PG [proteoglycan] synthesis in cartilage." The response to cyclic compressive loading is more variable.

Excessive loading may occur in certain athletes such as ice skaters, who repetitively jump and land on a hard surface in both practice and performance. Studies suggest that activities such as jumps should be interspersed with much longer periods of nonimpulsive loading to allow reconstruction of the cartilage following severe compression.

EFFECT OF EXERCISE

Exercise or motion in animals and humans has been shown to cause a swelling of articular cartilage. Prolonged exercise in animals was observed to produce hypertrophy of chondrocytes, an increase in the pericellular matrix, and an increase in the number of cells per chondron, particularly in the radial and transitional zones.[240] In rabbits, the superficial cells became more spherical for a transient period after brief exercise. This resulted in an overall change in the size of the cells.[241] Long-term exercise or loading produces more lasting enlargement. There was an increase in the volume of the nucleus but not in the overall size of the cells in the superficial layers. There also was an increase in the quantity of endoplastic reticulum and other cytoplasmic organelles.[242] These changes were observed in young rabbits given a nonstrenuous treadmill exercise program for 8 weeks. An increase in the size of chondrocytes in guinea pigs who did a running exercise has been reported.[243] Helminen and associates[244] observed an increase in the number but a decrease in both the volume and the volume density of chondrocytes after "strenuous" running in beagles. Following moderate running in young beagles, this Finnish group has also shown a positive change in articular cartilage proteoglycans[245] and no degeneration of the surface after a 15-week period.[246,247]

Other investigators have shown marked "wear and tear" type changes following exercise.[248,249] There were more degenerative surface changes in the femoral heads of rabbits with sudden maximal exercise compared with submaximal running.[249] Several in vitro studies have shown that the chondrocytic response to loading, particularly cyclic stresses, may vary with the length of the treatment. Palmoski and Brandt[235] subjected cartilage plugs to static and cyclic stresses that were equivalent to about 1.5 times body weight. They demonstrated a 38 percent increase in synthesis of GAGs with a cycle of 4 seconds on/11 seconds off but a decrease with a cycle of 60 seconds on/60 seconds off.[235] This varied response has been shown both in cell cultures and in chondrocyte cultures.[242] The response varied with the frequency of the pressure, duration of the application, and state of the cells. Application for 1.5 hours produced a strong inhibitory reaction, whereas 20-hour exposure produced stimulation of sulfate incorporation.[239] Response variability may relate to the observation that "complete aggrecan molecule synthesis takes about 1.5–2 hours."[239]

When cartilage explants were exposed to two different cycles of high frequency (2 seconds on/2 seconds off) and low frequency (60 seconds on/60 seconds off), there was a decrease in protein and proteoglycan synthesis with low frequency and static loading, whereas during the high-frequency cycle, there was a stimulatory effect on protein and proteoglycan synthesis.[251] Unloading restored the synthesis to the preloaded levels. Results of these studies suggest that in the early stages of rehabilitation, unloaded, quicker movements should be used. When static loading is introduced, time in unloaded conditions should follow and be of a longer interval. Research is needed to determine how different exercise regimens affect in vivo cartilage. Following review of in vivo and in vitro studies, van Kampen and van de Stadt[93] concluded that "nutrition of the tissue plays only a minor role in the processes" involved in articular cartilage's adaptation and response to under- or overloading.

It should be noted that in vitro studies expose the tissues to only one type of stress, with forces that are mostly lower than the physiologic levels experienced in vivo, such as at heel contact and toe-off in the gait cycle. Human hip and knee forces may reach four to seven times body weight during gait.[252,253] Quantitatively, contraction of muscles may result in greater forces across articular cartilage than does normal weight bearing.[16] For instance, although forces of four to five times body weight may be transmitted through the knee in walking, the force may be as much as 10 times body weight in squatting.[254] The compressive ankle joint reaction forces during running reach nine times body weight.[255] Similar reaction forces are estimated to occur in gymnastics (straight arm swing on rings: shoulder, 6.5 to 9.2 times body weight; takeoff vertical forces, 3.4 to 5.6 times body weight).[256] High transarticular forces can be predicted for all jumping activities. Studies show that joint surfaces can tolerate higher dynamic forces than static forces. Equipment can play a major role in damping joint forces. A new mat in gymnastics reduced tibia accelerations from 50 to 10 g and hip accelerations from 20 to 8 g.[256] Radin and colleagues[257] demonstrated negative effects on articular cartilage in weight-bearing joints in sheep that walked for long distances on concrete floors. Those that walked on wood chips did not show similar effects. It can be predicted that repetitive forces are considerably greater when a parachutist lands, or when an ice skater lands following a triple axle. If practice and performance jumping times are summed, these will result in high repetitive impulsive loading to joint surfaces. Microtrauma is cumulative.

If cartilage is exposed to unloading and is then loaded, there may be "gross functional failure of matrix."[258] This failure appears to be related to some defect in the ability of proteoglycans to re-form the hyaluronic acid–binding region of the aggregates. Various studies have shown that unloaded cartilage is less stiff. There is an impairment of the proteoglycan matrix that probably makes the cartilage more vulnerable to injuries if exposed to heavy loading. These results suggest that there is a need for programs of graduated weight bearing and activity after extended periods of non–weight bearing or casting. Tammi and associates[259] reviewed studies of various animal species involving "enhanced loading," which produced mixed results as to whether running exercise injures or does not injure articular cartilage. They suggested that one factor in the variability of results may be the rate at which the program is commenced. A conditioning period seems to be important. The Finnish group conducted many studies on articular cartilage both in vitro and in vivo, including immobilization, reloading, and moderate and strenuous exercise. It was concluded that the detrimental effects of unloading (loss of

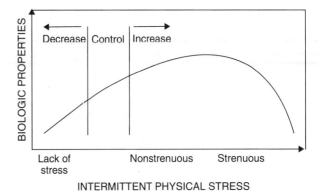

FIGURE 8–14. Hypothesis of the effect of intermittent physical stress on the biologic properties of articular cartilage. Tammi et al. suggested that atrophy or injury occurs in articular cartilage owing to suboptimal physical stresses, whereas stresses within physiologic limits stimulate the tissue to develop improved biologic properties. Increasing the stress beyond this physiologic boundary causes progressive deterioration of its biologic properties. (From Tammi M, et al: Joint loading-induced alterations in articular cartilage. *In* Helminen HJ, et al [eds]: Joint Loading. Bristol, Wright, 1987, p 82.)

stiffness, atrophy) can be reversed with a gentle, graduated program, but complete restoration was uncertain.[259] Enhanced loading in the form of moderate running has positive effects on articular cartilage, but these are reversed by strenuous running. It is not yet demonstrated whether the response to nonstrenuous exercising in human athletes is similar to that of animals. The limits of the "physiologic range" need to be determined, as well as how in vivo mature articular cartilage responds (Fig. 8–14). Studies suggest that exercise involving loading should be done gradually.

The knowledge of the response of articular cartilage to loading and to mechanical stimuli is growing. The results of studies over the last couple of decades appear to challenge the ancient dogma of "rest," since in unloaded joints, rest has proved to be detrimental to the health of articular cartilage. It is hypothesized that one of the objectives of physical therapy, particularly in mature clients who have been confined to bed for lengthy periods, such as in conservative treatment of a fractured femur, should be to provide loading experiences for the unaffected leg to maintain the health of articular cartilage. This could be as simple as a regimen of leg pushes against rubber bands or springs and bent leg and resisted pelvic raises. It may well be that *all* health care professionals should aim to minimize the unloaded period and, whenever possible, to allow at least partial weight bearing to provide some mechanical stimuli to the articular cartilage. Additionally, physical therapists must recognize that there is an unknown critical upper limit to the load that cartilage can bear without adverse effects. Following injury and periods of immobility, cartilage is less stiff and less capable of tolerating high loads.

SUMMARY

HAC is part of the load-bearing unit that consists of the HAC layer and the subchondral bone; it has important interactions with synovial fluid. Because it is avascular, healing is imperfect unless the defect involves the vascular subchondral bone. Although chondrocytes are active cells, their ability to reconstitute the tissue is very limited.

Nutrients to chondrocytes must traverse a long route from vessels in the subsynovial tissues through the joint space to cartilage. The vascular synovial lining tissues play a large role in the health of the joint and articular cartilage. These tissues can release, secrete, or allow passage of many substances with the capacity to degrade cartilage.

HAC functions to distribute and transmit loads to the subchondral bone, which undergoes significant deformation under loading. Both the collagen framework and the proteoglycan matrix are essential to the normal function of HAC. It is theorized that repetitive impulsive loading plays a major role in the degradation of HAC, producing microtrauma that is cumulative. Healing times for restoration of HAC's normal structure are lengthy and are not well defined in humans.

Despite extensive research, there is little definitive evidence to guide clinicians in rehabilitation programs, but load bearing appears to be essential to the existence of healthy HAC. High loads and static loading are less well tolerated and can be detrimental. Clinicians must consider the type, role, and quantity of load in treatment programs.

ACKNOWLEDGMENTS

My sincere thanks to Theresa Bidart for word processing and to publishers and authors for permission to use their copyright materials.

REFERENCES

1. Mankin HJ, Trasher AZ: Water content and binding in normal and osteoarthritic human cartilage. J Bone Joint Surg 1975; 57A:76–80.
2. Davies DV, Barnett CH, Cochrane W, Palfrey AJ: Electron microscopy of articular cartilage in the young adult rabbit. Ann Rheum Dis 1962; 21:11–21.
3. Warwick R, Williams PL: Gray's Anatomy, 35th ed. London, Longman, 1973, pp 210–211.
4. Wilsman NJ: Cilia of adult canine articular chondrocytes. J Ultrastructure Res 1978; 64:270–281.
5. Poole AR: Cartilage in health and disease. In McCarty DJ, Koopman WJ (eds): Arthritis and Allied Conditions, 12th ed, vol 1. Philadelphia, Lea & Febiger, 1993, pp 279–333.
6. Stockwell RA: Structure and function of the chondrocyte under mechanical stress. In Helminen HJ, Kiviranta I, Tammi M, et al (eds): Joint Loading: Biology of Articular Structures. Bristol, Wright, 1987, pp 126–148.
7. Caplan AI, Ordahl CP: Irreversible gene expression model control of development. Science 1978; 201:120–130.
8. Poole AR, Matsui Y, Hinek A, et al: Cartilage macromolecules and calcification of cartilage matrix. Anat Rec 1989; 224:167–179.
9. Brocklehurst R, Bayliss NT, Maroudas A: The composition of normal and osteoarthritic articular cartilage from human knee joints. J Bone Joint Surg 1984; 66A:95–106.
10. Castor CW: Regulation of connective tissue metabolism. In McCarty DJ, Koopman WJ (eds): Arthritis and Allied Conditions, 12th ed, vol 1. Philadelphia, Lea & Febiger, 1993, pp 245–262.
11. Rosenberg L: Structure and function of cartilage proteoglycans. In McCarty DJ, Koopman WJ (eds): Arthritis and Allied Conditions, 12th ed, vol 1. Philadelphia, Lea & Febiger, 1993, pp 229–243.
12. Fleischmajor R, Olsen BR, Kühn K: Structure, molecular biology and pathology of collagen. Ann N Y Acad Sci 1990; 580:1–592.
13. Miller EJ: The collagen of joints. In Sokoloff L (ed): The Joints and Synovial Fluid, vol 1. New York, Academic Press, 1988, pp 205–236.
14. Postlethwaite AE, Kang AH: Fibroblasts and matrix problems. In Gallin JI, Goldstein IM, Snyderman R (eds): Inflammation: Basic Principles and Clinical Correlates. New York, Raven Press, 1992, pp 747–773.
15. Prockop DJ, Williams CJ, Vandenburg P: Collagen in normal and diseased connective tissue. In McCarty DJ, Koopman WJ (eds): Arthritis and Allied Conditions, 12th ed, vol 1. Philadelphia, Lea & Febiger, 1993, pp 213–227.
16. Brandt KD, Mankin HJ: Osteoarthritis and polychondritis. In Kelley WN, et al (eds): Textbook of Rheumatology. Philadelphia, WB Saunders, 1993, pp 1355–1373.
17. Nimni ME: Collagen: its structure and function in normal and pathological connective tissues. Semin Arthritis Rheum 1974; 4:95–150.
18. Buckwalter JA, Cooper RR, Maynard JA: Elastic fibers in human intervertebral discs. J Bone Joint Surg 1976; 58A:73–76.
19. Cotta-Pereira G, Del-Caro LM, Nantes GS: Distribution of elastic system fibers in hyaline and fibrous cartilages of the rat. Acta Anat 1984; 119:80–85.
20. Walker JM: Age-related differences in the human sacro-iliac joint: a histological study; implications for therapy. J Orthop Sports Phys Ther 1986; 7:325–334.
21. Bowen V, Cassidy JD: Macroscopic and microscopic anatomy of the sacroiliac joint from embryonic life to the eighth decade. Spine 1981; 6:620–682.
22. Revell PA, Pirie C, Amir G, et al: Metabolic activity in the calcified zone of the cartilage; oxidations on tetracycline labelled articular cartilage in human osteoarthritic hips. Rheumatol Int 1990; 10:143–147.
23. Oettmeier R, Abendroth K, Oettmeier S: Analysis of the tidemark on human femoral heads. I. Histochemical, ultrastructural and microanalytical characterization of the normal structure of the intercartilaginous junction. Acta Morphol Hung 1989; 37:155–168.
24. Lane LB, Bullough PG: Age-related changes in the thickness of the calcified zone, the number of tidemarks in adult human articular cartilage. J Bone Joint Surg 1980; 62B:372–365.
25. Hamerman D, Rosenberg LC, Schubert M: Diarthrodial joints revisited. J Bone Joint Surg 1970; 52A:725–774.
26. Lane JN, Weiss C: Current comment: review of articular cartilage collagen research. Arthritis Rheum 1975; 18:553–562.
27. Mankin HJ, Radin EL: Structure and function of joints. In McCarty DJ, Koopman WJ (eds): Arthritis and Allied Conditions, 12th ed, vol 1. Philadelphia, Lea & Febiger, 1993, pp 181–197.
28. Poole CA, Flint MH, Beamont BW: Morphological and functional interrelationships of articular cartilage matrices. J Anat 1984; 138:113–138.
29. Stockwell RA: Cell density of human articular and costal cartilage. J Anat 1967; 101:753–763.
30. Kensora JE, Yosipovitch Z, Climcher MJ: The calcified cartilage zone of adult articular cartilage: a viable functional entity. Orthop Trans 1978; 2:101.
31. Meachim G, Stockwell RA: The matrix. In Freeman MAR (ed): Adult Articular Cartilage. New York, Grune & Stratton, 1972, pp 1–50.
32. MacConnaill MA: The movement of bones and joints. IV. The mechanical structure of articular cartilage. J Bone Joint Surg 1951; 33B:251–257.
33. Meachim G, Roy S: Surface ultrastructure of mature adult human articular cartilage. J Bone Joint Surg 1969; 51B:529–539.
34. Clarke IC: Articular cartilage: a review and scanning electron microscope study. J Bone Joint Surg 1971; 53B:732–750.
35. Weiss C, Rosenberg L, Helfet AJ: An ultrastructural study of normal young adult human articular cartilage. J Bone Joint Surg 1968; 50A:663–674.
36. Knets IV: Adaptation and remodelling of articular cartilage and

bone tissue. *In* Helminen HJ, et al (eds): Joint Loading. Bristol, Wright, 1987, pp 251–263.

37. Helminen HJ, Jurvelin J, Kiviranta I, et al: Joint loading effects on articular cartilage: a historical review. *In* Helminen HJ, et al (eds): Joint Loading. Bristol, Wright, 1987, pp 1–46.

38. Muir H, Bullough P, Maroudas A: The distribution of collagen in human articular cartilage with some of its physiological implications. J Bone Joint Surg 1970; 52B:554–563.

39. Moses MA, Sudhalter J, Langer R: Identification of an inhibitor of neovascularization from cartilage. Science 1990; 248:1408–1410.

40. Goodfellow JW, Bullough PG: The pattern of ageing of articular cartilage at the elbow joint. J Bone Joint Surg 1967; 49B:175–181.

41. Freeman MAR, Meachim G: Ageing, degeneration and remodeling of articular cartilage. *In* Freeman MAR (ed): Adult Articular Cartilage, 2nd ed. Tunbridge Wells, Pitman, 1979, pp 487–543.

42. Hall DA: A Biomedical Basis of Gerontology. Bristol, Wright, 1984.

43. Longmore RB, Gardner DL: Development with age of human articular cartilage surface structure. Ann Rheum Dis 1975; 34:26–37.

44. Verzar F: Lectures on Experimental Gerontology. Springfield, IL, Thomas, 1963.

45. Viidik A: Functional properties of collagenous tissues. Int Rev Connect Tissue Res 1973; 6:127–215.

46. Mankin HJ, Lippiello L: Biochemical and metabolic abnormalities in articular cartilage from osteoarthritic human hips. J Bone Joint Surg 1970; 52A:424–434.

47. Bollet AJ, Nance JL: Biochemical findings in normal and osteoarthritic articular cartilage. II. Chondroitin sulphate concentration and chain length, water and ash content. J Clin Invest 1966; 45:1170–1177.

48. Bonner WM, Jonsson H, Malanos C, Bryant M: Changes in the lipids of human articular cartilage with age. Arthritis Rheum 1975; 18:461–473.

49. Simunek Z, Muir H: Changes in the protein-polysaccharides of pig articular cartilage during prenatal life, development and old age. Biochem J 1972; 126:515–523.

50. Mankin HJ: The calcified zone (basal layer) of articular cartilage of rabbits. Anat Rec 1963; 145:73–87.

51. Tonna EA: Aging of skeletal-dental systems and supporting tissues. *In* Finch CE, Hayflick L (eds): Handbook of Aging. New York, Van Nostrand-Reinhold, 1977, pp 470–495.

52. Bonucci E, Dearden LC: Matrix vesicles in aging cartilage. Fed Proc 1976; 35:163–168.

53. Livne E, Weiss A, Silbermann M: Changes in growth patterns in mouse condylar cartilage associated with skeletal maturation in senescence. Growth Dev Aging 1990; 54:183–193.

54. Ziv I, Maroudas C, Robin G, Maroudas A: Human facet cartilage: swelling and some physicochemical characteristics as a function of age. Part 2. Age changes in some biophysical parameters of human facet joint cartilage. Spine 1993; 18:136–146.

55. Shrive NG, O'Connor JJ, Goodfellow JW: Load-bearing in the knee joint. Clin Orthop 1978; 131:279–287.

56. Fairbank TJ: Knee joint changes after meniscectomy. J Bone Joint Surg 1948; 30B:664–670.

57. Barnett CH, Davies DV, MacConnaill MA: Synovial Joints. London, Longman, 1961, p 131.

58. Van Sickle DC, Kincaid SA: Comparative arthrology. *In* Sokoloff L (ed): The Joints and Synovial Fluid, vol 1. London, Academic Press. 1978, pp 1–47.

59. Ghadially FN: Fine structure of joints. *In* Sokoloff L (ed): The Joints and Synovial Fluid. London, Academic Press, 1978, pp 105–176.

60. Bullough PG, Munuera L, Murphy J, et al: The strength of the menisci of the knee as it relates to the fine structure. J Bone Joint Surg 1970; 52B:564–570.

61. Arnoczky SP, Warren RF: Microvasculature of the human meniscus. Am J Sports Med 1982; 10:90–95.

62. Davies DV, Edwards DAW: The blood supply to synovial membrane. Ann R Coll Surg Engl 1948; 2:142–156.

63. Walker JM: Histological study of the fetal development of the human acetabulum and labrum: significance in congenital hip disease. Yale J Biol Med 1981; 54:255–263.

64. O'Brien SJ, Arnoczky SP: Inflammation and healing of meniscal injury. *In* Leadbetter WB, Buckwalter JA, Gordon SL (eds):

Sports-Induced Inflammation. Park Ridge, IL, American Academy of Orthopedic Surgeons, 1990, pp 225–255.

65. Mikic ZD: Detailed anatomy of the articular disc of the distal radioulnar joint. Clin Orthop 1989; 7:123–132.

66. Wirth CR: Meniscus repair. Clin Orthop 1981; 157:153–160.

67. Scott GA, Jolly BL, Henning CE: Combined posterior incision in arthroscopic intra-articular repair of the meniscus: an examination of factors affecting healing. J Bone Joint Surg 1986; 68A:847–861.

68. Arnoczky SP, Warren RF: The microvasculature of the meniscus and its response to injury: an experimental study in the dog. Am J Sports Med 1983; 11:131–141.

69. Holm SH, Urban JPG: The intervertebral disc: factors contributing to its nutrition and matrix turnover. *In* Helminen HJ, et al (eds): Joint Loading. Bristol, Wright, 1987, pp 187–226.

70. Happey F: Studies of the structure of the human intervertebral disc in relation to its functional and aging processes. *In* Sokoloff L (ed): The Joints and Synovial Fluid, vol 2. London, Academic Press, 1980, pp 95–139.

71. Inoue H, Takeda T: Three dimensional observations of collagen framework of lumbar intervertebral discs. Acta Orthop Scand 1975; 46:949–956.

72. Bernick S, Walker JM, Paule WJ: Age changes to the anulus fibrosus in human intervertebral discs. Spine 1990; 16:520–524.

73. Johnson EF, Berryman H, Mitchell R, Wood WB: Elastic fibres in the anulus fibrosus of the adult human lumbar intervertebral disc: a preliminary report. J Anat 1985; 143:57–63.

74. Maroudas A, Stockwell RA, Nachemson A, Urban J: Factors involved in the nutrition of the human lumbar intervertebral disc: cellularity and diffusion of glucose in vitro. J Anat 1975; 120:113–130.

75. Bernick S, Cailliet R: Vertebral end-plate changes with aging of human vertebrae. Spine 1982; 7:97–102.

76. Peereboom JWC: Some biochemical and histochemical properties of the age pigment in the human intervertebral disc. Histochemie 1973; 37:119–130.

77. Coventry MB: Anatomy of the intervertebral disk. Clin Orthop 1969; 67:9–15.

78. Naylor A: The biochemical changes in the human intervertebral disc and degeneration in nuclear prolapse. Orthop Clin North Am 1971; 2:343–358.

79. Urban JP, McMullin JF: Swelling pressure of the intervertebral disc: influence of proteoglycan and collagen contents. Biorheology 1985; 22:145–157.

80. Eyre DR, Muir H: The distribution of different molecular species of collagen in fibrous, elastic and hyaline cartilages of the pig. Biochem J 1975; 151:595–602.

81. Holm S, Maroudas A, Urban JPG, et al: Nutrition of the individual disc: solute transport and metabolism. Connect Tissue Res 1981; 8:101–119.

82. Bogduk N, Tynan W, Wilson AS: The nerve supply to the human lumbar intervertebral discs. J Anat 1981; 132:39–56.

83. Dee R: The innervation of joints. *In* Sokoloff L (ed): The Joints and Synovial Fluid, vol. 1. New York, Academic Press, 1978, pp 177–204.

84. Roofe PG: Innervation of the anulus fibrosus in posterior longitudinal ligament. Arch Neurol Psychiatry 1940; 44:110–123.

85. Taylor JR, Twomey LT: Innervation of lumbar intervertebral discs. Med J Aust 1979; 2:701–702.

86. Pedersen HE, Blunck CFJ, Gardner E: The anatomy of the lumbosacral posterior rami and meningeal branches of spinal nerves (sinu-vertebral nerves). J Bone Joint Surg 1956; 38A: 377–391.

87. Malinsky J: The ontogenic development of nerve terminations in the intervertebral discs of man. Acta Anat 1959; 38:96–113.

88. Peacock A: Observations on the postnatal structure of the intervertebral disc in man. J Anat 1952; 86:162–178.

89. Peereboom JWC: Age-dependent changes in the human intervertebral disc. Gerontologia 1971; 17:236–252.

90. Akeson WH, Amiel D, LaViolette D. The connective tissue response to immobility. A study of chondroitin 4 and 6 sulfate and dermatan sulfate changes in periarticular connective tissue of control and immobilized knees of dogs. Clin Orthop 1967; 51:183–197.

91. Salter B: Continuous Passive Motion (CPM): A Biological

Concept for the Healing and the Generation of Articular Cartilage, Ligaments, and Tendons: From Its Origination to Research to Clinical Applications. Baltimore, Williams & Wilkins, 1993.

92. Akeson WH, Amiel D, Woo SL-Y: Physiology and therapeutic value of passive motion. *In* Helminen HJ, et al (eds): Joint Loading. Bristol, Wright, 1987, pp 375–394.

93. van Kampen GPJ, van de Stadt JR: Cartilage and chondrocyte responses to mechanical loading in vitro. *In* Helminen HJ, et al (eds): Joint Loading. Bristol, Wright, 1987, pp 112–125.

94. Rodan GA, Bourret LA, Harvey A, et al: Cyclic AMP and cyclic GMP. Mediators of the mechanical effects on bone remodeling. Science 1975; 189:467–469.

95. Insall J: Patella pain. *In* Current concepts review. J Bone Joint Surg 1982; 64A:147–152.

96. Wyke BD: The neurology of joints. Ann R Coll Surg Engl 1967; 41:25–50.

97. Freeman MAR, Wyke BD: The innervation of the knee joint: an anatomical and histological study in the cat. J Anat 1967; 101:505–532.

98. Freeman MAR, Wyke BD: The innervation of the ankle joint: an anatomical and histological study of the cat. Acta Anat 1967; 68:321–333.

99. Hosokawa O: Histological study on the type and distribution of the sensory nerve endings in human hip joint capsule and ligament. J Jpn Orthop Assoc 1964; 38:64–79.

100. Wyke BD: Neurological aspects of low back pain. *In* Jayson MIU (ed): The Lumbar Spine and Back Pain. London, Sector Pulp, 1976, pp 189–256.

101. Wyke B: The neurology of joints: a review of general principles. Clin Rheum Dis 1981; 7:223–239.

102. Zimny ML: Mechanoreceptors in articular tissues. Am J Anat 1988; 182:16–32.

103. Johansson H, Sjölander P: Neurophysiology. *In* Wright V, Radin E (eds): Mechanics of Human Joints. Philadelphia, Marcel Dekker, 1993, pp 243–292.

104. Henderson B, Edwards JCW: The Synovial Lining in Health and Disease. London, Chapman and Hall, 1987, p xv.

105. McCarty DJ: Synovial fluid. *In* McCarty DJ, Koopman WL (eds): Arthritis and Allied Conditions, 12th ed, vol 1. Philadelphia, Lea & Febiger, 1993, pp 63–84.

106. Andersen H: Development, morphology and histochemistry of the early synovial tissue in human fetuses. Acta Anat 1964; 58:90–115.

107. Key JA: The synovial membrane of joints and bursae. *In* Special Cytology, II, 2nd ed. New York, Paul W. Hoeber, 1932, pp 1055–1076.

108. Ghadially FN: Fine Structure of Synovial Joints. London, Butterworth, 1983.

109. Knight AD, Levick JR: The effect of fluid pressure on the hydraulic conductance of the interstitium and fenestrated endothelium in the rabbit knee. J Physiol 1985; 360:311–332.

110. Davies DV: The lymphatics of the synovial membrane. J Anat 1946; 80:21–23.

111. Halata Z, Groth HP: Innervation of the synovial membrane of the cat's joint capsule. Cell Tissue Res 1976; 169:415–418.

112. Rodosky MW, Fu FH: Induction of synovial inflammation by matrix molecules, implant particles, and chemical agents. *In* Leadbetter WB, Buckwalter JA, Gordon SL (eds): Sports-Induced Inflammation. Park Ridge, IL, American Academy of Orthopaedic Surgeons, 1990, pp 357–381.

113. Gardner E: Physiology of movable joints. Physiol Rev 1950; 30:127–176.

114. Barland P, Novikoff AB, Hamerman D: Electron microscopy of the human synovial membrane. J Cell Biol 1962; 14:207–220.

115. Fox RI, Kang H: Structure and function of synoviocytes. *In* McCarty DJ, Koopman WJ (eds): Arthritis and Allied Conditions, 12th ed, vol 1. Philadelphia, Lea & Febiger, 1993, pp 263–278.

116. Chapman WW, Swaim R, Froshsin H Jr, et al: Degradation of human articular cartilage by neutrophils and synovial fluid. Arthritis Rheum 1993; 36:51–58.

117. Ghadially FN, Roy S: Ultrastructure of Synovial Joints in Health and Disease. London, Butterworth, 1969.

118. Henderson RN, Glyn LE, Chayen J: Cell division in the synovial lining in experimental allergic arthritis: proliferation of cells during the development of chronic arthritis. Ann Rheum Dis 1982; 41:275–281.

119. Ropes NW, Bauer W: Synovial Fluid Changes in Joint Disease. Cambridge, Harvard University Press, 1953.

120. Geborek P, Wollheim FA: Synovial fluid. *In* Wright V, Radin E (eds): Mechanics of Human Joints. New York, Marcel Dekker, 1993, pp 109–136.

121. Levick JR: Blood flow in mass transport in synovial joints. *In* Rankin EN, Michel CC (eds): Handbook of Physiology: The Cardiovascular System. IV. The Microcirculation, part 2. Bethesda, American Physiological Society, 1984, pp 917–947.

122. Swann DA, Slayter HS, Silver FH: The molecular structure of LGP-1, the boundary lubricant for articular cartilage. J Biochem 1981; 265:5921.

123. Simpkin PA: Synovial physiology. *In* McCarty DJ, Koopman WJ (eds): Arthritis and Allied Conditions, 12th ed, vol 1. Philadelphia, Lea & Febiger, 1993, pp 199–212.

124. Müller W: Über den negativen luftdrück in gelenkraum. Dtch Z Chir 1929; 218:395–401.

125. Jayson MIV, Dixon A St J: Intra-articular pressure in rheumatoid arthritis of the knee. Ann Rheum Dis 1970; 29:401–408.

126. Wood L, Ferrell WR, Baxendale RH: Pressures in normal and acutely distended human knee joints and effects on quadriceps maximum voluntary contractions. Q J Exp Physiol 1988; 73: 305–314.

127. Unsworth A, Dalcen D, Wright V: "Cracking joints": a bioengineering study of cavitation in the metacarpo-phalangeal joint. Ann Rheum Dis 1971; 30:348–358.

128. Levick JR: Synovial fluid dynamics. *In* Maroudas A, Holborow EJ (eds): Studies in Joint Disease, vol 2. London, Pitman, 1983, pp 153–240.

129. Ekholm R: Articular cartilage nutrition. Acta Anat (Basel) 1951; 15-2:1–76.

130. Brower TD, Akahoski Y, Orlic PL: The diffusion of dyes through articular cartilage in vivo. J Bone Joint Surg 1962; 44A:456–463.

131. McKibbin B, Holdsworth FW: The nutrition of immature joint cartilage in the lamb. J Bone Joint Surg 1966; 48B:793–803.

132. Mow VC, Holmes MH, Lai WM: Influence of load bearing on the fluid transport and mechanical properties of articular cartilage. *In* Helminen HJ, et al (eds): Joint Loading. Bristol, Wright, 1987, pp 264–286.

133. Koellar W, Meier W, Hartman F: Biomechanical properties of human intervertebral discs subjected to axial compression. Spine 1984; 9:725–733.

134. Tyrell AR, Reilly J, Tromp JDG: Circadian variations in stature and effects of spinal loading. Spine 1985; 10:161–164.

135. Wallis WJ, Simkin P, Nelp WB: Low synovial clearance of iodine provides evidence of hypoperfusion in chronic rheumatoid synovitis. Arthritis Rheum 1985; 28:1096–1104.

136. Simkin P: Biology of joints. *In* Wright V, Radin EL (eds): Mechanics of Human Joints. New York, Marcel Dekker, 1993, pp 3–23.

137. Unsworth A: Lubrication of human joints. *In* Wright V, Radin E (eds): Mechanics of Human Joints. New York, Marcel Dekker, 1993, pp 137–162.

138. Unsworth A: Tribology of human and artificial joints. Proc Inst Mech Eng [H] 1991; 205:163–172.

139. McCutchen CW: Lubrication of joints. *In* Sokoloff L (ed): The Joints and Synovial Fluid, vol 1. New York, Academic Press, 1978, pp 437–483.

140. Dintenfass L: Lubrication and synovial joints: a theoretical analysis—a logical approach to the problems of joint movements and joint lubrication. J Bone Joint Surg 1963; 45A:1241–1256.

141. MacConnaill MA: Function of intra-articular fibrocartilages with special reference to the knee and inferior-radio-ulnar joints. J Anat 1932; 66:210–227.

142. McCutchen CW: Sponge-hydrostatic and weeping bearings. Nature 1959; 184:1284–1285.

143. Mow BC, Mansour JM: The nonlinear interaction between cartilage deformation and interstitial fluid flow. J Biomech 1977; 10:31–39.

144. Dowson D, Jin Z-M: Micro-elastohydrodynamic lubrication of synovial joints. Eng Med 1986; 15:63–65.

145. Fein RS: Are synovial joints squeeze-film lubricated? Proc Inst Mech Eng [3J] 1966–67; 181:125–128.

146. Charnley J: The lubrication of animal joints. Inst Mech Engrs Symp Biomech 1959; 12–22.
147. Jones ES: Joint lubrication. Lancet 1934; 1:1426–1427.
148. Jones ES: Joint lubrication. Lancet 1936; 1:1043–1044.
149. Linn FC: Lubrication of animal joints. II. The mechanism. J Biomech 1968; 1:193–205.
150. Walker PS, Dowson D, Longfield MD, Wright V: "Boosted lubrication" in synovial joints by fluid entrapment and enrichment. Ann Rheum Dis 1968; 27:512–520.
151. Clarke IC, Contini R, Kenedi RN: Friction and wear studies of articular cartilage: a scanning electron microscopy study. J Lubr Tech 1975; 97:358–368.
152. Radin EL, Paul IL: A consolidated concept of joint lubrication. J Bone Joint Surg 1972; 54A:607–616.
153. Charnley J: How our joints are lubricated. Triangle 1960; 4:175–179.
154. Linn FC, Radin EL: Lubrication of animal joints. III. The effect of certain chemical alterations of the cartilage and lubricant. Arthritis Rheum 1968; 11:674–682.
155. Swann DA, Radin EL: The molecular basis of articular lubrication. I. Purification and property of the lubricating fraction from bovine synovial fluid. J Biochem 1972; 274:8069–8073.
156. Roberts BJ, Unsworth A, Mian N: Modes of lubrication in human hip joints. Ann Rheum Dis 1982; 41:217–224.
157. Unsworth A: The effects of lubrication in hip joint prostheses. Phys Med Biol 1978; 23:253–268.
158. Radin EL: Osteoarthrosis. In Wright V, Radin EL (eds): Mechanics of Human Joints. New York, Marcel Dekker, 1993, pp 341–354.
159. Zvaifler NJ: Etiology and pathogenesis of rheumatoid arthritis. In McCarty DJ, Koopman WJ (eds): Arthritis and Allied Conditions, 12th ed, vol 1. Philadelphia, Lea & Febiger, 1993, pp 723–736.
160. Krane SM: Mechanisms of tissue destruction in rheumatoid arthritis. In McCarty DJ, Koopman WJ (eds): Arthritis and Allied Conditions, 12th ed, vol 1. Philadelphia, Lea & Febiger, 1993, pp 763–780.
161. Hough AJ: Pathology of osteoarthritis. In McCarty DJ, Koopman WJ (eds): Arthritis and Allied Conditions, 12th ed, vol 1. Philadelphia, Lea & Febiger, 1993, pp 1699–1722.
162. Pinals RS: Traumatic arthritis and allied conditions. In McCarty DJ, Koopman WJ (eds): Arthritis and Allied Conditions, 12th ed, vol 1. Philadelphia, Lea & Febiger, 1993, pp 1521–1538.
163. Brandt KD, Mankin HJ: Pathogenesis of osteoarthritis. In Kelley WN, et al (eds): Textbook of Rheumatology, 4th ed, vol 2. Philadelphia, WB Saunders, 1993, pp 1355–1373.
164. Radin EL: Mechanically induced periarticular and neuromuscular problems. In Wright V, Radin EL (eds): Mechanics of Human Joints. New York, Marcel Dekker, 1993, pp 355–370.
165. Buckwalter JA, Rosenberg LC, Hunziker EB: Articular cartilage: composition structure, response to injury and methods of facilitating repair. In Ewing JJ (ed): Articular Cartilage and Knee Joint Function: Basic Science and Arthroscopy. New York, Raven Press, 1990, pp 19–56.
166. Radin EL, Ehrlich MGM, Chernack R, et al: Effect of repetitive impulse loading on the knee joints of rabbits. Clin Orthop 1978; 131:288–293.
167. Palmoski MJ, Colyer RA, Brandt KD: Joint motion in the absence of normal loading does not maintain normal articular cartilage. Arthritis Rheum 1980; 23:325–334.
168. Fassbender HG: Significance of endogenous and exogenous mechanisms in the development of osteoarthritis. In Helminen HJ, et al (eds): Joint Loading. Bristol, Wright, 1987, pp 352–374.
169. Havdrup T, Telhag H: Mitosis of chondrocytes in normal adult joint cartilage. Clin Orthop 1980; 153:248–252.
170. Sledge CB: Biology of the joint. In Kelley WN, Harris ED, Ruddy S, Sledge CB (eds): Textbook of Rheumatology, 4th ed, vol 1. Philadelphia, WB Saunders, 1993, pp 1–21.
171. Hulth A, Lindberg L, Telhag H: Mitosis in human osteoarthritic cartilage. Clin Orthop 1972; 84:197–199.
172. Landells JW: The reactions of injured human articular cartilage. J Bone Joint Surg 1957; 39B:548–562.
173. Crelin ES, Southwick WO: Changes induced by sustained pressure in the knee joint articular cartilage of adult rabbits. Anat Rec 1964; 149:113–133.
174. Havdrup T, Telhag H: Scattered mitosis in adult joint cartilage after partial chondrectomy. Acta Orthop Scand 1978; 48:424–429.
175. Mankin HJ, Brandt KD: Biochemistry and metabolism of cartilage in osteoarthritis. In Moskowitz RW, Hall DS, Goldberg VM, Mankin JH (eds): Osteoarthritis: Diagnosis and Management. Philadelphia, WB Saunders, 1984, pp 43–79.
176. Sokoloff L: In vitro culture of joints and articular tissues. In Sokoloff L (ed): The Joints and Synovial Fluid, vol 2. New York, Academic Press, 1980, pp 1–26.
177. O'Driscoll SW, Kelley FW, Salter RB: The chondrogenic potential of free autogenous periosteal grafts for biological resurfacing of major full thickness defects in joint surfaces under the influence of continuous passive motion: an experimental investigation in the rabbit. J Bone Joint Surg 1986; 68A:1017–1035.
178. O'Driscoll SW, Kelly FW, Salter RB: Durability of regenerated articular cartilage produced by free autogenous periosteal grafts in major full thickness defects in joint surfaces under the influence of continuous passive motion: a follow-up report at one year. J Bone Joint Surg 1988; 70A:595–604.
179. Buckwalter JS, Mow VC: Articular cartilage repair in osteoarthritis. In Howell DS, Mankin HJ, Moskowitz RW (eds): Osteoarthritis: Diagnosis and Management, 2nd ed. Philadelphia, WB Saunders, 1990, pp 71–107.
180. Convery FR, Akeson WH, Keown GH: The repair of large osteochondral defects: an experimental study in horses. Clin Orthop 1972; 82:253–262.
181. Caterson B, Buckwalter J: Articular cartilage repair and remodelling: overview. In Maroudas A, Kuettner K (eds): Methods in Cartilage Research. Boston, Academic Press, 1989, pp 311–318.
182. Byers PD, Brown RA: Reflections on the repair of articular cartilage. In Maroudas A, Kuettner K (eds): Methods in Cartilage Research. Boston, Academic Press, 1989, pp 319–321.
183. Radin EL, Maquet P, Park H: Rationale and indications for the "hanging hip" procedure: a clinical and experimental study. Clin Orthop 1975; 112:221–230.
184. Salter RB, Simmonds DF, Malcolm BW, et al: The biological effect of continuous passive motion on the healing of full-thickness defects in articular cartilage. J Bone Joint Surg 1980; 62A:1232–1251.
185. Salter RB, Simmonds DF, Malcolm BW, et al: The effects of continuous passive motion on the healing of articular cartilage defects. J Bone Joint Surg 1975; 57A:570 (Abstract).
186. O'Driscoll SW, Salter RB: The induction of neochondrogenesis in free intra-articular periosteal autografts under the influence of continuous passive motion: an experimental study in the rabbit. J Bone Joint Surg 1984; 66A:1248–1257.
187. Coutts RD, Woo SL, Amiel D, et al: Rib perichondral autografts in full-thickness articular cartilage defects in rabbits. Clin Orthop 1992; 275:263–273.
188. Amiel D, Coutts RD, Harwood FL, et al: The chondrogenesis of perichondral grafts for repair of full thickness articular cartilage defects in a rabbit model; a one year post-operative assessment. Connect Tissue Res 1988; 18:27–39.
189. Moran ME, Kim HK, Salter RB: Biological resurfacing of full-thickness defects in patella articular cartilage of the rabbit. Investigation of autogenous periosteal grafts subjected to continuous passive motion. J Bone Joint Surg 1992; 74B:659–667.
190. Elliott JP, Smith RL, Block CA: Time-varying magnetic fields: effects of orientation on chondrocyte proliferation. J Orthop Res 1988; 6:259–264.
191. Okihana H, Shimomura Y: Effect of direct current on cultured growth cartilage cells in vitro. J Orthop Res 1988; 6:690–694.
192. Brighton CT, Unger AS, Stambough JL: In vitro growth of bovine articular cartilage chondrocytes in various capacitatively coupled electric fields. J Orthop Res 1984; 2:15–22.
193. Aaron RK, Ciomber DM, Jolly G: Modulation of chondrogenesis and chondrocyte differentiation by pulsed electromagnetic fields. Trans Orthop Res Soc 1987; 12:272.
194. Aaron RK, Plaas AK: Stimulation of proteoglycan synthesis in articular chondrocyte cultures by a pulsed electromagnetic field. Trans Orthop Res Soc 1987; 12:273.
195. Lippiello L, Chakkalakal D, Connolly JF: Pulsing direct current–induced repair of articular defects. J Orthop Res 1990; 8:266–275.
196. Baker B, Becker OR, Spadaro J: A study of electrochemical enhancement of articular cartilage repair. Clin Orthop 1974; 102:251–267.
197. Armstrong PF, Brighton CT, Star AM: Capacitatively coupled

electrical stimulation of bovine growth plate chondrocytes grown in pellet form. J Orthop Res 1988; 6:265–271.

198. Wandhofer A, Bally GV, Kauffmann G, et al: Comparative morphological investigation on the rabbit's auricle after exposure to CO_2 and Nd:YAG-laser radiation. Arch Otorhinolaryngol 1977; 217:487–491.

199. Schultz RJ, Krishnamurthy S, Thelmo W, et al: Effects of varying intensities of laser energy on articular cartilage: a preliminary study. Lasers Surg Med 1985; 5:577–588.

200. Mitchell N, Shepard N: The resurfacing of adult rabbit articular cartilage by multiple perforations through the subchondral bone. J Bone Joint Surg 1976; 58A:230–233.

201. Ficat RP, Ficat C, Gedon P, et al: Spongilization: a new treatment for diseased patellae. Clin Orthop 1979; 144:74–83.

202. Ficat C: Spongilization and cartilage healing in the human. In Maroudas A, Kuettner K (eds): Methods in Cartilage Research. Boston, Academic Press, 1989, pp 324–327.

203. Robinson D, Halperin N, Nevo Z: Use of cultured chondrocytes as implants for repairing cartilage defects. In Maroudas A, Kuettner K (eds): Methods in Cartilage Research. Boston, Academic Press, 1989, pp 327–329.

204. Goto J, Goldberg V, Kaplan A: Osteochondral progenitor cells enhance repair of large defects in rabbit articular cartilage. Trans Orthop Res Soc 1992; 17:598.

205. Paletta GA, Arnoczky SP, Warren RF: The repair of osteochondral defects using an exogenous fibrin clot: an experimental study in dogs. Am J Sports Med 1992; 20:725–731.

206. Klompmaker J, Jansen HW, Veth RP, et al: Porous polymer implants for repair of full-thickness defects of articular cartilage: an experimental study in rabbit and dog. Biomaterials 1992; 13:625–634.

207. Muckle DS, Minns RJ: Biological response to woven carbon fiber pads in the knee: a clinical and experimental study. J Bone Joint Surg 1990; 72B:60–62.

208. Hart JAL: The use of carbon fibre implants for articular cartilage defects. J Bone Joint Surg 1989; 71B:162 (Abstract).

209. Buckwalter JA, Cruess R: Healing of musculoskeletal tissues. In Rockwood CA, Green DP, Bucholz RW (eds): Fractures in Adults, 3rd ed. Philadelphia, JB Lippincott, 1991, pp 181–222.

210. Frank CB, Hart DA: Cellular response to loading. In Leadbetter WB, Buckwalter JA, Gordon SL (eds): Sports-Induced Inflammation. Park Ridge, IL, American Academy of Orthopaedic Surgeons, 1990, pp 555–564.

211. Gravel C, McAllister D, Schachar N, et al: Non-uniform distribution of plasminogen activator expression and responsiveness to inflammatory mediators in bovine articular cartilage. Trans Orthop Res Soc 1989; 14:534.

212. McAllister D, Gravel C, Schachar N, et al: Heterogeneity of metabolic activity and responsiveness to inflammatory mediators in bovine articular cartilage. Trans Orthop Res Soc 1990.

213. Collins DH: The Pathology of Articular and Spinal Diseases. London, Arnold, 1949.

214. Eichelberger L, Miles JS, Roma M: The histochemical characterization of articular cartilages of poliomyelitis patients. J Lab Clin Med 1952; 40:284–296.

215. Akeson WH, Eichelberger L, Roma M: Biochemical studies of articular cartilage. II. Values following denervation of an extremity. J Bone Joint Surg 1958; 40A:153–162.

216. Threlkeld AJ, Smith SD: Unilateral hind paw amputation causes bilateral articular cartilage remodelling of the rat hip joint. Anat Rec 1988; 221:576–583.

217. Helminen HJ, Jurvelin J, Kuusela T, et al: Effects of immobilization for 6 weeks on rabbit knee articular surfaces as assessed by the semi-quantitative stereomicroscopic method. Acta Anat 1983; 115:327–335.

218. Jurvelin J, Helminen HJ, Lauritsalo S, et al: Influence of joint immobilization in running exercise on articular cartilage surfaces of young rabbits. Acta Anat 1985; 122:62–68.

219. Enneking WF, Horowitz M: The intra-articular effects of immobilization of the human knee. J Bone Joint Surg 1972; 54A:973–985.

220. Evans EB, Eggers GWN, Butler JK, et al: Experimental immobilization and remobilization of rat knee joints. J Bone Joint Surg 1960; 42A:737–758.

221. Hall MC: Articular changes in the knee of the adult rat after prolonged immobilization in extension. Clin Orthop 1964; 34:184–195.

222. Thompson RC, Bassett CAL: Histological observations on experimentally induced degeneration of articular cartilage. J Bone Joint Surg 1970; 52A:435–443.

223. Akeson WH, Woo SL-Y, Amiel D, et al: The connective tissue response to immobility: biochemical changes in periarticular tissue of the immobilized rabbit knee. Clin Orthop 1973; 93:356–362.

224. Trueta J: Osteo-arthritis: an approach to surgical treatment. Lancet 1956; 1:585–589.

225. Salter RB, Field P: The effects of continuous compression on living articular cartilage. J Bone Joint Surg 1960; 42A:31–49.

226. Trias A: Effect of persistent pressure on articular cartilage: an experimental study. J Bone Joint Surg 1961; 43B:376–386.

227. Hall MC: Cartilage changes after experimental immobilization of the knee joint of the young rat. J Bone Joint Surg 1963; 45A:36–44.

228. Ely LW, Mensor MC: Studies on the immobilization of the normal joints. Surg Gynecol Obstet 1933; 37:212–215.

229. Tomlinson N, Maroudas A: The effect of cyclic and continuous compression on the penetration of large molecules into articular cartilage. J Bone Joint Surg 1980; 62B:251 (Abstract).

230. Maroudas A: Biophysical chemistry of cartilaginous tissues with special reference to solute and fluid transport. Biorheology 1975; 12:233–248.

231. Sood SC: A study of the effects of experimental immobilization on rabbit articular cartilage. J Anat 1971; 108:497–507.

232. Gritzka TL, Fry LR, Cheesman RL, et al: Deterioration of articular cartilage caused by continuous compression in a moving rabbit joint. J Bone Joint Surg 1973; 55A:1698–1720.

233. Caterson B, Lowther DA:Changes in the metabolism of the proteoglycans from sheep articular cartilage in response to mechanical forces. Biochem Biophys Acta 1978; 540:412–422.

234. Veldhuijzen JP, Bourret LA, Rodan GA: In vitro studies of the effect of intermittent compressive forces on cartilage cell proliferation. J Cell Physiol 1979; 98:299–306.

235. Palmoski MJ, Brandt KD: Effects of static and cyclic compressive loading on articular cartilage plugs in vitro. Arthritis Rheum 1984; 27:675–681.

236. Tammi N, Kiviranta I, Peltonen L, et al: Effects of joint loading on articular cartilage collagen metabolism: assay of procollagen, prolyl 4-hydroxylase and galactosylhydroxylsyl glycosyltansfenase. Connect Tissue Res 1988; 17:199–206.

237. Simon MR, Holmes KR, Olsen AM: Effects of simulated increases in body weight on the growth of limb bones in hypophysectomized rats. Acta Anat (Basel) 1985; 121:1–6.

238. Repo RU, Finlay JB: Survival of articular cartilage after controlled impact. J Bone Joint Surg 1977; 59A:1068–1076.

239. Parkkinen JJ, Ikonen J, Lammi MJ, et al: Effects of cyclic hydrostatic pressure on proteoglycan synthesis in cultured chondrocytes and articular cartilage explants. Arch Biochem Biophys 1993; 300:458–465.

240. Engelmark VE: Functionally induced changes in articular cartilage. In Evans FG (ed): Biomechanical Studies of the Musculoskeletal System. Springfield, IL, Charles C Thomas, 1961, pp 3–19.

241. Ekholm R, Norbeck B: On the relationship between articular changes and function. Acta Orthop Scand 1951; 21:81–98.

242. Paukkonen K, Selkänaho K, Jurvelin J, et al: Cells and nuclei of articular cartilage chondrocytes in young rabbits enlarged after non-strenuous physical exercise. J Anat 1985; 142:13–20.

243. Sääf J: Effects of exercise on adult articular cartilage. Acta Orthop Scand Suppl 1950; 7:1–86.

244. Helminen HJ, Paukkonen K, Kiviranta I, et al: Decrease of chondrocyte volume and volume density but increase in their number in the canine articular cartilage after a strenuous training program. Scand J Rheumatol Suppl 1986; 60:114.

245. Säämänen A-M, Tammi M, Kiviranta I, et al: Moderate running increases but strenuous running prevents elevation of proteoglycan content in canine articular cartilage. Scand J Rheumatol Suppl 1986; 60:45.

246. Kiviranta I, Jurvelin J, Säämänen A-M, et al: Strenuous running exercise attenuates the increase of articular cartilage proteoglycans observed after moderate running program of young beagle dogs. Scand J Rheumatol Suppl 1986; 60:43.

247. Kiviranta I, Tammi M, Jurvelin J, et al: Moderate running exercise augments glycosaminoglycans and thickness of articular cartilage in the knee joint of young beagle dogs. J Orthop Res 1988; 6:188–195.

248. Vasan N: Effects of physical stress on the synthesis and degradation of cartilage matrix. Connect Tissue Res 1983; 12:49–58.

249. Candolin T, Videman T: Effects of running on the scanning electron microscopic appearance of joint surfaces of rabbits. Scand J Rheumatol Suppl 1986; 60:39.

250. Palmoski MJ, Perricone E, Brandt KD: Development and reversal of proteoglycan, aggregation defect in normal canine knee cartilage after immobilization. Arthritis Rheum 1979; 22:508–517.

251. Larsson T, Aspden RM, Heinegard D: Effects of mechanical loading on cartilage matrix biosynthesis in vitro. Matrix 1991; 11:388–394.

252. Hodge WA, Fijan RS, Carlson KL, et al: Contact pressures in the human hip joint measured in vivo. Proc Natl Acad Sci 1986; 83:2879–2883.

253. Finlay JB, Repo RU: Instrumentation and procedure for the controlled impact of articular cartilage. IEEE Trans Biomed Eng 1978; 25:34–39.

254. Sokoloff L: The Biology of Degenerative Joint Disease. Chicago, University of Chicago Press, 1969.

255. Rodgers MM: Biomechanics of the foot during locomotion. In Grabiner MD (ed): Current Issues in Biomechanics. Champaign, IL, Human Kinetics, 1993, pp 33–52.

256. Bruggemann GP: Biomechanics in gymnastics. Med Sci Sports 1987; 45:142–176.

257. Radin EL, Paul IL, Rose RM: Role of mechanical factors in pathogenesis of primary osteoarthritis. Lancet 1972; 1:519–522.

258. Palmoski M, Perricone E, Brandt K: Development and reversal of a proteoglycan aggregation defect in normal canine knee cartilage after immobilization. Arthritis Rheum 1979; 22:508–517.

259. Tammi M, Paukkonen K, Kiviranta I, et al: Joint loading induced alterations in articular cartilage. In Helminen HJ, et al (eds): Joint Loading. Bristol, Wright, 1987, pp 64–88.

CHAPTER 9

Articular Neurophysiology

PETER GRIGG *PhD*

Synovial joints are held together by soft tissue structures. Ligaments and joint capsule span the joint and couple the bones together. These tissues determine the types, and the magnitudes, of the rotation and translational motions of the joint. The constraints provided by the ligaments and capsule are passive; no active contractions of muscles are involved. Because of the location and properties of the capsule and ligaments, they are deformed by certain motions of the joint. The resulting tissue loads oppose these motions and thus restrict the movement of the joint. An intriguing aspect of these soft tissue structures is that they are innervated by sensory (afferent) neurons—neurons that are activated by mechanical or chemical stimuli applied to their receptive endings. When activated, these afferent neurons transmit action potentials into the central nervous system, where they evoke sensations or (potentially) cause reflex actions. In certain circumstances some afferents can function as efferents, releasing inflammatory mediators into inflamed tissues and promoting inflammation. This chapter deals with the properties of joint neurons and their role in proprioceptive sensations, in the regulation of the motor behavior of the limb, and in mediating inflammatory processes. The material presented mainly concerns the knee joint in cats, as that is the source of most of what is known about the innervation of joints.

A discussion of the sensory innervation of joints necessarily focuses primarily on the joint capsule, for that is where most of the sensory nerve processes are found. Although sensory nerve processes have been described in other components of the knee (notably in the ligaments), they appear to be a minor component of joint innervation and are covered separately.

THE JOINT CAPSULE

In order to understand the behavior of sensory neurons whose sensory processes reside in the joint capsule, it is necessary to understand the rudiments of the nature of the capsule and its mechanical behavior in joint motions.

A joint capsule is a sleeve of fibrous tissue that surrounds a synovial joint. A capsule is not necessarily uniform; it is made up of a set of structures that are coupled to each other and that together surround a joint. For example, the knee joint capsule technically includes the patellar tendon and the collateral ligaments as well as the broad sheet of tissue that covers the posterior of the joint. However, it is the thinnest and softest parts of the capsule that receive the bulk of the sensory innervation. In the knee, the ligaments and the patellar tendon are relatively poorly innervated. In contrast, the thin, broad sheet of capsule that covers the posterior of the joint is richly innervated. Figure 9–1[1] is a schematic view of the posterior side of the knee capsule (i.e., covering the femoral condyles) in the cat. The sensory innervation stems from the posterior articular nerve (PAN), which enters the posterior side of the knee.[2] Another region of the capsule with a significant innervation is the band of tissue on the anteromedial region of the joint (Fig. 9–2)[3] between the collateral ligament and the patellar tendon. It is innervated by the medial articular nerve (MAN).[2] Since the other components of the knee capsule—the patellar tendon and the collateral ligaments—are not very well innervated, they will be discussed only briefly.

When a joint, such as a knee, is rotated into extension, the capsule is stretched on one side and is relaxed on the

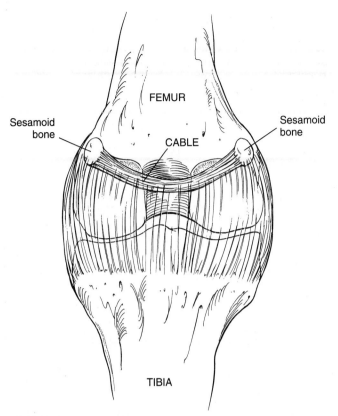

FIGURE 9–1. Posterior capsule of the cat knee. Sesamoid bones are also referred to as fabellar bones. Cable, the capsule thickening across the top of the capsule, is referred to in the text as the interfabellar ligament; it is called a cable because it acts as a suspension cable from which the capsule is suspended. LC, MC = area of capsule overlying the lateral and medial femoral condyles, respectively. (Reprinted from Grigg P, Hoffman AH: Calibrating joint capsule mechanoreceptors as in vivo soft tissue load cells. J Biomech 1989; 22: 781–785, with kind permission from Elsevier Science; Ltd.)

other side. The posterior ("flexion") side of the knee is stretched on extension and relaxed on flexion. It appears to be well adapted to stretching on extension, as it is made up of very soft material, and it is coupled to the femur at its top end through a system that functions like a suspension cable (see Fig. 9–1).[4] The suspension cable is made up of a capsule thickening (the interfabellar ligament, IFL) that is suspended from its ends, which attach to two sesamoid (fabellar) bones (S). The posterior capsule is a sheet of tissue attached along the bottom edge of the cable that covers the femoral condyles and is coupled along its bottom edge to the tibial plateau. When the knee is extended, the tibial plateau slides along the femoral surface, thus stretching the capsule along the long axis of the leg. The capsule pulls down along the length of the cable, creating tensile loads in the cable. The cable transmits those loads to the femur. The suspension system constitutes a compliant linkage between the capsule and the femur, sagging when the capsule sheet pulls down on it.[4] Another feature of this suspension system is that it causes the vertical stresses in the capsule to be very uniform across the joint.[5] The vertical stresses in the capsule are, at least in cat's knees, quite small. When the knee is fully extended, the capsule pulls down with a load of just 2

to 3 g per mm of length along the cable. Of the total moment applied to the leg, less than 2 percent is sustained by the capsule.[5] The balance of the applied moment (i.e., the remaining 98 percent) is opposed by loads in ligaments. Thus, the capsule plays only a small role in resisting rotation of the joint into extension, and it is not a major stabilizer of the knee.

The anteromedial part of the knee capsule, the thin strip of capsule material located between the patellar tendon and the collateral ligaments, referred to above, does not appear to sustain any major loading during knee rotations. It appears to be shielded from major tensile loading by virtue of its location between two major structural components of the knee, the patellar tendon and the medial collateral ligament.

The suspension cable system described above appears to be unique to small animals. The structure of human knee capsule is quite different, lacking the sesamoid bones and suspension cable system. Thus, the capsule structures studied in cats and described here do not have an exact homologue in humans. Nonetheless, the high degree of homology in structure and function between human and cat knees makes it unlikely that there are major differences in the mechanical role of the joint capsule between cats and humans.

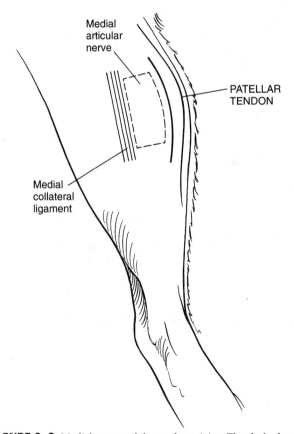

FIGURE 9–2. Medial aspect of the cat knee joint. The dashed area designates the anteromedial part of the capsule, lying between the medial collateral ligament and the patellar tendon, innervated by the medial articular nerve. (From Grigg P, Hoffman AH, Fogarty KE: Properties of Golgi-Mazzoni afferents in cat knee joint capsule, as revealed by mechanical studies of isolated joint capsule. J Neurophysiol 1982; 47: 31–40.)

THE INNERVATION OF THE JOINT

The majority of the sensory innervation of the joint is found in the joint capsule. As is the case with other somatic structures, two classes of sensory neurons make up the sensory innervation. There are (1) neurons with large-diameter, myelinated, group 2 axons; and (2) neurons with small-diameter, unmyelinated or thinly myelinated, groups 3 and 4 axons, also called fine or C-fiber afferents. Group 1 axons innervate only muscle sensors and thus are not found in joints.

The group 2 neurons innervate large, multicellular end-organ structures that are located in the capsule. These sensory units are mechanoreceptors; i.e., they are mechanically sensitive. They have low thresholds for activation by mechanical stimuli. For example, those that are sensitive to extension rotations are activated using very gentle extension stimuli. This is in contrast to the very forceful rotations that are required to activate sensors with fine (groups 3 and 4) axons, described later.

The small-diameter, groups 3 and 4 neurons have free nerve endings as terminals. They have high thresholds for mechanical activation. Intense, forceful indentational or rotational stimuli are required to activate them, and it is generally accepted that they are pain sensors (nociceptors). Under conditions of local inflammation, fine afferents can function as efferent fibers, releasing peptides that are inflammatory mediators. Together, fine afferents (groups 3 and 4) make up the overwhelming majority of the afferent fibers in the joint nerves (Table 9–1).[6,7]

NERVE ENDINGS WITH GROUP 2 AXONS

There are two types of end-organs innervated by group 2 axons.

RUFFINI ENDINGS

MORPHOLOGY. The parent axon enters the joint capsule and divides into multiple branches to form a spraylike ending (Fig. 9–3),[8] making large numbers of contacts with collagen fibers.[9] The nerve processes follow the direction of local collagen fibers, forming processes referred to as cylinders. The whole volume of an extended nerve process is encapsulated, with collagen fibers passing through the capsule at the ends of the cylinder. The directions of cylinders correspond to the directions of collagen fibers in the structure. Thus in the cable, which, like a ligament, is made up of parallel collagen fibers, the cylinders are aligned along the axis of the cable. In the sheet part of the posterior capsule, where different groups of collagen fibers are found to have different orientations, the two to six cylinders that make up the ending all have different orientations.[9]

DISTRIBUTION. Ruffini type endings are located in the capsule on the "flexion" side of joints, that is, the side that is stretched upon extension of the joint. In the knee they are found in the posterior capsule.[1,2]

MECHANICAL SENSITIVITY. The Ruffini endings are stretch sensors. A maintained stretch of the capsule produces a prolonged, slowly adapting response in the form of a train of action potentials.[1] It is generally accepted that the neuron is activated by stretching along the axis of one of the cylinders. Thus, the orientation of collagen fibers and of the cylinders will determine the direction of tissue stretch for which a given afferent will be most sensitive. When found in the suspension cable, which has the parallel fiber structure of a ligament, they are activated by uniaxial stretching along the direction of the fibers, i.e., the long axis of the cable.[10] When located in the capsule sheet, where collagen fibers have many orientations, a single afferent can be activated by stretching along many directions, reflecting the activity in many cylinders that have different orientations.[11]

It is somewhat unclear what mechanical states (i.e., local states inside the capsule) are responsible for activating Ruffini endings. In one study, Fuller et al.[12] showed that Ruffini endings were stress sensors. Axial stress and strain were decoupled by using dynamic stimuli applied to the knee joint capsule. The response of Ruffini neurons was best related to axial stress (the force applied to the tissue) rather than the strain (the deformation of the tissue). Thus the Ruffini afferents in the cable are a type of force sensor, detecting local stresses along the direction of the collagen fibers. When

---

TABLE 9–1

Composition of the Afferent Fibers in the Medial and Posterior Articular Nerves of the Cat's Knee

	Medial Articular Nerve (MAN)		Posterior Articular Nerve (PAN)	
	Number	*Percent*	*Number*	*Percent*
Group 1	0	0	27	4
Group 2	57	9	150	22
Group 3	132	21	85	12
Group 4	441	70	408	60
Total number of afferent fibers	630		680	
Percent that are fine (group 3 or group 4) afferents		91		74

The actual number of fibers varies between nerves. The numbers above are based on average numbers of fibers in the nerves and the relative proportions of fibers of different types. (Data from Heppelmann et al[6] and Langford and Schmidt.[7])

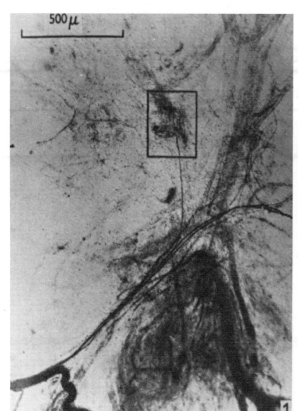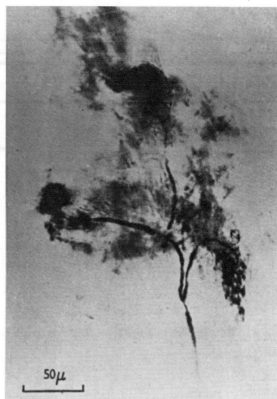

FIGURE 9–3. Photomicrographs of gold chloride–stained material from the fibrous capsule of the posterior cat knee joint, showing Ruffini type receptor processes. *Left panel,* low magnification; *right panel,* high magnification. The spraylike clusters are presumably components of different axis cylinders that make up the ending. (From Boyd IA: The histological structure of the receptors in the knee joint of the cat correlated with their physiological response. J Physiol [Lond] 1954; 124: 476–488.)

Ruffini neurons are studied using biaxial loading, very complex findings result. In the capsule sheet, both collagen fibers and the axis cylinders of the Ruffini ending have many orientations. Consequently, the neuron can be excited by stretching along any direction, although some stimuli are better than others. It was shown that if the capsule is stretched along different directions, and both stresses and strains were measured, the response of individual Ruffini endings was most closely related to the local strain energy density (Fig. 9–4).[11] Strain energy density is a scalar quantity that reflects the amount of elastic energy stored in a deformed structure. Ruffini endings have also been shown to be poorly activated by compression stimuli.

In joint rotations, Ruffini afferents respond only to movements of the joint into the limit of extension. At those positions, the capsule is loaded, which activates the neurons. Thus, these afferents serve as a limit detector.

It is possible to make Ruffini afferents discharge in positions at which they would otherwise be silent. For example, the response to extensional rotations is enhanced if the extended knee joint is also externally rotated.[13] Ruffini afferents are not activated by rotations of the joint through any ''intermediate'' angles of the joint, i.e., rotations in the flexion-extension direction with joint angles between the limits of flexion and extension. The minor exception to this statement

is that some afferents, depending on their location in the capsule, can be activated while the joint is at an intermediate angle of flexion and extension, if large isometric forces are initiated in the quadriceps muscles (Fig. 9–5).[14] This effect is seen in only a minority of afferents and, as shown in the figure, requires rather large loads in order to create the effect. Presumably, those loads either cause the joint to articulate in such a way as to load the capsule or directly deform or load the capsule through some coupling between the patellar tendon (i.e., the anterior capsule) and the posterior capsule. In summary, the sensory contributions made by Ruffini afferent neurons are almost entirely confined to extensional rotations, when the joint is in the limit of extension. In other joints, joint afferents would be activated by rotating the joint to its limit of movement.

LAMELLATED ENDINGS

MORPHOLOGY. The parent axon terminates in an elongated, thinly encapsulated structure with a lamellar interior that in some ways resembles a pacinian corpuscle (Fig. 9–6).[2,3,9] Lamellated endings have been referred to by various authors as Golgi-Mazzoni or paciniform endings. The author prefers the descriptive term ''lamellated,'' since referring to them as pacinian or paciniform implies that they are, like true

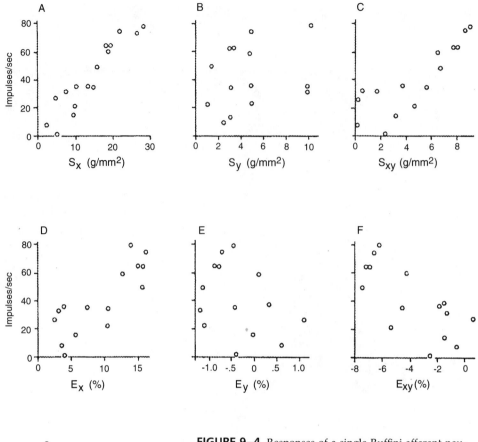

FIGURE 9–4. Responses of a single Ruffini afferent neuron, from knee joint capsule, plotted vs. the magnitudes of various states of stress and strain in the capsule. The neuron was recorded in a piece of isolated cat posterior capsule, in vitro, in response to biaxial stretching of the tissue. The tissue was stretched along both the Y (long axis of the leg) and the X (circumferential) directions. The same data points are plotted vs. seven different mechanical variables. S_x, S_y, S_{xy}: tensile stress along the X axis, Y axis, and shear stress. Ex, Ey, Exy: Strains along the X axis, Y axis, and shear strain. SED: Strain energy density. The neuron's response was positively correlated with each of the above variables but was best correlated with SED. (From Grigg P, Hoffman AH: Ruffini mechanoreceptors in isolated joint capsule: responses correlated with strain energy density. Somatosensory Research 1984; 2:149–162.)

pacinian corpuscles, vibration sensitive. There is no good evidence that the lamellated endings are vibration sensors.

DISTRIBUTION. Lamellated endings are found occasionally in the posterior side of the capsule[8] but mainly in the anterior parts of the knee joint.[2] They are located primarily in the subcapsular fibroadipose tissue rather than in the fibrous capsule itself.[2,3,9] They are also found in soft tissue structures (such as fascia) around the joint.[15,16]

MECHANICAL SENSITIVITY. The mechanical basis for activation of lamellated endings is not as clear as for the Ruffini endings. It has been hypothesized[8] that lamellated endings respond to vibrational stimuli. The connection between this ending and that response property is tenuous, however, being based mainly on the fact that in studies of afferents in the posterior capsule[8] both lamellated endings and rapidly adapting

units were infrequently observed. On the other hand, Grigg et al.[3] found endings with this morphology located under the fibrous capsule, in the anteromedial part of the capsule, having afferent axons in the medial articular nerve. The endings were located along the inside surface of the capsule, in the subcapsular fibroadipose tissue. Sensory neurons recorded in that region of the capsule were found to be compression sensitive (Fig. 9–7). Those endings had no sensitivity at all to axial stimuli (i.e., stretch) (Fig. 9–8). Using stress analysis, it was shown that the neurons that were compression sensitive resided along the inner surface of the fibrous capsule, corresponding to the location of the lamellated endings. Neurons in that region respond well to external compression stimuli (i.e., squeezing the joint). They also respond to increases in hydrostatic pressure in the joint (Fig. 9–9), which would create compressional stresses along the inside surface of the joint

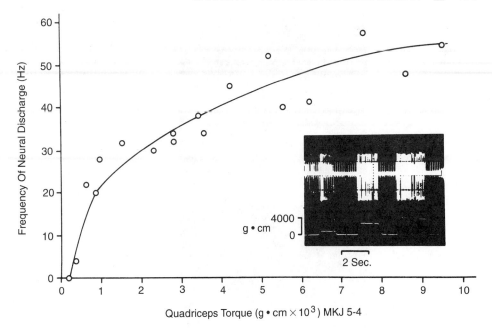

FIGURE 9–5. Activation of a joint capsule afferent neuron by force generated in the quadriceps muscles. The joint angle was fixed at 90 degrees, and the quadriceps muscles were contracted. The graph shows the response of the afferent in relation to the moment (torque) about the joint. The inset shows some of the raw data from which the graph was derived. (From Grigg P, Greenspan BJ: Response of primate joint afferent neurons to mechanical stimulation of knee joint. J Neurophysiol 1977; 40: 1–8.)

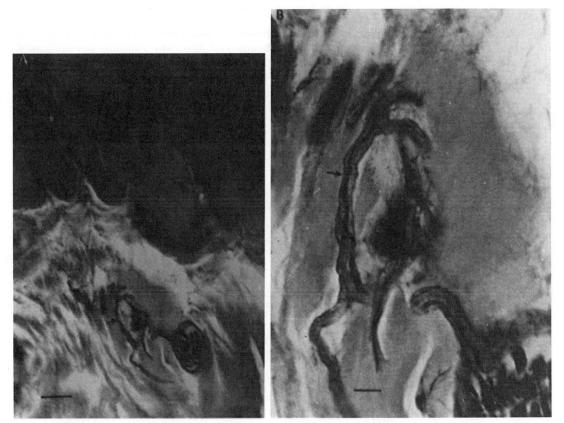

FIGURE 9–6. Photomicrographs of gold chloride–stained material from anteromedial joint capsule, in cat knee, showing fibrous capsule material and paciniform type receptor processes. *Left panel*, Low-power micrograph to show relationship between nerve processes *(arrow)* and the fibrous capsule *(darkly stained mass at top)*. Scale = 200 u. *Right panel*, High-power micrograph to show detail of the receptor process. Scale = 50 u. (From Grigg P, Hoffman AH, Fogarty KE: Properties of Golgi-Mazzoni afferents in cat knee joint capsule, as revealed by mechanical studies of isolated joint capsule. J Neurophysiol 1982; 47:31–40.)

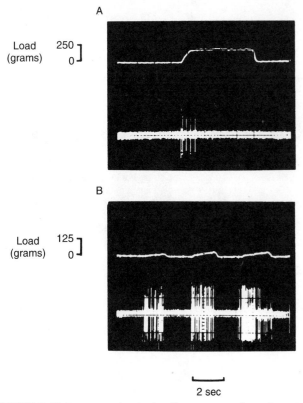

FIGURE 9–7. Response of a single afferent neuron from the medial articular nerve, recorded from a specimen of anteromedial capsule from the cat knee, in vitro, showing that afferents recorded in this preparation were compression sensitive and not tension sensitive. In *A*, the capsule specimen was stretched along the long axis of the leg; only transient responses result. In *B*, a probe was used to apply compressional stimuli to the inside (bone facing) surface of the capsule. The upper trace in *B* shows the axial load that resulted from the compression stimulus. (From Grigg P, Hoffman AH, Fogarty KE: Properties of Golgi-Mazzoni afferents in cat knee joint capsule, as revealed by mechanical studies of isolated joint capsule. J Neurophysiol 1982; 47: 31–40.)

capsule. In response to knee rotations, afferents located in the anteromedial part of the capsule are rather poorly activated by extension movements,[17] having a response that adapts to zero in about 10 seconds. It is unclear how this response is caused, since when MAN afferents are recorded in vitro, they have no response to tensile loading. In the final analysis, the lamellated endings appear to be compression sensors that may also be activated by extension rotations through mechanisms that are unclear. In summary, these neurons play no role in proprioception in the knee, but they appear to be responsible for the sensations of compression that result from applying external forces to the knee or from effusions of the knee.

AFFERENT NEURONS WITH GROUPS 3 AND 4 AXONS

Groups 3 and 4 afferents share many properties. They are presented and discussed together in this chapter, except for properties that are significantly different.

MORPHOLOGY. Group 3 axons are small in diameter and thinly myelinated. Group 4 axons are unmyelinated. The terminal process of both, however, is a fine, unmyelinated axon that branches and ends in fine tips having the lumpy appearance of a string of beads along the last 100 μ or so of each branch of the axon.[18] Each branch has an end-bulb the size of one of the beads at the tip. The enlargements that make up the string of beads and the end-bulb are believed to be separate receptive sites. The branching of the parent axon can result in multiple receptive endings that are separated by as much as 15 mm. About half of all C-fibers contain the peptide substance P (SP), and about half contain calcitonin gene–related peptide (CGRP).[19,20]

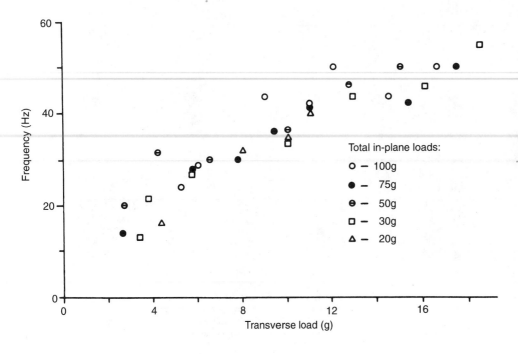

Total in-plane loads:
- ○ — 100g
- ● — 75g
- ◐ — 50g
- □ — 30g
- △ — 20g

FIGURE 9–8. Absence of response to axial loads in a compression-sensitive neuron recorded from the MAN, originating from the anteromedial capsule. Identical compression loads (horizontal axis) were applied while holding different axial (in-plane) loads, that ranged from 20 to 100 g. The response is independent of in-plane (tensile) loads. (From Grigg P, Hoffman AH, Fogarty KE: Properties of Golgi-Mazzoni afferents in cat knee joint capsule, as revealed by mechanical studies of isolated joint capsule. J Neurophysiol 1982; 47: 31–40.)

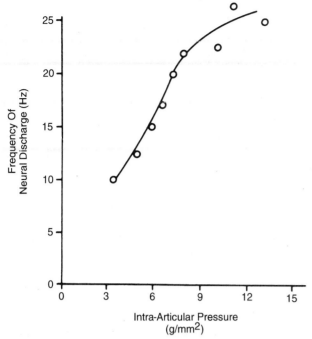

FIGURE 9–9. Afferent response to compressional stresses applied to the inside surface of the capsule. Response of a single afferent neuron from the MAN, originating from the anteromedial capsule while fluid is injected into the joint space, raising the intra-articular pressure. (From Grigg P, Hoffman AH, Fogarty KE: Properties of Golgi-Massoni afferents in cat knee joint capsule, as revealed by mechanical studies of isolated joint capsule. J Neurophysiol 1982; 47: 31–40.)

DISTRIBUTION. Sensory afferents with small-diameter ("fine") axons terminate in free nerve endings that are located in all the soft tissues of the joint, including the capsule, the collateral ligaments, and the patellar tendon.

MECHANICAL SENSITIVITY. Little was known about the properties of fine afferents in joints until the landmark studies of Hans Schaible and Robert Schmidt.[21,22] They showed that fine afferents in joints responded to very intense mechanical stimuli in the form of both indentations and joint rotations. A fundamental problem in doing experiments on anesthetized animals is that it is not clear what constitutes a noxious or painful stimulus. Sato et al.[23] concluded that the stimuli were noxious and that the fine afferents were nociceptors, because the stimuli that excited them were sufficiently noxious to cause changes in heart rate and blood pressure in anesthetized cats.

Responses to Indentations. Fine afferents can be directly stimulated by pushing on the appropriate location of the surface of the capsule using a blunt probe.[21] Rather high compression forces are necessary to initiate activity. The receptive fields of fine afferents are spotlike, and single afferent axons may have several sensitive spots (Fig. 9–10). The distribution of a sample of receptive spots in MAN afferents is shown in Figure 9–11. Individual endings are not activated by probing adjacent to the receptive field, indicating that the appropriate stimulus is compression and not tensile stresses that would be produced in the region of an indentation.

Responses to Joint Rotations. Most fine afferents can

also be excited by joint rotations. However, they are in general excited only by forceful rotations into the limits of movements, termed noxious rotations.[22] A given fine afferent may be excited by a variety of noxious rotations, such as external, internal, or extension rotations, at a variety of positions in flexion or extension (Fig. 9–12).

Sensitization of Fine Afferents. Sensitization refers to a decrease in the threshold of a neuron, typically caused by an inflammatory process. Characteristic of nociceptor neurons, fine afferents in the joint are sensitized by inflammation of the soft tissues of the joint. In-

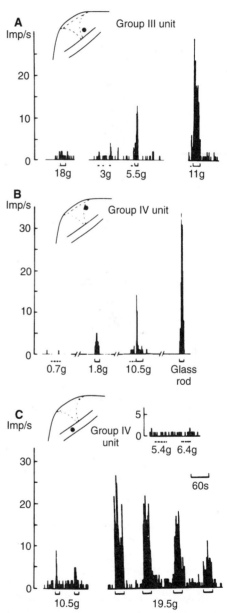

FIGURE 9–10. Response of one group 3 and two group 4 fibers in the MAN, originating from the anteromedial capsule. The location of the receptive field in relation to the gross features of the medial side of the cat knee is shown. Responses are shown as PST histograms. The responses are obtained by probing the receptive field using von Frey hairs that are calibrated to generate known compressional loads (shown). (From Schaible H-G, Schmidt RF: Activation of Groups III and IV sensory units in medial articular nerve by local mechanical stimulation of knee joint. Neurophysiol 1983; 49: 35–44.)

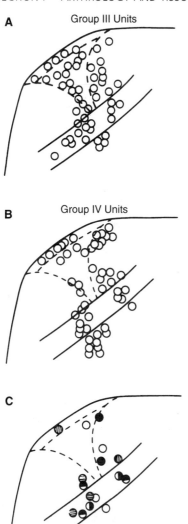

A   Group III Units

B   Group IV Units

C

◐ ⊖ ○ Group III Units
● ◐ ● Group IV Units

FIGURE 9–11. Locations of receptive fields of fine afferent neurons in the MAN in cat knee. *A,* Fifty-one receptive fields of 40 group 3 fibers; *B,* 50 receptive fields of 41 group 4 units. *C,* Locations of receptive fields of six units (both group 3 and group 4) with multiple receptive fields. (From Schaible H-G, Schmidt RF: Activation of Groups III and IV sensory units in medial articular nerve by local mechanical stimulation of knee joint. J Neurophysiol 1983; 49: 35–44.)

jecting kaolin and carrageenan into the joint causes inflammation,[24] which results in lowering the threshold for activation of fine afferents. Further, neurons lacking spontaneous discharge begin to discharge spontaneously. After sensitization, many neurons may be activated by rotating the joint into angles that were formerly benign (Fig. 9–13). Importantly, there is a large population of "silent" nociceptor afferents that are revealed (i.e., can be activated) only following inflammation.[25] These afferents are silent (i.e., unexcitable by any mechanical stimulus) in a normal, uninflamed joint. Following inflammation, they behave like standard nociceptors in an inflamed joint. Both the foregoing mechanisms—sensitization of nociceptors and recruitment of silent nociceptors—account for the increased pain sensations that are present after an injury to soft tissue components of joints.

NEUROGENIC INFLAMMATION

When a joint is inflamed, the sensory neurons that innervate it contribute to the generation and maintenance of the inflammatory process. This phenomenon has been studied in joints in which acute inflammatory processes are produced experimentally. When the agents carrageenan and kaolin are injected into a cat's knee joint, they cause an inflammation of the joint.[24] The joint swells and increases in temperature. Part of this inflammatory response is mediated by the C-fiber sensory afferents that innervate the joint. If C-fiber sensory neurons from the joint are interrupted,[26,27] the inflammation is reduced. If neural transmission in the spinal cord is blocked pharmacologically,[28,29] or if the dorsal roots are cut, the inflammation is also reduced. The process by which sensory neurons participate in generating and maintaining an inflammation is termed neurogenic inflammation. Neurogenic inflammation is caused by dorsal root reflexes (DRRs),[30] a mechanism through which sensory axons are depolarized at their synaptic terminations and caused to conduct antidromically (backward) (Fig. 9–14). The peripheral terminations of some C-fiber sensory neurons contain the peptides SP and CGRP. SP is held in sensory nerve endings in vesicular form, and it is released when the axon is backfired.[31] Both SP and CGRP are potent vasodilators.

DRRs are generated when an acute inflammatory process sensitizes (increases activity in) nociceptor afferents. Nociceptor afferents synapse with interneurons in the dorsal horn of the spinal cord, and the interneurons, in turn, become hypersensitized.[32] They have an increased response to all stimuli, and they respond to stimuli that were previously ineffective. The interneurons make synapses on, and depolarize, the terminals of other afferent fibers. This process is termed primary afferent depolarization (PAD); its normal function is to reduce the amount of transmitter released by the terminal, in which case the process is termed presynaptic inhibition. However, when the interneuron is in its sensitized state, the magnitude of the PAD can be great enough to result in initiating an action potential in the afferent fiber. The action potential is conducted backward along the axon, reaching the tissue in which the sensory ending lies and causing the local release of inflammatory peptides. Through this mechanism, an afferent fiber functions as an efferent, releasing vasoactive substances and contributing to the maintenance of the inflammation. Neurogenic inflammation is a major contributor to the acute inflammatory response that follows an injury process. The resulting neurogenic inflammation causes local hyperemia and hyperalgesia in areas that are distant to the initial, focal inflammation. Furthermore, stimuli that are distant from a focal inflammation can cause DRRs that release inflammatory peptides at the focus, thus maintaining the inflammation.

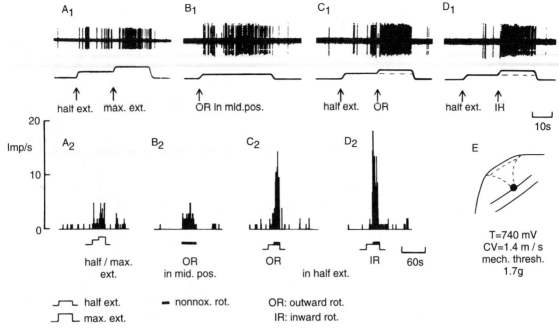

FIGURE 9–12. Responses of one fine afferent to a wide variety of rotational stimuli. A single group 4 neuron from the MAN is recorded in relation to passive movements of the knee. A_1–D_1 are raw data recorded in response to the type of rotation shown schematically below each record. OR = Outward (external) rotation of the knee; IR = inward (internal) rotation of the knee. The same data are shown as PST histograms in A_2–D_2. E, Sketch to show the location of the receptive field of the neuron at the anterior border of the medial collateral ligament. (From Schaible H-G, Schmidt RF: Responses of fine medial nerve afferents to passive movements of knee joints. J Neurophysiol 1983; 49: 1118–1126.)

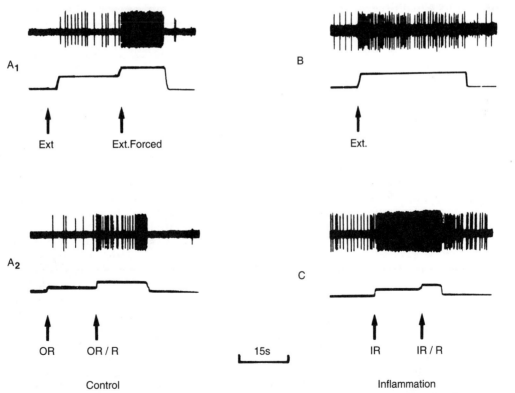

FIGURE 9–13. Recordings from single fine afferents in PAN from cat knee in the normal and inflamed conditions. A_1–A_2 show a modest response to extension (A_1) and outward rotation (A_2) in a normal (uninflamed) joint. B–C show increased responses to extension (B) and inward rotation (C) in the inflamed joint. (From Grigg P, Schaible H-G, Schmidt RF: Mechanical sensitivity of Groups III and IV afferents from posterior articular nerve in normal and inflamed cat knee. J Neurophysiol 1986; 55: 635–643.)

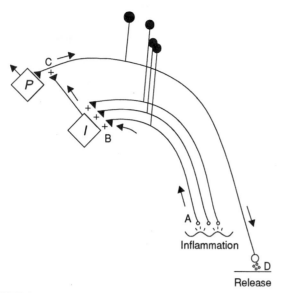

FIGURE 9–14. Schematic representation of neural elements subserving dorsal root reflexes. The fibers depicted are dorsal root primary afferent fibers, synapsing on an interneuron (I), and a projection neuron (P), whose axon enters the spinothalamic tract (not intended to be anatomically correct). *A,* Site of local inflammation; primary afferents are excited by the inflammation. *B,* Excitatory synapse between primary afferent fibers and interneuron. *C,* Depolarizing synapse produces PAD in afferent terminal, initiating action potential that is conducted backward. *D,* Peptides are released in peripheral tissue, causing local inflammation.

JOINT AFFERENTS IN PROPRIOCEPTION

Proprioception refers to the complex senses of position and movement of a joint. It arises from activity in populations of afferent neurons, in this case neurons located in and around the limb. Different mechanisms may be responsible for different components of proprioception. When a synovial joint is in a midrange position (the joint is freely moving and not at a limit of its movement range), the senses of movement and position arise from activity in muscle afferent neurons. A number of lines of evidence support this model. In experiments in human subjects, activation of muscle afferents, by vibrating muscles[33] or by stretching tendons,[34] creates illusions of movement. Tensing muscles, which increases the discharges of muscle receptors, increases the sensitivity for detecting changes in joint position.[35]

Joint afferents appear to play no role in proprioception when the joint is in the midrange of its position. For one thing, joint afferent neurons are not active at those positions and thus cannot contribute to sensations.[13,36] Second, Clark and colleagues,[37] in an experiment on human subjects, blocked joint afferents in the knee by filling it with local anesthetic; they found no change in the ability of the subjects to judge joint position (Fig. 9–15). Third, experiments using human subjects who have undergone joint replacement and capsulectomy find only slight changes in proprioceptive sensations.[38] For example, the ability to accurately position the hip (Fig. 9–16) was unchanged after total capsulectomy and replacement of joint surfaces; the ability to detect

threshold-level rotations was diminished, but only slightly.

Studies of the properties of joint afferents in animals, referred to earlier, show that joint afferents do not provide a signal to the central nervous system (CNS) that would be useful in determining joint positions. For example, Ruffini afferents signal the tensile stresses or strain energy in the capsule and in the interfabellar ligament. It is important to note that the posterior capsule sustains stresses (e.g., loads) only when the knee is rotated past 165 degrees into the limit of extension.[5] Therefore, the CNS could use the signal from Ruffini afferents only to recognize that the knee is in proximity to its limit of rotation in extension. In short, Ruffini afferents could serve as limit sensors in extension rotations.[1]

Lamellated endings, since they are sensitive to compression and not to rotational stimuli, are likewise poor candidates for a role in proprioception. Their role in joint sensory mechanisms is likely to be in subserving a sense of compression in the joint capsule.

Since a given fine afferent may be excited by a variety of noxious rotations, such as external, internal, or extension rotations, at a variety of positions in flexion or extension, fine afferents are poor candidates for a role in proprioception. Their properties are excellent ones for nociceptors, signaling very intense stimuli irrespective of joint position. However, this lack of angular specificity is a poor characteristic for a neuronal system used to encode joint angle. Thus, these neurons are unlikely to play a role in proprioceptive sensation.

Thus, in summary it is possible to rule out a role for joint afferents in the ordinary sense of joint position. One can argue logically for a role as a limit detector, but this role has not been demonstrated.

REFLEX CONNECTIONS MADE BY JOINT AFFERENT NEURONS

It is well known that the motion of a joint is constrained by the passive properties of the soft tissues that span it. The question addressed in this section is whether the motion of a joint may also be constrained by active, reflex mechanisms based on signals originating from neural sensors in joint tissues. The concept that certain aspects of limb mechanics may be actively controlled by the nervous system is widely accepted.[39] It is generally agreed that signals originating in peripheral sensors, such as muscle spindles, play a major role in limb stabilization. The evidence that shows that sensors in joint neurons do not play a major role in joint stabilization will be reviewed here.

If active stabilizing mechanisms around joints were based on joint afferent neurons, it should be possible to activate joint afferents and then look for changes in the activity of motor neurons that control the muscles acting around the joint. A number of investigators (see reference 13 for background) have observed that joint afferents make reflex connections with motoneurons innervating leg muscles. However, the methods used in many of these studies were so deeply flawed that little

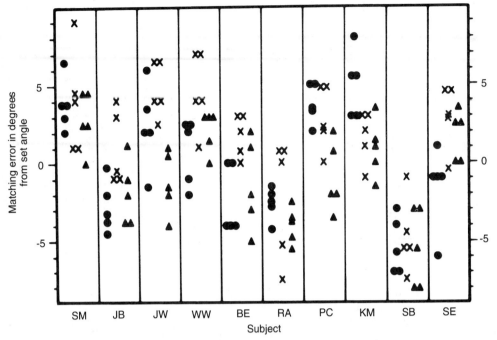

● PREINJECTION
✗ INJECTION
▲ POSTINJECTION

FIGURE 9–15. The effect of injecting a local anesthetic into the knee joint on the ability of the subject to match joint angles using the knee. One leg is moved passively, and the subject matches the angle by rotating the other knee. The vertical scale is the magnitude of mismatch observed. *Filled circles* = Before injection; X = during injection; triangles = after injection. (From Clark FJ, Horch KW, Bach SM, Larson GF: Contributions of cutaneous and joint receptors to static knee position sense in man. J Neurophysiol 1979; 42: 877–888.)

can be concluded from them. For example, certain anesthetics, used in some experiments, block inhibitory synaptic mechanisms. Thus, reflex effects observed in any such experiments are uninterpretable. Electrical stimulation of joint nerves may excite afferent nerves, causing reflex effects. However, electrical stimuli excite afferents in unnatural combinations, so that the results are not interpretable. It is therefore unclear how any results can be interpreted, beyond the statement that some neurons make some sort of reflex connection. Stimulating the joint with natural (i.e., rotational) stimuli is a better experimental strategy. First, the intensity of a stimulus can be controlled so that nociceptors are not involved. Second, by using a stimulus such as knee extension, it is possible to excite a specific subset of afferents without activating others. Using this experimental design, Grigg et al.[40] found that knee joint afferents made reflex connections onto knee motoneurons and that the reflex constituted a weak, positive feedback loop. Knee flexor (hamstring) motoneurons were weakly inhibited by knee extension, while knee extensors were weakly excited by knee extension stimuli (Fig. 9–17). This finding of positive feedback was confirmed by Ferrell et al.[41] They showed that activating PAN afferents by indenting the surface of the posterior capsule excited quadriceps motoneurons, consistent with the above finding.

In summary, reflex effects that are mediated by group 2 afferents do not have any important role in stabilizing joints or in movement control. For one thing, the reflex

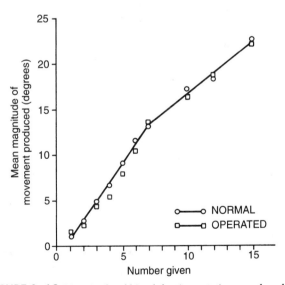

FIGURE 9–16. Magnitude of hip abduction rotations produced by a human subject with a normal hip on one side (normal) and a prosthetic joint replacement, with capsulectomy, on the other (operated). Abduction movements are scaled by the subject to be proportional in magnitude to a number given to the subject. Large numbers resulted in large abductions, small numbers in small abductions. The subject had one normal hip (normal) and one hip with a prosthetic joint and a capsulectomy (operated). (From Grigg P, Finerman GA, Riley LH: Joint-position sense after total hip replacement. J Bone Joint Surg 1973A; 55: 1016–1025.)

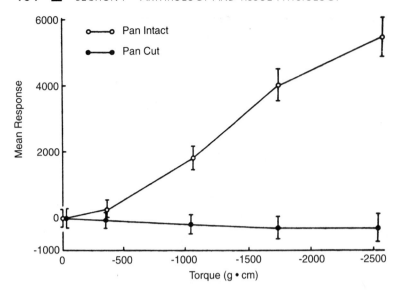

FIGURE 9–17. Magnitude of the electrically recorded monosynaptic reflex evoked in quadriceps motoneurons, in relation to rotation of the knee in extension. The moment applied to the knee is shown on the horizontal axis. The rotation stimulus was applied twice: one with the joint nerve (PAN) intact *(open circles)* and again with the PAN cut *(filled circles)*. This shows that quadriceps motoneurons are excited by extension of the knee joint, and the effect is mediated by neurons in the PAN. (From Grigg P, Harrigan EP, Fogarty KE: Segmental reflexes mediated by joint afferent neurons in cat knee. J Neurophysiol 1978; 41: 9–14.)

connections they make are quite weak. Second, the "sign" of the connection is wrong. Positive feedback, acting alone, would destabilize the joint rather than stabilize it.

Another way to test for the role of joint afferents in movement control is to eliminate their influence by cutting the joint nerves, and observing any subsequent changes in motor behavior. The most convincing use of this method was made by O'Connor et al.,[42] who found that surgically cutting all the nerves to a dog knee joint was without discernible effect. The authors surgically denervated one knee and allowed the dogs to recover for periods of up to 1 year. (Note: These dogs were the control group for an experiment on unstable joints that is described later.) During the year that the dogs survived, neither visual observation of their gait or motor behavior nor kinematic measures of their motor

behavior, made on a treadmill, revealed any effect of the neurectomy on any aspect of the dog's motor behavior.

Further evidence derives from observations made in human subjects who have had joint replacement surgery. Following joint replacement and capsulectomy, there is no change in the ability of patients to make accurate positioning movements of the affected joint (see Fig. 9–16).[38]

The reflex effects that are contributed by fine (nociceptor) afferents are difficult to evaluate. If a stimulus is sufficiently intense to excite nociceptor afferents, it will also excite group 2 (low-threshold) joint afferents. Thus, it is not possible to sort out which population of neurons is doing what. Schmidt and colleagues[43] attempted to bypass this problem using the following experimental design. They recorded from a single hindlimb flexor motor neuron in a cat. The activity of this neuron was

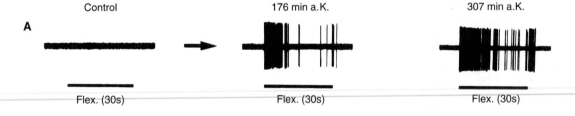

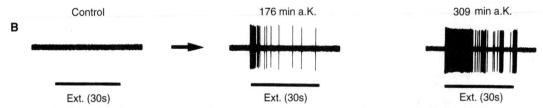

FIGURE 9–18. Responses of a single flexor (posterior biceps–semitendinosus) motoneuron, elicited by gentle rotations into flexion *(A)* and extension *(B)*. The stimuli are presented while the joint is uninflamed (control) and after inflammation (a.K.). Responses are shown before and approximately 3 and 5 min (176–179 sec, and 307–309 min) after inflammation. Before inflammation, the stimuli are without effect. After inflammation, the same rotations excite nociceptors and cause reflex excitation of the motoneuron. (From He X, Proske U, Schaible HG, Schmidt RF: Acute inflammation of the knee joint in cats alters responses of flexor motoneurons to leg movements. J Neurophysiol 1988; 59: 326–340.)

recorded in response to gentle rotations of the knee into flexion and extension. Figure 9–18 shows an example of this experiment: In the "control" records, neither flexion nor extension caused any response in a knee flexor (posterior biceps) motoneuron. The investigators then produced an inflammation of the knee by injecting it with carrageenan and kaolin. These agents caused the knee to become inflamed and increased the sensitivity of joint nociceptors. After the inflammation, the knee was rotated using the same gentle rotations as before. However, in the inflamed state, these gentle stimuli would excite nociceptor (fine) afferents. As shown in Figure 9–18, following inflammation, both flexion and extension stimuli excited the flexor motoneuron. The difference in response before and after inflammation was due to the fact that after inflammation, gentle flexion and extension rotations activate nociceptors. Importantly, the flexor motoneuron was excited irrespective of the direction of movement of the knee. This shows that the reflex effects made by fine afferents are consistent with the "flexor" reflex. In the flexor reflex, stimuli that are intense enough to excite nociceptors cause the stimulated limb to be withdrawn. Flexor motoneurons are excited, and extensor motoneurons are inhibited. Initiating the flexor reflex is a common role for nociceptors. In the present case, in the knee, the function of the reflex would be to flex the knee, thus protecting it by unloading it.

In summary, joint afferents do not have a role in active joint stabilization. The most important role appears to be that played by joint nociceptors. They do not actively stabilize the knee but protect it from intense stimuli by reflexly causing flexion of the joint, thus unloading it.

THE ROLE OF JOINT AFFERENT NEURONS IN AN UNSTABLE JOINT

Joint afferents play no role in the regulation of joint movement and only a minimal role in proprioception. They are, however, not without an important role. O'Connor et al.[42] have shown that joint afferents play a key role in protecting unstable joints from injury. They made dog knees unstable by surgically cutting the anterior cruciate ligament (ACL) unilaterally. The dogs were allowed to survive, moving about freely, for up to 1.5 years. They were then sacrificed and their knees

examined for evidence of osteoarthritis (i.e., cartilage lesions). All dogs whose ACL was cut eventually developed some degree of osteoarthritis. However, the degree of injury depended on whether the joint nerves were intact or cut. Cutting the nerves to an unstable joint increased the degree of cartilage injury. Leaving the joint nerves intact protected the joint, as the resulting cartilage damage was less severe (Table 9–2). These results indicate that the animal can use activity in joint afferents to detect extreme or potentially damaging stimuli, and that they can use this information to adopt movement strategies that minimize damage. Note that this model is consistent with what is known about both group 2 (Ruffini) and fine afferents. Ruffini afferents are activated when the joint is approaching the limit of its movement in extension. Fine afferents signal that the joint has been rotated into a "noxious" position. If the animal can reposition the joint, moving it so as to minimize signals from either or both types of afferents, it would result in protecting the joint. In subsequent experiments, O'Connor et al.[44] showed that the protective role of the joint innervation was apparent only in the period of time when the joint was made unstable. They removed afferent nerves at one of two times: (1) several weeks before making the joint unstable by ACL section, or (2) 52 weeks after ACL section. When the joint became unstable, and when it lacked afferent neurons, serious cartilage lesions resulted. Removing the same afferent neurons 52 weeks after the joint became unstable was without effect. The animal, in short, appears to use afferent signals from the joint to adapt or modify movement strategies in the limb. By using strategies that minimize afferent activity, tissue damage can be minimized. After 52 weeks, the nerves may be removed without effect, since by that time the animal has already acquired movement strategies appropriate for the unstable knee. It is most likely that this sensory function is subserved by the nociceptor afferents in the joint nerves. It is commonly accepted that the role for nociceptors is to signal stimuli intense enough to damage tissue. An animal confronted with persistent nociceptor activity from a part of its anatomy will take steps (i.e., acquire strategies) to minimize the pain. Once the new strategy is well learned, the afferent neurons are not required in order to sustain it. Understanding this role for joint afferent neurons is of great importance in the surgical treatment of unstable joints. If it is anticipated that a joint may be unstable, the

TABLE 9–2
Magnitudes of Cartilage Lesions Observed in Dog Knee Joints, 72 Weeks After Treatment

| Treatment | Severity of Cartilage Lesion | | | | | |
	0	1	2	3	4	5
Control	XX					
Joint nerves cut	XX					
ACL transected		XX	XX			
ACL transection plus joint nerves cut			X	X	XX	XX

Severity of lesions is ordered from 0 (normal cartilage) to 5 (fragmentation of the cartilage and exposure of the subchondral bone). (Adapted from O'Connor BL, Visco DM, Brandt KD: Neurogenic acceleration of osteoarthritis. J Bone Joint Surg 1992; 74A:367–376.)

preservation of its innervation should be an important priority in any surgical procedure.

MECHANORECEPTORS IN LIGAMENTS

Sensory nerve endings have been described in ligaments, notably the ACL.[45] There has been much speculation that these sensory neurons constitute the afferent limb of an important motor control system. Many of the hypotheses about a role for joint capsule afferents have recently been restated for ligament afferents. Regrettably, there is no evidence to support any of this vigorous speculation. Theories that are unfounded with regard to capsule afferents can now be said to be unfounded with regard to ligament afferents. This section reviews what is known about sensory processes in knee ligaments.

Joint ligaments are deformed during rotations, and it is known that there are groups 2, 3, and 4 sensory nerve endings in ligaments.[21,22,45] The nerve processes are morphologically similar to those found in capsule. Kraupse et al.[46] have recorded from group 2 afferent neurons originating in the ACL in cat knees. They showed that movement of the joint into any limiting position results in discharge of afferent mechanoreceptors (Fig. 9–19). These properties can be accounted for based on the known stretch sensitivity of Ruffini endings. The ACL is loaded when the joint is rotated to a limit of movement. Since Ruffini afferents respond to local tensile stresses or strain energy, they would be activated by stimuli that cause stress in the ACL. Movements of the knee through positions that do not load the ACL would be without effect on ACL afferents. The same model may be applied to stretch-sensitive afferents in the collateral ligaments.[47]

Do ligament afferents have a role in proprioception? Although ligament afferents have been proposed to serve a role in proprioception, they are unlikely to serve a major role, for the following reasons:

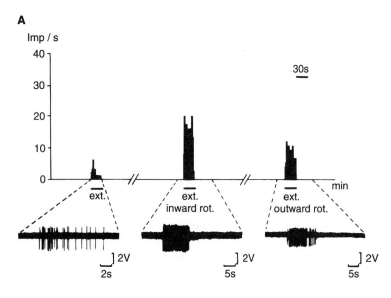

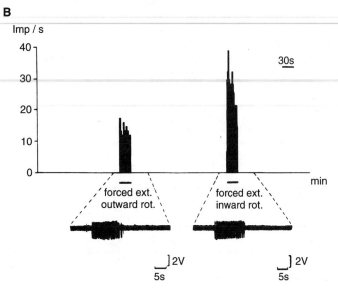

FIGURE 9–19. Responses of a single group 2 neuron originating from the anterior cruciate ligament, in cat knee. Responses are recorded in relation to extension, inward (internal) rotation, and outward (external) rotations. Responses are shown as raw data traces and PST histograms. This neuron responded to extension and inward and outward rotations. (From Kraupse R, Schmidt M, Schaible H-G: Sensory innervation of the anterior cruciate ligament. J Bone Joint Surg 1992A; 74: 390–397.)

TABLE 9–3
Summary of Properties of Sensory Neurons Found in Joints*

Location	Morphology	Axon Type	%†	Response to Local Stimuli	Response to Rotations	Role in Proprioception	Role in Motor Coordination	Other Features	Importance
Throughout soft tissues	Free nerve endings	Groups 3 and 4	84	Intense indentations	Nonspecific response to intense rotations	None; signal pain	Evoke flexion reflex	Sensitized by inflammation	Can promote inflammation through DRRs; protective role if joint is unstable
In fibrous capsule along 'flexion' side of joint	Ruffini corpuscle	Group 2	12	Tensile loads in collagen	Respond to extreme extensions	Hypothesized to be limit detectors	None	–	May play role in protecting unstable joint
Junction of fibrous capsule and subcapsular adipose	Golgi-Mazzoni corpuscle	Group 2	4	Compression of capsule	Poor; in extreme joint rotations only	None	None	–	None

*Listed in the order of the frequency of occurrence in knee joints.
†Percentage of the population of knee afferents that fall into this category.

1. *Paucity of nerve endings.* While there are a relatively large number of afferent neurons having endings in the joint capsule (i.e., the cat knee has approximately 200 group 2 fibers that originate in the capsule [see Table 9–1]), there appear to be no more than a few ligament afferents that originate in the ACL.

2. *Ligament afferents could serve only as nonspecific limit sensors.* Since ligament tension can be caused by a number of different types of rotations, the mechanoreceptors in them are a poor candidate to subserve proprioceptive sensations of movements in specific directions. Although neurons innervating the collateral ligaments are less well documented, they also appear to be tension sensitive and thus to be subject to the same reservations as those stated for ACL afferents.

Do knee ligament afferents have a role in motor control of the joint? Ligament afferent neurons have not been shown to serve a role in motor control. The same concerns that were stated previously, regarding reflex effects of capsule afferents, may be stated here for ligament afferents. Experiments were previously reviewed in which knee joints were rotated while reflex effects were sought in motoneurons acting around the knee.[40] In those experiments, the reflex effects that were observed were produced by afferent neurons in the PAN. Since the PAN is the source of afferent neurons for both the posterior capsule and the ACL, the reflexes that were described could be due to either capsule or ACL afferents, or to both. However, the reflex effects in those experiments were both very weak and positive in sign (i.e., destabilizing). Thus, ACL afferents do not mediate a reflex that has a role in coordinating limb movements.

SUMMARY

Soft tissue components of joints have a sensory innervation by both low-threshold group 2 mechanoreceptors and groups 3 and 4 nociceptors. Their properties and functions are summarized in Table 9–3. Low-threshold mechanoreceptors play a very small sensory role in proprioception. Ruffini afferents provide a limit of motion signal, that the joint is at or near a limit of its movement. Lamellated endings provide a sense of deep pressure. The role of low-threshold mechanoreceptors is strictly sensory; when activated, they do not mediate significant motor reflex actions. Joint nociceptors (groups 3 and 4) are activated by intense pressure stimuli or by forceful rotations, both of which can be considered to be noxious. They are sensitized by inflammation. They subserve sensations of pain originating from joints. When activated, these fine afferents evoke the flexion reflex at the joint. The principal functional role for the sensory innervation of the joint is to protect it in the event that it becomes unstable, by allowing the adoption of movement strategies that avoid damaging the unstable joint. Nociceptors in and around inflamed tissue can be activated antidromically in dorsal root reflexes. They then release inflammatory peptides in peripheral tissues and promote inflammations.

REFERENCES

1. Grigg P, Hoffman AH: Properties of Ruffini afferents revealed by stress analysis of isolated sections of cat knee capsule. J Neurophysiol 1982; 47: 41–54.
2. Freeman MAR, Wyke B: The innervation of the knee joint. An anatomical and histological study in the cat. J Anat 1967; 101: 505–532.
3. Grigg P, Hoffman AH, Fogarty KE: Properties of Golgi-Mazzoni afferents in cat knee joint capsule, as revealed by mechanical studies of isolated joint capsule. J Neurophysiol 1982; 47: 31–40.
4. Hoffman AH, Grigg P, Flynn DM: A biomechanical model of the posterior knee capsule of the cat. J Biomech Eng 1985; 107: 140–146.
5. Hoffman AH, Grigg P: Measurement of joint capsule tissue loading in the cat knee using calibrated mechanoreceptors. J Biomech 1989; 22: 787–791.
6. Heppelmann B, Heuss C, Schmidt RF: Fiber size distribution of myelinated and unmyelinated axons in the medial and posterior articular nerves of the cat's knee joint. Somatosens Res 1988; 5:273–281.
7. Langford LA, Schmidt RF: Afferent and efferent axons in the medial and posterior articular nerves of the cat's knee joint. Anat Rec 1983; 206: 71–78.
8. Boyd IA: The histological structure of the receptors in the knee-joint of the cat correlated with their physiological response. J Physiol (Lond) 1954; 124: 476–488.
9. Halata Z: The ultrastructure of the sensory nerve endings in the articular capsule of the knee joint of the domestic cat (Ruffini corpuscles and Pacinian corpuscles). J Anat 1977; 124: 717–729.
10. Grigg P, Hoffman AH: Calibrating joint capsule mechanoreceptors as in vivo soft tissue load cells. J Biomech 1989; 22: 781–785.
11. Grigg P, Hoffman AH: Ruffini mechanoreceptors in isolated joint capsule: responses correlated with strain energy density. Somatosens Res 1984; 2: 149–162.
12. Fuller MS, Grigg P, Hoffman AH: Response of joint capsule neurons to axial stress and strain during dynamic loading in cat. J Neurophysiol 1991; 65: 1321–1328.
13. Grigg P: Mechanical factors influencing response of joint afferent neurons from cat knee. J Neurophysiol 1975; 38: 1473–1484.
14. Grigg P, Greenspan BJ: Response of primate joint afferent neurons to mechanical stimulation of knee joint. J Neurophysiol 1977; 40: 1–8.
15. Strasmann T, Halata Z: Applications for 3-D image processing in functional anatomy—reconstruction of the cubital joint region and spatial distribution of mechanoreceptors surrounding the joint in Monodelphis domestica. Eur J Cell Biol 1989; 25: (Suppl 48) 107–110.
16. Strasmann T, Halata Z, Loo SK: Topography and ultrastructure of sensory nerve endings in the joint capsules of the Kowari (Dasyuroides byrnei), an Australian marsupial. Anat Embryol 1987; 176: 1–12.
17. Clark FJ: Information signaled by sensory nerve fibers in medial articular nerve. J Neurophysiol 1975; 38: 1464–1472.
18. Heppelmann B, Messlinger K, Neiss WF, Schmidt RF: Ultrastructural three-dimensional reconstruction of group III and group IV sensory nerve endings ("free nerve endings") in the knee joint capsule of the cat: evidence for multiple receptive sites. J Comp Neurol 1990; 292:103–116.
19. McCarthy PW, Lawson SN: Cell type and conduction velocity of rat primary sensory neurons with substance P–like immunoreactivity. Neuroscience 1989; 28: 745–753.
20. McCarthy PW, Lawson SN: Cell type and conduction velocity of rat primary sensory neurons with calcitonon gene–related peptide-like immunoreactivity. Neuroscience 1990; 34: 623–632.
21. Schaible HG, Schmidt RF: Activation of groups III and IV sensory units in medial articular nerve by local mechanical stimulation of knee joint. J Neurophysiol 1983; 49: 35–44.

22. Schaible HG, Schmidt RF: Responses of fine medial nerve afferents to passive movements of knee joints. J Neurophysiol 1983; 49: 1118–1126.

23. Sato A, Sato Y, Schmidt RF: Changes in blood pressure and heart rate induced by movements of normal and inflamed knee joints. Neurosci Lett 1984; 52: 55–60.

24. Coggeshall RE, Hong KAP, Langford LA, et al: Discharge characteristics of fine medial articular afferents at rest and during passive movements of inflamed knee joints. Brain Res 1983; 272: 185–188.

25. Grigg P, Schaible HG, Schmidt RF: Mechanical sensitivity of Group III and IV afferents from posterior articular nerve in normal and inflamed cat knee joint. J Neurophysiol 1986; 5: 635–643.

26. Levine JD, Dardick SJ, Roizen MF, et al: Contribution of sensory afferents and sympathetic efferents to joint injury in experimental arthritis. J Neurosci 1986; 6: 3423–3429.

27. Sluka KA, Lawand NB, Westlund KN: Joint inflammation is reduced by dorsal rhizotomy and not by sympathectomy or spinal cord transection. Ann Rheum Dis 1994; 53: 309–314.

28. Sluka KA, Westlund KN: Centrally administered non-NMDA but not NMDA receptor antagonists block peripheral knee-joint inflammation. Pain 1993; 55: 217–225.

29. Sluka KA, Willis WD, Westlund KN: Joint inflammation and hyperalgesia are reduced by spinal bicuculline. Neuroreport 1993; 5: 109–112.

30. Rees H, Sluka KA, Westlund KN, Willis WD: Do dorsal root reflexes augment peripheral inflammation? Neuroreport 1994; 5: 821–824.

31. Ferrell WR, Russell JW: Extravasation in the knee induced by antidromic stimulation of articular c fiber afferents of the anesthetized cat. J Physiol 1986; 379: 407–416.

32. Schaible H-G, Schmidt RF, Willis WD: Enhancement of the responses of ascending tract cells in the cat spinal cord by acute inflammation of the knee joint. Exp Brain Res 1987; 66:489–499.

33. Goodwin GM, McClosky DI, Matthews PBC: The contribution of muscle afferents to kinaesthesia shown by vibration induced illusions of movement and by the effect of paralysing joint afferents. Brain 1972; 95: 705–748.

34. Matthews PBC, Simmonds A: Sensations of finger movement elicited by pulling upon flexor tendons in man. J Physiol (Lond) 1974; 239: 27–28P.

35. Gandevia SC, McClosky DI, Burke D: Kinaesthetic signals and muscle contraction. Trends Neurosci 1992; 15: 62–65.

36. Burgess PR, Clark FJ: Characteristics of knee joint receptors in the cat. J Physiol (Lond) 1969; 203: 317–335.

37. Clark FJ, Horch KW, Bach SM, Larson GF: Contributions of cutaneous and joint receptors to static knee-position sense in man. J Neurophysiol 1979; 42: 877–888.

38. Grigg P, Finerman GA, Riley LH: Joint-position sense after total hip replacement. J Bone Joint Surg 1973; 55A: 1016–1025.

39. Hasan Z, Stuart DG: Animal solutions to problems of movement control: The role of proprioceptors. Ann Rev Neurosci 1988; 11: 199–223.

40. Grigg P, Harrigan EP, Fogarty KE: Segmental reflexes mediated by joint afferent neurons in cat knee. J Neurophysiol 1978; 41: 9–14.

41. Ferrell WR, Rosenberg JR, Baxendale RH, et al: Fourier analysis of the relation between the discharge of quadriceps motor units and periodic mechanical stimulation of cat knee receptors. Exp Physiol 1990; 75: 739–750.

42. O'Connor BL, Visco DM, Brandt KD: Neurogenic acceleration of osteoarthritis: the effects of prior articular neurectomy on the development of osteoarthritis after anterior cruciate ligament transection in the dog. J Bone Joint Surg 1992; 74A: 367–376.

43. He X, Proske U, Schaible HG, Schmidt RF: Acute inflammation of the knee joint in cats alters responses of flexor motoneurons to leg movements. J Neurophysiol 1988; 59: 326–340.

44. O'Connor BL, Visco DM, Brand KD, et al: Sensory nerves only temporarily protect the unstable canine knee joint from osteoarthritis. Arthritis Rheum 1993; 36: 1154–1163.

45. Haus J, Halata Z: Innervation of the anterior cruciate ligament. Int Orthop 1990; 14: 293–296.

46. Kraupse R, Schmidt M, Schaible H-G: Sensory innervation of the anterior cruciate ligament. J Bone Joint Surg 1992; 74A: 390–397.

47. Andrew BL: The sensory innervation of the medial ligament of the knee joint. J Physiol (Lond) 1954; 123: 241–250.

CHAPTER 10

Nerve: Structure, Function, and Physiology

D A V I D   B U T L E R   *B Phty, GDAMT*

All sensations and active movements are functions of the nervous system. Even during passive movement, the neural tissues must adapt to different joint angles and alterations in the position of the adjacent tissues. Thus, the status of neural tissue will always be a consideration in the management of any athletic injury. This chapter focuses on the peripheral nervous system, describing physiology and dynamics, pathophysiology and pathodynamics, and the clinical sequelae that may follow nerve injury. Athletes undoubtedly suffer peripheral nerve injuries, as recent reviews have shown,[1,2] with certain nerves vulnerable in particular sports (for example, the ulnar nerve at the elbow in throwing sports and the "burners" from brachial plexus injury in American football). However, the incidence of peripheral nerve injuries and their consequences may well be underestimated, as Sunderland,[3] Lundborg,[4] and Loeser[5] have argued. The focus in sports medicine is often on the target tissues of the nervous system, in particular muscles and joint tissue; perhaps the role of neurons in performance and injury has been belittled.

In addition to discussing more severe peripheral neuropathies such as nerve entrapment, this chapter also presents the case for the minor nerve injuries that clinicians are likely to encounter and that may be evident with testing, as outlined in Chapter 23 and elsewhere.[6]

NERVE FIBERS

The functional unit of the nervous system is the neuron. A neuron consists of a cell body and outgrowths, the Schwann cell–enveloped axon, and dendrites, which together are referred to as a nerve fiber. The neurons contributing to the peripheral nervous system exist in the cranial and spinal nerves, linking brain and spinal cord to peripheral tissues.

There are three functional types of nerve fibers in the major nerve trunks — afferent (sensory), autonomic (visceral efferent), and motor (somatic efferent). These fibers exist in varying quantities depending on the particular nerve. Neurology utilizes further classifications of fibers, based on their conduction velocity and axon diameter, although great care should be taken when classifying nerve fibers because of functional overlap. Alphabetical and numerical classifications exist and, unfortunately, do not always overlap. Commonly used classifications and the functions of the various types of fibers in peripheral nerve are presented in Table 10–1.

Note in Table 10–1 the different speeds of conduction of the fibers. The faster fibers are more concerned with speed and quality of human movement. Those related to pain, in particular the C-fibers conduct far more slowly. As discussed later, these fibers have functions

TABLE 10–1
Type, Function, and Speed of Peripheral Nerve Fibers

Type	Function	Diameter (μm)	Speed (m/sec)	Speed (mph)
Afferents				
Deep				
I	Input from muscle and tendon receptors	12–20	70–120	160–272
II	Afferents from muscle spindles	6–12	30–70	68–160
III	Pressure/pain afferents from joints and aponeuroses	2–6	12–30	27–68
IV	Pain	<2	0.5–2	1–4
Cutaneous				
Aα,β	Tactile receptors	6–12	30–70	68–160
A δ	Cold; "fast" pain	2–6	12–30	27–68
C	Warm; "tissue damage" pain	0.5–1.0	0.5–1.0	1.0–2.5
Efferents				
α	Extrafusal muscle fibers	12–20	60–100	135–225
γ	Intrafusal muscle fibers	2–8	10–30	23–68
B	Preganglionic autonomic	<3	3–30	6–68
C	Postganglionic autonomic	<1	0.5–2.0	1–4

other than the transmission of painful impulses. In myelinated fibers, there is a direct proportional relationship between fiber diameter and conduction velocity. Myelinated axons, such as the alpha-motor and the large-diameter sensory neurons, possess unmyelinated gaps (1 to 2 mm apart) called nodes of Ranvier. These allow faster conduction because impulses can "jump" from one node to the next in the process called saltatory conduction. Because impulse conduction in myelinated fibers can be six to eight times faster than in nonmyelinated fibers, many more impulses can be sent. Myelination is often altered in diseases and injury to peripheral nerves, either from mechanical distortion such as overstretch or compression or from loss of metabolic support.

A key element of nerve fibers is the Schwann cell (Fig. 10–1). Schwann cells are responsible for laying down myelin and "wrapping" it around axons. Where axons are unmyelinated, such as in the case of C-fibers, a Schwann cell will wrap around a group of fibers. A bilaminar plasma membrane, the axolemma or axon membrane, lies on the innermost aspect of the Schwann cell. This membrane ultimately surrounds the cytoplasm or axoplasm of the neuron. Ion channels are "pores" through the membrane that allow a transfer of ions across the membranes and give the neuron the property of excitability. The axons and Schwann cells are enclosed in a basement membrane (see Fig. 10–1) and then surrounded by a connective tissue sheath, discussed later in detail.

CENTRAL AND PERIPHERAL CONNECTIONS

An understanding of normal and abnormal peripheral nerve function requires some knowledge of the connections to the central nervous system (CNS) and to target tissues such as muscles, joints, and skin. Motor fibers emerge via rootlets from cells in the anterior horn of the spinal cord and then join with sensory fibers to form the spinal nerve and later the peripheral nerves.

Sensory fibers pass from peripheral nerve to the spinal cord via the dorsal roots. The large-diameter myelinated afferents (A alpha, beta) pass into the dorsal columns. The smaller diameter fibers (C and A delta) enter into the cord, perhaps travel up or down a segment or two in Lissauer's tract, and then pass into the laminated dorsal horn, particularly into laminae I, II, and V. Central nervous system neurons are particularly divergent, and one peripheral dendrite can make connections with hundreds of central axons. Interestingly, 30 percent of C-fibers join the spinal cord via the ventral roots.[7] The clinical consequences of this feature of peripheral neuroanatomy are unknown.

Preganglionic sympathetic fibers emerge from the lateral gray matter of spinal cord segments C8–L3 and then exit via the anterior horn and white rami communicantes to join the sympathetic trunk. These neurons pass up, down, or through the sympathetic trunk before forming a synapse, from which postganglionic fibers emerge to join the peripheral nerves and innervate nearly all the tissues in the body. Peripheral sympathetic neurons except those to the viscera, are efferent only and innervate glands, smooth muscle, and the connective tissue of peripheral nerves. The clinical sequelae of injury to these sympathetic pathways is poorly understood in comparison with somatic fibers.

At the distal end of peripheral nerve are the terminal boutons. These may be free nerve endings or specialized receptor endings responding to combinations of thermal, mechanical, and chemical stimuli, or the motor end-plate in the case of striated muscle.

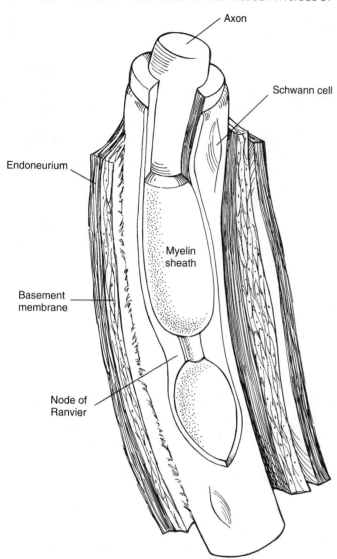

Axon

Schwann cell

Endoneurium

Myelin
sheath

Basement
membrane

Node of
Ranvier

FIGURE 10–1. Diagrammatic myelinated peripheral nerve fiber. (From Sunderland S: Nerves and Nerve Injuries, 2nd ed. Edinburgh, Churchill Livingstone, 1978.)

THE PERIPHERAL NERVE TRUNK

The nerve fibers, blood vessels, and connective tissues compose the nerve trunk. The connective tissues are quite specialized (Fig. 10–2). Around the basement membrane of each myelinated nerve fiber or group of unmyelinated fibers is an endoneurial tubule. Bundles of tubules are surrounded by layered perineurium to form fascicles, and these fascicles are held in internal epineurium and surrounded by external epineurium. The nerve trunk is then surrounded by a thin connective tissue membrane, the mesoneurium. This tissue facilitates sliding of nerve trunks next to adjacent tissues.[8] The epineurium, perineurium, and endoneurium provide a tough supporting framework for the contained nerve fibers. Collagen and a few elastin fibers interlace in all directions to form an irregular lattice pattern. Collagen fibers in the perineurium and endoneurium are about half the size of those in the epineurium. The perineurial layer is quite specialized. Perineurial cells are layered, which allows the perineurium to exert some influence over the tiny vessels that pass through it, forming a diffusion barrier (Fig. 10–3).

The endoneurium provides the intrafascicular packing and, by the tubular arrangement, also helps maintain the neuronal environment.[3,4]

Nerves are not homogeneous structures. Approximately 50 percent of a peripheral nerve is connective tissue, although this amount varies depending on the nerve and the level, from 80 percent (as in the sciatic nerve in the gluteal region) to as little as 22 percent (the ulnar nerve at the elbow.)[9] In addition to these variations, the fascicular arrangement differs. Fascicles spiral and form multiple links, allowing variable contributions of sympathetic, motor, and sensory fibers to branches off the parent nerve. The maximum length of a segment of nerve with a consistent fascicular pattern is 15 mm[3], although in distal segments of nerve there are fewer internal interconnections.[10] The fascicular patterns can range from one fascicle to many fascicles of varying sizes; usually the more fascicles, the greater the ratio of connective tissue to conducting tissue (Fig. 10–4).[3]

These structural variations are significant for the clinician. First, they mean that the sensorimotor outcome from injury depends on the site of injury and the

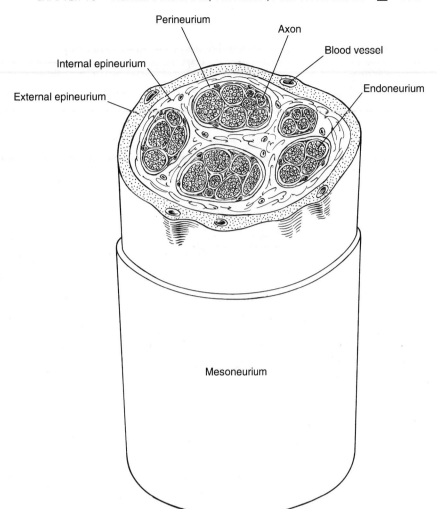

External epineurium

Internal epineurium

Perineurium

Axon

Blood vessel

Endoneurium

Mesoneurium

FIGURE 10–2. The peripheral nerve trunk. (From Butler DS: Mobilisation of the Nervous System. Melbourne, Churchill Livingstone, 1991.)

fascicular arrangement at that site. Second, it means that injury to, or forces placed on, a peripheral nerve in areas with less connective tissue may result in symptoms from long fibers, such as tingling or paralysis. In areas where there is more connective tissue, these symptoms are less likely. In this case, symptoms may come from connective tissue that is richly innervated. For example, entrapment/irritation of the ulnar nerve in the cubital tunnel at the elbow or banging the "funny bone" may result in tingling in the ulnar distribution, whereas entrapment/irritation of the same nerve in Guyon's canal at the wrist may result in pain, there being far more fascicles and connective tissue at the wrist compared with the elbow. Nerve injury will therefore not give a constant sensorimotor response—it depends on the site of injury as much as on the magnitude and kind of deforming forces (discussed below).

Neuroanatomic variations exist between nerve roots and nerve trunks. Nerve roots lack the epineurium and perineurium of peripheral nerve, making them more vulnerable to compressive forces from structures such as prolapsed disc or irritation by chemicals such as the byproducts of intervertebral joint injury in the intervertebral foramina. However, they can withstand considerable tensile force, as the peripheral nerve connective tissues dissipate forces to the dura mater

and the epidural connective tissues. The dural sleeve is a funnel, wider proximally than distally, and it may "plug" when pulled into the intervertebral foramen, thus preventing further elongation of the nerve root.[3] This funneling would occur in an outstretched arm position.

The neural connective tissues are self-innervated by the nervi nervorum.[11] This innervation, combined with a superb blood supply, makes the connective tissues of nerve particularly reactive. Branches form off primary afferent fibers and innervate the epineurium, perineurium, and endoneurium. There is also an extrinsic sympathetic innervation from fibers entering the nerve from the perivascular plexuses.[11,12] Mast cells exist in the epineurium, though few exist in the endoneurium.[13] With nerve injury, the number of mast cells in the endoneurium increases.[14] Mast cells release inflammatory mediators such as histamine and are a probable source of neurogenically mediated inflammation.[15] For the clinician, this means that nerves can be sources of pain, perhaps without alteration to the long fibers. The innervated connective tissues are the probable source of symptoms of the local, sometimes intense, pain when a nerve is palpated.[3] It also means that nerve injury does not have to be associated with paresthesia. The only symptom may be pain.

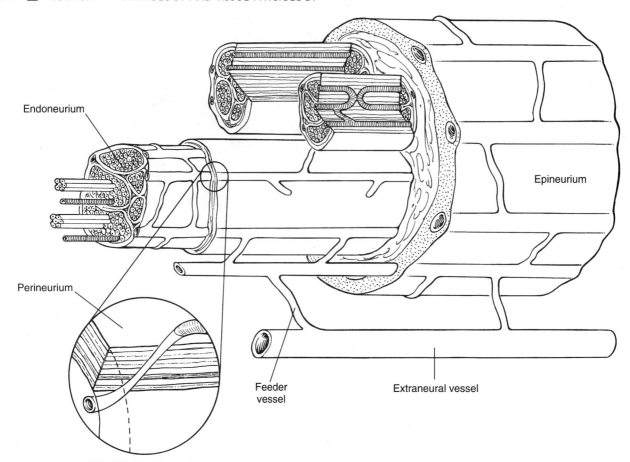

Endoneurium

Epineurium

Perineurium

Feeder
vessel

Extraneural vessel

FIGURE 10–3. The blood supply of a multifascicular segment of peripheral nerve. *Inset,* Blood vessel passing through the perineurial lamellae. (Adapted from Lundborg G: Nerve Injury and Repair. Edinburgh, Churchill Livingstone, 1988.)

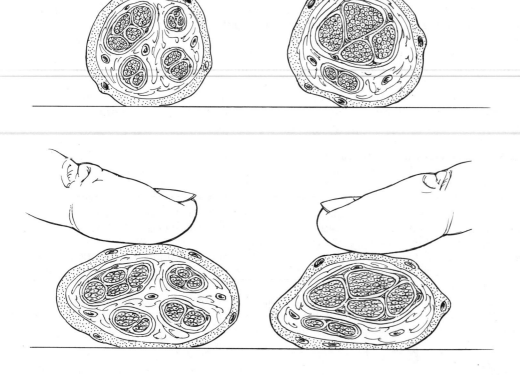

FIGURE 10–4. The effect of pressure on polyfascicular and oligofascicular peripheral nerve. Where a peripheral nerve is multifascicular, a greater pressure will be required to affect nerve fibers than where there is a small number of, or only one, fascicle. (From Butler DS: Mobilisation of the Nervous System. Melbourne, Churchill Livingstone, 1991.)

BASIC NEUROPHYSIOLOGY

ACTION POTENTIALS

A unique feature of neural tissues is that they can produce and propagate electrical messages. This function relates to the cell membrane. A difference in concentration exists across the cell membrane of potassium (K^+), sodium (Na^+) and chloride (Cl^-) ions. These ions can selectively permeate ion channels in the membrane so that an unequal distribution of net charge occurs. The resting membrane potential results from an internal negativity due to active transport of sodium from inside to outside the cell and potassium from outside to inside the cell. Membrane potential ranges between −70 mv and −90 mv. The generation of an action potential converts the negative resting potential into a positive depolarization of +40 mv.

Motor axons conduct action potentials peripherally toward the synaptic or neuromuscular junctions. Sensory neurons conduct toward the cell body. These conduction directions are referred to as orthodromic conduction. However, currents can travel in both directions along an axon. Antidromic impulses travel in an opposite direction to the orthodromic ones, and are the signal for the release of chemicals such as the neuropeptides stored in vescicles at the terminal boutons of C-fibers.

AXONAL TRANSPORT

Neurons are remarkable cells because they are so elongated. From dendrites in the dorsal horn to terminal boutons in the foot, for example, a neuron may be 4 ft long. Considering that the cell body in the dorsal root ganglion or in the anterior horn produces the axoplasm, the transport to the foot, passing over and through different structures and even receiving a different blood supply, is an exceptional feat. Mammalian axoplasm is quite viscous, about five times the viscosity of water,[16] and is thixotropic, meaning that it requires constant agitation and if it stops flowing, it will gel.[17] The energetics of axoplasmic flow require a system of neurofilaments, microtubules, and actin filaments. Mitochondria are located along the axon, providing a source of energy for the transport.

Within the axon cylinder, there is a bidirectional flow of axoplasm (Fig. 10–5). This is obvious, because compression will cause damming of axoplasm on both sides of the constriction. In antegrade transport (cell body outward) there are two rates of flow. Materials destined for the synapse, such as neurotransmitters, travel at up to 410 mm per day.[18] A slower flow carries material such as neurotubule constituents, in essence the cytoskeleton of the axon. This flow travels at no more than 30 mm per day.[19] There is also a flow back from nerve terminals to the cell body, called the retrograde flow, traveling quite rapidly at about 300 mm per day.[20] The axoplasm in this flow carries unused material from the antegrade flow and neuronotropic factors, proteins that can "inform" the cell body about the state of the axon and the target tissues.

Nerve growth factor, the most studied of these neuronotropic factors, can regulate the production of neuropeptides such as substance P and somatostatin.[21] Thus the material carried by the axoplasm is necessary for the health of the axon and the tissues that it innervates.

The action potential and the axoplasmic flow both require a source of energy; they access a common pool of adenosine triphosphate (ATP).[22] In an anoxic nerve, both axoplasmic flow and the action potential will stop within 15 minutes. The relationship between these electrical and chemical phenomena is further emphasized by the fact that the axoplasm carries essential materials for electrical conduction, such as axolemma constituents. Alteration in axoplasmic flow contributes to the double crush syndromes and neurogenic inflammation, as discussed below.

THE VASA NERVORUM AND DIFFUSION BARRIERS

Peripheral nerves possess a superb blood supply, which is necessary because peripheral nerve function is highly dependent upon adequate oxygenation. The vasa nervorum consists of a complex system of extraneural feeder vessels and an intrinsic longitudinal interconnected supply in all the neural connective tissues (see Fig. 10–3).[3,4] The intraneural system is extremely well developed and may still preserve nerve function if some extraneural feeders are damaged.[4] Intraneural blood vessels are sympathetically innervated[12,23]; the nerve supply to a particular blood vessel arises from the nerve trunk that the blood vessel supplies.[23] This arrangement probably allows an adjustable blood supply for functional demands on the nerve.

To maintain the neuronal environment, the endoneurial capillary bed and the perineurium have acquired specialized features. The endoneurial capillary bed is similar to the capillaries of the CNS, where there is a barrier to certain substances circulating in the blood that has been called (after the blood-brain barrier) the "blood-nerve barrier."[24,25] It is also clear that the perineurium presents a barrier to some external substances such as inflammatory agents and bacteria.[3,26] The barrier function also works from inside to outside as well as outside to inside, as no lymphatic channels cross it. Therefore, edema in the endoneurial space may take a long time to disperse.

It has been observed that peripheral nerves can pass through sites of infection without impairment of nerve function.[3,4] Although the perineurial barrier is quite resistant to ischemia[27] and mechanical deformation,[28,29] long-standing compression and pinching will breach it.[30] Once pathology becomes intrafascicular, because of the barrier, it may be difficult to move, and there may be irreversible aspects of the clinical picture such as persistent pain and muscle weakness.

The design of the vasa nervorum supports the mobile nervous system to ensure optimal neuronal function. Feeder vessels to peripheral nerve have some leeway so that the nerve can stretch and the feeder vessel is not

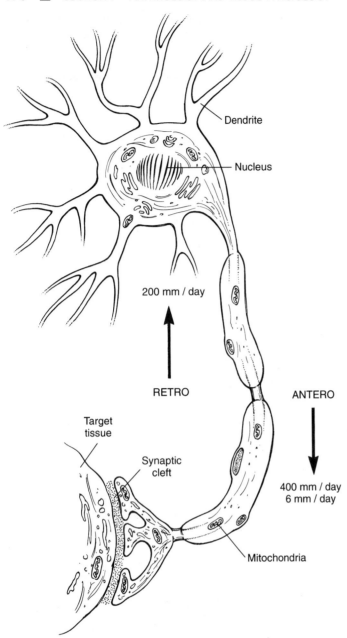

Dendrite

Nucleus

200 mm / day

RETRO

ANTERO

Target tissue

Synaptic cleft

400 mm / day
6 mm / day

Mitochondria

FIGURE 10–5. Bidirectional axoplasmic flow. (From Butler DS: Mobilisation of the Nervous System. Melbourne, Churchill Livingstone, 1991.)

overly stretched. The blood supply to nerve roots are in a spiraling "pigtail" formation[31] so that stretch does not hinder the flow and the nerve roots can move freely in the intervertebral foramina. In general, most blood vessels enter peripheral nerve around joints, where there is more protection and nerve movement in relation to surrounding tissues is not as extreme as in areas farther from the joints.

ENDONEURIAL FLUID PRESSURE

A fluid exists in the endoneurial spaces (the intrafascicular area). The pressure in this endoneurial fluid (endoneurial fluid pressure) is always slightly greater than in surrounding tissues such as muscle.[4,32] The endoneurial space lacks lymphatic channels, and the endoneurial fluid moves slowly in bulk. The pressure

gives nerves a stiffness and the perineurium an elasticity. Intraneural edema following nerve injury plays a major role in acute and chronic nerve lesions. Endoneurial fluid pressure increases following nerve trauma. Even moderate increases can interfere with the endoneurial capillary flow,[33] causing hypoxia and electrolyte imbalance. Because an endoneurial edema cannot escape rapidly owing to the perineurial diffusion barrier, it may persist and be subject to fibroblast invasion (discussed below).

AGING IN THE NERVOUS SYSTEM

After birth, no more neurons are formed, although synapses are continually formed. The nervous system appears to resist most of the forces of aging, and apparent aging may be the result of inevitable pathologies incurred throughout the years or of disuse. Conduction velocities reach adult values around the fifth year of life, and velocity slows in later years, by about 10 percent by the age of 60.[34] The amount of peripheral nerve connective tissue increases with age,[3] but it is not known whether there are alterations in physical properties. It is also not known whether this is the result of repeated minor injuries through life. The proportion of larger diameter peripheral fibers decreases with age,[3] and the sense of vibration may be absent in older people. Dura mater, however, does not appear to age, retaining its mechanical properties through life.[35] It would appear from surgical results that nerve injuries heal better in the young than in the older person.[3]

NEURODYNAMICS

Peripheral nerves are not only impulse and chemical conduits but also dynamic tissues, like muscles and joints. Along with the CNS, the peripheral nervous system is designed to function while stretching and sliding during a wide range and variety of body movement. In certain positions, such as a slump position,[6] neural tissue may physically limit the range of knee extension. The spinal canal is approximately 7 cm longer in flexion than in extension,[36,37] and nerves are located on opposite sides of joint axes. For example, during elbow flexion, the ulnar nerve at the elbow stretches while the radial and median nerves relax. Most neurodynamic studies have focused on the median nerve.[8,38,39] In 90 degrees of shoulder abduction, from wrist and elbow flexion to wrist and elbow extension, the median nerve has to adapt to a nerve bed nearly 20 percent longer.[8] The fate of the median nerve, and indeed all the peripheral nerves while they contend with body excursions, should be of interest to clinicians. With loss of movement or alterations in elasticity from pathologic changes from entrapment by surrounding tissues or with an intraneural fibrosis, for example, the normal mechanosensitivity of nerve may become enhanced during movement and thus provoke pain. Neurodynamics are probably underestimated, as is the link between neuropathodynamics and neuropathophysiology despite literature on the subject.[3,4,6,8,40]

PERIPHERAL NERVE COMPRESSION AND TENSION

When nerves are physically loaded by movement, they react by moving and by absorbing some of the pressure. Some studies emphasize this. McLellan and Swash[39] placed needles in the median nerve epineurium of the upper arms of 15 volunteers and measured the amount of nerve movement in relation to surrounding tissues during various upper limb movements. The results were impressive. Among them, wrist movement moved a needle positioned in the upper arm by 7 mm. In one volunteer, movements of 2 to 3 cm were noted, although, unfortunately, the position of the arm was not recorded. Similar amounts of movement have been recorded in a cadaver study[41]; on slim individuals, the median nerve may be observed or palpated moving in relation to surrounding tissue as the arm is actively or passively moved.

Lumbosacral nerve roots are drawn caudalward in relation to pelvic and spinal structures during a straight leg raise.[42,43] Movements in relation to adjacent tissues occur all the way to the foot.[44] Clinically and from some in vivo experiments, it appears that selective tension can be placed on a peripheral nerve.[6,45,46] In addition, the loading on the meninges and spinal cord will influence loading on the peripheral nervous system. In this regard, Breig's work on the biomechanics of the CNS[36] is highly recommended for clinicians.

Because of the connective tissue sheaths, nerves are strong structures, able to resist compression and tensile forces. The median nerve, for example, can sustain a maximal load of 70 to 220 N before breaking,[3] although damage will occur at forces much less than this. These figures equate to a length increase of 20 to 30 percent. During normal movement, as the nerve stretches the perineurium tightens, intraneural pressure increases, and intrafascicular capillaries stop flowing. This occurs at approximately 8 percent elongation,[47,48] with intraneural microcirculation ceasing at approximately 15 percent. Because the nervous system is dynamic, forces that temporarily disrupt circulation are easily handled and probably occur regularly with daily activities. For example, "hamstring" stretches probably load the sciatic nerve enough for temporary disruption. When loading persists, as it could from sustained unphysiologic postures or maintained local pressures from a swollen piriformis muscle, for example, damage may ensue.

In a peripheral nerve injury, any of the fiber types or parts of the fiber may be preferentially involved, with the potential for a vast array of sensorimotor deficits.

When tensile forces are placed upon nerve, the intraneural pressure increases. It is possible to quadruple the pressure in the ulnar nerve at the elbow in an ulnar nerve stress position.[49] Compression can also occur from alterations in interfacing tissues, such as changes in the size of a tunnel through which a nerve passes, and the introduction of foreign material, such as blood, into the nerve bed. A critical level for nerve function occurs with compression of 30 mm Hg.[50] Such pressures probably occur often during human movement but, if sustained, the viability of the nerve may be threatened[51] owing to edema formation. Thirty millimeters of mercury is enough pressure to slow the flow of axoplasm, with 80 mm Hg enough to stop intraneural circulation.[52] These alterations are usually reversible within a few hours. Injury will depend upon the magnitude of compression (or tension) and the duration of the loading. In an acute compartment syndrome, irreversible injury to nerve could be expected after 8 hours.[53]

With external compressive forces, if actual physical damage to neurons occurs, it will usually happen at the edge of the constriction,[4,54] where electron microscopy has revealed more myelin distortion and blood vessel damage than in the center of a compressive force. Tourniquets and plaster casts may be examples of such compressive forces. With either vascular or mechanically induced injury, larger diameter fibers, because of their higher metabolic demands, are usually the first affected.[55,56]

NEURAL/NON-NEURAL TISSUE RELATIONSHIPS

During movement, nerve takes its lead from the movement of joints and muscles, and it then has a dynamic relationship with all non-neural tissues. For example, it must slide through tunnels and muscles and through fascial openings and be compressed against various structures such as bone. The ulnar nerve, for example, will be pressed firmly onto bone at the elbow after 90 degrees of elbow flexion. This pressure will increase if the shoulder is abducted.[57] Some interfacing structures to nerve make the nervous system more vulnerable to injury. The bones and ligaments of the carpal tunnel are a well-known example; other vulnerable sites for the nervous system are listed below.

With abnormalities in these interfacing tissues, such as callus development, formation of bands of scar tissue, pressures from hematoma, or enlarging tumors and ganglia, peripheral nerve neurodynamics and therefore neurophysiology may be adversely affected. For clinicians treating nerve entrapment or irritation, examination and perhaps treatment of the interfacing structures will be necessary.

SYMPATHETIC NERVOUS SYSTEM NEURODYNAMICS

The sympathetic nervous system is part of the peripheral nervous system, and sympathetic neurons in peripheral nerves are subject to the same deformation and injury potential during movement as somatic neurons. Areas where the sympathetic nervous system is separate from the somatic system, i.e., in the trunk, rami, and ganglia, are also subject to deforming forces during movement.[58-60] Animal experiments have shown that sympathetic trunk stimulation has the potential to greatly reduce peripheral nerve blood flow and hence nerve function.[61] Recent research involving neurodynamics[62,63] has shown that commonly used tension tests, such as the Slump test, will induce sympathetic responses in humans. Clinicians are urged to consider the possibility that the structure and function of sympathetic neurons, either in the trunk or in peripheral nerve, may be adversely affected, particularly when injuries are long-standing or recurrent.

NEUROPATHOLOGY AND PAIN

Peripheral nerves are an undoubted source of pain and other symptoms, although a discussion of peripheral nerve pain patterns following pathologic changes must entail consideration of the pain phenomenon itself. "Pain is never the sole creation of our anatomy and physiology. It emerges only at the intersection of bodies, minds and cultures."[64] Important determinants of sporting performance such as anticipation, anxiety, reward potential, and aggression will all influence pain perception. With regard to anatomy and physiology, any peripherally evoked pain pattern observed will require notice of spinal cord, autonomic nervous system, and affective or emotional contributions to the pain as well as the injured peripheral nerve or root. Peripheral nerve injury is not a matter of whether the impulse goes through or not; it is more the creation of distorted and faulty sensations and perhaps movement alterations.[65] The almost inevitable involvement of the rest of the nervous system is probably the main reason that there is no constant pattern of pain or functional loss following nerve injury. In this regard, the reader is referred elsewhere.[7,66]

Nociceptive pain is that which arises from chemical or mechanically induced impulses from non-neural tissues. Peripheral neurogenic pain arises from the nerve trunks, plexuses, and roots, i.e., anywhere peripheral to the dorsal horn in the case of limb and trunk pain or the cervicotrigeminal nucleus in the case of facial pain. Pain from the connective tissues of nerve has never been classified, but, although physiologically it is nociceptive pain, injury and the ensuing pain patterns are difficult to consider apart from injury to the long fibers.

CATEGORIES OF NERVE INJURY

Nerve injuries have been classified according to severity by Seddon (neurapraxia, axonotmesis, neurotmesis)[67] and Sunderland (grades 1 to 5).[3] Similarities and differences of the classifications are summarized in Table 10–2.

For clinicians dealing with sports injuries, a peripheral neuropathy may exist in which the pathology is not as severe as in the categories shown in Table 10–2. Seddon and Sunderland's categorizations are based on gross pathology and functional loss and they do not register pain, sensory phenomena, or minor disturbances in motor function. These categories are more relevant to surgical states. A preneurapraxic state surely exists in both clinical and subclinical forms. Sunderland[3] refers to irritative lesions where conduction is normal, calling them "perversions of function." Jewett[68] refers to the need for a zero degree classification for similar reasons. Lundborg[4] defines two preneurapraxic categories. The first is an immediately reversible metabolic block; the second is a block occurring with intraneural edema, reversible in a few days or weeks. The variety of ectopic neural pacemakers (ENPs), such as neuroma or ephaptic synapses, as outlined by Devor,[65] are difficult to include in the Seddon and Sunderland classifications and are probably best considered "perversions of function." Connective tissue irritation and scarring that may involve the nervi nervorum cannot be classified along these classic lines.

TABLE 10–2
Categories of Nerve Injury

Seddon	Definition	Sunderland	Definition
Neurapraxia	Local conduction block; axon continuous and excitable; innervated tissue remains patent	Grade I	Local conduction block; axon continuous and excitable; innervated tissue remains patent
Axonotmesis	Loss of axonal continuity; some degeneration of distal axons; severe entrapment or traction injury may be etiology	Grade II	Loss of axonal continuity; some degeneration of distal axons; severe entrapment or traction injury may be etiology
Neurotmesis	Loss of continuity by severance or scar tissue.	Grade III	Loss of axonal and endoneurial continuity with perineurium intact
		Grade IV	Loss of perineurium with epineurium intact
		Grade V	Complete severance of nerve

THE VULNERABILITY OF THE NERVOUS SYSTEM

Despite the strength and arrangement of connective tissues, peripheral nerves are vulnerable to injury at certain sites. The demands of certain sports also place segments of peripheral nerve at a disadvantage; for example, the ulnar nerve in Guyon's canal at the wrist is vulnerable in cyclists,[69,70] and hyperextension of the hip injuring the femoral nerve has been described in dancers.[71]

Sites of peripheral nerve and nerve root vulnerability can be identified:

1. *Tunnels.* Where a nerve is in a tunnel, especially one with hard sides such as the carpal tunnel, spatial compromise of the nerve will be a greater possibility than elsewhere. Within a tunnel, the contained nervous system always has the potential to rub on the tunnel structure, creating friction. Trauma and alterations to tunnel structures, such as the intervertebral foramina, could mechanically or chemically compromise the neural structures contained within.
2. *Branches.* Where a nerve branches, it is more difficult for the nerve to move away from forces (e.g., radial nerve at the elbow, union of medial and lateral plantar nerves in the forefoot).
3. *Hard interfaces.* Where a nerve lies on bone or passes through fascia, it may be more readily compressed (e.g., radial nerve in the spiral groove of the humerus, cutaneous branches of the posterior primary rami of thoracic spinal nerves as they pass through fascia).
4. *Proximity to the surface.* Nerves such as the sensory radial nerve in the forearm or branches of the superficial peroneal nerve on the dorsum of the foot are vulnerable to external compression.
5. *Where nerves are fixed to interfacing structures.* Some areas of nerve are more firmly adherent to interfacing tissues than others, for example, the common peroneal nerve at the head of the fibula and the radial nerve at the elbow. It means that the adherent segment of nerve cannot move and slide next to adjacent tissues during movement.

Some nerves have a number of these vulnerable features. For example, at the ankle the tibial nerve branches into the medial and lateral plantar nerves in the posterior tarsal tunnel; it is superficial and lies on a hard interface.

Certain disease processes affect peripheral nerves and make them more vulnerable to injury. Generalized disease such as diabetes mellitus, hypothyroidism, alcoholism, immune deficiency syndromes, and rheumatoid arthritis adversely affect neuronal function. The peripheral nerves of diabetics are more susceptible to compression than are those of nondiabetics,[72] perhaps because of the greater ease of blocking axonal transport in diabetics. Texts on nerve entrapment invariably list vulnerable areas for particular nerves, and the reader is referred to more detailed sources.[3,69,73–75]

NERVE INJURY

Unlike the terminal boutons, dorsal root ganglia, and neuronal pools in the spinal cord, nerve trunks and roots are designed for impulse transmission rather than impulse generation. For a nerve to be a persistent source of pain, an ENP must develop along the nerve trunk, or the neural connective tissues must continually irritate endings of the nervi nervorum. The pathologies involved in an ENP are varied, and they arise via vascular and mechanical means. In the absence of frank trauma, it appears that the ultimate peripheral neuronal pathology is vascular in origin.[3,4]

PRESSURE GRADIENTS IN NERVE

Pressure gradients exist in nerves and in the tissues and fluids surrounding nerve. The carpal tunnel can be used as an example (Fig. 10–6). The pressure must be

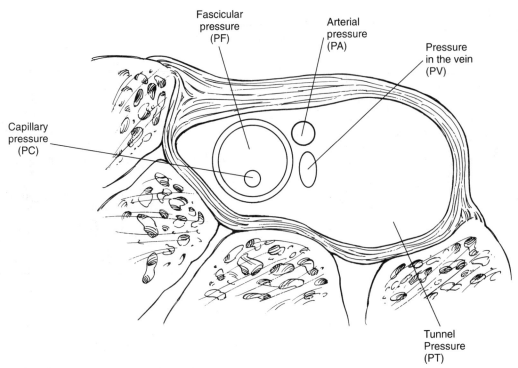

FIGURE 10–6. Diagrammatic representation of the pressure gradient in the carpal tunnel (transverse section). One fascicle is represented for ease of demonstration. For normal neural nourishment, the pressure gradient must be PA > PC > PF > PV > PT. (From Sunderland S: Nerves and Nerve Injury. Edinburgh, Churchill Livingstone, 1978.)

greatest in the epineurial arterioles and progressively less in capillaries, fascicles (endoneurial space), epineurial venules, and the tunnel around the nerve.[76] These pressure differences allow blood to flow into the tunnel, nourish the neurons, and then flow out again so fresh oxygenated blood can flow in. If the tunnel pressure increases to that greater than in the vein, venous drainage will be stopped. This stoppage can occur at pressures as low as 20 to 30 mm Hg.[51,52] Sunderland[76] detailed three stages that could ensue following persistent pressure around a nerve: hypoxia, edema, and fibrosis. Once venous stasis is present, nerve fiber nutrition will be impaired, and the resultant neuro-ischemia may cause pain and other symptoms such as paresthesia. If hypoxia continues, damage to the sensitive capillary endothelium follows, creating an edematous situation. The blood-nerve and perineurial barriers, so effective at protecting the nerve initially, are now a disadvantage. Endoneurial fluid pressure rises, intrafascicular pressure rises, and because there are no intrafascicular lymphatics, edema cannot disperse other than longitudinally along the trunk, and the nerve may swell. This edematous stage provides a superb environment for the proliferation of fibroblasts and the beginning of the intraneural fibrosis stage. If pathologic forces persist, the result will be intraneural fibrosis within the fascicle and in the epineurial tissues. Sunderland[76] refers to the segment's becoming a fibrous cord and that a further development may be friction fibrosis elsewhere along the nerve trunk, so that, for example, a patient with an ulnar nerve compromised in Guyon's canal at the wrist may complain of proximal symptoms,

perhaps at the elbow or neck. This spread of symptoms can be considered part of the double crush concept discussed below. Those who rely on nerve conduction tests should be aware that a nerve conduction test may be negative in the presence of neuropathy. The process described above could occur in one fascicle, and nerve conduction tests cannot be fascicle specific; therefore, the nerve conduction test may be testing a "good" fascicle.[53] In addition, nerve conduction tests cannot measure the involvement of the connective tissues.

Blood pressure, both local and general, is an important determinant in the pathogenesis of nerve lesions. The common night pain of nerve entrapment and the higher incidence of entrapment during pregnancy may, in part, reflect a lower blood pressure. The vascular originated pathologic process described starts within the nerve. Similar processes could occur with injury that affects nerve beds and tunnels, such as by blood or edema or scar strangling extraneural feeder vessels. Nerve damage may occur with rupture of extraneural blood vessels.[77] Some damage may follow if the nerve is adherent to the nerve bed and repetitive movement distorts the nerve. The under- or overactivity of the sympathetic nervous system with its effect on peripheral blood flow could also contribute to ischemic states.

MECHANICAL TRAUMA TO PERIPHERAL NERVE

Mechanical trauma takes the form of compression (e.g., tight plaster), stretch (e.g., "stinger"), or friction.

Acute compressive or tensile forces may damage nerve fibers and make any ischemic contribution to symptoms irrelevant. However, with a chronic compression, a vascular component is obvious, as the mechanical forces present may not be enough to deform nerve fibers.[78]

The connective tissues of nerve are easily injured. Slight trauma, such as mild compression or friction, may result in an epineurial edema.[79,80] Epineurial tears in the common peroneal nerve are common in ankle injuries, according to Nitz.[81] Owing to the perineurial diffusion barrier an epineurial injury is unlikely to affect conduction of the contained long nerve fibers unless it is severe enough to compress fascicles or is deeply placed in the internal epineurium.[82] It would seem that symptoms from neural connective tissue pathology would be more likely to be evoked by tensile than by compressive forces. For example, suppose that the connective tissues of peroneal nerve branches at the ankle were irritated or involved in post–ankle sprain scar. Although palpation of the nerves may provoke some symptoms, nerve stretch such as plantarflexion/inversion of the ankle plus a straight leg raise is likely to be more symptom evocative.

Compressive forces will distort myelin. Tourniquet experiments on primate nerves have shown that most nerve fiber injury occurs at the edge of the tourniquet. On analysis, the myelin sheaths of the compressed segments were found to be stretched on one side of the node of Ranvier and invaginated on the other side.[83,84] Such dysmyelination could easily be a source of symptoms. Vascular injury is also likely with such forces, and Schwann cell necrosis has been noted in similar experiments.[85] "Saturday night palsy" would be an example of such an injury.

ECTOPIC NEURAL PACEMAKERS

For a segment of nerve to become a persistent source of symptoms, a persistent pathology must be present. When a nerve or fascicle is damaged, symptoms may arise from damaged connective tissue, cut axons, demyelinated segments proximal to the injury, or dorsal root ganglion cells rendered hypersensitive from the injury, with the brain unaware of the true origin of the impulses.[65,86,87] The vast majority of nerve injuries occur in continuity; that is, the nerve is not cut. Ectopic neural pacemaker (ENP) pathologies may involve neuromas,[88] demyelination,[89] immature axon sprouts caught in scar,[89] cross-excitation (ephaptic synapses),[90] and chronic hypoxia.[91,92] In addition, these sites will probably be involved with endoneurial and perineurial tissue damage. ENPs are mechanosensitive and will be reactive to movement, particularly the neural loading techniques proposed in Chapter 23. They are also very sensitive to ischemia, which is even more likely to be induced by loading on the tissues. "Trigger points" may well be sites of ENPs.[65] This seems very feasible given that trigger points are commonly located over vulnerable segments of peripheral nerve as they pass through fascia or muscle tunnels. These pacemaker sites, particularly where peripheral, may be reactive to palpation,

thus assisting diagnosis of a particular neuropathic pain. Some cases of ectopia display spontaneous activity, although spontaneous activity is mainly confined to sensory axons.[92] The dorsal root ganglia are normally mechano- and chemosensitive segments of nerve, displaying rhythmic ectopic discharge, easily enhanced by mechanical probing and chemical stimulation.[92]

SEQUELAE OF NERVE INJURY

The nervous system is an electrochemical continuum. It is inevitable that a nerve injury, even a minor one, will have repercussions elsewhere along the neural continuum. The repercussions include the possibility of the original injury weakening the nervous system to allow the development of another injury (double crush), abnormal concentrations of neurotransmitters and modulators secreted into target tissues (neurogenic inflammation), altered responses of the receiving cells in the dorsal horn or cervicotrigeminal nucleus, and denervation changes in the target tissues. In addition, the sympathetic nervous system will react to all pain states and the patient will respond according to previous experiences of pain and his or her current psychologic status. Any or all of these states may exist in a sporting injury.

DOUBLE AND MULTIPLE CRUSH SYNDROMES

Many clinicians are aware that, after injury, pain will not always be localized to one spot. Often there will be pain or other symptoms elsewhere, some of which may be regarded by the patient as insignificant. When this pain is neurogenic, it may be part of a double crush mechanism. Upton and McComas[93] introduced this term to present their hypothesis that a proximal source of nerve compression would render the distal segment of nerve more vulnerable to compression. In their case, they described the association between carpal tunnel syndrome and cervical disc injury. Also noted was a link between thoracic outlet syndrome and cubital tunnel syndrome and between carpal tunnel syndrome and ulnar nerve compression at the elbow. Upton and McComas suggested that a neuron could become "sick," from compression or from a disease such as diabetes, and make the rest of the neuron more pathologically susceptible. These notions now have significant experimental support.[94–96] The causation for the second crush is that the axoplasmic flow is altered and that the ultrastructure of the neuron, including the axolemma, microtubules, and neurofilaments, is impaired. This enables previously resistible compressive forces to cause damage, usually at vulnerable areas of the nervous system. The second crush could also be a friction fibrosis as discussed above.

Double crush is an inadequate term because the second neuropathy can be a neuritis or friction injury. The term "double neuropathy" has been suggested[78] and appears to be more applicable, particularly with more minor injury. There is rapidly expanding literature on double crush injury, including tarsal tunnel syndrome and entrapment elsewhere in the leg,[97,98] brachial plexus lesions and carpal tunnel syndrome,[99] cervical injuries and carpal tunnel syndrome,[100,101] and bilateral carpal tunnel syndrome.[102] An excellent recent summary is available.[103]

A "reversed double crush"[4] seems likely when neurogenic symptoms occur initially in the periphery and then begin proximally. For example, shoulder symptoms following a carpal tunnel syndrome may well be neurogenic. "Multiple crush" has been proposed[7] when there are more than two sites of symptoms. In such cases, consideration should be given to the possibility that a subclinical generalized neuropathy, such as diabetes, may exist, in addition to the more likely effects of serial compression along an axon. Mackinnon[103] has proposed the clinically valuable concept of dynamic compression; i.e., there may be no pain at rest, but certain postures that usually involve stretch of nerve may evoke symptoms. The ulnar nerve provides a good example. For example, wrist pain experienced by a golfer at the end of the backswing could be coming from the ulnar nerve in or near Guyon's canal. This position loads the ulnar nerve.

These concepts of double neuropathy and multiple neuropathy provide an excellent reason for clinicians to evaluate along the nerve track when suspicious of a neurogenic lesion. For example, treatment of the piriformis muscle may be needed to alleviate neural symptoms at the foot, by altering a site of pressure contributing to altered axoplasmic flow at the foot. Clinicians should also consider the possibility of double crush mechanisms operating in even more minor pain situations, for example, a long distance runner with pain in the Achilles tendon and in the buttock.

NEUROGENIC INFLAMMATION

The terminals of primary afferent nociceptors, particularly the unmyelinated afferents (C-fibers), are sources of inflammatory mediators that are released into target tissues upon antidromic activation of the neuron.[104–106] The most studied of the neurogenic inflammatory mediators is substance P. This and other peptides are synthesized in the dorsal root ganglion and transmitted to the nerve terminals via the axoplasmic transport. The majority goes to the periphery, but some is also sent along dendrites into the CNS. Substance P is particularly vasoactive; its presence stimulates the release of histamine from mast cells[15] as well as inflammatory mediators such as leukotrienes. There are other proinflammatory peptides carried in C-fibers, such as the tachykinins (neurokinins A and B) and calcitonin gene–related peptide (CGRP), an extremely potent vasodilator.[107] These inflammatory mediators are essential for the health and healing of innervated tissues. However, with a chronic nerve injury, changes in material carried in the axoplasm or excessive antidromic stimulation could lead to a neu-

rogenically maintained target tissue inflammation (see Chapter 29).

Clinicians are urged to consider the possibility of concomitant nerve or nerve root injury in injuries that take longer to heal than expected. Reddening and maintained edema may be clues.

RESPONSES AT THE DORSAL HORN AND SYMPATHETIC NERVOUS SYSTEM

Every pain and sensation (including treatment responses) must in some way be electrochemically gated at the dorsal horn. Persistent barrages of ectopic impulses along unmyelinated primary afferents, or alterations in the axoplasmic flow, may lead to sensitization and, later, pathobiologic alterations in dorsal horn cells.[108,109] This situation may occur more readily in patients in whom descending pain control systems from the midbrain, brainstem, and dorsolateral funiculus are injured or altered, as may occur after mental depression. These same descending control systems may allow an athlete to suppress pain. With increasing sensitivity and alteration in central cell membranes, apparent peripheral motor and sensory responses may become more under the control of the CNS. The possibility exists for a peripheral injury to heal, but in a particular individual, pain may persist with its locus in the CNS. Symptoms such as allodynia (pain from normally innocuous stimuli), hyperalgesia (increased responses to normally painful stimuli), and summation (repetitive stimuli necessary to provoke pain) may ensue. Motor responses may include spasm, splinting of joints, and postural deviations. Zusman[110] has provided a review article relevant for clinicians.

In any pain state, there will be an autonomic nervous system response. Sometimes the sympathetic nervous system appears to play a disproportionate role in the pain presentation, for example, in causalgia and reflex sympathetic dystrophy. In many severe sympathetic stress states, there is no known reason for the sympathetic reaction that may follow entrapment, minor surgery, or injury. Both central and peripheral mechanisms are likely, with a positive feedback situation in which, following injury, sympathetic efferents continually activate somatic neurons.[111] Specific peripheral hypotheses include the development of ENPs along a nerve trunk, causing dorsal horn changes that influence sympathetic output; the development of adrenergic receptors on damaged primary sensory neurons,[65] creating nerve endings that are then sensitive to circulating epinephrine; and the injury-induced sensitization of nociceptive afferents, perhaps in neurogenically inflamed tissues.[65,111]

The role of the sympathetic nervous system in pain states is controversial and debated. Abnormalities in sympathetic function seem clear in the severe reflex sympathetic dystrophy states, but there are few data on more minor sympathetically related syndromes, although Wilson[112] considers some of the overuse injuries such as cumulative trauma disorders to have a sympathetic mechanism.

HEALING POTENTIAL OF PERIPHERAL NERVE

Compared with the CNS, peripheral nerves possess a far greater healing potential. When a nerve is cut or severely crushed and scarred, nerve fibers distal to the injury will degenerate, a process referred to as wallerian degeneration. The Schwann cell–myelin complex breaks up and macrophage activity occurs in the endoneurial tube, degrading the myelin to fat. Schwann cells proliferate, "waiting" for new axonal growth. Although the connective tissue sheaths remain intact, the result is a shrunken skeletal nerve with columns of Schwann cells. Regeneration attempts occur within hours in severance injury, or up to a week if a nerve has been badly crushed. Axon sprouts emerge from the proximal side of the injury and attempt to make contact with Schwann cells on the distal side. Once contact has been made, fine growth cones, or filopodia, anchor to the basement membrane and then enter into the endoneurial tubes. Results are never perfect. If sprouting axons fail to make Schwann cell contact, perhaps because they are blocked by scar or debris, a neuroma will form. Sometimes sprouts enter inappropriate endoneurial tubules of a different fiber type. Regeneration can be quite rapid, with an average rate of 1 to 2 mm per day. Even with total severance, skilled surgery can produce good results, although functional improvement may take many months.

With injury in continuity, similar degeneration-regeneration processes will be occurring, although in only one part of the nerve, perhaps a fascicle or part of a fascicle. There is neither literature nor data on the healing of injury to the connective tissue sheaths, but given that they are highly innervated and vascularized, it is assumed that they heal well. From what is known of the structure of nerve tissue, axoplasmic flow alterations and metabolically related action potential problems must also heal well. This may occur by simply removing mechanical stresses on the nervous system.

Recovery of function is extremely variable and depends on the kind and severity of injury and the postinjury management. As long as axonal continuity is preserved, complete functional recovery can be expected. Neurapraxias or Sunderland category 1 injuries (e.g., "stinger") have a very good chance for complete recovery in weeks or months,[4,113] depending on the area and severity of damage (see Chapter 23 for further details). Sometimes functional return and pain relief can be spontaneous after surgery or physical therapy treatments. This must be related to the instantaneous revascularization of fibers. In injuries in which myelin is damaged, healing takes longer.

MOBILIZATION AND IMMOBILIZATION

There is little literature on the effects of immobilization of nerve. The potential of ill effects following prolonged immobilization appears underconsidered, especially in postoperative cases. However, recently, early mobilization post peripheral nerve neurolysis has been encouraged,[53] and over the years there have been calls to mobilize nerve roots following spinal surgery.[37,39,114] Given the continuity of nerve, mobilization of neural tissue can be accomplished without movement or stress on neighboring tissues. For example, knee extension movements with the hip held in flexion will move and slide the neural tissues in the spine with minimal movement of the interfacing tissues. It means that early mobilization of neural tissue following spinal surgery or severe trauma is possible without adverse effects on neighboring tissues.

It is worth considering that it is nearly impossible to immobilize the nervous system. Even with a plaster cast immobilizing the wrist and elbow, movement of the shoulder and neck will still load neural tissues in the wrist. Likewise, the patient who wears a collar, post "stinger," will be able to move cervical neural tissues via shoulder and arm movements. Although a tension-free environment is best for nerve regeneration post suture,[115] the beneficial effects of gentle "microforces" to polarize the fibrin clot and guide regenerating axon sprouts should be considered.[4]

Clearly, peripheral nerve can be mobilized and during passive and active movements has always been mobilized, usually inadvertently. This becomes clear with knowledge of the structure of nerve — that a nerve has in-built design features that allow it to be mobilized, and if the design features cannot accommodate the loading placed on it, symptoms or, at worst, injury may ensue. Hamstring stretches, for example, mobilize many tissues, the sciatic tract being one of them. Shoulder stretches mobilize the brachial plexus, among other tissues. Indeed, neural mobilization techniques such as the "slump" have been shown to be worthwhile techniques for hamstring tears.[116] Techniques proposed to mobilize the nervous system are discussed elsewhere.[6,117]

SUMMARY

The primary function of neural tissue is to conduct impulses and to produce and convey a variety of neurochemicals to neural and non-neural connections. For optimal performance, these functions also require a mechanically sound nervous system. Because of the variety of tissues that constitute nerve, the kinds of trauma available, and neurochemical and electrical links to other tissues and neurons, injury management can present a formidable challenge to the clinician. Advances in science, particularly those related to pain, have created an awareness of the many possible sources and contributions to peripheral neurogenic pain. Some injuries do not fit into the classic categories of nerve injury, and the best management strategies may not yet have evolved. In addition, although nerve injuries are not regarded as common sports injuries, a close look at the structure of the neural tissues reveals that there is enormous potential for many minor injuries that could cause pain and affect the quality of movement and performance.

REFERENCES

1. Tsairis P: Peripheral nerve injury in athletes. *In* Jordan BD, Tsairis P, Warren RF (eds): Sports Neurology. Rockville, MD, Aspen Publishers, 1989.
2. Sicuranza MJ, McCue FC: Compressive neuropathies in the upper extremity of athletes. Hand Clin 1992; 8:263.
3. Sunderland S: Nerves and Nerve Injuries, 2nd ed, Edinburgh, Churchill Livingstone, 1978.
4. Lundborg G: Nerve Injury and Repair. Edinburgh, Churchill Livingstone, 1988.
5. Loeser JD: Pain due to nerve injury. Spine 1986; 10:232.
6. Butler D: Mobilisation of the Nervous System, Melbourne, Churchill Livingstone, 1991.
7. Fields H: Pain. New York, McGraw-Hill, 1987.
8. Millesi H: The nerve gap. Hand Clin 1986; 2:651.
9. Sunderland S, Bradley KC: The cross-sectional area of peripheral nerve trunks devoted to nerve fibers. 1949; Brain 96:865.
10. Jabaley ME, Wallace WH, Heckler FR: Internal topography of major nerves of the forearm and hand. Hand Surg 1980; 51B:1.
11. Hromada J: On the nerve supply of the connective tissue of some peripheral nervous system components. Acta Anat 1963; 55:343.
12. Thomas PK, Olsson Y: Microscopic anatomy and function of the connective tissue components of peripheral nerve. *In* Dyck PJ et al (eds): Peripheral Neuropathy, 2nd ed. Philadelphia, WB Saunders, 1984.
13. Makitie J, Teravainen H: Peripheral nerve injury and recovery after temporary ischaemia. Acta Neuropathol (Berlin) 1977; 37:55.
14. Nitz AJ, Dobner JJ, Matulionis DH: Structural assessment of rat sciatic nerve following tourniquet compression and vascular manipulation. Anat Rec 1989; 225:67.
15. Fitzgerald M: Capsaicin and sensory neurones—a review. Pain 1983; 15:109.
16. Haak RA, Kleinhaus FW, Ochs S: The viscosity of mammalian nerve axoplasm measured by electron spin resonance. J Physiol 1976; 263:115.
17. Baker PF, Ladds M, Rubinson KA: Measurement of the flow properties of isolated axoplasm in a defined chemical environment. J Physiol 1977; 269:10.
18. Droz B, Rambourg A, Koenig HL: The smooth endoplasmic reticulum: structure and role in the renewal of axonal membrane and synaptic vescicles by fast axonal transport. Brain Res 1975; 93:1.
19. Levine J, Willard M: The composition and organisation of axonally transported proteins in the retinal ganglion cells of the guinea pig. Brain Res 1980; 194:137.
20. Bisby MA: Retrograde axonal transport. *In* Hertz L, Federoff S (eds): Advances in cellular neurobiology. New York, Academic Press, 1980, pp 69–118.
21. Otten U: Nerve growth factor and the peptidergic sensory neurons. Trends Pharmacol 1984; 7:307.
22. Ochs S: Axoplasmic transport. *In* Tower DB (ed): The Nervous System, vol. 1. New York, Raven Press, 1975.
23. Appenzeller O, Dithal KK, Cowan T, et al: The nerves to blood vessels supplying blood nerves: the innervation of vasa nervorum. Brain Res 1984; 304:383.
24. Waksman BH: Experimental study of diphtheric polyneuritis in the rabbit and guinea pig III. The blood-nerve barrier in the rabbit. J Neuropathol Exp Neurol 1961; 21:35.
25. Olsson Y, Reese T: Permeability of vasa nervorum and perineurium in mouse sciatic nerve studies by fluorescence and electronmicroscopy. J Neuropathol Exp Neurol 1971; 30:105.
26. Lundborg G, Hansson HA: Recognition of peripheral nerve through a preformed tissue space. Preliminary observations on the reorganisation of regenerating nerve fibers and perineurium. Brain Res 1979; 179:573.
27. Lundborg G, Nordborg C, Rydevik B, Olsson Y: The effect of ischaemia on the permeability of the perineurium to protein tracers in rabbit tibial nerve. Acta Neurol Scand 1973; 49:287.
28. Rydevik B, Lundborg G, Nordborg C: Intraneural tissue reactions induced by internal neurolysis. Scand J Plast Reconstruc Surg 1976; 10:3.
29. Rydevik B, Lundborg G: Permeability of intraneural microvessels and perineurium following acute graded experimental nerve compression. Scand J Plast Reconstruc Surg 1977; 11:179.
30. Soderfeldt B, Olsson Y, Kristensson K: The perineurium as a diffusion barrier to protein tracers in human peripheral nerve. Acta Neuropathol 1973; 25:120.
31. Parke WW, Watanabe R: The intrinsic vasculature of the lumbosacral spinal nerve roots. Spine 1985; 10:508.
32. Myers RR, Powell HC, Costello ML, et al: Endoneurial fluid pressure: direct measurement with micropipettes. Brain Res 1978; 148:510.
33. Myers RR, Powell HC: Galactose neuropathy: impact of chronic endoneurial edema on nerve blood flow. Ann Neurol 1984; 16:587.
34. Wagman IH, Lesse H: Maximum conduction velocities of motor fibers of ulnar nerve in human subjects of various ages and sizes. J Neurophysiol 1952; 117:115.
35. van Noort R, Black MM, Martin TRP, et al: A study of the uniaxial properties of human dura mater preserved in glycerol. Biomaterials 1981; 2:41.
36. Breig A: Biomechanics of the Central Nervous System, Stockholm, Almqvist and Wiksell, 1960.
37. Louis R: Vertebroradicular and vertebromedullar dynamics. Anat Clin 1981; 3:1.
38. Zoech G, Reihsner R, Beer R, Millesi H: Stress and strain in peripheral nerves. Neuro-Orthop 1991; 10:73.
39. McLellan DC, Swash M: Longitudinal sliding of the median nerve during movements of the upper limb. J Neurol Neurosurg Psychiatry 1976; 39:566.
40. Rydevik B, Lundborg G, Skalak R: Biomechanics of peripheral nerve. *In* Nordin M, Frankel VH (eds): Basic Biomechanics of the Musculoskeletal System, 2nd ed. Philadelphia, Lea & Febiger, 1989.
41. Wilgis S, Murphy R: The significance of longitudinal excursions in peripheral nerves. Hand Clin 1986; 2:761.
42. Breig A, Troup JDC: Biomechanical considerations in the straight leg raising test. Spine 1979; 4:242.
43. Goddard MD, Reid JD: Movements induced by straight leg raising in the lumbosacral roots, nerves and plexuses and in the intra-pelvic section of the sciatic nerve. J Neurol Neurosurg Psychiatry 1965; 28:12.
44. Smith CG: Changes in length and posture of the segments of the spinal cord with changes in posture in the monkey. Radiology 1956; 66:259.
45. Kenneally M, Rubenach H, Elvey R: The upper limb tension test: the SLR of the arm. *In* Grant R (ed): Physical Therapy of the Cervical and Thoracic Spine. New York, Churchill Livingstone, 1988.
46. Butler D: The upper limb tension test revisited. *In* Grant R (ed): Physical Therapy of the Cervical and Thoracic Spine, 2nd ed. New York: Churchill Livingstone, 1994.
47. Lundborg G, Rydevik B: Effects of stretching the tibial nerve of the rabbit. A preliminary study of the intraneural circulation and barrier function of the perineurium. J Bone Joint Surg 1973; 55B:390.
48. Ogata K, Naito M: Blood flow of peripheral nerve: Effects of dissection, stretching and compression. J Hand Surg 1986; 11B:10.
49. Pechan J, Julis I: The pressure measurement in the ulnar nerve. A contribution to the pathophysiology of cubital tunnel syndrome. J Biomech 1975; 8:75.
50. Rydevik B, Lundborg G, Bagge U: Effects of graded compression on intraneural blood flow. J Hand Surg 1981; 6:3.
51. Lundborg G, Gelberman RH, Minteer-Convery M, et al: Median nerve compression in the carpal tunnel: functional response to experimentally induced control pressure. J Hand Surg 1982; 7:252.
52. Dahlin LB, Rydevik B, McLean WG, Sjostrand J: Changes in fast axonal transport during experimental nerve compression at low pressures. Exp Neurol 1984; 84:29.
53. Mackinnon S, Dellon AL: Surgery of the Peripheral Nerve. New York, Thieme, 1989.
54. Ochoa J, Fowler TJ, Gilliat RW: Anatomical changes in peripheral nerves compressed by a pneumatic tourniquet. J Anat 1972; 113:433.
55. Gasser HD, Erlanger J: The role of fibre size in the establishment of a nerve block by pressure or cocaine. Am J Physiol 1929; 88:581.
56. Ochoa J: Nerve fibre pathology in acute and chronic compression. *In* Omer GE, Spinner M (eds): Management of Peripheral Nerve Problems. Philadelphia, WB Saunders, 1980.

57. Macnicol MF: Mechanics of the ulnar nerve at the elbow. J Bone Joint Surg 1980; 62B:531.

58. Nathan H: Osteophytes of the spine compressing the sympathetic trunk and splanchnic nerves in the thorax. Spine 1986; 12:527.

59. Giles LGF: Paraspinal autonomic ganglion distortion due to vertebral body osteophytosis: a cause of vertebrogenic autonomic syndromes. J Manipulative Physiol Ther 1992; 15:551.

60. Breig A: Adverse Mechanical Tension in the Central Nervous System. Stockholm, Almqvist and Wiksell, 1978.

61. Selander D, Mansson LG, Karlsson L, et al: Adrenergic vasoconstriction in peripheral nerves of the rabbit. Anesthesiology 1984; 62:6.

62. Komberg C: The effect of neural stretching on sympathetic outflow to the lower limbs. J Orthop Sports Phys Ther 1992; 16:294.

63. Slater H, Vincenzino B, Wright A: "Sympathetic slump": The effects of a novel manual therapy technique on peripheral sympathetic function. J Man Manip Ther 2:156, 1995.

64. Morris DB: The Culture of Pain. Berkeley, University of California Press, 1991.

65. Devor M: Neuropathic pain and injured nerve: Peripheral mechanisms. Br Med Bull 1991; 47:619.

66. Wall PD, Melzack R: Textbook of Pain, 3rd ed. Edinburgh, Churchill Livingstone, 1994.

67. Seddon H: Three types of nerve injury. Brain 1943; 66:237.

68. Jewett DL: Functional blockade of impulse trains caused by acute nerve compression. In Jewett DL, McCarroll HR (eds): Nerve Repair and Regeneration. St. Louis, CV Mosby, 1980.

69. Mumenthaler M, Schliack H: Peripheral Nerve Lesions. New York, Thieme, 1991.

70. Noth JV, Dietz V, Mauritz KH: Cyclists palsy. J Neurol Sci 1980; 47:111.

71. Miller EH, Benedict FE: Stretch of the femoral nerve in a dancer: A case report. J Bone Joint Surg 1985; 67A:315.

72. Dellon AL, Mackinnon SE, Seiler WA: Susceptibility of the diabetic nerve to chronic compression. Ann Plast Surg 1988; 20:103.

73. Szabo RM: Nerve Compression Syndromes. Thorofare, NJ, Slack, 1989.

74. Kopell HP, Thompson WAL: Peripheral Entrapment Neuropathies. Baltimore, Williams & Wilkins, 1963.

75. Dawson DM, Hallett M, Millender LH: Entrapment Neuropathies. Boston, Little, Brown, 1983.

76. Sunderland S: The nerve lesion in carpal tunnel syndrome. J Neurol Neurosurg Psychiatry 1976; 39:615.

77. Nobel W: Peroneal palsy due to haematoma in the common peroneal nerve sheath after distal torsional fractures and inversion ankle sprains. J Bone Joint Surg 1966; 48A:1484.

78. Sunderland S: Nerve Injuries and Their Repair. A Critical Appraisal. Edinburgh, Churchill Livingstone, 1991.

79. Triano JJ, Luttges MW: Nerve irritation: a possible model of sciatic neuritis. Spine 1982; 7:129.

80. Rydevik B, Brown MD, Lundborg G: Pathoanatomy and pathophysiology of nerve root compression. Spine 1984; 9:7.

81. Nitz AJ, Dobner JJ, Kersey D: Nerve injury and Grade II and III ankle sprains. Am J Sports Med 1985; 13:177.

82. Rayan GM, Pitha JV, Wisdom P, et al: Histologic and electrophysiologic changes following subepiperineurial haematoma induction in rat sciatic nerve. Clin Orthop Rel Res 1988; 229:257.

83. Fowler TJ, Ochoa J: Unmyelinated fibres in normal and compressed peripheral nerves of the baboon: a quantitative electron microscopic study. Neuropathol Appl Neurobiol 1975; 1:247.

84. Ochoa J: Nerve fiber pathology in acute and chronic compression. In Omer GE, Spinner M (eds): Management of Peripheral Nerve Problems. Philadelphia, WB Saunders, 1980.

85. Powell HC, Myers RR: Pathology of experimental nerve compression. Lab Invest 1986; 55:91.

86. Devor M, Rappaport ZH: Pain and the pathophysiology of damaged nerve. In Fields H (ed): Pain Syndromes in Neurology. London, Butterworths, 1990.

87. Nordin M, Nystrom B, Wallin U, Hagbarth KE: Ectopic sensory discharges and paraesthesias in patients with disorders of peripheral nerves, dorsal roots and dorsal columns. Pain 1984; 20:231.

88. Wall PD, Gutnik M: Properties of afferent nerve impulses originating from a neuroma. Nature 1974; 248:740.

89. Calvin WH, Devor M, Howe JF: Can neuralgias arise from minor demyelination? Spontaneous firing, mechanosensitivity and afterdischarge from conducting axons. Exp Neurol 1982; 75:755.

90. Devor M: The pathophysiology of damaged peripheral nerves. In Wall PD, Melzack R (eds): Textbook of Pain, 3rd ed. Edinburgh, Churchill Livingstone, 1994.

91. Howe JF, Calvin WH, Loeser JD: Impulses reflected from dorsal root ganglia and from focal nerve injuries. Brain Res 1976; 116:139.

92. Howe JF, Loeser JD, Calvin WH: Mechanosensitivity of dorsal root ganglia and chronically injured axons: a physiological base for the radicular pain of nerve root compression. Pain 1977; 3:25.

93. Upton ARM, McComas AJ: The double crush in nerve entrapment syndromes. Lancet 1973; 2:259.

94. Dellon AL, Mackinnon SE: Chronic nerve compression model for the double crush hypothesis. Ann Plast Surg 1991; 26:259.

95. Dellon AL, Mackinnon SE, Seiler WA: Susceptibility of the diabetic nerve to chronic compression. Ann Plast Surg 1988; 20:117.

96. Nemoto K, Matsumoto N, Tazaki K, et al: An experimental study on the "double crush" hypothesis. J Hand Surg 1987; 12A:552.

97. Augustijn P, Vanneste J: The tarsal tunnel syndrome after a proximal lesion. J Neurol Neurosurg Psychiatry 1992; 55:65.

98. Sammarco GJ, Chalk DE, Feibel JH: Tarsal tunnel syndrome and additional nerve lesions in the same limb. Foot Ankle 1993; 14:71.

99. Dyro FM: Peripheral entrapments following brachial plexus lesions. Electromyog Clin Neurophysiol 1983; 23:251.

100. Massey EW, Riley TL, Pleet AB: Coexistent carpal tunnel syndrome and cervical radiculopathy (double crush syndrome) South Med J 1981; 74:957.

101. Murray-Leslie F, Wright V: Carpal tunnel syndrome, humeral epicondylitis and the cervical spine. A study of clinical and dimensional relations. Br Med J 1976; 5:1439.

102. Hurst LC, Weissberg D, Carroll RE: The relationship of double crush to carpal tunnel syndrome (an analysis of 1,000 cases of carpal tunnel syndrome). J Hand Surg 1985; 10B:202.

103. Mackinnon SE: Double and multiple crush syndromes. Hand Clin 1992; 8:369.

104. Buck SH, Walsh JH, Yamamura HT, et al: Neuropeptides in sensory neurones. Life Sci 1982; 30:1857.

105. Lembeck F, Holzer P: Substance P as neurogenic mediator of antidromic vasodilation and neurogenic plasma extravasation. Naunyn Schmiedebergs Arch Pharmacol 1979; 310:175.

106. Morton CR, Chahl LA: Pharmacology of the neurogenic oedema response to electrical stimulation of the saphenous nerve in the rat. Naunyn Schmiedebergs Arch Pharmacol 1980; 314:271.

107. Brain SD, William TJ, Morris HR, et al: Calcitonin gene related peptide is a potent vasodilator. Nature 1986; 313:54.

108. Woolf CJ: Generation of acute pain. Br Med Bull 1991; 47:523.

109. Wall PD: Neuropathic pain and injured nerve. Central mechanisms. Br Med Bull 1991; 47:631.

110. Zusman M: Central nervous system contribution to mechanically produced motor and sensory responses: Aust J Physiother 1992; 38:245.

111. McMahon SB: Mechanisms of sympathetic pain. Br Med Bull 1991; 47:584.

112. Wilson PR: Sympathetically maintained pain: diagnosis, measurement and efficacy of treatment. In Stantan-Hicks M (ed): Pain and the Sympathetic Nervous System. Norwell, Kluwer, 1990.

113. Rudge P, Ochoa J, Gilliat RW: Acute peripheral nerve compression in the baboon. J Neurol Sci 1974; 23:403.

114. Farhni WH: Observations on straight leg raising with special reference to nerve root adhesions. Can J Surg 1966; 9:44.

115. Millesi H, Meissl G: Consequences of tension at the suture line. In Gorio A, et al (eds): Post-traumatic Peripheral Nerve Regeneration: Experimental Basis and Clinical Implications. New York, Raven Press, 1981.

116. Kornberg C, Lew P: The effect of stretching neural structures on grade 1 hamstring injuries. J Orthop Sports Phys Ther 1989; 10: 481.

117. Elvey RL: Treatment of arm pain associated with abnormal brachial plexus tension. Aust J Physiother 1986; 32:225.

Physiology

of

Rehabilitation

CHAPTER 11

Physiological Principles of Conditioning

H A W E N G E R *PhD*

P F M c F A D Y E N *MSc*

R A M c F A D Y E N *BScPT*

Performance Principle	Stimulus Principle	Evaluation/Monitoring Principle
Fitness Principle	Rest Principle	Taper Principle
Individualization Principle	Loading/Unloading Principle	Preparation Principle
Optimization Principle	Maintenance Principle	Recovery Principle
Overload Principle	Interference Principle	Periodization Principle
Specificity Principle	Overtraining Principle	Conditioning Guidelines

This chapter will address the principles that form the foundation for designing conditioning programs. These principles provide guidelines for the prescription of exercise to enhance both physiological function and performance in different sports and activities. The application of these principles varies with the sport, athlete, stage of development, and time of year. The principles listed in Table 11–1 should be integrated into a training program to achieve both optimal physiological function and peak performance.

PERFORMANCE PRINCIPLE

There are many factors that contribute to or detract from performance (Fig. 11–1). The extent of the contribution of these factors varies in different individuals, in different sports, at different stages of development, and at different levels of competition. The importance of these factors must be identified, prioritized, assessed, and modified to elicit excellence in performance. At times some factors must be deemphasized to devote time to others that may be detracting from individual or team performance. It is important to be aware of the interactions of multiple factors and their impact on performance. Some factors can complement, supplement, or magnify the effects of other factors such that the entire effect is greater than the sum of the parts. Figure 11–1A portrays each performance factor as a gear in the machine (human body). For the performance

gear to function at optimal rates, each of the other gears must also be operating optimally. Often it is necessary to de-emphasize one gear in order to redevelop or strengthen a weaker one.

Different elite performers bring different strengths to each sport. Often exceptional development in one area has permitted elite performance, but at the expense of development in other areas. Therefore, it is necessary to evaluate the status of each of these factors and determine optimal combinations for peak performance in different athletes and at different stages of development. For example, in young athletes, it may be more important to focus on skill development and to use fun activities to build sufficient fitness to perform the skills. As the athlete matures, more and more emphasis can be placed on mental skills, tactics, and physiological development.

Figure 11–1 suggests an interaction between factors such that well-developed mental skills enhance the ability to train and develop physical fitness, and vice versa. Figure 11–1B illustrates some of the variables that affect physiology and demonstrates that for each of the major factors described in Figure 11–1A, there are many variables that influence its effectiveness in enhancing performance. The physiological factor is enhanced by proper balance of training, rest, and nutrition but can be impaired by injury, fatigue, or travel. Other factors such as skill, tactics, psychology, equipment, and environment each has its own set of variables that enhance or detract from

TABLE 11–1
Principles of Conditioning

1. Performance
2. Fitness
3. Individualization
4. Overload
5. Optimization
6. Specificity
7. Stimulus
8. Rest
9. Loading/unloading
10. Maintenance
11. Interference
12. Overtraining
13. Evaluation/monitoring
14. Taper
15. Preparation
16. Recovery
17. Periodization

the effectiveness of that factor in producing peak performance.

In most competitive sports, many players have highly developed skills that allow them to perform at elite levels in spite of low levels of development in other areas. For example, athletes may have high skill levels, but a poorly developed aerobic energy system can limit performance because of fatigue. Similarly, strength imbalances can predispose athletes to injury and loss of playing time. On the World Cup Ski circuit, many downhill skiers have well-developed tactical, technical, and physical skills. However, inappropriate equipment selection, such as the type of wax for skis, can lead to slower race times. Because many factors influence performance in both individual and team sports, it is important that the coach and the athlete prioritize the factors that most affect their performance and determine which variables must be altered to offset weaknesses or enhance strengths.

FITNESS PRINCIPLE

Physical fitness has many connotations in American society. Although it is often associated with the state of the cardiorespiratory system (aerobic fitness), it must embrace a wider, all-inclusive number of physical attributes (Fig. 11–2). The extent to which each of these attributes affects the specific fitness necessary for a particular athlete will depend on the sport, the strengths and weaknesses of the individual, his or her training background, the level of competition, and the competition and training schedule.

Figure 11–2 implies that physical fitness is a composite of many different components: energy systems, the cardiorespiratory system, the neuromuscular system, body composition, and flexibility. The level of development in each of these components varies based on the physical demands of the sport and the extent to which fitness affects performance, as shown in Figure 11–1.

ENERGY SYSTEMS. The power and capacity of the energy systems must be matched to the demands placed on the athlete by both the rigors of training and the requirements of competition. Different sports rely on different energy systems.[1] Also, recovery from high-intensity anaerobic exercise requires high levels of aerobic development to ensure high work volumes during both training and competitive efforts. Sports such as ice hockey, soccer, basketball, and field hockey all demand short bursts of high-intensity effort followed by periods of lower intensity work during which fuel stores are replenished and metabolites removed. Performance in these sports has a high reliance on anaerobic energy systems; however, recovery during competition, between competitions, and especially during training, demands a well-developed aerobic energy system, as this system is responsible for restoration of alactic stores and is instrumental in facilitating the removal of lactic acid.

CARDIORESPIRATORY SYSTEM. The need to develop the cardiorespiratory system, either centrally or peripherally, will depend on its importance for recovery, oxygen and fuel supply, removal of waste products, and heat dissipation or retention during both competition and training. Sports, which tax the aerobic energy supply system for extended periods of time and require the removal of waste products and maintenance of thermal balance, require highly developed levels of cardiorespiratory fitness. The single best measure of this fitness component is maximal oxygen consumption (VO_2max).[2] Cross-country skiing, middle and long distance running, and rowing are excellent examples of sports in which performance is dependent on a highly trained cardiorespiratory system (>70 ml/kg/min) for the uptake, delivery, and utilization of oxygen and fuels. High volumes of training are required to develop VO_2max and/or the ability to work at a high percentage of VO_2max. Other sports that require the cardiorespiratory system primarily for recovery, demand only an optimal level in this system rather than maximal levels; examples are intermittent team sports such as ice hockey and volleyball, in which a VO_2max of 60 ml/kg/min would be optimal to ensure adequate recovery during training and competition.

NEUROMUSCULAR SYSTEM. Adaptations in the neuromuscular system for enhanced strength, power, and endurance are mandatory in many sports. The neuromuscular system is important for overcoming external forces as well as accelerating loads relative to body mass. This system involves not only force and power production by the muscles, but also the precise application of force and power to simple and complex movements. Therefore, in some sports the neuromuscular system is developed to attain high levels of absolute strength, power, and endurance, whereas in others, strength, power, and endurance relative to body mass are the critical determinants of neuromuscular effectiveness. For weight lifters, interior linemen in football, participants in combative sports, and downhill skiers, high amounts of *absolute* strength and power are critical for peak performance. However, gymnastics, sprinting, jumping, and team sports that demand high

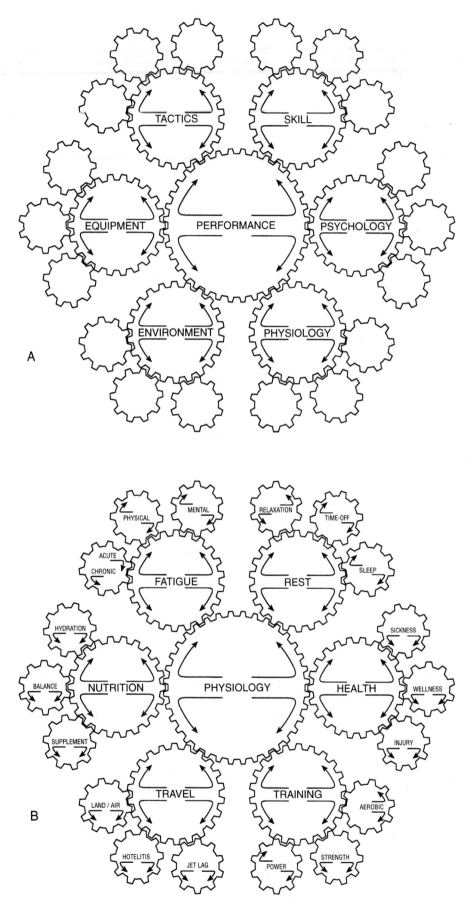

FIGURE 11–1. The performance factors.

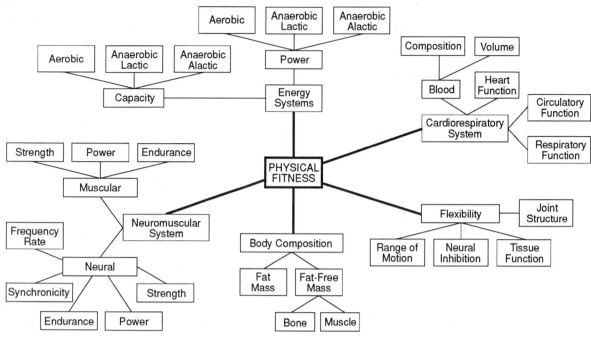

FIGURE 11–2. Components of physical fitness.

accelerations (e.g., soccer, tennis, and lacrosse) are more dependent on high levels of strength and power *relative* to body mass. Similarly, in sports such as weight lifting, shot-putting, and javelin throwing, the movements are fixed and relatively simple, whereas other sports involve "read-and-react" situations that create unpredictable applications of power and require coordinated multijoint movements. Thus, the acquisition of neuromuscular strength and power must be accomplished in settings where the nervous system is utilized specifically in the movement pattern necessary for performance (see "Specificity Principle").[3]

BODY COMPOSITION. The degree to which body composition—fat and fat-free mass—contributes to performance varies with different sports. Athletes in some sports require a high body mass for stability or inertia (e.g., offensive linemen in football and sumo wrestlers). In these instances the nature of the mass is not as critical as the amount. Similarly, in sports where body mass does not have to be moved or where it is supported, as in cycling and rowing, the nature of the mass is also not as critical as other variables. However, in sports in which body mass must be accelerated quickly or during rotations using strength and power, excess fat is detrimental. Because fat requires blood flow, the ability to effectively perfuse muscle during both exercise and recovery can be jeopardized when optimal levels of body fat are exceeded, and the insulative properties of fat can impair thermoregulation. Thus, with excess levels of body fat, performance and/or training can be compromised as a result of reduced muscle blood flow, ineffective recovery, overheating, and/or dehydration.

FLEXIBILITY. Flexibility involves the range of motion about a joint or series of joints and reflects the ability of the muscle-tendon units to elongate within the physical restrictions of the joint.[4] A causal relationship between flexibility and performance has not been clearly established, but athletes must move through the required range of motion to excel aesthetically or functionally. However, hypermobility or instability may make the joint more susceptible to injury in contact sports or when high speeds and forces are generated around the joint.

Therefore, a fitness profile must be developed for each athlete that matches the demands of his or her sport and individual goals. The relative importance of each of the preceding fitness components must be determined and then developed according to the guidelines described in all of the principles that follow.

INDIVIDUALIZATION PRINCIPLE

According to the individualization principle, each individual will respond uniquely to the same training stimulus. An individual's response is dependent on the following variables[5]: genetic endowment, biologic age, training state, health status, and fatigue state. To maximize the adaptation for each individual, the training programs must reflect a knowledge of that individual's genetic endowment, biologic age, training state, health status, and state of fatigue.

GENETIC ENDOWMENT. Each athlete has a given genetic potential that will limit the extent to which each component can be developed through physical training. The farther an individual is from the genetic limit, the larger will be the improvements to a given load (stimulus). As the individual gets closer to the limit, less improvement will be elicited, even with increases in the stimulus (Fig. 11–3).[5] If an athlete's genetic limit for VO_2max is 5 L/min and his or her present level is 3 L/min, large increases will occur during the initial 6 to 8 weeks of training. However, when VO_2max reaches

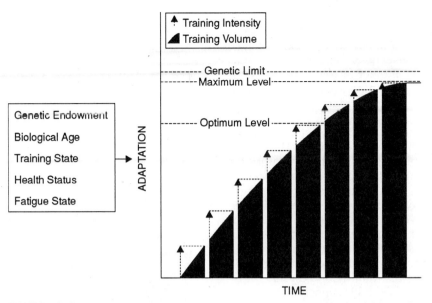

FIGURE 11–3. Physiological adaptations to progressive increases in the training stimulus.

4.5 L/min, less and less improvement will be elicited, even with greater and greater magnitudes of training. Although higher and higher intensities and volume of training are required as an individual approaches the genetic ceiling, coaches and athletes must be made aware of the risk of overuse injuries and/or overtraining (Overtraining Principle). Thus, periods of high-volume, high-quality loading must be interspersed with periods of unloading (Loading/Unloading Principle). Another implication of the genetic impact on physiological adaptations to training is that some individuals respond very early to a training stimulus, whereas others are late responders.[6] Therefore, for some athletes the training load should be increased frequently, while for others the steps should be more prolonged. Evaluation of progress (Evaluation/Monitoring Principle) must be planned throughout each training cycle to either determine or account for the differences in adaptation time.

BIOLOGIC AGE. The biologic age of an athlete can restrict the amount of adaptation that can be achieved to certain training stimuli, and furthermore, certain stimuli may even be detrimental or dangerous. For example, in prepubertal boys, the lack of testosterone will restrict the amount of muscle mass that can be developed with resistance training, and high loads may even damage the skeleton and/or impede growth. Strength can be increased with either increased muscle mass or enhanced neuromuscular adaptations (synchronicity or recruitment). Thus, when strength gains are desired in this population to permit skill development and/or provide protection, resistance protocols should focus on proper technique and low resistances to avoid the risks and facilitate neuromuscular adaptations.

TRAINING STATE. The state of training can determine the rate of improvement in most fitness variables. Individuals at low levels of fitness will respond with a higher rate and magnitude of adaptation than when they possess higher levels of fitness.[7] This is reflected in Figure 11–3 and outlined in the Optimization and Overload Principles.

HEALTH STATUS. The fact that the health status of an individual can affect both training and performance is obvious. During either sickness or injury, the amount of adaptive energy is reduced, along with the inability to perform at optimal intensities and volumes of work. Clearly then, during illness or when injured, the prescription of exercise and recovery must be altered to regain optimal health prior to reestablishing the training regimen.

FATIGUE STATE. Short-term fatigue brought about by depletion of fuels, substrates, accumulation of metabolites, heat stress, and/or dehydration will limit the ability to work at optimal intensities or durations. Therefore, to maximize the training stimulus—and thus maximize the training adaptation—recovery from fatigue should be accomplished with proper dietary, rehydration, and active and passive recovery strategies.

OPTIMIZATION PRINCIPLE

In many sports the factors that have the greatest influence on performance are skill level, tactics, equipment, environment, and/or mental skills (Performance Principle). In these sports it is not always necessary to develop maximum capabilities in each fitness component; instead, it is only necessary to attain optimal or sufficient levels to meet the demands of the sport, permit sufficient recovery to train and travel, and minimize the chance of injury. As reflected in Figure 11–3, the optimal levels of a fitness component are often less than the maximum that can be achieved. Because it may take less frequency, intensity, and time to achieve these optimal levels, time is allowed for developing other factors that can influence performance.

Different sports and positions have different energy requirements during competition.[1] For example, midfielders in soccer require 80 percent of their energy from the anaerobic energy systems and 20 percent from the aerobic energy supply, whereas cross-country skiers derive 85 percent of their energy from the aerobic system and only 15 percent from anaerobic sources. If the energy supply has high loading as a performance factor, then near maximal levels of those energy systems are necessary. However, if other factors such as skill or tactics are the predominant influence for success, then only optimal levels of the appropriate energy production systems are required. Even though competition in intermittent sports such as soccer, basketball, and ice hockey is predominantly anaerobic, a highly developed aerobic and cardiorespiratory system is mandatory for recovery from high-intensity work during breaks in play, between games, and throughout the season; during high volumes of training; and to deal with the added demands of travel. Although there is not a great deal of evidence that delineates a specific level of aerobic development sufficient to permit recovery in intermittent sports or to provide the recovery to handle high volumes of anaerobic training, a VO_2 max of 60 ml/kg/min for males and 56 ml/kg/min for females is often used. Because this fitness component is the baseline that permits sufficient time to develop other fitness components and both skill and tactics, it should be emphasized early during the training year (Periodization Principle). Once this optimal level is achieved, VO_2max can then be maintained (Maintenance Principle) and other fitness components or performance factors emphasized.

In addition to these requirements for optimal aerobic development, upper body strength may not be necessary in some sports to attain peak performance, but optimal levels of strength around the shoulder girdle and the abdominal and lower back areas can reduce the risk of injury during impact or during high training loads and allow training and performance to be uninterrupted.

OVERLOAD PRINCIPLE

Cells, tissues, organs, and systems adapt to loads that exceed what they are normally required to do (see Fig. 11–3). Adaptation to a stimulus takes many forms, from an increase in specific proteins, to cell division, to fuel storage, and to fluid shifts. Once an adaptation has taken place to a specific load or stimulus, then to get further changes, the load must be progressively increased.[8,9] This principle reflects the body's constant attempts to respond to different environmental strains. This process has been termed *homeostasis* and is illustrated in Figure 11–4. Figure 11–4A shows the equilibrium between physiological function and the demands imposed by daily physical loads. Figure 11–4B illustrates two concepts: the disturbance in equilibrium when the additional load is initially applied, and that same disturbance when the additional load acts as a stimulus for adaptation of physiological functions that were overloaded. Figure 11–4C shows that once the adaptation is complete, equilibrium is once again achieved. Therefore, to continually improve physiological function, progressive increases in load must be applied, to which adaptations will again occur (see Fig. 11–3).

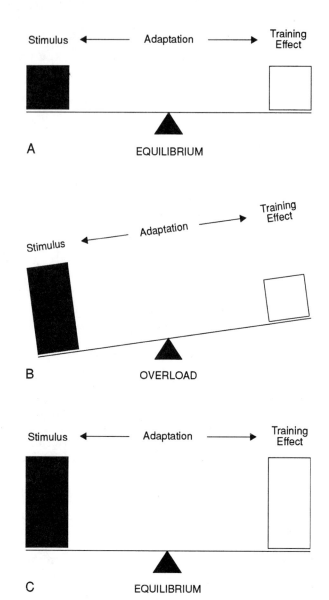

FIGURE 11–4. The effect of overload on stimulating adaptation to elicit an increased training effect.

When loads are applied, they should be specific to the desired effect (Specificity Principle), be appropriate to the individual (Individualization Principle), consider the time in the seasonal calendar (Periodization Principle), and be appropriate in terms of the type of stimuli (frequency, intensity, and duration) (Stimulus Principle). For example, when strength is being developed with resistance training, the prescription could consist of 8 to 12 repetitions for two to three sets, performed three times per week. For example, if bench press is a prescribed exercise and 150 lb permits the proper number of repetitions in the first set, then when 10 to 12 repetitions can be completed in the third set, the load should be increased by up to 5 percent to bring the number of repetitions back within the desired range to ensure overload. When aerobic power is being developed, the prescription should involve aerobic intervals of 1 to 3 minutes in duration with a 1:1 work-to-rest ratio at 90 to 100 percent of VO_2max performed with 6 to 10 repetitions.[10] The load can be progressed by

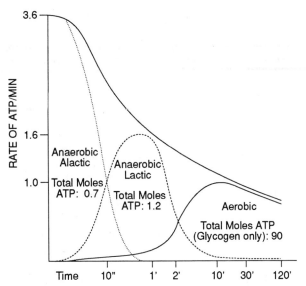

FIGURE 11–5. The maximal power and capacity of the three energy systems.

increasing the length of the work interval, decreasing the length of the rest interval, and/or increasing the number of repetitions.

It must be remembered that chronic overloading without sufficient rest (see "Rest Principle") and unloading (see "Loading/Unloading Principle") can result in overtraining (see "Overtraining Principle") and/or injury and therefore be counterproductive to training and/or performance.

SPECIFICITY PRINCIPLE

The adaptations that the body makes to exercise loads (training effect) are to a large degree specific to the structures and functions that are loaded. Training effects are specific to the energy supply systems that have been utilized, the locale of the stimulus (i.e., whether the central circulation or peripheral muscle has been loaded), the specific muscle groups, the joint action(s), the type of contraction (i.e., concentric, eccentric, or isometric), and the speed of contraction. This principle implies that overload results in adaptations specific to those cells, tissues, organs, or systems that have been overloaded. The adaptation that results depends on the type and amount of overload. As shown in Figure 11–5, the energy systems follow a continuum from the high-power, low-capacity (alactic) systems, to the moderate-power and -capacity (lactic) systems, and then to the low-power, high-capacity (aerobic) systems. The characteristics of these energy systems have been described in detail elsewhere.[1,2] In terms of development through specific conditioning programs, the power and/or capacity of each system must be challenged by a stimulus that overloads the specific energy component.

For example, because the maximum power of the alactic system occurs within the first 5 seconds (see Fig. 11–5), loads requiring maximal power in up to 5-second bursts will stimulate adaptations in the rate of energy supply from this system. Similarly, because the capacity of the lactic system extends from 45 to 180 seconds, exercise that challenges muscle maximally over this time frame will provide the optimal stimulus for adaptation. It should be noted that the power of the aerobic system is also challenged during the same time frame as lactic capacity. Thus, interval exercise designed to challenge the aerobic power can also stimulate significant adaptations of lactic capacity. This is consistent with the Specificity Principle, since these two portions of the energy supply systems are invoked by the same stimulus.

Prolonged stimulation of the cardiorespiratory (central) system results in changes in heart, vascular, and blood function. Changes to the central circulation enhance delivery of oxygen, fuels, hormones, and water; removal of metabolic wastes such as lactate, ammonia, and carbon dioxide; and maintenance of thermal balance. All of these adaptations improve prolonged performance in such activities as marathon running, cross-country skiing, rowing, and triathlons and/or recovery from high-intensity intervals during intermittent sports such as basketball, ice hockey, and soccer or during high-intensity resistance or interval training. The prolonged stimulus can be either continuous at moderate intensities or repeated intervals at intensities corresponding to VO_2max.

In skeletal muscle, different motor unit types (slow oxidative, fast oxidative-glycolytic, and fast glycolytic) are recruited with different intensities and duration of load and stimulus. The characteristics of these motor units and the nature of their recruitment patterns have been described in detail elsewhere.[11] During moderate-intensity prolonged exercise, slow-twitch motor units (type I) are primarily recruited. Once they begin to fatigue after an hour of activity, fast-twitch oxidative-glycolytic motor unit (type IIa) recruitment is increased, followed by the fast glycolytic pool (type IIb). However, high-intensity aerobic interval programs of 1 to 3 minutes' duration require a significant contribution from the fast-twitch motor units, thus stimulating aerobic changes in these muscles much sooner than would happen with continuous, prolonged low-intensity training. To enhance aerobic power, these programs must either be of very long duration (in excess of 1+ hours) or consist of high-intensity intervals to elicit maximal adaptations at the cellular level in all three fiber types.

The adaptation to skeletal muscle is also specific to both the muscle groups used and the joint action(s). For example, force overload achieved through biceps curls will challenge biceps brachii maximally when the forearm is supinated. When in the pronated position, less recruitment from the biceps is invoked, but greater demand is placed on the brachioradialis muscle. Similarly, in many actions, stabilizers for the surrounding or support-based muscles and synergists are also critical for both proper technique and optimal performance. Therefore, isolating single muscle groups during resistance training can be less effective for transferring strength to multijoint or complex movements than performing such movements under loaded conditions. For example, the strength of the leg extensions in rowing may be best achieved by a leg press or squat movement rather than by isolating each joint separately with free weights or machines, even though each individual joint action may become stronger from single joint training.

Similarly, the type of contraction (isometric, concentric, or eccentric) and the speed of contraction also affect the type of adaptation and, therefore, the ability to perform different types and speeds of movement. Therefore, when performance requires concentric movements in single or multijoint actions, then the training load should be applied concentrically for maximum return for the time invested. Likewise, when eccentric contractions contribute to muscular performance, then eccentric loads should be incorporated into the training prescription.[12] However, caution should be used in the prescription of eccentric exercise, since delayed-onset muscle soreness (DOMS), which occurs 24 to 72 hours later, can severely limit training time and enthusiasm.[13,14] Therefore, to minimize the effects of DOMS, eccentric loads should be applied gradually and used in combination with concentric contractions and proper preparation (Preparation Principle), and recovery strategies should be employed (Recovery Principle).

Even though significant tension can be imposed on muscle in isometric modes, the adaptations are specific to the joint angle trained, and less improvement is evident at joint angles further removed from the training angle. However, during rehabilitation, this type of training can elicit significant changes at points in the range of motion that are limiting performance owing to injury.

The velocity of contraction also elicits changes that are specific to the speed, such that resistance training at low velocity produces the greatest changes in low-velocity strength, whereas high-velocity training elicits maximum benefit at high-velocity contractions. The transfer of training from one speed to another is less clear, but it has been shown that high-velocity training provides more improvement at low velocity than vice versa. The neural mechanism behind this has yet to be determined. For maximum benefit in performance that involves speed- or velocity-specific requirements, the training stimulus should be applied at or above the required velocity.

STIMULUS PRINCIPLE

There are many characteristics of the exercise load that act as stimuli for both the type and magnitude of training effects. The characteristics are intensity (i.e., speed, resistance), duration of the exercise session, frequency (number of sessions per week), length (number of weeks or months), pattern (continuous versus interval), and mode (e.g., running, cycling).

The combination of these different stimuli has been addressed in a number of prescriptive programs. The fitness industry has adopted the FITT principle, which incorporates frequency (F), intensity (I), time (T), and type (T) of exercise to achieve optimal levels of health and fitness for the general public. These same stimuli are also the critical ingredients of the adaptive process for the highly trained athlete. The overload that achieves a training effect is a function of the combination of these stimuli. Progressions in the total load (volume) can be achieved by increasing intensity, time, or frequency, or a combination of the three. However, the nature of the adaptation will differ if the volume has been increased due to changes in intensity versus changes in time and frequency. The type of exercise will depend on the availability of equipment, the training location, and the specificity of the adaptation required for performance.

For changes in the aerobic energy system, intensities approaching VO_2max act as a stimulus for adaptations in aerobic power when the maximum rate of energy production from this system is critical. However, at these intensities, duration is limited to 5 to 10 minutes of continuous effort. Therefore, to increase the volume of this type of training, intermittent periods of recovery must be interspersed with work intervals of 1 to 3 minutes. The intensity of these VO_2max intervals can be monitored by measuring heart rate and ensuring it is maintained within 5 beats of maximum during the training interval. The heart rate during the recovery interval must be allowed to decrease to 30 beats/min below maximum heart rate.[1] In the early stages of this type of training, four to five intervals may be completed. The number of repetitions can be progressed to 8 to 10 over the training year. For training aerobic capacity, in which changes in the total volume of energy from the aerobic system, improvements in cardiovascular function, and high levels of caloric expenditure are desired, then lower intensity (70 to 85 percent maximum heart rate) and longer duration work (35+ min) is recommended, with a frequency of three to six times per week.[7]

The intensity component for challenging the anaerobic energy systems is altered by increasing either the speed of movement or the resistance. Therefore, short-term explosive actions at either high speed or high resistance will challenge the power of either the alactic or lactic energy supply, depending on the time interval during which these energy supply systems are designed to be operative (Fig. 11–5). The monitoring of these intensities is best achieved at present by the loads (speed or resistance) that permit maximal effort over the appropriate time. For example, 20-m sprints accomplished over 2.5 to 3 seconds at maximum velocity will challenge anaerobic alactic power. This same power can also be challenged by a maximal effort at a relatively slow pace against a high resistance using a leg press. If repeated intervals result in a decrease in the speed or load moved, then maximal alactic energy supply is no longer being challenged. Thus, sufficient recovery must be incorporated between intervals to permit maximum effort, usually in a 1:6 work-to-rest ratio (i.e., 5 seconds work to 30 seconds recovery). Recovery should consist of either rest or very low intensity exercise to permit replenishment of phosphogen stores.[1] This type of training should be done early in a training session when the athlete is well rested. Similarly, challenges to the lactic power should force maximal rates of energy supply from this system, which usually occurs at 15 to 25 seconds of all-out effort (see Fig. 11–5). Work-to-rest ratios of 1:3 or 1:4 are often prescribed to ensure sufficient training volume.

The intensity of the load required for optimal changes in muscular strength is dependent on the magnitude of the resistance offered to the muscle. Greater resistances require higher tension development in the muscle, which acts as the stimulus for changes in strength. Evidence suggests that loads that permit four to eight repetitions before failure invoke maximum strength changes without hypertrophy, whereas loads that permit 9 to 12 repetitions stimulate changes in both strength and muscle size.[15,16] When repetitions exceed these limits, the intensity (load) must be increased to provide the optimal stimulus.

The inverse relationship between intensity and duration has been outlined previously such that with high-intensity training, duration is reduced, and vice versa. The capacity (or volume) of energy that can be produced in any one of the systems is reflected in the amount of time that that system can produce its energy. Therefore, the stimulus for increasing the capacity of the alactic, lactic, and aerobic systems is an increased duration over which the specific system is required to provide its energy. To extend the capacity of alactic energy supply, intervals of all-out effort from 20 to 30 seconds in duration must be invoked. Similarly, the capacity of the lactic energy supply is challenged with work intervals that exceed 45 seconds. Aerobic capacity has its limits extended when intensity is reduced to a level sufficient to permit 1 to 2 hours of continuous activity involving large muscle groups.

Many activities require muscle groups to perform submaximal contractions for extended periods of time. This capability is often referred to as *strength endurance.* The stimulus is imposed by increasing the number of repetitions to meet the performance demands. The adaptation consists of increases in either force production (strength) or endurance (energy supply).

The frequency of training sessions is inversely related to both the intensity and the duration of the training loads. When particular cells, tissues, organs, or systems are overloaded with high-intensity training or long durations of training, they require extended times for adaptation, recovery, and regeneration. Therefore, application of repeated training sessions is an art as well as science that requires a sense of how effectively the athlete is adapting to the training loads. In general, training sessions of high intensity and/or long duration require 48 hours between sessions, but when the volume or intensity of training is reduced, the frequency can be increased to daily or twice-daily sessions. During periods in which the intensity, duration, and frequency are high, periods of unloading are mandatory (Loading/Unloading Principle) to avoid overtraining (Overtraining Principle).

The length of time (number of weeks) devoted to developing any one fitness component will depend on the importance of that component for either performing (Performance Principle) or training in a particular sport. It will also depend on the time of year, the competition schedule, the level of competition (Periodization Principle), and how readily the individual responds to the training stimulus (Individualization Principle).

The mode of training (type of activity) also dictates the extent to which adaptations will affect performance. For example, changes in the cardiorespiratory system can be achieved through proper stimuli in a variety of activities that involve large muscle masses (running, cycling, swimming, rowing, and skiing). These activities can be undertaken individually or combined in the same training session (cross-training). However, if changes are required in specific muscle groups and in specific modes (e.g., rowing) or maximum adaptation in that mode (rowing) is desired, then the stimulus should be specific to allow changes to both the central circulation and the specific peripheral muscles.

This principle provides the framework for deciding which exercise ingredients are necessary for the ideal training recipe.

REST PRINCIPLE

In response to a training stimulus, the components that were overloaded will undergo some breakdown at the subcellular, cellular, or tissue level, which will temporarily lower the functional ability of the cell, tissue, organ, or system. A rest period following exercise will allow the body to adapt by resynthesizing the protein associated with the components to a higher level than prior to the overload.[17] This building or synthesis process takes between 12 and 48 hours depending on the intensity (quality) of exercise and the volume (total amount) of load. Lower intensity and lower volume training sessions take as little as 12 hours of rest, while high-intensity training sessions can require more than 48 hours to build the training effect.

A rest period is also necessary to replenish muscle glycogen following prolonged exercise of a continuous or interval nature. The rate of replenishment differs depending on the extent of depletion, the type of exercise, and the amount of carbohydrate available, as well as the time of carbohydrate intake after exercise. If the rest phase between two training sessions is too long, the adaptation will plateau, and a stagnation in performance may occur. If the rest phase is too short, complete regeneration will not occur, and the athlete will train while fatigued. It is critical to establish a balance between work and rest to develop an effective training program. Rest days away from the rigors of training and competition are also important for emotional and psychologic well-being.

LOADING/UNLOADING PRINCIPLE

For the body to adapt effectively to periods of progressive overloading, it is necessary to allow the body a period of reduced load to ensure proper recovery, effective adaptations, and reduction in the risk of overtraining. There are a number of different ways to package the loading and unloading periods (cycles). A common format is three short periods (microcycles) of 1 week each in which the loads are progressively increased, followed by a 1-week microcycle of reduced volume and intensity (Fig. 11–6). This 4-week period has been termed a *mesocycle* and has specific objectives for development of a particular fitness component (Periodization Principle).[9] Additional mesocycles for further development of the same fitness component or a mesocycle for a transition into the development of another component will have their own microcycles of loading and unloading.

Although the principle of overload dictates that progression is necessary to achieve optimal adaptations (Optimization Principle), these progressions must be interspersed with short periods of unloading to facilitate the adaptive process through combining physiological, psychological, and emotional regeneration.

MAINTENANCE PRINCIPLE

The training effect is fragile. If the training stimulus is stopped, reduced, or altered, the training effect will decline. However, the training effect can be maintained, at least for a few months, if the frequency is reduced to one third and the intensity and duration are maintained.[18] For periods of 2 or 3 weeks, the effect can be maintained if the duration is reduced to two thirds but the intensity and frequency are maintained at the level that produced the training effect.[19] It is often necessary during the training and competitive year to change the focus of training either to some other fitness component or to optimizing performance for competition. During these periods of time, if previous development of a particular fitness component is ignored, then decrements will occur that can be detrimental to performance in the long term. Therefore, the ability to maintain established fitness levels through reduced frequency or duration will allow opportunities to emphasize the development of additional fitness components. For example, when aerobic power has been developed to an optimal level of 60 ml/kg/min through a training frequency of five times per week in an elite soccer player, VO_2 max can then be maintained by reducing the frequency to two times per week or reducing the number of aerobic intervals per training session to two thirds. This will then permit the athlete to focus on strength development while maintaining this critical level of aerobic power. Concomitantly, if strength changes are developed through a progressive resistance program three times per week, then the acquired levels can be maintained with these same reductions in either frequency or duration. An example of the reduced frequency required for maintenance of either aerobic power or strength is illustrated in days 15 through 28 in Figure 11–7.

INTERFERENCE PRINCIPLE

When training for two different types of adaptations (e.g., aerobic power and strength), the training stimuli can interfere with one another and result in less improvement in one or both of the effects. When attempting to train two different fitness components during a mesocycle, there is a risk of reducing the amount of adaptation when different stimuli are imposed during the same day or even on subsequent days. It seems that the adaptation to aerobic stimuli takes less time than the adaptation to higher intensity strength or power training, and the aerobic adaptation is not affected by the addition of a resistance stimulus. When strength loads are combined with aerobic training, the aerobic adaptation is not detrimentally affected, but there is a negative impact on strength development by the concurrent aerobic training.[20] When the strength and aerobic training occur on alternate days, the adaptations in strength are not impaired by the aerobic training on the previous or subsequent days over 8 weeks. However, over periods of time longer than 8 weeks, even interspersed days of aerobic and strength training can be detrimental to strength development.[21] When strength and aerobic training are blocked into separate mesocycles, there is no apparent interference effect. However, previously achieved aerobic effects are readily lost during subsequent strength training, but previously acquired strength gains are not as fragile when followed by a period of aerobic training.[22]

Therefore, separate periodized mesocycles for strength and aerobic benefits are the pattern of choice. However, if this is not possible, then alternate days of resistance and endurance loads are recommended. Although training both components on the same day will not be as effective as alternate-day training over similar time frames, aerobic training should occur early and resistance training later in the day to allow more adaptation time for the strength stimulus.

OVERTRAINING PRINCIPLE

Overtraining, also referred to as *overstress* or *staleness*, reflects an inability to recover from exercise, lowered resistance to injury, and chronic fatigue or exhaustion. Overtraining is caused by a loss in the body's adaptive

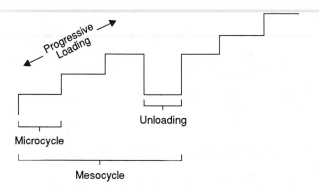

FIGURE 11–6. The sequencing of loading and unloading microcycles.

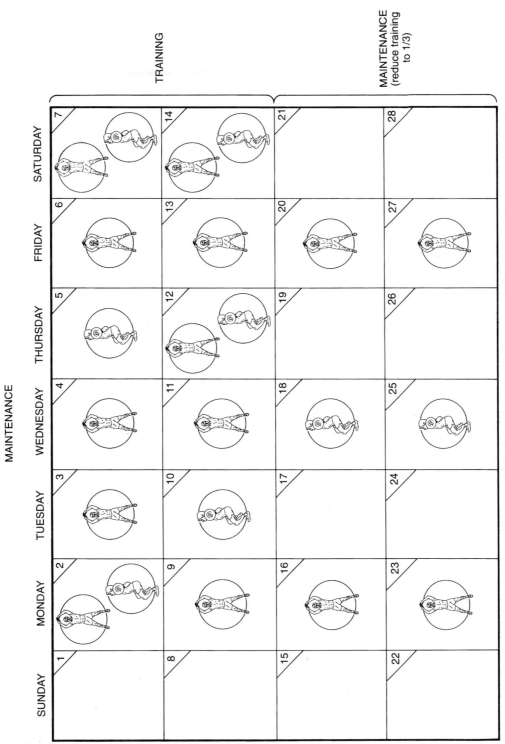

FIGURE 11–7. An example of the reduction in training frequency to maintain the training effect. Note that intensity and duration are maintained during the period of reduced frequency; only the number of sessions changes.

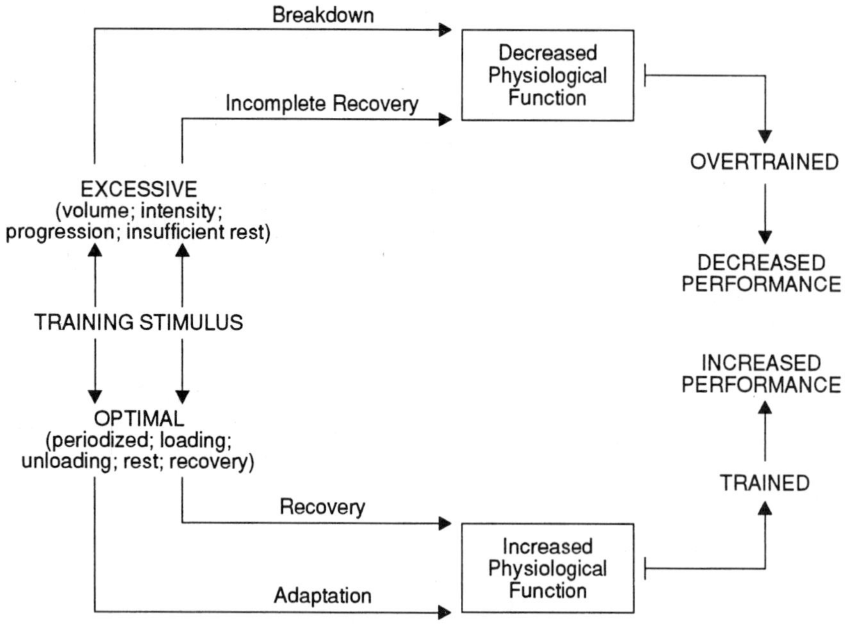

FIGURE 11–8. A model to describe the effects of excessive or optimal training stimuli.

capability after chronic high-volume loading or in response to a too-large increase in either duration or intensity of training. It is a poorly understood phenomenon that includes such symptoms as loss of appetite, inability to sleep, lethargy, muscle soreness, chronic fatigue, and declining performance.[22] It is not the acute fatigue associated with a single or a few training sessions that can be overcome by short rest, proper diet, and adequate nutrition. This syndrome can take from 3 weeks to several months to dissipate[23] and requires dramatically reduced training loads or no training at all.

As stated in the Overload Principle, individuals must overload their cells, tissues, organs, and systems to stimulate an adaptation. As a result of overload, fatigue occurs owing to many factors such as fuel or substrate depletion, buildup of metabolites, pH changes, or dehydration. This fatigue is short term, from a few hours to a few days. At the same time, the adaptation to the training stimulus (supercompensation) must also occur; during adaptation, protein is synthesized to build new structural and/or enzymatic protein so that the training effect can be expressed. The recovery and adaptive periods can take from a few hours to 2 days. To elicit maximal adaptations, a number of sports use an "overreaching" strategy to overload. This process involves applying training loads before recovery and adaptation to the previous load are completed. Because this overreaching process stresses the adaptive capability of the organism, a breakdown resulting in a mild staleness will ensue and, if continued, will result in the overtraining syndrome. The solution is to initiate the appropriate amount of rest (Rest Principle), recovery (Recovery Principle), unloading (Loading/Unloading Principle), and progression (Optimization Principle) in a periodized annual plan (Periodization Principle). The use of periodization to prevent overtraining has been reviewed by Fry et al.[24]

There have been a number of physiological predictors suggested for anticipating the overtrained state; these include increased resting morning heart rate, decreased body weight in the hydrated state, increased recovery heart rates after a maximal load, increased blood pressure, increased cortisol-to-testosterone ratios, and disturbed sleep patterns.[23, 25] The two most related variables are morning resting heart rate, either in the supine position or expressed as the difference between lying and standing heart rates,[23] and the recovery heart rate following maximal exercise. It has also been suggested that these measures should be obtained following a recovery period over which acute fatigue should have dissipated.[24] Although Figure 11–8 depicts only an inappropriate training stimulus contributing to the overtraining, other stressors (e.g., psychologic, sociologic, and economic factors) seem to add to the physical stress of training, which reduces the adaptive capability of the body.[26] Therefore, it is very important to try to keep nonphysical stressors to a minimum during periods of high loading or to be extra cautious of extended periods of high-volume loading when other stressors are present.

EVALUATION/MONITORING PRINCIPLE

Training programs are designed with specific objectives to be achieved. It is therefore necessary to regularly assess whether the programs have been effective so that they can be progressed or altered. This type of testing that brackets specific periods of time can consist of sophisticated laboratory testing with a high degree of precision or, at times, less rigorous but still effective field tests.[27] In either case it is necessary to take as much care as possible to make the conditions (e.g., time of day, testing location and environment, equipment, calibration, and personnel) as similar as possible at all testing sessions to ensure reliability.

An effective testing program provides an evaluation of the strength and weaknesses of an athlete as they pertain to the athlete's sport, baseline data at the onset of a particular phase in the training year, a measure of the effectiveness of the training program prescription, an index of the health status of the athlete, and a unique means for educating the athlete and coach about the athlete's physiological makeup and individual response to training.[27] Although a single test that provides a profile of the athlete's fitness level in selected components is often of interest, repeated tests that bracket specific training or competition periods throughout the training year or across many years will provide a more in-depth picture of the effectiveness of programs and the uniqueness of each individual's response to the training environment. To provide an objective means of quantifying training changes, testing and evaluations should be sport specific, valid and reliable, and administered by qualified personnel, and the results should be interpreted to both the coach and the athlete. Laboratory tests that isolate specific fitness components do not often permit evaluation in performance-specific modes of exercise. However, they do offer precision and an assessment of a specific physiological characteristic. When they are combined with performance-specific field tests, the two types of tests will provide a more complete picture of both the isolated components and their application in a sport-specific environment. However, where possible, the laboratory tests should utilize exercise modes that challenge the athlete's physiology as closely as possible to the sport-specific demands that the athlete will encounter. Specific examples of testing procedures for the different components of fitness have been documented.[28]

When choosing a testing battery, the location, facilities, cost, personnel, and information desired must be considered. Regardless of what types of tests are chosen, it is important to standardize the testing conditions at all testing sessions to ensure reliable results.

TAPER PRINCIPLE

Training sessions result in subcellular, cellular, and tissue breakdown as well as acute fatigue. Even though a training effect is being established in response to the training session, its expression as improved performance can be masked by short-term fatigue due to depletion of energy stores, dehydration, metabolite

accumulation, and/or acidity changes resulting from lactic acid and ammonia production. Therefore, it is difficult to produce high-quality performances during heavy training. However, if training is stopped to reduce fatigue, the training effect will also begin to decrease. Therefore, to elicit peak performance, the fatigue must be alleviated but the training effect maintained (Fig. 11–9). Fortunately, fatigue has a much faster decay time than the training effect.[29, 30] Thus, to remove the fatigue, the volume of training (duration and frequency) should be reduced while maintaining the training effect by holding the intensity of the training load constant.[31] The reduction in volume should be done progressively 7 to 14 days prior to competition (Fig. 11–10).[31,32] Volume should be decreased 50 to 75 percent over the taper, and the program should include high amounts of carbohydrate and fluid in the diet along with good sleep and rest.[33,34] Because this protocol reduces fatigue while attempting to hold the training effect at its present level, it does not build improvement. The taper is achieved at the expense of training, and therefore, priorities for tapering should be set for those competitions that are most important to permit both optimal training and peak performance.

This principle has been adapted in practice in those sports that have an extended competitive season (6 to 8 months) in which games or competition occur two to three times per week. The highest volumes of training are imposed as soon as possible after the previous performance. In the days approaching the next competition, the volume of work is then reduced while intensity is established at competition levels.

PREPARATION PRINCIPLE

It is important to be properly warmed up and stretched prior to training and competition. The purpose of the warm-up is to elevate the temperature of

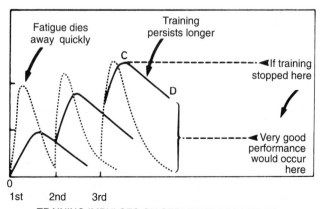

FIGURE 11–9. The growth and decay of fitness and fatigue in response to impulses of training on separate occasions.

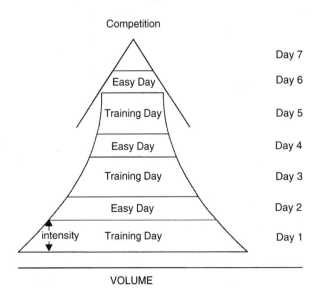

FIGURE 11–10. A figure that represents the reduction in training volume with the intensity varying (hard day/easy day) during a taper prior to competition.

muscle, blood, and connective tissue to both enhance performance and protect against soft tissue injury. Stretching also assists in relaxing the muscle to permit improved blood flow and neural activation.

A warm-up involves low-intensity exercise (<60 percent VO_2 max or 70 percent maximum heart rate) of relatively short duration (<15 minutes). The primary purpose of a warm-up is to increase core temperature (1° to 2° F) and muscle temperature (up to 5° F), which will[35,36]:

1. Enhance the rate of both muscular relaxation and contraction
2. Lower the viscous resistance in the muscle and therefore increase mechanical efficiency
3. Allow hemoglobin and myoglobin to dissociate more oxygen at the working tissue
4. Decrease the resistance in the vascular bed through vasodilation
5. Increase nerve conduction velocity
6. Decrease the risk of electrocardiogram (ECG) abnormalities
7. Increase metabolic processes

All of these physiological changes have the potential to enhance performance. However, if the exercise intensity is too high or the duration is too long, performance may be negatively affected by fatigue.

There are three main types of warm-up: passive, general, and specific. A passive warm-up involves increasing core temperature by external means such as a hot tub, shower, or massage. This type of warm-up does not produce a significant change in blood flow or blood redistribution to the working muscles but has been used by swimmers prior to a swimming event when a warm-up is not available.[36] A general (unrelated) warm-up involves performing movements that are not directly associated with the muscle movements and neural recruitment performed during the athletic activity.[37] A specific or related warm-up is the most common type. This procedure involves performing movements similar to the athletic activity. The type of warm-up chosen depends on the individual, event, type of competition, and facilities.

Stretching exercises are also performed during the preparation phase before training or competition. Stretching temporarily elongates the muscles, increases the range of motion about a joint, and stimulates neural activation. It is important to stretch the primary muscle groups prior to the exercise bout. In addition to being warmed up and stretched, it is necessary for the muscle to be properly hydrated and to ensure that fuel stores are replenished prior to competition or training. Adequate hydration will facilitate transportation of fuels, removal of wastes, and regulation of body temperature. Twenty-four hours before competition, 2 to 3 L of water should be ingested, with up to 2 L of water ingested 2 hours prior to the event.[38] Similarly, a well-balanced diet high in carbohydrates should be eaten 24 hours prior to competition to replenish energy stores, and a pregame meal should be eaten 4 hours prior to competition to supply additional energy during endurance events or prolonged intermittent work.[38]

RECOVERY PRINCIPLE

The purpose of a recovery phase is to restore the muscles and the body to pre-exercise levels. After training or competition, an active recovery will promote venous return and removal of metabolites from muscle, reestablish fluid balance, replace depleted fuel or energy reserves, and elicit relaxation in muscles that were active. Therefore, following exercise a short (5 to 10 minutes) low-intensity cool-down (30 to 65 percent VO_2 max) will assist in maintaining venous return and removal of metabolites,[39] ingestion of fluids (water, electrolytes, and up to 20 percent carbohydrate) will begin to reestablish fluid balance and fuels,[40] and carbohydrate-rich foods will assist in rapid replenishment of glycogen stores.[38]

Following prolonged continuous or intermittent work, supplementation of antioxidants such as ascorbic acid (vitamin C), α-tocopherol (vitamin E), and β-carotene (vitamin A) has been shown to be effective in removing waste products of oxidative stress (free radicals).[38,41]

Various modalities such as massage, hydrotherapy, and electrostimulation have been used for the purpose of enhancing recovery, with anecdotal but little scientific support.

Stretching techniques have been used to alter the range of motion (ROM) around a joint either acutely or chronically. In addition, they have been used after exercise to decrease muscle tension and facilitate recovery via increased blood flow. The three most common stretching techniques are ballistic stretching (rapid changes in length to the end of the ROM), static stretching (SS) (passive stretching to the end of the ROM), or proprioceptive neuromuscular facilitation (PNF). There are two types of PNF stretching: contract-relax (CR), in which the targeted muscle is contracted isometrically and then relaxed while it is stretched passively to the end of the ROM, and contract-relax–agonist contract (CRAC), in which CR stretching is performed as previously described, followed by contraction of the agonist muscles to assist in the stretching of the targeted muscles to the end of the ROM. In both PNF techniques the stretch torque is often increased by a trainer, therapist, or teammate. Ballistic stretching has been shown to be ineffective if not counterproductive,[42,43] whereas the SS technique has been shown to decrease muscle contraction on the electromyogram (EMG) to a greater extent than CR and CRAC.[44] Thus, for postexercise recovery, the SS is the technique that should be employed. It should be noted, however, that for acute increases in ROM, both SS and CRAC are equally effective, while the CRAC is most effective for long-term chronic increases in the ROM.[43] This is probably due to a reduction in other components of muscle stiffness other than the contraction as reflected by EMG. Therefore, for one-time increases in ROM prior to exercise, either SS or CRAC is preferred, whereas CRAC is the method of choice for absolute chronic increases in flexibility.

Recovery is a multidimensional process that requires the athlete to get plenty of rest, eat a balanced diet, and

Yearly Planning Instrument

Goals/Objectives for Year: ______________________________

Name of Athlete: ______________________ Level: __________ Date: ________ ______________________________

1.	Dates	Months																																																				
2.		Week Date																																																				
3.	Events	Dates																																																			
4.																																																					
5.	Details																																																				
6.																																																					
7.																																																					
8.	Training	Periods																																																				
9.		Phases																																																				
10.		Macrocycles																																																				
11.		Microcycles	1	2	3	4	5	6	7	8	9	10	11	12	13	14	15	16	17	18	19	20	21	22	23	24	25	26	27	28	29	30	31	32	33	34	35	36	37	38	39	40	41	42	43	44	45	46	47	48	49	50	51	52
12.	Dev. of skills	Techniques																																																				
13.																																																					
14.																																																					
15.																																																					
16.		Tactics/Strategies																																																				
17.																																																					
18.																																																					
19.	Mental Training	Stage 1 Positive Environment																																																				
20.		Stage 2 Emotional Control																																																				
21.		Stage 3 Attentional Control																																																				
22.		Stage 4 Strategies																																																				
23.		Stage 5 Application																																																				
24.		Assessment																																																				
25.	Physical Prep.	Aerobic																																																				
26.		Anaerobic																																																				
27.		Speed																																																				
28.		Strength																																																				
29.		Power																																																				
30.		Flexibility																																																				
31.		Nutrition																																																				
32.		Test, Monitor, Evaluation																																																				
33.																																																					
34.	Peaking Index	Volume* (H, M, L)																																																				
35.		Intensity* (H, M, L)																																																				
36.	% Emphasis	Physical																																																				
37.		Mental																																																				
38.		Techniques																																																				
39.		Tactics/Strategies																																																				
40.	Total Hours/Week																																																					

*H=High, M=Medium, L=Low

FIGURE 11–11. Yearly training model.

do a proper cool-down and stretching after an activity to facilitate faster restoration.

PERIODIZATION PRINCIPLE

The training and competitive periods within a year must be organized and sequenced with specific goals and objectives to permit effective development of the appropriate fitness components (Fitness Principle) as well as the other factors that determine performance (Performance Principle). This chapter focuses on the physiological factors, but the integration of all factors must be considered by the coach.

A yearly training program is divided into different phases characterized by changes in the goals, objectives, tasks, and contents, as well as training volume and intensity (Fig. 11–11). The classic model of periodization was developed by Mateveyev and incorporates the following training phases: preparation, competition, and transition. Each of these phases has been termed a *macrocycle*. Macrocycles outline the optimal training sequence for a 1-year program.[9,45] Each macrocycle has specific goals: the preparatory phase focuses on developing both general fitness and sport-specific training; the competition phase focuses on improving the athlete's performance and prepares him or her to peak for minor and major competitions; and the transition phase, which usually lasts between 2 and 6 weeks, allows both psychologic and physiological regeneration through rest and active recovery. When planning each of these cycles, the following factors should be considered:

1. Goals of the athlete, coach, and team
2. Length of the competition schedule and number of competitions
3. Stage of development of the athlete

By allotting the appropriate amount of time for each macrocycle, there will be adequate time to train all physiological components of the sport and peak for performance, although this may not be possible in a single training year.

Macrocycles are divided into smaller segments called *mesocycles*. Mesocycles allow the coach to structure periods of progressive overload by increasing training volume and incorporating periods of reduced training to facilitate regeneration. An average mesocycle lasts 2 to 5 weeks, during which specific training objectives are achieved. For example, for a track runner, one mesocycle may focus on improving aerobic power at the beginning of a season, and another mesocycle may focus on improving starts from the blocks. Mesocycles incorporate the Loading/Unloading Principle, with the first few weeks focusing on development, the next one on superloading, and the last week on recovery (see Fig. 11–6). Complete regeneration does not necessarily occur at the end of each mesocycle. The accumulation of fatigue over time can facilitate training adaptations but must not violate the Overtraining Principle. It is important to plan each cycle for each individual as well as for the team to allow time to make adaptations to the training stimulus and to make a smooth transition from one cycle to the next.

Mesocycles are subdivided further into *microcycles*.[9] Microcycles are training periods of up to 7 days in duration. Microcycles allow the coach to coordinate training in conjunction with all other factors that may influence training and performance (Performance Principle), as well as unforeseen occurrences in the everyday life of the athlete. The sequence of loading can change daily throughout the cycle, and the same microcycle may be repeated two to four times throughout a mesocycle. Incorporated into the microcycles are rest and recovery days (Rest Principle) to permit optimal adaptations to the training stimulus.

This terminology for the hierarchy of training cycles (i.e., macro-, meso-, and micro-) has been adapted by some training personnel, but the principles have not. Presently the traditional macrocycles are often termed *phases*, the term *macrocycle* is used to depict the 2- to 5-week specialized training periods, and the term *microcycle* is still used to describe up to 1-week training blocks.

CONDITIONING GUIDELINES

Listed below is a summary of the integration of the principles of conditioning.
1. Decide which factors (Fig. 11–1) affect performance in your sport (Performance Principle)
   • Prioritize these factors.
2. Based on the unique physical demands of your sport, decide on the specific fitness components (Fig. 11–2) that must be developed (Fitness Principle).
   • Prioritize each component.
3. Evaluate the status of your athlete(s) for each of the fitness components (Evaluation/Monitoring Principle).
4. Decide on the optimal level of fitness required in each fitness component (Overload Principle).
5. Periodize the yearly training calendar for competitions, including general and specific preparation (Periodization Principle).
6. For each microcycle, decide on the type of overload (Optimization Principle).
   • Decide on individual requirements (Individualization Principle).
   • Select the appropriate stimulus (Specificity and Stimulus Principles).
   • Remember to allow appropriate rest (Rest Principle), preparation (Preparation Principle), and recovery (Recovery Principle).
7. Decide on the progression to the next microcycle and the appropriate unloading within the mesocycle (Loading/Unloading Principle).
   • Be aware of the interference effect when training more than one fitness component (Interference Principle).
   • Remember that unloading is critical to avoid overtraining (Overtraining Principle).

8. Following each mesocycle, it is important to evaluate or monitor the components that wereemphasized (Evaluation/Monitoring Principle).
9. When training emphasis is shifted to another component, remember to maintain previously acquired effects (Maintenance Principle).
10. As competition approaches, remember to reduce the training volume (Taper Principle).
11. Apply your skills and art in coaching and rehabilitation to these scientific principles.

REFERENCES

1. Fox E, Bowers R, Foss M: The Physiological Basis for Exercise and Sport, 5th ed. Madison, WI, WCB Brown & Benchmark, 1993.
2. Green HJ: What do tests measure? In MacDougall JD, Wenger HA, Green HJ (eds): Physiological Testing of the High-Performance Athlete, 2nd ed. Champaign, IL, Human Kinetics, 1992.
3. Sale D, MacDougall D: Specificity in strength training: A review for the coach and athlete. Can J Appl Sport Sci 1981; 6(2):87–92.
4. Hubley-Kozey CL: Testing flexibility. In MacDougall JD, Wenger HA, Green HJ (eds): Physiological Testing of the High-Performance Athlete, 2nd ed. Champaign, IL, Human Kinetics, 1992.
5. Singh H: Principles of sports training. SNIPES J 1981; 4(4):14–28.
6. Bouchard C, Lortie G: Heredity and endurance performance. Sports Med 1984; 1:38–64.
7. Wenger HA, Bell GJ: The interactions of intensity, frequency, and duration of exercise training in altering cardiorespiratory fitness. Sports Med 1986; 3:346–356.
8. Fry RW, Morton AR, Keast D: Periodisation of training stress—a review. Can J Sport Sci 1992; 17(3):234–240.
9. Bompa T: Theory and Methodology of Training. Dubuque, Iowa, Kendall/Hunt, 1983.
10. MacDougall D, Sale D: Continuous vs. interval training: A review for the athlete and the coach. Can J Appl Sport Sci 1981; 6(2):93–97.
11. Saltin B, Henriksson J, Nygaard E, et al: Fiber types and metabolic potentials of skeletal muscle in sedentary man and endurance runners. Ann NY Acad Sci 1977; 301:3–29.
12. Hather BM, Tesch PA, Buchanan P, et al: Influence of eccentric actions on skeletal muscle adaptations to resistance training. Acta Physiol Scand 1991; 143:177–185.
13. Stauber WT, Clarkson PM, Fritz VK, et al: Extracellular matrix disruption and pain after eccentric muscle action. Med Sci Sport Exerc 1990;69(3):868–874.
14. Evans WJ, Cannon JG: The metabolic effects of exercise-induced muscle damage. Exerc Sport Sci Rev 1991; 19:99–125.
15. Tesch PA: Skeletal muscle adaptations consequent to long-term heavy resistance exercise. Med Sci Sport Exerc 1988; 20(5):S132–S134.
16. Tesch PA: Training for bodybuilding. In Komi PV (ed): Strength and Power in Sport. Oxford, Human Kinetics, 1991.
17. Lundin P: The monitoring of recovery in endurance athletes. JNSCA 1985; 7(6):41–42.
18. Hickson RC, Rosenkoetter MA: Reduced training frequencies and maintenance of increased aerobic power. Med Sci Sports 1981; 13(1):13–16.
19. Hickson RC, Kanakis C, Davis JR, et al: Reduced training duration effects on aerobic power, endurance, and cardiac growth. J Appl Physiol 1982; 53(1):225–229.
20. Hickson RC: Interference of strength development by simulta-

neously training for strength and endurance. Eur J Appl Physiol 1980; 45:255–263.
21. Bell GJ, Petersen SR, Wessel J, et al: Physiological adaptations to concurrent endurance training and low velocity resistance training. Int J Sports Med 1991; 12(4):384–390.
22. Bell GJ, Petersen SR, Wessel J, et al: Adaptations to endurance and low velocity resistance training performed in a sequence. Can J Sport Sci 1991; 16(3):186–192.
23. Roundtable. Overtraining of athletes. Phys Sports Med 1983; 11(6):93–109.
24. Fry RW, Morton AR, Keast D: Periodisation and the prevention of overtraining. Can J Sport Sci 1992; 17(3):241–248.
25. Dressendorfer RH, Wade C, Scaff JH: Increased morning heart rate in runners: A valid sign of overtraining? Phys Sports Med 1985; 13(8):77–86.
26. Selye H: The Stress of Life. London, Longmans Green, 1957.
27. MacDougall D, Wenger HA: The purpose of physiological testing. In MacDougall JD, Wenger HA, Green HJ (eds): Physiological Testing of the High-Performance Athlete, 2nd ed. Champaign, IL, Human Kinetics, 1992.
28. MacDougall JD, Wenger HA, Green HJ (eds): Physiological Testing of the High-Performance Athlete, 2nd ed. Champaign, IL, Human Kinetics, 1992.
29. Banister EW, Calvert TW: Planning for future performance: Implications for long term training. Can J Appl Sport Sci 1980; 5(3):170–176.
30. Fry RW, Morton AR, Keast D: Overtraining in athletes: An update. Sports Med 1991; 12(1):32–65.
31. Shepley B, MacDougall JD, Cipriano N, et al: Physiological effects of tapering in highly trained athletes. J Appl Physiol 1992; 72(2):706–711.
32. Costill DL, King DS, Thomas R, et al: Effects of reduced training on muscular power in swimmers. Phys Sports Med 1985; 13(2):94–101.
33. Houmard JA, Costill DL, Mitchell JB, et al: Reduced training maintains performance in distance runners. Int J Sports Med 1990; 11(1):46–52.
34. Neary J: Physiological adaptations of tapering. Sports Aider 1993; 9(2):10.
35. Shellock FG: Physiological benefits of warm-up. Phys Sports Med 1983; 11(10):134–139.
36. Ingjer F, Stromme SB: Effects of active, passive or no warm-up on the physiological response to heavy exercise. Eur J Appl Physiol 1979; 40:273–282.
37. deVries HA, Housch TJ: Physiology of Exercise for Physical Education, Athletics, and Exercise Science, 5th ed. Madison, WI, WCB Brown and Benchmark, 1994.
38. Bucci L: Nutrients as Ergogenic Aids for Sports and Exercise. Boca Raton, FL, CRC Press, 1993.
39. Belcastro AN, Bonen A: Lactic acid removal rates during controlled and uncontrolled recovery exercise. J Appl Physiol 1975; 34(6):932–936.
40. Gisolfi CV, Duchman SM: Guidelines for optimal replacement beverages for different athletic events. Med Sci Sport Exerc 1992; 24(6):679–687.
41. Keith RE: Vitamins in sport and exercise. In Hickson J, Wolinsky I (eds): Nutrition in Exercise and Sport. Boca Raton, FL, CRC Press, 1989.
42. Wallin D, Ekblom B, Grahn R, et al: Improvement of muscle flexibility: A comparison between two techniques. Am J Sports Med 1985; 13(4):263–268.
43. Hutton RS: Neuromuscular basis of stretching exercises. In Komi PV (ed): Strength and Power in Sport. Oxford, Blackwell Scientific, 1992.
44. Moore MA, Hutton RS: Electromyographic investigation of muscle stretching techniques. Med Sci Sport Exerc 1980; 12:322–329.
45. Harre D: Principles of Sports Training: Introduction to the Theory and Methods of Training. Berlin, Sportverlag, 1982.

CHAPTER 12

Physiological Principles of Resistance Training and Rehabilitation

JEFFREY E. FALKEL *PhD, PT, CSCS*
DANIEL J. CIPRIANI *MEd, PT*

One of the foremost aspects of rehabilitation after any injury is some form of resistance training in an attempt to provide the patient with an overloaded resistance by which to develop the necessary strength for functional and sport-related activities. It is critical that sports medicine clinicians understand the concepts, principles, and physiology of resistance training to provide the optimal exercise prescription for each of their patients. This chapter will provide the sports medicine clinician with an overview of the physiological principles and concepts of resistance training and how they apply to the art and science of rehabilitation.

Throughout this chapter the authors will use the term *resistance training* to describe any form of overload resistance specifically applied to enhance and develop muscular strength, endurance, and power. Resistance training utilizes several different types or modalities for strengthening, ranging from body weight to elastic rubber products, to conventional free weights and fixed-motion machines. Several other terms must be defined to clarify the concepts presented in this chapter (Table 12–1). *Strength* is the maximal force a muscle or muscle group can generate at a specified speed of contraction.[1] *Endurance* is the ability of a muscle to perform a particular number of contractions with proper form until muscle fatigue or degradation of proper technique. *Power* is the product of the force exerted on an object and the velocity of the object in the

direction in which the force is exerted.[2] With the exception of a single, maximal contraction, all exercise really involves the concept of power as it relates to force and velocity. Therefore, the velocity component of power should always be taken into consideration in the development of a resistance training program for rehabilitation.

Two other terms—intensity and volume of training—will be used throughout this chapter as they relate to resistance training. *Intensity* is the power output (rate of performing work) of the exercise.[3] In practical terms, intensity refers to the load or resistance under which the patient exercises. The *volume of training* is estimated by summing the total number of repetitions performed in a specified period of time.[3] Volume is calculated by adding the frequency and duration of rehabilitation or training sessions. It is suggested that the sports medicine clinician use these terms to describe and document the resistance training and rehabilitation programs that are established for each patient, for they provide objective and quantifiable documentation of progress.

BIOENERGETICS OF RESISTANCE TRAINING

Bioenergetics, or the flow of energy in a biologic system, is the conversion of food energy or chemical

TABLE 12–1
Critical Terms in Resistance Training

- Strength
- Endurance
- Power
- Intensity
- Volume of training

energy into biologically usable forms of energy and concerns the sources of energy for muscular contraction.[3,4] The breakdown or conversion of chemical bonds in the molecules of food, carbohydrates, fats, and protein releases energy to perform exercise involving muscular contractions.[4]

In an excellent review of bioenergetics,[4] Stone and Conley provide a model for the breakdown of large molecules into smaller molecules (catabolism) and the synthesis of larger molecules from smaller molecules by using the energy produced from catabolic reactions (anabolism). Figure 12–1 shows this model, and how exergonic (energy-releasing) reactions and endergonic reactions (reactions that require energy) form the general scheme of metabolism, which is the total of all catabolic/exergonic and anabolic/endergonic reactions in a biologic system.[4]

The final source of energy for muscular contraction is the adenosine triphosphate (ATP) molecule. An adequate supply of ATP is necessary for muscular contraction.[3] The catabolic breakdown of the chemical bonds of the ATP molecule provides the energy necessary to allow the myosin cross-bridges to pull the actin filaments across the myosin filaments, which results in the muscle contraction.[3,5,6] To accomplish muscle contraction of various intensities and durations, a source of ATP must be readily available to the muscle. The muscle cell has three sources of ATP available. ATP-phosphocreatine (ATP-PC) and lactic acid, which are formed without the need for direct sources of oxygen, are *anaerobic energy sources*. The third source of ATP for muscular contraction requires oxygen and is an *aerobic energy source*.[3] Table 12–2 provides an overview of the bioenergetics of maximal effort based on the duration of the exercise event. Although it is beyond the

scope of this chapter to provide the reader with a detailed description of biologic energy systems and supplies of ATP, a brief overview is necessary to appreciate the physiological justification for the utilization of resistance training in rehabilitation programs for athletes and patients alike. The reader is referred to several excellent sources for a detailed explanation of bioenergetics and energy metabolism.[4–6]

ENERGY SOURCES

ATP-PC. A limited amount of energy is available from the ATP-PC energy system for immediate use by the muscle for contraction. The ATP molecule is broken down into adenosine diphosphate (ADP), phosphorus (P), and energy for contraction. When PC is broken down to creatine, P, and energy, the energy from this reaction is used to "rebuild" ADP and P into ATP that can be used for additional muscular contraction.[3] Several studies have demonstrated that ATP-PC energy sources are exhausted in 30 seconds or less after an all-out exercise effort.[3,7,8] However, despite the limited amount of ATP-PC available for muscular contraction, there are two distinct advantages of this source of energy: it is an immediate source of energy for muscular contraction, and the ATP-PC energy source has a large power capacity in that it is capable of providing the muscle with a large amount of energy per unit of time.[3]

LACTIC ACID. Because of the constant need for energy to allow muscles to contract, the muscle has the capacity to store a form of carbohydrate called *glycogen.* Glycogen is formed by long strings of sugar molecules called *glucose,* and it is the splitting of glucose molecules into pyruvate that yields the energy needed to make ATP for muscular contraction.[3] Pyruvate is then transformed into lactic acid, and this entire process, performed without the need for oxygen, is called *anaerobic glycolysis,* as seen in Figure 12–2.[3,9]

The accumulation of lactic acid is probably most recognized in sport and resistance training by the initial sensation of "pins and needles" in the hands, fingers, or toes, followed by the sensation of pain in the local musculature as a result of lactate acid concentrations high enough to affect the nerve endings. As the intensity of the exercise continues and more lactic acid is produced,

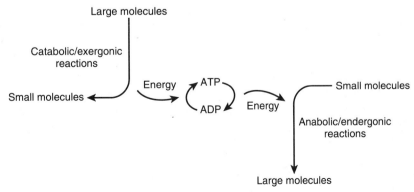

FIGURE 12–1. The general scheme of metabolism. (From Stone MH, Conley MS: Bioenergetics. *In* Baechle TR: Essentials of Strength Training and Conditioning. Champaign, IL, Human Kinetics, 1994. Copyright 1994 by the National Strength and Conditioning Association. Reprinted by permission.)

TABLE 12–2
Bioenergetics and Maximal Effort Duration

Primary System	Duration of Event
ATP-CP	0–10 sec
ATP-CP + anaerobic glycolysis	10–30 sec
Anaerobic glycolysis	30 sec–2 min
Anaerobic glycolysis + oxidative system	2 min–3 min
Oxidative system	>3 min and rest

From Stone MH, O'Bryant HS: Weight Training: A Scientific Approach. Minneapolis, Burgess International, 1987, p 32. An imprint of Burgess International Group, Edina, MN.

there is a change in the acidity of the muscle. Once the muscle pH drops below a certain level, phosphofructo-kinase (PFK), which is a rate-limiting enzyme in the process of glycolysis, shuts down, and local energy production then quickly ceases until replenished by oxygen stores. In addition, it has also been suggested that excess lactic acid in the muscle also interferes with calcium binding sites in the muscle, thus further limiting muscle contraction and useful power production.[10] Therefore, the amount of energy that can be produced by the lactic acid energy system is limited because of the various side effects of the accumulation of lactic acid in the muscle.[3]

However, the lactic acid system can still produce a larger amount of energy than the ATP-PC system, although it cannot supply the muscle with as much

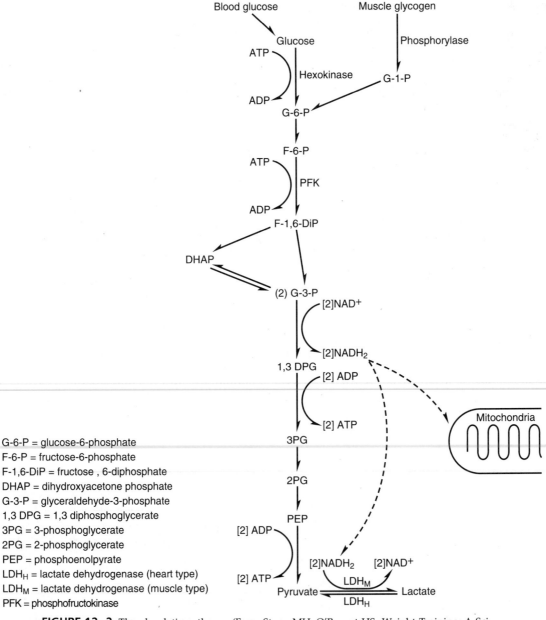

G-6-P = glucose-6-phosphate
F-6-P = fructose-6-phosphate
F-1,6-DiP = fructose , 6-diphosphate
DHAP = dihydroxyacetone phosphate
G-3-P = glyceraldehyde-3-phosphate
1,3 DPG = 1,3 diphosphoglycerate
3PG = 3-phosphoglycerate
2PG = 2-phosphoglycerate
PEP = phosphoenolpyrate
LDH_H = lactate dehydrogenase (heart type)
LDH_M = lactate dehydrogenase (muscle type)
PFK = phosphofructokinase

FIGURE 12–2. The glycolytic pathway. (From Stone MH, O'Bryant HS: Weight Training: A Scientific Approach. Minneapolis, Burgess International, 1987. An imprint of Burgess International Group, Inc., Edina, MN.)

energy per unit of time as does the ATP-PC system. Consequently, the lactic acid system is not as powerful as the ATP-PC system.[3] Lactic acid is the major energy source for providing the muscle with ATP in exercise bouts that last from 1 to 3 minutes (e.g., a long set of repetitions during resistance training, or running 400 to 800 m).

OXYGEN ENERGY SOURCE. The oxygen energy system is the major source of ATP for prolonged muscular contraction (i.e., for periods of exercise greater than 5 to 10 minutes). This energy system directly utilizes oxygen to produce energy and is thus considered to be the aerobic energy source.[3] The oxygen energy system has the ability to metabolize both carbohydrates and fats for energy production. The maximal amount of energy that can be supplied by the aerobic or oxygen energy system is determined by the ability of the body to obtain and utilize oxygen at the level of the local exercising tissues. Maximal aerobic power, or maximal oxygen consumption (VO_2 max), is the maximal amount of oxygen that can be supplied to the body and then utilized to allow for the continued aerobic production of oxygen.

Although it is well understood that aerobic activities such as long distance running, swimming, cycling, or rowing are the primary type of activities that stress the aerobic energy system, it has been shown that resistance training can also effectively place demands on the aerobic energy sources. Because of the large energy and caloric expenditure associated with aerobic exercise, most training programs designed to expend large amounts of calories for weight loss have focused on aerobic training. However, several studies have clearly shown that resistance training, particularly in the recovery period between sets, has the ability to cause the athlete to consume large amounts of oxygen and consequently can be effective in caloric reduction programs.[11-15] In fact, one study by Dohmeier et al.[13] demonstrated that heavy resistance training can provide a sufficient aerobic stimulus to elicit an aerobic adaptation similar to that seen with treadmill exercise.[9,13] The amount of the aerobic contribution to resistance training is dependent on several factors, such as intensity, rest interval, the volume or number of repetitions, and the duration of the resistance training session. Although the oxygen energy system is not normally considered a major contributor to the energy needs of resistance training, it does indeed contribute in some fashion that is specific to the type, intensity, and volume of the training.

SUMMARY. Table 12–3 provides a summary of the relative contributions of the anaerobic and aerobic energy systems based on the duration of the exercise bout and the relative intensity of the exercise.[4,16,17] It is important for sports medicine clinicians to have an understanding of the relative energy sources needed for the types, intensities, and volumes of exercise that they prescribe for the athletes and patients they treat. With this knowledge, they can more accurately and specifically design resistance training programs to meet the demands and requirements of specific sports and activities.

TABLE 12–3
Possible Factors Increasing Excess Postexercise Oxygen Consumption (EPOC)

- Resynthesis of ATP and creatine phosphate stores
- Resynthesis of glycogen from lactate (20 percent of lactate accumulation)
- Oxygen resaturation of tissue water
- Oxygen resaturation of venous blood
- Oxygen resaturation of skeletal muscle blood
- Oxygen resaturation of myoglobin
- Redistribution of ions within various body compartments
- Repair of damaged tissue
- Additional cardiorespiratory work
- Residual effects of hormone release and accumulation
- Increased body temperature

From Stone MH, Conley, MS: Bioenergetics. *In* Baechle TR: Essentials of Strength Training and Conditioning. Champaign, IL, Human Kinetics, 1994, p 77. Copyright 1994 by the National Strength and Conditioning Association. Reprinted by permission.

RECOVERY OR REPLENISHMENT OF ENERGY SOURCES

Recovery from an intense exercise bout, such as that seen with resistance training, is critical to the body's ability to continue training, both immediately and over the long term. After an intense exercise session, anaerobic energy sources must be replenished before they can be called on again to provide energy for muscular contraction.[3] The anaerobic energy sources of ATP-PC and lactic acid are ultimately replenished by the oxygen or aerobic energy system. The extra oxygen that is taken in to replenish the anaerobic energy sources after the cessation of the exercise effort has historically been termed the *oxygen debt.*[11] This oxygen recovery phase is currently more accurately referred to as *excess postexercise oxygen consumption* (EPOC),[12] which is the oxygen consumption above resting levels that is needed to restore energy sources.[4,12] There are numerous factors that might influence EPOC; these factors are listed in Table 12–4 and diagrammatically displayed in Figure 12–3.

TABLE 12–4
Contributions of Anaerobic and Aerobic Mechanisms to Maximal Sustained Effort

	Duration of Effort(s)			
	0–5	30	60	90
Exercise intensity (percentage of maximum power output)	100	55	35	31
Percent contribution of anaerobic mechanisms	96	75	50	35
Percent contribution of aerobic mechanisms	4	25	50	65

From Stone MH, Conley MS: Bioenergetics. *In* Baechle TR: Essentials of Strength Training and Conditioning. Champaign, IL, Human Kinetics, 1994, p 78. Copyright 1994 by the National Strength and Conditioning Association. Reprinted by permission.

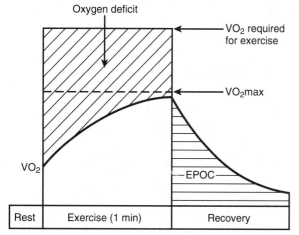

FIGURE 12–3. High-intensity, nonsteady state exercise metabolism at 80 percent of maximal power output. The required VO_2 is the oxygen uptake that would be required to sustain the exercise if such an uptake were possible to attain. Since it is not, the oxygen deficit lasts for the duration of the exercise. EPOC = excess postexercise oxygen uptake; VO_2max = maximal oxygen uptake. (From Stone MH, Conley MS: Bioenergetics. *In* Baechle TR: Essentials of Strength Training and Conditioning. Champaign, IL, Human Kinetics, 1994. Copyright 1994 by the National Strength and Conditioning Association. Reprinted by permission.)

Recovery from exercise takes place over time; the time required is based on the intensity and duration of the exercise. Low-level aerobic exercise has a very short EPOC, whereas heavy resistance training can result in a prolonged EPOC, well above resting oxygen consumption, for periods of greater than 30 minutes after the cessation of the exercise.[14,15]

From a practical standpoint, it is important in the design of resistance training programs to provide sufficient recovery time to allow for replenishment of anaerobic and aerobic sources of energy prior to the next exercise session. This takes on additional significance when resistance training is used as an adjunct to or part of the total conditioning and training program for an athlete. Elite-level power lifters, who are training only to develop maximal power in one of three events, sometimes have 7 to 10 days between training sessions to allow for adequate recovery of the muscles from the demands of the previous resistance training session.[18] When a resistance training session is only one of several training sessions in a given day for an athlete, it is critical that the relative intensity and volume of resistance training be taken into account in the total program design. Failure to allow for sufficient recovery from any training session, particularly resistance training exercise bouts, can result not only in system failure, but also in an increased probability of injury. The sports medicine clinician must work in close conjunction with the specific sport coach to ensure the proper design of not only the training program, but the recovery program as well.

RESISTANCE TRAINING FOR REHABILITATIVE PROGRAM DESIGN

Sports medicine clinicians may be involved in the development of resistance training programs from several perspectives. They should assist coaches in the design of specific resistance training programs to meet the demands of a given sport. They also must develop resistance training programs as part of the total rehabilitation program of an athlete after an injury. This section will address some of the basic adaptations that occur with resistance training, types of resistance training, methodology for documentation of resistance training, various systems of resistance training, and the design of individualized resistance and rehabilitation programs.

BASIC ADAPTATIONS THAT OCCUR WITH RESISTANCE TRAINING

The design of a resistance training program, either for sport-specific strength and conditioning or for rehabilitation of a sport-related injury, must facilitate systemic processes that allow for a physiological adaptation of the system over time.[19] The adaptation that occurs with resistance training is dependent on how much potential for adaptation exists in the athlete, as well as the process and design of the resistance training program.[19] Genetic and psychologic factors also determine the ultimate adaptation that occurs with resistance training and conditioning programs. Kraemer has found that a genetic ceiling exists for every physiologic function, and performance gains in most sports are related to the physiological adaptations in many systems.[19] Every athlete undertakes a strength and conditioning program, either for sport-specific training or rehabilitation, with his or her own genetic predisposition; potential for improvement; willingness to train appropriately; and with the underlying state of conditioning, deconditioning and injury pathomechanics that all interact to determine the adaptation that will occur as a result of resistance training and conditioning.[19] This section will focus on the adaptation that occurs within the musculoskeletal system with resistance training.

There have been several excellent and extensive reviews of the physiological effects of resistance training.[20–25] Table 12–5 provides a summary of the contrasting physiological adaptations that occur with resistance training and endurance training.[19] One of the major adaptations that occurs with resistance training is the alteration of muscle fibers. For many years it was thought that the initial adaptation to resistance training was a modification of the nervous system for the acquisition of a skill and maximal activation of the muscle.[26–28] It was speculated that the adaptations and changes in strength seen in the first 6 to 8 weeks were the result of these neural adaptations. However, Staron et al.[29] have demonstrated that skeletal adaptations can occur in various skeletal muscle fiber types in as little as 2 weeks if the training intensity is sufficiently high. Although a detailed description of human muscle physiology is beyond the scope of this chapter, the authors will review the basics of muscle fiber types and the alterations and transformations that occur in muscle fiber types with resistance training.

Skeletal muscle can best be described by two distinctly different fiber types that are classified by their contractile and metabolic characteristics.[30,31] Type I fibers (also referred to as *slow-twitch fibers*) are best suited for the performance of endurance or aerobic activities. These fibers contain large concentrations of mitochondria, myoglobin, and the enzymes necessary to allow the fibers to be fatigue resistant. Type II (or *fast-twitch*) fibers are more suited for anaerobic or power production requiring short, intense bouts of exercise. Type II fibers are larger and can fire with a faster velocity and develop greater force production. However, research from Staron et al.[29,32–35] has identified various subtypes of both type I and type II fibers, and it appears that much of the physiological adaptation that occurs with resistance training takes place in these subtypes.

There appears to be a continuum in the aerobic to anaerobic capabilities and qualities of skeletal muscle.[32] Along this continuum there are three identified subtypes: type A, which possess good aerobic and anaerobic characteristics; type B, which possess fair aerobic and poor anaerobic characteristics; and type C, which appear to be an intermediate alteration between type A and B fibers and are somewhat rare in humans.[32,33] There also appears to be an AB fiber type that serves as an intermediate step between type A and type B. These fiber types taken from a muscle biopsy sample are identified by histochemical and biochemical analyses of a muscle enzyme, myofibrillar adenosine triphosphatase (mATPase), and a total of six fiber types (I, IC, IIA, IIB, IIAB, IIC) can be distinguished based on their staining intensities and the pH level of the analyses.[32]

Figure 12–4 provides a schematic illustration of the staining intensities of the six fiber types at three pH levels.[32] It is important to know the pH level at which the fibers are tested, as type I fibers are stable in the acid ranges (staining dark) but labile in the alkaline ranges (staining light). Type II fibers are stable in the alkaline ranges (staining dark) but labile in the acid ranges (staining light). The three pH ranges are used to show transformations and fiber type conversions that occur with resistance training.[29]

Within this continuum of fiber types, there appears to be a consistent order of recruitment of fiber subtypes based on the intensity of the exercise, as follows[32,36]: type I fibers first, followed by IC, IIC, IIA, IIAB, and

---

TABLE 12–5
Comparison of Physiological Adaptations to Resistance Training and Aerobic Training

Variable	Result Following Resistance Training	Result Following Endurance Training
Performance		
Muscle strength	Increases	No change
Muscle endurance	Increases for high power output	Increases for low power output
Aerobic power	No change or increases slightly	Increases
Maximal rate of force production	Increases	No change or decreases
Vertical jump	Ability increases	Ability unchanged
Anaerobic power	Increases	No change
Sprint speed	Improves	No change or improves slightly
Muscle Fibers		
Fiber size	Increases	No change or increases slightly
Capillary density	No change or decreases	Increases
Mitochondrial density	Decreases	Increases
Fast heavy-chain myosin	Increases in amount	No change or decreases in amount
Enzyme Activity		
Creatine phosphokinase	Increases	Increases
Myokinase	Increases	Increases
Phosphofructokinase	Increases	Variable
Lactate dehydrogenase	No change or variable	Variable
Metabolic Energy Stores		
Stored ATP	Increases	Increases
Stored creatine phosphate	Increases	Increases
Stored glycogen	Increases	Increases
Stored triglycerides	May increase	Increases
Connective Tissue		
Ligament strength	May increase	Increases
Tendon strength	May increase	Increases
Collagen content	May increase	Variable
Bone density	No change or increase	Increases
Body Composition		
Percentage body fat	Decreases	Decreases
Fat-free mass	Increases	No change

From Kraemer WJ: General adaptations to resistance and endurance training programs. *In* Baechle TR: Essentials of Strength Training and Conditioning. Champaign, IL, Human Kinetics, 1994, p 131. Copyright 1994 by the National Strength and Conditioning Association. Reprinted by permission.

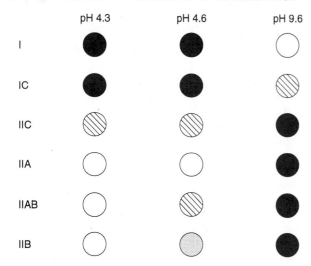

FIGURE 12–4. Schematic of histochemical fiber typing based on mATPase staining intensity following preincubation at various pH. (From Staron RS, Hikida RS: Histochemical, biochemical and ultrastructural analysis of single human muscle fibers with special reference to the C fiber population. J Histochem Cytochem 1992; 40:563–568.)

finally IIB fibers. The smaller motor units are recruited first because they are easiest to stimulate, and the larger motor units are stimulated based on the total amount of force necessary to perform the muscular contraction. Because the IIB fibers are recruited last, it has been *speculated* that the IIB fibers are the "strength" fibers and possess the greatest anaerobic potential.[30] However, the research from Staron et al. has shown that this IIB fiber is not the strength fiber, and its performance during exercise is inversely related to both aerobic and anaerobic conditioning.[37] However, because muscle is an extremely dynamic structure, fiber types can actually be transformed along the recruitment continuum. One of the primary and initial adaptations of strength training is a transformation of and reduction in the number of type IIB fibers.

Figure 12–5 presents data from a single subject before and after a high-intensity resistance training program.[29] Over time there was an adaptation in the size of the muscle fibers and a transformation of the type II fibers. High-intensity resistance training will cause a transformation of IIB fibers into IIAB and IIA fibers. In fact, in some of the subjects in this investigation and in another high-intensity resistance training study of women subjects,[36] no type IIB fibers could be found at the conclusion of the training program.[29,36] This adaptation of skeletal muscle to resistance training occurs rapidly with the initiation of high-intensity training, and as long as the athlete continues to incorporate some component of resistance training in his or her total strength and conditioning program, the adaptations will remain.

The other major adaptation that occurs in skeletal muscle with resistance training is the change in cross-sectional area of the muscle that results in hypertrophy of the muscle tissue. It appears that this increase in cross-sectional area results from an increase in the myofibrillar volume of the individual muscle fibers, not from an increase in the number of fibers per unit area.[19,24,30,38,39] There remains some debate over the muscle's ability to change the number of myofibrils (hyperplasia), with some investigators[40–42] supporting and some[43,44] rejecting the concept that the hyperplasia can be seen in humans.

The other primary forms of physiological adaptation that occur with resistance training are cellular, hormonal, connective tissue, and skeletal adaptations. Kraemer et al.[19,20] and Bandy et al.[24] provide excellent reviews of these systemic adaptations, which are summarized in Table 12–5.

Deconditioning, as might be expected, results in a reversal of many of the adaptations and training effects that are gained as the result of resistance training. Several studies have reported a reduction in cross-sectional area, a reduction in muscular enzymes, histochemical and biochemical alterations, and a regression of muscle fibers back toward control values.[45–50] Two investigations examined the effect of immobilization on the biochemical and cross-sectional areas of skeletal muscle after a period of heavy resistance training.[51,52] These studies found that the adaptations in skeletal muscle that occurred with heavy resistance training were negated and actually reversed after a period of immobilization-induced disuse; changes were particularly marked in type II fibers. Deconditioning is a significant problem for the sports medicine clinician, not only with regard to athletes who have to reduce or discontinue training as the result of an injury, but also (and perhaps more so) with regard to athletes who are just starting a conditioning program for fitness or some sporting activity. These latter individuals have been deconditioned for a significant amount of time, and the sports medicine clinician must use caution and care in the design of their resistance training program.

ADAPTATIONS TO RESISTANCE TRAINING IN SELECTED POPULATIONS

The physiological adaptations to resistance training have been well documented in healthy male subjects, both nonathletes and athletes. However, a growing number of pediatric, female, and elderly athletes have found a marked benefit in resistance training as it applies to their sports.

PEDIATRIC ATHLETES. Kraemer and Fleck[53] have extensively researched the area of resistance training for young athletes and have found it to be safe and effective if done properly. Children can improve strength and power, local muscular endurance, and balance and proprioception; prevent injuries; and develop a more positive body image and sport performance perspective with the use of appropriate resistance training. Table 12–6 provides some basic guidelines for resistance training for children.[53] It is important for the sports medicine clinician to realize that prior to puberty, the young athlete will gain significant strength and power without a concomitant increase in muscle hypertrophy. Until the child reaches puberty, he or she does not have sufficient hormonal levels to allow for the skeletal muscle hypertrophy that is seen in older resistance-trained athletes.[53,54]

Some of the most important considerations for allowing a young athlete to undertake a resistance training program are as follows:

1. Do not impose an adult training program on a child.

2. Make sure the resistance apparatus fits the child properly.
3. Do not let the child progress too quickly. It takes longer for children to adapt to resistance training loads.
4. Do not push children to get into resistance training: they are ready when *they* are ready.
5. Proper instruction in resistance training techniques is paramount.

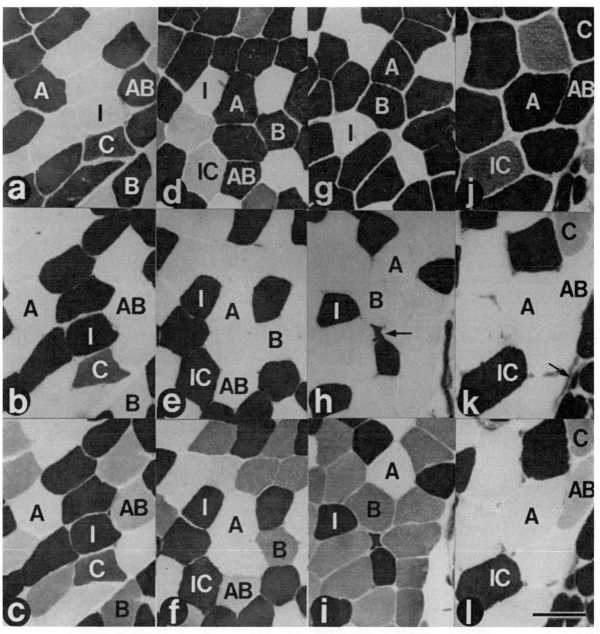

FIGURE 12–5. Serial cross-sections of muscle samples taken from male control subject at beginning *(a–c)* and end *(d–f)* of study and from male strength-trained subject at beginning *(g–i)* and after 8 weeks of high-intensity training *(j–l)*. Sections were assayed for myofibrillar ATPase activity after preincubation at pH values of 10.2 *(top row)*, 4.3 *(middle row)*, and 4.6 *(bottom row)*. Arrows = scattered atrophic fibers; I = type I; IC = type IC; C = type IIAC; A = type IIA; AB = type IIAB; B = type IIB; Bar = 100 μm. (From Staron RS et al: Skeletal muscle adaptations during early phase of heavy resistance training in men and women. J Appl Physiol 1994; 76:1247–1255.)

TABLE 12–6
Basic Guidelines for Resistance Exercise Progression in Children

Age (yr)	Considerations
≤7	Introduce child to basic exercises with little or no weight; develop the concept of a training session; teach exercise techniques; progress from body weight calisthenics, partner exercises, and lightly resisted exercises; keep volume low.
8–10	Gradually increase the number of exercises; practice exercise technique in all lifts; start gradual progressive loading of exercises; keep exercises simple; gradually increase training volume; carefully monitor toleration to the exercise stress.
11–13	Teach all basic exercise techniques; continue progressive loading of each exercise; emphasize exercise techniques; introduce more advanced exercises with little or no resistance.
14–15	Progress to more advanced youth programs in resistance exercise; add sport-specific components; emphasize exercise techniques; increase volume.
≥16	Move child to entry-level adult programs after all background knowledge has been mastered and a basic level of training experience has been gained.

Note: If a child of any age begins a program with no previous experience, start the child at beginning levels and move him or her to more advanced levels as exercise toleration, skill, amount of training time, and understanding permit.

From Kraemer WJ, Fleck SJ: Strength Training for Young Athletes. Champaign, IL, Human Kinetics, 1993, p 5. Copyright 1993 by William J. Kraemer and Steven J. Fleck. Reprinted by permission.

6. Adequate supervision to ensure proper lifting technique is critical.

FEMALE ATHLETES. Women have also significantly increased the amount of resistance training they do. Whether resistance training is used as a supplement to training for a particular sport or alone to enhance strength and muscle tone, women are becoming involved in resistance training in record numbers. Women are also involved in the competitive resistance training sports of body building, power lifting, and, most recently, Olympic lifting. Staron et al. have shown dramatically that women experience muscular adaptations similar to those seen in men, provided they are trained with a similar high-intensity resistance training program.[29,36] The National Strength and Conditioning Association (NSCA) has published a position paper on strength training for female athletes[55] providing 162 references that address the physiological and hormonal adaptations of women to resistance training, as well as considerations for resistance training program design for female athletes. This position paper is an excellent reference and would be invaluable for any sports medicine clinician who works with female athletes.

ELDERLY ATHLETES. Resistance training has also been studied with respect to the effects and adaptations of resistance training in the elderly. With the decline in strength in elderly individuals, there are concomitant increases in falls, functional decline, and impaired mobility.[56–58] Fiatarone et al.[59] studied the effects of resistance training on subjects over the age of 70 years. Their subjects trained for 45 minutes per day, 3 days per week, for 10 weeks at 80 percent of the established 1-repetition maximum (RM). This investigation found a significant increase in both muscular strength and muscle cross-sectional area. Grimby et al.[60] also used resistance training in a group of 78- to 84-year-old men and found significant increases in muscular strength and endurance in their subjects. As with any resistance training program, proper instruction, proper fit of the equipment, and proper supervision will allow resistance training to be an effective tool to increase muscular strength, endurance, and power, even in the very old.

TYPES OF RESISTANCE TRAINING

Figure 12–6 presents a strength model for the sports medicine clinician who designs resistance training programs for both athletes and nonathletes. As discussed earlier in the chapter, strength is traditionally defined as the maximal force a muscle or muscle group can generate at a specified speed of contraction.[1] Figure 12–6 divides strength into three components: maximal strength, explosive strength, and endurance strength. Athletic endeavors and specific sport skills require one or more of these types of strength, and a resistance training program must be designed to address one or all types of strengthening.

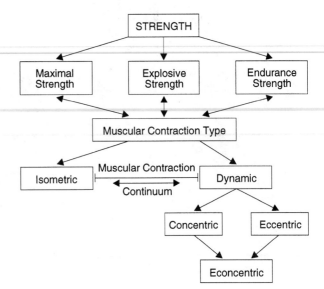

FIGURE 12–6. Theoretical model of strength and muscular contraction.

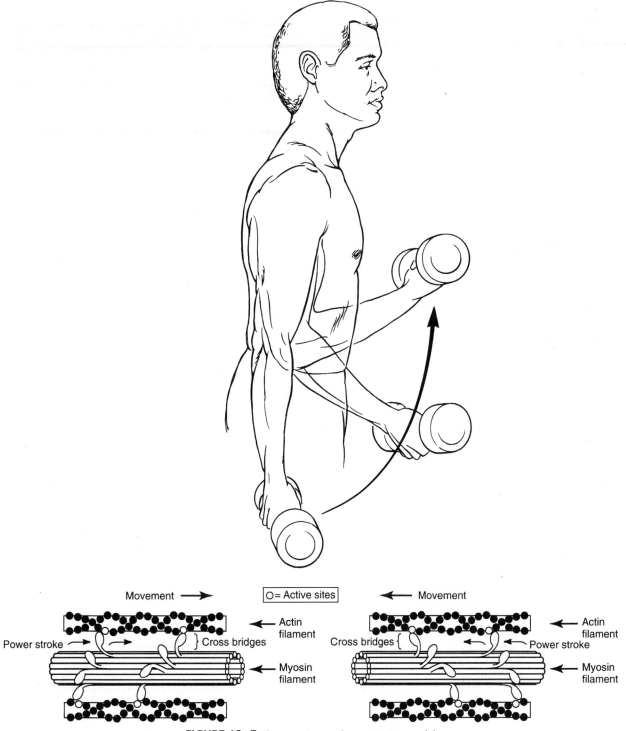

FIGURE 12–7. Concentric muscle contraction model.

TYPES OF MUSCLE CONTRACTION

Based on the amount of force needed for the strength application, the muscular contraction type will vary along a continuum from isometric to dynamic. Dynamic contractions are then further divided into three components: concentric, eccentric, and (a relatively new concept for the sports medicine clinician), econcentric muscular contractions. *Concentric* muscle contractions are defined as the shortening contraction in which tension develops as the insertion of the muscle moves toward the origin, as seen in Figure 12–7.[61] *Eccentric* contractions are those in which the muscle is lengthened under tension, when the insertion moves away from the origin, resisting or lowering the resistance against gravity, as seen in Figure 12–8.[61] It is commonly known that concentric contractions require significantly more motor units and thus more strength to move the same resistance than do eccentric contractions. Eccentric contractions require less energy expenditure, although they are thought to be related to some aspects of the postexercise muscle soreness that develops after a new or unfamiliar exercise is undertaken (see Chapter 6 for more information on postexercise muscle soreness).

Gray et al.[62] have introduced the concept of a muscular contraction that combines concentric and eccentric contraction, called an *econcentric* muscular contraction. Deusinger[63] identified a hypothetical, pseudoisometric muscle contraction that involves a controlled concentric contraction of a muscle with a concurrent eccentric muscle contraction of the same muscle as the movement occurs over two or more joints. This type of contraction is possible only for multiarticulate muscles. Because the ongoing concentric muscle contraction occurs at one joint simultaneously with the eccentric contraction over

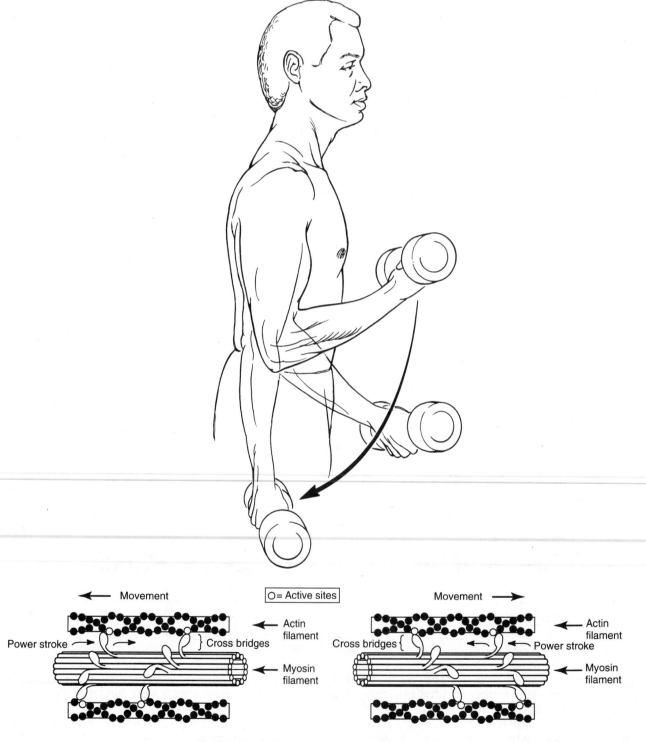

FIGURE 12–8. Eccentric muscle contraction model.

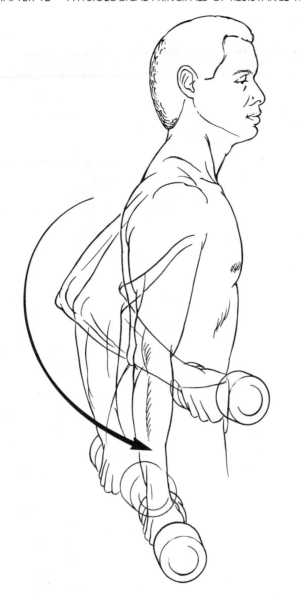

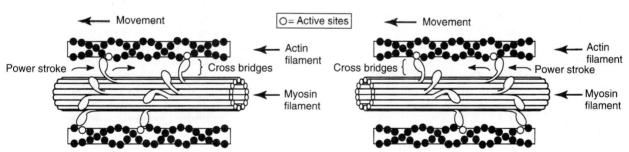

FIGURE 12—9. Econcentric muscle contraction model.

the second joint, Deusinger believed this type of contraction was due to an apparent lack of length in the multiarticulate muscle during activity. Gray et al.[62] redefined this type of contraction as econcentric, because it involves both an eccentric and a concentric contraction, but also because it is an economical type of muscular contraction in multiarticulate muscles.

Figure 12–9 presents the econcentric contraction model. The biceps brachii is a biarticulate muscle that crosses both the elbow and shoulder joints. The biceps is capable of producing flexion of either joint or controlling extension of either joint. During an activity such as lifting a dumbbell (see Fig. 12–9), the biceps works to concentrically flex the elbow, bringing the resistance close to the body. At the same time, the shoulder is extending from a forward flexed position to bring the dumbbell up in the shortest path. This shoulder extension is controlled eccentrically by the biceps at the shoulder. Thus, while the biceps is actively shorting at the elbow during flexion, it is actively lengthening at the shoulder during eccentric extension. In appearance, the biceps has not changed actual length, producing a pseudoisometric type of contraction.

In the lower extremity, contraction of the soleus during gait, either walking or running, is a prime example of an econcentric muscle contraction. The soleus is a two-joint muscle, crossing both the talocrural and subtalar joints. During the "transition period" of gait, or mid-stance, the soleus functions at the talocrural joint to decelerate the tibia eccentrically as it dorsiflexes over the fixed foot. At the same time, this same muscle tension works concentrically to create inversion of the calcaneus, assisting with the transition from pronation of the subtalar joint to supination. Again, the soleus works eccentrically at the ankle and concentrically at the subtalar joint, resulting in an econcentric contraction.

This concept of econcentrics becomes very important in the rehabilitation and training environments. Muscles and proprioceptors adapt as they are trained. Typical muscle rehabilitation and testing have relied on single joint motions and isolated evaluation and rehabilitation of a muscle at only one of its joints at a time. The dumbbell curl is a typical example: the biceps is normally rehabilitated only as it functions at the elbow. However, the biceps would be best served if it were rehabilitated as it functions at both the elbow and at the shoulder. Because most multijoint muscles are capable of pseudoisometric function, the rehabilitation and program design for resistance training should include econcentric exercises for these muscles. Specificity of training demands that the muscle be trained and rehabilitated econcentrically.

ISOMETRIC, ISOKINETIC, AND ISOTONIC TRAINING

Traditionally, three forms of muscular contractions have been used during resistance training exercises: isometric contractions, isokinetic contractions, and isotonic contractions.

ISOMETRIC TRAINING. Some of the early research in resistance training was done with isometric contractions. Isometric, or static, resistance training refers to a muscular contraction in which no apparent change in the length of the muscle takes place.[3] The muscle does not generate sufficient force against the resistance to result in movement of the resistance.

Isometrics were introduced in the early 1950s with the work of Hettinger and Muller,[64] and the definitive text on isometrics was written in 1961 by Hettinger.[65] Isometrics can result in gains of 5 to 30 percent in maximal voluntary contraction (MVC), depending on the percentage of MVC, the duration of the contraction, and the number of repetitions of the isometric contractions.[3,64–66] Strength gains with isometric contractions are limited to the specific angle of the exercise, and as a result, isometric training has not been viewed favorably as the method of choice for dynamic strengthening for sport and activity. However, one form of isometric training, functional isometrics, has specific implications in the design of the resistance training program of athletes. Functional isometrics consists of the application of isometric force and contraction at multiple angles through the functional range of motion. It has proven to be beneficial in providing strength gains at specific angles during a functional movement when the joint mechanics and muscle length relationships are less than optimal. Functional isometrics at these "sticking points" results in greater functional strength and can be used successfully as a component of a sport-specific resistance training program.[67] Figure 12–10 shows the use of functional isometrics at the sticking point of a bench press to gain strength and improve overall bench press strength.

ISOKINETIC TRAINING. Isokinetic resistance training refers to the performance of muscular contraction at some constant, predetermined speed of movement. Unlike other types of resistance training, there is no set resistance to meet; rather, the velocity of movement is set and any force applied against the equipment results in an equal reaction force.[3] The reaction force is similar to the force applied to the apparatus throughout any given range of motion, which would theoretically make it possible for a muscle to exert a continuous, maximal force throughout the predetermined range of movement.[3] Because of its accommodating resistance, isokinetics is frequently used in the rehabilitation of athletic injuries and in the testing of dynamic strength.

ISOTONIC TRAINING. Isotonic, or isodynamic, resistance training offers the sports medicine clinician the greatest flexibility and variability in the design of resistance training programs. In isotonic resistance training, the resistance stays the same, but as the resistance is moved through the range of motion, the relative force needed to move that resistance must vary. The speed of motion and the range of motion are controlled by the athlete, and these variables add to the variety of program design in isodynamic resistance training.

In isotonic (isodynamic) resistance training a variety of modalities can be used for the external resistance: free weights (dumbbells, barbells, medicine balls), body weight, or any of a plethora of machines for isolated muscle strengthening. Although isotonic or isodynamic machines are most popular in health clubs, they are very limiting in terms of range of motion, and unless they truly "fit" the individual properly, they are restricted in their ability to improve functional strengthening of the athlete. Free weights are truly free in that they do not restrict range of motion, speed of movement, or the use of multiplanar resistance training. Sport skills are rarely uniplanar or unidirectional and are rarely limited to a single joint movement or muscle function. Free weights therefore allow for the incorporation of sport-specific movement patterns and speeds of movement. With proper instruction and correct spotting techniques, free weight exercises can provide the athlete with an optimal resistance training program to address any form of strengthening that is required for a specific sport or activity.

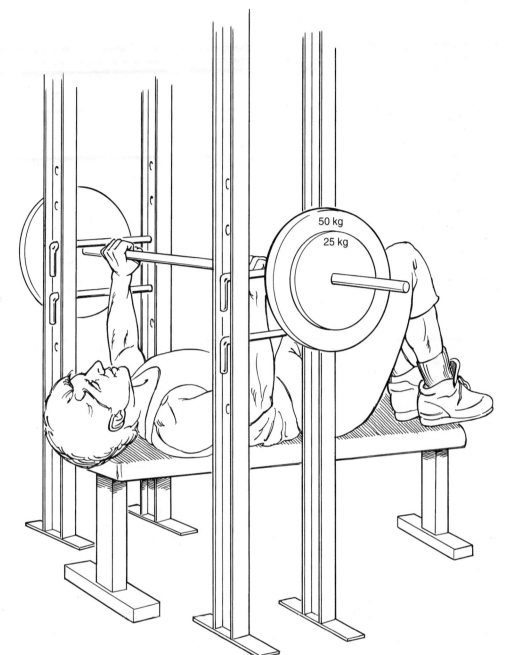

FIGURE 12–10. The use of functional isometrics at the sticking point in a bench press. (From Fleck SJ, Kraemer WJ: Designing Resistance Training Programs. Champaign, IL, Human Kinetics, 1987. Copyright 1987 by Steven J. Fleck and William J. Kraemer. Reprinted by permission.)

There are two competitive sports that utilize free weights as the resistance: power lifting and Olympic lifting.

Power Lifting. Power lifting events consist of three maximal lifts: the back squat, the bench press, and the deadlift. The squat and bench press are probably two of the most common lifts performed for any sport training and are used as a barometer of strength by many coaches. The squat, when done correctly, is a safe and excellent exercise to increase overall lower extremity and trunk strength. It is one of the most functional of our activities of daily living, and yet many sports medicine clinicians are fearful and concerned about using this lift in the resistance training programs of their athletes and patients. The NSCA has written a position statement and review of the literature on the squat as an

exercise in athletic conditioning.[68] This statement provides 69 references that support and substantiate the following nine points[68]:

1. Squats, when performed correctly and with appropriate supervision, are not only safe, but also may be a significant deterrent to knee injuries.
2. The squat exercise can be an important component of a training program to improve the athlete's ability to forcefully extend the knees and hips and can considerably enhance performance in many sports.
3. Excessive training, overuse injuries, and fatigue-related problems do occur with squats. The likelihood of such injuries and problems is substantially diminished by adherence to established principles of exercise program design.

4. The squat exercise is not detrimental to knee joint stability when performed correctly.
5. Weight training, including the squat exercise, strengthens connective tissue, including muscles, bones, ligaments, and tendons.
6. Proper form depends on the style of the squat and the muscles to be conditioned.
7. Although squatting results in high forces on the back, injury potential is low with appropriate technique and supervision.
8. Conflicting reports exist as to the type, frequency, and severity of weight training injuries. Some reports of a high injury rate may be based on biased samples. Other reports have attributed injuries to weight training, including the squat, that could have been caused by other factors.
9. Injuries attributed to the squat may result not from the exercise itself, but from improper technique, preexisting structural abnormalities, other physical activities, fatigue, or excessive training.

The squat is a safe and valuable exercise and should be included in the program design of most athletes. Proper instruction and technique can be learned from a variety of sources,[18,69] and sports medicine clinicians should learn proper techniques and applications of the squat and share them with their athletes and patients alike.

The deadlift is the third of the power lifts, and, like the squat, when done correctly and with proper form, is a valuable resistance training exercise and has many applications, not only to sport, but also to normal activities of daily living. Hatfield[18] and Garhammer[69] both provide excellent instruction in the technique and biomechanics of the deadlift, and the sports medicine professional should encourage the use of the deadlift as one of the core lifts of most resistance training programs.

Olympic Lifting. Olympic lifting is performed not just at the Olympics, but is one of the most popular international sports. The U.S. Weightlifting Federation in Colorado Springs, Colorado, has extensive literature not only on the sport, but also on training and coaching in proper technique.[70–74]

The two Olympic lifts are the snatch, in which the barbell is lifted from the floor to an overhead position in one movement, and the clean and jerk, in which the barbell is first lifted from the floor to the level of the shoulders and then is "jerked" overhead in a second movement. Figure 12–11 shows the sequential movements in the snatch, and Figure 12–12 presents the motions involved in the clean and jerk. The Olympic lifts are whole-body exercises, involving most of the major muscle groups and proprioceptors. They require extensive and integrated balance, coordination, speed, and control. They are excellent core lifts for most resistance training programs and provide superb speed, quickness, agility, and coordination training, as well as multijoint, multiplanar strength and endurance.

One of the most widely used modifications of the Olympic lifts in many resistance training programs is the power clean, a modification of the clean and jerk,

in which the barbell is quickly moved from the floor to the shoulders in one motion; this can be done in a progression from the mid-thigh (the clean pull), which allows for more rapid success and strengthening before the complete movement is attempted.[9,70,73]

The Olympic lifts require a great deal of coaching and technical instruction but can provide most athletes with an excellent strengthening and conditioning exercise.

PLYOMETRIC TRAINING

The term *plyometrics* (*plyo-* and *metrics,* meaning "measurable increases") was introduced in 1975 by Wilt,[75] who used it to describe what had been an Eastern European training technique known simply as *jump training.*[76] Plyometrics are exercises that enable a muscle to reach its maximal strength in as short a time as possible.[76,77] They allow exploitation of the muscles' cycle of lengthening and shortening to increase power.[77]

Plyometric exercises begin with rapid stretching of the muscle by an eccentric contraction, followed by a shortening of the same muscle in a concentric contraction.[77] These exercises are based on utilization of the serial elastic properties and the stretch-reflex properties of the muscle.[77] When a muscle is loaded during the eccentric contraction, there is an increase in muscle tension, which will allow for a greater concentric muscle contraction. The proprioceptors of the muscle spindles and ligaments and tendons surrounding a joint are also utilized during plyometric training, in that they play a role in presetting muscle tension and relaying sensory input from the rapidly stretching muscle for activation of the stretch reflex.[77–79]

Plyometric training is similar to any other form of resistance training in that it utilizes the overload principle to impose gradual adaptations to the muscles and joints.[78] Plyometrics can be done with the lower body, trunk, and upper body, but before a successful plyometric program can be implemented, the athlete or patient should develop a baseline level of strength.[76–79] Activities as basic and simple as walking and running incorporate plyometric principles, and as such, plyometrics should be included in all resistance training programs for both athletes and patients.

Because the demands of plyometric training are great, most strength and conditioning coaches recommend only one to three plyometric training sessions per week.[76,78] The intensity of plyometric exercise is almost always high, and therefore, progression of plyometric exercises should be from low-intensity exercises to in-place exercises, to medium-intensity exercises, and then to high-intensity exercise.[78,80] Recovery between sets, between exercises, and between training sessions is critical. Recovery between sets should be long enough to allow maximal effort on the next set (from 5–10 seconds to 2–4 minutes), and recovery between training sessions should be at least 2 days, and most often as long as 4 days.[78]

Plyometric exercises can and should be done in all three planes of motion, utilizing multiplanar movements as much as possible. Most sports skills involve at

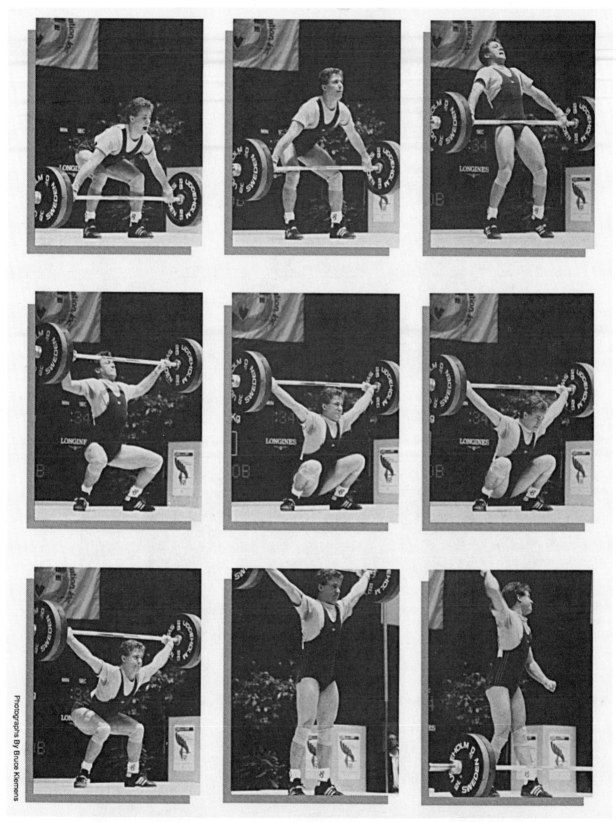

FIGURE 12–11. Sequential movements in the Olympic snatch lift. (Photographs by Bruce Klemens.)

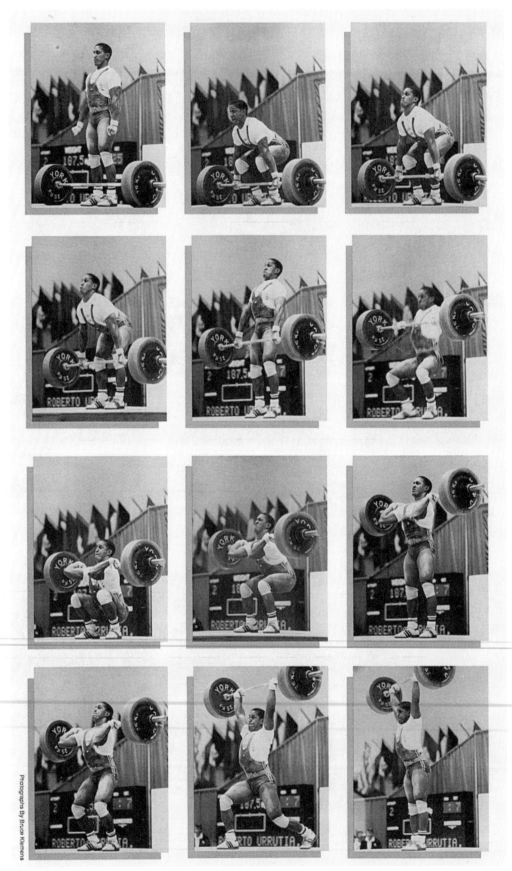

FIGURE 12–12. Sequential movements in the Olympic clean and jerk. (Photographs by Bruce Klemens.)

least two planes of movement, and therefore plyometric training should be done in at least two and preferably all three planes of movement.

One of the major goals of plyometric training is to maximize force in a minimal amount of time.[79] The transition phase between the eccentric landing and the concentric movement into the desired direction, or the amortization phase, should be as short as possible, so that more of the force is generated into the concentric phase to achieve greater distance and/or power.

PERIODIZATION OF RESISTANCE TRAINING

Vorobyev[81] and Matveyev,[82] two Eastern European physiologists, developed a model for year-round training of weight lifters called the *periodization model*. The theory behind this model was based in part on Selye's general adaptation syndrome and proposes that there are three phases of the body's adaptation when it is confronted with the stress stimulus of resistance training: shock, adaptation, and staleness.[3] In the first phase, new training results in soreness, and performance actually decreases. The body then adapts to the new stress and training stimulus, and performance then increases. In the third phase, the body has already adapted to the new stress, and no more adaptations are taking place. Periodization is utilized to avoid this staleness phase and to keep the exercise stress effective in creating new levels of performance and effective adaptation.[3,9,83]

The periodization model is made up of various cycles. A *microcycle*, the smallest period in the model, consists of one week of training. *Mesocycles* contain multiple microcycles, and the periodization model contains several distinct mesocycles. The largest cycle is the *macrocycle*, which usually refers to an entire training year. The number of mesocycles in a macrocycle is dependent on the goals of training, the number of major competitions, and the initial level of training and fitness of the athlete. Stone and O'Bryant[9] have adapted the Matveyev periodization model; their adaptation is shown in Figure 12–13 and Table 12–7.[9] The hypertrophy stage is an

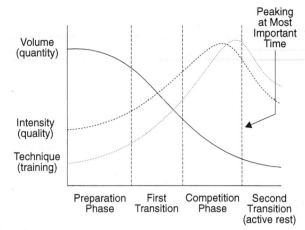

FIGURE 12–13. Matveyev's model of periodization (modified). (From Stone MH, O'Bryant HS: Weight Training: A Scientific Approach. Minneapolis, Burgess International, 1987. An imprint of Burgess International Group, Inc., Edina, MN.)

early preparation stage designed to allow the athlete to make the necessary physiological adaptations to prepare for the upcoming season. The volume of exercise is high, and the intensity is low; the emphasis on technique and technical aspects of the sport is also low.

The second stage is the basic strength stage, a later stage of preparation for the season, in which the emphasis is on near-maximal strength development, which serves as a foundation for the upcoming stages of power development. Volume starts to decrease, while intensity and technique take on larger and more important roles.

The third stage is the power/strength stage, which acts as a transition period between the preparatory and competition phases. The emphasis in this stage is generation of maximal power; thus, volume is decreased to prevent fatigue and overtraining, and the intensity and technical aspects are very high and of utmost importance.

The fourth phase is the competition or peaking/maintenance phase, in which the stress is on preparing for the competitive effort, maximizing technique, and keeping volume low to prevent injury and fatigue. The

TABLE 12–7
Theoretical Model of Strength Training (Associated with Matveyev's Periodization Model)

Phase	Preparation		Transition 1: Strength and Power	Competition: Peaking or Maintenance*	Transition 2: Active Rest
	Hypertrophy	*Basic Strength*			
Sets†	3–10	3–5	3–5	1–3	Athlete does other
Repetitions	8–12	4–6	2–3	1–3	activities dur-
Days/week	3–4	3–5	3–5	1–5	ing this period
Times/day	1–3	1–3	1–2	1	
Intensity cycle (weeks)‡	2–3/1	2–4/1	2–3/1	—	
Intensity	Low	High	High	Very high to low	
Volume	High	Moderate to high	Low	Very low	

*Peaking for sports with a definite climax or maintenance for sports with a long season such as football.
†Does not include warm-up sets.
‡Ratio of number of heavy training weeks to light training weeks.
From Stone MH, O'Bryant HS: Weight Training: A Scientific Approach. Minneapolis, Burgess International, 1987, p 123. An imprint of Burgess International Group, Inc., Edina, MN.

fifth phase, which was added to the original Matveyev model, is the active rest phase. In the current competitive environment, there really is no off-season, but the athlete needs some time to pursue other athletic interests and to "get away" from the rigors of training. Active rest is designed to allow the athlete to maintain some level of fitness, strength, and power by participating in other sports or activities unrelated to his or her competitive sport.

The concepts of periodization should be incorporated into the design of every training program, for both athletes and nonathletes. The sports medicine professional must work closely with the coach and physician in designing the necessary microcycles and mesocycles to assist the athlete or nonathlete to be maximally prepared for the competitive season or for return to work and the normal activities of daily living. The periodization model may have to be modified to fit the individual needs of the athlete or nonathlete, but the basics of the model can be adapted to fit each individual as needed.

METHODOLOGY FOR DOCUMENTATION OF RESISTANCE TRAINING EXERCISES

With the specificity of training and the need for individualization of training programs, it becomes imperative that a method of documentation of resistance training exercises be established for each athlete. The documentation system should be one that any sports medicine clinician can interpret, understand, and use to direct the individual athlete or nonathlete in the proper technique and execution of his or her resistance training program.

Gray has established a documentation system for resistance training exercises that provides information about posture, equipment, volume, intensity, body positions, exercise motions, and planes of movement[84]; the documentation chart used in this system is seen in Figure 12–14. To use this form of documentation, several definitions must be established:

1. *Anatomic position* is the reference relative to the plane of movement and starting position.
2. The *free weight motion* can be parallel with gravity, perpendicular to gravity, or a combination of these two motions.
3. The *posture* is prone, supine, side-lying, kneeling, sitting, standing, stride stance, single-leg stance, wide stance, or narrow stance.
4. The *equipment* is any apparatus that facilitates the posture to be used, such as an incline bench, preacher curl bench.
5. The *amount of weight* is the poundage being used for whatever type of equipment is being used in the exercise.
6. The *type of weight* can, for example, be a dumbbell, barbell, medicine ball, body weight, or any combination.
7. The *fixed positions* are positions other than anatomic position and should be described in increments of 20, 45, 70, 90, 110, and 135 degrees.
8. When describing motion/exercise, *movements occur from proximal to distal and from inferior to superior.*
9. *Combination movements* are documented with a slash (/) (e.g., shoulder flexion/abduction/external rotation).
10. *Transitional movements* are documented with an arrow (→) (e.g., elbow flexion → shoulder flexion).

By applying these simple rules to the documentation of resistance training exercises, any exercise can be documented and, more importantly, reproduced or replicated by another sports medicine professional who might supervise the athlete or nonathlete during a resistance training session. With its emphasis on and the importance of reproducible and accurate documentation of exercise, this system provides a simple, easy, and reproducible documentation system for any sports medicine professional.

SYSTEMS OF RESISTANCE TRAINING

Most sports medicine students have been introduced to the DeLorme system of resistance training, developed by DeLorme and Watkins in 1948, in which the athlete determines his or her 10-repetition maximum (10-RM).[85] The first set consists of 10 repetitions at 50 percent of the 10-RM resistance, the second set consists of 10 repetitions at 75 percent of the 10-RM, and the third set consists of 10 repetitions at 100 percent of the 10-RM. Although this system of resistance training has proven to be effective in the development of strength and endurance, there exist a multitude of other systems of resistance training. This section will present and describe a variety of resistance training systems to give the sports medicine professional more choices in the design of resistance training programs and allow the athlete to go beyond "three sets of 10."

A modification of the DeLorme system, developed by Knight,[86,87] is called the *Daily Adjustable Progressive*

FREE WEIGHT EXERCISE CHART © Gary Gray and Associates Physical Therapy Clinic, Inc.			
Posture/ Equipment	# / Type	Positions	Motions/ Exercise

FIGURE 12–14. Free weight exercise chart. (From Gray GW: Chain Reaction. Fort Wayne, IN, Wynn Marketing, 1993.)

Resistance Exercise (DAPRE) *System*. The DAPRE program ensures that the athlete works at or near optimal capacity for each set, thus gaining gradual adaptation to the resistance training stimulus.

The DAPRE system consists of four sets. The first set of 10 repetitions is with the "working weight," which is an estimate based on the stage of conditioning or of reconditioning after an injury. The resistance is adjusted in the second set so that six repetitions are completed against approximately 75 percent of the working resistance. The third and fourth sets are against the full working resistance, and this is where the daily adjustment of the progressive resistance takes place. In the third set, a maximal number of repetitions is attempted, and based on the number of repetitions completed, the working weight is either increased or decreased to allow approximately five to six repetitions in the fourth set. The resistance is thus adjusted daily based on performance. The DAPRE program has been successful in producing significant strength gains in a patient population.[87]

Fleck and Kraemer[3] have written the definitive text on designing resistance training programs, describing in detail a number of systems of resistance training that have proven successful in both the research and athletic environments. This section will describe some of the more popular systems of resistance training. For more detail, and for scientific references about these systems, the reader is referred to the Fleck and Kraemer text.[3]

The most popular systems of resistance training are as follows:

1. *Single-Set System:* Only one set per exercise is performed, with 8 to 12 repetitions maximum.
2. *Multiple-Set System:* Two to three warm-up sets are performed with increasing resistance, followed by two to five sets at 5 to 6 RM. This system seems to yield optimal results for increases in strength.
3. *Light-to-Heavy System:* This is the DeLorme system (see previous discussion).
4. *Heavy-to-Light System:* After a warm-up set, a set of three to six repetitions is performed with heavy weight, followed by sets with lighter weight, keeping the number of repetitions the same with each successive set.
5. *Triangle or Pyramid Program:* A warm-up set of ten repetitions is followed by successive sets in which the resistance is increased and the number of repetitions is decreased. Once 1 RM is achieved, this is reversed, with weight decreased and repetitions increased until the starting resistance and 10 to 12 repetitions are reached.
6. *Super Sets:* Two distinct exercises are performed with the same body part, one right after the other, with no rest between the two exercises.
7. *Circuit Program:* This is a series of resistance training exercises performed one right after the other with only minimal rest (10 to 15 seconds) between sets. Ten to 15 repetitions are normally performed in each set at approximately 40 to 60 percent of

the established 1 RM. The exercises in the circuit can be done per some time factor (e.g., 30 seconds of exercise, 15 seconds of rest), and the circuit is normally repeated two to four times.

8. *Peripheral Heart Action Program:* This is a variation of the circuit program in which there are several sets of five to six exercises, each for a different body part. The training session consists of four to six sequences, each containing different exercises for each body part.
9. *Tri-Set System:* Three exercises for the same body part are performed in succession, with little or no rest between the three exercises.
10. *Multi-Poundage System:* This system requires two spotters to assist with removing a set amount from the bar after each set of repetitions. The athlete does as many repetitions as possible at the given resistance, the spotters remove some of the resistance, and another set is attempted.
11. *Blitz Program:* This system exercises only one body part in one exercise session (e.g., back on Monday, chest on Wednesday, legs on Saturday, etc.).
12. *Exhaustion Set System:* The objective of this system is to perform each set to exhaustion or to degradation of proper form, rather than to a given number of repetitions.
13. *Forced Repetition System:* After completion of a set to exhaustion, a spotter assists the lifter with just enough help to allow for several more repetitions.

These are just a few systems of resistance training. The key to designing a resistance training system is to provide an adequate stimulus to elicit training adaptation, based on the needs and demands of the athlete or nonathlete. The sports medicine clinician must understand the progression and modification of a resistance training program to prevent the athlete or nonathlete from getting stale, injured, or bored with the training program. By modifying the resistance training programs or systems, variety and adaptation can be maintained, and the athlete or nonathlete will continue to make progress and enjoy the resistance training program.

INDIVIDUALIZATION OF RESISTANCE TRAINING PROGRAMS

Before the sports medicine professional can design a resistance training program for an athlete or nonathlete, he or she first must conduct a "needs analysis" to determine the exercise movements needed for the specific sport skill, the metabolic system needed for energy supplies, and appropriate exercises for injury prevention or rehabilitation.[3] The needs analysis will be different for each athlete. A key role of the sports medicine clinician is to assist the sport coach in designing individualized, specific resistance training programs for each person. All too often, an entire team performs the same resistance training workout, with no modification of volume or intensity. This is similar to all injured patients undertaking a given protocol as part of rehabilitation after an injury or surgery. Each patient progresses, heals, and responds differently to the stress of the injury. Forcing a patient to progress too rapidly may risk further damage or complications; conversely, preventing a patient from progressing more rapidly will prolong the rehabilitation process and yield a less than optimal result. Resistance training and rehabilitation programs should not be set up in protocol formats, but should have general guidelines such as when to progress, add exercises, increase volume and intensity. In this way the resistance training program is custom designed for the individual, who will then get the most out of the resistance training program.

One final consideration in the design of a sport-specific or activity-specific resistance training program: In terms of designing strengthening exercises for the lower extremities, the sports medicine clinician must assess muscle function as it pertains to the gait activities of that sport or activity. Because of the strong influence of specificity of exercise, lower extremity muscles and movements must be strengthened and trained based on their functions during gait. The term *gait-abilitation* was introduced to encourage clinicians and sports medicine professionals to design exercises for the lower extremity based on muscle function during the different stance/swing phases of gait.[88] More specifically, gait-abilitation is designed to train muscles to work in the ranges in which they will be working during the gait of the sport or activity.

The gait function of the gluteus medius is an example of a need for specificity of training. During gait, the gluteus medius functions eccentrically to stabilize the pelvis in the frontal plane.[89] This muscle function occurs during the initial loading of early stance, as well as during mid-stance. The range of motion in which the gluteus medius functions is approximately 5 to 10 degrees of hip adduction. However, in a clinical or sports medicine setting, the hip is typically strengthened in a position of abduction through a range of 0 to 20 degrees of abduction. With regard to the actual function of the gluteus medius, it has a reverse muscle action on the pelvis during gait. During the stance phase, the gluteus medius controls the frontal plane drop of the pelvis at the hip by stabilizing the pelvis. The gluteus medius must be trained to stabilize the pelvis on the femur, not to abduct the femur at the hip.

Strengthening muscles and joints based on gait simply follows the concept of specificity of exercise. Lower extremity muscles must be trained in terms of their function (e.g., walking, running, jumping) and in the ranges they will function during these activities. The sports medicine clinician is encouraged to closely examine the biomechanics of gait of the athlete's sport or activity of daily living and to design exercises that closely replicate these functions. This requires a thorough appreciation and understanding of joint kinematics and joint positions during gait. Keeping gait in mind can ensure specificity of training as an adjunct to resistance training and rehabilitation programs.

SUMMARY

The sports medicine clinician has a major responsibility to the athlete and coach in the design of a specific and appropriate resistance training program to maximize the athlete's abilities and potential. With consideration of the bioenergetics of muscle contraction, the physiology and adaptation of muscle during resistance training, and the implementation of a sport-specific, individualized resistance training program, the athlete or nonathlete will get the most out of a resistance training program and will have maximal functional abilities.

REFERENCES

1. Knuttgen HG, Kraemer WJ: Terminology and measurement in exercise performance. J Appl Sport Sci Res 1987; 1:1–10.
2. Harman E: The biomechanics of resistance training. *In* Baechle TR (ed): Essentials of Strength Training and Conditioning. Champaign, IL, Human Kinetics, 1994, p 29.
3. Fleck SJ, Kraemer WJ: Designing Resistance Training Programs. Champaign, IL, Human Kinetics, 1987.
4. Stone MH, Conley MS: Bioenergetics. *In* Baechle TR (ed): Essentials of Strength Training and Conditioning. Champaign, IL, Human Kinetics, 1994, p 67.
5. Astrand PO: Textbook of Work Physiology. New York, McGraw-Hill, 1986.
6. O'Shea JP: Scientific Principles and Methods of Strength Fitness. Reading, MA, Addison-Wesley, 1976.
7. Goldspink G, Larson RE, Davies RE: The immediate energy supply and cost of maintenance of isometric tension for different muscles in the hamster. Z Verg Physiol 1970; 66:389–397.
8. Meyer RA, Terjung RL: Differences in ammonia and adenylate metabolism in contracting fast and slow muscle. Am J Physiol 1979; 237:C11–C18.
9. Stone MH, O'Bryant H: Weight Training: A Scientific Approach. Minneapolis, Burgess International, 1987.
10. Nakamura Y, Schwartz S: The influence of hydrogen ion concentration calcium binding and release by skeletal muscle sarcoplasmic reticulum. J Gen Physiol 1972; 59:22–32.
11. Magaria R, Edwards HT, Dill DB: The possible mechanism of contracting and paying oxygen debt and the role of lactic acid in muscular contraction. Am J Physiol 1933; 106:687–714.
12. Brooks GA, Fahey TD: Exercise Physiology: Human Bioenergetics and Its Applications. New York, Wiley, 1984.
13. Dohmeier TE, Farrel PA, Foster C, Greenisen M: Metabolic responses to submaximal and maximal timed interval squats. Med Sci Sport Exerc 1984; 16:126.
14. Scala D: Oxygen uptake, oxygen debt and energy cost of high volume non-circuit Olympic style weight lifting. Master's thesis, Auburn University, 1984.
15. Stone MH, Wilson GD, Blessing D, Rozenek R: Olympic weight-lifting: Metabolic consequences of a workout. *In* Science of Weightlifting. Del Mar, CA, Academic, 1979, pp 54–67.
16. Vandewalle H, Peres G, Monod H: Standard anaerobic exercise tests. Sports Med 1976; 4:268–289.
17. Withers RT, Sherman WM, Clark DG, et al: Muscle metabolism during 30, 60 and 90 seconds of maximal cycling on an airbraked ergometer. Eur J Appl Physiol 1991; 63:354–362.
18. Hatfield FC: Powerlifting, A Scientific Approach. Chicago, Contemporary Books, 1981.
19. Kraemer WJ: General adaptations to resistance and endurance training programs. *In* Baechle TR (ed): Essentials of Strength Training and Conditioning. Champaign, IL, Human Kinetics, 1994, p 127.
20. Kraemer WJ, Dechenes MR, Fleck SJ: Physiological adaptations to resistance exercise. Sports Med 1988; 6:246–256.
21. Kraemer WJ, Fleck SJ, Dechenes MR: Factors in exercise prescription of resistance training. NSCA J 1988; 10:36–41.

22. Kraemer WJ, Daniels WL: Physiological effects of training. *In* Bernhardt DB: Sports Physical Therapy. New York, Churchill Livingstone, 1986, p 29.

23. Stone MH, Fleck SJ, Triplett NT, Kraemer W: Health and performance related potential of resistance training. Sports Med 1991; 11:210–231.

24. Bandy WD, Lovelace-Chandler V, McKitrick-Bandy B: Adaptation of skeletal muscle to resistance training. J Orthop Sports Phys Ther 1990; 12:248–255.

25. Costill DL, Coyle EF, Fink WF, et al: Adaptations in skeletal muscle following strength training. J Appl Physiol 1979; 46:96–99.

26. Enoka RM: Muscle strength and its development. Sports Med 1988; 6:146–168.

27. Jones DA, Rutherford OM, Ward A: Physiological changes in skeletal muscle as a result of strength training. Q J Exp Physiol 1989; 74:233–256.

28. Moritani T: Time course of adaptations during strength and power training. *In* Komi PV (ed): Encyclopedia of Sports Medicine: Strength and Power in Sports. London, Blackwell Scientific, 1992, p 266.

29. Staron RS, Karapondo DL, Kraemer WJ, et al: Skeletal muscle adaptations during early phase of heavy resistance training in men and women. J Appl Physiol 1994; 76:1247–1255.

30. McArdle WD, Katch FI, Katch VL: Exercise Physiology: Energy, Nutrition and Human Performance. Philadelphia, Lea & Febiger, 1991.

31. Armstrong RB: Muscle fiber recruitment patterns and their metabolic correlates. *In* Horton ES, Terjung RL: Exercise Nutrition and Energy Metabolism. New York, Macmillan, 1988.

32. Staron RS, Hikida RS: Histochemical, biochemical and ultrastructural analyses of single human muscle fibers with special reference to the C fiber population. J Histochem Cytochem 1992; 40:563–568.

33. Staron RS, Malicky ES, Leonardi MJ, et al: Muscle hypertrophy and fast fiber conversion in heavy resistance trained women. Eur J Appl Physiol 1990; 60:71–79.

34. Staron RS, Johnson P: Myosin polymorphism and differential expression in adult human skeletal muscle. Comp Biochem Physiol B Comp Biochem 1993; 106:463–475.

35. Staron RS: Correlation between myofibrillar ATPase activity and myosin heavy chain composition in single human muscle fibers. Histochemistry 1991; 96:21–24.

36. Staron RS, Leonardi MJ, Karapondo DL, et al: Strength and skeletal muscle adaptations in heavy resistance trained women after detraining and retraining. J Appl Physiol 1991; 70:631–640.

37. Prince FP, Hikida RS, Staron RS, et al: A morphometric analysis of human muscle fibers with relation to fiber types and adaptations to exercise. J Neurol Sci 1981; 49:165–179.

38. Luithis JM, Howald H, Claasen H, et al: Structural changes in skeletal muscle tissue with heavy resistance exercise. Int J Sports Med 1986; 7:123–127.

39. MacDougall JD, Sale DG, Elder GCB, et al: Ultrastructural properties of human skeletal muscle following heavy resistance training and immobilization. Med Sci Sports 1976; 8:72.

40. Schoutens A, Laurent E, Poortmans JR: Effects of inactivity and exercise on bone. Sports Med 1989; 7:71–81.

41. MacDougall JD, Sale DG, Elder GCB, et al: Muscle ultrastructure characteristics of elite powerlifters and bodybuilders. Med Sci Sports Exerc 1980; 2:131.

42. Tesch PA, Larson L: Muscle hypertrophy in bodybuilders. Eur J Appl Physiol 1982; 49:310.

43. MacDougall JD, Sale DG, Alway SE, et al: Muscle fiber number in biceps brachii in bodybuilders and control subjects. J Appl Physiol 1984; 57:1399–1403.

44. Chi MY, Hintz CS, Coyle EF, et al: Effects of detraining on enzymes of energy metabolism in individual human muscle fibers. Am J Physiol 1983; 244:C276–C287.

45. Staron RS, Hagerman FC, Hikida RS: The effects of detraining on an elite power lifter. J Neurol Sci 1981; 51:247–257.

46. Graves JE: Effect of reduced training frequency on muscular strength. Int J Sports Med 1988; 9:316–319.

47. Thorstensson A: Observations on strength training and detraining. Acta Physiol Scand 1977; 100:491–493.

48. Hakkinen K, Komi PV: Electromyographic changes during strength training and detraining. Med Sci Sports Exerc 1983; 15:455–460.

49. Simoneau JA, Lortie G, Boulay MR, et al: Effects of two high intensity intermittent training programs interspaced by detraining on human skeletal muscle and performance. Eur J Appl Physiol 1987; 56:516–521.

50. Moore RL, Hutton RS: Effect of training/detraining on submaximal exercise response in humans. J Appl Physiol 1987; 63:1719–1724.

51. MacDougall JD, Elder GCB, Sale DG, et al: Biochemical adaptation of human skeletal muscle to heavy resistance exercise and immobilization. J Appl Physiol 1977; 43:700–703.

52. MacDougall JD, Ward GR, Sale DG, et al: Effects of strength training and immobilization on human muscle fibers. Eur J Appl Physiol 1980; 43:25–34.

53. Kraemer WJ, Fleck SJ: Strength Training for Young Athletes. Champaign, IL, Human Kinetics, 1993.

54. Kraemer WJ, Fry AC, Frykman PN, et al: Resistance training and youth. Pediatr Exerc Sci 1989; 1:336–350.

55. National Strength and Conditioning Association: Position paper on strength training for female athletes. Lincoln, NE, NSCA, 1990.

56. Fiatarone MA, Evans WJ: Exercise in the oldest old. Top Geriatr Rehab 1990; 5:63–77.

57. Bendall MJ, Bassey EF, Pearson MB: Factors affecting walking speed of elderly people. Age Ageing 1989; 18:327–332.

58. Vellas B, Baumgartner RN, Wayne SJ: Relationship between malnutrition and falls in the elderly. Nutrition 1992; 8:105–108.

59. Fiatarone MA, O'Neill EF, Ryan ND, et al: Exercise training and nutritional supplementation for physical frailty in very elderly people. N Engl J Med 1994; 330:1769–1775.

60. Grimby G, Aniansson A, Hedberg M, et al: Training can improve muscle strength and endurance in 78–84 year old men. J Appl Physiol 1992; 73:2517–2523.

61. Edington DW, Edgerton VR: The Biology of Physical Activity. Boston, Houghton Mifflin, 1976.

62. Gray GW, Cipriani DJ, Falkel JE: Econcentrics—a theoretical model for muscle function. J Orthop Sport Phys Ther. Submitted for publication.

63. Deusinger RH: Biomechanics in clinical practice. Phys Ther 1984; 64:1860–1868.

64. Hettinger R, Muller E: Muskelleistung und muskeltraining. Arbeits Physiol 1953; 15:111–126.

65. Hettinger R: Physiology of Strength. Springfield, IL, Charles C Thomas, 1961.

66. Petrofsky JS: Isometric Exercise and Its Clinical Implications. Springfield, IL, Charles C Thomas, 1982.

67. Jackson A, Jackson T, Hnatek J, et al: Strength development: Using functional isometrics in an isotonic strength training program. Res Q 1985; 56:234–237.

68. National Strength and Conditioning Association: The squat exercise in athletic conditioning: A position statement and review of the literature. Lincoln, NE, NSCA, 1992.

69. Garhammer J: Weight lifting and training. *In* Vaughn CL (ed): Biomechanics of Sport. Boca Raton, FL, CRC Press, 1989.

70. U.S. Weightlifting Federation: Coaching Manual. Volume I: Technique. Colorado Springs, CO, USWF, 1986.

71. U.S. Weightlifting Federation: Coaching Manual. Volume II: General Physical Training for the Weightlifter. Colorado Springs, CO, USWF, 1986.

72. U.S. Weightlifting Federation: Coaching Manual. Volume III: Training Program Design. Colorado Springs, CO, USWF, 1986.

73. U.S. Weightlifting Federation: Coaching Accreditation Course Manual. Colorado Springs, CO, USWF, 1991.

74. U.S. Weightlifting Federation: Safety Manual. Colorado Springs, CO, USWF, 1990.

75. Wilt F: Plyometrics—what it is and how it works. Athlet J 1975; 55:89–90.

76. Chu DA: Jumping into Plyometrics. Champaign, IL, Human Kinetics, 1992.

77. Chu DA: Plyometric Exercises with the Medicine Ball. Livermore, CA, Bittersweet, 1989.

78. Allerheiligen WB : Speed Development and Plyometric Training. *In* Baechle TR (ed): Essentials of Strength Training and Conditioning. Champaign, IL, Human Kinetics, 1994, p 314.

79. Radcliffe JC, Farentinos RC: Plyometrics: Explosive Power Training. Champaign, IL, Human Kinetics, 1985.

80. Allerheiligen WB: Poke Power Training Manual. Ft. Collins, CO, 1992.
81. Vorobyev AN: A Textbook of Weightlifting. Budapest, International Weightlifting Federation, 1978.
82. Matveyev L: Fundamentals of Sport Training. Moscow, Progress Press, 1981.
83. Wathan D: Periodization: Concepts and applications. *In* Baechle TR (ed): Essentials of Strength Training and Conditioning. Champaign, IL, Human Kinetics, 1994, p 459.
84. Gray GW: Chain reaction. Fort Wayne, IN, Wynn Marketing, 1993.
85. DeLorme TL, Watkins AL: Techniques of progressive resistance exercise. Arch Phys Med 1948; 29:263–273.
86. Knight KL: Knee rehabilitation by the daily adjustable progressive resistive exercise technique. Am J Sports Med 1979; 7:336–337.
87. Knight KL: Quadriceps strengthening with the DAPRE technique: Case studies with neurological implications. Med Sci Sports Exerc 1985; 17:646–650.
88. Cipriani DJ: Gait Re-Defined. Gait-Abilitation: A Basic Approach to Rehabilitation. Toledo, OH, MCO, 1994.
89. Winter D: The Biomechanics and Motor Control of Human Gait. Waterloo, ONT, Waterloo Press, 1988, p 46.

CHAPTER 13

Return to Competition: Functional Rehabilitation

M A R K   A .   A N D E R S O N   *PhD, PT, ATC*
T E R R I   L .   F O R E M A N   *MS, PT, SCS*

The ultimate goal of rehabilitation of an injured athlete is the restoration of function to the greatest possible degree in the shortest possible time, thus allowing the athlete to safely and quickly return to athletic competition. Although it is virtually impossible to speed up the normal healing process following an injury, much can be done to optimize the healing environment, ensuring that nothing impedes the progress of healing. In order for this to occur, injured athletes must participate in an appropriately designed functional rehabilitation program. Such a program must take into account the normal phases of healing while addressing the specific needs of individual athletes in terms of preparing them for the physical demands they will encounter when they return to competition. Failure to address both normal healing parameters and sports-specific requirements will delay the successful completion of the rehabilitation program and ultimately place athletes at risk for reinjury or diminished performance.

CLINICAL VERSUS FUNCTIONAL REHABILITATION GOALS

In order to return the athlete to competition, the sports rehabilitation team, consisting of the physician, the physical therapist, the athletic trainer, the athlete, and the coach, must identify both clinical and functional goals for the athlete (Table 13–1). The successful attainment of all clinical goals is in no way an indication that the athlete is ready to return to competition. The athlete must also successfully meet all functional goals set by the sports rehabilitation team before clearance is given to return to full sports activity.

THE GOAL-ORIENTED APPROACH TO REHABILITATION

Athletes are goal oriented, and it is often difficult to limit their activities long enough to allow injuries to heal. Because of this, the rehabilitation program for injured athletes must also be goal oriented and designed to return them to their previous level of competition as quickly as possible. The most frequently asked question by injured athletes is "When can I return to training?" When the answer is given in terms of a specific time period, for example, a certain number of days or weeks, the athlete may be returned to sports competition either too soon or not soon enough. By establishing sequential rehabilitation goals that an athlete must meet before progressing in the rehabilitation program, the sports rehabilitation team can be assured that an injured athlete is ready to return to competition as quickly and as safely as possible.

The use of the goal-oriented approach to rehabilitation has other advantages.[1] It establishes goals that athletes can understand and shows them the role that they must play in the process. Involving athletes in the planning of these goals increases their involvement in the rehabilitation process. The goal-oriented approach also builds short-term success into the long rehabilitation process. This is important, because it improves the athletes' mental outlook and decreases the amount of discouragement they feel about being unable to participate in athletics. By setting a series of attainable goals for the athlete, a therapist or trainer is able to establish guidelines for re-evaluation as well as avoid the "time trap"—when an athlete complains, "You said that I would be back to training in 2 weeks." Finally, the goal-oriented approach to rehabilitation ensures consistency of information and understanding among the physician, the therapist, the trainer, the athlete, and often the coach.

In order to attain selected goals, the rehabilitation process must be designed in a sequential, step-by-step progression, with each step requiring slightly more skill or demanding slightly more ability and more involvement on the part of the athlete than the previous level. The type and severity of each athletic injury will dictate where this progression will begin. However, the last step, in most instances, will be resumption of sports activity.

In order to design an appropriate individualized rehabilitation program, one must understand the demands placed on individual athletes by their sport or event. With such an understanding, it is possible to design and implement a rehabilitation program based on the SAID (specific adaptation to imposed demands) principle. Such a program attempts to prepare athletes, through the rehabilitation process, to meet the specific demands of their sport or event (Table 13–2).

What might be considered "normal" strength, range of movement, and endurance for most patients in rehabilitation would probably be considered inadequate for most athletes.[2] The use of a sports parameter rating scale, as developed by Kibler,[3] may be helpful in determining the relative contribution of these performance factors in various sporting activities (Table 13–3). By placing athletes undergoing rehabilitation in controlled environments that mimic the requirements of their sport, the chances for reinjury after return to sports participation are lessened.

ASSESSING AND TREATING THE INJURY

The formulation of initial clinical goals and consequent management of any athletic injury begin with assessment and treatment. The injury may be significant enough to produce typical signs and symptoms of acute inflammation, or it may be subclinical, producing no overt signs or symptoms. In either case, following tissue repair, functional biomechanical deficits in the injured and surrounding tissue may persist, producing altered mechanics and substitution patterns. Rehabilitation, therefore, should not be solely symptom based. It should be assumed that injured athletes have a functional disability until they complete a rehabilitation program designed to address all factors necessary for successful return to competition. Failure to address these problems will result in performance drop-off, recurrent injury, or both.[4]

Initial treatment during the acute phase of healing should be directed toward alleviating the signs and symptoms of acute injury. This may be accomplished by following the acronym PRICED, which stands for protection, rest, ice, compression, elevation, and drugs.[5]

Protection is utilized to prevent reinjury or to keep an injury from becoming worse. It may involve the use of padding, shock attenuation material, or external supports for the injured area. Rest may also be necessary in the acute management of an injured athlete. However, to tell a serious athlete to stop exercising is ineffective. Therefore, when dealing with athletes, rest should never mean inactivity. Instead, the concept of early protected motion should be introduced. This is a physiologically sound principle that is helpful in meeting the goals of rehabilitation (Table 13–4).[4,6,7]

In cases in which full weight bearing will increase the severity of the injury, such as with a grade II ankle sprain, rest may involve the use of crutches or other assistive devices to allow healing of the injured part. However, nothing precludes the athlete from exercising the uninvolved extremities to maintain strength, flexibility and cardiovascular fitness until weight-bearing activities in the injured extremity can be initiated safely.

TABLE 13–1
Clinical versus Functional Rehabilitation Goals

Clinical Goals

Measurable goals that can be met in a clinical setting
May relate to parameters such as strength, range of motion, swelling, pain, cardiovascular endurance, or muscular endurance

Functional Goals

Goals that relate to the factors required for the athlete to successfully return to athletic competition
May relate to parameters such as speed, agility, power, and sport- or position-specific endurance

---

TABLE 13–2
Sport-Specific Demands

- Specific biomechanical demands
- Level of strength
- Muscular endurance
- Cardiovascular endurance
- Amount of range of movement
- Skill level necessary for successful performance

TABLE 13–3
Sports Parameter Rating Scale

Sport	Flexibility	Strength	Speed	Anaerobic	Aerobic
Football	3	4	4	3	2
Halfbacks	3	4	4	4	3
Basketball	3	3	4	4	4
Baseball	3	3	4	4	2
Tennis	4	2	4	4	3
Swimming	4	4	3	2	4
Sprinters	4	4	2	4	2
Long-distance running	3	2	2	2	4
Sprinting	3	3	2	4	2
Golf	3	4	3	2	1
Soccer	3	2	3	4	4
Bicycling	3	3	4	3	4
Ice skating	3	2	4	3	4
Skiing	3	3	4	3	2
Volleyball	3	2	4	4	2
Cheerleading	3	3	4	2	2

4, maximally required for optimum performance (aerobic endurance in running, strength in football); 3, synergistic for optimum performance (flexibility in basketball, speed [power] in tennis); 2, necessary for injury reduction (strength in tennis, aerobic endurance in football); 1, minimally needed (aerobic endurance in golf).
From Kibler WB: The Sports Preparation Fitness Examination. Champaign, IL, Human Kinetics, Publishers. Copyright 1990 by W. Ben Kibler. Reprinted by permission.

TABLE 13–4
Potential Advantages of Early Motion[4,6,7]

- Decreased disuse effects
- Stimulation of collagen fiber growth and realignment
- Limitation of adhesion and contracture formation
- Maintenance of articular cartilage
- Better maintenance of joint proprioception

Rest may also mean modification of activities or alternative activities that give the injury an opportunity to heal. Allowing athletes to participate in activities that permit near normal function but do not interfere with the healing process means that functional athletic skills will usually return more quickly.[8] Activity modification may be implemented by decreasing the amount of activity, such as decreasing mileage for a runner, to allow an injury to heal. For other athletes, changing both the amount and the intensity of activity may be required to relieve the symptoms, such as decreasing a runner's mileage as well as changing to a softer surface.

For some athletes, due to the nature of their injuries, activity modification may not be the solution. For these athletes, specific athletic participation, regardless of where or how it is done, may be the cause of the problem. In such cases, in order to allow healing to occur and to avoid the effects of inactivity, alternative activities must be suggested. Preferably, these alternative activities should be bilateral and reciprocal in nature, should allow the athlete to maintain cardiovascular fitness, and should not increase or aggravate the athlete's injury.

There are many activities that can be used as an alternative form of exercise for injured athletes. Early in the rehabilitation of lower extremity injuries, it is critical to develop leg control. This may be accomplished by initiating bilateral mini-squats and calf raises.[9,10] As rehabilitation progresses, lunges (Fig. 13–1) or lateral step-ups (Fig. 13–2) may be added to the program.

Bicycling is one of the most commonly used forms of alternative exercise. Cycling is a freewheeling, open system that enables the foot to be in pedal contact with a resistive force but without impact loading. The therapist or trainer may utilize either an upright or a recumbent bicycle in the rehabilitation program. It is believed that the recumbent bicycle changes the way the quadriceps and hamstring work in the traditional upright bicycle, due to the change in lower extremity position.[11] Such a position may closer mimic functional activities for some athletes. Cycling intensity may be varied, depending on the terrain and gear ratio. In the traditional upright bicycle, if motion of a particular weight-bearing joint needs to be controlled due to pain or restricted motion, hip, knee, and ankle range of movement can be somewhat influenced by seat height position. However, the bicycle should not be used to forcefully gain lower extremity motion because of the increased risk of reinjury to healing tissues.[12] Other variable parameters include length of lever arm to the pedal, angulation of the pedal, and resistance of

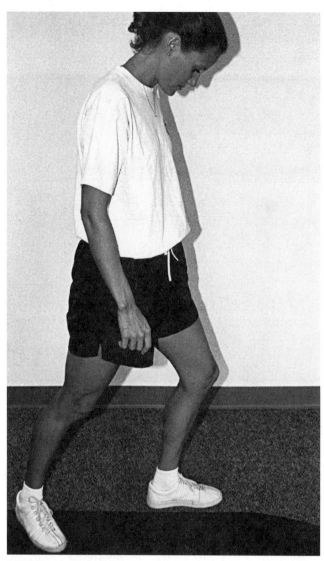

FIGURE 13–1. Lunges.

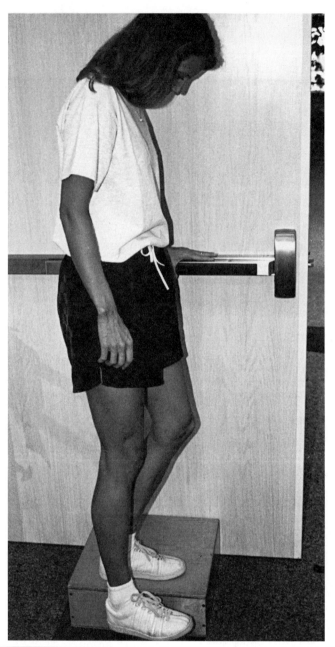

FIGURE 13–2. Lateral step-ups.

motion.[11] If pain or restriction of motion makes it impossible for an injured athlete to cycle using both extremities, unilateral cycling on a bicycle ergometer may be used to help the athlete maintain some degree of cardiovascular endurance.

Another alternative exercise involves retrorehabilitation. Retrorehabilitation is the performance of certain activities in a reverse direction.[11] The most common forms are retrowalking (Fig. 13–3) and retrorunning. Compared with forward walking or running, retrorunning has been shown to decrease knee joint loading while increasing quadriceps strength and power.[13,14] In addition, retrorunning has been shown to be a good method for stimulating isometric and concentric oblique vastus medialis and vastus lateralis muscle action, which would be helpful in clinical rehabilitation programs designed to strengthen the knee extensors.[15]

If it is unnecessary to restrict an athlete's weight bearing but the therapist or trainer wishes to control or minimize the ground reaction forces transmitted to an injured area, there are several forms of alternative exercise that may be utilized. Indoor cross-country ski machines, exercise cycles, and skating machines are useful in helping to maintain cardiovascular fitness. Roller skates, roller blades, or ice skates may be used by an athlete to help maintain fitness while minimizing potentially harmful ground reaction forces. Reciprocal climbers, either vertical climbers or stair climbers, are also useful and may be used by an athlete during the rehabilitation process.

Many therapists employ pool therapy or water exercise during rehabilitation.[9,10,16,17] Swimming is an excellent way to exercise all extremities while providing support for the injured part. The buoyancy provided by the water minimizes the stress placed on the injured part; resistance for other parts may be facilitated by increasing drag forces through the use of paddles or flotation devices, increasing the body surface area in contact with the water, or increasing the velocity of movement of a part through the water. Swimming, however, is not a very sport-specific exercise for athletes other than swimmers. For injured athletes who wish to continue to exercise in a sport-specific manner, a flotation vest may be used to allow them to exercise in deep water without sinking or touching the bottom. Injured athletes may also exercise in waist- to chest-high water without a flotation device if their injuries allow. This allows the motion of running without the stress and impact loading associated with ground running. Athletes may do endurance work, such as interval work in the pool, or they may incorporate other sport-specific motions such as hopping, kicking, or cycling into their pool programs.[16,17] Again, the principles of buoyancy and drag may be utilized to the advantage of the athlete. It must be remembered, however, that skin friction is 790 times greater in water than in air, thus significantly increasing resistance to all movements as well as significantly increasing energy expenditure by the athlete.[18]

The final principles of acute management—ice, compression, elevation, and drugs—are the cornerstone for managing the signs and symptoms of acute inflammation. Whenever possible, they should be used concurrently for maximum benefit and results and to facilitate a quick but safe progression to more functional activities. It has been shown that pain and effusion inhibit muscle activation and decrease strength. Control of both these factors increases the effectiveness of rehabilitation by allowing comfortable, coordinated motion with the avoidance of substitute patterns of movement.[7,19]

Because of its ability to relieve pain and decrease muscle spasm, ice may be used in conjunction with therapeutic exercise (cryokinetics) to facilitate early mobilization and minimize the effects of immobilization. The use of cryokinetics should be restricted to the clinic, where exercise intensity can be controlled and monitored.

To further assist athletes in the management of an acute injury, the use of nonsteroidal anti-inflammatory drugs (NSAIDs) may be beneficial.[20] Although the inflammatory process is part of normal healing, prolonged or chronic inflammation may be deleterious to athletes who are trying to achieve the goal of a safe and speedy return to athletic participation. By helping to control the pain and swelling associated with inflammation, anti-inflammatory medications may allow athletes to progress to functional activities more quickly in their rehabilitation programs.[4] Some concerns have been expressed regarding the use of NSAIDs during the acute inflammatory stage of healing. They may interfere with tissue repair and remodeling,[21] and if they are used, dosage, timing, and potential side effects should be considered.[4]

Following injury and the subsequent management of the acute signs and symptoms, rehabilitation should involve a variety of factors designed to prepare the athletes for their ultimate return to athletic competition.

These factors include strength, flexibility, muscular and cardiovascular endurance, proprioception, power, speed, agility, and other sport-specific skills (Fig. 13–4).

CLINICAL REHABILITATION GOALS

STRENGTH

The maintenance or redevelopment of strength in an injured athlete is the primary step in the rehabilitation progression. Initial treatment is directed at the tissues directly affected by the injury, but it must be remembered that the goal is to rehabilitate the athlete, not just the injury.

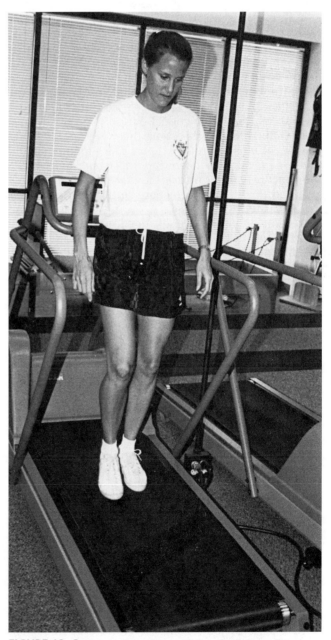

FIGURE 13–3. Retrowalking (Accumill Treadmill, Pacer Fitness Systems, Inc., Belton, TX).

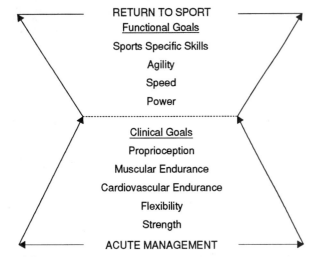

FIGURE 13–4. Rehabilitation factors from acute management to return to competition.

The concept of specificity continues to be of paramount importance when beginning this phase of the rehabilitation program. Therefore, strengthening exercises should be as functional or sport-specific as possible. Individual muscle actions must be integrated into functional muscle group actions. The program should address the athletes' needs in terms of specific exercise movements (specific muscles used, range of movement required, type of contraction, and loading needs), primary metabolism utilized during the sport, and correction or prevention of functional biomechanical deficits.[18,22]

Gambetta[23] described strength as a continuum, moving from general strength to special strength to specific strength. General strength is gained with traditional weight training exercises such as the bench press, squat, or military press; these do not attempt to imitate specific sports skills. Movement with resistance that takes into account the joint dynamics of a particular sport, such as the use of weighted balls in a throwing program, is used to develop special strength. Specific strength is developed through the use of exercises such as a walk-jog-run program, with specificity regarding the mechanics and speed as well as the imitation of the specific joint action of a desired skill.

With this philosophy, increasing measurable strength does not lead to improved sports performance or more effective rehabilitation. These can be accomplished only by developing functional strength. The development of functional strength requires that the athlete be able to control body weight, for example, through the use of pull-ups, dips, step-ups, or other similar exercises, before external resistance is added. Developing functional strength helps develop balance, proprioception, and synergistic muscle action required for more sport-specific activities. Functional strength exercises also utilize functional movement patterns, incorporating multiplane and multijoint movements instead of isolated muscle or joint exercises. The use of dumbbells and free weights is one of the best methods for increasing functional strength, because they allow for

unilateral and bilateral functional movement patterns. They do, however, require the athlete to have good unilateral and bilateral strength in order to control the weight.

A typical progression for an athlete such as an offensive lineman involved in a functional strength training program might be bench press for the development of general strength, heavy blocking dummy for the development of special strength, and use of the two-man sled for specific strength. A track sprinter might progress from lunges to bounding to towing to develop functional strength, whereas a basketball player might go from squatting with weights to body weight squats to squat jumps. Throwers and athletes involved in racket sports might progress from pullovers to two-arm medicine ball throwing to weighted ball throws or racket swings for specificity.[23] Strength training follows a planned, progressive sequence as outlined in Figure 13–5.

Early in the rehabilitation program, isometric exercises may be initiated for the involved extremity to regain strength lost due to injury or disuse. This helps establish a base of strength on which athletes can build. Because of the joint angle specificity of isometric strengthening, multiple-angle isometric contractions every 20 degrees may be used to achieve strength throughout the range of motion.[24]

The injured athlete may progress from isometric to isotonic exercise, with the goal of developing dynamic concentric and eccentric strength. In this way, isotonic exercise is more functional than isometric exercise, because the demands placed on the muscle are similar to those placed on it during functional activity. An isotonic exercise program may be implemented using free weights (barbells, dumbbells, cuff weights), rubber tubing or some other elastic material, closed chain activities, or various types of exercise machines. There are many different isotonic protocols for rehabilitation, but no one combination of sets and repetitions has been shown to be optimal for building strength.[22] The one consistent factor identified for the facilitation of optimal strength improvement has been the use of maximal voluntary contractions. However, when dealing with injured athletes, maximal voluntary contractions may not be possible. Fortunately, isotonic exercise using submaximal voluntary contractions has also been shown to significantly increase strength and may be used effectively during rehabilitation.[25]

Manual resistive exercises through the use of proprioceptive neuromuscular facilitation (PNF) may be incorporated into the athlete's strengthening program. Appropriate use of PNF techniques enables the therapist or trainer to control the part being facilitated, thus eliminating or correcting substitution patterns of movement. PNF techniques also accommodate for positions in the range of movement where pain or weakness may be a problem, allowing exercises to be individualized.

PNF techniques may be used to obtain a variety of muscle actions in a single exercise session, such as isometric, concentric, and eccentric actions, which may be utilized early in the rehabilitation program and may be applied through any portion of the available range of movement, in functional planes of movement, and in many different patient positions.[12,26] PNF techniques eliciting reciprocal contractions and co-contractions may be used to simulate activities such as walking or running so that the exercises become more functional.[6,12] Resistance may also be provided throughout the PNF pattern or in functional movement patterns by incorporating elastic cords or bands into the exercise program.

The importance of the eccentric component of isotonic exercise is often overlooked but may be critical in the rehabilitation of some athletic injuries. Serious tendon injuries, such as ruptures, appear to occur during instances of high eccentric loading to the tendon.[27] The force generated by an eccentric contraction of a muscle is nearly always greater than that generated by a concentric contraction of the muscle. It is thought by some that this combination of high-magnitude force during a sudden eccentric contraction of the muscle-tendon unit is an important causative factor in tendinitis, particularly in repetitive loading situations such as running.[28,29] For the rehabilitation program to follow the SAID principle, the exercise must prepare athletes to meet and withstand the imposed demands—in this case, an eccentric load placed on a tendon. To do this, the tendon must be exercised eccentrically during the rehabilitation process, progressing from slow to fast movements at each resistance before progressing on to a greater resistance.

The frequent use of the stretch-shortening cycle by athletes in sporting activities is also an important factor to remember when implementing a functional rehabilitation program. In the stretch-shortening cycle, the muscle is placed on a quick eccentric stretch immediately before generating a strong concentric contraction, such as when an athlete squats before jumping or winds up before throwing. By preloading the muscle, the stretch-shortening cycle facilitates a stronger concentric action by the muscle. This functional eccentric pattern usually involves multiple joint segments moving in multiple planes and, as such, may not be enhanced through training techniques that involve open-chain, single-joint, single-plane eccentric movement patterns.[18]

With isokinetic exercise, joint movement is performed at a constant angular velocity. Resistance to that movement is provided by the isokinetic equipment and is equal to the force generated by the exercising muscle throughout the range of movement. Theoretically, this provides continual, maximal resistance to the muscle through the exercised range. Maximal strengthening of the muscle should therefore be accomplished throughout the entire range. Although isokinetic exercise has been shown to be an effective way of strengthening muscles, it must be remembered that there are no functional sports activities that are isokinetic in nature; therefore, specificity is limited to the speed of muscle contraction and not the type of muscle contraction.

Speed specificity is an important factor when rehabilitating athletes. Angular velocity of the lower extremities during normal walking ranges from 240 to 270 degrees per second, whereas in a skilled sprinter, angular velocity approaches 700 degrees per second.[30] In order to make the rehabilitation program as sport specific as possible, exercise in the later stages of rehabilitation should incorporate high-velocity training. Research substantiates this, as it has been shown that motor performance in the 40-yard dash increased with fast-speed isokinetic training more than it did with slow-speed isokinetic training.[31] Isokinetic exercise allows exercise to be done in a controlled, quantitative, and reproducible manner, but it must be remembered that isokinetic machines do not allow exercise in a functional position or at functional speeds.

Positioning of athletes on the isokinetic device is also an important consideration in terms of specificity. During running, as the knee reaches its maximum flexion of 125 to 130 degrees after toe-off, the hip is in approximately 40 degrees of flexion. Just prior to heel strike, when the knee is rapidly extending to its position of approximately 40 to 45 degrees flexion, the hip is still flexed 50 to 55 degrees. If one is trying to rehabilitate a runner with a quadriceps strength deficit in a functional position, the athlete should be positioned on the isokinetic device with the hip flexed 45 to 50 degrees instead of the more traditional 80 to 90 degrees.[5]

FLEXIBILITY

The second primary step in the rehabilitation process for an injured athlete is the development of sport-specific muscle flexibility and joint range of motion. It should be remembered that both injury and disuse or inactivity may result in shortening of connective tissue and muscle. For an athlete, muscle groups that need to exhibit adequate flexibility are often sport or position specific and must be identified and treated if a lack of flexibility or range of motion exists.

There are two general types of flexibility: static and dynamic. Static flexibility involves the actual range of movement about a joint and the muscle's ability to lengthen or deform, with no relationship to speed of movement. Dynamic flexibility is the ability to use that range of joint movement by overcoming the resistance to movement during the performance of an activity, at the normal speed of that activity.[32] Both must be considered if sport-specific flexibility is to be regained or maintained.

The two most common exercises used to increase flexibility are static stretching exercises and ballistic or dynamic stretching exercises. Static stretching involves the use of isometric, controlled, or slow stretch of muscle and soft tissue. This type of exercise has generally been considered safe and effective in increasing static flexibility.[32] Static stretching should be incorporated into the athlete's early-season conditioning program as the initial modality to increase flexibility. However, as conditioning improves, the proportion of dynamic stretching exercises used to increase flexibility should be increased.[33]

Dynamic flexibility may be developed using the Progressive Velocity Flexibility Program (PVFP) (Table 13–5). This program takes the muscle being stretched

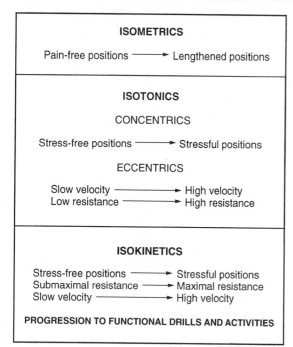

FIGURE 13–5. Exercise progression. (From Zachazewski JE: Flexibility in sports. *In* Sanders B [ed]: Sports Physical Therapy. East Norwalk, CT, Appleton and Lange, 1990, p 229.)

TABLE 13–5
Progressive Velocity Flexibility Program
• Static stretching
• SSER—slow short-end range stretching
• SFR—slow full-range stretching
• FSER—fast short-end range stretching
• FFR—fast full-range stretching

From Zachazewski JE: Flexibility in sports. *In* Sanders B (ed): Sports Physical Therapy. East Norwalk, CT, Appleton & Lange, 1990, p 228.

through a reciprocal antagonist to agonist action, requiring athletes to work on their neuromuscular coordination during this activity. The goal of the PVFP is to facilitate a motor learning response as the muscle stretches at higher velocities over time, simulating movement and integrating functional activities required for sport.[33]

Depending on the status of the athlete (postinjury or requiring prophylactic stretching), the PVFP may take days or weeks to complete. Following warm-up and static stretching, the athlete begins with slow short-end ballistic stretching exercises, followed by slow full-range stretching, progressing to fast short-end stretching and fast full-range stretching. This allows a progression from a controlled, slow-velocity activity to a high-velocity, simulated functional activity (Fig. 13–5). With the PVFP, both control and range are the responsibility of the athlete, and no outside force is exerted by anyone.[33]

MUSCLE ENDURANCE

For an injured athlete, another important step in the rehabilitation process is the development and maintenance of both local muscular endurance and cardiovascular endurance. Local muscular endurance may be defined as the ability or capacity of a muscle group to perform repeated contractions against a load.[34] Muscular endurance usually takes much longer than strength to return, and many athletes do not regain their normal endurance until they reverse the muscle atrophy that accompanies a musculoskeletal injury.[35] Activities that are used to promote the development of endurance are usually high repetition and low load. Again, it is very important to have

the athlete exercise at speeds that simulate the speed of athletic performance as closely as possible, because the development of muscular endurance is also speed specific. Isokinetic exercise, therefore, is an excellent clinical means of developing local muscular endurance.

CARDIOVASCULAR ENDURANCE

As previously mentioned, during rehabilitation, it is important to include exercises that help maintain the athlete's cardiovascular endurance. This is known as cross training. Cross-training exercises for cardiovascular endurance, such as the ones mentioned earlier, may be used successfully. It has been shown that over a 6-week period, runners who cannot run due to soft tissue injury may maintain a VO₂max and 2-mile run performance similar to that achieved with running training through the use of cycling or water running cross-training methods.[36] However, although cross training can produce a similar cardiovascular effort as the original sport, it does not necessarily produce the same musculoskeletal effects.[37] This cross-training effect becomes even more critical as the athlete prepares to return to competition. Although sport-specific cardiovascular and local muscular endurance required for optimum athletic performance can be accomplished only by actually training and competing, the less deconditioning that takes place during the rehabilitation process, the quicker the injured athlete may return to peak performance.[4]

PROPRIOCEPTION

Proprioception is a neuromuscular position sense that orients individuals as to body or body part position in relation to space or other objects. Following an injury, this position sense diminishes or is lost.[38] In order to re-establish normal proprioception, specific exercises must be utilized to retrain this sense. Although range of motion exercises and progressive resistive exercises help re-establish joint proprioception, they are not as functional or effective as exercises in a weight-bearing position that help the athlete redevelop joint proprioception.

Proprioceptive exercises must be done in a controlled environment where the affected joint or joints are moving in a functional relationship to each other and to the same degree as in normal functional activities, including sports activities.[11] This is why direct therapist or trainer supervision of the injured athlete is critical: to prevent overstress of healing tissues, resulting in reinjury. The goal of proprioceptive exercises should be to reduce the time between neural stimuli and muscular response, thus reducing the stress on the injured joint during functional activities.[39]

Proprioceptive exercises may be started early in the rehabilitation program, even before the athlete has achieved full weight-bearing status.[7,10] The athlete may progress from partial weight bearing in a seated position, to weight bearing on both extremities, to weight bearing on each extremity with weight shifting, to unilateral weight bearing. Devices such as mini-trampolines, balance boards or balls, and wobble boards may be used to increase the difficulty of proprioceptive activities and thus progress the athlete toward return to sports activities.[40,41]

The use of a mini-trampoline changes the weight-bearing surface from hard to soft and provides an element of instability, thus requiring more control in the weight-bearing lower extremity for stability. While on the apparatus, athletes may be progressed from a single leg stance (Fig. 13–6), to a single leg stance with partial squat, to a single leg stance while performing sport-specific upper extremity skills such as dribbling or throwing.

Balance boards utilize varying sizes of dowel rods under a 2 to 2½ foot long, 2- by 12-inch board (Fig. 13–7). By placing the dowel rods either parallel or perpendicular to the board, the athlete may work on single-plane balance in either a frontal or a sagittal plane. Exercise difficulty may be progressed by changing from bilateral to unilateral standing, by increasing the size of the dowel rod under the board, or by adding lower extremity motion or upper extremity

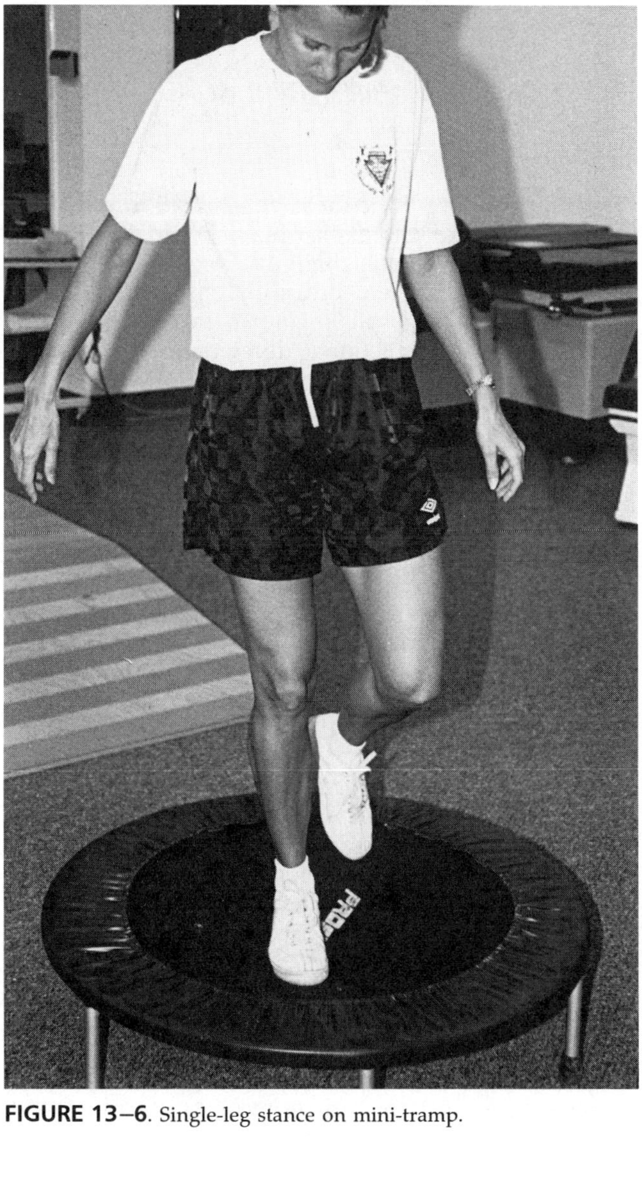

FIGURE 13–6. Single-leg stance on mini-tramp.

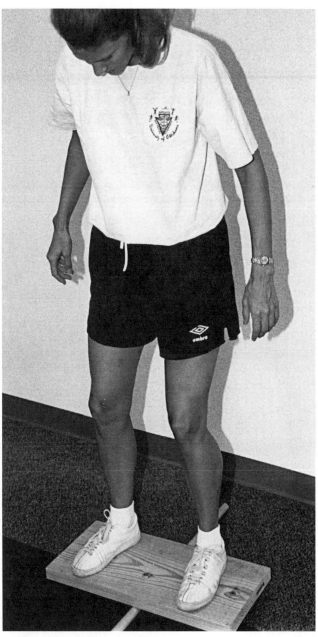

FIGURE 13–7. Balance board.

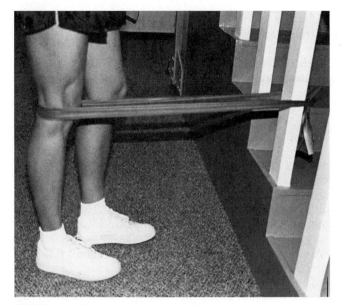

FIGURE 13–9. Closed chain knee extension.

extremity sport-specific skills may be added as the athlete progresses.

FUNCTIONAL REHABILITATION GOALS

CLOSED-CHAIN EXERCISES

As part of the functional rehabilitation program, closed kinematic chain exercises should be emphasized. Closed kinematic chain exercises are performed with the distal segment of an extremity fixed, allowing motion to occur at segments proximal.[11] These exercises provide functional deceleration training for large lower extremity muscle groups as well as enhanced neuromuscular training benefits of speed, balance, and coordination.[7] Closed-chain exercises also contribute to increased joint stability through greater joint congruency and enhanced muscle action around the joint.[40]

Because of the functional nature of closed-chain exercises, they are, in many cases, replacing the more traditional isotonic exercises in rehabilitation programs.[12,42] These exercises may begin with partial squats (Fig. 13–8), leg presses, step-ups, lunges, or closed-chain terminal knee extension (Fig. 13–9). As symptoms subside and function improves, athletes may begin to use other closed-chain exercise devices such as reciprocal (vertical or stair) climbers, lateral slide boards (Fig. 13–10), treadmills, cross-country ski simulators, the Biomechanical Ankle Platform System (BAPS) (Camp International, Inc., Jackson, MI) (Fig. 13–11), the Fitter (Fitter International, Calgary, Canada) (Fig. 13–12), elastic resistance cords (Fig. 13–13), or mini-trampolines.[7,9,11,12,40,42–44]

Devices such as wobble or balance boards, balls, or the Fitter may also be used to develop or re-establish upper extremity proprioception. By placing the athlete in a closed-chain, weight-bearing position on the device (Fig. 13–14), the athlete receives proprioceptive

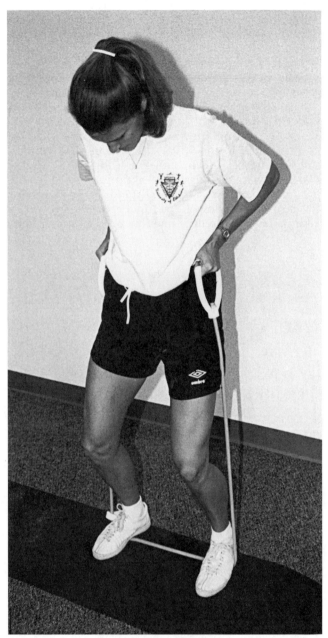

FIGURE 13–8. Partial squat with resistance.

skills to the exercise routine, as with the mini-trampoline.

Wobble boards are made up of an 18- to 24-inch disc with half a sphere fixed to the center of the disc. The size of half sphere may vary from small (less than 1-inch diameter) to large (up to 6-inch diameter), depending on the difficulty desired. Athletes stand on the disc and rotate it around its edge, both clockwise and counterclockwise. This allows them to work on multiplane balance in a weight-bearing position. The exercise may be progressed by changing from bilateral standing to unilateral standing, by varying the amount of upper extremity support allowed, by increasing the size of the sphere, or by changing the surface on which the board is placed from soft (e.g., carpet) to hard (e.g., tile). As with the mini-trampoline and the balance boards, upper

input into the joints of the upper extremities, helping to develop proximal stability as well as distal mobility.

Along with the closed-chain exercises, athletes should be progressed through a walk-jog-run program. These activities combine both open- and closed-chain components. The stance phase of gait, when the foot is on the ground, is considered closed chain, whereas the swing phase of gait is open chain.[11] Although walking and running activities contain both open- and closed-chain components, their functional nature requires a controlled progression from one to another. Athletes may progress from walking 20 minutes to jogging, progressing in quarter-mile increments, and then to running, progressing from half to full speed. If the running program is initiated on an oval track, the athlete should begin running with the involved limb toward the outside of the track to help control any additional stress that might be placed on the knee while running the curve. The criterion for progressing from one stage to another should be no increase in signs and symptoms related to the original injury, especially pain and swelling.[45]

The final three steps in the rehabilitation progression—power, speed, and agility—are more sport-specific skills. These activities help the injured athlete relearn or reacquire sport-specific neurophysiologic skill patterns known as coordination engrams.[7] Coordination engrams are thought to represent neurologic organization, accounting for the memory of preprogrammed, highly skilled movement patterns, and are formed only by thousands of repetitions of the precise movement pattern. The goal of this stage of rehabilitation is to redevelop the coordination engrams of the athlete's sport.[7] By working on power, speed, and agility skills, the injured athlete is re-establishing those engrams and progressing from meeting clinical goals to

meeting functional goals in preparation for returning to athletics.[41]

POWER

Power, speed, and agility are all dependent on the return of strength following an injury. Power is the ability of the muscle to exert a large amount of force at a fast rate.[46] As such, an increase in strength, in speed of muscle shortening, or in both may produce greater power output. For all athletes, power is required to maximally accelerate the body, and training must be performed at both the force and the velocity specific

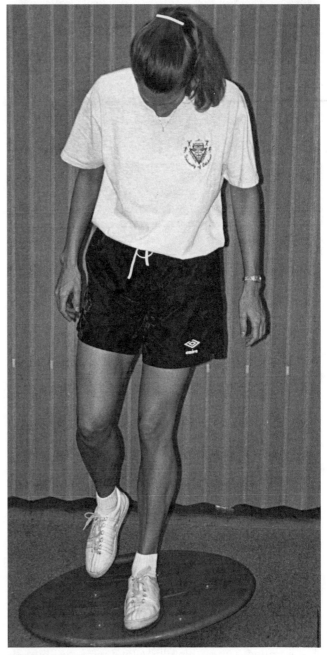

FIGURE 13–11. BAPS training (Camp International, Inc., Jackson, MI).

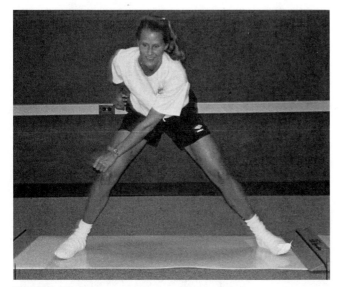

FIGURE 13–10. Lateral slide board (Euroglide, Improve Human Performance, Inc., Baltimore, MD).

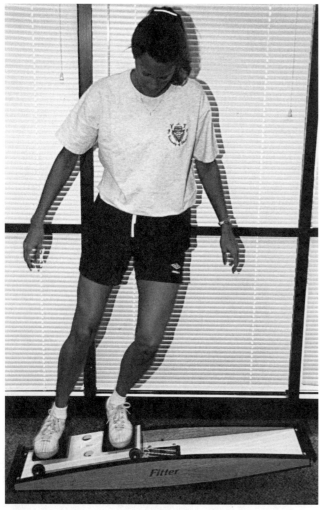

FIGURE 13–12. Fitter—lower extremity exercise (Fitter International, Inc., Calgary, Alberta, Canada).

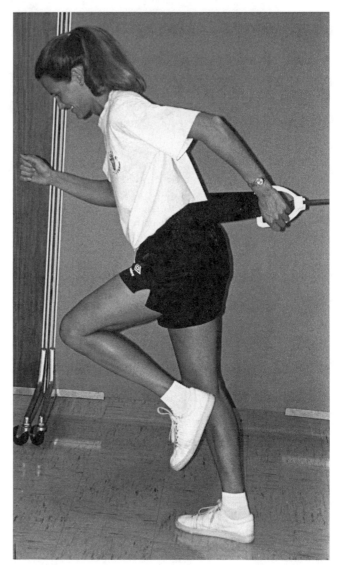

FIGURE 13–13. Elastic resistance cords—forward running.

for the given requirements of an athletic event. Training at 100 percent maximal voluntary contraction (MVC) has been shown to improve force but not velocity.[47] However, training done at 30 to 60 percent MVC has been shown to improve both the force and the velocity of the contraction and may be used to develop power.[47]

Plyometric exercises are also helpful in the development of muscular power. Plyometric exercises utilize the stretch-shortening cycle to elicit a more forceful concentric contraction. Because these exercises require muscle to rapidly change from eccentric to concentric action, they theoretically help develop reciprocal reflex training, which may be useful in injury prevention.[12] Athletes may begin a plyometric exercise program once they have completed their initial strength and proprioception training and have initiated closed-chain and minimal functional activities. Plyometrics are performed two to three times per week to allow for soft tissue repair and recovery from fatigue; they are discontinued if the athlete develops pain, swelling, or other signs of overuse.[12]

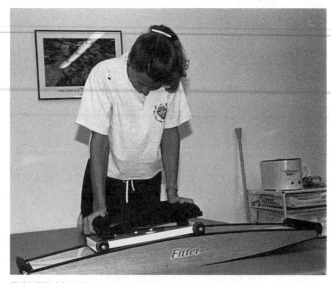

FIGURE 13–14. Fitter—upper extremity exercise.

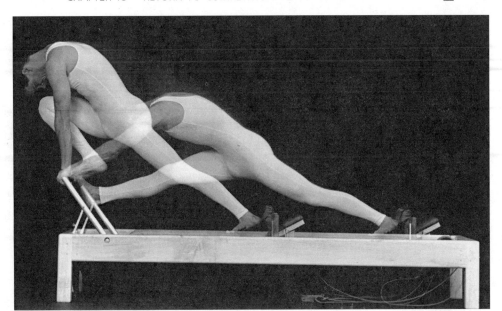

FIGURE 13–15. Pilates (Pilates, Inc., New York, NY).

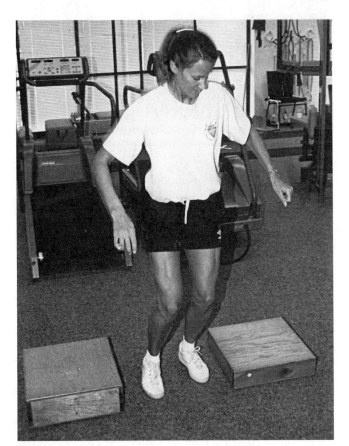

FIGURE 13–16. Plyometric exercise with 4-inch box.

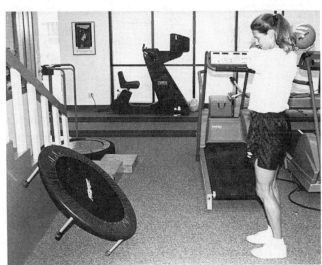

FIGURE 13–17. Upper extremity plyometric exercise with medicine ball.

A plyometric exercise program may begin with the athlete on a supine rebounder, such as the Pilates (Fig. 13–15). Effort and intensity may be increased by adding resistance with elastic cords or by progressing from bilateral to unilateral bounding. From the Pilates, the athlete may be progressed to plyometric exercise on the mini-trampoline to control excessive ground reaction forces. As strength, pro-

prioception, and lower extremity control improve, the athlete may begin hopping or jumping activities, beginning with jumping from a 4-inch platform to the floor and back up to the platform (Fig. 13–16). The platform height may be increased 2 to 4 inches per week, up to 10 inches or higher, depending on the functional demands required of the athlete.

Athletes may perform three to five sets of 15 to 20 repetitions per exercise session. Difficulty of the exercises may be increased by having the athlete turn 90 to 180 degrees in the air during the jump, by performing the plyometric exercises on a multiple slant board, or both. Theoretically, these modifications help increase spatial awareness and train the body to prepare for a safe landing.[12] Single or double leg bounding may also be used as plyometric training to develop lower extremity speed and power. Athletes who require enhanced upper extremity power and who are exposed

TABLE 13–6
Criteria for Progression[51]

A subjective assessment from the therapist or trainer that the athlete is able to use the injured extremity well
The athlete's ability to demonstrate enough self-confidence to fully participate in these activities without experiencing pain, swelling, or giving way

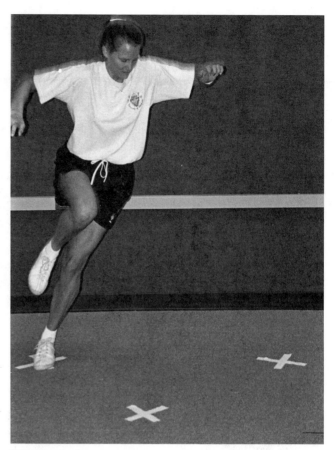

FIGURE 13–19. Hop stress test.

SPEED

Speed is utilized to some degree by every athlete. The muscular force generated by the lower extremities is important to accelerate the athlete quickly. The ability of the athlete to move quickly may be lost after an injury due to a failure of the mechanoreceptor feedback mechanism. Therefore, activities that emphasize regaining proprioceptive coordination and muscle recruitment in order to facilitate rate of acceleration and maximal running speed should be initiated at this time.[41]

AGILITY

Agility is the ability to change direction of the body and its parts quickly.[49] It is a combination of many different athletic traits such as reaction time, speed, coordination, power, and strength.[41] For athletes, agility allows them to avoid contact with other athletes on the field or to avoid obstacles or pitfalls in their way, and it may be sport or position specific.[50] There are many activities that help promote the development of agility.[9,40,41,45] Athletes may begin with activities such as running figure of eights, zigzags, shuttle runs, cariocas, and retrorunning, with progression from half to full speed. They may then progress to more difficult activities such as lateral and cross-over cutting and sport-specific drills. Difficulty of these activities may be increased by progressing from half to full speed, by

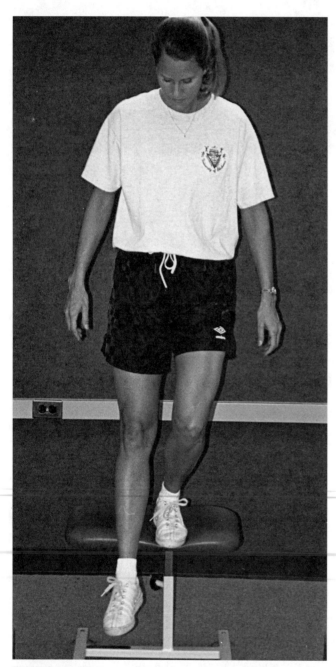

FIGURE 13–18. Twenty-four-inch step for leg control.

to significant deceleration forces may utilize an upper extremity plyometric program. Upper extremity plyometric exercises may use a plyoball or medicine ball (Fig. 13–17), resistive elastic tubing, or a wall.[41,48]

TABLE 13–7
Sports-Specific Drills

Sports	Name of Drill	Position	Drill	Repetitions
Baseball	Sprints		Start at home. Go to following positions and return home:	
			First base	15 sec: 2–5 reps
			Left field fence	60 sec: 2–5 reps
			Pitcher's mound	15 sec: 2–5 reps
			Second base	15 sec: 2–5 reps
			Center field fence	75 sec: 2–5 reps
			Third base	15 sec: 2–5 reps
			Right field fence	75 sec: 2–5 reps
			Pitcher's mound	15 sec: 2–5 reps
			Second base	20 sec: 2–5 reps
			All bases	20 sec: 2–5 reps
	Slides		Run to one base, slide to next. Slide with noninvolved leg first, then involved.	
	Catching fly balls		From infield and move progressively into outfield. Ball hit to patient. Ball hit to right or left or patient.	
Basketball	Post-ups solo	Offense faces away from basket in post		10 in each direction
	One-on-one (single team) post-up	As above	Receive pass, pivot R or L, square up to basket, shoot.	10 in each direction
	Double team post-up	As above	As above. Defenseman is behind patient and tries to deny post-up position.	10 in each direction
	Shooting off the pick	Offense away from basket	As above. One defender at post, one defender on patient's involved side.	10 in each direction
	Shooting off the dribble	Offense	Runs from post off a pick/screen, receives pass, squares up, shoots.	10 in each direction
	Jump shot	Offense	Receives ball, dribble, stop and shoot.	10 in each direction
	Defended jump shot		As above. Defender faces patient and tries to block shot.	10 in each direction
	Rebounding	Defense. Faces away from basket. In post	Ball is shot from outside.	
	Rebounding	Offense	Patient turns and blocks (boxes out) the offensive player.	
	Game situation	Patient-specific	Patient attempts rebound. Patient shoots ball from outside, tries to make rebound from one or two defenders. One-on-one, 1/2 court and progress to two-on-one, two-on-two, three-on-three. Goal: full court.	

Criterion: Performs agility drill without symptoms.
Goals: No recurrence of symptoms, normal running gait, involved limb not favored.
(Fron Eifert-Mangine M, et al: Patellar tendinitis in the recreational athlete. Orthopedics 1992; 15: 1366

TABLE 13–8
Interval Throwing Program

45 Degree Phase	90 Degree Phase	150 Degree Phase
Step 1: Warm-up throwing 45' (25 throws) Rest 15 minutes Warm-up throwing 45' (25 throws)	Step 5: Warm-up throwing 90' (25 throws) Rest 15 minutes Warm-up throwing 90' (25 throws)	Step 9: Warm-up throwing 150' (25 throws) Rest 15 minutes Warm-up throwing 150' (25 throws)
Step 2: Warm-up throwing 45' (25 throws) Rest 10 minutes Warm-up throwing 45' (25 throws) Rest 10 minutes Warm-up throwing 45' (25 throws)	Step 6: Warm-up throwing 90' (25 throws) Rest 10 minutes Warm-up throwing 90' (25 throws) Rest 10 minutes Warm-up throwing 90' (25 throws)	Step 10: Warm-up throwing 150' (25 throws) Rest 10 minutes Warm-up throwing 150' (25 throws) Rest 10 minutes Warm-up throwing 150' (25 throws)

60 Degree Phase	120 Degree Phase	180 Degree Phase
Step 3: Warm-up throwing 60' (25 throws) Rest 15 minutes Warm-up throwing 60' (25 throws)	Step 7: Warm-up throwing 120' (25 throws) Rest 15 minutes Warm-up throwing 120' (25 throws)	Step 11: Warm-up throwing 180' (25 throws) Rest 15 minutes Warm-up throwing 180' (25 throws)
Step 4: Warm-up throwing 60' (25 throws) Rest 10 minutes Warm-up throwing 60' (25 throws) Rest 10 minutes Warm-up throwing 60' (25 throws)	Step 8: Warm-up throwing 120' (25 throws) Rest 10 minutes Warm-up throwing 120' (25 throws) Rest 10 minutes Warm-up throwing 120' (25 throws)	Step 12: Warm-up throwing 180' (25 throws) Rest 10 minutes Warm-up throwing 180' (25 throws) Rest 10 minutes Warm-up throwing 180' (25 throws)
		Step 13: Warm-up throwing 180' (25 throws) Rest 10 minutes Warm-up throwing 180' (25 throws) Rest 10 minutes Warm-up throwing 180' (50 throws)
		Step 14: Begin throwing off the mound or return to respective position.

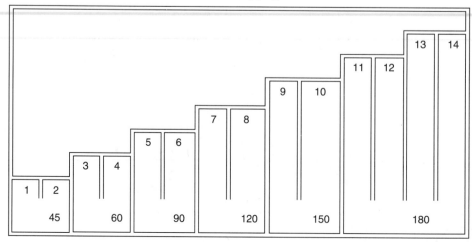

Interval throwing program

From Wilk KE, Andrews FR: Rehabilitation following arthroscopic subacromial decompression. Orthopedics 1992, 16: 356–358.

TABLE 13–9
Interval Tennis Program

First Week	Second Week	Third Week	Fourth Week
Monday 12 FH 8 BH 10-min rest 13 FH 7 BH	*Monday* 25 FH 15 BH 10-min rest 25 FH 15 BH	*Monday* 25 FH 25 BH 10 OH 10-min rest 30 FH 25 BH 10 OH	*Monday* 30 FH 30 BH 10 OH 10-min rest Play 3 games 10 OH 10 BH 5 OH
Wednesday 15 FH 10 BH 10-min rest 15 FH 10 BH	*Wednesday* 30 FH 20 BH 10-min rest 30 FH 20 BH	*Wednesday* 30 FH 25 BH 15 OH 10-min rest 30 FH 25 BH 15 OH	*Wednesday* 30 FH 30 BH 10 OH 10-min rest Play set 10 FH 10 BH 5 OH
Friday 15 FH 10 BH 10-min rest 15 FH 10 BH	*Friday* 30 FH 25 BH 10-min rest 30 FH 15 BH 10 OH	*Friday* 30 FH 30 BH 15 OH 10-min rest 30 FH 15 OH 10-min rest 30 FH 30 BH 15 OH	*Friday* 30 FH 30 BH 10 OH 10-min rest Play 1½ sets 10 FH 10 BH 3 OH

BH, backhand stroke; FH, forehand ground stroke; OH, overhead shot.
Ice after each day of play.
From Wilk KE, Andrews FR: Rehabilitation following arthroscopic subacromial decompression. Orthopedics 1992; 16:356–358.

increasing the angle of cutting from 45 to 90 degrees, and by moving from cutting at predetermined sites to cutting on demand. The use of a mini-trampoline for progressive cutting activities has also been reported in the literature.[40]

PROGRESSION TO SPORT-SPECIFIC ACTIVITIES

Criteria that would permit the athlete to progress to more sport-specific activities should be established (Table 13–6).[51] Specific tests, which place stress on specific joints, may also be used to determine the readiness of the athlete to progress to more functional activities. Having the athlete slowly descend a high (18- to 24-inch) step with the involved leg controlling the descent (Fig. 13–18) may be used to assess knee control.[52] The hop stress test (Fig. 13–19), requiring the athlete to perform a series of jumps forward, backward, and side-to-side on a single involved limb, places significant stress on the rehabilitated ankle or knee.[53]

For athletes, the best exercises to promote functional power, speed, and agility are sport-specific activities (Table 13–7). This may involve different training methods such as sprinting, throwing, jumping, sport-specific agility drills, or other sport-specific skills such as rebounding, blocking, or base running. It should be remembered that the training should reflect the demands placed on the athletes during their activity. There are many sports skill progression programs designed to gradually return athletes safely to their sports, such as throwing programs (Table 13–8),[16,48,54–56] tennis programs (Table 13–9), and golf programs (Table 13–10).

RETURN TO UNRESTRICTED ACTIVITY

In order for an injured athlete to return to unrestricted sports activities, the functional rehabilitation program must continue to be sequential, with the ultimate goal of safely returning to competition as quickly as possible. The sequence will differ, depending on the needs of the athlete, but the overall plan remains the same. Each step should demand slightly more from the athlete until the final step, which should mimic the conditions of competition or performance. Athletes whose sports require running may be progressed from walk-jog to jog-run to full run without restriction.

Athletes whose sports require throwing may be progressed from short lobs to long lobs and from one-half to three-quarter to full-speed throwing. It is important to note that functional progression activities are frequently neglected when nonspecific instructions are given to the athlete. Therefore, specific instructions in terms of those variables that can be modified must be given to the athlete. Frequency (exercise bouts per week or per day), intensity (maximal or submaximal effort), repetitions (number of throws, distance run, and so on), and rest (amount of time between exercise bouts) are the variables that may be modified, depending on the needs of the athlete. However, the athlete's progress must still be monitored and the workout modified if any signs or symptoms of the original injury or a new injury appear.

Once athletes have successfully completed a functional rehabilitation program, they must still meet certain criteria before they are allowed full return to sports activities. These criteria may vary somewhat, depending on the athlete, the sport, and the recommendations of the sports rehabilitation team. However, certain crite-

| | TABLE 13–10 | | |
| | Interval Golf Program | | |
Week	**Monday**	**Wednesday**	**Friday**
First	10 putts	15 putts	20 putts
	10 chips	15 chips	20 chips
	5-min rest	5-min rest	5-min rest
	15 chips	25 chips	20 putts
			20 chips
			5-min rest
			10 chips
			10 short irons
Second	20 chips	20 chips	15 short irons
	10 short irons	15 short irons	10 medium irons
	5-min rest	10-min rest	10-min rest
	10 short irons	15 short irons	20 short irons
		15 chips	15 chips
Third	15 short irons	15 short irons	15 short irons
	15 medium irons	10 medium irons	10 medium irons
	10-min rest	10 long irons	10 long irons
	5 long irons	10-min rest	10-min rest
	15 short irons	10 short irons	10 short irons
	15 medium irons	10 medium irons	10 medium irons
	10-min rest	5 long irons	10 long irons
	20 chips	5 woods	10 woods
Fourth	15 short irons		
	10 medium irons		
	10 long irons	Play 9 holes	Play 9 holes
	10 drives		
	15-min rest		
	Repeat		
Fifth	Play 9 holes	Play 9 holes	Play 18 holes

Do flexing exercises before hitting; use ice after play.
chips = pitching wedge
short irons = w, 9, 8
medium irons = 7, 6, 5
long irons = 4, 3, 2
woods = 3, 5
drives = driver
From Wilk KE, Andrews JR: Rehabilitation following arthroscopic subacromial decompression. Orthopedics 1992; 16:356–358.

TABLE 13–11
Criteria for Full Return to Sports Activities[4,6,40,57]

The athlete should have complete resolution of acute signs and symptoms related to the injury

The athlete should have full, dynamic range of motion of all joints, with adequate strength and proprioception to be able to perform expected skills successfully

There should be no alteration of the athlete's normal mechanics, which might predispose him or her to subsequent reinjury

The athlete must be able to successfully perform sport-specific activities at or above preinjury level

TABLE 13–12
Functional Test Criteria

Functional tests should be both valid and reliable

Functional tests should evaluate conditioning (e.g., strength, endurance, and flexibility) and sport-specific skills

Functional testing should be conducted under strictly controlled conditions

Functional tests should be repeatable at specified intervals to allow for valid comparisons and program modification

Functional tests should provide practical information for the sports rehabilitation team, including the coach and the athlete

The purpose, procedures, and inherent risks of functional testing should be clearly defined and fully explained to the athlete

ria should be addressed (Table 13–11).[4,6,40,57] Failure to address each of these parameters in a functional rehabilitation program puts the athlete at risk and leaves questions unanswered as to his or her readiness to return to competition.

THE USE OF FUNCTIONAL TESTS IN ATHLETICS

Functional tests are tests that evaluate neuromuscular control, strength, power, and functional ability.[12] How an athlete performs on such tests may be used to determine the readiness or ability of that athlete to perform specific sports-related skills. The tests used in a functional testing program should meet certain standards (Table 13–12).[58]

USEFULNESS OF A TEST

The functional utility of a test lies in its ability to accurately compare and consequently differentiate specified parameters (i.e., skills and abilities) among samples of a defined population. A population is that set of individuals for which the examiner would like to compare test measures. This could be based on variables such as gender, age, or sport. It could also be based on more discrete characteristics such as medical diagnosis or rank in sport (beginner, intermediate, advanced, or elite). Frequently, the examiner desires to evaluate performance based on a combination of characteristics, such as males aged 18 to 21 playing college baseball.

Since it is often impossible to actually test all members of a given population, a portion of the population is evaluated and comparisons are made with a sample of the population. A sample is a subset of the defined population to be evaluated and serves as representative of the population for a given characteristic or set of characteristics.[59] The sample must be an appropriate representative of the population. Therefore, defining the important characteristics can be a difficult task when selecting the sample.

In the medical field, diagnostic tests are used to discriminate among various diagnoses that present with a similar clinical picture. If test subjects are selected solely on the basis of whether or not they have the disorder in question, test discrimination may not be accurately assessed.[60] Instead, the examiner should select individuals who represent differing levels of dysfunction for a given disorder. For example, an examiner interested in assessing the ability of individuals with anterior cruciate ligament (ACL) deficiency to successfully return to sports might include the following groups in the study: asymptomatic patients with ACL deficiency, patients with symptoms only during high-level sport activity, patients with symptoms during recreational sport activity, patients with symptoms during activities of daily living, and persons without a history of ACL trauma. In addition, the examiner might include patients with knee dysfunction due to conditions other than ACL deficiency (e.g., posterior cruciate, medial collateral, or lateral collateral ligament deficiency) in order to evaluate the test's ability to discriminate for use with the ACL-deficient population.

When defining a population, the greater the degree of specificity, the more accurate the comparisons can be. If an examiner sought to evaluate the maximum weight an athlete was able to squat for use as a criterion in determining fitness for participation, it would be important to define not only the sport (football vs. basketball) but also the position in that given sport (running back vs. lineman). When available normative data do not specify the criterion utilized, the sample comparisons may or may not be accurate. In addition, there must be a satisfactory number of subjects tested in the sample population in order to achieve statistical power. Normative data without an adequate number of subjects are of limited utility for comparison.

CONCEPTS OF STANDARDIZATION, VALIDITY, AND RELIABILITY

A test has three important characteristics that should not be violated: standardization, validity, and reliability. Standardization pertains to rules for administration of the test. A standardized test is one in which the equipment, method of procedure, and scoring are invariant. This allows for comparison of outcomes in different settings as well as testing at different time intervals. With standardized test administration, an examiner is able to compare outcomes derived from the same individual on different occasions for the purpose of assessing progress or decline in function. This is true of clinical measures of strength and range of motion as well as functional testing. It also allows for comparison between individuals in varied centers. In addition, standardization helps limit experimental error in testing.

Validity is the degree to which a test measures what it purports to be measuring. If the test does, in fact, appropriately measure what the examiner intends, it has utility. For example, if examiners wish to determine fitness for return to sports participation and use only clinical measures of assessment (e.g., range of movement, degree of joint laxity, isokinetic test outcomes), they may fail to accurately assess true functional capacity. Functional tests must incorporate some of the more dynamic physical characteristics required for sports, such as dynamic muscle control, agility, coordination, and power. If a functional test has predictive validity, then one can conclude that individuals who perform well on the test have a high probability for a successful return to competition.[61]

Reliability is the degree to which a test consistently measures the defined characteristic. It is a measure of test accuracy in generating consistent measures between raters (inter-rater reliability) and over time (test-retest reliability). For example, an isokinetic measure of quadriceps strength should be relatively constant across time unless there is an actual change in muscle strength, as opposed to change caused by motor learning. Reliability does not, however, ensure validity.

Diagnostic tests have been employed for various purposes. According to Feinstein,[60] diagnostic tests are used for the purposes of discovery, confirmation, and exclusion. A discovery test is utilized when examining an apparently healthy population to imply the presence of a particular disorder. Preseason screening tests fall into the category of discovery tests. A confirmation test is utilized for verification in situations where there is a strong suspicion that a disorder is present. An exclusion test is utilized to rule out a certain disorder when its presence is suspected.

Tests of discovery and exclusion must have high sensitivity for detection, whereas confirmation tests require high specificity. The terms *sensitivity* and *specificity* have been applied to a variety of tests used in the identification of clinical conditions.[60] Sensitivity indicates the ability of a test to make an accurate diagnosis in confirmed positive cases of a disorder. Test specificity indicates the capacity for correct diagnosis in confirmed negative cases. The sensitivity and specificity of a test can be determined by the use of a binary table and associated equations as described by Feinstein[60] and utilized by Barber et al.[62] in their study of patients with ACL-deficient knees and normal subjects.

HOP TESTS

Various hop tests have been used over the years to measure the lower limb power and functional ability of athletes. The tests most commonly employed include the vertical jump (both single and double limb), bilateral

TABLE 13–13
Studies Showing Significant Relationships Between Strength and Functional Performance

Author	Results
Bangerter[65]	Significant gains in vertical jump by strengthening knee and/or hip extensors
Berger & Henderson[66]	Measures of lower extremity isometric and isotonic strength were highly correlated to vertical jump
McClements[67]	Significant correlations of isometric extension strength and power scores as measured by vertical jump
Wiklander & Lysholm[68]	Significant correlations between lower extremity isokinetic strength and functional jump tests in runners (standing long jump, five-step jump, and vertical jump)
Häkkinen[69]	Maximal leg extension force correlated significantly with vertical jump height in male and female basketball players
Miyashita & Kanehisa[70]	Significant relationship between knee extensor peak torque and 50-meter-dash speed
Davis et al.[71]	Simulated firefighting tasks were major predictors of physical work capacity

TABLE 13–14
Studies Showing no Significant Relationship Between Strength and Functional Performance

Author	Results
Considine & Sullivan[72]	Low to moderate relationships between selected leg strength and leg power variables
Viitasalo[73]	No significant correlations between maximal leg and trunk strength and various vertical jump measures in elite male volleyball players
Smith[74] & Clark[75]	No significant correlation between isometric strength measures and vertical jump scores
Anderson et al.[76]	No significant correlation between concentric and eccentric measures of quadriceps and hamstring strength and vertical jump

broad jump for distance, single leg hop for distance, and single leg hop for time. The vertical jump and broad jump tests were initially designed for bilateral performance; however, these tests have been converted to single leg tests to allow for right-to-left comparison following injury (with the uninvolved limb being used as the control). Although there is controversy in the literature as to whether the vertical jump and broad jump tests are true measures of power,[63,64] they appear to have value, particularly for sports requiring jumping and sprinting.

Attempts to relate traditional strength measures to functional performance have yielded varied results. Numerous authors have found significant positive relationships between strength measures and functional test performance (Table 13–13).[65–71] However, there appears to be an equal number of investigators who have found no significant correlations (Table 13–14).[73–76]

One problem inherent in these studies is the use of open-chain, slow-speed, single-plane strength measures for comparison with closed-chain, high-speed functional tests requiring contribution from multiple muscles, vast proprioceptive input, and movement in all three planes. Functional tests assess not only strength but also other factors that may contribute to physical outcomes, namely, pain, edema, ligament integrity, flexibility, coordination, agility, power, and proprioception (neuromuscular function).

Barber et al.[62] conducted a study to evaluate the ability of five tests to assess functional deficiencies in an ACL-deficient population. In addition, they evaluated normal subjects in order to determine acceptable values for lower extremity symmetry. Data collected on the normal group showed no effect of gender, sports activity level, or dominance on limb symmetry. Tests employed included the single leg hop for distance, single leg vertical jump, single leg timed hop, and shuttle run with and without pivot. They utilized an 85 percent symmetry score as the criterion for normal limb symmetry, since 92 to 93 percent of the normal population scored at this level or above for the hop tests. Results of testing showed that a relatively large percentage of normal subjects fell outside the normal limb symmetry range for the vertical jump. For this reason, the authors concluded that the vertical jump test should not be utilized for detection of lower extremity functional limitations.

Results of the single leg hop for distance showed a large difference between the symmetry scores of normal and ACL-deficient populations (the ACL-deficient population showed a mean difference of 25.2 cm between limbs, and the normal population a 0.71 cm difference).[62] It should be noted, however, that 50 percent of the ACL-deficient population scored in the normal symmetry range. Symmetry scores of those with ACL deficits were much lower than those of the normal population for all three hop tests. In addition, statistically significant relationships were found between abnormal symmetry scores in each of the three hop tests; subjective limitations in sprinting, jumping-landing, and cutting-twisting activities; and quadriceps

weakness at 60 degrees per second. The authors advised that a minimum of two function tests be used to assess functional limitation, since the range of abnormal performance increased with the addition of a second test.

In a second study, Noyes et al.[77] evaluated the single leg hop for time and the single leg hop for distance tests with a larger sample size to determine whether higher sensitivity ratings would be found. They also added the triple hop and the cross-over hop tests. Results of the study showed no significant differences between the single leg hop test and the timed hop test for abnormal limb symmetry (52 and 49 percent, respectively). They also determined that the single hop and timed hop tests could be classified only as confirmation tests (confirmation of lower limb functional limitation), since they were unable to determine which of the many variables necessary to lower limb functioning was deficient (neuromuscular coordination, strength, ligament integrity).

When evaluating all four hop tests, Noyes et al.[77] found that no single combination of tests yielded a significant increase in the number of patients with abnormal limb symmetry over other combinations. In addition, the sensitivity rates and false-positive rates of the cross-over hop test and the triple hop test were reported to be similar to the rates found for the single hop and timed hop tests. They concluded that any of the four tests, or any combination of tests, could be used to provide information concerning lower extremity limitations, when used in conjunction with other clinical assessment techniques.

Lephart et al.[78] conducted a study to assess the relationship between conventional physical measures and functional performance tests in two groups of athletes with ACL-deficient knees. They compared the functional capacities of athletes able to return to preinjury levels of activity and those unable to return to preinjury activities. Functional performance tests utilized were a co-contraction semicircle maneuver, a carioca run, and a shuttle run. Results of their study showed that conventional physical measures correlated poorly with functional test performance. In addition, they found that athletes who were able to return to preinjury levels of competition performed significantly better on the functional performance tests than those who were unable to return. They recommended the use of functional performance tests and the athlete's self-assessment as the criteria for an athlete's readiness to return to preinjury activities.

Giambelluca et al.[79] evaluated the ability of knee function tests to identify dysfunction related to ACL deficiency. Results showed that the ACL-deficient group scored significantly lower on the single leg triple jump when compared with the normal group. The authors concluded that the single leg triple jump for distance was a moderately valid objective measure of knee function.

Delitto et al.[80] conducted a study of the relationship between concentric and eccentric quadriceps strength and work measures to the vertical jump and single leg hop in active individuals without knee pathology. They found strong positive relationships between concentric quadriceps peak torque and work to the single leg hop, moderately strong positive relationships between eccentric quadriceps peak torque and work to the single leg hop and between concentric quadriceps peak torque and work to the vertical jump, and a weak positive relationship between eccentric quadriceps peak torque and work to the vertical jump. However, the investigators also reported weak positive relationships between quadriceps peak torque and work to the single leg hop and vertical jump in subjects following ACL reconstruction.

VERTICAL JUMP

The vertical jump was first described by D. A. Sargent[81] in 1921 as "the physical test of a man." Modifications have been made to the original test over the years. Although the basic components of the test are fairly standard, there are minor alterations to the test procedure found in the literature (bilateral vs. single leg jump, countermovement vs. static squat start, approach steps vs. stationary start, and use of the upper extremities for propulsion vs. restricted use of the upper extremities). Regardless of the technique employed, the vertical jump test remains a basic measure of anaerobic power.

RELIABILITY. There are good test-retest reliability scores for vertical jump tests reported in the literature, with a range of 0.90 to 0.99.[72,73,82]

VALIDITY. Johnson and Nelson[82] reported a validity coefficient of 0.78 based on comparison of the vertical jump to a sum of four power events in track and field. In addition, they reported construct validity of jumping ability.

METHOD. Minimal equipment is required to conduct the vertical jump test. Necessary equipment includes a wall with a high ceiling and adequate floor space for safe landing, a measuring tape, gymnastic chalk to mark the reach and jump height, and an accurate scale to measure the weight of the subject at the time of testing.

The subject should undergo a warm-up period, which might include activities such as biking, stretching, and submaximal jumping or plyometrics. Testing begins with a measure of reach height. The subject stands erect with the dominant side next to the wall and feet flat on the floor. Chalk is applied to the fingers, and the subject is instructed to reach as high as possible on the wall, with the highest point reached being marked and recorded.

The subject should take two or three practice jumps; this enhances reliability by allowing the subject to become familiar with the environment and testing procedures. Chalk is reapplied to the fingers prior to the test jumps. Once the test is ready to commence, the subject is not allowed to move the feet. When ready, the subject makes the jump and reaches to touch the wall, placing a second mark at the peak of the jump. Jump height is scored as the difference between the standing reach height and the peak height achieved in jumping. Measurement should be made to the nearest 1 cm or ½ inch.[83] The best jump distance of three trials is recorded and used for calculation.

The traditional vertical jump test is performed bilaterally, but this test can be conducted with a single leg jump for assessment of limb symmetry. If limb symmetry scores are desired, the subject would perform the jump three times on each leg. Whereas the takeoff is performed with a single leg, it is recommended that landing occur bilaterally, as this is a more functional movement pattern and lessens excessive stress on the lower extremity. As with bilateral jumping, the best jump distance is recorded and used for calculation of limb symmetry scores.

The vertical jump can be performed with or without a preceding countermovement. Although some investigators employ the use of a static squat jump,[81,84] the use of a quick countermovement with activation of the stretch-shortening cycle is more functional and sport specific and is, therefore, recommended. Komi and Bosco[85] examined vertical jump performance with different stretch loads imposed on the leg extensor muscles. Experimental conditions included the squat jump from a static starting position, the countermovement jump from a freestanding position with preparatory countermovement, and the drop jump from various heights. Results showed that the squat jump was significantly the least efficient condition as compared with performance in the countermovement or drop jumps in all groups studied. In addition, there was no significant difference in performance between the countermovement jump or drop jump in all groups studied. Furthermore, Bosco et al.[86] found that mechanical efficiency observed in rebound (countermovement) jumps was greater than that observed in no rebound jumps due to the recoil of elastic energy within the tissue.

A second vertical jump variation concerns the use of the upper extremities during jumping. Lower vertical jump scores have been reported during testing with the dominant upper extremity maintained in the elevated position.[87] This method is employed to limit contribution from the upper extremities and better isolate the lower extremity muscles. However, use of the upper extremities for propulsion is a normal movement pattern for jumping, whereas restricted use of the upper extremities is abnormal and awkward. If one is interested in simulating athletic movement for testing, it seems logical to permit normal use of the upper extremities. In addition, if testing is conducted with single leg jumps for bilateral comparison, the upper extremity movement would be a constant variable and should not affect the results. Power calculations for the vertical jump can be derived from the equation found in Table 13–15.[88] Calculation of lower extremity sym-

---

TABLE 13–15
Power Calculations for the Vertical Jump[88]

Power (kg/s) = 2.21 × wt $\sqrt{D}$

Where 2.21 is a constant, wt is equal to the subject's body weight at the time of testing, and D is equal to the distance between reach height and jump height in meters.

TABLE 13–16
Calculation of Lower Extremity Symmetry[89]

$$\text{Symmetry value} = \frac{\text{Involved limb score}}{\text{Uninvolved limb score}} \times 100$$

---

metry is made by dividing the score of the involved limb by the score of the uninvolved limb.[89] The result is then multiplied by 100 for the percentage score of lower extremity symmetry (Table 13–16).

NORMS. Norms for the bilateral vertical jump can be found in the literature (Table 13–17).[68,88,90] However, it should be noted that most of the norms are based on a relatively small sample size, and caution must be advised in their use.

SINGLE LEG HOP FOR DISTANCE

Daniel et al.[91] were the first to describe the single hop test. This test measures the distance covered in one hop for use in the evaluation of lower extremity symmetry. The original test used a single hop, but Noyes et al.[77] used both the triple hop for distance and the cross-over hop for distance and found no significant difference between the test results for limb symmetry scores and sensitivity ratings. Test construction is basically the same whether the single or triple hop is used; minor variation is required for the cross-over hop test.

RELIABILITY. Hu et al.[92] conducted a study to evaluate the reliability of the one-legged vertical jump and standing hop tests. They determined that the one-legged vertical jump and standing hop test with or without use of the upper extremities were reliable measures for lower extremity bilateral comparisons in the clinic. Reported interclass correlation coefficients ranged from 0.79 to 0.96.

VALIDITY. Validity for the various unilateral hop tests has not been established.

METHOD. Minimal equipment is required for the single or triple hop for distance. Necessary equipment includes a floor with adequate space to cover potential distances jumped, tape to mark the starting line and center lines, gymnastic chalk to mark the bottom of the shoes, and a tape measure long enough to extend the length of the jump site.

Prior to testing, the subject should go through an adequate warm-up period. In addition, the subject

---

TABLE 13–17
Norms for Vertical Jump Based on Performance of College Basketball Players

Position	Vertical Jump (in.)	
	Male	*Female*
Center	30	19
Forward	32	21
Guard	33	23

---

should be allowed to practice the hopping technique until it can be done correctly in order to enhance test reliability and validity.

Subjects stand behind the starting line on the limb to be tested and are instructed to jump as far as possible, landing on the same limb. No restrictions are placed on the upper extremities. The evaluator measures the distance between the starting line and the chalk mark left by the heel. Measurements are made to the nearest 1 cm or ½ inch. Subjects are given three trials, and the best of three jumps is used in the calculation. The triple hop for distance is essentially the same except that the subject makes three consecutive hops on the same limb. The evaluator measures the distance between the starting line and the third heel mark.

The cross-over hop for distance adds a frontal plane stress to this predominantly sagittal plane activity. Noyes et al.[77] utilized a 15-cm strip extending approximately 6 meters in length. Subjects were instructed to perform three consecutive hops, crossing over the center line with each hop. Although the basic test design used by Noyes is acceptable, it is recommended that four consecutive hops be incorporated for testing; this allows an equal number of medial and lateral stresses to be applied to the limb. In addition, change in the width of the center strip provides varied challenges for the subjects. For all these single leg hop tests, calculation of lower extremity symmetry may be made using the equation provided in Table 13–16.

NORMS. To the best of my knowledge, there are no known norms for the single leg hop for distance test.

SINGLE LEG HOP FOR TIME

The single leg hop for time is another measure of anaerobic power. At present, there are no consistent standards for test construction in the literature. Therefore, the 6-meter distance utilized by Barber et al.[62] was selected for this description. Validity and reliability for this test are unknown or unavailable.

METHOD. Equipment required for testing includes a level floor with tape to mark the starting line and 6-meter finish, a stopwatch for precise time measurement to the nearest one hundredth of a second, and a calibrated scale to weigh the subject if power measures are desired.

Prior to testing, subjects go through an adequate warm-up period. In addition, subjects should be allowed practice trials to become familiar with the test, allowing for enhanced reliability and validity. Subjects are instructed to hop as fast as possible over the 6-meter distance. The evaluator begins the stopwatch as soon as the subject initiates forward movement. The subject hops across the 6-meter distance on a single limb. The upper extremities are permitted to move naturally. The watch is stopped when the subject crosses the finish line. Subjects are given three trials on each limb, with the best of the three trials used for calculation of limb symmetry and power scores.

Risberg and Ekeland[93] utilized a cross-over hop test for time as part of a battery of functional tests for patients following ACL reconstruction. This test is conducted like the cross-over hop test for distance,[77] covering a 6-meter distance. However, the center strip is 30 cm wide. Test construction is the same as the straight-plane single leg hop for time, except that the subject crosses the center line with each successive hop. This places an additional side-to-side stress on the extremity during the procedure. The test may be further modified by having the athlete move medially or laterally while hopping forward and backward across the line for a distance of 6 meters. Calculation of lower extremity symmetry for these single leg hop tests for time may be made by using the equation provided in Table 13–16. To the best of my knowledge, there are no known norms available for the single leg hop for time tests.

WINGATE BIKE TEST

The Wingate bike test was designed by Bar-Or[94] to evaluate muscular work with primary energy contribution from anaerobic sources. This test can be used to assess both peak anaerobic power and anaerobic capacity.

RELIABILITY. High rates of test-retest reliability have been reported by Bar-Or,[94] Evans and Quinney,[95] and Kaczkowski et al.,[96] with a range of 0.95 to 0.98 for reported scores.

VALIDITY. Kaczkowski et al. found a significant relationship between both peak anaerobic power and anaerobic capacity when compared with fast-twitch fiber percentage and area. In addition, they found a high relationship (r = −0.91) between anaerobic capacity and time for the 50-meter dash.[96] Tharp et al.[97] found that the Wingate test was able to differentiate between sprint and distance running ability in elite males aged 10 to 15 years when scores were expressed relative to body weight.

METHOD. Required equipment for testing includes a bicycle ergometer on which specific loads can be set and a stopwatch to monitor 5-second intervals and 30-second test duration.

The test is initiated with a 5-minute low-intensity warm-up period, which includes four to five intervals of maximal sprints for a 5-second duration against the prescribed load.[88] The load is calculated using the following equation and is reported to represent a task requiring approximately 85 percent anaerobic function:[95]

$$\text{Force (kg)} = \text{Body weight (kg)} \times 0.075$$

A 2- to 5-minute recovery period should be granted following the warm-up and prior to test initiation.

The test begins with a 15-second acceleration period. The subject cycles for 10 seconds at one third the prescribed load and then for 5 seconds with a progressive increase in resistance to the desired force setting. One technician is needed to make the necessary adjustments in the resistance setting while additional technicians monitor time and revolution counts. One technician monitors the time for each 5-second interval and the overall 30 second test du-

---

TABLE 13–18
Calculation of Peak Anaerobic Power and Anaerobic Capacity

- Peak anaerobic power: (kg/5 s) = Max revolutions × 6 M × force (kg)
- Anaerobic capacity: (kg/30 s) = Total revolutions × 6 M × force (kg)

---

ration. Other technicians are used to count and record pedal revolutions.

The force-setting technician initiates the test with the command "go" once the prescribed force has been reached. The subject is instructed to pedal at maximal capacity and remain seated on the bike throughout the test. The technician timing the test shouts the elapsed time every 5 seconds while the counters record the number of pedal revolutions for each interval. Upon completion of the 30-second test, the timer shouts "stop," the force is reduced to a low level, and the subject pedals comfortably for a 1- to 2-minute recovery period.

The two work measurements calculated include peak anaerobic power and anaerobic capacity. Peak anaerobic power is calculated by multiplying the maximal number of revolutions achieved among the 5-second intervals by the prescribed force setting (kg). This total is then multiplied by 6, which is the distance (in meters) the wheel travels for each revolution.

The second calculation is for anaerobic capacity, which is a measure of the total work accomplished during the 30-second test. Anaerobic capacity is calculated by multiplying the total number of revolutions by 6 meters to obtain the total distance covered. The distance is then multiplied by the prescribed force to obtain total work. The equations for calculating both peak anaerobic power and anaerobic capacity are found in Table 13–18.

In order to convert the above measures to watts, peak anaerobic power must be multiplied by 2 and anaerobic capacity must be divided by 3 (using the conversion factor: 6 kg/min = 1 watt).[89] Relative power can be calculated by dividing the power score by body weight. In addition, the fatigue index can be determined by subtracting the lowest power score from the peak power, divided by the peak power score (Table 13–19).

NORMS. Maud and Schultz[98] produced a table of normative standards for peak anaerobic power and anaerobic capacity of men and women aged 18 to 28 (Table 13–20). MacDougall et al.[99] present these norms for various sports.

TABLE 13–19
Fatigue Index Calculation

$$\frac{\text{Peak power} \times \text{lowest power score}}{\text{Peak power score}} \times 100$$

MARGARIA-KALAMEN POWER TEST

The Margaria-Kalamen test was designed to measure maximum anaerobic power or work performance.[100] The test requires a brief burst of maximal power output involving a large percentage of the body's muscle mass, but no particular skill or training is required of the subject.

RELIABILITY. Margaria et al.[100] reported a variation of 4 percent within the same test session and a variability of less than 2 percent when testing two subjects on multiple occasions over a 5-week period.

VALIDITY. Margaria et al.[100] reported equivalent anaerobic power values between treadmill running and the stair-climb test. In addition, they found high individual variability in the data, with athletes scoring significantly higher than nonathletes. Johnson and Nelson[82] reported that sprinters have higher scores than distance runners.

METHOD. Equipment requirements are minimal. The test utilizes a staircase of 12 to 16 stairs measuring 15 to 20 cm in height. Margaria conducted experiments to determine whether power measures could be influenced by step height. Results of testing revealed an optimal height value of 35 cm for stepping, which corresponds with two steps of an ordinary staircase. However, step heights of 30 to 38 cm resulted in values that were within 5 percent of the optimum. Although the use of electric switch mats is preferable, Johnson and Nelson[82] reported that reliable results are obtained with an accurate stopwatch sensitive to one hundredth of a second. An accurate scale is needed to measure body weight of the subject at the time of testing.

There are multiple variations of this test.[100–102] The basic test entails a brief sprint to the staircase and up the stairs as rapidly as possible while the speed of the climb is measured for a specified number of steps. The subject should warm up satisfactorily before testing. The warm-up should include practice trials to allow for familiarization with the test procedures. The subject stands either 2 meters[82] or 6 meters[101,103] in front of the staircase. Once ready, the subject sprints to the staircase and climbs the stairs at a maximal velocity. In Margaria's

TABLE 13–20
Norms for Peak Anaerobic Power and Anaerobic Capacity for the Wingate Anaerobic Test

Percentile Rank	Watts		W · kgBW^{-1}		W · kgBM^{-1}	
	Male	Female	Male	Female	Male	Female
95	676.6	483.0	8.63	7.52	9.30	9.43
90	661.8	469.9	8.24	7.31	9.03	9.01
85	630.5	437.0	8.09	7.08	8.88	8.88
80	617.9	419.4	8.01	6.95	8.80	8.76
75	604.3	413.5	7.96	6.93	8.70	8.68
70	600.0	409.7	7.91	6.77	8.63	8.52
65	591.7	402.2	7.70	6.65	8.5	8.32
60	576.8	391.4	7.59	6.59	8.44	8.18
55	574.5	386.0	7.46	6.51	8.24	8.13
50	564.6	381.1	7.44	6.39	8.21	7.93
45	552.8	376.9	7.26	6.20	8.14	7.86
40	547.6	366.9	7.14	6.15	8.04	7.70
35	534.6	360.5	7.08	6.13	7.95	7.57
30	529.7	353.2	7.00	6.03	7.80	7.46
25	520.6	346.8	6.79	5.94	7.64	7.32
20	496.1	336.5	6.59	5.71	7.46	7.11
15	484.6	320.3	6.39	5.56	7.28	7.03
10	470.9	306.1	5.98	5.25	6.83	6.83
5	453.2	286.2	5.56	5.07	6.49	6.70
M	562.7	380.8	7.28	6.35	8.11	7.96
SD	66.5	56.4	.88	.73	.82	.88
Minimum	441.3	235.4	4.63	4.53	5.72	5.12
Maximum	711.0	528.6	9.07	8.11	9.66	9.66

From Maud PJ, Shultz BB: Norms for the Wingate anaerobic test with comparison to another similar test. Res Q Exerc Sports 1989; 60;144–151. Reproduced with permission from the American Alliance for Health, Physical Education, Recreation and Dance. Reston, VA 22091.

TABLE 13–21
Calculation of Power Output for the Margaria-Kalamen Power Test

$$\text{Power (kg/s)} = \frac{\text{Work}}{\text{Time}} = \frac{\text{Force (kg)} \times \text{Distance (M)}}{\text{Time (s)}}$$

Where force is equal to body weight, distance is the vertical height between the initial and final test steps, and time is the measure of duration required to cover the specified distance

---

original description of the test, the subject was instructed to run up two steps (17.5 cm each) at a time while the time required to cover an even number of steps was recorded. The time was measured from the fourth to the sixth step (70 cm height) for calculation of the power measurement. Fox and Matthews[102] described the test with the subject being instructed to run up three steps at a time, measuring the time between the third and ninth steps. Either method can be used, as long as the sum of the steps falls in the 30- to 38-cm range.

The clock starts as the subject steps on the initially selected step and stops as the last step is reached. Time to cover the distance between the designated steps is recorded to the nearest one hundredth of a second by the use of switch mats or a stopwatch. The best of three trials is recorded for computation of power output. Power output is computed with the product of body weight and total vertical distance being divided by the time in seconds (Table 13–21).

NORMS. Johnson and Nelson[82] reported normative data for high school and college aged men.

ANAEROBIC STEP TEST

Adams[88] defines the anaerobic test as a long anaerobic power test. It is a modification of aerobic step tests[104,105] and an anaerobic step test described by Manahan and Gutin[106] in 1971. The primary differences between the

---

TABLE 13–22
Calculation of Peak Anaerobic Power and Anaerobic Capacity for the Anaerobic Step Test

Peak anaerobic power: $\text{(kg/s)} = \dfrac{\text{Force} \times \text{Distance} \times 1.33}{\text{Time}}$

Where force equals the weight of the subject (kg), distance equals 0.40 M × the number of completed steps in 15 seconds, time equals 15 seconds, and 1.33 is a factor used to convert positive work to total work

Anaerobic capacity: $\text{(kg/min)} = \dfrac{\text{Force} \times \text{Distance} \times 1.33}{\text{Time}}$

Where force equals body weight (kg), distance equals 0.40 M × number of completed steps in 60 seconds, and time equals one

---

TABLE 13–23
Norms for Step Test Anaerobic Capacity[88]

Percentile	Male Power (W)	Female Power (W)
99	730	490
95	608	407
90	584	391
85	554	370
80	536	358
75	520	348
70	507	339
65	495	331
60	483	322
55	472	315
50	460	307
45	448	299
40	438	292
35	425	283
30	413	275
25	400	266
20	384	258
15	366	244
10	336	223
5	312	207

anaerobic and aerobic step tests are that there is no prescribed cadence, the anaerobic test is conducted unilaterally, and the subject stands beside the step rather than facing the step.

RELIABILITY. Adams[88] reported a test-retest reliability value of 0.96 with testing of 30 university students on two occasions within a 1-week period. Manahan and Gutin[106] reported reliability coefficients of 0.95 for the two-count anaerobic step test.

VALIDITY. Manahan and Gutin[106] reported that correlations between the 1-minute anaerobic step test and 600-yard run time were fairly high (r = −0.824).

METHOD. The only equipment requirements are a bench or step with a recommended height of 40 cm (15.75 in.), a stopwatch, and an accurate scale to measure body weight at the time of testing.[88]

The athlete should go through an adequate warm-up, which includes practice of the stepping technique. The stepping technique places the majority of the work on the stepping leg. The athlete stands beside the bench (step) and places the foot of the test leg on the top of the bench. The contralateral leg need not touch the bench during the course of the test. With each step, the body is raised to the level of the top of the step as the test leg fully extends. The contralateral limb dangles in an extended position throughout the ascent but may be used for support and push-off when the foot comes in contact with the floor. The back is to remain straight throughout the course of the test. The upper extremities may be used for balance but are not to be used vigorously in an attempt to assist the test limb. There is a two-count cadence, which includes the ascent and descent.

The subject is instructed to perform the test at maximal effort for the 60-second test. The clock is started with the initial upward movement of the subject. A step is counted each time the test leg fully extends and returns to the starting position. Credit for a step is not granted if the leg does not fully extend or if the back is flexed. The number of completed steps is recorded at 15, 30, and 60 seconds.

The count at 15 seconds is used to calculate peak anaerobic power (assumed to be the highest step count). The count at 30 seconds can be used for comparison with the Wingate bike test. The count at 60 seconds is used to calculate anaerobic capacity. Equations for the calculation of peak anaerobic power and anaerobic capacity for the anaerobic step test are found in Table 13–22. Peak power is converted to watts (true power unit) by multiplication with the conversion factor 1 kg/s = 9.81 W. Anaerobic capacity is converted to watts by dividing with the conversion factor 1 W = 6.12 kg/min.

NORMS. I was unable to locate norms for peak anaerobic power. Adams [88] presented a table of norms for anaerobic capacity of active men and women aged 18 to 30 years (Table 13–23).

AGILITY TESTS

There is a paucity of literature concerning standardization, reliability, and validity issues for functional tests of agility. When the literature is analyzed, it becomes readily apparent that investigators have utilized various tests of agility; therefore, it is difficult to compare the studies.

Tegner et al.[107] conducted a performance test using the single leg hop, a figure-of-eight run, a spiral staircase run, and a slope run to evaluate dysfunction following ACL injury. Separate times were recorded for the turn running and straight running on the figure-of-eight course. Results of the study showed that ACL-deficient subjects were significantly slower than the uninjured subjects around the turn, but no significant differences were found in straight running. In addition, significant differences were found in stair running and slope running.

Anderson et al.[76] used a multiple figure-of-eight course to assess the relationship between various quadriceps and hamstring forces. Eccentric hamstring force at 90 degrees per second was found to be the best predictor of agility run time.

Barber et al.[62] evaluated the effectiveness of the shuttle run with and without pivot for determination of lower limb functional limitations in ACL-deficient knees. It was found that more than 90 percent of the ACL-deficient population scored within the normal limb symmetry range for both shuttle run tests. Therefore, it was concluded that the shuttle run should not be utilized for detection of lower extremity functional limitations.

Giambelluca et al.[79] used a 25-yard shuttle run and a 25-yard figure-of-eight run in addition to the single leg triple jump to identify dysfunction in an ACL-deficient population. Results of the study showed no significant difference between the healthy group and the ACL-deficient group for either the shuttle run or the figure-of-eight run.

FIGURE-OF-EIGHT

Figure-of-eight runs have been advocated throughout the literature for use as a functional (sport-specific) drill to be utilized in the final stages of rehabilitation. However, there is no standardized figure-of-eight run in the literature for testing purposes.

RELIABILITY. Anderson et al.[76] were the only authors to present reliability values for a figure-of-eight test of agility. They reported a test-retest reliability score of 0.90 for the multiple figure-of-eight course described in their study.

VALIDITY. To the best of my knowledge, there are no validity values for figure-of-eight tests available in the literature.

METHOD. Necessary equipment to conduct a figure-of-eight test is minimal. Three accurate stopwatches measuring to the nearest one hundredth second are needed if symmetry scores are desired. Additional equipment includes cones around which the subject can run, tape to mark the floor, and sufficient floor space to accommodate the desired course.

The figure-of-eight course can be set up in various lengths and widths, depending on the degree of difficulty desired. Tegner et al.[107] utilized a 10-meter straight run with narrow turns, whereas Reid[108] presented various figure-of-eight patterns that can be run on a basketball court.

Several timers should be employed. One timer measures the overall time required to complete the figure-of-eight run. Limb symmetry can be evaluated by placing timers at each turn in order to measure time required to run the turn. To evaluate limb symmetry, separate time measures are taken for turns to the left and turns to the right. Tape marks should be placed at the start and finish of the turns to enhance accuracy in timing. The subject should be granted an adequate warm-up period, which includes trials of the run at a submaximal velocity.

The subject starts the test stationed at the beginning of the straight run portion of the course (at the line marking the finish of the turn). The test begins with the command "go." The subject runs as fast as possible through the figure-of-eight course. Three trials should be given, with the best time being used in symmetry calculations. Each timer clocks a specified portion of the run. Right-to-left symmetry scores are calculated using the equation found in Table 13–16.

NORMS. To the best of my knowledge, normative data for the figure-of-eight run are unavailable.

TABLE 13–24
Norms for Barrow Zigzag Run Test

T-Score	Grade				
	7	**8**	**9**	**10**	**11**
80	20.1 down	17.8 down	20.2 down	21.6 down	21.5 down
75	21.4–20.2	19.5–17.9	21.3–20.3	22.7–21.7	22.6–21.6
70	22.7–21.5	21.2–19.6	22.4–21.4	23.8–22.8	23.7–22.7
65	24.0–22.8	22.8–21.3	23.5–22.5	24.8–23.9	24.7–23.8
60	25.2–24.1	24.5–22.9	24.6–23.6	25.8–24.9	25.8–24.8
55	26.5–25.3	26.2–24.6	25.7–24.7	26.9–25.9	26.8–25.9
50	27.8–26.6	27.8–26.3	26.8–25.8	27.9–27.0	27.8–26.9
45	29.0–27.9	29.5–27.9	27.9–26.9	28.9–28.0	28.9–27.9
40	30.3–29.1	31.2–29.6	29.9–28.0	29.9–29.0	29.9–29.0
35	31.6–30.4	32.8–31.3	30.1–29.1	31.0–30.0	31.0–30.0
30	32.8–31.7	34.5–32.9	31.2–30.2	32.1–31.1	32.0–31.1
25	34.1–32.9	36.2–34.6	32.3–31.3	33.1–32.2	33.0–32.1
20	34.2 up	36.3 up	32.4 up	33.2 up	33.1 up

From Johnson BL, Nelson JK: Practical Measurements for Evaluation in Physical Education, 4th ed. Needham Heights, MA, Allyn & Bacon, 1986. Reprinted by permission.

BARROW ZIGZAG RUN

The Barrow zigzag run is a measure of agility. It assesses the athlete's ability to rapidly change direction with cutting and turning maneuvers as well as to accelerate and decelerate with control.

RELIABILITY. Gentile et al.[109] reported ICC (intraclass correlation) values ranging from 0.90 to 0.95 (p < .01) for Barrow's zigzag run. In addition, reliability generalized over time and session was 0.90 (p < .05).

VALIDITY. To the best of my knowledge, there are no available measures of validity for the Barrow zigzag run test.

METHOD. Equipment needs are minimal and include a stopwatch to measure time to the nearest tenth of a second, five cones, and adequate space to accommodate the 16- by 10-foot course.[82] Five cones are set up, one in each corner and one in the center of the course (Fig. 13–20). The subject should be granted an adequate warm-up period, which includes submaximal runs through the course for familiarization with the running pattern. The subject runs the course as rapidly as possible without touching the standards. The stopwatch is started when the command "go" is given and stopped when the athlete crosses the finish line.

Lower extremity symmetry scores may be determined by having the subject repeat the run in the opposite direction (starting on the righthand side of the course). The best of three trials is recorded and used for calculation of limb symmetry or comparison with norms. Calculation of lower extremity symmetry can be made using the equation in Table 13–16.

NORMS. Johnson and Nelson[82] presented a copy of Barrow's norms for high school and junior high school boys (Table 13–24). No additional normative data could be found.

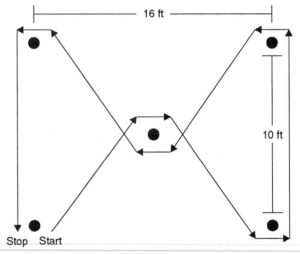

FIGURE 13–20. Barrow zigzag run test. (Drawn from test description in Johnson BL, Nelson JK [eds]: Practical Measurements for Evaluation in Physical Education, 4th ed. New York, Macmillan College Publishing, 1986.)

LINE DRILL

The line drill test is purported to be a measure of speed and anaerobic capacity.[110,111] In addition, it can be classified as an agility test, since it requires rapid directional change, cutting, pivoting, and sudden accelerations and decelerations. To the best of my knowledge, there are no measures of reliability or validity for the line drill test in the literature.

METHOD. Equipment needs are minimal. The course is designed to be run on a basketball court, with cones marking the correct distances (Fig. 13–21). The five cones are arranged as follows: (1) near baseline (point A), (2) near free-throw line (point B), (3) halfcourt line (point C), (4) far free-throw line (point D), and (5) far baseline (point E). In addition, two stopwatches capable of measuring to one tenth of a second are required—one to monitor elapsed time of the run and one to monitor the rest period. The athlete should undergo an adequate warm-up prior to testing. The athlete should be given an explanation of the test procedure and allowed submaximal trial runs as needed to become familiar with the course.

The athlete starts the test from the near baseline (point A). On the command "go," the athlete makes four continuous roundtrips: (1) from the near baseline to the near free-throw line and return (A to B to A), (2) from the near baseline to the halfcourt line and return (A to C to A), (3) from the near baseline to the far free-throw line and return (A to D to A), and (4) from the near baseline to the far baseline and return (A to E to A). The athlete must touch each line with his or her foot during the shuttle run.

The first timer stops the watch as the athlete completes the course. At the same time, the second timer starts a stopwatch to monitor the 2-minute rest period. The original test requires the course to be repeated for a total of four repetitions.

The original test directs that the four run times be averaged for comparison to target times. However, additional test methods and scores can be gleaned from the basic test. For example, the degree of fatigue can be evaluated by comparing the time of the first run with

TABLE 13–25
Calculation of Fatigue for the Line Drill Test

$$\text{Percent fatigue} = \frac{\text{Time of last run} - \text{time of first run} \times 100}{\text{Time of first run}}$$

the time of the fourth (Table 13–25). Also, limb symmetry can be evaluated by directing the subject to run the course pivoting only with the uninvolved limb. After adequate rest, the test would be repeated pivoting only from the involved limb. A minimum of two trials should be granted, with the best time of both limbs being used in the calculations of limb symmetry (see Table 13–16).

NORMS. The only normative data available in the literature are a list of target times found in National Strength and Conditioning Association journals (Table 13–26).[110,111]

BALANCE TESTS

Balance may be defined as the ability to maintain a state of equilibrium in which the body's center of gravity is over the base of support.[112] Balance incorporates visual, vestibular, and proprioceptive information and requires the ability to coordinate these sources of stimulation.[113] In addition, Berg[114] described balance as the ability to maintain a position, to move voluntarily, and to react to a perturbation.

Balance is an essential element for participation in sports, since athletes commonly function at the outer edge of their base of support.[115] Although the need for balance is readily apparent in activities such as gymnastics and ballet, it is also required for any activity in which athletes must control their bodies against the force of gravity. This includes even uncomplicated activities such as walking, which entails a continuous series of losing and regaining balance.

Although balance control is necessary in sports, there is a paucity of research concerning the assessment of balance in athletic populations. The majority of balance studies found were conducted with adults and children with central nervous system or vestibular system disorders.[116–121] In addition, numerous authors[122–125] utilized sophisticated and costly equipment such as stabilometers, force platforms, and motion analysis systems, which is impractical for most clinicians.[121]

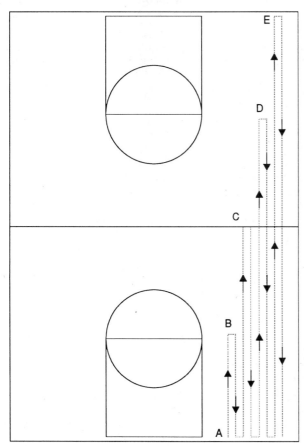

FIGURE 13–21. Line drill test.

TABLE 13–26
Norms for Line Drill Test Based on Performance of College Basketball Players[111]

Position	Time(s) Male	Female
Center	30	35
Forward	28	33
Guard	26	30

The two basic forms of balance tests are static and dynamic.[82] Static balance tests evaluate the ability of an individual to maintain a stationary position within the base of support. Dynamic balance tests evaluate the ability of an individual to maintain balance while in motion, such as while walking on a balance beam, reaching, or hopping from one spot to another.

The single leg balance test is a form of static balance assessment. This test is both simple and inexpensive to administer. In addition, variations can be added to the test to address specific needs of individual athletes.

RELIABILITY. Johnson and Nelson[82] reported a reliability value of 0.87 for the stork stance test when the best trial of the first test session was compared with the best trial of a second test session conducted on separate days. Atwater et al.[126] reported moderate to high test-retest reliability coefficients when the scores for left and right feet were combined in both eyes-open and eyes-closed test conditions.

VALIDITY. Estep[127] reported a positive relationship between static equilibrium and ability in gross motor performance. Subjects who rated high in motor ability in sports also rated high in static equilibrium.

METHOD. The only equipment required for the standing balance test is a stopwatch and possibly a metronome, foam support, or mini-trampoline. The athlete should be given several practice repetitions in order to ensure that the correct test position can be easily assumed.

The athlete is instructed to assume a unilateral stance position and maintain balance as long as possible without using the upper extremities, trunk, or contralateral lower extremity for counterbalancing. The hands should be placed on the pelvis and the athlete should look straight ahead at a selected target.

The watch is started when the unsupported foot is lifted from the floor. The watch is stopped when the raised foot touches the floor, the hands are removed from the pelvis, or the supporting foot is moved from its original position.[119]

The same test is repeated with the eyes closed. The subject is instructed to close the eyes when balance has been established. Timing is started once the eyes are closed. Timing is stopped for the same conditions listed above, in addition to the athlete's opening the eyes. However, a blindfold may be utilized to ensure that visual input has been eliminated.

Three trials are conducted, with the greatest length of time the athlete is able to maintain balance being recorded as the timed balance score. The best performance on each foot and under each testing condition is recorded.

The single leg balance test can be duplicated with a variation in the testing surface. Since there are varied playing surfaces encountered in athletics, the evaluator may wish to assess an athlete's balance on a surface specific to the sport in which he or she is involved. A variation in testing might include the use of a mini-trampoline or a foam surface to provide a greater perturbance to balance.[119]

Finally, the single leg balance test can be combined with contralateral hip movements to provide for stress in the three cardinal planes. Contralateral hip flexion-extension, hip abduction-adduction, and pelvis rotation can provide stress in the sagittal, frontal, and transverse planes, respectively. The clinician can use a metronome to establish a consistent cadence or establish a specified range of motion (ROM) through which the athlete is instructed to move the limb.

The watch is started once the athlete achieves the specified cadence or ROM. The watch is stopped for the same reasons listed above, in addition to a drop in cadence or a reduction in the ROM below the set standard. The length of time the athlete is able to maintain balance is recorded. The best time over three trials is used for calculation. The percentage deficit of the involved limb is calculated using the equation in Table 13–16.

NORMS. Oberg et al.[128] used the single leg stance as one test in a battery of functional tests used to evaluate dysfunction of the lower extremities in patients with osteoarthritis of the hip and knee. A time of 40 to 60 seconds was reported in the group who experienced no reduced function. Atwater et al.[126] reported a mean time of 25 seconds with the eyes-open condition for normally developed children aged 4 through 9 years. No norms could be found for the single leg balance test in athletic populations.

SUMMARY

There is a paucity of literature on well-controlled and well-designed studies concerning the validity and reliability of functional testing. Most of the available research has attempted to correlate clinical measures such as strength, range of motion, or balance to some functional skill or performance variable. Of the functional tests being utilized, few have established values for validity or reliability. There is also very little standardization of these tests, which makes comparison of results difficult if not impossible.

In order to make functional tests more "functional" in terms of prediction of performance or readiness to return to competition, these tests must be developed using sport-specific skills necessary for satisfactory participation in given sports activities. No one would argue that performance of sports activities is multifactorial, and it appears unreasonable to expect to be able to predict performance based on only one component of that performance.

Functional tests should be selected on the basis of their ease of administration, equipment needs, expense, and incorporation of skills required as a component of sport. Some variation in test administration is acceptable if it is required to meet the athlete's needs. However, consistency of test administration must be ensured from one test session to the next, and the exact method of testing must be specified to allow for replication of the test at a later date or by other individuals.

There is still much that needs to be done with regard to functional testing. Currently, there are no known valid and reliable functional tests for the upper extremities or trunk. Norms must be established for those tests that are currently being used. The validity and reliability of currently used functional tests as well as newly developed tests must be established. Sports medicine professionals will be unable to adequately assess an athlete's capacity to return to competition on the basis of unproven or nonfunctional tests.

REFERENCES

1. Garrick JG: A practical approach to rehabilitation. Unpublished handout.
2. Kegerreis S: The construction and implementation of functional progressions as a component of athletic rehabilitation. J Orthop Sports Phys Ther 1983; 5:14–19.
3. Kibler WB: The Sports Preparticipation Fitness Examination. Champaign, IL, Human Kinetics, 1990.
4. Herring SA: Rehabilitation of muscle injuries. Med Sci Sports Exerc 1990; 22:453–456.
5. Anderson MA: Postinjury rehabilitation in the runner. Techniques Orthop 1990; 5:64–75.
6. Kibler WB, Chandler TJ, Pace BK: Principles of rehabilitation after chronic tendon injuries. Clin Sports Med 1992; 11:661–671.
7. Lutz GE, Stuart MJ, Sim FH: Rehabilitative techniques for athletes after reconstruction of the anterior cruciate ligament. Mayo Clin Proc 1990; 65:1322–1329.
8. DeLee J, Allman F, Howe J, et al: Therapeutic exercise modalities. In Drez D (ed): Therapeutic Modalities for Sports Injuries. Chicago, Year Book Medical Publishers, 1989, p 59.
9. DeCarlo MS, Shelbourne KD, McCarroll JR, et al: Traditional versus accelerated rehabilitation following ACL reconstruction: a one-year follow-up. J Orthop Sports Phys Ther 1992; 15:309–316.
10. Mangine RE, Noyes FR, DeMaio M: Minimal protection program: advanced weight bearing and range of motion after ACL reconstruction—weeks 1 to 5. Orthopedics 1992; 15:504–515.
11. Gray GW: Rehabilitation of running injuries: biomechanical and proprioceptive considerations. Top Acute Care Trauma Rehabil 1986; 1:67–78.
12. DeMaio M, Mangine RE, Noyes FR, et al: Advanced muscle training after ACL reconstruction: weeks 6 to 52. Orthopedics 1992; 15:757–766.
13. Threlkeld AJ, Horn TS, Wojtowicz JG, et al: Kinematics, ground reaction force, and muscle balance produced by backward running. J Orthop Sports Phys Ther 1989; 11:56–63.
14. Mackie JW, Dean TE: Running backwards training effects on upper leg musculature and ligamentous instability of injured knees. Med Sci Sports Exerc 1984; 16:151.
15. Flynn TW, Soutas-Little RW: Mechanical power and muscle action during forward and backward running. J Orthop Sports Phys Ther 1993; 17:108–112.
16. Croce P, Gregg JR: Keeping fit when injured. Clin Sports Med 1991; 10:181–195.
17. Kulund DN: The injured runner. Va Med 1985; 112:565–580.
18. Styer-Acevedo J, Cirullo JA: Integrating land and aquatic approaches with a functional emphasis. Orthop Phys Ther Clin North Am 1994; 3:165–178.
19. Garrett WE, Malone TR: The modality of therapeutic exercise. Instr Course Lect 1993; 42:453–459.
20. Roy S, Irvin R: Sports Medicine: Prevention, Evaluation, Management, and Rehabilitation. Englewood Cliffs, NJ, Prentice-Hall, 1983, pp 502–503.
21. Kellett J: Acute soft tissue injuries—a review of the literature. Med Sci Sports Exerc 1986; 18:489.
22. Fleck SJ, Kraemer WJ: Designing Resistance Training Programs. Champaign, IL, Human Kinetics, 1987.
23. Gambetta V: Strength in motion. Training & Conditioning 1993; 3:12–16.
24. Knapik JJ, Mawdsley RH, Ramos MU: Angular specificity and test mode specificity of isometric and isokinetic strength training. J Orthop Sports Phys Ther 1983; 5:58–65.
25. Berger RA, Hardage B: Effect of maximum loads for each of ten repetitions on strength improvement. Res Q 1967; 38:715–718.
26. Engle RP, Canner GG: Proprioceptive neuromuscular facilitation (PNF) and modified procedures for anterior cruciate

27. ligament (ACL) instability. J Orthop Sports Phys Ther 1989; 11:230–236.
27. Stanish WD, Curwin S, Rubinovich M: Tendinitis: the analysis and treatment for running. Clin Sports Med 1985; 4:593–609.
28. Clancy WG (ed): Running injuries. Part II. Evaluation and treatment of specific injuries. Am J Sports Med 1980; 80:287–289.
29. Smart GW, Taunton JE, Clement DB: Achilles tendon disorders in runners—a review. Med Sci Sports Exerc 1980; 12:231–243.
30. Cooper JM, Glassow RB: Kinesiology, 4th ed. St. Louis, CV Mosby, 1976.
31. Smith MJ, Melton P: Isokinetic versus isotonic variable resistance training. Am J Sports Med 1981; 9:275–279.
32. Alter MJ: Science of Stretching. Champaign, IL, Human Kinetics, 1988.
33. Zachazewski JE: Flexibility for sports. In Sanders B (ed): Sports Physical Therapy. Norwalk, CT, Appleton & Lange, 1990, pp 201–238.
34. Bergfield JA, Anderson TE: Achieving mobility, strength, and function of the injured knee. In Hunter LY, Funk FJ (eds): Rehabilitation of the Injured Knee. St. Louis, CV Mosby, 1984, pp 288–297.
35. Leach RE: Overall view of rehabilitation of the leg for running. In Mack RP (ed): AAOS Symposium on the Foot and Leg in Running Sports. St. Louis, CV Mosby, 1982, pp 160–161.
36. Eyestone ED, Fellingham G, George J, et al: Effect of water running and cycling on maximum oxygen consumption and 2-mile run performance. Am J Sports Med 1993; 21:41–44.
37. Clancy WG: Specific rehabilitation for the injured recreational runner. Instr Course Lect 1989; 38:483–486.
38. Freeman MAR, Wybe B: Articular contributions to limb muscle reflexes: the effects of a partial neurectomy of the knee joint on postural reflexes. Br J Surg 1966; 53:61.
39. Ihara H, Nakayama A: Dynamic joint control training for knee ligament injuries. Am J Sports Med 1986; 14:309–315.
40. Blair DF, Wills RP: Rapid rehabilitation following anterior cruciate ligament reconstruction. Athl Training 1991; 26:32–43.
41. Scott SG: Current concepts in the rehabilitation of the injured athlete. Mayo Clin Proc 1984; 59:83–90.
42. Beckman M, Craig R, Lehman RC: Rehabilitation of patellofemoral dysfunction in the athlete. Clin Sports Med 1989; 8:841–860.
43. Galik C: Link by link: understanding the closed kinetic chain. Training & Conditioning 1993; 3:4–11.
44. Steadman JR, Forster RS, Silferskiold JP: Rehabilitation of the knee. Clin Sports Med 1989; 8:605–627.
45. Eifert-Mangine M, Brewster C, Wong M, et al: Patellar tendinitis in the recreational athlete. Orthopedics 1992; 15:1359–1367.
46. Kreighbaum E, Barthels KM: Biomechanics—A Qualitative Approach for Studying Human Movement. Minneapolis, Burgess, 1985.
47. deVries HA: Physiology of Exercise, 3rd ed. Dubuque, William C. Brown, 1980.
48. Wilk KE, Andrews JR: Rehabilitation following arthroscopic subacromial decompression. Orthopedics 1993; 16:349–358.
49. Jensen CR, Fisher AG: Scientific Basis of Athletic Conditioning, 2nd ed. Philadelphia, Lea & Febiger, 1979.
50. Holden DL, Eggert AW, Butler JE: The nonoperative treatment of grade I and II medial collateral ligament injuries to the knee. Am J Sports Med 1983; 11:340–344.
51. Curl WW, Markey KL, Mitchell WA: Agility training following anterior cruciate ligament reconstruction. Clin Orthop Rel Res 1983; 172:133–136.
52. Delitto A, Lehman RC: Rehabilitation of the athlete with a knee injury. Clin Sports Med 1989; 8:805–840.
53. Ryan JB, Hopkinson WJ, Wheeler JH, et al: Office management of the acute ankle sprain. Clin Sports Med 1989; 8:477–495.
54. Anderson TE, Ciolek JS: Specific rehabilitation programs for the throwing athlete. Instr Course Lect 1989; 38:487–491.
55. Carson WG: Rehabilitation of the throwing shoulder. Clin Sports Med 1989; 8:657–689.
56. Seto JL, Brewster CE, Randall CC, et al: Rehabilitation following ulnar collateral ligament reconstruction of athletes. J Orthop Sports Phys Ther 1991; 14:100–105.
57. Clancy WG: Knee symposium: functional rehabilitation of isolated medial collateral ligament sprains. Am J Sports Med 1979; 7:206–209.
58. MacDougall JD, Wenger HA, Green HJ: Physiological Testing of the Elite Athlete. New York, Mouvement Publications, 1983.

59. Howell DC: Statistical Methods for Psychology. Boston, PWS-Kent, 1987.

60. Feinstein AR: Clinical biostatistics XXXI: on the sensitivity, specificity & discrimination of diagnostic tests. Clin Pharmacol Ther 1975; 17:104–116.

61. Payton OD: Research: The Validation of Clinical Practice. Salem, MA, FA Davis, 1989.

62. Barber SD, Noyes FR, Mangine RE, et al: Quantitative assessment of functional limitations in normal and anterior cruciate ligament-deficient knees. Clin Orthop 1990; 225:204–214.

63. Glencross DJ: The nature of the vertical jump test and the standing broad jump. Res Q 1966; 37:353–359.

64. McArdle WD, Katch FI, Katch VL: Exercise Physiology: Energy, Nutrition and Human Performance. Philadelphia, Lea & Febiger, 1991.

65. Bangerter BL: Contributive components in the vertical jump. Res Q 1968; 39:432–436.

66. Berger RA, Henderson JM: Relationship of power to static and dynamic strength. Res Q 1966; 37:9–13.

67. McClements LE: Power relative to strength of leg and thigh muscles. Res Q 1966; 37:71–78.

68. Wiklander J, Lysholm J: Simple tests for surveying muscle strength and muscle stiffness in sportsmen. Int J Sports Med 1987; 8:50–54.

69. Häkkinen K: Force production characteristics of leg extensor, trunk flexor and extensor muscles in male and female basketball players. J Sports Med Phys Fit 1991; 31:325–331.

70. Miyashita M, Kanehisa H: Dynamic peak torque related to age, sex and performance. Res Q 1979; 50:249–255.

71. Davis PO, Dotson CO, Santa Maria DL: Relationship between simulated fire fighting tasks and physical performance measures. Med Sci Sports Exerc 1982; 14:65–71.

72. Considine WJ, Sullivan WJ: Relationship of selected tests of leg strength and leg power on college men. Res Q 1973; 44:404–416.

73. Viitasalo JT: Anthropometric and physical performance characteristics of male volleyball players. Can J Appl Sport Sci 1982; 7:182–188.

74. Smith LE: Relationship between explosive leg strength and performance in the vertical jump. Res Q 1961; 32:405–408.

75. Clark HH: Relationships of strength and anthropometric measures to physical performances involving the trunk and legs. Res Q 1957; 28:223–232.

76. Anderson MA, Gieck JH, Perrin D, et al: The relationship among isometric, isotonic and isokinetic concentric and eccentric quadriceps and hamstring force and three components of athletic performance. J Orthop Sports Phys Ther 1991; 14:114–120.

77. Noyes FR, Barber SD, Mangine RE: Abnormal lower limb symmetry determined by function hop tests after anterior cruciate ligament rupture. Am J Sports Med 1991; 19:513–518.

78. Lephart SM, Perrin DH, Fu FH, et al: Relationship between selected physical characteristics and functional capacity in the anterior cruciate ligament-insufficient athlete. J Orthop Sports Phys Ther 1992; 16:174–181.

79. Giambelluca G, Nicholson GG, Gossmen MR, et al: Evaluation of knee function tests: a pilot study. Phys Ther 1993; 73:S53 (Abstract).

80. Delitto A, Irrgang JJ, Harner CD, et al: Relationship of isokinetic quadriceps peak torque and work to one legged hop and vertical jump in ACL reconstructed subjects. Phys Ther 1993; 73:S85 (Abstract).

81. Sargent DA: The physical test of a man. Am Phys Educ Rev 1921; 26:188–194.

82. Johnson BL, Nelson JK: Practical Measurements for Evaluation in Physical Education, 4th ed. New York, Macmillan College Publishing, 1986.

83. Henry FM: Influence of measurement error and intra-individual variation on the reliability of muscle strength and vertical jump tests. Res Q 1959; 30:155–159.

84. Harman E: The importance of testing power output. Natl Strength Cond Assoc J 1991; 13:72–73.

85. Komi PV, Bosco C: Utilization of stored elastic energy in leg extensor muscles by men and women. Med Sci Sports 1978; 10:261–265.

86. Bosco C, Ito A, Komi PV, et al: Neuromuscular function and mechanical efficiency of human leg extensor muscles during jumping exercises. Acta Physiol Scand 1982; 114:543–550.

87. Gray RK, Start KB, Glencross DJ: A test of leg power. Res Q 1962; 33:44–50.

88. Adams GM: Exercise Physiology Laboratory Manual. Dubuque, William C. Brown, 1990.

89. Barber SD, Noyes FR, Mangine R, et al: Rehabilitation after ACL reconstruction: function testing. Orthopedics 1992; 15:969–974.

90. Semenick D: Basketball bioenergetics. Natl Strength Cond Assoc J 1985; 7:45, 72–73.

91. Daniel DM, Malcom LL, Stone ML, et al: Quantification of knee stability and function. Contemp Orthop 1982; 5:83–91.

92. Hu HS, Whitney SL, Irrgang J, et al: Test-retest reliability of the one-legged vertical jump and the one-legged standing hop test. J Orthop Sports Phys Ther 1992; 15:S51 (Abstract).

93. Risberg MA, Ekeland A: Assessment of functional tests after anterior cruciate ligament surgery. J Orthop Sports Phys Ther 1994; 19:212–217.

94. Bar-Or O: A new anaerobic capacity test: characteristics and applications. Proceedings of the 21st World Congress in Sports Medicine. Brasilia, September 1978.

95. Evans JA, Quinney HA: Determination of resistance settings for anaerobic power testing. Can J Appl Sport Science 1981; 6:53–56.

96. Kaczkowski W, Montgomery DL, Taylor AW, et al: The relationship between muscle fiber composition and maximal anaerobic power and capacity. J Sports Med Phys Fitness 1982; 22:407–413.

97. Tharp GD, Johnson GO, Thorland WG: Measurement of anaerobic power and capacity in elite young track athletes using the Wingate test. J Sports Med 1984; 24:100–105.

98. Maud PJ, Shultz BB: Norms for the Wingate anaerobic test with comparison to another similar test. Res Q 1989; 60:144–151.

99. MacDougall JD, Wenger HA, Green HJ: Physiological Testing of the High-Performance Athlete. Champaign, IL, Human Kinetics, 1991.

100. Margaria R, Aghemo P, Rovelli E: Measurement of muscular power (anaerobic) in man. J Appl Physiol 1966; 21:1662–1664.

101. Kraemer WJ, Fleck SJ: Anaerobic metabolism and its evaluation. Natl Strength Cond Assoc J 1982; 4:20–21.

102. Fox EL, Matthews DK: The Physiological Basis of Physical Education and Athletics. Chicago, Saunders College, 1981.

103. McArdle WD, Katch FI, Katch VL: Exercise Physiology: Energy, Nutrition, and Human Performance. Philadelphia, Lea & Febiger, 1991.

104. Sharkey BJ: Physiology of Fitness. Champaign, IL, Human Kinetics, 1984.

105. Skubik V, Hodgkins J: Cardiovascular efficiency tests for girls and women. Res Q 1963; 34:191–198.

106. Manahan JE, Gutin B: The 1-minute step test as a measure of 600-yard run performance. Res Q 1971; 42:173–177.

107. Tegner Y, Lysholm J, Lysholm M, et al: A performance test to monitor rehabilitation and evaluate anterior cruciate ligament injuries. Am J Sports Med 1986; 14:156–159.

108. Reid DC: Sports Injury Assessment and Rehabilitation. New York, Churchill Livingstone, 1992.

109. Gentile PA, Irrgang JT, Whitney SL: Reliability of functional performance tests designed to identify functional deficits in anterior cruciate deficient athletes. Phys Ther 1993; 73:S50 (Abstract).

110. Semenick D: Anaerobic testing: practical applications. Natl Strength Cond Assoc J 1984; 6:45, 70–73.

111. Semenick D: Tests and measurements: the line drill test. Natl Strength Cond Assoc J 1990; 12:47–49.

112. Horak FB: Clinical measurement of postural control in adults. Phys Ther 1987; 67:1881–1885.

113. Shumway-Cook A, Horak FB: Assessing the influence of sensory interaction on balance: suggestion from the field. Phys Ther 1986; 66:1548–1550.

114. Berg K: Balance and its measure in the elderly: a review. Physiother Can 1989; 41:240–246.

115. Irrgang JJ, Whitney SL, Cox ED: Balance and proprioceptive training for rehabilitation of the lower extremity. J Sport Rehabil 1994; 3:68–83.

116. Bohannon PW, Larkin PA, Cook AC, et al: Decrease in timed balance test scores with aging. Phys Ther 1984; 64:1067–1070.

117. Flores AM: Objectives measurement of standing balance. Neurology Report 1992; 16:17–21.

118. Kantner RM, Rubin AM, Armstrong CW, Cummings V: Stabilometry in balance assessment of dizzy and normal subjects. Am J Otolaryngol 1991; 12:196–204.

119. Nashner LM, Black FO, Wall C: Adaptation to altered support and visual conditions during stance: patients with vestibular deficits. J Neurosci 1982; 2:536–544.

120. Di Fabio RP, Badke MB: Relationship of sensory organization to balance function in patients with hemiplegia. Phys Ther 1990; 70:542–548.

121. Cohen H, Blatchly CA, Gombash LL: A study of the clinical test of sensory interaction and balance. Phys Ther 1993; 73:346–354.

122. Tropp H, Ekstrand J, Gillquist J: Stabilometry in functional instability of the ankle and its value in predicting injury. Med Sci Sports Exerc 1990; 16:64–66.

123. Grabiner MD, Lundin TM, Feuerbach JW: Converting Chattecx balance system vertical reaction force measurements to center of pressure excursion measurements. Phys Ther 1993; 73:316–319.

124. Nashner L: Analysis of movement control in man using the movable platform. *In* Desmedt JE (ed): Motor Control Mechanisms in Health and Disease. New York, Raven Press, 1983, pp 607–619.

125. Friden T, Zatterstrom R, Lindstrand A, et al: A stabilometric technique for evaluation of lower limb instabilities. Am J Sports Med 1989; 17:118–122.

126. Atwater SW, Crowe TK, Deitz JC, Richardson PR: Interrater and test-retest reliability of two pediatric balance tests. Phys Ther 1990; 70:79–84.

127. Estep DO: Relationship of static equilibrium to ability in motor activities. Res Q 1957; 28:5–12.

128. Oberg U, Oberg B, Oberg T: Validity and reliability of a new assessment of lower-extremity dysfunction. Phys Ther 1994; 74:70–80.

CHAPTER 14

Environmental Considerations for Exercise

SCOTT J. MONTAIN *PhD*
BEAU J. FREUND *PhD*

Exercise testing and physical training are integral components in the physical rehabilitation process. Regular physical exercise is also an essential component in any preventive medicine program. The stress imposed by the exercise intensity, however, is only one consideration in the exercise testing and prescription process. An equally important stress to consider is that imposed by the environment (i.e., heat, cold, altitude, and air quality). The environment can alter the physiologic responses of the muscular, cardiovascular, and thermoregulatory systems and, either singly or in combination with exercise, induce potentially hazardous health conditions.

The purpose of this chapter is to provide the reader with information on the physiologic responses that occur when humans are exposed to heat, cold, altitude, and air pollution. The chapter focuses on the impact that each environmental extreme has on the physiologic responses to exercise, exercise performance, and exercise prescription. In each section, special considerations are discussed that can modify the physiologic responses to the environment, as well as effective ways to prevent, recognize, and treat illnesses arising from environmental exposure.

TEMPERATURE REGULATION AND ENERGY BALANCE

Humans, like other homeothermic animals, must maintain body temperature within a relatively narrow

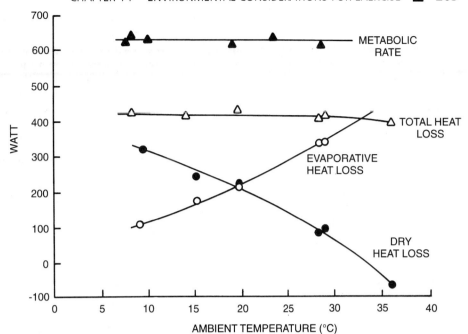

FIGURE 14–1. Avenues of heat exchange during exercise over a wide range of ambient air temperature. (Modified from Nielsen M: Die Regulation der Körpertemperatur bei Muskelarbeit. Skand Arch Physiol 1938; 79:193.)

range in order to function optimally and/or survive. Deviations in body temperature ±4°C from 37°C (normal resting core temperature) are known to reduce physical and cognitive performance, and deviations of +6°C or −12°C are usually lethal.[1]

Body temperature is physiologically regulated by integrating both thermal and nonthermal information within the anterior and preoptic areas of the hypothalamus and sending the appropriate efferent signals to alter heat loss and gain. Thermal signals include afferent input from temperature-sensitive nerve endings located in the brain, body core, and skin. Nonthermal signals include afferent information from the cardiopulmonary and arterial baroreceptors and osmoreceptors. Passive heat transfer properties also affect heat movement within the body. These passive properties include body mass, body mass–surface area ratio, and body composition.

Despite its complex nature, body temperature regulation can be viewed simply as the process of balancing heat production with heat loss. This is accomplished by physiologic processes that control the rate of heat production, the transfer of metabolic heat from the body core to the skin surface, and the transfer of heat from the skin surface to the surrounding environment. Deep body (core) temperature remains stable whenever body heat production equals body heat loss. Core temperature increases when heat production exceeds heat loss and falls when heat losses exceed heat production.

During exercise, metabolic substrates are broken down to provide energy for cellular metabolism. However, only 20 to 23 percent of the substrate's energy is used to accomplish work. The remaining 77 to 80 percent becomes heat that must be dissipated to prevent dangerous elevations in core temperature. Heat production, which can increase 20 times the basal rate, can be conveniently estimated from the measured oxygen

uptake and the useful work that is accomplished. The magnitude of heat storage (i.e., increase in body core temperature) depends on the magnitude of heat production, the ability to transfer the heat to the skin surface, and the capacity of the environment to accept heat from the skin surface. In hot environments, the heat produced during exercise may be compounded by heat gained from the environment and further raise core temperature. In cold environments, the heat produced by exercise or involuntary rhythmic contractions of skeletal muscle (shivering) may be needed to attenuate reductions in body temperature.

The majority of heat generated within the body is convected from the inner core to the skin's surface via the circulation. Heat is then dissipated to the environment by three primary means: radiation, convection, and evaporation. The relative contribution of each pathway is dependent on the environmental conditions, as summarized in Figure 14–1. Any imbalance between the rate of heat dissipation and the rate of heat production results in a change in heat storage or heat debt. To better understand the different pathways for heat loss, a brief description of each is provided.

Radiation is the heat gained or lost at the skin surface due to the arrival or release of energy in the infrared and related portions of the electromagnetic energy spectrum from or to the surrounding radiant surfaces. Radiant heat exchange is independent of ambient air temperature, depending on the temperature gradient between the emitting and receiving surfaces.

Convection is the heat lost or gained due to the mass transfer or conduction of heat at the boundary layer of air (or water) moving past the skin's surface. In thermoneutral conditions and still air, convection accounts for 12 to 15 percent of total heat loss. However, convective heat loss increases rapidly with air movement. Water is approximately 40 times more effective in convecting heat from the body than is air. As a consequence, cold exposure combined with body surface wetting causes substantial heat loss and is more likely to result in hypothermia than is cold air alone.

Evaporation is the heat lost by vaporization of water from the skin surface. Evaporation is the most effective means of heat loss in terms of absolute quantities of heat, and it is the most important route of heat loss during exercise-heat stress. Evaporation is dependent on the water vapor pressure gradient between the skin and the air and the air velocity moving over the skin surface. It does not require a positive skin–to–ambient air temperature gradient. Thus, under conditions in which there is a positive water vapor pressure gradient between the skin and the ambient air, secreted sweat will evaporate, removing heat from the body. In high ambient humidity conditions, the evaporative capacity is reduced, and secreted sweat will drip from the skin surface without dissipating body heat.

HEAT EXPOSURE

CORE TEMPERATURE RESPONSES TO EXERCISE-HEAT STRESS

During physical exercise in ambient conditions that allow steady-state heat balance, core temperature initially increases rapidly and then increases more slowly until heat loss equals heat production (Fig. 14–2). The initial increase in core temperature is due to a lag in the activation of the heat dissipation mechanisms (i.e., sweating, cutaneous vasodilatation). The magnitude of increase in core temperature is proportional to the metabolic rate (e.g., the exercise intensity) and is nearly independent of environmental conditions within a range of climatic conditions termed the *prescriptive zone* (Fig. 14–3).[2–6] The prescriptive zone refers to a range of ambient air conditions in which there is little or no difference in steady-state exercise core temperature despite varying ambient air conditions. During exercise in climatic conditions above the prescriptive zone, the steady-state core temperature is elevated in proportion to the climatic conditions. Therefore, steady-state body core temperature will be similar during exercise in a temperate (20 to 28°C) environment but will be elevated

when performing the same exercise in hot environments. Equally important, Figure 14–3 also illustrates that the upper end of the prescriptive zone is shifted to a lower ambient temperature condition with increasing exercise intensity. This means that core temperature will begin to be affected by environmental conditions at a lower ambient temperature when performing high-intensity exercise than during moderate or low-intensity exercise.

The core temperature increase during endurance exercise does not reflect a failure of the temperature control system. On the contrary, core temperature is finely regulated even under extremes of exercise and environmental temperature. During exercise, the core temperature increase is the result of integrated physiologic responses that optimize skeletal muscle perfusion and heat transport without compromising arterial blood pressure. Under conditions in which skin blood flow is compromised (e.g., dehydration, high exercise intensity), the core temperature increase widens the temperature gradient between the body core and the skin, preserving heat transport to the peripheral circulation despite lower skin blood flow.

There are climatic conditions, however, in which steady-state core temperature values cannot be attained. Whenever heat production exceeds the environment's capacity to accept heat, core temperature progressively increases, and persons are at increased risk for heat exhaustion and heatstroke. Athletes, race organizers, and trainers must evaluate the ambient weather conditions prior to beginning exercise and modify the exercise intensity and duration, as well as fluid requirements, to reduce the risk of heat injury. The American College of Sports Medicine has recommended that endurance athletic events be rescheduled when the ambient wet bulb globe temperature (WBGT = $0.7*T_{wb} + 0.2*T_g + 0.1*T_{db}$; where T_{wb} = wet bulb temperature, T_g = black globe temperature, and T_{db} = dry bulb temperature) exceeds 28°C.[7]

CARDIOVASCULAR RESPONSES TO EXERCISE-HEAT STRESS

When exercising is done in warm or hot ambient temperatures, the cardiovascular system is challenged

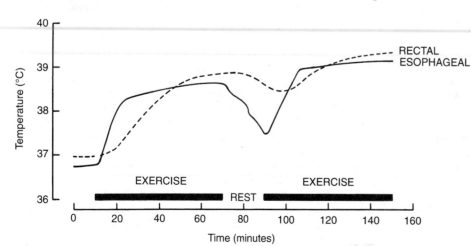

FIGURE 14–2. Esophageal and rectal temperature responses to rest and exercise during compensable heat stress. (From Sawka MN, Wenger CB: Physiological responses to acute exercise–heat stress. *In* Pandolf KB, Sawka MN, Gonzalez RR [eds]: Human Performance Physiology and Environmental Medicine at Terrestrial Extremes. Indianapolis, Benchmark Press, 1988, p 110.)

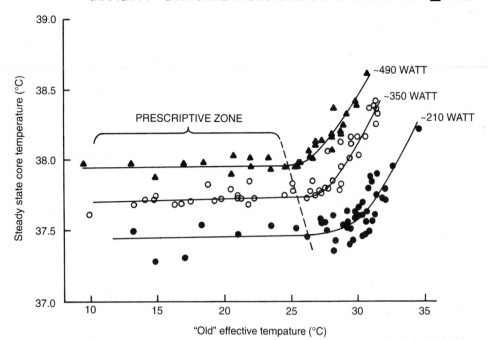

FIGURE 14–3. Relationship of steady-state core temperature responses and the "old" effective air temperature at three metabolic rates. Effective air temperature derived from dry and wet bulb temperature, and wind speed. (Modified from Lind AR: A physiological criterion for setting thermal environmental limits for everyday work. J Appl Physiol 1963; 18:51.)

with simultaneously delivering sufficient muscle blood flow to support metabolism and sufficient cutaneous blood flow to support heat loss from the body while still maintaining blood pressure. Because the blood flow demand to these vascular beds can exceed the cardiovascular system's capacity, reductions in blood flow to the skin and/or muscle may be necessary to preserve cardiovascular stability.

Several adjustments occur during exercise-heat stress to optimize the balance between cutaneous and skeletal muscle blood flow. First, blood flow to the splanchnic organs and kidneys is reduced, with the magnitude of reduction proportional to the exercise intensity and environmental heat stress.[8] The lower blood flow to these organs reduces their blood volume, helping to maintain central blood volume, cardiac filling pressure, and arterial blood pressure. Second, at the onset of exercise, a generalized venoconstriction occurs in proportion to the severity of exercise.[9,10] The venoconstriction acts to reduce skin blood volume, enhancing central blood volume and cardiac filling.[8]

The cardiovascular system has finite limits to its ability to distribute blood volume during exercise-heat stress. The redistribution of blood into the cutaneous circulation during heat stress can compromise cardiac filling, cardiac output, and blood pressure. Figure 14–4 illustrates the cardiovascular responses of six subjects during graded exercise in a neutral (25.6°C) and hot (43.3°C) environment.[8] When exercising in the hot environment, the subjects had higher heart rates but lower central blood and stroke volumes, compared with the neutral environment. Although the subjects' cardiac output was similar in the hot and neutral environments during the two lower exercise intensities, cardiac output was lower in the hot environment at the two higher exercise intensities. The lack of ability to redistribute sufficient blood volume to preserve cardiac output during heat stress is further evidenced by the 5 to 8 percent lower maximal oxygen uptake during exercise

in hot environments.[11–15] The greater cardiovascular strain can reduce exercise tolerance and impair endurance exercise performance.

METABOLIC RESPONSES TO EXERCISE-HEAT STRESS

Whether heat stress increases the caloric requirement to perform a specific task remains unclear. Although several investigators have reported elevated metabolic rates with exercise-heat stress,[16–20] others have reported no change or lower metabolic rates.[21–24] One explanation for the discrepancy may be contributions of anaerobic metabolism to total energy cost, as the investigations reporting similar or lower metabolic rates during exercise-heat stress also reported increased plasma or blood lactate concentration.[22–24]

The impact of exercise-heat stress on muscle blood flow and metabolism has been examined in several studies. Exercise-heat stress does not appear to impair either blood flow or oxygen delivery to the working muscle. Two recent studies reported similar leg blood flow and leg oxygen uptake during moderately intense exercise in hot (40°C) and temperate (20–23°C) climates.[20,25] Exercise-heat stress also appears to have little impact on muscle glycogen utilization.[20,24,26] Therefore, there is little evidence to suggest that hot ambient air temperatures impair oxygen delivery to skeletal muscle or increase skeletal muscle glycogenolysis during exercise.

SKELETAL MUSCLE STRENGTH AND FATIGABILITY

Several investigations have reported that sprinting and jumping performance improves after warming skeletal muscle.[27,28] Bergh and Ekblom[27] found that

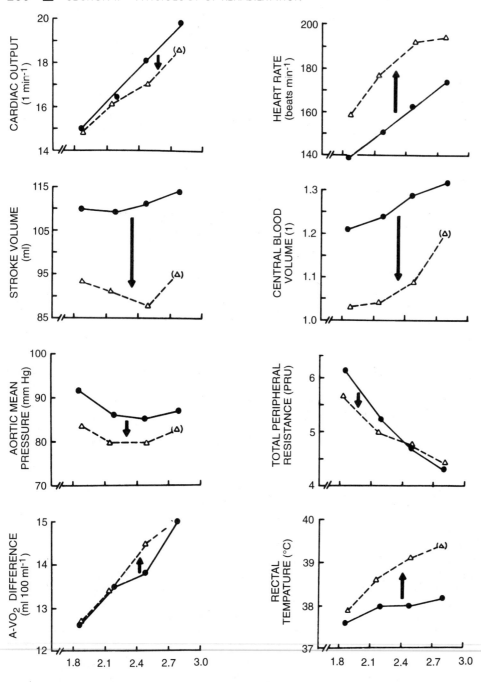

FIGURE 14–4. Summary of cardiovascular responses to graded upright exercise in neutral (25.6°C, *solid circles*) and hot (43.3°C, *open triangles*) environments. Heat stress reduced cardiac output at the two higher workloads and depressed stroke volume and central blood volume at all levels of exercise. Each data point is the average of multiple measurements during each 15-minute exercise period from six men. The data points in parentheses show where data from one subject are missing. (From Rowell LB: Human Circulation: Regulation during Physical Stress. New York, Oxford University Press, 1986, p 379.)

maximal torque and power output during knee extensor exercise were positively related to muscle temperature, with each measure changing about 5 percent per degree Celsius change over a muscle temperature range of 30 to 39°C. Other investigators reported no difference in maximal isometric force[29–31] or a reduction in submaximal isometric endurance[29,32–34] following skeletal muscle heating. One explanation for these disparate findings may be the magnitude of increase in muscle temperature accrued with heating, as there is an optimal skeletal muscle temperature for isometric endurance.[32–34] Therefore, muscle performance can be compromised if its temperature becomes excessively elevated during exercise-heat stress.

SPECIAL CONSIDERATIONS

ACCLIMATIZATION

Physical tasks that are relatively easy to perform in cool weather can become extremely difficult to complete during initial exposures to hot weather. Depending on the exercise intensity and accompanying physiologic strain, heat exposure may result in higher core temperature, a more rapid heart rate, narrowed pulse pressure, headache, dizziness, cramps, dependent edema, flushing of face and neck, and orthostatic hypotension.[35–37] In addition, these symptoms may be accompanied by a feeling of lassitude and increased fatigue. Fortunately, repeated exposure to hot environments produces adaptations that improve an individual's work capacity during subsequent heat exposures. The physiologic adjustments that improve work capacity in the heat are collectively termed *heat acclimatization*.

As depicted in Figure 14–5, most heat acclimatization occurs during the first week of heat exposure, and acclimatization to a given environmental condition is virtually complete after 10 days of exposure. Heat acclimatization leads to marked reductions in exercise heart rate, core temperature, skin temperature, and the core temperature at which cutaneous vasodilatation and sweating begin.[38] There appears to be little change in cardiac output, mean arterial pressure, pulse pressure, or total vascular conductance with acclimatization.[38]

The reductions in heart rate and core temperature are greater and occur more quickly with the combination of exercise and heat stress as opposed to heat stress alone.[39] Furthermore, heat acclimatization occurs only when an individual is "stressed" by the environment. Little acclimatization to the hot midday weather occurs if an individual trains in the cool hours of the morning or evening and spends the rest of the day in an air-conditioned room.

Regular exercise in a cool environment has been shown to improve one's ability to thermoregulate during exercise-heat stress.[40,41] The exercise-induced "internal" heat stress (e.g., increased core temperature) stimulates adaptation of the peripheral circulation and evaporative capacity, similar to that which occurs with heat exposure. As a result, aerobically trained persons store less body heat during exercise than untrained persons. However, regular exercise in a cool environ-ment does not fully acclimatize an individual to exercise in a hot environment, as regular training in a hot environment can further reduce the thermal and cardiovascular strain associated with exercise in a hot environment.[42–45] Therefore, if exercise is to be performed in hot weather, it is optimal to acclimatize to that climate.

DEHYDRATION

Dehydration, or body water deficits, occurs during exercise-heat stress if sufficient fluids are not ingested to offset sweat losses. Dehydration results in elevated body core temperature and heart rate during exercise,[41,46–48] with the magnitude of these increases graded in proportion to the amount of dehydration (Fig. 14–6).[41,47] Dehydration negates the thermoregulatory advantage of heat acclimatization and aerobic training.[49,50] Dehydration also increases the perception of effort[47] and reduces endurance exercise performance.[41,46,51] In addition, a recent study showed that dehydrated subjects incurred exhaustion from heat strain at lower core temperatures than did normally hydrated subjects during uncompensable heat stress, suggesting that dehydrated persons have a reduced tolerance to exercise-heat strain.[52]

To minimize dehydration, fluids should be ingested during prolonged exercise. The increase in core temperature during exercise is smallest when fluid intake most closely matches sweat loss and no dehydration occurs.[47,53] In hot climates, this may require persons to drink 1.0 to 1.5 liters of fluid per hour. The timing of rehydration during exercise is not critical to thermoregulation if the volume of fluid intake is adjusted

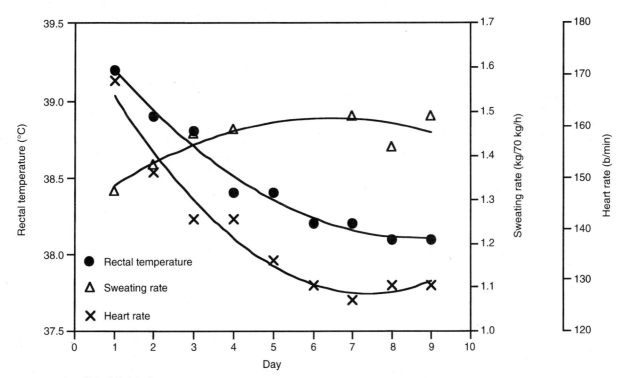

FIGURE 14–5. Rectal temperature, sweating rate, and heart rate responses over 9 consecutive days of exercise–heat stress. Each data point is the average response of three men after 100 minutes of exercise in a desert climate (49°C$_{db}$, 17% rh). (Modified from Lind AR, Bass DE: Optimal exposure time for development of acclimatization to heat. Fed Proc 1963; 22:704.)

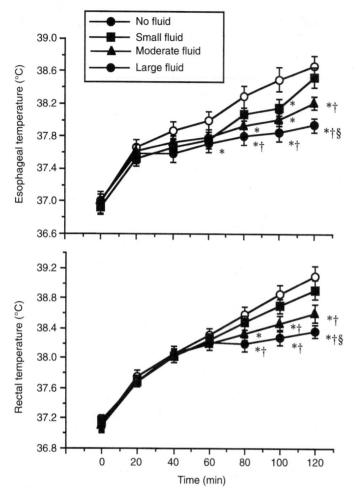

FIGURE 14–6. Influence of dehydration on esophageal and rectal temperature during 2 hours of moderately intense exercise. (From Montain SM, Coyle EF: Influence of graded dehydration on hyperthermia and cardiovascular drift during exercise. J Appl Physiol 1992; 73:1340.)

accordingly; the rise in core temperature is dependent on the magnitude of fluid loss and not the timing of fluid intake.[54] The composition of the fluid replacement solution can vary as well. Commercial carbohydrate-electrolyte solutions with up to 8 percent carbohydrate appear to be equally effective as water for attenuating increases in core temperature and heart rate during prolonged exercise.[55]

Although dehydration produces graded increments in core temperature during exercise-heat stress and can impair endurance performance, it remains unclear whether drinking large volumes of fluid to prevent dehydration actually improves athletic performance. Drinking large volumes of fluid during prolonged exercise may force athletes to slow to consume the beverage, and subsequent race pace may be compromised due to gastric bloating and discomfort.[56] Each athlete needs to determine whether the time lost as a result of drinking larger volumes of fluid is compensated for by the physiologic benefits obtained by attenuating dehydration during prolonged exercise.

AGING

Studies have documented that older populations have a greater incidence of heat intolerance compared with younger adults.[57] The elderly also exhibit a larger than normal basal body temperature fluctuation com-

pared with younger adults.[58] This latter liability appears to be largely due to a reduced circulatory effectiveness in controlling heat transport between the body core and the cutaneous circulation. Research suggests, however, that aging per se is not responsible for the greater incidence of heat intolerance in the elderly.[59,60] When matched for activity and aerobic fitness, and when exercise is performed at the same relative percentage of maximal aerobic capacity, older and younger adults have similar increases in core temperature. In addition, aging per se does not impair the ability to acclimatize to hot environments.[59,60] The greater incidence of heat intolerance observed in the elderly is now thought to result from functional changes accompanying a more sedentary lifestyle, obesity, a reduced sweating response, cardiovascular insufficiency, and the effects of medication.[57]

GENDER

Both men and women have similar thermoregulatory responses during exercise and moderate heat stress when matched for fitness and training.[61–63] Yet differences between genders do exist. Women appear to sweat more efficiently than men in humid climates, as more of their secreted sweat is evaporated and less sweat drips from the body prior to evaporation.[63,64] The menstrual cycle produces regular fluctuations in basal body temperature. During the luteal phase of the menstrual cycle, basal body temperature is roughly 0.4°C higher than during the follicular phase.[65] Whether the phase of the menstrual cycle alters the ability to regulate body temperature remains unresolved. Although several investigations reported that the luteal phase simply produces a graded increase in steady-state core temperature during exercise, compared with exercise during the follicular phase,[65,66] a separate investigation found that women were unable to achieve a steady-state core temperature during the luteal phase.[67] The ability of women to effectively train and compete throughout the menstrual cycle, however, suggests that body temperature is adequately regulated during the luteal phase, albeit at a higher core temperature.

CLOTHING

Clothing impairs the ability to dissipate heat during exercise-heat stress, as it creates a barrier for the transfer of heat between the skin and the environment. The properties of the clothing, such as its insulation properties and air and vapor permeability, as well as the proportion of the body surface covered, determine the impact of clothing on body temperature regulation and exercise-heat tolerance. Warm-weather clothing should be loose fitting to permit free circulation of air between the skin and the environment. Further, it should be light colored to reflect radiant light and minimize radiant heat gain in sunny weather. The protective clothing worn by firefighters and soldiers on the chemical-biologic battlefield greatly increases the thermal and cardiovascular strain of exercise and reduces physiologic tolerance to heat strain.[68,69]

EXERCISE TRAINING IN HOT ENVIRONMENTS

Exercise training can be conducted safely in hot environments if precautions are taken to minimize the risk of heat illness. Persons exercising in hot environments should attempt to attenuate dehydration by drinking fluids before and during exercise. Individual fluid requirements can be estimated from body weight lost during exercise. Proper clothing should be worn to minimize added heat stress during the exercise bout. Finally, persons exercising in the heat should adjust the exercise intensity to accommodate circulatory strain accompanying exercise in hot environments.

Heart rate remains a reliable indicator of cardiovascular strain during exercise-heat stress. Using the exercise heart rate to set the exercise intensity is a good method for reducing thermal strain in hot climates. However, it should be realized that this method reduces the training stimulus placed on skeletal muscle.

POPULATIONS SUSCEPTIBLE TO HEAT INTOLERANCE

Although the etiology of heat intolerance is poorly understood, there are a number of congenital and acquired risk factors that have been associated with reduced heat tolerance (Table 14–1). The identification of susceptible persons is important for reducing the risk of heat injury during work in hot weather.

Congenital anomalies underlying heat intolerance usually impair the ability to produce and secrete sweat onto the skin surface. Ectodermal dysplasia is the most common form of congenital anhidrosis. It is attributed to an autosomal dominant or X-linked recessive trait and therefore affects only males.[70] The sweat glands of those afflicted are either absent, functionally impaired, or histologically present but not innervated. Patients with cystic fibrosis and Parkinson's disease have altered neural sweat gland regulation, which may predispose them to heat intolerance during environmental heat stress.[71–73]

Several skin disorders, such as miliaria rubra (heat rash), impede heat transfer, increase heat storage, and impair performance.[74–76] Psoriatic patients have been shown to have reduced sweating and elevated core

TABLE 14–1
Factors Associated with Heat Intolerance

Functional-Physiologic Factors

Dehydration
Low physical fitness/activity
Lack of acclimatization
Surface area–to–mass ratio
Age
Fatigue

Concurrent Disease

CNS lesions
Cardiovascular disease
Sweat gland dysfunction
Infectious diseases
Psychiatric illness
Diabetes mellitus
Extensive skin burns
Hyperthyroidism
Parkinsonism
Pheochromocytoma

Congenital Abnormalities

Ectodermal dysplasia
Linear skin dystrophy
Idiopathic anhidrosis
Cystic fibrosis
Scleroderma

Drugs

Drug abuse
Medications
Alcohol

Other

Clothing
Previous heatstroke

Data from Epstein Y: Heat intolerance: predisposing factor or residual injury? Med Sci Sports Exerc 1990; 22:29.

TABLE 14–2
Diagnosis and Treatment of Heat Disorders

Disorder	Cause/Predisposing Factor	Clinical Features and Diagnosis	Treatment	Prevention
Heat Cramps	Heavy and prolonged sweating Inadequate salt intake	Low serum sodium and chloride Muscle twitching, cramps, and spasms in arms, legs, and abdomen	Severe cramps: intravenous saline infusion Mild cramps: oral administraton of 0.1% salt solution Rest in cool environment Eat salty foods	Ensure acclimatization Provide extra salt at meals and with fluids
Heat Exhaustion	Inability of the cardiovascular system to meet demands of thermoregulatory, muscular and visceral blood flow Water and/or salt depletion due to heavy prolonged sweating Inadequate fluid and/or salt intake Polyuria or diarrhea Vomiting Inadequate acclimatization Heat production exceeds environmental heat-loss capacity	Fatigue, orthostatic dizziness, ataxia, hypotension Syncope Nausea and vomiting Tingling in hands and feet Wrist and/or ankle spasm Dyspnea Elevated skin and core temperatures High hematocrit, serum protein, and sodium Dry tongue and mouth Excessive thirst Weak, disconsolate, uncoordinated, and mentally dull	Rest supine in cool environment Intravenous saline infusion Sponge with cool water Provide small quantities of semiliquid food Keep record of body weight, water and salt intake, and body temperature Avoid exercise-heat stress for 24–48 h	Provide adequate fluids Ensure acclimatization Provide opportunity for intermittent cooling and adequate rest Reduce work rate when exercising in hot temperatures and high-humidity climates
Heatstroke	Distinguished from heat exhaustion by the presence of tissue injury	Collapse Severe encephalopathy and hyperthermia Dehydration Rhabdomyolysis Myoglobinuria Diarrhea and vomiting	Active cooling IV dextrose-saline infusion Isoproterenol, dopamine, or dobutamine as needed Maintain airway Monitor and treat hyperkalemia Monitor and treat acute renal injury Keep record of core temperature Treat secondary disorders Avoid exercise-heat stress until clinical recovery is complete	Provide adequate fluids Ensure acclimatization Provide opportunity for intermittent cooling and adequate rest Reduce work rate when exercising in hot temperatures and high-humidity climates
Heat Syncope	Inability to maintain blood pressure Peripheral vasodilatation and pooling of blood Circulatory instability and loss of vasomotor tone Hyperventilation Inadequate acclimatization Infection	Weakness and fatigue Hypotension Increased venous compliance Blurred vision Pallor Syncope Elevated skin and core temperatures	Place supine and elevate legs Rest in cool environment Provide oral saline if conscious and resting Keep record of blood pressure and body temperature	Ensure acclimatization Avoid sustained upright static work
Miliaria Rubra, Miliaria Profunda	Local inflammation caused by occlusion of the sweat gland	Pruritic, inflamed papulovesicular skin eruptions High ambient humidity	Cool and dry affected skin Avoid re-exposure until lesions have healed Control for infection	Wear loose-fitting clothing Good hygiene

emperatures during heat stress.[76] Burn victims have an impaired ability to sweat, and heat tolerance is negatively correlated to the burnt skin area.[57] Conversely, mild sunburn does not seem to increase the thermal strain accompanying exercise in hot climates.[77]

Obese individuals appear to be less tolerant to heat stress.[78,79] The lower heat tolerance in this population may be due to their lower cardiovascular fitness compared with lean individuals (as evidenced by a higher heart rate at rest and during exercise) as well as their lower surface area–to–body mass ratio.[57]

Spinal cord–injured persons cannot dissipate body heat as effectively as able-bodied persons during exercise-heat stress. They cannot redistribute blood flow as effectively as able-bodied persons, and their maximal whole-body sweat rate is impaired due to insensate skin. The magnitude of this impairment is dependent on the level of the spinal lesion.

Patients with multiple sclerosis typically demonstrate adverse reactions to heat exposure. External heat, in the form of either climatic conditions or therapeutic modalities, may exacerbate clinical symptoms and induce fatigue.[80]

Various pharmaceutical agents impair heat transfer to the environment.[81–83] For example, anticholinergic drugs, such as atropine, increase core temperature and reduce exercise tolerance time when working in hot environments.[84] Acute amphetamine poisoning commonly leads to hyperpyrexia and fatal heat stroke.[57] Neuroleptic drugs such as chlorpromazine can also impair heat transfer.[81]

HEAT ILLNESS

There are several illnesses that may occur during exercise-heat stress (Table 14–2). The clinical features and treatment of these illnesses have been discussed in detail elsewhere.[85,86]

HEAT CRAMPS. This condition can arise after heavy and prolonged sweating. The etiology is unknown but is associated with low serum electrolyte concentration. It is characterized by skeletal muscle twitching, cramps, and spasm. It generally occurs in the arms, legs, and abdomen. The incidence of heat cramps can be minimized by ensuring acclimatization and inclusion of salt supplementation at mealtime.

HEAT EXHAUSTION. This disorder is the most common form of heat illness. It is a "functional" illness and is not associated with organ damage. Heat exhaustion arises when the cardiovascular system is unable to meet the competing demands of thermoregulatory skin blood flow and skeletal muscle and vital organ blood flow. Individuals become fatigued, with orthostatic dizziness and ataxia. Common features include dyspnea and tingling in hands and feet. Persons may be disconslate, uncoordinated, and mentally dull. Acute management should be focused on reducing cardiovascular demand and reversing water and salt deficits.

HEATSTROKE. At presentation, the distinction between heat exhaustion and heatstroke is difficult to make. Heatstroke is distinguished from heat exhaustion by the presence of tissue injury. The degree of injury appears to be dependent on both the magnitude of core temperature elevation and the duration of exposure. Pre-existing conditions (e.g., hypokalemia, endotoxemia, tissue ischemia) probably have a role in the evolution of heatstroke. It is a serious illness that requires medical attention. If heatstroke is suspected and temperature is elevated, active cooling should be initiated, and the person should be transported to medical facilities.

MILIARIA RUBRA AND MILIARIA PROFUNDA. Miliaria rubra (heat rash or prickly heat) is a papulovesicular skin eruption that can arise when active eccrine sweat glands become occluded by organic debris. It generally occurs in humid climates or to skin that is sufficiently encapsulated by clothing to produce high-humidity conditions. It is treated by cooling and drying the skin, treating itching symptoms, and controlling for infection. Exercise-heat exposure should be avoided until the rash has disappeared.

Miliaria that becomes generalized and prolonged is termed miliaria profunda. It can lead to anhidrotic heat exhaustion, as the occluded sweat glands no longer produce sweat for evaporation. The lesions are truncal, noninflamed, and papular. They are also asymptomatic. Persons with miliaria profunda are less heat tolerant compared with the general population.

HEAT TETANY. This is a rare condition that occurs in individuals acutely exposed to overwhelming heat stress. It appears to be caused by hyperventilation. Patients present with respiratory alkalosis, carpopedal spasm, and syncope. They should be removed from the heat and treated for hyperventilation.

COLD EXPOSURE

THERMOREGULATION IN COLD CLIMATES

Cold weather need not be a deterrent for outdoor exercise. Physical exercise can be performed safely in extremely cold conditions if sufficient clothing is worn to maintain body core temperature and protect the skin from cold injury. It does require special consideration for the exercise participant, however, as inadequate clothing can lead to rapid reductions in body temperature and commensurate impairment of exercise performance.

Behavioral thermoregulation (e.g., seeking shelter and wearing warm clothing) is the most effective means of tolerating cold exposure. Cold-weather clothing adds an insulation layer between the body core and the ambient air or water, enabling persons to tolerate extremely cold ambient temperatures without becoming cold. The amount of clothing necessary to maintain thermal balance is inversely related to metabolic rate.

Humans have two primary physiologic responses to cold exposure, both of which attempt to prevent or minimize a fall in body core temperature. The initial response is cutaneous vasoconstriction. This reduces blood flow to the periphery and increases insulation. The second response is to increase metabolic heat production by shivering and/or physical activity.

PERIPHERAL VASOCONSTRICTION. Cutaneous vasoconstriction is sympathetically mediated. It reduces heat transfer from the core to the periphery and adds an insulative layer between the body core and the environment. Depending on the magnitude of cold and the duration of exposure, cold exposure can also induce limb skeletal muscle vasoconstriction.[87] Peripheral vasoconstriction is initiated with the onset of skin cooling, but muscle blood flow is maintained until cold strain is severe enough to compromise the core temperature.[87]

In many individuals, the hands and feet demonstrate cyclic blood flow when exposed to cold. This phenomenon, often referred to as the "hunting reflex," is now more commonly termed cold-induced vasodilatation (CIVD). It occurs due to rhythmic cycling of sympathetic vasoconstrictor stimulation. The cyclic warming and cooling of these peripheral tissues is generally thought to be beneficial for preventing peripheral cold injuries and improving manual dexterity. It is not observed in all persons, however, and can be highly variable within an individual.

Exercise can modify peripheral vasoconstriction. If exercise heat production exceeds the rate of heat loss, peripheral vasoconstriction will attenuate, and cutaneous blood flow will increase. During moderate cold stress, exercise can completely abolish the peripheral vasoconstriction. However, the peripheral vasoconstrictor drive will persist if the heat produced during exercise is lower than the rate of heat loss.

THERMOGENESIS. At rest, humans increase heat production primarily through shivering, which is the involuntary contraction of skeletal muscle. Shivering is stimulated when cold stress reduces skin and/or core temperature. The magnitude of shivering is dependent on the relative intensity of the cold stress, as shivering is proportional to the decrement in body temperature.[88,89] To support shivering, oxygen uptake increases up to a value of about $1.5\ 1 \cdot min^{-1}$ as body temperature declines.[87–89] Some heat may also be released from other metabolic but nonshivering sources, such as digestion, although the contribution appears to be limited.[90]

Physical exercise can produce substantial heat and offset heat loss in cold weather. As discussed, physical activity can increase metabolic heat production 15-fold. During competition, endurance-trained athletes may exercise for several hours at metabolic intensities that produce 700 to 800 watts of heat.[47,54] This rate of heat production enables these individuals to exercise comfortably with minimal clothing in cold air temperatures.

CARDIOVASCULAR AND METABOLIC RESPONSES TO EXERCISE DURING COLD STRESS

The peripheral vasoconstriction induced by cold exposure redistributes blood from the periphery to the body core. As a result of this redistribution of blood, end-diastolic volume and stroke volume are elevated during cold exposure. Cardiac output at a given oxygen uptake remains unchanged, however, as heart rate is reduced during cold exposure.[91] Diastolic blood pressure is increased about 10 torr as a consequence of peripheral vasoconstriction.[87]

Cold exposure can increase caloric expenditure during submaximal exercise. However, the impact of cold exposure on metabolic rate is dependent on exercise intensity and the effect of cold exposure on core temperature. At rest and during low-intensity exercise, it is not uncommon for oxygen uptake to be elevated compared with oxygen uptake under temperate conditions.[91–93] During more intense exercise, oxygen uptake is generally similar in cold and temperate conditions. This relationship is likely due to the additive energy cost imposed by shivering during low-intensity exercise.

Cold-weather clothing and winter terrain (e.g., snow and slush) increase caloric expenditure during exercise or other activity. Bulky and heavy cold-weather clothing can increase the energy cost of exercise from 10 to 20 percent,[94,95] depending on the number of clothing layers and the exercise task. Similarly, walking or running through snow increases the caloric cost compared with exercise on a smooth, firm surface.[96] As illustrated in Figure 14–7, walking in moderately deep snow at 2.5 mph increases the energy cost approximately threefold compared with walking on pavement.

EFFECT OF BODY COOLING ON PHYSICAL PERFORMANCE

Some studies report no reduction in physical performance during cold exposure, but it should be noted that the individuals tested often were not cold. It is only when body core and/or muscle temperatures are reduced that decrements in physical performance occur.

Whole-body cooling can reduce maximal oxygen uptake.[93,97–100] Experiments that have lowered core temperature 0.5 to 2.0°C have reported 10 to 20 percent reductions in maximal oxygen uptake. The reduction may result from reduced maximal cardiac output,[86] as maximal heart rate is 10 to 30 beats per minute lower after body cooling.[87,91] In addition, blood temperature reductions shift the oxygen dissociation curve to the right, reducing oxygen delivery to the cells.

Body cooling has been shown to reduce endurance exercise performance.[97,101,102] This may be due to increased metabolic strain, as blood lactate begins to accumulate at lower workloads and the rate of accumulation is greater during incremental exercise in the cold.[99,100] In addition, since maximal oxygen consumption is reduced in the cold, any given submaximal intensity represents a higher percentage of maximal oxygen consumption and, therefore, a greater relative exercise intensity.

The discomfort of severe cold stress may be, in part, responsible for reduced tolerance to exercise-cold stress. Adolph and Molnar[103] found that their subjects became confused and stuporous when resting or working in the cold. They speculated that the pain and discomfort accompanying cold exposure were important causes for termination. Similarly, Doubt[104] reported that 14 of 63 trials in which subjects were immersed for 6 hours in 5°C water were terminated prematurely because of the intolerable discomfort associated with low finger and toe temperatures.

Cold exposure can impair muscle strength, power, and fatiguability. Investigations have found that peak power output, sprint performance, and jumping ability are lowered by muscle cooling.[27,105] Similarly, during the initial minutes of recovery from sustained cold-water immersion, there is a reduction in maximal isometric strength and faster time to fatigue during submaximal isometric contractions.[29,34,106] Cooling might reduce muscle strength and endurance by interfering with muscle relaxation.[106] However, there is also evidence that cooling impairs muscle excitation-coupling, as supramaximal stimulation of motor nerves produces no muscle action potential when skin temperatures are reduced below 6°C.[107,108] Regardless of the mechanisms, muscle performance may be impaired immediately following cold exposure if it has lowered muscle temperature.

During recovery from muscle cooling, strength can be higher compared with that in temperate conditions. Johnson and Leider[109] examined the impact of cold exposure on muscle strength by measuring maximal handgrip strength prior to immersing the forearm in 10° to 15°C water for 30 minutes and during a 3-hour recovery period. They reported a significant reduction in maximal handgrip strength immediately following cold exposure. However, maximal handgrip strength was 17 to 21 percent higher than control measures 100 to 180 minutes into recovery. In similar experiments, Oliver et al.[110] observed an acute reduction in plantar flexion strength after precooling the calf in 10°C water for 30 minutes. During a 3-hour recovery period, plantar flexion strength became 33 to 40 percent higher than control measures 120 to 180 minutes into recovery. This muscle strength increase occurred despite the fact that muscle temperature remained below baseline levels during recovery. The mechanisms responsible for these strength gains remain unclear. Limb cooling is known to decrease muscle spindle discharge and the monosynaptic reflex.[111,112] Possibly, the sensitivity of the spindles is suppressed by limb cooling, enabling potentiation of muscle force production during recovery and rewarming.

SPECIAL CONSIDERATIONS

AMBIENT WEATHER CONDITIONS

The magnitude of environmental cold stress is determined by the ambient temperature, wind velocity, and wetness. The rate of body cooling is inversely related to the air temperature at temperatures below the critical temperature at which heat production cannot balance heat loss. The addition of air motion accelerates body cooling, as the movement of air past the skin surface replaces the warmer insulating air surrounding the body with colder air. As a consequence of air movement, body cooling can occur rapidly in relatively mild ambient air temperatures. The windchill index (Table 14–3) provides a useful index for the combined effects of ambient temperature and air velocity on subjective comfort and the potential for peripheral cold injury. Skin wetness increases the effective windchill and the rate of body heat loss.

Water immersion increases the rate of body cooling compared with ambient air exposure. Water has a 25-fold greater heat transfer coefficient compared with air. As a consequence, body cooling occurs much more quickly, and begins at a higher absolute temperature, in water than in air. Low-intensity exercise in water can actually speed the development of hypothermia, as physical movement increases conductive heat transfer from the active limb muscles to the water, with little

FIGURE 14–7. Effect of terrain on energy expenditure at various walking speeds. (Modified from Pandolf KB: Predicting energy expenditure with loads while standing or walking very slowly. J Appl Physiol: Respir Environ Exerc Physiol 1977; 43:577.)

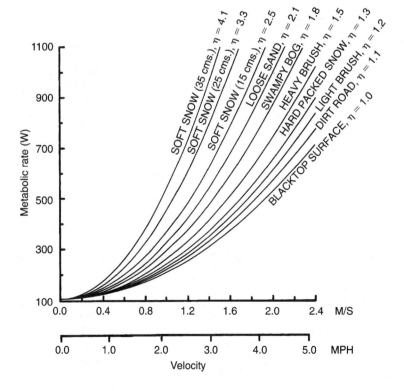

TABLE 14–3
Windchill Chart*

Wind Speed (mph)	Actual Temperature (°F)											
	50	40	30	20	10	0	−10	−20	−30	−40	−50	−60
	Equivalent Chill Temperature (°F)											
Calm	50	40	30	20	10	0	−10	−20	−30	−40	−50	−60
5	48	37	27	16	6	−5	−15	−26	−36	−47	−57	−68
10	40	28	16	3	−9	−21	−33	−46	−58	−70	−83	−95
15	36	22	9	−5	−18	−32	−45	−58	−72	−85	−99	−112
20	32	18	4	−10	−25	−39	−53	−67	−82	−96	−110	−124
25	30	15	0	−15	−29	−44	−59	−74	−89	−104	−118	−133
30	28	13	−2	−18	−33	−48	−63	−79	−94	−109	−125	−140
35	27	11	−4	−20	−35	−51	−67	−82	−98	−113	−129	−145
40	26	10	−6	−22	−37	−53	−69	−85	−101	−117	−132	−148
(Wind speeds greater than 40 mph have little additional effect)	Little Danger (Exposed dry skin may freeze in less than 5 hr, greatest hazard from false sense of security)				Increasing Danger (Exposed flesh may freeze within 1 min)				Great Danger (Exposed skin may freeze within 30 s)			

*To determine the windchill temperature, enter the chart at the row corresponding to the wind speed and read right until reaching the column corresponding to the actual air temperature.

metabolic heat left to warm the body core.[113] However, moderate-intensity exercise (heat production approximately 400 watts) can retard or prevent the reduction in core temperature that occurs when resting in 20° to 26°C water.[114]

CLOTHING

Clothing is an effective method for attenuating body heat loss during cold exposure. By choosing clothing with high insulation, humans can remain comfortably warm even in extreme cold conditions. For optimal effectiveness, the insulative value of the clothing should be balanced with metabolic heat production. It is important not to wear too much clothing during cold exposure, as this can lead to increases in body core temperature and the stimulation of sweating. Profuse sweating is not advisable in cold climates, as many clothing materials lose their insulative properties when wet, and peripheral cold injury is more likely when skin is wet. Similarly, if too little clothing is worn, hypothermia and its consequences can occur. It is generally recommended that individuals wear several layers of clothing during cold exposure. This method of dressing enables the individual to add or remove clothing as exercise intensity and weather conditions dictate.

As discussed, the energy cost of exercise can be 10 to 20 percent higher when wearing cold-weather clothing. The greater energy cost means that exercise at the same work rate requires a greater percentage of a person's maximal oxygen uptake. The greater relative exercise stress may shorten time to fatigue.

BODY MORPHOLOGY

Both body morphology (e.g., mass, surface area) and composition affect the body cooling rate during cold stress. Persons with small body mass and/or high surface area–to–mass ratios cool faster than larger persons with similar body morphology.[114,115] Similarly, persons with thicker layers of subcutaneous fat, and therefore greater peripheral insulation, cool more slowly than those with less fat.[91,92,116,117] A thick subcutaneous fat layer also enables individuals to tolerate lower ambient temperatures before initiating shivering.[118] Differences in body size and composition are considered to be largely responsible for much of the interindividual variability in physiologic responses to cold exposure.

GENDER

Whether gender alters the ability to defend body temperature during cold stress remains unresolved. Although there are well-documented differences between men and women during cold stress, these differences may not be due to differences between the genders per se but rather due to differences in body mass, body composition, surface area, and aerobic power. To date, no study examining the physiologic responses to cold exposure has matched men and women for weight, fitness, body surface area, and fatness.

During cold-water immersion, women generally lose heat at a faster rate than men.[92] This can be explained, in part, by females having a smaller body mass and a greater surface area–to–body mass ratio. However, women show less increase in metabolic rate for the same magnitude of body cooling,[119] suggesting that they have a blunted response to reductions in core temperature.

During cold-air exposure, women generally maintain body core temperature as effectively as men.[119] They accomplish this by maintaining a lower skin temperature compared with men during cold stress.[119] The lower skin temperature not only reduces heat transfer to the periphery but also serves to increase the insulative barrier between the body core and the environment.

AEROBIC FITNESS AND TRAINING

The physiologic adaptations that occur with regular physical activity can improve tolerance to cold environments. Because endurance exercise training increases maximal aerobic power and endurance performance, trained individuals can sustain relatively high exercise intensities for prolonged periods. This ability is of great value when high rates of heat production are necessary to prevent hypothermia during cold exposure.

It is controversial whether exercise training produces adaptations that improve thermoregulatory responses during cold exposure. There is evidence that endurance-trained persons have a reduced sensitivity to cold stress, as suggested by a delayed onset of shivering during body cooling.[120] However, Bittel et al.[121] found that aerobically fit persons had greater metabolic heat production during cold exposure as well as an increased shivering sensitivity; that is, the onset of shivering began at warmer skin temperatures. Similarly, skin temperatures during cold exposure have been reported to both increase[113,122] and decrease[123] after physical training. Young et al.[124] recently showed that aerobic training improves the vasoconstrictor response to cold exposure. Obviously, more study is needed to clarify the role of fitness and training on the physiologic responses to cold exposure.

AGING

The risk of hypothermia is widely considered to be greater in older compared with younger adults, and hypothermia is thought to contribute to the increased winter mortality rate in the elderly.[125–127] Studies have found that older persons are less able than younger adults to defend body temperature during cold stress.[128] This has been attributed to a reduced ability to vasoconstrict peripheral arterioles during cold exposure[129,130] and a smaller rise in heat production during cold stress.[131] Older persons have also been reported to have less CIVD response than younger persons.[132] The difference between the older and younger adults in these studies may not have been due to aging per se but to other factors such as differences in body morphology, fitness, and health. When these confounding variables are experimentally controlled, the rate of body cooling appears to be similar between old and young adults in some[133,134] but not all studies.[135]

NUTRITIONAL STATUS

Persons who become hypoglycemic during cold exposure have a reduced tolerance to cold stress and are more susceptible to cold injury.[136–138] Those with hypoglycemia exhibit either attenuated shivering or no shivering during cold stress,[137–139] and they therefore have lower rates of heat production. Interestingly, Gale et al.[139] demonstrated that intravenous glucose infusion restored shivering, within seconds, after euglycemia was restored in persons rendered hypoglycemic during cold stress. The restoration of shivering occurred even in a limb removed from circulation by arterial occlusion. These findings suggest that hypoglycemia affects temperature regulation through a central rather than peripheral mechanism. Regardless of the mechanism, hypoglycemia can have traumatic consequences for persons working in cold environments and should be prevented whenever possible.

Both carbohydrate and fat are oxidized to meet the metabolic cost of shivering. The increase in plasma catecholamine concentration that typically occurs with cold exposure facilitates the mobilization of both glycogen and triglyceride stores.[140] Debate exists, however, whether muscle glycogen is an important substrate during shivering; some studies[141–143] report reductions in muscle glycogen concentration after cold exposure, but others do not.[144]

ACCLIMATIZATION

Cold acclimatization has been examined in a variety of populations. Studies of individuals who have a lifetime of repeated cold exposure indicate that cold acclimatization can occur in humans. For example, Australian aborigines, African Bushmen, and women breath-holding divers of Korea have different whole-body thermoregulatory responses during cold stress compared with persons unaccustomed to cold climates.[90,145,146] Similarly, persons whose occupations require repeated limb exposure to cold temperatures have made peripheral adjustments (e.g., enhanced CIVD response) to attenuate the impact of cold during exposure.[147,148] The magnitude of physiologic adaptation to cold exposure appears to be modest, however, when compared with the marked physiologic adaptations associated with heat acclimatization.

CHRONIC DISEASE OR DISABILITY

Individuals with chronic diseases and disabilities may be at more risk for cold-induced injury. Spinal cord–injured persons cannot vasoconstrict peripheral arterioles in the insensate skin and have a blunted shivering response during cold exposure. Both of these factors cause their core temperature to decline during even moderate cold stress.[149] Therefore, care must be taken to ensure that these people wear adequate clothing during cold exposure to protect against cold injury and hypothermia.

Persons with cardiovascular disease are at more risk of having angina during cold exposure, since cold increases blood pressure and myocardial oxygen demand. The positive relationship between the incidence of stroke and myocardial infarction and sudden reductions in air temperature is well recognized.[150]

Cold exposure can elicit asthma-like symptoms. It was generally thought that cold exposure increased respiratory resistance due to intrathoracic airway cooling. Evidence now suggests that the increased pulmonary resistance is due to respiratory tract dehydration.[151] Medication can prevent the asthma-like symptoms in most sufferers.[151]

Persons with multiple sclerosis have improved motor coordination after moderate levels of body cooling. Therefore, cold exposure may be an effective method of temporarily reducing spasticity in this population. Cold appears to exert its effects on motor control by reducing muscle spindle firing and gamma spasticity.[111,112] These cold-induced effects decrease the strength of the stretch reflex and reduce resistance to passive movement. The improvements in motor control may persist for several hours following cold exposure.

DRUGS

Alcohol can predispose persons to cold injury.[136,152,153] Alcoholic beverages, for example, can induce hypoglycemia, which in turn suppresses shivering.[136–138,152] Several prescription medications, such as barbiturates, phenothiazines, reserpine, and narcotics, act directly on the hypothalamus and interfere with normal temperature control.[154]

COLD DISORDERS

ACCIDENTAL HYPOTHERMIA. This condition can occur whenever body heat loss exceeds body heat production. Predisposing factors include insufficient clothing, inadequate nutrition and fluid intake, infection, and alcohol and drug use.[155] Persons with mild hypothermia (core temperature 32 to 35°C) have the ability to spontaneously rewarm and generally do not present with cardiac arrhythmias. Clinical features include persistent shivering; cool, pale skin; bradycardia; and hypotension. Peripheral pulses are weak, and hypopnea may be present. Persons may be withdrawn and irritable, confused and lethargic. Acute treatment should be directed at warming the individual. Since persons may be hypoglycemic, warm, sweet beverages are recommended. Those with severe hypothermia (core temperature < 28°C) require active rewarming and immediate medical attention.

FREEZING INJURY (FROSTBITE). Frostbite occurs when skin tissue freezes. It primarily afflicts the digits, ears, and exposed facial tissue. Initially, the frozen tissue is cold, hard, and bloodless. The severity of frostbite is classified by the depth of the injury. First-degree frostbite afflicts the epidermal tissue. After thawing, the skin may become wheal-like, red, and painful. It may become edematous but does not blister.

Second-degree frostbite affects the superficial dermis and is characterized by blister formation. Third-degree frostbite extends to the reticular layer. It is characterized by edema with hemorrhagic bullae. Permanent tissue loss is possible. Fourth-degree frostbite involves the full thickness of skin. Thawing does not restore muscle function, and the affected area shows early necrotic change. There will be permanent tissue and functional loss. The affected area should be warmed gradually (temperatures greater than 39°C can aggravate injury). During initial treatment, affected areas should be protected from physical injury and excessive cold or heat exposure. The tissue should be elevated to reduce swelling. The risk of frostbite can be minimized by wearing proper clothing, ensuring adequate diet and hydration, and avoiding unduly prolonged cold exposure.

NONFREEZING INJURIES. Sustained exposure to cold-wet conditions can induce skin injury. Chilblain is a skin condition that primarily affects the hands and feet. Patients present with red, swollen, tender areas on the dorsum of the extremities between the joints. The affected area should be warmed and carefully dried. Persons should be treated for infection, and re-exposure should be avoided until the affected region is healed. Trench foot can occur with prolonged exposure to wet-cold conditions when circulation is restricted. The tissue becomes pale, anesthetic, pulseless, and immobile. The skin is frequently macerated and slightly edematous. After warming, there is marked hyperemia, pain, and blister formation. Immersion foot can occur after prolonged immersion in cold water. The clinical features are similar to trench foot. Acute treatment for both trench foot and immersion foot is directed at warming (passively) the affected feet, protecting the area from physical injury, controlling for infection, and treating concomitant hypothermia and dehydration. Nonfreezing injuries can be reduced by frequent hand and foot inspection and by regularly warming and drying exposed limbs.

Table 14–4 summarizes the diagnosis and treatment of cold disorders.

HIGH TERRESTRIAL ALTITUDE

Improved access to mountainous areas has increased the number of people visiting and living at high altitude. It is now possible for travelers to fly to a major airport and quickly drive to a high-altitude destination. In the mountain states of Utah, Colorado, Wyoming, and New Mexico, for example, major roads reach 12,000 feet (3650 meters), some towns are located above 10,000 ft (3050 meters), and lodges are at 9000 feet (2750 meters) and higher. In these states, approximately 7 million people ascend to altitudes above 8500 feet (2590 meters) each year.[156]

Most people who ascend to high altitude are unaware of the physiologic impact that altitude exposure can have on exercise performance and health. Altitude exposure impairs exercise performance and can produce debilitating illness and death. It has been esti-

TABLE 14–4
Diagnosis and Treatment of Cold Disorders

Disorder	Cause/Predisposing Factor	Clinical Features and Diagnosis	Treatment	Prevention
Accidental hypothermia	Body heat loss exceeds body heat production Insufficient clothing Inadequate nutrition and fluid intake Alcohol and drug use Infection	Mild hypothermia (core temperature 32–35°C): ability to spontaneously rewarm; no cardiac arrhythmias Severe hypothermia (core temperature <28°C): active rewarming required, high risk of ventricular fibrillation In conscious victim: Persistent shivering Cool, pale skin Withdrawal and irritability Confusion, lethargy, and obtundation Bradycardia and hypotension Weak peripheral pulse Hypopnea	Measure core temperature Warm afflicted individual; remove wet clothing Mild hypothermia: warm, sweet oral fluids Moderate to severe hypothermia: IV fluid for dehydration and hypovolemia Maintain airway Medical management if suspect hypoglycemia, alcohol or opiate intoxication Manage secondary complications, e.g., pneumonia, pancreatitis, rhabdomyolysis, and renal failure	Proper clothing for weather conditions Ensure adequate nutritional and hydration state Seek warm shelter at the earliest suspicion of hypothermia
Freezing injury (frostbite)	Freezing of skin tissue Predominantly afflicts digits, ears, and exposed facial skin	Frozen tissue is cold, hard, and bloodless Classified by depth of injury (see below)	Warm affected areas; temperatures >39°C will aggravate injury Protect affected areas from physical injury and excessive cold or heat exposure Treat coincident medical problems—hypothermia, dehydration Elevate tissue to reduce swelling Prophylactic antibiotics for postinjury infection Whirlpool débridement for 2°–4° injuries	Proper clothing Ensure adequate diet and hydration Avoid unduly prolonged cold exposure
First-degree frostbite	Epidermal injury Post-thawing is wheal-like, red, and painful Affected area may become edematous but has no blister formation			
Second-degree frostbite	Affects superficial dermis Some initial limits on range of motion Edema with blister formation			
Third-degree frostbite	Affects dermis to reticular layer Edema with hemorrhagic bullae Swelling restricts range of motion Permanent tissue loss possible			
Fourth-degree frostbite	Involves full thickness of skin Thawing does not restore muscle function, and skin reperfusion is poor Affected area shows early necrotic change Permanent tissue and functional loss			
Nonfreezing injuries Trench foot Immersion foot	Prolonged exposure of extremities to wet-cold conditions Restricted circulation Prolonged immersion in cold water	Initially, afflicted area is pale, anesthetic, pulseless, and immobile Skin is frequently macerated and slightly edematous After warming: marked hyperemia, proximal burning pain, and blister formation Classifed by degree of severity	Warm (passively) and dry feet Protect affected area from physical injury Treat for infection and pain Treat concomitant hypothermia and dehydration Avoid weight-bearing activity until healing is complete	Frequent foot inspection Regular warming and drying of feet during exposure Boots and socks should not be replaced until feet are warm, with normal feeling
Chilblain	Sustained exposure to cold-wet conditions Primarily afflicts hands and feet	Red, swollen, tender areas on dorsum of extremities between joints Itching Chronic lesions may be turgid, with blister formation	Warm and dry afflicted skin areas Treat for infection Avoid re-exposure until affected region is healed	Frequent foot and hand inspection Frequent breaks to warm and dry feet and/or hands Boots, socks, and/or gloves should not be replaced until limbs are warm, with normal feeling

mated that 25 percent of travelers to altitudes greater than 8200 ft (2500 meters) develop acute mountain sickness,[157] a short-duration, debilitating illness that can ruin a long-planned vacation. Fortunately, the human body can adapt to the stress of high altitude, and preventive measures are available for many of the altitude-induced illnesses.

PHYSICAL IMPACT OF ALTITUDE EXPOSURE

Ascent to high altitude impairs the ability to transport oxygen to the cell. With ascent from sea level to altitude, the partial pressure of oxygen (PO_2) declines proportionately to the reduction in barometric pressure. The lower atmospheric PO_2 not only reduces the volume of oxygen inspired at a specific pulmonary ventilation but also reduces the PO_2 at each step of the oxygen transport chain. The result is an impaired ability to transport oxygen to the cell and the development of hypoxia. Typical reductions in PO_2 at several steps of the oxygen transport chain are presented in Table 14–5. Secondary problems accompanying altitude exposure are the reduction in air temperature and humidity, decreased ability to sleep, reduced appetite, dehydration, and increased exposure to ultraviolet radiation.

PULMONARY VENTILATION AT HIGH ALTITUDE

One of the first observable physiologic responses to hypoxia is an increase in pulmonary ventilation. The increased ventilation serves to increase alveolar PO_2 and reduce the alveolar partial pressure of carbon dioxide (PCO_2), thereby improving arterial oxygen saturation. The increased ventilatory volume is achieved through an increased tidal volume, but the respiratory rate may also increase. The increase in ventilation can be detected when the inspired PO_2 drops below 110 mm Hg or the arterial PO_2 is less than 60 mm Hg.[158,159] The increase in pulmonary ventilation is considered by many to be the most important response to hypoxia.[156]

The magnitude of hyperventilation is dependent on competing signals. The initial increase in ventilation is stimulated by peripheral chemoreceptors within the aortic and carotid bodies, as total denervation of the carotid and aortic bodies significantly attenuates or abolishes the ventilatory response to acute hypoxia.[158] The increase in ventilation, however, produces hypocapnia and arterial alkalosis, which act to brake further elevations in ventilation.

Altitude acclimatization produces additional increases in minute ventilation, reaching maximum after 4 to 7 days at the same altitude (Fig. 14–8).[160] One mechanism facilitating this adaptation is the elimination of excess bicarbonate by the kidneys during the initial days at altitude. By removing excess bicarbonate, the kidneys attenuate the arterial alkalosis and the accompanying hypoventilatory drive. It has also been suggested that there may be an increased sensitivity to hypoxia during the initial weeks at altitude.[161]

Hyperventilation not only improves arterial oxygen saturation but also facilitates transport of oxygen to the peripheral tissues. The systemic alkalosis accompanying hypocapnia increases oxygen affinity to hemoglobin, promoting binding of oxygen at the lung. In addition, hypoxia and alkalosis activate the glycolytic enzyme phosphofructokinase, leading to an increased synthesis of 2,3-diphosphoglycerate (2,3-DPG). 2,3-DPG helps oxygen dissociate at the tissue level by decreasing hemoglobin's affinity to oxygen.

CIRCULATORY RESPONSES AT HIGH ALTITUDE

Hypoxia alters the cardiovascular responses both at rest and during exercise. Acute exposure to altitude produces a mild increase in blood pressure, moderate increase in heart rate and cardiac output, and increased venous tone.[156] Heart rate at rest may initially rise 20 percent or more.[157] Initially, cardiac output is elevated secondary to tachycardia, with normal stroke volume, but cardiac output becomes similar to or lower than control values after approximately 1 week of exposure.

TABLE 14–5							
Typical Acute Reduction in Arterial Oxygen Partial Pressure and Saturation With Increasing Altitude for Unacclimatized Men							
Elevation							
m	ft	P_B (torr)	$P_{I}O_2$ (torr)	$P_{A}O_2$ (torr)	P_aO_2 (torr)	$P_{A}CO_2$ (torr)	S_aO_2 (%)
0	0	760	149	104	96	40	96
1600	5248	627	122	82	69	36	94
3100	10,169	522	100	62	57	33	89
4300	14,104	448	84	53	40	30	84
5500	18,000	379	70	38	35	27	75

P_B, barometric pressure; $P_{I}O_2$, inspired oxygen partial pressure; $P_{A}O_2$, alveolar oxygen partial pressure; P_aO_2, arterial oxygen partial pressure; $P_{A}CO_2$, alveolar carbon dioxide partial pressure; S_aO_2, arterial oxygen saturation.
Modified from Fulco CS, Cymerman A: Human performance and acute hypoxia. *In* Pandolf KB, Sawka MN, Gonzalez RR (eds): Human Performance Physiology and Environmental Medicine at Terrestrial Extremes. Indianapolis, Benchmark Press, 1988, p. 471.

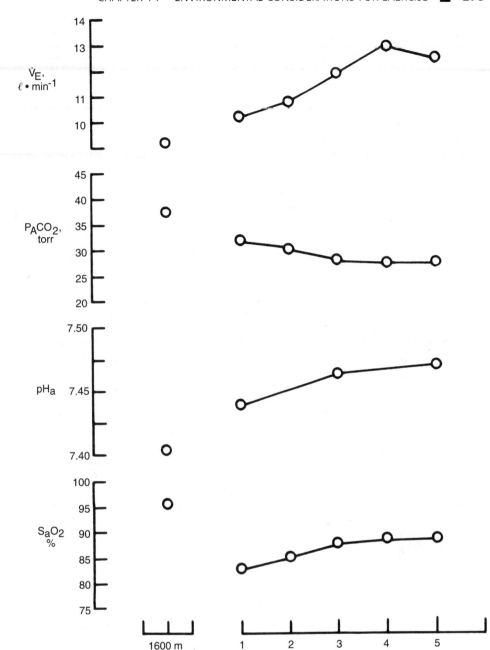

FIGURE 14–8. Changes in resting minute ventilation ($\dot{V}_E$), alveolar P_{CO_2} ($P_{A_{CO_2}}$), arterial pH (pH_a) and arterial saturation of hemoglobin (S_aO_2) in 12 lowland residents during the first 5 days at 14,000 feet (4300 m). (Modified from Huang SY, Alexander JK, Grover JT, et al: Hypocapnia and sustained hypoxia blunt ventilation on arrival at high altitude. J Appl Physiol 1984; 56:602.)

The decline in cardiac output occurs due to reductions in stroke volume.[162–165] The pulmonary circulation is also affected by hypoxia, as pulmonary vascular resistance and pulmonary arterial pressure are elevated with acute altitude exposure.[166]

During acclimatization, two additional circulatory adaptations occur to enhance oxygen transport. The first adaptation is an increase in hemoglobin concentration secondary to reduced plasma volume. The hemoconcentration is apparent within 1 to 2 days of exposure and persists for several weeks. It arises as a consequence of the diuresis of excess bicarbonate,[167] and plasma volume may be reduced as much as 10 to 20 percent (300 to 600 ml).[161] The trade-off to this mechanism, however, is that the lower blood volume reduces stroke volume, increasing circulatory and thermoregulatory strain during exercise.[168] A later adaptation is an increase in red cell volume. Within 2 hours of hypoxemia, plasma erythropoietin concentration is elevated, stimulating red blood cell production in the bone marrow. Within 4 to 5 days of stimulation, new red blood cells are in the circulation.[156] Over a period of weeks to months, red cell mass increases.[161,169]

Maximal oxygen uptake is not measurably altered between sea level and 4900 feet (1500 meters). Above 4900 feet (1500 meters), however, there is a linear decline in maximal oxygen uptake at a rate of 10 percent per 1000 meters.[170] At 14,100 feet (4300 meters), maximal oxygen uptake is reduced approximately 27 to 28 percent.[171] There appears to be no gender influence on this response.[172] Although there is evidence that individuals with a high aerobic capacity have larger decrements in maximal oxygen uptake with altitude,[171] there is large interindividual variability in response to hypoxia. Acute hypoxia appears to reduce maximal oxygen uptake by impairing maximal oxygen carrying capacity, as maximal values for heart rate, stroke volume, cardiac output, venous oxygen content, and ventilation are not reduced from sea-level values.[164,173–175] The magnitude of reduction in maximal oxygen uptake is similar to the reduction in arterial oxygen content.[173,175]

Altitude acclimatization has little effect on maximal oxygen uptake. Studies generally report either no change in maximal oxygen uptake or only modest increases (3 to 5 percent) following short-term altitude acclimatization.[161,165,176–180] The modest results may be due, in part, to detraining, as training time and intensity are reduced due to acute mountain sickness and hypoxia. It may also be due to a lower maximal cardiac output, as maximal heart rate is reduced following acclimatization to high altitude,[181,182] and this is not completely reversed either by breathing normoxic air or with atropine infusion.[181]

The reduced oxygen carrying capacity at high altitude also affects the physiologic responses during submaximal exercise. At high altitude, the same absolute power output elicits a greater percentage of maximal oxygen uptake than at sea level (Fig. 14–9). As a consequence of the lower maximal oxygen uptake at altitude, heart rate, ventilation, and lactate concentration are higher during hypoxia than at sea level at the same power output.[174,175] During exercise at the same percentage of environment-specific maximal oxygen uptake, however, heart rate, ventilation, and lactate concentration are similar under hypoxia and sea-level conditions.[183–186]

EXERCISE PERFORMANCE AT HIGH ALTITUDE

Acute exposure to hypoxia impairs endurance performance. Hypoxia reduces the time to exhaustion during exercise at a given absolute power output, with the magnitude of decrement proportional to the magnitude of hypoxia. Reducing the workload to elicit the same percentage of environment-specific maximal oxygen uptake results in similar time to exhaustion during high-altitude and sea-level exercise.[165,186]

Acclimatization to high altitude can dramatically improve time to exhaustion during submaximal exercise[165,186,187] as well as athletic performance during sporting events.[178] For example, Maher et al.[186] reported a 45 percent increase in time to exhaustion during cycle exercise between the second and twelfth day at 4300 meters, and Horstman et al.[165] found a 60 percent increase in treadmill running time between the second and sixteenth day of acclimatization at the same altitude.

The improved endurance performance appears to be due, at least in part, to altered substrate utilization and less disturbance of cellular homeostasis. Following high-altitude acclimatization, there is less reliance on anaerobic energy metabolism, as evidenced by lower plasma ammonia and lactate concentrations,[186,188,189] less glycogen utilization,[188] and reduced lactate production.[189] There is also less disturbance of cellular homeostasis, as the ATP-ADP ratio is higher and the inorganic phosphate concentration lower after high-altitude acclimatization.[190] Since intracellular acidosis (which accompanies lactic acid formation) and elevations in inorganic phosphate concentration have been shown to induce fatigue in skeletal muscle,[191] less reliance on anaerobic metabolism should enhance endurance performance.

An improved intracellular buffering capacity may be another possible mechanism for the improved endur-

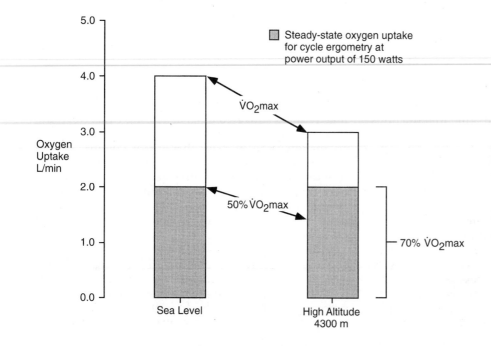

FIGURE 14–9. Effect of high altitude on the relationship between absolute power output, oxygen uptake ($\dot{V}O_2$) and relative exercise intensity (% maximal oxygen uptake, % $\dot{V}O_2$max). (Modified from Young AJ, Young PM: Human acclimatization to high terrestrial altitude. *In* Pandolf KB, Sawka MN, Gonzalez RR [eds]: Human Performance Physiology and Environmental Medicine at Terrestrial Extremes. Indianapolis, Benchmark Press, 1988, p 510.)

ance performance following high-altitude acclimatization. Mizuno et al.[187] reported that 2 weeks of exercise training at altitude (8850 ft; 2700 meters) produced a 6 percent increase in vitro skeletal muscle buffer capacity. In addition, they reported a strong relationship (r = 0.83) between improved skeletal muscle buffer capacity and short-duration (range 240 to 380 seconds) running endurance time (average improvement of 17 percent) after high-altitude acclimatization.

Ascent to high altitude does not impair skeletal muscle strength but does increase fatiguability of skeletal muscle during small muscle mass activity.[172,192] Acclimatization to high altitude, however, improves skeletal muscle endurance capacity,[192] presumably due to improved oxygen delivery and less disturbance of intracellular homeostasis.

NEUROPSYCHOLOGIC BEHAVIOR AT HIGH ALTITUDE

Acute hypoxia exposure can impair neuropsychologic function. Relatively small reductions in arterial oxygen saturation significantly impair mental and motor coordination, personality, and judgment.[193] The ability to do mathematical calculations, make decisions, and perform coding and conceptual reasoning tasks is reduced when inspired Po_2 is reduced below 110 torr. Short-term memory begins to be affected at inspired Po_2 below 118 to 127 torr, declining progressively with further reductions in oxygen saturation.

Several of the perceptual and motor decrements associated with acute altitude exposure are lessened with acclimatization. Decrements in ability to perform simple mental tasks, such as coding, are attenuated with as little as 4 days of exposure. Perception of effort during exercise at a given percentage of maximal oxygen uptake is lower following acclimatization to altitude. However, it has been suggested that the improvements may be related to recovering from mountain sickness rather than acclimatization per se.[161]

SPECIAL CONSIDERATIONS AT HIGH ALTITUDE

EXERCISE TRAINING

Because high altitude reduces maximal oxygen uptake and results in elevated heart rate at a given oxygen uptake, exercise prescriptions based on tests at sea level need modification. Heart rate remains a reliable indicator of cardiovascular stress during exercise, but exercise at a given heart rate provides less absolute stress to skeletal muscle. Therefore, to provide the same overoad to skeletal muscle, exercise must be performed at a greater absolute heart rate.

Optimal training for improving athletic performance at altitude depends on the altitude of residence and the athletic event. For aerobic activities (events lasting longer than 3 to 4 minutes) at altitudes above 2000 meters, acclimatization for 10 to 20 days is necessary for maximal performance.[156] Highly anaerobic activities at intermediate altitudes require only arrival at the time of the event.[156]

The effects of high-altitude training on sea-level athletic performance remain controversial.[194] Studies have suggested that sea-level performance can be improved by living and training at altitude.[176,180,187,195] These studies, however, often lacked a control group performing similar training at sea level. Studies containing the proper control groups have not found altitude training to be superior to sea-level training with regard to sea-level performance.[177,179,196] Regardless, any benefit appears to be dependent on choosing an altitude that maximizes physiologic stress but minimizes the detraining that is inevitable when maximal oxygen uptake is limited (altitudes greater than 4900 to 6550 feet [1500 to 2000 meters]). Levine and Stray-Gundersen[194] reported that athletes train faster and at greater oxygen uptakes at low altitude (3900 feet, 1200 meters) than at higher altitude (9150 feet, 2800 meters), suggesting that altitude exposure may compromise training overload. They also found that athletes who lived at altitude but trained near sea level had improved maximal aerobic power (5 percent) and 5000-meter running time (30 seconds) compared with a control group who lived and trained near sea level. Levine and Stray-Gundersen[194] suggested that living at altitude stimulates beneficial changes for athletic performance, and training near sea level provides optimal exercise training.

CHRONIC DISEASES

There is little information on the impact of altitude on the health of people with chronic diseases, nor is much known about the impact of medicines during hypoxia. The first 5 to 10 days at altitude are the most dangerous period for those with cardiovascular disease. It is known that patients with coronary artery disease have decreased exercise tolerance and earlier onset of angina and ST-segment changes during exercise at altitude.[197–199] Those who can achieve 9 minutes on the Bruce protocol without anginal symptoms will probably be safe at altitude.[157] Those with severe angina and limitation of effort at sea level should not go to altitude, as hypoxia will increase cardiac energy demand and precipitate anginal episodes. Those afflicted should choose an itinerary with access to easy descent and medical help. A good suggestion is to simulate the activity at moderate altitudes before attempting a specific activity at higher altitudes.

Individuals with mild to moderate lung disease may tolerate modest altitudes but have a higher incidence of acute mountain sickness.[200] Patients with primary pulmonary hypertension do not do well at altitude. Diabetics may experience problems regulating their insulin doses because of varying energy expenditure and food intake. More frequent insulin dosing may be needed, as well as more frequent blood glucose determinations. The presence of sickle cell disease is a contraindication for ascent to altitude, as ascent to altitudes as low as 6320 feet (1925 meters) is associated with an increased incidence of clinical symptoms.[157]

HIGH-ALTITUDE ILLNESS

ACUTE MOUNTAIN SICKNESS. This is a common illness that arises after rapid ascent (<24 hours) to altitudes above 8200 feet (2500 meters), with symptoms beginning within hours to days after exposure. Persons often present with headache, anorexia, insomnia, nausea, and malaise.[156,157,201] In moderate forms, there may be vomiting, unrelieved headache, and decreased urine production. Severe mountain sickness produces altered consciousness, localized rales, cyanosis, and ataxia. It is most common among those who ascend quickly and those who have a past history of acute mountain sickness. Vigorous physical activity during ascent or within 24 hours of ascent increases the incidence and severity of symptoms. Whether physical fitness attenuates the symptoms remains questionable. Mountain sickness is most likely to occur in those who retain fluid at altitude and have a blunted ventilatory response.[167, 202] The symptoms typically improve over a few days if hypobaric stress is not increased.

HIGH-ALTITUDE PULMONARY EDEMA. This illness occurs in 5 to 10 percent of those with acute mountain sickness and has a high mortality rate.[157] It often occurs the second night after ascent to altitude and is thought to be due to hypoxia-induced pulmonary hypertension and increased permeability of the pulmonary capillary endothelium. It is characterized by elevated pulmonary artery pressures and marked ventilation-perfusion mismatch; a patchy edema is typically seen on chest roentgenograms. The bronchoalveolar fluid has a high protein content and contains increased numbers of macrophages, leukotrienes and evidence of complement activation. Features include decreased exercise performance, dry cough, fatigue, tachycardia, rales in the middle right lobe, and tachypnea. Later, cyanosis, extreme weakness, productive cough, and dyspnea may be present at rest. Mental confusion, irrational behavior, and coma can also occur. It is most common in people who ascend rapidly, perform strenuous exercise upon arrival, are obese, are male, and have a previous history of pulmonary edema. High-altitude pulmonary edema is a medical emergency requiring rapid descent and medical attention. Acute treatment should be directed at increasing oxygen availability and decreasing pulmonary artery pressure.

HIGH-ALTITUDE CEREBRAL EDEMA. This illness usually occurs several days after the onset of mild acute mountain sickness and arises as a result of increased brain cell volume. Symptoms include impaired judgment, inability to make decisions, irrational behavior, severe headache, nausea and vomiting, truncal ataxia, severe lassitude, and progression to coma. Cerebral edema is most common in people who ascend rapidly to significant altitudes; it rarely occurs at altitudes below 10,000 feet. High-altitude cerebral edema is a medical emergency requiring rapid descent and medical attention. Acute treatment should be directed at increasing oxygen availability and reducing cerebral edema.

HIGH-ALTITUDE PERIPHERAL EDEMA. Altitude-related edema of the hands and face may occur in up to one third of travelers to high altitude.[201] It is thought to be due to hypoxia-induced retention of sodium and water. The condition is benign but may cause enough discomfort to degrade physical performance. It occurs most often in women and in those with a previous history of high-altitude peripheral edema. The condition can be treated successfully with diuretic therapy. Descent is the definitive treatment.

Table 14–6 summarizes the diagnosis and treatment of high-altitude illnesses.

AIR POLLUTION

There are several chemical compounds present in the atmosphere that can directly impact on our health. These compounds, collectively termed air pollutants, have been classified as either primary or secondary pollutants. Primary pollutants are those emitted directly into the environment. They are produced primarily from the combustion of petroleum-based fuels and include carbon monoxide, sulfur oxides, nitrogen oxides, hydrocarbons, and particulates. Secondary pollutants are those that develop from the interaction of the primary pollutants with the environment and include ozone, peroxyacetyl nitrate, sulfuric acid, aldehydes, and sulfates. The smog or brown cloud associated with large metropolitan areas usually contains both primary and secondary pollutants.

The quantity of air pollution inhaled during exercise is determined by several factors. The concentration of both primary and secondary air pollutants is influenced by the season, the ambient weather conditions, and the topography of the region. Ozone typically reaches peak concentration in the late morning and early afternoon in summer and is lowest at night during the winter months. The highest carbon monoxide concentrations are typically during peak traffic periods. The geography of the region also affects the dispersion of air pollutants. The relatively high ozone concentrations in the inland valleys of Los Angeles, for example, are the result of prevailing sea breezes pushing the pollutants inland against the mountain ranges that surround the city. Additional factors that determine whether air pollutants will impact our health are whether breathing is done nasally or orally and the quantity of air inspired. Oral ventilation removes fewer air pollutants than nasal breathing, resulting in greater exposure to air pollutants per unit time. Since physical exercise increases the rate and depth of inspiration, more air pollutants are inspired during exercise than at rest.

Certain individuals are more susceptible to the adverse effects of air pollutants. It is well documented that subthreshold concentrations of air pollutants for healthy adults can compromise respiratory and cardiovascular function in children and the elderly, persons with respiratory disorders (e.g., those with asthma or chronic obstructive pulmonary disease), and persons with ischemic heart disease.[203–206]

TABLE 14–6
Diagnosis and Treatment of High-Altitude Illnesses

Disorder	Cause/Predisposing Factor	Clinical Features and Diagnosis	Treatment	Prevention
Acute mountain sickness	Hypoxia-induced sub-clinical cerebral edema Lack of acclimatization to high altitude Rapid ascent (<24 h) to altitudes greater than 6000 ft	Symptoms typically begin 3–24 h after ascent Headache and nausea Anorexia, vomiting, and general malaise Dizziness and oliguria	Descend to lower elevation Supplemental oxygen Acetazolamide therapy Analgesic for headache symptoms Condition self-limited	Ascend in stages and/or graded manner Acetazolamide prophylaxis High-carbohydrate diet (>70% of total Kcal)
High-altitude pulmonary edema	Combination of hypoxia-induced hypertension and increased permeability of pulmonary capillaries Lack of acclimatization to high altitude Rapid ascent (<24 h) to high altitude	Symptoms typically begin within 2–4 days after ascent Early: nonproductive cough and a few rales; as edema progresses, cough becomes productive and rales become numerous Dyspnea on exertion; fatigue and weakness Resting tachycardia and tachypnea Cyanosis	Immediate passive descent Supplemental oxygen Nifedipine Transport to medical facility	Ascend in stages and/or graded manner Nifedipine prophylaxis Acetazolamide prophylaxis
High-altitude cerebral edema	Edema of the brain associated with high altitude Increased permeability of the blood-brain barrier or alteration of cell fluid regulation Lack of acclimatization to high altitude Rapid ascent (<24 h) to altitudes greater than 12,000 ft Acute mountain sickness Prior history	Time of symptom onset is highly variable; generally several days after ascent Severe headache, nausea, vomiting, and lassitude Truncal ataxia Ataxic gait Mental confusion, disorientation, drowsiness Social withdrawal Cyanosis	Immediate passive descent Supplemental oxygen Portable hyperbaric chamber Dexamethasone Transport to medical facility	Staged or graded ascent High-carbohydrate diet Acetazolamide prophylaxis
High-altitude peripheral edema	Hypoxia-induced retention of sodium and water More frequent in females	Primarily afflicts hands and periorbital areas of the face Associated with decreased urine output and weight gain Most evident upon awakening	Descent to lower altitudes Diuretic therapy	Salt prophylaxis Acetazolamide prophylaxis

In many regions of the country, the air quality meets the national air quality standards (Table 14–7). However, in many areas of southern California, the concentration of air pollutants often exceeds national air quality standards. For example, in Los Angeles County, California, each of the 16 Environmental Protection Agency (EPA) testing stations exceeded the national standard for ozone (0.12 ppm for 1 hour) on one or more occasions during a 2-year period spanning 1991–1993, with several locations exceeding the national standard 50 days or more during the calendar year. Similar results have been reported for the other counties along the coast of southern California.

Unfortunately, although there has been a great deal of research on the impact of individual air pollutants on pulmonary function and the ability to tolerate the stress of exercise, relatively few studies have investigated the interaction of these pollutants with exercise performance. There is even less information addressing the effect of air pollutants and other environmental stress-

TABLE 14–7
National Air Quality Standards

Pollutant	Averaging Time	Concentration,* $\mu g \cdot m^{-3}$	ppm
Sulfur Dioxide	1 year	80	0.03
	24 hours	365	0.14
	3 hours	1300	0.05
Particulate Matter	1 year	50	—
	24 hours	150	—
Carbon Monoxide	8 hours	10,000	9
	1 hour	40,000	35
Ozone	1 hour	250	0.12
Nitrogen Dioxide	1 year	100	0.05

*Corrected for standard conditions at sea level and 25°C.

ors (e.g., heat, cold, altitude) on pulmonary function and exercise performance. The goal of this section is to discuss the physiologic impact of several major air pollutants, both alone and in combination.

CARBON MONOXIDE

Carbon monoxide is the most frequently occurring air pollutant in urban environments. It is released primarily from auto emissions but is also a byproduct of industrial combustion and cigarette smoke. Carbon monoxide impacts our health and physiologic function by reducing the oxygen carrying capacity of the blood, as hemoglobin has a 200-fold greater affinity for carbon monoxide than for oxygen. Thus, when the carboxyhemoglobin (COHb) concentration is elevated, there is less hemoglobin available to transport oxygen for cell respiration.

Normal resting COHb concentration is approximately 1 percent, but many behaviors can significantly increase COHb concentration. Driving with an open window during peak traffic hours, for example, can raise the COHb concentration to 5 percent.[205] Aerobic exercise under similar conditions can further increase COHb, as the greater minute ventilation increases the amount of carbon monoxide inhaled per unit time. Nicholson and Case[207] reported that 30 minutes of running in New York City resulted in COHb concentrations of 4 to 5 percent. Smoking three cigarettes over a short time can increase COHb to approximately 5 percent.[45]

During light- to moderate-intensity aerobic exercise (30 to 75 percent maximal oxygen uptake), healthy individuals can tolerate COHb concentrations of up to 20 percent with no reduction in physical performance.[208–210] However, during exercise at 70 to 75 percent maximal oxygen uptake, individuals with elevated COHb have increased heart rates, greater respiratory distress, and higher blood lactate concentrations compared with control conditions.[208,211] In addition, there is evidence that high COHb (25 to 35 percent)

concentrations may result in higher core temperatures during prolonged exercise.[212]

Carbon monoxide exposure appears to have little effect on maximal oxygen uptake up to 4 percent COHb.[213] Beyond this apparent threshold, however, maximal oxygen uptake declines approximately 0.9 percent with every 1 percent increase in COHb up to 35 percent COHb.[214] Carbon monoxide appears to reduce maximal oxygen uptake by reducing blood oxygen transport capacity. Maximal cardiac output is unaffected by carbon monoxide exposure.[213]

Persons with cardiovascular or pulmonary disease have a reduced ability to perform exercise when COHb is acutely elevated. Several investigators have reported that patients with angina have a decreased exercise time to angina onset; systolic blood pressure and heart rate are lower at the onset of angina, suggesting that angina occurs at a lower myocardial oxygen uptake.[205,206,215–217] Carbon monoxide exposure has also been shown to reduce the exercise tolerance of persons with chronic bronchitis, emphysema,[218] and anemia.[219]

SULFUR OXIDES

Sulfur oxides are products of fossil fuel combustion and are upper respiratory tract irritants that can cause reversible bronchoconstriction and increased airway resistance. The dominant forms of sulfur oxides are sulfur dioxide, sulfuric acid, and sulfate, with 98 percent of the sulfur released into the atmosphere in the form of sulfur dioxide.[203]

In healthy adults, sulfur dioxide does not impair pulmonary function until the concentration exceeds 1 to 3 ppm.[220] However, in asthmatics and others with pulmonary hyperactivity, the threshold for airway restriction is less than 1 ppm,[221–224] with one study reporting progressive bronchoconstriction with exposure to 0.1 to 0.5 ppm sulfur dioxide.[223] To these authors' knowledge, no study has evaluated whether sulfur dioxide exposure impairs either endurance exercise performance or maximal oxygen uptake.

Repeated exposure to sulfur dioxide does induce adaptation. Industrial workers routinely exposed to 10 ppm sulfur dioxide retain normal pulmonary function when exposed to 5 ppm sulfur dioxide.[225] Andersen et al.[226] conducted studies investigating the physiologic responses that occur when subjects breathe 1, 5, or 25 ppm sulfur dioxide for 6 hours. They reported that the subjects tolerated each concentration of sulfur dioxide "very well," but investigators who occasionally entered the climatic chamber reported that the 25-ppm sulfur dioxide concentrations were "almost intolerable." These adaptations to sulfur dioxide occur in both healthy and asthmatic individuals.[227]

NITROGEN OXIDES

Nitrogen oxides develop from high-temperature combustive processes involving nitrogen and oxygen.

The concentration of nitrogen oxides is elevated during peak traffic periods, at airports, and in the smoke accompanying cigarette smoking and fire fighting. There are several forms of nitrogen oxides, including nitrous oxide, nitric oxide, nitrogen dioxide, dinitrogen dioxide, dinitrogen pentoxide, and nitrate ions. Nitrogen dioxide is known to be harmful to health; acute exposure to high nitrogen dioxide levels (200 to 4000 ppm) can cause severe pulmonary edema and death.[228] At lower concentrations (2 to 5 ppm), nitrogen dioxide increases airway resistance and reduces pulmonary diffusion capacity.[229,230] Fortunately, the ambient air concentration of nitrogen dioxide is generally less than 1 ppm.

For healthy persons, nitrogen dioxide concentrations of less than 0.7 ppm appear to have no adverse affects on pulmonary function or exercise performance.[220,231] Aging does not appear to reduce tolerance to nitrogen dioxide.[232] However, people with chronic obstructive pulmonary disease and, presumably, other respiratory diseases have reduced pulmonary function when exposed for 4 hours to 0.3 ppm nitrogen dioxide.[232]

PRIMARY PARTICULATES

Primary particulates include dust, soot, and smoke.[203,233] These pollutants are of physiologic importance because they can impair pulmonary function after they are inhaled into the lungs. The fine dust from charcoal[234] and cigarette smoke[235] has been shown to increase airway resistance and reduce forced expiratory volume. The lung depth reached by the dust is determined by the particle size. The dispersion of dust within the lung is influenced by the tidal volume, frequency of breathing, and whether the particle was inhaled nasally or orally.[220] Because aerobic exercise increases ventilation and oral inhalation, it is likely that exercise increases the effective dose of this pollutant.

Unfortunately, there is little information on the physiologic consequences of particulate inhalation during exercise. Klausen et al.[235a] suggested that inhalation of particulates may reduce endurance exercise time. In their study, subjects performed a maximal exercise test under control conditions after inhalation of the smoke of three cigarettes and after sufficient carbon monoxide inhalation to raise their COHb concentration the same magnitude as when they smoked three cigarettes. Interestingly, Klausen and colleagues found that raising the COHb concentration produced a 7 percent reduction in maximal oxygen uptake in both treatment groups, but endurance time during the maximal oxygen uptake test was reduced 20 percent after smoking and only 10 percent after carbon monoxide inhalation. They interpreted the results to suggest that the decrease in maximal oxygen uptake after smoking or carbon monoxide inhalation was due to reduced oxygen carrying capacity of the blood, whereas the decrease in endurance time was a combined effect of the carbon monoxide concentration and the increased cost of breathing caused by the smoke particulates.

OZONE

Ozone is produced in oxygen-containing atmospheres primarily from the interaction of hydrocarbons and nitrogen dioxide in the presence of solar ultraviolet radiation. As a consequence, ozone is most prevalent in urban areas and reaches its highest concentration during the midday hours.

Ozone is a potent airway irritant, causing reflex bronchoconstriction in upper airways. The most common subjective symptoms are a cough, substernal soreness, and dryness of the upper respiratory passages. These symptoms can occur after brief exposures to low concentrations of ozone (0.05 to 0.10 ppm) and can persist for several hours after exposure.[203] Furthermore, there may be heightened sensitivity to ozone during the initial hours following ozone exposure.[236]

During light- to moderate-intensity exercise, exposure to ozone in the range of 0.2 to 0.4 ppm reduces pulmonary function and enhances subjective discomfort[237] but does not appear to impair exercise performance. These ozone concentrations can produce cough, substernal pain, wheezing, and malaise during exercise,[238] with the incidence of symptoms increasing in proportion to the ozone concentration.[239,240]

During high-intensity aerobic exercise (75 to 85 percent maximal oxygen uptake), ozone inhalation can impair endurance exercise performance. Schelegle and Adams[241] evaluated the effect of 0, 0.12, 0.18, or 0.24 ppm ozone exposure on the endurance performance of 10 highly trained athletes during 60 minutes of simulated competition (the last 30 minutes were at 86 percent of maximal oxygen uptake). All subjects completed the protocol when breathing 0 ppm ozone, whereas one, five, and seven subjects did not complete the exercise when exposed to 0.12, 0.18, and 0.24 ppm ozone, respectively. Folinsbee et al.[242] reported that inhalation of 0.21 ppm ozone during 60 minutes of exercise at 75 percent of maximal oxygen uptake induced significant reductions in pulmonary function, and six of seven subjects developed subjective distress (symptoms included tracheal irritation, substernal soreness, chest tightness, and shortness of breath). Adams and Schelegle[243] also documented decrements in pulmonary function and subjective discomfort. In addition, they reported that 4 of 10 subjects could not complete the exercise trials when breathing 0.35 ppm ozone. Similarly, Gibbons and Adams[244] reported that 3 of 10 subjects discontinued exercise prematurely when exposed to 0.3 ppm ozone during 60 minutes of moderate-intensity (66 percent maximal oxygen uptake) exercise in a 35°C environment.

Ozone inhalation can reduce maximal oxygen uptake. Folinsbee et al.[245] reported a 10 percent reduction in maximal oxygen uptake in those exposed to 0.75 ppm ozone. Similarly, Gong et al.[240] reported that 0.20 ppm ozone reduced maximal oxygen uptake (−16 percent), maximal ventilation (−18 percent), and exercise tolerance time (−30 percent) during a graded exercise test following 1 hour of exercise. Not all investigators have reported reductions in maximal oxygen uptake after ozone exposure.[246,247] One explanation for these divergent findings may be the duration of ozone exposure prior to initiating the maximal exercise test, as the studies reporting no change in maximal oxygen uptake exposed the subjects to ozone only during the exercise test.

There is evidence that repeated ozone exposure produces adaptations that attenuate ozone-induced reductions in pulmonary function[237,248–256] and decrements in maximal oxygen uptake and exercise time to exhaustion.[257] This adaptation generally occurs within 2 to 5 days of repeated exposure[237,251–256,258] and persists for 7 to 20 days upon discontinuation of exposure,[255,258] with the least persistent adaptation occurring in persons sensitive to ozone. However, acclimatization to ozone does not attenuate decrements in pulmonary function when subjects are exposed to higher ozone concentrations.[254] The time course of adaptation is similar between genders.[237]

INTERACTIONS BETWEEN VARIOUS AIR POLLUTANTS

Because polluted atmospheres contain many contaminants, it is important to investigate whether combinations of various pollutants interact to affect pulmonary function and exercise performance in an additive, synergistic, or subtractive manner. The majority of research has focused on the interaction of various air pollutants with ozone. Although the early work of Hazucha and Bates[259] suggested that exposure to 0.37 ppm ozone and 0.37 ppm sulfur dioxide resulted in synergistic reductions in pulmonary function, subsequent investigations found only additive effects.[248,260–262] Koenig et al.[263] reported that asthmatic patients who received prior exposure to ozone had a greater decrement in pulmonary function during subsequent exposure to sulfur dioxide at dosages that were subthreshold for normal subjects. They concluded that ozone exposure made the asthmatic subjects more susceptible to low concentrations of sulfur dioxide.

Experiments that have evaluated the interaction of nitrogen dioxide and ozone suggest that there is no interaction between the two compounds; the effects of the combination produced no greater effects than exposure to ozone alone.[238,239,264] The combination of nitrogen dioxide and sulfur dioxide appears to produce only additive effects. Pulmonary resistance is increased abruptly after sulfur dioxide exposure, with no persistent effects; nitrogen dioxide has a more delayed and persistent effect.[265] Combining subthreshold doses of nitrogen dioxide (0.5 ppm) and sulfur dioxide (0.3 to 0.5 ppm) during 2 hours of light-intensity exercise does not induce deficits in pulmonary function in either healthy or asthmatic subjects.[222]

Particulates interact with carbon monoxide to produce greater reductions in endurance time than carbon monoxide alone.[45] However, particulates do not appear to accentuate the effects of ozone on pulmonary function in either normal subjects or asthmatics.[266–268]

INTERACTIONS BETWEEN ENVIRONMENTAL STRESSORS

COLD AND ALTITUDE

Ascent to high altitude is typically accompanied by reductions in ambient temperature and humidity and increased wind velocity. These added environmental stressors exacerbate the physiologic stress of hypoxia, potentially compromising exercise performance and/or health. Since temperature typically falls about 10°C with every 1500-meter rise in elevation, even moderate increases in elevation can significantly magnify the degree of cold stress.[269] Therefore, persons traveling to high altitudes should bring adequate clothing to protect themselves against environmental cold stress.

The combined effects of cold and hypoxia on injury and exercise performance remain poorly understood, due to a lack of experimental information. However, it is likely that the combined stress of cold and altitude exposure predisposes persons to injury and premature fatigue, because (a) both body cooling and hypoxia impair mental function and decision-making ability; (b) the lower maximal oxygen uptake at altitude reduces a person's ability to increase heat production and defend core temperature; (c) both cold and hypoxic stress are associated with hemoconcentration and peripheral vasoconstriction, which may contribute to peripheral cold injury; and (d) since both cold and hypoxia increase blood lactic acid concentration at a given exercise intensity, premature fatigue may occur during exercise.

AIR POLLUTION AND HEAT

Since elevated concentrations of air pollutants are often associated with excessive heat and humidity,[270] which are known to impair exercise performance, it is likely that the combined stresses of excessive heat, humidity, and poor air quality further impair exercise performance. Gibbons and Adams[244] found that subjective symptoms increased when ambient temperature was 35°C rather than 25°C and subjects were exposed to either 0.15 or 0.30 ppm ozone during 60 minutes of moderately intense exercise. Furthermore, they reported that 3 of 10 subjects were unable to complete the 1-hour exercise bout (66 percent maximal oxygen uptake) when heat and/or ozone was present. Similarly, Folinsbee et al.[271] reported greater reductions in pulmonary function when subjects were exposed to 0.5 ppm ozone during exercise in a hot climate compared with a cool climate. However, the same primary investigator subsequently found no temperature interaction when subjects were exposed to 0.5 ppm ozone and 0.5 ppm nitrogen dioxide.[264]

Rather surprisingly, there is no evidence that hot ambient temperatures and carbon monoxide produce either additive or synergistic effects on maximal oxygen uptake or performance. Since both hot ambient conditions and increased COHb have individually been shown to reduce maximal oxygen uptake, it would be expected that the combination would produce additive reductions on maximal oxygen uptake and performance. The only studies to date, however, reported no additive effect on maximal oxygen uptake when heat and carbon monoxide were combined.[272–274]

AIR POLLUTION AND COLD OR ALTITUDE

Exercise in cold environments can induce reflex bronchoconstriction and cold-induced asthma in approximately 12 percent of the population.[275,276] Unfortunately, no studies have evaluated the interaction of cold temperatures and pollution exposure on exercise performance in this population.

Several studies have examined the impact of carbon monoxide at high altitude.[220,277,278] Carbon monoxide exposure at altitude further lowers oxygen transport capacity. The effect appears to be additive, however, as a given COHb at altitude and sea level produces a similar decrement in endurance tolerance time and maximal oxygen uptake at both altitudes.[278] But since it takes a smaller concentration of carbon monoxide at high altitude to elicit the same COHb concentration,[220] persons at high altitude are more sensitive to the effects of carbon monoxide.

REFERENCES

1. Hardy JD: Physiology of temperature regulation. Physiol Rev 1961; 41:521.
2. Gonzalez RR, Berglund LG, Gagge AP: Indices of thermoregulatory strain for moderate exercise in the heat. J Appl Physiol 1978; 44:889.
3. Lind AR: A physiological criterion for setting thermal environmental limits for everyday work. J Appl Physiol 1963; 18:51.
4. Nielsen M: Die Regulation der Körpertemperatur bei Muskelarbeit. Skand Arch Physiol 1938; 79:193.
5. Nielsen M: Heat production and body temperature during rest and work. In Hardy JD, Gagge AP, Stolwijk JAJ (eds): Physiological and Behavioral Temperature Regulation. Springfield, IL, Charles C. Thomas, 1970, p 205.
6. Stolwijk JAJ, Saltin B, Gagge AP: Physiological factors associated with sweating during exercise. Aerospace Med 1968; 39:1101.
7. American College of Sports Medicine: The prevention of thermal injuries during distance running. Med Sci Sports Exerc 1987; 19:529.
8. Rowell LB: Human Circulation: Regulation During Physical Stress. New York, Oxford University Press, 1986.
9. Bevegård BS, Shepherd JT: Reaction in man of resistance and capacity vessels in forearm and hand to leg exercise. J Appl Physiol 1966; 21:123.
10. Hanke D, Schlepper M, Westermann K, et al: Venentonus, hut-und mskeldurchblutung an uterarm und hand bei beinarbeit. Pflugers Arch 1969; 309:115.
11. Klausen K, Dill DB, Phillips EE Jr, et al: Metabolic reactions to work in the desert. J Appl Physiol 1967; 22:292.
12. Rowell LB, Murray JA, Brengelmann GL, et al: Human cardiovascular adjustments to rapid changes in skin temperature during exercise. Circ Res 1969; 24:711.
13. Saltin B, Gagge AP, Stolwijk JAJ: Body temperatures and sweating during thermal transients caused by exercise. J Appl Physiol 1970; 28:318.
14. Sawka MN, Young AJ, Cadarette BS, et al: Influence of heat stress and acclimation on maximal aerobic power. Eur J Appl Physiol 1985; 53:294.
15. Saltin B, Gagge AP, Bergh U, et al: Body temperatures and sweating during exhaustive exercise. J Appl Physiol 1972; 32:635.
16. Consolazio CF, Matoush LO, Nelson RA, et al: Environmental temperature and energy expenditure. J Appl Physiol 1963; 18:65.
17. Consolazio CF, Shapiro R, Masterson JE, et al: Energy requirements of men in extreme heat. J Nutr 1961; 73:126.
18. Dimri GP, Malhotra MS, Sen Gupta J, et al: Alterations in aerobic-anaerobic proportions of metabolism during work in heat. Eur J Appl Physiol 1980; 45:43.
19. Fink WJ, Costill DL, Van Handel WJ: Leg muscle metabolism during exercise in the heat and cold. Eur J Appl Physiol 1975; 34:183.
20. Nielsen B, Savard G, Richter EA, et al: Muscle blood flow and muscle metabolism during exercise and heat stress. J Appl Physiol 1990; 69:1040.
21. Brouha L, Smith PE Jr, De Lanne R, et al: Physiological reactions of men and women during muscular activity and recovery in various environments. J Appl Physiol 1960; 16:133.
22. Petersen ES, Vejby-Christensen H: Effect of body temperature on steady-state ventilation and metabolism in exercise. Acta Physiol Scand 1973; 89:342.
23. Williams CG, Bredell GAG, Wyndham CH, et al: Circulatory and metabolic reactions to work in heat. J Appl Physiol 1962; 17:625.
24. Young AJ, Sawka MN, Levine L, et al: Skeletal muscle metabolism during exercise is influenced by heat acclimation. J Appl Physiol 1985; 59:1929.
25. Savard G, Nielsen B, Laszczynska I, et al: Muscle blood flow is not reduced in humans during moderate exercise and heat stress. J Appl Physiol 1988; 64:649.
26. Yaspelkis BB III, Scroop GC, Wilmore KM, et al: Carbohydrate metabolism during exercise in hot and thermoneutral environments. Int J Sports Med 1993; 14:13.
27. Bergh U, Ekblom B: Influence of muscle temperature on maximal muscle strength and power output in human skeletal muscles. Acta Physiol Scand 1979; 107:33.
28. Davies CTM, Young K: Effect of heating on the contractile properties of triceps surae and maximal power output during jumping in elderly men. Gerontology 1985; 31:1.
29. Petrofsky JS: Isometric Exercise and Its Clinical Implications. Springfield, IL, Charles C Thomas, 1982.
30. Clarke RSJ, Hellon RF, Lind AR: The duration of sustained contractions of the human forearm at different muscle temperatures. J Physiol 1958; 143:454.
31. Barter TJ, Clarkson PM, Melchionda A: The relationship of forearm flexion isometric strength, endurance, and fiber composition: and the effect of heating. Int J Sports Med 1982; 3:159.
32. Petrofsky JS, Burse HL, Lind AR: The effect of deep muscle temperature on the cardiovascular responses of man to static effort. Eur J Appl Physiol 1981; 47:7.
33. Petrofsky JS, Lind AR: Insulative power of body fat on deep muscle temperatures and isometric endurance. J Appl Physiol 1975; 39:639.
34. Edwards RHT, Harris RC, Hultman E, et al: Effect of temperature on muscle energy metabolism and endurance during successive isometric contractions, sustained to fatigue, of the quadriceps muscle in man. J Physiol 1972; 220:335.
35. Bean WB, Eichna LW: Performance in relation to environmental temperature: reactions of normal young men to simulated desert environment. Fed Proc 1993; 2:144.
36. Eichna LW, Bean WB, Ashe WF, et al: Performance in relation to environmental temperature: reactions of normal young men to hot, humid (simulated jungle) environment. Bull Johns Hopkins Hosp 1945; 76:25.
37. Machle W, Hatch TF: Heat: man's exchanges and physiological responses. Physiol Rev 1947; 27:200.
38. Wenger CB: Human heat acclimatization. In Pandolf KB, Sawka MN, Gonzalez RR (eds): Human Performance Physiology and Environmental Medicine at Terrestrial Extremes. Indianapolis, Benchmark Press, 1988, p 153.
39. Armstrong LE, Maresh CM: The induction and decay of heat acclimatization in trained athletes. Sports Med 1991; 12:302.
40. Gisolfi CV, Wilson NC, Claxton B: Work-heat tolerance of distance runners. In Milvy P (ed): The Marathon: Physiological, Medical, Epidemiological, and Psychological Studies. New York, New York Academy of Sciences, 1977, p 139.

41. Armstrong LE, Pandolf KB: Physical training, cardiorespiratory physical fitness and exercise-heat tolerance. *In* Pandolf KB, Sawka MN, Gonzalez RR (eds): Human Performance Physiology and Environmental Medicine at Terrestrial Extremes. Indianapolis, Benchmark Press, 1988, p 199.

42. Avellini BA, Shapiro Y, Fortney SM, et al: Effects on heat tolerance of physical training in water and on land. J Appl Physiol 1982; 53:1291.

43. Adams WC, Fox RH, Fry AJ, et al: Thermoregulation during marathon running in cool, moderate, and hot environments. J Appl Physiol 1975; 38:1030.

44. Piwonka RW, Robinson S, Gay VL, et al: Preacclimatization of men to heat by training. J Appl Physiol 1965; 20:379.

45. Piwonka RW, Robinson S: Acclimatization of highly trained men to work in severe heat. J Appl Physiol 1967; 22:9.

46. Ladell WSS: The effects of water and salt intake upon the performance of men working in hot and humid environments. J Physiol 1955; 127:11.

47. Montain SJ, Coyle EF: Influence of graded dehydration on hyperthermia and cardiovascular drift during exercise. J Appl Physiol 1992; 73:1340.

48. Sawka MN, Young AJ, Francesconi RP, et al: Thermoregulatory and blood responses during exercise at graded hypohydration levels. J Appl Physiol 1985; 59:1394.

49. Buskirk ER, Iampietro PF, Bass DE: Work performance after dehydration: effects of physical conditioning and heat acclimatization. J Appl Physiol 1958; 12:189.

50. Sawka MN, Toner MM, Francesconi RP, et al: Hypohydration and exercise: effects of heat acclimation, gender, and environment. J Appl Physiol 1983; 55:1147.

51. Below PR, Coyle EF: Fluid and carbohydrate ingestion individually benefit intense exercise lasting one-hour. Med Sci Sports Exerc 1993; 25:S3.

52. Sawka MN, Young AJ, Latzka WA, et al: Human tolerance to heat strain during exercise: influence of hydration. J Appl Physiol 1992; 73:368.

53. Rothstein A, Towbin EJ: Blood circulation and temperature of men dehydrating in the heat. *In* Adolph EF (ed): Physiology of Man in the Desert. New York, Interscience, 1947, p 172.

54. Montain SJ, Coyle EF: Influence of the timing of fluid ingestion on temperature regulation during exercise. J Appl Physiol 1993; 75:688.

55. Coyle EF, Montain SJ: Carbohydrate and fluid ingestion during exercise: are there tradeoffs? Med Sci Sports Exerc 1992; 24:671.

56. Mitchell JB, Voss KW: The influence of volume on gastric emptying and fluid balance during prolonged exercise. Med Sci Sports Exerc 1991; 23:314.

57. Epstein Y: Heat intolerance: predisposing factor or residual injury? Med Sci Sports Exerc 1990; 22:29.

58. Exton-Smith AN: Accidental hypothermia. Br Med J 1973; 4:727.

59. Pandolf KB, Cadarette BS, Sawka MN, et al: Thermoregulatory responses of matched middle-aged and young men during dry-heat acclimation. J Appl Physiol 1988; 65:65.

60. Seals DR: Influence of aging on autonomic-circulatory control at rest and during exercise in humans. *In* Gisolfi CV, Lamb DR, Nadel ER (eds): Perspectives in Exercise Science and Sports Medicine, vol 6. Exercise, Heat, and Thermoregulation. Dubuque, Wm. C. Brown, 1993, p 257.

61. Kolka MA, Stephenson LA, Gonzalez RR: Depressed sweating during exercise at altitude. J Thermal Biol 1989; 14:167.

62. Kolka MA, Stephenson LA, Rock PB, et al: Local sweating and cutaneous blood flow during exercise in hypoxic environments. J Appl Physiol 1987; 62:2224.

63. Frye AJ, Kamon E: Responses to dry heat of men and women with similar aerobic capacities. J Appl Physiol 1981; 50:65.

64. Avellini BA, Kamon E, Krajewski JT: Physiological responses of physically fit men and women to acclimation to humid heat. J Appl Physiol 1980; 49:254.

65. Stephenson LA, Kolka MA: Thermoregulation in women. *In* Holloszy JO (ed): Exercise and Sport Sciences Reviews, vol 21. Baltimore, Williams & Wilkins, 1993, p 231.

66. Carpenter AJ, Nunneley SA: Endogenous hormones subtly alter women's response to heat stress. J Appl Physiol 1988; 65:2313.

67. Pivarnik JM, Marichal CJ, Spillman T, et al: Menstrual cycle phase affects temperature regulation during endurance exercise. J Appl Physiol 1992; 72:543.

68. Montain SJ, Sawka MN, Quigley MD, et al: Physiological tolerance to uncompensable heat stress: effect of exercise intensity, protective clothing and climate. J Appl Physiol 1994; 77:216.

69. Speckman KL, Allan AE, Sawka MN, et al: Perspectives in microclimate cooling involving protective clothing in hot environments. Int J Industrial Ergonomics 1988; 3:121.

70. Cage GW, Sato K, Schwachman N: Eccrine glands. *In* Fitzpatrick TB, Eisen AZ, Wolff K, et al (eds): Dermatology in General Medicine. New York, McGraw-Hill, 1987, p 691.

71. Davis PB, di Sant'Agnese PA: Diagnosis and treatment of cystic fibrosis: an update. Chest 1984; 85:802.

72. Matthews LW, Drotar D: Cystic fibrosis—a challenging long-term chronic disease. Pediatr Clin North Am 1984; 31:133.

73. De Marinis M, Stocchi F, Testa SR, et al: Alterations in thermoregulation in Parkinson's disease. Funct Neurol 1991; 6:279.

74. Pandolf KB, Griffin TB, Munro EH, et al: Persistence of impaired heat tolerance from artificially induced miliaria rubra. Am J Physiol 1980; 239:R226.

75. Pandolf KB, Griffin TB, Munro EH, et al: Heat intolerance as a function of percent of body surface involved with miliaria rubra. Am J Physiol 1980; 239:R233.

76. Leibowitz E, Seidman DS, Laor A, et al: Are psoriatic patients at risk of heat intolerance? Br J Dermatol 1991; 124:439.

77. Pandolf KB, Gange RW, Latzka WA, et al: Human thermoregulatory responses during heat exposure after artificially induced sunburn. Am J Physiol 1992; 262:R610.

78. Bar-Or O, Lundegren H, Buskirk ER: Heat tolerance of exercising obese and lean women. J Appl Physiol 1969; 26:403.

79. Buskirk ER, Lundegren H, Magnusson L: Heat acclimation patterns in obese and lean individuals. Ann N Y Acad Sci 1965; 131:637.

80. O'Sullivan SB, Schmitz TJ: Physical Rehabilitation: Assessment and Treatment. Philadelphia, FA Davis, 1988.

81. Clark WG, Lipton JM: Drug-related heatstroke. *In* Schönbaum E, Lomax P (eds): Thermoregulation: Pathology, Pharmacology, and Therapy. New York, Pergamon Press, 1991, p 125.

82. Lomax P: Drug induced changes in the thermoregulatory system. *In* Khogali M, Hales JRS (eds): Heat Stroke and Temperature Regulation. New York, Academic Press, 1983, p 197.

83. Lomax P: Drug abuse and heatstroke. *In* Lomax P, Schönbaum E (eds): Thermoregulation: Research and Clinical Applications. Basel, Karger, 1988, p 42.

84. Levine L, Cadarette BS, Gonzalez RR, et al: Atropine and thermoregulation in man (a report of three studies). US Army Research Institute of Environmental Medicine 1985; T12/85.

85. Burr RE: Heat illness: a handbook for medical officers. US Army Research Institute of Environmental Medicine 1991; Tech. Note 91-3.

86. Haymes EM, Wells CL: Environment and Human Performance. Champaign, IL, Human Kinetics, 1986.

87. Pendergast DR: The effect of body cooling on oxygen transport during exercise. Med Sci Sports Exerc 1988; 20:S171.

88. Hong S-I, Nadel ER: Thermogenic control during exercise in a cold environment. J Appl Physiol: Respir Environ Exerc Physiol 1979; 47:1084.

89. Nielsen B: Metabolic reactions to changes in core and skin temperature in man. Acta Physiol Scand 1976; 97:129.

90. Young AJ: Human adaptation to cold. *In* Pandolf KB, Sawka MN, Gonzalez RR (eds): Human Performance Physiology and Environmental Medicine at Terrestrial Extremes. Indianapolis, Benchmark Press, 1988, p 401.

91. McArdle WD, Magel JR, Lesmes GR, et al: Metabolic and cardiovascular adjustments to work in air and water at 18, 25 and 33° C. J Appl Physiol 1976; 40:85.

92. McArdle WD, Magel JR, Gergley TJ, et al: Thermal adjustment to cold water exposure in exercising men and women. J Appl Physiol 1984; 56:1572.

93. Nadel ER, Homer I, Bergh U, et al: Energy exchanges of swimming man. J Appl Physiol 1974; 36:465.

94. Amor AF, Vogel JA, Worsley DE: The energy cost of wearing multilayer clothing. Army Personnel Research Establishment Report, 1973; 18/73.

95. Teitlebaum A, Goldman RF: Increased energy cost with multiple clothing layers. J Appl Physiol 1972; 32:743.

96. Pandolf KB, Givoni B, Goldman RF: Predicting energy expenditure with loads while standing or walking very slowly. J Appl Physiol: Respir Environ Exerc Physiol 1977; 43:577.

97. Bergh U, Ekblom B: Physical performance and peak aerobic power at different body temperatures. J Appl Physiol 1979; 46:885.

98. Davies M, Ekblom B, Bergh U, et al: The effects of hypothermia on submaximal and maximal work performance. Acta Physiol Scand 1975; 95:201.

99. Dressendorfer RH, Morlock JF, Baker DG, et al: Effect of head-out water immersion on cardiorespiratory responses to maximal cycling exercise. Undersea Biomed Res 1976; 3:177.

100. Holmér I, Bergh U: Metabolic and thermal response to swimming in water at varying temperatures. J Appl Physiol 1974; 37:702.

101. Patton JF, Vogel JA: Effects of acute cold exposure on submaximal endurance performance. Med Sci Sports Exerc 1984; 16:494.

102. Faulkner JA, White TP, Markley JM: The 1979 Canadian ski marathon: a natural experiment in hypothermia. In Nagle FJ, Montoye HJ (eds): Exercise in Health and Disease—Balke Symposium. Springfield, IL, Charles C. Thomas, 1981, p 184.

103. Adolph EF, Molnar GW: Exchanges of heat and tolerances to cold in men exposed to outdoor weather. Am J Physiol 1946; 146:507.

104. Doubt TJ: Physiology of exercise in the cold. Sports Med 1991; 11:367.

105. Asmussen E, Bonde-Peterson F, Jorgensen K: Mechano-elastic properties of human muscles at different temperatures. Acta Physiol Scand 1976; 96:83.

106. Bigland-Ritchie B, Thomas CK, Rice CL, et al: Muscle temperature, contractile speed, and motoneuron firing rates during human voluntary contractions. J Appl Physiol 1992; 73:2457.

107. Marshall HC: The effects of cold exposure and exercise upon peripheral function. Arch Environ Health 1972; 24:325.

108. Vanggaard L: Physiological reactions to wet-cold. Aviat Space Environ Med 1975; 46:33.

109. Johnson DJ, Leider FE: Influence of cold bath on maximum handgrip strength. Percept Mot Skills 1977; 44:323.

110. Oliver RA, Johnson DJ, Wheelhouse WW, et al: Isometric muscle contraction response during recovery from reduced intramuscular temperature. Arch Phys Med Rehabil 1979; 60:126.

111. Michalski WJ, Séguin JJ: The effects of muscle cooling and stretch on muscle spindle secondary endings in the cat. J Physiol 1975; 253:341.

112. Eldred E, Lindsley DF, Buchwald JS: The effect of cooling on mammalian muscle spindles. Exp Neurol 1960; 2:144.

113. Keatinge WR: The effect of work and clothing on the maintenance of body temperature. Q J Exp Physiol 1961; 46:69.

114. Toner MM, McArdle WD: Physiological adjustments of man to the cold. In Pandolf KB, Sawka MN, Gonzalez RR (eds): Human Performance Physiology and Environmental Medicine at Terrestrial Extremes. Indianapolis, Benchmark Press, 1988, p 361.

115. Toner MM, Sawka MN, Pandolf KB: Thermal responses during arm and leg and combined arm-leg exercise in water. J Appl Physiol 1984; 56:1355.

116. Park VS, Pendergast DR, Rennie DW: Decreases in body insulation with exercise in cold water. Undersea Biomed Res 1984; 11:159.

117. Veicsteinas A, Ferretti GT, Rennie DW: Superficial shell insulation in resting and exercising man in cold. J Appl Physiol 1982; 52:1557.

118. Smith RM, Hanna JM: Skinfolds and resting heat loss in cold air and water: temperature equivalence. J Appl Physiol 1975; 39:93.

119. Graham TE: Thermal, metabolic, and cardiovascular changes in men and women during cold stress. Med Sci Sports Exerc 1988; 20:S185.

120. Baum E, Bruck K, Schwennicke HP: Adaptive modifications in the thermoregulatory system of long-distance runners. J Appl Physiol 1976; 40:404.

121. Bittel JHM, Nonotte-Varly C, Livecchi-Gonnot GH, et al: Physical fitness and thermoregulatory reactions in a cold environment in men. J Appl Physiol 1989; 65:1984.

122. Kollias J, Boileau R, Buskirk ER: Effects of physical conditioning in man on thermal responses to cold air. Int J Biometeorol 1994; 16:389.

123. Adams T, Heberling EJ: Human physiological responses to a standardized cold stress as modified by physical fitness. J Appl Physiol 1958; 13:226.

124. Young AJ, Sawka MN, Latzka WA, et al: Effect of aerobic fitness on thermoregulation. Med Sci Sports Exerc 1993; 25:S62 (Abstract).

125. Vaisrub S: Accidental hypothermia in the elderly. J Am Med Soc 1978; 239:1888.

126. Taylor G: The problem of hypothermia in the elderly. Practitioner 1964; 193:761.

127. Horvath SM, Rochelle RD: Hypothermia in the aged. Environ Health Perspect 1977; 20:127.

128. Young AJ: Effects of aging on human cold tolerance. Exp Aging Res 1991; 17:205.

129. Collins KJ, Dore C, Exton-Smith AN, et al: Accidental hypothermia and impaired temperature control homeostasis in the elderly. Br Med J 1977; 1:353.

130. Collins KJ, Easton JC, Exton-Smith AN: Shivering thermogenesis and vasomotor responses with convective cooling in the elderly. J Physiol 1981; 320:76.

131. Horvath SM, Radcliffe CE, Hutt BK, et al: Metabolic responses of old people to a cold environment. J Appl Physiol 1955; 8:145.

132. Spurr GB, Hutt BK, Horvath SM: The effects of age on finger temperature responses to local cooling. Am Heart J 1955; 50:551.

133. Mathew L, Purkayastha SS, Singh R, et al: Influence of aging in the thermoregulatory efficiency of man. Int J Biometeorol 1986; 30:137.

134. Wagner JA, Robinson S, Marino RP: Age and temperature regulation of humans in neutral and cold environments. J Appl Physiol 1974; 37:562.

135. Falk B, Bar-Or O, Smolander J, et al: Response to rest and exercise in the cold: effects of age and aerobic fitness. J Appl Physiol 1994; 76:72.

136. Freund BJ, O'Brien C, Young AJ: Alcohol ingestion and temperature regulation during cold exposure. Wildern Med 1994; 5:88.

137. Haight JSJ, Keatinge WR: Failure of thermoregulation in the cold during hypoglycemia induced by exercise and ethanol. J Physiol 1973; 229:87.

138. Graham T, Dalton J: Effect of alcohol on man's response to mild physical activity in a cold environment. Aviat Space Environ Med 1980; 32:1704.

139. Gale EAM, Bennett T, Green JH, et al: Hypoglycaemia, hypothermia and shivering in man. Clin Sci 1981; 61:463.

140. Wagner JA, Horvath SM: Influences of age and gender on human thermoregulatory responses to cold exposure. J Appl Physiol 1985; 58:180.

141. Jacobs I, Tiit T, Kerrigan-Brown D: Muscle glycogen depletion during exercise at 9° C and 21° C. Eur J Appl Physiol 1985; 54:35.

142. Martineau L, Jacobs I: Muscle glycogen utilization during shivering thermogenesis in humans. J Appl Physiol 1988; 65:2046.

143. Blomstrand E, Essén-Gustavsson B: Influence of reduced muscle temperature on metabolism in type I and type II human muscle fibres during intensive exercise. Acta Physiol Scand 1987; 131:569.

144. Young AJ, Sawka MN, Neufer PD, et al: Thermoregulation during cold water immersion is unimpaired by low muscle glycogen levels. J Appl Physiol 1989; 66:1809.

145. Hong SK, Rennie DW, Park YS: Cold acclimatization and deacclimatization of Korean woman divers. In Pandolf KB (ed): Exercise and Sport Sciences Reviews, vol 14. New York, Macmillan, 1986, p 231.

146. LeBlanc J: Man in the Cold. Springfield, IL, Charles C. Thomas, 1975.

147. Nelms JD, Soper DJG: Cold vasodilation and cold acclimatization in the hands of British fish filleters. J Appl Physiol 1962; 17:444.

148. LeBlanc J: Local adaptation to cold of the Gaspé fishermen. J Appl Physiol 1962; 17:950.

149. Claus-Walker J, Halstead LS, Carter RE, et al: Physiological responses to cold stress in healthy subjects and in subjects with cervical cord injuries. Arch Phys Med Rehabil 1974; 55:485.

150. Teng HC, Heyer HD: The relationship between sudden changes in weather and the occurrence of acute myocardial infarction. Am Heart J 1955; 49:9.

151. Anderson SD: Issues in exercise-induced asthma. J Allergy Clin Immunol 1985; 76:763.

152. Kalant H, Le AD: Effects of ethanol on thermoregulation. Pharmacol Ther 1984; 23:313.

153. Kortelainen MJ: Drugs and alcohol in hypothermia and hyperthermia related deaths: a retrospective study. J Forensic Sci 1987; 32:1704.

154. Paton BC: Accidental hypothermia. In Schönbaum E, Lomax P (eds): Thermoregulation: Pathology, Pharmacology and Therapy. New York, Pergamon Press, 1991, p 397.

155. Burr RE: Medical aspects of cold weather operations: a handbook for medical officers. US Army Research Institute of Environmental Medicine 1993; Tech. Note 93-4.

156. Hackett PH, Roach RC, Sutton JR: High altitude medicine. In Auerbach PS, Geehr EC (eds): Management of Wilderness and Environmental Emergencies. St. Louis, CV Mosby, 1989, p 1.

157. Bezruchka S: High altitude medicine. Med Clin North Am 1992; 76:1481.

158. Dempsey JA, Forester HV: Mediation of ventilatory adaptations. Physiol Rev 1982; 62:262.

159. Laciga P, Koller EA: Respiratory, circulatory, and ECG changes during acute exposure to high altitude. J Appl Physiol 1976; 41:159.

160. Huang SY, Alexander JK, Grover RF, et al: Hypocapnia and sustained hypoxia blunt ventilation on arrival at high altitude. J Appl Physiol 1984; 56:602.

161. Young AJ, Young PM: Human acclimatization to high terrestrial altitude. In Pandolf KB, Sawka MN, Gonzalez RR (eds): Human Performance Physiology and Environmental Medicine at Terrestrial Extremes. Indianapolis, Benchmark Press, 1988, p 497.

162. Alexander JK, Hartley LH, Modelski M, et al: Reduction of stroke volume in man following ascent to 3,100 m altitude. J Appl Physiol 1967; 23:849.

163. Vogel JA, Hansen JE, Harris CW: Cardiovascular responses in man during exhaustive work at sea level and high altitude. J Appl Physiol 1967; 23:531.

164. Vogel JA, Hartley LH, Cruz JC, et al: Cardiac output during exercise in sea level residents at sea level and high altitude. J Appl Physiol 1974; 36:169.

165. Horstman D, Weiskopf R, Jackson RE: Work capacity during 3-week sojourn at 4300 m; effects of relative polycythemia. J Appl Physiol 1980; 49:311.

166. Lockhart A, Saiag B: Altitude and the human pulmonary circulation. Clin Sci 1981; 60:599.

167. Milledge JS: Salt and water control at altitude. Int J Sports Med 1992; 13(suppl 1):S61.

168. Fortney SM, Nadel ER, Wenger CB, et al: Effect of blood volume on sweating rate and body fluids in exercising humans. J Appl Physiol 1981; 51:1594.

169. Hannon JP: Comparative altitude adaptability in young men and women. In Folinsbee LJ, Wagner JA, et al (eds): Environmental Stress. New York, Academic Press, 1978, p 335.

170. Buskirk ER: Decrease in physical work capacity at high altitude. In Hegnauer AH (ed): Biomedicine of High Terrestrial Elevations. Natick, MA, US Army Research Institute of Environmental Medicine, 1969, p 204.

171. Young AJ, Cymerman A, Burse RL: The influence of cardiorespiratory fitness on the decrement in maximal aerobic power at high altitude. Eur J Appl Physiol 1985; 54:12.

172. Fulco CS, Cymerman A: Human performance and acute hypoxia. In Pandolf KB, Sawka MN, Gonzalez RR (eds): Human Performance Physiology and Environmental Medicine at Terrestrial Extremes. Indianapolis, Benchmark Press, 1988, p 467.

173. Gleser MA: Effects of hypoxia and physical training on hemodynamic adjustments to one-legged cycling. J Appl Physiol 1973; 34:655.

174. Grover RF, Weil JV, Reeves JT: Cardiovascular adaptation to exercise at high altitude. In Pandolf KB (ed): Exercise and Sport Sciences Reviews. New York, Macmillan, 1986, p 269.

175. Stenberg J, Ekblom B, Messin R: Hemodynamic response to work at simulated altitude, 4000 m. J Appl Physiol 1966; 21:1589.

176. Faulkner JA, Daniels JT, Balke B: Effects of training at moderate altitude on physical performance capacity. J Appl Physiol 1967; 23:85.

177. Hansen JR, Vogel JA, Stelter GP, et al: Oxygen uptake in man during exhaustive work at sea level and high altitude. J Appl Physiol 1967; 26:511.

178. Buskirk ER, Kollas J, Akers RF, et al: Maximal performance at altitude and on return from altitude in conditioned runners. J Appl Physiol 1967; 23:259.

179. Adams WC, Bernauer EM, Dill DB, et al: Effects of equivalent sea level and altitude training on VO2max and running performance. J Appl Physiol 1975; 39:262.

180. Dill DB, Adams WC: Maximal O_2 uptake at sea level and at 3,090 m altitude in high school champion runners. J Appl Physiol 1971; 30:854.

181. Saltin B: Limitations to performance at altitude. In Sutton JR, Houston CS, Coates G (eds): Hypoxia: The Tolerable Limits. Indianapolis, Benchmark Press, 1988, p 9.

182. Reeves JT, Groves BM, Sutton JR, et al: Cardiac function with prolonged hypoxia. In Sutton JR, Houston CS, Coates G (eds): Hypoxia: The Tolerable Limits. Indianapolis, Benchmark Press, 1988, p 195.

183. Bouissou P, Peronnet F, Brisson G, et al: Metabolic and endocrine responses to graded exercise under acute hypoxia. Eur J Appl Physiol 1986; 55:290.

184. Escourrou P, Johnson DG, Rowell LB: Hypoxemia increases plasma catecholamine concentrations in exercising humans. J Appl Physiol 1984; 57:1507.

185. Knuttgen HG, Saltin B: Oxygen uptake, muscle high-energy phosphates, and lactate in exercise under acute hypoxic conditions in man. Acta Physiol Scand 1973; 87:368.

186. Maher JT, Jones LG, Hartley LH: Effects of high altitude exposure on submaximal endurance capacity of man. J Appl Physiol 1974; 37:895.

187. Mizuno M, Juel C, Bro-Rasmussen T, et al: Limb skeletal muscle adaptation in athletes after training at altitude. J Appl Physiol 1990; 68:496.

188. Young AJ, Evans WJ, Cymerman A, et al: Sparing effect of chronic high-altitude exposure on muscle glycogen utilization. J Appl Physiol 1982; 52:857.

189. Brooks GA, Butterfield GE, Wolfe RR, et al: Decreased reliance on lactate during exercise after acclimatization to 4,300 m. J Appl Physiol 1991; 71:333.

190. Green HJ, Sutton JR, Wolfel EE, et al: Altitude acclimatization and energy metabolic adaptations in skeletal muscle during exercise. J Appl Physiol 1992; 73:2701.

191. Cooke R, Pate E: The effects of ADP and phosphate on the contraction of muscle fibers. Biophys J 1985; 48:789.

192. Fulco CS, Cymerman A, Muza SR, et al: Adductor pollicis muscle fatigue during acute and chronic altitude exposure and return to sea level. J Appl Physiol 1994; 77:179.

193. Crow TJ, Kelman GR: Psychological effects of mild acute hypoxia. Br J Anaesth 1973; 45:335.

194. Levine BD, Stray-Gundersen J: A practical approach to altitude training: where to live and train for optimal performance enhancement. Int J Sports Med 1992; 13(suppl 1):S209.

195. Daniels J, Oldridge N: The effects of alternated exposure to altitude and sea level on world-class middle-distance runners. Med Sci Sports Exerc 1970; 2:107.

196. Levine BD, Engfred K, Friedman DB, et al: High altitude endurance training: effect on aerobic capacity and work performance. Med Sci Sports Exerc 1990; 22:S35.

197. Brammell H, Morgan B, Niccoli S, et al: Exercise tolerance is reduced at high altitude in patients with coronary artery disease. Circulation 1988; 55(suppl 2):371.

198. Neill W, Hallenhauer M: Impairment of myocardial O_2 supply due to hyperventilation. Circulation 1975; 52:854.

199. Ziolkowski L, Wojcik-Ziolkowska E: Ischemic alterations in electrocardiogram and hemodynamic insufficiency during physical exercise in the mountain environment in patients after myocardial infarction. Przegl Lek 1987; 44:400.

200. Graham WG, Houston CS: Short-term adaptation to moderate altitude—patients with chronic obstructive pulmonary disease. JAMA 1978; 240:1491.

201. Cymerman A, Rock PB: Medical problems in high mountain environments: a handbook for medical officers. US Army

Research Institute of Environmental Medicine 1994; Tech. Note 94-2.

202. Rathat C, Richalet JP, Herry JP, et al: Detection of high-risk subjects for high altitude diseases. Int J Sports Med 1992; 13(suppl 1):S76.

203. McCafferty WB: Air Pollution and Athletic Performance. Springfield, IL, Charles C. Thomas, 1981.

204. Raven PB: Heat and air pollution: the cardiac patient. In Pollock ML, Schmidt DH (eds): Heart Disease and Rehabilitation. Boston, Houghton Mifflin, 1979, p 563.

205. Aronow WS, Harris CN, Isbell MW, et al: Effect of freeway travel on angina pectoris. Ann Intern Med 1972; 77:669.

206. Aronow WS, Isbell MW: Carbon monoxide effect on exercise-induced angina pectoris. Ann Intern Med 1973; 79:392.

207. Nicholson JP, Case DB: Carboxyhemoglobin levels in New York City runners. Phys Sports Med 1983; 11:135.

208. Ekblom B, Huot R: Response to submaximal and maximal exercise at different levels of carboxyhemoglobin. Acta Physiol Scand 1972; 86:474.

209. Gliner JA, Raven PB, Horvath SM, et al: Man's physiological response to long-term work during thermal and pollutant stress. J Appl Physiol 1975; 39:628.

210. Pirnay F, Dujardin J, Deroanne R, et al: Muscular exercise during intoxication by carbon monoxide. J Appl Physiol 1971; 31:573.

211. Vogel JA, Gleser MA: Effect of carbon monoxide on oxygen transport during exercise. J Appl Physiol 1972; 32:234.

212. Nielsen B: Exercise temperature plateau shifted by a moderate carbon monoxide poisoning. J Physiol (Paris) 1971; 63:362.

213. Horvath SM, Raven PB, Dahms TE, et al: Maximal aerobic capacity at different levels of carboxyhemoglobin. J Appl Physiol 1975; 38:300.

214. Horvath SM: Impact of air quality in exercise performance. In Miller DI (ed): Exercise and Sport Science Reviews, vol 9. Philadelphia, Franklin Institute Press, 1981, p 265.

215. Anderson EW, Andelman RJ, Strauch JM, et al: Effect of low-level carbon monoxide exposure on onset and duration of angina pectoris: a study in ten patients with ischemic heart disease. Ann Intern Med 7993; 79:46.

216. Allred EN, Bleecker ER, Chaitman BR, et al: Short-term effects of carbon monoxide exposure on the exercise performance of subjects with coronary artery disease. N Engl J Med 1989; 321:1426.

217. Adams KF, Koch G, Chatterjee B, et al: Acute elevation of blood carboxyhemoglobin to 6% impairs exercise performance and aggravates symptoms in patients with ischemic heart disease. J Am Coll Cardiol 1988; 12:900.

218. Calverley PM, Leggett RJ, Flenley DC: Carbon monoxide and exercise tolerance in chronic bronchitis and emphysema. Br Med J 1981; 283:878.

219. Aronow WS, Schlueter WJ, Williams MA, et al: Aggravation of exercise performance in patients with anemia by 3% carboxyhemoglobin. Environ Res 1984; 35:394.

220. Pandolf KB: Air quality and human performance. In Pandolf KB, Sawka MN, Gonzalez RR (eds): Human Performance Physiology and Environmental Medicine at Terrestrial Extremes. Indianapolis, Benchmark Press, 1988, p 591.

221. Kirkpatrick MB, Sheppard D, Nadel JA, et al: Effect of the oronasal breathing route on sulfur-dioxide-induced bronchoconstriction in exercising asthmatic subjects. Am Rev Respir Dis 1982; 125:627.

222. Linn WS, Jones MP, Bailey RM, et al: Respiratory effects of mixed nitrogen dioxide and sulfur dioxide in human volunteers under simulated ambient exposure conditions. Environ Res 1980; 22:431.

223. Sheppard D, Saisho A, Nadel JA, et al: Exercise increases sulfur dioxide–induced bronchoconstriction in asthmatic subjects. Am Rev Respir Dis 1981; 123:486.

224. Sheppard D, Wong WS, Uehara CF, et al: Lower threshold and greater bronchomotor responsiveness of asthmatic subjects to sulfur dioxide. Am Rev Respir Dis 1980; 122:873.

225. Amdur MO, Melvin WW Jr, Drinker P: Effects of inhalation of sulfur dioxide in man. Lancet 1953; 1:758.

226. Andersen I, Lundqvist GR, Jensen PL, et al: Human response to controlled levels of sulfur dioxide. Arch Environ Health 1974; 28:31.

227. Sheppard D, Epstein J, Bethel RA, et al: Tolerance to sulfur dioxide–induced bronchoconstriction in subjects with asthma. Environ Res 1983; 30:412.

228. Lowry T, Schuman LM: "Silo-filler's disease"—a syndrome caused by nitrogen dioxide. JAMA 1956; 162:153.

229. von Nieding G, Krekeler G, Fuchs H, et al: Studies of the acute effects of NO_2 on lung function: influence of diffusion, perfusion, and ventilation in the lungs. Int Arch Arbeitsmed 1973; 31:61.

230. von Nieding G, Wagner M, Krekeler G, et al: Minimum concentrations of NO_2 causing acute effects on the respiratory gas exchange and airway resistance in patients with chronic bronchitis. Int Arch Arbeitsmed 1971; 27:338.

231. Horvath SM, Folinsbee LJ: The Effect of Nitrogen Dioxide on Lung Function in Normal Subjects. Research Triangle Park, NC, US Environmental Protection Agency, 1978.

232. Morrow PE, Utell MJ, Bauer MA, et al: Pulmonary performance of elderly normal subjects and subjects with chronic obstructive pulmonary disease exposed to 0.3 ppm nitrogen dioxide. Am Rev Respir Dis 1992; 145:291.

233. Pierson WE, Covert DS, Koenig JQ: Air pollutants, bronchial hyperreactivity, and exercise. J Allergy Clin Immunol 1984; 73:717.

234. Widdicombe JG, Kent DC, Nadel JA: Mechanism of bronchoconstriction during inhalation of dust. J Appl Physiol 1962; 17:613.

235. Nadel JA, Comroe JH Jr: Acute effects of inhalation of cigarette smoke on airway conductance. J Appl Physiol 1961; 16:713.

235a. Klausen K, Andersen C, Nandrop S: Acute effects of cigarette smoking and inhalation of carbon monoxide during maximal exercise. Eur J Appl Physiol 1983; 51:371–379.

236. Schonfeld BR, Adams WC, Schelegle ES: Duration of enhanced responsiveness upon re-exposure to ozone. Arch Environ Health 1989; 44:229.

237. Dimeo MJ, Glenn MG, Holtzman MJ, et al: Threshold concentration of ozone causing an increase in bronchial reactivity in humans and adaptation with repeated exposures. Am Rev Respir Dis 1981; 124:245.

238. Hackney JD, Linn WS, Mohler JG, et al: Experimental studies on human health effects of air pollutants II: four-hour exposure to ozone alone and in combination with other pollutant gases. Arch Environ Health 1975; 30:379.

239. Hackney JD, Linn WS, Law DC, et al: Experimental studies on human health effects of air pollutants III: two-hour exposure to ozone alone and in combination with other pollutant gases. Arch Environ Health 1975; 30:385.

240. Gong H, Brandley PW, Simmons MS, et al: Impaired exercise performance and pulmonary function in elite cyclists during low-level ozone exposure in a hot environment. Am Rev Respir Dis 1986; 134:726.

241. Schelegle ES, Adams WC: Reduced exercise time in competitive simulations consequent to low level ozone exposure. Med Sci Sports Exerc 1986; 18:408.

242. Folinsbee LJ, Bedi JF, Horvath SM: Pulmonary function changes after 1 h continuous heavy exercise in 0.21 ppm ozone. J Appl Physiol 1984; 57:984.

243. Adams WC, Schelegle ES: Ozone and high ventilation effects on pulmonary function and endurance performance. J Appl Physiol 1983; 55:805.

244. Gibbons SI, Adams WC: Combined effects of ozone exposure and ambient heat on exercising females. J Appl Physiol 1984; 57:450.

245. Folinsbee LJ, Silverman F, Shephard RJ: Decrease of maximum work performance following ozone exposure. J Appl Physiol 1977; 42:531.

246. Savin WM, Adams WC: Effects of ozone inhalation on work performance and VO_2max. J Appl Physiol 1979; 46:309.

247. Horvath SM, Gliner JA, Matsen-Twisdale JA: Pulmonary function and maximum exercise responses following acute ozone exposure. Aviat Space Environ Med 1979; 50:901.

248. Bell KA, Linn WS, Hazucha M, et al: Respiratory effects of exposure to ozone plus sulfur dioxide in southern Californians and eastern Canadians. Am Ind Hyg Assoc J 1977; 38:696.

249. Hackney JD, Linn WS, Karuza SK, et al: Effects of ozone exposure in Canadians and southern Californians: evidence for adaptation? Arch Environ Health 1977; 32:110.

250. Hackney JD, Linn WS, Mohler JG, et al: Adaptation to short-term respiratory effects of ozone in men exposed repeatedly. J Appl Physiol 1977; 43:82.

251. Folinsbee LJ: Effects of ozone exposure on lung function in man: a review. Rev Environ Health 1981; 3:211.

252. Folinsbee LJ, Bedi JF, Gliner JA, et al: Concentration dependence of pulmonary function adaptation to ozone. *In* Mehlman MA, Lee SD, Mustafa MG (eds): The Biomedical Effects of Ozone and Related Photochemical Oxidants. Princeton Junction, NJ, Princeton Scientific Publishers, 1983, p 175.

253. Folinsbee LJ, Bedi JF, Horvath SM: Respiratory responses in humans repeatedly exposed to low concentrations of ozone. Am Rev Respir Dis 1980; 121:431.

254. Gliner JA, Horvath SM, Folinsbee LJ: Preexposure to low ozone concentrations does not diminish the pulmonary function response on exposure to higher ozone concentrations. Am Rev Respir Dis 1983; 127:51.

255. Horvath SM, Gliner JA, Folinsbee LJ: Adaptation to ozone: duration of effect. Am Rev Respir Dis 1981; 123:496.

256. Farrell BP, Kerr HD, Kulle TJ, et al: Adaptation in human subjects to the effects of inhaled ozone after repeated exposure. Am Rev Respir Dis 1979; 119:725.

257. Foxcroft WJ, Adams WC: Effects of ozone exposure on four consecutive days on work performance and VO_2max. J Appl Physiol 1986; 61:960.

258. Linn WS, Medway DA, Anzar UT, et al: Persistence of adaptation to ozone in volunteers exposed repeatedly for six weeks. Am Rev Respir Dis 1982; 125:491.

259. Hazucha M, Bates DV: Combined effect of ozone and sulphur dioxide on human pulmonary function. Nature 1975; 257:50.

260. Bedi JF, Folinsbee LJ, Horvath SM, et al: Human exposure to sulfur dioxide and ozone: absence of a synergistic effect. Arch Environ Health 1979; 34:233.

261. Bedi JF, Horvath SM, Folinsbee LJ: Human exposure to sulfur dioxide and ozone in a high temperature-humidity environment. Am Ind Hyg Assoc J 1982; 43:26.

262. Folinsbee LJ, Bedi JF, Horvath SM: Pulmonary response to threshold levels of sulfur dioxide (1.0 ppm) and ozone (0.3 ppm). J Appl Physiol 1985; 58:1783.

263. Koenig JQ, Covert DS, Hanley QS, et al: Prior exposure to ozone potentiates subsequent response to sulfur dioxide in adolescent asthmatic subjects. Am Rev Respir Dis 1990; 141:377.

264. Folinsbee LJ, Bedi JF, Gliner JA, et al: Combined effects of ozone and nitrogen dioxide on respiratory function in man. Am Ind Hyg Assoc J 1981; 42:534.

265. Abe M: Effects of mixed NO_2-SO_2 gas on human pulmonary functions. Bull Tokyo Med Dent Univ 1967; 14:415.

266. Avol EL, Linn WS, Shamoo DA, et al: Acute respiratory effects of Los Angeles smog in continuously exercising adults. J Air Pollut Control Assoc 1983; 33:1055.

267. Avol EL, Linn WS, Venet TG, et al: Comparative respiratory effects of ozone and ambient oxidant pollution exposure during heavy exercise. J Air Pollut Control Assoc 1984; 34:804.

268. Linn WS, Jones MP, Bachmayer EA, et al: Short-term respiratory effects of polluted ambient air: a laboratory study of volunteers in a high-oxidant community. Am Rev Respir Dis 1980; 121: 243.

269. Ward M: Mountain Medicine: A Clinical Study of Cold and High Altitude. London, Crosby Lockwood Staples, 1975.

270. Ellis FP: Mortality from heat illness and heat-aggravated illness in the United States. Environ Res 1972; 5:1.

271. Folinsbee LJ, Horvath SM, Raven PB, et al: Influence of exercise and heat stress on pulmonary function during ozone exposure. J Appl Physiol 1977; 43:409.

272. Raven PB, Drinkwater BL, Horvath SM, et al: Age, smoking habits, heat stress, and their interactive effects with carbon monoxide and peroxyacetylnitrate on man's aerobic power. Int J Biometeorol 1974; 18:222.

273. Drinkwater BL, Raven PB, Horvath SM, et al: Air pollution, exercise and heat stress. Arch Environ Health 1974; 28:177.

274. Raven PB, Drinkwater BL, Ruhling RO, et al: Effect of carbon monoxide and peroxyacetyl nitrate on man's maximal aerobic capacity. J Appl Physiol 1974; 36:288.

275. Katz RM: Prevention with and without the use of medications for exercise-induced asthma. Med Sci Sports Exerc 1986; 18:331.

276. Strauss RH, McFadden ER, Ingram RH Jr, et al: Enhancement of exercise-induced asthma by cold air. N Engl J Med 1977; 297: 743.

277. Wagner JA, Horvath SM, Andrew GM, et al: Hypoxia, smoking history, and exercise. Aviat Space Environ Med 1978; 49:785.

278. Weiser PC, Morrill CG, Dickey DW, et al: Effects of low-level carbon monoxide exposure on the adaptation of healthy young men to aerobic work at an altitude of 1,610 meters. *In* Folinsbee LJ, Wagner JA, Borgia JF, et al (eds): Environmental Stress: Individual Human Adaptations. New York, Academic Press, 1978, p 101.

CHAPTER 15

The Use of Ergogenic Aids in Athletics

ARNOLD T. BELL PhD, PT, SCS, ATC

In the complex world of sporting activity today, many individuals involved with organized competitive athletics, such as athletes and coaches, are in a continuous search for methods of gaining a competitive advantage to improve athletic performance. The slightest improvement in athletic performance often means the difference between "the thrill of victory and the agony of defeat." According to deVries,[1] athletes value small improvements in performance, but these improvements are often difficult to obtain through traditional training methods. Coaches as well as athletes utilize special aids to performance known as ergogenic aids to enhance athletic performance.

An ergogenic aid is any agent, substance, or technique that improves physical performance through its particular effect on the human body. Specifically, the term *ergogenic aid* also refers to any substance, process, or procedure that may enhance or is perceived to improve performance through improvement of strength, speed, response time, or endurance of the athlete. An ergogenic aid may hasten recovery time after stress or injury.[2] These aids are also thought to enhance perfor-

mance above levels anticipated under normal conditions. When competition is taken seriously, athletes may seek and utilize these substances or methods in an attempt to gain the aforementioned competitive edge.

Ergogenic aids are used routinely at almost all competitive levels of organized sports. Use of certain types of ergogenic aids is very common among athletes of different age groups and levels of competition. Unfortunately, some of those who abuse the more dangerous or harmful types of ergogenic aids to performance seem to be getting younger, according to media accounts. The habitual use of some types of ergogenic aids (e.g., pharmacologic agents) may lead to dependency or addiction, and they often produce harmful effects on the human body, adversely affecting athletic performance. It is common knowledge among sports medicine practitioners in many disciplines that some types of ergogenic aids are unquestionably acceptable as adjuncts to athletic performance enhancement, whereas others are questionable, potentially harmful to the athlete, or illegal. Additionally, many aids have been condemned, banned, or declared illegal by

TABLE 15–1
Ergogenic Aids: Acceptable, Questionable or Potentially Harmful, and Illegal Practices and Substances

Acceptable Practices and Substances

- Amino acids, proteins
- Sports drinks
- Vitamin E
- Relaxation techniques
- Carbohydrate approaches (loading, feeding, replenishment)
- Water (prehydration, hydration, rehydration)
- Minerals
- Liquid food supplements
- Psychologic approaches

Questionable or Potentially Harmful Practices and Substances

- Caffeine
- Alcohol
- Nicotine—tobacco
- Oxygen utilization (before, during, after performance)
- Bee pollen
- Marijuana
- Bicarbonate ingestion

Illegal Practices and Substances

- Anabolic steroids
- Barbiturates
- Diuretics
- Cocaine
- Blood doping (red blood cell reinfusion)
- Amphetamines
- β-blockers
- Human growth hormone
- Dimethyl sulfoxide

TABLE 15–2
Major Types of Ergogenic Aids to Performance

Classification	Examples
Pharmacologic	Anabolic steroids, amphetamines, human growth hormone, β-blockers, iron supplementation, barbiturates, diuretics
Nutritional	Amino acids, protein supplements, carbohydrate supplementation, minerals, water, sports drinks, wheat germ oil
Physiologic	Red blood cell reinfusion (blood doping), oxygen use
Psychologic	Relaxation, imagery, hypnosis
Miscellaneous	Alcohol, caffeine, cocaine, nicotine, marijuana, buffering solutions, lactate ingestion, phosphate ingestion, dimethyl sulfoxide (DMSO)

national and international sports governing bodies, sports medicine organizations, and medical societies. Certain ergogenic substances can have severe deleterious side effects both physiologically and psychologically, and their use should not be condoned under any circumstances.[3] Table 15–1 provides a differentiation of ergogenic aids (substances and practices) that are acceptable, questionable, and illegal.

The United States Olympic Committee (USOC) Drug Education and Doping Control Program is a resource for details on legal and illegal ergogenic aids, providing guidelines for banned medications and practices as defined by the International Olympic Committee.

Included among ergogenic aids to performance is a wide variety of practices and substances used to improve an athlete's performance, such as nutritional supplements, drugs, blood doping, dietary manipulation, and psychologic methods such as visualization and imagery. Table 15–2 classifies and provides examples of the different ergogenic aids to performance.

It is important for sports health care practitioners, regardless of discipline, to have a thorough knowledge of the effects and side effects, as well as advantages and disadvantages, of various types of ergogenic aids to performance. The purpose of this chapter is to focus attention on the different types of ergogenic aids most commonly used in athletics and to review some of the evidence regarding their performance-enhancing characteristics.

A HISTORICAL NOTE

The use of ergogenic aids to boost performance is not a new phenomenon. It dates back to ancient Greece and Rome, where those participating in athletic competitions and in battle ate raw meat to increase muscle strength and endurance. Greek athletes also ingested mushrooms in an attempt to improve athletic performance.[4] The first reported fatality from a performance-enhancing drug occurred in 1886, when an English cyclist died from an overdose of trimethyl.[5]

The media have been full of accounts of athletes, both amateur and professional, who have abused performance-enhancing agents, resulting in countless numbers of scandals, fines, suspensions, and tragedies. The most-abused substances include anabolic steroids, cocaine, amphetamines, alcohol, and marijuana. Although all these substances have received attention regarding their use and abuse in sports, the most attention has been given to the use and abuse of anabolic steroids.

The first reported use of anabolic steroids to increase strength, weight, and power occurred in Russian athletes in the mid-1950s.[6,7] It was not long before anabolic steroids were perceived to be beneficial in sports, as the Soviet Union and other Eastern-bloc countries adopting this practice began to dominate the sports world in international competition. This was the impetus for the advent of anabolic steroid use and abuse among athletes from Western countries.[8]

In the 1960s, a dramatic increase in the use of ergogenic aids, especially pharmacologic ones, occurred as a result of the reported success of this practice in

Europe and the belief by society that drugs could cure almost any condition. Sports became deeply involved in the drug culture, and athletes, coaches, and even some physicians began to look at ergogenic aids, particularly the pharmacologic ones, as shortcuts to success.

Many performance-enhancing substances and techniques have now been discredited, but athletes still use them, often with greater frequency and greater knowledge than previously. We still witness athletes being disqualified and stripped of medals at international sports competitions; college athletes banned from participation in intercollegiate games, matches, and meets; and professional athletes who utilize questionable or illegal performance-boosting practices or substances. A discussion of the underlying motives for using and perhaps unknowingly abusing supposedly performance-enhancing substances and practices is warranted prior to the examination of the various types of ergogenic aids to performance.

RATIONALE FOR ERGOGENIC AID UTILIZATION: USE OR ABUSE?

Questions have been raised about certain ergogenic aids to performance and whether their use constitutes abuse. Additional concerns have been expressed regarding the motives behind utilization of ergogenic aids that are perceived to improve physical work capacity, physiologic function, or athletic performance.[9] Is use of such a substance based on the athlete's desire to excel, peer pressure, a coaching decision or encouragement, or any number of other factors?

Some ergogenic aids are clearly acceptable for the improvement of performance. Certain practices, such as ingestion of water for fluid replenishment and prehydration, and carbohydrate loading and other nutritional approaches to boosting performance, may be neither questionable nor harmful to the athlete and may have practical application. The use of certain pharmacologic agents, such as amphetamines, anabolic steroids, barbiturates, diuretics, and β-blockers, is illegal and banned in national and international competitions and often does more harm than good. These substances may even be life-threatening to the athlete if they are used chronically and continually or if the athlete uses excessive amounts or develops an addiction to them.

Perceived improvement of performance, easy access, peer acceptance, direct exposure, and selling and marketing styles of salespeople with regard to the different types of ergogenic aids are sometimes used to defend the utilization of performance-boosting approaches.[10] A list of some of the common reasons for using ergogenic aids is presented in Table 15–3.

Many of the ergogenic aids, especially some of the pharmacologic approaches, may be perceived as mechanisms to reduce stress and anxiety as well as to boost athletic performance.[11] In considering ergogenic aids to performance, one must take into account the psychologic stresses that competitive athletes encounter and the perceived psychologic as well as physiologic benefits of ergogenic aids.

ERGOGENIC AIDS: PHARMACOLOGIC APPROACH

The pharmacologic approach to ergogenic aids involves drug compounds taken orally or injected into the body to bring about a perceived and desired effect. The use of pharmacologic agents and drugs as ergogenic aids has raised many questions as well as ethical, legal, and clinical concerns. This discussion of pharmacologic approaches to ergogenic aids focuses on anabolic-androgenic steroids, amphetamines, barbiturates, β-blockers, diuretics, and human growth hormone.

ANABOLIC-ANDROGENIC STEROIDS

Anabolic-androgenic steroids are synthetic derivatives of the male hormone testosterone; they were originally developed to hasten tissue repair in severely debilitated patients.[12] These synthetic compounds are similar to endogenous steroid hormones and are thought to have muscle-building properties. They are used by athletes in the hope of increasing muscle strength, power, endurance, and lean body mass. The effects of synthetic derivatives are anabolic (protein building) and androgenic (masculinizing or producing male secondary sex characteristics).[13]

It is believed that anabolic-androgenic steroids directly affect the muscle cell by increasing the content of skeletal muscle protein as a result of raising the activity of RNA-polymerase in skeletal muscle nuclei.[14] The steroid binds with special receptor sites in the muscle cell, and protein synthesis is stimulated.[15] With the alteration of the genetic machinery of muscle, especially at the cell nucleus, RNA is produced at a faster rate, which results in more protein. Two of these proteins are actin and myosin, which are force-producing contractile proteins.[16,17]

In the early 1950s, European weight lifters started using anabolic-androgenic steroids, and this practice quickly spread to North America. A decade later, use of anabolic-androgenic steroids was widespread in competitive sports at national and international levels. The theoretical rationale for the use of anabolic-androgenic steroids is that they increase muscle size and strength,

TABLE 15–3
Rationales for Use of Ergogenic Aids

- Greater success and greater potential in sport
- Accessibility of and exposure to ergogenic aids
- Performance enhancement
- Marketing influences by sales personnel
- Peer pressure and peer acceptance
- Pressure by coach, trainer, or physician
- Legality of substance or technique
- Shortcut to goal attainment
- Pressure to win or excel in sport or event
- Ease of administration
- Lack of fear of potential adverse health effects
- Perception of gaining a competitive edge
- Performance stress relief

TABLE 15–4
Commonly Used Oral and Injectable Anabolic Steroids

Generic Name	Trade Name
Oral	
Oxymethalone	Anadrol
Ethylestrenol	Maxobolin
Stanozolol	Winstrol
Oxandrolone	Anavar
Methyltestosterone	Android
Norethandrolone	Nilevar
Fluoxymesterone	Hasotestin
Injectable	
Nandrolone deconate	Deca-Durabolin
Nandrolone phenpropionate	Durabolin
Testosterone enanthate	Delatestryl
Testosterone cypionate	Depo-Testosterone
Methenolone enanthate	Primobolan
Testosterone nicotinate	Bolfortan
Stenbolone acetate	Anatrofin
Phenproprionate	Durololin

leading to improvement in performance.[18] Currently, anabolic steroids are prescribed for a variety of medical problems, including insufficient testosterone levels in males and different types of anemias.

The merits of anabolic-androgenic steroid use are continually debated in our society. There is no other ergogenic aid that has been as controversial or as abused, especially in sports that put a premium on body size and weight.[19] Anabolic-androgenic steroids may be taken orally or injected. Table 15–4 presents some of the more common anabolic-androgenic steroids. One great concern about the use of anabolic-androgenic steroids is that so many of them are purchased illegally as black-market drugs, and over $100 million is spent annually on steroids.[20] It is an alarming phenomenon that steroid users and abusers are getting younger and younger, as determined by recent surveys of high school athletes.[21–23]

The major focus on anabolic-androgenic steroids initially centered on the physiologic effects of these drugs and whether they can really boost performance. Early studies of the effects of anabolic-androgenic steroids sought to determine whether these drugs have an impact on strength and endurance, especially when taken in conjunction with a strength development program, with or without protein augmentation. The conflicting scientific data produced many moral and ethical issues related to the use of anabolic-androgenic steroids. There is some evidence and concern that athletes using anabolic steroids may develop life-threatening complications as a result of exceeding the recommended dosage for therapeutic purposes, which is 5 to 20 mg per day.[24] Dosages of anabolic steroids above this level have been found to produce detrimental side effects, especially in nonmedically supervised users.[24]

Athletes frequently use a progressively increasing combination of oral and injectable forms of anabolic steroids at dosages higher than the recommended therapeutic dosage. This technique is called "stacking," and an athlete may experiment with different numbers of anabolic steroids and gradually reduce usage as he or she gets closer to competition to avoid detection if drug testing is necessary. Some early studies found enhancement of muscular mass, strength, and endurance performance,[25–28] whereas others yielded conflicting results.[29,30]

Since the advent of anabolic-androgenic steroid use and abuse, the number of females using these drugs has increased dramatically.[31,32] Despite warnings to athletes and the banning of these drugs from national and international competitions, athletes still use them, taking serious risks. Clement[33] surveyed 220 Canadian athletes of international caliber and found 11 athletes who admitted using anabolic steroids, including two weight lifters, a basketball player, a rower, and seven athletes who remained anonymous.

Although some athletes abusing anabolic-androgenic steroids may experience only minor side effects, according to scientific evidence and personal testimonials from abusers, others may suffer severe and potentially life-threatening effects.[17] Despite warnings, athletes frequently ignore the dangers of these drugs, having witnessed the astounding physical results among their peers. However, they do not take into consideration the well-documented adverse long-term effects. The potentially harmful medical side effects greatly outweigh any performance-boosting benefits these drugs may offer. Clearly, anabolic-androgenic steroids should not be utilized as ergogenic aids to performance. (A summary of the major side effects of anabolic-androgenic steroids appears in Table 15–5.)

Due to the masculinizing effects of anabolic-androgenic steroids, females taking these drugs often develop hirsutism (increased body and facial hair), decreased breast size, menstrual irregularities, and decreased libido.[32] The drugs also cause hormonal alterations in males, and prolonged use can result in decreased sperm production, decreased testicular size and function, decreased libido, increased irritability and aggressive behavior, gynecomastia (enlarged, palpable breast tissue), and an increased concentration of estradiol, a major female hormone.[34–36]

Additional side effects of anabolic-androgenic steroid use are documented psychologic changes and aggressive behavior, which may eventually result in psychiatric problems. Pope and Katz[37] alluded to these mood changes and aggressive behavior and found that the drugs have a euphorogenic effect that influences the athlete's attitude toward training and training quality. By increasing competitiveness and aggression, the athlete can train harder, longer, more frequently, and with less fatigue. A potential danger of this type of aggression is that it can often lead to psychiatric manifestations, including psychotic symptoms, manic episodes, major depression, and acute schizophrenia.[38–41]

Much attention has also been focused on some of the metabolic manifestations and adverse effects that target vital organs, such as the liver and kidneys. The literature documents early evidence of the adverse effects of anabolic-androgenic steroids on the liver,[24] and liver tumors have been found in users.[40,42] Another side effect is peliosis hepatis, a condition characterized by blood-filled liver cysts.[6] Kidney tumors—especially Wilms' tumor, a rare kidney malignancy—have also been associated with anabolic steroid use.[43]

Additional problems presented by anabolic andro genic steroid use and abuse involve adverse effects on the immune system,[44] including AIDS acquired by sharing needles for anabolic steroid injections.[45] Premature closure of the epiphyseal growth plates in the bones of adolescents and children who abuse steroids has also been reported.[34] Prostate problems, including prostate adenocarcinoma,[46] may occur.

Much attention has also been focused on the adverse effects of anabolic-androgenic steroids on the cardiovascular system, especially detrimental blood lipid changes. Weight lifters, bodybuilders, and other sports participants consuming a high level of anabolic-androgenic steroids have shown a consistent tendency to develop high total cholesterol readings, with low to very low blood levels of high-density lipoproteins (HDL) and high levels of low-density lipoproteins (LDL), a pattern associated with high risk for premature coronary artery disease.[47–52] It is interesting to note that when subjects stopped using steroids for a period of time, HDL cholesterol levels rebounded to normal within 3 to 6 weeks.[50] Manifestations of this adverse effect on the cardiovascular system include possible impairment of left ventricular function,[53,54] myocardial infarction,[55] and cardiomyopathy and cerebrovascular accident in long-term abusers.[56]

Strong, continuous efforts should be made by sports medicine personnel in every athletic discipline to educate athletes, coaches, the general public, and others associated with athletes about the inconsistent effects of anabolic steroids and their potentially harmful side effects. The potential dangers of taking these substances for long periods in large doses should be made abundantly clear. Further, the use of anabolic-androgenic steroids is considered illegal by sports governing bodies, as these drugs are taken with the intent of unfair performance enhancement. The International Olympic Committee outlawed the use of anabolic steroids starting with the 1976 Olympic Games, and testing procedures were instituted for detecting anabolic steroids in urine.

Sports medicine organizations have also presented statements and position papers on the use and abuse of anabolic-androgenic steroids for the enhancement of performance. In 1977, the American College of Sports Medicine carefully searched and scrutinized the worldwide literature regarding claims made both for and against the use of anabolic steroids.[57] Its position statement was the first and has served as a guideline for others. The major points of the position statement include the following:

1. Anabolic-androgenic steroids in the presence of an adequate diet can contribute to increases in body weight.
2. Gains in muscular strength achieved through high-intensity exercise and proper diet can occur by the increased use of anabolic-androgenic steroids in some individuals.
3. Anabolic-androgenic steroids do not increase aerobic power or capacity for muscular exercise.
4. Anabolic-androgenic steroids have been associated with adverse effects on the liver, cardiovascular system, reproductive system, and psychologic status in therapeutic trials and in limited research on athletes. Until further research is done, the potential hazards of the use of anabolic-androgenic steroids in athletes must include those found in therapeutic trials.
5. Use of anabolic-androgenic steroids by athletes is contrary to the rules and ethical principles of athletic competition as set forth by many sports governing bodies. The American College of Sports Medicine supports these ethical principles and deplores the use of anabolic-androgenic steroids by athletes.

In 1985, the National Strength and Conditioning Association released its own position paper on the use and abuse of anabolic-androgenic steroids, based on an extensive scrutiny of worldwide literature on the topic and citing over 200 references.[58] Among the salient

---

TABLE 15–5
Major Adverse Side Effects of Anabolic-Androgenic Steroid Use

General

- Liver dysfunction
- Alopecia (hair loss)
- Immune system dysfunction
- Wilms' tumor (kidney malignancy)
- Peliosis hepatis (liver cysts filled with blood)
- Decreased high-density lipoproteins (HDL)
- Increased low-density lipoproteins (LDL)
- Aggressive behavior (explosive rages)
- Psychiatric problems (depression, suicidal thoughts, psychoses)
- Premature epiphyseal closure in children
- Liver and kidney tumors
- Hypercholesterolemia
- Migraine headaches

In Males

- Testicular atrophy
- Prostate gland problems (enlargement, adenocarcinoma)
- Gynecomastia (breast development)
- Increased sexual aggressiveness initially, but impotence with prolonged use
- Acne
- Abnormally low sperm count

In Females

- Enlarged clitoris
- Masculinizing effect
- Menstrual irregularities (dysmenorrhea, amenorrhea)
- Hirsutism (excessive hairiness of face, body)
- Deepening of voice

points presented in the position paper are the following:

1. Steroids alone do not increase performance, strength, or body weight.
2. Steroids in conjunction with weight training increase mass and may increase maximum strength and power.
3. Steroids are a threat to major body systems, including the cardiovascular system, the endocrine and immunologic systems, and the liver.
4. Athletes should be educated regarding the benefits and potential risks of steroid use.
5. Athletes at all levels of competition should be tested if drug testing is to be a deterrent to use.
6. Research on the long- and short-term effects of steroid use is actively supported by the National Strength and Conditioning Association.
7. The National Strength and Conditioning Association condemns the use of anabolic steroids on the basis of ethics and rules of fair play.

The technique of "stacking"[59] and other uses of anabolic-androgenic steroids should be strongly discouraged due to the potentially damaging effects of these drugs on the human body. Anabolic-androgenic steroids are extremely dangerous and should not be utilized by athletes as ergogenic aids. They have been condemned not only for their deleterious side effects but also because using them is unfair and unsporting.

AMPHETAMINES

Amphetamines are synthetic alkaloids usually taken in tablet form and are structured to mimic epinephrine and norepinephrine, thus serving as central nervous system stimulants. These drugs have become attractive to athletes who seek to improve their endurance by suppressing the sensations of muscle fatigue and by increasing alertness, aggressiveness, and concentration, all of which are perceived to increase one's competitive edge, especially in sports such as cycling and football. Publicity regarding the use of amphetamines by professional football players in the National Football League over the past few decades has focused on the drugs' ability to allay fatigue.[60,61] The data supporting enhancement of physical performance by amphetamine use are limited, however.

Chandler and Blair[62] found improvements in muscle strength and endurance tasks, but they also found that there was a significant increase in lactate production associated with increased endurance, suggesting that amphetamine use may mask fatigue symptoms, allowing for prolonged endurance. Conversely, a study by Williams and Thompson[63] found that there was no beneficial effect of varying dosages of amphetamines on time to exhaustion. Thus, the premise on which this pharmacologic ergogenic aid is based may have only a psychologic foundation. Therefore, its use in sports for the reduction of fatigue cannot be condoned.[64] With continuous use and abuse of amphetamines, many types of side effects become manifest.[65–67] Table 15–6

TABLE 15–6 Amphetamines
Commonly Utilized
• Benzedrex
• Benzedrine
• Dexedrine
• Desyphed
• Tuamine
Adverse Side Effects
• Restlessness
• Depression
• Poor judgment
• Insomnia
• Paranoia
• Tremors
• Psychosis
• Abdominal cramps
• Nervousness (prolonged use)
• Agitation and overaggression
• False sense of well-being or euphoria
• Masking of pain symptoms
• Dizziness
• Hallucinations
• Hostility
• Confusion
• Seizures
• Nausea
• Headaches
• Hematuria

presents some of the different types of amphetamines and the side effects and complications of acute and chronic use.

Among the reported side effects of amphetamine use are agitation, overaggression, hostility, poor judgment, possible hallucinations, confusion, paranoia, insomnia, dizziness, and depression.[65] Additional side effects include vomiting, abdominal pain, weight loss, and excessive diaphoresis.[65] Anorexic effects have been reported among sporting participants concerned with weight and weight classes, and amphetamines have been used by wrestlers, boxers, jockeys, and dancers to lose weight prior to competition.[66] Seizures have also been reported in users due to central nervous system hyperexcitability effects.[67] A particular danger of the use and overuse of amphetamines is that they may mask pain and lead to further aggravation of a pre-existing injury. Further, a tolerance may be built up for amphetamines; consequently, larger and larger doses are needed to produce the same feeling of euphoria. Athletes often take barbiturates or other depressants after a competitive event to serve as a "downer" from the effects of amphetamines. This can be a dangerous practice, as barbiturate ingestion may induce an adverse drug interaction with the amphetamine. Athletes, coaches, and the general public need educational programs to expose and emphasize the potential physiologic and psychologic dangers of this deceptive pharmacologic ergogenic aid.

BARBITURATES

Barbiturates traditionally are not considered an ergogenic aid to athletic performance, but more and more athletes are presenting personal testimonials regarding the perceived benefit of taking them, especially for relaxation purposes and in sports requiring a steady hand. Barbiturates are very effective in the reduction of tremor[68,69] and may be utilized where hand steadiness is essential to executing a skill (e.g., archery, shooting, weight events in track and field). The athlete may also take these drugs when preparing for the stress of athletic participation.

An early study of the effects of barbiturates on athletic performance was done by Smith and Beecher,[70] who found a significant improvement in maximum and mean distances achieved by field event throwers taking barbiturates as opposed to a placebo. Seemingly, the calming effect in athletes whose events require hand steadiness is the only positive factor, as reaction time, cognitive function, attention span, and visual tracking are adversely affected by barbiturates.[71]

Although not used frequently by athletes, barbiturates have an abuse potential, especially in athletes who use them for relaxation and hand steadiness prior to competition. A potential danger with the utilization of barbiturates is addiction, often induced by athletes who perceive that there are potential benefits of overutilizing the drug. This may lead to overdose, resulting in accidental or intended suicide. Education regarding this class of drugs also needs to be presented to athletes.

β-BLOCKERS

β-Adrenergic blocking agents, or β-blockers, are pharmacologic agents used therapeutically to produce blocking of the β-adrenergic receptors. They are commonly used for patients with cardiac arrhythmias, angina pectoris, and hypertension. The effects of decreasing the heart rate and cardiac output have become attractive to sports participants for limited purposes.

β-Blockers produce bradycardia as well as antitremor and antianxiety effects prior to competition.[69,72] They are utilized in sports such as golf, archery, and riflery to promote hand steadiness. They have also been found to be beneficial to skiers to reduce tachycardia and anxiety, especially before ski jumps.[73]

Due to the adverse effects on exercise tolerance reported in the literature,[74–79] these agents should not be used in highly trained athletes or sporting participants who train and compete for prolonged periods of time.[79] Other types of antihypertensive medications (e.g., calcium channel blockers) should be prescribed for athletes with primary or essential hypertension, as they have been found to be more suitable and do not cause excessive impairment of exercise capacity.[80] It should be noted that these agents are banned from use in competition by the National Collegiate Athletic Association and the International Olympic Committee.

DIURETICS

Traditionally, diuretics are used as antihypertensive therapy and for patients with fluid retention problems. Athletes in sports such as wrestling, boxing, judo, weight lifting, and horse racing often use these drugs in an attempt to lose weight to qualify for a certain weight class for competition. Athletes often take diuretics as a "washout" drug following the use of anabolic steroids.

Diuretics act to reduce fluid in the body, but the potential dangers of electrolyte imbalance and dehydration make use of these agents a dangerous and questionable practice.[81] With prolonged, chronic use of diuretics, electrolytes such as potassium, magnesium, calcium, and phosphorus—essential for regulating normal body processes—may be depleted to dangerously low levels. Athletes also use these agents in attempts to reduce the concentration of certain drugs in the urine, especially banned substances, through rapid diuresis.[80] Common side effects of abuse include muscle cramps due to reduced potassium levels.

Another population of athletes using diuretics more frequently now is female athletes, especially gymnasts and dancers, because of pressure from peers, coaches, and others to remain thin. Abuse of these pharmacologic agents may have adverse effects and can lead to eating disorders.[82] Another sad and dangerous scenario that occurs with all types of athletes involves using diuretics in combination with other short-term practices such as exhaustive exercise, steam saunas, starvation, fluid deprivation, and induced vomiting in an attempt to lose weight quickly.[83–85] The potential complications and adverse side effects of this pharmacologic approach, especially dehydration, warrant discouragement of its use as an ergogenic aid. Diuretics are also on the list of drugs banned from use in competition by the International Olympic Committee and the National Collegiate Athletic Association.

HUMAN GROWTH HORMONE

The use of human growth hormone (HGH) is becoming an increasingly popular pharmacologic approach to ergogenic aids to performance. HGH has been used clinically to stimulate growth in children lacking sufficient amounts of growth hormone, in an attempt to help them grow to normal height.[86] The theory and rationale behind the use of HGH are that it stimulates growth by increasing the transport of amino acids into cells of the body, especially in muscle and the liver.[86,87] It stimulates the production of protein in muscle cells and the release of energy from the breakdown of fats. There is also some evidence that HGH accelerates fat mobilization and catabolism.[87] It is generally agreed that a certain amount of this hormone is normally present in the body.

HGH is now prepared synthetically and has become increasingly available to athletes.[88] Some athletes use HGH due to their perception and peer acknowledgment that it improves physical and physiologic qualities, most notably muscle strength. Actually, these perceived improvements may be nonexistent. There has been limited research about the effects of HGH on athletic performance.[89–91] However, Crist and associates[89] found beneficial effects of HGH on eight well-trained men in a resistance training program. There were positive changes in body composition, including decreased body fat and increased lean body mass.

HGH is often used in combination with anabolic steroids for muscle growth, and HGH has become popular because of the difficulty of detecting its presence through traditional drug testing procedures. An athlete may believe that he or she can get the benefits of anabolic steroids in terms of muscle growth without the associated side effects, complications, and drug detection risks. The hormone has its risks, however, including the possible development of gigantism in children and acromegaly in adults, if it is used excessively.[90,91] HGH use is condemned and banned by the National Collegiate Athletic Association, the USOC, and the International Olympic Committee.

ERGOGENIC AIDS: NUTRITIONAL APPROACHES

The relationship between nutrition and athletic performance has become a popular topic in recent years, along with the subtopics of dietary fads, supplementation, and variations that are supposed to provide fuel for improving athletic performance. Nutrition and its role in the improvement of athletic performance receive much attention, but some practices of nutritional supplementation and variation, as well as dietary fads, lack scientific merit due to incomplete or inconclusive research.

Athletes are utilizing some of these approaches as ergogenic aids to performance, regardless of the questionable quality and minute quantity of scientific evidence that the approaches are sound. Presented briefly in this section are common nutritional supplements and practices that may be used as ergogenic aids to performance by athletes. Further insight into the basic nutritional concerns, needs, and problems of athletes may be found in Chapter 39.

AMINO ACIDS AND PROTEINS

There has been considerable debate over the issue of amino acids and protein needs in athletes, and whether dietary supplementation is necessary to meet the recommended daily allowance (RDA) for protein. The practice of protein supplementation dates back to the Roman Empire, when gladiators and athletes ate raw meat to prepare for battle and athletic competition. The belief was that this practice would provide greater strength for meeting the physical demands imposed on them.

Proteins are the main structural component of tissue and organs and are needed for the growth and repair of cells. Chemicals composed of carbon, oxygen, hydrogen, and nitrogen form basic molecules known as amino acids, which are in turn synthesized by living organisms into large, complex molecules known as proteins.[92] There are 20 amino acids found in the body, assisting a wide variety of bodily functions. Eight of these amino acids (known as essential amino acids) cannot be made by the body and must be obtained from a balanced diet. The nonessential amino acids are manufactured by the body and need not be constituents of the foods one eats. The major controversy surrounding athletes and protein is whether protein and amino acid supplements should be taken in addition to eating a diet that contains the recommended daily protein requirements for the individual's age and activity level.

The debatable issues surrounding this topic are primarily whether additional dietary protein is necessary in athletes as opposed to nonathletes, and whether different types of athletic endeavor (e.g., strength vs. endurance) require different amounts of protein. Athletes use amino acid and protein supplementation for different reasons, believing that it is an ergogenic aid to performance. Among the perceived benefits of amino acid supplementation are increased muscle bulk and energy utilization and stimulation of endogenous growth hormone release.[93] Some of these questions and concerns have been investigated, and attempts have been made to clarify them with relevant research.

Studies have found evidence of decreased protein synthesis[94,95] as well as increased protein degradation[96,97] during and after exercise. Additionally, there is some indirect evidence that, as duration of exercise increases, there is occasional utilization of protein as an energy source,[98] especially in the presence of depleted glycogen stores.[99] There is also significant evidence that amino acid and protein supplements are not necessary for exercise and exert little influence on protein requirements.[100,101]

Scientific information regarding the benefits of protein and amino acid supplementation is unclear and inconclusive in the literature, and most experts concur that a well-balanced diet containing the recommended daily protein requirement supplies all the essential amino acids.[92] If an athlete still desires additional protein, it is recommended that he or she increase protein intake within a well-balanced meal.[101] Precautions should be taken when using amino acid supplements due to numerous reported side effects, including dehydration, liver and kidney damage, gout, frequent urination, decreased urinary calcium, and suppressed amino acid absorption.[92,100]

CARBOHYDRATES

The importance of dietary carbohydrates and their value during prolonged exercise have received much attention in recent years. Carbohydrates are macronutrient molecules consisting of carbon, hydrogen, and oxygen that are found in sugars and starches in cereals and vegetables, which are sources of dietary carbohydrates.[102] Ingested carbohydrates are converted by digestive enzymes into glycogen, which is stored in the liver, muscles, and fat and become a fuel that is readily available for muscle contraction. Thus, carbohydrates are the most important nutrients for athletic performance.

The amount of glycogen stored in a given muscle determines the endurance of that muscle, and athletes engaging in sports or competitions, especially of an aerobic nature, need significant glycogen stores to resist fatigue.[103] When energy-providing glycogen stores are depleted, fatigue results, and the athlete cannot continue to exercise intensely. Some athletes fail to incorporate adequate amounts of carbohydrates into their diets or to appreciate carbohydrates' important role, especially in endurance activities.[104,105] Costill[106] reported that 55 to 65 percent of the calories supplied by training diets for prolonged exercise should come from carbohydrates.

Although an in-depth analysis of carbohydrates is beyond the scope of this section, carbohydrate approaches to improving athletic performance are discussed briefly.

CARBOHYDRATE USE BEFORE EXERCISE

Athletes engaging in sports or competitions of an intense aerobic nature for prolonged periods need extra stores of muscle glycogen to continue to perform maximally and to resist fatigue.[107] The storing of glycogen seems to be of value, and elevation of muscle glycogen above normal resting levels can be brought about prior to an endurance activity. This technique is known as glycogen supercompensation or carbohydrate loading.[102,107,108]

There are several variations of this nutritional approach to training, and the technique involves regulation or adjustment of diet and training components for maximum utilization of glycogen stores a few days before a prolonged, intense, competitive event. The most practical approach to carbohydrate loading includes training intensively up until 5 or 6 days before the competition, then gradually decreasing training intensity as the competition approaches, as well as eating meals high in carbohydrates for 3 days prior to the competition to increase glycogen stores.[102] It is recommended that during this period of carbohydrate loading, 70 percent of the total caloric intake should consist of carbohydrates.[109] Benefits of high-carbohydrate precompetition meals have been reported, and high-carbohydrate meals eaten within 6 hours of competition have been found to be beneficial in adding glycogen stores to the liver and muscles.[110] However, athletes should avoid high-carbohydrate feedings shortly before competition to prevent a rapid decrease in blood glucose levels during exercise, caused by possible elevation of blood insulin levels.[111]

CARBOHYDRATE USE DURING EXERCISE

Carbohydrate utilization during exercise, or carbohydrate feeding, is occurring more frequently as athletes and researchers find out more about its effectiveness. After several hours of continuous exercise, athletes tire due to glycogen depletion. Fatigue can be delayed by ingesting carbohydrates, such as a glucose solution or solid sucrose with water, ensuring that sufficient glycogen will be present during later stages of exercise.[112] It is believed that carbohydrate feedings during exercise allow muscles to rely on blood glucose for energy after prolonged exercise.[112] Without carbohydrate feeding, fatigue may occur because blood glucose is insufficient to compensate for depleted muscle glycogen.[113,114] Carbohydrates have also been found to be beneficial during long-duration intermittent exercise (e.g., soccer, lacrosse, tennis).[115]

CARBOHYDRATE USE AFTER EXERCISE

Another focus in recent years has been dietary carbohydrates and muscle glycogen resynthesis or replenishment after exercise or between training sessions. Athletes undergoing intense training on a regular basis should eat diets rich in carbohydrates to replenish energy stores lost or depleted during training sessions.

Total replenishment or restoration of the body's muscle glycogen stores is estimated to take approximately 20 hours, especially after exhaustive exercise.[116] An athlete's nutrition between training sessions and after an exhaustive competition is of primary importance and should include a diet rich in carbohydrates. Some athletes, however, might not want to eat during these periods. A recommended alternative to solid food may be a carbohydrate beverage, such as electrolyte-glucose solutions or glucose solutions, to help muscle glycogen resynthesis and aid in rehydration.[117] The method of carbohydrate replenishment (solid food vs. liquid) does not make a difference, and any of several modes may be used for this purpose. Unresolved concerns regarding the use of sugar drinks include their effect on the speed of digestion, which types of drinks are optimal for hydration, and whether they compromise intestinal fluid intake.

MINERALS

Mineral supplements are sometimes perceived as ergogenic aids by athletes, and their use is becoming more popular and frequent among competitive athletes. Currently, there is little evidence that mineral supplementation has beneficial effects on the enhancement of performance, provided the athlete is getting the normal RDA of minerals.[118,119]

Minerals are chemical elements that must be present in the diet to regulate normal body functions and to maintain homeostasis. At least 13 minerals are essential to health. It should be noted, however, that some mineral elements may have harmful effects when taken in excess.

SODIUM AND POTASSIUM

Both sodium and potassium deservedly receive much attention. In particular, there is concern over the loss of these minerals with profuse sweating. Among the functions of sodium and potassium are regulating fluid balance and fluid exchange in the body's fluid compartments and allowing for proper electrical gradients across cell membranes, especially in nerves and muscles.

Dietary supplementation of sodium through the use of salt tablets has been recommended for many years; however, this is not necessary, and most athletes can replenish sodium lost during exercise through proper nutrition.[120] Potassium deficiencies may occur with exercise, but maintenance of potassium levels can be accomplished with diets rich in potassium and by drinking citrus juices to replace potassium lost in sweat.[121] There is little scientific documentation to support dietary supplementation of these minerals beyond normal dietary RDAs.

CALCIUM

Calcium, a mineral found in great abundance in the body, plays a vital role in muscle contraction, bone formation, nerve impulse transmission, enzyme activation, and homeostasis. It is also essential for bone and tooth development. Attention has focused on the relationship between calcium levels in the body and bone density, and on the question of whether there is a correlation between low bone density and stress fractures caused by amenorrhea in female endurance athletes.[122,123] It is unclear whether calcium supplementation is beneficial in retarding bone loss, especially if the cause of calcium loss is unknown. Attention has also focused recently on the need for adequate dietary calcium intake in active older women to guard against bone loss and the onset of osteoporosis.[124]

ZINC

Zinc is a trace element that is essential for normal carbohydrate metabolism, tissue repair, blood cell reproduction, protein synthesis, growth, and reproduction. Research on how exercise affects this mineral and whether zinc supplementation is needed has been limited. There is some evidence that exercise may place a strain on the body's content of this trace mineral,[125,126] but whether zinc supplementation would be beneficial and warranted is still unclear. It has been noted, however, that prolonged, excessive intake of zinc (usually through supplements) may interfere with intestinal absorption of iron and copper, eventually causing negative side effects.

IRON

Iron, along with hemoglobin in the red blood cells, functions to increase the oxygen-carrying capacity of the blood. Iron is also the major structural component of myoglobin, which aids in the storage and transport of oxygen within the muscle cells. Females need more iron than males to resynthesize red blood cells lost during menstruation. The increased participation of women in sports, especially in endurance activities, has focused a great deal of attention on the effects of intense physical training on the body's iron stores.[126]

Iron-deficiency anemia resulting from inadequate iron intake occurs frequently in physically active women,[127] and the worst combination for iron deficiency is a physically active endurance athlete who is menstruating and not eating a balanced diet. The major discussion regarding iron and exercise focuses on whether iron supplementation is warranted.

Iron supplementation in female athletes with sufficient dietary iron does not always lead to increases in hemoglobin content or hematocrit.[128] The majority of the literature supports the use of the RDA with a balanced diet to maintain proper levels of iron in the body. If the hemoglobin is normal, there is no need for iron supplementation.[128,129] In the presence of a definite iron deficiency or iron-deficiency anemia, dietary iron supplementation is effective and acceptable for the restoration of depleted iron stores.[128,130] Based on scientific evidence, however, there is no justification for all female athletes to ingest oral iron supplements as a widespread practice.

WATER

Loss of body water is a serious consequence of excessive sweating, especially during exercise. Factors such as environmental temperature, relative humidity, and exercise intensity, are some determinants of the amount of water lost during profuse sweating. Physical activity increases the need for fluid replenishment in the body tissues. Water for prehydration, hydration, and rehydration before, during, and after exercise is used as an ergogenic aid and warrants brief discussion.

Heat illness is a potential problem for athletes who exercise in high environmental temperatures or humidity. Water loss from sweating occurs in great amounts, and failure to replace the lost water can result in decreased circulating blood volume, which may lead to various heat illnesses. Adequate fluids should be made available to athletes, especially during prolonged exercise in heat, to prevent the debilitating effects of dehydration. Water consumption in adequate amounts before, during, and after workouts, training sessions, and competition should be encouraged to counteract dehydration and heat illness, which may have severe physical consequences.

SPORTS DRINKS

A variety of commercial sports drinks are now on the market as an alternative or addition to water for fluid and electrolyte replenishment. In long endurance events, these carbohydrate- and sodium-containing drinks may be the mechanism for replacing lost glycogen and improving performance.[131] Although some sports drinks are better than others, athletes should be warned that overzealous salespeople may try to overwhelm them with the benefits of their respective products without any scientific evidence and may succeed by unscrupulously exploiting public ignorance.

Choices of sports drinks should be made with care. A major consideration is the electrolyte and carbohydrate constituency of the sports drink. Although studies regarding the effectiveness of sports drinks have been inconclusive, several researchers have found that carbohydrate percentages of 6 to 8 percent, along with sodium and potassium, are most beneficial due to efficient gastric-emptying and intestinal absorption qualities, resulting in rapid fluid absorption[132-134] and maintenance of circulatory and thermoregulatory functions during exercise.[135]

The benefits of drinking fluids during vigorous exercise are obvious, but the debate over which sports drink to consume continues. There is a surprisingly large variety of commercial fluid replacement beverages. Table 15–7 presents a comparison of sports drinks and their ingredients.

LIQUID FOOD SUPPLEMENTS

Liquid food supplements are often used by athletes as substitutes for adequate nutritional intake. Pregame meals may be rejected because of gastrointestinal upset resulting from precompetition tension. Liquid supplements afford energy and can also serve as additional sources of fluid. Moreover, these meals leave the stomach quickly and allow for completion of digestion, usually in time for the competition.

Athletes may perceive liquid food supplements as ergogenic aids. Proper guidance in the use of these supplements should be provided to the athlete through proper nutritional and dietary counseling.

ERGOGENIC AIDS: SPORTS TRAINING AND PHYSIOLOGIC APPROACHES

Sports training and physiologic approaches to enhancing athletic performance are becoming increasingly popular. These approaches utilize agents and techniques designed to alter body systems positively, especially the cardiovascular and respiratory systems, to bring about changes perceived to boost performance. Among these approaches are blood doping, or induced erythrocythemia, and supplementary oxygen.

BLOOD DOPING

The practice of blood doping, also known as blood packing, blood boosting, or red blood cell reinfusion, and scientifically referred to as induced erythrocythemia, began to receive much attention in the 1970s as an approach to enhancing athletic performance. The practice involves the removal, storage, and subsequent intravenous reinfusion of a certain amount of blood from an endurance athlete and is designed to enhance the ability of the blood to carry, transport, and deliver oxygen to tissues, thus increasing aerobic power and maximum oxygen consumption.

Blood doping was first reported in the late 1940s,[136] and there has been much debate and many questions about the ethics of this practice. In the 1976 Olympics in Montreal, many athletes reported voluntarily that this approach is commonly used to boost performance.[137,138] In 1985, the International Olympic Committee added blood doping to its list of banned substances and procedures. This was followed by statements and positions from the USOC prohibiting this practice and a statement from the American College of Sports Medicine citing blood doping as an unethical and unjustifiable practice to enhance athletic performance.[139] The practice is also banned by the National Collegiate Athletic Association.

The rationale for the use of this approach as an ergogenic aid is that blood volume, red blood cells, and hemoglobin are major determinants of efficient oxygen transport, and if these are enhanced, an augmented oxygen transport system and oxygen-carrying capacity of the blood will result, thereby producing an increase in aerobic endurance capabilities. Early studies on blood doping were contradictory, some finding that the technique was beneficial for enhancing endurance performance[140-143] and others reporting no beneficial effects.[144-146] Many of the early studies conflicted due to research design flaws and inconsistency in blood storage techniques. Recent studies tend to support the belief that blood doping improves athletic performance, despite its controversial nature.[147-150] All these recent studies found that blood doping increased aerobic power and improved endurance performance. The practice of blood doping has been used primarily by athletes engaged in sports of an aerobic nature (e.g., cycling, cross-country skiing, long-distance running, rowing) in an attempt to increase transport of oxygen to the working muscles, thus increasing total aerobic power.

Procedures involved in the withdrawal, storage, and reinfusion of stored blood may vary according to when, where, and by whom the procedure is done. Autologous approaches involve the removal of a certain volume of blood from an individual, separation and storage of blood cells for a certain amount of time, and subsequent reinfusion; homologous approaches involve removing blood from a donor, storing it, and then transfusing it into a recipient.[151] Optimally, blood removal occurs 6 to 10 weeks before the anticipated competition.[138] Red blood cells are separated from plasma and preserved by means of an expensive freezing technique known as glycerol freezing.[152,153] This technique is necessary due to strict regulations in North America concerning maximum refrigeration storage time of blood—3 weeks. The athlete should continue to train during the 6- to 10-week period to attempt to re-establish normal hemoglobin and red blood cell status and efficient aerobic capacity prior to reinfusion.[138,153]

Several days before the competition, the frozen red blood cells are reinfused after thawing and special treatment with saline.[153,154] Gledhill[138,151] acknowledged that when the stored cells are reinfused, the red

TABLE 15–7
Beverage Comparison Chart

Beverages	Flavors	Carbohydrate Ingredient	Carbohydrate Concentration (%)	Sodium (mg) per 8 oz serving	Potassium (mg) per 8 oz serving	Other Minerals and Vitamins
Gatorade® Thirst Quencher Quaker Oats Company	Lemon-lime, lemonade, fruit punch, orange, citrus cooler, tropical fruit, grape, iced tea cooler	Powder: sucrose/ glucose Liquid: sucrose/ glucose Syrup solids	6	110	25	Chloride, phosphorus
PowerAde® Coca-Cola	Lemon-lime, fruit punch, orange	High-fructose corn syrup, maltodextrin	7.9	73 or less	33	Chloride
AllSport® Pepsico	Lemon-lime, orange, fruit punch	High fructose corn syrup	8–9	55	55	Chloride, phosphorus, calcium
10-k® Beverage Products, Inc.	Lemon-lime, orange, fruit punch, lemonade, iced tea, pink lemonade, apple	Sucrose, glucose, fructose	6.3	52	26	Vitamin C, chloride, phosphorus
Nautilus®	Lemon-lime, orange, fruit punch	None	Less than 1.0	50	50	Calcium, magnesium
Snap-up® Snapple	Lemonice tea, fruit punch, lemon-lime, orange	Glucose polymers/ fructose	20	58	49	Chloride
Quickick® Cramer Products, Inc.	Lemon-lime, fruit punch, orange, grape, lemonade	Fructose/ sucrose	4.7	116	23	Calcium, chloride, phosphorus
Sqwincher® The Activity Drink Universal Products, Inc.	Lemon-lime, fruit punch, lemonade, orange, grape, strawberry, grapefruit	Glucose/ fructose	6.8	60	36	Vitamin C, chloride, phosphorus, calcium, magnesium
Exceed® Energy Drink Ross Laboratories	Lemon-lime, orange	Glucose polymers/ fructose	7.2	50	45	Calcium, magnesium, phosphorus, chloride
Endura® Unipro	Orange, lemon-lime	Glucose polymers/ fructose	6	92	180	Calcium, chloride, magnesium, chromium
1st Ade Daily's™	Lemon-lime, orange, fruit punch	High-fructose corn syrup/ sucrose	6	110	25	Phosphorus
Hydrafuel™ Twin Labs	Orange, fruit punch, lemon-lime	Glucose polymers	7	25	50	Chloride, magnesium, chromium, phosphorus, vitamin C
Cytomax®	Apple	Fructose/corn syrup solids/ sucrose	7–11	~50	~100	Chrominum, magnesium
Gookinaid® Gookinaid ERG	Lemon, fruit punch, orange	Glucose	12	70	70	Vitamins C, A; calcium, iron
Soft drinks	Cola, non-cola	High-fructose corn syrup/ sucrose	10.2–11.3	9.2–28	Trace	Phosphorus
Diet soft drinks	All	None	0	0–25	Low	Phosphorus
Water	—	—	0	Low	Low	Low

For applicable research, see Costill,[106] Bjorkman et al.,[225] Davis et al.,[226] Greenleaf,[227] Gisolfi et al.,[228] Lamb and Brodowicz,[229] Murray,[230] Murray et al.[231] and Sherman and Lamb.[232]
Courtesy of Gatorade Sports Science Institute, Chicago, 1988.

blood cell count is increased, and hemoglobin may be increased by as much as 10 percent. The amount of blood removed is usually 900 to 1000 mL, and the critical factors associated with success in this approach include the total volume of red blood cells reinfused, the time interval between blood withdrawal and reinfusion, and the blood storage method.[138]

Despite the apparent benefits of this approach, blood doping can be dangerous. There are many associated risks and side effects. Utilization of this technique by nonmedical personnel is potentially hazardous, as the approach involves invasive techniques. The hazards include conditions associated with the infusion and reinfusion of blood, such as air emboli, blood infections, transfusion reactions, thrombosis, blood incompatibilities, metabolic shock, allergic reactions, and AIDS.[155] Due to these risks, blood doping cannot be condoned or recommended at any level of competition. Use of blood doping is in violation of guidelines set forth by national and international sports governing bodies, as well as by scientific sports medicine organizations.

OXYGEN

A frequently observed practice is athletes' use of an oxygen-enriched or hyperoxic gas mixture, usually on the bench or sidelines, commonly with the perceived notion that it will speed recovery from exhaustive bouts of exercise. One often witnesses a football player breathing oxygen after making a touchdown as a result of a long running play. Although the use of oxygen is popular with athletes, the reality is that the physiologic benefits of this practice are questionable. There has been limited research in this area, but the use of oxygen before, during, and after exercise has been briefly investigated.

There have been few reports regarding beneficial effects of oxygen-enriched gas used prior to exercise. An early study by Karpovich[156] found that oxygen utilization prior to exercise had a beneficial effect on performance if the exercise involved holding one's breath. A later study, however, found that the use of oxygen prior to activity where the breath is not held had little effect on performance.[157] An athlete utilizing this technique prior to exercise for perceived physiologic benefits, such as enhanced oxygen-carrying capacity, thus has no scientific justification for doing so, and its benefits remain unproven.

The practice of breathing supplemental oxygen during exercise has been found to have a beneficial effect on exercise, especially endurance exercise, and leads to enhanced performance.[158,159] However, no practical method of delivering an oxygen-enriched gas mixture during exercise or athletic performance has been found so far.

Finally, research regarding the effects of oxygen as an adjunct to hastening recovery after exercise has been inconclusive,[157,160,161] and no real benefits have been shown. This practice is more a psychologic than a therapeutic tradition—there is no scientifically documented benefit.

ERGOGENIC AIDS: RELAXATION AND PSYCHOLOGIC APPROACHES

In the complex microcosm of organized sports, a common problem is competitive athletes' low arousal level. A greater challenge is presented when athletes also have high levels of anxiety and tension. Athletes and coaches often try to boost arousal levels and depress heightened anxiety states that may be present before practice or competition. The services of a sports psychologist may be utilized for this purpose.

This section focuses on types of relaxation techniques, including Jacobson's progressive relaxation, autogenic training, transcendental meditation, and biofeedback, as well as psychologic approaches (cognitive strategies) such as imagery, goal setting, and hypnosis, which are designed to help the athlete alter existing levels of arousal and anxiety.

JACOBSON'S PROGRESSIVE RELAXATION

This relaxation technique was developed in the early twentieth century by Edmund Jacobson.[162] It is a progressive, systematic relaxation procedure that involves tensing, then relaxing, specific muscles and muscle groups in a predetermined order. The rationale for this type of relaxation is that when muscles are completely relaxed, it is impossible to be nervous or tense, and with skeletal muscle relaxation, nervousness and tension of involuntary muscles can be reduced.[162]

The technique for Jacobson's progressive relaxation involves having the subject assume the supine position with the arms at the sides. The subject tenses individual muscles and then relaxes them to ascertain the difference between tension and relaxation. The subject should eventually be able to relax a limb without initial tensing of the muscles. The goal of this technique is to achieve progressive relaxation to reduce tension and anxiety, which may result in improved performance.

AUTOGENIC TRAINING

Autogenic training was developed in the late 1950s by Johannes Schultz, a German physician.[163] This technique emphasizes how the limbs and body parts feel after tensing and relaxing the muscles in a manner similar to that used in Jacobson's technique. There are six exercises in the training technique, and each one must be practiced until the subject achieves the desired level. The subject can then progress to the next exercise. The goal is to relax specific parts of the body while experiencing feelings of heaviness in each limb. Mastering the technique of autogenic training allows an athlete to apply it to stressful situations for the reduction of anxiety and tension.

TRANSCENDENTAL MEDITATION

This meditation technique is popular with athletes and nonathletes in Western society to reduce anxiety and tension. One meditates while focusing on breathing, visualization, muscle relaxation, and the silent repetition of a "mantra"—a simple sound selected by the teacher for mental concentration (e.g., "Om"). The subject usually assumes a cross-legged sitting position on the floor, and the combination of positioning, deep breathing, and silent mantra repetition induces a relaxation response.[164] It is unclear whether this practice is beneficial or practical in reducing tension and anxiety in athletic performance, and it would be difficult to measure.

BIOFEEDBACK

Biofeedback training techniques are now being used by athletes who suffer from excessive anxiety or arousal problems, and benefits have been reported in different populations of athletes.[165,166] In biofeedback training, various types of instrumentation (e.g., electromyography, echoencephalography, skin temperature thermometers) are used to measure responses of the autonomic nervous system that the subject learns to control voluntarily through different types of cues or thoughts. Skin temperature, heart rate, muscle tension, and brain waves are some of the common responses that the subject can learn to control. Eventually, it is desirable to remove the instrumentation, thus allowing the subject to control the desired response without monitoring. The drawback of this type of relaxation technique is the expense of the equipment.

IMAGERY

Imagery, or visualization, is a popular cognitive strategy used by professionals to prepare an athlete for competition. The subject uses visualization to imagine an experience in the mind that can be created or recreated.[167] Mahoney and Avener[168] identified two distinct methods of imagery related to sport performance. Internal or kinesthetic imagery is characterized by visualization in which athletes perceive that they are within their own bodies while performing and concentrate on feeling themselves performing. External or visual imagery involves athletes' pretending to watch themselves perform from the outside and is more of a visual phenomenon.

Imagery is useful for practicing and learning sports skills and strategies, problem solving, increasing sport perception, and controlling physiologic responses.[167] Green[169] proposed that imagery may be beneficial during injury recovery and rehabilitation, as it helps develop an awareness of injury and creates a mind-set for recovery. Although positive results have been described in the literature,[168,170,171] other studies have presented speculative doubt about the effectiveness of imagery for anxiety reduction in sports.[172,173] Despite this conflict, imagery is a widely used technique that has much potential for anxiety reduction in athletes.

GOAL SETTING

Goal setting is becoming a popular training strategy to help athletes perform maximally and to produce positive changes in psychologic states such as anxiety, confidence, and motivation.[174] Setting specific, well-defined, realistic goals for specific days, weeks, or months can be very beneficial, especially in injury recovery.[175] Goal setting has also been found to affect the speed of injury recovery; injured athletes who set goals heal more quickly.[176] Further, attainment of long-term goals seems more realistic when short-term goals are also set, when the goals are realistic and capable of being evaluated, and when a specific plan is outlined for meeting the goals.

HYPNOSIS

Hypnosis is another approach used by trained professionals (e.g., professional hypnotists or psychologists) in attempting to alter or influence arousal and anxiety states in competitive athletes. Traditionally, hypnosis is referred to as an altered state of consciousness, but it should be thought of as an alternative state of consciousness. This implies that the individual being hypnotized is still in a natural, albeit alternative, state of mind.[177] Heterohypnosis is hypnosis that is brought about by another person, usually a trained professional; autohypnosis is self-induced.[178]

There is still conflict over what happens during hypnosis. Is the subject in a "hypnotic trance," or is the basis for hypnosis a cortical inhibition known as a hemispheric shift, in which there is dominant activity by the nondominant hemisphere and inhibition of functions in the dominant hemisphere?[177] Any positive effect of hypnosis on athletic performance is still unproven, and there is some evidence that it may be harmful and cannot improve performance.[179]

ERGOGENIC AIDS: MISCELLANEOUS APPROACHES

This section focuses on some miscellaneous approaches and substances commonly used by athletes to enhance performance or that may be perceived to improve athletic abilities. Some of these substances are not only banned by both national and international sports governing bodies but are also against the law. Discussed in this section are alcohol, caffeine, cocaine, tobacco, marijuana, dimethyl sulfoxide (DMSO), bee pollen, sodium bicarbonate, and vitamin E.

ALCOHOL

Alcohol abuse and alcoholism still plague our society, particularly because alcohol is a socially and legally acceptable drug. Yet alcohol has been identified as the number one abused drug in the United States.[180] Reports are rampant regarding athletes' abuse of alcohol, at both amateur and professional levels, and sometimes the abuse results in tragedy. Athletes are often more susceptible to alcohol abuse than others due to its use by peers, teammates, coaches, boosters, and others affiliated with sports. Alcohol is available if the athlete is over a state's legal drinking age, and alcohol consumption is socially acceptable when done in moderation. Due to the legality of alcohol, strict policies regarding its use by athletes are sometimes difficult to enact and enforce. Alcohol has not been identified as an ergogenic aid and should not be utilized for this purpose.[181]

Alcohol in very small amounts has been used for its antitremor effects and has been found to be superior to β-blockers in reducing tremors prior to competition in sports such as riflery and pistol shooting.[182] Athletes should avoid this practice, however, as alcohol use for this purpose is banned by the National Collegiate Athletic Association and the International Olympic Committee. Furthermore, alcohol has definite adverse effects on various psychomotor skills such as reaction time, hand-eye coordination, accuracy, balance, and complex coordination tasks.[183–185] Alcohol may be erroneously perceived by an athlete to improve athletic performance, but in reality, it does not.[182] Athletes may endanger themselves, teammates, and opponents by ingesting alcohol prior to athletic competition.

CAFFEINE

Caffeine is a stimulant found in tea, coffee, cola drinks, cocoa, chocolate, and some over-the-counter medications. Caffeine has been used by athletes primarily in endurance events in attempts to enhance exercise performance.[186] Renewed interest in the effects of caffeine as an aid to athletic performance was evoked by researchers at Ball State University. An initial study by Costill et al.[187] and a subsequent study by Ivy et al.[188] found significant improvement in cycling endurance following caffeine ingestion in moderate amounts.

The ergogenic effects of caffeine are believed to occur as a result of glycogen sparing, thus delaying glycogen depletion and fatigue as well as promoting utilization of fat as a fuel for exercise, especially during prolonged exertion.[189,190] There have been some research studies supporting the ergogenic effects of caffeine ingestion, especially on endurance, and supporting the fat utilization–glycogen sparing theory.[189,191–193] Other studies have found no improvement in endurance performance.[194–197] There is also some evidence that caffeine may exert a beneficial effect directly on muscle, but the mechanism is not known.[198] Currently, evidence is insufficient to state that caffeine is either beneficial or detrimental to endurance performance.[181] Moreover, because it can improve short-term athletic performance, caffeine has been included in the list of drugs banned in sports competitions.[199] The International Olympic Committee and the National Collegiate Athletic Asso-

ciation allow limited urinary caffeine levels; above these levels, an athlete may be accused of doping. Side effects of caffeine may include nervousness, irritability, insomnia, elevated blood pressure, cardiac arrhythmias, and diuresis.

COCAINE

The use of cocaine unfortunately continues to escalate, especially in the world of professional sports. However, its use is becoming more common among athletes at other levels as well. Use and abuse of cocaine are evident, regardless of the stiff penalties one can incur. Additionally, cocaine-related deaths occasionally stun the sports world, such as the death of Len Bias in 1986. Cocaine has no valid ergogenic qualities but is used by athletes as a recreational drug. As a central nervous system stimulant, cocaine causes a sense of euphoria.

Cocaine may also be used by an athlete to mask pain, which may lead to further injury. Continual cocaine use can lead to severe adverse side effects, addiction, and bizarre personality and behavioral changes, including hallucinations and paranoid behavior.[200] Cocaine and its stimulating effects also destroy nasal tissues and often cause conflict in interpersonal relationships.[201] Widespread cocaine abuse has necessitated periodic drug testing by the National Collegiate Athletic Association and International Olympic Committee for this agent.[202]

NICOTINE AND TOBACCO

Nicotine, ingested through cigarette smoking and the use of smokeless tobacco, and its effects on athletic performance have not been investigated thoroughly. Nevertheless, enough detrimental evidence exists regarding both of these practices to state that they do not possess ergogenic qualities.

There has been very little research specifically targeted at the effects of cigarette smoking on exercise performance. Most athletes, especially endurance athletes, disdain cigarettes as a hindrance to efficient performance. Smoking increases peripheral airway resistance,[203] and early studies found that it severely impaired exercise tolerance.[204] Further observations have found impaired physiologic function during exercise after smoking,[205] including decreased lung function, decreased pulmonary compliance, and reduced lung capacity. From the limited research available, it is readily apparent that cigarette smoking hinders rather than enhances athletic performance.

The use of smokeless tobacco is often presented by advertising as a safe and desirable alternative to smoking. However, it is neither safe nor ergogenic, and chronic use can be devastating. Athletes use smokeless tobacco more than the general population does,[206] ignorant of the potential medical problems and its inability to enhance performance.[207] First-time users are becoming younger,[208] and often the motivation for trying smokeless tobacco is its use by a parent, coach, friend, or sports figure who is seen as a role model.[209] The adverse effects of smokeless tobacco include bad breath, stained teeth, tooth sensitivity to temperature extremes, cavities, gum recession, irritated gums, tooth and bone loss, and various forms of oral cancer.[210] A massive education program is needed regarding the adverse effects of smokeless tobacco.

MARIJUANA

Marijuana is often erroneously presented as a harmless substance whose use has no detrimental effects. Marijuana comes from the plant *Cannabis sativa;* its leaves are rolled into cigarettes and smoked. Among the adverse effects of marijuana are impaired pulmonary function and performance; cardiovascular impairment, including tachycardia and electrocardiogram changes; male reproductive system effects, including lowered sperm count; short-term memory loss; and adverse behavioral and psychologic effects (coordination, tracking, perceptual tasks).[211]

Other problems associated with marijuana include diminished judgment, poor focus and attention span, and slower thought processes. Although an athlete may perceive that marijuana benefits performance by increasing mental awareness, the actual impairment of perception makes this a dangerous substance to use as an ergogenic aid. Marijuana has no ergogenic effects.

DIMETHYL SULFOXIDE

Athletes are using dimethyl sulfoxide (DMSO) with alarming frequency as a topical agent to promote healing after injury. This substance, illegal for use on humans except in two states, is a strong industrial solvent that has excellent penetration capabilities through the skin and is quickly absorbed. There is still controversy regarding the use of DMSO as a topical anti-inflammatory agent, and the mechanism by which it functions is still not completely understood.

DMSO is commonly used by veterinarians as a topical anti-inflammatory medication for horses that have suffered traumatic injuries. It is available in gel and solution forms. It quickly reduces soft tissue swelling and inflammatory reaction to acute trauma. DMSO has been approved by the Food and Drug Administration for use only in horses as a topical agent for the treatment of acute swelling and inflammation. Athletes, coaches, fitness personnel, and others who work with athletes sometimes obtain DMSO by illegal means and use it to hasten recovery from injury. Until more is known about this agent—its physiologic effects and its possible complications, especially in humans—DMSO must be considered potentially hazardous. The Food and Drug Administration has banned the use of this agent in humans.

BEE POLLEN

Bee pollen, a nutrient supplement composed of vitamins, minerals, and proteins, has been advertised as an ergogenic aid that is essential for athletic performance. It is often marketed to augment the RDA for vitamins, minerals, and proteins, especially when these nutritional components are inadequate.

There have been only a few controlled investigations of the effects of bee pollen on physical performance, and no enhancement has been reported.[212–214] Until further well-controlled research is done on bee pollen and its effects on performance, claims that it is a significant ergogenic aid cannot be substantiated.

SODIUM BICARBONATE

The use of buffering solutions, namely sodium bicarbonate, has attracted some attention in recent years, especially among athletes involved in sports that rely on anaerobic metabolism. The use of sodium bicarbonate is also referred to as bicarbonate loading or bicarbonate doping and involves the ingestion of a sodium bicarbonate solution (usually baking soda and water) prior to athletic competition. The rationale for this technique, according to Williams,[215] is that the sodium bicarbonate serves as a natural buffer in the body that assists in the neutralization of metabolic acids, especially lactic acid, to maintain a normal acid-base balance.

In exhaustive exercise of a short-term nature, when energy transfer is accomplished primarily by anaerobic means, there is a concomitant increase in the accumulation of lactic acid and a concurrent decrease in intracellular pH value. There is speculation that in the presence of intense, short-duration exercise of an aerobic nature, this increased acidity may eventually have an inhibitory effect on energy transfer and may render the contractile capabilities of the active muscle fibers ineffective.[216] The ingestion of sodium bicarbonate prior to exercise is believed to increase extracellular buffering by facilitating hydrogen ion efflux from working muscle cells, thus delaying decreases in intracellular pH, increases in lactic acid, and the consequent onset of muscle fatigue.[217] The use of sodium bicarbonate is believed to increase the body's bicarbonate reserve prior to exercise and to enhance short-term anaerobic exercise by delaying the onset of muscle fatigue.

Studies regarding the effects of bicarbonate loading have produced conflicting results.[218–221] Although bicarbonate loading has been found to have benefits in certain anaerobic athletic endeavors—namely, short-term, high-intensity exercise—more research needs to be done on its effectiveness. The use of bicarbonate loading may also cause unpleasant complications, such as diarrhea and gastrointestinal disturbances. Although the use of sodium bicarbonate is not banned by the various athletic governing bodies, ethical considerations discourage its use as an ergogenic aid.

VITAMIN E

Tocopherol (vitamin E) is an antioxidant that functions in the body to prevent cell membrane damage and helps in the formation of muscle, red blood cells, and other tissues.[222] Sources of vitamin E include salad oils, margarine, whole-grain products, fruits, and leafy green vegetables. Vitamin E is also commercially available in capsule form and can be bought at health food stores and pharmacies.

The use of vitamin supplements is common among athletes, and vitamin E is sometimes taken by athletes who believe the exaggerated claims that it protects the cardiovascular system.[222] Some athletes claim that tocopherol boosts their performance, but scientific studies have not concluded that large doses of vitamin E enhance athletic performance.[223,224]

ETHICAL AND LEGAL CONSIDERATIONS

In today's complex world of sports, we have witnessed athletes at many levels of competition use different types of ergogenic aids, with or without concern about whether the technique or substance was legal. The major emphasis in sports today is winning, and the athlete or coach may seek ways of gaining the "competitive edge." Many questionable ergogenic aids are sought, purchased illegally, ingested, and used, in spite of the possibility of being detected. Many athletes seemed to be unconcerned about the long-term effects of many of these agents and are willing to accept the risks in their pursuit of optimal athletic achievement.

Being detected and exposed for use or abuse of a banned ergogenic substance or technique can be embarrassing, humiliating, and shameful to the athlete, coaches, teammates, country or organization represented, and family. The stripping of a medal, forfeiture of a victory, or returning of a trophy as a result of detection of a banned ergogenic technique or substance may eventually cause the athlete much psychologic pain, especially after he or she has worked so hard to achieve a particular athletic goal. Some of the questions an athlete should ask himself or herself when pondering the use of ergogenic aids include the following:

1. What are the benefits of using ergogenic aids, and have they been scientifically proved to improve performance?
2. What are the adverse side effects and long-term effects of utilization on my health?
3. What is the position of the applicable sports governing body regarding its use?
4. Will use of the ergogenic aid constantly be on my conscience?
5. Can utilization of this ergogenic aid pose a danger to me or my opponent in competition?
6. If I use the aid, will my opponent experience competition against his or her real opponent?

TABLE 15–8
Some Ethical Concerns Athletes Should Have About Ergogenic Aids Usage

- Benefits of utilization (True? False? Speculative?)
- Side effects, long-term effects on health
- Sports governing body position regarding use
- Potential disciplinary actions against me for use
- Violation of code of ethics for respective sport
- Jeopardization of respect and regard others may have for me
- Effects on career/eligibility if caught and exposed
- Long, complicated recovery if addiction occurs
- Embarrassment and humiliation factors
- Criminal record potential
- Fear of being caught
- New drug testing procedures detecting previously undetectable substances
- Effects of utilization on conscience

---

7. What are the consequences of being caught and exposed if I use a banned ergogenic aid?
8. Is using the ergogenic aid a violation of the code of ethics governing this sport?
9. How will the detection and consequences imposed affect my status as a role model to others?
10. How will my eligibility or career be affected if I am caught using illegal substances?

Although these are not all the questions an athlete should ask, they represent the major concerns regarding the use, adverse side effects, and long-term effects of ergogenic aids, as well as some important matters of ethics and morals. Legal concerns must also be considered. A list of ethical concerns that athletes should have regarding the use of ergogenic aids may be found in Table 15–8.

Athletes who abuse ergogenic aids and drugs will look for flaws in policy and due process in an attempt to escape punitive measures and discipline. Increasing numbers of substance abuse cases involving athletes are litigated in the courts every year and involve various circumstances, such as invasion of privacy, drug testing, informed consent, and rehabilitation and recovery.

SUMMARY

Various approaches to the use of ergogenic aids designed and perceived to enhance athletic performance have been presented here. Athletes at many levels of competition use or abuse ergogenic aids on a daily basis through pharmacologic, nutritional, sports training and physiologic, psychologic, and miscellaneous approaches that are supposed to provide the "competitive edge." Sports medicine practitioners, regardless of discipline, should be thoroughly knowledgeable about the different approaches and their components in order to educate athletes and associates about the pros and cons of their use.

REFERENCES

1. deVries H: Physiology of Exercise for Physical Education and Athletics, 3rd ed. Dubuque, William C. Brown Publishers, 1980, p 534.
2. Fox E, Bowers R, Foss M: The Physiological Basis for Exercise and Sport, 5th ed. Dubuque, Brown and Benchmark, 1993, p 614.
3. Arnheim D: Modern Principles of Athletic Training, 6th ed. St. Louis, Times Mirror/Mosby College Publishing, 1985, p 172.
4. Puffer J: Use of drugs in swimming. Clin Sports Med 1986; 5(1):77.
5. Dyment PJ: Drugs and the adolescent athlete. Pediatr Ann 1981; 13:602.
6. Houpt HA, Rovere GD: Anabolic steroids: a review of the literature. Am J Sports Med 1984; 12:469.
7. Perlmutter G, Lowenthal DT: Use of anabolic steroids by athletes. Am Fam Physician 1985; 32:208.
8. Wade NA: Anabolic steroids: doctors denounce them but athletes aren't listening. Science 1972; 176:1399.
9. McArdle WD, Katch FI, Katch VL: Exercise Physiology: Energy, Nutrition, and Human Performance, 3rd ed. Philadelphia, Lea & Febiger, 1991, p 520.
10. Hossler P, Kleinschmidt D, McCormick M, et al: Ergogenic aids: the athletic trainer's perspective. Sports Sci Exch Roundtable 1991; Fall:2.
11. Wadler GI, Hainline B: Drugs and the Athlete, 1st ed. Philadelphia, FA Davis, 1989, p 14.
12. Gregg D: Anabolic steroids: the debate builds up. Clin Update Sports Med 1984; 1:3.
13. Prentice B: Pharmacologic considerations for sports medicine. In Malone T (ed): Physical and Occupational Therapy: Drug Implications for Practice, 1st ed. Philadelphia, JB Lippincott, 1989, p 279.
14. Rogozkin V: Metabolic effects of anabolic steroids on skeletal muscle. Med Sci Sports Exerc 1979; 11:160.
15. Sweeney GD: Drugs: some basic concepts. Med Sci Sports Exerc 1981; 13:250.
16. Wilson JD: Androgen abuse by athletes. Endocr Rev 1988; 9:188.
17. Lamb D: Abuse of anabolic steroids in sport. Sports Sci Exch 1989; 2:3.
18. Millar AL: Ergogenic aids. In Saunders B (ed): Sports Physical Therapy, 1st ed. Norwalk, Appleton & Lange, 1990, p 79.
19. Noble BJ: Physiology of Exercise and Sport, 1st ed. St. Louis, Times Mirror/Mosby College Publishing, 1986, p 500.
20. Cowart V: Some predict increased steroid use in sports despite drug testing and crackdown on suppliers. JAMA 1987; 257:3025.
21. Buckley WE: Estimated prevalence of anabolic-androgenic steroid use among male high school seniors. JAMA 1980; 260:241.
22. Windsor R, Dumitriv D: Prevalence of anabolic steroid use by male and female adolescents. Med Sci Sports Exerc 1989; 21:494.
23. Strauss RH: Drug abuse in sports: a three-pronged response. Phys Sports Med 1988; 16:47.
24. Johnson FL: The association of oral androgenic steroids and life-threatening disease. Med Sci Sports 1975; 7:284.
25. Stamford B, Moffat R: Anabolic steroid: effectiveness as an ergogenic aid to experienced weight trainers. J Sports Med Phys Fitness 1974; 14:191.
26. Ward P: The effect of anabolic steroids on strength and lean body mass. Med Sci Sports 1973; 5:207.
27. Johnson L, Fisher G, Sylvester L, et al: Anabolic steroid: effects on strength, body weight, oxygen uptake, and spermatogenesis upon mature males. Med Sci Sports 1972; 4:54.
28. Bowers RW, Reardon JP: Effects of Dianabol on strength development and aerobic capacity. Med Sci Sports 1972; 4:54.
29. Golding LJ, Freydinger J, Fishel S: Weight, size, and strength—unchanged with steroids. Phys Sports Med 1974; 2:39.
30. Fahey TD, Brown CH: The effects of anabolic steroids on strength, body composition, and endurance of college males when accompanied by a weight training program. Med Sci Sports 1973; 5:272.
31. Duda M: Female athletes: targets for drug abuse. Phys Sports Med 1988; 16:16–17.
32. Strauss RH, Liggett MT, Lanese RR: Anabolic steroid use and perceived effects in ten weight trained women athletes. JAMA 1985; 253:2871.
33. Clement DB: Drug use survey: results and conclusions. Phys Sports Med 1983; 11:65.
34. Strauss RH, Wright J, Finerman GA, et al: Side effects of anabolic steroids in weight trained men. Phys Sports Med 1983; 11:87.
35. Friedl KE, Yesalis CS: Self treatment of gynecomastia in body builders who use anabolic steroids. Phys Sports Med 1989; 17:67.
36. Alén M: Response of serum hormones to androgen administration in power athletes. Med Sci Sports Exerc 1985; 17:354.
37. Pope HG, Katz DL: Body builders' psychosis. Lancet 1987; 145:865.
38. Pope HG, Katz DL: Affective and psychotic symptoms associated with anabolic steroid use. Am J Psychiatry 1988; 145:487.
39. Annito WJ, Layman WA: Anabolic steroids and acute schizophrenia episode. J Clin Psychiatry 1980; 41:143.
40. MacDougall D: Anabolic steroids. Phys Sports Med 1983; 11:95.
41. Taylor WN: Synthetic anabolic-androgenic steroids: a plea for controlled substance status. Phys Sports Med 1987; 15:140.
42. Creagh TM, Rubin A, Evans EG: Hepatic tumors induced by anabolic steroids in the athlete. J Clin Pathol 1988; 41:441.
43. Pratt J: Wilms' tumor in an adult associated with androgen abuse. JAMA 1977; 237:2322.
44. Calabrese LH: The effects of anabolic steroids and strength training on the human immune response. Med Sci Sports Exerc 1985; 21:386.
45. Sklarek HM: AIDS in a body builder using anabolic steroids. N Engl J Med 1984; 311:1701.
46. Roberts JT, Essenhigh DM: Adenocarcinoma of the prostate in a 40-year-old body builder. Lancet 1984; 142:742.
47. Hurley BF, Seals OR, Hagberg JM: High-density lipoprotein cholesterol in body builders vs. power lifters. JAMA 1984; 252:507.
48. Kantor MA, Bianchiani A, Bernier D: Androgens reduce HDL-2 cholesterol and increase hepatic triglyceride lipase activity. Med Sci Sports Exerc 1985; 17:462.
49. Cohen JC, Faber WM, Spinnler AJ, et al: Altered serum lipoprotein profiles in male and female power lifters ingesting anabolic steroids. Phys Sports Med 1986; 14:131.
50. Costill DL, Pearson DR, Fink WJ: Anabolic steroid use among athletes: changes in HDL-C levels. Phys Sports Med 1984; 12:113.
51. Peterson GE, Fahey TD: HDL-C in five elite athletes using anabolic-androgenic steroids. Phys Sports Med 1984; 12:120.
52. Webb OL: Severe depression of high density lipoprotein cholesterol levels in weight lifters and body builders by self administered exogenous testosterone and anabolic-androgenic steroids. Metabolism 1984; 33:11.
53. Pearson AC, Schiff M, Mirasek D, et al: Left ventricular diastolic function in weight lifters. Am J Cardiol 1975; 58:1254.
54. Salke RC, Rowland TW, Burke EJ: Left ventricular size and function in body builders using anabolic steroids. Med Sci Sports Exerc 1985; 17:701.
55. McNutt RA, Ferenchick GS, Kirlin PC, et al: Acute myocardial infarction in a 22 year old world class weight lifter using anabolic steroids. Am J Cardiol 1988; 62:164.
56. Mochizuki RM, Richter KJ: Cardiomyopathy and cerebrovascular accident associated with anabolic-androgenic steroid abuse. Phys Sports Med 1988; 16:109–114.
57. American College of Sports Medicine: Position statement on use and abuse of anabolic-androgenic steroids in sports. Med Sci Sports 1977; 9:xi–xii.
58. National Strength and Conditioning Association: Position Paper on Anabolic Drug Use by Athletes. Lincoln, NE, 1985.
59. Burkett LN, Falduto MT: Steroid use by athletes in a metropolitan area. Phys Sports Med 1984; 12:69.
60. Bell AJ, Doege CT: Athletes' use and abuse of drugs. Phys Sports Med 1984; 15:99.
61. Mandell AJ, Stewart KD, Russo PV: The Sunday syndrome: from kinetics to altered consciousness. Fed Proc 1981; 31:2693.
62. Chandler JV, Blair SN: The effect of amphetamines on selected physiological components related to athletic success. Med Sci Sports Exerc 1980; 12:65.
63. Williams MH, Thompson J: Effect of variant dosages of amphetamine upon endurance. Res Q Exerc Sport 1973; 44:417.
64. Cooter GR: Amphetamines and sports performance. J Phys Ed Rec 1980; 51:63.

65. Strauss RH: Drugs in sports. *In* Strauss RH (ed): Sports Medicine, 1st ed. Philadelphia, WB Saunders, 1984, p 481.

66. Beckett AH: The doping problem. *In* Dirix A, Knuttgen HG, Tittel K (eds): The Olympic Book of Sports Medicine, 1st ed., vol 1. Oxford, Blackwell Scientific Publications, 1988, p 660.

67. Schuster C, Fischman M: Amphetamine toxicity: behavioral and neuropathological indexes. Fed Proc 1984; 34:1850.

68. Baruzzi A: Phenobarbital and propranolol in essential tremor: a double blind controlled clinical trial. Neurology 1983; 33:296.

69. Findley LJ, Koller WC: Essential tremor: a review. Neurology 1987; 37:1194.

70. Smith GM, Beecher HK: Amphetamine sulfate and athletic performance: objective effects. JAMA 1959; 197:542.

71. Truijens C, Trumbo D, Wagenaar W: Amphetamine and barbiturate effects on two tasks performed singly and in combination. Acta Psychol 1976; 40:233.

72. Brantigan CO, Brantigan CO, Joseph N: Effect of beta-blockade and beta-stimulation on stage fright. Am J Med 1982; 72:88.

73. Videmon T, Sonc KT, Janne J: The effects of beta-blockade in ski jumpers. Med Sci Sports Exerc 1979; 11:266.

74. vanBaak MA, Bohm RO, Arends BG, et al: Long term antihypertensive therapy with beta blockers: submaximal exercise capacity and metabolic effects during exercise. Int J Sports Med 1987; 8:342.

75. Ades PA, Gunther PG, Meacham C, et al: Hypertension, exercise, and beta-adrenergic blockade. Ann Intern Med 1988; 109:629.

76. Chick TW, Halperin AK, Gaeck EM: The effect of antihypertensive medications on exercise performance: a review. Med Sci Sports Exerc 1988; 20:447.

77. Kalis JK, Freund BJ, Joyner MJ, et al: Effect of beta-blockade on the drift in oxygen consumption during prolonged exercise. J Appl Physiol 1988; 64:753.

78. Joyner MJ, Freund BJ, Jilka SM, et al: Effects of beta-blockade on exercise capacity of trained and untrained men: a hemodynamic comparison. J Appl Physiol 1986; 60:1429.

79. Wilmore JH, Joyner MJ, Freund BJ, et al: Beta-blockade and response to exercise: influence of training. Phys Sports Med 1985; 13:63.

80. Eichner ER: Ergolytic drugs. Sports Sci Exch 1989; 2:3.

81. Armstrong LE, Costill DL, Fink WJ: Influence of diuretic-induced dehydration on competitive running performance. Med Sci Sports Exerc 1985; 17:456.

82. Rosen LW, Hough DO: Pathogenic weight-control behaviors of college gymnasts. Phys Sports Med 1988; 16:140.

83. Horstman DH, Horvath SM: Cardiovascular adjustments to progressive dehydration. J Appl Physiol 1973; 35:501.

84. Ribisl PM, Hervert WG: Effects of rapid weight reduction and subsequent rehydration upon the physical work capacity of wrestlers. Res Q Exerc Sport 1970; 41:536.

85. Cauldwell JE, Ahonen E, Nousiainen U: Differential effects of sauna, diuretic, and exercise induced hypohydration. J Appl Physiol 1984; 57:1018.

86. Spilliotis EB, August GD, Hung W, et al: Growth hormone neurosecretory dysfunction. JAMA 1984; 252:2223.

87. Millar AL: Ergogenic aids in athletes. *In* Saunders B (ed): Sports Physical Therapy, 1st ed. Norwalk, Appleton & Lange, 1990, p 82.

88. Murray TH: Human growth hormone in sports?—No. Phys Sports Med 1986; 14:29.

89. Crist DM, Peake GT, Egan PA, et al: Body composition response to exogenous growth hormone during training in highly conditioned athletes. J Appl Physiol 1988; 54:366.

90. Cowart VS: Human growth hormone: the latest ergogenic aid? Phys Sports Med 1988; 16:175.

91. Underwood LE: Report of the conference on uses and possible abuses of biosynthetic human growth hormone. N Engl J Med 1984; 311:606.

92. Sargent RG, Hohn E: Protein needs for the athlete. Natl Strength Cond Assoc J 1988; 10:54.

93. Wadler GI, Hainline B: Drugs and the Athlete, 2nd ed. Philadelphia, FA Davis, 1989, p 166.

94. Booth FW, Watson PA: Control of adaptations in protein levels in response to exercise. Fed Proc 1985; 44:2293.

95. Laurent GJ, Miliward DJ: Protein turnover during skeletal muscle hypertrophy. Fed Proc 1980; 39:42.

96. Kasparek GJ, Dohm GL, Barakat HA, et al: The role of lysosomes in exercise-induced hepatic protein loss. Biochem J 1982; 202:218.

97. Kasparek GJ, Snider RD: Increased protein degradation after eccentric exercise. Eur J Appl Physiol 1985; 54:30.

98. Haralambie G, Berg A: Serum urea and amino nitrogen changes with exercise duration. Eur J Appl Physiol 1976; 36:39.

99. Lemon PW, Nagle FJ, Mullin JP: Effects of initial muscle glycogen on protein catabolism during exercise. J Appl Physiol 1980; 48:624.

100. Slavin JL, Lanners G, Engstrom M: Amino acid supplements: beneficial or risky? Phys Sports Med 1988; 16:221.

101. Layman DK: How much protein does an athlete need? Phys Sports Med 1987; 15:181.

102. Coyle EF: Carbohydrates and athletic performance. Sports Sci Exch 1988; 1:1.

103. Burke LM, Read RS: Diet patterns of elite Australian male triathletes. Phys Sports Med 1987; 15:140.

104. Peters AJ, Dressendorfer RH, Dimar J, et al. Diets of endurance runners competing in a 20-day road race. Phys Sports Med 1986; 15:63.

105. Welch PK, Zager KA, Endres J: Nutrition education, body composition, and dietary intake of female college athletes. Phys Sports Med 1987; 15:73.

106. Costill DL: Carbohydrates for exercise: dietary demands for optimum performance. Int J Sports Med 1988; 9:1–18.

107. Applegate L: Fad diets and supplement use in athletics. Sports Sci Exch 1988; 7:1.

108. Jetté M: The nutritional and metabolic effects of a carbohydrate-rich diet in a glycogen supercompensation regimen. Am J Clin Nutr 1978; 31:2140.

109. Sherman WM, Costill DL, Fink WJ, et al: Effect of exercise and diet manipulation on muscle glycogen and its subsequent utilization during performance. Int J Sports Med 1991; 2:114.

110. Coyle EF, Coggan AR, Hemmart MK, et al: Substrate usage during prolonged exercise following a pre-exercise meal. J Appl Physiol 1985; 59:429.

111. Bonen J, Malcolm RD, Kilgour KP: Glucose ingestion before and during intense exercise. J Appl Physiol 1981; 55:776.

112. Coggan AR, Coyle EF: Reversal of fatigue during prolonged exercise by carbohydrate infusion or ingestion. J Appl Physiol 1987; 63:5.

113. Coyle EF, Coggan AR, Hemmert AK: Muscle glycogen utilization during prolonged strenuous exercise when fed carbohydrate. J Appl Physiol 1986; 61:165.

114. Coyle EF, Hagberg JM, Hurley BF, et al: Carbohydrate feeding during prolonged strenuous exercise can delay fatigue. J Appl Physiol 1983; 55:230.

115. Hargreaves M, Costill DL, Coggan AR, et al: Effects of carbohydrate feeding on muscle glycogen utilization and exercise performance. Med Sci Sports Exerc 1984; 16:219.

116. Costill DL, Sherman WM, Fink WJ, et al: The role of dietary carbohydrates in muscle glycogen resynthesis after strenuous running. Am J Clin Nutr 1981; 34:1831.

117. Reed MJ: Muscle glycogen storage post-exercise: effect of mode or carbohydrate administration. J Appl Physiol 1989; 66:720.

118. Aronson V: Vitamins and minerals as ergogenic aids. Phys Sports Med 1986; 14:209.

119. Weight LM, Myburgh KH, Noakes TD: Vitamin and mineral supplementation: effect on the running performance of trained athletes. Am J Clin Nutr 1988; 47:192.

120. Herker MA: Salt replacement by natural methods. Ath Train 1985; 20:25.

121. Costill DL: Dietary potassium and heavy exercise: effects on muscle water and electrolytes. Am J Clin Nutr 1982; 36:266.

122. Lloyd T, Triantafyllow SJ, Baker ER, et al: Women athletes with menstrual irregularity have increased musculoskeletal injuries. Med Sci Sports Exerc 1986; 18:374.

123. Drinkwater BL, Nilson K, Chestnut CH, et al: Bone mineral content of amenorrheic and eumenorrheic athletes. N Engl J Med 1984; 311:277.

124. Lee CJ: Effects of supplementation of the diets with calcium and calcium-rich foods on bone density of elderly females with osteoporosis. Am J Clin Nutr 1981; 34:819.

125. Lulaski HC: Physical training and copper, iron, and zinc status of swimmers. Am J Clin Nutr 1990; 51:1093.

126. Nickerson JH, Tripp HJ: Iron deficiency in adolescent cross-country runners. Phys Sports Med 1983; 11:60.

127. Clement DB, Asmundson RC: Nutritional intake and hematological parameters in endurance runners. Phys Sports Med 1982; 10:37.

128. Pate R: Dietary iron supplementation in women athletes. Phys Sports Med 1979; 7:16.

129. Pate R: Sports anemia: a review of the literature. Phys Sports Med 1983; 11:15.

130. Van Swearingen JV: Iron deficiency in athletes: consequence or adaptation in strenuous activity. J Orthop Sports Phys Ther 1986; 7:192.

131. Owens M: Nutritional concerns. In Sanders B (ed): Sports Physical Therapy, 1st ed. Norwalk, Appleton & Lange, 1990, p 126.

132. Davis JM, Lamb DR, Burgess WA, et al: Carbohydrate-electrolyte drinks: effects on endurance-cycling in the heat. Am J Clin Nutr 1988; 48:1023.

133. Murray R: Fluid replacement, gastrointestinal function, and exercise. Ath Train 1988; 23:215.

134. Seiple RS, Vivian VM, Fox EL: Gastric-emptying characteristics of two glucose-polymer electrolyte solutions. Med Sci Sports Exerc 1983; 15:366.

135. Coleman E: Sports drink update. Sports Sci Exch 1988; 1:1.

136. Pace N: The increase in hypoxia tolerance of normal men accompanying polycythemia induced by transfusion of erythrocytes. Am J Physiol 1947; 148:152.

137. Gledhill N: The ergogenic effect of blood doping. Phys Sports Med 1983; 11:97.

138. Gledhill N: Blood doping and related issues: a brief review. Med Sci Sports Exerc 1982; 14:193.

139. American College of Sports Medicine: Blood doping as an ergogenic aid: ACSM position stand. Med Sci Sports Exerc 1987; 19:540–543.

140. Ekblom B, Goldberg AN, Gullbring B: Response to exercise after blood loss and reinfusion. J Appl Physiol 1972; 33:175.

141. Ekblom B, Wilson G, Astrand PO: Central circulation during exercise after venesection and reinfusion of red blood cells. J Appl Physiol 1976; 40:379.

142. Frye A, Ruhling R: Red blood cell infusion, exercise, hemoconcentration and VO_2. Med Sci Sports 1977; 9:69.

143. Robertson RR, Gilcher R, Metz K: Effect of red blood cell reinfusion on endurance exercise performance in female distance runners. Med Sci Sports 1978; 10:48.

144. Pate R, McFarland J, Van Wyk J: Effect of blood reinfusion on endurance exercise performance in female distance runners. Med Sci Sports 1978; 11:97.

145. Williams MH, Lindhiem M, Schuster R: The effect of blood-infusion upon endurance capacity and ratings of perceived exertion. Med Sci Sports 1978; 10:113–118.

146. Videman T: Effect of blood removal and autoinfusion on heart rate response to a submaximal workload. J Sports Med 1977; 17:387.

147. Buick FJ: Effect of induced erythrocythemia on aerobic work capacity. J Appl Physiol 1980; 48:636.

148. Williams MH: The effect of induced erythrocythemia upon 5-mile treadmill run time. Med Sci Sports Exerc 1981; 13:169.

149. Spriet LL: Effect of graded erythrocythemia on cardiovascular and metabolic responses to exercise. J Appl Physiol 1986; 61:1942.

150. Sawka MN: Erythrocyte reinfusion and maximum aerobic power: an examination of modifying factors. JAMA 1987; 257:1496.

151. Gledhill N: Blood doping and performance. In Torg JS, Shephard RJ, Welsh RP (eds): Current Therapy in Sports Medicine—2, 1st ed., vol 2. Toronto, BC Decker, 1990, p 59.

152. Brien AJ, Simon TL: The effects of red blood cell infusion on 10-km race time. JAMA 1987; 257:2761.

153. Wilmore JH: Blood doping. Sports Med Digest 1987; 9:6.

154. Eichner ER: Blood doping: implications of recent research. Sports Med Digest 1987; 9:4.

155. Dirix A: Doping and doping control: classes and methods. In Dirix A, Knuttgen HG, Tittel K (eds): The Olympic Book of Sports Medicine, 1st ed., vol 1. London, Blackwell Scientific Publications, 1988, p 674.

156. Karpovich P: The effect of oxygen inhalation on swimming performance. Res Q Exerc Sport 1959; 5:24.

157. Elbel E, Ormond D, Close D: Some effects of breathing oxygen before and after exercise. J Appl Physiol 1961; 16:48.

158. Wilson GD, Welch HG: Effects of hyperoxic gas mixtures on exercise tolerance in men. Med Sci Sports 1975; 7:48.

159. Allen PD, Pandolf KB: Perceived exertion associated with breathing hyperoxic mixtures during submaximal work. Med Sci Sports 1977; 9:122.

160. Bjorgum RK, Sharkey BJ: Inhalation of oxygen as an aid to recovery after exertion. Res Q Exerc Sport 1966; 37:462.

161. Hagerman FC, Bowers RW, Fox EL: The effects of breathing 100 percent oxygen during rest, heavy work, and recovery. Res Q Exerc Sport 1968; 39:965.

162. Jacobson E: Progressive Relaxation. Chicago, University of Chicago Press, 1929.

163. Schultz JH, Luthe W: Autogenic Training: A Psychological Approach in Psychotherapy. New York, Grune & Stratton, 1959.

164. Wallace RK, Benon H, Wilson AF: The physiology of meditation. Sci Am 1972; 226:85–90.

165. Dewitt DJ: Cognitive and biofeedback training for stress reduction with university athletes. J Sport Psych 1980; 2:288–294.

166. Daniels FS, Landers DM: Biofeedback and shooting performance: a test of disregulation and systems theory. J Sport Psych 1981; 3:271–282.

167. Vealey RS: Imagery training for performance enhancement. In Williams J (ed): Applied Sport Psychology: Personal Growth to Peak Performance, 1st ed. Palo Alto, Mayfield, 1986, pp 209–224.

168. Mahoney MJ, Avener M: Psychology of the elite athlete: an exploratory study. Cognitive Ther Res 1977; 1:135–141.

169. Green FB: The use of imagery in the rehabilitation of injured athletes. In Pargman D (ed): Psychological Bases of Sport Injuries, 1st ed. Morgantown, WV, Fitness Information Technology, 1993, p 204.

170. Hale BD: The effects of internal and external imagery on muscular and ocular concomitants. J Sport Psych 1982; 4:379–387.

171. Ryan ED, Simons J: Cognitive demand, imagery, and frequency of mental rehearsal as factors influencing acquisition of motor skills. J Sport Psych 1981; 3:35–45.

172. Epstein MF: The relationship of imagery and mental rehearsal to performance of a motor task. J Sport Psych 1980; 2:211–220.

173. Rotella RJ, Gansneeder B, Ojala D: Cognitive and coping strategies of elite skiers: an exploratory study of young developing athletes. J Sport Psych 1980; 2:350–354.

174. Gould D: Goal setting for peak performance. In Williams JM (ed): Applied Sport Psychology: Personal Growth to Peak Performance, 1st ed. Palo Alto, Mayfield, 1986, pp 133–148.

175. Ievleva L, Orlick T: Mental paths to enhanced recovery from a sports injury. In Pargman D (ed): Psychological Bases of Sport Injuries, 1st ed. Morgantown, WV, Fitness Information Technology, 1993, pp 218–245.

176. Ievleva L: Psychological factors in knee and ankle injury recovery: an exploratory study. Master's thesis, University of Ottawa, 1988.

177. Unestahl LE: Self-hypnosis. In Williams JE (ed): Applied Sport Psychology: Personal Growth to Peak Performance, 1st ed. Palo Alto, Mayfield, 1986, pp 285–300.

178. Cox RH: Sport Psychology, 1st ed. Dubuque, William C. Brown, 1985, p 130.

179. Johnson WR: Hypnosis and muscular performance. J Sport Med Phys Fitness 1961; 1:71–79.

180. Wells J: Alcohol: the number one drug of abuse in the United States. Ath Train 1982; 17:172.

181. Williams MH: Alcohol and sports performance. Sports Sci Exch 1992; 4:1.

182. Kuller WC, Biary N: Effect of alcohol on tremors: comparison with propranolol. Neurology 1984; 34:221.

183. Collins W, Schroeder D, Gibson R: Effects of alcohol ingestion on tracking performance during angular acceleration. J Appl Physiol 1971; 55:559.

184. Belgrave BE: The effect of cannabidiol, alone, and in conjunction with ethanol on human performance. Psychopharmacology 1979; 64:243.

185. Gustafson R: Alcohol and vigilance performance: effect of small doses of alcohol on simple visual reaction time. Percept Mot Skills 1986; 62:683.

186. Rogers CC: Cyclists try caffeine suppositories. Phys Sports Med 1985; 13:38.
187. Costill DL, Dalsky GP, Fink WJ: Effects of caffeine ingestion on metabolism and exercise performance. Med Sci Sports 1978; 10:155.
188. Ivy JL, Costill DL, Fink WJ, et al: Influence of caffeine and carbohydrate feedings on exercise performance. Med Sci Sports Exerc 1979; 11:6.
189. LeBlanc J: Enhanced metabolic response to caffeine in exercise-trained human subjects. J Appl Physiol 1985; 59:832.
190. Wilcox AR: Caffeine and endurance performance. Sports Sci Exch 1990; 3:2.
191. Essig D, Costill DL, Van Handel PJ: Effects of caffeine ingestion on utilization of muscle glycogen and lipid during leg ergometer cycling. Int J Sports Med 1980; 1:86.
192. Erickson MA, Schwartzkopf RJ, McKenzie RD: Effects of caffeine, fructose, and glucose ingestion on utilization of muscle glycogen utilization during exercise. Med Sci Sports Exerc 1987; 19:579.
193. Sasaki H, Takaoka I, Ishiko T: Effects of sucrose and caffeine ingestion on running performance and prolonged strenuous running. Int J Sports Med 1987; 8:261.
194. Casal DC, Leon AS: Failure of caffeine to affect substrate utilization during prolonged exercise. Med Sci Sports Exerc 1985; 17:174.
195. Powers SK, Dodd S, Woodyard J: Caffeine alters ventilatory and gas exchange kinetics during exercise. Med Sci Sports Exerc 1986; 18:101.
196. Sasaki H, Takaoka I, Ishiko T: Effects of sucrose and caffeine ingestion on running performance and biochemical responses to endurance running. Int J Sports Med 1987; 8:205.
197. Slavin JL, Joensen DJ: Caffeine and sports performance. Phys Sports Med 1985; 13:191.
198. Lopes JM: Effect of caffeine on skeletal muscle function before and after fatigue. J Appl Physiol 1983; 54:1303.
199. Clayman CB (ed): The American Medical Association: Home Medical Encyclopedia, vol 1. New York, Random House, 1989, p 223.
200. Cregler LI, Mark H: Medical complications of cocaine abuse. N Engl J Med 1986; 315:1495.
201. Bell AJ, Doege CT: Athletes' use and abuse of drugs. Phys Sports Med 1986; 15:99.
202. Duda M: Cocaine deaths may increase drug tests. Phys Sports Med 1986; 14:37.
203. Nakamura M: Acute effects of inhalation of cigarette smoke on airway resistance. J Appl Physiol 1985; 58:27.
204. Rode A, Shephard RJ: The influence of cigarette smoking upon oxygen cost of breathing in near-maximal exercise. Med Sci Sports 1971; 3:51.
205. Rotstein A, Sagiv M: Acute effect of cigarette smoking on physiologic response to graded exercise. Int J Sports Med 1986; 7:322.
206. Glover ED, Edmundson SW, Edwards EW: Implications of smokeless tobacco use among athletes. Phys Sports Med 1986; 14:94.
207. National Cancer Institute: Spitting into the Wind: Facts about Dip and Chew. Wilmington, Fox, 1993, p 1.
208. Boyd GM: Use of smokeless tobacco among children and adolescents in the United States. Prev Med 1987; 16:402.
209. Marty PJ, McDermott RJ, Williams T: Patterns of smokeless tobacco use in a population of high school students. Am J Public Health 1986; 76:190.
210. Schroeder KL, Soller HA, Chen MS, et al: Screening for smokeless tobacco lesions: recommendations for the dental practitioner. J Am Dent Assoc 1988; 116:37.
211. Biron S, Wells J: Marijuana and its effect on the athlete. Ath Train 1983; 18:297–298.
212. Steben RE, Wells JC, Harless IL: The effects of bee pollen tablets on the improvement of certain blood factors and performance of male collegiate swimmers. J Natl Ath Train Assoc 1976; 11:124.
213. Steben RE, Boudreaux P: The effects of pollen and protein extracts on selected blood factors and performance of athletes. J Sports Med 1978; 18:221.
214. Woodhouse ML, Williams M, Jackson C: The effects of varying doses of orally ingested bee pollen extract upon selected performance variables. Ath Train 1987; 22:26.
215. Williams M: Bicarbonate loading. Sports Sci Exch 1992; 4:1.
216. Parkhouse WS, McKenzie DC: Possible contribution of muscle buffers to enhanced anaerobic performance: a brief review. Med Sci Sports Exerc 1984; 16:328.
217. Wilkes K, Gledhill N, Smyth R: Effect of acute induced metabolic acidosis on 800-meter racing time. Med Sci Sports Exerc 1983; 15:277.
218. Costill DL: Is sodium bicarbonate an aid to sprint performance? Sports Med Digest 1988; 10:4.
219. Horswill CA, Costill DL, Fink WJ: Influence of sodium bicarbonate on sprint performance: relationship to dosage. Med Sci Sports Exerc 1985; 20:566.
220. Jones NL: Effect of pH on cardiorespiratory and metabolic response to exercise. J Appl Physiol 1977; 43:959.
221. Katz A: Maximal exercise tolerance after induced alkalosis. J Sports Med 1984; 5:107.
222. Smith NJ: Nutrition and the athlete. Orthop Clin North Am 1983; 14:220.
223. Shephard RJ, Campbell D, Pimm P: Do athletes need vitamin E? Phys Sports Med 1974; 2:57–60.
224. Sherman IM, Dawn MG, Sen RN: The effects of vitamin E on physiological function and athletic performance in adolescent swimmers. Br J Nutr 1971; 26:265–276.
225. Bjorkman O, Sahlin K, Hagenfeldt L, Wahren J: Influence of glucose and fructose ingestion on the capacity for long-term exercise in well-trained men. Clin Physiol 1984; 4:483–494.
226. Davis JM, Lamb DR, Burgess WA, Bartoli WP: Accumulation of deuterium oxide in body fluids after ingestion of D20-labeled beverages. J Appl Physiol 1987; 63:2060–2066.
227. Greenleaf JE: Environmental issues that influence intake of replacement beverages. In Marriott, B (ed): Fluid Replacement and Heat Stress. Washington, DC, National Academy of Sciences Press, 1991, p XV 1–25.
228. Gisolfi CV, Summer RW, Schedl HP, et al: Human intestinal water absorption: direct vs. indirect measurements. Am J Physiol 1990; 258:G216–G222.
229. Lamb DR, Brodowicz GR: Optimal use of fluids of varying formulation to minimize exercise-induced disturbances in homeostasis. Sports Med 1986; 3:247–274.
230. Murray R: The effects of consuming carbohydrate-electrolyte beverages on gastric emptying and fluid absorption during and following exercise. Sports Med 1987; 4:322–351.
231. Murray R, Eddy DE, Murray T, et al: The effect of fluid and carbohydrate feedings during intermittent cycling exercise. Med Sci Sports Exerc 1987; 19:597–604.
232. Sherman WM, Lamb DR: Nutrition and prolonged exercise. In Lamb DR, Murray R (eds): Perspectives in Exercise Science and Sports Medicine, vol 1, Prolonged Exercise. Indianapolis: Benchmark Press, 1988.

Applied

Sport

Biomechanics

in

Rehabilitation

CHAPTER 16

Biomechanics of Swimming

MARILYN M. PINK *PhD, PT*
FRANK W. JOBE *MD*

Swimming is a sport enjoyed by all ages. Approximately 100 million Americans consider themselves swimmers,[1] making swimming the most popular sport in the United States. Some of these people swim competitively, others swim for fitness, and others for recreation. Swimming can be done safely by people with musculoskeletal systems that cannot withstand the impact forces found in running, jogging, or jumping. Swimming is also highly regarded as an aerobic activity.

Most sports are performed as a closed chain; that is, the feet push into the ground. Strong ground reaction forces are found in pitching, running, golfing, batting (unpublished data, Centinela Hospital Medical Center [CHMC] Biomechanics Laboratory), and cycling.[2] In swimming, the arms are the powerhouse of propulsion. Thus, the shoulder is particularly vulnerable to injury.

Competitive swimmers may cover 10,000 to 14,000 meters a day (6 to 8 miles), 6 to 7 days a week. Some distance swimmers may swim up to 24,000 meters a day. This equates to 16,000 shoulder revolutions per week. Comparably, in competition, there are approximately 1000 shoulder revolutions per week for a professional tennis player or baseball pitcher, 300 revolutions per week for a college javelin thrower, and 200 per week for a professional touring golfer.[1] These examples demonstrate the strain on the shoulder caused by the high repetition rate, the extremes of range of motion (ROM), and the force required for propulsion. Microtrauma is inevitable and can lead to injury. Shoulder problems are reported in 66 percent of elite swimmers, 57 percent of professional pitchers, 44 percent of college volleyball players, 29 percent of college javelin throwers,[1] and 7 percent of professional golfers (unpublished data, CHMC Biomechanics Laboratory).

The purpose of this chapter is to describe the vulnerabilities and mechanics in the four competitive swimming strokes. Joint laxity in the swimmer is discussed first, followed by a description of swimmer's characteristics and associated injuries, a review of stroke mechanics and muscle activity in the shoulder during the four competitive swim strokes, and finally a discussion of injury prevention and rehabilitation exercise programs.

LAXITY

Competitive swimmers are frequently described as being hyperlax. Their body position when standing typically consists of a forward head, rounded shoulders, lordotic back, and hyperextension of the knee.[3] The laxity is assumed to enable swimmers to undergo the large degree of ROM required for the strokes. Indeed, vigorous stretching programs have been recommended for swimmers to attain or maintain ROM.[4] An underlying question is whether swimming causes the hyperlaxity, or whether individuals with hyperlaxity select swimming because they can excel. This is analogous to the age-old question of what came first, the chicken or the egg. Another question stemming from this concept is whether the laxity predisposes swimmers to injury. Obviously, as clinicians, the

317

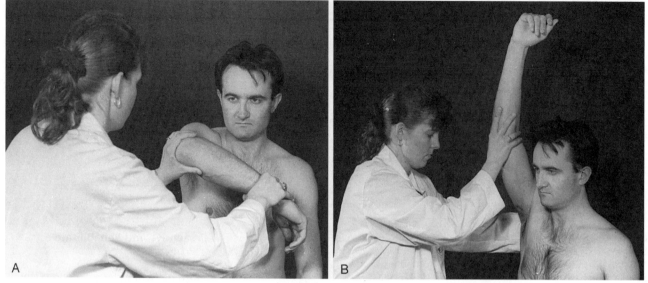

FIGURE 16–1. Clinical tests for classic impingement. *A*, Hawkins test. *B*, Neer test.

follow-up is for us to ask what can be done to minimize the risk of injury.

To answer this question, a study was designed that measured joint laxity and clinical signs of shoulder pathology in 154 competitive high school, collegiate, and master swimmers. An additional 21 nationally ranked swimmers (hereafter called elite swimmers) were measured. One hundred fifty matched controls (nonoverhead athletes) were also measured. Thus, the total sample was 325 subjects (unpublished data, CHMC Biomechanics Laboratory).

All four competitive swimming groups (high school, college, elite, and master) demonstrated significantly more knee recurvation than did the matched controls. The collegiate, elite, and master swimmers revealed more elbow recurvation, and the collegiate and master groups also exhibited more laxity in their digits. From these findings, one could generalize that competitive swimmers do have an inherent predisposition to joint laxity, and perhaps people with joint laxity elect to participate in the sport of swimming.

Very few swimmers (less than 5 percent) demonstrated anterior, inferior, or posterior instability of the shoulder during clinical examination. Likewise, less than 2 percent of the controls evidenced instability. One conclusion that can be drawn is that shoulder joint laxity does not necessarily mean instability (instability can be thought of as symptomatic laxity).

Looking at the issue of instability from a biomechanical point of view and considering the larger population of overhead athletes, one begins to see some logical distinctions between swimmers and throwers. Generally, the most common type of instability in throwing athletes is anterior instability. This finding makes sense, since the late cocking phase of throwing is similar to the position of the anterior instability test (abduction to 90 degrees and maximal external rotation). Hence, the repetitive stress to the anterior structures when throwing could lead to instability. New research has shown that the pain elicited during the relocation test (i.e., the

test for anterior instability) comes from a pinching of the undersurface of the rotator cuff on the posterosuperior glenoid labrum (personal communication, Christopher Jobe, MD). This pinching causes undersurface rotator cuff tears.

In swimming, however, the shoulder is not typically placed in the vulnerable position of abduction and external rotation, which leads to instability. Hence, the mechanical wear and tear of the rotator cuff tendons on the posterosuperior glenoid labrum is not present, and swimmers do not appear to be inordinately at risk for anterior instability.

Swimmers exhibited a higher incidence of positive Hawkins tests (Fig. 16–1A) than did the control group, but the elite swimmers were the only population that exhibited a significantly higher frequency of positive Neer tests (Fig. 16–1B). Thus, swimmers more frequently exhibit positive Hawkins tests than positive Neer tests.

Traditionally, both the Hawkins and the Neer tests were thought to be tests for impingement of the rotator cuff tendon under the anterior third of the acromion.[5,6] New cadaver research has demonstrated slightly different mechanics of injury, however (personal communication, Christopher Jobe, MD). With forced humeral flexion, the impingement is on the undersurface of the rotator cuff tendon on the anterosuperior glenoid rim. This is consistent with the surgical findings of undersurface rotator cuff fraying. The same research project performed cadaver cross-sections, with the humerus in the position of 90 degrees forward flexion and maximal internal rotation (the position of the Hawkins test). In this position, the rotator cuff is compressed beneath the anterior portion of the acromion.

Thus these two examination tools appear to be testing for two different types of shoulder problems—one being a pinching of the cuff undersurface on the anterosuperior glenoid rim (the Neer test), and one being a compression of the tendons under the acromion (Hawkins test). The implication of more swimmers with positive Hawkins tests than positive Neer tests is that swimmers tend to have compression of the tendons under the acromion rather than undersurface tears. Obviously, this is an area for future research.

As will be discussed later, one of the key findings in muscle firing of swimmers with painful shoulders is that the serratus anterior muscle shuts down.[7] If the serratus anterior does not function to upwardly rotate and protract the scapula, the acromion most certainly would also lack upward rotation and hence could mechanically compress the rotator cuff tendons. It has been found that exercise to strengthen the scapular and shoulder muscles frequently eliminates the need for surgery in swimmers. This finding not only reinforces the need for exercise programs but also implies that the progression of injury can be halted before anatomic damage occurs.

Interestingly, the hand entry position during the freestyle stroke is a frequent point of pain in swimmers with dysfunctional shoulders, and the position at hand entry is halfway between the positions of the Neer and the Hawkins tests. Obviously, more mechanical and anatomic research needs to be done on this issue, as this information is breaking new ground.

Thus, competitive swimmers with normal shoulders reveal a predisposition to laxity, but they do not demonstrate a significant increase in clinical signs of instability. There is a higher incidence of positive Hawkins tests than positive Neer tests in this population. These findings may relate to the mechanics of potential injury in competitive swimmers.

SWIMMER'S CHARACTERISTICS AND ASSOCIATED INJURIES

As mentioned earlier, 66 percent of elite swimmers have reported shoulder injuries at some time during their swimming careers.[1] The populations that most clinicians are involved with, however, are competitive collegiate or master-level swimmers. To explore the characteristics of swimmers and the injuries in competitive collegiate and master swimmers, a survey was conducted by Stocker et al.[8]

Five hundred thirty-two collegiate swimmers and 395 master swimmers returned the survey. Table 16–1 describes the two populations.

Interestingly, 47 percent of the collegiate and 48 percent of the master swimmers had a history of three or more weeks of shoulder pain that forced them to alter or decrease their training schedules. Of these swimmers, 55 percent of the college group and 39 percent of the master group sought medical attention. Only 10 percent of the college swimmers and 12 percent of the master swimmers were advised to have surgery. The majority of the swimmers returned to their prior levels of competitive swimming following treatment consisting of ice, rest, anti-inflammatory medication, and exercise. Half of the injured swimmers thought that their injuries were correlated with intensity or duration of workouts. Fifty-eight percent of the college students had a recurrence of the injury that was perceived to be due to

intensity and distance of training, whereas 68 percent of the master group reported a recurrence. Approximately 20 percent of the injured swimmers used hand paddles at the time of injury, yet statistical tests revealed that there was no statistical probability of association between hand paddle usage and shoulder pain.

One of the points of information from this survey by Stocker et al[8] is that the incidence of injury was the same for the two groups. Hence, age, years swimming, and age at which swimming began do not appear to relate to the incidence of injury. The injuries in the collegiate group may have been more severe (or their livelihood as competitive swimmers was deemed more important) than in the master group, in that 55 percent of the college-age swimmers sought medical attention, whereas only 39 percent of the master group did so. Fortunately, the majority of the swimmers were able to return to their sport with noninvasive intervention. Of those swimmers who had had an injury and continued to compete, only 10 to 12 percent had had surgery. (This sample of swimmers was taken from a group of current competitors, so these values may be skewed in that some of those who had surgery may have ceased to swim.)

Unfortunately, over half of the shoulder injuries recurred. Hence, the long-term intervention needs to be evaluated. Some clues as to the causes of injury recurrence may be in the intensity and duration of workouts.

STROKE MECHANICS

The rest of the chapter is based on a fine-wire electromyography (EMG) and high-speed film study done on 34 competitive swimmers while they were swimming each of the four swim strokes.[7,9–13]

TABLE 16–1
Population Description of Survey of Competitive Swimmers

	Collegiate Swimmers	Master Swimmers
Sample size	532	395
Average age (years)	19.5	41.5
Average age competitive swimming begun (years)	9.1	22.5
Continuous period of competitive swimming (years)	10.1	12.1
Number of workouts/week	8.6	4.0
Number of weeks/year trained	40.6	42.0
Percent of workout with 70% or more freestyle stroke	60	60
Percent of swimmers using hand paddles	46	28
Percent currently using hand paddles	71	73

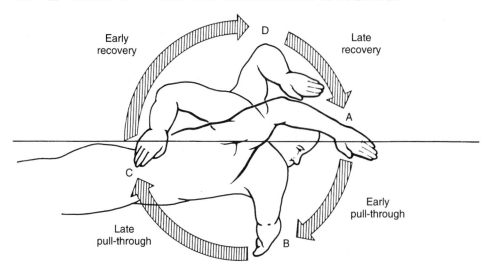

FIGURE 16–2. Phases of the freestyle swimming stroke. (From Pink M, Perry J, Browne A, et al: The normal shoulder during free-style swimming. Am J Sports Med 1991; 19:569–576.)

FREESTYLE STROKE

MECHANICS

The arm motion in the freestyle stroke is reciprocal, and the arm position marks the different phases of the freestyle stroke (Fig. 16–2). The portion of the phase in which the hand is underwater is called pull-through. The hand enters the water forward of, and lateral to, the head and medial to the shoulder. The elbow is flexed and positioned above the hand, so that the fingers are the first to enter the water. The hand then reaches forward under the water and the palm begins to rotate down. At the point of maximal elbow extension, the hand initiates an S-shaped pattern of pulling, which is called early pull-through (Fig. 16–3). During the most propulsive portion of the phase, the humerus power-fully adducts and the hand crosses under the chest. The point at which the humerus is perpendicular to the body is called mid pull-through. Subsequent to this point is late pull-through. The hand continues and then travels laterally and passes under the pelvis until it exits the water, leading with the little finger.

The amount of time spent in the recovery phase (the portion of the phase when the hand is above the water) is much shorter than the amount of time spent in the pull-through phase. The purpose of this phase is simply to bring the arm into position to pull once again. The humerus is internally rotated as it lifts out of the water. It then abducts and externally rotates to a small degree in order to swing the forearm forward. The arm is then brought into position for hand entry once again.

During the freestyle stroke, the lower extremities do a reciprocal diagonal sweep called the flutter kick. The flutter kick can be used for both propulsion and stabilization. Multiple studies have found that kicking causes a demonstrable increase in the energy cost of swimming.[15–18] Hence, distance swimmers may want to minimize the effort of kicking in order to reduce fatigue. The legs can then be used for the final sprint.

Swimmers encounter less resistance when their bodies are streamlined horizontally and laterally. This streamlining diminishes the drag on the swimmer. Good alignment can be obtained by rolling the body

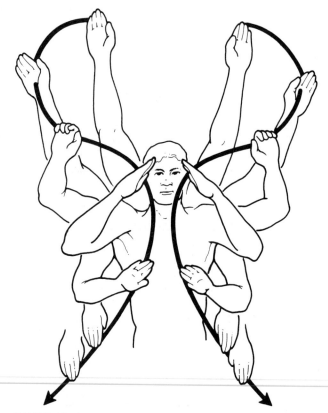

FIGURE 16–3. S-shaped pull of the freestyle swimming stroke. From Pink M, Perry J, Browne A, et al: The normal shoulder during freestyle swimming. Am J Sports Med1991; 19–569 576.)

from side to side to coincide with the movement of the arms. Swimmers roll to the left once the left arm reaches mid pull-through, and to the right when the right arm reaches mid pull-through.

There are several breathing patterns used during the freestyle stroke. The most common in recreational and fitness swimmers is to roll the head to the side of the dominant arm as the arm exits the water. Many competitive swimmers prefer to breath alternately on the right and left sides during every third hand exit.

The shoulder is the primary area of interest to clinicians working with freestyle swimmers because of its vulnerability to injury. Hence, the muscle firing patterns are discussed in freestyle swimmers with normal shoulders and likewise in swimmers with painful shoulders. In that the freestyle stroke is the most common stroke, it is described in detail. The other three strokes (butterfly, backstroke, and breaststroke) are summarily described.

MUSCLE ACTIVITY

THE NORMAL SHOULDERS. Swimmers with normal shoulders have a definable pattern of hand entry and hand exit (Fig. 16–4). During hand entry and forward reach, the upper trapezius elevates the scapula while the rhomboids retract it. The serratus anterior is active in order to protract and upwardly rotate the scapula (Fig. 16–5A). The force couple formed by these scapular muscles firmly tethers this broad, flat bone (scapula) at every corner. This muscle action positions the glenoid fossa for the humeral head as the arm is abducted and flexed by the supraspinatus and the anterior and middle deltoids when the hand reaches forward in the water. The force couple formed by the supraspinatus and the two heads of the deltoid is important, as the supraspinatus inserts closer to the axis of rotation than does the deltoid. Without the supraspinatus, the deltoids could lever the humeral head within the glenoid fossa.

The actual pulling of the body over the arm begins after the forward reach. The pectoralis major is responsible for the initial and powerful humeral adduction and extension. The pectoralis major also causes internal rotation of the humerus; thus the teres minor fires with the pectoralis major to provide an antagonistic external rotation force to balance the greater pectoral rotational forces (Fig. 16–5B). The teres minor inserts closer to the axis of rotation than does the pectoralis major, hence it keeps the head of the humerus congruent with the glenoid. The teres minor is a more likely component of the force couple than is the infraspinatus, in that the angle of the fibers in the teres minor contributes to humeral extension.

After the phasic peak of activity from the pectoralis major and teres minor, the humerus crosses the point of mid pull-through, and the latissimus dorsi has the mechanical advantage. Thus, the latissimus dorsi becomes the primary muscle of propulsion after mid pull-through. The subscapularis (another internal rotator) forms a force couple with the latissimus dorsi. The subscapularis, which inserts closer to the axis of rotation, keeps the humeral head approximated in the joint.

Throughout the propulsive motions of the pectoralis major and latissimus dorsi, the serratus anterior is also active as it pulls the body over the arm and through the water. The serratus anterior maintains the scapula in a position of upward rotation and also assists with joint congruency of the humerus and glenoid.

The posterior deltoid becomes active after the latissimus dorsi reaches its peak. The posterior deltoid is a "transition" muscle. By virtue of its extension component, it contributes to the final part of pulling while it begins to lift the humerus out of the water.

As the hand begins to exit the water, the group of muscles that were active at hand entry once again begins to function. The middle deltoid is active to abduct and continue lifting the arm. The supraspinatus forms a force couple once again with the deltoids. The anterior deltoid abducts and begins to flex the humerus. The scapular force couple forms again as the upper trapezius upwardly rotates the scapula, while the rhomboids retract the medial superior border and the serratus anterior assists with rotation and protraction.

The muscles that function at hand exit continue with their activity during recovery. In addition, the infraspinatus depresses and slightly rotates the humerus externally as the forearm swings around, and the subscapularis is active to control the degree of humeral rotation.

Throughout the freestyle stroke, the serratus anterior and subscapularis continually fire above 20 percent of their maximum. The serratus anterior is active to stabilize the scapula, which provides a stable base for

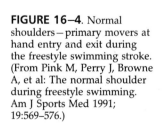

FIGURE 16–4. Normal shoulders—primary movers at hand entry and exit during the freestyle swimming stroke. (From Pink M, Perry J, Browne A, et al: The normal shoulder during freestyle swimming. Am J Sports Med 1991; 19:569–576.)

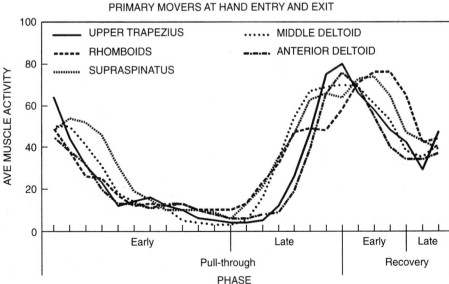

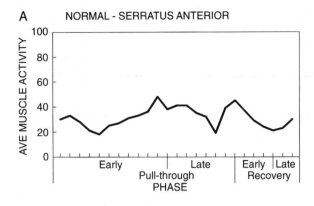

A   NORMAL - SERRATUS ANTERIOR

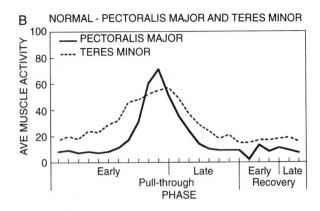

B   NORMAL - PECTORALIS MAJOR AND TERES MINOR

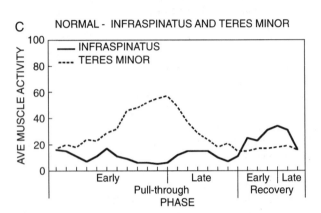

C   NORMAL - INFRASPINATUS AND TERES MINOR

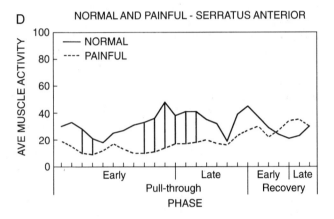

D   NORMAL AND PAINFUL - SERRATUS ANTERIOR

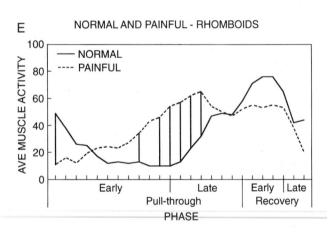

E   NORMAL AND PAINFUL - RHOMBOIDS

FIGURE 16–5. *A,* Normal shoulders—muscle activity in the serratus anterior during the freestyle stroke. *B,* Normal shoulders—muscle activity in the pectoralis major and teres minor during the freestyle swimming stroke. *C,* Normal shoulders—muscle activity in the infraspinatus and teres minor during the freestyle swimming stroke. (From Pink M, Perry J, Browne A; et al: The normal shoulder during freestyle swimming. Am J Sports Med 1991; 19: 569–576.) *D,* Normal and painful shoulders—muscle activity in the serratus anterior during the freestyle swimming stroke. *E,* Normal and painful shoulders—muscle activity in the rhomboids during the freestyle swimming stroke. (From Scovazzo ML, et al: In Post M, Morrey BF, Hawkins RJ (eds): Surgery of the shoulder. St. Louis, Mosby–Year Book, 1989.)

the humerus. If the scapula were allowed to "float" without this stability, impingement would likely occur. The subscapularis is continually active, as the humerus is predominantly in internal rotation throughout the stroke. Only for a brief period during mid-recovery is the humerus positioned to a slight degree of external rotation as the forearm swings forward. Monad[19] demonstrated that 15 to 20 percent of a muscle's maximal voluntary contraction is the highest level at which sustained activity can be performed without fatigue. Thus these two muscles, the serratus anterior and subscapularis appear to be susceptible to fatigue.

Another important clinical point is the different activity patterns of the teres minor and the infraspinatus (Fig. 16–5C). Because of their anatomic proximity and shared insertion on the humerus, one might be led to believe that they function similarly. However, this is not the case. The infraspinatus depresses and externally rotates the humerus during mid-recovery, whereas the teres minor is active during pull-through, when it forms a force couple with the greater pectoral.

PAINFUL SHOULDERS. Swimmers with painful shoulders exhibit several differences in muscle activity when compared with swimmers with normal shoulders. The most notable difference is a significant decrease in activity in the serratus anterior during mid pull-through, while the rhomboids significantly increase their activity (Fig. 16–5D and E). Quite likely, the serratus anterior fatigues in swimmers with painful shoulders, producing a "floating" scapula. In order to compensate, the rhomboids contract to stabilize the scapula. It is of interest that these two muscles function antagonistically. When the serratus anterior cannot perform, there is no muscle that can assist by doing a similar action. The only way the body can stabilize the scapula is to call upon antagonistic muscles, the rhomboids, which attempt to substitute for a deficient anterior serratus. Thus, the optimum synchrony of firing seen in normal scapular rotation is disturbed at the time of propulsion.

Another interesting trade-off is the decrease in activity of the subscapularis during mid-recovery and an overall general increase in activity of the infraspinatus muscle. Here again, opposing muscles (an internal and an external rotator) change the intensity of their activity — the subscapular decreases and the infraspinatus increases. Like the serratus anterior, the subscapularis is susceptible to fatigue because of its continual activity in swimmers with normal shoulders. Swimmers with painful shoulders may have fatigued their subscapularis. Also, the subscapularis may diminish its function in order to avoid the painful extremes of internal rotation, whereas the infraspinatus increases its activity to externally rotate the humerus for the same end goal.

During hand entry, there is also a decrease in activity in the anterior and middle deltoids and in the upper trapezius and rhomboids. At hand exit, there is a kindred diminution of activity in the two heads of the deltoid. This finding is in keeping with the dropped elbow that coaches sometimes see in swimmers. Coaches commonly respond by telling the swimmers to "keep their elbows up" or to "stop being lazy." Yet the truth is that this altered position may be a subtle sign of injury. The "lower" elbow means that the swimmer is entering the water with a wider hand entry to avoid the painful impingement. The normal position of hand entry in swimmers with normal shoulders is similar to a position between the Neer and Hawkins impingement tests. Thus, a wider hand entry avoids the impingement.

There is no significant difference in the muscle firing of the primary muscles of propulsion (the pectoralis major, latissimus dorsi, and posterior deltoid) when comparing swimmers with normal and painful shoulders. Nor is there a significant difference in the muscle firing of the teres minor in swimmers with normal and painful shoulders. Hence the pectoralis major and teres minor force couple is intact. The supraspinatus muscle also functions normally as it approximates the head of the humerus in the glenoid.

This work leads us to believe that the key muscle to focus on for injury prevention and rehabilitation in competitive freestyle swimmers is the serratus anterior. A stable scapula is paramount in preventing shoulder injuries, and the serratus anterior is the muscle that constantly fires in order to provide the necessary stability. There is no other muscle that can substitute for the serratus anterior and still provide the same synchronous pattern of muscle firing. The rhomboids contract when the serratus anterior fails, but the direction of pull is directly opposed to that of the serratus anterior. Thus, asynchronous firing commences.

The subscapularis is another muscle to focus on, as it inserts close to the humeral axis of rotation, precisely holding the head in the fossa. It forms the first layer of the muscular "anterior wall" for joint protection. The changes in muscle firing patterns in the anterior and middle deltoids, the upper trapezius, and the infraspinatus appear to be the result of a pain-avoidance pattern.

BUTTERFLY STROKE

MECHANICS

Today's butterfly stroke is similar to the freestyle stroke. It has been suggested that the same muscle groups and mechanics are used in the two strokes.[20] Indeed, many of today's premier butterfliers are also known for their aptitude in the freestyle. They train largely with the freestyle and have excellent carryover into the butterfly stroke. The phases of early and late pull-through and recovery are marked by the same positions of the hand and humerus in the two strokes. The S-shaped pattern of pulling is present in both strokes but is a bit wider and shorter in the butterfly. The most marked difference between the strokes is that the butterfly is a bilateral activity and the freestyle is a reciprocal, unilateral pattern. During the butterfly, the arms stroke simultaneously, and the legs kick simultaneously. This simultaneous movement means that there is no body roll during the butterfly stroke. Breathing occurs by lifting the head up and out of the water rather than rolling the head to the side. Also, the hand entry is wider in the butterfly, and the hands exit the water earlier.

The body motion in the butterfly stroke is an undulating motion. The principle of propulsion is much like that of an eel, with a transfer of motion from the lower extremities to the upper extremities.[21] The kick is called a dolphin kick, in that the legs move together, similar to the tail of a dolphin. The legs move up then down for two cycles during each complete arm cycle. When the arms begin the actual pulling, the legs kick upward. The body is kept as level as possible to reduce the drag. The first downkick is rather shallow yet sufficiently strong to be propulsive as it moves the hips up and forward through the surface. The force of the second kick should keep the hips at the surface without pushing them beyond the surface. To push them beyond the surface would interfere with arm recovery.[21]

MUSCLE ACTIVITY

NORMAL SHOULDERS. During the butterfly stroke, the patterns of muscle activity in swimmers with normal shoulders were quite similar to those of the freestyle stroke. The rhomboids, upper trapezius, serratus anterior, supraspinatus, and the anterior and middle deltoids all exhibit a peak of muscle activity during hand entry. However, the peak is just a little bit later than that in the freestyle stroke. This later peak is due to the fact that hand entry is wider in the butterfly stroke, and the humerus is not flexed as much initially. Thus the posterior deltoid is also active during the butterfly stroke because of the abduction component. The subscapularis is active at hand entry because the arm is in a relative degree of internal rotation. As the hands move outward in preparation for pulling, the infraspinatus and teres minor fire to externally rotate the humerus.

The pattern of muscle activity during the pull in the butterfly stroke is identical to that in the freestyle stroke. However, there are some notable differences in intensity of muscle activity. There is slightly more activity during the butterfly in the pectoralis major, teres minor, and rhomboids; a decrease in the latissimus dorsi and subscapularis, and relatively the same amplitude in the serratus anterior and posterior deltoid. As the activity increases in the pectoralis major during the butterfly stroke (relative to the freestyle stroke), it also increases in its companion muscle (i.e., the force couple), the teres minor. A similar relationship is demonstrated for the decrease in the latissimus dorsi and its companion muscle, the subscapularis. This increased activity can be accounted for by the shorter late pull-through phase in the butterfly stroke. Thus, more of the pull comes from the early half of the phase (pectoralis major and teres minor) than from late pull-through (latissimus dorsi and subscapularis). The increased activity in the rhomboids is due to the excessive scapular retraction in the butterfly. This excessive retraction is necessary to lift the arm out of the water in the absence of the lateral body roll, which is present in the freestyle stroke.

At hand exit, the upper trapezius has more activity in the butterfly stroke than in the freestyle stroke. This is probably due to the excessive scapular elevation needed to replace the lateral body roll of the freestyle and to clear the hand above the water. The deltoid and supraspinatus activity patterns were similar, yet the level of activity is much higher in the butterfly. As with the upper trapezius, this excessive activity is probably the means to lift the hand out of the water in the absence of lateral body roll. The activity of the serratus anterior is similar for both strokes in pattern as well as intensity. The subscapularis, however, has higher activity during the butterfly stroke. This higher activity again prompts the question whether the subscapularis will fatigue and thus show depressed activity in swimmers with painful shoulders during the butterfly stroke.

During the early recovery phase of the butterfly stroke, there is more activity in the posterior deltoid and infraspinatus and less activity in the supraspinatus and subscapularis. These differences are related to the wider arm position, which produces an outward rather than upward position of the elbow and an accompanying increase in external rotation. The outward position of the elbow may be attributed to an increase in posterior deltoid activity and a decrease in supraspinatus activity. The increase in external rotation may be attributed to increased infraspinatus activity, with decreased activity of the subscapularis.

There is slightly less muscle action in the upper trapezius, rhomboids, and anterior and middle deltoids during late recovery in the butterfly stroke as compared

with the freestyle stroke. This decreased activity is the result of the arm preparing for an entry that is more lateral and more abducted.

Interestingly, the serratus anterior and subscapularis both have the same constant level of relatively high activity as that expressed during the freestyle stroke. As explained earlier, this higher level of activity leaves these muscles vulnerable to fatigue. Thus, it is important that these two critical muscles, the subscapularis and serratus anterior be in the best possible condition in order to avoid fatigue and the resultant potentially damaging substitution patterns. The upper trapezius and teres minor also reveal relatively high and consistent levels of activity; thus, they also need to be considered.

The carryover of the force couples of the pectoralis major and teres minor, the latissimus dorsi and subscapularis, and the supraspinatus and anterior and middle deltoids also deserves clinical consideration. In each of these cases, a small rotator cuff muscle teams up with a large power or positioning muscle in order to keep the humerus congruent with the glenoid. By virtue of the rotator cuff insertions (which are closer to the axis of rotation than are the larger muscles), the rotator cuff prevents the head of the humerus from subluxating and therefore protects the joint from ensuing injury.

PAINFUL SHOULDERS. When comparing the results of normal and painful shoulders during the butterfly and freestyle strokes, marked similarities are seen. In both strokes, the latissimus dorsi and pectoralis major have the same patterns of enhanced activity, but with no significant differences between painful and normal shoulders. The infraspinatus, upper trapezius, and serratus anterior have not only similar patterns of activity but also similar patterns of significant differences.

The subscapularis demonstrates an overall trend for enhanced activity during the butterfly stroke in swimmers with painful shoulders during the early part of pulling. For only one brief moment does it demonstrate significantly greater activity. This action is in keeping with the pattern of enhanced activity of the latissimus dorsi, which is the companion muscle of the subscapularis.

In the freestyle stroke, the anterior and middle deltoids demonstrate significant differences when comparing normal shoulders with painful shoulders. The posterior deltoid is the portion that demonstrates differences during the butterfly stroke. This difference may be attributed to the more flexed humeral position during the freestyle stroke, specifically affecting the anterior and middle deltoids. The wider hand entry with greater humeral abduction and extension during the butterfly affects the posterior deltoid.

During the butterfly stroke, the supraspinatus has a brief moment of difference in normal and painful shoulders. However, since this difference is between 1 and 5 percent of its maximum potential output, no clinical inference can be made.

The teres minor and rhomboids interchange their patterns of significant differences between painful and

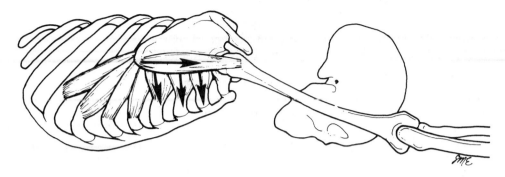

FIGURE 16–6. With a floating scapula during the butterfly stroke, there is no stable base, and the teres minor and serratus anterior cannot function adequately.

normal shoulders in the butterfly and freestyle strokes. In the butterfly, the teres minor exhibits a large duration of significantly less activity in the painful group during pull-through, in conjunction with the decrease of activity in the serratus anterior. With an unstable scapula, due to the decrease of activity in the serratus anterior, the teres minor is unable to control the humeral rotation caused by the pectoralis major during the powerful pull-through phase. Thus, the serratus anterior and teres minor, both of which attach to the scapula, lack the synergistic interplay to assist with propulsion and balance of humeral rotatory motion (Fig. 16–6). In the freestyle stroke, the rhomboids increase the muscle activity during pull-through to stabilize the scapula and compensate for the decreased activity in the serratus anterior. The rhomboids and teres minor in these two strokes both appear to be responding to the deficient serratus anterior: the rhomboids increase activity in the freestyle stroke to attempt to stabilize the scapula, and the teres minor decreases activity in the butterfly stroke because the scapula is not acting as a stable base.

During the butterfly stroke, four muscles demonstrate high electrical activity throughout all phases in normal shoulders: the subscapularis, serratus anterior, teres minor, and upper trapezius. Thus, these four muscles may be susceptible to fatigue and require specific endurance training.

Swimmers using the butterfly stroke do not put in the same yardage as those swimming freestyle without resting between sets. Therefore, the concern is not as great for fatigue in the butterfly stroke. Yet the fact that the involved muscles showed significant differences between normal and painful shoulders, and the fact that many butterfliers actually train largely with the freestyle stroke, cannot be overlooked. The factor of fatigue must be considered. With that in mind, exercises to prevent and rehabilitate injuries in swimmers who do the butterfly stroke must pay particular attention to this high level of muscle activity.

BACKSTROKE

MECHANICS

Today, the backstroke is similar to the freestyle stroke, except that it is performed supine. The arms stroke reciprocally and the legs do a reciprocal, diagonal flutter kick. The phases are the same for the two strokes: hand entry marks the beginning of pull-through, the humerus perpendicular to the body is mid pull-through and differentiates early from late pull-through, hand exit is the beginning of early recovery, and the humerus perpendicular to the water is the start of late recovery. The face is above the water throughout the backstroke, hence there is no specific body motion pattern to accommodate breathing. The body is held in horizontal alignment with the water, and there is only a slight bend at the waist. The body rolls in the direction of the arm that is entering the water in order to minimize the lateral motion of the legs and hips.

MUSCLE ACTIVITY

NORMAL SHOULDERS. In swimmers with normal shoulders, the three heads of the deltoid have a similar pattern (with differing intensities of activity) during hand entry and exit to place the arm in position. At hand entry, the posterior and middle deltoids are in the optimal position and therefore have higher intensities of activity. At hand exit, the anterior deltoid is positioned optimally and thus is more electrically active. In addition, the posterior deltoid contributes to the propulsive motion as it pulls the body over the arm in mid pull-through.

The rotator cuff muscles have separate and distinct patterns of activation. As with the previously described strokes, the supraspinatus functions in synchrony with the deltoids. Hence, its role in abduction is more apparent than its role in external rotation. The infraspinatus is minimally active throughout the stroke, which is in contrast to the constantly active teres minor. Thus, the unique pattern of each of these external rotators of the rotator cuff is again demonstrated in the backstroke.

The subscapularis has a pattern much like that of the teres minor. These two muscles appear to be forming a force couple to control the motion of the humeral head and to protect the joint from subluxation. The only difference between these two muscles is during late recovery, when the subscapularis has a small peak of activity and the teres minor does not. This difference is due to the shift in humeral rotation from neutral to internal rotation as hand entry is made with the little finger leading. Both the subscapularis and teres minor are constantly active at an intensity that would make them vulnerable to fatigue.

The scapular muscles function together just before hand entry and as the hand exits the water. As with the aforementioned strokes, these muscles tether each corner of the scapula in order to position it in a way that minimizes impingement of the rotator cuff muscles on the acromion while maximizing congruency of the glenoid and humeral head. In addition, the rhomboids have a third peak of muscle action during mid pull-through, when they are isolated from the other scapular rotators to retract the scapula as the body is pulled over the humerus. This peak is simultaneous with the isolated peak of the posterior deltoid.

Because the backstroke is done supine, the latissimus dorsi has the mechanical advantage over the pectoralis major in bringing the trunk in line with the humerus as the arm pulls the body over the arm. This advantage is reflected in the intensity of muscle activation, as the latissimus dorsi is much more active than the pectoralis major.

From this information, the muscles can be divided into two functional groups: positioners and pullers. The three heads of the deltoid, along with the supraspinatus and the scapularis, are primarily responsible for placing the shoulder girdle in position for hand entry and exit. The latissimus dorsi, rhomboids, posterior deltoid, subscapularis, and teres minor are active during the propulsive phase of the backstroke. The pectoralis major and infraspinatus are minimally active throughout the stroke and thus cannot be placed in either group.

PAINFUL SHOULDERS. Backstroke swimmers with painful shoulders demonstrate a decrease of muscle activity in the supraspinatus, teres minor, and subscapularis during pull-through. This decreased activity may be due to the pain of impingement (secondary to instability) or to fatigue. As these critical muscles diminish their firing, they are unable to depress the humeral head as necessary during the extreme range of motion required for the backstroke. In order to compensate, the pectoralis major and latissimus dorsi increase their muscle activity. These two large muscles attempt to depress the humeral head when the rotator cuff is unable to fulfill that role. Because the latissimus dorsi and pectoralis major are large muscles with origins and insertions further away from the joint axis, their ability to depress the humeral head is much less precise.

During hand exit, the infraspinatus increases its action in swimmers with painful shoulders. This increased activity is another compensatory move as the infraspinatus attempts to depress the humeral head and externally rotate it in order to relieve the impingement found with internal rotation.

Another difference in muscle activity in backstroke swimmers with normal and painful shoulders is that those with painful shoulders have less activity in the posterior deltoid and rhomboids during recovery. This decreased activity is due to the lower, wider, and more passive arc of recovery.

From this information, it appears that the important muscles in competitive backstroke swimmers are the teres minor, subscapularis, and supraspinatus. If these muscles fail to function, the latissimus dorsi and

pectoralis major attempt to substitute, but neither is accurate in its attempt to depress the humeral head.

BREASTSTROKE

MECHANICS

The breaststroke is the oldest of all competitive swim strokes, and it is unique in that the arms do not exit the water. It uses a bilateral arm motion in which the arms reach forward and then sweep outward (the beginning of the pull-through), and the elbows begin to bend. When the hands are in line with the mid-chest, the hands move inward and upward until they are thrust forward (recovery) once again.

The kicking motion most frequently used in competition is the whip kick, but some less competitive swimmers may use a frog kick. Both forms of kicking use a symmetric, bilateral action.

There are two styles of body motion in the breaststroke. The first is a flat style in which the body is held horizontal and breathing is done by lifting and lowering the head. In the wave style, the head and shoulders come out of the water when the swimmer breathes, and the hips are lower when the legs glide back to the extended position.[21]

MUSCLE ACTIVITY

NORMAL SHOULDERS. In breaststroke swimmers with normal shoulders, the pectoralis major is responsible for the powerful humeral adduction and extension to provide propulsion. As the pectoralis major pulls, it also internally rotates the humerus. Once again, a force couple is formed with the teres minor to control the degree of rotation, thus balancing the rotation and maintaining congruency of the humeral head in the glenoid fossa.

The latissimus dorsi assists the pectoralis major and forms a force couple with the subscapularis. This is another repeated pattern of coactivation throughout the different swim strokes.

The posterior deltoid also assists with the humeral extension and pulling. The serratus anterior is active throughout pull-through as it stabilizes the scapula and pulls the body over the arm.

The three heads of the deltoid fire sequentially during recovery in order to position the arms forward. The supraspinatus is active at the same time as it optimizes the position of the humeral head in the glenoid while the forward reach occurs.

The serratus anterior remains active throughout recovery to stabilize, protract, and upwardly rotate the scapula for the forward reach. The upper trapezius functions at the same time as it elevates and rotates the scapula.

PAINFUL SHOULDERS. During pull-through, breaststroke swimmers with painful shoulders have increased activity in the subscapularis and latissimus dorsi. The increased subscapularis activity, along with a decrease in action of the teres minor, leads to a relative increase in internal rotation. Increased internal rotation places the arm in a position that is vulnerable to impingement. The increase in activity in the latissimus dorsi may assist with humeral head depression in order to relieve the impingement.

The overall muscle activity pattern of the serratus anterior throughout pull-through was depressed in swimmers with painful shoulders. Thus, there is a lack of scapular stabilization and upward rotation. The upper trapezius increases its activity, perhaps in an attempt to compensate for the serratus anterior and avoid impingement.

During recovery, there is a decrease in activity in the supraspinatus and upper trapezius, with reciprocally increased activity in the infraspinatus and latissimus dorsi. The diminished activity in the supraspinatus disrupts the force couple formed with the deltoid and may lead to the mechanics of injury. The increase in activity of the infraspinatus may be a response to the increase in internal rotation during the pull-through phase in swimmers with painful shoulders. This increased activity may reflect a need to increase external rotation in recovery in order to bring the humerus back to the original starting position for pull-through. The increase in infraspinatus activity may also be a response to the increase in latissimus dorsi activity. This increased activity occurs as the latissimus dorsi attempts to depress the humeral head in compensation for the diminished supraspinatus activity. The latissimus dorsi is less effective at this function because of its more distal humeral insertion. Thus, the increase in activity leads to relatively more internal rotation than depression. This internal rotation needs to be balanced by an increase in external rotation provided by the infraspinatus.

During recovery, the middle deltoid and then the upper trapezius have decreased activity in swimmers with painful shoulders. This decreased activity is correlated with swimmers who drop their elbows and limit abduction in order to avoid impingement. As the upper trapezius diminishes its activity, impingement could occur, since the scapula would have less upward rotation and elevation. With this information in mind, the muscles to focus on for competitive breaststroke swimmers are the teres minor, supraspinatus, and serratus anterior.

PREVENTIVE AND REHABILITATIVE PROGRAMS

The purpose of understanding the mechanics of swimming is to determine the tissues at risk for injury and then design effective and efficient preventive and rehabilitative exercise programs. This section pulls together the information just described and applies it to the development of a stretching and strengthening program for swimmers.

STRETCHING

Because swimmers have a tendency for hyperlaxity, and because hyperlaxity leaves individuals vulner-

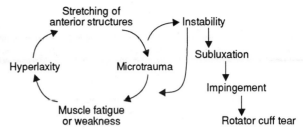

FIGURE 16–7. The instability continuum.

able to the instability continuum and resultant shoulder injury, stretching must be done judiciously (Fig. 16–7).

Since the majority of shoulder problems are due to anterior instability, swimmers definitely do not want to stretch any of the anterior structures. They should stretch the pectoral area, however, as swimmers frequently have rounded, forward shoulders. In order to stretch the pectoral region without endangering the anterior wall structures, the individual lies supine on the floor in the crook-lying position with the arms abducted to 90 degrees. He or she lets the knees fall to one side, turns the head in the opposite direction, and holds the position for 20 to 30 seconds (Fig. 16–8A). The knees and head are then brought back to neutral, and the stretch is repeated in the other direction.

Stretching of the inferior and posterior shoulder structures can be executed as well, unless the swimmer demonstrates signs of extreme laxity or multidirectional instability.

After the shoulder stretches are done, the swimmer can do a gentle warm-up on the deck. Shoulder circles can be performed, but it is advised to avoid a vigorous attack at the extremes of range.

Swimmers might want to stretch their backs and lower extremities. One good back stretch is the "cat and the cow" stretch. For this stretch, the individual gets into the quadriped position, and lets the back drop into a swayback position (the cow) then reciprocally arches the back (the cat) (Fig. 16–8B and C). Also, swimmers can go into the long-leg sitting position and try to lean over to touch their toes (or at least grasp the lower leg) (Fig. 16–8D). This position stretches not only the back but also the hamstrings. The quadriceps can be effectively stretched by standing (facing) a few feet from a wall, leaning one hand against the wall for stability, and with the other hand reaching behind to grasp the ipsilateral foot as the knee is maximally flexed and the foot is near the buttocks. While keeping the pelvis stable, the hip is then hyperextended.

It is important for swimmers to stretch the ankle dorsiflexors, as the most effective kicking is executed with the ankle in plantar flexion. Women tend to be better kickers than men, and this is probably partially due to the fact that women tend to be more flexible. One way to stretch the dorsiflexors is to sit on the ground with the knees maximally bent and the lower leg in contact with the ground and directly under the thigh. The ankle is directly under the thigh and is in maximal

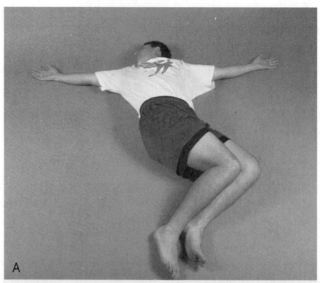

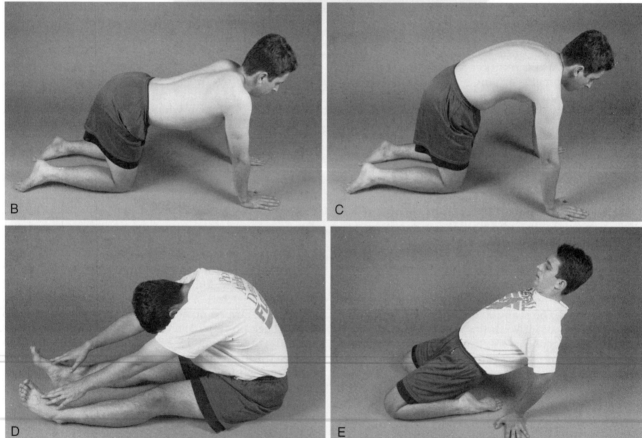

FIGURE 16–8. *A,* Pectoral stretch. *B–C,* Back stretch. *D,* Hamstring and back stretch. *E,* Dorsiflexor stretch.

plantar flexion (Fig. 16–8*E*). It is important to stretch the ankle as opposed to the forefoot.

This stretching program is specifically designed to protect swimmers' innate propensity to hyperlaxity while preparing them for a workout. The omission of anterior capsule stretching is crucial to prevent injury; however, because swimmers have done such stretching for years, it may be a difficult habit to break. Experience has shown that educating the swimming population as to why not to do anterior capsule stretching and why to do the other stretches leads to the greatest compliance and the best results.

STRENGTHENING

The goal of a strengthening exercise program is threefold. First and most obviously, it is to strengthen the muscles that are key to the specific swim strokes that the swimmer performs. Second, the endurance of the critical muscles needs to be built up. Third, restoration of the force couples specific to the swim stroke needs to occur. In general, the muscles that require a focus for strengthening and endurance are the rotator cuff muscles and the serratus anterior. The force couples of interest are the supraspinatus and the deltoids, the subscapularis and the latissimus dorsi, and the teres minor and the pectoralis major. Given this as background, the specific exercises for each stroke are discussed.

FREESTYLE. Based on fine-wire EMG studies during freestyle swimming, the two muscles to focus on for both strengthening and endurance are the serratus anterior and the subscapularis. Separate EMG studies have determined the optimal exercises for these muscles.[23,24]

The push-up with a plus is the optimal exercise for the serratus anterior. This exercise is similar to a standard push-up. When at the top of the push-up, exaggerated scapular protraction is added so that a little arch occurs between the shoulder blades (Fig. 16–9). The exaggerated scapular protraction is the best way to strengthen the serratus anterior. If the athlete is initially not strong enough to do a push-up in the hands and toes position, the position can be altered so that weight bearing is on the elbows, the knees, or both.

The upper extremity ergometer (UBE™) is ideal for endurance training of the serratus anterior. When using a UBE, the athlete makes certain that the seat is back far enough for exaggerated scapular protraction to occur and that the protraction is an active motion instead of the contralateral arm actively pulling the pedal toward the body. Also, because the serratus anterior is a broad muscle and all components of the muscle need endurance training, the seat height needs to be varied. When the seat height is high, the arms are pitched down and the horizontal fibers are most active. When the seat height is low, the arms are pitched upward and the upper and lower fibers are active.

The subscapularis is strengthened with humeral internal rotation. To do this exercise, the athlete lies on the involved side with the elbow bent to 90 degrees just in front of the trunk. The hand holds a weight and rotates the arm toward the trunk (Fig. 16–10). The activity is begun with relatively low weights. After the internal rotation is at least a "good" strength, the endurance component can begin with isokinetic training.

BUTTERFLY. The four muscles that appear to be most vulnerable during the butterfly stroke are the serratus anterior, subscapularis, teres minor, and upper trapezius. The specific exercises for the serratus anterior and subscapularis are described above.

Fine-wire EMG has demonstrated that the highest level of activity in the teres minor is when the humerus is abducted. A recommended exercise to isolate and optimize the teres minor is to have the athlete lie prone on a table with the humerus abducted to about 50 degrees and supported on the table while the forearm is off the edge. The hand holds a weight, and the athlete externally rotates his or her arm (Fig. 16–11). Once the

strength of external rotation reaches a strength grade of "good," isokinetic training can begin. The isokinetic training begins at low speeds and builds up to high speeds for endurance training.

Rowing is an exercise that optimally strengthens the upper trapezius.[24] To perform this exercise, the athlete is prone with the arm off the edge of the surface. The hand holds a weight. The humerus is raised toward the ceiling and the elbow bends (Fig. 16–12). As the humerus is elevated, the scapula is retracted.

BACKSTROKE. The teres minor, subscapularis, and supraspinatus all appear to be critical muscles for swimmers who perform the backstroke. The exercises for the teres minor and subscapularis are described above. The supraspinatus is optimally strengthened by performing humeral elevation in the scapular plane, which is called scaption.[23] To do this exercise, the athlete stands with the arms at the sides in the scapular plane (30 degrees forward of abduction). The hands can hold a light weight, and the thumbs are pointed downward. The athlete then elevates the arms in the scapular plane up to about 80 degrees (Fig. 16–13). If the athlete is allowed to elevate to 90 degrees and beyond with the humerus in internal rotation, impingement could occur. Thus, an athlete in a rehabilitation program does not proceed beyond 80 degrees. An athlete who is performing this exercise prophylactically, however, is asked to externally rotate while elevating the humerus and can then proceed with elevation to approximately 120 degrees. Between the arc of 90 and 120 degrees, the highest level of EMG activity is attained. In an athlete with a normal shoulder, the strength and sequence of muscle activity in the humeral rotators and depressors

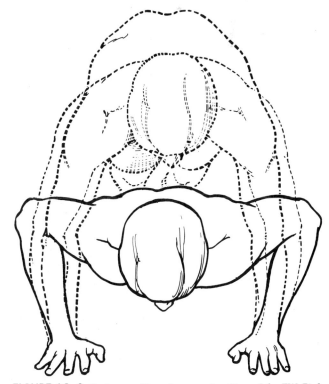

FIGURE 16–9. Push-up with a plus exercise. (From Jobe FW, Pink M: shoulder injuries in the athlete. J Hand Thera. April–June 1991.

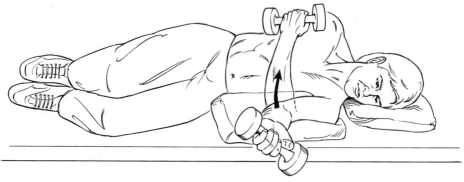

FIGURE 16—10. Humeral internal rotation exercise. (From Jobe FW, et al: Impingement Syndrome in overhand athletes. Part II. Surgical Rounds for Orthopaedics, Sept. 1990.)

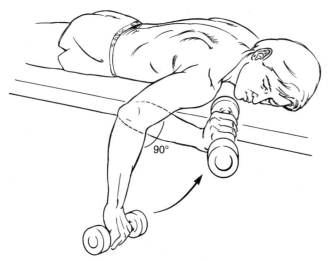

FIGURE 16—11. Teres minor exercise. (From Jobe FW, et al: Impingement Syndromes in overhand athletes. Part II. Surgical Rounds for Orthopaedics, Sept. 1990.)

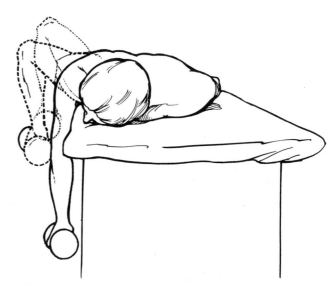

FIGURE 16—12. Rowing exercise. (From Jobe FW, Pink M: Shoulder injuries in the athlete. J Hand Ther. April–June 1991.)

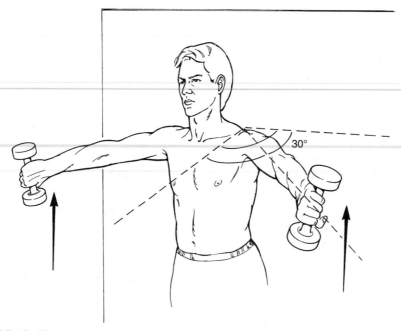

FIGURE 16—13. Scaption (scapular plane elevation) exercise with humeral internal rotation. (From Jobe FW, Bradley JP: The diagnosis and nonoperative treatment of shoulder injuries in athletes. Clin Sports Med 1959; 8:419–438.)

are adequate to add the external rotation and the higher degree of elevation.

There are other exercises that have been recommended for the supraspinatus.[24-26] Although not harmful, these exercises are done at the isometric end range, and the optimal electrical activity was defined by the peak-to-peak amplitude. The scaption exercise mentioned above was defined by integrating and normalizing the EMG, and the exercise optimizes the muscle throughout the range of motion.

BREASTSTROKE. The teres minor, supraspinatus, and serratus anterior are important muscles to strengthen for swimmers who do the breaststroke. Exercises for each of these muscles are discussed above.

SUMMARY

To optimally treat swimmers, one must have a sound understanding of the vulnerabilities and mechanics during the swim strokes. Each stroke is unique in relation to the care of the athlete. By understanding this information, a thought process is developed that enables health care providers and coaches to problem solve for a specific athlete. Ideal prevention and rehabilitation programs can be designed. Stretching, strengthening, and endurance training all need to be considered in a prevention and rehabilitation program. With such a program, injury can be minimized and performance can be optimized.

REFERENCES

1. Johnson D: In swimming, shoulder the burden. Sportcare and Fitness 1988; May–June:24–30.
2. Patterson RP, Moreno MI: Bicycle pedalling forces as a function of pedalling rate and power output. Med Sci Sports Exerc 1990; 22:512–516.
3. Becker TJ: The athletic trainer in swimming. Clin Sports Med 1986; 5:9–24.
4. Anderson B: Stretching. Bolinas, CA, Shelter Publications, 1980.
5. Hawkins RJ, Kennedy JC: Impingement syndrome in athletes. Am J Sports Med 1980; 8:151–158.
6. Neer CS, Welsh RP: The shoulder in sports. Orthop Clin North Am 1977; 8:583–591.
7. Scovazzo ML, Browne A, Pink M, et al: The painful shoulder during freestyle swimming: an electromyographic and cinematographic analysis of twelve muscles. Am J Sports Med 1991; 19:577–582.
8. Stocker D, Pink MM, Jobe FW: Comparison of shoulder injury in collegiate and masters level swimmers. Clin J Sports Med 1995; 5:4–8.
9. Pink M, Perry J, Browne A, et al: The normal shoulder during freestyle swimming. Am J Sports Med 1991; 19:569–576.
10. Pink M, Jobe FW, Perry J, et al: The normal shoulder during the butterfly stroke: An electromyographic and cinematographic analysis of twelve muscles. Clin Orthop Rel Res 1993; 288:48–59.
11. Pink M, Jobe FW, Perry J, et al: The painful shoulder during the butterfly stroke: An electromyographic and cinematographic analysis of twelve muscles. Clin Orthop Rel Res 1993; 288:60–72.
12. Pink M, Jobe FW, Perry J, et al: The normal shoulder during the backstroke: An EMG and cinematographic analysis of twelve muscles. Clin J Sport Med 1992; 2:6–12.
13. Perry J, Pink M, Jobe FW, et al: The painful shoulder during the backstroke: An EMG and cinematographic analysis of twelve muscles. Clin J Sport Med 1992; 2:13–20.
14. Ruwe PA, Pink M, Jobe FW, et al: The normal and painful shoulder during the breaststroke: An EMG and cinematographic analysis of twelve muscles. Am J Sports Med 1993; 6:709–796.
15. Adrian M, Singh M, Karpovich P: Energy cost of the leg kick, arm stroke and whole stroke. J Appl Physiol 1966; 21:1763–1766.
16. Astrand P: Aerobic power in swimming. *In* B Erickson, B Furberg (eds): International Series on Sports Sciences, vol 6. Baltimore, University Park Press, 1978, pp 127–131.
17. Charbonnier JP, Lacour JP, Rigffal J, Flandrois R: Experimental study of the performance of competitive swimmers. J Appl Physiol 1975; 34:157–167.
18. Holmer I: Energy cost of the arm stroke, leg kick and the whole stroke in competitive swimming style. J Appl Physiol 1974; 33:105–118.
19. Monad H: Contractility of muscle during prolonged static and static dynamic activity. Ergonomics 1985; 28:81.
20. Counsilman JE: The Science of Swimming. Englewood Cliffs, NJ, Prentice-Hall, 1968, pp 67–68.
21. Persyn U, DeMaeyer J, Vervaecke H: Investigation of hydrodynamic determinants of competitive swimming strokes. *In* LeWillie L, Clarys JP (eds): Swimming II, vol 2. Baltimore, University Park Press, 1975, p 217.
22. Maglischo EW: Swimming Even Faster. Mountain View, CA, Mayfield Publishing, 1993.
23. Townsend H, Jobe FW, Pink M, Perry J: Electromyographic analysis of the glenohumeral muscles during a baseball rehabilitation program. Am J Sports Med 1991; 19:264–272.
24. Moseley JB, Jobe FW, Pink M, et al: EMG analysis of the scapular muscles during a shoulder rehabilitation program. Am J Sports Med 1992; 20:128–134.
25. Blackburn TA, McLeod WD, White B, Wofford L: EMG analysis of posterior rotator cuff exercises. Athl Train 1990; 25:40–45.
26. Worrell TW, Corey BJ, York SL, Santiestaban J: An analysis of supraspinatus EMG activity and shoulder isometric force development. Med Sci Sports Exerc 1992; 24:744–747.

CHAPTER 17

Biomechanics of Throwing

GLENN S. FLEISIG *PhD*
RAFAEL F. ESCAMILLA *PhD*
JAMES R. ANDREWS *MD*

Biomechanics is a function of both kinematics and kinetics. Kinematics describes *how* something is moving without stating the causes behind the motion. Specifically, it quantifies linear and angular displacement, velocity, and acceleration—the *effects* of the motion. Kinetics explains *why* an object moves the way it does; it quantifies both the forces and the torques that *cause* the motion.

One of the most demanding activities on the arm in sports is the throwing motion. The prevalence of overuse injury due to throwing is well documented.[1-6] Most of these overuse throwing injuries occur due to repetitive trauma to the shoulder and elbow. A proper understanding and application of throwing mechanics can help maximize performance as well as minimize injuries, which are often due to faulty throwing mechanics.

In this chapter, the kinetic chain concept, rotational inertia, and angular momentum are discussed relative to the throwing motion. The biomechanics of each phase of the throwing motion is then presented in detail. Finally, common injuries caused by throwing are presented, followed by implications for rehabilitation.

THE KINETIC CHAIN CONCEPT

It is important to understand that the entire body is used during the throwing motion. In order to maximize performance and minimize internal forces at the shoulder and elbow, an athlete's body should function as a "kinetic chain." The kinetic chain mechanism involves neuromuscular coordination (i.e., sequential movements of body segments) in such a manner as to transfer energy up the body from the legs to the hips, trunk, upper arm, forearm, hand, and finally the ball.[7-9] The more body segments that sequentially contribute to the total force output, the greater the potential velocity at the distal end where the object is released.

The principle of the kinetic chain can be illustrated using roller skating as an example (Fig. 17–1A). When a number of roller skaters hold hands in a line and try to maximize the speed of the last skater, they take turns applying force to the person next to them. The first skater, who represents a base segment, "whips" the second skater, followed immediately by the second skater "whipping" the third skater. This sequence continues until the last skater (the distal segment) is "whipped." Each skater is whipped a little faster than the preceding skater, transferring energy to the next skater. The overall effect is that the last skater attains the greatest velocity. An analogy that can be drawn is that each skater represents a segment of a thrower's body (e.g., thigh, trunk, arm) and that hands held between adjacent skaters represent joints on the thrower's body (e.g., hip, shoulder, elbow) (Fig. 17–1B).

During throwing activities, movements are initiated from the larger base segments and terminate with the smaller distal segments. There are seven segments that have both angular and linear movements during the throw: lower extremity, pelvis, trunk, shoulder girdle, upper arm, forearm, and hand. These segments rotate

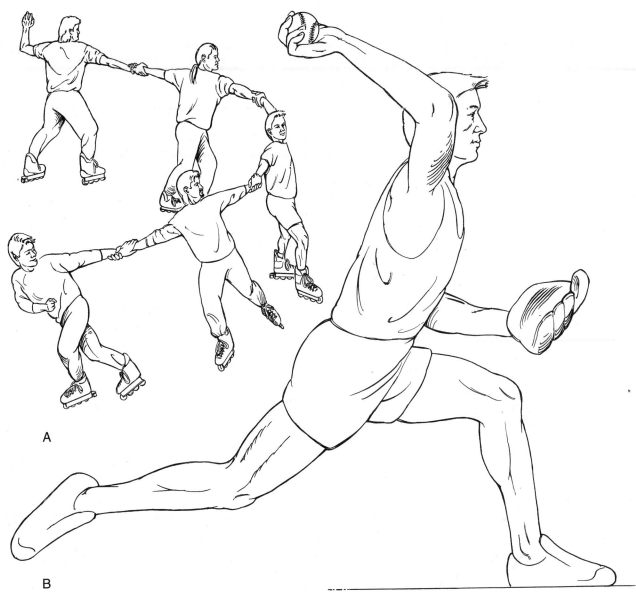

FIGURE 17–1. Examples of kinetic chains. *A*, A chain of roller skaters executing a whip maneuver; *B*, the body segments of a baseball pitcher.

about axes through the ankle, knee, hip, intervertebral, sternoclavicular, shoulder, elbow, radioulnar, and wrist joints.

ROTATIONAL INERTIA

To rotate a body segment, an athlete applies a torque, or twisting force, at a joint. How much angular acceleration can be generated for a body segment by an applied torque is directly proportional to the segment's rotational inertia (i.e., a segment's resistance to rotation). Rotational inertia is related to how much mass a body segment has and the distance between that segment's mass and its axis of rotation. For any given muscle torque, the greater the mass of a segment and the further that mass is distributed away from its rotational axis, the greater that segment's rotational

inertia will be; consequently, as a segment's rotational inertia increases, angular acceleration of that segment decreases proportionately.

In throwing, the lower extremity, pelvis, and trunk are the larger base segments that produce the muscular torques needed to accelerate the smaller distal segments (i.e., the shoulder girdle, upper arm, forearm, and hand). These base segments have greater rotational inertia, thus they generate smaller angular velocities as they rotate. The smaller distal segments have less rotational inertia; therefore, they move with greater angular velocities.

CONSERVATION OF ANGULAR MOMENTUM

The kinetic link principle can be illustrated further utilizing the law of conservation of angular momentum.

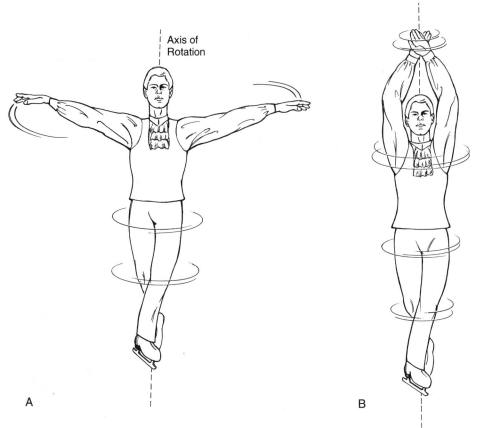

FIGURE 17–2. Angular velocity of an ice skater varying with changes in rotational inertia. *A*, Slow velocity due to large inertia; *B*, large velocity due to small inertia.

This law states that the total angular momentum (the product of rotational inertia, *I*, and angular velocity, ω) of a system remains constant if there is no net torque acting on the system (i.e., *I*ω = constant). An ice skater can be used to illustrate this principle. With both arms abducted, a skater can rotate about an imaginary vertical axis through the body (Fig. 17–2*A*). In this case, rotational inertia is high and angular velocity is low, since mass is being distributed further away from the axis of rotation. To generate more angular velocity, the skater can bring both arms in closer to the axis of rotation, thus reducing rotational inertia (Fig. 17–2*B*). Since there is no net torque acting on the body (ice friction is negligible), angular momentum must be conserved. Therefore, a decrease in rotational inertia corresponds with an increase in angular velocity.

A simplified three-segment throwing model of the pelvis, trunk, and arm can be used to illustrate how angular momentum is conserved in throwing. When the athlete applies force to the ground, an equal but opposite force is applied by the ground to the athlete. This external force applies both force and torque to the athlete, accelerating the athlete and adding both linear and angular momentum to the system. Subsequently, the trunk flexors and trunk rotators impart an internal torque (equal but opposite torques exerted on each segment, thus a net torque of zero) between

the pelvis and trunk segments, thus decelerating the pelvis segment and accelerating the trunk segment. Since angular momentum is conserved, the angular momentum lost by the pelvis segment is gained by the trunk segment. Similarly, the intersegmental muscles between the trunk and the arm impart an internal torque between these two segments, decelerating the trunk segment and accelerating the arm segment. Angular momentum is conserved, and the angular momentum lost by the trunk is gained by the arm. As this process is continued, angular momentum is finally transferred to the hand segment, which releases the ball. As angular momentum is transferred from the larger base segments to the smaller distal segments, rotational inertia decreases and angular velocity increases, thus conserving angular momentum. This conservation can be illustrated as shown in Figure 17–3.

As seen in Figure 17–3, the rotational inertia is large in the more massive base segments and becomes progressively smaller as angular momentum is transferred to the smaller distal segments. Conversely, angular velocity is small in the base segments and progressively increases as angular momentum is transferred to the distal segments.

Although the human model of throwing and angular momentum transfer is more complex than the model just illustrated, this simplified model provides some insight into segmental interactions and coordination. More biomechanical studies need to be conducted to determine not only which muscles are acting on the segments but also the quantity and time occurrence of the muscle firing patterns. Slight changes in timing may result in a drastic reduction in performance as well as increased forces generated at the elbow and shoulder joints.

Elastic properties of muscle and connective tissue can also affect joint torques, as they enhance recoil tendencies after a segment has been placed on stretch. As proximal segments are accelerated forward, distal segments "lag back" and are placed on stretch. An evoked stretch reflex and stored elastic energy (i.e., from series and parallel elastic components such as connective tissue, tendon, and muscle) can further enhance voluntary muscle force throughout the sequential movements.

GENERAL THROWING MOTION

The general throwing motion is similar among various sports, including baseball, softball (except underhand pitching), football, team handball, javelin, and water polo. Even the overhead serve in tennis, the badminton smash, and the serve or spike in volleyball have similar mechanics. In order to rehabilitate athletes and minimize injury potential, a thorough understanding of throwing biomechanics is needed.

Baseball pitching and football passing are used throughout this chapter to represent a general throwing model. Ranges presented throughout this section are primarily for baseball pitching, with some ranges also presented for football passing. Baseball pitching and football passing parameters are contrasted in Table 17–1. Ranges given throughout this chapter are those values commonly seen in high school, college, and professional baseball pitchers and football quarterbacks. Kinematic and kinetic parameters are reported for pitchers and quarterbacks who weigh approximately 85 to 90 kg (185 to 200 lbs). The quantification of other throwing movements is similar to these two types of throws.

To better understand the total motion, throwing can be divided into phases. The throwing motion has previously been divided into six phases (Fig. 17–4): windup, stride, arm cocking, arm acceleration, arm deceleration, and follow-through.[10–12]

WINDUP

The objective of the windup phase is to put the thrower in a good starting position. The windup begins when the athlete initiates the first motion and ends with maximum knee lift of the stride leg. For pitching, the time from when the stance foot pivots to when the knee has achieved a maximum height and the pitcher is in a balanced position is typically between 0.5 and 1.0 s.

In pitching, the athlete typically begins with the weight evenly distributed on both feet. The stance foot then pivots to a position parallel with the rubber (Fig. 17–4A). The lead leg is lifted by concentric contractions of the hip flexors (rectus femoris, iliopsoas, sartorius, pectineus), and the lead side (left side for a right-handed thrower) faces the target. Except during pitching, the leg lift is usually not very high. The stance leg bends slightly, controlled by eccentric contractions from the quadriceps muscle, and remains in a fairly fixed position due to isometric contractions of the quadriceps until a balanced position is achieved (Fig. 17–4B). The hip abductors (gluteus medius and minimus and tensor fasciae lata) of the stance leg must also contract isometrically to prevent a downward tilting of the opposite-side pelvis, and the hip extensors of the stance leg contract both eccentrically and iso-

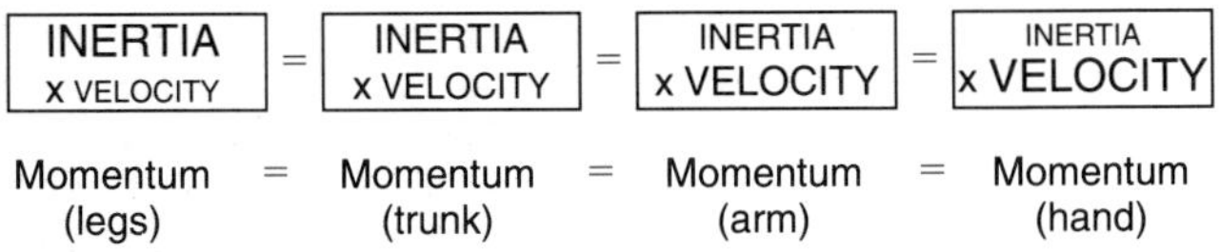

INERTIA x VELOCITY	=	INERTIA x VELOCITY	=	INERTIA x VELOCITY	=	INERTIA x VELOCITY
Momentum (legs)	=	Momentum (trunk)	=	Momentum (arm)	=	Momentum (hand)

FIGURE 17–3. Conservation of angular momentum.

D E F I N I T I O N S

PHASES OF THROWING

1. WINDUP PHASE: From first movement until the hands separate. As the lead leg lifts up, causing the hip and knee to flex, all the weight is placed on the stance leg. A balanced position just prior to hand separation.
2. STRIDE PHASE: From hand separation until the lead foot contacts the ground. If the lead foot lands to the right of the stance foot (left for a left-handed pitcher), a closed stance results. Conversely, if the lead foot lands to the left of the stance foot (right for a left-handed pitcher), an open stance results.
3. ARM COCKING PHASE: From foot contact until maximum shoulder external rotation.
4. ARM ACCELERATION PHASE: From maximum shoulder external rotation until ball release.
5. ARM DECELERATION PHASE: From ball release until maximum shoulder internal rotation (approximately zero degrees of rotation).
6. FOLLOW-THROUGH: From maximum shoulder internal rotation until a balanced position is achieved.

LOADS OF FORCES AND TORQUES AT ELBOW AND SHOULDER JOINTS

1. INTERNAL ROTATION TORQUE: The torque produced to stop shoulder external rotation and start shoulder internal rotation.
2. VARUS TORQUE: The torque produced to stop valgus rotation, or valgus extension, at the elbow and start varus rotation.
3. ANTERIOR SHEAR FORCE: The force produced either to prevent the upper arm from translating posteriorly or to move it anteriorly.
4. POSTERIOR SHEAR FORCE: The force produced either to prevent the upper arm from translating anteriorly or to move it posteriorly.
5. COMPRESSIVE FORCE: The force produced to prevent distraction.

TABLE 17–1
Mean Values of Baseball Pitching and Football Passing Kinematic Parameters

Parameter	Baseball (n = 23)	Football (n = 14)
Foot contact (degree)		
Elbow flexion*	80 ± 21	105 ± 13
Shoulder external rotation*	65 ± 29	88 ± 36
Shoulder abduction	103 ± 13	105 ± 17
Shoulder horizontal adduction	−11 ± 24	−2 ± 17
Lead knee flexion	48 ± 11	43 ± 11
Delivery		
Angular variables (degree)		
Maximum elbow flexion*	96 ± 12	115 ± 9
Maximum external rotation*	175 ± 12	168 ± 12
Angular velocity (degree)		
Maximum elbow extension*	2340 ± 351	1716 ± 193
Maximum internal rotation*	7365 ± 1503	4586 ± 843
Maximum shoulder horizontal adduction	657 ± 266	519 ± 165
Maximum upper torso*	1180 ± 294	1017 ± 177
Maximum pelvis*	662 ± 148	518 ± 97
Trunk tilt*	377 ± 76	260 ± 71
Release (degree)		
Elbow flexion*	24 ± 6	56 ± 28
Shoulder external rotation*	124 ± 22	145 ± 25
Shoulder abduction*	99 ± 8	114 ± 15
Shoulder horizontal adduction*	10 ± 8	21 ± 10
Lead knee flexion*	42 ± 17	32 ± 6
Trunk tilt forward*	57 ± 9	72 ± 9
Trunk tilt lateral	117 ± 17	113 ± 6
Ball velocity (mph)*	74 ± 5	46 ± 4
Duration of throw(s)*	.15 ± .03	.20 ± .03

*Significant difference p ≤ .05.
Adapted from Wick H, Dillman CJ, Werner S, et al: A kinematic comparison between baseball pitching and football passing. Sports Med Update 1991; 6:13–16.

metrically to stabilize hip flexion.[13] The shoulders are partially flexed and abducted and are held in this position by the anterior and medial deltoids, the supraspinatus, and the clavicular portion of the pectoralis major. [14,15] In addition, elbow flexion is maintained by isometric contraction of the elbow flexors (biceps, brachialis, and brachioradialis).[13,16] Normally, low forces, torques, and muscle activity occur in the throwing arm during this phase.

STRIDE

The stride phase begins at the end of the windup, when the lead leg begins to fall and move toward the target and the two arms separate from each other (Fig. 17–4C). This phase, which ends when the lead foot first contacts the ground (Fig. 17–4F), lasts between 0.50 and 0.75 s when pitching (Fig. 17–5) and between 0.25 and 0.50 s when throwing a football.

As the phase begins, the lead leg strides toward the target as the stance leg remains in contact with the ground. Eccentric contraction of the hip flexors controls the lowering of the lead leg, while concentric contraction from the stance leg hip abductors helps lengthen the stride. In pitching, it is still unclear how much of the stride is due to pushing off the rubber and how much

is simply from "falling" off the rubber. In either case, the forward movement is probably initiated to some degree by hip abduction, followed by knee and hip extension from the stance leg. As the lead leg falls downward and forward, the lead hip begins to rotate externally (initiated by the gluteus maximus, the sartorius, and the six deep external hip rotators), and the stance hip begins to rotate internally (initiated by the gluteus medius and minimus and tensor fasciae lata).[17] The stance hip also extends due to concentric contractions from the hip extensors (gluteus maximus muscle and hamstrings).[13] Throughout the stride phase, the trunk is tilted slightly sideways—away from the target.

The stride length, when measured from ankle to ankle at lead foot contact, varies considerably, depending on the type of throw. In pitching, it is approximately 70 to 80 percent of the athlete's height; a quarterback's stride during the throw is approximately 55 to 65 percent of height. At foot contact (see Fig. 17–4F), the lead foot should be pointed slightly inward (i.e., closed). For a right-handed pitcher, the left foot would point to the right, and for a left-handed pitcher, the right foot would point to the left. This closed foot position is usually between 5 and 25 degrees deviation from the foot pointing straight ahead toward home plate (Fig. 17–6). This position helps the lead leg act as a stable brace over which the upper body can rotate. The lead knee is flexed approximately 45 to 55 degrees at foot contact. The placement and position of the lead foot are very important in throwing. The lead foot should land either directly in front of the rear foot toward the

direction of the throw or a few centimeters closed (lead foot to the right of the stance foot in right-handed throwing) or open (lead foot to the left of the stance foot in right-handed throwing). However, if the foot posi-

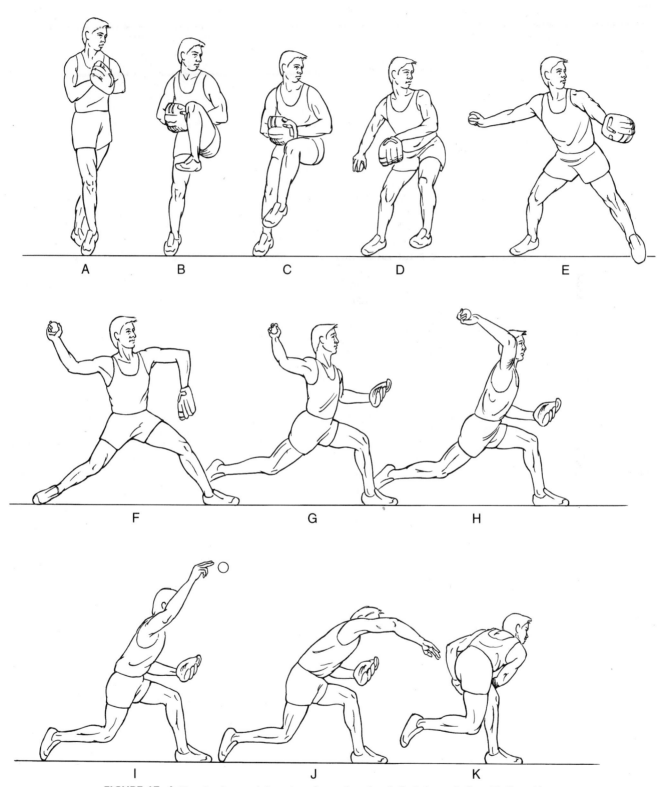

FIGURE 17–4. The six phases of throwing, shown for a baseball pitcher: wind-up (A–C); stride (C–F); arm cocking (F–H); arm acceleration (H–I); arm deceleration (I–J); and follow-through (J–K). (Modified from Werner SL, Fleisig GS, Dillman CJ, Andrews JR: Biomechanics of the elbow during baseball pitching. J Orthop Sports Phys Ther 1993; 17:274–278.)

tion is excessively closed, pelvic rotation can be impeded and the athlete ends up "throwing across the body," which minimizes the contribution of the lower body to the force of the throw. Conversely, if the foot is positioned excessively open, pelvic rotation occurs too early. This results in improper timing, causing energy from pelvic rotation to be applied to the upper trunk too early. Consequently, one ends up throwing with too much "arm," since the energy generated from the pelvic rotation is dissipated instead of being applied to the arm. The elastic energy generated in the legs, trunk, and arms during the stride phase is transferred to subsequent phases of the throw.

During the stride, both shoulders abduct, externally rotate, and horizontally abduct owing to concentric muscle action (see Fig. 17–4E). At lead foot contact, shoulder abduction is approximately 80 to 100 degrees. The deltoid and supraspinatus are responsible for abducting and holding the arm in this position; the supraspinatus has an additional job of maintaining proper humeral head position within the glenoid fossa. The upper trapezius and serratus anterior upwardly rotate and position the glenoid for the humeral head; this action is extremely important, since an improperly positioned scapula can lead to impingement and shoulder control problems.[18] Muscular activity during the stride phase is shown in Table 17–2.

During the stride phase, the throwing arm is positioned slightly behind the trunk (i.e., horizontally abducted) during pitching and slightly in front of the trunk during football passing. The posterior deltoid, latissimus dorsi, teres major, and posterior rotator cuff muscles (infraspinatus and teres minor) are responsible for horizontally abducting the shoulder while the rhomboids and middle trapezius retract the scapula.[19]

Elbow flexion of the throwing arm at foot contact is approximately 80 to 100 degrees while the forearm is rotated up, approaching a vertical position (see Fig. 17–4F). Quarterbacks have slightly greater elbow flexion

and shoulder external rotation at lead foot contact as compared with pitchers (see Table 17–1). In both cases, the elbow flexor muscles of the throwing arm contract eccentrically and isometrically in controlling elbow flexion, while the supinator and biceps muscles supinate the forearm as the shoulder abducts and externally rotates. Electromyography has shown that the wrist and finger extensors have very high activity during this phase, causing the wrist to move from a position of slight flexion to a position of hyperextension.[19] These muscles contract concentrically as they work against gravity, with the throwing palm and ball facing downward and the shoulder abducting. Consequently, they must overcome the mass of both the hand and the ball.

ARM COCKING

Arm cocking begins at lead foot contact and ends at maximum shoulder external rotation. In the arm cocking phase, which lasts between 0.10 and 0.15 s (see Fig. 17–5), the upper body is rotated to face the target. The quadriceps of the lead leg initially contracts eccentrically to decelerate knee flexion and then contracts isometrically to stabilize the lead leg during the arm cocking phase. At this time, the thrower's body should be stretched out in the direction of the target. In pitching, the ankle of the stance leg plantar flexes as it leaves contact with the rubber. This motion usually occurs concurrent with pelvic rotation, just after lead foot contact.

The pelvis continues its transverse rotation as both hips internally rotate. In baseball pitching, the pelvis achieves a maximum rotation of approximately 400 to 700 degrees/s. Maximal pelvic rotation occurs approximately 0.03 to 0.05 s after foot contact, which is approximately 30 percent into the arm cocking phase. As the hips rotate to face the target, the trunk rotators are placed on stretch, which produces a recoil effect for

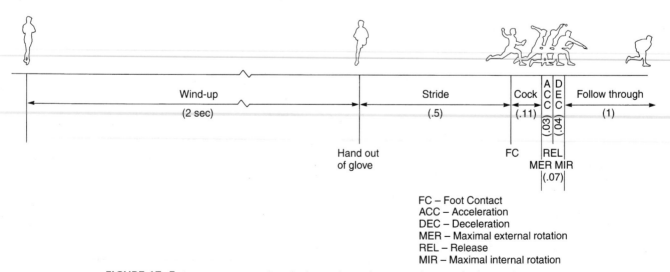

FIGURE 17–5. Approximate time lengths for pitching phases: wind-up, stride, arm cocking (COCK), arm acceleration (ACC), arm deceleration (DEC), and follow-through. Events shown separating phases: hand out of glove, foot contact (FC), maximum shoulder external rotation (MER), ball release (REL), and maximum internal rotation (MIR).

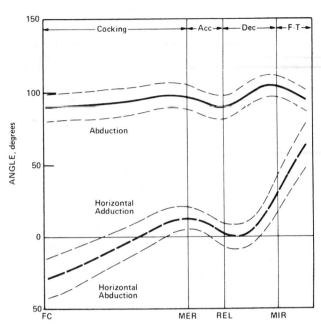

FIGURE 17–7. Shoulder abduction and horizontal adduction. FC = time of foot contact; MER = maximum shoulder external rotation; REL = ball release; MIR = maximum internal rotation; Cocking = arm cocking; Acc = arm acceleration; Dec = arm deceleration; F-T = follow-through. (From Dillman CJ, Fleisig GS, Andrews JR: Biomechanics of pitching with emphasis upon shoulder kinematics. J Orthop Sports Phys Ther 1993; 18:402–408.)

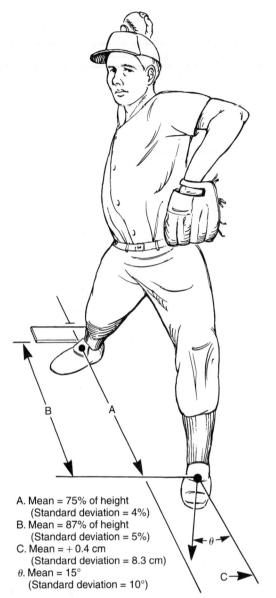

A. Mean = 75% of height
   (Standard deviation = 4%)
B. Mean = 87% of height
   (Standard deviation = 5%)
C. Mean = + 0.4 cm
   (Standard deviation = 8.3 cm)
θ. Mean = 15°
   (Standard deviation = 10°)

FIGURE 17–6. The stride during baseball pitching. (Modified from Dillman CJ, Fleisig GS, Andrews JR: Biomechanics of pitching with emphasis upon shoulder kinematics. J Orthop Sports Phys Ther 1993; 18:402–408.)

the subsequent shoulder rotation. Shortly after the pelvis begins its rotation, the upper torso begins transverse rotation about the spinal column (see Fig. 17–4G); consequently, the anterior trunk now faces the target. Maximum upper torso angular velocity of approximately 900 to 1300 degrees/s (approximately twice as large as pelvis angular velocity) is achieved (see Table 17–1). This action occurs 0.05 to 0.07 s after lead foot contact, which is approximately 50 percent into the arm cocking phase. The abdominal and oblique musculature is also placed on stretch due to the hyperextension of the lumbar trunk that occurs as the upper torso rotates.

As the larger base segments of the pelvis and torso rotate about the longitudinal vertebral axis, a great deal of energy is imparted to the system. Subsequently, this energy is transferred to the smaller, more distal seg-

ments if the motion is done correctly. The sequence of attaining maximal pelvic rotation prior to maximal upper torso rotation is important in establishing proper timing and coordination for subsequent portions of the throw.

As the trunk rotates to face the target, the throwing shoulder horizontally adducts, moving from a position of 20 to 30 degrees of horizontal abduction at lead foot contact to a position of 15 to 20 degrees of horizontal adduction at the time of maximum shoulder external rotation (Fig. 17–7).[10] During this time, a maximum shoulder horizontal adduction velocity (relative to the trunk) of approximately 500 to 650 degrees/s is obtained. The pectoralis major and the anterior deltoid are the primary shoulder horizontal adductors. These muscles initially contract eccentrically as the trunk rotates to face the target, thus limiting shoulder horizontal abduction. It is still unclear how much these muscles act isometrically as arm stabilizers to allow the arm to move with the trunk, and how much they function concentrically to provide dynamic horizontal adduction at the shoulder. Undoubtedly, both functions are performed in varying degrees throughout this phase.

The shoulder girdle muscles (levator scapulae, serratus anterior, trapezius, rhomboids, and pectoralis minor) are also important during the arm cocking phase. The serratus anterior is the most active, as it provides both stabilization and protraction to the scapula.[19] The middle trapezius and rhomboids, which oppose the scapular motion created by the serratus anterior, have also been shown to be quite active (see Table 17–2). The levator scapula also displays high muscle activity (see Table 17–2). These muscles work together, helping to stabilize the scapula and provide position of the glenoid for subsequent action of the humeral head. Dysfunction of these scapula muscles may cause additional stress to the anterior shoulder stabilizers. During late arm cocking, the serratus anterior is important in providing upward rotation and protraction of the scapula, allowing the scapula to move with the horizontally adducting humerus.

Throughout the arm cocking phase, the shoulder remains abducted approximately 80 to 100 degrees (see Fig. 17–7). The forearm and hand segments lag behind the rapidly rotating trunk and shoulder, producing a maximum shoulder external rotation of approximately 165 to 180 degrees (Fig. 17–8). The forearm now lies in a horizontal position approximately 90 degrees backward from its vertical position obtained at or just after lead foot contact. Because of the way shoulder external rotation is measured in biomechanical research, this apparent abnormal position of the throwing arm is not totally due to external rotation at the glenohumeral joint. Some of the "external rotation" measurement is from shoulder girdle movement at the scapulothoracic interface, and some is due to hyperextension of the lumbar trunk. Nevertheless, shoulder external rotation appears to be very important in throwing, for this parameter influences the range of motion that ensues during the rapid acceleration phase. Electromyography has shown that as the shoulder externally rotates, the wrist and finger extensors have very high activity, placing the wrist in a hyperextended position.[19]

Throwers with inadequate shoulder flexibility may need to perform various shoulder stretching and strengthening exercises to improve their range of motion and increase the motion available at the glenohumeral joint. Repetitive throwing tends to increase shoulder capsule laxity and shoulder flexibility. It is not unusual for a baseball pitcher to possess 10 to 15 degrees more external rotation in the throwing shoulder compared with the nonthrowing shoulder.[20] This extra range of motion may help maximize performance and minimize injury potential at the shoulder by allowing a greater range of motion in which force can be generated. However, having too much shoulder flexibility can

TABLE 17–2
Muscle Activity During Pitching*

Muscle	N	Windup	Stride	Arm Cocking	Arm Acceleration	Arm Deceleration	Follow-Through
Scapular							
Upper trapezius	11	18 ± 16	64 ± 53	37 ± 29	69 ± 31	53 ± 22	14 ± 12
Middle trapezius	11	7 ± 5	43 ± 22	51 ± 24	71 ± 32	35 ± 17	15 ± 14
Lower trapezius	13	13 ± 12	39 ± 30	38 ± 29	76 ± 55	78 ± 33	25 ± 15
Serratus anterior (sixth rib)	11	14 ± 13	44 ± 35	69 ± 32	60 ± 53	51 ± 30	32 ± 18
Serratus anterior (fourth rib)	10	20 ± 20	40 ± 22	106 ± 56	50 ± 46	34 ± 7	41 ± 24
Rhomboids	11	7 ± 8	35 ± 24	41 ± 26	71 ± 35	45 ± 28	14 ± 20
Levator scapulae	11	6 ± 5	35 ± 14	72 ± 54	77 ± 28	33 ± 16	14 ± 13
Glenohumeral							
Anterior deltoid	16	15 ± 12	40 ± 20	28 ± 30	27 ± 19	47 ± 34	21 ± 16
Middle deltoid	14	9 ± 8	44 ± 19	12 ± 17	36 ± 22	59 ± 19	16 ± 13
Posterior deltoid	18	6 ± 5	42 ± 26	28 ± 27	68 ± 66	60 ± 28	13 ± 11
Supraspinatus	16	13 ± 12	60 ± 31	49 ± 29	51 ± 46	39 ± 43	10 ± 9
Infraspinatus	16	11 ± 9	30 ± 18	74 ± 34	31 ± 28	37 ± 20	20 ± 16
Teres minor	12	5 ± 6	23 ± 15	71 ± 42	54 ± 50	84 ± 52	25 ± 21
Subscapularis (lower third)	11	7 ± 9	26 ± 22	62 ± 19	56 ± 31	41 ± 23	25 ± 18
Subscapularis (upper third)	11	7 ± 8	37 ± 26	99 ± 55	115 ± 82	60 ± 36	16 ± 15
Pectoralis major	14	6 ± 6	11 ± 13	56 ± 27	54 ± 24	29 ± 18	31 ± 21
Latissimus dorsi	13	12 ± 10	33 ± 33	50 ± 37	88 ± 53	59 ± 35	24 ± 18
Elbow and forearm							
Triceps	13	4 ± 6	17 ± 17	37 ± 32	89 ± 40	54 ± 23	22 ± 18
Biceps	18	8 ± 9	22 ± 14	26 ± 20	20 ± 16	44 ± 32	16 ± 14
Brachialis	13	8 ± 5	17 ± 13	18 ± 26	20 ± 22	49 ± 29	13 ± 17
Brachioradialis	13	5 ± 5	35 ± 20	31 ± 24	16 ± 12	46 ± 24	22 ± 29
Pronator teres	14	14 ± 16	18 ± 15	39 ± 28	85 ± 39	51 ± 21	21 ± 21
Supinator	13	9 ± 7	38 ± 30	54 ± 38	55 ± 31	59 ± 31	22 ± 19
Wrist and fingers							
Extensor carpi radialis longus	13	11 ± 8	53 ± 24	72 ± 37	30 ± 20	43 ± 24	22 ± 14
Extensor carpi radialis brevis	15	17 ± 17	47 ± 26	75 ± 41	55 ± 35	43 ± 28	24 ± 19
Extensor digitorum communis	14	21 ± 17	37 ± 25	59 ± 27	35 ± 35	47 ± 25	24 ± 18
Flexor carpi radialis	12	13 ± 9	24 ± 35	47 ± 33	120 ± 66	79 ± 36	35 ± 16
Flexor digitorum superficialis	11	16 ± 6	20 ± 23	47 ± 52	80 ± 66	71 ± 32	21 ± 11
Flexor carpi ulnaris	10	8 ± 5	27 ± 18	41 ± 25	112 ± 60	77 ± 42	24 ± 18

*Means and standard deviation, expressed as a percentage of the maximal manual muscle test.
Adapted from DiGiovine NM: An electromyographic analysis of the upper extremity in pitching. J Shoulder Elbow Surg 1992; 1:15–25.

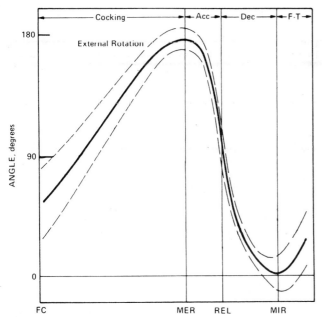

FIGURE 17–8. External/internal rotation. FC = time of foot contact; MER = maximum shoulder external rotation; REL = ball release; MIR = maximum internal rotation; Cocking = arm cocking; Acc = arm acceleration; Dec = arm deceleration; F-T = follow-through. (From Dillman CJ, Fleisig GS, Andrews JR: Biomechanics of pitching with emphasis upon shoulder kinematics. J Orthop Sports Phys Ther 1993; 18:402–408.)

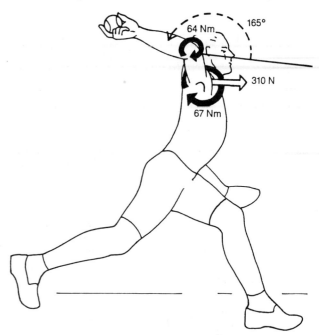

FIGURE 17–9. Shortly before maximum external rotation is achieved, a critical instant occurs; at this instant, a pitcher's shoulder is externally rotated 165 degrees and the elbow is flexed 95 degrees. Among the loads generated at this time are 67 N-m of internal rotation torque, 310 N of anterior force at the shoulder, and 64 N-m of varus torque at the elbow. (From Fleisig GS, Dillman CJ, Andrews JR: Kinetics of baseball pitching with implications about injury mechanisms. Am J Sports Med 1995; 23:233–239.)

be as detrimental as or worse than having too little. Excessive stretching may exacerbate shoulder capsule laxity, which, over time, may lead to shoulder instability. Injuries to the capsulolabral complex and rotator cuff muscles often accompany shoulder instability. Stretching of the shoulder complex should therefore be closely monitored by a trainer or therapist and should be individualized after shoulder flexibility has been properly assessed.

In a study comparing amateur pitchers and professional pitchers, Gowan[21] showed that the muscle activity of the subscapularis during arm cocking is approximately twice as great in professional pitchers as in amateur pitchers. However, muscle activity of the biceps, serratus anterior, supraspinatus, and pectoralis major pectforalis major was approximately 50 percent greater in the amateur pitchers. This may be due to better throwing efficiency by professional pitchers, necessitating less muscle recruitment.

Shoulder joint forces and torques generated during the arm cocking phase are quite high. A maximum compressive force of approximately 550 to 770 N (approximately 80 percent body weight) is needed to resist distraction due to rapid pelvic and upper torso rotation.[12] This compressive force is generated largely by high activity from the rotator cuff muscles (supraspinatus, infraspinatus, teres minor, and subscapularis) (see Table 17–2), which help keep the humeral head properly centered within the glenoid fossa. Furthermore, the posterior rotator cuff muscles apply a posterior force to the humeral head to resist anterior humeral head translation that occurs as the shoulder externally rotates.[14,22] Eccentric internal rotation torque is pro-

duced to decelerate shoulder external rotation. In pitching, a peak shoulder internal rotation torque of approximately 55 to 80 N-m is generated just prior to maximum shoulder external rotation (Fig. 17–9),[12] due to strong eccentric contractions from the shoulder internal rotators (pectoralis major, latissimus dorsi, anterior deltoid, teres major, and subscapularis). In addition, a maximum shoulder anterior shear force of approximately 290 to 470 N (Fig. 17–10) and a shoulder horizontal adduction torque of approximately 80 to 120 N-m (Fig. 17–11) are produced at the shoulder to resist posterior translation at the shoulder and keep the arm moving with the trunk.[12] Shoulder anterior force is greatest when throwing a fastball (Table 17–3). Football passing generates significantly less shoulder joint force and torque compared with baseball pitching.[23]

Elbow joint forces and torques are also generated throughout the arm cocking phase. Maximum elbow extensor torques of approximately 20 to 40 N-m have been reported during the arm cocking phase (Fig. 17–12).[11,12,24] Consequently, the elbow flexors show some activity, but primarily during the middle third of the arm cocking phase.[11,16,19] A large valgus torque is produced at the elbow, caused in part by the large amount of shoulder external rotation. To resist valgus torque, a maximum varus torque of approximately 50 to 75 N-m is generated shortly before maximum shoulder external rotation (see Fig. 17–9).[12] The flexor and pronator muscle mass of the forearm displays moderate to high activity, which contributes to varus torque (see Table 17–2).[19] Since these muscles originate at the medial epicondyle, they contract to help stabilize the elbow. Large tensile forces on the medial aspect of the elbow result from the valgus torque placed on the arm. Repetitive valgus loading may eventually lead to injury to the ulnar collateral ligament (UCL); furthermore, inflammation of the medial epicondyle or adjacent tissues may also occur (i.e., medial epicondylitis).

An in vitro study by Morrey and An[25] showed that the UCL contributes approximately 54 percent of the resistance to valgus. Assuming that the UCL produces 54 percent of a 64-N-m varus torque generated by an elite pitcher, the UCL would then provide 35 N-m of the varus torque.[12] This is similar to the 32-N-m failure load of the UCL reported by Dillman et al.[26] Thus, during baseball pitching, the UCL appears to be loaded near its maximum capacity.[12] However, this result is only an approximation of the UCL's contribution in throwing, because the cadaveric research does not account for muscle contributions. Muscle contraction during this phase may reduce the stress on the UCL by compressing the joint and adding stability.[11]

Valgus torque can also cause high compressive force on the lateral elbow, which can lead to lateral elbow compression injury.[12] Specifically, valgus torque can cause compression between the radial head and the humeral capitellum.[1] According to the in vitro study by Morrey and An,[25] 33 percent of the varus torque needed to resist valgus torque applied by the forearm is supplied by joint articulation. Thirty-three percent of the 64-N-m maximum varus torque generated during pitching is 21 N-m. Assuming that the distance from the axis of valgus rotation to the compression point between the radial head and the humeral capitellum is approximately 4 cm, the compressive force generated between the radius and humerus to produce 21 N-m of varus torque is approximately 500 N.[12] Muscle contraction about the elbow or loss of joint integrity on the medial side of the elbow can cause this compressive force to increase. Excessive or repetitive compressive force can result in avascular necrosis, osteochondritis dissecans, or osteochondral chip fractures.[1]

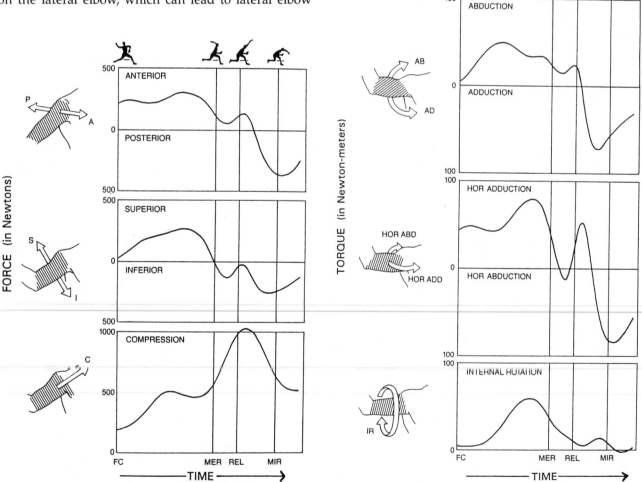

FIGURE 17–10. Forces applied to a pitcher's arm at the shoulder in anterior-posterior (AP), superior-inferior (SI), and compression (C) directions. The instants of foot contact (FC), maximum shoulder external rotation (MER), ball release (REL), and maximum internal rotation (MIR) torque are shown. (From Fleisig GS, Dillman CJ, Escamilla RF, et al: Kinetics of baseball pitching with implications about injury mechanisms. Am J Sports Med 1995; 23:233–239.)

FIGURE 17–11. Torques applied to a pitcher's arm at the shoulder in abduction-adduction (AB-AD), horizontal adduction-abduction (HOR ADD, HOR ABD), and internal rotation (IR) directions. The instants of FC, MER, REL, and MIR torque are shown. (From Fleisig GS, Dillman CJ, Escamilla RF, et al: Kinetics of baseball pitching with implications about injury mechanisms. Am J Sports Med 1995; 23:233–239.)

TABLE 17–3
Elbow and Shoulder Biomechanics of Different Pitches

Phase	Fastball	Curveball	Change-up	Slider
Arm cocking				
Elbow medial force (N)	290	270	240	240
Shoulder anterior force (N)	370	330	320	330
Arm acceleration				
Elbow extension velocity (degree/s)	2400	2400	2100	2400
Shoulder internal rotation velocity (degree/s)	7700	7000	6400	7300
Arm deceleration				
Elbow compressive force (N)	790	730	620	780
Shoulder compressive force (N)	890	820	760	920

Adapted from Escamilla RF, Fleisig GS, Alexander E, et al: A kinematic and kinetic comparison while throwing different types of baseball pitches. Med Sci Sports Exerc 1994; 26:S175.

In addition to a varus torque, a 240- to 360-N medial force is applied by the upper arm onto the forearm to resist lateral translation of the forearm at the elbow (Fig. 17–13). This force is significantly greater when throwing a fastball or curveball than when throwing a slider or change-up (see Table 17–3). The greater medial force during arm cocking in the curveball compared with the change-up or slider may put the medial elbow at greater risk when throwing the curveball. More research is needed to address this issue. The forearm is supinated more during the arm cocking phase for a curveball compared with a fastball, which may also be related to the risk of injury.[27]

Other forces are also produced at the elbow during arm cocking. A maximum anterior elbow force of approximately 100 to 220 N is applied by the upper arm onto the forearm to resist posterior translation of the forearm at the elbow (see Fig. 17–13). In addition, a maximum elbow compressive force of approximately 250 to 350 N is applied by the upper arm to the forearm to resist distraction of the forearm at the elbow (see Fig. 17–13).

The elbow achieves maximum flexion of approximately 80 to 90 degrees about 30 ms before maximum shoulder external rotation (see Fig. 17–12).[11,12] Maximum elbow flexion appears to be controlled by the triceps muscle, which shows moderate activity during the last third of the arm cocking phase.[11,19] This hypothesis is supported by data from Roberts[28] that show that if the triceps muscle is paralyzed by a radial nerve block, the elbow "collapses" and continues flexing near its limit (approximately 145 degrees). This collapse is caused by a centripetal flexion torque at the elbow, which is created by the rapidly rotating upper torso and arm. The triceps muscle apparently contracts eccentrically and then isometrically in resisting the centripetal elbow flexion torque that occurs during late arm cocking. At about the time that the elbow reaches maximum elbow flexion (i.e., approximately 30 ms prior to maximum shoulder external rotation), the triceps contracts concentrically to aid in elbow extension.[11,12] The interaction between muscle activity, elbow joint torque, and elbow extension can be seen in Fig.17–12.

ARM ACCELERATION

Arm acceleration begins at maximum shoulder external rotation (see Fig. 17–4H) and ends at ball release (see Fig. 17–4I). The acceleration phase is very rapid, lasting approximately 0.03 to 0.04 s (see Fig. 17–5). The acceleration phase has been shown to have fairly low muscle activity, even though the arm accelerates forward both linearly and angularly.[14,15]

Just prior to maximum shoulder external rotation, elbow extension begins. This movement is followed immediately by the onset of shoulder internal rotation. The initiation of elbow extension before shoulder internal rotation allows the thrower to reduce the rotational inertia about the arm's longitudinal axis, therefore allowing greater internal rotation velocity to be generated. The shoulder internal rotators contract concentrically to help produce an extremely high maximal internal rotation velocity of approximately 7000 to 8000 degrees/s in pitching and 4000 to 5000 degrees/s in football passing (see Table 17–1). Maximal shoulder internal rotation angular velocity, which occurs at approximately ball release, is greatest during the fastball and least during the change-up (see Table 17–3). Electromyographic data show that the subscapularis is the most active of the shoulder internal rotators, followed by the latissimus dorsi and pectoralis major.[18,19,21,29]

As the elbow extends and the shoulder internally rotates, the trunk flexes forward from its hyperextended position to a neutral position at ball release. High muscle activity from the trunk flexors (rectus abdominis and obliquus) has been demonstrated during the acceleration phase.[30] Forward trunk tilt achieves a maximal angular velocity of approximately 300 to 450 degrees/s for pitchers and 200 to 325 degrees/s for quarterbacks (see Table 17–1). Forward flexing of the trunk is enhanced by the lead knee beginning to straighten, providing a stable base for the trunk to rotate about. At ball release, the lead knee has approximately 30 to 40 degrees of flexion, which is slightly less that seen at foot contact (see Table 17–1). This is due to a straightening of the lead leg, which occurs during the latter portion of the acceleration phase. Forward trunk

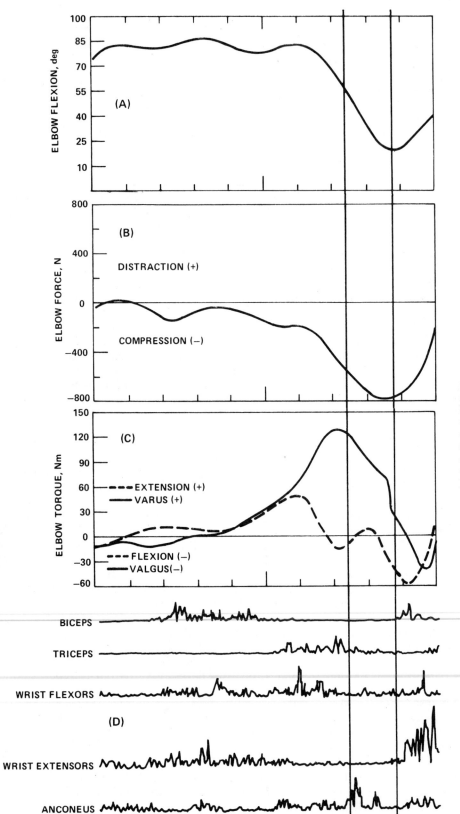

FIGURE 17–12. Time-matched measurements during the baseball pitch: elbow flexion (*A*); force applied at the elbow (*B*); torque applied at the elbow (*C*); and electromyographic muscle activity (*D*). (From Werner SL, Andrews JR, Fleisig GS, et al: Biomechanics of the elbow during baseball pitching. J Orthop Sports Phys Ther 1993; 17:274–278.)

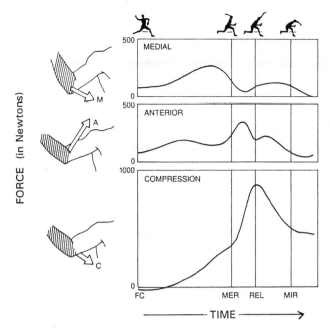

FIGURE 17–13. Forces applied to a pitcher's forearm at the elbow in the medial (M), anterior (A), and compression (C) directions. The instants of FC, MER, REL, and MIR torque are shown. (From Fleisig GS, Dillman CJ, Escamilla RF, et al: Kinetics of baseball pitching with implications about injury mechanisms. Am J Sports Med 1995; 23:233–239.)

tilt may be hindered if the lead knee continues flexing and moving forward. At release, the trunk of a baseball pitcher is normally flexed forward from a vertical position approximately 25 to 40 degrees, with quarterbacks usually having less forward flexion than pitchers (see Table 17–1). The throwing shoulder remains abducted approximately 80 to 100 degrees throughout the acceleration phase (see Fig. 17–7), which implies that this is a strong position for the shoulder. This is true regardless of the type of throwing pattern that occurs—sidearm, three-quarters, or overhand.[31,32] It is the trunk tilt that changes with varying types of deliveries; and an overhand thrower tilts the trunk sideways (away from the throwing arm) more than a sidearm thrower, whose trunk is close to vertical. In throwing, trunk tilt normally deviates from a vertical position 20 to 30 degrees away from the throwing arm (see Table 17–1).

The rotator cuff muscles, trapezius, serratus anterior, rhomboids, and levator scapula all demonstrate high levels of activity during the acceleration phase.[19] This implies that humeral head control and scapula stabilization are crucial during this phase. However, Gowan[21] demonstrated that rotator cuff activity is significantly different between professional and amateur pitchers. Muscle activity of the infraspinatus, teres minor, supraspinatus, and biceps was two to three times higher in amateur pitchers. In contrast, the muscle activity of the subscapularis, serratus anterior, and latissimus dorsi was much greater in professional pitchers. These findings may imply that professional pitchers better coordinate the movements of their body segments to increase throwing efficiency. This improved efficiency

may minimize glenohumeral instability during the arm cocking and arm acceleration phases, thus less rotator cuff muscle activity is needed. These findings also seem to support the results of previous electromyographic studies.[14,15]

Maximum elbow angular velocity during pitching occurs at approximately halfway through the acceleration phase and reaches a peak of approximately 2100 to 2400 degrees/s (see Tables 17–1 and 17–3).[11] This rapid elbow extension may be due to centrifugal force acting at the elbow as the trunk and arm rotate, for it is unlikely that the elbow extensors can shorten fast enough to generate the high angular velocity measured at the elbow.

Several studies have examined the role of the triceps in extending the elbow during the acceleration phase of throwing. Roberts[28] reported that a pitcher with a paralyzed triceps due to a differential nerve block was able to throw a ball at over 80 percent of the speed attained prior to paralysis. This seems to support the concept that triceps contraction does not generate all the elbow extension velocity and that centrifugal force is a major factor. Electromyography has shown high triceps and anconeus activity during the arm acceleration phase, suggesting that the triceps probably initiates or contributes some of the angular velocity generated during this phase.[11,15,16,19] However, these muscles may function more as arm stabilizers than as accelerators.[24]

Toyoshima et al.[33] compared "normal throwing" (using the entire body) to throwing using only the forearm to extend the elbow. The latter "forearm throw" involved a maximum voluntary effort to extend the elbow with the upper arm immobilized. If it is assumed that the triceps muscle shortened as fast as voluntarily possible during the forearm throw, the resulting elbow angular velocity would be the maximum that could be generated with maximum triceps contraction alone. The results from this study showed that normal throwing generated about twice the elbow angular velocity that could be achieved during forearm throwing. It was concluded that the elbow was swung open like a whip when the entire body was involved in the throw, and that the elbow angular velocity that occurred during normal throwing was due more to the rotary actions of other parts of the body—such as the hips, trunk, and shoulder—than to the elbow-extending capabilities of the triceps. It was further stated that in normal throwing, the elbow contributed less than 43 percent to ball velocity, and that a larger contribution to ball velocity resulted from body rotation.

Ahn[34] used computer simulations and optimization techniques to compare theoretical data with experimental data. His data showed that hand velocity at ball release was approximately 80 percent of the experimental result when the resultant elbow joint torque was set to zero, approximately 95 percent of the experimental value when the resultant wrist joint torque was set to zero, and approximately 75 percent of the experimental value when both the resultant elbow and wrist joint torques were set to zero. Consequently, he concluded that ball velocity at release was generated primarily by body segments other than the upper extremity—namely, the legs, hips, and trunk.

At ball release, the elbow is almost fully extended and is positioned slightly anterior to the trunk. At release, the elbow is flexed approximately 20 to 30 degrees, and shoulder horizontal adduction is approximately 5 to 20 degrees (see Table 17–1). In football passing (compared with pitching), the elbow is flexed more at ball release and is positioned more anteriorly to the trunk.

Shoulder internal rotation torque and elbow varus torque decrease during the arm acceleration phase as the arm begins rotating forward and generating speed. By the time the arm has reached its maximum velocity, near the time of ball release, low forces and torques are generated at the shoulder and elbow joints (see Figs. 17–10 to 17–13).[11,31,32,35] However, resisting valgus stress at the elbow can result in a wedging of the olecranon against the medial aspect of the trochlear groove and the olecranon fossa. This impingement leads to osteophyte production at the posterior and posteromedial aspects of the olecranon tip and can cause chondromalacia and loose body formation.[6] Figure 17–12 shows that substantial varus torque is generated throughout the arm cocking and arm acceleration phases in order to resist valgus torque. During these phases, the elbow extends from approximately 85 degrees elbow flexion to 20 degrees elbow flexion (see Fig. 17–12).[12] This combination of elbow extension and resistance to valgus torque supports the "valgus extension overload" mechanism described by Wilson.[6] In addition, Campbell et al.[36] found greater valgus torque (normalized by body weight × height) in 10-year-old pitchers than in professional pitchers at the instant of ball release, which they thought might be related to "Little League" elbow syndrome in young pitchers.

A maximum elbow compressive force of approximately 600 to 900 N is produced at the elbow to prevent distraction of the forearm due to the centrifugal force acting on the forearm (see Fig. 17–12).[12] In addition, a maximum elbow flexor torque of approximately 50 to 60 N-m is generated by low to moderate activity from the elbow flexors (see Fig. 17–12).[11,12,16,19] Contraction of the elbow flexors in this phase adds compressive force for joint stability and also controls the rate of elbow extension.

The final segment to impart force to the ball is the hand, which moves from a hyperextended wrist position at maximum shoulder external rotation to a neutral wrist position at ball release. The wrist flexors have been shown to be active during this phase of throwing (see Table 17–2). Their activity may initially be eccentric in order to slow down the hyperextending wrist at the beginning of the acceleration phase; however, as they continue to fire, they concentrically contract and flex the wrist as ball release is approached. The pronator teres is also active during this phase to pronate the forearm. Mean ball velocity for college and professional football passers is approximately 45 to 55 mph, whereas college and professional pitchers average approximately 75 to 85 mph (see Table 17–1).

ARM DECELERATION

This phase, which lasts between 0.03 and 0.05 s (see Fig. 17–5), goes from ball release to maximum shoulder internal rotation (Fig. 17–4J). The trunk and hips continue to flex, and the lead knee and throwing elbow continue to extend until almost full extension is reached. The stance leg now starts moving upward in reaction to the flexing trunk and hips. Internal shoulder rotation continues until it reaches approximately 0 degrees (i.e., neutral position). Pronation also occurs at the radioulnar joint during this phase, but it is difficult to quantify the magnitude of pronation, since there are no known studies in the literature that have quantitatively studied forearm pronation during throwing. The moving of the arm forward, down, and across the body may be a natural occurrence in throwing to minimize injury potential at the elbow and shoulder.[37]

Large eccentric loads are needed at both the elbow and the shoulder joints to decelerate the arm. Fisk[38] demonstrated that the pronator teres is quite active as the forearm pronates during the deceleration phase. The biceps and supinator muscles are also eccentrically loaded to decelerate the rapidly pronating forearm. Table 17–2 shows that the brachialis is also active during this phase. The similar firing patterns of the biceps and brachialis suggest that the primary function of the biceps during this phase is to decelerate elbow extension. Elbow extension terminates when the elbow is flexed approximately 15 to 25 degrees. The triceps has been shown to be active after ball release.[15] Since all three heads of the triceps fire in similar sequence and activity, the triceps may affect the elbow more than the shoulder, since only the long head crosses both joints.

The posterior muscles of the shoulder have been identified as having a paramount role in resisting shoulder distraction and anterior subluxation forces.[13–15,18,22,32,35,39,40] Specifically, these muscles include the infraspinatus, supraspinatus, teres major and minor, latissimus dorsi, and posterior deltoid.[13] Contraction of the teres major, latissimus dorsi, and posterior deltoid also helps decelerate the shoulder abduction that occurs during this phase. The lower trapezius, rhomboids, and serratus anterior have all been shown to be quite active, thus providing stability to the scapula (see Table 17–2). The teres minor, which is often an isolated source of rotator cuff pain, has demonstrated the highest activity of all the glenohumeral muscles during this phase, providing a posterior restraint that may limit humeral head anterior translation, horizontal adduction, and shoulder internal rotation.[14,18,19]

In comparing professional and amateur pitchers, Gowan[21] found that amateur pitchers had over twice as much muscle activity in the biceps and posterior deltoid. This may imply that amateur pitchers incur greater posterior shoulder stress due to a less efficient throwing pattern.

The wrist and finger flexors had very high muscle activity during this phase (see Table 17–2). These muscles continue contracting and flexing the wrist. In addition, the wrist and finger extensor muscles demon-

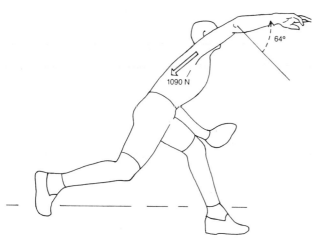

FIGURE 17–14. Shortly after ball release, a second critical instant occurs; at this instant, a pitcher's shoulder is externally rotated 64 degrees and the elbow is flexed 25 degrees. Among the loads generated at this time are 1090 N of compressive force at the shoulder. (From Fleisig GS, Dillman CJ, Escamilla RF, et al: Kinetics of baseball pitching with implications about injury mechanisms. Am J Sports Med 1995; 23:233–239.)

strate low to moderate activity, perhaps being eccentrically active to decelerate the flexing wrist and fingers.

Large shoulder and elbow forces and torques are needed during arm deceleration to slow the rapidly moving arm. Maximum compressive forces of approximately body weight are needed at both the elbow (800 to 1000 N) and the shoulder (1000 to 1200 N) to prevent distraction at these joints (see Figs. 17–10, 17–12, and 17–14).[12] These compressive forces, which are two to three times greater than other shoulder and elbow forces generated during throwing, are greatest during a fastball or slider and least during a change-up (see Table 17–3). Compressive forces are 15 to 20 percent greater in pitchers than in quarterbacks.

A maximum shoulder posterior force of approximately 310 to 490 N and a maximum shoulder horizontal abduction torque of approximately 75 to 125 N-m are applied to the arm in order to resist shoulder horizontal adduction and anterior humeral head translation (see Figs. 17–10 and 17–11).[12] In addition, a maximum shoulder inferior force of approximately 230 to 390 N and a maximum shoulder adduction torque of approximately 60 to 110 N-m are produced to resist shoulder abduction and superior humeral head translation (see Figs. 17–10 and 17–11).[12]

FOLLOW-THROUGH

The follow-through phase begins at the time of maximum shoulder internal rotation and ends when the arm completes its movement across the body and a balanced position is obtained. In the follow-through phase, energy in the throwing arm continues to be dissipated back through the kinetic chain. A long arc of deceleration from the throwing arm, as well as sufficient forward tilting of the trunk, allows energy to be absorbed by the large musculature of the trunk and legs. This absorption helps reduce the stress placed on the

throwing arm. All the body's weight is now borne by a straight or almost straight lead leg. The trunk and hips continue flexing, and the stance leg continues moving upward (see Fig. 17–4K).

As in the deceleration phase, the posterior shoulder muscles continue to be eccentrically active throughout the follow-through, continuing to decelerate the horizontally adducting shoulder. Shoulder and elbow joint forces and torques generated during the follow-through are generally lower than joint forces and torques generated during the deceleration phase.

The serratus anterior has demonstrated the highest activity of all scapular rotators in this phase, contracting either concentrically or isometrically (see Table 17–2); however, the middle trapezius and rhomboids are eccentrically loaded to decelerate scapula protraction. As in the deceleration phase, electromyography has shown that the wrist and finger extensor muscles have low to moderate activity during the follow-through, implying that they are eccentrically loaded to decelerate the flexing wrist (see Table 17–2).

COMMON SHOULDER INJURIES IN THROWING

Most shoulder injuries in throwing involve soft tissues, including muscles, tendons, ligaments, capsule bursae, and fibrocartilaginous tissue. Both static (capsulolabral complex) and dynamic (rotator cuff and scapular rotators) stabilizers control the movement and stability of the humeral head within the glenoid cavity. The subacromion impingement syndrome, in which the rotator cuff muscles and long biceps tendon are intimately involved, is the most common soft tissue injury seen in throwing. The rotator cuff muscles generate shear and compressive forces to depress, rotate, and center the humeral head within the glenoid fossa. Consequently, they help prevent superior translation of the humeral head caused largely by deltoid activity. When these muscles function abnormally, such as when a partial or complete rotator cuff thickness tear occurs or due to muscle fatigue and weakness, superior translation of the humeral head occurs, and the upper surface of the rotator cuff muscles and tendons is abraded against the undersurface of the acromion. Owing to its intimate relationship with the rotator cuff muscles, the long biceps tendon is often impinged as well.

Anterior shoulder instability is also common in throwers, especially baseball pitchers. Glousman et al.[41] reported that muscle activity in pitchers with normal shoulder stability and those with abnormal shoulder stability differed significantly during each pitching phase (Fig. 17–15A through G). The greatest differences in muscle activity were seen during the arm cocking, acceleration, and follow-through phases. Interestingly, the muscle activity patterns of pitchers with normal shoulder stability are very similar to the patterns observed in the professional pitchers studied by Gowan.[21] Furthermore, pitchers with abnormal shoulder stability exhibited muscle activity patterns similar to those observed in amateur pitchers.

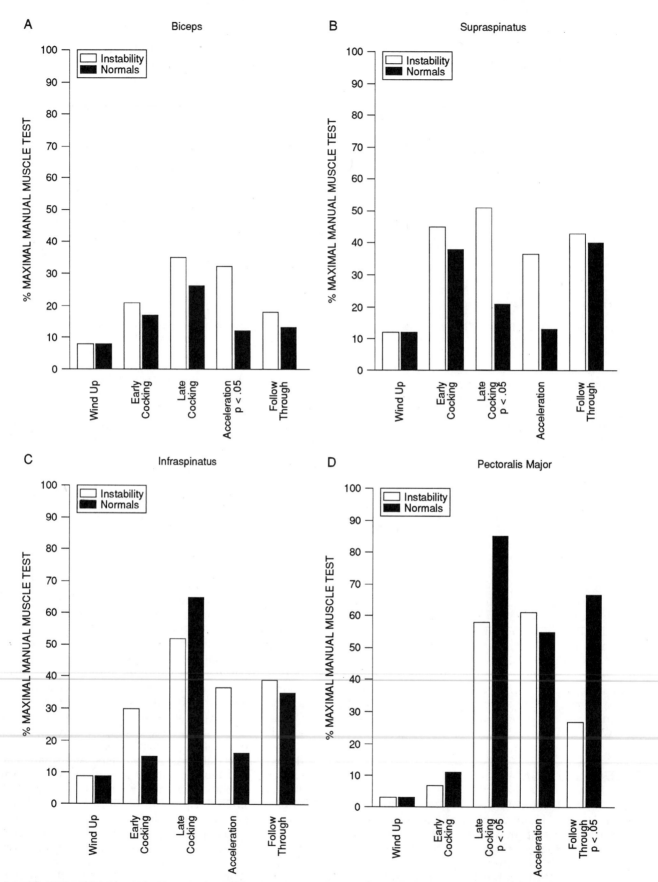

FIGURE 17–15. *A,* Comparison of activity in the biceps brachii in an unstable shoulder as compared with a normal shoulder. A statistically significant difference between the groups (p < 0.05) is indicated. *Note:* Wind-up, early cocking, late cocking, acceleration, and follow-through correspond to wind-up, stride, arm cocking, arm acceleration, and arm deceleration, respectively, in the text. *B,* Comparison study in the supraspinatus in an unstable shoulder as compared with a normal shoulder. A statistically significant difference between the groups (p < 0.05) is indicated. *C,* Comparison of activity in the infraspinatus in an unstable shoulder as compared with a normal shoulder. *D,* Comparison of activity in the pectoralis major in an unstable shoulder as compared with a normal shoulder. A statistically significant difference between the groups (p < 0.05) is indicated.

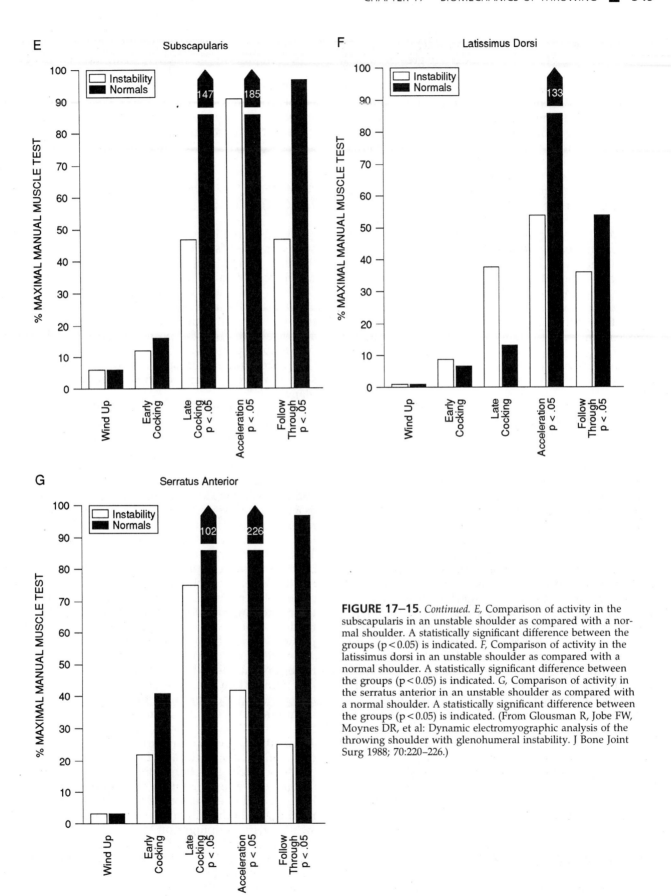

FIGURE 17–15. *Continued. E,* Comparison of activity in the subscapularis in an unstable shoulder as compared with a normal shoulder. A statistically significant difference between the groups (p < 0.05) is indicated. *F,* Comparison of activity in the latissimus dorsi in an unstable shoulder as compared with a normal shoulder. A statistically significant difference between the groups (p < 0.05) is indicated. *G,* Comparison of activity in the serratus anterior in an unstable shoulder as compared with a normal shoulder. A statistically significant difference between the groups (p < 0.05) is indicated. (From Glousman R, Jobe FW, Moynes DR, et al: Dynamic electromyographic analysis of the throwing shoulder with glenohumeral instability. J Bone Joint Surg 1988; 70:220–226.)

Muscle imbalances between the internal and external shoulder rotator muscles can exacerbate the impingement problem. This is true for at least two reasons: (1) the internal rotators of the shoulder are greater in both number and strength compared with the shoulder external rotators; and (2) most weight training programs emphasize muscles that internally rotate the shoulder and de-emphasize those muscles that externally rotate the shoulder.

Impingement can also occur as the subacromion space becomes smaller. An inflamed subacromion bursa or swollen rotator cuff muscle and biceps tendon can decrease the volume of the subacromion space. The subacromion space can also diminish as the shoulder joint musculature and the humerus hypertrophy. These latter conditions are often the result of an overload response that occurs in muscles and connective tissue. Baseball pitchers, for example, may throw several thousand pitches per year. Consequently, this repetitive microtrauma can increase injury potential.

Different phases of the throw affect shoulder structures differently. During the windup and stride, the stresses and muscle activity generated at the shoulder are fairly low; shoulder stress is much greater during the arm cocking, arm acceleration, arm deceleration, and follow-through phases.

ARM COCKING PHASE

The rotator cuff muscles are very active during the arm cocking phase, both to stabilize the humeral head within the glenoid fossa and to control the large external rotation of the shoulder that occurs. Due to the rapid transverse rotation of the trunk, eccentric muscle loading by the horizontal adductors and internal rotators of the shoulder is very high. As the shoulder proceeds into horizontal abduction and external rotation, the humeral head tends to sublux first posteriorly and then anteriorly against the anterior capsule; consequently, tendinitis of the anterior muscle tendons (especially the pectoralis major and latissimus dorsi) is quite common.[3,4,22,42] Muscle imbalances, such as overpowering anterior shoulder muscles and weak posterior shoulder muscles, can also contribute to the humeral head being pulled forward within the glenoid. Repeated stretching of the anterior capsule can further stress the joint, leading to chronic inflammation and damage to the anterior capsular structures and anterior labrum. Hyperlaxity or laxity within the joint can exacerbate this problem, resulting in further anterior shoulder instability. In Glousman's study comparing anterior shoulder instability and normal shoulder stability, he found that the supraspinous muscle showed significantly greater activity in pitchers with anterior shoulder instability (see Fig. 17–15B).[41]

ARM ACCELERATION PHASE

Humeral distraction and translation during the arm acceleration or deceleration phases introduce an in-

creased risk of labrum degeneration. This is due to humeral motion coupled with rapid internal rotation of the humerus, causing a "shoulder grinding factor."[5]

In comparison to pitchers with normal shoulder stability, pitchers with anterior shoulder instability had significant increases in muscle activity of the biceps (see Fig. 17–15C and E). In contrast, pitchers with normal shoulder stability had significantly greater muscle activity in the subscapular, latissimus dorsi, and serratus anterior (see Fig. 17–15E and G).

ARM DECELERATION AND FOLLOW-THROUGH PHASES

Owing to the large eccentric loads on the posterior shoulder muscles during the deceleration and follow-through phases, these muscles are frequently injured during throwing. If the rotator cuff muscles and other posterior shoulder muscles are weak, fatigued, or injured, the humeral head will distract and anteriorly translate out of the glenoid fossa. This action can place abnormal stress on the posterior capsule and lead to "posterior capsule syndrome."[3,4] Repeated abrasions of the posteroinferior capsule structures have been described as creating an exostosis of the posteroinferior glenoid.[43–45]

Although the biceps has been considered to function primarily at the elbow, the biceps also contributes to shoulder abduction and flexion, especially when the shoulder is externally rotated and the forearm is supinated.[46,47] Biceps activity, especially the long head, has been shown to be a significant contributor to shoulder abduction and flexion in a compromised shoulder, such as a torn rotator cuff.[41] Since the biceps long head originates at the anterosuperior glenoid labrum, its contraction could abnormally stress this portion of the labrum. This is especially true in throwing, since the biceps has been shown to eccentrically contract in decelerating the rapidly extending elbow. Andrews[48] arthroscopically observed 73 throwing athletes who had labrum tears in their throwing shoulders. The long head of the biceps tendon appeared to have pulled the anterosuperior portion of the labrum off the glenoid. This observation was verified arthroscopically by electrically stimulating the biceps muscle. When stimulated, the tendinous portion became taut near its attachment to the labrum and actually lifted the labrum off the glenoid.[48]

Another injury that occurs during the deceleration and follow-through phases is a "snapping scapula." This pathology, which can be quite painful, is the result of an inflamed bursa located beneath the medial border of the scapula. This bursa provides lubrication as the scapula moves in relation to the thorax. During repetitive use and overuse conditions, bursitis can develop, resulting in both pain and a "snapping" sound as the swollen tissue impinges on the thorax. A good follow-through can help minimize the injury potential of the shoulder. A long arm arc of deceleration and sufficient forward trunk tilt (trunk approximately in a horizontal position) both help minimize stress on the shoulder complex.

The pectoralis major, subscapularis, latissimus dorsi, and serratus anterior muscles are all active during arm deceleration. Muscle activity is significantly greater in pitchers with anterior shoulder instability (see Fig. 17–15E and G).

COMMON ELBOW INJURIES IN THROWING

Musculotendinous, joint, and neural injuries are the most common problems that occur in the throwing elbow. These pathologies can be compartmentalized into four areas.

ANTERIOR COMPARTMENT

The anterior elbow is the least commonly injured region; however, anterior capsular sprains, flexor-pronator strains, bicipital tendinitis, and intra-articular loose bodies are problems that may occur in the anterior elbow.[49] In a throwing athlete, these pathologies can lead to incomplete elbow extension, especially during the acceleration phase of the throw.

Anterior pain can also result from neural injuries, such as radial nerve entrapment. Repetitive supination and pronation movements, such as those occurring during the throwing motion, can lead to entrapment. For example, anterior pain can occur when the median nerve is entrapped between the two heads of the pronator teres. This is referred to as pronator teres syndrome and occurs due to the repetitive forearm pronation that is seen during throwing.

POSTERIOR COMPARTMENT

The posterior region of the elbow is injured more than the anterior region but less than the medial and lateral regions. Due to overuse, the triceps tendon can be injured (triceps tendinitis) at its insertion on the olecranon. It may even partially avulse off the olecranon.

Due to repetitive extension of the elbow during throwing, the olecranon is continually and forcefully driven into the olecranon fossa. Consequently, a stress fracture of the olecranon or a hypertrophic olecranon may develop. Valgus stress that occurs during late arm cocking and early acceleration may exacerbate the problem by forcing the olecranon against the medial olecranon fossa (i.e., valgus extension overload).[6] Due to the repetitive trauma of the olecranon being forced against the olecranon fossa, osteophytes may form and migrate anteriorly. Loose bodies can also arise due to a shearing off of osteocartilaginous fragments.

MEDIAL COMPARTMENT

Medial musculotendinous injuries are quite common, especially involving the muscles that originate at the medial epicondyle (medial epicondylitis). These mus-

cles, which are collectively referred to as the flexor-pronator mass, comprise primarily the pronator teres, radial flexor of the wrist, superficial flexor of the fingers, and ulnar flexor of the wrist. During throwing, pain and tenderness can occur in the medial epicondyle region. The flexor-pronator mass is greatly stressed as a result of tensile force during the late arm cocking and early acceleration phases of throwing. These dynamic contractile structures must apply a varus torque to the forearm to resist the valgus stress created by the throwing motion. Valgus stress is greatest as the forearm approaches maximum shoulder external rotation during the arm cocking phase. An excessive or repetitive valgus stress can also create abnormal tension on the medial capsule.

Capsular and ligamentous tensile stress on the ulna and humerus may lead to osteophyte formation. These osteophytes usually form distally at the ulnar attachment. Since the ulnar nerve lies near the medial capsule and ulnar collateral ligament (UCL), these osteophytes may compress the nerve. Furthermore, the repetitive valgus stress of the medial elbow during throwing can excessively stretch the ulnar nerve, contributing to ulnar neuritis. The UCL, which also originates at the medial epicondyle, helps reinforce the medial elbow capsule. The UCL is most susceptible to injury when the flexor-pronator muscle mass weakens and fatigues owing to repetitive throwing and overuse.

In order to protect a previously injured elbow, an athlete may try to alter his or her mechanics; specifically, he or she may "lead with the elbow" and increase elbow flexion and shoulder horizontal adduction. Such modification in throwing mechanics may indeed reduce the load on the medial aspect of the elbow but may increase the load and injury probability at other locations, such as the shoulder complex. Leading with the elbow may also decrease performance, since throwing velocity is lower. Leading with the elbow seems to occur naturally in Little League pitchers or pitchers who have injured their arms and may be afraid to throw 100 percent.

LATERAL COMPARTMENT

In contrast to medial musculotendinous injuries, lateral musculotendinous injuries involve the wrist and finger extension musculature. These muscles, which all originate at or near the lateral epicondyle, can cause lateral epicondylitis when abnormally stressed. These muscles are rapidly stretched and eccentrically loaded during the deceleration and follow-through phases in pitching.

Whereas the medial elbow is subject to high tensile stresses, the lateral region is subject to high compressive forces. These compressive forces occur between the radial head and the humeral capitellum. Degenerative changes in the articular cartilage of these structures can result from the repetitive compressive stress across the radiocapitellum joint. Consequently, loose body formations can occur as the articular cartilage fragments break off into the joint. Osteochondrosis of the radiocapitellum joint may also occur in preadolescent athletes before physeal closure.

IMPLICATIONS FOR REHABILITATION

Because of the involvement of the full body in the throwing motion, it is important to condition the musculature of both the upper and the lower body to maximize performance and minimize the risk of injury. The principle of the kinetic chain implies that weakness in any segment may result in a deficiency in performance. When an athlete with a deficiency in one section of the kinetic chain tries to compensate by increasing the demands on other segments, injury can result.

It is especially important to evaluate a thrower's mechanics after rehabilitation from an injury. Improper mechanics may be related to either the cause of the initial injury or modifications resulting from the initial injury. In either case, improper mechanics should be corrected to prevent reinjury.

Joint flexibility and high-speed, controlled motion are essential for throwing and should be emphasized in a rehabilitation program. Constrained exercises that include limited ranges of motion and joint speeds are useful during rehabilitation, but they have certain limitations. Another important concept in the design and selection of a rehabilitation program for a throwing athlete is that joint loads in throwing are largely eccentric. These eccentric loads occur primarily in the arm cocking, acceleration, and deceleration phases. Exercises emphasizing eccentric contractions should therefore be performed with appropriate ranges of motion and speeds of movement. The best exercise for throwing rehabilitation is throwing. Under the guidance of a therapist or trainer, an athlete should include throwing in the rehabilitation program as soon as possible. An interval throwing program or other moderate throwing program may be appropriate. Joint loads do not reach maximum values during the acceleration phase, where velocity is maximum, but rather during the arm cocking and deceleration phases of the throw. In accordance with Newton's second law of motion, it is the acceleration of a segment, not the velocity, that is proportional to the net force acting on that segment. The analogy of a skater can be used again. A skater who wishes to skate quickly for a short distance needs to generate significant force to start the motion, minimal force to move at a fast speed, and significant force to stop the motion.

SUMMARY

Throwing is a highly dynamic activity in which body segments move through large ranges of motion and high speeds of movement; consequently, large joint forces and torques are generated, especially at the elbow and shoulder. A proper understanding of the throwing mechanism is helpful to physicians, therapists, trainers, and coaches in recommending appropriate treatment and conditioning.

REFERENCES

1. Atwater AE: Biomechanics of overarm throwing movements and of throwing injuries. Exerc Sport Sci Rev 1979; 7:43–85.
2. DeHaven KE: Throwing injuries of the elbow in athletes. Orthop Clin North Am 1973; 4:801–808.
3. Jobe F, Kvitne R: Shoulder pain in the overhand or throwing athlete: the relationship of anterior instability and rotator cuff impingement. Orthop Rev 1989; 18:963–975.
4. McLeod WD, Andrews JR: Mechanisms of shoulder injuries. Phys Ther 1986; 66:1901–1904.
5. McLeod WD: The pitching mechanism. In Zarins B, Andrews JR, Cheson WG: Injuries to the Throwing Arm. Philadelphia, WB Saunders, 1985, pp 22–29.
6. Wilson FD: Valgus extension overload in the pitching elbow. Am J Sports Med 1983; 11:83–88.
7. Feltner ME, Dapena J: Three-dimensional interactions in a two-segment kinetic chain. Part I. General model. Int J Sport Biomech 1989; 5:403–419.
8. Feltner ME, Dapena J: Three-dimensional interactions in a two-segment kinetic chain. Part II. Application to the throwing arm in baseball pitching. Int J Sport Biomech 1989; 5:420–450.
9. Dillman CJ: Proper mechanics of pitching. Sports Med Update 1990; 5:15–18.
10. Dillman CJ, Fleisig GS, Andrews JR: Biomechanics of pitching with emphasis upon shoulder kinematics. J Orthop Sports Phys Ther 1993; 18:402–408.
11. Werner SL, Fleisig GS, Dillman CJ, Andrews JR: Biomechanics of the elbow during baseball pitching. J Orthop Sports Phys Ther 1993; 17:274–278.
12. Fleisig GS, Dillman CJ, Andrews JR: Kinetics of baseball pitching with implications about injury mechanisms. Am J Sports Med 1995; 23:233–239.
13. Jacobs P: The overhand baseball pitch: a kinesiological analysis and related strength-conditioning programming. NCSA 1987; 9:5–13.
14. Jobe FW, Moynes DR, Tibone JE, Perry J: An EMG analysis of the shoulder in throwing and pitching: a preliminary report. Am J Sports Med 1983; 11:3–5.
15. Jobe FW, Moynes DR, Tibone JE, Perry J: An EMG analysis of the shoulder in pitching: a second report. Am J Sports Med 1984; 12:218–220.
16. Sisto DJ, Jobe FW, Moynes DR: An electromyographic analysis of the elbow in pitching. Am J Sports Med 1987; 15:260–263.
17. Fleisig GS, Dillman CJ, Andrews JR: Proper mechanics for baseball pitching. Clin Sports Med 1989; 1:151–170.
18. Bradley JP: Electromyographic analysis of muscle action about the shoulder. Clin Sports Med 1991; 10:789–805.
19. DiGiovine NM: An electromyographic analysis of the upper extremity in pitching. J Shoulder Elbow Surg 1992; 1:15–25.
20. Brown LP, Niehues SL, Harrah A: Upper extremity range of motion and isokinetic strength of internal and external shoulder rotators in major league baseball players. Am J Sports Med 1988; 16:577–585.
21. Gowan ID: Comparative electromyographic analysis of the shoulder during pitching. J Sports Med 1987; 15:586–590.
22. Cain PR: Anterior stability of the glenohumeral joint. Am J Sports Med 1987; 15:144–148.
23. Wick H, Dillman CJ, Werner S, et al: A kinematic comparison between baseball pitching and football passing. Sports Med Update 1991; 6:13–16.
24. Feltner M, Dapena J: Dynamics of the shoulder and elbow joints of the throwing arm during a baseball pitch. Int J Sport Biomech 1986; 2:235–259.
25. Morrey BF, An KN: Articular and ligamentous contributions to the stability of the elbow joint. Am J Sports Med 1983; 11:315–319.
26. Dillman CJ, Smutz C, Werner S: Valgus extension overload in baseball pitching. Med Sci Sports Exerc 1991; 23(suppl 4): S135.
27. Sakurai S, Ikegami Y, Dkamato A: A three-dimensional cinematographic analysis of the baseball pitch. In Proceedings from the 6th International Symposium on Biomechanics in Sports. Bozeman, MT, 1990.

28. Roberts TW: Cinematography in biomechanical investigation: selected topics in biomechanics. *In* CIC Symposium on Biomechanics. Chicago, Athletic Institute, 1971, pp 41–50.
29. Moynes DR: Electromyography and motion analysis of the upper extremity in sports. Phys Ther 1986; 66:1905–1911.
30. Watkins RG, Dennis S, Dillin WH: Dynamic EMG analysis of torque transfer in professional baseball pitchers. Spine 1989; 14:404–408.
31. Dillman CJ, Fleisig GS, Werner SL: Biomechanics of the shoulder in sports: throwing activities. *In* Postgraduate Studies in Sports Physical Therapy. Rosemont, IL, Forum Medicum, 1991, pp 621–633.
32. Fleisig GS, Dillman CJ, Andrews JR: Biomechanics of the shoulder during throwing. *In* Andrews JR, Wilk KE (eds): The Athlete's Shoulder. New York, Churchill Livingstone, 1994, pp 355–368.
33. Toyoshima S, Hoshikawa T, Miyashita M: Contributions of the body parts of throwing performance. *In* Nelson RC, Morehouse CA (eds): Biomechanics IV. Baltimore, University Park Press, 1974, pp 169–174.
34. Ahn BH: A model of the human upper extremity and its application to a baseball pitching motion. East Lansing, MI, Michigan State University, 1991.
35. Fleisig GS, Dillman CJ, Andrews JR: A biomechanical description of the shoulder joint during pitching. Sports Med Update 1991; 6:10–15.
36. Campbell KR, Hagood SS, Takagi Y: Kinetic analysis of the elbow and shoulder in professional and little league pitchers. Med Sci Sports Exerc 1994; 26:S175.
37. Dillman CJ, Fleisig GS, Werner SL: Biomechanics of the shoulder in sports: throwing activities. *In* Matsen FA (ed): The Shoulder: A Balance of Mobility and Stability. American Academy of Orthopaedic Surgeons, Rosemont, IL, 1993, pp 621–633.
38. Fisk CS: Dynamic function of skeletal muscles of the forearm: an electromyographical and cinematographical analysis. Indiana University, 1976.
39. Tullos HS, King JW: Throwing mechanism in sports. Orthop Clin North Am 1973; 4:709–720.
40. Howell SM, Kraft TA: The role of the supraspinatus and intraspinatus muscles in glenohumeral kinematics of anterior shoulder instability. Clin Orthop Rel Res 1991; 263:128–134.
41. Glousman R, Jobe FW, Tibone JE: Dynamic electromyographic analysis of the throwing shoulder with glenohumeral instability. J Bone Joint Surg 1988; 70A:220–226.
42. Harryman DT: Translation of the humeral head on the glenoid with passive glenohumeral motion. J Bone Joint Surg 1990; 72A:1334–1343.
43. Colachis SC, Strohn BR: Effects of suprascapular and axillary nerve blocks on muscle force in upper extremity. Arch Phys Med Rehabil 1971; 52:22–29.
44. Doody SG, Freedman L, Waterland JC: Shoulder movements during abduction in the scapular plane. Arch Phys Med Rehabil 1970; 51:595–604.
45. Dvir Z, Berme N: Shoulder complex in elevation of the arm: a mechanism approach. J Biomech 1978; 11:219–225.
46. Basmajian JV: Integrated actions and functions of the chief flexors of the elbow: a detailed electromyographic analysis. J Bone Joint Surg 1957; 39A:1106–1118.
47. Furlani J: Electromyographic study of the m. biceps brachii in movements of the glenohumeral joint. Acta Anat 1976; 96:270–284.
48. Andrews JR: Glenoid labrum tears related to the long head of the biceps. Am J Sports Med 1985; 13:337–341.
49. Andrews JR: Common elbow problems in the athlete. J Orthop Sports Phys Ther 1993; 17:289–295.
50. Escamilla RF, Fleisig GS, Alexander E: A kinematic and kinetic comparison while throwing different types of baseball pitches. Med Sci Sports Exerc 1994; 26:S175.

CHAPTER 18

Applied Sports Biomechanics in Rehabilitation: Running

T H O M A S   G.   M C P O I L   *PhD, PT, ATC*
M A R K   W.   C O R N W A L L   *PhD, PT*

The evaluation and management of running injuries present a tremendous challenge to the health care provider. When evaluating the client with a running injury, the clinician must be aware of the numerous differences in anatomic alignment and mechanics that occur during running in comparison to walking. Furthermore, the activity of running causes an increase in ground reaction forces and pressures acting on the plantar surface of the foot. These variations in anatomic alignment, ground reaction force, and plantar pressures can significantly magnify abnormalities in lower extremity alignment and result in overuse or repetitive trauma to body tissues. Successful treatment is dependent on the ability of the clinician to recognize those biomechanical factors that can lead to excessive tissue stress.

Numerous surveys have been conducted to determine the most common running injuries. One of the first epidemiologic studies on running injuries was conducted by James et al. in 1978.[1] They reported that 30 percent of all injuries occurred in the knee, with another 13 percent of patients having shin splints, and an additional 7 percent diagnosed with plantar fasciitis. Lutter reported similar results in a survey of 171 runners, with 50 percent of all injuries occurring in the foot and 29 percent in the knee.[2] A subsequent survey of 540 runners conducted by Kerner and D'Amico in 1983 found that 28 percent had shin splints and 25 percent had knee pain.[3]

The results of these epidemiologic surveys indicate that the most common problem affecting the runner is injury of the knee complex, followed by lower leg and foot injuries. Based on the findings of these studies, it becomes obvious that the clinician must evaluate the entire lower extremity when treating the injured runner. To highlight those anatomic and mechanical factors that can result in overuse injuries during running, this chapter will first describe the kinematic or movement patterns associated with the running cycle. The electromyographic activity of lower extremity musculature as well as the ground reaction force and plantar pressure patterns that occur during running will then be discussed. Finally, variations in lower extremity alignment that can cause abnormal movement patterns of the lower extremity during running and lead to overuse injuries will be reviewed.

BIOMECHANICS OF RUNNING

RUNNING KINEMATICS

THE RUNNING CYCLE. Running is basic to almost every athletic activity. The primary objective of running is to move the body rapidly over the ground. This is accomplished by repeatedly propelling the body forward through the alternating movements of each lower extremity.

The running cycle has been previously described by numerous authors,[4-8] who have broken the act of running into a series of strides or cycles. Each stride is further divided into a support phase and a flight or recovery phase. Thus, a support and a flight/recovery phase for the same extremity constitutes one stride. The periods of support and flight have been further divided into six separate components, or subphases (Fig. 18–1).

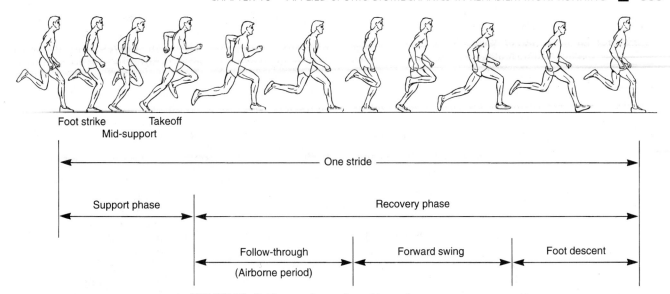

Foot strike   Takeoff
          Mid-support

One stride

Support phase

Recovery phase

Follow-through

(Airborne period)

Forward swing

Foot descent

FIGURE 18–1. The running cycle and its various components.

The three components of the support phase are foot strike, mid-support, and takeoff. The three components of the recovery phase are follow-through, forward swing, and foot descent.

The support phase begins with foot strike. Foot strike occurs when the foot initially contacts the ground and continues until the plantar surface of the foot is fully plantigrade to the support surface. The mid-support component of the support phase starts from the point at which the foot is in full contact with the ground and continues until the heel starts to leave the ground. The final component of the support phase is takeoff, which begins when the heel starts to leave the ground and continues until the toes are completely free of the supporting surface. The primary purposes of the support phase are to (1) re-establish contact with the supporting surface; (2) provide a stable base of support for the advancing opposite limb in its flight phase; and (3) reverse the retarding influence of the early stance phase, as well as accelerate the runner's mass forward to the next cycle.

The initial component of the flight or recovery phase is follow-through. Follow-through starts at the end of takeoff, when the trailing foot leaves the ground, and continues until that foot stops any posterior or backward motion. The second component of the flight or recovery phase is termed *forward swing*. Forward swing begins with the initiation of forward movement of the foot and stops when the foot reaches the most forward position. The final component of the flight or recovery phase is foot descent. Foot descent starts at the point of maximal hip flexion, with the foot at its most forward position. Foot descent continues until foot strike, at which time a new cycle is initiated. The primary purpose of the flight or recovery phase is to add momentum to the center of mass by means of the swinging limb.

During the flight or recovery phase, the airborne period occurs. This is the period in which neither foot is in contact with the ground. Because neither foot is in contact with the ground, when the swinging foot recontacts the ground at foot strike, the magnitude of ground reaction force is substantially increased in comparison with walking. Various studies have indicated that the ground reaction force during running may be as much as two to three times greater than when walking.[9,10] This increase in the magnitude of ground reaction force is an example of Newton's second law of motion, which states that force is equivalent to mass times acceleration. If an individual's mass remains constant and he or she accelerates his or her mass, then the ground reaction forces at foot strike will be increased. This is certainly the case when going from walking to running. Furthermore, a byproduct of this change in ground reaction force is an increase in both the amplitude and the rate of foot pronation during the support phase of running. These factors, which are unique to running, can combine to result in an injury that would not occur during walking.

JOINT MOVEMENTS DURING RUNNING. A summary of joint movements in the lower extremity during running is found in Table 18–1. The amount of joint movement that occurs in the hip, knee, and ankle during the running cycle is different from that that occurs during the walking cycle. From foot strike to the mid-support period of the support phase, hip joint flexion decreases from 45 degrees to 20 degrees, while knee joint flexion increases from 20 degrees to 40 degrees. The position of the ankle (talocrural) joint at foot strike is 5 degrees plantar flexed, with progression to 10 degrees dorsiflexion by the mid-support phase.

One of the major differences between running and walking is the position of the knee joint when the foot makes contact with the ground. During walking, the knee joint is either completely extended or flexed approximately 5 degrees at the time of heel strike. At the instant of foot strike in running, the knee joint is already in at least 20 degrees of flexion. This flexed position of the knee is important to assist the runner in attenuating impact forces that are being applied through the lower extremity. Unfortunately, this greater degree of knee flexion also causes increased compressive forces be-

TABLE 18–1
Typical Range-of-Motion Values for the Lower Extremities During Running

Running Phase	Joint	Motion
Foot strike* to mid-support†	Hip	45°–20° flexion at mid-support
	Knee	20°–40° flexion by mid-support
	Ankle	5° plantar flexion to 10° dorsiflexion
Midsupport to take-off‡	Hip	20° flexion to 5° extension
	Knee	40°–15° flexion
	Ankle	10°–20° dorsiflexion
Follow-through	Hip	5°–20° Hyperextension
	Knee	15°–5° flexion
	Ankle	20°–30° plantar flexion
Forward swing‖	Hip	20°–65° flexion
	Knee	5°–130° flexion
	Ankle	30° plantar flexion to 0°
Foot descent¶	Hip	65°–40° flexion
	Knee	130°–20° flexion
	Ankle	0°–5° dorsiflexion to 5° plantar flexion

*Foot strike begins when the foot first touches the ground and continues until the foot is firmly fixed.

†Mid-support starts when the foot is fixed and continues until the heel leaves the ground.

‡Take-off begins when the heel starts to rise and continues until the toes leave the ground.

§Follow-through begins as the trailing foot leaves the ground and continues until the foot ceases rearward motion. It includes the airborne period.

‖Forward swing starts with forward motion of the foot and stops when the foot reaches its most forward position.

¶Foot descent starts after the recovering foot has reached it most forward position, reverses direction, and then terminates with foot strike.

tween the patella and femur. This is an important factor, considering the extremely high incidence of knee injuries, particularly to the patellofemoral joint, in runners. This flexed position of the knee joint at foot strike also implies that flexibility of the soleus muscle is just as important as flexibility of the gastrocnemius when assessing range of motion in runners.

From mid-support to takeoff, the hip joint moves from 20 degrees of flexion to a 5-degree extended position, helping to propel the runner's mass forward in preparation for the next foot strike. The knee joint decreases the amount of its flexion by moving from a 40-degree to a 15-degree position. Finally, the talocrural joint moves from a 10-degree dorsiflexed position to a 20-degree plantar flexed position. During the flight or recovery phase, the swinging limb assists in increasing the forward momentum of the runner, thereby improving efficiency. From takeoff to forward swing, the hip joint will move from 5 degrees of extension to 20 degrees of flexion. The knee joint starts in a 15-degree flexed position and moves to within 5 degrees of full extension. The talocrural joint moves from a 20-degree

plantar flexed position to approximately 30 degrees of plantar flexion. As was previously mentioned, during forward swing, the hip joint moves into its most maximally flexed position. Thus, the hip joint moves from a 20-degree extended position to a 65-degree flexed position. At the same time, the knee joint undergoes 125 degrees of motion, moving from a 5-degree flexed position to almost 130 degrees of flexion. This amount of knee joint motion is significantly greater than that during walking, which is only 65 to 70 degrees, and, as previously mentioned, is related to the greater momentum generated by the lower limbs during running. Finally, the talocrural joint will move from 30 degrees of plantar flexion to a position of neutral (i.e., neither dorsiflexed nor plantar flexed). During foot descent, the hip joint will move from a 65-degree flexed position to 40 degrees of flexion, whereas the knee joint moves from 130 degrees of flexion to 20 degrees of flexion in preparation for foot strike. The talocrural joint will move from 0 to 5 degrees of dorsiflexion to 5 degrees of plantar flexion in preparation for foot strike.

STRIDE LENGTH CHARACTERISTICS. A major issue when evaluating a client's running cycle is the optimal stride length for that individual runner, as well as variations in stride length that can occur with different speeds of running. In general, stride length increases as the speed of running increases. However, there will be variations depending on whether the person is running on level ground, uphill, or downhill. Cavanagh[11] notes that when running uphill, stride length decreases, whereas during downhill running, stride length is typically increased. Landry and Zebas noted that improved running performance was generally associated with increased stride rate, but not necessarily with increased stride length.[12] Cavanagh and Williams demonstrated that at a specific running speed, each individual has a stride length that appears to be optimal in terms of utilizing the most efficient metabolic energy necessary for running.[13] Their study further showed that forcing an individual to lengthen or shorten his or her stride could possibly increase energy cost by 1 to 2 percent. This is an important point for clinicians to remember when they are considering advising runners to reduce or increase their stride length. Although it might seem impractical to suggest that runners change their self-selected stride length because of the possibility of increasing energy costs, certain injuries may dictate a recommendation to modify stride length. For example, the individual who is having heel pain might be advised to reduce or shorten his or her stride length. By shortening his or her stride, the runner with a diagnosis of plantar fasciitis can enhance the possibility of contacting the ground with the midfoot rather than with the rearfoot, thereby decreasing impact stress to the heel tissues.

FOOT PLACEMENT DURING RUNNING. Another factor that differs between walking and running is a variation in the base of gait, or the distance between the midpoints of the heels. Murray et al. reported that in walking, the typical base of gait for both men and women was approximately 2 to 4 inches.[14,15] In running, however, this value approaches 0.[11] The implications of this are that in running, instead of having the feet fall 1 to 2 inches on either side of the line of progression, both feet actually fall on the same line of progression. The reason for this decrease in base of gait during running is because of an increase in the functional limb varus of the entire support leg. Functional limb varus is defined as the angle between the bisection of the lower leg and the floor. An increase in functional limb varus results during the period of single limb support when the pelvis is shifted laterally over the single supporting lower extremity. During running, the entire center of mass of the body must be placed over the single support foot. During walking, however, even though there is a period of single limb support, the movement of the body's center of mass is not usually displaced completely over the single support foot. Bogdan et al. were the first to report that there was an increase in functional limb varus during running.[16] In their report, Bogdan and colleagues noted that there was an approximate 10-degree increase in functional limb varus in running compared with walking.

McPoil and Cornwall assessed five female and five male cross country runners using two-dimensional videography to determine the change in functional limb varus during running in comparison with walking.[17] They found that the average increase in functional limb varus when going from walking to running was approximately 5 degrees. Figure 18–2 illustrates the increase in functional limb varus in a runner while walking and running.

Recognition of this increase in functional limb varus by the clinician is important when evaluating the runner, as a change in alignment can increase both valgus stress at the knee and foot pronation. The clinician should attempt to evaluate the change in the angle of the lower leg to the floor when evaluating runners with lower extremity injuries. This is accomplished by having the individual shift his or her weight laterally while standing with both feet in contact with the ground (Fig. 18–3A) and then assuming a position of single limb support (Fig. 18–3B). We have found that the average increase in single limb varus when shifting from standing on both feet to standing on a single limb is approximately 5 degrees.

The clinician must also consider the effect of functional limb varus on foot movement. If the amount of functional limb varus increases during running, a greater degree of foot pronation is required to allow the foot to remain plantigrade to the supporting surface. Thus, even if the runner does not excessively pronate during walking, the increase in functional limb varus during the running cycle will cause a greater degree of pronation during running. This increased amount of foot pronation may lead to excessive soft tissue stress in the lower extremity and foot. The end result of this excessive tissue stress may be the development of plantar fasciitis, shin splints, or knee pain. Because a greater amount of foot pronation is expected to occur during running, clinicians should counsel their clients to use running shoes that have adequate rearfoot stabilization. Running shoes with enhanced rearfoot stabilization features can assist in controlling excessive foot pronation, thereby reducing soft tissue stress while running.

REARFOOT MOTION DURING RUNNING. Of major interest to the clinician treating a runner is the effect of the running cycle on the pattern of foot motion. The preceding section discussed the fact that the increase in functional limb varus will cause increased foot pronation in order to allow the plantar surface of the foot to fully contact the supporting surface. Several investigations have studied the pattern of rearfoot motion during the running cycle[18–20] and have reported that the

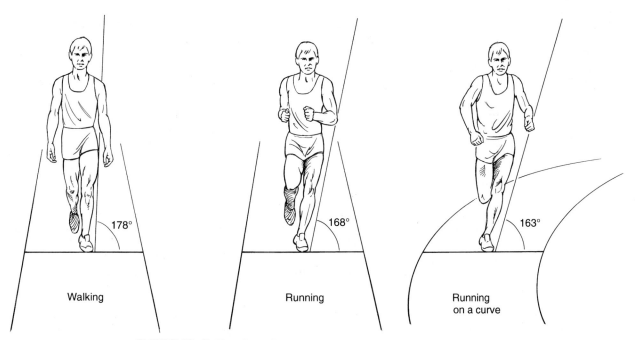

178°   Walking

168°   Running

163°   Running on a curve

FIGURE 18–2. The effect of walking and running on functional limb varus.

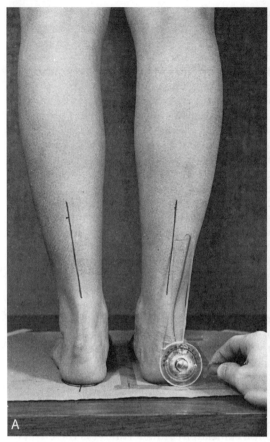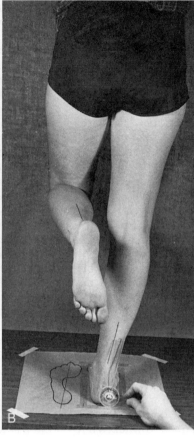

FIGURE 18–3. Static assessment of functional limb varus. Bilateral limb stance assessment *(A)* and single limb stance assessment *(B)*.

period of pronation is longer during running than walking. Other studies have also shown that the magnitude of foot pronation is also greater during running than during walking. Another factor that affects rearfoot motion during running is the increase in ground reaction forces, which can cause greater acceleration of foot pronation.

Studies that have analyzed rearfoot motion have used both two- and three-dimensional analysis techniques.[19–27] In general, these studies have defined rearfoot motion as the movement of the calcaneus in relation to the lower one third of the leg. Three-dimensional rearfoot analysis has been shown to be significantly different from two-dimensional analysis during running. These differences are caused primarily by projection errors onto the plane of a single camera placed behind the subject.[19,20] In 1990 Areblad et al. compared two-dimensional and three-dimensional measurement of rearfoot inversion/eversion during running and found that as the alignment angle between the foot and camera axis increased, so did the differences between the two measurement methods.[19] They advised the use of a three-dimensional model when studying motion between the foot and lower leg during running. Soutas-Little and colleagues also made a comparative study of two- and three-dimensional analysis of foot motion during running.[20] Although they found that projection errors did occur when measuring foot inversion and eversion with two-dimensional analysis techniques, the rearfoot motion determined from two-dimensional measurements approximated

that determined from three-dimensional measurements during much of the running cycle support phase.

Although several authors have attempted to look not just at rearfoot and midfoot motion during walking, no studies to date have attempted to assess both rearfoot and midfoot motion during the running cycle. Based on published rearfoot motion studies, the clinician should expect the rate or speed of pronation, as well as the total magnitude of pronation, to increase during the running cycle. Thus, appropriate shoes and the use of foot orthoses must be considered if the clinician desires to control or modify the amount and speed of rearfoot pronation as part of the management program.

MUSCLE ACTIVITY DURING RUNNING

In general, investigations of muscle action during running have demonstrated increased magnitudes of electromyographic (EMG) activity in comparison with walking.[28] In addition, the duration of EMG activity has been found to be longer during the support phase of running in comparison to the stance phase of walking.[28] However, the reader should be aware that the majority of researchers have used surface electrodes, rather than indwelling or fine wire electrodes, to study EMG activity because of the velocity and intensity of the motions required for running.

HIP JOINT. Hip joint flexors have been shown to have a greater period of EMG activity during the forward swing of running than during the swing phase of walking. The rectus femoris muscle is active during the early support phase and then diminishes toward the end of the support phase.[29–31] The lack of appreciable activity during the late support and early swing phases shows that muscle contraction is not responsible for limiting hip extension. The hip joint extensors, specifically the gluteus maximus, demonstrate EMG activity early in the foot descent period, and this activity continues through the first 40 percent of the support phase.[8] While the hip joint abductors demonstrate similar EMG activity in both walking and running, the adductors show increased EMG activity throughout the entire support phase.

KNEE JOINT. At the time of foot strike, the quadriceps muscle is very active in preparation for the rapid loading that occurs at this time. The quadriceps muscle group reaches peak activity during the early support phase.[29–31] Quadriceps muscle activity during this period of the running cycle facilitates the shock attenuation process as the hip, knee, and ankle joints undergo flexion to create a shortening of the lower extremity. The hamstring muscles have been shown to be active from before foot strike until the hip joint completes its period of extension later in the support phase.[30,31] The activity reported before foot strike is responsible for slowing the rapidly extending knee in preparation for loading.[30–32] The later activity helps to propel the runner's body mass forward.

ANKLE JOINT. The tibialis anterior muscle is active at the instant of foot strike so as to provide a stable base of support by co-contracting with the triceps surae muscles.[30–32] The muscle's activity during the early portion of the support phase is much more variable than at other times in the running cycle. The tibialis anterior muscle has been shown to be both active as well as absent from foot strike until the foot is plantigrade to the ground.[30,31,33,34] The observed absence of tibialis anterior activity might be caused by the variation in foot placement at contact by different runners. A rearfoot striker may need the tibialis anterior muscle to contract eccentrically to allow smooth plantar flexion after foot strike. A midfoot striker, however, would already be in a plantigrade position and therefore would not need the muscular contraction for support.[35] Finally, during the swing phase of running, there is a small amount of activity to prevent the toes from contacting the ground.[30–32] As mentioned earlier, co-contraction of the triceps surae and tibialis anterior muscles has been reported at the instant of foot strike. Continued high activity during early support helps to control the eccentric dorsiflexion that is occurring at this time.[30,31,33,34] During the later portion of the support phase, activity in the triceps surae muscles continues and helps propel the runner's body into the air.[30,31] Mann and Hagy[33] demonstrated that triceps surae muscle activity ceased before toe-off when running at speeds of 2.7 m/s. If the running speed increased to 5.4 m/s, the muscle was found to be active all the way until toe-off.

In summary, the phasic muscle activity of muscles during running is very similar to that during walking, except that the magnitude of activity is increased during running.[36] As the speed of running increases, so does the integrated EMG activity.[31,36–39] Ito et al.[40] showed that integrated EMG activity increased during the swing phase but remained constant during the contact phase as running speed increased from 3.7 to 9.3 m/s. To date, there has been very little research on what effect, if any, orthotic devices or footwear have on muscular activity in the foot and lower extremity during running.

RUNNING KINETICS

INFLUENCE OF GROUND REACTION FORCES. During walking, the vertical component of the ground reaction force acting through the lower extremity throughout the stance phase is approximately 125 percent of body weight. The vertical component of the ground reaction force is typically greater during the latter half of the walking cycle when the propulsion period is occurring. Several studies have shown that the vertical component of ground reaction force during distance running is usually 150 percent to 200 percent greater than during slow walking.[41,42] Cavanagh and LaFortune noted that the typical distance runner who runs approximately 130 km (80.8 miles) a week subjects each lower extremity to approximately 40,000 such impacts over a 7-day period.[41] Drez states that vertical force values of two to three times body weight can occur at foot strike during running and jogging.[43] He further notes that there are about 800 foot strikes on each foot in a 1-mile run. Thus, if a 150-lb (68.2-kg) man were running 1 km, each foot would endure about 120 tons (1.1 million N) of force. During a 26-mile (41.8 km) marathon, each foot would then endure approximately 3000 tons (2.65 million N) of force. Drez further notes that for this reason, adequate midsole cushioning in a running shoe is necessary to help the body attenuate or lessen the effect of these impact forces.

To lessen or attenuate the increased ground reaction forces that occur during running, the body must provide a mechanism similar to the shock absorber used in a car. The shock absorber is designed to attenuate forces acting on the car by shortening to absorb energy. The shock absorber consists of two solid cylinders, one smaller in diameter than the other, and a spring that is positioned between the two cylinders. At rest, the spring is in its normal, or fully lengthened, position. When the car travels over a bump, the smaller cylinder moves within the larger diameter cylinder and the spring compresses, absorbing energy. Thus, the spring goes from a state of potential energy at rest to a state of kinetic energy when the car encounters a bump in the road (Fig. 18–4A).

To provide a system similar to the automobile shock absorber, the lower extremity must also permit shortening and absorption of energy. During the support phase of running, simultaneous movements of the hip, knee, and ankle joints cause a shortening of the lower extremity. To function as the spring in the automobile shock absorber, the muscles surrounding the hip, knee, and ankle articulations contract eccentrically during the early support phase.[44] Thus, shock attenuation during

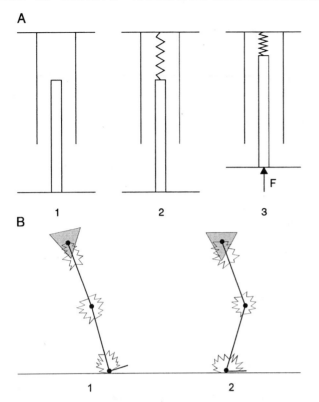

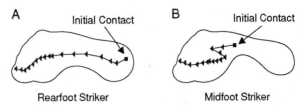

FIGURE 18–5. Center of pressure paths for a rearfoot and midfoot striker.

FIGURE 18–4. Shock attenuation model. *A*, Diagram 1 illustrates a simple plunger and cylinder system. Diagram 2 depicts the system with a shock attenuation spring added. Diagram 3 shows the system compressed under some compressive load (F). *B*, Diagrams 1 and 2 illustrate the shock attenuation model applied to the lower extremities during walking. See text for further explanation.

running is created by movements of the lower extremity articulations, which cause a shortening of the lower limb and energy absorption via contraction of the muscles surrounding the joints of the lower extremity (Fig. 18–4*B*). Theoretically the effectiveness of this anatomic shock absorber could be reduced by muscle fatigue or loss of flexibility, which may explain the occurrence of stress reactions or fractures in highly trained athletes during the middle or later part of their competitive season. It could also be hypothesized that a loss of shock absorption could occur if the runner has not undergone appropriate muscular endurance training for the distance he or she intends to run.

Another factor that affects the magnitude of the vertical force component of the ground reaction force is variation in running speed. The results of a study done by Hamill et al. indicate that although the events in ground reaction force curves occurred at the same relative time, an increase in magnitude of both vertical force and relative impulses at greater speeds was observed.[45] Relative impulse was defined as the amount of time the force was applied over the areas of the foot.

Cavanagh and LaFortune, in studying ground reaction forces that occurred during distance running, observed that runners could be classified by the first point of ground contact made by their foot.[41] Based on the part of the shoe contacting the ground at foot strike,

those individuals who made contact with the posterior one third of the shoe were classified as rearfoot strikers, whereas those runners whose initial contact with the ground was in the middle one third of the shoe were classified as midfoot strikers. The plots of the center of pressure and three-dimensional wire diagrams illustrate the differences observed in the patterns of initial contact between rearfoot and midfoot strikers (Figs. 18–5 and 18–6). Rearfoot strikers demonstrate a double-peak vertical force component of the ground reaction force, whereas midfoot strikers have a single-peak vertical force component (Fig. 18–7). Nigg noted that the large initial spike in the vertical force component pattern of the rearfoot striker occurred just as the heel was making contact with the ground and referred to this as the *impact peak*.[46] Nigg also found that in most rearfoot runners, this peak occurred at approximately 20 ms after the initiation of ground contact. Cavanagh has stated that if any muscular activity is instituted to help reduce impact forces, it must be initiated before foot strike in rearfoot strikers, since the impact peak occurs very quickly.[11]

Heil has reported that runners who make initial contact with the forefoot experienced a reduced ground reaction force when compared with rearfoot strikers.[47] Heil states that this is because the calf muscles act as a shock-absorbing system to help reduce impact loads. However, forefoot contact also causes a significant increase in the tensile loading of the Achilles tendon. Becker has noted that midfoot strikers keep the knee and hip in a slight degree of flexion and thus absorb the shock of contact in a more elastic fashion.[48] McMahon and colleagues reported that running with the knees bent reduces the magnitude of vertical ground reaction forces and diminishes the transmission of mechanical shock through the lower extremity and foot.[49] They also reported, however, that this style of running produces an increased force in the muscles of the leg and can require as much as a 50 percent increase in the rate of oxygen consumption. They referred to this increased oxygen requirement as the "cost of cushioning." Becker has also reported that in both heel and forefoot strikers, impact forces are decreased by the degree of pronation, which he notes is principally controlled by the anterior and posterior tibial muscles.[48]

The recommendation of proper footwear as well as the prescription of foot orthoses are partially dependent on whether the runner is a midfoot or rearfoot striker. The individual who is a midfoot striker will not benefit from a foot orthosis that has been fabricated with a rearfoot wedge, as the purpose of the wedge is to affect foot function from foot strike to the mid-support phase.

In addition, a midfoot striker using footwear that has special cushioning features only in the posterior one third of the midsole will obtain less than optimal function from the shoe. Midfoot strikers should be counseled to purchase footwear that has more cushioning in the forefoot. However, as Cavanagh and LaFortune[41] have noted, running shoe companies have paid little attention to providing more cushioning in a shoe that would be designed specifically for midfoot or forefoot strikers.

FOOT PLANTAR PRESSURES DURING RUNNING. Another factor that must be considered when evaluating the runner is how the plantar surface of the foot contacts the supporting surface and the resulting plantar pressures that occur. To illustrate the significance of plantar pressures, if two runners have equal body weight, equal height, and the same style of running, including identical stride length, then these two runners theoretically would generate similar magnitudes of ground reaction force when running at identical speeds. However, if one of these runners has a high-arch foot structure and the other runner has a low-arch foot structure, the pressures applied to the plantar surface of their feet will be different. Because pressure is equal to force divided by area, the runner with the low-arch foot structure will have greater surface area in contact with the ground in comparison with the runner with the high-arch foot structure and thus will experience lower pressures on the plantar surface of the foot.

Nachbauer and Nigg evaluated the effect of arch height of the foot on ground reaction forces in running.[50] They found that impact forces were not significantly different for low-arch and high-arch individuals, even though a link has been suggested between running injuries and type of foot arch. However, it is important to realize that even though ground reaction forces may not be significantly different, the pressures acting through the plantar surface of the foot may be different. The runner with a more mobile or pronatory foot type that allows increased plantar surface area of the foot to make contact with the ground will experience less overall pressure than the person with a less mobile, or supinatory, foot type, as he or she has decreased plantar surface area in contact with the ground. Figure 18–8 shows the area in contact with the ground for two different individuals, a person with a low arch and a person with a high arch. As can be seen in the runner with the high-arch foot structure, only the supporting surface of the heel and forefoot make contact. Unlike the person with the low-arch foot structure, there is no midfoot contact with the ground, and thus plantar surface area is reduced, causing increased plantar pressures under the foot.

This has important implications for the clinician when prescribing footwear. The individual with a pes cavus, or high-arch, foot structure may be using a running shoe that has good midsole cushioning properties, but he or she will still have reduced plantar surface area contacting the shoe. In the management of these individuals, some type of foot orthosis or accommodative arch support should be placed within the shoe to increase the total area of contact within the running shoe and reduce plantar pressures.

SUMMARY. To effectively evaluate and treat the runner, not only must the pattern of joint motion during the running cycle be considered, but the effect of muscle activity, ground reaction forces, and plantar pressures acting on the lower extremity and foot must also be taken into account. These kinematic and kinetic factors, as well as their effect on the lower extremity during running, have been reviewed. If abnormalities exist in lower extremity alignment, the changes in the pattern of joint motion, muscle activity, ground reaction forces,

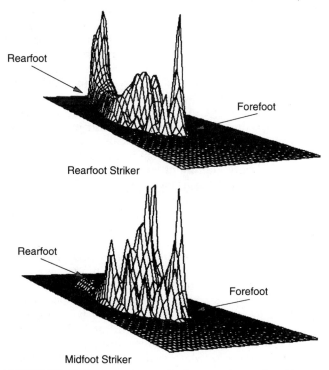

FIGURE 18–6. Plantar pressure plot for a rearfoot and midfoot striker.

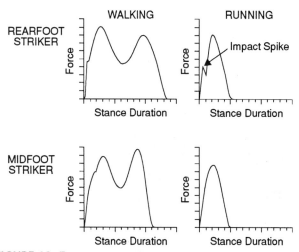

FIGURE 18–7. Typical vertical ground reaction force patterns for rearfoot and midfoot strikers during walking and running.

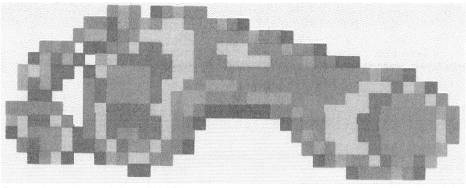

A   Low Arch

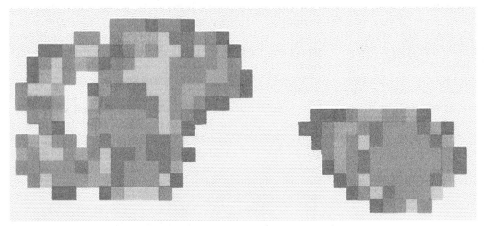

B   High Arch

FIGURE 18–8. Surface area in a high-arch and a low-arch individual.

and plantar pressures associated with running can exacerbate the already increased level of stress on soft tissues as well as dynamic muscle stabilizers and contribute to the development of overuse injuries.

PATHOMECHANICS

Numerous abnormalities in the anatomic alignment of the lower extremity and foot, as well as limitations in soft tissue mobility, have been identified as etiologic factors in lower extremity overuse running injuries. These various abnormalities will be discussed relative to lower extremity malalignment and foot pronation.

LOWER EXTREMITY MALALIGNMENT

Root et al. identified several structural abnormalities in the lower extremity as factors extrinsic to the foot that were compensated for by abnormal foot pronation.[51] These extrinsic factors included tibial varus, internal and external tibial or malleolar torsion, internal and external femoral torsion, as well as leg length discrepancies. Root et al. also noted that limitations in the normal degree of flexibility of the calf, hamstring, and iliopsoas muscles could cause or accentuate abnormal lower extremity alignment during activity. Excessive pronation in the foot has also been identified as one of

the factors that causes excessive stress to the patellofemoral joint. Excessive pronation of the foot can cause the lower leg to be maintained in a prolonged period of internal rotation. This prolonged period of lower leg internal rotation can alter the normal patellar tracking pattern during both walking and running.

Numerous authors have reported a strong link between knee pain and excessive subtalar joint pronation.[47,52–54] Heil has indicated that various extrinsic factors, including genu varum, genu valgum, coxa vara, coxa valga, and abnormal internal and external rotations of the tibia and the femur, can lead to excessive pronation because of a change in the normal foot and lower extremity alignment.[55]

In a study that examined the etiologic factors associated with patellofemoral pain in runners, Messier et al. noted that the only significant discriminatory anthropometric variable that was identified from numerous measurements, including isokinetic assessments, was an increased Q angle.[56] Arch index, leg length, and ankle and knee range of motion were not found to be significant discriminators. Moss and colleagues found that heavy subjects and those with a larger static quadriceps Q angle were more likely to have patellofemoral stress syndrome.[57] Because an activity such as running involves numerous repetitions of knee extension, Moss and colleagues[57] noted that it was possible for a small variation in the Q angle to cause symptoms.

A more recent study, however, conducted by Caylor et al. found no significant difference in the Q angle between 52 patients with anterior knee pain syndrome and a control group of 50 subjects without anterior knee pain syndrome.[58] The intratester reliability for the determination of the Q angle was quite good, but increased Q angles were not responsible for anterior knee pain syndrome in this group of patients.

FOOT PRONATION

Foot pronation has been identified as a major cause of foot and lower leg running injuries, including plantar fasciitis and shin splints. Schuster, in describing the influence of the environment on the foot of long distance runners, indicated that foot deformities, such as rearfoot varus, tibial varus, and forefoot varus, were a common cause of extreme structural imbalance within the foot, causing excessive pronation.[59] Excessive pronation of both the rearfoot and midfoot during running causes increased stress on the soft tissues surrounding the various joints of the foot, including the capsule, ligaments, and plantar fascia. More importantly, there can be an overreliance on lower leg and foot musculature in an attempt to control excessive foot mobility and provide a more stabile foot structure. Thus, a thorough evaluation to determine whether these various foot abnormalities exist appears to be a sound method to predict which individuals might develop foot or lower leg problems, including plantar fasciitis and shin splints.

In a study that attempted to determine the etiologic factors associated with selected running injuries, Messier and Pittala collected anthropometric and motion data on runners affected with iliotibial band friction syndrome, shin splints, or plantar fasciitis.[60] The groups studied consisted of a control group of 19 healthy subjects, a shin splint group (17 subjects), a plantar fasciitis group (15 subjects), and an iliotibial band group (13 subjects). All of the runners underwent an evaluation that included foot prints, determination of plantar flexion and dorsiflexion range of motion, hamstring and lower leg flexibility testing, and assessment of Q angle and leg length. The authors also determined total rearfoot motion and time from maximal pronation to maximal supination by analyzing film records. The results of their study indicated that the only significant discriminator between the plantar fasciitis group and the control group was that the fasciitis group had greater plantar flexion range of motion. No other significant differences could be validated statistically. They did note, however, that the iliotibial band friction syndrome group had a significantly higher arch foot structure than the control group, and the shin splint and iliotibial band friction groups had less ankle dorsiflexion range of motion than the control group. The results of this study seem to question the accepted theory that structural deformities in the foot cause a deviation in alignment leading to the development of foot problems.

Ross and Schuster conducted a similar study in which they attempted to predict injuries in distance runners.[61] They evaluated 63 runners, measuring inversion and eversion of the subtalar joint, the position of the subtalar joint (to determine whether a varus or valgus deformity of the hindfoot existed), forefoot varus or valgus, and the amount of available dorsiflexion at the ankle with the knee joint both flexed and extended. They also performed two weight-bearing measurements: resting calcaneal stance position and neutral calcaneal stance position. Based on their results and considering the etiology of lower extremity injuries studied, the authors could not conclude that there was a single "cause-and-effect" factor responsible for running injuries.

Warren and Jones attempted to determine those anatomic factors that could be used to predict plantar fasciitis, in long distance runners.[62] Forty-two runners were classified as (1) having no history of plantar fasciitis, (2) currently having plantar fasciitis, or (3) having recovered from plantar fasciitis. Various measurements were taken on each subject, including leg length, degree of pronation from neutral, arch height of the foot, and dorsiflexion and plantar flexion of the ankle. The results of the study were extremely interesting in that the control group who had never had a history of plantar fasciitis actually had a greater degree of pronation than both of the other two groups. These authors noted that perhaps plantar fasciitis was caused by excessive overuse stress rather than faulty biomechanics. Little has been written regarding the runner with a high-arch and hypomobile foot structure. Schuster noted that runners with high-arch foot structure had an extremely rigid foot, and their joint ranges of motion were usually less than average.[59] He further noted, as has been previously discussed, that they had a much smaller weight-bearing pattern and difficulty in attenuating impact forces. Thus, the runner with limited rearfoot motion could be classified as having decreased shock attenuation and increased plantar pressures, especially in the forefoot, secondary to limited midfoot loading.

USE OF THE LOAD-DEFORMATION CURVE TO EXPLAIN RUNNING INJURIES

Although numerous factors have been outlined as possible causes of overuse injuries in the lower extremity and foot, it does not appear that any study to date has been able to accurately predict which individuals will develop lower extremity overuse injuries. Furthermore, the literature strongly suggests that it is extremely difficult to pinpoint the actual cause of an overuse injury. Often individuals who exhibit the most profound lower extremity and foot malalignments are asymptomatic, whereas those individuals with an "ideal" runner's alignment—including symmetric hip rotation, no evidence of external or internal malleolar torsion, and a "normal" foot structure with minimal pronation—can be highly susceptible to overuse injuries. Because of these problems, we believe that a tissue stress model that is based on the load-deformation curve can assist the clinician in understanding the effect of lower extremity and foot malalignments on the development of overuse injuries in runners.

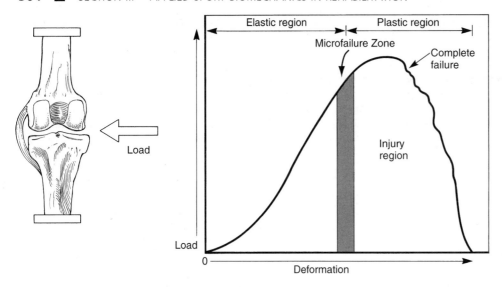

FIGURE 18-9. Schematic of the load-deformation principle of soft tissue.

Each individual runner has his or her own level of tolerance for the amount of tissue stress that can be withstood during the activity of running. The importance of this individual level of tissue stress tolerance can be illustrated using the load-deformation curve (Fig. 18–9). The load-deformation curve consists of two regions or zones: an elastic region and a plastic region.[63] A load-deformation curve is commonly used by material engineers to explain the degree of deformation that occurs when a load is applied to an object. The region or area separating the elastic and plastic regions is termed the *microfailure zone*. Although deformation occurs when the load is applied, the object being tested can completely recover from the deformation, provided the deformation does not exceed the microfailure zone. If deformation of the object exceeds the microfailure zone and enters the plastic region, then permanent, nonrecoverable deformation will occur.

The deforming force may be from a single load or the summation of several loadings. To illustrate the effect of loads applied to soft tissue during running, using the load-deformation curve, the elastic region represents the normal "give and take" of soft tissues as the foot is loaded and unloaded during the running cycle. As long as the runner maintains the level of tissue stress within this elastic region, the amount of soft tissue stress will most likely be tolerated and an overuse injury will be avoided.

The various factors that contribute to excessive tissue stress include the amount of stress applied to the soft tissues, the amount of extrinsic and intrinsic muscle activity required to enhance foot stability, and the degree of abnormal lower extremity and foot alignment. If these factors can be balanced so that the tissues never go beyond the elastic range and enter the microfailure zone, then injury will be avoided. If runners increase their running speed or the training distance is accelerated too quickly, soft tissues may enter the microfailure zone, resulting in an overuse stress injury. If the runner does not rest the injured tissues when microtrauma is present, the stressed tissues can eventually be taken beyond the microfailure zone and into the plastic range,

with the result being a breakdown of soft tissues, muscle guarding, and pain. The load-deformation curve also provides a model to explain the effectiveness of footwear and foot orthoses in precluding excessive tissue stress by restricting excessive motion and preventing soft tissues from entering the microfailure zone.

SUMMARY

Clearly, research to date indicates that the etiology of running injuries is a multifactorial problem. Although clinicians often emphasize abnormal anatomic alignment as a primary cause of running injuries, anatomic malalignment can be considered only one of numerous factors leading to injury. Because running injuries are often the result of repetitive stress over an extended duration, management of the individual with a running injury requires the clinician to have a thorough understanding of joint kinematics, ground reaction forces, muscle activity, and plantar pressures affecting the body while running. To effectively treat the runner with an overuse injury of the lower extremity and foot, the clinician must understand normal running mechanics so that he or she can determine the causes of repetitive trauma and inflammation secondary to tissue stress. Only then will the runner be provided with optimal treatment and a rehabilitation program that will lead to a return to full activity.

REFERENCES

1. James SL, Bates BT, Osternig LR: Injuries to runners. Am J Sports Med 1978; 6:40.
2. Lutter LD: Injuries in the runner and jogger. J Am Podiatr Med Assoc 1980; 70:45.
3. Kerner JA, D'Amico JC: A statistical analysis of a group of runners. J Am Podiatr Med Assoc 1983; 73:160.
4. Slocum DB, James SL: Biomechanics of running. JAMA 1968; 205:97.
5. James SL, Brubaker CE: Biomechanics of running. Orthop Clin North Am 1973; 4:605.

6. Adrian MJ, Kreighbaum E: Mechanics of distance-running during competition. *In* Jokl E (ed): Biomechanics III. Baltimore, University Park Press, 1973, p 354.

7. Deshon DE, Nelson RC: A cinematographical analysis of sprint running. Res Q 1964; 35:451.

8. Mann RA, Hagy J: Biomechanics of walking, running and sprinting. Am J Sports Med 1980; 8:345.

9. Roy B: Caracteristiques biomecaniques de la course d'endurance. Can J Appl Sports Sci 1982; 7:104.

10. Sprague P, Mann RV: The effects of muscular fatigue on the kinetics of sprint running. Res Q Exerc Sport 1983; 54:60.

11. Cavanagh PR: The biomechanics of lower extremity action in distance running. Foot Ankle 1987; 7:197.

12. Landry M, Zebas CJ: Biomechanical principles in common running injuries. J Am Podiatr Med Assoc 1985; 75:48.

13. Cavanagh PR, Williams KW: The effect of stride length variation on oxygen uptake during distance running. Med Sci Sports Exerc 1982; 14:30.

14. Murray MP, Drought AB, Kory RC: Walking patterns of normal men. J Bone Joint Surg 1964; 46A:335.

15. Murray MP, Kory RC, Sepic BS: Walking patterns of normal women. Arch Phys Med Rehabil 1970; 51:637.

16. Bogdan RJ, Jenkins D, Hyland T: The runner's knee syndrome. *In* Rinaldi RR, Sabia M (eds): Sports Medicine. Mount Kisco, NY, Futura Publishing, 1978, p 159.

17. McPoil TG, Cornwall MW: Influence of running on functional limb varus. Unpublished data, 1992.

18. Bates BT, Osternig LR, Mason BR, et al: Functional variability of the lower extremity during the support phase of running. Med Sci Sports Exerc 1979; 11:328.

19. Areblad M, Nigg BM, Ekstrand J, et al: Three-dimensional measurement of rearfoot motion during running. J Biomech 1990; 23:933.

20. Soutas-Little RW, Beavis GC, Verstraete MC, et al: Analysis of foot motion during running using a joint co-ordinate system. Med Sci Sports Exerc 1987; 19:285.

21. Engsberg JR, Andrews JG: Kinematic analysis of the talocalcaneal/ talocrural joint during running support. Med Sci Sports Exerc 1987; 19:275.

22. Rodgers MM, LeVeau BF: Effectiveness of foot orthotic devices used to modify pronation in runners. J Orthop Sports Phys Ther 1982; 4:86.

23. Nigg BM, Herzog W, Read LJ: Effect of viscoelastic shoe insoles on vertical impact forces in heel-toe running. Am J Sports Med 1988; 16:70.

24. Nigg BM, Morlock M: The influence of lateral heel flare of running shoes on pronation and impact forces. Med Sci Sports Exerc 1987; 19:294.

25. Stacoff A, Reinschmidt C, Stussi E: The movement of the heel within a running shoe. Med Sci Sports Exerc 1992; 24:695.

26. Clarke TE, Frederick EC, Hamill CL: The effects of shoe design parameters on rearfoot control in running. Med Sci Sports Exerc 1983; 15:376.

27. Reinschmidt C, Stacoff A, Stussi E: Heel movement within a court shoe. Med Sci Sports Exerc 1992; 24:1992.

28. Boden F, Volkert R, Menke W, et al: Computer-assisted electromyographic running studies of athletic shoes with various sole configurations. *In* Segesser B, Pforringer W (eds): The Shoe in Sport. Chicago, Year Book Medical, 1989.

29. Brandell BR: An analysis of muscle coordination in walking and running gaits. *In* Jokl E (ed): Biomechanics III. Baltimore, University Park Press, 1973, p 278.

30. Elliott BC, Blanksby BA: A biomechanical analysis of the male jogging action. J Hum Movement Stud 1979; 5:42.

31. Elliott BC, Blanksby BA: The synchronization of muscle activity and body segment movements during a running cycle. Med Sci Sports Exerc 1979; 11:322.

32. Frigo C, Pedotti A, Santambrogio G: A correlation between muscle and ECG activities during running. *In* Terauds J, Dale G (eds): Science in Athletics. Del Mar, CA, Academic Press, 1979, p 61.

33. Mann RA, Hagy JL: The function of the toes in walking, jogging, and running. Clin Orthop 1994; 142:24.

34. Dietz V, Schmidtbleicher D, Noth J: Neuronal mechanisms of human locomotion. J Neurophysiol 1979; 42:1212.

35. Williams KR: Biomechanics of running. Exerc Sports Sci Rev 1985; 13:389.

36. Miyashita M, Matsui M, Miura M: The relation between electrical activity in muscle and speed of walking and running. *In* Vredenbregt J, Wartenweiler JW (eds): Biomechanics II. Baltimore, University Park Press, 1971, p 192.

37. Hoshikawa T, Matsui H, Miyashita M: Analysis of running pattern in relation to speed. *In* Jokl E (ed): Biomechanics III. Baltimore, University Park Press, 1973, p 342.

38. Komi PV: Biomechanical features of running with special emphasis on load characteristics and mechanical efficiency. *In* Nigg B, Kerr B (eds): Biomechanical Aspects of Sport Shoes and Playing Surfaces. Calgary, Alberta, Canada, University of Calgary, 1983, p 134.

39. Knuttgen HG: Oxygen uptake and pulse rate while running with undetermined and determined stride lengths at different speeds. Acta Physiol Scand 1961; 52:366.

40. Ito A, Fuchimoto T, Kaneko M: Quantitative analysis of EMG during various speeds of running. *In* Winter DA, Normal RW, Wells RP, et al (eds): Biomechanics IX. Champaign, IL, Human Kinetics Publishers, 1985.

41. Cavanagh PR, LaFortune MA: Ground reaction forces in distance running. J Biomech 1980; 13:397.

42. Dickinson JA, Cook SD, Leinhardt TM: The measurement of shock waves following heel strike while running. J Biomech 1985; 18:415.

43. Drez D: Running footwear: Examination of the training shoe, the foot, and functional orthotic devices. Am J Sports Med 1980; 8:140.

44. Dillman CJ: A kinetic analysis of the recovery leg during sprint running. *In* Cooper J (ed): Biomechanics. Chicago, Athletic Institute, 1971, p 137.

45. Hamill J, Bates BT, Knutzen KM, et al: Variations in ground reaction force parameters at different running speeds. Hum Movement Sci 1983; 2:47.

46. Nigg BM: Biomechanics of Running Shoes. Champaign, IL, Human Kinetics Publishers, 1986.

47. Heil B: Lower limb biomechanics related to running injuries. Physiotherapy 1992; 78:400.

48. Becker N-L. Specific running injuries and complaints related to excessive loads: Medical criteria of the running shoe. *In* Segesser B, Pforringer W (eds): The Shoe in Sport. Chicago, Year Book Medical, 1987, p 16.

49. McMahon TA, Valiant G, Frederick EC: Groucho running. J Appl Physiol 1987; 62:2326.

50. Nachbauer W, Nigg BM: Effects of arch height of the foot on ground reaction forces in running. Med Sci Sports Exerc 1992; 24:1264.

51. Root ML, Orien WP, Weed JH: Clinical Biomechanics, Vol 2. Normal and Abnormal Function of the Foot. Los Angeles, Clinical Biomechanics Corporation, 1977, p 175.

52. McConnell J: The management of chondromalacia patellae: A long term solution. Aust J Physiother 1986; 32:215.

53. James SL: Chondromalacia of the patella in the adolescent. *In* Kennedy JC (ed): The Injured Adolescent Knee. Baltimore, Williams & Wilkins, 1979, p 205.

54. Buchbinder MR, Napora NJ, Biggs EW: The relationship of abnormal pronation to chondromalacia of the patella in distance runners. J Am Podiatr Med Assoc 1979; 69:159.

55. Heil B: Running shoe design and selection related to lower limb biomechanics. Physiotherapy 1992; 78:406.

56. Messier SP, Davis SE, Curl WW, et al: Etiologic factors associated with patellofemoral pain in runners. Med Sci Sports Exerc 1991; 23:1008.

57. Moss RI, DeVita P, Dawson ML: A biomechanical analysis of patellofemoral stress syndrome. J Athletic Training 1992; 27:64.

58. Caylor D, Fites R, Worrell TW: The relationship between quadriceps angle and anterior knee pain syndrome. J Orthop Sports Phys Ther 1993; 17:11.

59. Schuster RO: Foot types and the influence of environment on the foot of the long distance runner. Ann NY Acad Sci 1977; 301:881.

60. Messier SP, Pittala KA: Etiologic factors associated with selected running injuries. Med Sci Sports Exerc 1988; 20:501.

61. Ross CF, Schuster RO: A preliminary report on predicting injuries in distance runners. J Am Podiatr Med Assoc 1983; 73:275.

62. Warren BL, Jones CJ: Predicting plantar fasciitis in runners. Med Sci Sports Exerc 1986; 19:71.

63. Cornwall MW: Biomechanics of noncontractile tissue: A review. Phys Ther 1984; 64:1869.

ADDITIONAL SUGGESTED READINGS

Bates BT, Osternig, LR, Mason B, et al: Lower extremity function during the support phase of running. In Asmussen E, Jorgensen K (eds): Biomechanics VI-B. University Park Press, Baltimore, 1978.

Blair SN, Kohl HW, Goodyear NN: Rates and risks for running injuries: Studies in three populations. Res Q 1987; 58:221.

Brubaker CE, James SL: Injuries to runners. J Sports Med 1974; 2:189.

Clancy WG: Runners' injuries: Part I. Am J Sports Med 1980; 8:137.

Clancy WG: Runners' injuries: Part II. Evaluation and treatment of specific injuries. Am J Sports Med 1980; 8:287.

Claremont AD, Hall SJ: Effects of extremity loading upon energy expenditure and running mechanics. Med Sci Sports Exerc 1988; 20:167.

Clement DB, Taunton JE, Smart GW, et al: A survey of overuse running injuries. Phys Sports Med 1981; 9:47.

Cureton TK: Mechanics of track running: Review of the research that has been done to determine factors in running efficiency. Scholastic Coach 1935; 4:7.

Dal Monte A, Fucci S, Manoni A: The treadmill used as a training and a simulator instrument in middle- and long-distance running. In Cerquiglini S, Vernarando A, Wartenweiler J (eds): Biomechanics III. Basel, Switzerland, Karger, 1973, p 359.

D'Amico JC, Rubin M: The influence of foot orthoses on quadriceps angle. J Am Podiatr Med Assoc 1986; 76:337.

Dillman CJ: Kinematic analyses of running. In Wilmore JH, Keogh JF (eds): Exercise and Sport Sciences Reviews. New York, Academic Press, 1975, p 193.

Dyson GHG: The Mechanics of Athletics. New York, Holmes & Meirer, 1977.

Elliott BC, Blanksby BA: A cinematographic analysis of overground and treadmill running by males and females. Med Sci Sports Exerc 1976; 8:84.

Elliott BC, Blanksby BA: Optimal stride length considerations for male and female recreational runners. Br J Sports Med 1979; 13:15.

Hamill J, Bates BT: A kinetic evaluation of the effects of in vivo loading on running shoes. J Orthop Sports Phys Ther 1988; 10:47.

Hamill J, Freedson PS, Boda W, et al: Effects of shoe type on cardiorespiratory responses and rearfoot motion during treadmill running. Med Sci Sports Exerc 1988; 20:515.

Hoffman K: The relationship between the length and frequency of stride, stature and leg length. Sport VIII 1965; 3:11.

Ikai M: Biomechanics of sprint running with respect to the speed curve. In Jokl E (ed): Biomechanics I. Basel, Switzerland, Karger, 1968, p 282.

Jones RE: A kinematic interpretation of running and its relationship to hamstring injury. J Health Phys Ed Rec 1970; 41:83.

Lilletvedt J, Kreighbaum E, Phillips RL: Analysis of selected alignment of the lower extremity related to the shin splint syndrome. J Am Podiatr Med Assoc 1979; 69:211.

Luhtanen P, Komi PV: Mechanical factors influencing running speed. In Asmussen E, Jorgensen K (eds): Biomechanics VI-B. Baltimore, University Park Press, 1978, p 23.

Mann RA, Baxter DE, Lutter LD: Running symposium. Foot Ankle 1981; 1:190.

Mero A, Komi PV: Force-, EMG-, and elasticity-velocity relationships at submaximal, maximal and supramaximal running speeds in sprinters. Eur J Appl Physiol 1986; 55:553.

Miura M, Kobayashi K, Miyashita M, et al: Experimental studies on biomechanics in long distance running. In Matsui H (ed): Review of Our Researches, 1970–1973. Nagoya, Japan, Department of Physical Education , University of Nagoya, 1973, p 46.

Montgomery L, Nelson F, Norton J, et al: Orthopedic history and examination in the etiology of overuse injuries. Med Sci Sports Exerc 1989; 21:237.

Nelson RC, Brooks CM, Pike NL: Biomechanical comparison of male and female distance runners. Ann NY Acad Sci 1977; 301:793.

Nelson RC, Gregor RJ: Biomechanics of distance running: A longitudinal study. Res Q 1976; 47:417.

Nilsson J, Thorstensson A, Halbertsma J: Changes in leg movements and muscle activity with speeds of locomotion and mode of progression in humans. Acta Physiol Scand 1985; 123:457.

Noble CA: Iliotibial band friction syndrome in runners. Am J Sports Med 1980; 8:232.

Payne AH: A comparison of the ground forces in race walking with those in normal walking and running. In Asmussen E, Jorgensen K (eds): Biomechanics VI-A. Baltimore, University Park Press, 1978, p 293.

Robbins SE, Gouw GJ, Hanna AM: Running-related injury prevention through innate impact-moderating behavior. Med Sci Sports Exerc 1989; 21:130.

Robbins SE, Hanna AM, Gouw GJ: Overload protection: Avoidance response to heavy plantar surface loading. Med Sci Sports Exerc 1988; 20:85.

Rubin BD, Collins HR: Runner's knee. Phys Sports Med 1980; 8:49.

Sinning WE, Forsyth HL: Lower-limb actions while running at different velocities. Med Sci Sports Exerc 1970; 2:28.

Slocum DB, Bowerman W: The biomechanics of running. Clin Orthop 1962; 23:39.

Smart G, Taunton J, Clement D: Achilles tendon disorders in runners—a review. Med Sci Sports Exerc 1980; 4:231.

Smith WB: Environmental factors in running. Am J Sports Med 1980; 8:138.

Stanton P, Purdam C: Hamstring injuries in sprinting—the role of eccentric exercise. J Orthop Sports Phys Ther 1989; 10:343.

Warren B: Anatomical factors associated with predicting plantar fasciitis in long-distance runners. Med Sci Sports Exerc 1984; 16:60.

CHAPTER 19

Biomechanics of Cycling

ROBERT J. GREGOR PhD
EILEEN FOWLER PhD, PT

Common Cycling Injuries
Cycling Kinematics
   Muscle Length Changes
Muscle Activity During Cycling

Cycling Kinetics
   Pedal Reaction Forces
   Pedal Pressure Distribution
   Lower Extremity Joint Kinetics

Knee Joint Reaction Forces
Muscle Moments
Pedal Torsion Measurements
Mechanical Work and Power

Cycling is a competitive sport associated with specific injuries, as well as a popular form of exercise used for musculoskeletal and aerobic conditioning and rehabilitation. In the competition setting, the primary focus is on maximum performance; the rider assumes a position on the bicycle designed to minimize wind resistance and maximize energy input to the bicycle. Research on elite competitive cyclists usually focuses on factors such as bicycle components (e.g., frame and pedal design), safety features (e.g., helmet design), aerodynamic clothing, and physiologic and mechanical response to changes in load, body position, and frame setup. In an aerobic exercise setting, the primary focus is usually on comfort, safety, and the ability to regulate resistance in accommodating a broad range of individual demands. The stationary bicycle is commonly used as a form of aerobic exercise for weight loss and cardiac rehabilitation.

Cycling is also used in the rehabilitation of athletes from a variety of sport settings and with a wide spectrum of proficiency. In this rehabilitation setting the primary focus is on providing a safe environment that appropriately challenges each patient. In designing a rehabilitation program, the physical therapist must have specific knowledge of the injury or disability as well as an understanding of cycling mechanics so that demands placed on the patient will improve his or her condition yet not induce further trauma.

The bicycle is commonly used for (1) nonsurgical rehabilitation following musculoskeletal injuries to the lower extremity, (2) postoperative rehabilitation following surgery (usually of the knee), and (3) maintenance of cardiovascular conditioning for athletes until healing is sufficient for them to resume their more rigorous training program. The bicycle uniquely combines lower extremity strengthening, range of motion, and cardiovascular conditioning while controlling joint, musculotendinous, and ligament stress. Parameters can be adjusted to precisely meet the requirements of an individual at his or her stage of rehabilitation. The degree of lower limb loading, which can be regulated by the resistance setting on the bicycle, and the speed of joint movement, which can be regulated by pedaling cadence and seat height changes, offer the potential for objective measurements to document progress and gradually increase intensity. Outdoor cycling is also an option; however, in outdoor cycling it is difficult to control the amount of muscular effort and stress due to the high inertial loads that may be generated, for example, in propelling the bike up a hill. Despite this, outdoor cycling is less "boring" and perhaps more challenging and thus may be a matter of choice for the athlete who has reached an advanced stage of rehabilitation. A person undergoing rehabilitation, however, should receive careful guidance to ensure that the benefit exceeds the risks that may otherwise be introduced.

The primary focus of this chapter is to provide information on the mechanics of the interface between the rider and the bicycle. Specific emphasis will be placed on the lower extremities, as they assume the primary role in the production and transmission of power to the bicycle and, as a consequence, endure the largest loads and the most profound chronic injuries. We will begin with a review of common chronic injuries incurred in the lower extremity as a result of cycling, followed by a discussion of lower extremity kinematics and an understanding of how changes in bike setup affect movement patterns. The contribution of lower extremity musculature will be explored in a discussion of electromyography (EMG) patterns reported for the

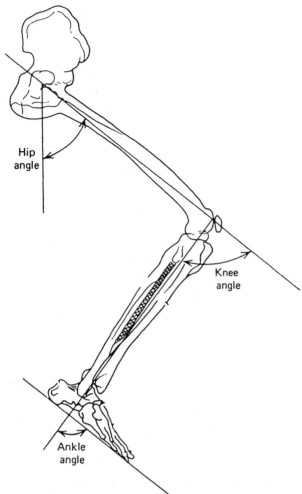

FIGURE 19–1. Sketch of the right lower extremity showing reference angles for the hip, knee, and ankle. An angle of 0 degrees at the hip is the vertical reference, with a positive angle representing hip flexion; 0 degrees at the knee is full extension, and 0 degrees at the ankle is the anatomic position.

major joint flexors and extensors in the leg. This information will lead to a review of the understanding of lower extremity kinetics and the generation and transmission of power to the bicycle.

COMMON CYCLING INJURIES

Most of the adjustments made to a bicycle are performed to obtain a comfortable riding position and proper range of motion for the lower extremities. With a limited understanding of the interactive forces involved, each rider makes adjustments to the frame, which include alterations in seat height, handlebar height, and distance from the seat; pedal type; and crank length, as well as inclusion of a reasonable selection of gears. The objective is to provide enough flexibility to prevent the occurrence of overuse injuries from repeated stress during extended periods of training.

The incidence of overuse injuries to the ankle/foot complex is low and usually related to the interface between the foot and pedal. Factors such as shoe design, pedal design, and even seat height should be examined

if discomfort occurs. Shoe design is an important factor and must incorporate foot support and comfort as well as effective transmission of force.[1] Shoes should be sufficiently stiff to distribute pressure but flexible enough to permit natural foot motion. The manner in which the foot is secured to the pedal is also related to the type of injuries observed. Compression of the digital nerves of the foot, resulting in numbness and temporary paresthesia, has been reported with toe-strap and cleat designs. This condition is easily relieved by periodic loosening of shoes and straps. Cleat designs, especially those with smaller shoe-pedal contact surface area, may cause metatarsalgia and soft tissue injury as a result of high pressure concentration on the plantar surface of the foot. Achilles tendinitis and/or plantar fasciitis may occur as a result of excessive dorsiflexion due to a low seat height.[2]

Francis[3] described foot structural malalignments, including forefoot and rearfoot varus and valgus malalignments, but inferred that these problems may have greater influence on knee kinematics and subsequent knee pain than on specific foot/ankle injuries. No discussion of pedal interface was presented; only the potential for orthotics placed in the shoe to benefit knee function.

Knee pain, which results from improper mechanics and the accumulation of insult through repetitive loading, is the most common overuse problem across all levels of cycling participants. Injuries include chondromalacia patella, quadriceps tendinitis, patellar tendinitis, iliotibial band syndrome, retropatellar or prepatellar bursitis, pes anserinus bursitis, infrapatellar fat pad syndrome, medial capsule strain and inflammation of the synovial plica, and medial or lateral collateral ligament sprain.[4–8] The primary factor influencing knee joint dynamics and subsequent tissue strain is the "fit" between the rider and bicycle. This includes shoe-cleat alignment on the pedal, seat height, and fore-aft adjustment, as well as the assumption of various aerodynamic positions. Secondary factors include individual pedaling technique, structural variations among cyclists, and anatomic asymmetry in the same cyclist. These structural asymmetries necessitate individual variations in bike setup and selective modifications of equipment components.

In a report by Holmes et al.,[7] cycling patients were evaluated for complaints of chronic knee pain over a 5-year period. They found that 64 percent of the patients in the professional and advanced amateur categories had anterior knee pain, specifically chondromalacia patella and patellar tendinitis, and attributed this problem to intense training loads and high mileage. In a cycling knee pain survey conducted for the U.S. Olympic Committee at the UCLA Biomechanics Laboratory,[5] overuse injuries and shoe/pedal type data were collected from 168 experienced racers. Sixty percent of the respondents reported anterior knee pain, especially retropatellar pain, followed by lateral and medial knee pain.

Bohlmann[4] listed the hip as the most common site of all crash-related superficial abrasions. Overuse hip injuries, however, are rare and consequently are not well documented in the literature. Mellion[2] suggests that trochanteric bursitis can develop in cyclists from an irritation of the fascia lata on the greater trochanter, and iliopsoas tendinitis can occur when the seat is set too high. It is our experience that very few cyclists are set up with excessively high seat positions for extended periods of time, and this may partially account for the lack of reported cases of related chronic hip ailments.

While the information presented on injuries is specific to competitive cyclists, it seems the knee is the primary joint targeted by excessive training and overuse. Consequently, any alterations made to the bicycle in an effort to adjust the bike to the rider must be made with caution. In the clinical setting, proper adjustments must be made to provide the range of motion necessary to strain all muscles and supportive connective tissue structures within appropriate limits (i.e., to prevent any further damage to injured tissues targeted by the rehabilitation program), yet "push the envelope" to regain normal range of motion.

CYCLING KINEMATICS

Kinematic, kinetic, and muscle activity patterns during cycling are most often described relative to the angle of the crank, with 0 or 360 degrees representing top dead center (TDC) and 180 degrees representing bottom dead center (BDC). The power, or propulsive, phase takes place between TDC and BDC. During this time, the contralateral limb is in the recovery phase between BDC and TDC.

Most reports on cycling kinematics have been limited to sagittal plane motion: hip and knee flexion and extension and ankle dorsiflexion and plantar flexion. Displacements, velocities, and accelerations of the thigh, shank, and foot are most affected by cadence and

bicycle geometry (e.g., seat height, crank length, and foot position on the pedal). The complex interactions between bicycle geometry and rider kinematics and attempts at "optimizing" the bicycle-rider system have been the subjects of many studies that systematically varied rider kinematics by changing bicycle configuration, pedaling cadence, or both.[9] Peak flexion and extension of the lower extremity joints will vary depending on the seat height and fore-aft adjustments. However, once the constrained cyclic movement of the lower extremity is established for comfort by each rider at a selected seat position and crank length, lower extremity kinematic patterns remain quite consistent.

Faria and Cavanagh[10] studied sagittal plane kinematics and reported a total excursion of 45 degrees for the thigh, 75 degrees for the knee, and 20 degrees for the ankle. These values were measured at a seat height chosen for comfort by the cyclist. Using an angle convention similar to the one employed by Faria and Cavanagh,[10] (Fig. 19–1), data from the laboratory at UCLA[11] (Fig. 19–2) demonstrate the effect of seat height changes on hip and knee range of motion as seat height varied from 100 percent to 115 percent of pubic symphysis height (height measured from the pubic symphysis, or crotch, to the floor). This range of seat heights is considered somewhat extreme, since the comfortable range chosen by most competitive riders usually varies from 106 percent to 109 percent of pubic symphysis height.

A striking feature of the hip and knee patterns is the increase in peak knee extension (approximately 30 degrees) as seat height increased, coupled with much smaller increases in peak hip extension (less than 10 degrees). The general shape and timing of each joint's kinematic curve, however, remained fairly similar across the four seat height conditions. In all conditions peak

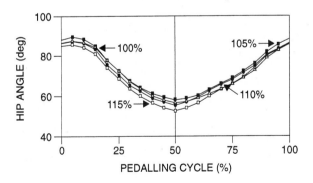

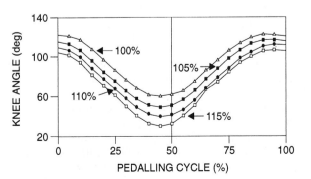

FIGURE 19–2. Angular displacement of the hip and knee for one pedaling cycle at four different seat heights: 100, 105, 110, and 115 percent of leg length. Angle convention is presented in Figure 19–1.

hip flexion and extension occurred at approximately 10 degrees and 180 degrees of the pedaling cycle, respectively, while peak knee flexion and extension occurred at approximately 350 degrees and 170 degrees of the pedaling cycle. In a subsequent investigation[11] (unpublished data), we employed a lower range of seat height conditions (96 to 108 percent of pubic symphysis height) and found almost identical results at the knee and hip, while the ankle joint demonstrated a marked increase in plantar flexion around BDC in the 108 percent condition (approximately 18 degrees above the 96 percent condition). In all studies, however, the knee was the joint most affected by changes in seat height.

Ericson et al.[12] also reported changes in range of motion at the hip, knee, and ankle during stationary cycling in what was referred to as "low," "middle," and "high" seat height conditions with the pedal spindle almost directly under the arch of the foot. Data from this study are summarized in Table 19-1.

Although comparative values for absolute seat heights were not available, these data also indicate that the knee is the joint most affected by changes in seat height. Total knee joint excursion increased from 20 degrees to 80 degrees as the seat was raised from the low to the high position. In addition, the knee proceeds into a greater degree of flexion at the low seat height and to a greater degree of extension (less flexion) at the high seat height. Although the hip range of motion displayed less dramatic changes, the thigh is generally in a more extended position at the high seat height, placing both the hip and the knee and their surrounding musculature in a different range of operation (e.g., operating in a different absolute range of muscle length while shortening and/or lengthening). These differing absolute ranges of motion affect the force production capabilities of the muscles by placing them in a different area of their length-tension and force–velocity curves; implications for these changes in the absolute range of motion experienced by each body segment on the individual joints and surrounding musculature will be discussed in a subsequent section of this chapter.

Efforts to more completely describe lower extremity kinematics involve three-dimensional analyses, including movement in the transverse and frontal planes. For example, internal and external rotation of the tibia about its long axis, knee translation in the frontal plane, and considerable movement of the lower extremity outside the sagittal plane have all been reported.[6] Movement of the knee in the frontal plane has been reported by McCoy,[13] Ruby et al.,[14] and Boutin et al.,[15] and results indicate that the joint center can move as much as 6 cm in the mediolateral direction during one pedaling cycle. Beginning at TDC, the femur internally rotates and adducts as the lower extremity proceeds through the power phase. In addition, as the knee moves medially with respect to the pedal, the tibia inwardly rotates as the foot pronates. Rotational components are difficult to measure, but allowing these natural movements to take place with minimal constraint may have a marked affect on joint forces and tissue stress.

Addressing another aspect of this issue — that is, how much movement should be allowed to minimize

TABLE 19–1 Joint Excursion (in degrees)			
	Seat Height		
	Low	*Middle*	*High*
Hip	40–80	32–70	20–65
Knee	65–125	46–112	25–105
Ankle	5 PF–25 PF	2 DF–22 PF	12 DF–20 PF

DF, Dorsiflexion; PF, plantar flexion.

load on muscle and connective tissue structures— Hannaford et al.[6] reported that subjects without knee problems showed less transverse and frontal plane movement than did riders with a history of knee pain. In support of this finding, Francis,[3] using qualitative video analysis, reported less knee movement in the frontal plane in elite cyclists who used in-shoe orthotics. Using trial-and-error adjustments in pedal cant and video feedback to reduce frontal plane movement seemed to decrease knee pain in elite cyclists. The issue of how much to limit natural movement of lower extremity structures remains open to discussion.

McCoy[13] investigated the effects of different seat positions on lower extremity kinematics and kinetics in the frontal plane. Seat height was varied from 94 to 106 percent of leg length, a range comparable to that used in the unpublished data previously discussed.[11] Results indicated the knee was medial of the pedal center of pressure throughout the power phase. The greatest magnitude of deviation occurred at approximately 90 degrees of crank rotation in the low seat height condition (94 percent of pubic symphysis height) and at 150 degrees of crank rotation at the medium and high seat heights (100 and 106 percent of pubic symphysis height, respectively). Data presented in Figure 19–3 represent average patterns for 150 pedal revolutions from five subjects riding at 200 W at the three seat height conditions just mentioned. The zero line is corrected for natural excursion of the pedal center of pressure, with the data showing the knee moving from a position medial to the center of pressure during the power phase to one lateral to the center of pressure during recovery. Although their measurements were referenced to the center of the pedal and not the center of pressure, similar data have been presented by Ruby et al.[16] Despite the fact that no seat height changes were reported, the significance of these data lies in the fact that the lower extremity displays considerable movement in the frontal plane, and variation in seat height has a marked effect on the amount of actual movement.

Clinically, the stationary bike is often used to provide gentle knee range-of-motion exercises during the initial stages of a rehabilitation program. Seat height can be set relatively high if the patient has limited knee flexion and low if knee extension is limited so that the patient can perform a full pedal revolution. In addition, some companies manufacture telescoping cranks that can be adjusted for the involved or injured side. These attachments, however, may move the foot to a position that is more lateral to the knee than the standard pedal position and should be carefully considered in the patient where medial joint distraction must be minimized (e.g., after medial collateral ligament strain). Permanent adjustments can be made to the crank to customize the patient's bicycle for chronic conditions such as arthritis; this can also be of great benefit in pediatrics. As stated earlier, a minimum knee flexion range of approximately 110 degrees is necessary to permit a complete crank revolution for a middle seat height position without adjusting the crank. Initially, a patient could power the bicycle with the contralateral limb to perform passive range-of-motion exercises, with pedaling rate and resistance gradually increased to tolerance.

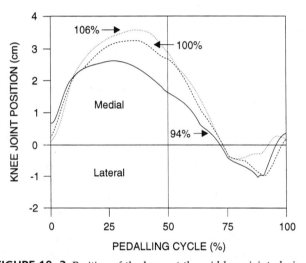

FIGURE 19–3. Position of the knee, at the mid-knee joint, during the pedaling cycle with respect to the pedal center of pressure at three different seat heights: 94, 100, and 106 percent of leg length. Each curve is an average of 150 pedal revolutions (10 subjects × five trials) at 200 W and 80 rpm. (From McCoy RW: The Effect of Varying Seat Position on Knee Loads During Cycling. Unpublished doctoral dissertation, University of Southern California Department of Exercise Science, 1989.)

MUSCLE LENGTH CHANGES

Changes in limb kinematics will naturally affect the length-tension and force-velocity relationship of separate muscle-tendon units, as well as the performance of muscle groups (e.g., quadriceps and hamstrings). Consequently, knowledge of muscle length, velocity, previous history (e.g., muscle stretch), muscle architecture, and activation—all variables that affect the muscle's ability to produce force—is important. Range-of-motion information is also significant when applied to a situation when the muscle-tendon unit sustains an injury, since it is important to know what type of length changes (both active and passive) the rehabilitation program imposes. Following acute injuries, rehabilitation should begin with exercises that minimize muscle length changes, especially in active muscle, as muscle length changes would increase tension on healing structures. Cycling is an especially gentle exercise following injuries that commonly occur to two-joint muscles of the lower extremity (e.g., hamstrings, gastrocnemius, and rectus femoris). Hip and knee angular changes have opposing effects on muscle length (increasing vs. decreasing), resulting in minimal length change in these muscles. For example, hip extension acts to decrease hamstring length, while knee extension acts to increase it during the propulsive phase. During the recovery phase, hip flexion acts to increase hamstring length, while knee flexion acts to decrease it.

Using hip, knee, and ankle joint angular kinematics and lower extremity anatomy, estimates of length changes for all major lower extremity muscle-tendon units have been made.[15] Exemplar data are presented for different seat height conditions in Figures 19–4 and 19–5 for the vasti and hamstring muscle groups at seat heights of 100, 105, 110, and 115 percent of leg length.[11] These data were obtained from the kinematic data previously discussed at these same four conditions. The zero line in each case is referenced to the hip and knee positioned at 90 degrees. Results clearly indicate that changes in seat height have a marked effect on muscle

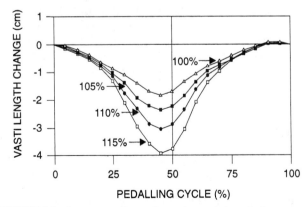

FIGURE 19–4. Patterns of muscle-tendon unit length changes during the pedaling cycle for the vasti group (vastus lateralis and medialis) at four different seat heights: 100, 105, 110, and 115 percent of leg length. The zero line represents the muscle length with the hip and knee at 90 degrees. Negative slopes indicate muscle-tendon unit shortening.

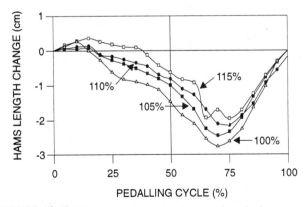

FIGURE 19–5. Patterns of muscle-tendon unit length changes during the pedaling cycle for the hamstring group (all biarticular muscles) at four different seat heights: 100, 105, 110, and 115 percent of leg length. The zero line represents the length with the hip and knee at 90 degrees. Negative slopes indicate muscle-tendon unit shortening.

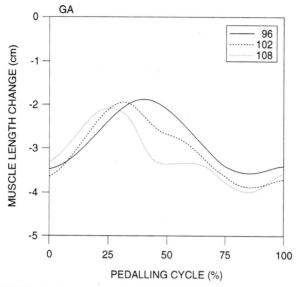

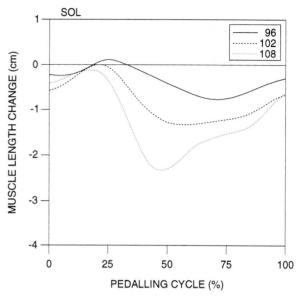

FIGURE 19–6. Patterns of muscle-tendon unit length changes during the pedaling cycle for the gastrocnemius muscle (both medial and lateral head) at three different seat heights: 96, 102, and 108 percent of leg length. The zero line represents the length in the anatomic position. Negative slopes indicate muscle-tendon unit shortening.

FIGURE 19–7. Patterns of muscle-tendon unit length changes during the pedaling cycle for the soleus muscle at three different seat heights: 96, 102, and 108 percent of leg length. The zero line represents the length in the anatomic position. Negative slopes indicate muscle-tendon unit shortening.

length patterns and further imply that as seat height increases, muscle-tendon unit shortening and lengthening velocities increase. For example, as seat height increases at a constant cadence, the vasti muscles experience greater shortening as the knee extends toward BDC. Total shortening approaches 4 cm in the 115 percent condition but less than half of that (1.5 cm) in the 100 percent condition. In contrast, the biarticular hamstrings show initial lengthening prior to shortening, less shortening in the 115 percent than in the 100 percent condition, and qualitatively similar velocities in each condition. In addition, for all cases, cyclic patterns of lengthening and subsequent shortening appear in each muscle group during a complete pedaling cycle.

Data for the gastrocnemius and soleus muscles are presented in Figures 19–6 and 19–7 and indicate that changes in seat height appear to affect the soleus more than the gastrocnemius. These data were obtained from the unpublished kinematic data previously discussed using the seat height conditions of 96 percent to 108 percent of pubic symphysis height.[11] The gastrocnemius displays essentially the same pattern at each seat height condition, lengthening markedly during the first 90 degrees of crank rotation (about 1.5 cm), then shortening about 2 cm, only to lengthen again prior to TDC. In contrast, the soleus muscle displays very different patterns at the separate seat height conditions, lengthening slightly during the early stages of propulsion and then markedly shortening as the crank approaches BDC. The muscle then lengthens again during the second half of the pedaling cycle (180 to 360 degrees). Although the magnitude of initial lengthening is about the same for each seat height, the magnitude of shortening dramatically increases from less than 1 cm at the 96 percent condition to approximately 2.5 cm at the 108 percent condition. Shortening velocities apparently in-

crease as well. Although magnitudes will vary from experiment to experiment because of different seat height conditions, similar patterns for all four muscles presented as examples in this chapter have been demonstrated in the literature.[15,17,18] The general conclusion drawn from these data is that biarticular muscles display less total length change than do their uniarticular synergists and also appear to be less affected by variations in seat height. These facts make cycling an excellent form of exercise during the acute stages of rehabilitation following a muscle-tendon injury to biarticular muscle.

MUSCLE ACTIVITY DURING CYCLING

To rehabilitate a patient after injury or appropriately condition an athlete, knowledge of muscle activation patterns, considering both intensity and duration, is important. Activation should be maximized in muscles that are weak and minimized in muscles whose action may stress healing tissue. Muscle recruitment patterns during cycling have been reported for major lower extremity muscles using both surface and fine-wire EMG.[19–23] Activity patterns are also most commonly described relative to the angle of the crank. In general, the greatest activity occurs in the leg that is in the propulsive phase between TDC and BDC, when almost all of the energy needed to drive the bicycle is imparted from the rider to the bicycle. At this time the opposite-side limb is in the recovery phase between BDC and TDC and substantially less muscle activity is observed. During this recovery phase, any observable muscle activity usually results in unloading the pedal and minimizing resistance to the propulsive demands.

Representative data from 18 experienced cyclists riding at 90 rpm and 250 W on their own bicycles are

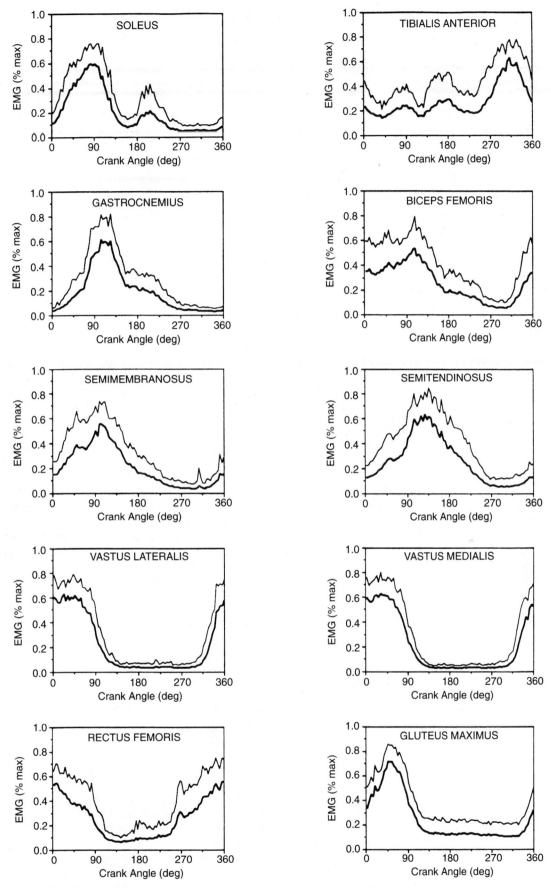

FIGURE 19–8. Mean patterns of muscle activation during the pedaling cycle for ten muscles in the lower extremity. The dark lower curve is the average pattern from 15 pedaling cycles across 18 subjects (270 cycles), and the lighter upper curve is one standard deviation above the mean. Magnitudes are normalized to maximal activation. (From Ryan MM, Gregor RJ: EMG profiles of lower extremity muscles during cycling at constant workload and cadence. J Electromyogr Kinesiol 1992; 2:69–80.)

shown in Figure 19–8.[23] During the propulsive phase, power is imparted to the bicycle via forceful hip and knee extension, with the gluteal (e.g., gluteus maximus) and quadriceps muscles heavily recruited during this time. For example, onset of activity for the gluteus maximus occurs just before TDC, with peak activity observed at approximately 55 degrees of crank rotation. Both medial and lateral vasti muscles exhibit a rapid onset and cessation with relatively constant activity in between, while the rectus femoris demonstrates a more gradual rise and decline. Rectus femoris activity onset occurs before the vasti and declines earlier in the power phase, most likely due to its biarticular function at the hip. EMG activity ceases shortly after 90 degrees in all three quadriceps muscles, essentially ending their role as significant contributors to the work necessary to drive the bicycle.

Major ankle extensors are also active during the propulsive phase and, although not considered major power producers, are important in providing a stable link between the pedal, foot, and the more proximal joints so that the total amount of energy produced in lower extremity musculature can be transmitted to the pedal. The soleus is recruited just prior to the gastrocnemius; both muscles are active before TDC, with peak activity occurring before 90 degrees in the pedaling cycle. The gastrocnemius is recruited shortly after the soleus, and peak activity occurring at an average of 107 degrees, declining gradually during recovery, and ending at approximately 270 degrees of crank rotation. This phase shift in the soleus relative to gastrocnemius onset may be related to two factors: First, peak stretch occurs later in the gastrocnemius than in the soleus (see Figs. 19–6 and 19–7), and in both muscles peak EMG activity seems to occur just prior to peak stretch. Second, a delayed peak in the activation of the gastrocnemius would help contribute to the knee flexor moment consistently observed after 90 degrees in the pedal cycle. Force enhancement may occur due to the presence of active stretch prior to muscle shortening in both the gastrocnemius and the soleus muscles.[17] In addition, the anterior tibial muscle is active during the propulsive phase in many individuals, and coactive with the ankle extensors, and may be used to enhance ankle stability during propulsion and force transmission to the pedal.

The hamstring muscles are also active during the power phase of cycling and most likely function to extend the hip during simultaneous knee extension. The semimembranosus and semitendinosus muscles are recruited after TDC, with peak activity occurring at or slightly after 90 degrees, when activity in the gluteal and vasti muscles is rapidly declining. Peak activity in the semitendinous muscle occurs slightly after that of the semimembranous, with biceps femoris activity being the most variable of the hamstring group. In some individuals timing of the biceps femoris is similar to that in the semimembranous and semitendinous muscles, while in others the biceps femoris is already maximally active at TDC and declines throughout propulsion.[23] Finally, continued activation of the hamstrings for the remainder of the power phase contributes to the knee flexor moment, especially in the absence of any quadriceps activity after 90 degrees of crank rotation.[24]

During recovery, the recovery limb flexes to lessen resistance to the crank as the propulsive limb provides power. Initially (between 180 and 235 degrees of the pedal cycle), the hamstrings and gastrocnemius, already active, provide a major component to flex the knee. Later in the recovery phase, between 235 and 360 degrees, the anterior tibial muscle acts to dorsiflex the ankle, and the rectus femoris (also a knee extensor) acts to flex the hip. Although no reports are available, it is assumed that the iliopsoas is also active during hip flexion. In some subjects there is a smaller soleus burst during the recovery phase, whereas for all subjects the primary tibial burst occurs during recovery, between 270 and 360 degrees. Ideally, the net flexion of the lower extremity during recovery would require just enough energy to match the acceleration of the crank between 180 and 360 degrees of the cycle. If this were the case, no counter torques would be present to resist crank rotation or the efforts of the propulsive limb, and the recovery limb would not be "pulling up" on the crank, actively adding to crank rotation. In short, there should be a fine balance during recovery to provide just enough energy to lift the limb. More energy would actively lift the crank and possibly be an inefficient contribution to crank rotation, while less energy would be counterproductive and force the limb to provide excess energy during propulsion to both drive the bicycle and lift the recovery limb.

Almost all of the data presented on EMG patterns in the lower extremity during cycling, have been collected using surface electrodes, and although good agreement has been found between surface and fine-wire electrodes in the evaluation of large muscles, evidence of cross-talk has been reported when using surface electrodes to evaluate smaller muscles such as the gracilis, sartorius, and tensor fasciae latae. In studies that used fine-wire electrodes, it has been reported that gracilis activity seems to begin just prior to BDC and to end just before TDC. Tensor fasciae latae activity begins at about 240 degrees and ends at approximately TDC, while sartorius activity begins approximately at BDC and ends approximately at TDC.

In normal subjects there are no dramatic changes in the timing of muscle activity relative to pedal position with changes in bicycle configuration, pedal speed, or rider position on the bicycle. As seat height increases, there seems to be a slight shift in the timing of muscle activity: the major muscles appear to begin activation later in the cycle and remain active for a longer period of time.[19] The significance of this shift to cycling performance is currently unknown. Increases in work load appear to affect the intensity of activation but not the timing.

In summary, the major points regarding muscle activation during the cycling task are:

1. Coactivation of knee flexors and extensors appears during the first 90 degrees of the pedaling cycle, while the hamstrings and gastrocnemius muscle

continue activation through the second quadrant and past BDC.

2. Single-joint muscle activity is very consistent across subjects, while biarticular muscle activity is significantly more variable.

3. Almost all muscles begin activity during muscle stretch, and some end before the muscle has completed its shortening.

CYCLING KINETICS

PEDAL REACTION FORCES

A kinetic analysis of lower extremity function requires knowledge of the interactive forces between the rider and the bicycle. Newton's third law of motion essentially states that forces act in pairs that are equal and opposite in direction. Therefore, when the foot applies a force to the pedal, it will be met with a reaction force that is equal in magnitude and opposite in direction. These forces, called *pedal reaction forces,* act on the lower limb during cycling and have been quantified with the use of specially instrumented pedals.[25] These pedals are similar to force platforms widely used to measure ground reaction forces during gait. Force components perpendicular to the pedal surface (Fz) and shear forces tangential to the pedal surface, both mediolateral (Fx) and anteroposterior (Fy) (Fig. 19–9A), have been measured, and from these components a center of pressure (Fig. 19–9C, Ay and Ax), or point of force application, can be calculated. Finally, a rotational moment about an axis perpendicular to the surface of the pedal (Fig. 19–9B, Mz) and positioned at the center of pressure may also be quantified. This rotational moment will be discussed in a later section of this chapter.

Patterns representing the perpendicular component of the pedal reaction force were first reported in 1896[26]; however, it was not until 1968 that patterns of this component were presented again.[27] Subsequent to these reports, results of a two-dimensional force pedal analysis were reported in which patterns for both perpendicular and tangential pedal reaction force components were presented.[28] Numerous studies have reported the use of pedal force transducers[9] in the study of lower extremity mechanics during cycling.

As observed in Figure 19–9, peak force perpendicular to the pedal surface is approximately 350 N, or 60 percent of the subject's body weight. This percentage is about the same for all seated cycling under steady-state conditions. These reaction forces will, of course, increase as resistance increases, but they rarely exceed body weight unless the subject stands up. In addition, although riders often feel they pull up on the pedals during recovery, this is rare as well. Pulling up on the pedal is not essential to efficient cycling technique, and competitive riders reserve this action for climbing or sprinting. Finally, symmetry in pedaling technique is also rare. This is true for both highly competitive cyclists and recreational cyclists. Depending on power requirements, individual conditioning, and bike setup, bilateral asymmetry can be large.

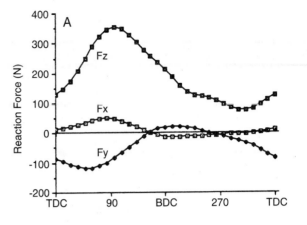

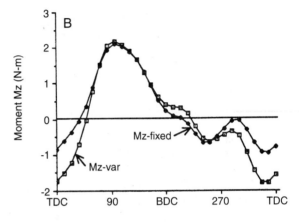

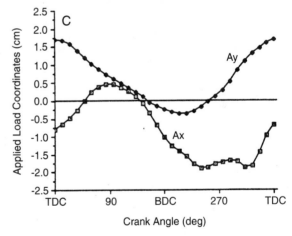

FIGURE 19–9. Mean patterns for five pedal revolutions for the pedal reaction force *(A)*, applied moment *(B)*, and center of pressure patterns *(C)* during one pedaling cycle (top dead center [TDC] at 0 degrees to TDC at 360 degrees). *A*, Fz is the component orthogonal to the pedal surface, Fy is anteroposterior (AP) shear, and Fx is the medial/lateral shear. *B*, The applied moment (Mz) about an axis orthogonal to the pedal surface when this axis is through the center of pressure (Mz-var) or through the center of the pedal (Mz-fixed). *C*, Coordinates of the applied load in the x (Ax) and y (Ay) directions. (From Broker JP, Gregor RJ: A dual piezoelectric element force pedal for kinetic analysis of cycling. Int J Sport Biomech 1990; 6:394–403. Copyright 1990 by Human Kinetics Publishers, Inc. Reprinted by permission.)

Although the magnitude of the pedal reaction force is important, the orientation of the resultant vector (Fr) with respect to the lower extremity is also important and will markedly influence how the leg musculature

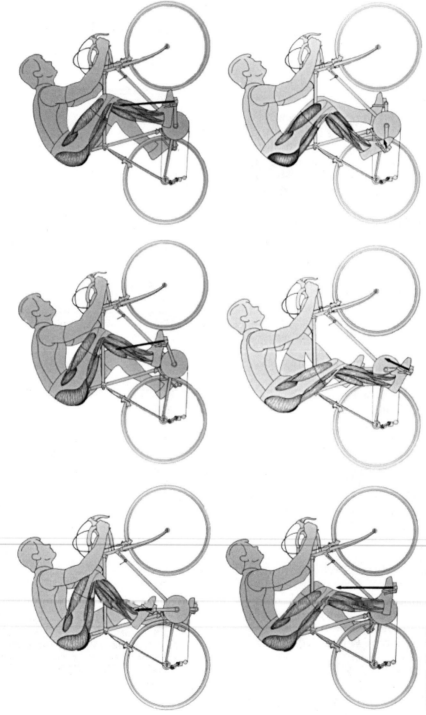

FIGURE 19–10. Resultant pedal reaction force with respect to the right lower extremity for six separate locations during the pedaling cycle. The length of the arrow indicates increases and decreases in magnitude.

responds to various environmental demands. An exemplar pattern of the resultant pedal reaction force measured at six intervals during the pedaling cycle is presented in Figure 19–10, together with the relationship between the resultant vector and the right lower extremity. The objective of any rehabilitation program is to effectively transmit power to the bicycle; make sure these reactive loads are oriented in such a way as to use lower extremity musculature in an efficient and effective manner; and ensure that unusually high loads, which may result in overuse injuries to the legs, are kept to a minimum.

The angle of the pedal reaction force with respect to each segment in the frontal plane (e.g., the knee) is important, and several published reports[13,14,29] indicate, for example, that a varus load is applied to the knee during the power phase (0 to 180 degrees; Fig. 19–11) when the largest magnitude of the pedal reaction force is observed. This is obviously a result of the reaction force passing medial to the knee, despite the fact that the knee appears to be medial to the pedal center. The applied moment of the pedal reaction force will vary according to the magnitude of the pedal force and the distance the force vector passes either medial or lateral to the knee joint center. Values reported in the literature for peak varus load moments at the knee range from 6 to 25 N-m. Both Ericson et al.[29] and Ruby et al.[14] assumed the reaction force was located in the center of the pedal, but McCoy[13] employed a system that calculated movement of the center of pressure in the frontal plane during the pedaling cycle and described the position of the vector with respect to the knee (see Fig. 19–11) for three seat height conditions: 94, 100, and 106 percent of leg length.

Translation of pedal force components to "effective" crank rotation can be accomplished with the additional knowledge of pedal and crank position. LaFortune and Cavanagh[30] first presented the concept of pedaling effectiveness by calculating the effective force on the crank—i.e., the force component perpendicular to the crank. This force is responsible for turning the crank and providing the angular impulse necessary to power the bicycle (Fig. 19–12). In addition, they calculated the component parallel to the crank and considered it to be the ineffective force, a component inherent in cycling dynamics but one that does not contribute to crank rotation. An index of effectiveness has also been presented; this is the ratio between the effective and ineffective components.

Developing an "optimal" pedaling pattern has long been the objective of coaches and competitive cyclists with training programs designed to develop and maintain an effective pattern of force application. Broker et al.[31,32] examined the effect of visual feedback on the ability to produce a more effective pattern of force application during cycling. Although all subjects were able to follow the "ideal" pattern presented on a computer monitor, concurrent feedback was found to be just as effective as summary feedback in a 2-week and a 2-month retention test for producing an effective force pattern on the crank. In addition, Perell[33] reported the use of an effective force pattern in feedback presented to stroke patients for the purpose of enhancing gait symmetry. Improvements in symmetry were variable between the feedback and no-feedback groups, but use of the effective force pattern as the feedback parameter was found to be difficult for the impaired stroke patients to follow and understand.

Browning[34] examined the index of effectiveness when elite triathletes assumed an aerodynamic versus an advanced aerodynamic position on the bicycle and concluded there was no change in force effectiveness between the two positions. It seems that as the riders assumed a more forward advanced aerodynamic position—one in which they are in a very low position out over the handlebars—the effective force pattern simply rotated forward, or clockwise, offering the same

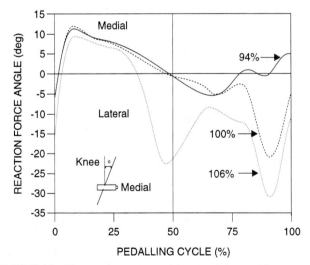

FIGURE 19–11. Position of the pedal reaction force with respect to the knee during the pedaling cycle in the frontal plane. Each curve is an average of 150 pedal revolutions (ten subjects × five trials) at 200 W and 80 rpm. Separate patterns are an average at three seat conditions: 94, 100, and 106 percent of leg length. (From McCoy RW: The Effect of Varying Seat Position on Knee Loads During Cycling. Unpublished doctoral dissertation, University of Southern California Department of Exercise Science, 1989.)

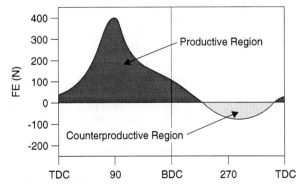

FIGURE 19–12. Effective force profile during one pedal revolution. The productive region is positive work done to drive the crank; the counterproductive region during recovery represents an extra load that the contralateral limb must work against during its power phase (TDC to BDC).

mechanically efficient kinetics regardless of the rider's position. These results are of great practical value and support the conclusion that as the rider assumes an aerodynamic position to minimize wind drag, there are minimal losses in cycling efficiency, with very similar patterns of effective force on the crank. Wheeler et al.[35] reported that regardless of the pedal design chosen (toe-strap and cleat, clipless fixed, or clipless float), power transmitted to the bicycle, as measured by effective crank force patterns, was not compromised. These results are also significant because there has been some speculation that current clipless pedal designs permitting "float" result in a reduction in power transferred to the bike.

Collectively, data on effective force patterns on the crank are also useful in the clinical setting. Although aerodynamics and shoe-pedal interface designs are not a major concern in a clinical environment, kinematics of the ankle, methods of securing a patient's foot to the pedal on either an upright or recumbent stationary bike, and any other factors related to the control of the position of a patient's lower extremity during a selected rehabilitation protocol warrant consideration, since strategies developed by each patient to energize the bike focus on his or her ability to effectively transmit forces to the crank in a manner intended to maximize the use of surrounding musculature and minimize further trauma to injured tissue (e.g., ligaments and bone).

PEDAL PRESSURE DISTRIBUTION

Forces acting on the bottom of the foot can also be quantified by examining pressure (force per unit area), and such quantification is a useful measure to examine injuries related to the interface between the foot and the pedal. Sanderson and Cavanagh[36] studied the variations in pressure distribution throughout the pedaling cycle using a specially designed insole with 256 discrete force measuring elements (Fig. 19–13). They reported that the majority of foot pressure was localized in the forefoot directly over the pedal, especially in the head of the first metatarsal and hallux. More recently, Sanderson and Hennig[37] used a shoe insert with 12 separate pressure transducers to measure the distribution during steady-state cycling and found that pressures were more evenly distributed across the sole of rigid cycling shoes than across the sole of running shoes (see Fig. 19–13). Pressure distributions were measured by Amoroso et al.[38] across different cadences and by Hennig and Sanderson[39] across different power outputs; both found an increased relative pressure assumed by the anteromedial structures of the forefoot, the first metatarsal and hallux, with increased resultant pedal force. The implications to injury and rehabilitation were not addressed by these authors except for the observation that cycling shoes are preferred probably because of the more evenly distributed pressure afforded by the rigid soles.

The ability to measure the distribution of pressure offers an additional perspective on the shoe-pedal

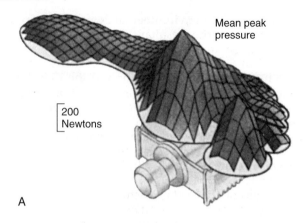

A

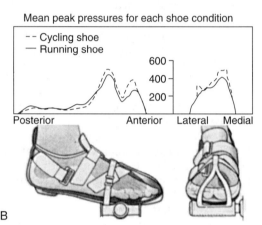

B

FIGURE 19–13. Pattern of pressure distribution on the sole of the cycling shoe, including data from a subject using a cycling shoe and a running shoe. (From Sanderson DJ: The biomechanics of cycling shoes. Cycling Sci 1990; Sept.: 27–30.)

interface critical to the understanding of lower extremity kinetics during cycling. The center of pressure reported earlier offered the opportunity to investigate the effects of changes in this variable and subsequent effects on the calculation of lower extremity loads during the cycling task. However, application of a pressure measurement system may be more valuable in evaluating clinical cases in which specific shoe-pedal systems are suspected to be the source of individual foot pain or, in combination with orthotics, in correcting lower extremity dynamics related to injury.

LOWER EXTREMITY JOINT KINETICS

KNEE JOINT REACTION FORCES

Although knowledge of joint reaction forces is significant to our understanding to lower extremity function, little data are available on the magnitude and direction of these calculated values for the cycling task. Data specific to each joint are critical to our understanding of joint function and rehabilitation. Even though all segments are of interest, for the most part the data that are available describe knee joint loads, because the knee is the joint most often under rehabilitation in a cycling exercise program. Vector components specific to the knee joint are schematically presented in Figure 19–14, with a positive Fy_k (tensile-compressive component) and positive Fx_k (anteroposterior component; the mediolateral component is orthogonal to this vector) described with respect to the tibial plateau.

Ericson et al.[40] calculated anteroposterior shear forces across normal, noninjured tibiofemoral joints during ergometer cycling and found that they reflected both an external joint reaction force and an estimated force component due to extensor activity at the knee. Tests were conducted at 60 rpm, 120 W of power, and a seat height of 113 percent ischial tuberosity–to–medial malleolus length (a bit different from the measurements used in the previous section on lower extremity kinematics). With use of a forward foot/pedal position (i.e., with the lateral malleolus over the pedal spindle), Ericson et al.[40] reported shear forces posteriorly directed for the first 80 degrees of the pedaling cycle at a time when the knee was extending from approximately 110 to 75 degrees (0 degrees is full extension). Shear forces then became anteriorly directed from 80 to 140 degrees of crank rotation as the knee continued to extend from 75 to 48 degrees. The peak anterior shear force was only 37 N (0.05 times body weight) and occurred at about 104 degrees of the pedaling cycle and at a knee angle of approximately 68 degrees. Shear forces then shifted posteriorly again from 135 to 180 degrees in the pedaling cycle. These shear forces were less than 10 N and fluctuated from anteriorly to

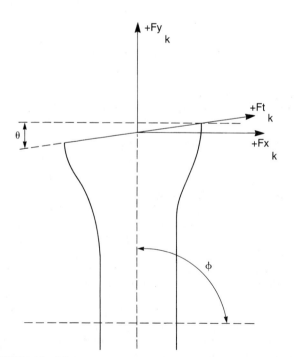

FIGURE 19–14. Sagittal plane view of the proximal tibia and the orientation of the posterior tilt angle of the tibial plateau with respect to the horizontal axis of the tibia. Ft_k is the AP shear joint reaction force component, Fx_k is the horizontal shear component, and Fy_k is the vertical knee reaction force component; θ is the posterior tilt angle and ϕ is the shank angle. (From Furumizo SH: A Biomechanical Analysis of Anterior/Posterior Shear Joint Reaction Forces in the ACL-Deficient Knee During Stationary Cycling. Unpublished master's thesis, UCLA Department of Kinesiology, 1991.)

posteriorly directed forces for the remainder of the recovery phase (180 to 360 degrees of crank rotation). Finally, these authors found that use of a posterior foot position (i.e., the ball of the foot over the pedal spindle) and increased pedaling speed increased the magnitude of the anteriorly directed shear force component, while changes in seat height had little effect on the shear force component.

McCoy and Gregor[41] also reported knee joint reaction forces in an investigation of ten male cyclists riding at 200 W and 80 rpm. Results are reported for three seat height conditions: 94, 100, and 106 percent of leg length. The vector calculated along the tibial shaft was compressive throughout the entire pedaling cycle at all seat conditions and reached values of 207 N at 92 degrees in the pedaling cycle for the 106 percent seat condition and 209 N at 110 degrees in the pedaling cycle at the 94 and 100 percent seat conditions (Fig. 19–15A). The most noticeable effect of seat height was the rapid change in compressive load at the 106 percent condition. After reaching a peak at approximately 90 degrees in the pedaling cycle, the compressive load decreased to about 15 N at about 160 degrees in the pedaling cycle. In contrast, the pattern of compressive loading was essentially the same for the other two seat height conditions.

The anteroposterior shear force component, perpendicular to the tibial shaft, was anteriorly directed during the power phase, with peak values observed near 90 degrees for all seat height conditions (Fig. 19–15B). The peak magnitude at the lowest seat height condition (129.8 N) was significantly larger ($P < .05$) than the values obtained at the middle and highest seat height conditions (115.6 N and 113.1 N, respectively). Similar to the compressive joint reaction force, the anterior joint reaction force decreased at a greater rate at the highest seat height position than at the other two seat height conditions and actually became posteriorly directed at 150 degrees in the pedaling cycle. The appearance of a posteriorly directed shear force component at this phase of the pedaling cycle is consistent with the data presented by Ericson et al.[29] and support the hypothesis that changes in seat height can have a marked effect on the direction of the shear force component at the knee and subsequently have direct relevance, for example, in rehabilitation of anterior cruciate ligament (ACL)-deficient patients using a cycling task in the rehabilitation program.

The joint reaction force in the mediolateral direction was laterally directed during the power phase, with peak values observed just after 90 degrees into the pedaling cycle for all seat height positions (Fig. 19–15C).[41] Values obtained during the highest seat height condition (46.3 N) were significantly smaller ($P < .05$) than the peak lateral force calculated at the middle and lowest seat height conditions (49.8 N and 52.4 N, respectively). Medially directed forces occurred during the recovery phase of the pedaling cycle, with values being smaller and more variable than the laterally directed forces. Values obtained during the lowest seat height condition were significantly larger than the values observed at the middle seat height condition, with peak values of 31.3 N and 21.0 N, respectively.

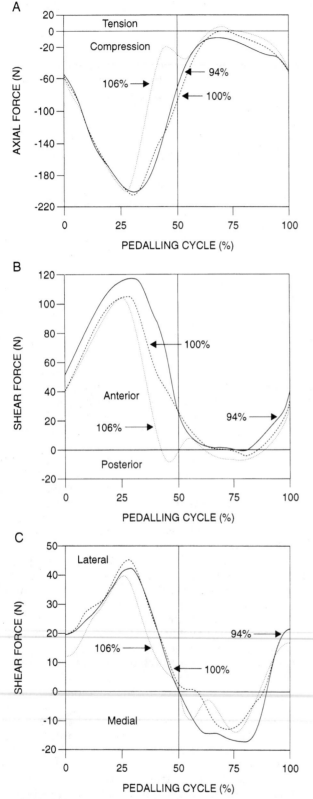

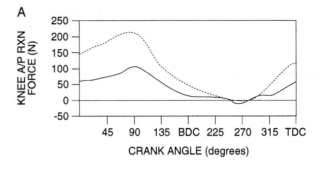

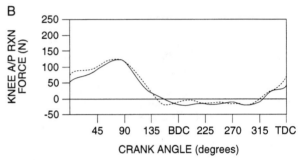

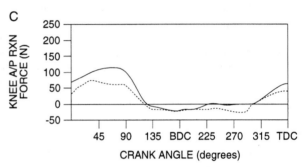

FIGURE 19–16. Anteroposterior knee joint reaction force profiles for three anterior cruciate ligament (ACL)–deficient patients. The solid line represents the ACL-deficient limb, and the dashed line represents the contralateral limb. (From Furumizo SH: A Biomechanical Analysis of Anterior/Posterior Shear Joint Reaction Forces in the ACL-Deficient Knee During Stationary Cycling. Unpublished master's thesis, UCLA Department of Kinesiology, 1991.)

ANTERIOR CRUCIATE LIGAMENT IMPLICATIONS. In an investigation of ACL-deficient patients, Furumizo[42] studied three patients and three control subjects riding at 70 to 90 rpm at a power output of 250 W in a stationary ergometer. Postoperative time at testing varied from 3 to 9 months. Although a standard approach in Newtonian mechanics was used to solve for joint forces and moments, the orientation of the shear component of the knee joint reaction force was corrected for an 8-degree posterior tilt of the tibial plateau (see Fig. 19–14, Ft$_k$). All three control subjects displayed an anteriorly directed shear force (positive values) at the knee during the first 135 degrees of crank rotation, with two of the three subjects continuing this pattern up to at least 230 degrees in the pedaling cycle. ACL-deficient patients displayed essentially the same patterns (anteriorly directed shear forces until at least 135 degrees in the cycle) but showed considerable variance between the involved and contralateral limbs (Fig. 19–16). Axial loads were not reported in this study,

FIGURE 19–15. Knee joint reaction force components averaged for 150 pedal revolutions (ten subjects × five trials) at 200 W and 80 rpm for three seat height conditions: 94, 100, and 106 percent of leg length. *A,* The axial component along the shaft of the tibia. *B,* The anteroposterior shear force component. *C,* The medial/lateral shear force component. (From McCoy RW: The Effect of Varying Seat Position on Knee Loads During Cycling. Unpublished doctoral dissertation, University of Southern California Department of Exercise Science, 1989.)

since the primary purpose was to study shear loads in ACL-deficient patients.

The relationship between muscle activity and forces applied to connective tissue structures is an important one to consider in rehabilitation. Skeletal muscle contractions produce both compressive and shear force components, as well as rotation. For example, when the quadriceps contracts with the knee in an extended position, an anterior shear force is produced. The magnitude of this force is related to the strength of the contraction and the precise joint angle. Smidt[43] and Yasuda and Sasaki[44] studied the effects of isometric quadriceps and hamstring contractions on anterior tibial displacement. Shear force calculations included both an external joint reaction and an estimated muscle force component. Smidt[43] reported anteriorly directed shear forces for the first 60 degrees of knee flexion, with a peak force of 340 N (43 percent of body weight) at a knee angle of 15 degrees. A posteriorly directed shear force was reported at 75 and 90 degrees of knee flexion. Yasuda and Sasaki[44] found maximum anterior shear forces at 5 degrees of knee flexion; these decreased with increasing knee joint angle and shifted to a posterior shear force at 45 degrees (± 12 degrees). In both studies posterior shear forces were observed during maximal isometric hamstring contractions; these increased with greater knee joint angles from 5 to 90 degrees. A maximum force of 1479 N was reported by Smidt[43] and 785 N $\pm$ 108 N by Yasuda and Sasaki.[44] Yasuda and Sasaki[45] also studied the effect of simultaneous quadriceps and hamstring isometric contractions on anterior tibial shear force. A maximum anterior shear force was again found at 5 degrees but this was transitioned to a posteriorly directed shear force at an average of 7.4 degrees (± 5 degrees). All of these studies were performed under non–weight-bearing conditions. Yack et al.[46] studied anterior tibial translation during progressive loading of the ACL-deficient knee during both weight-bearing and non–weight-bearing isometric exercise and found that anterior tibial translation was substantially less during weight-bearing exercises and did not increase with increased loading. In contrast, non–weight-bearing exercise resulted in anterior tibial translation that was proportional to the knee extensor moment. Some degree of weight bearing must occur during knee extension during the propulsive phase of cycling, minimizing anterior tibial translation.

In vivo data reported by Henning et al.[47] support the presence of very low anterior shear forces during cycling. ACL strains were studied in two subjects with grade II ACL sprains. Relative to the strain produced during a Lachman test with an external load of 353 N imposed on the same knee, anterior tibial displacement was 7, 36, -7, and between 87 and 107 percent during stationary cycling, overground walking, isometric hamstring contractions, and isometric quadriceps contractions (0 degrees flexion), respectively.

In a report by Ruby et al.,[14] three-dimensional knee joint loading during seated cycling was studied in 11 male subjects cycling at their chosen seat height at 90 rpm and 225 W. Data indicate a compressive load during the entire pedaling cycle, with a peak plateau of about 240 N at between approximately 80 and 100 degrees in the pedaling cycle. Anteroposterior shear forces were anteriorly directed during the entire pedaling cycle, reaching a peak of about 125 N at about 70 degrees, while mediolateral forces were laterally directed during the first half of the pedal cycle, peaking at approximately 50 N at around 90 degrees; medially directed forces were present up to about 320 degrees, and laterally directed forces were present for the remainder of the pedal cycle. McCoy[41] reported similar patterns with laterally directed forces (also affected by seat height; see Fig. 19–15C) observed in the power phase, medially directed forces observed up to about 320 degrees, and laterally directed forces seen for the remainder of the cycle.

Information concerning calculated knee joint reaction force components, when combined with kinematic and EMG data, indicates that cycling is an excellent form of rehabilitation for patients after ACL injury and surgical repair. Although the EMG data presented in Figure 19–8 are from normal subjects, Furumizo[42] found similar quadriceps and hamstring EMG patterns in ACL-deficient knees. From TDC to approximately 90 degrees of the pedal cycle, the knee is relatively flexed, with coactivation of the quadriceps and hamstring muscles. Beyond this point, quadriceps activity sharply declines, and by the time the crank is at BDC, or in peak knee extension, only the hamstrings are active. By positioning the seat at a low height, the clinician can ensure that the knee is in a greater degree of knee flexion throughout the pedaling cycle. As the rehabilitation program progresses and weight bearing increases, anterior tibial strain will not increase as it would in the case of non–weight-bearing exercise. Caution should be taken, however, when using cycling to rehabilitate the patient with an injured posterior cruciate ligament, as posteriorly directed shear forces may be present throughout the pedaling cycle.

PATELLOFEMORAL JOINT. The patellofemoral joint reaction force is critical to knee function during cycling, and two reports have studied this joint as it relates to cycling and knee rehabilitation.[48,49] Pevsner et al.[48] reported that normal mechanics of patellar motion may lead to eventual age-dependent degeneration of the patellofemoral joint in many individuals. Although cycling was not specifically discussed, a range of studies were reviewed, all of which relate to the compromised knee, rehabilitation, and important considerations regarding strengthening of the knee, range of motion, and progressive resistance exercise.

Ericson and Nisell[49] estimated patellofemoral joint forces generated during pedaling a bicycle ergometer. Using a specially designed force pedal and high-speed cinematography, six males were studied at 0, 120, and 240 W, pedaling at 40, 60, 80, and 100 rpm at three different seat heights. Two foot positions on the pedal were employed, and all data supported previous statements that cycling is an excellent form of exercise and rehabilitation because of the low loads and tissue strains imposed on the knee. The magnitude of patellofemoral joint forces appeared to be independent of body weight, pedaling rate, and foot position but was greatly influenced by load and seat height. These data are specifically useful for knee pain patients and patients with chondromalacia patella.

MUSCLE MOMENTS

Muscle moments may be calculated for the cycling task using a linked segment model and equations of motion with kinematic, pedal reaction force, center of pressure, and anthropometry (mass and moment of inertia of each of the segments) data used as input. External moments may be computed for each joint, and these external demands must be met by internal moments produced by muscle and/or connective tissue forces acting about the same joint axis of rotation. For example, when an external flexor moment is produced about the knee joint, an internal knee extensor muscle moment, presumed to be dominated by the quadriceps muscles, must be generated. In the case of an external knee abductor moment, an internal knee adductor muscle moment, dominated by the medial collateral ligament and vastus medialis, must be generated. This internal muscle moment represents the sum of *all* active and passive structures acting about a joint producing moments in response to external demands. An internal knee flexor muscle moment, for example, does not mean that the knee extensor muscles are not active but that the net result of all forces results in a flexor muscle moment.

SAGITTAL PLANE. Sagittal plane muscle moments, in particular large hip and knee extensor moments, create crank rotation during the propulsive phase of cycling. During the recovery phase, flexor moments may act to unload the pedal, potentially minimizing resistance to the contralateral limb. Hip, knee, and ankle extensor and flexor moments are the most important in powering the bicycle. Investigations using a force pedal system to evaluate lower extremity kinetics during cycling have produced a great deal of information on muscle moment patterns during normal, steady-state cycling. These data have demonstrated, as first reported by Gregor[50] (Fig. 19–17), that the muscle moments at the hip, knee, and ankle have *fairly repeatable patterns*, despite variations in loading conditions, subject population, and bike setup. Magnitudes will increase in response to increased demands, and some timing features may be affected by cadence, but in almost all cases the general patterns remain the same.

As can be seen in the data presented in Figure 19–17, the hip and knee perform very different actions during the propulsive phase of cycling (i.e., the hip consistently produces an extensor moment, while the knee yields an extensor and then a flexor moment prior to attaining 180 degrees, or BDC in the pedaling cycle). This switch from a knee extensor to a knee flexor moment during knee extension in the power phase has been supported in several studies and has stimulated additional research on the coordinated function of the three linked segments in the lower extremity during the constrained cycling task.[24,40,51–54] Gregor et al.[24] discussed the

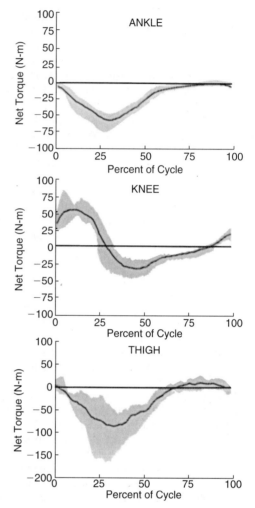

FIGURE 19–17. Muscle moment patterns for the ankle, knee, and thigh (hip) during the pedaling cycle. Patterns represent the average of 25 pedaling cycles (five subjects × five trials) at approximately 260 W and 84 rpm. (Reprinted from Gregor RJ, Cavanagh PR, LaFortune M: Knee flexor moments during propulsion in cycling—a creative solution to Lombardi's paradox. J Biomech 1985; 18:307–316, with kind permission from Elsevier Science, Ltd.)

moment reversal at the knee during propulsion with reference to the paradoxical behavior of biarticular muscles, in that a two-joint muscle may act as an extensor of the joint of which it is a flexor.[55] The muscles in question here are the hamstrings and quadriceps, antagonists at the hip and knee. Andrews[51] redefined "paradoxical" muscle action during cycling and based his conclusions on the fact that any explanation of two-joint muscle function in a kinetic analysis of the lower extremity during cycling may depend on the method of classification employed in the study. Van Ingen Schenau[56] further described the role of flexors and extensors in the production and distribution of energy between adjacent joints during cycling. He essentially concluded that the uniarticular muscles were "power producers" and the biarticular muscles were "power distributors" in the coordinated action of the lower extremity segments during the cycling task. In other words, the vasti muscles and gluteus maximus provide a great deal of the power needed during propulsion, while the rectus femoris and hamstring muscles may distribute some of the energy needed at joints unable to meet the power demands during certain portions of the pedaling cycle.

As discussed in the kinematics section, seat height changes affect lower extremity function. Browning et al.[52] reported that the ankle muscle moment, although being almost entirely plantar flexor throughout the pedaling cycle, increased in peak magnitude as seat height decreased from 108 to 96 percent of pubic symphysis height. In addition, seat height affected the magnitude of peak knee extensor moments, as higher peak magnitudes were observed at the 96 percent than at the 108 percent pubic symphysis height condition, which was consistent with the significant difference reported by McCoy[13,41] between his low (94 percent) and high (106 percent) seat height conditions. Browning et al.[52] also showed that knee flexor muscle moments occurred earlier in the pedaling cycle (at approximately 100 degrees) at 108 percent pubic symphysis height and later in the pedaling cycle (at approximately 145 degrees) at 96 percent pubic symphysis height. Furthermore, peak knee flexor magnitudes were higher at 108 percent pubic symphysis height than those reported at either 96 or 102 percent, a finding also supported by McCoy.[13,41]

Changing seat height also affected the peak hip moment. A hip extensor moment of approximately 55 N-m occurred at 108 percent, compared with 45 N-m at both the 96 percent and 102 percent pubic symphysis height conditions. Hip moment patterns displayed high intersubject variability; in fact, some cyclists exhibited hip flexor moments during isolated regions of the power phase. Hip flexor muscle moments during the power phase seem counterintuitive, but intersegmental dynamics indicate that large knee extensor moments occurring early in the power phase may necessitate coincidentally large hip flexor moments. In summary, then, it appears that *as seat height increases, peak ankle moments decrease, peak knee extensor moments decrease, peak knee flexor moments increase, and peak hip extensor moments increase.*

FRONTAL PLANE. Motion in the frontal plane occurs to varying degrees at the hip, knee, and ankle during cycling and appears to be most influenced by bike setup, rider position, and load. Because large frontal plane knee moments may result in injury and the bike is commonly employed in the rehabilitation of medial collateral ligament injuries, the greatest amount of data reported has been concerned with the knee.

Frontal plane muscle moments generated at the knee in response to the varus load moment from the pedal force oriented medial to the knee begin as a valgus moment, with values ranging between 6 and 7 N-m across seat positions[13,41] (Fig. 19–18). Magnitudes then appear to increase and reach a peak value near 90 degrees of crank rotation for all seat positions studied by McCoy and Gregor.[41] The lowest valgus moment (−16 N-m) was observed at the highest seat height (106 percent of leg length). The valgus muscle moment at the knee subsequently decreased to zero near BDC (180 degrees in the pedaling cycle), where it became a varus muscle moment for most of the recovery phase. The

peak varus muscle moment was significantly smaller ($P < .05$) for the middle seat position (4 N-m at 100 percent of leg length) when compared with the lowest (6 N-m at 94 percent of leg length) and highest (7 N-m at 106 percent of leg length) seat height conditions.[13,41] A second study by Ruby et al.[16] suggested that since external loads are applied to the foot during pedaling, anatomic variations in the foot may contribute to the loads transmitted to the knee and, subsequently, to joint injury. They concluded that a varus-applied moment occurs during the power phase and a valgus-applied moment occurs during recovery, suggesting that if knee injuries result from varus/valgus moments, then lateral knee structures may be injured during the power phase, whereas medial knee structures may be injured during the recovery phase.

These findings suggest the bicycle is a relatively benign environment for some structures in the knee but places potentially significant demands on others. With loads lower than those observed during walking, a varus moment applied to the knee as a result of a medially directed pedal reaction force places strain in the lateral structures of the knee, especially during the power phase. Valgus muscle moments generated in response to the pedal loads, however, are also lower than those observed during walking. With proper feedback and control, the bicycle may offer a valuable exercise paradigm designed to meet specific demands imposed in a clinical setting.

PEDAL TORSION MEASUREMENTS

Knowledge of torsion, or rotation of segments about a long axis through the center of the segment, is significant to understanding musculoskeletal function and mechanisms of injury. With function and potential injury in mind, Francis[57] and Sanderson[1] discussed the

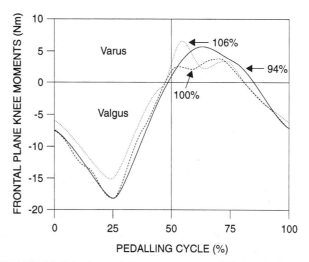

FIGURE 19–18. Knee muscle moment patterns in the frontal plane averaged for 150 pedal revolutions (ten subjects × five trials) at 200 W and 80 rpm for three seat height conditions: 94, 100, and 106 percent of leg length. (From McCoy RW: The Effect of Varying Seat Position on Knee Loads During Cycling. Unpublished doctoral dissertation, University of Southern California Department of Exercise Science, 1989.)

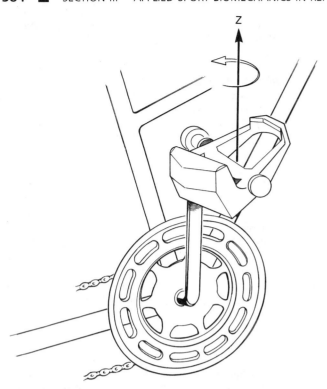

FIGURE 19–19. Sketch of the applied moment (Mz) about an axis orthogonal to the pedal surface.

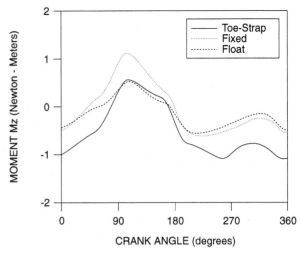

FIGURE 19–20. The applied moment (Mz) pattern during the pedal cycle averaged across 27 subjects using three separate shoe-pedal interface designs: a standard toe-strap and cleat, a clipless fixed design, and a clipless float design. A positive moment indicates an inwardly applied moment against the pedal surface (heel out). (From Wheeler JB, Gregor RJ, Broker JP: The effect of clipless float design on shoe/pedal interface kinetics: Implications for overuse injuries during cycling. J Appl Biomech 1995; 11:119–141. Copyright 1995 by Human Kinetics Publishers, Inc. Reprinted by permission.)

pathomechanics of tibial internal rotation and valgus knee position during the propulsive phase of cycling and compared this situation to running kinetics during midstance. It is during these phases of running and cycling that the greatest loads are imposed on the lower extremities. Several similarities were found.

The applied moment at the pedal surface about an axis perpendicular to the pedal surface (Mz) is a kinetic parameter that has been suggested to be directly related to knee loads and subsequent overuse knee pain.[5,14,58,59] In an effort to further understand pedal loads, specifically the twisting forces on the pedal, a dual piezoelectric transducer force pedal system was designed at the Biomechanics Laboratory at UCLA and is schematically presented in Figure 19–19. Use of the system demonstrated that the center of pressure varied throughout the pedaling cycle (data previously discussed) and that it influenced the calculation of twisting moment, or Mz, at the pedal. In fact, Ruby et al.[14] calculated knee loads from force pedal data, sagittal plane kinematics, and frontal plane knee motion and reported that the moment, Mz, about the axis orthogonal to the pedal surface was a significant contributor to Mz' at the knee, or the twisting moment at the knee.

The twisting moment, Mz, at the pedal relates directly to the "float" pedal designs currently on the market, since the claim of many of these designs is that if movement is allowed, strain is minimized and injury is reduced. The dual transducer force pedal system was adapted for compatibility with several available popular pedal systems (toe-clip and strap, Shimano, and Time) with and without float features. Preliminary data demonstrated that individual peak

Mz applied to the pedal surface was attenuated with the use of clipless float designs (Fig. 19–20). Further tests were conducted across different pedal systems and with different workloads and used subjects with and without cycling-related knee pain, with the primary focus on the Mz pattern throughout the pedaling cycle. Applied internal moments (+Mz) about the z-axis correspond to a shoe force exerted onto the pedal surface tending to rotate the toe in and heel out. Applied external moments (−Mz) correspond to a shoe force exerted onto the pedal surface tending to rotate the toe out and heel in (see Fig. 19–20). Gregor and Wheeler[5] reviewed the biomechanical factors associated with the shoe-pedal interface and reported the following:

1. The applied moment Mz was external for approximately the first 60 degrees of the pedaling cycle.
2. An internally applied moment dominated the remainder of the power phase, with a peak value monitored at about 105 degrees in the cycle.
3. An externally applied moment occurred throughout the recovery phase (180 to 360 degrees).
4. The peak internally applied moment (+Mz) increased significantly with increased workload (e.g., an increase from 150 W to 350 W nearly doubled the magnitude of peak +Mz value), while externally applied moments (−Mz) changed very little with workload.
5. The use of clipless float systems decreased both the internal and external Mz peaks, especially when compared to a clipless system that permitted very little rotation.
6. Asymmetric moment patterns were observed, but general patterns were consistent within subjects without knee pain.

7. Knee pain subjects exhibited distinctly different moment patterns.
8. Cyclists with chronic anterior knee pain, the most common type reported by cyclists, demonstrated exaggerated internally applied peak moments, increased rates of loading (dMz/dt), and longer duration of the applied internal moment during the power phase of the pedaling cycle (0 to 180 degrees) (Fig. 19–21).

"Clipless" pedal designs have been developed that permit the cyclist to rotate the foot on the pedal (about an axis orthogonal to the pedal surface), with the intent of minimizing stress on the knee and ankle. Little is known, however, about the degree of rotation of the foot at the pedal surface or of the shank and thigh during cycling with this type of design. Gregor and Wheeler[5] reviewed the literature regarding clipless pedal designs and concluded that permitting the foot to rotate at the pedal surface markedly attenuated the loads experienced by the joints in the lower extremity, especially the knee. Actual magnitudes of rotation were not recorded, but data implied that releasing constraints on the foot permitted normal movement of the bones in the leg and minimized trauma to the lower extremity. Unfortunately, only kinematic data and/or kinetic calculations were provided, leaving only inferences to bone movement, and as previously discussed, the issue of movement allowance remains open to debate.

Wooten and Hull[60] presented another pedal system designed to study the shoe-pedal interface and its effect on overuse injuries at the knee. Their setup permitted systematic variation in inversion/eversion and abduction/adduction, either separately or in combination, and movements could be free or resisted by spring assem-blies. However, no data were presented directly relating movement allowed by the pedal design to knee pain, and the design of the system precludes its use "on the road." Ruby and Hull[61] investigated the significance of permitting relative motion between the shoe-pedal interface with regard to the effects on three-dimensional knee loads as modeled by Ruby et al.[14] Their study employed a clipless pedal interface with four separate conditions: fixed condition, mediolateral translation, adduction/abduction rotation (equivalent to the previously discussed internal/external rotation about the z-axis), and inversion/eversion rotation. Ruby and Hull[61] found that, relative to the fixed platform condition, (1) permitting mediolateral translation did not significantly decrease intersegmental knee load quantities; (2) both rotation platforms significantly decreased many of the predicted knee load quantities and did not significantly increase any of the knee loads; (3) permitting adduction/abduction rotation significantly reduced axial and varus/valgus knee moments; and (4) permitting inversion/eversion rotation only decreased varus/valgus knee moments. Specifically, the internal axial knee moments (+Mz) exerted by the tibia onto the femur were attenuated during the power phase (0 to 180 degrees) of the pedaling cycle when rotational movements were permitted at the pedal surface. These data, in conjunction with the exaggerated Mz patterns demonstrated by cyclists with knee pain,[5] make a strong argument for the benefits of pedal float systems in reducing knee load and preventing injury. It appears that cyclists with chronic knee pain, especially the most common patellofemoral anterior syndromes, would benefit from using float systems. Cyclists who have not yet developed knee pain would probably benefit from floating shoe-pedal systems as a preventive measure. An added piece of information useful to riders is that regardless of the pedal design chosen (toe-clip and strap, fixed, or float), energy imparted to the bicycle, as measured by the force effectiveness pattern, is not compromised.[35] As in the study by Browning,[34] it seems that the elite riders and triathletes maintain the ability to effectively impart power to the bike using a range of pedal systems and aerodynamic riding positions.

MECHANICAL WORK AND POWER

Ultimately, the lower extremities are responsible for generating and transmitting power to the bicycle. Although this mechanical transmission involves elements on the bicycle (e.g., gear selection, crank length, etc.), the focus of this final section is on the human "machine" and how effectively it operates within the constraints imposed by the personally established bicycle geometry.

Mechanical work and power are biomechanical variables reported in the literature in studies related to power transmission to the bicycle, as well as in studies related to performance efficiency and physiologic cost of cycling at selected workloads. In an effort to address load sharing among the hip, knee, and ankle joints

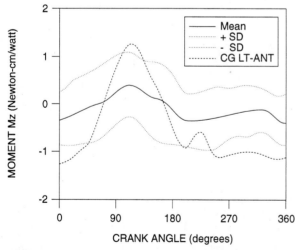

FIGURE 19–21. The mean applied moment (Mz) pattern (±1 SD) during the pedaling cycle for 27 subjects using a clipless float shoe-pedal interface design and the mean pattern for one knee pain patient. A positive moment indicates an inwardly applied moment against the pedal surface (heel out). (From Wheeler JB, Gregor RJ, Broker JP: The effect of clipless float design on shoe/pedal interface kinetics: Implications for overuse injuries during cycling. J Appl Biomech 1995; 11:119–141. Copyright 1995 by Human Kinetics Publishers, Inc. Reprinted by permission.)

during cycling and the possibility of energy transfer between segments, Broker[62] used a clipless pedal design to study the management of mechanical energy in the lower extremities of 12 elite cyclists. Power delivered to the bicycle was calculated from pedal reaction forces and kinematics at 200, 250, and 300 W and at 90, 100, and 110 rpm; Newtonian equations were used in a sagittal plane model of the right lower extremity to calculate joint muscle powers (the product of the muscle moment and angular velocity for each joint) and hip joint force power (the product of the hip joint reaction force and velocity of the estimated center of rotation of the hip) for all riders at all conditions. It has been suggested by Ericson et al.[40] and Van Ingen Schenau[56] that more than 80 percent of the energy generated at the joints in the lower extremity can be delivered to the pedals as useful energy to drive the bicycle. This is in contrast to the results of similar analyses on running and walking, where the mechanical efficiency of the task is much lower. Broker and Gregor[63] reported the use of three energy models to further study the issue of energy production and transmission during cycling. Because it is now generally considered that single-joint muscles, such as the vastus lateralis, produce energy, and biarticular muscles, such as the hamstrings, can transfer, or distribute, energy from one joint to another, the three models ranged from one in which only hypothetical single-joint muscles acted (no transfer) to one in which multijoint muscles acted and permitted unlimited transfer. The latter model has no basis in anatomic function and was purely hypothetical. A third model apportioned joint muscle powers to single- and two-joint muscles and muscle groups in accordance with minimum energy expenditure criteria. During the cycling task, the third model—which has a sound basis in anatomic function and is consistent with reported EMG patterns in the lower extremity during cycling—resulted in the appropriate transfer of energy across two-joint muscles and limited the energy dissipated to nontransferable sources to less than 6 J per limb during cycling. The muscles primarily responsible for the appropriate transfer of energy were the hamstrings, modeled as a group, and the gastrocnemius muscle.

Joint muscle power is shown in Figure 19–22, and regions in the cycle where the transfers are possible are summarized as follows:

1. Energy absorbed at the knee during the second quadrant (90 to 180 degrees) can be transferred to the ankle by the active gastrocnemius and to the hip by the active hamstrings.
2. Energy absorbed at the ankle and hip during the third quadrant can be transferred to the knee by the active gastrocnemius and active hamstring muscles, respectively.

In summary, the cycling task presents a unique opportunity to the lower extremity through the use of appropriate two-joint muscle action to conserve mechanical energy and effectively deliver power to the bicycle. Unlike in walking and running, the stretch-

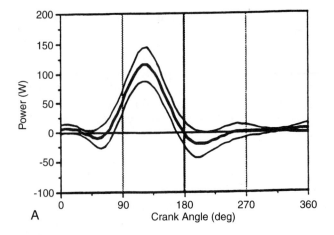

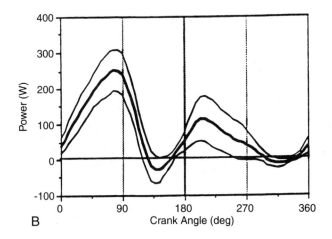

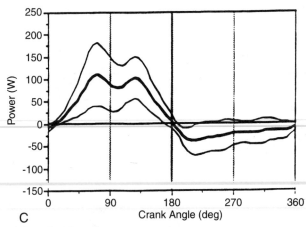

FIGURE 19–22. Mean (±1 SD) patterns of muscle power (calculated as the product of the muscle moment and angular velocity for each joint) during the pedaling cycle for 12 subjects riding at 250 W and 100 rpm. The top trace is the ankle, the middle trace is the knee, and the bottom trace is the hip. (From Broker JP, Gregor RJ: Mechanical energy management in cycling: Source relations and energy expenditure. Med Sci Sports Exerc 1994; 26:64–74.)

shorten cycle of muscle action is not necessary to reduce mechanical energy expenditure. The presence of the active stretch-shorten cycle in many muscles of the lower extremity, then, appears to be most important to the metabolic and physiologic function of the muscle and not necessarily its mechanical output. Finally, knowledge of lower extremity kinetics at the level of intersegmental dynamics and load sharing among all segments (thigh, leg, and foot) responsible for the coordination of energy delivery to the crank is important in the clinical setting where certain areas of the lower extremity are impaired. For example, how does the contralateral leg adapt to the loss of the involved leg when energizing the bicycle during rehabilitation in a unilateral stroke patient? How do the hip and knee adapt in a unilateral below-knee amputee? How does each lower extremity adapt in a patient after ACL reconstruction? A great deal of work is needed in applying existing biomechanical analysis procedures to clinical problems.

REFERENCES

1. Sanderson DJ: The biomechanics of cycling shoes. Cycling Sci 1990; Sept.: 27–30.
2. Mellion MB: Common cycling injuries: Management and prevention. Sports Med 1991; 11:52–70.
3. Francis PR: Injury prevention for cyclists: A biomechanical approach. In Burke ER (ed): Science of Cycling. Champaign, IL, Human Kinetics Books, 1986, pp 145–184.
4. Bohlmann JT: Injuries in competitive cycling. Phys Sports Med 1981; 9:117–124.
5. Gregor RJ, Wheeler JB: Knee pain: Biomechanical factors associated with shoe/pedal interfaces: Implications for injury. Sports Med 1994; 17:117–131.
6. Hannaford DR, Moran GT, Hlavac HF: Video analysis and treatment of overuse knee injury in cycling: A limited clinical study. Clin Podiatr Med Surg 1986; 3:671–678.
7. Holmes JC, Pruitt AL, Whalen NJ: Cycling knee injuries. Cycling Sci 1991; June: 11–14.
8. Pruitt AL: The cyclist's knee: Anatomical and biomechanical considerations. In ER Burke, B Newsom (eds): Medical and Scientific Aspects of Cycling. Champaign, IL, Human Kinetics Books, 1988, pp 17–24.
9. Gregor RJ, Broker JP, Ryan MM: The biomechanics of cycling. Exerc Sport Sci Rev 1991; 19:127–169.
10. Faria E, Cavanagh PR: The Physiology and Biomechanics of Cycling. ACSM Series. New York, John Wiley & Sons, 1978.
11. Rugg SG, Gregor RJ: The effect of seat height on muscle lengths, velocities and moment arm lengths during cycling. J Biomech 1987; 20:899.
12. Ericson MO, Nisell R, Nemeth G: Joint motions of the lower limb during ergometer cycling. J Orthop Sports Phys Ther 1988; 9:273–278.
13. McCoy RW: The Effect of Varying Seat Position on Knee Loads During Cycling. Unpublished doctoral dissertation, University of Southern California, Department of Exercise Science, 1989.
14. Ruby P, Hull ML, Hawkins D: Three-dimensional knee loading during seated cycling. J Biomech 1992; 25:41–53.
15. Boutin RD, Rab GT, Hassan IAG: Three dimensional kinematics and muscle length changes in bicyclists. Proceedings 13th Annual Meeting ASB. Burlington, VT, UVM Conferences, 1989, pp 94–95.
16. Ruby P, Hull ML, Kirby KA, Jenkins DW: The effect of lower-limb anatomy on knee loads during seated cycling. J Biomech 1992; 25:1195–1207.
17. Gregor RJ, Komi PV, Browning RC, Jarvinen M: Comparison between the triceps surae and residual muscle moments at the ankle during cycling. J Biomech 1991; 24:287–297.
18. Hawkins D, Hull ML: Muscle-tendon kinematics of the lower extremity during cycling. In Torsilli PA, Friedman MH (eds): Proceedings Biomechanics Symposium, vol 98, July 9–12, 1989. Applied Mechanics Division, ASME.
19. Desipres M: An electromyographic study of competitive road cycling conditions simulated on a treadmill. In Nelson, Morehouse (eds): Biomechanics IV. Champaign, IL, Human Kinetics Publishers, 1974, pp 349–355.
20. Ericson MO, Nisell R, Arborelius UP: Muscular activity during ergometer cycling. Scand J Rehabil Med 1985; 17:53–61.
21. Houtz SJ, Fischer FJ: An analysis of muscle action and joint excursion during exercise on a stationary bicycle. J Bone Joint Surg 1959; 41A:123–131.
22. Jorge M, Hull ML: Analysis of EMG measurement during bicycle pedaling. J Biomech 1986; 19:683–694.
23. Ryan MM, Gregor RJ: EMG profiles of lower extremity muscles during cycling at constant workload and cadence. J Electromyogr Kinesiol 1992; 2:69–80.
24. Gregor RJ, Cavanagh PR, LaFortune M: Knee flexor moments during propulsion in cycling—a creative solution to Lombard's paradox. J Biomech 1985; 18:307–316.
25. Broker JP, Gregor RJ: A dual piezoelectric element force pedal for kinetic analysis of cycling. Int J Sport Biomech 1990; 6:394–403.
26. Sharp A: Bicycles and Tricycles. Cambridge, MA, MIT Press, 1977, pp 267–270.
27. Hoes JJ, Binkhorst RA, Smeekes-Kuyl AE, Vissers AC: Measurement of forces exerted on pedal and crank during work on a bicycle ergometer at different loads. Int Zeitschrift Ang Physiol 1968; 26:33–42.
28. DalMonte A, Manoni A, Fucci S: Biomechanical study of competitive cycling. In Cerquiglini S, Venerando A, Wartenweiler J (eds): Biomechanics III. Basel, Karger, 1973, pp 434–439.
29. Ericson MO, Nisell R, Ekholm J: Varus and valgus loads on the knee joint during ergometer cycling. Scand J Sports Sci 1984; 6:39–45.
30. LaFortune MA, Cavanagh PR: Effectiveness and efficiency during bicycle riding. In H Matsui, K Kobayashi (eds): Biomechanics VIII-B. Champaign, IL, Human Kinetics Publishers, 1983, pp 928–936.
31. Broker JP, Browning RC, Gregor RJ, Whiting WC: Effect of seat height on force effectiveness in cycling. Med Sci Sports Exerc 1988; 20:S83.
32. Broker JP, Gregor RJ, Schmidt RA: Extrinsic feedback and the learning of kinetic patterns in cycling. J Appl Biomech 1993; 9:111–123.
33. Perell KA: Force Summary Feedback Training on the Bicycle in Patients With Unilateral Cerebrovascular Accidents. Unpublished doctoral dissertation, UCLA, 1994.
34. Browning RC: Lower Extremity Kinetics During Cycling in Elite Triathletes in Aerodynamic Cycling. Unpublished masters thesis, UCLA Department of Kinesiology, 1991.
35. Wheeler JB, Gregor RJ, Broker JP: The effect of clipless float design on shoe/pedal interface kinetics: Implications for overuse injuries during cycling. J Appl Biomech. 1995; 11:119–141.
36. Sanderson DJ, Cavanagh PR: An investigation of the in-shoe pressure distribution during cycling in conventional cycling shoes or running shoes. In B Jonsson (ed): Biomechanics X-B. Champaign, IL, Human Kinetics Publishers, 1987, pp 903–907.
37. Sanderson DJ, Hennig EM. In-shoe pressure distribution in cycling and running shoes during steady-rate cycling. Proceedings of The Second North American Congress on Biomechanics, Chicago, August 24–28, 1992, pp 247–248.
38. Amoroso AT, Hennig EM, Sanderson DJ: In-shoe pressure distribution for cycling at different cadences. Proceedings of The Second North American Congress on Biomechanics, Chicago, August 24–28, 1992, pp 249–250.
39. Hennig EM, Sanderson DJ: In-shoe pressure distribution for cycling at different power outputs. Proceedings of The Second North American Congress on Biomechanics, Chicago, August 24–28, 1992, pp 251–252.
40. Ericson MO, Bratt A, Nisell R, et al: Load moments about the hip and knee joints during ergometer cycling. Scand J Rehabil Med 1986; 18:165–172.
41. McCoy RW, Gregor RJ: The effect of varying seat position on knee loads during cycling. Med Sci Sports Exerc 1989; 21:S79.
42. Furumizo SH: A Biomechanical Analysis of Anterior/Posterior Shear Joint Reaction Forces in the ACL-deficient Knee During Stationary Cycling. Unpublished masters thesis, UCLA Department of Kinesiology, 1991.

43. Smidt GL: Biomechanical analysis of knee flexion and extension. J Biomech 1973; 6:79–92.

44. Yasuda K, Sasaki T: Exercise after anterior cruciate ligament reconstruction: The force exerted on the tibia by separate isometric contractions of the quadriceps or hamstrings. Clin Orthop 1987; 220:276–283.

45. Yasuda K, Sasaki T: Muscle exercise after anterior cruciate ligament reconstruction: Biomechanics of the simultaneous isometric contraction method of the quadriceps and the hamstrings. Clin Orthop 1987; 220:266–274.

46. Yack JH, Riley LM, Whieldon TR: Anterior tibial translation during progressive loading of the ACL-deficient knee during weight-bearing and non-weight-bearing isometric exercise. J Orthop Sports Phys Ther 1994; 20:247–253.

47. Henning CE, Lynch MA, Glick KR: An in vivo strain gauge study of elongation of the anterior cruciate ligament. Am J Sports Med 1985; 13:22–26.

48. Pevsner DE, Johnson JPG, Blazina ME: The patellofemoral joint and its implications in the rehabilitation of the knee. Phys Ther 1979; 59:869–874.

49. Ericson MO, Nisell R: Patellofemoral joint forces during ergometric cycling. Phys Ther 1987; 67:1365–1369.

50. Gregor RJ: A Biomechanical Analysis of Lower Limb Action During Cycling at Four Different Loads. Unpublished doctoral dissertation, The Pennsylvania State University, 1976.

51. Andrews JG: The functional roles of the hamstrings and quadriceps during cycling: Lombard's paradox revisited. J Biomech 1987; 20:565–575.

52. Browning RC, Gregor RJ, Broker JP, Whiting WC: Effects of seat height changes on joint force and moment patterns in experienced cyclists. J Biomech 1988; 21:871.

53. Jorge M, Hull ML: Biomechanics of bicycle pedaling. *In* T Terauds, K Barthels, E Kreighbaum, et al (eds): Sports Biomechanics. Del Mar, CA, Research Center for Sports, 1984, pp 233–246.

54. Redfield R, Hull ML: On the relation between joint moments and pedaling rates at constant power in bicycling. J Biomech 1986; 19:317–329.

55. Lombard WP: The action of two-joint muscles. Am Phys Ed Rev 1903; 8:141–145.

56. Van Ingen Schenau GJ: From rotation to translation: Constraints on multi-joint movements and the unique action of bi-articular muscles. Hum Move Sci 1989; 8:301–337.

57. Francis PR: Pathomechanics of the lower extremity in cycling. *In* E Burke, B Newsom (eds): Medical and Scientific Aspects of Cycling. Champaign, IL, Human Kinetics Books, 1988, pp 3–16.

58. Hull ML, Davis RR: Measurement of pedal loading in bicycling: I. Instrumentation. J Biomech 1981; 14:843–855.

59. Wheeler JB, Gregor RJ, Broker JP: A dual piezoelectric bicycle pedal with multiple shoe/pedal interface compatibility. Int J Sports Biomech 1992; 8:251–258.

60. Wooten D, Hull ML: Design and evaluation of a multi-degree-of-freedom foot/pedal interface for cycling. Int J Sports Biomech 1992; 8:152–164.

61. Ruby P, Hull ML: Response of intersegmental knee loads to foot/pedal platform degrees of freedom in cycling. J Biomech 1993; 26:1327–1340.

62. Broker JP: Mechanical Energy Management During Constrained Human Movement. Unpublished doctoral dissertation, UCLA, 1991.

63. Broker JP, Gregor RJ: Mechanical energy management in cycling: Source relations and energy expenditure. Med Sci Sport Exerc 1994; 26:64–74.

Clinical Considerations and Management

CHAPTER 20

Head Injuries

JAMES J. KINDERKNECHT MD

Head injuries in athletes, although most commonly associated with collision sports such as football, hockey, and boxing, occur in all sports (Table 20–1). The potential severity of these injuries causes a great deal of concern. All individuals, be it physicians, athletic trainers, physical therapists, or nurses, who care for athletes must be well versed in the recognition and management of head injuries.

The magnitude of head injuries varies widely, from scalp lacerations and soft tissue contusions to concussions, subdural hematomas, epidural hematomas, cerebral contusions, intracranial hemorrhages, closed skull fractures, and open skull fractures. Caring for athletes with head injuries involves several, often difficult, clinical decisions. What is the extent of the injury? Can the athlete return to activity, and when?

Fortunately, head injuries associated with death or significant morbidity are rare in sports, but the so-called minor traumatic brain injuries occur commonly. The advent of the National Football Head and Neck Injury Registry in 1975 has allowed more accurate and thorough data collection of injuries related to American football. The registry recorded 123 cases of intracranial hemorrhage and 72 cases of craniocerebral deaths from 1975 to 1984.[1] It has been estimated that an average of eight deaths occur yearly as a result of head injuries in football. There were 335 boxing-related deaths recorded from 1945 to 1979.[2]

Most sports-related head injuries are concussions. It is estimated that 250,000 concussions occur yearly in football alone. It has been reported that concussions make up 4.5 percent of all high school sports injuries and 19 percent of all high school football injuries.[3,4] However, despite the frequent occurrence of concussions, there is no universally accepted system for their classification and management. The concern is to recognize those athletes who are at risk of developing second-impact syndrome or those in whom the injury is not transient but may involve a degree of organic brain damage. The potential cumulative effects of "minor" head trauma also are a concern. These clinical decisions are made difficult by the desire to not unnecessarily limit the athlete's activities if the individual can safely participate. This desire is coupled by the fact the patients are typically highly motivated to return to activity and often conceal or minimize their injury.

ANATOMY

Knowledge of the anatomy of the head is essential; however, a review of facial anatomy will not be included here. The osseous cranium, the supporting structure, is made up of eight tightly joined bones: the temporal bones (2), frontal bone, parietal bones (2), occipital bone, ethmoid bone, and sphenoid bone. The first layer covering the cranium is the thick fibrous glia, which is the periosteum. This is further covered by the scalp, consisting (from the superficial to deep layers) of the hair, skin, the superficial fascia, and the galea aponeurotica, which is a strong, dense, fibrous layer.

The brain is contained and protected by the cranium. It is completely encased except for the foramen magnum. Essentially, the brain is a fixed volume of tissue enclosed in a nonexpandable vault. The meninges are three distinct layers that line the inner cranial vault and cover the brain. The outermost layer is the dura, which in turn consists of two layers. These layers in most areas cannot be separated by dissection. They do, however,

TABLE 20–1
Classification of Sports

Contact		Noncontact		
Contact/Collision	*Limited Contact/Impact*	*Strenuous*	*Moderately Strenuous*	*Nonstrenuous*
Boxing	Baseball	Aerobic dance	Badminton	Archery
Field hockey	Basketball	Crew	Curling	Golf
Football	Bicycling	Fencing	Table tennis	Riflery
Ice hockey	Diving	Field (discus, javelin,		
Lacrosse	Field (high jump, pole	shot put)		
Martial arts	vault)	Running/track		
Rodeo	Gymnastics	Swimming		
Soccer	Horseback riding	Tennis		
Wrestling	Skating (ice, roller)	Weight lifting		
	Skiing (cross country,			
	downhill, water)			
	Softball			
	Squash/handball			
	Volleyball			

From the American Academy of Pediatrics, Committee on Sports Medicine: Recommendations for participation in competitive sports. Reproduced by permission of Pediatrics 1988; 81(5):737–739. Copyright 1988.

divide to form the venous sinuses superiorly and laterally. There are three sites where the dura is folded inward, creating fibrous dividers within the cranial cavity: the tentorium cerebelli, the falx cerebri, and the falx cerebelli. The next layer is the arachnoid layer, which is loosely adherent to the cortex of the brain. It creates a subarachnoid space between the fibrous cortex layer and the brain's surface that contains approximately 150 ml of cerebrospinal fluid. Tightly attached to the brain is the pia layer (Fig. 20–1).

The brain consists of several distinct entities. The largest of these is the cerebral hemispheres, which are partially separated by the falx cerebri. The hemispheres are attached together by a band of fibers, the corpus callosum. The cerebrum is divided into the frontal, temporal, parietal, and occipital lobes. There are also cerebrospinal fluid–containing cavities within the cerebrum that are termed *ventricles*. The cerebellum is positioned posteriorly, essentially under the occipital lobe of the cerebrum. The midbrain (mesencephalon) and the smaller diencephalon are positioned below the cerebral hemispheres. The medulla oblongata is the uppermost portion of the spinal cord exiting through the foramen magnum (Fig. 20–2).

In understanding head trauma, it is important to be aware of the anatomic location of the vessels. The

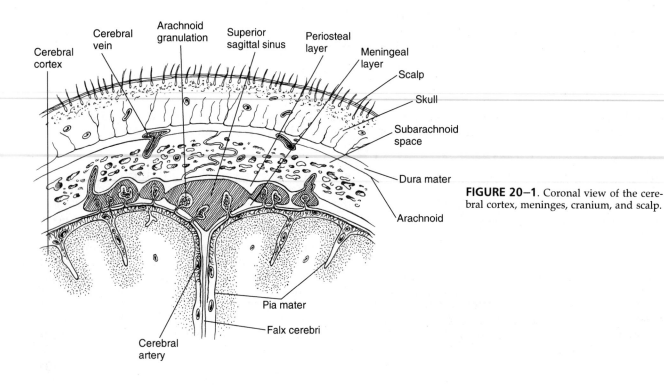

FIGURE 20–1. Coronal view of the cerebral cortex, meninges, cranium, and scalp.

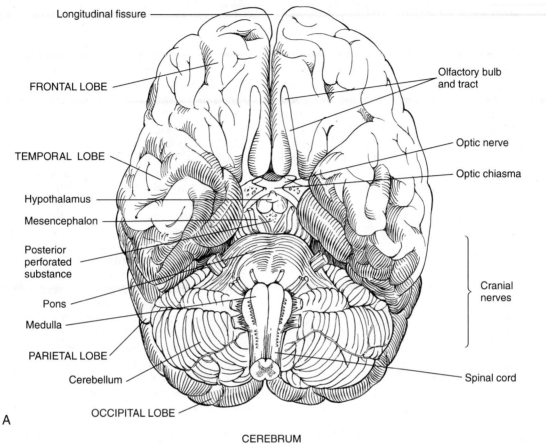

A

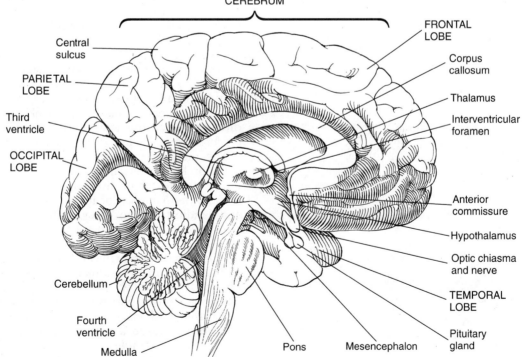

B

FIGURE 20–2. *A,* Inferior surface of the brain. *B,* Sagittal view of the brain.

meningeal arteries are firmly attached to the surface of the dura, lying between it and the cranium. This renders the vessels susceptible to laceration during injury; such laceration is often associated with skull fractures. The largest is the middle meningeal artery, which courses along the temporal region of the skull (Fig. 20–3). Several bridging veins from the brain pass through the subarachnoid space into the subdural sinuses.

The blood supply to the brain originates from the internal carotid arteries anteriorly and the vertebral arteries posteriorly. The internal carotid artery then gives rise to the anterior and middle cerebral arteries. The vertebral arteries connect to form the basilar artery, which then forms the right and left posterior cerebral arteries. Arterial branches connect the posterior cerebral artery with the internal carotid artery, forming the "circle of Willis" (Fig. 20–4).

Twelve cranial nerves are attached to the brain. Each of these has a specific function (Table 20–2).

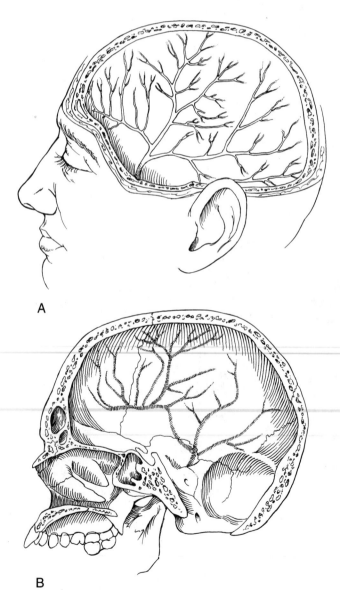

A

B

FIGURE 20–3. The middle meningeal artery along the cerebral cortex (*A*) and the inner table of the skull (*B*).

BIOMECHANICS

The biomechanics of athletic head injuries are extremely complex. The severity as well as the location of the injury is dependent on several features. The magnitude and direction of the impact of the force, the position of the head and its direction of movement at impact, and the structural features of the skull are all determinants of the severity of the injury. The forces applied to the skull can be either direct or indirect. The injury is usually related to the response of the brain and skull to the force, not to the force itself.

Direct injuries can be produced by two different mechanisms. The first involves a moving object striking a fixed or slowly moving head, as occurs in sports such as boxing, baseball, ice hockey, field hockey, or soccer. The second direct mechanism of injury involves a moving head striking a fixed or slowly moving object (the "contrecoup" injury). This type of injury is seen in football, ice hockey, rugby, skiing, and equestrian sports. An additional mechanism of injury is cumulative trauma. Such injuries have been termed the *punch drunk syndrome* and are most commonly recognized in boxers.

Trauma produces acceleration and deceleration forces. These can be considered translational (straight) or angular (rotational) (Fig. 20–5) and produce a shearing effect on the blood vessels or on the nerve fibers (axons). It has been demonstrated that these forces may cause either localized less severe injuries or widespread axonal trauma to the white matter of the brain. The bridging veins may also be injured, resulting in subdural hematomas. Gennarelli, in experiments with primates, was unable to induce a cerebral concussion with a pure translational force, but was easily able to induce one with a rotational force.[5]

Less commonly, the impact can cause a direct injury at the site to the skull, scalp, or brain. Skull fractures are uncommon in sports but may result in severe brain injuries when they do occur. Temporal skull fractures may lacerate the middle meningeal artery, resulting in an epidural hematoma. Focal cortical injuries may occur directly under the site of the impact, resulting in cerebral contusions or intracranial hemorrhage.

The mechanism of injury may also be indirect, a situation known as *impulsive loading.* A force impacting on another part of the body is transferred to the cranium, as in the case of an ice skater or gymnast falling and landing on the coccyx. This type of force also produces deceleration and acceleration to the skull and its contents.

Injuries to the brain may also be viewed as primary or secondary. Primary trauma may be related to either the impact (direct blow) or the impulse of the injury (shearing force). Secondary injury, which includes hemorrhage, edema, brain swelling, hypoxia, or release of neurotoxic substances, can then occur in either setting. For example, a bridging vein that is torn through a shear force is a primary injury; the resulting subdural hematoma is the secondary injury. Although the secondary injury is usually the most life threatening and may lead to irreversible damage, it is also the most preventable and treatable part of the trauma.

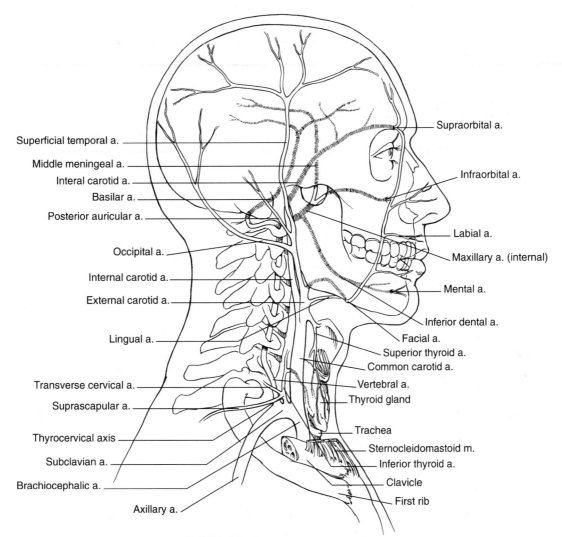

FIGURE 20–4. Cerebral vascular supply.

Brain swelling may occur with a diffuse brain injury or with focal trauma. Again, this is a secondary response to the injury. Swelling may be acute or delayed. The pathophysiology of brain swelling is poorly understood and is not synonymous with a brain edema, which is an increase in extravascular fluid. Animal models have demonstrated autoregulatory dysfunction creating vascular congestion of the brain.[6] It has been proposed that repeated concussions can make an individual susceptible to cerebrovascular congestion, which may be fatal. This has been termed the *second-impact syndrome*.[7,8]

EVALUATION

Evaluation of an injured athlete with known or suspected head trauma occurs in two settings: on the field (the on-field, or on-site evaluation) and in the physician's office (the office evaluation, which occurs several hours to several days after the injury).

A systematic and rehearsed evaluation of the athlete with a head injury or a suspected head injury is essential. Individuals who potentially could be required

	TABLE 20–2 Cranial Nerve Function	
Cranial Nerve		**Function**
I	Olfactory	Smell
II	Optic	Vision
III	Oculomotor	Eye movements, pupillary response
IV	Trochlear	Upward movement of eye
V	Trigeminal	Mostly sensory function of face
VI	Abducent	Lateral movement of eye
VII	Facial	Mostly motor function of face
VIII	Vestibulocochlear	Equilibrium and hearing
IX	Glossopharyngeal	Sensation of taste on the posterior third of tongue
X	Vagus	Several functions, laryngeal muscles
XI	Accessory	Motor to trapezius and sternomastoid muscles
XII	Hypoglossal	Motor function of the tongue

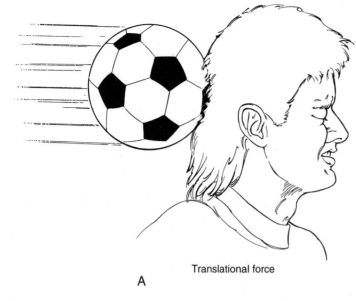

Translational force

A

FIGURE 20–5. Mechanism of injury. Forces applied to the head are either translational *(A)* or angular *(B)*.

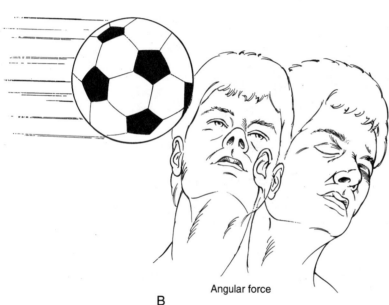

Angular force

B

to make an initial assessment and treat an individual with a head injury must establish a protocol to follow. This requires a knowledge base as to the types of potential injuries, symptoms or signs warranting emergent action or careful observation, and the necessary equipment to perform these tasks. A yearly rehearsal of different mock situations involving head injuries is also extremely valuable. The evaluation is obviously a very individualized procedure for each patient, but a standard framework is beneficial.

The on-site evaluation of an athlete begins with an assessment of the patient's airway, respiratory effort, and circulation. An adequate airway must be obtained emergently if not present and ventilation supported. In addition, appropriate cardiac resuscitation must be emergently instituted if required (Fig. 20–6).

A neurologic assessment is vital in determining the type and the severity of injury. An initial examination

should be performed immediately on the "field." A quick screening using the Glasgow Coma Scale will determine the athlete's eye-opening response, best motor response, and best verbal response (Table 20–3).[9] This score has both diagnostic and prognostic importance. The individual who has experienced a transient or sustained loss of consciousness requires careful and close neurologic examination for signs of a significant injury. If the loss of consciousness is greater than 60 seconds, it is usually most appropriate to transport the patient to a hospital for further evaluation and to include neuroimaging studies. In this setting, unless a cervical spine injury can be completely ruled out, the standard cervical spine precautions should be used during transportation. In a football injury, if the player's helmet is on, it should not be removed until a cervical spine injury has been eliminated, which often requires a radiographic assessment. However, the helmet's facemask should be removed to allow access to the airway and a partial evaluation.

The assessment of the injured athlete should then continue in the appropriate setting based on the suspected severity of injury. It may be appropriate for such assessment to take place on the sideline or in the locker room, but transporting the athlete may be necessary.

Evaluation of the athlete demands a thorough neurologic examination. If the individual has not been rendered unconscious, the clinician must take precautions to not underestimate the injury. The athlete's mental status must be assessed, including his or her orientation, memory, speech, and retrograde or posttraumatic awareness; the presence and time of amnesia

must also be determined. A thorough history to determine the presence of headache, visual changes (diplopia or visual field defect), tinnitus, dizziness, nausea, and previous history of concussions is critical.

During the physical examination of the injured athlete, evidence of musculoskeletal trauma is initially sought. The head and neck should be inspected and palpated for evidence of external trauma. The scalp should be examined for lacerations, localized areas of tenderness or swelling, or palpable depressions. Areas are inspected for ecchymosis, with particular attention paid to the retromastoid (Battle sign) and periorbital regions ("raccoon eyes" indicative of basilar skull fracture), and for otorrhea/rhinorrhea, which is consistent with cerebrospinal fluid leakage. The examiner should always remember to perform a detailed evaluation of the cervical spine.

The examination must then continue with a screening neurologic evaluation. Cranial nerve function can be tested to assess neuro-ophthalmologic function (i.e., pupillary size, shape, and reactivity to light; extraocular movements; nystagmus; visual fields to confrontation; and gross visual acuity). Further cranial nerve evaluation includes assessment of facial sensory and motor function, gross hearing, and tongue movements. Extremity motor function (strength) and sensation (light touch, pin prick, vibratory sense, and position sense) are then assessed (Table 20–4). Deep tendon reflexes are tested, with particular attention paid to long tract signs (i.e., Babinski reflex). Coordination and gait may then be evaluated with the finger-nose-finger test, the heel-shin test, and checks for tandem gait and the Romberg sign.

Athletes who have sustained a head injury and have any of the above symptoms or positive findings on physical examination must be observed carefully. This observation entails frequent questioning and repetition of the neurologic examination. Individuals who are unconscious for more than 60 seconds and those who have signs of increased intracranial pressure (i.e., pupillary asymmetry, intractable vomiting, prolonged altered mental status, seizures, or severe headache) or signs of cerebral injury (i.e., focal or lateralizing features) require immediate transfer to the hospital. Immediate transfer is also required for anyone with a Glasgow Coma Scale score of 13 or less. Any patients who experience deterioration of their level of consciousness or progression of neurologic findings should be transported emergently.

Management of the athlete with a severe head injury (Glasgow Coma Scale score of 3 to 8) requires emergent action. A trained paramedic team should be immediately summoned. If the appropriate personnel and equipment are available, the patient should be intubated and hyperventilated to prevent aspiration as well as reduce cerebral arterial carbon dioxide tension. Bag-mask ventilation should be performed at a rate of 24 breaths per minute with 100 percent oxygen to reduce intracranial pressure. Other measures to reduce intracranial pressure should be considered in patients who are cardiovascularly stable but have lateralizing neurologic signs (i.e., asymmetric pupil size, hemipa-

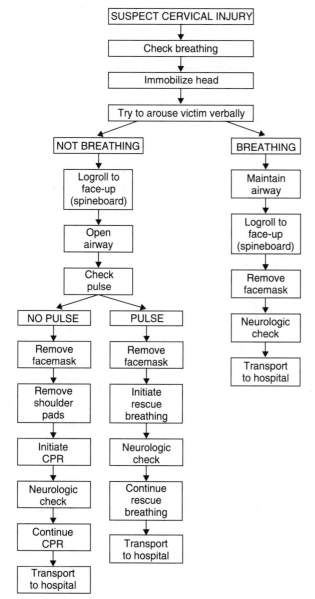

FIGURE 20–6. On-field evaluation of the unconscious athlete. (Redrawn from Torg JS (ed): Athletic Injuries to the Head, Neck and Face. Philadelphia, Lea & Febiger, 1982, p 43.)

TABLE 20-3
Glasgow Coma Scale

		Response	Score	Time 1 ( )	Time 2 ( )
Eyes	Open	Spontaneously	4		
		To verbal command	3		
		To pain	2		
		No response	1	_____	_____
Best motor response	To verbal command	Obeys	6		
	To painful stimulus*	Localizes pain	5		
		Flexion—withdrawal	4		
		Flexion—abnormal (decorticate rigidity)	3		
		Extension (decerebrate rigidity)	2		
		No response	1	_____	_____
Best verbal response†		Oriented and converses	5		
		Disoriented and converses	4		
		Inappropriate words	3		
		Incomprehensible sounds	2		
		No response	1	_____	_____
Total			3–15		

*Apply knuckles to sternum: observe arms.
†Arouse patient with painful stimulus if necessary.

The Glasgow Coma Scale, based on eye opening, verbal, and motor responses, is a practical means of monitoring changes in level of consciousness. If response on the scale is given a number, the responsiveness of the patient can be expressed by summation of the numbers. The lowest score is 3, and the highest is 15.

From Magee DJ: Orthopedic Physical Assessment, 2nd ed. Philadelphia, WB Saunders, 1992.

TABLE 20-4
Neural Watch Chart

Unit		Time 1 ( )	Time 2 ( )	Time 3 ( )
I Vital signs	Blood pressure			
	Pulse			
	Respiration			
	Temperature			
II Conscious and	Oriented			
	Disoriented			
	Restless			
	Combative			
III Speech	Clear			
	Rambling			
	Garbled			
	None			
IV Will awaken to	Name			
	Shaking			
	Light pain			
	Strong pain			
V Nonverbal reaction to pain	Appropriate			
	Inappropriate			
	"Decerebrate"			
	None			
VI Pupils	Size on right			
	Size on left			
	Reacts on right			
	Reacts on left			
VII Ability to move	Right arm			
	Left arm			
	Right leg			
	Left leg			
VIII Sensation	Right side (normal/abnormal)			
	Left side (normal/abnormal)			
	Dermatome affected (specify)			
	Peripheral nerve affected (specify)			

From Magee DJ: Orthopedic Physical Assessment, 2nd ed. Philadelphia, WB Saunders, 1992.

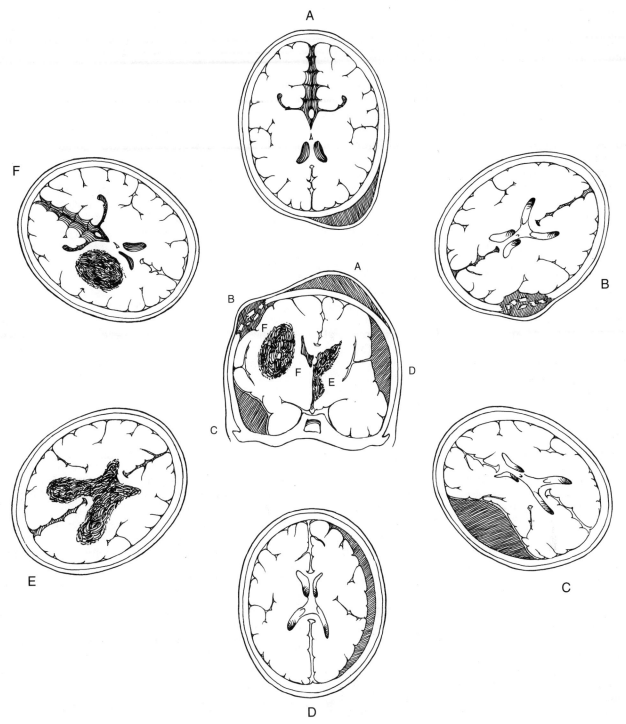

FIGURE 20–7. Types of head injuries. *A,* Subgaleal hematoma. *B,* Depressed skull fracture. *C,* Epidural hematoma. *D,* Subdural hematoma. *E,* Intraventricular hematoma. *F,* Intracerebral hematoma. (Redrawn from Lehman LB, Ravich SJ: Closed head injuries in athletes. Clin Sports Med 1990; 9: 249.)

resis, or abnormal posturing); such measures include intravenous mannitol drip (0.25 mg to 1.0 g/kg) administered over 15 to 30 minutes. The benefit of corticosteroids is controversial. Hypotension must be aggressively treated if it occurs concomitantly with administration of intravenous fluids.

Further evaluation and management will be discussed as they pertain to each clinical entity.

CLINICAL INJURIES

The spectrum of head injuries varies widely, from injuries associated with a high mortality rate to transient injuries with quick and complete recovery. The following discussion reviews skull fractures, epidural hematomas, subdural hematomas, cerebral contusions, and concussions (Fig. 20–7).

SKULL FRACTURES

Skull fractures anecdotally are an unusual injury in athletes. Fractures of the skull typically require a large force over a small area with rapid dissipation of the energy. Skull fractures are classified as linear, comminuted, or depressed. Like other bones, the skull fails when exposed to tensile stress, not when exposed to compression. If a ball strikes a person's skull with enough magnitude to fracture it, the site of injury will vary relative to the thickness of the skull. In areas where the bone is thin, the outer table is compressed, and the inner table fails under tension, creating a fracture at the site of impact. However, if the bone is thick, the force creates very little in-bending, and the surrounding bone bends out, creating tension on the outer table, which can then produce a skull fracture not directly at the site of impact.

There are some common fracture patterns. Impact on the forehead or supraorbital areas creates a fracture line along the thin cribriform plate at the base of the skull or along the orbital roofs. This can propagate to the base of the skull and to the anterior cranial fossa. Frontolateral impacts that create a fracture often involve the thin inferolateral skull in the area of the temporal bone and orbital roofs. Impacts above and behind the ear travel along the lines of least resistance, resulting in fractures of the thinnest portion of the temporal bone, causing the fracture to propagate from the site of impact to the middle cranial fossa. Posterior trauma may cause a fracture that extends through the occipital bone to the foramen magnum. If a large force is dissipated quickly over a small area, comminution of the bone may occur.

Linear skull fractures cause concern for the secondary injuries that may potentially occur. Fractures in the temporoparietal region are frequently associated with middle meningeal artery lacerations and an epidural hematoma. Linear fractures may also extend to a sinus cavity, resulting in an increased risk of infection. As with all fractures, skull fractures may be open (i.e., they may communicate with the environment). It is important to realize that because of the mobility of the scalp over the skull, a laceration may not overlie its associated fracture at the time of the physical examination.

Basilar skull fractures may be considered open fractures because of the communication with a sinus. Clinical findings of basilar skull fractures include bilateral periorbital ecchymosis ("raccoon eyes"), ecchymosis behind the ear (Battle sign), hemotympanum, cerebrospinal fluid (CSF) otorrhea or rhinorrhea, seventh or eighth nerve palsies, or blood in the ear canal. Watery rhinorrhea that tests positive for glucose (a urinalysis strip works well) is consistent with a CSF leak.

Management of basilar skull fractures associated with a CSF leak involves careful and persistent monitoring. Signs of infection including fever, elevated white blood cell (WBC) count, or altered mental status must be monitored. Prophylactic antibiotics are not recommended, as they have not been shown to be effective in preventing meningitis and may select out more resistant organisms.[10] The majority of CSF leaks resolve spontaneously.[11]

The utility of skull radiographs for the evaluation of head injuries has been debated. Physical examination can be misleading because of scalp movement at the time of impact. In addition, soft tissue swelling can either mimic a palpable "step-off" or conceal a skull depression. A panel of experts has published guidelines for obtaining radiographs in patients with head trauma[12]; these are outlined in Table 20–5. Most moderate-risk and all high-risk patients warrant neurologic imaging with a computed tomography (CT) scan.

Depressed skull fractures have a higher risk of complications than do linear fractures. Eighty-five percent of depressed skull fractures are open. A compound depressed skull fracture is a neurosurgical emergency. Also, the osseous fragments and the force of impact creating the depression may traumatize the brain. Intracranial hematomas requiring neurosurgical intervention occur in 7 percent of depressed skull fractures. In addition, 11 percent of depressed skull fractures have long-term neurologic sequelae.[13]

Skull fractures, if uncomplicated, rarely influence management decisions.[14] However, when fractures of the skull are recognized, because of the risk of severe complications, neurosurgical consultation is appropriate.

EPIDURAL HEMATOMA

Epidural hematomas, although not common, require a high index of suspicion to enable early intervention. Epidural hematomas occur in 1 percent of all patients sustaining a head injury but make up 5 percent to 15 percent of fatal head injuries.[10] If this condition is recognized early, before secondary injury to the brainstem occurs from elevated intracranial pressure, it can usually be surgically corrected. However, even with early diagnosis and aggressive treatment, epidural hematomas carry a mortality rate of 8 percent.[15]

The "classic" presentation of an epidural hematoma occurs in about one third of all cases. This clinical picture consists of an initial loss of consciousness at the time of injury, followed by a lucid interval in which the patient feels nearly normal. A decline in mental status then occurs, with associated deterioration in the neurologic examination involving pupillary dilatation on the side of the epidural hematoma in 30 percent to 50 percent of cases and contralateral extremity weakness or decerebrate posturing in 50 percent to 75 percent of cases. Bradycardia is present in 25 percent of patients.[14] One third of patients do not recover from the initial loss of consciousness, and in another third, loss of consciousness never occurs or occurs late in the course of injury.

Ninety percent of epidural hematomas are associated with a skull fracture.[10] The force creating the fracture, if located in close proximity to a blood vessel will lacerate the vessel. The meningeal arteries are susceptible to such injury, because they run along the inner table of the skull and are often imbedded in bony grooves. The

TABLE 20–5
Management Strategy for Radiographic Imaging in Patients With Head Trauma*

Low-Risk Group	Moderate-Risk Group	High-Risk Group

Possible findings:
  Asymptomatic
  Headache
  Dizziness
  Scalp hematoma
  Scalp laceration
  Scalp contusion or abrasion
  Absence of moderate-risk or high-risk criteria
	Possible findings:
	  History of change of consciousness at the time of injury or subsequently
	  History of progressive headache
	  Alcohol or drug intoxication
	  Unreliable or inadequate history of injury
	  Age less than 2 yr (unless injury very trivial)
	  Posttraumatic seizure
	  Vomiting
	  Posttraumatic amnesia
	  Multiple trauma
	  Serious facial injury
	  Signs of basilar fracture†
	  Possible skull penetration or depressed fracture‡
	  Suspected physical child abuse
		Possible findings:
		  Depressed level of consciousness not clearly due to alcohol, drugs, or other cause (e.g., metabolic and seizure disorders)
		  Focal neurologic signs
		  Decreasing level of consciousness
		  Penetrating skull injury or palpable depressed fracture

Recommendations:
  Observation alone: discharge patients with head injury information sheet (listing subdural precautions) and a second person to observe them.
	Recommendations:
	  Extended close observation (watch for signs of high-risk group).
	  Consider CT examination and neurosurgical consultation.
	  Skull series may (rarely) be helpful, if positive, but do not exclude intracranial injury if normal.
		Recommendations:
		  Patient is a candidate for neurosurgical consultation or emergency CT examination or both.

*Physician assessment of the severity of injury may warrant reassignment to a higher risk group. Any single criterion from a higher risk group warrants assignment of the patient to the highest risk group applicable.
†Signs of basilar fracture include drainage from ear, drainage of cerebrospinal fluid from nose, hematotympanum, Battle sign, and "raccoon eyes."
‡Factors associated with open and depressed fracture include gunshot, missile, or shrapnel wounds; scalp injury from firm, pointed object (including animal teeth); penetrating injury of eyelid or globe; object stuck in the head; assault (definite or suspected) with any object; leakage of cerebrospinal fluid; and sign of basilar fracture.
From Masters SJ, McClean PM, Arcarese JS: Skull x-ray examinations after head trauma. N Engl J Med 1987; 316:84–91. Reprinted by permission. Copyright 1987. Massachusetts Medical Society. All rights reserved.

middle meningeal artery can be traumatized with temperoparietal skull fractures, as previously described. This accounts for 60 percent to 70 percent of epidural hematomas, which are located in the middle fossa. Other common locations of epidural hematomas are the frontal area (11 percent), occipital (6 percent), and posterior fossa (12 percent).[14]

CT is the best diagnostic test for the evaluation of epidural hematomas. Any patient with a loss of consciousness of more than 60 seconds, focal neurologic findings, progression or persistence of symptoms, or headache with confusion or disorientation greater than 1 hour should undergo a CT scan. If the patient has a normal neurologic examination and minimal symptoms but the injury is a high-risk one, then skull radiographs should be obtained. This again underscores the need for careful and frequent observation with repetitive examination of all patients with head injuries.

The treatment of epidural hematomas consists of surgical evacuation. Intracranial pressures are then carefully monitored. Although this has not been specifically addressed in the literature, individuals who sustain an epidural hematoma should not be permitted to return to collision or contact sports unless cleared by a neurosurgeon.

SUBDURAL HEMATOMA

Subdural hematomas occur at approximately three times the rate of epidural hematomas in all head injuries.[16] In fact, subdural hematomas make up 26 percent to 63 percent of severe head injuries.[17] All subdural hematomas are a result of the acceleration forces of the head and not the impact of the force. They are classified as acute or chronic and simple or complicated.

Simple subdural hematomas are a collection of blood in the subdural space and involve no underlying cerebral injury. During the injury bridging and surface vessels are torn, resulting in bleeding in the subdural space. Athletes with simple subdural hematomas are less likely to be rendered unconscious. These individuals do not usually demonstrate a decline in level of consciousness, and only 13 percent will have a lucid interval. This simple type accounts for 45 percent of acute subdural hematomas and has a 21 percent mortality rate.[16]

The complicated type of subdural hematoma involves the underlying brain. Not only is there a subdural blood collection, but the shear force related to head acceleration also involves the cerebral cortex, which in turn produces intracerebral swelling and intracranial pressure elevation. It is not the mass occupying lesion that produces the injury, but the increase in intracerebral pressure. The mortality rate in complicated subdural hematomas is 53 percent.[16] Patients sustaining an acute subdural hematoma with associated brain injury are usually unconscious. The initial neurologic condition at the time of injury correlates highly with outcome. Pupillary dilatation is common, and retinal changes are often present. Focal neurologic findings are seen in approximately 50 percent of cases at admission.[18] Again, a CT scan is the best imaging tool to diagnose subdural hematomas and evaluate the cortical injury.

Diagnosis of subdural hematomas early in the course of severe head injuries is vitally important. Surgical treatment of subdural hematomas less than 4 hours after the injury has been determined to result in a mortality rate of less than 40 percent. However, the mortality rate increases to 80 percent to 90 percent if surgery is delayed beyond 4 hours.[19] Surgical evacuation is not indicated in all subdural hematomas, but intracranial pressure monitoring is required. Return to sports is not recommended. In fact, it is unusual for these individuals to return to work.

CEREBRAL CONTUSIONS

Cerebral contusions represent a focal injury to the brain, but although the injury is focal, it is not a mass occupying lesion. Instead, it involves microhemorrhages of the brain, resulting in bleeding. This bleeding is seen on the CT scan as an area of high-density blood interspersed with brain tissue.

Cerebral contusions are usually the result of an impulse injury. The typical scenario is that of an athlete striking the occiput as the result of a fall and sustaining an injury to the frontal lobe. The tips of the frontal lobes and the inferior frontal lobes are susceptible to this type of injury because of their close anatomic relationship to prominent bony ridges. The contusions may occur in any portion of the cortex, the brainstem, or the cerebellum. The contusions occasionally coalesce to form a hematoma, which may need surgical drainage.

Clinically individuals who sustain a cerebral contusion may have very different clinical presentations. Most patients will have experienced a loss of consciousness. Subsequently these individuals may become very alert and conversant, or they may become comatose. Results of the neurologic examination may also vary widely. Diagnosis is made with CT scans, which should be obtained in all individuals with an abnormal neurologic examination. The hallmark of patients who have a cerebral contusion but a normal neurologic examination is the persistence of symptoms. These individuals will have persisting headaches, dizziness, or nausea, which should lead to further evaluation, including a CT scan.

Return to activities following a cerebral contusion is not specifically addressed in the literature. These individuals should be referred to a neurosurgeon for an opinion as to when they may resume activities. The patient obviously should be asymptomatic, and a repeat CT scan of the brain should be normal.

CONCUSSIONS

Concussion has been defined by the Congress of Neurological Surgeons as a clinical syndrome characterized by immediate and transient posttraumatic impairment of neural function owing to mechanical forces.[20] Despite the fact that concussions are extremely common injuries in athletes, occurring in all levels and potentially in any sport, the variation in dealing with these injuries is extremely widespread. There are various classifications of concussions, some of which are clinically difficult to apply. There is also a wide range of clinical practice in assessing and treating concussions. Furthermore, there is debate as to whether this injury is truly a transient reversible injury and what the implications are of repeated concussions. The question that must be answered in every case is, "Can the athlete safely return to activities, and when?"

A favored definition of concussions is "a traumatically induced alteration in mental status." It is imperative to understand that concussions do not always involve loss of consciousness. A concussion should not be considered universally transient. Concussed athletes often demonstrate impaired cognitive abilities, despite a completely normal neurologic examination. Concussions may also lead to a more chronic condition, posttraumatic concussion syndrome. Rimel and colleagues followed more than 400 patients who sustained "minor" head injuries.[21] Such injuries were defined as an initial Glasgow Coma Scale score of 13 to 15, unconsciousness of less than 20 minutes, and hospitalization of less than 48 hours. Three months after injury, 79 percent had persisting headaches and 59 percent had subjective difficulties with memory. Mild impairment on neuropsychological testing was also evident in a majority of the patients tested.

The pathophysiology of concussions is best understood as a diffuse brain injury. This diffuse injury is produced by acceleration forces (either impact or impulse) to the head related to the shear forces generated. Rotational acceleration produces the greatest shear forces and thus a higher magnitude of injury. These injuries have been demonstrated to occur at the periphery and at sites of structural change in the brain. The degree of trauma at the site of impact is minimal.

Gennarelli[5] divided diffuse brain injuries into four categories on a continuum in which there is a direct relationship between the acceleration forces and the injury: the higher the acceleration forces are, the more severe the diffuse brain injury. In *mild concussion* the force creates a disturbance in cortical function but does not alter the communication between the cerebral cortex and the brainstem activating system. Therefore, memory is affected, but there is no loss of consciousness.

In *classic cerebral concussion,* the cerebral hemispheres are disconnected from the brainstem reticular activating system, resulting in a loss of consciousness. This disconnection does not involve a structural lesion, and the unconsciousness is transient. *Diffuse injury* applies to individuals with a loss of consciousness for more than 24 hours. This injury is attributed to axonal disruption within the cortex, resulting in a higher severity of injury. Patients in this group demonstrate some residual deficits, if not significant deficits. Rimel and coworkers[22] studied patients with moderate head injuries (Glascow Coma Scale Score of 9 to 12). Of the patients who had undergone a CT scan, 79 percent had a diffuse injury, and of these patients, 56 percent had a moderate or severe disability; the mortality rate was 4 percent.[22]

The most severe type of diffuse injury is the *shearing injury.* In this type of injury, many axons are disrupted, with extension into the brainstem. Death occurs in 55 percent of patients, but the clinical course is dictated by the degree of axonal injury. Thirty-six percent of patients will remain in a vegetative state.[21] However, patients in this group do have a potential for recovery, and this potential is thought to be proportional to the number of axons that are injured. Microscopically, torn axons are seen diffusely throughout the cerebral white matter.

CONCUSSION CLASSIFICATION SYSTEMS

The classification of concussions based on clinical presentation and course is extremely difficult. The symptoms and physical findings in concussions are dependent on the severity of injury. Several guidelines have been presented for classification of concussions based on the symptoms and signs.[23–27] These classifications delineate subgroups of concussions, which in turn guide management. The difficulty in establishing a classification system is encompassing all clinical presentations and dividing them into separate groups. The ability to then meaningfully categorize evaluated patients is needed. Despite numerous attempts to design a system, none has been universally accepted (Table 20–6).

The Colorado Medical Society (CMS) has developed a classification system defining levels of injury and recommended management. As with previous guidelines, loss of consciousness and whether amnesia is present are the major determinants as to the grade of injury. CMS divides the injuries into three grades, with the first two involving confusion without loss of consciousness. Grade I injury is without amnesia, and grade II injury involves amnesia. Grade III injuries include any injury with a loss of consciousness. However, difficulty arises when trying to apply this to all individuals sustaining head trauma. This classification does not divide the groups based on the length of amnesia or the duration of unconsciousness, as do other previously published guidelines.

Kulund[26] and Cantu[27] also divided concussion into three groups: mild, moderate, and severe. Cantu defines a severe concussion as loss of consciousness greater than 5 minutes. Moderate concussions involve a loss of consciousness for less than 5 minutes. In mild concussions, no loss of consciousness is rendered, but intellectual function is impaired. Kulund's classification is similar, with severe concussions involving prolonged loss of consciousness (no specific time is given). A moderate concussion involves loss of consciousness with associated mental confusion and retrograde amnesia that resolves rapidly. With a mild injury, the athlete is stunned or dazed but feels well in 1 to 2 minutes.

Torg's[25] classification system contains six groups. Grade 6 is death, and grade 5 is a paralytic coma. Grade 4 patients are rendered unconscious for less than a few minutes and have a component of confusion with amnesia (posttraumatic and/or retrograde). A grade 3 injury is characterized by retrograde amnesia and no loss of consciousness. Torg defines grade 2 concussions as involving posttrauamtic amnesia and confusion. Grade 1 injuries do not involve amnesia, but the patient may be confused or dazed, and the gait may be unsteady. In addition, the grade 1 patient may have vertigo, headaches, or photophobia that are transient (less than 15 minutes).[23]

Nelson's classification of concussions seems to be the most applicable, as most athletic injuries do not involve a loss of consciousness. Nelson also creates five different groupings (grades 0 to 4) that apply to most of the injuries seen. A grade 0 injury involves the athlete "taking a hit," without any initial symptoms. Later, a headache develops, or there may be difficulty concentrating. These patients usually present with complaints after activities. A grade 1 injury is similar, but the patient is dazed or stunned initially, with his or her sensorium clearing in less than 1 minute; this is the typical "I got my bell rung" injury. In a grade 2 injury, there is no loss of consciousness, but the athlete's sensorium is altered for more than 1 minute. The usual symptoms are headache, visual changes, nausea, tinnitus, dizziness, confusion, and amnesia. This category is similar to CMS grade 2 concussions, but in the CMS classification, these individuals have a component of amnesia, whereas in Nelson's system, amnesia may or may not be present. For grade 3 concussions, loss of consciousness occurs for less than 1 minute. Unconsciousness of more than 1 minute is a grade 4 concussion.

Evaluation of the athlete with a suspected concussion is identical to the initial evaluation previously outlined. The length of unconsciousness, if present, should be noted. After the patient has been found to be clearly stable with regard to cardiopulmonary and neurologic status, careful questioning to determine the symptoms is performed. Orientation and memory are assessed. The presence of a headache, tinnitus, balance disturbance ("I feel spongy"), visual disturbance (diplopia, a visual field deficit, or decreased acuity), amnesia (posttraumatic or retrograde), or nausea is determined. Again, a thorough neurologic examination is critical.

MANAGEMENT

Management is best determined based on the grade of the concussion. The Nelson classification seems to be the most applicable. Figure 20–8 shows a flow chart that

TABLE 20–6
Concussion Classifications

Nelson	Colorado Medical Society	Torg	Kulund	Cantu
Grade 0 Head struck or moved rapidly Not stunned or dazed Develops headache and difficulty concentrating			**Mild** Dazed No confusion or unsteadiness Well in 1–2 min	
Grade 1 Stunned or dazed No loss of consciousness or amnesia Sensorium clears quickly (<1 min)	**Grade 1** Confusion No amnesia No loss of consciousness	**Grade 1** Transient confusion Unsteady gait Dazed No amnesia No loss of consciousness	**Moderate** Loss of consciousness Retrograde amnesia Confusion	**Grade 1** No loss of consciousness Posttraumatic amnesia <30 min
Grade 2 Headache, cloudy sensorium >1 min No loss of consciousness May have tinnitus, amnesia, irritability, confusion, dizziness	**Grade 2** Confusion Amnesia No loss of consciousness	**Grade 2** Confusion Posttraumatic amnesia only No loss of consciousness	**Severe** Longer loss of consciousness Amnesia	**Grade 2** Loss of consciousness <5 min Posttraumatic amnesia >30 min
Grade 3 Loss of consciousness <1 min Not comatose Grade 2 symptoms	**Grade 3** Loss of consciousness	**Grade 3** Confusion Posttraumatic and retrograde amnesia No loss of consciousness		
Grade 4 Loss of consciousness >1 min Not comatose		**Grade 4** Loss of consciousness seconds to minutes		
		Grade 5 Paralytic coma		
		Grade 6 Death		

can be followed. Athletes with grade 0 and grade 1 concussions are allowed to return to activities after the sensorium clears completely and the athlete is completely asymptomatic, with a normal neurologic examination. It is prudent to observe most athletes for at least 10 minutes before allowing them to return to activities. The CMS guidelines recommend at least a 20-minute observation. Repetition of the examination to discover the presence of symptoms such as headache, visual changes, nausea, or balance disturbance is important. If any symptoms are present or the physical examination is abnormal, the patient must be removed from activity.

Athletes with Nelson grade 2 concussions must be removed from activity per their guidelines. Again, this is similar to a CMS grade 2 concussion. These individuals should be frequently questioned and examined, looking for progression of symptoms. The decision of when to allow the athlete to return to activity is difficult. If there is no amnesia, the patient may be allowed to return to activities in 24 to 48 hours after being completely asymptomatic, similar to grade 0 to 1 concussions. The initial return to activity should involve no contact for 24 hours and can then advance to full activities if the patient remains asymptomatic.

Athletes with grade 2 concussions with a degree of amnesia often present the most difficult clinical decisions. These athletes are removed from activity and should be closely observed and monitored. It is worth restating that if symptoms persist for more than 24 to 48 hours without improvement or progress, then CT imaging or neurosurgical consultation is warranted. The CMS guidelines recommend prohibiting activities for 1 week following the resolution of symptoms. Nelson recommends no return until the patient is asymptomatic, with no specifications made regarding the time interval from the resolution of symptoms. Clinically, although not discussed in the literature, it appears that return to activity varies with the length of posttraumatic amnesia (PTA). It should again be emphasized, however, that the neurologic examination in such patients is normal. If PTA is less than 10 to 20 minutes, then the athlete can return to noncontact activities 48 hours after he or she is asymptomatic. An individual with a persisting headache is *not* asymptomatic! Conversely, if the PTA is greater than 20 minutes, a CT scan of the head is required. Assuming the CT scan is normal, the athlete is allowed to return to activities 72 hours to 1 week after injury, taking into account the entire clinical picture. On return to activity, contact is avoided for the initial 24 to 48 hours. Any recurrence of symptoms during this phase requires removing the individual from activity and considering further evaluation.

The higher grade concussions (Nelson grade 3 and grade 4; CMS grade 3) involve loss of consciousness. Nelson recommends transporting patients with grade 4 concussions to the nearest hospital (preferably a trauma center), as the CMS recommends for patients with grade 3 concussions. Nelson's recommended management for patients with grade 3 concussions is similar to that recommended by the CMS for CMS grade 2 concussions. These individuals are removed from activity and

observed closely. If there is any progression of symptoms or the neurologic examination is abnormal, the athlete is immediately transported to the hospital.

Return to activity after loss of consciousness is variable. Nelson defers this decision to the neurosurgeon for patients with grade 3 or 4 concussions. The CMS recommends return to participation only after 2 full weeks without symptoms. Nelson's guidelines should be followed when determining when an athlete may return to activity. If an individual is rendered unconscious for less than 60 seconds (grade 3) and that individual's symptoms clear in 24 to 48 hours without progression, then that individual may return to activity, similar to patients with grade 2 concussions. Nelson recommends return to activity after neurosurgical consultation. Clearance to return to activity should be made by a qualified physician who is knowledgeable in head injuries. Patients with grade 4 concussions (loss of consciousness for more than 60 seconds) should be transported to the nearest hospital and neurosurgical consultation obtained. Athletes who subsequently are found to have a reversible transient injury are then allowed to return to activity based on the neurosurgical opinion. Again, this is an area of variation compared with the CMS guidelines. The CMS recommendations are to remove an athlete from activity for 2 weeks, but it is not uncommon in clinical practice to see these individuals cleared to return to activities in less than 1

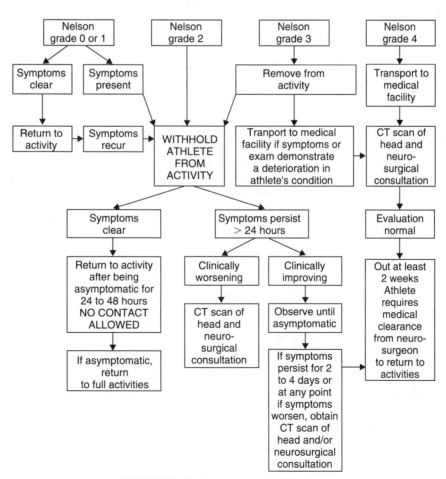

FIGURE 20–8. Management of concussions.

TABLE 20–7
Guidelines for Return to Play After Concussion

	First Concussion	Second Concussion	Third Concussion
Grade 1 (mild)	May return to play if asymptomatic* for 1 wk	Return to play in 2 wk if asymptomatic at that time for 1 wk	Terminate season; may return to play next season if asymptomatic
Grade 2 (moderate)	Return to play after asymptomatic for 1 week	Minimum of 1 mo; may return to play then if asymptomatic for 1 wk; consider terminating season	Terminate season; may return to play next season if asymptomatic
Grade 3 (severe)	Minimum of 1 mo; may then return to play if asymptomatic for 1 wk	Terminate season; may return to play next season if asymptomatic	

*No headache, dizziness, or impaired orientation, concentration, or memory during rest or exertion. (From Cantu RC: Guidelines for return to contact sports. The Physician and Sportsmedicine, October 1986. Copyright 1986. Reproduced with permission of McGraw-Hill, Inc.)

week. The approach to these patients is individualized to the injury and the patient's response to that injury. That is why universal guidelines often fall short in establishing treatment algorithms. It is important to keep in mind that these guidelines are simply a framework to aid in management of patients.

Recurrent concussions also involve difficult clinical decisions. Currently Cantu's guidelines are the only ones in the literature to specifically address patients who experience more than one concussion in a season (Table 20–7). As previously mentioned, there are three grades of concussions (see Table 20–6). Cantu's grade 1 concussion would encompass Nelson's grades 0 through 2. Recommendations are to remove the athlete from activity for at least 2 weeks after a second concussion of this grade and to make sure the athlete is asymptomatic for at least 1 week prior to return to activity. A third concussion of this type requires termination of activities for the season. A second concussion of Cantu grade 2 (equivalent to Nelson grade 3) requires eliminating activity for at least 1 month, with strong consideration given to terminating the season. A third concussion of this grade would be season ending. A second Cantu grade 3 concussion (Nelson grade 4) would terminate the season. Policy and decision-making criteria concerning recurrent concussions in either the same season or different seasons should be established.

Communication with all members of the staff is vitally important. This communication should involve not only medical personnel, but also the entire team. For example, the individual who is most knowledgeable regarding equipment needs should be alerted to investigate the possibility of a football helmet not fitting properly. Coaches should be encouraged to observe the athlete's techniques (overutilization of the head), as this may be putting the athlete at higher risk for head trauma.

"PUNCH DRUNK SYNDROME"

The cumulative effects of concussions have been well documented. The so-called punch drunk syndrome has

been recognized mainly in boxers, often several years after participation.[28] However, it may be seen in any sport in which there is repetitive "mild" head trauma. Another consideration that Lehman terms *sports synergy* is when an athlete may be exposed to head trauma in more than one sport.[29] Typical features of the syndrome include slurring of speech, tremor, and impairment of balance and coordination. Intellectual dysfunction has been demonstrated to occur. Gronwall and Wrightson studied 20 young adults after a second concussion.[30] This group, although they were not considered to be the typical "punch drunk" patients, demonstrated an impaired ability to process information when compared with a control group who had sustained only one concussion.

POSTTRAUMATIC HEADACHES

Posttraumatic vascular headaches may occur in athletes and may be confused with a mild concussion or a postconcussive headache. The vascular headache is a result of cerebral vasospasm, as in the case of a migraine headache. Vasospasm is directly related to head trauma. It may be difficult to determine the difference, but the vascular headache usually occurs not at impact, but shortly afterward. Prodromal symptoms such as visual scotomata are often noted.

POSTCONCUSSION SYNDROME

Postconcussion syndrome may develop after a concussion. This can be seen after even a low-grade concussion. It is characterized by persisting headaches, inability to concentrate, irritability, and fatigue. Typically these individuals will often undergo a CT scan of the head because of persisting symptoms, but this scan is generally normal. The symptoms may be extremely debilitating, especially at school, or cause job impairment at work. Symptoms can start from the time of injury to 48 hours after the trauma and last several weeks to months after injury. There is no definitive treatment other than symptomatic measures to control the headache. It is also important to limit the athlete's activities, and he or she should not be allowed to return to activity until the symptoms resolve.

CONCLUSION

Head injuries are the most feared of all injuries in sports because of the catastrophic consequences that may occur with them. Although head injuries are inevitable in several sports, those who care for athletes must seek ways to minimize the risks. There has been a great deal of refinement of the equipment used to protect against injuries to the head. Further advances must continue along these lines. In addition, several rule changes in individual sports have decreased the incidence of head injuries. In 1976 the "no spearing" rule making use of the head illegal as the initial point of contact in football reduced the number of fatal head injuries. The sports medicine field must continue to determine ways to make sports safer.

The approach to the athlete who sustains a head injury must be comprehensive and skillful. This requires no "weak links in the chain," from the person making the initial assessment to the point of the definitive care. A thorough understanding of the head injuries discussed, as well as the evaluation and treatment of these injuries, is vital for those caring for athletes.

REFERENCES

1. Torg JS, Vegso JJ, Sennett B, et al: The national football head and neck registry 1971–1984. JAMA 1985; 254:3439–3443.
2. Lehman LB. Nervous system sports-related injuries. Am J Sports Med 1987; 15:494–499.
3. Garrick JG, Requa RK: Medical care and injury surveillance in the high school setting. Phys Sports Med 1981; 9:115.
4. Gerberich SG, Priest JD, Boen JR, et al: Concussion incidence and severity in secondary school varsity football players. Am J Public Health 1983; 73(12):1370–1375.
5. Gennarelli TA: Cerebral concussion and diffuse brain injuries. In Torg JS (ed): Athletic Injuries to the Head, Neck and Face. Philadelphia, Lea & Febiger, 1982, pp 93–104.
6. Moody RA, Ruamsuke S, Mullan SF: An evaluation of decompression in experimental head injuries. J Neurosurg 1968; 29:586–590.
7. Saunders RL, Harbaugh RE: The second impact in catastrophic contact-sports head trauma. JAMA 1984; 252:538–539.
8. Wilberger JE Jr, Maroon JC: Head injuries in athletics. Clin Sports Med 1989; 8:1–9.
9. Teasdale G, Jennett B: Assessment of coma and impaired consciousness. Lancet 1974; 2:81–84.
10. Ingelzi RJ, VanderArk GD: Analysis of the treatment of basilar skull fractures with and without antibiotics. J Neurosurg 1975; 43:721–726.
11. Geisler FH, Greenberg J: Management of the acute head-injury patient. In Salcman M (ed): Neurologic Emergencies, 2nd ed. New York, Raven Press, 1990, pp 135–165.
12. Masters SJ, McClean PM, Arcarese JS, et al: Skull x-ray examinations after head trauma. N Engl J Med 1987; 316:84–91.
13. Levin HS, Benton AI, Grossman RG, eds: Neurobehavioral Consequences of Closed Head Injury. New York, Oxford University Press, 1982.
14. Cooper PR, Ho VH: Role of emergency skull x-ray films in the evaluation of the head-injured patient. A retrospective study. Neurosurgery 1983; 13:136–140.
15. Jamieson KG, Yelland JDN: Extradural hematoma: Report of 167 cases. J Neurosurg 1968; 29:13–23.
16. Bruno LA: Focal intracranial hematoma. In Torg JS (ed): Athletic Injuries to the Head, Neck, and Face. Philadelphia, Lea & Febiger, 1982, pp 105–121.
17. Jamieson KG, Yelland JDN: Surgically treated traumatic subdural hematomas. J Neurosurg 1972; 37:137–149.
18. Plum F, Posner JR: The Diagnosis of Stupor and Coma, 3rd ed. Philadelphia, FA Davis, 1980.
19. Seelig JM, et al: Acute subdural hematoma: Major mortality reduction in comatose patients treated within four hours. N Engl J Med 1981; 304:1511–1518.
20. Committee on Head Injury Nomenclature of the Congress of Neurological Surgeons. Glossary on head injury. Clin Neurosurg 1966; 12:338.
21. Rimel RW, Giordani B, Barth JT, et al: Disability caused by minor head injury. Neurosurgery 1981; 9:221–228.
22. Rimel RW, Giordani B, Barth JT, et al: Moderate head injury: Completing the clinical spectrum of brain trauma. Neurosurgery 1982; 11:344–351.
23. Nelson WE, Jane JA, Grick JH. Minor head injury in sports: A new system of classification and management. Phys Sports Med 1984; 12:103–107.
24. Colorado Medical Society: Report of the Sports Medicine Committee: Guidelines for the Management of Concussion in Sports (Revised). Denver, Colorado Medical Society, 1991.
25. Vegso JJ, Bryant MH, Torg JS: Field evaluation of head and neck injuries. In Torg JS (ed): Athletic Injuries to the Head, Neck and Face. Philadelphia, Lea & Febiger, 1982, pp 39–52.
26. Kulund DN: The Injured Athlete. Philadelphia, JB Lippincott, 1982.
27. Cantu RC: Guidelines for return to contact sports after a cerebral concussion. Phys Sports Med 1986; 14:75–83.
28. Casson IR, Siegel O, Sham R, et al: Brain damage in modern boxers. JAMA 1984; 251:2663–2667.
29. Lehman LH: Nervous system sports-related injuries. Am J Sports Med 1987; 15:494–499.
30. Gronwall D, Wrightson P: Cumulative effect of concussion. Lancet 1975; 995–997.

CHAPTER 21

Traumatic Injuries to the Cervical Spine

JAMES E. ZACHAZEWSKI MS, PT, SCS, ATC
GARY GEISSLER MS, PT, SCS, ATC
DONALD HANGEN MD

OVERVIEW OF THE PROBLEM

Millions of people participate each year in organized and recreational athletics, placing themselves at risk for possible injury.[1,2] The majority of individuals participate without suffering from significant injury or disability. Most injuries that do occur are relatively minor, allowing the participant to return to desired recreational activities and lifestyle without incident. Unfortunately, catastrophic injuries do sometimes occur from participation in organized or recreational athletic activity. Such catastrophic, and potentially fatal, injuries involve fractures and fracture-dislocations of the cervical spine.

Epidemiologic studies reviewed by Keenen and Benson[3] reveal that up to 11,000 new traumatic spinal cord–injured patients each year require medical intervention, and approximately 5000 other patients die prior to arrival at the hospital. While involvement in athletic activity accounts for only 15 percent of all spinal cord injuries yearly (Fig. 21–1), a high percentage of athletics-related traumatic cervical spine injuries that do cause some type of *significant* neurologic deficit result in quadriplegia (92 percent). Most of these athletics-related cases of quadriplegia are associated with diving accidents. As a comparison, quadriplegia is a consequence in 54 percent of traumatic cervical spine injuries that result in significant neurologic deficit as a result of motor vehicle accidents.[3]

Clinicians involved in sports medicine are in a position to influence the prevention, management, and outcome of these injuries. The role that providers play differs depending on the level of organization of the sport (youth league, interscholastic, intercollegiate, or professional), and the clinician's level of involvement with the team or athlete.

The makeup of the sports medicine team varies depending on the situation. In organized athletics, physicians, athletic trainers, physical therapists, paramedics, and emergency medical technicians (EMTs) specifically trained in the management of acute cervical injuries are often present when injury occurs and are available to assist. In recreational athletics, however, a paramedic or EMT is often called on to manage an acute cervical injury after it has occurred.

In organized athletics, the overall responsibility of the sports medicine team is to establish the policy and procedures for the emergency management of catastrophic injuries. All personnel must be appropriately trained and aware of their role. Communication links

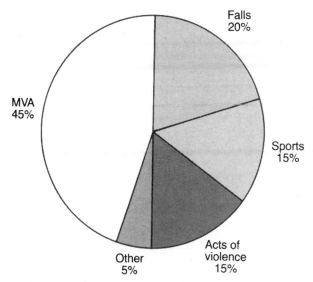

FIGURE 21–1. Etiology of spinal cord injuries. MVA, Motor vehicle accidents. (From Keenen TL, Benson DR: Initial evaluation of the spine injured patient. *In* Browner BD, Jupiter JB, Levine AM, Tafton PG (eds): Skeletal Trauma. Philadelphia, WB Saunders 1992, pp 585–603.)

must be established with all other appropriate medical personnel, such as paramedics and EMTs. The sports medicine team has the responsibility to (1) provide oversight and coverage of appropriate practices and competition, (2) make sure equipment fits well and is well maintained and appropriate for the sport, and (3) ensure that training and conditioning methods minimize the risks to the athlete. The sports medicine team must implement the policies and procedures for handling these injuries prior to the occurrence of injury. If injury occurs, policies and procedures must be carried out in an efficient, expedient manner.

NATIONAL FOOTBALL HEAD AND NECK INJURY REGISTRY

The National Football Head and Neck Injury Registry (NFHNIR) was established in 1975 in Philadelphia by Joseph S. Torg, MD. The purpose of the registry is to track athletics-related head and neck injuries in the United States. Dr. Torg initially established the registry to determine whether injuries sustained by 12 players in 1975 reflected a national trend toward catastrophic neurotrauma related to football.[4] The registry has built on work initiated by Schneider and reported on from the years 1959 through 1963.[5,6] Retrospective data were compiled from 1971 through 1975, and data continue to be collected each year.

Through this tracking and surveillance mechanism, recommendations have been made for changes in rules, coaching and training practices, and equipment that have resulted in a decrease in the incidence of cervical spine injuries. The most apparent of these rules changes was adopted in 1976. Preliminary data analysis in 1975 demonstrated that the majority of serious cervical spine football injuries were caused by cervical flexion and axial loading. Because of these data, a rule change was implemented by the National Collegiate Athletic Association (NCAA) and the National Federation of High School Athletic Associations (NFHSAA) that prohibited spearing, or using the crown of the helmet as the initial contact point when tackling. This change has resulted in a significant decrease in the incidence of cervical spine injury and quadriplegia (Fig. 21–2).[7] The registry continues to provide valuable information on which to base recommendations for changes.

EPIDEMIOLOGY

TYPES OF INJURY

BRACHIAL PLEXUS INJURIES

The signs and symptoms of all types of brachial plexus injuries usually sustained in athletics include sharp, burning pain in the neck and shoulder. Pain and paresthesia may radiate into the upper extremity. Weakness may be present as an additional symptom. Signs and symptoms are usually unilateral. Statistically these injuries are infrequent in athletics, with the exception of American football.[8,9] A full discussion of these injuries and their management is presented in Chapter 23.

Brachial plexus injuries, often termed *burners,* are most commonly incurred in collision sports such as football. The football rules change instituted in 1976 as a result of the efforts of the NFHNIR required a return to shoulder blocking and tackling. Because of this change, an increase in the frequency of brachial plexus injuries might have been anticipated, since a common mechanism causing these injuries in football is shoulder depression during blocking and tackling. However, a review of data collected on collegiate athletes from 1975 through 1978 by the National Athletic Injury Reporting System (NAIRS) did not demonstrate this to be the case.

The burner is the most common neural injury sustained by football players. Clancy has reported that a significant number of (33 of 67) collegiate football athletes studied sustained at least one burner during their collegiate careers.[10,11] No studies to date have been completed and published in the literature concerning the incidence of these injuries in the high school or club setting.

SPRAINS AND STRAINS

Minor injuries to the cervical spine that are a result of trauma are usually termed *sprains* or *strains.* Trauma is imposed by some means of acceleration, deceleration, or contact with an object such as the ground, an opponent, or the ball. This is probably the most common type of injury to the cervical spine in athletics, although no reports are available in the literature detailing the specific incidence of this injury.

Clinically, the athlete may complain of "jamming" his or her neck. Pain is most often localized to the area of the upper trapezius and cervical spine. Pain may radiate

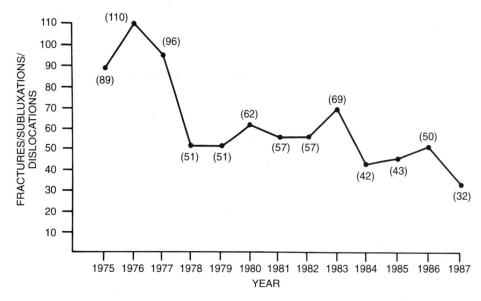

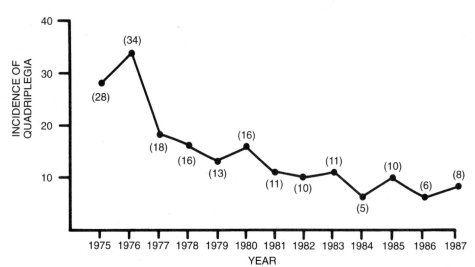

FIGURE 21–2. *A,* Yearly incidence of cervical spine fractures/dislocations/subluxations for all levels of participation (1975–1987) decreased markedly in 1978 and continued to decline during the remaining 9 years as a direct result of the rule changes instituted in 1976 banning headfirst blocking, tackling, and spearing. *B,* Yearly incidence of permanent cervical quadriplegia for all levels of participation (1975–1987) decreased dramatically in 1977 after initiation of rule changes prohibiting use of headfirst tackling and blocking techniques. The number of injuries continued to decline until 1984, after which the dramatically lowered levels were maintained. (From Torg JS, Vegso JJ, O'Neil J, et al: The epidemiologic, pathologic, biomechanical and cinematrographic analysis of football induced cervical spine trauma. Am J Sports Med 1990; 18:50–57.)

down one or both upper extremities if a nerve root is involved or inflamed, but this is not usually the case. Symptoms usually consist of pain, with or without radiation or paresthesia. Cervical range of motion may be limited. The clinical neurologic examination is usually negative for reflex or sensory changes. Weakness of the cervical musculature may be present as a result of pain and spasm. If the injury was a result of contact, a radiographic examination should be performed as a precaution to rule out fracture. Noncontact injuries without radicular symptoms do not necessarily mandate radiologic examination. The injured or involved structures may include the muscles, tendons, ligaments, intervertebral disc, or intervertebral joints.

Treatment considerations vary based on the stage of healing and the symptoms present. In the very acute period, the goal is to reduce the inflammatory response. The athlete should be instructed to use ice and counseled on appropriate positions of comfort. Nonsteroidal anti-inflammatory agents or analgesics may be utilized as indicated based on symptoms. Soft cervical

collars are of no biomechanical use in restraining motion; however, they may serve as a "reminder" that injury has occurred and that the head and neck should not be moved too vigorously during various activities of daily living (ADLs). Therapeutic modalities may be used as appropriate to assist in providing symptomatic relief. As the athlete's condition progresses, various forms of therapeutic exercise and manual therapy techniques may be initiated to facilitate regaining range of motion and strength. The athlete should not be allowed to return to participation until full range of motion and strength have returned. Individuals participating in collision sports should not be allowed to return until they are able to hold their body weight in all directions when positioned at a 45-degree angle (Fig. 21–3).

FRACTURES, SUBLUXATIONS, AND DISLOCATIONS

Fractures, subluxations, and dislocations constitute the type of injury that may result in the greatest degree of morbidity. They may be divided into injuries that occur in the upper (C1–C2), middle (C3–C4), or lower (C5–C7) cervical spine. A full description of the pathomechanics involved in fractures and fracture-dislocations will be presented later in this chapter.

UPPER CERVICAL SPINE (C1–C2). These injuries are rare in athletics. Injuries in this region of the cervical spine include fractures of the atlas and the odontoid.[12] Injuries to both of these anatomic structures occur as a result of a vertical compressive force to the head. A burst fracture of the atlas may occur as force is transmitted to the occipital condyles and lateral masses of C1. A flexion or extension force associated with this vertical compressive force may result in fractures of one or more of the arches of the atlas (anterior, posterior, or both) or a fracture of the odontoid. The mechanism of odontoid fractures is less well understood. Atlantoaxial dislocations may occur as a result of ruptures of the transverse and alar ligaments. These injuries may be associated with a flexion mechanism of injury.

MIDDLE CERVICAL SPINE (C3–C4). Traumatic injuries to the middle cervical spine associated with athletics were rare and infrequently reported until documented by NFHNIR in 1979 and 1986.[13,14] These injuries are the result of axial loading. The frequency of bony fracture is low, which makes these injuries unique.[15] From 1971 through 1988, the NFHNIR documented 1062 cervical injuries in athletics that resulted in a fracture, subluxation, or dislocation. Twenty-five of these, or 2.4 percent, involved the C3–C4 level.[16]

LOWER CERVICAL SPINE (C5–C7). Injuries at these levels account for most of the fractures and dislocations seen in athletics. The most common level of injury is C5–C6.[17] Again, axial loading is the most common mechanism of injury, although six common patterns of injury have been reported in the literature.[18] These patterns are compressive flexion, vertical compression, distractive flexion, compressive extension, distractive extension, and lateral flexion. Each of these patterns may be further subdivided into stages based on the degree of ligamentous injury and osseous damage. These stages and their medical and surgical management have been fully reviewed by Leventhal.[19]

CERVICAL SPINE STENOSIS WITH CORD NEURAPRAXIA AND TRANSIENT QUADRIPLEGIA

This syndrome was originally reported by Torg et al. in 1986[20] and has since been reviewed by Torg and Fay based on their research and the few reported cases of transient quadriplegia in the literature.[21]

Torg et al. reported that the incidence rate for transient paresthesia in all four extremities was 6 per 10,000 exposures in football, and the rate for paresthesia associated with transient quadriplegia was 1.3 per 10,000 exposures in the survey of a single season.[20] Symptoms of transient paresthesia include sensory changes that may be associated with motor paresis involving both arms, both legs, or all four extremities. This very acute, transient neurologic episode is of cervical cord origin. Findings are *always* bilateral and should not be confused with root or brachial plexus injuries, which are unilateral. This syndrome may follow forced hyperflexion, hyperextension, or axial loading of the spine. Routine radiographs are negative for fracture or dislocation. Developmental cervical spine narrowing is often apparent, either as an isolated finding or associated with congenital fusion, disc disease, or ligamentous instability.[20]

The diagnosis of cervical spine stenosis is based on the size of the vertebral canal relative to the vertebral body, as originally described in 1986 by Torg et al.[20] A group of 24 football players with transient quadriplegia attributed to neurapraxia of the cervical spinal cord was studied. All demonstrated vertebral canal–to–vertebral body ratios of less than 0.80 (Fig. 21–4). This ratio was thought to indicate significant spinal stenosis, as the ratio in a group of controls was 0.98.[22] Since the original description and the development of the Torg "ratio," other conflicting studies have questioned the use of this ratio as an absolute value to be used as criteria for significant spinal stenosis.[23,24] Odor et al. demonstrated that 74 of 224 asymptomatic professional and rookie football players (33 percent) demonstrated a Torg ratio of less than 0.80 at one or more levels between C3 and C6[23] while Herzog et al. examined 80 symptomatic professional football players and reported an abnormal Torg ratio in 49 percent.[24] The Torg ratio was also

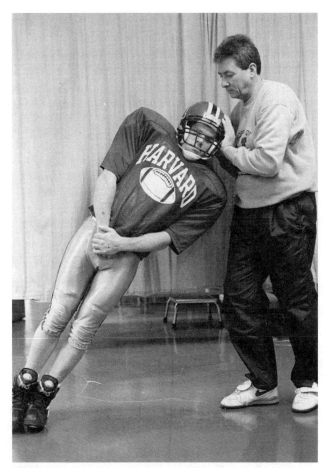

FIGURE 21–3. Athletes involved in collision sports such as football should be able to support their body weight with the cervical spine in neutral in all directions when positioned at a 45-degree angle.

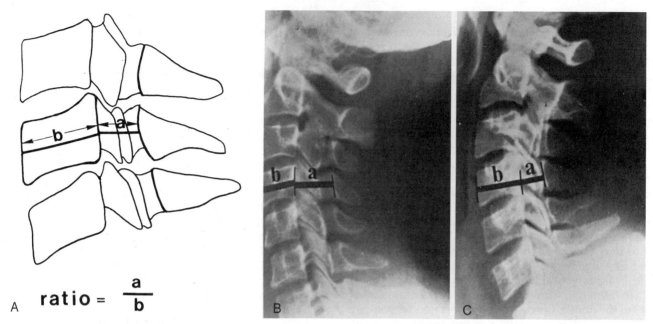

$$\text{ratio} = \frac{a}{b}$$

FIGURE 21–4. *A,* The spinal canal–to–vertebral body ratio is the distance from the midpoint of the posterior aspect of the vertebral body to the nearest point on the corresponding spinolaminar line (a) divided by the anteroposterior width of the vertebral body (b). *B* and *C,* Comparison between the spinal canal–to–vertebral body ratio in a "normal" control subject with that in a stenotic patient demonstrated on lateral radiographs of the cervical spine. The ratio is 1:1 (1.00) in the control subject (B) compared with 1:2 (0.50) in the stenotic patient (C). (From Torg JS, Pavlov H, Genuario S, et al: J Bone Joint Surg 1986; 68A:1354–1370.)

stated to be highly unreliable in Herzog et al.'s study, demonstrating a positive predictive value of only 12 percent. Thus, the Torg ratio may be abnormal in individuals with and without a transient quadriplegic episode. Given some of the conflict in the current literature, further evaluation of the Torg ratio and other factors may have to be considered prior to diagnosing a significant spinal stenosis and determining whether an athlete may continue to play. Each case must be evaluated on an individual basis.

SPORT-SPECIFIC INCIDENCE

FOOTBALL

Trauma to the cervical spine in football that produces significant injuries are infrequent but often catastrophic. Torg, in a retrospective review of the years 1971 through 1975,[25] demonstrated that the rate of fractures, subluxations, or dislocations of the cervical vertebrae *increased* 204 percent to 4.14 per 100,000 exposures, and the rate of cervical injuries associated with quadriplegia *increased* 116 percent to 1.58 per 100,000 exposures compared with data reported by Schneider and Kahn for the years 1959 through 1963.[26] Over this same period, a *decrease* in the rate of intracranial hemorrhages (66 percent) and craniocerebral deaths (42 percent) was noted (Fig. 21–5).[25] This shift in injury patterns—a decrease in significant head injuries and an increase in cervical spine injuries—is probably attributable to changes in protective equipment used from the early 1960s to the early 1970s.

During this period, better protection of the face and head were afforded by a change in facemask designs and helmet technology. The protection provided by improved helmet designs and materials decreased the incidence and severity of injury; however because of this, players may have felt at greater liberty to hit with their head as the initial point of contact, increasing the incidence of catastrophic cervical spine injuries (Fig. 21–6).

Most cervical spine injuries occur during the act of tackling an opposing player. The player who suffers the injury is usually the player who is doing the tackling, and consequently, the highest percentage of these injuries are suffered by defensive players making open field tackles.[13]

Because of the rise in cervical injuries documented and reported by Torg in 1976, the NCAA and NFHSAA adopted rule changes that stated "no player shall intentionally strike a runner with the crown or the top of the helmet or deliberately use his helmet to butt or ram a player." These rule changes decreased the use of the head as the initial point of contact in blocking and tackling in football.

Traumatic cervical spine fractures, subluxations, and dislocations have continued to progressively decrease since the 1976 rule change. Between 1976 and 1987, the rate of severe cervical spine injuries decreased 70 percent at the high school level and 65 percent at the collegiate level. The largest rate change took place in 1977 and 1978, 2 years after the rule change took effect. Injuries continued to decline until approximately 1984 and remained the same over the next 3 years. Data for the years 1988 to 1995 have not yet been published (see Fig. 21–2).[27]

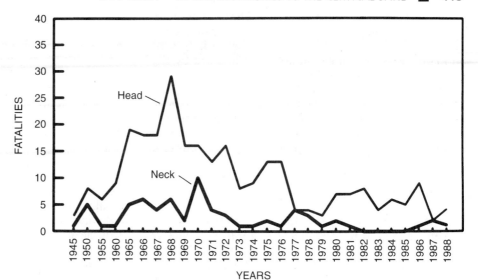

FIGURE 21–5. Intracranial and cervical spine injury fatalities, 1945–1988. (From Clarke KS: An epidemiologic view. *In* Torg JS (ed): Athletic Injuries to the Head, Neck and Face, 2nd ed., St. Louis, Mosby–Year Book, 1991, pp 5–28.)

ICE HOCKEY

Tator reviewed the literature available and documented a total of 117 cervical spine and spinal cord injuries between 1966 and 1987.[28] Spinal cord injuries incurred as a result of playing ice hockey were rare until approximately 1980. Prior to 1980, there was an average of two to three injuries per year. From 1982 to 1987, approximately 15 injuries per year were reported. Seventy percent of the injuries occurred when a player collided with the boards. Seventy-three percent of these injuries occurred during games, when the intensity of competition and checking from behind were the highest. Tator also attributes the increase in incidence since 1980 to better reporting mechanisms, physical factors related to players (increased weight and speed of skating), social and psychological factors among young hockey players (increased aggression and willingness to take risks), coaching attitudes and techniques (insufficient emphasis on conditioning, the risks of hockey, and methods of protecting the spine from injury; overemphasis on body contact), and small rinks with rigid boards. Unlike in football, Tator has stated that he has found no evidence that the increased use of helmets and facemasks, which have decreased the incidence of facial injuries, has increased the incidence of cervical spine injury.

WINTER SPORTS

Considering the number of individuals who participate in winter sports, the incidence of injury is surprisingly low. Reid and Saboe have reviewed spine injuries specific to sports in Canada. Of 202 injuries reviewed, 25 percent (n = 48) occurred from participation in winter sports.[29] Snowmobiling accounted for 10 percent, tobogganing for 6 percent, alpine skiing for 6 percent, and ice hockey for 3 percent.

Cervical spine injuries account for approximately 25 percent of all spine fractures that occur in relation to snowmobiling. Injuries are often related to driving a snowmobile at night; being under the influence of

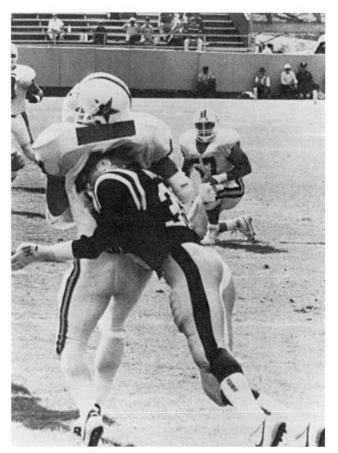

FIGURE 21–6. Inappropriate tackle that resulted in a catastrophic cervical spine injury. Note the position of slight cervical flexion, which enables axial loading to be produced when a tackler is spearing. (From Torg JS, Sennett B, Pavlov H, et al: Spear tackler's spine. Am J Sports Med 1993; 21:640–649.)

alcohol; being unfamiliar with the terrain; or various operator errors, such as becoming airborne, colliding with objects, or tipping over.

Injuries are equally divided between novice skiers and experienced skiers. The most common mechanisms of injury include attempting a jump and landing poorly, or losing control and hitting a tree. Other factors are collisions with other skiers or objects. All of these factors are related directly or indirectly to errors in judgment and control, which often cannot be influenced by the health care professional.

Toboggan injuries frequently involve younger individuals. Approximately one third of the cervical spine fractures in tobogganing occur in individuals under the age of 15. Like skiing, collisions with objects, becoming airborne, and demonstrating poor judgment account for most mechanisms of injury.

WATER SPORTS

Between 1964 and 1974, 152 of 1600 patients (9.5 percent) admitted to the Spinal Cord Injury Service at Rancho Los Amigos Hospital were injured during recreational activities. Eighty-two of these patients (54 percent) had been injured while diving. The average depth of water into which these individuals were diving was 5 feet. Surfing accounted for 29 injuries, and water skiing for seven.[30] All of these individuals were injured by striking the head on the bottom of the pool, lake, river, or ocean. As the head struck, the body continued to progress forward, resulting in an axial loading injury. A typical vertical compression load may result, although opinions vary.[31]

RUGBY

Rugby is gaining in popularity in the United States, as evidenced by club and varsity level competition for men and women at universities and numerous recreational leagues. Injury data must be drawn from the British Commonwealth countries, where it is played on a large scale.

Retrospective data are available for Australia and England. Between 1960 and 1985, 107 injured patients were admitted to spinal cord centers in Australia,[32] while 82 injuries occurred in England from 1959 through 1987.[33] Injuries usually occurred from a collapsing scrum or from tackling. Forwards were the most often injured players in amateur play because of their position and its requirements during play. A rule change was initiated in England in 1983 that reduced injuries from 10 the previous season to five between 1986 and 1987. This change kept players on their feet and in a more upright position in the scrum and the maul. Silver and Gill described the mechanisms of injury during rugby as the head being driven into the ground or a blow to the head.[33]

GYMNASTICS/TRAMPOLINE

Significant cervical spine injuries associated with gymnastics are predominantly associated with the use of the trampoline as a training device. Seventy-one percent of permanent spinal cord injuries to female gymnasts from 1973 through 1975 were associated with the trampoline. Other pieces of apparatus may be involved, however. During the same period, 33 percent of men's injuries were associated with the trampoline,

22 percent with the floor exercise and high bar, and 11 percent with the rings and mini-trampoline.[34] More than 114 catastrophic injuries have been attributed to the use of a trampoline since the initial report by Ellis in 1960. These injuries are usually associated with a somersault and an uncontrolled landing.[35]

The incidence of injury led to a position paper by the American Academy of Pediatrics in 1977.[36] This paper caused the American Alliance for Health, Physical Education and Recreation (AAHPER) and the NCAA Committee on Competitive Safeguards and Medical Aspects of Sports to issue guidelines making use of the trampoline optional and voluntary and specifically detailing safety and maintenance standards. Since 1978 a distinct decrease has been observed in all catastrophic gymnastic injuries and, more specifically, in injuries resulting from the use of trampolines and mini-trampolines.[35]

LEGAL CONSIDERATIONS

Catastrophic injuries to the cervical spine impose a severe emotional shock, pain and suffering, potential financial ruin, and anger on the injured athlete and family. A desperate need to shift responsibility outside the family is often felt. A member of the medical team often becomes the target of this shift. Any time members of the team are in a position to manage a catastrophic and potentially fatal injury, they may be at risk of being accused of incompetence or negligence. Patterson[37] and Heck et al.[38] provide an excellent, concise discussion of the legal aspects of athletic injuries to the cervical spine.

General claims against the athletic staff usually concern instruction in proper technique, the condition and appropriateness of equipment, the matching of participants based on size and skill, supervision, and/or postinjury care. Defensive responses to these claims include the assumption of risk by the competitor, statutory immunity, a release or waiver signed by the participant or parents, and the standard of reckless disregard.[38] Whether such defenses are successful in exonerating the medical team of legal liability depends on the facts of each particular case and the law of the state in which the legal action is brought.

To be better positioned to both avoid and defend such legal claims, the medical team must take reasonably prudent precautions to minimize the risk of injury for the participant during practice or competition and to minimize their own risk should catastrophic injury and the possibility of litigation occur. To minimize the athlete's risk, all equipment should be in good repair, comply with standards set by the National Operating Committee on the Safety of Equipment in Athletics (NOCSEA), and be fit by appropriately trained personnel only (athletic trainer, equipment manager, coach). All athletes should undergo a preseason physical that specifically includes questions relevant to previous cervical spine injuries and examination and screening of the cervical spine if the athlete is involved in a collision sport. The medical staff must make sure that the appropriate equipment is available, readily positioned, and in good repair to allow for appropriate management of catastrophic cervical spine injuries. All personnel involved in caring for the injured athlete must be properly trained and practice such training regularly. Training in the management of catastrophic injuries should be reviewed yearly. Recognized policies and procedures should be in place and agreed upon by all medical personnel, athletic administrators, and coaches.

In addition, questionnaires and statements of acknowledgment of risk, informed consent, and medical release should be on file prior to the start of any practice or competition. Both coaches and athletes should sign statements to document that (1) correct techniques outlining the dangers of initial contact with the head while involved in a collision sport have been reviewed, understood, and implemented; (2) rules and procedures to minimize exposure will be enforced continuously; and (3) appropriate strength and flexibility programs are included in conditioning drills.

MECHANICS AND PATHOMECHANICS

MECHANISM OF INJURY

Multiple mechanisms of injury may be responsible for cervical fractures, subluxations, or dislocations. Over time, numerous theories have been proposed regarding the mechanism of injury that is usually associated with athletics. Purported mechanisms of injury must withstand the scrutiny of research and critical review. Although mechanisms such as hyperflexion and hyperextension are feasible, they have not withstood such scrutiny. Even though injury may be possible from hyperflexion, hyperextension, or lateral bending/rotation, most of the force of these energies is absorbed by the cervical spine range of motion, strength of the musculature, intervertebral discs, and, to a lesser extent, the ligaments. Injuries that occur from these forces are most often sprains, strains, or brachial plexus injuries, generally not fractures, subluxations, or dislocations.

Attempts have been made to associate equipment specific to football with these mechanisms. It has been stated that the facemask may cause hyperflexion with the ground or an opponent; however, this was not reported to be the factor in the more than 200 injuries that occurred between 1971 and 1975.[39] Various authors and researchers have also demonstrated that the so-called guillotine effect of the helmet (the posterior rim of the helmet impact the cervical spine during tackling or contact with another player) is not implicated in football-related cervical spine fractures and dislocations.[14,15,40,41]

Current theory and evidence demonstrate that the most commonly acknowledged mechanism responsible for fracture-dislocation of the cervical spine in athletics is that of axial loading in flexion. The factor of axial loading is a common thread presented earlier in this chapter concerning the sport-specific incidence of injury.

When the cervical spine is placed in a position of slight flexion, there is a reduction of cervical lordosis,

and the cervical spine is straightened (Fig. 21–7). When an axial load is applied in this position (as may be the case with spearing in football or diving into a shallow pool) (Fig. 21–8), the energy-absorbing and energy-dissipating mechanisms afforded to the cervical spine through flexion, extension, and lateral bending/rotation are reduced. Load thus occurs on a segmented vertical column. When this load exceeds the energy-absorbing capacity of the vertebral bodies, intervertebral discs, posterior elements or ligaments, failure and injury result. Injuries incurred may be crush fractures of the cervical vertebrae, buckling (which produces an acute flexion dislocation at one level), or a combination of these two modes. The numerous anatomic and analytical modeling studies confirming this mechanism of injury have been reviewed by Otis et al.[39]

Because of the mechanics just described, it should be obvious that the majority of cervical spine injuries in athletics that produce cervical fracture or fracture-dislocation, with or without neurologic involvement, are caused by cervical flexion with axial loading. Proper technique is critical in the prevention of injury. Tackling or contact with the head in any collision sport (e.g., football, rugby), or diving into shallow water, striking the crown of the head, may produce catastrophic injury. These injuries are prevented not by equipment, but by adherence to appropriate technique and common sense.

EMERGENCY MANAGEMENT

PRACTICE/COMPETITION SITE

The emergency medical management of any athlete who has suffered a catastrophic cervical spine injury is the combined responsibility of the sports medicine team present at the practice or competition site. The makeup of this team may vary depending on the setting (professional, college, high school, or recreational). Regardless of the setting, an action plan should be developed and agreed on prior to the start of the season. Teamwork is critical to ensure safe, efficient management of these injuries.

In the organized athletic setting, the medical team usually comprises the team physician, athletic trainers, and/or physical therapists and emergency medical services (EMS) personnel. In the well-organized, well-funded setting, there may often be a greater number of physicians, trainers, and therapists in comparison with EMS personnel making up this team. In many other settings, EMS personnel may make up a greater percentage of this team for the management of this type of injury.

Duties and lines of communication should be determined prior to the start of the season. Members of the sports medicine staff should meet with local EMS personnel to work out specific logistics of access to facilities, transport, and responsibilities. Not all EMS agencies are capable of delivering advanced life support measures, nor is 911 service available in all regions of the United States or Canada.[42] Prior to the start of the

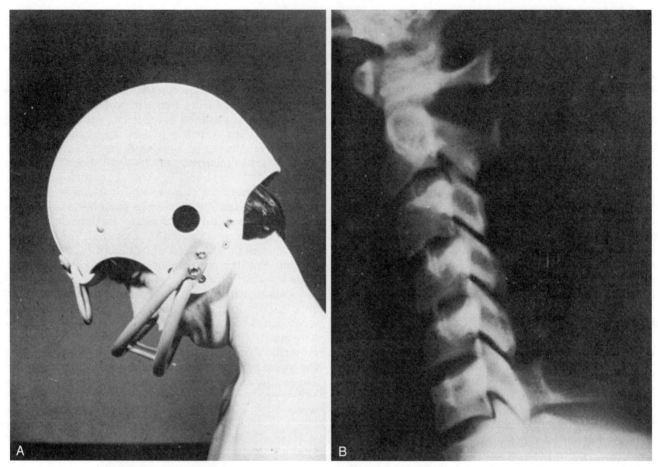

FIGURE 21–7. When the neck is flexed approximately 30 degrees *(A)*, the cervical spine becomes straight from the standpoint of force, energy absorption, and effect on tissue deformation and failure. The straightened cervical spine, when axially loaded, acts as a segmented column *(B)*. (From Torg J: National Football Head and Neck Injuries Registry: Report on the cervical quadriplegia from 1971–1975. Am J Sports Med 1979; 7:127.)

season, it should be decided who has primary responsibility to direct all facets of emergency care, immobilization, and transport of the athlete who has suffered a cervical spine injury: the physician, athletic trainers/therapists, or EMS personnel? How will the process differ depending on who is present? If responsibilities cannot be predetermined, trauma triage guidelines (Fig. 21–9) and legal regulations must be followed regarding lines of authority. Above all, communication is the key factor. All professionals involved in this situation have the same primary goal: the safe, efficient management of a traumatic situation.

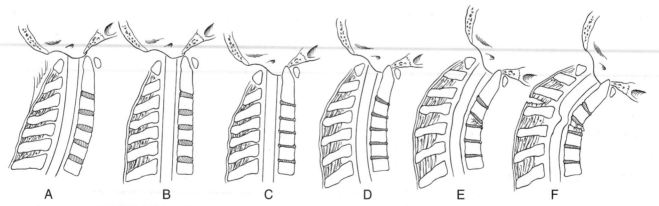

FIGURE 21–8. Axial load applied to a segmented column initially results in deformation by compression. If the axial load is large enough, more marked deformation occurs. Absorption of excessive amounts of energy during this axially applied load may result in buckling, with resultant fracture or dislocation of the segmented column.

Prior to the start of the season, all protective equipment and emergency care equipment must be checked to make sure that it is in good operational condition. Some members of the team may be uncomfortable with the evaluation and management of the cervical spine owing to the severity of the consequences of significant injury or the potential for further damage if mishandled. Training sessions should be scheduled with all members of the sports medicine staff and local EMS personnel, if possible. These training sessions should assist in easing lack of confidence in handling specific situations. Hypothetical injury situations should be utilized so that techniques of immobilization and transport may be practiced and everyone knows his or her role. Ensuring proper training of staff and communication among all personnel involved is the best way to guarantee appropriate management of this type of injury. On-the-job training at the time of the emergency is unacceptable.

On-field management consists of injury recognition and triage, situation management and immobilization of the cervical spine, and transport. Only a small percentage of sports-induced cervical spine injuries are significant and result in permanent neurologic deficit. However, a lesion without neurologic deficit can easily become one with a neurologic deficit if it is improperly handled.[43] Figure 21–9 summarizes an action plan for significant cervical spine injury.

Suspicion of cervical spine injury may occur through observation of the position of the head and neck at the time of the injury. If the mechanism of injury was not observed, observing whether the athlete is moving immediately following the injury will provide significant information about the severity of the injury. Most

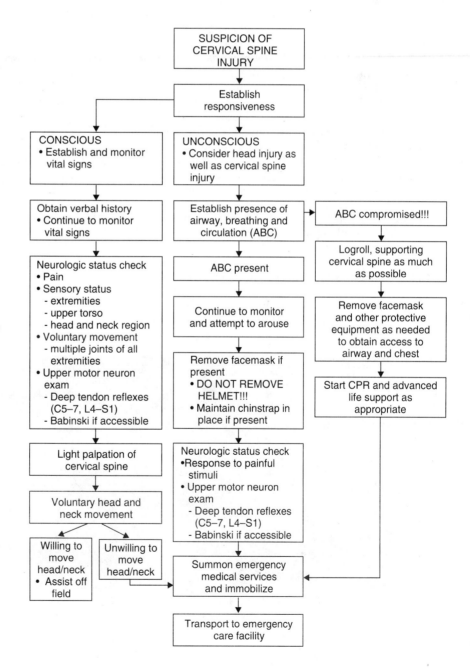

FIGURE 21–9. Algorithm for suspicion of cervical spine injury.

athletes will move after injury if they are able. An athlete lying completely still following injury is an indication that a potentially significant injury has occurred. Teammates of the injured athlete should be instructed not to move or touch the athlete until the clinician has determined exactly what is wrong.

On getting to the injured athlete, the clinician's initial duty is to establish the responsiveness of the athlete. The athlete should not be moved while doing this. Responsiveness and consciousness determine the next sequence of events.

UNCONSCIOUS ATHLETE. If the athlete is unconscious, the possibility of cervical injury as well as head injury must be considered. All unconscious athletes must be treated as if a significant cervical injury has occurred until determined otherwise. Establishing that the athlete has a viable airway, is breathing, and has a pulse (circulation) are critical; this is known as the *ABCs* of cardiopulmonary resuscitation (CPR). If the athlete is not breathing or does not have a pulse, the local EMS system should be activated and the athlete placed in a supine position appropriate for the administration of rescue breathing or CPR. If possible, care should be taken to attempt to logroll the individual to minimize trauma to the cervical spine (see "Immobilization"). If the athlete is wearing a facemask, as is common in sports such as football, hockey, or lacrosse, it should be removed. Facemasks may be removed without significant motion of the cervical spine by cutting the plastic pieces that hold the mask in place while stabilizing the head and neck (Fig. 21–10). The uniform and straps that hold shoulder pads in place may also have to be cut to allow access to the chest if the administration of CPR is required. *The helmet should not be removed.* This will be discussed in depth later in this chapter. CPR and/or advanced life support should be started as appropriate. When appropriate, the athlete should be immobilized and transported to an appropriate emergency medical facility.

If the athlete is unconscious but is breathing and has a pulse, the clinician should continue to monitor his or her vital signs and attempt to gently arouse the athlete without movement of the athlete. If a facemask is present, it should be removed at this time without moving the athlete and while stabilizing the head and neck. (Removal of the facemask at this time will allow access to the airway if necessary. The helmet should not be removed, as stated earlier). If the facemask cannot be removed without moving the athlete, this step is delayed until one is ready to immobilize the athlete. Airway, breathing, and circulation are continuously monitored. A neurologic check is then initiated. This check incorporates a response to painful stimuli (e.g., a sharp or dull instrument or pulling on extremity hair) and assessment of deep tendon reflexes related to C5–C7 and L5–S1. The Babinski sign may be elicited if the sole of the foot is readily accessible. Once the examination is completed, the athlete should be immobilized and transported. Immobilization will be described in detail later in this chapter.

CONSCIOUS ATHLETE. If the athlete is conscious after determining responsiveness, the clinician must continue to monitor his or her vital signs. Removal of the facemask is considered, as stated earlier. A history should be obtained from the athlete in a slow, firm, confident voice. Composure by the physician, trainer, therapist, or EMS personnel at the scene will assist the injured athlete in maintaining his or her composure, reduce anxiety, and help to control the situation at hand. During this portion of the examination, the athlete should not be moved but should be kept calm and quiet. Memory and recollection of the event of the injury should be established. The athlete may be able to describe the mechanism of injury and what he or she felt at the time of injury. Attention should be paid to the quickness, comprehensiveness, and confidence of the athlete's response and the clarity of his or her speech, as these will assist the clinician in determining the possibility of head injury in conjunction with cervical injury. While one member of the sports medicine team monitors the athlete's vital signs and level of consciousness, another member of the team begins a neurologic check.

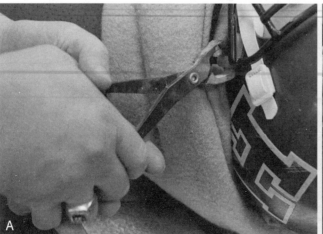
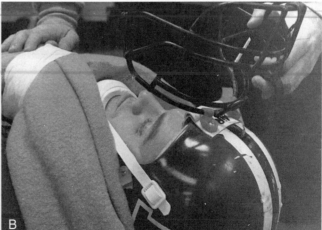

FIGURE 21–10. Plastic pieces that hold facemasks in place may be cut with a razor knife or other commercially available product to allow the facemask to swing out of the way, enabling access to the athlete's airway without removal of the helmet.

Pain is assessed as stated previously. Dermatome sensation is assessed for all four extremities, as well as for exposed areas of the face, neck, and torso. Attention is paid to the ability of the athlete to perceive which body part or parts are being touched. The ability to perceive light touch as well as sharp or dull sensation should be assessed. Extremity movement and strength are assessed by movement of multiple joints of each extremity. The athlete's ability to follow directions and comprehension are also important at this time. If sensation and movement are compromised in any extremity or dermatome, a complete neurologic examination, including assessment of deep tendon reflexes and the Babinski sign as described earlier, should be completed. On completion of the neurologic check, light, gentle palpation of the cervical spine and upper shoulders is performed. Pain, spasm, and any type of asymmetry of the cervical musculature or spinal erector muscles are noted. Particular attention is paid to any finding of point tenderness and abnormal alignment of the spinous processes of the cervical spine. If all components of the examination described previously are normal, the athlete may then attempt to move his or her head and neck. If there is any unwillingness or hesitancy of the athlete to move the head and neck, the athlete is immobilized. If the athlete is willing to move the head and neck, he or she is assisted off the field.

IMMOBILIZATION. A well-coordinated group effort is required to safely and efficiently immobilize an athlete with a suspected cervical spine injury. As mentioned previously, the specific technique to be used should be practiced prior to the start of any season. If members of the sports medicine team have not had opportunity to practice these techniques or are not familiar with them, only trained EMS personnel should be involved with the immobilization procedure.

Having the appropriate equipment readily available to immobilize the cervical spine is mandatory for collision sports such as football, hockey, or lacrosse, or other sports in which there is significant risk, such as gymnastics. Immobilization of the spine traditionally has been carried out by using a full-length spine board (Fig. 21–11). These boards are usually fabricated from wood or aluminum and may be purchased commercially from various emergency medical equipment manufacturers. The board must be designed to allow multiple positions for using strap systems to immobilize the injured athlete. Recently vacuum form splinting and immobilization systems have been developed that allow total body immobilization (Plasco MDI, 3849 Swanson Court, Gurnee, IL; telephone: 800-323-9035; or Hartwell Medical Corp., 6352 Corte del Abeto, Suite J, Carlsbad, CA, 92009; telephone: 800-633-5900). These systems offer the advantage of being lightweight and easily transportable.

As stated previously, on reaching the injured athlete, responsiveness, airway, breathing, and circulation must be established. Removal of the facemask is completed.

There is disagreement in the literature regarding whether the helmet should be removed.[43–48] We concur with the most recent publication from the American Academy of Orthopaedic Surgeons[48] that the

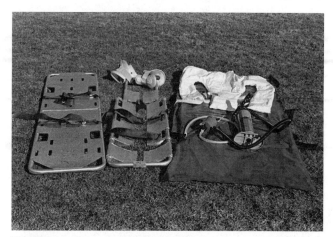

FIGURE 21–11. *Left to right,* Aluminum backboard, scoop stretcher, and vacuum backboard system.

helmet *should not* be removed, except in the following instances:

- when the facemask or visor interferes with adequate ventilation or with the clinician's ability to restore an adequate airway (*Authors' note:* If removal of the facemask or visor does not allow adequate access to the airway, then the helmet must be removed if warranted by the situation at hand.)
- when the helmet is so loose that securing it to the spinal immobilization device will not provide adequate immobilization of the athlete's head
- when life-threatening hemorrhage under the helmet can be controlled only by its removal
- when, because of the size of the helmet, using it as part of the spinal immobilization will cause extreme flexion of the neck. This situation usually occurs in children. (*Authors' note:* This does not tend to occur when the injured athlete is wearing shoulder pads as well as a helmet, because the shoulder pads will assist in keeping the torso in line with the head and cervical spine. However, it may occur when the athlete is wearing a helmet without using shoulder pads.)

Because helmets are usually used in conjunction with shoulder pads in athletics, removal of the helmet without removal of all other protective padding from the chest up may alter head and neck position when immobilizing the spine on a backboard. Radiologically, Swenson et al.[49] and Hulstyn et al.[49a] have demonstrated no significant difference in sagittal cervical alignment in subjects immobilized with and without football helmet and shoulder pads. A significant increase in cervical lordosis was demonstrated when subjects were immobilized in a supine position with shoulder pads but without a helmet. From these studies it may be concluded that immobilization on a backboard with helmet and shoulder pads left in place will maintain cervical sagittal alignment in a position most closely approximating normal. The removal of the helmet and shoulder pads should be an "all or none" proposition. Any attempt to remove the helmet should be delayed until both the helmet and shoulder pads can be removed in a controlled setting such as the emergency department.

After establishing vital signs and responsiveness, preventing further injury is the single most important objective.[43] The member of the medical team who is at the head of the injured athlete and who established vital signs and responsiveness is responsible for directing the emergency management of the injured athlete. At this time, the head should be immobilized by holding it in the position in which it lies. Once the head is immobilized manually, it is not released until the body and head are fully immobilized on the spinal board or vacuum splint system.[50] Because this may be a lengthy process, the individual who is manually immobilizing the head and neck should choose his or her position of comfort carefully.

If the injured athlete is in a face-down position, he or she must be rolled to a face-up position. This is done by using a logrolling technique, as demonstrated in Figure 21–12. The leader of the team applies gentle longitudinal support to the head and neck.[50] An adequate number of assistants (usually at least three) are required to logroll the injured athlete without compromising the athlete's condition or safety. These assistants should be stationed at the shoulders, pelvis, and legs. A greater number of assistants may be required to roll a larger or heavier athlete. The member of the team who is manually immobilizing the cervical spine is responsible for coordination of the logroll procedure through direct commands. A smooth coordinated pull is accomplished by the assistants stationed as just described. The assistants should *always* roll the injured athlete toward them.[43,50] The injured athlete may be rolled directly onto the spine board or vacuum splint. Any facemask, if not already removed, is removed once the athlete is in a supine position. Removal of the facemask may be accomplished by using a razor knife or any of a number of commercially available clippers.

Often it is difficult to logroll an injured player who is wearing protective equipment such as a helmet and shoulder pads directly onto a spine board or vacuum mattress and into the correct position for immobilization. It is not as difficult to obtain the correct position with athletes who are not wearing protective equipment. If the player must be moved from his or her initial position to obtain proper immobilization, it must be done with extreme caution. A well-coordinated effort is required to lift the injured athlete and reposition the spine board or vacuum mattress. At least three assistants should be stationed on each side of the injured player. The team leader is still responsible for immobilization and control of the head and neck. Another assistant is responsible for repositioning the board or vacuum mattress under the athlete. The athlete is lifted and lowered on command of the leader to a height sufficient to allow the spine board or vacuum mattress to be

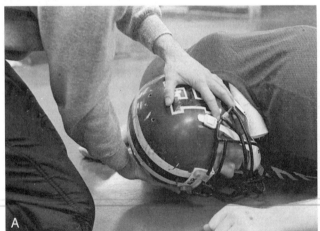
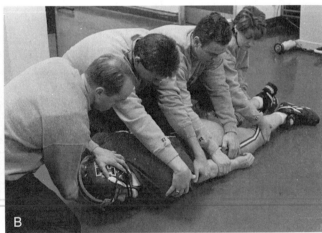
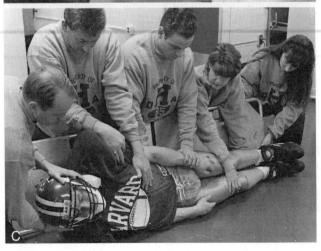

FIGURE 21–12. *A*, Appropriate grasp and immobilization of the athlete's head and neck. The member of the team immobilizing the head and neck must make sure that when the athlete is rolled into a supine position, his hands are not crossed and he is able to maintain appropriate support for the duration of the time required to fully immobilize the athlete. *B* and *C*, Appropriate logrolling technique. Sufficient support of the entire body with assistance in placing the backboard in the best position is needed to prevent moving the athlete a second time to place him or her in the center of the board.

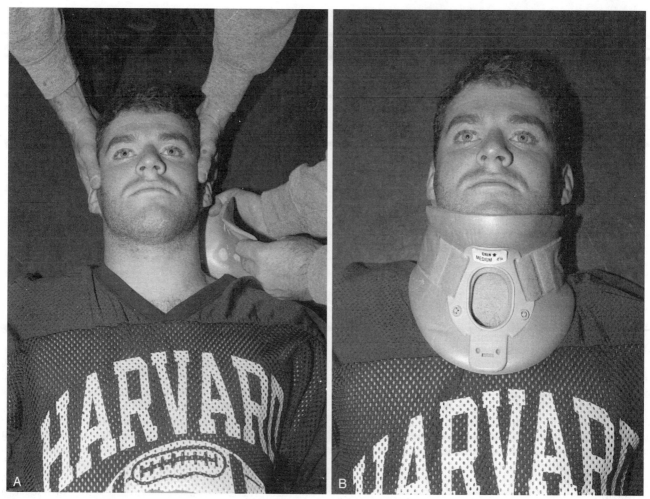

FIGURE 21–13. Application of an extrication collar with the athlete in a supine position.

repositioned under the athlete by another assistant. *The spine board or vacuum mattress is moved relative to the athlete; the athlete is not moved in any direction other than vertically.* This minimizes movement of the athlete and the potential for complications.

The athlete's vital signs, level of consciousness, and neurologic status are monitored by the team leader throughout the procedure of positioning the athlete on the spine board or vacuum mattress. At this time, an extrication collar should be applied to assist in immobilization of the head and neck if the athlete is not wearing a helmet (Fig. 21–13).[50] Commercially available cervical collars may not fit if an athlete is wearing a helmet and/or shoulder pads. In this situation, a towel or blanket roll should be substituted if a spine board is used.[44] The towel roll or blanket is slid under the athlete's neck and the ends are brought together and secured. After some type of cervical support is applied as described earlier, the athlete's torso is secured to the spine board prior to securing the head.[48] Areas around the athlete's legs and in the lumbar area are padded to remove any room between the athlete and strapping system when using a spine board. This minimizes any movement of the athlete's torso relative to the board. After the athlete's torso is secured, the head and neck

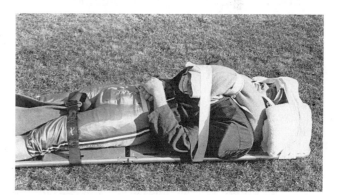

FIGURE 21–14. Athlete secured to backboard with a towel/blanket roll appropriately placed around the head and neck.

are secured. A foam block, a rolled-up blanket, or towels are placed around the head when securing the athlete to a spine board to assist in immobilization (Fig. 21–14).

When using a vacuum splint/mattress system, the head may be sufficiently immobilized without use of the towel or blanket roll. This additional padding is not necessary when using the vacuum mattress system and vacuum cervical collar, as they may be brought in close proximity to the athlete prior to removing the air from

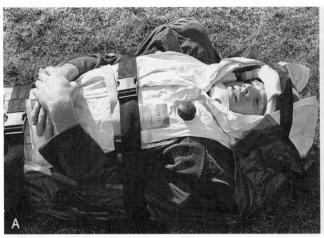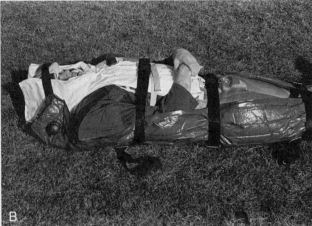

FIGURE 21–15. Athlete immobilized in a vacuum cervical collar and mattress.

the system. Together these create a rigid support (Fig. 21–15). As with any system of spine immobilization, sufficient personnel are required to carry out the task, minimizing the chances of further injury to the athlete. Care is taken to maintain appropriate access to the athlete's airway, should it be required.

Throughout the procedure of applying an extrication collar, blanket roll, or vacuum immobilization system, longitudinal support and control of the head are maintained by the team leader. Only after the athlete's head and neck are secured to the immobilization device does the team leader relinquish control of the head and neck. Once the athlete has been secured, he or she is lifted using the immobilization device and transported to the appropriate emergency medical facility for further management.

EMERGENCY DEPARTMENT MANAGEMENT

The goals of emergency department management of athletes with suspected cervical spine trauma are to (1) avoid, if present, further damage to the spinal cord; (2) prevent injury to uninjured tissues; (3) assess the athlete for neurologic injury; and (4) image the cervical spine for the presence of fractures, dislocations, instability, or disc herniations. The dictum of "do no harm" certainly applies. Early pharmacologic treatment can be instituted and the appropriate neurosurgical and orthopaedic consultations obtained for definitive treatment and stabilization.

It is important to maintain a high suspicion for cervical spine injury and obtain a prompt diagnosis. In one series,[51] a delay in diagnosis of spine trauma led to a 10 percent incidence of secondary neurologic deficits. Patients with a spine injury diagnosed on initial evaluation had a much lower (1.5 percent) incidence of secondary neurologic injury. Reasons for a delay in diagnosis included failure to obtain a radiograph, missing a fracture on a radiograph, or failure of the athlete to seek medical attention. Other reasons included polytrauma and altered levels of consciousness. The incidence of a delay in diagnosis of trauma in the cervical spine is estimated to be approximately 30

percent. It should also be noted that approximately 50 to 60 percent of spine-injured patients have an associated nonspinal injury.[52]

It has been estimated that 5 to 10 percent of spinal cord injuries occur in the immediate postinjury period.[53] Extreme care must be exercised when moving and transporting athletes with possible cervical trauma. Immobilization of the cervical spine must be maintained during examination and imaging until an unstable cervical spine injury is ruled out. This immobilization includes a spine board, cervical collar, or other appropriate stabilization devices. If a helmet is in place, it should remain on during transport unless it has a nonremovable facemask that is obstructing ventilation or access to the injured athlete's airway. In such a case, the face shield should be removed with the aid of a razor knife, bolt cutters, or other similar means. The helmet can be useful in assisting with stabilization of the cervical spine during transport. In addition, removal of the helmet requires significant motion of the cervical spine. Therefore, it is best to exclude unstable fractures prior to removal, if possible. In the presence of cervical spine injury, the helmet should be removed only in the emergency department setting by personnel trained in the care of such injuries.

PHYSICAL EXAMINATION

Cervical spine–injured athletes should be considered trauma patients and undergo a trauma evaluation, including the ABCs and cervical spine as part of the initial survey. A complete physical examination should be performed that literally involves an examination from head to toe. The entire spine should be inspected for wounds and ecchymosis and palpated for any point tenderness or any step deformity. A thorough neurologic examination is necessary and includes motor testing of the upper and lower extremities. Motor testing is conducted by nerve root level and is graded using the 0-to-5 Oxford scale, in which 0 is no contraction, 1 is a trace contraction without motion, 2 is motion with gravity eliminated, 3 is motion against gravity, 4 is motion against resistance but diminished strength, and 5 is normal motor strength. With cervical spine injuries, diaphram motion indicates function to the C4 root level, and patients with complete injuries proximal to this level generally do not survive. Injury to the C5 level is indicated by altered deltoid and biceps function; to C6, by weakness of the short and long radial wrist extensors; to C7, by weakness of the triceps and finger extensors; to C8, by weakness of the finger flexors; and to T_1, by intrinsic hand muscle weakness.

Sensory examination of all dermatomes is completed using pin-prick sensation and proprioception. Care is used in examining the anal and perineal regions. The skin in these regions is innervated by sacral nerve roots, and sensation in these areas may indicate an incomplete lesion in an otherwise insensate patient. Deep tendon stretch reflexes at multiple nerve root levels should be assessed. Reflexes involving cervical nerve roots include the biceps (C5), brachioradialis, (C6), and triceps (C7). Additional important reflexes include the Babinski reflex in the foot and the bulbocavernosus reflex. If the latter reflex is absent, the patient may be in spinal shock, and the neurologic level of injury cannot be determined until the reflex returns. The unconscious athlete presents a more difficult examination problem, although much information can be obtained from examination of rectal tone, reflexes, and responses to painful stimuli.

There are various patterns of neurologic injury in spinal cord–injured athletes based on anatomic areas of injury. Not all athletes fit into a single category, but it is important to document the patterns as accurately as possible because of the prognostic importance that various patterns have for neurologic recovery and return to function. Spinal shock is defined as a nonstructural dysfunction of the spinal cord that occurs soon after injury and usually ends within 24 hours. The end of spinal shock is determined by return of the bulbocavernosus reflex, and it is at this time that the degree of spinal cord injury can be evaluated. Injuries can be classified as either complete (no function below the level of injury) or incomplete (some neurologic function persists caudal to the level of injury). Incomplete injury patterns include the central cord syndrome, the most common type of incomplete injury, which presents with sacral sparing (perianal sensation, rectal motor tone, and great toe flexor activity) and carries a relatively good prognosis for the return of functional activity. The anterior cord syndrome, which presents with complete motor and sensory loss (with the exception of some retained deep pressure and proprioception), carries a poor prognosis. The posterior cord syndrome, a rare injury, presents with the loss of only deep pressure, pain, and proprioception. The Brown-Séquard syndrome presents with an ipsilateral motor deficit and a contralateral pain and temperature deficit, indicating unilateral cord injury.

RADIOLOGIC EXAMINATION

The standard plain film radiologic examination of the cervical spine is made up of five views: a cross-table lateral, an anterioposterior view of the atlantoaxial segments done through an open-mouth projection, an anterioposterior view of the remainder of the cervical spine, and left and right oblique projections. *The cross-table lateral view, anteroposterior views, and open-mouth projections should be completed prior to removal of the helmet, if possible.* Completion prior to helmet removal allows the physician to visualize obvious trauma and deformity and make an initial assessment of the extent of trauma. If complete visualization of the spine is not possible with the helmet or any other protective equipment on, then the helmet and other protective equipment (shoulder pads) should be removed and the radiologic examination repeated.

The cross-table lateral cervical spine radiograph should show the entire cervical spine from the occiput to the top of T1. It should be remembered that a normal lateral view does not "clear" the cervical spine but rather serves to identify or exclude grossly unstable cervical spine fractures and to check for the presence of prevertebral soft tissue swelling. Cervical spine alignment is determined by four parallel lines running along the anterior surface of the vertebral bodies, the posterior border of the vertebral bodies, the posterior surface of the facet joints, and the spinolaminar interfaces.[54] The lateral view is also used to assess vertebral body height and disc spaces, as well as the spinal canal diameter and the atlas-dens interval.

The open-mouth view is used specifically to examine the atlantoaxial vertebrae for fractures or abnormal relationships that may indicate rotary subluxation. The other anteroposterior view is used to visualize from C3 to C7. This view demonstrates the tracheal air shadow (which should be in midline) and the alignment of the pedicles, spinous processes, and articular masses. Oblique projections are used to give additional information about the facet joints and to image neural foramen. Readers are referred to the text by Harris for a complete description of evaluation cervical spine films, which is beyond the scope of this chapter.[55]

Other imaging studies include tomograms, which can be used to look for subtle fractures in areas of superimposed bony structures. Computed tomography (CT) provides axial images that can be used to better evaluate subtle fractures and to image areas not well visualized on plain radiographs. In addition to axial images, three-dimensional reconstructions can be done to image complex fractures. Myelography alone or in combination with CT scans can be used to evaluate for any cord or nerve root compression. Magnetic resonance imaging (MRI) techniques can be used to obtain sagittal, axial, and coronal views of bony elements, intervertebral discs, the spinal cord, cerebrospinal fluid, ligaments, and other anatomic structures.

Flexion and extension lateral views of the cervical spine can be obtained to look for ligamentous instability. These views should be obtained only after an unstable fracture pattern has been excluded and should be done with voluntary motion. They are contraindicated in patients with neurologic injury and those with altered states of consciousness. These views are useful in assessing not only acute ligamentous instability, but also late cervical spine instability following traumatic injury. White and Punjabi have defined stability of the lower cervical spine as "the ability of the spine to limit

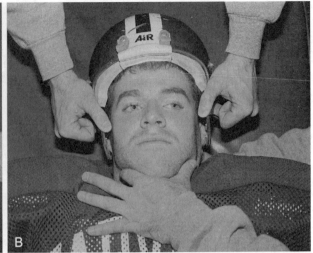

FIGURE 21–16. Helmet removal. Care is taken to manually support and immobilize the head and cervical spine. The cheek pads are carefully removed and the helmet is spread laterally prior to removal.

the patterns of displacement under physiologic stress so as not to damage or irritate the spinal cord or nerve roots."[56] Radiographically, this displacement has been defined as angular displacements of 11 degrees more than visualized in adjacent vertebral segments, or sagittal plane displacements of one segment in relationship to another of greater than 3.5 mm.

HELMET AND SHOULDER PAD REMOVAL

This procedure is often required to obtain full radiographic evaluation and has been well summarized by Denegar and Saliba.[44] Manual stabilization of the player's head and neck should be reapplied as the head is released from the spine board or vacuum immobilization. This is accomplished by having an assistant place his or her fingers on each side of the mandible around the helmet. At this time the head and neck are stabilized by placing one hand behind the athlete's neck and exerting pressure along the occiput, and placing the other hand along the mandible. The helmet is removed by unsnapping the cheek pads and expanding it laterally to clear the ears. After it is removed, longitudinal manual stabilization should be maintained by placing one hand on each side of the head with the fingers under the angle of the mandible and in the proximity of the mastoid process (Fig. 21–16). The shoulder pads may then be removed by cutting all straps and slipping them off the athlete, being careful not to disturb the position of the head and neck. Cervical spine films are repeated if appropriate visualization was not obtained with the helmet and shoulder pads in place.

INTERVENTION

When spinal cord injury is present, prompt consideration should be given to early pharmacologic treatment. Although there has been much controversy about the safety and efficacy of various treatments, animal studies and clinical trials have demonstrated the value of some agents. A randomized controlled clinical trial of methylprednisolone, a corticosteroid, demonstrated some efficacy of this agent following acute spinal cord injury.[57] Patients in this study were given a 30-mg/kg dose of methylprednisolone, followed by 5.4 mg/kg/hr given by continuous drip for a total of 23 hours. Theoretically, steroids will reduce the degree of edema in injured spinal cord tissues. Other drugs that may be of possible benefit to spinal cord–injured patients include opiate antagonists such as thyrotropin-releasing hormone and opiate receptor antagonists such as naloxone.

Once an unstable cervical spine injury is detected, prompt involvement of specialists trained in definitive management of such injuries is instituted. Although the individuals involved vary among institutions, generally an orthopaedic surgeon manages further stabilization and a neurosurgeon is involved if significant neurologic injury is present. Stabilization procedures completed in the emergency department include applying traction through either a halo ring or the more rapidly applied Gardner-Wells tongs. In some cases traction may be the definitive treatment, or it may be preliminary to surgical stabilization. The halo ring can also be connected to a vest apparatus for long-term immobilization.

SUMMARY

Injuries to the cervical spine associated with athletics have the potential to cause severe spinal cord trauma or quadriplegia; they may even prove to be fatal. It is therefore imperative that the sports medicine team be well skilled in on-field emergent care management, immobilization, transportation, and emergency department management of these injuries. Management of the injury by the sports medicine team, in whom the injured athlete is placing his or her trust, must be efficient and flawless to minimize the consequences of traumatic cervical spine injuries. Policies, procedures, and protocols for the management of these injuries should be in place for all organized athletic teams and organizations. The sports medicine team should practice techniques involved in on-field emergent care, immobilization, and transportation at least once each year.

REFERENCES

1. Nicholas JA: What sports medicine is all about. *Commun Med* 1975; 42:4.

2. Requa RK: The scope of the problem: The impact of sport related injuries. *In* Proceedings: Sports Injuries in Youth Surveillance Strategies. Publication no. 93-3444. Washington, DC, National Institutes of Health, 1992; pp 19–25.

3. Keenen TL, Benson DR: Initial evaluation of the spine injured patient. *In* Browner BD, Juputer JB, Levine AM, Tafton PG (eds): Skeletal Trauma. Philadelphia, WB Saunders, 1992; 585–603.

4. Torg JS, Quedenfeld TC, Bustein A, et al: National Football Head and Neck Injury Registry: Report on cervical quadriplegia 1971–1975. *Am J Sports Med* 1979; 7:127–132.

5. Schneider RC: Serious and fatal neurosurgical football injuries. *Clin Neurosurg* 1966; 12:226–236.

6. Schneider RC: Head and Neck Injuries in Football. Baltimore, Williams & Wilkins, 1973.

7. Clarke KS: An epidemiologic view. *In* Torg J (ed): Athletic Injuries to the Head, Neck and Face. St. Louis, Mosby–Year Book, 1991, pp 15–27.

8. Hirasawa Y, Sakakida K: Sports and peripheral nerve injury. *Am J Sports Med* 1983; 11:420–426.

9. Takazawa H, Sudo N, Akoi K, et al: Statistical observation of nerve injuries in athletes. (In Japanese) Brain Nerve Injury 1971; 3:11–17.

10. Clancy WG, Brand RL, Bergfeld JA: Upper trunk brachial plexus injuries in contact sports. *Am J Sports Med* 1977; 5:209–214.

11. Clancy WG: Brachial plexus and upper extremity peripheral nerve injuries. *In* Torg JS (ed): Athletic Injuries to the Head, Neck and Face. Philadelphia, Lea & Febiger, 1982, pp 215–220.

12. Glasgow SG: Upper cervical spine injuries (C1-C2) *In* Torg J (ed): Athletic Injuries to the Head, Neck and Face. St. Louis, Mosby–Year Book 1991, pp 457–468.

13. Torg JS, Treux R, Quedenfeld TC, et al: The National Football Head and Neck Injury Registry: Report and conclusions 1978. *JAMA* 1979; 241:1477–1479.

14. Torg JS, Vegso JJ, Sennett B, et al: The National Football Head and Neck Injury Registry: 14 year report on cervical quadriplegia, 1971–1984. *JAMA* 1986; 254:3439–3443.

15. Torg JS, Treux RC, Marshall J, et al: Spinal injury at the third and fourth cervical vertebrae from football. *J Bone Joint Surg* 1977; 59A:1015–1019.

16. Torg JS, Pavlov H: Middle cervical spine injuries (C3 and C4). *In* Torg JS (ed): Athletic Injuries to the Head, Neck and Face. St. Louis, Mosby–Year Book, 1991, pp 469–490.

17. Shields CL, Fox JN, Stauffer ES: Cervical cord injuries in sports. *Phys Sports Med* 1978; 6:71–76.

18. Allen BL, Ferguson RL, Lehmann TR, et al: A mechanistic classification of closed, indirect fractures and dislocations of the lower cervical spine. *Spine* 1982; 7:1–5.

19. Leventhal MR: Management of lower cervical spine injuries. *In* Torg J (ed): Athletic Injuries to the Head, Neck and Face. St. Louis, Mosby–Year Book, 1991, pp 491–515.

20. Torg JS, Pavlov H, Genuario SE, et al: Neurapraxia of the cervical spinal cord with transient quadriplegia. *J Bone Joint Surg* 1986; 68A:1354–1370.

21. Torg JS, Fay CM: Cervical stenosis with cord neurapraxia and transient quadriplegia. *In* Torg J (ed): Athletic Injuries to the Head, Neck and Face. St. Louis, Mosby–Year Book, 1991, pp 533–552.

22. Pavlov H, Torg JS, Robie B, et al: Cervical spinal stenosis: Determination with vertebral body ratio method. *Radiology* 1987; 164:771–774.

23. Odor JM, Watkins RG, Dillin WH, et al: Incidence of cervical spinal stenosis in professional and rookie football players. *Am J Sports Med* 1990; 18:507–509.

24. Herzog RG, Wiens JJ, Dillingham MF, et al: Normal cervical spine morphometry and cervical spinal stenosis in asymptomatic professional football players. *Spine* 1991; 16:178–186.

25. Torg JS: Epidemiology, biomechanics and prevention of cervical spine trauma resulting from athletics and recreational activities. *Oper Tech Sports Med* 1993; 1:159–168.

26. Schneider RC, Kahn EA: Serious and fatal neurosurgical football injuries. *Clin Neurosurg* 1966; 12:226–236.

27. Torg JS, Vegso JJ, O'Neill J, et al: The epidemiologic, pathologic, biomechanical and cinematographic analysis of football induced cervical spine trauma. *Am J Sports Med* 1990; 18:50–57.

28. Tator CH: Injuries to the cervical spine and spinal cork resulting from ice hockey. *In* Torg J (ed): Athletic Injuries to the Head, Neck and Face. St. Louis, Mosby–Year Book, 1991, pp 124–132.

29. Reid DC, Saboe LA: Spine injuries resulting from winter sports. *In* Torg J (ed): Athletic Injuries to the Head, Neck and Face. St. Louis, Mosby–Year Book, 1991, pp 142–156.

30. Shields CW, Fox JM, Stouffer ES: Cervical cord injuries in sports. *Phys Sports Med* 1978; 6:71–76.

31. Torg JS: Injuries to the cervical spine and cork resulting from water sports. *In* Torg J (ed): Athletic Injuries to the Head, Neck and Face. St. Louis, Mosby–Year Book, 1991, pp 157–173.

32. Taylor TKF, Coolican MRJ: Spinal cord injuries in Australia football, 1960–1985. *Med J Aust* 1987; 147:112–118.

33. Silver JR, Gill G: Injuries of the spine sustained during rugby. *Sports Med* 1988; 5:328–334.

34. Clarke K: Survey of spinal cord injuries in schools and college sports, 1973–1975. *J Safety Res* 1977; 9:140.

35. Torg JS: Trampoline induced cervical quadriplegia. *In* Torg J (ed): Athletic Injuries to the Head, Neck and Face. St. Louis, Mosby–Year Book, 1991, pp 85–96.

36. American Academy of Pediatrics, Committee on Accident and Poison Prevention: Trampolines. Evanston, IL, American Academy of Pediatrics, September 1977.

37. Patterson D: Legal aspects of athletic injuries to the head and cervical spine. *In* Torg J (ed): Athletic Injuries to the Head, Neck and Face. St. Louis, Mosby–Year Book, 1991, pp 198–209.

38. Heck FJ, Weiss MP, Gartland JM, et al: Minimizing liability risks of head and neck injuries in football. *J Athletic Training* 1994; 29:128–139.

39. Otis JC, Burstein AH, Torg JS: Mechanisms and pathomechanics of athletic injuries to the cervical spine. *In* Torg J (ed): Athletic Injuries to the Head, Neck and Face. St. Louis, Mosby–Year Book, 1991, pp 438–456.

40. Virgin H: Cineradiographic study of football helmets and the cervical spine. *Am J Sports Med* 1980; 8:310.

41. Carter DR, Frankel VH: Biomechanics of hyperextension injuries to the cervical spine in football. *Am J Sports Med* 1980; 302.

42. Feld F: Management of the critically injured football player. *J Athletic Training* 1993; 28:206–212.

43. Vegso JJ, Torg JS: Field evaluation and management of cervical spine injuries. *In* Torg J (ed): Athletic Injuries to the Head, Neck and Face. St. Louis, Mosby–Year Book, 1991, pp 426–438.

44. Denegar C, Saliba E: On field management of the potentially cervical spine injured athlete. *J Athletic Training* 1989; 24:108–111.

45. Feld F, Blanc R: Immobilizing the spine injured football player. *J Emerg Med Serv* 1987; 12:38–40.

46. Feld F: Management of the critically injured football player. *J Athletic Training* 1993; 28:206–212.

47. Segan RD, Cassidy C, Bentkowski J: A discussion of the issue of football helmet removal in suspected cervical spine injuries. *J Athletic Training* 1993; 28:294–305.

48. Heckman JD: Emergency Care and Transportation of the Sick and Injured, 5th ed., Rosemont, IL, American Academy of Orthopaedic Surgeons, 1993, pp 334–349.

49. Swenson TM, Lauerman WF, Donaldson WF, et al: Cervical spine position in the immobilized football player—radiographic analysis before and after helmet removal. *Med Sci Sports Exerc* 1994; 26(suppl):S148.

49a. Hulstyn MS, Palumbo MA, Fadale PD, et al: The effect of protective football equipment on alignment of the injured cervical spine: Radiographic analysis in a cadaveric model. Presented at American Orthopaedic Society of Sports Medicine, Toronto, Canada, July 1995, Abstracts, p. 27.

50. Heckman JD: Emergency Care and Transportation of the Sick and Injured, 5th ed. Rosemont, IL, American Academy of Orthopaedic Surgeons, 1993, pp 670–700.

51. Reid DC, Henderson R, Saboe et al: Etiology and clinical course of missed spine fractures. J Trauma 1987; 27:980–986.

52. Benson DR, Keenen TL, Antony J: Unsuspected associated lesions in the fractured spine. Presented at the Orthopaedic Trauma Association Meeting, Dallas, October 1988.

53. Castelano V, Bocconi FL: Injuries of the cervical spine with spinal cord involvement (myelic fractures): Statistical considerations. Bull Hosp Joint Dis 1970; 31:188–194.

54. Pavlov H, Potter HG: Imaging techniques applicable to athletically induced cervical spine trauma. Oper Tech Sports Med 1993; 1:169–182.

55. Harris JH: The Radiology of Acute Cervical Spine Trauma, 2nd ed. Baltimore, Williams & Wilkins, 1987.

56. White AA, Punjabi MM: Clinical Biomechanics of the Spine. Philadelphia, JB Lippincott, 1978.

57. Bracken MB, Shepard MJ, Collins WF, et al: A randomized controlled trial of methylprednisolone or naloxone in the treatment of spinal cord injury. N Engl J Med 1990; 322:1405–1411.

CHAPTER 22

Maxillofacial Injuries

J O H N P. K E L L Y *DMD, MD, FACS*

Even though the widespread use of improved protective devices, such as helmets, facemasks, eye shields, and mouthguards, has significantly reduced the incidence of injury to the head and neck region, such use has not eliminated the common occurrence of both major and minor injuries to the critical structures of this anatomic area. In fact, concerns have been expressed that in some sports, improvements in protective headgear have given athletes a false sense of invulnerability, leading to more dangerous play and transference of the site of injury from the face to the central nervous system or the cervical spine, as discussed in the preceding chapters. Nevertheless, the large numbers of athletes participating in sports in which facial protection is not customary or is not complete and the occurrence of injuries despite full headgear make a thorough knowledge of maxillofacial trauma important to physicians, physical therapists, and athletic trainers who work with such athletes.

INITIAL MANAGEMENT PRIORITIES

Fortunately, most maxillofacial injuries in sports occur as isolated injuries. However, the potential for serious injury must not be overlooked. The types of trauma suffered in athletic competition (excluding auto racing) tend to be "low-energy" wounds with relatively few associated injuries. However, both the apparently trivial bruise to the chin and the dramatically bleeding scalp laceration can be indicative of potential serious injury to the intracranial vault or the cervical spine. Injuries such as these must always be suspected and ruled out.

As with major trauma, the highest priority must be given to the adequacy of the patient's airway. Blows to the neck resulting in a fracture of the larynx are most likely to produce serious compromise of the airway and require emergency treatment, as discussed later. Difficulty with breathing as a result of oral, nasal, or pharyngeal bleeding is rarely a problem in low-energy trauma, but positioning the patient on his or her side or in a prone position may be necessary for comfortable air exchange until hemorrhage is controlled.

After management of the airway and breathing, control of bleeding is the next priority in the initial treatment. Direct pressure applied with sterile gauze sponges or any clean, absorbent cloth is the mainstay of primary therapy for wounds of the head, face, and neck. Rarely in athletic injuries will the amount of blood loss result in acute circulatory embarrassment. It is generally not necessary or desirable to attempt ligation of bleeding vessels in the field. Specific management of bleeding will be covered in the discussion of particular injuries in the following pages.

The athlete's pertinent past medical history must be confirmed. Of particular importance to those responsible for emergency care are the existence of drug allergies, current use of medications, and the history of tetanus immunization (Table 22–1).

AIRWAY INJURIES

The most dangerous of all maxillofacial injuries encountered in athletics is that resulting from a blow to the neck by a hockey stick, puck, or other such equipment (Fig. 22–1). Careful attention and observa-

TABLE 22–1
Prophylaxis Against Tetanus

Immunization Status	Wound Condition	
	Clean and Minor	*Grossly Contaminated*
Previously immunized		
Within 6 yr	No treatment required	0.5 ml tetanus toxoid booster
More than 6 yr	0.5 ml tetanus toxoid booster	0.5 ml tetanus toxoid booster; 250 U human immunoglobin; antibiotics
Not previously immunized	0.5 ml tetanus toxoid; repeat in 4–6 wk and 6–12 mo	0.5 ml tetanus toxoid booster; 250 U human immunoglobulin; antibiotics

tion of even seemingly minor injury to the larynx is critical because of the potential for progressive worsening to life-threatening airway obstruction as edema progresses in the postinjury period.[1]

For a patient with a history of blunt trauma to the neck, the significant signs and symptoms of laryngeal injury include hoarseness, difficulty breathing, pain (including pain on swallowing), tenderness, subcutaneous emphysema, hematoma, and hemoptysis. On examination, the voice quality may be described as muffled, hoarse, or "breathy," depending on the specific location of injury in the laryngotracheal area. At the scene of injury it is primarily important to recognize a *change* in voice quality. Fracture of the thyroid or cricoid cartilage may be suggested by a flattening or loss of normal prominence in the anterior neck, although these structures may be difficult to evaluate if there has been sufficient time for edema or hematoma to obscure the anatomic features. A critical finding is the presence of subcutaneous emphysema, which signifies loss of integrity of the upper aerodigestive tract and requires urgent attention.

All patients with suspected laryngeal injury, based on the above signs and symptoms, should be referred immediately for endoscopic examination and definitive therapy. Minor airway symptoms will usually require only observation, and return to full activity can be anticipated in several days. When airway compromise is present, obtaining a clear airway is critical. Some controversy exists as to whether endotracheal intubation or tracheostomy is the preferred emergency measure for such patients. The preponderance of opinion favors tracheostomy, as intubation may cause additional trauma to the already injured larynx. An emergency tracheostomy in the field is an extremely uncommon event in the context of athletic injuries.

SOFT TISSUE INJURIES

The most common injuries to the head and face involve trauma to the soft tissues, resulting in contusions, abrasions, or lacerations.

In all locations, a contusion from contact with a blunt object requires attention to the possibility of injury to a deeper, bony structure. In the absence of such damage, the bruised area needs little more than ice for comfort and pressure to inhibit the development of a hematoma.

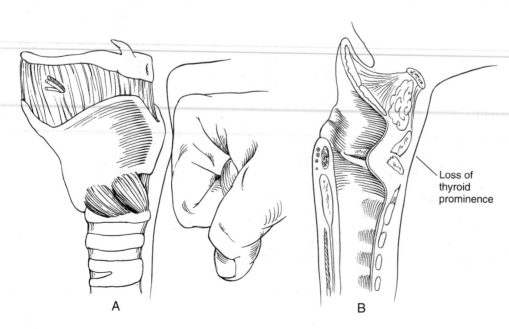

A   B

Loss of thyroid prominence

FIGURE 22–1. *A,* External trauma to larynx over prominence of thyroid cartilage ("Adam's apple"). *B,* Fracture of the larynx, as seen on the lateral view, produces narrowing of airway and disruption of the vocal cords. Airway compromise is worsened as tissues become edematous.

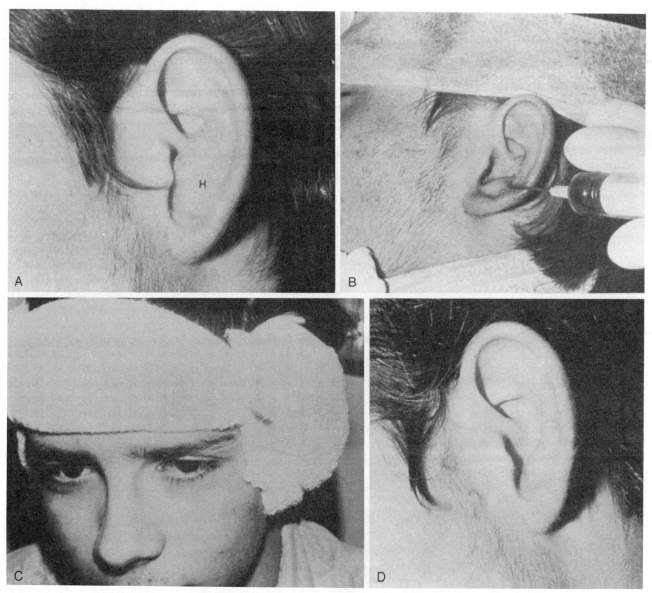

FIGURE 22–2. "Cauliflower ear." *A,* Hematoma (H) of the auricle caused by a wrestling injury. *B,* Hematoma being aspirated. *C,* Contoured head dressing to force perichondrium back against auricular cartilage. *D,* Good result 4 weeks after injury. (From Handler SD: Diagnosis and management of maxillofacial injuries. *In* Torg J (ed): Athletic Injuries to the Head, Neck and Face. St. Louis, Mosby–Year Book, 1991, pp 611–634.)

Special consideration, however, must be given to a contusion to the external ear. In such an injury, any accumulated blood beneath the skin surface should be aspirated or drained to prevent permanent deformation of the underlying auricular cartilage ("cauliflower ear") (Fig. 22–2). This condition is quite common in wrestlers and is easily prevented with the use of appropriate protective headgear. With trauma, fluid accumulates between the skin and the cartilage. If the fluid is not evacuated fibrosis and keloid formation result.

Aspiration can usually be carried out without anesthesia, but formal incision and drainage may require infiltration of local anesthesia. A small amount of lidocaine with epinephrine is injected into the hematoma, and the area is gently massaged. The lidocaine

and hematoma are then removed. A form-fitting compression dressing is applied after the procedure and left in place for 48 to 72 hours. Return to activity is strictly a matter of the athlete's comfort.

Abrasions occur when the integrity of the skin surface is lost as a result of falls or collisions with hard or rough surfaces. Careful, gentle cleansing of the abraded surface should be carried out, and particular attention must be paid to any embedded foreign bodies, such as dirt or asphalt; such material must be meticulously removed so as to prevent permanent "tattooing" of the abraded area. Small areas of abrasion are readily treated immediately and require only a simple antibiotic ointment dressing. Larger areas or areas with deeply embedded foreign material may require local or general anesthesia for adequate debridement. Flushing the affected area with sterile saline under pressure, utilizing a 30-ml syringe, is an effective method of cleansing for all abrasions. Scrubbing the area with a sterile brush is usually reserved for deeper wounds or those with extensive foreign material.

Lacerations of the face, scalp, and neck may be accompanied by brisk bleeding initially, which reflects the area's rich blood supply. This blood supply is greatly beneficial in terms of quick healing and resistance to infection. Control of acute bleeding is the first priority and is accomplished by simple pressure over the wound with sterile gauze. Placement of absorbable cellulose gauze (Surgicel) into the wound may assist with hemostasis until definitive treatment can be accomplished.

LACERATIONS

TYPES

Simple *linear lacerations* result from contact of the skin with sharp objects such as skates or sticks. *Stellate lacerations* have the appearance of a bursting of the skin and usually result from a blunt object striking skin that overlies bone (Fig. 22–3). In either case, it is not uncommon for large lacerations to give the appearance of tissue loss owing to retraction of the wound edges along the lines of skin tension; however, careful inspection and reapproximation of the wound edges will frequently reveal no loss of tissue. *Avulsive wounds*

actually do result in loss of tissue and require more complex methods of repair.

CLEANSING AND DEBRIDEMENT

The most favorable repair of lacerations occurs when early cleansing is carried out and debridement of all foreign material is accomplished. This is particularly important for wounds that are grossly contaminated with dirt, grass, gravel, and the like, as foreign material may promote subsequent wound infection. Effective cleansing, debridement of foreign material, and prompt skin closure are the most effective means of promoting good healing in the absence of infection, making antibiotic use rarely necessary for simple facial lacerations.

Inspection of the wound prior to closure is essential for identification of devitalized tissue whose retention will contribute to the promotion of later wound infection. However, the excellent blood supply of this region allows the surgeon to be very conservative in the debridement of tissue. Compromised tissue, whether it be contused or jagged, can and should be preserved in most facial wounds; only skin that is definitively necrotic should be sacrificed at the time of initial repair. It is not necessary to shave hair at the site of a laceration on the scalp or face. In fact, shaving of the eyebrows is contraindicated, both because a vital landmark for alignment of the laceration is lost and because regrowth of the eyebrow cannot be assured. Other specific anatomic landmarks for the alignment of lacerations are the gray line of the eyelid and the vermillion border of the lip (Fig. 22–4).

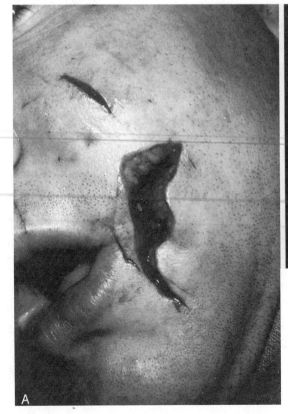

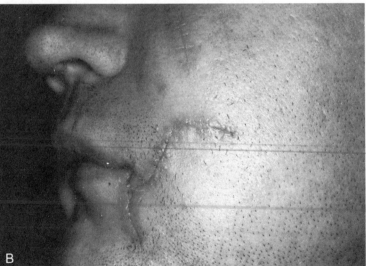

FIGURE 22–3. Linear and stellate type lacerations before (*A*) and after (*B*) skin closure.

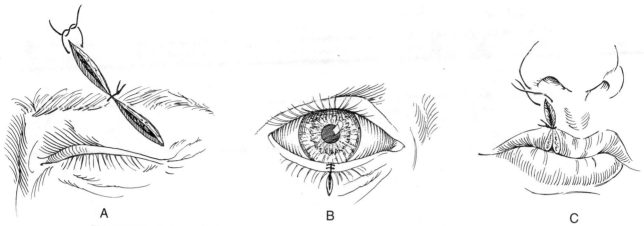

FIGURE 22—4. Anatomic landmarks for alignment of lacerations. *Left,* Eyebrow. *Middle,* Gray line of eyelid. *Right,* Vermillion border of lip.

ANESTHESIA

For all but the most extensive lacerations, local anesthesia is the preferred method of management. Although regional nerve blocks of the supraorbital, infraorbital, or mental nerves may be employed, infiltration of the wound edges with a solution of 2 percent lidocaine containing 1:100,000 epinephrine will provide excellent anesthesia and aid in hemostasis of the wound. However, care must be taken not to distort the wound by excessive infiltration, as vital clues to perfect alignment of the skin edges can be lost.

SPECIAL STRUCTURES

The specialized anatomy of facial structures requires careful attention in the course of treatment of lacerations. Both deep and surface structures must be taken into account.

FACIAL NERVE. Deep lacerations of the cheek, posterior to a vertical line from the lateral canthus of the eye, place the main branches of the facial nerve at risk (Fig. 22–5). Examination of a patient with such an injury requires that attention be paid to the patient's ability to raise the eyebrow, furrow the forehead, close the eyes tightly, and smile and pucker the lips. Any deficit in these facial animations in the presence of a laceration in the described location suggests an injury to a branch of the facial nerve, which can and must be repaired primarily. For lacerations occurring anterior to that line, facial nerve reanastomosis is not necessary, because the nerve has branched sufficiently that animation of the involved muscles can be anticipated to return without surgical intervention. Facial nerve repair generally requires that the athlete be transferred to a hospital where an operating microscope is available.

PAROTID DUCT. The salivary duct from the parotid gland, which opens into the mouth through the buccal mucosa adjacent to the upper molar teeth, runs along a course externally identified by a line from the tragus of the ear to the alar base of the nose. Any deep laceration of the posterior cheek that traverses this line must be inspected carefully for identification of the duct. If the

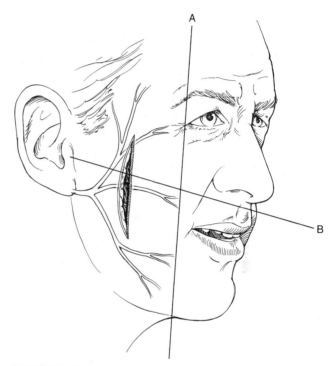

FIGURE 22—5. Landmarks for identification of critical area for facial nerve injury (A) and parotid duct laceration (B).

duct is severed, it will require direct suture repair along with placement of a plastic catheter within its lumen for a period of 7 to 10 days.

EYEBROWS. As mentioned earlier, the eyebrows provide an excellent cue to proper alignment of lacerations in that area. Failure to repair the wound with excellent alignment of the eyebrow will result in a very noticeable cosmetic deformity that is difficult to repair at a later date.

EYELIDS. As will be discussed shortly, a through-and-through laceration of the eyelid requires careful examination to rule out injury to the globe itself. Repair of the eyelid must be carried out with attention to alignment and repair of the deep structures (the orbicularis oculi muscle, the levator muscle of the upper lid, the orbital

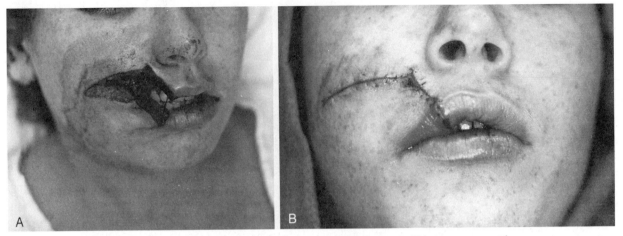

FIGURE 22–6. Laceration of the lip that involves the orbicularis oris. This structure must be repaired prior to closure of the skin. Note how the vermillion border of the lip is precisely aligned following repair.

septum, and the tarsal plate) and the surface anatomy (the lashes and the "gray line" of the lid edge) (see Fig. 22–4B). Both cosmetic and functional impairment can be the result of inattention to the anatomic details in this area.

EARS AND NOSE. Deep lacerations of the ear and nose share the common problem of laceration of underlying cartilage, which must be repaired or debrided prior to skin closure, lest the cosmetic result be unfavorable.

LIPS. Like the eyelid, the lips must be carefully repaired after lacerations to preserve function and appearance. Through-and-through lacerations of the lips, which are frequently the result of external blows that drive the teeth through the lip, must be inspected for the presence of any tooth fragments that may have been dislodged by the external blow. The circumferential muscle of the lip, the orbicularis oris, must be repaired with sutures prior to closure of the skin or the mucosa. Any laceration that crosses the vermilion border of the lip, where the mucosa meets the skin, requires precise alignment of the vermilion border before any other sutures are placed (Fig. 22–6).

TONGUE. Most lacerations of the tongue result from external force that causes the patient's teeth to bite the tongue. Most tongue lacerations are minor and do not necessitate suture closure. However, if there is persistent bleeding or there is a large flap defect of the tongue, suturing is recommended and will allow for prompt return to full activity.

SUTURING

Although many minor facial lacerations might be managed successfully by approximating the wound edges with adhesive strips, such indirect measures may not be adequate for the athlete seeking a quick return to activity. Suture repair of even small lacerations provides hemostasis and skin integrity to allow the athlete to return to competition immediately. A dressing of collodion is often more effective than any

attempts to protect the facial or scalp wound with bandaging; small areas may simply be dressed with an antibiotic ointment. Facial sutures can be safely removed in 4 or 5 days, with the longer time being favored for the athlete whose wound will be at risk for reopening by continued competition.

ANTIBIOTICS

Systemic antibiotics are not generally indicated for treatment of facial or scalp lacerations that have received prompt attention and careful cleansing and debridement. The exception to the rule may be the common use of penicillin (or erythromycin for those allergic to penicillin) for intraoral lacerations of the tongue, lips, or cheeks and for through-and-through wounds involving the lips and cheeks. Such use is not universally accepted, however, and many clinicians reserve it for severe wounds or for wounds in which there is high risk of contamination by external debris. There is no evidence that the use of antibiotics adds to the success of treatment when the wound has been properly cared for.

OCULAR INJURIES

An estimated 100,000 ocular injuries occur annually in the United States as a result of athletic activities.[2] The use of protective equipment in sports such as football and amateur hockey has caused a significant reduction in such injuries, but the large number of players who are unprotected—in baseball, basketball, racket sports, and professional hockey, for example— results in a significant risk for devastating injury. Even an apparently trivial injury can be vision threatening, making early recognition, appropriate emergency care, and prompt referral for definitive ophthalmologic treatment essential priorities for all who care for athletes.

ANATOMY

Knowledge of the anatomy of the eye is fundamental to the evaluation of injuries (Figs. 22–7 and 22–8).

The visible anatomy of the eye consists of the *cornea* through which light must pass to reach the retina. This outermost layer of the eye is fully translucent and allows visualization of the iris and pupil beneath it. Continuous with the cornea is the *sclera*, the tough, white, fibrous outer layer of the globe that surrounds the entire eye to become continuous with the dura overlying the optic nerve posteriorly. The junction of the cornea and the sclera is the *limbus*. Anteriorly, the sclera is covered by the loose layer of tissue known as the *conjunctiva*, which attaches to the upper and lower lids. Posteriorly, the loose covering over the sclera is known as *Tenon's capsule*. The *iris*, the colored part of the eye that opens and closes as a diaphragm, allows light to pass through the pupil. The *ciliary body* produces the aqueous fluid of the anterior chamber of the eye and regulates the focusing of the lens within the eye. The *choroid* carries the blood supply to the *retina*, the inner coating of the eye and a highly specialized tissue that converts light impulses to electrical signals, which are then transmitted by the optic nerve to other portions of the brain.

The anatomy of the eye must further be understood in terms of the compartments or chambers into which it is organized. The anterior chamber, containing aqueous fluid, extends from the cornea to the iris. The posterior chamber contains the lens by which light is focused and extends from the iris to the vitreous space. The latter is the largest compartment of the eye and is filled with a clear gel that maintains the shape of the eye and the retina while transmitting focused light to the retina.

External to the eye are the six extraocular muscles, which extend from the orbit to the sclera and move the eyes in coordinated fashion in all directions. The lacrimal system, responsible for the production of tears that lubricate and cleanse the anterior surface of the cornea, consists of the lacrimal gland in the upper lateral portion of the orbit and the collecting ducts at the lower, inner side of the lid.

Any alteration in the integrity of this delicate system can result in loss of vision. Alteration may involve loss of clarity of the light-transmitting portions of the visual tract, loss of alignment of the focusing elements, loss of shape of the light-receiving retina, loss of blood supply to the retina, or loss of integrity of the transmitting optic nerve.

EXAMINATION

In the absence of effective prevention of eye injury, the priorities for those with initial responsibility for management involve recognition of the injury, limitation of progression of the injury's severity, and arranging for prompt referral for specialized care.[3]

Evaluation begins with a pertinent history of how the injury occurred, what struck the eye, the symptoms experienced by the patient, and the patient's use of contact lenses or corrective eyewear.

Visual acuity is the most important aspect of assessment of any traumatized eye. Any deviation from normal must be documented, as must any progressive change in acuity over time. The athlete's best visual response is recorded concerning his or her ability to

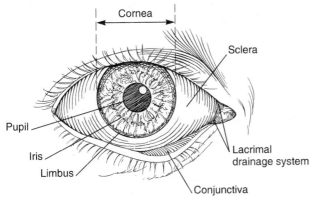

FIGURE 22–7. Landmarks of surface anatomy of the globe.

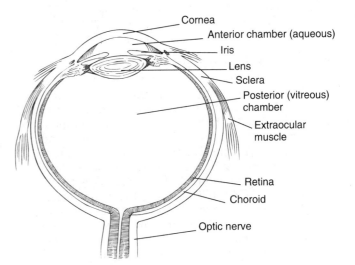

FIGURE 22–8. Cross-sectional anatomy of the globe.

read, count fingers, detect hand motion, and perceive light. Partial loss of vision and the visual field defects that may be produced are also recorded. More sophisticated evaluation of acuity is reserved for the ophthalmologic setting.

The lids and orbital rims are palpated to assess any irregularities that might suggest fractures or foreign bodies. Gentle palpation of the globe through the lid allows for gross assessment of elevated intraocular pressure or softening.

A simple penlight examination can be carried out to determine normal pupillary response and clarity and gross integrity of the cornea, the anterior chamber, and the lens. Visual inspection of the conjunctiva and the sclera is also done at this time. Protrusion of the eye (a result of increased pressure behind the globe) or retraction of the globe (resulting from increased orbital volume with fractures into the adjacent sinuses) should also be noted.

When complaints of pain and foreign body sensation suggest the possibility of corneal abrasion, examination of the eye with a blue light after instillation of fluorescein dye on moistened strips is essential in this initial evaluation.

In the field, examination of the posterior chamber and the vitreous is usually confined to observation of a red reflection (the "red reflex") seen when light is shone onto the retina. Absence of such a reflection from the retina may indicate bleeding into the vitreous fluid or detachment of the retina. In either case, ophthalmologic consultation is essential for full examination of the retina with dilation of the pupils.

By asking the patient to move the eye in all directions, assessment of the functions of the extraocular muscles can be readily carried out. Impairment in motion may be the result of direct injury to the muscles or injury to the cranial nerves supplying the muscles.

ANTERIOR SEGMENT INJURIES

FOREIGN BODIES. Foreign bodies, including displaced contact lenses, are probably the most common and the most benign of the emergency problems that athletes encounter. Care must be taken not to allow the athlete to rub the eye, because this may cause a corneal abrasion. The simple sensation of a foreign body, occasionally accompanied by tearing and scleral redness in the area of the foreign object, requires that the lids be everted to search for the object. Copious irrigation with normal saline is usually sufficient to remove the offending agent, and the athlete can return to activity immediately. If the article is embedded such that it cannot be flushed away, referral for ophthalmologic consultation is preferable to attempted instrumentation and risk of corneal abrasion. If the athlete must be transported for consultation, *both eyes* should be covered to minimize any movement of the injured eye.

CORNEAL ABRASION. When there has been a glancing blow to the eye, a scratch, or a persistent foreign body, the likelihood of corneal abrasion is high. The patient usually has exquisite pain; photophobia and tearing are common accompaniments. A fluores-

cein-impregnated strip can be moistened and touched to the conjunctival fold between the sclera and the lower lid. Examination with a blue light will then demonstrate the corneal defect as a green stain or streak. Once the diagnosis is made, the eyelid should be closed and patched and the patient sent for ophthalmologic referral. Definitive care usually includes cycloplegic eyedrops, topical antibiotics, and patching for several days. In the absence of other accompanying injury, the athlete can return to full competition as soon as the patch is removed.

SUBCONJUNCTIVAL HEMORRHAGE. Bright red blood overlying the sclera in the plane beneath the conjunctiva may occur spontaneously (often in scuba divers) or as the result of a minor blow to the eye. In the absence of other symptoms or signs, no treatment is required, and the individual can return to full activity immediately, with the expectation that the bloody discoloration will resolve in a week or two.

Chemosis, or edema of the conjunctiva, seen in association with subconjunctival hemorrhage mandates a thorough investigation for more significant injury, either to the orbit or to the globe itself. Diffuse chemosis and subconjunctival hemorrhage may indicate actual corneal laceration or perforation of the globe; such serious injury may have no other signs or symptoms initially but must be suspected. Should these findings be made after trauma, a plastic or metal shield should be placed over the eye while prompt referral for ophthalmologic care is made.

HYPHEMA. Bleeding into the anterior chamber of the eyes, ranging from small streaks visible beneath the cornea to complete filling of the anterior chamber that obliterates the view of the iris and pupil, is known as *hyphema.* This type of injury is vision threatening, even with the smallest amount of blood, not only because of the high risk of rebleeding within 3 or 4 days and the significant risk of developing posttraumatic glaucoma (i.e., increased intraocular pressure), but also because one third of patients with hyphema have other significant eye injuries that must be diagnosed and treated. Such injuries may occur readily in sports such as squash and hockey, where small, hard projectiles or sticks can injure the unprotected eye. Suspicion or evidence of this injury demands prompt referral, with the eye protected by a shield in the interim. Patients with sickle cell disease are at higher risk for the secondary complications of hyphema.

POSTERIOR SEGMENT INJURIES

Even in the absence of grossly visible injury to the anterior portions of the eye, blunt trauma can result in severe damage to the posterior segments of the eye. Such injuries include lens dislocation, retinal edema, retinal tears or detachment, vitreous hemorrhage, choroidal rupture, and optic nerve injury. Various degrees of alteration of vision, ranging from minor blurring to loss of visual fields to complete loss of vision, signify the presence of such injuries after trauma. The absence of a red reflex when a light is shone through the pupil may be noted with such injuries, but the symptoms of visual loss alone are sufficient to warrant that the athlete be withdrawn from activity and referred for specialized examination and treatment. Again, a shield that protects the eye from pressure should be placed while the patient is in transit.

PREVENTION OF EYE INJURIES

As noted earlier, most eye injuries in sports can be prevented by appropriate equipment. The virtual elimination of serious eye injuries in hockey with the use of full face shields has been well documented; in contrast, the use of visors to protect the eye has resulted in several serious injuries when sticks have been lodged between the visor and the eye. Similarly, an awareness of the value of eye protection has increased in those who play racket sports or sports such as baseball and basketball, which theoretically do not involve contact.[4] Those involved in the care of athletes must continue to campaign for prevention of eye injuries by insisting on the use of effective protective gear at all levels of sports.

FACIAL FRACTURES

NASAL FRACTURES

Given its "leading" position on the face, the nose is frequently traumatized in any sport involving contact.

Simple nosebleed, or epistaxis, is the most common result of blunt trauma to the nasal area. External compression of the nose performed by squeezing the nostrils shut is usually successful in stopping the bleeding. Persistence or recurrence of hemorrhage may require the placement of intranasal petrolatum-gauze packs or the use of silver nitrate cauterization under direct vision. Careful intranasal examination must be carried out to rule out a septal hematoma with accumulation of blood beneath the mucosa overlying the septal cartilage of the nose. Such hematomas must be drained and evacuated because of the high risk of infection and septal necrosis associated with this injury if it is not treated promptly.

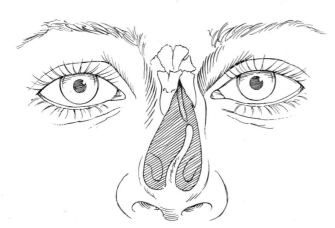

FIGURE 22–9. Nasal bone fracture with deviation of septum and obstruction of the airway.

Examination of the traumatized nose is directed first at the external appearance to determine the presence of deviation of the tip or the dorsum of the nose (Fig. 22–9). Next the nose is palpated to determine whether crepitus, step deformities, or bony asymmetries are present. Finally, the patency of each nostril is assessed by having the patient breathe through each nostril separately. Visual inspection of the interior nasal anatomy is performed to evaluate whether there is deviation of the septum.

This physical examination of the traumatized nose, focusing on external deformity and airway patency, will usually determine the need for any treatment. X-ray studies are rarely of significant help in the management of isolated nasal fractures.

Treatment of nasal fractures requiring reduction is usually carried out right away, using local anesthesia in most instances. If edema prevents adequate evaluation of the deformity, treatment may be delayed by as much as 7 days without compromising the outcome. Beyond that time, a formal rhinoplasty procedure will usually be required to correct the posttraumatic deformity.

Closed reduction of the nasal fracture generally requires placement of intranasal packing and application of an external splint. The packing is left in place for 3 to 7 days; during this time the athlete's breathing ability is significantly compromised, and exertion is not recommended. The external splint is removed in 7 to 10 days, although it can be left in place longer for protection of the nose of the athlete who is returning to competition. When return to full activity is not crucial, a period of 2 to 3 weeks away from endangering competition would be prudent. Athletes who return to competition should wear some type of protective facemask (see Chapter 42).

ZYGOMATIC FRACTURES

Collisions involving heads, fists, elbows, rackets, and projectiles are so common in athletic competition that fractures of the cheeks are frequently seen (Table 22–2).

The zygoma is the most likely of the midfacial bones to be fractured in the context of injuries related to athletics. The more complicated midfacial fractures (Fig. 22–10) are high-energy injuries and are rarely seen in ordinary athletic trauma. Blows to the cheeks or the

TABLE 22–2
Location and Cause of Injury Resulting in Facial Bone Fractures for a Professional Hockey Team, 1991–1994

Location of Fracture	Cause
Mandibular symphysis	Errant puck
Mandibular symphysis	Penalized high stick
Mandibular body/condyle	Penalized elbow contact
Zygoma/orbit	Errant puck
Nose	Penalized punch
Nose	Legal check
Zygomatic arch	Errant puck (practice)

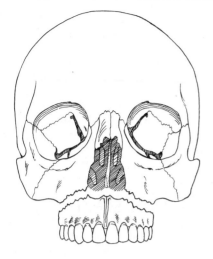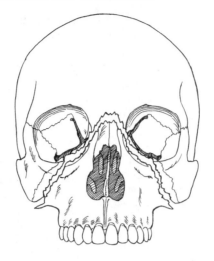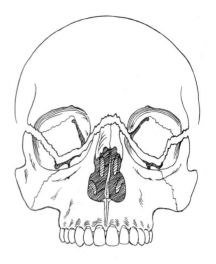

LeFort I   LeFort II   LeFort III

FIGURE 22–10. LeFort classification for midface fractures. LeFort I: A horizontal maxillary fracture at the level of the nasal floor. LeFort II: A pyramidal fracture, with the base of the pyramid being the palate and upper teeth and the apex of the pyramid at the nasal bone. LeFort III: Complete separation of the midface from the base of the skull.

orbit, on the other hand, frequently result in fracture of the zygoma and its attachments to the frontal, temporal, and maxillary bones; because of the zygoma's important contribution to the structure of the orbital rim and floor, fractures involving this bone may have significant consequences relative to vision. An additional important relationship is that of the arch of the zygoma, which forms the lateral portion of the cheek, to the underlying temporal muscle and the coronoid process of the mandible to which the muscle attaches.

Diagnosis of maxillary or zygomatic fractures by physical examination can be difficult shortly after the injury because of the development of edema. Prompt physical examination is necessary. Possible physical findings from this examination are listed in Table 22–3 and illustrated in Figure 22–11.

When the fracture involves the floor of the orbit, double vision (diplopia), inability to move the eye in an upward gaze, and enophthalmus or sunken eye may be observable. Fractures confined to the arch of the zygoma present with localized depression of the cheek over the arch and painful limitation of motion of the mandible owing to impingement of the arch on the temporal muscle as it attaches to the mandible. Observation of cerebrospinal fluid leaking from the nose or ear or blood coming from the ear often signifies a major LeFort type fracture and requires specialized study and treatment.

Nondisplaced zygomatic fractures do not require treatment, but careful ocular examination is essential to rule out associated injury to the globe.

The indications for surgical repair of displaced fractures of the zygomatic complex are related to functional problems (visual disturbance, limitation of mandibular motion, or infraorbital nerve dysfunction) or to cosmetic deficits. Evaluation of the latter often requires waiting several days for edema to subside. Repair can safely be delayed for 7 to 10 days without compromising the result.

TABLE 22–3
Physical Examination Findings:
Maxillary and Zygomatic Fractures

1. Facial asymmetry
2. Loss of cheek prominence
3. Palpable steps
   - Infraorbital rim (zygomaticomaxillary suture)
   - Lateral orbital rim (frontozygomatic suture)
   - Root of zygoma intraorally
   - Zygomatic arch between ear and eye (zygomaticotemporal suture)
4. Hypoesthesia/anesthesia
   - Cheek, side of nose, upper lip, and teeth on the injured side
   - Compression of infraorbital nerve as it courses along floor of the orbit to exit into the face via the foramen beneath the orbital rim

---

Return to full athletic activity after midfacial fractures is dependent on resolution of double vision, pain, and edema. The resolution of double vision is of most obvious importance. Participation without protective headgear should be avoided for at least 6 weeks when there is high likelihood of repeated trauma.

MANDIBULAR FRACTURES

Fractures of the lower jaw may be seen in any sport with the possibility of collision of bodies or equipment. Even athletes with apparent facial protection (i.e., with helmet and facemask) are subject to mandibular fractures from blows directed from below the facemask.

The key symptoms of such fractures are *malocclusion* (inability to bring the teeth easily into the preinjury position, as subjectively reported by the injured athlete) and *pain* on movement of the jaw. Signs for the examiner include deviation of the jaw, visible maloc-

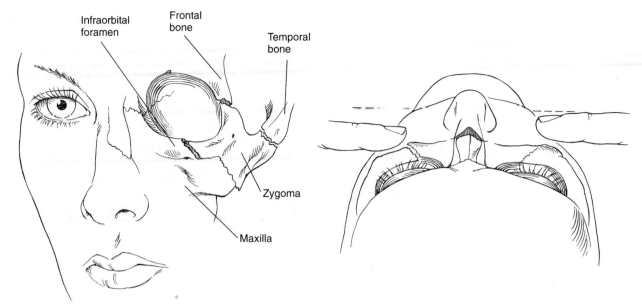

FIGURE 22–11. Zygomatic fractures. Inspection from above with palpation of the cheek demonstrates asymmetry and depression of the fractured zygoma.

clusion (occlusion that differs from the patient's normal bite, as indicated by wear facets on the teeth), crepitus (palpable steps along the inferior border of the jaw), mobility of segments of the tooth-bearing portions of the jaw relative to one another (as distinct from mobility of individual teeth or segments of teeth that are mobile independent of the jaw), and the presence of bleeding or bruising between teeth or in the floor of the mouth adjacent to the jaw (Fig. 22–12).

Particular attention must be paid to examination of the condyles, especially when the trauma has been directed at the point of the chin. Neither pain in the joints nor malocclusion can be used to definitively diagnose a condylar fracture, since traumatic effusion (bleeding into the joint as a result of a blow to the chin) can produce either finding without the presence of a fracture. On the other hand, a fracture usually produces both preauricular pain and malocclusion and is accompanied by limitation of jaw motion and deviation of the jaw on mouth opening in the direction toward the fractured side. On physical examination, palpation of the condyle by placing a finger just anterior to the ear or in the ear canal will reveal an absence of movement by the fractured condyle when the jaw is opened.

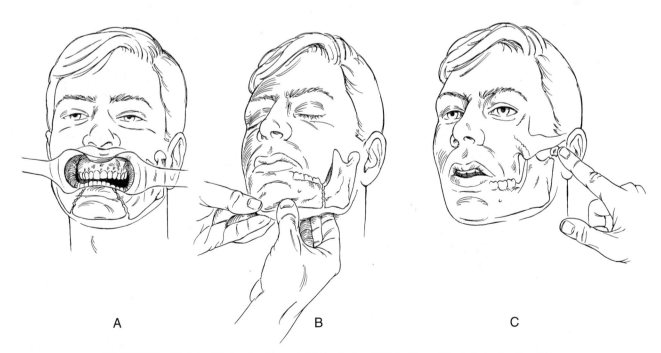

A   B   C

FIGURE 22–12. Mandibular fractures. *A,* Malocclusion. *B,* Palpation of the inferior border of the mandible. *C,* Palpation of the mandibular condyle.

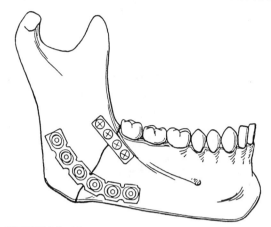

FIGURE 22–13. Rigid plating of a mandibular fracture.

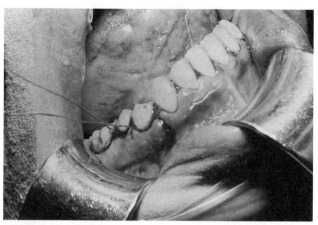

FIGURE 22–15. Multiple teeth loosened as an independent segment as a result of blunt trauma.

Fracture of the mandible must be distinguished from traumatic dislocation or subluxation of the jaw. Dislocation is accompanied by a fixed opening of the jaw, with the patient unable to close. Palpation of the condyles will show an absence of condyles in the usual position immediately anterior to the tragus of the ear and the presence of a bony prominence 1 to 2 cm anterior to the normal position of the joint.

Early reduction of the dislocated jaw is most effective, as delayed reduction is complicated by the development of pain and muscle spasm, which may necessitate pharmacologic muscle relaxation or anesthesia. In the acute phase, the jaw is relocated as follows:

1. The clinician faces the patient, who is seated in a sturdy chair.
2. The clinician's thumbs are placed in the mouth lateral to the posterior teeth (never on the teeth), with the fingers grasping the lower border of the jaw externally.

3. A rotational force is applied to bring the posterior jaw downward while the chin is brought forward.
4. When the condyle is rotated sufficiently to clear the anterior margin of the joint, the jaw will passively retrude, and the teeth can gently be brought together.

The athlete must be cautioned to limit jaw-opening width for several days, and anti-inflammatory medication is recommended to reduce the joint effusion that follows such an injury.

When a jaw fracture is diagnosed, referral for specialty care is required. Treatment ranges from a soft diet and analgesics for patients with undisplaced or incomplete fractures to surgical reduction and fixation for patients with more significant injuries. Although many fractures of the lower jaw can be treated

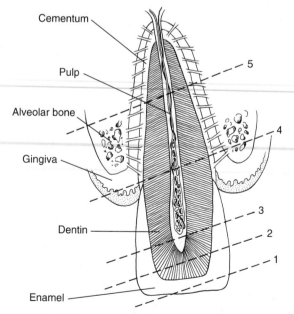

FIGURE 22–14. Anatomic classification of dental injuries. 1, Enamel fracture. 2, Fracture exposing the dentin. 3, Fracture exposing the pulp. 4, Fracture extending below the gingiva. 5, Root fracture.

Cementum
Pulp
Alveolar bone
Gingiva
Dentin
Enamel

TABLE 22–4
Guidelines for Initial Treatment of an Avulsed Tooth

I. Extraoral Time
  A. One of the most critical factors affecting prognosis
  B. If possible, replant the tooth immediately at the time of injury. If contaminated, rinse with water before replanting.
    1. If notified by telephone, instruct patient, parent, or involved party on replantation technique.
    2. Stress importance of seeing a dentist immediately for follow-up splinting and treatment.
II. Transport media—When immediate replantation is not possible, place tooth in the best transport medium possible.
  A. Buccal vestibule (in saliva between cheek and gum, but patient must be conscious because of the possibility of aspiration or swallowing, especially if a small child.
  B. Hank's Balanced Salt Solution (H.B.S.S.)
  C. Milk
  D. Saline
  E. If none of the above is readily available, use water.

TABLE 22–5
Treatment of the Avulsed Permanent Tooth:
Recommended Guidelines of the American Association of Endodontists

I. Management at Site of Injury
   A. Replant immediately, if possible. If contaminated, rinse with water before replanting.
   B. When immediate replantation is not possible, place tooth in the best transport medium available.
II. Transport Media
   A. Hank's Balanced Salt Solution (H.B.S.S.)
   B. Milk
   C. Saline
   D. Saliva (buccal vestibule)
   E. If none of the above is readily available, use water.
III. Management in the Dental Office
   A. Replantation of Tooth
      1. If extraoral **dry** time is less than one hour with or without storage in a physiological medium (such as Hank's Balanced Salt Solution, milk, or saline), replant immediately.
      2. If extraoral **dry** time is greater than one hour, soak tooth in an accepted dental fluoride solution for 20 minutes, rinse with saline, and replant.
   B. Management of the Root Surface
      1. Keep the tooth moist at all times.
      2. Do not handle the root surface (hold tooth by the crown).
      3. Do not scrape or brush the root surface or remove the tip of the root.
      4. If the root appears clean, replant as is after rinsing with saline.
      5. If the root surface is contaminated, rinse with H.B.S.S. or saline (use tap water if above are not available). If persistent debris remains on root surface, gently use cotton pliers to remove remaining debris and/or gently brush off debris with a wet sponge.
   C. Management of the Socket
      1. Gently aspirate without entering the socket. If a clot is present, use light irrigation with saline.
      2. Do not curette the socket.
      3. Do not vent socket.
      4. Do not make a surgical flap unless bony fragments prevent replantation.
      5. If the alveolar bone is collapsed and prevents replantation, carefully insert a blunt instrument into the socket to reposition the bone to its original position.
      6. After replantation, manually compress (if spread apart) facial and lingual bony plates.
   D. Management of Soft Tissues—tightly suture any soft tissue lacerations, particularly in the cervical region.
   E. Splinting (indicated in most cases)
      1. Use acid-etch/resin alone or with soft arch wire, or use orthodontic brackets with passive arch wire. Suture in place only if alternative splinting methods are unavailable. (Circumferential wire splints are contraindicated.)
      2. Splint should remain in place for 7–10 days; however, if tooth demonstrates excessive mobility, splint should be replaced until mobility is within acceptable limits.

      3. Bony fractures resulting in mobility usually require longer splinting periods (2–8 weeks).
      4. Home care during splinting period should encompass:
         a. No biting on splinted teeth
         b. Soft diet
         c. Maintenance of good oral hygiene
IV. Adjunctive Drug Therapy Considerations
   A. Systemic antibiotics
   B. Referral to physician for tetanus consultation within 48 hours
   C. Chlorhexidine rinses
   D. Analgesics
V. Endodontic Treatment
   A. Tooth with open apex (divergent apex) and less than one hour extraoral dry time:
      1. Replant in an attempt to revitalize the pulp.
      2. Recall patient every 3–4 weeks for evidence of pathosis.
      3. If pathosis is noted, thoroughly clean and fill the canal with calcium hydroxide (apexification procedure).
   B. Tooth with open apex (divergent apex) and greater than one hour extraoral dry time:
      1. Thoroughly clean and fill canal with calcium hydroxide.
      2. Recall the patient in 6–8 weeks.
      3. Because of poor prognosis, consider alternative treatment options.
   C. Tooth with partially to completely closed apex and less than one hour extraoral dry time:
      1. Biomechanically clean the root canal system in 7–14 days.
      2. Medicate the canal with calcium hydroxide for as long as practical, usually 6–12 months.
      3. Then, obturate canal with gutta percha and sealer unless complications are apparent.
   D. Tooth with partially to completely closed apex and greater than one hour extraoral dry time:
      1. Perform root canal therapy either intraorally or extraorally.
      2. Prior to replantation, remove tissue tags from the root surface and soak the tooth in an accepted dental fluoride solution.
VI. Restoration of the Avulsed Tooth
   A. Recommended Temporary Restorations (placed prior to final obturation)
      1. Reinforced zinc oxide eugenol
      2. Acid etch/composite resin
   B. Recommended Permanent Restorations
      1. Dentin bonding agent
      2. Acid etch/composite resin
VII. Additional Considerations
   A. Avulsed primary teeth should not be replanted.
   B. Avulsed permanent teeth require follow-up evaluations for a minimum of 5 years to determine the outcome of therapy.
   C. Inflammatory resorption, replacement resorption, ankylosis and tooth submergence are potential complications when avulsed teeth are replanted.

By permission of American Association of Endodontists, Chicago, IL.

successfully with closed reduction, such treatment requires immobilization of the jaw by wiring the upper and lower teeth to one another for a period of 4 or more weeks. This treatment clearly compromises the athlete's ability to compete, both because of nutritional difficulties and because of the inability to engage in mouth breathing during exertion. An alternative to closed reduction is surgical repair with rigid plating of the fractured bone (Fig. 22–13). Although this is more complex surgically, the patient's jaw can be mobilized early, nutrition and breathing are greatly improved, and early return to competition (based on resolution of pain and swelling and the use of protective headgear) can be anticipated.

DENTAL INJURIES

The mandatory use of mouthguards by high school and college football players (since 1962 and 1973, respectively) has significantly reduced the incidence of oral injuries for these athletes, but injuries to the teeth remain a significant problem for players of most other sports.[5]

The simplest trauma to teeth is a concussive injury. The tooth is neither loosened nor fractured, but the blow may lead to necrosis of the pulp and a subsequent need for endodontic (root canal) therapy. Only discoloration and darkening of the tooth give a clue to the developing abnormality.

Direct trauma to a tooth may result in a fracture of the substance of the tooth (Fig. 22–14). A simple chip of the enamel will be asymptomatic, but any sharp edges will have to be smoothed or recontoured to avoid uncomfortable abrasion of the lip or tongue. When the fracture involves a deeper layer of tooth structure and dentin is exposed, there may be sensitivity to thermal changes or to touching of the exposed surface with the tongue, but routine restorative dentistry can salvage the tooth.

A tooth whose pulp is exposed as a result of coronal fracture will be exquisitely tender to touch and to exposure to cold air. On inspection, the pulp is visible as a pink area within the white surrounding dentin. Acute dental treatment is required and involves either "capping" of the exposed pulp or extirpating the pulp in preparation for root canal treatment.

When the fracture line of the crown extends below the gingival level, consultation with a dentist is necessary to determine whether the tooth can be restored or must be removed.

A tooth that is loosened by trauma must be carefully evaluated to differentiate a tooth with a fractured root from one that is partially dislodged from its socket. Repositioning of the tooth and splinting it to adjacent teeth is the preferred treatment in either case.

When several teeth are loosened as an independent segment, fracture of the alveolar bone is to be expected (Fig. 22–15). Radiographic evaluation is essential, and splinting of the segment to adjacent stable teeth is required after repositioning of the segment.

Indirect injury to teeth, as when a blow from below the chin forces the teeth sharply together, can cause vertical fracture of posterior teeth. Diagnosis is made by visual inspection and palpation of a split tooth or by extreme tenderness to biting pressure on the tooth. Referral for dental treatment is necessary.

Occasionally a vertical force on an anterior tooth will intrude the tooth beneath the gingiva. This is particularly likely to occur in younger patients with immature root formation. No treatment is necessary, as the tooth will normally re-erupt.

Avulsion or loss of a tooth from its socket is a common injury among athletes of all ages. The success of replantation of the tooth is directly related to the length of time that the tooth is out of its socket. *Survival of the tooth decreases precipitously after 1 hour.* Hence, the tooth should be recovered and replaced promptly. Only gentle rinsing of the tooth with saline or water should be performed before replantation. The root surface should be handled minimally and should not be scrubbed. If the tooth cannot be replaced in its socket immediately, the best transport vehicle is the patient's mouth. Obviously, the patient must be conscious and capable of holding the tooth in the cheek without swallowing it while awaiting definitive dental care. If necessary, the tooth may be transported in media listed in Table 22–4. After replantation, the tooth requires splinting to adjacent teeth for a period of 1 week. Dental follow-up is necessary to determine whether such a tooth will require root canal treatment (Tables 22–4 and 22–5).

Both custom-made and self-adapted mouthguards afford significant protection against dental injury in athletes, and their use should be strongly encouraged, if not mandated. Custom-made mouthguards are easily constructed by the patient's dentist, and such appliances offer more comfort and better acceptance for the wearer, although self-adapted guards have the advantage of lower cost.

CONCLUSION

Prevention of maxillofacial injuries in athletics remains the best treatment. Wearing of protective eyewear, mouthguards, and effective facemasks and enforcement of the rules of play will reduce even further the incidence of injuries. Effective treatment and prompt rehabilitation of the facially injured athlete are a function of effective initial diagnosis and treatment, as outlined here, and prompt referral for consultation with the appropriate maxillofacial, ophthalmologic, or dental specialist.

REFERENCES

1. Schaefer SD. The treatment of acute external laryngeal injuries: State of the art. Arch Otolaryngol Head Neck Surg 1991; 117:35–39.
2. Stock JG, Cornell FM. Prevention of sports-related eye injury. Am Fam Physician 1991; 44:515–520.
3. Shingleton BJ. Eye injuries. N Engl J Med 1991; 325:408–413.
4. Zagelbaum BM, Hersh PS, Donnenfeld ED, et al. Ocular trauma in major league baseball players. N Engl J Med 1994; 330:1021–1023.
5. DeYoung AK, Robinson E, Godwin WC. Comparing comfort and wearability: Custom-made vs. self-adapted mouthguards. J Am Dent Assoc 1994; 125:1112–1118.

CHAPTER 23

Peripheral Nerve Injuries

CAROLINE DRYE MS, PT
JAMES E. ZACHAZEWSKI MS, PT, ATC, SCS

Peripheral nerve injuries are infrequent in comparison with the multitude of other injuries with which the physician, physical therapist, or athletic trainer must contend. Because they are infrequent, they may be overlooked in the process of differential diagnosis. The authors' purpose in writing this chapter is to alert clinicians who treat athletes to a class of injuries that, although infrequent, can have potentially devastating functional implications.

There is a paucity of literature available documenting the epidemiologic factors concerning peripheral nerve injuries specifically related to athletics, with the exception of brachial plexus injuries in American football. The largest available reports are from the Japanese. Takazawa et al.[1] reviewed 9550 injuries treated over a 95-year period at the clinic of the Japanese Athletic Association. During that period, only 28 cases of peripheral nerve injuries were documented. Hirasawa and Sakakida[2] reviewed 18 years of experience with peripheral nerve injuries and reported that only 5.7 percent (66 of 1167 cases) were associated with athletes. In the injuries associated with athletics, the brachial plexus was involved most often, accounting for 24.2 percent of injuries (16 of 66). These studies did not include high-contact sports such as American football.

ETIOLOGY

Injury to a peripheral nerve can occur via several mechanisms in sports: stretch, compression (sustained compression or blunt trauma), friction, inflammation, or laceration. The clinical results of stretch or compression of the nerve will vary depending on whether the insult is of rapid onset or the result of a gradual change over time. A sudden insult does not allow for any adaptive change in the connective tissue of the nerve and is more likely to cause acute disruption of the nerve's blood supply or connective tissue. Conversely, the nerve can adapt amazingly well to a slow increase in compressive forces, such as that brought on by a growing osteophyte.[3] A classification of peripheral nerve injuries that was originally developed by Seddon is presented in Table 23–1.[4,5]

Compression of the nerve can occur from external sources or from swelling in a rigid compartment, such as the carpal tunnel at the wrist or the anterior compartment of the lower leg.[6] In 1973 Upton and McComas[7] theorized that compression at one point along the nerve trunk increased the vulnerability of distal points along the nerve to the effects of compression. They hypothesized that the proximal compression disrupted axonal transport of vital nutrients and pos-

TABLE 23–1
Seddon's Classification of Nerve Injuries[4,5]

Type of Injury	Possible Causes	Resolution
Neuropraxia: Nerve is temporarily not functioning due to a transient physiologic block	Electrolyte imbalances Mechanical deformation of the myelin sheaths Ischemia due to compression or traction	Recovery occurs within minutes, hours, or days if the lesion was due to anoxia or ionic imbalances. Failure to recover over several weeks indicates a mechanical compression or stretch. Recovery takes much longer due to the need for the nerve to undergo demyelination and remyelination after injury.
Axonotmesis: Total disruption of the nerve and its myelin sheath so that peripheral degeneration occurs. The connective tissue elements of the nerve remain intact.	Compression	Wallerian degeneration occurs along the entire nerve distal to the point of compression. The length of time for regeneration of the nerve and recovery of function will depend on the distance of the injury from the end of the nerve.
Neurotmesis: Occurs when the nerve has been severed or severely disorganized by intraneural scarring so that there is no possibility of regeneration.	Compression Traction Laceration	Surgical resection and repair are the only chances for recovery, with full recovery unlikely. Factors that affect the level of recovery include the nerve injured, the level at which it is damaged, the extent of the injury, the time passed since the injury, and the age of the patient.

sibly the blood supply to the nerve and termed this type of lesion a *double-crush lesion.* They also noted that nerves with some other type of preexisting physiological disturbance (i.e., diabetic peripheral neuropathy) would be more vulnerable to any compressive lesion.

Friction over a nerve trunk can cause inflammation and fibrosis of the nerve's connective tissue elements. Fibrosis of the nerve trunk decreases its extensibility. Loss of extensibility at one site along the nerve trunk may cause other portions of the nerve to bear increasing tensile loads when the nerve bed is elongated,[8] leading to a mechanical form of a double-crush syndrome.[3] *Because of the mechanical and physiological effects of compression on a nerve, the presence of a second lesion along a nerve trunk should always be explored as a contributing factor to peripheral nerve injuries.*

Injury to tissues adjacent to nerve trunks can cause extensive scarring around the nerve trunk, which could impair the nerve's ability to move relative to its interfacing tissue or compress the nerve if it is enclosed in a rigid space.[3]

Finally, laceration injuries can sever the nerve.

INJURIES TO THE CERVICAL NERVE ROOTS AND BRACHIAL PLEXUS

ETIOLOGY

Brachial plexus injuries are the most common nerve injuries in athletics, although they are infrequent except

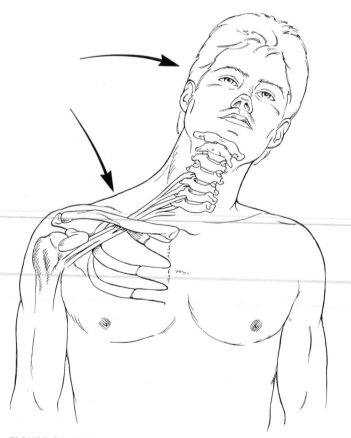

FIGURE 23–1. The combination of shoulder depression and contralateral cervical side flexion can lead to a traction injury to the brachial plexus. This is commonly referred to as a *burner.*

in American football. Clancey et al.[9] reported that 33 of 67 college football players studied had sustained at least one significant brachial plexus injury. Markey et al.[10] have reported that 18 of 261 cadets (6.9 percent) involved in football (236 intramural; 25 varsity) at the U.S. Military Academy had signs and symptoms indicative of brachial plexus injuries from football at the time of preparticipation physical examinations. Over a 4-year period, the incidence of brachial plexus injuries was as high as 15 percent (40 of 266). Although none of these individuals stated that their symptoms were significant enough to prohibit their participation in football, 17 (42.5 percent) demonstrated weakness, and 15 (37.5 percent) demonstrated an abnormal electromyogram (EMG).

To obtain a thorough understanding of epidemiologic factors associated with brachial plexus injuries in football, the incidence as well as the mechanism of injury must be considered along with player position and other biomechanical and physical factors.

Three distinct mechanisms of injury have classically been described in the literature: (1) head and neck lateral flexion with shoulder depression, causing a traction injury to the brachial plexus. (Fig. 23–1)[11–18]; (2) a direct blow to the supraclavicular region in the area of Erb's point, causing direct compression of the brachial plexus at its most superficial point (Fig. 23–2)[10–12,15]; and (3) cervical hyperextension and lateral flexion, causing ipsilateral compression of the nerve roots within the foraminae (Fig. 23–3).[10,13,19–21] Cumulative trauma from multiple minor compression sprains such as these may lead to chronic inflammation and secondary narrowing of the foraminae where nerve roots exit.[19]

A relationship of cervical spinal stenosis has been demonstrated to be associated with brachial plexus injuries, which are caused by the extension and compression mechanism described earlier.[19] Thirty-four of the 40 players (85 percent) who suffered brachial plexus injuries over a 4-year period (N = 266 total players studied) were injured through an extension-compression mechanism, whereas only six (15 percent) suffered from brachial plexus injuries through a stretch or traction mechanism. The mean Torg ratio (see Chapter 22) was significantly smaller (0.8) in 47.5 percent of the players who suffered brachial plexus injuries. No players with a stretch injury to the plexus had a mean Torg ratio of less than 0.8, but 20.6 percent of the players injured via the extension-compression mechanism did. Players with a Torg ratio less than 0.8 had three times the risk of incurring brachial plexus injuries in this study.

CLINICAL PRESENTATION

Brachial plexus injuries in American football are usually a result of tackling or blocking. Because of this,

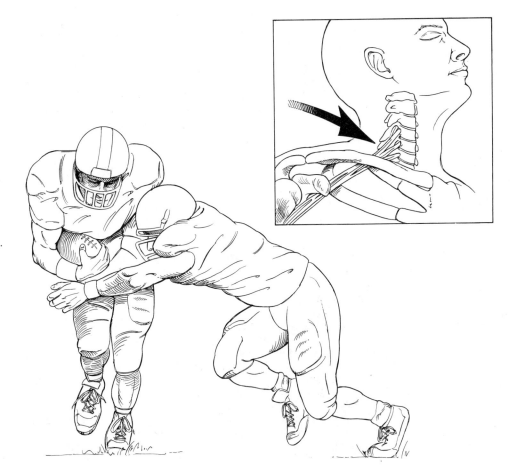

FIGURE 23–2. A second mechanism for a burner is a direct blow to the base of the neck (Erb point). This leads to a compression injury to the trunks of the brachial plexus.

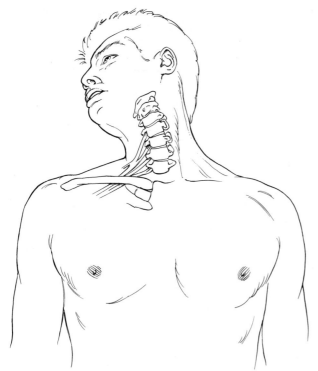

FIGURE 23–3. A third mechanism for injury in the burner syndrome is cervical extension combined with side flexion to the same side. This leads to compression of the cervical nerve roots in the neural foramina.

the incidence is highest in defensive players such as linemen, linebackers, and defensive backs.[22] This injury is commonly referred to as a *burner* or *stinger*. The athlete experiences transient weakness of the shoulder musculature accompanied by upper extremity paresthesia. In the acute syndrome, symptoms usually last several seconds to a few minutes and are followed by complete recovery. Neck pain may or may not be present.[16,23]

The injury usually affects the upper trunks of the plexus (C5 and C6 nerve roots).[11–13,25] Immediately after injury, weakness can be found in the biceps, deltoid, supraspinatus, and infraspinatus muscles. Deep tendon reflexes of the biceps may also be diminished. Symptoms can often be reproduced by cervical extension and

side flexion toward the involved extremity or lateral flexion away from the extremity.[17,23] Any restriction of cervical movement or spinal pain should alert the examiner to the possibility of cervical spine injury. True "burners" rarely involve restricted cervical mobility.[22] Restriction of shoulder range of motion should alert the clinician to the possibility of a clavicular fracture or acromioclavicular separation.

The injury to the nerve is usually considered a neuropraxic lesion, as it recovers almost immediately.[16,23] A thorough neurologic examination will help to differentiate spinal cord trauma from injury to the nerve root or plexus (Table 23–2). Neurologic status should be closely monitored over the next several days after injury to accurately determine the level of recovery. Athletes with persistent weakness or sensory loss should be referred to a physician for follow-up evaluation for possible axonotmesis or neurotmesis. EMG studies will not differentiate denervation from wallerian degeneration for 10 to 20 days after injury.[17] Therefore, EMG studies are generally not performed until a minimum of 2 to 3 weeks after injury. Garrick and Webb[16] suggest that EMG studies be performed 6 weeks after injury. Clinically, Speer and Bassett[15] have demonstrated that strength deficits at 72 hours after injury equaled those at 4 weeks after injury.

Acute management mainly involves resting the extremity. If strength and function return completely in 1 to 2 minutes, the athlete can return to play.[23] If any neurologic deficits persist after this time, the athlete should not be allowed to continue participation until full strength, range of motion, and sensation are restored in the cervical spine and extremity. Wroble et al.[23] advocate the use of ice, transcutaneous electrical nerve stimulation (TENS), ultrasound, and anti-inflammatory medications if there is persistent pain and tenderness of the cervical spine and shoulder. Neck and shoulder strengthening exercises are prescribed to address any residual weakness.[22]

The athlete returning to play should be advised of the increased risk of reinjury and the likelihood of more severe injury with further trauma. With chronic plexus injuries, the athlete may experience symptoms with subsequent trauma from a much smaller force. They may show postural changes (e.g., a dropped shoulder),

		TABLE 23–2	
		Neurologic Evaluation of Brachial Plexus Injury	
Lesion	**Motor Findings**		**Sensory Findings**
Root level:	Motor examination: resisted tests:		Sensory examination: light touch or pin prick
C4	Upper trapezius: shoulder elevation		Top of shoulders
C5	Supraspinatus and deltoid: shoulder abduction		Lateral upper arm or distal radius
C6	Biceps: elbow flexion		Lateral forearm, thumb
C7	Triceps: elbow extension		Index and middle fingertips
C8	Extensor pollicis longus: extension of distal phalanx of thumb		Fourth and fifth fingers and hypothenar eminence
T1	Intrinsics of hand: abduction/adduction of fingers		Medial forearm
Suspected spinal cord lesions	Diffuse motor loss, bilateral weakness, lower extremity motor loss		Diffuse paresthesia or numbness, bilateral sensory loss (nondermatomal)

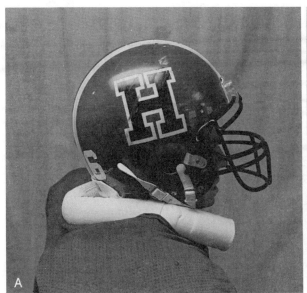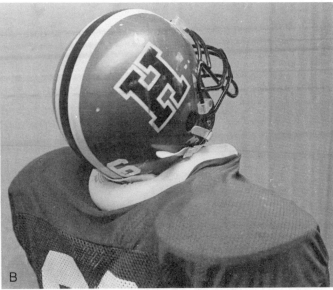

FIGURE 23–4. Neck rolls are often used to prevent excessive lateral flexion of the cervical spine during tackling in American football. *A*, Proper placement of the neck roll close to the helmet and cervical spine. *B*, Appropriate restriction of motion of the head and cervical spine.

atrophy of the shoulder muscles, or both.[10] Clearly, more severe neurologic losses and longer periods of time needed to recuperate indicate that it is less advisable for the athlete to return to play.[23]

Padded neck rolls and shock-absorbing shoulder pads may be of some assistance in preventing recurrent "burner" injuries in football players.[15,17] However, Garrick and Webb[16] regarded most currently used neck rolls as inadequate for the prevention of side flexion injuries because of their size. The roll may need to be larger or have extra padding placed in strategic locations to prevent excessive motion. An appropriately fitted collar should be worn close to the neck and should restrict cervical extension and side bending (Fig. 23–4). Fitted properly the collar will not restrict cervical rotation. Often the athlete wears the neck roll too low

on the shoulder pads in an effort to be able to move the head and neck and see the football easier. This renders the neck roll ineffective (Fig. 23–5). *At no time* should straps running from the shoulder pads to the helmet be used to prevent head and neck movement. Use of straps may predispose the cervical spine to excessive axial loading and resultant fracture or fracture-dislocation by preventing movement of the cervical spine. The U.S. Military Academy has designed augmented shoulder pads that add buffer padding to the neck in an effort to prevent compressive injuries to the plexus (Fig. 23–6).

Cervical nerve root avulsion injuries can occur with more severe traction injuries in collision sports such as football. The athlete presents with complete motor loss in muscles innervated by the affected nerve root levels, and spontaneous recovery does not occur (neu-

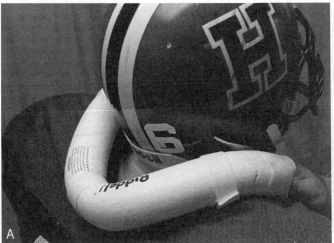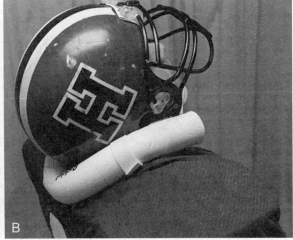

FIGURE 23–5. The position of padding will also determine the effective protection of the spine. *A*, Improper placement of the neck roll too far away from the helmet and cervical spine. *B*, Ineffective restriction of motion of head and cervical spine.

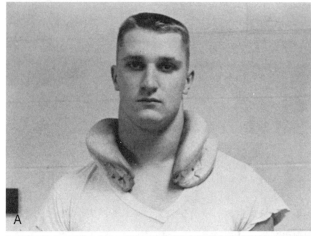

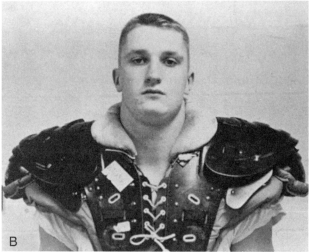

FIGURE 23–6. *A*, Orthosis currently in use at the United States Military Academy. *B*, Interval pad adds a buffer to the neck opening of football shoulder pads. (From Markey KL, DiBenedetto M, Curl WW. Upper trunk brachial plexopathy: The stinger syndrome. Am J Sports Med 1993; 21(5):650–655.)

rotmesis). Diagnostic findings may include fractures of the transverse processes on cervical radiographs.[22] Rehabilitation consists of maintaining range of motion in the extremity and reconstructive surgery to restore as much function as possible.

ACUTE BRACHIAL NEUROPATHY

Acute brachial neuropathy is a rare syndrome characterized by acute or subacute intense shoulder pain, accompanied by weakness and wasting of various muscles of the shoulder and proximal arm. There is no clear pattern of motor nerve or brachial plexus involvement. Denervation may be limited to one muscle supplied by a peripheral nerve (e.g., normal infraspinatus muscle with denervation of the supraspinatus muscle). Sensory loss is usually limited. Most reported cases occur in the dominant upper extremity.[24,25] The cause of acute brachial neuropathy is unknown.

Management in the acute phase includes rest and analgesics. The athlete begins rehabilitation as soon as the pain subsides.[22] The prognosis is generally good for a return to athletics. It is common, however, to have residual weakness for several months or years after diagnosis. It is an important diagnosis to consider as a part of the differential diagnosis of shoulder joint, muscle, and peripheral nerve injuries.

PERIPHERAL NERVE INJURIES IN THE UPPER QUARTER

THORACIC OUTLET SYNDROME

Thoracic outlet syndrome (TOS) is a controversial diagnosis consisting of neural and/or vascular compression in the thoracic outlet (Fig. 23–7). There are a variety of clinical manifestations depending on the site of compression and the neurovascular structures involved. Vascular symptoms are less frequent than neurogenic symptoms. The most common neurogenic signs arise from compression of the lower trunk of the brachial plexus, leading to symptoms such as pain and paresthesias of the medial arm and hand, upper extremity fatigue, and muscle atrophy. This syndrome may occur in athletes with excessive shoulder girdle depression[26] or overly developed trapezius and neck musculature or in sports requiring repetitive overhead use of the upper extremity. Swimmers may develop symptoms as a result of hypertrophy of the pectoralis minor muscle. Tennis and baseball players may develop symptoms owing to either greater muscular development of the dominant arm or increased scapular depression as a result of failure to maintain adequate scapular stabilization with repetitive motions.[16,27] Tennis and baseball players may complain of difficulty gripping a racket or bat because of intrinsic muscle weakness in the hands.

Because the exact diagnosis of TOS is difficult to confirm, symptoms in the upper extremity should always be carefully evaluated to differentiate true TOS from shoulder instabilities, cervical radiculopathies, and other peripheral nerve injuries. Treatment is directed at restoring posture and muscle balance of the upper trunk and shoulder girdle. Modification of technique or avoidance of some activities may be necessary to prevent recurrence of symptoms.[16]

SPINAL ACCESSORY NERVE INJURY

The spinal accessory nerve innervates the sternocleidomastoid muscle and the trapezius. It is vulnerable to injury from blunt trauma (e.g., a blow from a hockey or lacrosse stick) or a traction injury.[22] Injury can result in paralysis and atrophy of the trapezius muscle. Weakness usually develops soon after the injury and is accompanied by a persistent ache about the shoulder girdle.[28,29] If the nerve does not recover, scapular stabilizing procedures or transfer of the leva-

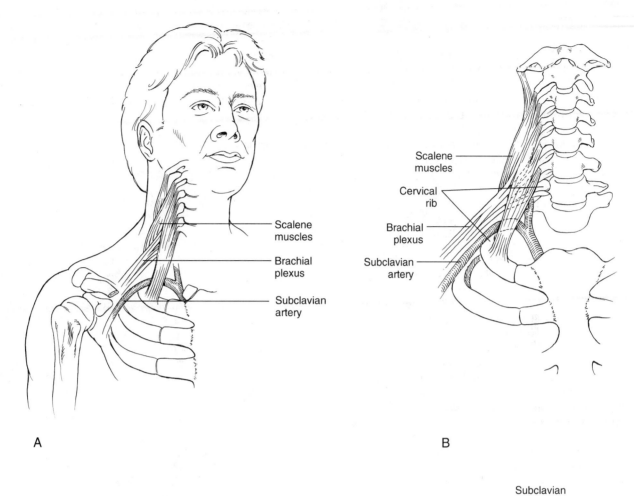

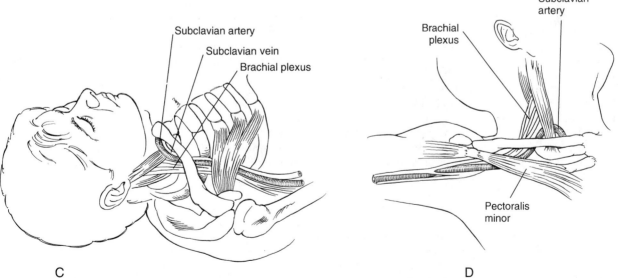

FIGURE 23–7. Sites of compression in thoracic outlet syndrome (TOS). *A*, Scalenus anterior syndrome. *B*, A cervical rib or a fibrous band can obstruct the neurovascular bundle. *C*, Compression can occur between the clavicle and first rib. *D*, Hyperabduction compresses the neurovascular bundle under the pectoralis minor tendon.

tor scapulae can be performed surgically. The prognosis for full return to athletics, however, is usually poor.[28]

LONG THORACIC NERVE INJURY (BACKPACKER'S PALSY)

The long thoracic nerve originates from the C5–C7 nerve roots and innervates the serratus anterior muscle, which is essential for scapular stabilization and protraction. The nerve is vulnerable to blunt trauma as it passes from the brachial plexus across the base of the neck and, more distally, where it lies against the chest wall. It is commonly injured by traction or compression from the strap of a backpack. Paralysis of the serratus anterior has also been reported as an overuse injury in sports such as archery, basketball, bowling, cycling, golf, rope skipping, weightlifting, and tennis.[28] White and Witten[30] reported one incidence of a stretch injury to the long thoracic nerve in a male ballet dancer from aggressive warm-up stretches. The presenting complaint is usually difficulty elevating the arm and winging of the scapula, often accompanied by aching or burning around the shoulder or scapula.[28]

The prognosis is good if the injury is the result of overuse. The injury is treated with rest and exercise to maintain range of motion. Closed injuries have a more guarded prognosis; if the injury was caused by compression, prognosis will depend on how long the compression has been applied. If strength and endurance do not fully recover with conservative management over 24 months, the scapula may have to be stabilized surgically.[28]

AXILLARY NERVE INJURY

The axillary nerve is formed from fibers of C5 and C6 nerve roots. It arises from the posterior cord of the brachial plexus and innervates the deltoid and teres minor muscles. It also provides sensory innervation for a small area of skin over the lateral deltoid. The most common mechanism of injury is an acute anterior shoulder dislocation or its reduction.[28,29] Other mechanisms of injury include blunt trauma to the shoulder, compression by a hematoma, irritation by osteophytes

of the glenoid margin, and compression as the nerve passes through the quadrilateral space.[28] Trauma may also occur during many surgical procedures on the shoulder.[28,31]

If EMG findings show incomplete denervation, the prognosis for recovery is generally good. Fortunately, the supraspinatus and infraspinatus muscles can compensate for some of the loss of abduction and external rotation after axillary nerve injury.[28]

SUPRASCAPULAR NERVE INJURY

The suprascapular nerve innervates the suprapinatus and infraspinatus and provides sensory branches to the posterior glenohumeral joint and the acromioclavicular joint. The five potential sites of trauma along the nerve[28,32] are outlined in Table 23–3.

The mechanism of injury may be direct trauma, such as a fall on the shoulder or acute dislocation, or traction and friction to the nerve as it passes through the suprascapular notch. Rapid stretching of the accompanying artery may contribute to ischemic injury of the nerve.[32] Volleyball players, swimmers, and other athletes who perform repetitive overhead motions are vulnerable to this injury. It has frequently been reported in baseball players, especially pitchers,[28,32,33] owing to the extreme angular velocities and torque forces acting on the shoulder during the phases of pitching or throwing.[32,34] Injury to the nerve in the spinoglenoid notch will lead to denervation of the infraspinatus alone. This lesion often remains asymptomatic, even in competitive athletes.[28,33]

The onset of symptoms is often insidious, beginning with a vague shoulder ache and weakness without paresthesia or numbness.[28,32] Visible atrophy and EMG changes may be present without noticeable impairment in athletic performance.[28,33] However, weakness of the supraspinatus and infraspinatus may lead to a loss of functional control of the humeral head and imbalance of force couples around the shoulder, placing other shoulder structures at risk of impingement.

If the nerve lesion fails to recover spontaneously, surgical exploration is indicated to see if the nerve is entrapped by ligaments across the suprascapular notch or the spinoglenoid notch or is compressed by a lipoma or cyst.[18,28,32,33]

TABLE 23–3
The Suprascapular Nerve (C4, C5, C6): Potential Sites of Injury[27]

1. Spinal roots and upper trunk of plexus between fascia of anterior and middle scalenes	Signs and symptoms:
	   Vague ache or weakness of the shoulder girdle
	   Visible muscle atrophy

2. Nerve trunk in the fascia of the subclavius and omohyoid muscles	Injury in spinoglenoid notch will give selective atrophy of infraspinous muscle
3. Suprascapular notch as nerve trunk passes inferior to the transverse scapular ligament	Mechanism of injury:
4. The fascial compartment between the supraspinous and the base of the coracoid process	Direct trauma from fall or dislocation Insidious or repetitive injury
5. Spinoglenoid notch as the nerve enters the infraspinous fossa	

TABLE 23–4
The Radial Nerve (C6–T1): Potential Sites of Injury in the Radial Tunnel[5,39]

Cause/Site	Signs and Symptoms
1. Anterior to the radial head, as the nerve enters the tunnel, it may be tethered by a fibrous band.	Elbow pain reproduced wth active supination in elbow flexion
2. Blood vessels can compress the nerve as they fan across it in the tunnel.	Increased symptoms during exercise
3. The arcade of Frohse, a fibrous band of the superficial head of the proximal supinator muscle, may cause friction or compression against the nerve.	Weakness of finger extensors and ulnar extensor muscle of the wrist. Pain with full passive pronation and wrist flexion and resisted supination
4. The tendinous margin of the radial extensor muscle of the wrist may extend medially and compress the nerve.	Pain with full passive pronation and wrist flexion

MUSCULOCUTANEOUS NERVE INJURY

The musculocutaneous nerve is derived from the C5 and C6 nerve roots and occasionally the C7 nerve root. It arises from the lateral cord of the brachial plexus and provides motor innervation to the biceps, brachialis, and coracobrachialis muscles and sensory innervation to the radial side of the forearm. It may be injured during acute anterior shoulder dislocations[28] or closed clavicle fractures[35] or during surgery to repair a recurrent shoulder dislocation.[31] Mendoza and Main[28] cite several cases from the literature of injuries to the nerve during athletic activities such as rowing, throwing a football, or weightlifting. However, injury to this nerve rarely occurs in isolation.

RADIAL NERVE INJURY

The radial nerve arises directly from the posterior cord of the brachial plexus and innervates the triceps, brachialis, brachioradialis, supinator, and extensor muscles of the wrist and fingers.[36] The radial nerve is vulnerable to compression at several places along the nerve trunk. Proximally, it is vulnerable to compression as it passes under the lateral head of the triceps in the upper arm.[5,18,37] Strong contraction of the triceps, as may occur during throwing or weight training,[18] can compress the nerve, causing weakness in the forearm extensors.[37] Trauma such as radial head dislocation or fracture or elbow hyperextension may result in injury to the interosseous branch of the radial nerve as it crosses anteriorly to the elbow.[38]

Lesions of the posterior interosseus branch of the radial nerve in the radial tunnel (Table 23–4) can mimic the common symptoms of "tennis elbow" (lateral epicondylitis), or the two conditions may exist in combination. Chronic inflammation of the common extensor tendons at the elbow can lead to a reactive synovitis of the annular ligament involving the radial nerve. Fibrosis and local edema from overuse of the tendons may also increase the compression on the nerve as it passes under the radial extensor muscle of the wrist.[39] Both conditions will usually respond to conservative treatment, which includes anti-inflammatory medication, rest, ice, and muscle stretching and strengthening.[5,18,39] In true radial tunnel syndrome, the most effective treatment is usually surgical decompression of the nerve.[5,39]

Differential diagnosis of lesions to this nerve also must include the possibility of cervical radiculopathy. Gunn and Milbrandt[40] examined the cervical spines of individuals with a history of tennis elbow who had failed to respond to treatment directed at their elbows. All 42 patients in their study had EMG findings "consistent with early radiculopathy or neuropathy of the affected myotomes," and all had increased resistance to passive motion of the C5 and C6 apophyseal joints. Treatment was directed to the cervical spine and included spinal mobilization, traction, various treatment modalities, and isometric exercises. Such treatment of the cervical spine was followed by good or satisfactory relief of symptoms in 86 percent of their patients in an average of 5.25 weeks.

The positive response to treatment of the cervical spine in Gunn and Milbrandt's study[40] does not necessarily indicate that all the symptoms came from a cervical lesion. It is more likely that treatment directed to the cervical spine removed one component of a double-crush lesion involving both the cervical spine and the radial nerve at the elbow. The interplay of proximal and distal components of nerve irritation, as well as the local effects on the nerve of joint and muscle inflammation, may help to explain why the differential diagnosis and treatment of lateral epicondylitis are often difficult.

Butler[3] describes this complex interplay between cervical joints and muscle tightness, elbow joint and soft tissue signs, and neural tension tests and neurologic findings in the management of a patient with lateral elbow pain. He has devised a test known as the *upper limb tension test 2 with a radial nerve bias* (ULTT 2), in which mechanical tension is applied to the radial nerve throughout its course. This test consists of a combination of shoulder depression, elbow extension, medial rotation of the extremity, pronation of the forearm, wrist flexion, thumb and finger flexion, and ulnar deviation of the hand (Fig. 23–8). If symptoms have not been provoked by this point in the test, shoulder abduction is performed. Cervical lateral flexion away from the extremity will also increase the tension on the brachial plexus,[41] further sensitizing the test. The final forearm position in this test (pronation, wrist flexion and ulnar

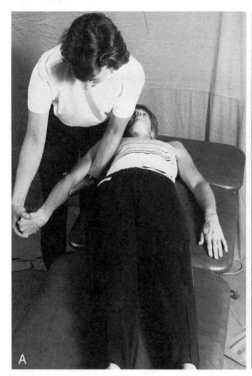
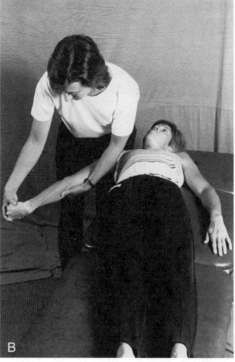

FIGURE 23–8. The upper limb tension test (ULTT) 2 with a radial nerve bias is designed to place traction on the radial nerve.[3] *A,* The upper extremity is placed sequentially in elbow extension; forearm pronation; upper arm internal rotation; wrist, finger, and thumb flexion; and ulnar deviation. *B,* The test is further sensitized with the addition of shoulder depression and abduction and contralateral side flexion of the cervical spine. Symptoms are monitored at each position of the test.

deviation, and thumb flexion) is a position that is commonly used to test flexibility of the common extensor muscles. Pain from muscle stretching in this position can be differentiated from pain from neural structures by the addition of shoulder abduction or cervical lateral flexion. Both of these maneuvers increase tension through the nerve tract without increasing tension in the extensor muscles.

Yaxley and Jull[42,43] have studied this test in normal subjects and in those with tennis elbow. In young, healthy subjects the test provoked a stretching pain over the radial aspect of the forearm.[42] This response to the test was compared with that in 20 subjects with unilateral tennis elbow. Both groups had symptoms in similar areas of the arm, but the symptoms were reported as more intense in the symptomatic arms.[43] Yaxley and Jull observed a statistically significant

difference in available range of shoulder abduction in the symptomatic arms of their subjects (12.45 degrees less than the asymptomatic side). They recommend routine inclusion of this test as a part of the differential diagnosis of lateral epicondylitis.

The superficial radial nerve provides cutaneous innervation to the posterolateral forearm and hand. It may be compressed proximally if it runs through the radial extensor muscle of the wrist instead of over it. It can also be compressed at the wrist after fracture or as a result of a tight watchband or bracelet.[44]

ULNAR NERVE INJURY

The ulnar nerve arises from the medial cord of the brachial plexus. It is most vulnerable to athletic injury at

TABLE 23–5
The Ulnar Nerve (C7–T1): Cubital Tunnel Lesions[45,46]

Cause/Site:	Signs and Symptoms:

1. Traction injuries due to increased valgus forces
  a. Prior fracture or injury to growth plate
  b. MCL disruption
2. Entrapment under:
  a. Thickened arcuate ligament
  b. Hypertrophy of the medial triceps, anconeus, or ulnar flexor muscle of the wrist
3. Irregularities in the ulnar groove due to osteophytes may prevent sliding of the ulnar nerve
4. Subluxation or dislocation of the nerve over the medial epicondyle (usually due to laxity of soft tissue restraints) leads to a friction fibrosis
	1. Medial elbow pain radiating to the medial forearm
	2. Numbness and tingling in the ulnar aspect of the forearm and hand

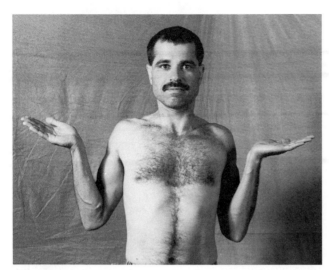

FIGURE 23–9. The elbow flexion test for ulnar nerve irritation in the cubital tunnel.[48] A positive response is the production of paresthesias along the ulnar border of the forearm and hand.

two sites: the cubital tunnel at the elbow and in or near Guyon's canal at the wrist.[44–46] The four major etiologic factors for injury of the nerve at the elbow are outlined in Table 23–5. Injury is most common in athletes who perform repeated throwing motions.[45,46] There is a normal rise in pressure in the nerve in the cubital tunnel as the elbow is flexed in combination with wrist extension and shoulder abduction, which is the upper extremity position at the beginning stage of throwing.[47] Entrapment or inflammation of the nerve accentuates this phenomenon.

Most cases of ulnar neuritis at the cubital tunnel have an insidious onset of medial elbow pain radiating down the medial forearm and numbness and tingling in the ulnar aspect of the forearm and hand. Symptoms are aggravated by continued use.[45]

Various tests for lesions along the path of the ulnar nerve have been described in the literature. Buehler and Thayer[48] suggested using the elbow flexion test as a clinical test for cubital tunnel syndrome (Fig. 23–9). A positive response to the test consists of reproduction of paresthesias along the ulnar border of the forearm and hand. Butler's upper limb tension test with an ulnar nerve bias (ULTT 3) (Fig. 23–10) is similar but increases the tensile stress on the brachial plexus and proximal portion of the ulnar nerve by adding shoulder girdle depression, glenohumeral abduction, and external rotation.[3] Although the test was originally described with the forearm in supination, pronation of the forearm will often make the test more provocative of symptoms. Cervical lateral flexion away from the extremity being tested can also be added.

Responses to Butler's ULTT 3 have been studied in normal patients[49,50] and in symptomatic patients.[50] In most normal subjects, symptoms of tingling or stretching occurred in the medial forearm and hand. Subjects also frequently reported a sensation of stretching or pressure at the medial elbow. Several arms tested in one study[50] had no symptomatic response to the test. This study also tested the response to the test in 18 subjects with a variety of upper extremity or cervical spine symptoms and found that all subjects had some response to the test. As a group, they also had more frequent reports of medial upper arm pain (44 percent

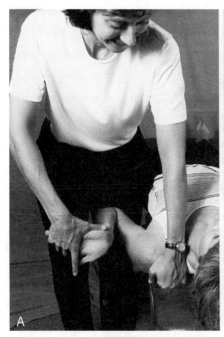
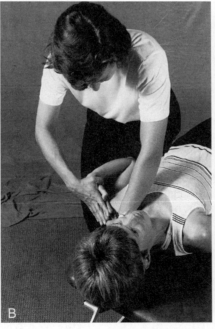
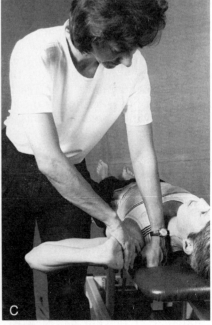

FIGURE 23–10. The ULTT 3[3] was designed to place tensile stress on the ulnar nerve. The test consists sequentially of shoulder depression, wrist and finger extension (A), supination or pronation (B) of the forearm, and elbow flexion. C, The shoulder is then externally rotated and abducted. Contralateral lateral flexion of the cervical spine further sensitizes the test.

TABLE 23–6
The Median Nerve (C5–T1): Sites of Compression in the Pronator Syndrome[5]

Cause/Site	Signs and Symptoms
1. Swelling due to trauma can compress the nerve in the fibro-osseus tunnel created by the ligament of Struthers as it passes between the supracondylar process and the medial epicondyle.	Pain with resisted forearm pronation.
2. Abnormal thickness of the bicipital aponeurosis can compress the nerve during resisted elbow flexion.	Pain is aggravated by resisted elbow flexion.
3. A fibrous band on the superficial head of the pronator teres muscle may compress the nerve where it passes between the superficial and deep heads.	Pain is aggravated by resisted forearm pronation and flexion.
4. The nerve can be compressed under the fibrous arch on the proximal margin of the superficial flexor muscles of the fingers.	Pain with resisted flexion of the superficial tendon of the third finger.

vs. 18 percent in healthy subjects) and occasional symptoms in the contralateral extremity.

Another important finding in that study was that 9 of 36 arms (25 percent) tested in the patient group had onset of symptoms prior to the addition of shoulder abduction, something that never occurred in healthy subjects. When range of shoulder abduction at the onset of symptoms in the remaining symptomatic arms was compared with that in healthy subjects, the difference in range was not statistically significant. Clinically, this seems to indicate that provocation of symptoms in the early stages of the ULTT 3 or with the elbow flexion test is a better measure of the presence of abnormality than the degree of abduction available prior to the onset of symptoms in the ULTT 3. Unfortunately, there were not enough subjects with unilateral symptoms in this study to compare the difference in symptom reproduction in the symptomatic and asymptomatic extremities in the same individual.

Treatment for cubital tunnel syndrome consists initially of rest, ice, and anti-inflammatory medications. The athlete should also be examined for any problems in the cervical spine or shoulder that may be contributing to the symptoms or increasing stresses on the medial elbow by altering the mechanics of throwing.

If conservative treatment fails, surgical treatment should be considered. Surgical options include (1) transposition of the ulnar nerve to the anterior surface of the elbow joint and (2) removal of the medial epicondyle.[44–46] Rettig and Ebben[51] retrospectively reviewed the cases of 20 athletes who underwent anterior subcutaneous transfer of the ulnar nerve. The average length of time between surgery and return to sports was 12.6 weeks (range, 6 to 43 weeks), and 19 of 20 athletes returned to their preinjury level of athletic activity.

Compression of the ulnar nerve at the wrist is a common problem for cyclists.[25,52,53] Fernald[52] studied the incidence of overuse injuries in elite cyclists and found that 21 percent had sensory changes in their upper extremities. The compression can cause sensory disturbances and motor weakness in the intrinsic muscles of the hand.[44,53] The abnormality may result from acute or chronic compression of the nerve in Guyon's canal as a result of prolonged weight bearing on the hands or a fall. It also can be caused by traction on the nerve produced by the extended wrist position on the handlebars.[25,53] Normally a cyclist bears approximately 45 percent of his or her weight on the upper extremities,[52] so the combination of compression and vibration from the road increase the likelihood of neurogenic symptoms.

Strategies to prevent irritation to the nerve at the wrist include frequent changing of the position of the hands while riding, using padded gloves and handlebars, and adjusting the overall "fit" of the bike to decrease weight bearing on the hands.[52,53]

Digital nerves in the hand are vulnerable to compression and friction injuries. Bowlers are susceptible to compression of the ulnar digital nerve to the thumb produced by direct pressure from the hole in the bowling ball.[54] Rettig reported a case of digital neuritis in a cheerleader from repetitive clapping.[54]

MEDIAN NERVE INJURY

The median nerve arises from the medial and lateral cords of the brachial plexus. There are three common compression syndromes involving this nerve: the pronator syndrome, the interosseous syndrome, and the carpal tunnel syndrome. Sites of compression in the pronator syndrome are outlined in Table 23–6.[5]

The anterior interosseous syndrome occurs when the nerve is compressed by a fibrous band of the superficial flexor muscle of the fingers or by anomalous tendons of the forearm. Weakness is confined to the long flexor muscle of the thumb, the deep flexor muscle of the second and third fingers, and the pronator quadratus muscle.[44]

Carpal tunnel syndrome is by far the most common form of compression of the median nerve. In athletes it occurs as a result of weight bearing on the hands in cycling[25,53] and with repetitive gripping, throwing, or wrist flexion and extension. It can also occur after trauma.[54] Conservative management for cyclists has been previously described. Splinting may be necessary to facilitate rest. Other adjunct procedures include icing, steroid or lidocaine injection, and resection of the transverse retinacular ligament.[53,54]

Differential diagnosis of median nerve compression syndromes includes ruling out cervical radiculopathies. As with radial and ulnar nerve abnormality, the possibility of a mechanical or physiological double-crush lesion must always be considered. Murray-Leslie and Wright[55] found a positive correlation between the incidence of carpal tunnel syndrome and a decrease in the size of the anteroposterior measurements of the cervical spinal canal at C5 and C6 and a decrease in cervical disc height when subjects were compared with age-matched controls.

It has been the authors' clinical experience that symptoms may be present in the median nerve distribution that appear to be due to adverse mechanics along the course of the nerve, frequently occurring in the absence of EMG abnormalities. A similar observation led Elvey[41] to develop what is currently considered the first upper limb tension test (ULLT 1) (Fig. 23–11). His cadaveric studies demonstrated that the C5–C7 nerve roots moved laterally during shoulder abduction if the shoulder was prevented from elevating. Elbow extension and wrist extension increased the tension on these structures as well as on the brachial plexus and median nerve. Other studies have confirmed the motion of the median nerve with shoulder abduction, elbow extension, and wrist extension.[8]

Kenneally et al.[56] tested symptomatic response to the ULTT 1 in 100 asymptomatic subjects and demonstrated that in the final position, the test provoked a deep, sometimes painful stretch over the anterior shoulder, elbow, and the lateral forearm. It also provoked a mild

to moderate amount of tingling in the thumb and first two fingers. His findings support Elvey's belief that the test predominantly stresses the median nerve and the C5 and C6 nerve roots.

Butler's variation on the ULTT 1 also stresses the median nerve. It utilizes the same components of motion as Elvey's test but in a differing order. Butler developed the ULTT 2 (Fig. 23–12) to more closely replicate the functional movements that reproduced the patient's symptoms.[3] The final position of the test is similar to the backswing of a forehand shot in tennis.

Richards[57] examined the ULTT 2 in 80 normal subjects and found symptoms to occur along the distribution of the median nerve. The symptoms provoked were similar to those found by Kenneally et al.[56] for the ULTT 1.

All of the ULTTs described are useful in helping to determine whether abnormal neurobiomechanics are contributing to persistent symptoms. Treatment can then focus on mobilization or release/decompression of the neural tissues involved. These tests should be carried out routinely if apparent muscular or tendinous lesions fail to resolve with treatment to local structures.

COMBINED LESIONS

Injury to the radial, median, and ulnar nerves can occur as a result of compression in the axilla or upper arm from the misuse of crutches during rehabilitation of lower extremity injuries.[5,44] The median and ulnar nerves are always vulnerable at the wrist during activities requiring weight bearing on extended wrists.[25]

FIGURE 23–11. The ULTT 1 was developed by Elvey.[41] It places tensile stress on the brachial plexus and median nerve throughout its course. The test consists sequentially of (A) shoulder depression, abduction, external rotation, and wrist and finger extension, followed by (B) elbow extension and contralateral cervical lateral flexion.

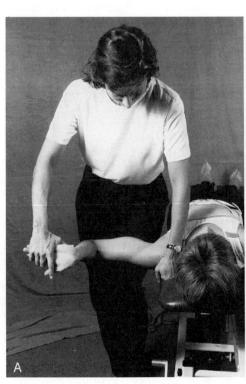
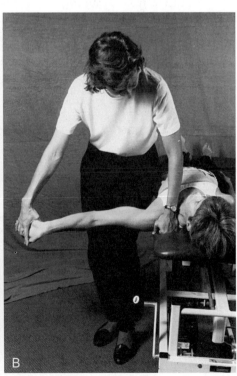

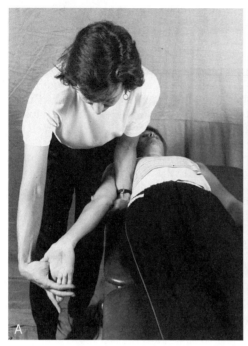
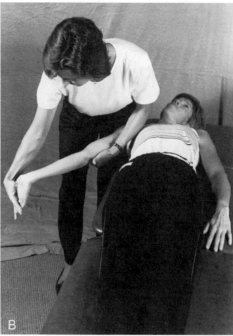

FIGURE 23–12. The ULTT 2 was developed by Butler[3] as an alternative test of the median nerve tract. It consists of *(A)* shoulder depression, external rotation, supination of the forearm, wrist and finger extension, and *(B)* shoulder abduction. Contralateral cervical lateral flexion further sensitizes the test.

PERIPHERAL NERVE INJURIES IN THE LOWER QUARTER

SCIATIC NERVE INJURY

The sciatic nerve (Table 23–7) is formed by the peroneal and tibial nerves and contains contributions from the L4–S3 nerve roots. The nerve can be irritated as it passes under or through the piriformis muscle in the buttocks.[58] Pain may be due to spasm or scarring of the muscle from straining or overuse.[44] Clinically, pain may radiate down the posterior leg (sciatica). Tenderness will be located over the muscle belly. The athlete will complain of pain with resisted hip abduction and external rotation. Full passive internal rotation can also compress the nerve under the piriformis muscle. The pain is usually not associated with neurologic loss.[44]

The hamstring syndrome results from entrapment of the sciatic nerve by tight tendinous bands near the lateral origin of the hamstrings at the ischial tuberosity.[58] It is often found in sprinters or hurdlers. Pain is felt at the ischial tuberosity and may radiate down the posterior thigh. Symptoms are aggravated with sitting, stretching, or running. Neurologic and straight-leg raising tests are usually negative. Surgical release of the tendinous bands is usually successful in relieving symptoms.[58]

Pain from a torn hamstring muscle must be differentiated from irritation of the lumbar nerve roots and the sciatic nerve. The slump-sitting test helps to differentiate pain arising from neural or muscular structures (Fig. 23–13). The test combines full neck and trunk flexion, knee extension, ankle dorsiflexion, and hip flexion in a sitting position.[3,59] It places tensile stress on the neural tissues throughout the spinal canal and the sciatic

TABLE 23–7	
The Sciatic Nerve (L4–S3): Areas of Entrapment/Irritation	
Cause/Site	**Signs and Symptoms**
1. Compression as nerve runs under or through the piriformis in the buttocks	Tenderness over the piriformis muscle belly Pain with resisted hip abduction and external rotation Pain with full passive internal rotation or hip adduction in hip flexion
2. Entrapment in the fibers of the origin of the hamstrings at the ischial tuberosity	Pain from ischial tuberosity to posterior thigh Neurologic and straight-leg–raising tests are negative Symptoms provoked with stretching, sitting, or running

3. In association with hamstring tear	Differentiation:
	   Hamstring tear alone: Pain with palpation of muscle with or without bruising; slump test negative
	   Sciatic nerve or nerve root involved: slump test positive (see Fig. 23–13)

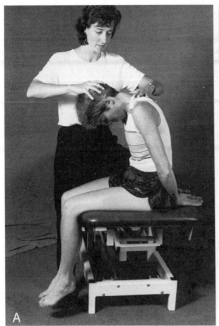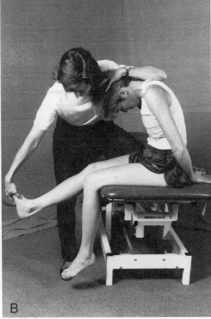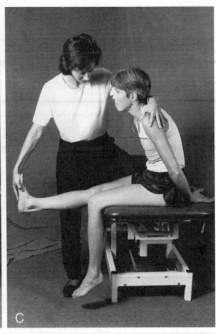

FIGURE 23–13. The slump test was developed by Maitland[59] to stress the neural structures in the spinal canal and along the course of the sciatic nerve. The test consists of trunk flexion, neck flexion, (A), knee extension (B), and, as needed, dorsiflexion of the ankle and hip flexion, adduction, or internal rotation. If knee extension increases or symptoms decrease when the neck flexion component is released (C), the test is considered positive.

nerve. Pain from a stretch on the neural tissue can be differentiated from muscular pain from the hamstrings if the leg is maintained in the same degree of knee extension that reproduces the muscle pain and the head and neck are extended. If the pain is decreased, neural structures are implicated, as the muscle length has not been changed and the tension on the neural tissues has decreased.

Kornberg and Lew[60] have demonstrated that use of the slump-sitting test as a treatment technique facilitates faster return to play in Australian football players with grade I hamstring tears, indicating that in some cases motion of the sciatic nerve must be impaired as it passes through the muscle either before the tear or from the inflammation and exudate surrounding the nerve after injury.[3] Butler[3] advocates early but gentle motion of the muscle and nerve to prevent scarring and adhesion formation between the muscle and nerve.

TIBIAL NERVE INJURY

The tibial nerve (Table 23–8) usually descends vertically through the popliteal space, where it may be vul-

TABLE 23–8 Tibial Nerve (L4–S3): Sites of Entrapment or Irritation	
Cause/Site	**Signs and Symptoms**

1. Popliteal space:
  a. Compression by a Baker cyst
  b. Entrapment in proximal portion of medial gastrocnemius
	Posterior knee pain, possibly radiating to calf

2. Tarsal tunnel:
  a. Space occupying lesion (osteophyte, ganglion, etc.)
  b. Eversion strain (acute or repetitive)
	Pain from medial malleolus to heel, sole of foot, and occasionally to calf; worse at night or with walking or running; positive Tinel test at tarsal tunnel

3. Medial plantar nerve distal to tarsal tunnel or in hypertrophic abductor muscle of the thumb	Pain and paresthesias in the medial 3½ toes with weight bearing under load or with running
4. Lateral plantar nerve distal to tarsal tunnel	Pain in the lateral foot and lateral two toes; may cause persistent medial heel pain

5. Interdigital neuromas:
  a. Compression from callous formation under the metatarsal heads
  b. Stretching of nerve under the deep transverse tarsal ligament
	Pain and paresthesias at the metatarsal heads that may radiate proximally or to toes

nerable to compression by a Baker's cyst.[36,44] Ekelund[61] reported one case of a female athlete who presented with entrapment of the nerve in the proximal portion of the medial gastrocnemius muscle. Her main complaint was posterior knee pain with training. She had tenderness over the nerve on palpation. Surgical release relieved her symptoms completely.

Entrapment of the tibial nerve in the tarsal tunnel usually occurs as a result of alteration in the size or shape of the tunnel owing to fracture, dislocation, trauma, lipoma, tendon sheath cyst, or direct pressure. It can also occur from acute or chronic eversion.[44,62,63] The classic symptoms include pain at the medial malleolus radiating to the sole of the foot, the heel, and sometimes the calf; paresthesia; worsening of the symptoms at night, with walking or running, or with dorsiflexion; and weakness of toe flexion. Pain is reproduced with the Tinel test over the nerve in the tarsal tunnel.[62]

The nerve splits into the medial and lateral plantar nerves within the tarsal tunnel. Entrapment of the medial plantar nerve will usually cause paresthesia or pain in the medial 3½ toes.[62,63] The medial plantar nerve can also be entrapped in a hypertrophic or fibrous abductor muscle of the great toe.[44] The repetitive nature of running combined with altered mechanics of the foot and ankle places the nerve at risk for stretch injuries in the tarsal tunnel. Ironically, symptoms may also be provoked by pressure placed on the medial arch by new arch supports.[27] Johnson et al.[64] reported similar problems in a competitive weightlifter owing to the large weight-bearing loads on the foot.

Entrapment of the lateral plantar nerve will cause similar symptoms in the lateral foot and lateral two toes. Branches of this nerve supply the medial heel and calcaneus and the long plantar ligament. Irritation of the calcaneal branch of this nerve is a potential source for persistent heel pain.[62,63]

Butler[3] believes that many cases of "plantar fasciitis" may be of neurogenic origin. An important part of differential diagnosis of neurogenic and fascial pain includes the use of tests for adverse tension of the nerves. To differentiate the cause of pain, the foot and ankle are positioned in a pain-provoking position for plantar fasciitis (dorsiflexion of the foot and toes), and movement of a proximal part of the limb is superimposed, increasing the tension on the tibial nerve (Fig. 23–14). The plantar fascia is not stressed further by straight-leg raising. Therefore, if symptoms increase in response to the test, they are likely to have at least a partial neurogenic origin.[3]

Interdigital neuromas most commonly occur in runners and dancers owing to repetitive dorsiflexion of the metatarsophalangeal joints. The nerve is stretched under the deep transverse metatarsal ligament. Compression can also occur as a result of increased pressure on the nerve from callus formation under the metatarsal heads. Pain and paresthesia are felt at the metatarsal heads and may radiate proximally or to the toes.[63] Treatment usually consists of rest, modification of footwear, corticosteroid injection, or surgical excision of the neuroma. Mobilization of the intermetatarsal joints may help alter the mechanical interface among the nerve, the metatarsal heads, and the transverse ligament[3] (Fig. 23–15).

PERONEAL NERVE INJURY

The peroneal nerve (Table 23–9) is formed from fibers from L4–S2 nerve roots. It diverges from the sciatic nerve in the upper part of the popliteal space.

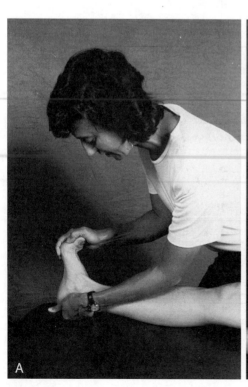
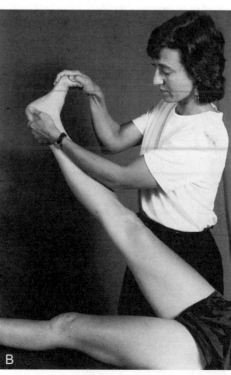

FIGURE 23–14. *A,* Maximal toe extension and dorsiflexion place tensile stress on the plantar fascia. *B,* The position shown in *A* is maintained while the lower extremity is raised in a straight-leg raise. If symptoms increase with the addition of straight-leg raising, then neural structures are implicated, as there has been no change in the tension on the plantar fascia.

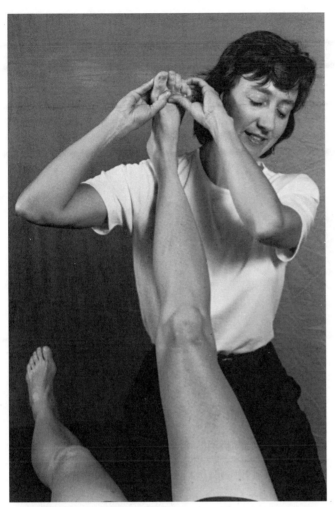

FIGURE 23–15. Mobilization of the intermetatarsal joints may decrease stress on a digital neuroma. Mobilization is depicted here in a straight-leg raising position, which places the nerve under increased tensile loading.

Nobel[65] described two patients who developed a hematoma of the nerve just distal to the bifurcation from the sciatic nerve after an inversion sprain of the ankle or fracture of the lower leg. He hypothesized that the blood vessels supplying the nerve were

ruptured by abrupt longitudinal traction on the nerve. Evacuation of the hematoma relieved the patients' discomfort completely.

The peroneal nerve is vulnerable to compression injuries from a direct blow, a lower leg cast, or sustained pressure at the point where the nerve passes around the head of the fibula (e.g., a race car driver leaning his leg against a car door).[18] Leach et al.[66] have found this area to be a common site of entrapment in runners. They found the nerve entrapped in musculofascial bands at various points around the fibular head. The main symptoms reported were progressive lateral leg and foot pain and paresthesia and weakness of the ankle evertors and toe extensors. Runners seem to be especially vulnerable to irritation at this site because of repetitive stretching of the nerve during inversion and plantar flexion. One other important observation from Leach et al.'s study was the fact that many of the patients had normal neurologic findings or EMG studies when examined in the office. However, if the patients returned to the office immediately after a long run, the neurologic findings and EMG changes were much more pronounced.

Peroneal nerve injury should also be considered as a probable sequela of grade III ankle sprains or fractures. Grade III sprains involve disruption of the lateral ligaments, the deltoid ligament, and the distal anterior talofibular ligament. Nitz et al.[67] found a high incidence of peroneal and tibial nerve injuries in patients with this type of sprain. Thirty-one of 36 patients (86 percent) had evidence of peroneal nerve injuries, and 30 of 36 (83 percent) had tibial nerve injuries; 19 patients in this group also had sensory losses. Of 30 patients with grade II sprains (lateral ligaments and deltoid ligaments torn), five had peroneal nerve injuries and three had tibial nerve injuries.

The superficial peroneal nerve can be entrapped as it exits from the deep fascia in the lower leg to cross the dorsolateral ankle.[63] Entrapment of this nerve causes numbness or tingling over the dorsum of the foot. The deep peroneal nerve can be injured as it crosses the dorsum of the ankle under the extensor retinaculum, where it is vulnerable to compression from ill-fitting boots or shoes or from swelling or osteophytes after a

TABLE 23–9	
Peroneal Nerve (L4–S2): Areas of Entrapment/Irritation	
Cause/Site	**Signs and Symptoms**
1. Traction injury at bifurcation from sciatic nerve	Acute-onset severe lateral leg pain from hematoma formation within nerve after ankle fracture or inversion sprain
2. Fibular head: compression from a blow or entrapment	Pain and/or paresthesias of the lateral leg and foot; EMG may not be positive in entrapment unless symptoms have been provoked by a long run
3. Dorsolateral ankle following a sprain	Lateral foot and ankle pain/paresthesias; possible EMG findings, positive straight-leg–raising test with plantar flexion/inversion of foot and ankle
4. Dorsolateral ankle: superficial or deep peroneal nerve compressed by fascial bands, swelling, or ill-fitting boots or shoes	Pain and/or paresthesias in the dorsolateral foot and ankle; symptoms provoked with palpation of nerve at site of lesion

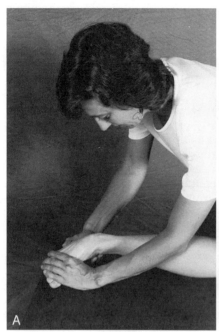
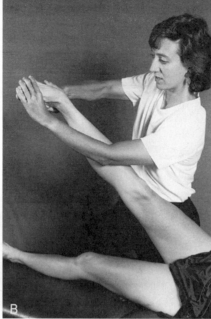
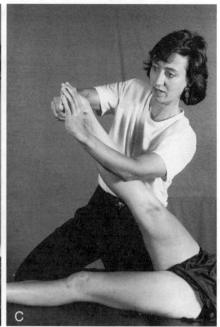

FIGURE 23–16. Lateral ankle pain from ligament sprain or nerve irritation can be differentiated using the following test. *A*, The ankle is placed in the pain-provoking position of inversion and plantar flexion. *B*, Straight-leg raising is then performed, increasing tensile stresses on the peroneal nerve but not on the ankle joint and ligaments. *C*, Hip adduction and internal rotation place further tension on the lumbosacral nerve roots and peroneal nerve.

fracture. It is also vulnerable at this site to traction from repetitive ankle sprains.[18] Both sites of injury are most common in runners.[63]

A modification of the straight-leg–raising test can be used to differentiate neurogenic causes from ligament or joint causes of persistent lateral foot and ankle pain.[3] The test is similar to the test described earlier for plantar foot pain. In this case, the foot and ankle are held in the pain-provoking position of inversion and plantar flexion, and the entire lower extremity is raised into a straight-leg raise (Fig. 23–16). Symptoms caused by abnormality along the peroneal nerve tract will increase with this test. Symptoms caused by joint and/or ligament abnormality will not change.

flexion. This position is similar to that used in the prone knee-bending test for tension on the femoral nerve and L3–L4 nerve roots[3] (Fig. 23–17).

OBTURATOR NERVE INJURY

The obturator nerve is derived from the anterior divisions of the lumbar plexus (L2–L4). It emerges from the medial border of the psoas near the brim of the pelvis and passes through the obturator foramen to the medial side of the thigh.[36] Although injury to the nerve has not been reported in the sports medicine literature,

FEMORAL NERVE INJURY

The femoral nerve is formed from the posterior branches of the L2–L4 nerve roots.[36] Different mechanisms can cause injury to the nerve. Compression may occur in the iliac compartment as a result of a hematoma and should be considered in anyone on anticoagulant therapy or with hemophilia.[44] The nerve is vulnerable to compression as it passes under the inguinal ligament in athletes who must squat for long periods of time or wear protective clothing that compresses this area. It may also be vulnerable to injury during gynecologic or hip surgery.[44]

Sammarco and Stephens[68] described one case of femoral nerve palsy in a modern dancer. The apparent mechanism of injury was traction from dance positions that required simultaneous hip extension and knee

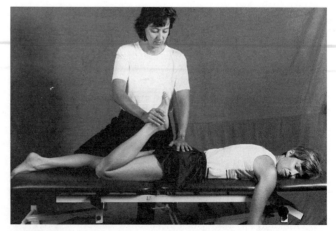

FIGURE 23–17. Prone knee bending is a common test for tension on the femoral nerve and L3 and L4 nerve roots.

such injury can occur from pelvic tumors, obturator hernias, or pelvic and proximal femoral fractures.[36] The nerve supplies the great adductor and external obturator muscles, as well as part of the sensory innervation for the hip joint and medial thigh.

Butler[3] suggests that entrapment of the obturator nerve may contribute to complaints of persistent groin pain in an athlete with an adductor muscle strain. He suggests modifying the slump-sitting test to examine for nervous system involvement by positioning the patient in a sitting position with the leg abducted to the point where groin symptoms are felt. If subsequent alteration of trunk or neck flexion or side flexion alters the groin pain, then there may be a neurogenic component to the disorder.

SENSORY NERVE INJURY

Meralgia paresthetica is a condition caused by irritation of the lateral cutaneous nerve of the thigh, which provides sensation over the anterolateral portion of the thigh.[36] The nerve is formed from the L3 and L4 nerve roots. It is vulnerable to compression or kinking as it passes from the pelvis through the fascia to the thigh or as it passes under the inguinal ligament. In athletes it may be compromised by pressure from protective equipment (e.g., a tight belt used to hold up heavy and bulky hockey pants) or, more commonly, from weight belts that are worn too tight. This nerve injury is more common in diabetic, pregnant, or obese patients.[36,44]

The sartorial nerve is a cutaneous branch of the obturator nerve and provides sensation to the medial knee joint.[36,69] It is vulnerable to injury from valgus stresses at the knee and during surgical procedures to the medial knee.[69]

The saphenous branch of the femoral nerve may be entrapped in the adductor canal of the medial thigh. Compression will increase during strong muscular contraction, as during squats or knee extension exercises.[27] The athlete may complain of medial knee pain

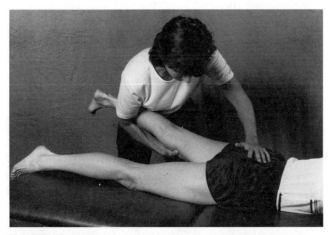

FIGURE 23–18. Tension can be placed on the saphenous nerve by placing the lower extremity in hip extension, external rotation, knee extension, and hip abduction.[3]

or paresthesias in the medial lower leg. Butler[3] has devised a modified femoral nerve stretch test to test for adverse tension along the saphenous portion of the femoral nerve (Fig. 23–18).

The sural nerve, derived from branches of the tibial and peroneal nerves, provides cutaneous innervation to the lateral lower leg and foot[36] and should be considered as a source of lateral foot and calf pain. The nerve emerges from the fascia of the leg approximately 16 cm proximal to the lateral malleolus. It can be palpated laterally in the foot and proximal to the malleolus.[3] Like the peroneal nerve, this nerve is vulnerable to injury from repetitive inversion sprains of the ankle or compression from ill-fitting shoes.[3,63]

DIFFERENTIAL DIAGNOSIS OF PERIPHERAL NERVE INJURIES

"When in doubt, do a history and physical."[70] This advice is critical in the differential diagnosis of peripheral nerve injuries. The subjective examination must delineate the specific type and area of the athlete's symptoms. Paresthesia or sensory losses should be mapped out to determine whether the symptoms are in a dermatomal or peripheral nerve distribution.[3] The precipitating injury or predisposing factors from overtraining or biomechanical abnormalities should give clues as to which nerves might have been injured. A nerve injury should always be suspected if the athlete experiences sensory changes in addition to weakness and/or pain.

Important components of objective testing include reflex, strength, and sensory testing; a Tinel test over the nerve trunks; and palpation along the course of the nerve[3] (Fig. 23–19). EMG is an important component of the evaluation of peripheral nerve injuries. As mentioned earlier, the timing of the examination is critical. Abnormalities in the sensory nerve action potentials (SNAPs) and combined motor action potentials (CMAPs) will not be evident for 7 to 10 days after injury. Fibrillations resulting from denervation of muscles will not be evident for 3 to 5 weeks,[25,70] which makes it difficult to distinguish between an axonotmesis and a neurotmesis in the first few days and weeks after an injury. Wilbourn[25] believes that EMG examination is most useful when performed between 3 weeks and 3 to 6 months after injury.

In addition to tests of neural conductivity, several tests have been described that check for mechanical tension along nerve trunks. These are useful in identifying pathomechanics of neural structures and their contribution to symptoms. Butler details the applications and variations of these tests in his text on mobilization of the nervous system.[3] The tests are thought to be clinically significant when there is a difference in any of the following variables when the symptomatic side is compared with the asymptomatic side: available range of motion, resistance to motion as perceived by the clinician, symptom reproduction, or a deviation from the established symptomatic responses in normals. The tests are considered particularly rel-

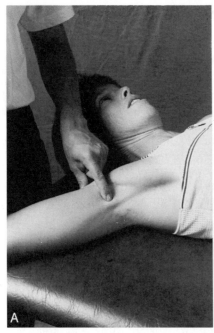
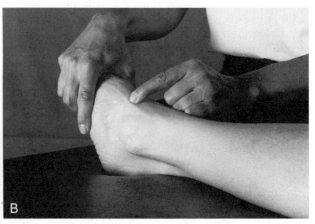

FIGURE 23–19. Palpation of the nerves is an important part of the examination. Nerves are often tender to touch at the site of a lesion. *A,* The brachial artery and median and ulnar nerves can be readily palpated in the axilla. *B,* The superficial peroneal nerve is visible at the dorsolateral ankle.

evant if the exact symptoms that the athlete has been complaining of are reproduced during testing.[3]

Measurement of compartment pressures after exercise will help to rule out compartment syndromes. A compartment syndrome occurs when tissue pressures increase within a confined space, compromising circulation and muscle function and potentially causing injury to the peripheral nerves that traverse the compartment. The compartment may be limited from expanding by the surrounding fascia or skin or by an external constraint such as a dressing or cast. The source of increased tissue pressure can be a hematoma occurring after injury or hypertrophy of the muscles within the compartment.[6] Injury to the nerve can occur as a result of ischemia or direct mechanical compression. Compartment pressures will not be elevated in other peripheral nerve entrapment syndromes.[6,67]

Compartment syndromes are far more common in the lower extremities of athletes. The athlete will typically complain of increased pain and cramping or weakness with increasing activity. Symptoms subside when activities stop. [6]

MANAGEMENT

Management of acute nerve injuries depends on the location and severity of the injury; specific management of several lesions has already been described in the text. Rest of the injured part as well as anti-inflammatory measures (e.g., appropriate medication and icing) may facilitate the initial stages of healing.[5,22,28,46] Corticosteroid or lidocaine injections may be of some use

therapeutically and in confirming the location of the neural lesion.[51]

Butler[3] advocates early intervention after injury, beginning with mobilization of the structures surrounding the neural tissue. Gentle mobilization of neural tissues should begin away from the site of the lesion, imparting only gentle movement or tensile loads across the injured nerve. The goal of early mobilization is to prevent scarring between the nerve and the nerve bed or within the connective tissue of the nerve itself as the nerve heals. Care must be taken to avoid tensile loads on a nerve if there is acute neurologic loss suggesting the possibility of an axonotmesis or neurotmesis. If the symptoms are more chronic in nature, all of the neural tension tests described previously can be used in various ways as mobilization techniques. The goal of this type of treatment is to improve the mobility of the nerve relative to adjacent tissues and to stretch the connective tissue elements of the nerve to improve its tolerance to tensile forces. The reader is referred to Butler's text[3] for guidelines on the use of these techniques in treatment.

Persistent weakness owing to nerve injury can be addressed with strength training programs.[16,17,23,24] Particular care should be taken to include strengthening exercises that will help to lessen the potential for reinjury. For example, with injuries to the brachial plexus, the muscles of the cervical spine and shoulders must be strengthened to increase resistance to injury.[15,17] The authors recommend that an athlete in high-risk sports should be able to support his or her body with the body at a 45-degree angle from the head (Fig. 23–20). This may be used as a criterion for athletes' preseason physicals as well as for returning to participation.

Muscle imbalances of the shoulder or forearm may lead to poor technique in throwing sports, which puts the athlete at risk for rotator cuff and labral injuries. In addition, as a result of the change in tensile stresses on neural tissues, a number of nerve injuries throughout the shoulder girdle and upper extremity may be exacerbated.[6,28,33,46] Therefore, rehabilitation of the throwing athlete must include appropriate strength training and careful monitoring of technique. Communication among the athletic trainer, physical therapist, and weight training coaches is important to ensure that compensatory techniques during weight training do not promote further muscle imbalances.

Another biomechanical problem in the throwing athlete is ligamentous laxity of the medial collateral ligament at the elbow, in which the increased valgus mobility places excessive stresses on the ulnar nerve in the cubital tunnel. Surgical intervention may be necessary to correct this problem.

Biomechanical factors that contribute to nerve injuries in the lower extremity include excessive pronation of the feet, compressive footwear, or ill-fitting protective clothing. These should be addressed by conservative means as previously indicated.

If conservative measures fail to restore normal neurologic function, then surgery may be indicated to decompress,[6,54,66] transpose,[46,51] or repair a segment of the nerve.[71] The optimal time for repair of most closed nerve injuries is about 3 months after injury.[71] By that time, it is clear whether the nerve will recover spontaneously (neurapraxia), and in the case of a more severe injury (axonotmesis), swelling has had time to decrease. An interdigital neuroma of the foot is often treated successfully by surgical excision.[63] A laceration of a nerve can be surgically repaired immediately.[71]

PREVENTION

By far the most important part of the management of peripheral nerve injuries in athletics is prevention. Protective equipment and splints used in any sport should be carefully padded to avoid compression over vulnerable nerves such as the lateral femoral cutaneous nerve at the inguinal ligament and the peroneal nerve as it passes around the fibular head. Care should also be taken when applying ice over superficial nerves. Bassett et al.[72] reported five cases of cryotherapy-induced nerve injuries. They recommend that ice be applied for no more than 20 minutes at a time and in a manner that cannot compress a peripheral nerve. Green et al.[73] reported long-term peroneal nerve injury in one patient after icing for only 20 minutes. They hypothesized that the injury in this case may have been more severe because of the addition of a compressive wrap over the ice pack and the ectomorphic body type of the athlete. They cautioned that the athlete should be checked 5 to 10 minutes after the ice is applied for signs of paresthesia or numbness distal to the site of application of the ice and compressive wrap.

CONCLUSIONS

The potential for injury to the nervous system occurs every time an ankle ligament is sprained,[67] a shoulder joint dislocates,[28] or a hamstring muscle is torn.[60] Physicians, athletic trainers, coaches, and physical therapists must work to prevent injuries to the peripheral nerves by screening athletes for biomechanical faults, strength deficits, and poor technique for their sports. Careful monitoring of training programs should help to prevent overuse injuries to the musculoskeletal and nervous systems. Early recognition of nerve injuries after any trauma should help to ensure that the athlete receives appropriate acute management, rehabilitation, and advice regarding continued athletic participation.

ACKNOWLEDGMENTS

The authors wish to thank Michael Jhon for assistance in photography for many of the figures in this chapter and Carol Jo Tichenor, MA, PT, for her editorial insights.

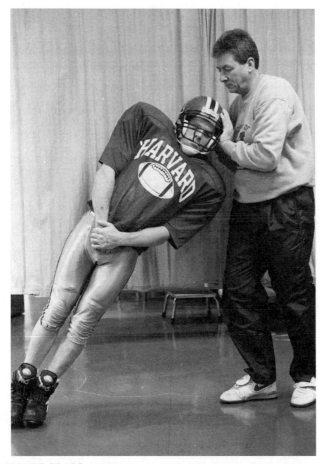

FIGURE 23–20. In an effort to prevent injuries to the cervical spine in sports such as football, the athlete should develop adequate cervical strength to support his body weight at a 45-degree angle in the supine, prone, and side-lying positions while maintaining the head and neck in midline.

REFERENCES

1. Takezawa H, Sudo N, Akoi K, et al: Statistical observation of nerve injuries in athletes (in Japanese). Brain Nerve Injury 1971; 3:11–17.
2. Hirasawa Y, Sakakida K: Sports and peripheral nerve injury. Am J Sports Med 1983; 11:420–426.
3. Butler D: Mobilisation of the Nervous System. New York, Churchill Livingstone, 1991.
4. Seddon HJ: Three types of nerve injury. Brain 1943; 66:237.
5. Posner MA: Compressive neuropathies of the median and radial nerves at the elbow. Clin Sports Med 1990; 9:343–363.
6. Black KP, Lombardo JA: Suprascapular nerve injuries with isolated paralysis of the infraspinatus. Am J Sports Med 1990; 18:225–228.
7. Upton ARM, McComas AJ: The double crush in nerve entrapment syndromes. Lancet 1973; 2:359–362.
8. McMellan DL, Swash M: Longitudinal sliding of the median nerve during movements of the upper limb. J Neurol Neurosurg Psychiatry 1976; 39:566–570.
9. Clancey WG, Brand RL, Bergfield JA: Upper trunk brachial plexus injuries in contact sports. Am J Sports Med 1977; 5:209–214.
10. Markey KL, Di Benedetto M, Curl WW: Upper trunk brachial plexopathy: The stinger syndrome. Am J Sports Med 1993; 21:650–655.
11. Albright JP, McAuley E, Martin RK, et al: Head and neck injuries in college football: An eight year analysis. Am J Sports Med 1985; 13:147–152.
12. Bateman JE: Nerve injuries about the shoulder in sports. J Bone Joint Surg 1967; 49A:785–792.
13. Watkins, RG: Neck injuries in football players. Clin Sports Med 1986; 5:215–246.
14. Christman OD, Snook GA, Stanitis JM, et al: Lateral flexion injuries in athletic competition. JAMA 1965; 192:117–119.
15. Speer KP and Bassett FH: The prolonged burner syndrome. Am J Sports Med 1990; 18:591–594.
16. Garrick J, Webb D: Sports Injuries: Diagnosis and Management. Philadelphia, WB Saunders, 1990.
17. Harrelson GL: Evaluation of brachial plexus injuries. Sports Med Update 1989; 4(4):3–8.
18. Mendell JR: The nervous system. In Strauss RH (ed): Sports Medicine. Philadelphia, WB Saunders, 1989.
19. Meyer SA, Schulte KR, Callagnan JJ, et al: Cervical spinal stenosis and stingers in college football players. Am J Sports Med 1994; 22:158–166.
20. Funk FJ, Wells RE: Injuries of the cervical spine in football. Clin Orthop 1975; 109:50–58.
21. Wroble RR, Albright JP: Neck and low back injuries in wrestling. Clin Sports Med 1986; 5:295–325.
22. Hershman EB: Brachial plexus injuries. Clin Sports Med 1990; 9:311–329.
23. Wroble R, Hoegh J, Albright J: Wrestling in sports medicine. In Reider B (ed): The School Aged Athlete. Philadelphia, WB Saunders, 1992.
24. Hershman EB, Wilbourn AJ, Bergfeld JA: Acute brachial neuropathy in athletes. Am J Sports Med 1989; 17:655–659.
25. Wilbourn AJ: Electrodiagnostic testing of neurologic injuries in athletes. Clin Sports Med 1990; 9:229–245.
26. Karas SE: Thoracic outlet syndrome. Clin Sports Med 1990; 9:297–310.
27. Bojanic I, Pecina MM, Markiewitz AD: Tunnel syndrome in athletes. In Pecina MM, Krmptoti E, Nemanic JL, Markiewitz AD (eds): Tunnel syndromes. Boca Raton, FL, CRC Press, 1991.
28. Mendoza FX, Main K: Peripheral nerve injuries of the shoulder in the athlete. Clin Sports Med 1990; 9:331–342.
29. Vegso JJ, Torg E, Torg JS: Rehabilitation of cervical spine, brachial plexus and peripheral nerve injuries. Clin Sports Med 1987; 6:135–158.
30. White SM, Witten CM: Long thoracic nerve palsy in a professional ballet dancer. Am J Sports Med 1993; 21(4):626–628.
31. Richards RR, Hudson AR, Bertoia JT, et al: Injury to the brachial plexus during Putti-Platt and Bristow procedures. Am J Sports Med 1987; 15:374–380.
32. Ringel SP, Treihaft M, Carry M, et al: Suprascapular neuropathy in pitchers. Am J Sports Med 1990; 18:80–86.
33. Liverson JA, Bronson MJ, Pollack MA: Suprascapular nerve lesions at the spinoglenoid notch: Report of three cases and review of the literature. J Neurol Neurosurg Psychiatry 1991; 54:241–243.
34. Fleisig GS, Dillman CJ, Andrews JR: A biomechanical description of the shoulder joint during pitching. Sports Med Update 1991; Fall/Winter:10–15.
35. Bartosh RA, Dugdale TW, Nielsen R: Isolated musculocutaneous nerve injury complicating closed fracture of the clavicle: A case report. Am J Sports Med 1992; 20(3):356–359.
36. Chusid JG: Correlative Neuroanatomy and Functional Neurology. 17th ed. Los Altos, CA, Lange Medical Publications, 1979.
37. Mitsunaga MM, Nakano K: High radial nerve palsy following strenuous muscular activity, Clin Orthop 1988; 234:39–42.
38. Hoffman DF: Elbow dislocations: Avoiding complications. Phys Sports Med 1993; 21(11):56–67.
39. Lutz FR: Radial tunnel syndrome: An etiology of chronic lateral elbow pain. JOSPT 1991; 14:14–17.
40. Gunn CC, Milbrandt WE: Tennis elbow and the cervical spine. Can Med J 1976; 8:803–809.
41. Elvey R: The clinical relevance of signs of adverse brachial plexus tension. In Proceedings: International Federation of Manipulative Therapists Congress, Cambridge, England, 1988.
42. Yaxley GA, Jull GA: A modified upper limb tension test—an investigation of responses in normal subjects. Aust J Physiother 1991; 37:143–152.
43. Yaxley GA, Jull GA: Adverse tension in the neural system. A preliminary study of tennis elbow. Aust J Physiother 1993; 39:15–22.
44. Stewart JD, Aguayo AJ: Compression and entrapment neuropathies. In Dyck PJ, Thomas PK, Lambert EH, Bunge R (eds): Peripheral Neuropathy. Vol II. Philadelphia, WB Saunders, 1984.
45. Allman FL: Overuse Injury in the throwing sports. In Torg J, Welsh RP, Shepherd RJ (eds): Current Therapy and Sports Medicine. Vol 2. Philadelphia, BC Decker, 1985.
46. Glousman RE: Ulnar nerve problems in the athlete's elbow. Clin Sports Med 1990; 9:365–377.
47. Pechan J, Julis I: The pressure measurement in the ulnar nerve. A contribution to the pathophysiology of the cubital tunnel syndrome. J Biomech 1975; 8:75–79.
48. Buehler MJ, Thayer DT: The elbow flexion test: A clinical test for the cubital tunnel syndrome. Clin Orthop 1988; 233:213–216.
49. Flanagan M, Bell A: The normal response to the ulnar nerve bias upper limb tension test. Poster presentation. Manipulative Physiotherapy Association of Australia, 8th Biennial Conference, Perth, West Australia, 1993.
50. Drye C: The upper limb tension test 3: An investigation of the intrarater and interrater reliability and the subjective response to the test. Unpublished master's thesis. MGH Institute of Health Professions, Boston, MA, 1993. Copyright Caroline Drye, 1993.
51. Rettig AC, Ebben JR: Anterior subcutaneous transfer of the ulnar nerve in the athlete. Am J Sports Med 1993; 21(6):836–840.
52. Fernald D: Incidence of upper extremity "overuse" injuries in elite cyclists. Unpublished master's thesis. MGH Institute of Health Professions, Boston, MA, 1988.
53. Mellion MB: Common cycling injuries: Management and prevention. Sports Med 1991; 11:52–70.
54. Rettig AC: Neurovascular injuries in the wrists and hands of athletes. Clin Sports Med 1990; 9:389–417.
55. Murray-Leslie CF, Wright V: Carpal tunnel syndrome, humeral epicondylitis, and the cervical spine: A study of clinical and dimensional relations. Br Med J 1976; 1:1439–1442.
56. Kenneally M, Rubenach H, Elvey R: The upper limb tension test: The SLR test of the arm. Clin Phys Ther 1988; 17:167–194.
57. Richards J: The upper limb tension test 2: An investigation of the responses and reliability in testing asymptomatic subjects. Unpublished thesis. University of Alabama, Birmingham, AL, 1991.
58. Puranen J, Orava S: The hamstring syndrome. Am J Sports Med 1988; 16:517–521.
59. Maitland GD: The slump test: Examination and treatment. Aust J Physiother 1985; 31(6):215–219.
60. Kornberg C, Lew P: The effect of stretching neural structures on grade I hamstring injuries. JOSPT 1989; June:481–487.
61. Ekelund AL: Bilateral nerve entrapment in the popliteal space. Am J Sports Med 1990; 18:108.

62. Jackson DL, Haglund B: Tarsal tunnel syndrome in athletes. Am J Sports Med 1991; 19:61–65.

63. Schon LC, Baxter DE: Neuropathies of the foot and ankle in athletes. Clin Sports Med 1990; 9:489–509.

64. Johnson ER, Kirby K, Lieberman JS: Lateral plantar nerve entrapment: Foot pain in a power lifter. Am J Sports Med 1992; 20(5):619–620.

65. Nobel W: Peroneal palsy due to hematoma in the common peroneal nerve sheath after distal torsional fractures and inversion ankle sprains. J Bone Joint Surg 1966; 48A(8):1484–1495.

66. Leach RE, Purnell MB, Saito A: Peroneal nerve entrapment in runners. Am J Sports Med 1989; 17(2):287–291.

67. Nitz AJ, Dobner JJ, Kersey D: Nerve injury and grades II and III ankle sprains. Am J Sports Med 1985; 13:177–182.

68. Sammarco GJ, Stephens MM: Neuropraxia of the femoral nerve in a modern dancer. Am J Sports Med 1991; 19:413–414.

69. Arthornthurasook A, Gaew-Im K: The sartorial nerve: Its relationships to the medial aspect of the knee. Am J Sports Med 1990; 18:41–42.

70. Leffert R: Clinical diagnosis, testing, and electromyographic study in brachial plexus traction injuries. Clin Orthop 1988; 237:24–31.

71. Elul BL: Treatment of traumatic peripheral nerve injuries. Am Fam Pract 1991; 43:897–905.

72. Bassett FH, Kirkpatrick JS, Engelhardt DL, Malone T: Cryotherapy-induced nerve injury. Am J Sports Med 1992; 20(5):516–518.

73. Green GA, Zachazewski JE, Jordan SE: Peroneal nerve palsy induced by cryotherapy. Phys Sports Med 1989; 17(9):66–70.

CHAPTER 24

Injuries to the Thoracolumbar Spine and Pelvis

DANIEL A. DYREK MS, PT
LYLE J. MICHELI MD, FAAOS, FACSM
DAVID J. MAGEE BPT, PhD

Many clinicians view injury to the spine in sports as not so much an athletic injury as a orthopaedic injury. Seldom is an injury to this area seen in a similar light as a medial collateral ligament sprain or a hamstring strain. However, these injuries do occur to athletes; reports in the literature show that 10 to 50 percent of athletes suffer a back injury during their sporting career, depending on the sport.[1] Athletes often do not complain of low back pain unless it limits their performance, because they often consider low back pain to be a common and normal result of training. These so-called nontraumatic back problems are often the result of poor posture or poor body mechanics, similar to those seen in the general population. In addition, there are other predisposing factors that may lead to injury to the thoracolumbopelvic region.[2] These may include intrinsic or extrinsic factors as shown in Table 24–1. Some of these intrinsic factors may be age related, inherited, or acquired. Extrinsic factors may include sport-specific demands, cumulative overload, and training errors.[3,4] In addition, the athlete who already has a spinal anomaly, which is common, can be put at further risk of injury.[3,5,6] Such predisposing spinal conditions include scoliosis, spondylolysis, and spondylolisthesis; lumbosacral asymmetry; excessive lumbar lordosis or poor posture; poor reciprocal muscle strength of the muscles controlling the pelvis and spine; degenerative disc disease (spondylosis); spina bifida occulta; facet tropisms; and Scheuermann's disease. However, traumatic injuries involving high-velocity microtrauma or macrotrauma may set the athlete apart from the general population. In addition, some sports have a higher potential for causing spinal injury. For example, equestrian sports, weight lifting, gymnastics, jogging, water ski jumping, and aerobics impose higher than normal vertical loading forces on the spine. Sports such as diving, football, gymnastics, hockey, aerobics, and high jumping (especially using the "Fosbury flop" technique) put extensive flexion-extension force loads on the spine, particularly the lumbar spine. Sports such as aerobics, golf, and racket sports cause increased rotational forces to be applied to the thoracic and lower spine as well as the pelvis.[3]

Thus, numerous intrinsic and extrinsic factors contribute to injuries within the thoracolumbopelvic region. The clinician must suspect all possible contributions during the examination process. The injury may have a slow, insidious onset, as in the endurance athlete, or a sudden onset secondary to a high-energy lesion of known cause, such as a spinal injury resulting from a collision of two hockey players. Basically, when injuries of the neuromusculoskeletal system occur in sports, they are the result of a deficit in the tissue deformation characteristics of the involved structure. This deficit can be the result of insufficient strength of the passive connective tissue component of the structure of the muscle–tendon unit. The deficit results in the inability to sustain or generate sufficient tissue strength to

465

TABLE 24–1
Intrinsic and Extrinsic Predisposing Factors to Thoracolumbar Pathology

Intrinsic Factors	Extrinsic Factors
Scoliosis	Environment (e.g., competing surfaces)
Spondylolysis	Equipment
Lumbosacral asymmetry	Technique/biomechanics of activity
Excessive lumbar lordosis	Speed of activity
Obesity	Society demands (e.g., win at all costs, aggressiveness,
Spondylosis (degenerative disc disease)	"he-man" attitude)
Muscle imbalance (especially of muscles controlling the	Load applied
pelvis)	Range of motion/flexibility required of the activity
Hypomobility	Overuse
Hypermobility	Coaching
Spinal anomalies	Cumulative overload (training errors)
Scheuermann's disease	Low- or high-energy trauma
Athlete's size	
Growth spurt	
Age and age-related changes	
Disease	
Leg length inequality	
Deconditioning	

withstand the load or stress created within a structure, which subsequently leads to injury.

The thoracolumbopelvic region serves an important dual role in the transmission of loads within the body, providing stability to support the weight of the upper body during upper extremity function while simultaneously providing sufficient mobility and stability to absorb and transmit ground reaction forces from the lower extremities. It is this simultaneous dual role that renders the region especially susceptible to injuries during sporting activities.

EPIDEMIOLOGY

In a review of the literature, Alexander concluded that the type of injury to the thoracolumbopelvic region depended on the direction, magnitude, and point of application of the force to the spine.[7] He found that the most common types of low back injuries were muscle strains, ligament sprains, lumbovertebral fractures, intervertebral disc injuries, and neural arch fractures. Sward et al.[8] reported that athletes who put great demands on their backs were prone to increased risk of symptomatic damage to the spine. Tall and DeVault[1] estimated that the incidence of spinal injury in sports was 10 to 15 percent. Of these, 0.6 to 1.0 percent had associated neurologic involvement. The most common serious injury was determined to be the neural arch fracture or spondylolysis involving the pars interarticularis. The sports that represent the greatest risk to low back pain were gymnastics (spinal extension loading), weight lifting (high magnitude of shear loads on the spine), and football (sudden application of hyperextension loads, as experienced by a lineman).

Jackson et al.[9] reported an 11 percent incidence of pars interarticularis defects and a 6 percent incidence of spondylolisthesis in female gymnasts. This incidence was four times that expected in a general white female population and about two times higher than that expected in a general young male population. Other studies have shown an increase in spinal anomalies, including abnormalities of the anterior portion of the vertebral ring apophysis, that occurred only in athletes, especially gymnasts and wrestlers.[10] The incidence of these anomalies increases with increased age.[11]

Ohlen et al.[12] reported that increased lordosis as measured with an inclinometer was an indication of potential low back pain. They found that female gymnasts suffering from low back pain tended to have an increased lordosis relative to those who complained of no stiffness or low back pain. However, a correlation between total lumbar mobility and low back pain was not demonstrated. Likewise, Kirby et al.[13] reported no correlation between flexibility and symptomatology of low back pain.

Weight lifting, regardless of whether the individual is simply lifting a weight or object or participating in weight lifting as a sport, increases the load on the spine and, thus, the potential for injury. Brown and Kimball[14] reported that 50 percent of all injuries in teenage powerlifters were low back injuries. The increased load (up to six to ten times body weight) may be due to the biomechanical forces applied in lifting the load itself, the rise in intra-abdominal pressure during the lifting, or both, and often depends on the technique used.[15–17] In fact, if the lower back has been injured, the rise in intra-abdominal pressure may be greater than normal, making a more significant contribution to the pain.[15] Several studies[18–20] have reported that the use of a weight belt enables the athlete to increase intra-abdominal pressure, thus adding support to the trunk and enabling the abdominal cavity to take up to 50 percent of the load.[20] It may also reduce the compressive force on the disc and thus make lifting safer.[19] Without the weight belt, rise in intra-abdominal pressure is dependent on proper coordinated action among the diaphragm, oblique abdominal muscles, and pelvic floor muscles.[21]

When examining football players, Semon and Sprengler[22] reported that 27 percent of college football linemen had low back pain at some time in their career, with 57 percent having mild transient symptoms. In addition, 43 percent of 506 players studied had some radiographic findings of degeneration in the lumbar spine, with 12 athletes having spondylolysis and two having grade 1 spondylolisthesis. Semon and Sprengler concluded, however, that skeletally mature football players were able to successfully take part in football despite having lumbar spondylolysis, as slipping was seen more commonly in the skeletally immature. McCarroll et al.[23] reported in a prospective x-ray study of 145 freshmen that 13 percent of college football athletes had positive radiographic findings for spondylolysis or spondylolisthesis, and 21 percent had low back pain. They found that 16 athletes had spondylolysis and six had spondylolisthesis, primarily a grade 1, at L5–S1. However, only 2.4 percent developed spondylolysis while playing college football. They believed the cause of the low back pain was repetitive shear stress from blocking, which caused an extension type injury. In addition, they found five athletes with spina bifida occulta, eight with transitional vertebrae (two with low back pain), and three with degenerative disc disease (two with low back pain). It is interesting to note that most of these individuals had spinal anomalies and no obvious symptoms. This finding has been supported by other studies that showed the presence of scoliosis, S1 lumbarization, L5 sacralization, anomalous ribs, spondylolysis, and spina bifida occulta.[24] These investigators also believed that weight lifting and other training techniques could contribute to the low back pain.

Gymnastics, weight lifting, and football are not the only sports in which athletes complain of back pain. Just as the general population suffers back pain from activity, so do athletes. For example, it has been shown that the majority of joggers, cross-country skiers, and tennis players complain of some low back pain.[25–27] Several studies have shown that running activities decrease the vertical height of the spinal column regardless of age.[28–31] This loss in height, which results in potential transient functional instability of the spine, combined with the flexibility often seen in athletes' spines and a lack of good muscular control of the pelvis and spine, may explain the symptoms of low back pain in these individuals.

Only a very weak positive association between disc herniation and participation in sports has been demonstrated.[32,33] Some authors[34] believe that weight lifting by football linemen rather than playing football is the cause of lost playing time, at least in some cases. Perhaps a contributing factor is the greater weights generally lifted by linemen, or the problem may lie in the type of training rather than participation in the sport itself. In one study, if other spinal problems (for example, Scheuermann's disease, spondylolysis) were present, secondary disc degeneration was evident, especially in older athletes.[33] Degeneration due to aging can contribute to the low back pain experienced by athletes in the long term.[35,36]

Although less frequently studied than the spine, the pelvis has been shown to contribute to low back pain in athletes. A case report of four athletes illustrated sports-related stress reactions of the sacroiliac joint as diagnosed by bone scintigraphy.[37] The athletes represented the sports of tennis, track, and shot putting, with one individual participating in gymnastics and ballet. Cross-country skiers have demonstrated sacroiliac joint dysfunction that was thought to be the result of asymmetric ski-skating techniques utilized in the sport.[27]

Lloyd-Smith et al.[38] reported that the most common pelvic injuries seen in their study of 204 patients were sacroiliac sprains (10.3 percent), pelvic and femoral neck stress fractures (8.1 percent), and osteitis pubis (6.3 percent). Most of these injuries were seen in runners, and the largest percentage (82 percent) were due to overuse. They believed the sacroiliac sprain was due to poor hip muscle control, especially the abductors and adductors, leading to excessive up-and-down tilt of the pelvis and increasing the shearing stress on the sacroiliac joints.

ASSESSMENT

The thoracolumbopelvic region can be visualized as having anterior, posterior, superior, and inferior boundaries. The lumbar spine, at a minimum, should be considered to extend superiorly to the T10 or T11 segment and inferiorly to include the sacrum, sacroiliac joints, and symphysis pubis, based on segmental innervation patterns of the spine, spinal mechanics, and continuous innervation patterns of spinal nerves within the region. Similarly, the thoracic spine assessment must include the lower cervical spine and upper lumbar spine. The segmental innervation pattern of the spine is complex and involves an overlapping pattern of the posterior primary rami with neighboring segments. The posterior primary rami can innervate as many as two segments above and up to three segments below the segment of origin. For example, the posterior primary rami arising from the T12–L1 segment will innervate in a proximal direction to the T10–T11 segment and distally to the L3–L4 segment. Therefore, the clinician must consider examining the lower thoracic segments as well as the lumbar spine when the athlete presents with low back pain, as the T10–T11 segment is capable of referring pain to the more distal area.

The spinal biomechanics of the distal thoracic spine are similar to those of the lumbar spine owing to the orientation of the posterior zygapophyseal or facet joints. The middle and superior lumbar segments have their facet joint orientation in the sagittal plane. This pattern continues into the lower thoracic spine until the more distal joint or transitional level of the thoracic spine is reached, where the facet joints assume a coronal-oblique orientation. Although the typical transition segment for this change in facet orientation occurs at the T11–T12 level, the change can occur at the T10–T11 level.[39,40] Therefore, because facet orientation influences that quantity of the different segmental motions that exist, the inferior thoracic levels function similar to the lumbar spine.[39,41] Also, related to the above discussion, a key "stress junction" exists at the junction of the mobile thoracolumbar spine and the more stable thoracic spine along with its associated ribs, predisposing this area to injury in a similar fashion to the stress junction that occurs between the lumbar spine and the sacrum. Likewise, in the upper thoracic spine, which is relatively stable because of the ribs, there is a transition from the stable thoracic spine to the more mobile cervical spine.

The origin of superficial cutaneous nerves that arise from the inferior thoracic region to travel into the lumbopelvic area must be recognized as creating the potential for a thoracic lesion that refers symptoms to common locations for low back pain. These nerves, sometimes referred to as the *cluneal nerves,* are extensions of the lateral branches of the posterior primary ramus arising from T11, T12, and L1 and may also receive contributions from the T10 and L2 nerves.[41] These nerves form anterior, posterior, and lateral branches in the periphery. The anterior branch extends laterally and inferiorly from its origin to innervate the dermis within the inguinal area; the posterior branch descends to the posterior iliac crest, where it innervates the dermis of the posterosuperior buttock; and the lateral branch innervates the region of the greater trochanter. Because the posterior primary ramus innervates the paravertebral tissues and facet joints of the thoracic region, lesions within that area can refer symptoms to the distal sites of the dermal innervation. Therefore, the clinician must be aware of the potential contribution of the inferior thoracic segments to symptoms in the lumbopelvic complex. Likewise, the cervical spine (see Chapter 21) may be the cause of symptoms in the upper thoracic spine, referring pain into the scapular and chest region. In the cervical region, the dorsal scapular nerve arises from the fifth cervical nerve (the C4–C5 segment) and extends distally to the thoracic paravertebral region, where it innervates the rhomboid muscle.[40] The clinician must differentiate pain in the rhomboid muscle area as being pain from the myotendon unit itself, referred pain from a C4–C5 segmental lesion creating the radiculopathy, pain from another underlying muscle, or pain of ligamentous or articular origin.[42] Although less commonly involved, the long thoracic nerve, arising from the fifth, sixth, and sometimes the seventh cervical nerves to innervate the serratus anterior muscle, may be involved when dysfunction of the serratus anterior results in pain within the posterior scapular region of the thorax. Therefore, the C4–C5, C5–C6, and C6–C7 segments will require, at a minimum, examination to thoroughly assess all origins of thoracic symptoms.

Further definition of the boundaries requires consideration of the superior aspect of the region—in other words, the upper thoracic spine. The thoracic region proper can be considered to extend from the level of the transitional mortise segment at which point the true ribs

T1–T10 are present, superiorly to the T1–T2 segment. The presence of the ribs with their costovertebral and costosternal articulations and accompanying musculature provide for a stable thoracic region. The amount of segmental mobility of the thoracic region proper is generally less than that of the neighboring cervical and thoracolumbar spinal regions.[39] The junctions of the mobile superior cervical and inferior thoracolumbar regions with the stable thoracic region create stress on the surrounding tissues and structures, which commonly results in lesions at these locations. The clinician, however, must not be misled into thinking that the thoracic region proper is so stable that it is a nonmobile area and therefore not capable of producing signs and symptoms. The region requires a thorough examination, just like other spinal regions.

The posterior wall of the thoracolumbopelvic region should be considered to be the skin. The dermal tissue is capable of developing mechanical deformation impairments secondary to underlying dysfunction and requires examination as a component of the region and treatment when it is found to contribute to the patient's diagnosis.[39,43,44] The anterolateral wall of the region is the abdominal musculature, which must be considered to function in concert with the intrinsic transversospinal muscles, the erector spinae muscles, and the thoracolumbar fascia with its muscle attachments.[44,45] The integrated function of these groups provides dynamic stability and mobility to the region.[46] The inferior portion of the region is the pelvis, including the hip articulations and accompanying soft tissue.

The lowest common denominator at which one can examine and manage injuries involving the spine is the functional segmental unit (FSU). The FSU is defined as the inferior half of the superior vertebra combined with the superior half of the inferior vertebra and includes all tissue within these boundaries (Fig. 24–1). The FSU can be further delineated into an anterior and posterior column. The anterior column comprises the vertebral

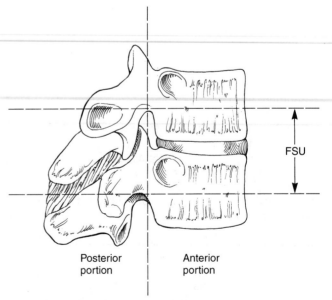

FIGURE 24–1. Functional segmental unit (FSU).

TABLE 24–2
Motions, Axes, Types, and Locations of Loads on the Functional Segmental Unit (FSU)

Segmental Spinal Motion	Axis	Type and Location of Load
Forward bend	Junction of middle ⅓ to posterior ⅓ of disc	Compression on anterior ⅔ of anterior FSU column Tensile load on posterior ⅓ of anterior FSU column and on tissues and structures of the entire posterior column
Backward bend	Junction of middle ⅓ to posterior ⅓ of disc	Tensile load on anterior ⅔ of anterior FSU column Compression load on posterior ⅓ of anterior FSU column and on structures of the entire posterior column
Lateral side bend*	Junction of the lateral ⅓ to middle ⅓ of disc on the convex side of the lateral side bend	Compression on the ⅔ of the anterior column and the posterior column on the concave side of the motion Tensile load on the ⅓ of the anterior column and on the posterior column on the convex side of the motion
Rotation*	Junction of the middle ⅓ to posterior ⅓ of the disc	Compression of the anterior column, primarily the intervertebral disc, and on the posterior column on the side opposite of the rotation Tensile load on tissues of the posterior column on the ipsilateral side of the rotation

*Lateral side bend and rotation will occur together as coupling motions in the spinal segment.

body, cartilaginous end-plate, intervertebral disc, and anterior and posterior longitudinal ligaments. The posterior column comprises the pars interarticularis, zygapophyseal (facet) joints, spinous and transverse processes, the associated musculotendinous units of the paravertebral region, and the ligamenta flava and the supraspinous and interspinous ligaments. The central canal with its spinal cord or cauda equina (depending on the spinal level under consideration), dura, and blood vessels, belongs to both the anterior and posterior columns, as it is subjected to the influence from both areas.

The FSU provides a model for understanding loads or stresses placed on tissues that result in injury. The anterior and posterior columns of the FSU provide a reference point to understand where and what type of load is being placed on the tissues and the structures of the segment during normal motions. The clinician can then extrapolate from this understanding to interpret the nature of the injury. Table 24–2 identifies the types of spinal motion, the axes on which they occur, and the basic interpretation of the locations and types of load they place on the FSU. For example, trunk flexion creates a forward bending movement at the segmental level and places a compression load on the anterior intervertebral disc, cartilaginous end-plate, and vertebral body and a tensile load on the posterior wall of the disc. It produces primarily a tensile load to the tissues and structures of the posterior column. Thus, the load could create a compression fracture of the vertebral body and/or a strain of the posterior intrinsic myotendinous units of the spinal segment. The clinician must have a detailed understanding of spinal biomechanics to successfully make clinical decisions regarding the diagnosis and management of the athletic patient.[39,41,46–49]

The key to a clinical diagnosis for the spectrum of injuries occurring in the thoracolumbopelvic region is (1) recognition of the important points related by the athlete in the history, (2) identification of precipitating or perpetuating factors, and (3) careful examination and palpation of the structures generating the pain.[50] The clinician must approach the physical examination of the thoracolumbopelvic region with the goal of examining each tissue and structure of the region to the maximum extent allowed by current knowledge, physical examination skills, medical imaging, and laboratory tests. Physical examination of the thoracolumbopelvic region in the athlete is a challenging process, because the clinician must be prepared to examine for a wide spectrum of potential lesions and across several regions. For example, to properly assess the region, gait as well as leg length must be assessed to determine if these or other factors are causing or leading to problems in the spine or pelvis. A clinician can be challenged by identifying the source of the problems; sources range from the obvious findings of a gross neural lesion resulting in compromise of myotome strength, sensory loss, and absence of deep tendon reflexes to more obscure, subtle findings in the neuromusculoskeletal system, such as a contracture of the adductors of the hip or hypomobility in the ribs, that may be responsible for the pain or impaired function. The clinician is further challenged in the examination process by considering the natural sequelae of degenerative events, so common in the athlete, that can follow the initial stimulus of a neuromusculoskeletal lesion. The clinician must screen for premorbid impairments that may have predisposed the region to injury and enabled the current complaint to evolve. In addition, although the athlete has many potential athletic sources of injuries to the thoracolumbopelvic region, the clinician must also be aware that back pain, especially if it is progressive and worse at night, may be due to other, more insidious causes. With these symptoms, the clinician must also consider tumors or infection as potential causes.[51]

The primary factors to be included in assessment are the mode of onset, primary etiology of the chief complaint, the diagnosis, the stage of symptoms, and contributing factors to the primary etiology; once these have been identified, prognosis and therapeutic measures and the projected duration and frequency of treatment can be determined.[52]

The goal of the examination process is to determine a diagnosis that will explain the cause of the athlete's complaints. The diagnosis is an integration of normal and abnormal findings to establish a specific identification of the source of the patient's primary complaint.[53,54] The purpose of the diagnosis is to (1) identify the specific lesion responsible for the chief complaints; (2) assess the integrity and performance of the involved tissues and structures; and (3) determine the athlete's functional ability to perform daily training, competition, and occupational activities. A detailed description of examination of the thoracolumbar and pelvic regions can be found elsewhere.[53–55] However, there are specific points regarding assessment that the clinician must especially be aware of. For example, in a normal population, when performing the straight-leg raise or testing for the Lasègue sign, maximum deformation of the nerve roots normally occurs before 70 degrees.[55] However, in hypermobile athletes, true positive symptoms when performing this test may not be seen until 90 to 120 degrees of hip flexion.[56] Thus, the clinician should not assume that pain in the 90- to 120-degree range is only the result of hamstring tightness. Leg pain in this range should be tested with neck flexion and/or foot dorsiflexion to rule out a neural cause.

The position of the pelvis plays a major role in determining the forces and stresses that will be applied to the thoracolumbopelvic region. If the lumbar spine is properly "balanced" on the pelvis and the pelvis is properly "balanced" on the legs through the hips with sufficient spinal segmental and pelvic articular alignment and mobility, and good reciprocal muscle strength and flexibility of the flexor (abdominals and iliopsoas) and extensor muscles of the spine, as well as good mobility and strength of the hamstring and hip flexors (iliopsoas and rectus femoris), then the forces and stresses applied to the spine will be less (Fig. 24–2).[40,57] If, however, the load on or posture of the spine is altered (for example, increased lordosis in the lumbar spine or increased kyphosis in the thoracic spine), then the load placed on the spine will increase with various athletic activities.

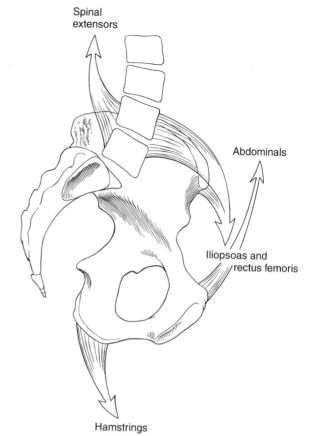

FIGURE 24–2. Muscles "balancing" the pelvis.

Radiographic examination involves plain radiographs (anteroposterior [AP], lateral, and oblique views) to ensure visualization of the transverse processes, spinous processes, disc spaces, vertebral body, pedicles, laminae, facet joints, and pars interarticularis. In some cases, motion (flexion-extension) views may be taken if instability is suspected. The clinician should also watch for congenital anomalies such as spina bifida occulta, facet asymmetry, and transitional vertebra.[58] Bone scans or radionuclide imaging may be used if a stress fracture or stress reaction is suspected.[59] Computed tomography (CT) is best for assessing bony configuration and structure and can be used along with magnetic resonance imaging (MRI) to visualize soft tissue such as ligaments, discs, nerve roots, and fat.[59] Both of these last two techniques should be used primarily to confirm the diagnosis, not as a tool for primary diagnosis.[2,60] Interestingly, disc herniations visible on MRI may not be pathologic, and care must be taken when noting their occurrence. Often more than one MRI must be taken over time to show any changes (expansion or contraction) in the disc, which may then require a modification in treatment.

The physical examination process culminates with the identification of the source — that is, the diagnosis of the athlete's complaints of pain and functional limitations. Secondary contributing factors to the primary diagnosis that will affect the management of the athlete should be included in the assessment. The assessment is a correlation of the normal and abnormal examination findings compared against a knowledge base of possible etiologies that would explain the athlete's symptoms and problems.

The establishment of a prognosis will be assisted by determining the length of time since the onset of symptoms or recurrence of trauma in the athlete's presentation in the clinic. The prognosis is more favorable when less time has lapsed between the initial onset and the seeking of medical attention so the sequelae of musculoskeletal lesions have less time to evolve. Also, the variables of mode of onset, extent and type of tissue involvement, tissue reactivity, effective prior treatment, and clarity of the diagnosis will affect the formulation of a prognosis.

INJURIES TO THE THORACIC SPINE

Injuries to the thoracic spine are rare in sports, although fractures, primarily the compression type, may be seen. Orthopaedic conditions, however, can affect sports participation but should not necessarily preclude it. For example, an individual who has scoliosis may take part in noncontact sports if he or she wears a brace and the activity is within the ability of the athlete. After scoliosis surgery, any contact sports or sports involving violent rotation should be attempted only if cleared by the surgeon. If the athlete has Scheuermann's disease in the active phase, activity should be decreased or stopped until the active phase has passed.

INJURIES TO THE STERNUM

Injuries to the sternum are relatively rare in sports except in high-speed sports such as automobile racing. The lower portion of the sternum is more flexible and has more "give" than the upper portion. Manubriosternal dislocations from a direct blow (for example, from a football helmet or elbow) have been reported and are often accompanied by forced flexion of the cervicothoracic junction.[61–64] Contusions to the sternum can also occur from a direct blow and are sometimes associated with rib fractures.[61] Stress fractures of the sternum have also been reported.[65] A fracture or fracture-dislocation may be distinguished from a simple contusion by inspiration that is painful and is accompanied by anterior chest wall pain. Crepitus and deformity may also be present. On palpation, the deformity or "step-off" may be evident. With these severe injuries, the clinician must always be aware of the possibility of pulmonary contusion, pneumothorax, or vascular injury.[61]

RIB INJURIES

The true ribs, T1 through T10, have anterior and posterior articulations that can be responsible for clinical signs and symptoms. Given the high-energy trauma (e.g., boarding in hockey, piling on in football and rugby) some athletes are exposed to during training and competition, the ribs and their articulations should be considered a source of pain and functional impairment. Each true rib has an anterior costal cartilage that extends to the sternum. The junction of the osseous portion of the rib with its cartilage is the costochondral junction; this is covered with periosteum.[40] Given the "articulation" of the osseous rib with the cartilage and the resulting difference in deformation characteristics, this junction is subject to trauma and can produce symptoms. The anterior articulations of the costal cartilage with the sternum, referred to as the *sternocostal joints,* are of mixed types.[40] Each rib articulating with the sternum has a cartilaginous extension of the bone connecting with the sternum. The articulation of the costal cartilage of the first rib to the sternum is a synchondrosis, whereas the remaining true ribs articulate as synovial joints.

Two posterior rib articulations with the vertebra exist: the costotransverse joint (the articulation of the rib with the transverse process) and the costovertebral joint (the articulation of the rib with the posterolateral border of two adjacent vertebral bodies and the intervertebral disc). An exception exists for the first, tenth, eleventh, and twelfth ribs, which articulate with a single vertebra.[40] The costotransverse and costovertebral articulations have fibrous capsules and numerous ligaments that provide the area with stability.[66,67] However, the region remains susceptible to trauma resulting in soft tissue strains and sprains. Horner[68] reported that stress fractures of the lower ribs can occur from overexertion, and in some cases, pain is referred into the low back.

Differential diagnosis of rib abnormality can be made with a careful history, localized tenderness over the ribs, and pain on respiration, a sign not often seen with true low back pain. The intercostal musculature must also be considered as a source of symptoms. The musculotendinous unit could be a source of pain and dysfunction owing to an intrinsic lesion, such as a strain or adhesion, or it could be a secondary source of symptoms accompanying a primary sprain of the posterior costovertebral and costotransverse joints.[69,70] Pain originating from the rib articulations tends to follow the course of the rib.

Like rib–vertebra injuries, costochondral or sternochondral separations are usually caused by a sharp, direct blow; a sudden twisting; rib cage compression; or the arm being pulled to one side, stretching the costochondral junction.[71] Signs and symptoms include possible deformity caused by overriding of bone or cartilage; sharp pain at the site, especially on inspiration and movement; point tenderness; and possible popping or clicking.[72] Interestingly, these injuries often take longer to heal than true rib (bone) fractures, as the blood supply to the costal cartilage is not as plentiful as that to the bone.

Rib fractures generally occur from the same mechanisms of injury that cause costochondral separations.[73] Fractures usually occur at the weakest point (posterior angle). They may also occur as stress fractures from chronic overload[74–80] or from repeated pulling of the serratus anterior muscle.[74,78] Thus, scapular control exercises can play a large part in the rehabilitation process for this injury. Without careful management, these fractures may show delayed union or nonunion.[81] Such injuries have been seen in athletes who place the upper limb under repeated stress (e.g., pitchers, gymnasts, and rowers). Signs and symptoms are similar to those of costochondral separations, so palpation plays a significant role in diagnosis, as does radiologic examination.[80] With traumatic rib fractures, the clinician must always be aware of the possibility of a pneumothorax or hemothorax if the rib has fractured.[72,82] Such fractures occur when a force is applied against the lateral aspect of the rib, causing the rib to protrude into the thoracic cavity.[83] Ribs may also be fractured by a strong muscle contraction, especially the upper ribs, because of the anatomy of the attachment of the neck (scalene) muscles.[73,76,77,81,84-86] Care must be taken when assessing these injuries, as pain is often located over the shoulder and neck, which may lead the clinician away from the true area of injury.

THORACIC DISC LESIONS

Disc lesions can occur in the thoracic spine, but they are rare (1 per 1 million population).[87] Symptoms may result from compression on the spinal cord or from pressure on the anterior spinal artery affecting the spinal cord's blood supply. Patients complain of thoracic back pain, which may spread to several dermatomes in a "girdle" distribution or into one or both lower limbs. Burning pain and/or unpleasant paresthesia may be present. Patients may complain of lower limb weakness, and interestingly, upper as well as lower motor neurone signs may be present.[87,88]

SCHEUERMANN'S DISEASE

Scheuermann's disease, a condition seen in immature athletes,[89] involves the ring epiphysis of the vertebral body, resulting in anterior wedging of the affected vertebrae. Usually at least three levels are affected, and the anterior wedging is due to axial or flexion overload of the anterior vertebral body. The visible result is a kyphosis of the thoracic spine.[90,91] Clinically, activity increases the pain, especially if forward flexion is involved. Forward flexion is limited, but muscle spasm is minimal. Radiographs will show wedging of two or more vertebrae, the presence of Schmorl's nodes, decreased intervertebral disc space, epiphyseal ring fragmentation, and sclerosis of adjacent vertebral margins.[89] The condition may be aggravated by the athlete's sport. For example, Wilson and Lindseth[92] reported on three swimmers whose backache was aggravated by the butterfly stroke. Even though the athletes were found to have Scheuermann's disease, they were encouraged to continue swimming (but not the butterfly stroke), as the body's weight on the spine was eliminated by the water. Bracing is usually part of active conservative treatment, which includes a controlled progressive conditioning program.[89] Sward et al.[10] reported that trauma can lead to damage of the anterior vertebral ring apophysis. This type of injury is reported most commonly in wrestlers and female gymnasts and should not be confused with Scheuermann's disease.[10]

Fractures in the thoracic spine are rare because of the thoracic spine's inherent stability and support. However, compression fractures have been reported to occur in sports.[93]

INJURIES TO THE LUMBAR SPINE

MUSCLE STRAINS AND LIGAMENT SPRAINS

The lumbar spine may suffer from muscle strains and ligament sprains caused by a direct blow, sustained posture, activity overload, poor technique, or muscle imbalance.[94-96] In the young athlete, the condition may represent a transient "overgrowth" syndrome in which the soft tissue elements of the spine do not adapt quickly enough to the changing bony elements during the second growth spurt, resulting in hypomobile soft tissues.[97,98] The injury is often due to a sudden extension contraction on an overloaded, unprepared, or underdeveloped spine, especially if a rotary component is involved.[99] Chronically weak muscles and tight muscles (hyperlordosis) often contribute to the problem.[98] Athletes with these conditions usually complain of pain of sudden onset that may be in the midline or to one side. The injury may be due to poor conditioning, overuse, or lack of control at the speed at which the activity was performed.[50] Diagnosis is often arrived at by ruling out discogenic and bony injury.[100] In addition, the clinician must consider other causes of back pain, especially if there is no history of trauma. These include visceral causes (e.g., kidney stones, bladder infection), vascular causes (e.g., abdominal aortic aneurysm), tumors, and infections.[91] Often this aching pain is aggravated by movement, especially flexion, and relieved by rest. Referred pain into the buttock and/or posterior thigh indicates irritation of the nerve root. Most of these conditions can be treated with proper postural correction, strengthening exercises, and stretching techniques. Depending on the postural or biomechanical correction needed, Williams flexion exercises (Fig. 24–3)[2,94,101,102] or McKenzie extension exercises (Fig. 24–4)[2,103] may be given. Pain-relieving modalities such as transcutaneous electrical nerve stimulation (TENS) coupled with ice and/or ultrasound may give some relief.[104,105] If hypomobility results, mobilization techniques may be used.[106,107] Nonsteroidal anti-inflammatory drugs (NSAIDs), analgesics, and muscle relaxants are sometimes prescribed in the acute phase.[108]

As the patient improves, he or she should be advanced to a phase in which functional control to maintain a "balanced" spine and pelvis becomes the primary focus. Saal[109] advocated controlled strengthening of the muscles of the spine and pelvis to "brace" the spine and to control the forces applied to the spine. He stressed abdominal exercises to support the ligamentous structures, quadriceps and hamstring exercises, balancing exercises for the muscles of the pelvis to

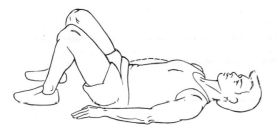

1. Pelvic tilt. Lie on your back with knees bent, feet flat on floor. Flatten the small of your back against the floor, without pushing down with the legs. Hold for 5 to 10 seconds.

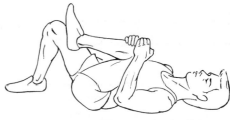

2. Knees to chest. Lie on your back with knees bent and feet flat on the floor. Slowly pull your right knee toward your shoulder and hold 5 to 10 seconds. Lower the knee and repeat with the other knee.

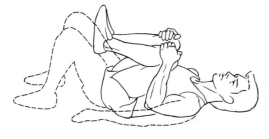

3. Double knee to chest. Begin as in the previous exercise. After pulling right knee to chest, pull left knee to chest and hold both knees for 5 to 10 seconds. Slowly lower one leg at a time.

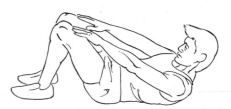

4. Partial sit-up, straight version. Do the pelvic tilt (exercise 1) and, while holding this position, slowly curl your head and shoulders off the floor. Hold briefly. Return slowly to the starting position.

FIGURE 24–3. Examples of Williams flexion exercises. (From Harvey J, Tanner S: Low back pain in young athletes—a practical approach. Sports Med 1991; 12:404.)

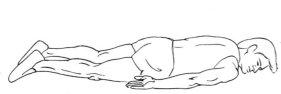

1. Prone lying. Lie on your stomach with arms along your sides and head turned to one side. Maintain this position for 5 to 10 minutes.

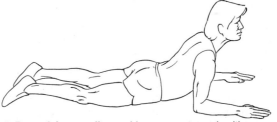

2. Prone lying on elbows. Lie on your stomach with your weight on elbows and forearms and your hips touching the floor or mat. Relax your low back. Remain in this position 5 to 10 minutes. If this causes pain, repeat exercise 1, then try again.

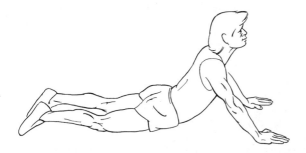

3. Prone press-ups. Lie on your stomach with palms near your shoulders, as if to do a standard pushup. Slowly push your shoulders up, keeping your hips on the surface and letting your back and stomach sag. Slowly lower your shoulders. Repeat 10 times.

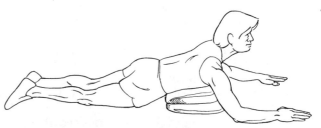

4. Progressive extension with pillows. Lie on your stomach and place a pillow under your chest. After several minutes, add a second pillow. If this does not hurt, add a third pillow after a few more minutes. Stay in this position up to 10 minutes. Remove pillows one at a time over several minutes.

FIGURE 24–4. Examples of McKenzie extension exercises. (From Harvey J, Tanner S: Low back pain in young athletes—a practical approach. Sports Med 1991; 12:404.)

control the center of gravity, exercises for the gluteus maximus to control anterior translation, spinal extensor muscle strength and flexibility exercises to control anterior shear stress, and latissimus dorsi exercises to help control the lumbodorsal fascia. "Balancing" the pelvis involves maintaining a "corset-like" effect on the lumbar spine, resulting in stabilization.[110] Thus, the clinician must ensure good muscular control strength at activity speed, as well as sufficient mobility and flexibility in the muscles controlling the pelvis to decrease the chance of reinjury when the athlete returns to activity. Stability exercises thus progress from prone or supine to kneeling, then to standing, and finally to controlled activity transition movements, always ensuring proper technique and control. The use of stabilization exercises using a large gymnastic ball (approximately 3 ft in diameter) is also very effective in teaching this control.[111,112] The athlete is then taught to control pelvic movement during actual activities such as cycling, running, or swimming. The need for control, flexibility, and proper technique cannot be overstressed.[113]

Postural pain syndrome is similar to that seen in the general population. Poor flexibility may lead to any condition in which cumulative overload is an accompanying factor. There may be poor force dissipation and abnormal biomechanics, which lead to breakdown. Poor posture and poor flexibility may be the sole cause of the pain in some cases but almost always will exacerbate pain that is caused by another condition. In some cases the problem may be due to hypomobility in one direction and hypermobility in the opposite direction. The treatment is the same as that required for lumbar sprains and strains.

There is also the problem of athletes having a rapid growth spurt in which the growth of bony elements outstrips the growth of soft tissue elements. In such cases the tissues are often overstressed in a cumulative overload. This overload is often characterized by tight lumbosacral fascia, tight hamstrings, increased lordosis, decreased abdominal strength, and a compensating kyphosis without any underlying disease process. Generally the pain is aggravated at the end of range of motion, for no apparent reason. Treatment again revolves around stabilizing the pelvis and spine and ensuring normal flexibility.

Surgical interventions for sports injuries to the thoracolumbar spine are relatively uncommon[114]; immediate surgical intervention for sports-related injuries to these structures is particularly unusual. Forces generated by sport participation, even in contact sports, are rarely of a magnitude to cause derangement of the structures of the thoracolumbar spine or peripelvic region sufficient to threaten neuromuscular function, particularly the neural elements of the spine. This is, of course, in contrast to high-velocity injuries occurring in other walks of life (e.g., motor vehicle accidents).

SPONDYLOLYSIS AND SPONDYLOLISTHESIS

Spondylolysis, which is a break or discontinuity in a vertebra, is being reported with increasing frequency in athletes. Spondylolysis has been reported as a stress or fatigue fracture of the pars interarticularis caused by recurring trauma resulting from repeated flexion and hyperextension and twisting. These repetitive movements cause a shearing stress to the vertebra, resulting in the stress fracture.[2,50,99,100,115–123] Hoshina thought a development defect might contribute to the problem.[116] Stress fractures adjacent to this area have also been reported.[124] The developing instability that results can then be exacerbated by sporting activities such as gymnastics, diving, and football.[3] If a separation begins to occur at the defect, spondylolisthesis results, so that there is actual slippage of one vertebra forward on another.[125] This condition is more likely to be seen during the rapid growth spurt of early adolescence.[99] If the displacement or slip is 25 percent or less (grade 1), then sports are allowed if the athlete is asymptomatic, although in a skeletally immature individual, a brace may be required.[3,125] Commonly the athlete will show all the signs of low back abnormality: back pain, sometimes referred into the leg; muscle spasm; loss of the lordotic curve; and limited straight-leg raise. There is demonstrable muscle spasm in the lumbosacral region and flattening of the lumbosacral curve, but there are usually no sciatic nerve symptoms. Spasm (tightness) of the hamstrings may also be evident, which may decrease anterior pelvic inclination with flexed hips and knees.[126] Volski et al.[127] also noted tightness in the iliotibial band. The stork, or one-leg hyperextension, test may be positive on the affected side.[115] Definitive diagnosis is made by an oblique radiograph showing a "Scottie dog with a collar" pattern (spondylolysis) or a "Scottie dog decapitated" pattern (spondylolisthesis).[55] Caution is advised, however, as Jackson et al.[9] reported that gymnasts reporting with low back pain initially had negative radiographs that progressed to evident defects in the pars interarticularis. Thus, a bone scan to show potential "hot spots" is appropriate. In dancers, pain on doing an arabesque should increase the examiner's suspicion for spondylolysis. If the pain the athlete has experienced is of less than 10 months' duration, it should be treated as a fracture. These lesions often take up to 16 months to heal. This type of injury is common in weight lifters who perform the standing overhead press; gymnasts; football linemen; and anyone performing activities such as pitching, weight lifting, tennis serving, shooting a rifle in a standing position, and pole vaulting.[9,115,116,128,129] It may also be seen in volleyball, hurdling, diving, and swimming.[9] Often the athlete is under the age of 20, and the pain is exaggerated by flexion-extension stress rather than rotation. The majority of spondylolisthesis patients, especially if the grade of slip is less than or equal to 2, can be successfully treated conservatively.[130] Conservative treatment consists of rest, intermittent traction, a spinal orthosis (brace), exercises to strengthen and stabilize the muscles controlling the pelvis (e.g., flexion routine, ball stabilization exercises, abdominal strengthening), and hamstring stretching similar to that used for lumbar muscle strains.[131,132] A lumbosacral orthosis is often prescribed, as it decreases lumbar lordosis, lessens axial loading on the spine by increasing intra-abdominal pressure, and limits pelvic torsion.[131] The brace should be worn about

23 hours a day for at least 3 to 6 months.[125] Up to 1 year may be required for conservative treatment.[115,130]

An acute injury of the lumbar or thoracolumbar spine that results in disruption of the pars interarticularis in most instances, is a stable fracture that does not require acute intervention to prevent further neural injury. In such instances of acute disruption of the pars interarticularis—and certainly in other instances of more chronic segmental instability resulting from stress fractures of the pars interarticularis—functional disability, recurrent episodes of acute back syndrome, or severe pain with moderate levels of athletic activity may require consideration of surgical intervention.

In our experience, nonoperative techniques have been highly successful in relieving symptoms and usually allow ongoing athletic participation in conditions such as spondylolysis or spondylolisthesis. In particular, the adolescent-onset spondylolysis stress fracture, even when it has not been successfully immobilized to the point where healing has occurred, may be a source of intermittent painful episodes and back spasms but does not result in true instability of the lumbar spine. In such cases, lysis of the pars interarticularis may result in a low-grade forward listhesis at the segmental level in question. We have never convincingly seen a spondylolysis of this type progress to a spondylolisthesis greater than the second degree (Fig. 24–5).[133]

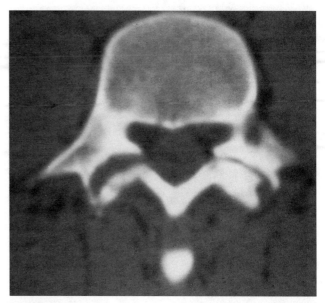

FIGURE 24–6. Axial computed tomography (CT) scan of the lumbar spine showing bilateral fracture nonunions of the pars interarticularis.

When conservative management has been unsuccessful in controlling symptoms and in cases of spondylolysis or spondylolisthesis in athletes that results in recurrent severe pain and dysfunction, consideration may be given to surgical stabilization with spinal fusion (Fig. 24–6).

The traditional technique used for stabilization of a painful spondylolysis is posterolateral fusion, in which no attempt is made to actually attain direct bony fusion of the pars defect itself, but instead, a bone graft is placed in the posterolateral margins across the vertebral bodies in question in an attempt to attain posterolateral fusion. Interestingly, in such cases of posterolateral fusion for spondylolysis, long-term studies have suggested that up to 80 percent of the pars defects then also go on to bony union once posterolateral fusion has been attained (Fig. 24–7).[134]

A number of authors have described attempts to directly stabilize and attain fusion of the fractured pars interarticularis segment itself. In such cases the area of pars nonunion is exposed, and the hypertrophic scar tissue and cartilaginous tissue at the site of nonunion are excised. Cancellous bone graft is then packed in place at the level of the pars defect, and stabilization across the pars segment is then attained either by a cerclage wire encircling the base of the transverse process and the base of the spinous process at the site of defect or by a pedicle screw from the posterior element across the site of nonunion and into the adjacent pedicle.[135] As with any attempted fusion of the elements of the lumbar spine, a period of 6 to 12 months is necessary before fusion can be expected (Fig. 24–8).

It must be noted that in any attempt at fusion of the lumbar spine with autogenous iliac crest bone graft, the most optimistic reviews have found a rate of failure of fusion or nonunion of at least 10 percent. In such instances, a second surgery may be required for further bone grafting. Alternatively, electrical fields can be

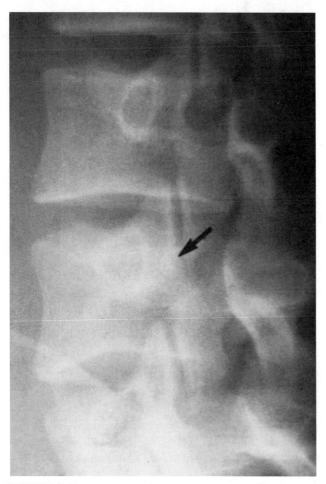

FIGURE 24–5. Oblique radiograph of lumbar spine demonstrates a pars fracture of L4.

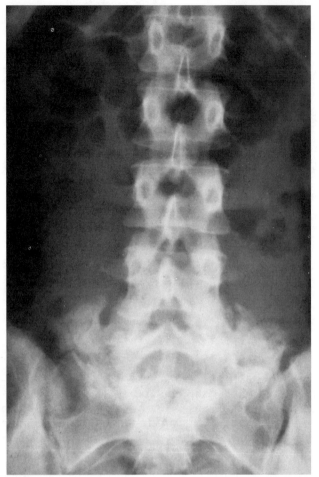

FIGURE 24–7. Anteroposterior (AP) radiograph of the lumbar spine after posterolateral in situ fusion of L5 to the sacrum.

pected range of motion.[56] Often a positive SLR test is not seen until 90 to 110 degrees of hip flexion.

Nonsurgical treatment for discogenic pain is the treatment of choice for these individuals. The treatment is aggressive, involving manual treatment of adverse mechanical neural tension, correction of underlying segmental and myotendon impairments, aerobic conditioning, spinal strength and stabilization exercises, and functional stabilization control in sports and daily activities.

The treatment of adverse mechanical neural tension involves treating abnormal restriction and/or excessive tension on neurologic elements (e.g., dura, spinal nerve roots, spinal cord, peripheral nerve) and is based on the work of Butler.[136–138] These techniques may involve Maitland's posteroanterior central or unilateral pressures; lumbar rotation mobilization; and a modified hold-relax straight-leg raise involving hip rotation and progressing to hip adduction, internal rotation, and ankle dorsiflexion. Improvement will be slow and should be relatively painless. At the same time, the athlete is taught to control the trunk. Farrell and Drye[136] report that the idea is to teach the athlete to find the

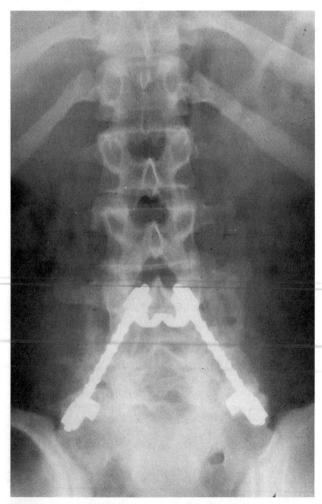

FIGURE 24–8. AP radiograph of the lumbar spine showing posterolateral fusion from L3 to the sacrum with Harrington spinal instrumentation and bone graft.

directed from skin surface electrodes to induce a bioelectric environment about the site of nonunion; this has been shown to result in late union in certain cases.

LUMBAR DISC LESIONS

Lumbar discogenetic pain has become more and more frequent in sports due to higher and higher stress loads being placed on the athlete and hypermobility of the lumbar spine combined with lack of muscular control.[128] Disc herniation, especially in the posterolateral direction, is the result usually of torsion and compression, not just compression.[25,120] The cause of these injuries may be repeated microtrauma or macrotrauma or a combination of both, in addition to high torque and cumulative overload. Discogenic pain tends to be sharp or burning and often shoots into the lower leg. Neurologic tension tests are commonly positive, and myotomic weakness is often evident. Abnormal sensation in the affected dermatomes may also be seen.[108] Generally, athletes demonstrate asymmetric tight hamstrings, and the condition is aggravated by poor posture or by activity or anything that increases disc pressure. Interestingly, many of these athletes present with a straight leg-raising (SLR) test within the normal, ex-

lumbopelvic position that is most stable and pain free. They called this the *spinal functional position.* The athlete is taught to maintain this position while imposing extremity movements to enhance the strength of the lumbar stabilizers. Progression is made to bridging activities on a stable surface and then to bridging activities using a large (3-ft diameter) ball (ball stabilization exercises).[111,112] Once the athlete is able to control the spinal functional position in these positions, he or she progresses to learning to control the position while doing sport-specific drills and, finally, during practices and games.

Surgical intervention for disc herniation in athletes should be extremely conservative. There is tremendous potential, particularly in younger athletes, for healing and shrinkage of herniated disc material, even when early acute symptoms are severe. In a series of 12 athletes with significant disc herniations undergoing a period of conservative management that included bracing, exercises, and progressive return to sports activities, the senior author (LJM) found that subsequent magnetic resonance imaging (MRI) found dissolution and resolution of the disc herniation by MRI criteria.

The criteria for surgical intervention for disc herniation include (1) uncontrollable sciatic pain in association with the herniation that is not mitigated or resolved with 3 to 6 months of nonoperative management, including medications, exercises, bracing, and even corticosteroid injection; (2) persistent motor loss of the lower extremity in conjunction with the disc herniation that does not resolve with 3 to 6 months of conservative management; and (3) cauda equina syndrome in which there is measurable derangement of bladder and/or bowel function (an absolute indication for early discectomy and decompression). In the last condition, a delay of as little as 12 hours may result in irreversible loss of bladder or bowel function. This is a *true emergency of the lumbar spine.* Again, although this is relatively rare, it may be encountered in all cases of disc herniation and must be appreciated as a true surgical emergency.[139]

Since the mid-1980s, advances in surgical technique and instrumentation have made lumbar disc excision a much more benign procedure. The use of microscopic surgical techniques, in particular, has enabled disc excision to be done with a relatively small incision and with minimal injury to associated muscular elements posteriorly.[140–142] In many instances the athlete may go home the same day or within 24 hours.[143]

It is extremely important to educate the athlete as to the expected outcomes from this type of intervention and surgery. Although surgical discectomy may be sufficient to relieve acute or ongoing impingement on the nerve roots and usually will be quite successful in relieving sciatica, it in no way reverses the progressive degeneration of the disc elements that has already occurred prior to the herniation in almost every instance. Thus, while the acute leg pain may be relieved, the athlete may in future years be subject to subsequent symptoms related to progressive disc narrowing, alteration of facet and foraminal mechanics in the posterior

elements, and anterior and posterior derangements of the spinal segment.

It is rarely necessary for intervertebral discectomy to be accompanied by segmental fusion. Although this was much more common in past years, more recent experience has suggested that discectomy alone followed by a carefully directed rehabilitation and exercise program can provide sufficient stabilization to the segments without the need for this type of surgical fusion. The addition of fusion significantly increases the morbidity and dysfunction of this intervention and may result in a lasting inability to perform athletic functions at the level enjoyed prior to the surgical intervention, thus rendering it much more problematic for the serious amateur and certainly for the professional or elite class athlete.[144]

LUMBAR FACET INJURIES

Injury to the facet joints (facet syndrome) may occur, usually as a result of high-velocity or high-torque extension-type movement associated with rotation.[2,145] Because the facet joints are well innervated, the pain may be localized or referred down the leg (often to the thigh or groin) owing to the close association of the facet joint to the nerve root.[146–149] Typically, the pain is unilateral and sharp and may cause paraspinal muscle spasm and a scoliosis-type posture. Often the pain may be incapacitating and may be indistinguishable from pain due to a disc problem. However, pain is relieved with ambulation.[105] There may be trophic abnormalities, sclerotic changes, or narrowing evident on radiographs. Generally, the pain increases with extension, compression and rotation, and returning from flexion. The symptoms are very similar to a ligament sprain or muscle strain, with the exception of the incapacitation with possible postural deformity and deviation of the movement pattern. Anesthetic facet block usually causes complete relief of symptoms; however, because of the innervation pattern it has been found that the adjacent facets may also have to be injected.[105,146,147,150,151]

Some athletes have complained of a dull, constant ache localized to the posterior portion of one iliac crest and are able to point to a specific area of pain. Hirschberg et al.[152] referred to this condition as *iliolumbar syndrome,* and a characteristic finding is pain on lateral bending, usually away from the affected side, with increased symptoms into the low back. Hirschberg et al. report that with this syndrome, the SLR-test, hip flexion test with the knee flexed, and the Patrick test will all be positive to pain at or near the posterior iliac crest. A positive diagnosis is confirmed by injecting the iliolumbar ligament with anesthetic.

SPINAL FRACTURES

Spinal fractures are most commonly divided into stable or unstable fractures. In a stable fracture, the anatomic disruption is such that there is little chance of injury to neural elements or progressive deformity with physiologic loads on the spine.[153] Examples of stable fractures that can occur in sports settings include compression fractures of the thoracolumbar junction. These stable compression fractures generally result in less than 10 degrees of angular compression of the anterior portions of the vertebral body. These types of fractures may be seen in winter sports such as snow-mobiling and tobogganing.[99] The posterior element ligamentous structures and facet complexes are mechanically intact, and treatment is often symptomatic, employing first aid techniques, followed by progressive strengthening and range-of-motion exercises. On occasion, a thermoplastic or even a cloth brace may be used to assist in symptomatic improvement and early function of the athlete.

Unstable fractures at the thoracolumbar junction or lumbar spine are extremely rare in a sports setting.[154] Such fractures might occur in pole vaulters or during falls in the course of competition, such as in mountain biking or triathletes who fall from a roadway or over a precipice.

At the time of initial assessment, a very careful neurologic assessment is required to determine whether there has been complete or incomplete neural injury at this site of bony disruption. Even in the event of neurologic stability without compromise, an unstable fracture may be present, and mobilization or resumption of activity too early might result in late bony deformity or neural compromise.

Following initial physical examination to determine the status of the neural system, careful radiographs, including initial plain radiographs consisting of antero-posterior (AP), lateral, and oblique views of the lumbar or thoracolumbar spine are necessary. These initial plain radiographs can give an early indication as to whether the spine has been sufficiently injured to render it mechanically unstable (Fig. 24–9).

Quite often additional imaging studies, including computerized tomography (CT) or even myelography combined with CT, must be obtained to determine the exact extent of injury to the posterior and/or anterior elements. An example of such an unstable lesion would be a Chance fracture, which results from a combination of flexion and rotation at the thoracolumbar junction, such as in a seat belt injury. The fracture line travels through the posterior elements, often splitting the spinous process and lamina, and then extends out into the anterior elements, producing a shearing injury to the vertebral body with disruption of both the anterior and posterior longitudinal ligaments of the spine.[155]

In the event that the spinal injury in question meets criteria for radiographic instability, stabilization of the spine with metallic instrumentation is usually required.[156] This instrumentation may involve fixation screws through the anterior elements, posterior elements, or both. Most commonly, two vertebral elements are stabilized proximal and distal to the site of vertebral instability (Fig. 24–10). This instrumentation is usually accomplished by decortication of the posterior elements of the spine across the area of instability, removal of any intervening disc material anteriorly, and packing of the posterior and anterior elements as indicated with iliac

crest bone graft obtained from a donor site in the patient's own ilium.

After stabilization with instrumentation and bone grafting, additional external immobilization, including the use of special frame beds or rigid braces, may be required until bony union has been attained. This may take from 6 to 12 months following injury.

LATERAL SPINAL STENOSIS

When the diagnosis of lateral stenosis of neural elements has been made in association with back pain in the athlete, every attempt is made to manage the impingement with nonoperative techniques. Unfortunately, at times a herniated lateral disc or a narrowing of the intervertebral foramina caused by osteophytes on the margins of the facet joints may be unresponsive to dynamic stabilization. In such instances, an operative intervention is performed in which the osteophytes or disc material is removed and the foramina opened wide.[157]

If, in the course of lateral element decompression, sufficient posterior elements have been removed to render the segments at risk for subsequent segmental instability, decompression may be accomplished by fusion across the level of decompression. Again, this is

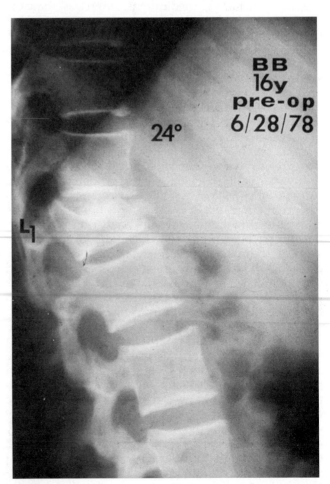

FIGURE 24–9. Unstable spinal fracture at the thoracolumbar junction in a young rider.

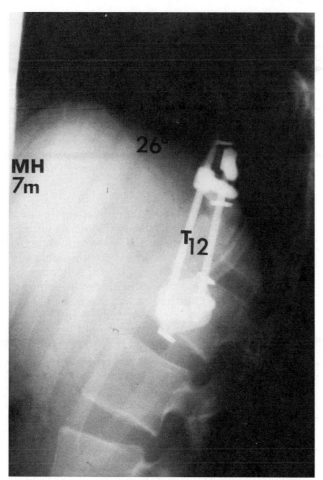

FIGURE 24–10. Anterior spinal instrumentation and fusion for an unstable thoracolumbar fracture.

done using iliac crest bone graft, most commonly applied to the posterolateral structures of the spine, particularly over the transverse processes and posterior elements of the spine.

In athletes who have undergone foraminotomy and osteophyte excision for lateral spinal stenosis without accompanying fusion, very rapid mobilization and return to functional activity may be accomplished in combination with an appropriate spinal strengthening and mobilization regimen. If spinal fusion is required in association with decompression, a sufficient period of immobilization (6 to 12 months) is necessary until bony fusion has been attained across the level of decompression.

CENTRAL SPINAL STENOSIS

Central stenosis of the thoracolumbar or lumbar spine is relatively uncommon in younger athletes. However, as regular fitness activities, including sports activities, become part of healthy living as well as health maintenance in older populations, greater numbers of people who ultimately are determined to be suffering from central spinal stenosis are presenting to sports medicine clinics. When the condition is first detected, the patient with central spinal stenosis should be directed toward a regimen that includes exercises and/or bracing techniques in an attempt to increase the capacity and the volume of the neural canal. Properly instituted and supervised exercises can often relieve the majority of the symptoms of spinal stenosis.

At times, however, spinal stenosis may be associated with a genetic shortening of the pedicles of the spine. In such cases, even in young athletes, a small amount of facet hypertrophy or posterior central disc herniation may be sufficient to result in unremitting spinal stenosis symptoms.[158]

An additional adjunct in the nonoperative management of spinal stenosis includes epidural corticosteroid injection. To be effective, this intervention should be done under fluoroscopic control by a skilled anesthesiologist or physician comfortable with the anatomy of the thoracolumbar and lumbar spine. Used in conjunction with an exercise regimen and bracing regimen, we have found corticosteroid injection to be highly successful in relieving symptoms and allowing a return to sports activities in a great number of these patients.

In athletes with spinal stenosis that is unresponsive to conservative management, neural decompression may be required. As with lateral stenosis, if it is necessary to remove portions of the posterior elements, including laminae, facets, and even pedicles, to provide a satisfactory decompression of the neural elements of the spine, then segmental posterolateral spinal fusion may be required in conjunction with decompressive resection surgery for the central stenosis.

In ideal circumstances, the major site of stenosis may be localized to one or perhaps, at the most, two of the segmental elements of the spine. With a single level of spinal stenosis compression, posterior and, in some cases, associated anterior decompression may be sufficient to remove the pressure on the neural elements without resulting in instability of the segment, and spinal fusion surgery is not required.

When more than two elements of the spine have been decompressed or when, in a one- or two-element decompression, there is potential instability to the spine because of excessive removal of facet joints or posterior elements, the resultant need for bone graft and fusion will necessitate a prolonged period of immobilization (again, 6 to 12 months), often supplemented by external bracing techniques. As in cases of lateral spinal stenosis, athletes have successfully returned to sports activities, particularly recreational sports activities such as golf or tennis, following surgical decompression for central spinal stenosis.

More recently, in situ iliac crest bone grafting to attain bone fusion has been supplemented by metallic instrumentation, including screws passed through the pedicles to provide early rigid stabilization and, hopefully, to increase the rate of bony fusion.

BACK SURGERY

The scope and role of surgical intervention for back pain and back injuries in athletes is quite narrow. At one extreme, there may be rare cases in which immediate surgery is necessary, such as in unstable fractures of the thoracic or lumbar spine resulting from high-energy trauma. In the case of a herniated disc, onset of cauda equina syndrome with compromise of bladder and bowel function is certainly another emergency situation in which immediate intervention is necessary. In the remainder of cases in which back pain with or without associated sciatica is encountered in the athletic population, very careful surgical indications must be used.

In particular, the potential for sustaining a high degree of musculoskeletal function, particularly at the level demanded by the sport in question, must be entertained when making a decision as to whether surgical intervention is necessary. In the case of a deteriorated disc with herniation, it must be well understood by the athlete that although it is a very reasonable expectation that the referred sciatic pain may resolve after surgery, there may indeed be episodes of ongoing back pain due to persistent deterioration of the disc, which cannot, of course, be addressed at this time with any type of disc replacement or revitalization.

In addition, in any surgical intervention in the spine in which bone fusion has been necessary, it must be emphasized to the athlete that the fusion results in a loss of segmental motion that may compromise athletic function. In addition, the time required for a fusion to occur, at a minimum in the range of 6 to 12 months, may result in a deconditioning process and subsequent dysfunction that may also contribute to a compromise in the level of athletic participation previously enjoyed.

The best way to ensure that excessive dysfunction and erosion of athletic performance do not occur after surgical intervention is to have a careful and coordinated rehabilitation procedure in place in which the therapist and surgeon work together at every step to coordinate progressive increased levels of strength and flexibility within the ranges of safety.

INJURIES TO THE PELVIS

OSTEITIS PUBIS

Osteitis pubis is a condition in which there is an injury to the insertion of the adductor muscles into the symphysis pubis. It is common in distance running, soccer (kicking sports), football, and wrestling and is due to the repetitive pull of the adductor muscles on the symphysis pubis.[159–162] This repeated minor trauma from excessive repetitive biomechanical shearing stresses leads to injury, which may be confused with an adductor strain or hernia. On examination the clinician will find painful abduction owing to stretch or stress on the symphysis pubis, with point tenderness on the pubic tubercles. Situps and squats may also be painful.[163] Usually there is a gradual onset of localized pubic pain and tenderness over the pubic ramus that may radiate to the groin or lower abdomen.[164] The insertions of the rectus abdominis and adductor muscles and of the inguinal ligament may be tender in the ischeopubic region. There may be intense pain or sudden contraction of the muscles on particular movements. The pain is often aggravated by pivoting in one leg, kicking a ball, sprinting, "pumping" the legs against the chest, climb-

ing stairs, sitting up, sneezing, or coughing.[164] Radiographs will show periosteal reaction, sclerosis, and, in advanced cases, demineralization of the cortical bone that may extend to the subcortical bone.[74,164] Irregularity of the symphyseal margins will be demonstrated, as will widening of the symphysis, especially in the lower one half to two thirds of the joint. These changes may be asymmetric. It should be understood that radiographic changes lag behind the clinical features by several months. Symmetric bone reabsorption of the medial ends of the pubic bones and instability of the symphysis pubis may be seen on the films during weight bearing (flamingo views). A bone scan will demonstrate areas of increased radionucleotide activity that may be unilateral or bilateral.[165] Generally these conditions persist for long periods even with treatment, which involves minimizing stress to the pubic bone. Because true complete rest is often the treatment of choice, compliance may be difficult for the athlete. If cycling does not bother him or her, it may be used as a fitness tool.[160]

Liebert et al.[166] reported instability of the symphysis pubis in an athlete who suffered three traumatic forced abduction injuries to the pelvis. The pain felt by the athlete was similar to that described by patients with osteitis pubis. Treatment involves rest, followed by strengthening and flexibility routines for the muscles of the hip (abductors, adductors, hamstrings, and quadriceps).

SACROILIAC JOINT SPRAIN

Sacroiliac joint sprain, although not a common injury, must be considered as a possible source of back pain, especially when the mechanism of injury involves a loaded torsion injury while weight bearing, or a fall on the buttock.[167–169] It may also occur as a result of repetitive muscle action that puts abnormal stress on the joint.[37] Generally there is unilateral dull pain over the affected sacroiliac joint that may be referred to the lumbar spine area, buttock, or to the leg (lateral aspect of greater trochanter or groin).[170] Muscle spasm is not often seen, and other neurologic tests are negative.[170] Stress tests for the sacroiliac joint are helpful in the diagnosis.[55] The athlete may complain of tenderness over the posterior superior iliac spine and "heaviness" of the lower limb or tightness of the hamstring on the affected side. Standing on one leg and climbing stairs may increase the pain. An up-slip of the ilium on the affected side may be present, and there may be asymmetry of the gluteal folds with decreased internal rotation on the affected side.[55,171,172] Treatment of the condition includes heat, ultrasound, pelvic stabilization exercises, and mobilization of the affected sacroiliac joint. In severe cases a pelvic binder may be required to stabilize the joint.[172]

PELVIC STRESS FRACTURES

Pelvic stress fractures may occur to the ischeum or the inferior pubic ramus. These are overuse injuries and, in the conditioned athlete, may be due to changes in training techniques, mileage, or footwear. It may take up to 3 months following the change for the fracture to actually occur.[173] Satterfield et al.[174] reported a stress fracture of the ischial tuberosity brought on by excessive backward running (retrorunning). These types of fractures often take 2 to 5 months to heal and on assessment demonstrate groin discomfort during activity (e.g., running makes the pain severe).[175] Pain, which may be severe on flamingo standing and deep palpation, will reveal exquisite nauseating tenderness on the pubic ramus.[175] A similar stress reaction has been reported[37,176] in the area of the sacroiliac joints, which we speculate was due to a sudden increase in activity. Because pain is usually referred to the lumbar spine area, care must be taken to ensure a correct diagnosis.

AVULSION FRACTURES

Avulsion fractures may also occur to the pelvic area, commonly to the various apophyses in the adolescent.[177] The most common sites of occurrence include the iliac crest, the ischeal tuberosity at the insertion of the hamstrings and the adductors, the anterosuperior iliac spine (the insertion of the sartorius and tensor fascia lata), the anteroinferior iliac spine (the insertion of the rectus femoris), the ischial tuberosity at the hamstrings insertion, and the symphysis pubis, where the adductors insert.[50,178–180] These types of injuries are due to a failure of the bone as the result of an application of a sudden tensile force (e.g., kicking) across an open apophysis or to sudden excessive passive lengthening.[177] Often the fragment is fairly stabilized, as it is prevented from migrating by other soft tissue attachments. This type of injury is more likely to be seen in children than in adults. Initial treatment involves placing the athlete on crutches. The athlete is allowed to progress according to symptoms moving from achieving full range of motion, to progressive resistance, to resisted functional activity, and finally to return to activity when full strength and flexibility are restored.[177] Activities are usually resumed after 6 to 8 weeks.[178]

CONCLUSION

Because the thoracolumbopelvic region is such a major component of the human kinetic chain as it is used in sport, training and competition can be quickly interrupted by the presence of an injury in this area. Often these injuries, especially in the spine, become chronic or long-lasting, which can further add to the problem because of the strong psychological effect of chronic injuries. These injuries must be handled with care and proper attention to ensure that the athlete is able to return to competition with maximum effectiveness.

REFERENCES

1. Tall RL, DeVault W: Spinal injury in sport: Epidemiologic considerations. Clin Sports Med 1993; 12:441–448.
2. Harvey J, Tanner S: Low back pain in young athletes—a practical approach. Sports Med 1991; 12:394–406.
3. Stanish WL: Low back pain in the athlete: An overuse syndrome. Clin Sports Med 1987; 6:321–344.
4. Micheli LJ: Low back pain in the adolescent: Differential diagnosis. Am J Sports Med 1979; 7:362–364.
5. Gillespie HW: The significance of congenital lumbosacral anomalies. Br J Radiol 1949; 22:270–275.
6. Mahlamaki S, Soimakallio S, Michelsson JE: Radiological findings in the lumbar spine of 39 young cross country skiers with low back pain. Int J Sports Med 1988; 9:196–198.
7. Alexander MJL: Biomechanical aspects of lumbar spine injuries in athletes: A review. Can J Appl Sport Sci 1984; 10(1):1.
8. Sward L, Hellstrom M, Jacobson B, Peterson L: Back pain and radiographic changes in the thoraco-lumbar spine in athletes. Spine 1990; 15:124–129.
9. Jackson DW, White LL, Circincione RJ: Spondylolysis in the female gymnast. Clin Orthop 1976; 117:68–73.
10. Sward L, Hellstrom M, Jacobsson B, Karlsson L: Vertebral ring apophysis injury in athletes: Is the etiology different in the thoracic and lumbar spine? Am J Sports Med 1993; 21(6):841–845.
11. Goldstein JD, Berger PE, Windler GE, et al: Spine injuries in gymnasts and swimmers: An epidemiological investigation. Am J Sports Med 1991; 19(5):463.
12. Ohlen G, Wredmark T, Spangfort E: Spinal sagittal configuration and mobility related to low back pain in the female gymnast. Spine 1989; 14:847–850.
13. Kirby RL, Simms FC, Symington VJ, Garner JB: Flexibility and musculoskeletal symptomatology in female gymnasts and age-matched controls. Am J Sports Med 1982; 9:160–164.
14. Brown EW, Kimball RG: Medical history associated with adolescent powerlifting. Pediatrics 1983; 72:636–643.
15. Fairbank JC, O'Brien JP, Davis PR: Intraabdominal pressure rise during weight lifting as an objective measure of low back pain. Spine 1980; 5:179–184.
16. Cholewicki J, McGill SM, Norman RW: Lumbar spine loads during the lifting of extremely heavy weights. Med Sci Sports Exerc 1991; 23:1179–1186.
17. Cappozzo A, Felici F, Figura F, Gazzani F: Lumbar spine loading during half squat exercises. Med Sci Sports Exerc 1985; 17:613–620.
18. Lander JE, Simonton RL, Giacobbe JK: The effectiveness of weight-belts during the squat exercise. Med Sci Sports Exerc 1990; 22:117–126.
19. Harman EA, Rosenstein RM, Frykman PN, Nigro GA: Effects of a belt on intraabdominal pressure during weight lifting. Med Sci Sports Exerc 1989; 21:186–190.
20. Lander JE, Hundley JR, Simonton RL: The effectiveness of weight belts during multiple repetitions of the squat exercise. Med Sci Sports Exerc 1992; 24:603–609.
21. Hemberg B, Moritz U, Lowing H: Intra-abdominal pressure and trunk muscle activity during lifting. Scand J Rehabil Med 1985; 17:25–37.
22. Semon R, Sprengler J: Significance of lumbar spondylolysis in college football players. Spine 1981; 6:172–174.
23. McCarroll JR, Miller JM, Ritter MA: Lumbar spondylolysis and spondylolisthesis in college football players: A prospective study. Am J Sports Med 1986; 14:404–406.
24. Mahlamaki S, Soimakallio S, Michelsson JE: Radiological findings in the lumbar spine of 39 young cross-country skiers with low back pain. Int J Sports Med 1988; 9:196.
25. Marks MR, Haas SS, Wiesel SW: Low back pain in the competitive tennis player. Clin Sports Med 1988; 7:277–287.
26. Frymoyer JW, Pope MH, Clements JH, et al: Risk factors in low back pain. J Bone Joint Surg 1983; 65A:213–218.
27. Lindsay DM, Meeuwisse WH, Vyse A, et al: Lumbosacral dysfunctions in elite cross-country skiers. J Orthop Sports Phys Ther 1993; 18(5):580.
28. White TL, Malone TR: Effects of running on intervertebral disc height. J Orthop Sports Phys Ther 1990; 12(4):139.
29. Carrigg SY, Hillemeyer LE: The effect of running-induced intervertebral disc compression on thoracolumbar vertebral column mobility in young healthy males. J Orthop Sports Phys Ther 1992; 16(1):19.
30. Ahrens SF: The effect of age on intervertebral disc compression during running. J Orthop Sports Phys Ther 1994; 20(1):17.

31. Howell DW. Musculoskeletal profile and incidence of musculoskeletal injuries in lightweight women rowers. Am J Sports Med 1984; 12:278–282.

32. Mundt DJ, Kelsey JL, Golden AL, et al: An epidemiologic study of sports and weight lifting as possible risk factors for herniated lumbar and cervical discs. Am J Sports Med 1993; 21:854–860.

33. Tertti M, Paajanen H, Kujala U, et al: Disc degeneration in young gymnasts—a magnetic resonance imaging study. Am J Sports Med 1990; 18:206–209.

34. Day AL, Friedman WA, Indelicato PA: Observations on the treatment of lumbar disc disease in college football players. Am J Sports Med 1987; 15:72–75.

35. Granhed H, Morelli B: Low back pain among retired wrestlers and heavyweight lifters. Am J Sports Med 1988; 16(5):530.

36. Aggrawal ND, Kaur R, Kumar S, Mathur DN: A study of changes in the spine in weightlifters and other athletes. Br J Sports Med 1979; 13:58–61.

37. Marymont JV, Lynch MA, Henning CE: Exercise-related stress reaction of the sacroiliac joint: An unusual cause of low back pain in athletes. Am J Sports Med 1986; 14(4):320.

38. Lloyd-Smith R, Clement DB, McKenzie DC, Taunton JE: A survey of overuse and traumatic hip and pelvic injuries in athletics. Phys Sports Med 1985; 18(10):131–141.

39. Grieve GP: Common Vertebral Joint Problems. New York, Churchill Livingstone, 1981.

40. Warwick R, Williams PL (eds): Gray's Anatomy, 35th ed. Philadelphia, WB Saunders, 1973.

41. White AA, Panjabi MM: Clinical Biomechanics of the Spine. Philadelphia, JB Lippincott, 1978.

42. Wyke B: The neurological basis of thoracic spinal pain. Rheum Phys Med 1970; 10(7):356.

43. Maigne R: Manipulation of the spine. In Rogoff JB (ed): Manipulation, Traction and Massage. Baltimore, Williams & Wilkins, 1980.

44. Porterfield JA, DeRosa C: Mechanical Low Back Pain: Perspectives in Functional Anatomy. Philadelphia, WB Saunders, 1991.

45. Gracovetsky S, Farfan H, Helleur C: The abdominal mechanism. Spine 1985; 10(4):317.

46. Bogduk N, Twomey LT: Clinical Anatomy of the Lumbar Spine. New York, Churchill Livingstone, 1991.

47. Kapandjii IA: The Physiology of the Joints, vol 3: The Trunk and the Vertebral Column. New York, Churchill Livingstone, 1974.

48. Yong-Hing K, Kirkaldy-Willis WH: The pathophysiology of degenerative disease of the lumbar spine. Orthop Clin North Am 1983; 14(3):491.

49. Farfan HF, Gracovetsky S: The nature of instability. Spine 1984; 9(7):714.

50. Stanitski CL: Low back pain in young athletes. Phys Sports Med 1982; 10(10):77–91.

51. Clark A, Stanish WD: An unusual cause of back pain in the young athlete—a case report. Am J Sports Med 1985; 13:51–54.

52. Dyrek DA: Assessment and treatment planning strategies for musculoskeletal deficits. In O'Sullivan SB, Schmitz TJ (eds): Physical Rehabilitation: Assessment and Treatment. Philadelphia, FA Davis, 1994.

53. Eddy DM, Clanton DH: The art of diagnosis: Solving the clinicopathological exercise. N Engl J Med 1982; 306(21):1263.

54. Balla JI: The Diagnostic Process: A Model for Clinical Teachers. New York, Cambridge University Press, 1985.

55. Magee DJ: Orthopedic Physical Assessment. Philadelphia, WB Saunders, 1992.

56. Day AL, Friedman WA, Indelicato PA: Observations on the treatment of lumbar disc disease in college football players. Am J Sports Med 1987; 15:72–75.

57. Jorgensson A: The iliopsoas muscle and the lumbar spine. Austr J Physiother 1993; 39:125–131.

58. Thomas JC: Plain roentgenogram of the spine in the injured athlete. Clin Sports Med 1986; 5:353–371.

59. Greenan TJ: Diagnostic imaging of sports-related spinal disorders. Clin Sports Med 1993; 12:487–505.

60. Eismont FJ, Kitchel SH: Thoracolumbar spine. In DeLee JC, Drez D (eds): Orthopedic Sports Medicine. Philadelphia, WB Saunders, 1994.

61. Lyons FR, Rockwood CA: Fractures of the sternum. In DeLee JC, Drez D (eds): Orthopedic Sports Medicine—Principles and Practice. Philadelphia, WB Saunders, 1994.

62. Johnson CD, MacKenzie JW, Zawadsky JP: Manubriosternal dislocation in a football player. Surg Rounds Orthop 1989; 2:45–50.

63. DeTarnowsky G: Contrecoup fracture of the sternum. Ann Surg 1905; 41:253–264.

64. Woo CC: Traumatic manubriosternal joint subluxations in two basketball players. J Manip Physiol Ther 1988; 11:433–437.

65. Keating TM: Stress fracture of the sternum in a wrestler. Am J Sports Med 1987; 15:92–93.

66. Andriacchi T, Schultz A, Belytschko T, et al: A model for studies of mechanical interactions between the human spine and rib cage. J Biomech 1974; 7:497.

67. Valencia F: Biomechanics of the thoracic spine. In Grant R (ed): Physical Therapy of the Cervical and Thoracic Spine. New York, Churchill Livingstone, 1988.

68. Horner DB: Lumbar back pain arising from stress fractures of the lower ribs. J Bone Joint Surg 1964; 46A:1553–1556.

69. Wyke B: Morphological and functional features of innervation of the costovertebral joints. Folia Morph 1975; 23:296–305.

70. Wyke B: The neurological basis of thoracic spinal pain. Ann Phys Med 1969; 10:356–367.

71. Widner PE: Thoracic injuries: Mechanisms, characteristics, management. Athletic Training 1988; 23:148–151.

72. Floyd RT, Tew M: Injury on impact—thoracic injuries due to sport-related contact. Sports Med Update 1991; 6(1):10–15.

73. Lyons FR, Rockwood CA: Fractures of the rib. In DeLee JC, Drez D (eds): Orthopedic Sports Medicine. Philadelphia, WB Saunders, 1994.

74. Holden DL, Jackson DW: Stress fracture of the ribs in female rowers. Am J Sports Med 1985; 13:342–348.

75. McKenzie DC: Stress fracture of the rib in an elite oarsman. Int J Sports Med 1989; 10:220–222.

76. Curran JP, Kelly DA: Stress fracture of the first rib. Am J Orthop 1966; 8:16–18.

77. Sacchetti AD, Beswick DR, Morse SD: Rebound rib: Stress-induced first rib fracture. Ann Emerg Med 1983; 12:177–179.

78. Lord MJ, Carson WG: Multiple rib stress fractures—a golfer overdoes it. Phys Sports Med 1993; 21(5):81–91.

79. Lankenner PA, Micheli LJ: Stress fracture of the first rib—a case report. J Bone Joint Surg 1985; 67A:159–160.

80. Gurtler R, Pavlov H, Torg JS: Stress fracture of the ipsilateral first rib in a pitcher. Am J Sports Med 1985; 13:277–279.

81. Mikawa Y, Kobori M: Stress fracture of the first rib in a weightlifter. Arch Orthop Trauma Surg 1991; 110:121–122.

82. Brown HR, Indelicato PA: Isolated first rib fracture in a football player: A case report. Clin J Sports Med 1991; 1:255–258.

83. Vaccaro PS: Thoracic and vascular injuries in athletics. Athletic Training 1987; 22:290–292.

84. Moore RS: Fracture of the first rib: An uncommon throwing injury. Br J Accid Surg 1991; 22:149–150.

85. Mintz AC, Albano A, Reisdorff EJ, et al: Stress fracture of the first rib from serratus anterior tension: An unusual mechanism of injury. Ann Emerg Med 1990; 19:411–414.

86. Fruh JM: Fracture of the first rib in a collegiate soccer player. J Sports Rehabil 1993; 2:196–199.

87. Shaw NE: The syndrome of the prolapsed thoracic intervertebral disc. J Bone Joint Surg 1975; 57B:412.

88. Benson MK, Byrnes DP: The clinical syndromes and surgical treatment of thoracic intervertebral disc prolapse. J Bone Joint Surg 1975; 57B:471–477.

89. Wilcox PG, Spencer CW: Dorsolumbar kyphosis or Scheuermann's disease. Clin Sports Med 1986; 5:343–351.

90. Timm KE, Malone TR: Back Injuries and Rehabilitation. Baltimore, Williams & Wilkins, 1990.

91. Keene JS: Low back pain in the athlete from spondylogenic injury during recreation or competition. Postgrad Med 1983; 74:209–217.

92. Wilson FD, Lindseth RD: The adolescent "swimmer's back." Am J Sports Med 1982; 10:174–176.

93. Elattrache N, Fadale PD, Fu FH: Thoracic spine fracture in a football player—a case report. Am J Sports Med 1993; 21:157–160.

94. Rovere GD: Low back pain in athletics. Phys Sports Med 1987; 15(1):105–117.

95. Locke S, Allen GD: Etiology of low back pain in elite boardsailors. Med Sci Sports Exerc 1992; 24:964–966.

96. Kujala UM, Salminen JJ, Taimela S, et al: Subject characteristics and low back pain in young athletes and non athletes. Med Sci Sports Exerc 1992; 24:627–632.
97. Micheli LJ: Low back pain in the adolescent: Differential diagnosis. Am J Sports Med 1979; 7:362–364.
98. Micheli LJ: Back injuries in dancers. Clin Sports Med 1983; 2:473–484.
99. Alexander MJ: Biomechanical aspects of lumbar spine injuries in athletics: A review. Can J Appl Sports Sci 1984; 10:1–20.
100. Micheli LJ: How I manage low back pain in athletes. Phys Sports Med 1993; 21(3):182–194.
101. Williams PC: Examination and conservative treatment for disc lesion of the lower spine. Clin Orthop 1955; 5:28–39.
102. MacNab I, McCulloch J: Backache. Baltimore, Williams & Wilkins, 1990.
103. McKenzie RA: The Lumbar Spine—Mechanical Diagnoses and Therapy. Waikanae, NZ, Spinal Publications Ltd, 1981.
104. Saal JA: Rehabilitation of football players with lumbar spine injury (part 1). Phys Sports Med 1988; 16(9):61–74.
105. Spencer CW, Jackson DW: Back injuries in the athlete. Clin Sports Med 1983; 2:191–215.
106. Maitland GD: Vertebral Manipulation. London, Butterworths, 1986.
107. Grieve GP: Mobilization of the Spine. Edinburgh, Churchill Livingstone, 1991.
108. Borenstein DG, Wiesel SW, Boden SD: Low Back Pain—Medical Diagnosis and Comprehensive Management. Philadelphia, WB Saunders, 1995.
109. Saal JA: Rehabilitation of football players with lumbar spine injury (part 2). Phys Sports Med 1988; 16(10):117–125.
110. Norris CM: Spinal stabilization. Physiotherapy 1995; 81:61–79.
111. Konerding MA, Sedelmaier A: Exercises with the Gymnastic Ball. Temecula, CA, Sissel Products, 1992.
112. Watkins RG: Trunk Stabilization Program. Los Angeles, Kerlan-Jobe Orthopedic Clinic, 1992.
113. Gelabert R: Dancers' spinal syndromes. J Orthop Sports Phys Ther 1986; 7:180–191.
114. Micheli LJ: Sports following spinal surgery in the young athlete. Clin Orthop 1985; 198:152–157.
115. Jackson DW, Wiltse LL, Dingeman RD, Hayes M: Stress reactions involving the pars interarticularis in young athletes. Am J Sports Med 1981; 9:304–312.
116. Hoshina H: Spondylolysis in athletes. Phys Sports Med 1980; 8(9):75–79.
117. Johnson RJ: Low back pain in sports—managing spondylolysis in young patients. Phys Sports Med 1993; 21(4):53–59.
118. Hensinger RN: Spondylolysis and spondylolisthesis in children and adolescents. J Bone Joint Surg 1989; 71A:1098–1107.
119. Fredrickson BE, Baker D, McHolick WJ, et al: The natural history of spondylolysis and spondylolisthesis. J Bone Joint Surg 1984; 66A:699–707.
120. Kahler DM: Low back pain in athletics. J Sports Rehabil 1993; 2:63–78.
121. Ichikawa N, Ohara Y, Marishita T, et al: An etiological study on spondylolysis from a biomechanical aspect. Br J Sports Med 1982; 16:135–141.
122. Teitz CC: Sports medicine concerns in dance and gymnastics. Clin Sports Med 1983; 2:571–593.
123. Stinson JT: Spondylolysis and spondylolisthesis in the athlete. Clin Sports Med 1993; 12:517–528.
124. Fehlandt AF, Micheli LJ: Lumbar facet stress fracture in a ballet dancer. Spine 1993; 18:2537–2539.
125. Kraus DR, Shapiro D: The symptomatic lumbar spine in the athlete. Clin Sports Med 1989; 8:59–69.
126. Barash HL, Galante JO, Lambert CN, Day RD: Spondylolisthesis and tight hamstrings. J Bone Joint Surg 1970; 52A:1319–1328.
127. Volski RV, Bourguignon GJ, Rodriguez HM: Lower spine screening in the shooting sports. Phys Sports Med 1986; 14(1):101–106.
128. Jackson DW: Low back pain in young athletes: Evaluation of stress reaction and discogenic problems. Am J Sports Med 1979; 7:364–366.
129. Gainor BJ, Hagen RJ, Allen WC: Biomechanics of the spine in the polevaulter as related to spondylolysis. Am J Sports Med 1983; 11:53–57.
130. Pizzutillo PD, Hummer CD: Nonoperative treatment for painful adolescent spondylolysis or spondylolisthesis. J Pediatr Orthop 1989; 9:538–540.
131. Micheli LJ, Hall JE, Miller ME: Use of modified Boston brace for back injuries in athletics. Am J Sports Med 1980; 8:351–355.
132. Weber MD, Woodall WR: Spondylogenia disorders in gymnasts. J Orthop Sports Phys Ther 1991; 14:6–13.
133. Steiner ME, Micheli LJ: Treatment of symptomatic spondylolysis and spondylolisthesis with the modified Boston brace. Spine 1985; 10:937–943.
134. O'Neill DB, Micheli LJ: Postoperative radiographic evidence for fatigue fracture as the etiology of spondylolysis. Spine 1989; 14:1342–1355.
135. Buck JE: Direct repair of the defect in spondylolysis. Preliminary report. J Bone Joint Surg 1970; 52B:432–436.
136. Farrell JP, Drye CD: The young patient. Spine: State of the Art Rev 1991; 5:379–389.
137. Butler D, Gifford L: The concept of adverse mechanical tension in the nervous system. Part I: Testing for dural tension. Physiotherapy 1989; 75:631–636.
138. Butler D, Gifford L: The concept of adverse mechanical tension in the nervous system. Part II: Examination and treatment. Physiotherapy 1989; 75:629–636.
139. Floman Y, Wiesel SW, Rothman RH: Cauda equina syndrome presenting as a herniated lumbar disc. Clin Orthop 1980; 147:234–237.
140. Sakou T, Masuda A, Yone K, Nakagawa M: Percutaneous discectomy in athletes. Spine 1993; 18:2218–2221.
141. Matsunaga S, Sakou T, Taketomi E, Ijiri K: Comparison of operative results of lumbar disc herniation in manual labourers and athletes. Spine 1993; 18:2222–2226.
142. Cooney FD: Percutaneous lumbar discectomy. Clin Sports Med 1993; 12:557–568.
143. Kahanovitz N: Surgical disc excision. Clin Sports Med 1993; 12:579–585.
144. Wright A, Ferree B, Tromanhauser S: Spine fusion in the athlete. Clin Sports Med 1993; 12:599–602.
145. Jackson RP: The facet syndrome—myth or reality. Clin Orthop 1992; 279:110–121.
146. Schellinger D, Wener L, Ragodale B, Patronas N: Facet joint disorders and their role in the production of back pain and sciatics. RadioGraphics 1987; 7:923–942.
147. Mooney V, Robertson J: The facet syndrome. Clin Orthop 1976; 115:149–156.
148. Helbig T, Lee CK: The lumbar facet syndrome. Spine 1988; 13:61–64.
149. Hourigan CL, Bassett JM: Facet syndrome: Clinical signs, symptoms, diagnoses and treatment. J Manip Physiol Ther 1989; 12:293–297.
150. Lynch MC, Taylor JF: Facet joint injection for low back pain—a clinical study. J Bone Joint Surg 1986; 68B:138–141.
151. Moran R, O'Connell D, Walsh MG: The diagnostic value of facet joint injections. Spine 1988; 13:1407–1410.
152. Hirschberg GG, Froetscher L, Naeim F: Iliolumbar syndrome as a common cause of low back pain: Diagnosis and prognosis. Arch Phys Med Rehabil 1979; 60:415–419.
153. Roaf R: A study of the mechanics of spine injuries. J Bone Joint Surg 1960; 42B:810–823.
154. Denis F: The three column spine and its significance in the classification of acute thoracolumbar spine injuries. Spine 1983; 8:817–831.
155. Chance C: Note on a type of flexion fracture of the spine. Br J Radiol 1948; 21:452–456.
156. Aebi M, Thalgott JS: Fractures and dislocations of the thoracolumbar spine treated by the interval spinal skeletal fixation system. In Proceedings of the North American Spinal Society, 1987, p 68.
157. Wiltse LL, Kirkaldy-Willis WH, McIvor GW: The treatment of spinal stenosis. Clin Orthop 1976; 115:83–91.
158. Hackley DR, Wiesel SW: The lumbar spine in the aging athlete. Clin Sports Med 1993; 12:465–468.
159. Harris NH, Murray RO: Lesions of the symphysis in athletes. Br Med J 1974; 4:211.
160. Koch RA, Jackson DW: Pubic symphysitis in runners—a report of two cases. Am J Sports Med 1981; 9:62–63.

161. Wiley JJ: Traumatic osteitis pubis: The gracilis syndrome. Am J Sports Med 1983; 11:360–363.

162. Gamble JG, Simmons SC, Freedman M: The symphysis pubis—anatomic and pathologic considerations. Clin Orthop 1986; 203:261–272.

163. Hanson PG, Angevine M, Juhl JH: Osteitis pubis in sports activities. Phys Sports Med 1978;6(10):111–114.

164. Harris NH, Murray RO: Lesions of the symphysis in athletes. Br Med J 1974; 4:211–214.

165. Pearson RL: Osteitis pubis in a basketball player. Phys Sports Med 1988; 16(7):69–74.

166. Liebert PL, Lombardo JA, Belhobek GH: Acute post traumatic pubic symphysis instability in an athlete. Phys Sports Med 1988; 16(4):87–90.

167. Cassidy JD: The pathoanatomy and clinical significance of the sacroiliac joints. J Manip Physiol Ther 1992; 15:41–42.

168. DonTigny RL: Dysfunction of the sacroiliac joint and its treatment. J Orthop Sports Phys Ther 1979; 1:23–35.

169. Anderson MK, Hall SJ: Sports Injury Management. Baltimore, Williams & Wilkins, 1995.

170. LeBlanc KE: Sacroiliac sprain: An overlooked cause of back pain. Am Fam Physician 1992; 46:1459–1463.

171. Gitelman R: A chiropractic approach to biomechanical disorders of the lumbar spine and pelvis. *In* Haldeman S (ed): Modern Developments in the Principles and Practice of Chiropractic. New York, Appleton-Century-Crofts, 1980.

172. Wilson DJ: Diagnosis and treatment of sacroiliac joint dysfunction. Physiotherapy 1989; 75:500–501.

173. Latshaw RF, Kantner TR, Kalenak A, et al: A pelvic stress fracture in a female jogger—a case report. Am J Sports Med 1981; 9:54–56.

174. Satterfield MJ, Yasumura K, Abreu SH: Retro runner with ischial tuberosity enthesopathy. J Orthop Sports Phys Ther 1993; 17:191–194.

175. Noakes TD, Smith JA, Lindenberg G, Wills CE: Pelvic stress fractures in long distance runners. Am J Sports Med 1985; 13:120–123.

176. Atwell EA, Jackson DW: Stress fractures of the sacrum in runners—two case reports. Am J Sports Med 1991; 19:531–533.

177. Metzmaker JN, Pappas AM: Avulsion fractures of the pelvis. Am J Sports Med 1985; 13:349–358.

178. Miller ML: Avulsion fracture of the anterior superior iliac spine in high school track. Athletic Training 1982; 17:57–59.

179. Weiker GG: How I manage hip and pelvis injuries in adolescents. Phys Sports Med 1993; 21(12):72–82.

180. Zenteno BC: Avulsion fracture of the pelvis in a high jumper: Case report. Clin J Sports Med 1993; 3:268–270.

GENERAL REFERENCES

Anderson SJ: Evaluation and treatment of back pain in children and adolescents. J Back Musculoskel Rehabil 1991; 1:49.

Barrett GR, Shelton WR, Wiles JW: First rib fractures in football players. Am J Sports Med 1988; 16:674–676.

Goodman CE: Low back pain in the cosmetic athlete. Phys Sports Med 1987; 15(8):97–104.

Lee D: Manual Therapy for the Thorax. Delta, BC, DOPC, 1994.

Maffulli N, Pintore E: Stress fracture of the sixth rib in a canoeist. Br J Sports Med 1990; 24:247.

Maigne R: Low back pain of thoracolumbar origin. Arch Phys Med Rehabil 1980; 61:1987.

Micheli LJ: Sports injuries in children and adolescents. *In* Nudel DB (ed): Pediatric Sports Medicine. New York, PMA Publishing, 1989.

Panjabi MM, Krag MH, Chung TQ: Effects of disc injury on mechanical behavior of the human spine. Spine 1984; 9:707.

Press JM, Berkowitz M, Wiesner SL: The medical history and low back pain. J Back Musculoskel Rehabil 1991; 1:7.

Proffer DS, Patton JJ, Jackson DW: Nonunion of a first rib fracture in a gymnast. Am J Sports Med 1991; 19:198–201.

Schnute WJ: Osteitis pubis. Clin Orthop 1961; 20:187–192.

Wooden MJ: Preseason screening of the lumbar spine. J Orthop Sports Phys Ther 1981; 4:6–10.

CHAPTER 25

Abdominal and Thoracic Injuries

ANDREW W. NICHOLS MD

The abdomen and chest are frequent sites of injury during athletic competition and training. The prompt recognition and appropriate initial management of such injuries are often vital. The types of injuries that occur in the two regions differ significantly because of the presence of circumferential bony protection for the thorax but not for the abdomen. This lack of defense predisposes the abdomen to soft tissue traumatic injury, particularly in contact sports. Seven to ten percent of all athletic injuries affect the abdomen, the most commonly injured abdominal organs being the spleen, liver, and kidney.[1,2] Unlike thoracic injuries, abdominal injuries typically are not immediately life-threatening, unless a major exsanguination has occurred.

Thoracic injuries often result from high-velocity sports, from accidents, or from the use of inadequate protective equipment. The severity of these injuries may escalate rapidly and become life-threatening if not accurately assessed and treated. One quarter of all trauma-induced deaths result from chest injuries, although proper initial treatment results in only 15 percent of isolated chest injuries requiring surgical intervention. This high morbidity and mortality associated with thoracic trauma are due to tissue hypoxia, which develops secondary to cardiopulmonary system compromise.

ABDOMINAL INJURIES

INJURIES OF THE ABDOMINAL WALL

ABDOMINAL WALL CONTUSION

Abdominal wall muscular contusion is a common injury affecting athletes involved in contact sports. This injury is rarely serious because of the compressive, blow-cushioning effect of the soft abdominal contents. Differentiation from intra-abdominal injury may be difficult, however, underlining the importance of making a proper early diagnosis.

Abdominal wall contusions tend to manifest clinically with localized tenderness over the area of impact, pain caused by actively contracting (and relieved by relaxing) the underlying muscles, and the absence of referred pain. Muscle contusions over the iliac crest, at the insertion of the abdominal muscles, also known as "hip pointers," are often particularly debilitating injuries. This condition may adversely affect athletic performance to a greater degree than the seriousness of the injury would indicate. The presence of any contusion of the upper abdominal wall should prompt consideration of concurrent injury to the lower anterior floating ribs (Fig. 25–1).

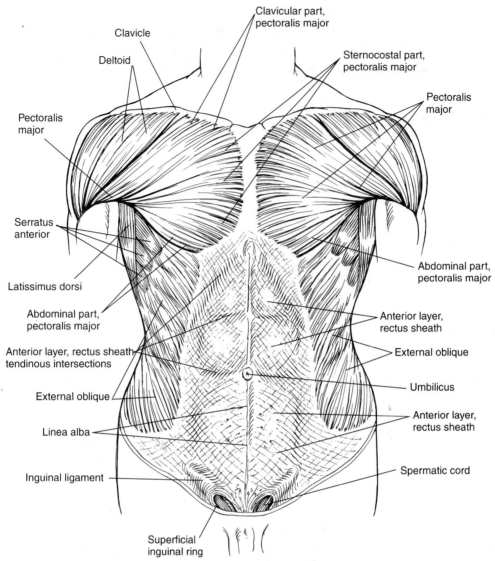

FIGURE 25–1. Superficial anatomy of the abdominal and thoracic wall.

BLOW TO THE SOLAR PLEXUS. A traumatic blow to the abdomen of an athlete whose abdominal muscles are not tensed is the usual mechanism of the often frightening sensation of "having the wind knocked out." The clinical presentation is that of an inability to catch one's breath. The initial management includes ruling out airway obstruction by objects such as the mouthguard, tongue, or turf from the field. Once a clear airway is confirmed and if symptoms persist, the hip belt should be loosened and the athlete placed in the supine position with the knees and hips flexed in an attempt at relaxation. Paradoxical as it may seem, asking the athlete to take a deep breath and hold it, and to repeat several times, often restores the athlete's breath more quickly. Additionally, a cold towel may be applied to the forehead, and the athlete should be assured that symptoms will be short-lived. The presence of concurrent intra-abdominal injury must be suspected, however. Table 25–1 helps to differentiate among the signs and symptoms of a blow to the solar plexus, an abdominal wall injury, and an intra-abdominal injury.

ABDOMINAL MUSCLE STRAIN

Strains of the abdominal muscles are extremely common athletic injuries. Symptoms depend on the size and location of injury. The most commonly injured abdominal muscle, the rectus abdominis, may be damaged at the musculotendinous junction adjacent to the lower anterior rib origin, at the pubic insertion, or at the horizontal fibrous bands within the muscle itself.

The potential mechanisms of injury include a sudden, violent muscular contraction or recurrent microtrauma from overuse, such as that commonly occur in soccer or in other sports requiring repetitive abdominal contractions. The physical findings consist of localized tenderness with muscle spasm at the site of injury and pain during active muscle contraction or stretching. Again, it is important to differentiate this injury from damage to the intra-abdominal organs.

Certain forms of abdominal muscle strain, especially those that occur at the ribs, pubis, or iliac crest, may

TABLE 25–1
Differentiation of Intra-abdominal Injury From Abdominal Wall Injury From Blow to the Solar Plexus

	Intra-abdominal Injury	Abdominal Wall Injury	Blow to Solar Plexus
Mechanism:	Blunt or penetrating trauma	Direct trauma	Blow to untensed abdominal muscle
Pain location:	Initially localized, often becomes diffuse	Localized	Minimal pain
Symptoms:	Pain which increases	Steady pain	Inability to catch breath
Duration:	Prolonged	Moderate to prolonged	Brief
Pain with tensing muscles?:	Often	Yes	No
Referred pain:	Often	No	No
Physical examination:	Guarding, rebound, rigidity, quiet BS	Localized tenderness	Minimal to no tenderness
Laboratory studies:	Abnormal	Normal	Normal

BS = bowel sounds.

result in chronic symptoms. Initial treatment should include relative rest and protection of the injured muscle. Activity should be limited by pain. An avulsed fragment of iliac crest is often reattached surgically, although surgery has little role in the treatment of proximal or midsubstance tears. A recent report identified a group of soccer players with chronic groin pain and the absence of preoperatively identifiable inguinal hernias, who at the time of surgical exploration were found to have various irregularities of the abdominal wall, including inguinal hernias, and microscopic tears or avulsions of the internal oblique muscle. These individuals were successfully treated with herniorrhaphy and were able to return to play within 3 months.[3]

RECTUS ABDOMINIS INTRAMUSCULAR HEMATOMA. The rectus abdominis muscle receives its blood supply from branches of the underlying inferior epigastric arteries. Sudden severe motions, such as an abrupt twisting of the trunk, a sudden contraction of the abdominal muscles, or a sudden extension of the spine, may produce a tear in the rectus abdominis muscle. The resultant shearing forces may rupture the supplying artery, resulting in intramuscular hematoma formation.

The onset of symptoms is generally abrupt, with localized pain, muscle guarding, and nausea and vomiting. Pain may be provoked by straight-leg raising or hyperextension of the back. A palpable mass, which becomes fixed when the a muscle is contracted, is often identifiable. A bluish discoloration of the periumbilical area, known as the Cullen sign, may appear. Computed tomography (CT) helps to confirm the diagnosis and outline the extent of hematoma formation.[4]

Most cases of rectus abdominis hematoma may be treated nonoperatively. Treatment includes application of ice during the first 48 hours after injury, followed by heat. Strengthening of the abdominal muscles should be instituted with isometric exercises and should progress to sit-ups, crunches, and other exercises as pain permits. If active bleeding persists, however, surgical ligation of the inferior epigastric artery and hematoma evacuation

may be required. Percutaneous drainage of the hematoma is rarely successful because of early clot organization.

HERNIA

A hernia is a protrusion of an anatomic structure, via a passageway or weakened area of the body wall, through which it should not normally pass. Common types include inguinal (direct and indirect), femoral, ventral, umbilical, and epigastric hernias. Approximately 1.5 percent of Americans are estimated to have hernias.[5] Table 25–2 lists the relative occurrence rates of various forms of hernias.[6] It is notable that 81 percent of hernias are located in the groin, 86 percent of these occurring in men. Although 84 percent of all femoral hernias affect women, inguinal hernias still occur more commonly than femoral hernias in women.[6]

It seems unlikely that hernias are ever exclusively caused by athletic participation, although they may be aggravated by activities that increase intra-abdominal pressure, such as weight-lifting and rowing. Some surgeons believe that the earlier a hernia is detected and

TABLE 25–2
Frequency of Various Types of Hernias

Hernia Type	Frequency (%)
Indirect inguinal	50
Direct inguinal	25
Ventral	10
Femoral	6
Umbilical	3
Epigastric	3
Esophageal	1
Miscellaneous	2

repaired, the stronger the repair will be.[7] Early repair is also advocated to avoid the potentially serious complications of hernia incarceration and strangulation. Incarceration occurs when a loop of bowel is caught in a hernial "ring," and it cannot be "reduced" or replaced into the abdominal cavity. Strangulation results from a compromise of blood flow to the bowel segment, which ultimately leads to bowel necrosis (Fig. 25–2). Absolute recommendations as to the appropriate timing of surgery for hernias are difficult. Decisions are best made on a case-by-case basis, depending on the type of hernia, the presence of symptoms, and the level of sports participation. It is clear, however, that individuals with symptomatic hernias should undergo immediate surgical repair or cease the offending activity. Generally, athletes at the nonprofessional level should undergo immediate repair of even asymptomatic hernias. Elite athletes who wish to delay repair must be made aware of the potential complications associated with continued participation in sports. These athletes should be followed throughout the season with serial physical examinations for the development of symptoms. They should be instructed to avoid wearing a truss, because this may mask worsening symptoms while providing little protection from injury. Participants in contact sports must have additional padding to the area, and hernia repair should be performed as soon as the season ends.

INGUINAL HERNIAS. Inguinal hernias, which are often discovered on routine physical examination, are the most common type of hernia in young athletes. As many inguinal hernias are asymptomatic, their identification includes a thorough examination by the physician in addition to questioning the athlete about the presence of pain or bulging in the groin. The

examination is performed by checking for an inguinal bulge, followed by insertion of the examiner's finger through the external ring of the inguinal canal while asking the athlete to cough. An inguinal hernia, if present, may produce a tap against the examiner's finger.

Indirect inguinal hernias, which are common in childhood, are treated by simple high ligation of the hernia sac. The treatment of adult indirect hernias is more difficult, usually requiring sac ligation in addition to repair of the inguinal canal floor. Direct hernias, which represent protrusions through the weakened floor of the inguinal canal, require more extensive repairs than indirect hernias. The recurrence rate of direct hernias is 13 percent compared with less than 5 percent for indirect hernias.[7]

Inguinal hernias may produce groin pain in the absence of an identifiable inguinal hernia on physical examination. In one study, eight such individuals were treated with herniorrhaphy, and all were able to return to full activity by 12 weeks postoperatively.[3] Inguinal hernia as must be considered as a potential source of chronic groin pain, even in the absence of hernia on physical examination.

OTHER ABDOMINAL HERNIAS. Femoral hernias, which occur far more commonly in women, are often difficult to detect. The hernia protrudes through the femoral ring, beneath the inguinal ligament, just medial to the femoral vein at the fossa ovalis. Surgical repair should be carried out as early as possible so as to avoid incarceration or strangulation, which are common sequelae of this hernia type.

Umbilical hernias are common in infants and children. Ten percent of Caucasian newborns, and 40 to 90 percent of black newborns are born with umbilical hernias. The great majority are small and close spontaneously by the age of 2 years, thus requiring no specific treatment. If surgical repair is necessary, the procedure is relatively simple in children but is more complicated in adults.

Epigastric hernias are located in the linea alba, or abdominal midline, superior to the umbilicus, and generally contain only a small amount of preperitoneal fat. Epigastric hernias are often asymptomatic and not recognized, as autopsy studies reveal their presence in five percent of normal adults.[6] Surgery is indicated only if enlargement or pain develops, in which case repair is relatively simple.

Ventral hernias, which are typically complications of previous midline abdominal surgery, are uncommon in athletes. Repair of ventral hernias may be quite difficult, especially when they are of large size, occur in obese individuals, or are associated with vertical incisions. The recurrence rate is high at 15 percent.[7] Table 25–3 provides useful guidelines for the timing of return to activity after the surgical repair of various hernia types and other abdominal surgical procedures.

"STITCH" IN THE SIDE

A "stitch" in the side, or "side-ache," is characterized by sharp pains in the runner's upper abdominal side

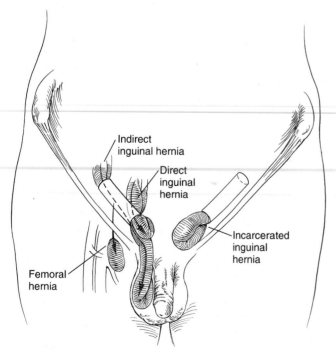

FIGURE 25–2. Diagram showing courses of inguinal hernias and incarcerated inguinal hernia.

TABLE 25–3
Hernia Repair and Abdominal Surgery: Return-to-Activity Guidelines

Procedure	Return to Classes	PRE* and Conditioning	Noncontact	Full Activity
Inguinal hernia				
Indirect (children)	1 wk	2 wk	3 wk	4 wk
Indirect (adult)	1 wk	3 wk	7 wk	8–10 wk
Direct	1 wk	3 wk	8 wk	12 wk
Femoral hernia	1 wk	3 wk	8 wk	12 wk
Umbilical hernia				
Children	1 wk	2 wk	3 wk	3 wk
Adults	1 wk	2 wk	4–6 wk	8 wk
Epigastric hernia	1 wk	2 wk	3–4 wk	6 wk
Ventral hernia	2 wk	8 wk	3–6 mo	?Avoid
Appendectomy	1 wk	3 wk	4 wk	6 wk
Other uncomplicated abdominal operations	2 wk	4 wk	8 wk	12 wk

*Progressive resistance exercise.
Adapted from Haycock CE: How I manage hernias in the athlete. Phys Sports Med 1983, 11:77–79; Olsen WR: Abdominal trauma in the athlete. *In* Schneider RC, Kennedy JC, Plant ML (eds): Sports Injuries—Mechanisms, Prevention, and Treatment. Baltimore, Williams & Wilkins, 1985, pp 809–817.

behind the lower ribs. Potential causes include trapped colonic gas bubbles, localized diaphragmatic hypoxia with spasm, liver congestion with stretching of the liver capsule, and poor conditioning. Poorly conditioned athletes commonly experience stitches, with a reduction in their frequency as fitness improves. An athlete may be able to "run through" a stitch by exhaling steadily and forcefully through pursed lips. Alternative means of relieving stitches include lying on the back with the arms extended overhead or flexing the trunk so that the chest nears the thighs. Once the discomfort of a stitch has abated, a workout may usually be completed without further recurrences.

SURGICAL WOUNDS

Physical activity produces an increase in intra-abdominal pressure, which may exert stress on surgical wounds and consequently delay or prevent healing. Skin wounds heal rapidly, whereas deep tissues heal much more slowly, increasing the risk of wound dehiscence. Douglas has demonstrated that aponeurosis tissue regains only 50 percent of its previous tensile strength at 2 months after surgery (Fig. 25–3).[8] Table 25–3 provides useful guidelines for the timing of returning athletes to various levels of physical activity after abdominal surgery.[7,9]

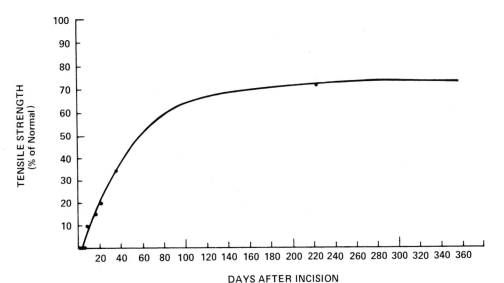

FIGURE 25–3. Tensile strength of healing wounds versus time. (From Olsen WR: Abdominal trauma in the athlete. *In* Schneider RC, Kennedy JC, Plant ML (eds): Sports Injuries—Mechanisms, Prevention, and Treatment. Baltimore, Williams & Wilkins, 1985, pp 809–817.)

INTRA-ABDOMINAL INJURIES

EVALUATION OF THE INJURED ATHLETE

Abdominal injuries occur in two forms: penetrating trauma and blunt trauma. Common forms of penetrating injury include knife, gunshot, or impalement wounds, which may occur accidentally in certain sporting events such as the javelin throw. Penetrating injuries due to large foreign objects should initially be managed by leaving the impaled object in place during transport to a surgical operating room unless the airway is compromised.[10] If the size of the object interferes with transport, a portion of the exposed object may be cut away. The application of direct pressure around the impaled object and the avoidance of placing traction on the object will help control bleeding from the entrance and exit wounds.[10] Removal of the object should take place only after large-bore needle intravenous access has been obtained and blood is available for emergent transfusion in the case of major exsanguination at the time of removal.

Blunt trauma is by far the most common type of athletic abdominal injury. The unprotected abdomen is struck by an opposing force, and the abdominal organs are compressed against the vertebral column. The severity of symptoms resulting from blunt abdominal trauma varies widely, ranging from severe pain in the presence of significant bleeding and peritoneal irritation to only mild tenderness. Peritoneal irritation, which is caused by bacterial or chemical intra-abdominal contamination, may occur after injury to the stomach, gallbladder, pancreas, small intestine, or colon. Localized tenderness may represent the only initial symptom, but soon the manifestations of generalized peritonitis, known as the peritoneal signs, including abdominal rigidity, guarding, referred pain, and loss of bowel sounds, may ensue. Referred pain deserves special mention, in that diaphragmatic irritation due to liver injury, spleen damage, or subdiaphragmatic fluid collection may produce pain that is referred to the corresponding shoulder. Table 25–1 helps to differentiate the signs and symptoms of intra-abdominal visceral injury from abdominal wall injury and a solar plexus blow.

The initial evaluation of an awake and alert individual who has sustained acute blunt abdominal injury begins with a careful history of injury and complete physical examination. Fig. 25–4 illustrates the major

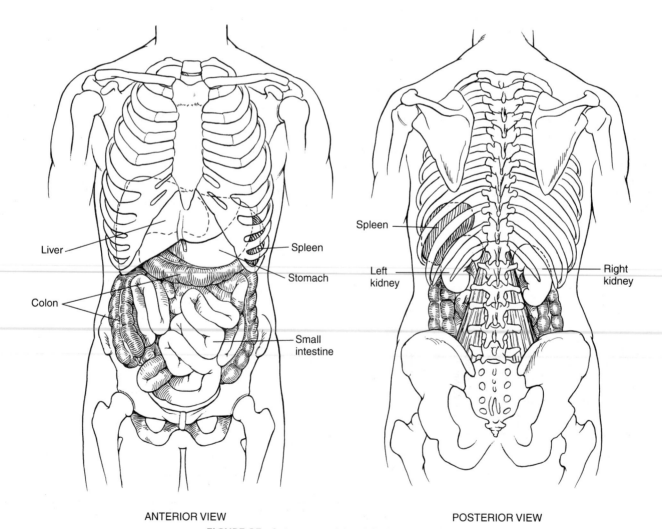

ANTERIOR VIEW   POSTERIOR VIEW

FIGURE 25–4. Anatomy of the abdominal cavity.

TABLE 25–4
Physical Examination of the Abdomen After Blunt Trauma Frequently Is Misleading

Signs of Visceral Injury on Initial Abdominal Examination	Percent of Patients	Incidence of Significant Intraabdominal Injury (%)
Obvious	22	80
Equivocal	46	35
Negative	12	43
Unreliable because of head or spine jury	19	35

From Olsen WR: Abdominal trauma in the athlete. *In* Schneider RL, Kennedy JC, Plant ML (eds): Sports Injuries—Mechanisms, Prevention, and Treatment. Baltimore, Williams & Wilkins, 1985, pp 809–817.

TABLE 25–5
Organs of the Three Abdominal Regions

Intrathoracic Abdomen
- Spleen
- Liver
- Diaphragm

"True" Abdomen
- Small intestines (most of)
- Colon (most of)
- Bladder (most of)
- Uterus
- Fallopian tubes
- Ovaries

Retroperitoneal Abdomen
- Retroperitoneal colon
- Retroperitoneal duodenum
- Pancreas
- Kidneys
- Retroperitoneal bladder

organs of the abdominal cavity. Depending on the findings, it is often possible to avoid extensive laboratory, radiographic, and invasive procedures. Suspicion must be maintained, since up to 43 percent of individuals who have a significant intra-abdominal injury initially present with a negative physical examination (Table 25–4).[9,11] Moreover, it has been reported that 20 percent of subjects with a retroperitoneal hematoma appear to have an initially benign abdominal examination.[12] The presence of multiple body system injuries, or an impaired ability to respond to painful stimuli, however, should prompt the clinician to perform additional diagnostic studies.

Diagnostic peritoneal lavage (DPL), having a sensitivity of 98.5 percent, is a useful test in the evaluation of an individual with multiple system injuries or an impaired level of consciousness. The procedure involves pericentesis with abdominal cavity saline lavage. An aspirate that reveals an elevated number of red blood cells is highly predictive for significant intra-abdominal injury and should prompt surgical exploration. The accuracy of DPL, however, is limited by its inability to specify the source of bleeding, poor results in the detection of retroperitoneal bleeding, risk associated with its invasiveness, and controversy over the management of intermediate results (e.g., 20,000 to 999,999 red blood cells/mm^2). A negative peritoneal lavage in the presence of other suspicious physical or laboratory findings should prompt the clinician to pursue the workup further with other diagnostic modalities such as computed tomography (CT). CT has recently gained widespread usage in the initial evaluation of intra-abdominal trauma. It is extremely accurate in the identification of significant intra-abdominal injury, including liver, spleen, and kidney lacerations, as well as retroperitoneal hematomas.[13] CT is particularly valuable in avoiding unnecessary exploratory laparotomies, which may have previously been performed on the basis of equivocal DPL results. Shortcomings of CT include its limited ability to detect hollow viscus injuries, its time-consuming nature, and the expertise required to accurately interpret subtle findings.

The initial treatment decision in the presence of intra-abdominal injury is whether to operate or not. The presence of obvious intra-abdominal bleeding, penetrating trauma to the abdomen or the thorax, or a mechanism and physical findings in an injury that is strongly suggestive of a "surgical abdomen" indicates the need for urgent laparotomy. Such individuals should not be observed for an extensive period of time, because these injuries may result in sudden and rapid deterioration.

An approach to the initial evaluation of the acutely injured abdomen begins with observation of the entire exposed anterior and posterior abdomen, flanks, lower chest, buttocks, and perineum for evidence of contusions, abrasions, lacerations, and penetrating wounds. Contusions may not appear for several hours after trauma has occurred. The abdomen should then be auscultated to assess the frequency and quality of bowel sounds. The presence of bacteria, blood, or chemical irritants in the abdomen may result in an ileus, or paralysis of the intestines, manifested by absent or reduced bowel sounds. This finding, however, is extremely nonspecific and should prompt further evaluation. The ab-

TABLE 25–6
Usefulness of Diagnostic Evaluation Methods by Abdominal Region

Region	Palpation	DPL	CT
Intrathoracic	1+	2+	3+
"True"	3+	2+	3+
Retroperitoneal	1+	1+	3+

CT = Computed tomography; DPL = diagostic peritoneal lavage.

domen should then be examined for physical signs of peritoneal irritation, including rebound tenderness, muscle guarding, tenderness with percussion, or pain with coughing.

The complete examination of the abdomen must include careful evaluation of the three regions of the abdomen: the intrathoracic abdomen, the "true" abdomen, and the retroperitoneal abdomen. The organs located in each region are listed in Table 25–5. The intrathoracic abdomen, which is difficult to palpate since it lies protected by the bony thorax, is susceptible to injury from blows to the lower or midabdomen, which direct forces upward. The true abdomen is more accessible to examination by palpation, whereas the retroperitoneal abdomen is often extremely difficult to evaluate by physical examination. Hematomas are a common finding in the retroperitoneal space, and CT is often required for a diagnosis. Table 25–6 summarizes the usefulness of the various diagnostic modalities in the evaluation of each abdominal region.

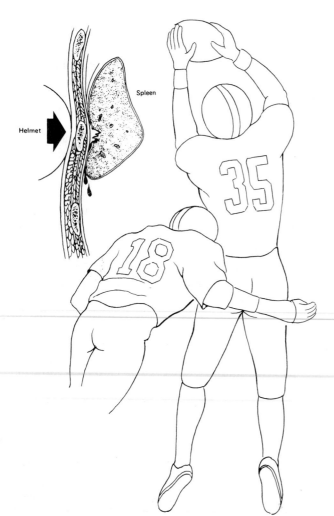

FIGURE 25–5. Mechanism of spleen injury by direct blunt trauma. (From Olsen WR: Abdominal trauma in the athlete. *In* Schneider RC, Kennedy JC, Plant ML (eds): Sports Injuries—Mechanisms, Prevention, and Treatment. Baltimore, Williams & Wilkins, 1985, pp 809–817.)

SPLENIC INJURY

The spleen, located deep to the left ninth through eleventh ribs, is the most commonly injured organ in the abdomen. Laceration or rupture may occur as a result of blunt trauma to the left upper abdomen or lower chest wall, or secondary to overlying rib fractures (Fig. 25–5). The clinical features of splenic injury are often insidious in onset, because symptoms develop secondary to bleeding. Significant and rapid bleeding occurs in as much as 85 percent of cases of frank rupture. Subcapsular hematoma formation results in less bleeding, although rupture with resumption of bleeding may occur from even minor recurrent trauma for up to several weeks later. Symptoms of splenic injury include left upper quadrant or diffuse abdominal pain, left shoulder pain caused by diaphragmatic irritation, and shock.[9]

Splenic injury may be fatal if not promptly diagnosed or if appropriate treatment is delayed. The diagnosis may be readily confirmed by CT, which has the advantage over diagnostic peritoneal lavage in its greater than 95 percent accuracy, information provided regarding the location and severity of the splenic damage, quantity of hemoperitoneum, and ability to identify associated injuries. Buntain and colleagues have provided a useful classification of splenic injury based on CT appearance to assist with management decisions (Fig. 25–6).[14,15]

The spleen was once considered an expendable organ that played little physiologic role in adults. Recently, however, the treatment of splenic injuries has taken a major shift toward the preservation of splenic tissue. Splenectomy results in the loss of an invaluable reticuloendothelial filter of the blood, reduced immune function with lowered levels of IgG and IgM immunoglobulins and T-cells, and an increased risk of overwhelming bacterial infection. The encapsulated organisms *Streptococcus pneumoniae, Haemophilus influenzae,* type B, and *Neisseria meningitides,* are particularly virulent for splenectomized individuals.

The criteria for nonoperative management of splenic injuries include hemodynamic stability, a nonenlarging splenic defect, and stable peritoneal findings. All nonoperative patients should be treated in the hospital with observation, serial examinations, and hematocrit levels to detect any hemodynamic instability. Up to 90 percent of classes 1 and 2 injuries can be treated nonoperatively, without blood transfusions, and can be ready for discharge in less than 7 days.[14] Hospitalization is particularly important, given the risks of delayed rupture or hemorrhage.

Surgical exploration and treatment are indicated in cases in which conservative management fails or is deemed inappropriate. Total splenectomy should be avoided if at all possible. Splenorrhaphy, consisting of debridement, suturing, partial resection, and the application of a hemostatic agent to preserve functioning splenic tissue, is the procedure of choice.

Return-to-play decisions after splenic injury require great prudence. Classes 1 and 2 injuries may heal

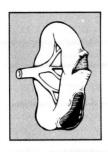
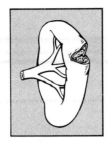
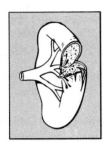
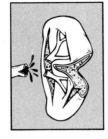

FIGURE 25–6. CT-based classification of splenic injury:

Class 1: Subcapsular hematoma or localized capsular disruption without significant parenchymal injury.

Class 2: Single or multiple capsular and parenchymal disruptions, transverse or longitudinal, that do not extend into the hilum or involve major blood vessels. Intraparenchymatous hematoma may or may not coexist.

Class 3: Deep fractures, single or multiple, transverse or longitudinal, extending into the hilum and involving the major blood vessels.

Class 4: Completely shattered or fragmented spleen, or separated from its normal blood supply at the pedicle (may or may not have associated intra- or extra-abdominal injury).

(Text reprinted with permission from Buntain WL, Gould HR, Maull KI: Predictability of splenic salvage by computed tomography. J Trauma 28(1):24–34, 1988. Illustrations from Affect TP: Severe sports-related spleen injury. The Physician and Sports Medicine 1992; 20:109–123. Reprinted by permission of McGraw-Hill, Inc.)

completely within 6 to 8 weeks without surgery.[14] Two weeks of endurance training should be instituted before return to even noncontact sports. Return to contact sports should be delayed for another 2 to 3 weeks following the healing period. More severe injuries may be followed with serial CT scans or ultrasonograms on a monthly or bimonthly basis until complete healing is confirmed. A similar recovery pattern, with two to three weeks of endurance training followed by return to noncontact sports and ultimately return to contact sports, is advisable.

INFECTIOUS MONONUCLEOSIS AND SPLENIC DAMAGE. Infectious mononucleosis, a viral infection caused by the Epstein-Barr virus, commonly affects adolescents and young adults. Clinical manifestations include sore throat, fever, cervical adenopathy, splenomegaly, and hepatomegaly. Splenic enlargement occurs in up to 70 percent of individuals with infectious mononucleosis between days 4 and 21 of the illness. This period coincides with the time of maximal risk for splenic rupture, which complicates 0.1 to 0.2 percent of cases. Individuals with splenomegaly who participate in contact sports are at increased risk for splenic rupture. Vigorous physical activity should be

curtailed until splenomegaly resolves. A spleen that is palpable during abdominal physical examination, is at least two to three times its normal size. It may take as long as 3 weeks from the time that the splenic tip is no longer palpable for splenomegaly to completely resolve.

The management of mononucleosis-induced splenomegaly includes examinations of the abdomen on at least a weekly basis. Radiographs, ultrasonograms, and CT may also be helpful to confirm resolution of splenomegaly before allowing the athlete to return to activity. Low-impact endurance training should be resumed initially, whereas high-impact activity and contact sports should be avoided for an additional 2 to 3 weeks.[16,17] Corticosteroids may be useful in the treatment of upper airway obstruction, which is often associated with infectious mononucleosis, although they have not been shown to reduce the prevalence or severity of splenomegaly.

LIVER INJURY

The liver is the second most commonly injured organ of the abdominal cavity, accounting for 4.4 to 4.9 percent of athletic injuries.[1] The most common mechanism of injury is a blunt blow to the right abdomen or lower chest. A recent case report, however, described liver injury after a blow to the left abdomen.[18] Symptoms of liver injury vary with the severity of damage but may include right upper quadrant pain, diffuse abdominal pain, or peritoneal irritation signs, if heavy bleeding is present. Liver injuries, unlike splenic injuries, rarely progress to serious hemorrhage.

Hepatic contusions result in mild right upper quadrant abdominal pain, occasional nausea and vomiting, hemodynamic stability, and an absence of peritoneal signs. Treatment includes bed rest with observation and avoidance of athletic activities for at least 2 to 3 weeks, at which time endurance activities may be gradually reintroduced.[19]

Hepatic lacerations range from minor tears producing little bleeding, to more severe, deeper parenchymal bleeding, which may result in hemodynamic instability and require surgical intervention and repair. Eighty percent of liver injuries involve the right hepatic lobe because of its larger volume, proximity to the lower ribs, and the location of the falciform ligament.[19] Most liver lacerations result in subcapsular hematoma formation or intraparenchymal tears. Associated hemorrhage is typically minimal, with 70 percent having stopped bleeding by the time of laparotomy.[20,21] The amount of hemoperitoneum detected by CT, rather than the degree of liver damage, correlates well with the need for operative intervention.[18] Liver trauma may be managed nonoperatively in the presence of hemodynamic stability and the absence of peritoneal signs or significant extrahepatic injury. Surgical management is indicated if hemodynamics are unstable, the abdomen distends, and the hematocrit continues to fall or fails to respond to blood transfusions. Clinical recovery is best assessed by the use of serial CT, which will demonstrate early healing within 2 to 4 weeks. Complete healing must be confirmed before permitting an athlete to return to full activity, which usually takes 3 to 6 months.[22]

INTESTINAL TRACT INJURY

RUPTURED HOLLOW VISCUS. Rupture of a hollow viscus is an uncommon injury but has been reported in athletes who have sustained blunt abdominal trauma.[18,23,24] The specific segments of bowel that are fixed to the abdominal wall appear to be most susceptible to rupture. These include the duodenum, proximal jejunum, terminal ileum, and any areas attached by adhesions. The mechanism of injury is not known, although it is suspected that the bowel is crushed against the spine, resulting in rupture or hematoma formation.[24] The duodenum seems to be particularly vulnerable to injury where it crosses the spine.

The symptoms of bowel rupture include severe abdominal pain, nausea, vomiting, and muscle spasm. The quality of abdominal pain is typically diffuse, and "gripping" or "crampy" in nature. Injury to various portions of the intestinal tract may refer pain to other locations in the abdomen as follows: stomach or duodenum to the epigastrium, small bowel to the umbilical area, and colon to the suprapubic region. The physical examination may reveal rebound tenderness consistent with peritoneal irritation, an absence of bowel sounds, and abdominal rigidity.

The diagnosis of bowel rupture may be suspected by the presence of free air under the diaphragm on an upright abdominal radiograph and may be confirmed by CT with contrast, magnetic resonance imaging (MRI), or exploratory laparotomy. The treatment of a ruptured hollow viscus is surgical, with immediate repair of damage, irrigation of the abdominal cavity, and appropriate treatment of peritonitis.

INTRAMURAL HEMATOMA. Intestinal intramural hematoma has been reported as a result of contact in an adolescent football player.[23] The duodenum is particularly susceptible to injury, given the presence of a transitional area between the portion that is tightly anchored to the abdominal wall and the loosely tethered segment attached to mesentery. This area becomes particularly stressed during sudden deceleration, which commonly occurs in football, bicycling, and equestrian sports. The resultant forces may cause the submucosal vessels to be sheared against the muscularis mucosa, with bleeding into the duodenal wall, between the muscularis and submucosal layers. Partial to complete lumenal obstruction may ensue. The mechanism of this injury is severe deceleration rather than blunt trauma.[23]

KIDNEY INJURY

The kidney is the most commonly injured intraabdominal organ in sports participants.[1] Glenn and Harvard found that renal trauma was the cause of hospitalization in 19 percent of all injured athletes who required hospitalization for sports trauma.[25] Additionally, 15 to 50 percent of all renal injuries have been found to be a result of sports-related trauma.[1,26] Football produces the largest number of kidney injuries in the United States, although soccer, rugby, lacrosse, basketball, boxing, hockey, and wrestling are also frequently associated with renal trauma.[1] Most injuries result from blunt blows to the flank or abdomen. The upper one third of the right kidney and the upper one half of the left kidney lie above the twelfth rib, within the thorax. Three layers of anterior abdominal muscles, retroperitoneal fat, the psoas muscles, and the paravertebral muscles provide further renal protection, particularly when the muscles are tensed. Children are at increased risk of renal damage because of the absence of fatty anatomic padding. Kidney injury may be severely painful, particularly if damage has occurred within the substance of the kidney with resultant bleeding into the collecting system. Occult hematuria without radiographic evidence of injury is a common finding in boxers, football players, basketball players, and longdistance runners.

Kidney damage must be suspected when an athlete has sustained a blow to the flank, abdomen, or lower chest. Signs and symptoms of renal damage include flank pain, tenderness, ecchymosis, and hematuria (blood in the urine). The quantity of hematuria correlates poorly with the degree of renal injury. An example of a susceptible body position for renal injury occurs when the body is extended, and the abdominal muscles are relaxed, as when a football player is leaping for a pass.[27] Hematuria may also occur secondary to repeated microtrauma, resulting in cumulative damage to the urinary tract. Long-distance runners are particularly prone to this condition as a result of shock transmission from repeated footstrikes, as are boxers who sustain recurrent punches to the torso.

Types of kidney injuries include contusion, subcapsular hematoma, parenchymal rupture into the renal pelvis, rupture across the capsule, and laceration (Fig. 25-7).[2] Renal contusion, the most common type of kidney injury, typically results from a shock transmitted to the kidney after a blow to the torso. These injuries are usually self-limited, although extravasated blood under the capsule may be problematic if it becomes infected. Increasing forces may produce more serious kidney damage, such as capsular rupture, perirenal hematoma formation, and subcapsular hemorrhage with progression to kidney necrosis. The severity and clinical manifestations of renal rupture depend on the extent and area of injury. Extrinsic hemorrhage may trigger symptoms of localized pain, back and flank muscle spasm, and painful muscle functioning.

A differential diagnosis of hematuria is offered in Table 25-7. The medical evaluation of an athlete with hematuria who has sustained trauma to the abdomen, back, or lower chest should include a complete history and physical examination, urinalysis, complete blood count, plain film radiograph of the abdomen, and CT scan or intravenous pyelogram (IVP). Plain x-ray films may disclose associated injuries, such as lower rib or lumbar vertebral fractures, as well as loss of the psoas muscle and renal outlines, if retroperitoneal bleeding is present. Contrast-enhanced CT, if available, is generally preferable to IVP, since it is quicker to perform, noninvasive, and has greater accuracy in predicting the

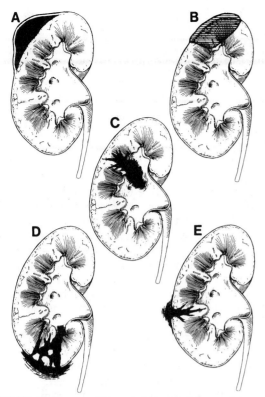

FIGURE 25–7. Common kidney injuries: *A*, Subcapsular hematoma. *B*, Contusion. *C*, Parenchymal rupture into renal pelvis. *D*, Rupture across capsule. *E*, Laceration. (From Diamond DL: Sports-related abdominal trauma. Clin Sports Med 1:91, 1989.)

quantity of blood loss, extent of damage, and presence of urinary extravasation. CT has the additional advantage of assessing damage to other organs.[28] IVP has a lower specificity, and is inadequate in the diagnosis of vascular injuries, which may necessitate the use of arteriography.

The absence of red blood cells on a single urinalysis, does not exclude the possibility of renal damage. If the clinical presentation and mechanism of injury provide one with a strong suspicion of renal damage, successive urine specimens should be collected. If continued concern exists, contrast CT or IVP should be performed.

The treatment of renal injuries depends on the type and extent of damage. The great majority of cases will heal without complications when treated with complete bed rest until hematuria clears. Hospitalization is indicated to monitor for continued bleeding, the development of shock, hematoma expansion, or continued free extravasation of urine on IVP or contrast CT scan. These conditions warrant surgical intervention. Generally, contusions, small cortical lacerations, and caliceal lacerations do not require surgical treatment, whereas complete ruptures and pedical injuries demand prompt operative management.

The athlete who has sustained a relatively minor renal injury should avoid strenuous sports activity for at least 4 weeks. This reduces the risk of rebleeding, since it takes 15 to 21 days for clots to dissolve. The recovery phase of more significant renal trauma should include serial monitoring of the blood pressure, urinalysis, and CT or IVP every 3 months for 1 year. These measures

will help identify the late-developing complications of hydronephrosis, transient hypertension, reduced renal function, infection, and renal calcification. The athlete who has sustained extensive injury should be allowed to return to play only after contrast CT confirms complete healing, which often takes 6 or more months.[29]

URETERAL INJURY

The ureter is the least commonly injured portion of the urinary tract. Avulsion of the ureter has been reported after a severe blow to a hyperextended back, which may occur during a fall from a horse or during a motor vehicle accident. The most common symptom of ureteral rupture is nondescript back pain, often in conjunction with signs of severe abdominal injuries and peritoneal irritation. The diagnosis may be confirmed by IVP, and the treatment is surgical.

BLADDER INJURY

The urinary bladder is infrequently injured in sports because of its location deep to the pubic bones, within the protective pelvic ring. Moreover, injury to an empty bladder is rare, because of the collapsed configuration that reduces its susceptibility to macrotraumatic injury. As a preventive measure, it is wise to have contact sport athletes use the bathroom prior to competition.

Bladder contusion, the most common bladder injury, typically results from abdominal or pelvic trauma. The presentation is hematuria with indefinite suprapubic tenderness and an absence of peritoneal signs, such as abdominal rigidity and rebound tenderness. Bladder rupture is a rare but extremely serious condition that necessitates prompt recognition and surgical treatment. The symptoms of bladder rupture include severe suprapubic pain, which often progresses rapidly to peritoneal signs, and shock. An individual who is unable to void after abdominal or pelvic trauma, should undergo a cystogram. Any extravasation of contrast on cystography accurately depicts the site of injury. If urethral damage is suspected, retrograde urethrography should precede blind catheterization to avoid inducing further damage to the urethra.

"Runner's hematuria" must be considered in the evaluation of an athlete with hematuria. Macrohema-

TABLE 25–7
Differential Diagnosis of Hematuria

- Trauma
- Infection
- Urinary tract stones
- "Runner's hematuria"
- Neoplasms (benign and malignant)
- Prostatitis
- Glomerulonephritis
- Analgesic nephropathy
- Sickle cell anemia
- Disorders of coagulation
- Thrombocytopenia

turia or microhematuria, often with dysuria and suprapubic pain, has been reported in up to 18 percent of runners at the conclusion of a marathon race.[30] Cystoscopic studies have identified the presence of a mucosal contusion at the bladder base that involves the trigone, from the internal meatus to the interureteric ridge, and a mirror image contusion lesion on the posterior bladder wall.[31] It is suspected that the repetitive impact of running results in the bladder mucosal contusion, especially if the bladder is empty. Hematuria typically resolves rapidly with rest.

PANCREATIC INJURY

Athletics-related injury to the pancreas is uncommon because of its relatively protected anatomic location, deep in the retroperitoneum. An extremely forceful abdominal blow that compresses the organ against the spine is usually necessary to produce pancreatic damage. Because of the vital physiologic nature of the pancreas, the severity of trauma necessary to induce damage to the pancreas, and the corrosive nature of pancreatic contents, injuries to the pancreas are often life-threatening.

The signs and symptoms of pancreatic injury include mild-to-severe midabdominal pain, which often radiates to the back, nausea and vomiting, signs of peritoneal irritation, and shock. Damage to the pancreas may occur in the form of a contusion with pseudocyst development, traumatic pancreatitis, laceration, or transection. Incidental pancreatitis, such as that occurring with excessive alcohol intake or cholelithiasis, must also be considered in the differential diagnosis of pancreatic abnormalities. The diagnosis is made by CT or MRI. Serum amylase determination may serve as a useful screening test, but a level in the normal range does not exclude the possibility of pancreatic damage. The treatment of a traumatic pancreatic injury is determined by the severity of the injury. Conservative care includes bed rest, bowel rest, and fluid replacement, whereas severe injury may require surgical intervention, including distal pancreatectomy.

INJURIES TO THE GENITALIA AND PERINEUM

TESTICULAR AND SCROTAL INJURY

Groin trauma is relatively common in sports that use hard implements, such as hockey, baseball, softball, and lacrosse. Many of these sports use protective cups to safeguard this area, and thus, fortunately, serious injury occurs only rarely. The symptoms of testicular or scrotal injury, which include localized pain, scrotal swelling, and ecchymosis, are relatively nonspecific (Fig. 25–8). The early identification of serious injuries, such as testicular rupture or torsion, however, is essential for the preservation of the injured testicle.

Testicular rupture, the most serious groin injury, is uncommon because of the mobility of the testes. Rupture usually results from high-velocity sports, such as bicycling, when a testis is compressed between the bicycle saddle and the pubic bones. The tunica vaginalis, which covers the tubular and vascular components of the testis, ruptures after impact. The symptoms include pain and bleeding into the scrotum with massive swelling. The treatment is emergent surgical testicular repair and drainage of the scrotum.

Blunt groin trauma may cause a rapid accumulation of blood in the scrotum, known as a hematocele, caused by rupture of the pampiniform plexus venous network of the spermatic cord. Treatment for a hematocele involves bed rest, application of ice, and elevation of the scrotum with the possibility of surgical ligation of

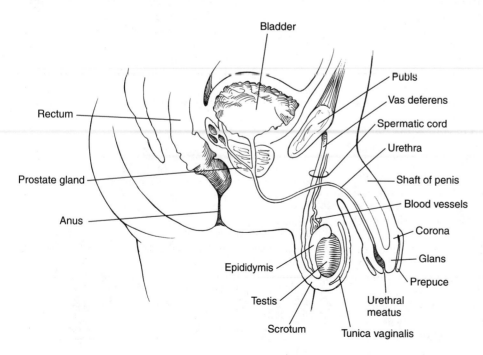

FIGURE 25–8. Anatomy of the male genitalia.

bleeding vessels in case the hematoma continues to accumulate rapidly. Individuals with varicoceles, a condition characterized by chronic engorgement of the pampiniform plexus, seem to be at increased risk of developing a hematocele.

Contusions of the testicle or scrotum are the most common groin injuries. They are most accurately evaluated in the period immediately following the injury, before swelling develops. Initial treatment should include bed rest, the application of ice packs, scrotal elevation, and oral analgesics. Ambulation is permitted once pain has resolved and swelling has stabilized. A scrotal support should then be worn for several days.[32]

Torsion of the spermatic cord may occur spontaneously, after a blow to the scrotum, or as a result of forceful contraction of the cremasteric muscle, which draws the testis superiorly over the pubis and twists the cord. Torsion is unlikely if a supporter is worn. This injury must be suspected, particularly in the young athlete who experiences sudden or slowly progressive abdominal or groin pain with no history of trauma. The physical examination may reveal poor definition of the scrotal structures. The diagnosis is suggested further by a radionuclide scan that shows reduced uptake in the involved testicle, an indication for prompt surgical intervention.

Other conditions that must be considered in the evaluation of an athlete with groin pain include epididymitis and neoplasms. Epididymitis typically manifests with a gradual onset of scrotal pain in young males. A soft, nontender testis adjacent to a discretely tender, swollen epididymis, is noted on physical examination. Pyuria may be apparent on urinalysis. Testicular carcinomas are relatively common neoplasms in young men and must be considered in the evaluation of any scrotal masses.

The workup and evaluation of scrotal and testicular injuries always should begin with a thorough history of injury. The physical examination may be best performed with the individual in the supine position so as to help relieve discomfort and reduce the tug of gravity on the testicle. The anatomic structures should be palpated systematically with an attempt to identify each testis, epididymis, and spermatic cord. The presence of scrotal swelling or fullness should prompt the use of transillumination to help differentiate between a hydrocele, which does transilluminate and produces a testicular shadow, and a hematocele or testicular mass that does not transilluminate. A Doppler probe evaluation is useful if one suspects torsion of the cord, and the presence of a spermatic artery pulse at the hilum of the testis helps to rule out torsion. Ultrasonography provides the most useful noninvasive imaging assessment of the scrotal contents. It helps to identify hematoceles, testicular masses, epididymal swelling, and testicular integrity. Ultrasonography may be limited, however, by available equipment and the expertise of the individual ultrasonographer. Diagnostic percutaneous needle aspiration of scrotal fluid should generally be avoided, to reduce the risk of introducing infection and because of the technical difficulty of the procedure. Aspiration

may be appropriate, however, in the presence of a tensely swollen scrotum.[32] As a general rule, if groin trauma results in a nonpalpable testicle and a non-transilluminable scrotum, testicular rupture must be considered, and urgent urologic consultation should be sought.

PENILE AND URETHRAL INJURY

The penis is rarely injured when the athlete wears an athletic supporter. Bicycle racers commonly experience a traumatic irritation of the pudendal nerve as a result of prolonged episodes of direct pressure from the hard bicycle saddle on the pudendal nerve. Symptoms, which may include localized penile numbness, priapism, and ischemic neuropathy, typically resolve after the bicycle race. The condition is usually preventable by using a longitudinally furrowed saddle and by avoiding squeezing the saddle during hill-climbing.

The urethra is a rarely injured structure in athletics. Men are generally affected more commonly than women. The mechanism of injury is often a straddle injury, which most frequently occurs in bicycling or equestrian events. The bulbous portion of the urethra is most often involved, since the penile urethra is usually protected by the supporter, and the posterior urethra by the pubic bones. A serious blow to the perineum, pelvic diastasis, or the presence of blood at the urethral meatus should prompt further diagnostic investigation with retrograde urethrography. If urethral injury is suspected, retrograde urethrography should always be done before passing a urethral catheter. Extravasation of contrast during the retrograde urethrogram accurately delineates the location and extent of urethral damage. The treatment is surgical repair, with a suprapubic cystostomy placed for urinary diversion. Urethral stricture is a common complication.

PERINEUM INJURIES

HEMATOMA. Women athletes occasionally sustain sports-related trauma to the vulva and labia, resulting in edema and hematoma formation. Appropriate treatment includes ice application and protection. Vaginal lacerations rarely accompany such injuries, but their prompt recognition and treatment are necessary to avoid infection or long-term dysfunction.

VAGINAL WATER INJECTION INJURIES. The female reproductive organs are fortunately well protected by the pubis and thus not very frequently injured. Water skiing, however, may result in "water injection" damage to the vagina, uterus, and fallopian tubes. A novice skier may have difficulty standing and consequently assumes a squatting position, which may enable water to enter the vagina. Vaginal damage, incomplete abortions, and salpingitis may occur. Salpingitis manifests with signs of an acute abdomen and sepsis. However, symptoms do not generally appear clinically until after 3 days, at which time the athlete may not associate the injury with the infection. Vaginal injection of water injuries may be avoided by wearing neoprene shorts or wetsuits.

THORACIC INJURIES

INJURIES OF THE CHEST WALL

RIB INJURIES

Twelve pairs of ribs articulate with the twelve corresponding thoracic vertebrae. Strong ligaments firmly attach each rib to its analogous vertebra and to those located immediately above and below. Additional capsular ligaments hold each rib tightly against the vertebral body and transverse process at each level, while other ligaments extend vertically from the transverse process of the vertebrae above, to the upper aspect of the rib below. The strength of these ligamentous attachments makes sprains uncommon. The anatomy of the ribcage is presented in Figure 25–9.

Each rib-costocartilage pair, the corresponding vertebra, and the sternum form a ring structure that is smallest and most circular in the superior thorax and becomes progressively larger and more oval in shape, inferiorly to the seventh rib. The orientation of the ribs is nearly horizontal at the top, gradually becomes increasingly oblique lower in the thorax, and approaches verticality at the inferior end. The upper seven ribs are attached directly to the sternum by costocartilage. The costocartilage of the eighth through tenth ribs does not attach immediately to the sternum, but instead joins the costocartilage of the rib above. The eleventh and twelfth ribs, known as the "floating ribs," are engulfed by abdominal musculature anteriorly, with no bony attachment. The undersurface of each rib has a groove through which traverse the intercostal neurovascular structures.

The ribs lie subcutaneously in the anterior chest. This places them at greater risk for damage from direct trauma than the deeper-positioned posterior aspects of the ribs, which are better protected by the heavy musculature of the back and paraspinal muscles. The ribs are elevated by the intercostal and other accessory muscles during inspiration, with a resultant increase in the anterior-posterior diameter of the lower thorax. Adjacent ribs are further secured by fascial extensions from the external intercostal muscles between ribs. The abdominal muscles stretch from the lower anterior ribs to the pelvic brim, providing the anterior connection between the thorax and the pelvis.

CONTUSION. A direct blow to the anterior chest often leads to contusion of the subcutaneously located ribs, whereas a similar blow to the posterior chest is more likely to cause paraspinal muscular injury. The most common symptom of a rib contusion occurring from direct trauma is localized pain during deep inspiration. The physical examination reveals localized tenderness over the injury without the crepitation which is sometimes noted with a rib fracture. The clinical differentiation of a rib fracture from a contusion is difficult, but the elicitation of injury site pain when the examiner compresses the chest by placing one hand on the back of the hemithorax and the other on the front is indicative of fracture. Additionally, manipulation of the affected rib at a site distant to the injury should not induce injury site pain. A rib contusion should be treated symptomatically. Once the possibility of an

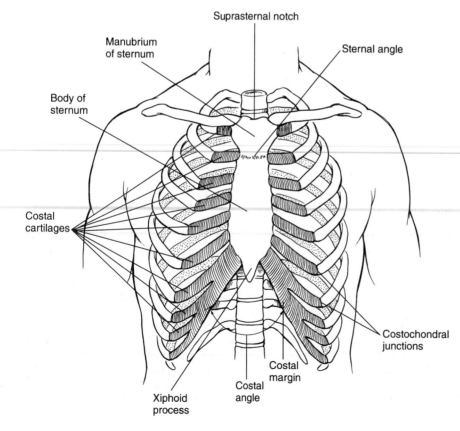

Suprasternal notch

Manubrium of sternum

Sternal angle

Body of sternum

Costal cartilages

Costochondral junctions

Xiphoid process

Costal angle

Costal margin

FIGURE 25–9. Anatomy of the ribcage, sternum, and costochondral joints.

occult fracture has been eliminated, the athlete may be allowed to return to participation with padding over the injury site.

SPRAIN, SUBLUXATION, OR DISLOCATION OF THE VERTEBRAL ATTACHMENTS. Damage to the ligaments and joints of the rib may occur posteriorly at the vertebral attachment or anteriorly at the costochondral junction. Sprains of the vertebral attachment are uncommon, although they may be identified by point tenderness over the injured ligament complex. Mild sprain is characterized by an absence of discomfort during inspiration, whereas a more severe sprain results in pain on inspiration. The treatment of vertebral attachment sprains is symptomatic, including initial cold application, followed by heat, mobilization, and protection against motion at the injured joint by use of a rib belt or strapping of the lower chest.

Subluxation of the rib-vertebral attachment may occur, but dislocation is thought to be rare. Most cases of subluxation have spontaneously reduced by the time a physician is consulted. The diagnosis of a rib-vertebral subluxation or reduced dislocation is made by the identification of a localized tender spot that corresponds to the site of injury and the complete resolution of symptoms when local anesthetic is injected into the joint. If the subluxation has reduced, the athlete may return to sports participation in 7 to 10 days with lower chest strapping.

Occasionally, dislocations remain unreduced at the time of evaluation. Pain is typically more severe, and physical findings reveal localized tenderness, muscle spasm, and joint motion. Associated damage to the neurovascular bundle often causes neuritis symptoms in the distribution of the costal nerve. Unreduced dislocations should be manually reduced to prevent complications of long-term degenerative joint disease. Reduction may be accomplished by hyperextending the spine and allowing the shoulders and arms to fall backward, and then applying direct pressure to the posterior dislocated segment while simultaneously applying pressure against the anterior chest.

ACUTE COSTOCHONDRAL INJURIES. The anterior attachment of the rib is far more frequently injured than the vertebral junction. Direct sternal trauma or lateral compression of the chest may produce costochondral joint sprain, subluxation, or dislocation. The diagnosis is made based on the presence of tenderness at the costochondral junctions, which are located one to two finger-breadths lateral to the costosternal junctions. The severity of the injury is determined by the amount of tenderness, localized swelling, and hematoma formation over the injury site. More severe sprains are associated with pain during deep inspiration. Persistent joint dislocation is readily apparent clinically as a step-off at the joint site, which may reduce with an audible click, as direct pressure is applied over the rib end. Radiographs are of little use in diagnosing costochondral separations, since the costocartilage is radiolucent.

Acute costochondral separation without displacement or a palpable click involves an at least partially intact ligamentous complex. The treatment is to prevent further injury and relieve discomfort with injection of a long-acting local anesthetic. In the presence of a palpable step-off or audible click, the treatment should be directed toward preventing recurrence. A direct pressure pad should be applied over the anterior end of the rib rather than over the costochondral joint. A rib belt or strapping may be used to hold the pad in place. Union of acute costochondral separation occurs slowly, typically taking 6 to 8 weeks. Participation in contact sports should be withheld for 3 to 4 weeks.

CHRONIC COSTOCHONDRAL INJURIES. Costochondral subluxation becomes chronic when an athlete fails to seek medical evaluation until after multiple episodes of subluxation have occurred. The treatment of this condition is determined by the amounts of instability and pain. In the presence of joint stability, when pain is the major complaint, local injections with anesthetics and corticosteroids may be employed. If some degree of pain relief is not achieved after repeated injections over the first 3 to 4 days, it is unlikely that further injections will be effective. If pain is severe and disabling with or without instability, surgery may be considered. Surgery involves the resection of adequate opposing joint surfaces so that they no longer rub together. Given the inherent stability of the rib even after resection of the costochondral junction and the difficulty in fusing rib to cartilage, the rib end is generally not internally fixated. Chronic instability or dislocation alone does not justify surgery, but if localized pain, swelling, and muscle spasm occur, surgery may become necessary. Surgery in such cases involves the resection of a portion of chondrocartilage or the rib end to avoid painful impingement.

Fortunately, given the common occurrence of costochondral injuries, few are severe enough to require the discontinuation of athletics. It is important, however, to treat acute injuries with reduction, pad application, and strapping to avoid chronic symptoms. Union of a separated costochondral junction takes 8 weeks, during which time contact sports should be avoided.

FRACTURE. Rib fractures are common, generally benign, and usually self-limited injuries in athletes. The first through third ribs are well protected by the shoulder girdles, making superior rib fractures rare. The presence of upper rib fractures should suggest the possibility of coexisting injuries to the aorta, great vessels, and airways. Arteriography may be considered if clinically appropriate. A special type of stress fracture of the first rib has also been reported; it is discussed later.

The fourth through ninth ribs are the most commonly fractured ribs, as a result of their greater exposure to direct trauma and rigid anterior and posterior fixations. The mechanism of such injuries may involve direct chest trauma, which may occur from a pitched baseball, or a blunt blow to the chest. The tenth through twelfth ribs, or floating ribs, are extremely mobile, lacking anterior bony attachments, and thus are less susceptible to injury. The presence of a lower rib fracture should prompt a search for associated upper abdominal visceral damage.

Fractures may be nondisplaced or displaced. Nondisplaced fractures are generally uncomplicated, whereas displaced fractures are often accompanied by complications that may be far more serious than the rib injury itself. The mechanisms of most rib fractures are either direct blows or compressive forces. Ribs typically break at the point of impact or at the rib's weakest point, the posterior angle. Fortunately, the bones of young athletes are often soft and pliable enough so as not to splinter. Potential complications of displaced splintering rib fractures include penetration of the lung with development of a pneumothorax, hemothorax, or subcutaneous emphysema; penetration of the pericardium with development of a pericardial effusion or tamponade; damage to the internal mammary artery; and injury to the intercostal neurovascular bundle, which may produce marked swelling, hematoma, and neuritis symptoms. These complications are discussed later in the chapter.

The symptoms of a rib fracture include pleuritic pain aggravated by coughing, deep inspiration, and chest movement at the site of injury. Pain tends to be most severe during the first 3 to 5 days following injury, at which time it gradually subsides, and it ultimately disappears after 3 to 6 weeks. The physical examination discloses localized tenderness and may reveal crepitance if displacement is present. The diagnosis may be confirmed by a positive rib x-ray film, but up to 50 percent of rib fractures are not apparent radiographically during the first 10 to 14 days after injury. The subsequent formation of callus eventually results in radiographic identifiability of most fractures.[33] The early identification of acute rib fractures in a patient with trauma-induced chest pain has been shown not to affect medical management.[34] However, the important reason to obtain radiographs in cases of suspected rib fractures, is to detect associated complications such as pneumothorax or pleural fluid collection, which may indicate the presence of a hemothorax. Serial chest films at 24 and 48 hours may be helpful in the detection of the delayed development of pneumothorax or hemothorax.

The management of rib fractures should initially ensure full recovery from any associated dyspnea. If respiratory distress, cyanosis, or shock is present, a thorough investigation for underlying visceral injury should be undertaken.

Pain and muscle spasm of an uncomplicated fracture may be treated with analgesics and local anesthetic infiltration into the intercostal nerve region. The location of needle insertion should be at the inferior edge of the affected rib, at least one handsbreadth proximal (toward the spine) from the fracture. The syringe plunger should be drawn back prior to the injection, to avoid intravascular injection. In addition to the affected rib, the two ribs above and the two ribs below may also require intercostal nerve blocks, to achieve complete pain control.

A rib fracture may cause the individual to "splint" with respirations, in an attempt to protect the injured area. As a consequence, respiratory function may be compromised, which predisposes to atelectasis and pneumonia. Deep breathing exercises, incentive spirometry, and early ambulation should be encouraged to reduce the risk of such complications.

The use of rib belts, rib strapping, and rib binding in the treatment of mid to lower rib fractures is controversial. Some experts advocate circumferential strapping, from the lower chest to the top of the xiphoid, by use of a four- to six-inch rib belt, adhesive tape, or elastic wrap. Other authorities strongly oppose the use of rib binders out of concern for the potential development of pulmonary complications. A rib binder is not indicated for upper rib fractures, where pain is better managed by limiting shoulder and neck motion with a sling or strapping over the shoulder to limit elevation of the shoulder girdle when raising the arms overhead.

If an athlete is allowed to return to contact sports participation, a local rigid protective pad should be worn over the injured area for 6 weeks, at which time healing should be complete. The pad may be secured with a rib belt. Under no circumstances should an acute rib fracture be injected with anesthetics to allow sports participation.

More than 300 cases of stress fractures of the first rib, in athlete participants in overhead or throwing sports have been described.[35] Golfers, baseball pitchers, rowers, tennis players, weight lifters, and gymnasts have all been reported with the condition.[35] The fracture occurs as a result of repetitive, indirect, shearing forces at the relatively weak subclavian sulcus of the first rib rather than direct trauma. This area constitutes a border between opposing upward and downward forces. The scalene, intercostal, and serratus muscles exert conflicting forces during activities such as throwing a ball, serving a tennis ball, and pressing a barbell overhead, which may result in fracture. The symptoms of first-rib stress fractures range from dull, aching pain along the distribution of the first intercostal nerve to a pleuritic, knifelike pain. Radiographs are typically negative until at least 14 days after the injury, although bone scans may identify the fracture earlier. The treatment involves avoidance of the offending mechanism, usage of an arm sling, and a graduated exercise program. In rare cases, a surgical emergency may develop if the subclavian artery is acutely torn.

Stress fractures of other ribs have been reported in elite female athletes who participate in rowing, tennis, golf, and gymnastics. Symptoms include pain in the posterolateral scapular region of the thorax. Clinical symptoms have typically been present for 2 to 6 months prior to the establishment of a diagnosis. Plain radiographs often fail to identify stress fractures, but bone scans can provide an early diagnosis. The treatment is avoidance of the causative activity.

THORACIC MUSCLE STRAIN

The muscles of the chest wall may be injured either by violent exertional forces or overstretching of the chest muscles. A discussion of thoracic muscle strains should actually be included in a review of shoulder injuries, since most of the injured thoracic muscles are associated with the upper extremity. However, given the location of pain and to aid in the differentiation from other chest injuries, these strains are included in this section.

Thoracic muscle strains typically involve muscles that connect the chest to another body part. Examples include the rhomboids, which connect the scapula to the thorax; the serratus muscles, which connect the upper extremity to the chest; and the abdominal rectus muscles, which connect the pelvis to the thorax. The intercostal muscles rarely experience isolated injury, since they are protected by superficial muscular structures and are generally unable to contract with sufficient force to rupture muscle fibers.

Muscle strains occurring at the rib attachments are likely to be more painful than disabling. The often considerable muscle spasm that may accompany such injuries may result in respiratory "splinting," with the risk of pulmonary complications and decreased ability to train. The treatment of thoracic muscle strains is determined by the specific muscle or group of muscles that are injured. Local injection is often difficult because of the broad thoracic muscle insertions. Ice should be applied initially, followed by heat and gradual rehabilitation. If the injured muscle is attached to the scapula, a sling may be worn to promote rest and recovery. Similarly, if an abdominal muscle has been injured, bed rest, with the head of the bed and the knees elevated to completely relax the abdominal muscles, may be prescribed.

STERNUM

The sternum, which protects the vital anatomic structures of the mediastinum, is made up of three bones: the upper manubrium, the middle body; and the lower xiphoid (Fig. 25–9). The first rib and the upper portion of the second rib usually inserts onto the manubrium. The lower portion of the second rib and the third through sixth (and sometimes seventh) ribs insert on the sternal body. The seventh rib usually inserts on the xiphoid. The newborn has six unfused sternal segments, which gradually fuse through the late teenage years to form the three-bone adult sternum. Persistent prefusion lines should not be mistaken for fractures when radiographically evaluating children and adolescents.

CONTUSION. The subcutaneous location of the sternum makes it susceptible to contusions. Participants in contact sports that do not require the use of protective sternal pads or that involve high-velocity objects are particularly vulnerable to sternal injury. A direct blow to the sternum typically produces superficial edema, ecchymosis, periosteal reaction, and a severe "shock reaction," in which the athlete transiently senses difficulty with respiration. Deep inspiration will not typically aggravate pain in the absence of complications.

Mild-to-moderate sternal contusions are treated with ice, followed by heat application. If pain is severe, however, the area of injury may be injected with local anesthetics. A protective pad should be applied before permitting the athlete to return to contact sports.

Football shoulder pads generally provide excellent sternal protection.

SPRAIN, SUBLUXATION, AND DISLOCATION. A direct sternal blow may also result in sternal joint sprain, subluxation, or dislocation. The ligaments between the manubrium and body are quite firm and thus are rarely damaged. When joint subluxation or dislocation does occur, however, reduction is usually spontaneous. Clinical symptoms include pain and tenderness at the manubrium-body junction without pain during ordinary breathing. But severe pain is produced when direct compressive pressure is placed on the manubrium or sternal body.

The treatment of a sprain or spontaneously reduced subluxation entails avoidance of sports participation for a minimum of 7 to 10 days, followed by usage of a hollowed plastic sternal pad. If chronic pain symptoms persist, injections of local anesthetics with corticosteroids may be considered.

On rare occasions, sternal injury produces a complete dislocation. These injuries should be reduced as soon as possible. Closed reduction, under general anesthesia, may initially be attempted, although open reduction with wire loop internal fixation may be required. As with any severe chest injury, the presence of subluxation or dislocation should alert the clinician to the possibility of underlying visceral injury.

Sprains are uncommon at the junction of the sternal body and xiphoid as a result of the free anterior-posterior movement of this joint. Sternal body–xiphoid dislocations are rare.

FRACTURE. Sternal fractures may also result from direct trauma. Most fractures occur in the upper portion of the sternal body, caused by direct pressure driving the body backward, relative to the first and second ribs, which are fixed to the manubrium. Fractures may be complete or incomplete and displaced or nondisplaced.

The history of injury is a direct sternal blow and immediate loss of breath. Severe pain is provoked only with deep inspiration if the fracture is incomplete, but pain occurs during normal respiration if the fracture is complete. The diagnosis may be confirmed with plain radiographs, which should include a lateral view to establish the presence of displacement.

The treatment of an undisplaced sternal fracture includes cold application, followed by heat. Chest compression with a rib binder may be used to provide comfort. A displaced fracture typically results in fragments that are caught or locked on each other. Reduction usually must be accomplished under anesthesia. Participation in contact sports should be restricted for at least a few weeks after reduction, unless the athlete is completely pain-free during deep inspiration and with chest compression.

The presence of a sternal fracture indicates a major injury, which may be associated with visceral injuries such as pneumothorax, hemothorax, subcutaneous emphysema, damage to the great vessels, hemopericardium, and cardiac contusion. These complications may take several hours to develop clinically, and thus individuals with sternal fractures should be admitted to the hospital for bed rest, observation, and serial radiographic studies.

PECTORALIS MAJOR INJURY

Rupture of the pectoralis major muscle is a relatively uncommon event, although it has recently been reported with increasing frequency in male weight lifters.[36–38] Early reports of this injury occurred when an individual would extend the arms so as to break a fall.[39]

The pectoralis major muscle originates from the medial clavicle, the first six ribs, and the aponeurosis of the external oblique muscle. The strong tendon actually twists before inserting onto the proximal humerus. The clavicular and upper sternal portions insert distally, and the lower and abdominal portions cross over these fibers to insert more proximally on the humerus (Fig. 25–10). The primary action of the pectoralis major muscle is to adduct the humerus. It additionally contributes to forward flexion and internal rotation.

Pectoralis major muscle rupture may occur as a result of a direct blow to the chest or excessive tension on the pectoralis muscle in activities such as weight lifting in the bench press or football.[36,37] Most ruptures occur within the muscle itself, at the musculotendinous junction, or with an avulsion of the tendon from the humerus.[27] Wolfe demonstrated that the relatively short muscle fibers of the inferior portion of the pectoralis muscles must lengthen disproportionately during the final 30 degrees of humeral extension in the

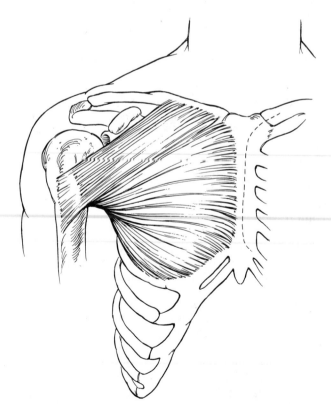

FIGURE 25–10. Anatomy of the pectoralis major muscle. (From Wolfe SW, Wickiewicz TL, Cavanaugh JT: Ruptures of the pectoralis major muscle. Am J Sports Med 21:475–477, 1992.)

bench press. These fibers are placed at a mechanical disadvantage, which, in conjunction with the high-load eccentric forces of the lift, causes rupture.[37]

The symptoms of acute pectoralis major muscle rupture are severe anterior chest pain, which may radiate to the shoulder or upper arm, a "snapping" or "popping" sound, ecchymosis, and swelling. The diagnosis may be difficult to confirm unless the injury is seen immediately after rupture, because of nonspecific swelling and extreme pain. Repeated physical examinations are often necessary. Characteristic physical findings include weakness of upper arm adduction, flexion, internal rotation and bulging of the torn pectoralis muscle during forced adduction. Additionally, if the tear occurs with an avulsion of the tendon, a palpable defect may be noted in the anterior axillary fold. A tear localized at the musculotendinous junction may however be inapparent to palpation and inspection because of the integrity of the fascial covering. A clue to the diagnosis is an absent pectoralis major shadow on the frontal chest radiograph.

The treatment of complete pectoralis major rupture is generally nonsurgical for elderly or sedentary individuals. Incomplete tears are also typically treated nonoperatively. Injuries that go unrepaired will however leave the individual with a significant strength deficit, compared with the uninvolved side. Immediate surgical repair is the treatment of choice for young or athletic individuals.[38] Pectoralis major ruptures that are repaired surgically result in comparable muscular torques and work measurements relative to the uninvolved sides.[37] Immediate surgical repair is optimal, because this reduces the development of adhesions, muscle retractions, atrophy, and any delays in return to athletic competition. But individuals with chronic tears, who may be identified by serial examinations, strength-testing, and magnetic resonance imaging (MRI), have undergone successful operative repair. The common surgical procedure involves a deltopectoral incision, evacuation of hematoma, and reattachment of the tendon to bone, using any remaining attachment to reinforce the tendon. A sling is generally used for 4 weeks postoperatively, followed by progressive resistance exercise, and institution of resistive exercise after the twelfth week.

MRI has been promoted as an early diagnostic tool to assist in the diagnosis and management of pectoralis major ruptures.[36] To help prevent ruptures, it seems sensible to change the arc of the bench press exercise to limit hyperextension of the arm and the resultant passive stretch of the muscle fibers. Additionally, despite denials of anabolic steroid usage in weight lifters who had sustained pectoralis major ruptures, the possibility of an association must be considered.[36]

BREAST INJURY

Athletic female breast injury has become an increasingly common occurrence as the number of women participating in sports at all levels has increased. Breast injury may occur as a result of direct trauma or repetitive microtrauma from inadequate breast support. One report revealed that 56 percent of physically active female subjects had experienced previous sports-related breast discomfort or pain.[40]

Direct trauma to the breast may produce fat necrosis or hematoma formation, both of which are painful and may result in the formation of a focal breast mass. Mammographic appearance of these lesions is often indistinguishable from that of malignancy. The treatment of direct breast trauma is cold application, followed by heat application, breast support, and protection with padding. Sports participation should be limited until inflammation has subsided.

Running causes the female breasts to bounce vertically, and slap against the chest wall, producing breast contusions and soreness. Women with large breasts are especially at risk for running-induced breast injury. Inadequate breast support may also result in stretching of the Cooper ligaments, the structures that attach the breast to the chest wall. Chronic lack of breast support may exacerbate ptosis, or sagging, of the breasts. Sports brassieres have been shown to help prevent breast ptosis by limiting breast motion during running and by holding the breasts against the chest wall.

Many different sports bras are available to the consumer. Large-breasted women generally require more rigidity in the bra construction than do smaller breasted athletes. Athletes who compete in sports that require overhead arm activities require elastic shoulder straps to avoid the bra's riding up. Runners who engage in little overhead activity are better served by wide, nonstretch shoulder straps. In addition to the shoulder straps, support should come from lift provided below the breasts. The bra fabric should contain adequate cotton to allow absorbency, whereas elasticity should be minimized but sufficient to permit easy respirations. Insertable protective cup pads are desirable for participants in contact sports. The bra design should avoid irritating seams or fasteners and should include nonslip shoulder straps, rounded cup shapes that hold the breasts firmly against the body, and firm, durable construction. Better support may be achieved, with breast motion reduced by 50 percent, when a 4-inch elastic binder wrap is worn over a sports bra.[41]

Injuries to the male breast are similar to those affecting female breasts, occurring in the form of contusions secondary to direct trauma. Symptoms include inflammation around the nipple and areola, erythema, tenderness, and a serous nipple discharge. Treatment is heat application and protective pads. On occasions, a painful, fibrous nodule, which may require surgical excision persists.[42]

Both women and men athletes may experience nipple skin friction, or "runner's nipples," from a running shirt. This may be avoided by wearing a noncotton synthetic shirt or by applying a protective Band-Aid or dab of petroleum jelly over the nipple.

INTRATHORACIC INJURIES

EVALUATION OF THE INJURED ATHLETE

Tissue hypoxia is the critical pathologic condition responsible for the high morbidity and mortality associated with chest injuries. Hypoxia and metabolic acidosis may result from various mechanisms, including hypoventilation, hypoxemia, respiratory alkalosis, reduced cardiac output, and pulmonary shunting. The clinician's initial evaluation of the athlete with an isolated chest injury should include assessments of the airway, breathing, and circulation. This should identify the presence of any acutely life-threatening conditions, such as airway obstruction, massive hemothorax, cardiac tamponade, tension pneumothorax, flail chest, open pneumothorax, and massive tracheoesophageal air leakage, and allow for their appropriate management.

The airway should be checked for obstruction by listening for air movement at the mouth and nose, observing for intercostal and supraclavicular muscle retractions, monitoring the respiratory rate and pattern, and recognizing the presence of cyanosis. To properly assess breathing, the chest must be completely exposed, and respirations should be observed, palpated, and auscultated. Circulation is evaluated by monitoring the rate, regularity, and quality of the pulse and the width of the pulse pressure. The neck veins should be examined for distention, and the peripheral circulation must be judged by skin temperature and color.

Upper airway obstruction results in an ashen, gray, or cyanotic skin color; an absence of normal breath sounds, often with gurgling or stridor; and the use of accessory respiratory muscles. The presence of paradoxical respiratory chest movements may be due to a flail chest, which should be apparent, if the chest has been properly exposed. Sucking wounds of the chest should be evident by their characteristic sound. A large hemothorax may be suspected by the presence of dullness to percussion over the affected lung field. A tension pneumothorax results in absent breath sounds on the affected side with tracheal deviation contralaterally. Cardiac tamponade produces a narrowed pulse pressure and distended neck veins.

PULMONARY INJURY

CONTUSION. Most cases of pulmonary contusion result from motor vehicle accidents, although athletes may experience blunt chest trauma of sufficient force to cause the condition. Trauma-induced alveolar capillary damage with interstitial and intra-alveolar hemorrhage leads to pulmonary parenchymal edema and hemorrhage, atelectasis, and copious tracheobronchial secretions, which may impair pulmonary function.

Initial chest radiographs are often normal, but unilateral or bilateral, patchy, ill-defined pulmonary infiltrates may develop within 4 to 6 hours of injury. Thus, if a pulmonary contusion is suspected, the athlete should be admitted to the hospital, and serial chest x-ray films should be obtained. The symptoms of a mild contusion include tachypnea, tachycardia, the presence of rales on auscultation of the lung fields, and a cough with abundant blood-tinged secretions. The treatment of mild pulmonary contusion incorporates pulmonary physical therapy, nasotracheal suctioning, analgesics, humidified oxygen supplementation, bronchodilators as needed, and appropriate antibiotic therapy or prophylaxis. Severe pulmonary contusions often occur in conjunction with extrathoracic injuries, which may detract from the danger of the pulmonary damage. A severe contusion results in an increased alveolar-to-arterial oxygen gradient and reduced PaO_2 while breathing 100 percent oxygen, in addition to the presence of frankly bloody tracheobronchial secretions and progressive respiratory failure. Despite aggressive treatment with mechanical ventilation, tracheobronchial suctioning, bronchodilators, and diuretics to reduce pulmonary edema, this condition is often fatal.

PNEUMOTHORAX. Pneumothorax is the most common complication of rib fractures. A fractured rib edge may puncture the pleura and lung to cause a leakage of air into the intrapleural space. A simple pneumothorax may also occur in the absence of rib fractures. Mechanisms of injury include sudden compression of the chest while the glottis is closed with resultant alveolar blow-out and spontaneous bleb rupture. Most episodes of simple pneumothorax are self-limited in that the apposition of the lung and pleural surfaces tends to seal the air leak. The findings of dyspnea, cyanosis, and progressive respiratory collapse are consistent with severe cases. Signs of pulmonary insufficiency may be absent, however, in young, athletic individuals because of their large functional cardiopulmonary reserve. The physical examination may reveal tachypnea, decreased breath sounds to auscultation, and hyperresonance to percussion. Chest radiography often confirms the presence of a pneumothorax, and the sensitivity is improved further by obtaining upright inspiration and expiration films (Fig. 25–11).

The treatment of a simple pneumothorax is dependent on the percentage of lung volume that is lost, the severity of pulmonary compromise, and the need for general anesthesia to address associated injuries. The

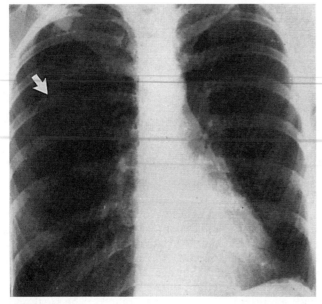

FIGURE 25–11. Chest radiograph of a pneumothorax. (From Orringer MB: Chest injuries in the athlete. *In* Schneider RC, Kennedy JC, Plant ML (eds): Sports Injuries—Mechanisms, Prevention, and Treatment. Baltimore, Williams & Wilkins, 1985, pp 818–829.)

size of a pneumothorax is estimated as a percentage of volume loss within a hemithorax, by viewing the chest radiograph. Generally, a pneumothorax of 30 percent or less without respiratory distress or the need for general anesthesia may be treated without a chest tube. Serial chest radiographs should be obtained to confirm improvement. A pneumothorax should resorb by approximately 1 percent volume per day. Physical activity should be restricted during recovery.

A pneumothorax occupying 30 percent or more of the hemithorax, associated with pulmonary compromise or in conjunction with other injuries that may require general anesthesia for treatment, should be treated with a chest tube. The chest tube is generally inserted in the third intercostal space at the anterior axillary line and is connected to underwater seal drainage, with or without suction. Re-expansion of the lung occurs relatively rapidly when a chest tube is placed, since the leak becomes sealed as a result of apposition of the visceral and parietal pleurae. The chest tube is removed once the leak has been eliminated for 24 hours. Return to vigorous athletic participation should be restricted for 2 to 3 more weeks.

Spontaneous pneumothorax, in the absence of trauma, may occur in individuals with a congenital predisposition for pulmonary bleb rupture. Onset of symptoms may be insidious to acute. Surgical resection of a nest of pulmonary apical blebs is often recommended after a third pneumothorax has occurred.

TENSION PNEUMOTHORAX. Tension pneumothorax is a severe, life-threatening form of pneumothorax. This may develop secondary to a rib fracture that produces a tangential tear in the pulmonary parenchyma, resulting in a flap-valve mechanism that permits air to enter the pleural space during inspiration. The evolution of positive intrapleural pressure relative to the atmosphere may cause the mediastinum to shift away from the injured side, compression of the vena cava, reduced cardiac diastolic filling, and decreased cardiac output. If untreated, a tension pneumothorax may rapidly progress to fatal hypoxia and acidosis. The symptoms of tension pneumothorax include acute respiratory distress, restlessness, and agitation. The physical examination reveals tachypnea, hypotension, tachycardia, respiratory distress, absent breath sounds to auscultation, hyperresonance to percussion of the involved hemithorax, and tracheal deviation toward the uninvolved side.

Early treatment of a tension pneumothorax is crucial, and thus confirmation with chest radiographs is usually not possible. The immediate treatment involves the insertion of a 14- to 18-gauge needle into the pleural cavity through the second intercostal space in the midclavicular line (Fig. 25–12). The needle should pass over the superior edge of the third rib, so as not to damage the neurovascular bundle. If the correct diagnosis has been made, the puncture should produce a rush of air, and immediate clinical improvement. This procedure converts a tension pneumothorax into a much less serious simple pneumothorax. It is far better to produce a pneumothorax while erring on the side of aggressiveness in relieving

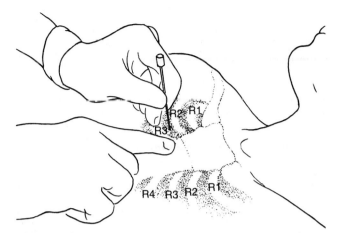

FIGURE 25–12. Emergent needle decompression of a tension pneumothorax is achieved by inserting a 14 to 18 gauge needle into the second intercostal space (at the level of the angle of Louis) in the midclavicular line. The needle should be inserted over the superior aspect of the rib to avoid injury to the intercostal vessels that course along the inferior edge of the rib. As extrapulmonary intrathoracic air under pressure is evacuated through the needle, the tension pneumothorax is converted to a simple pneumothorax, which is far better tolerated physiologically and can then be treated with a chest tube.

a tension pneumothorax than to allow the progression of respiratory collapse.

HEMOTHORAX. Hemothorax, a collection of blood within the thoracic cavity, is a common sequela of blunt chest trauma. The source of bleeding may be from a rib fracture–induced lung laceration, or from a compression "blow-out" injury. Bleeding from the lung tends to be self-limited because of the relatively low pulmonary vasculature pressure. If an intercostal artery is lacerated, however, the bleeding may be brisk and severe. Symptoms associated with a large hemothorax (400 ml or more) may include hypotension, hypovolemia, reduced cardiac output, hypoxia, compression of the ipsilateral lung, and deviation of the mediastinum away from the involved side. A small hemothorax of less than 400 ml is often asymptomatic.

The physical examination reveals dullness to percussion over the hemothorax, reduced or absent breath sounds, less tactile fremitus, and mediastinal shift toward the uninvolved side. A chest x-ray film will show blunting of the costophrenic angles with as little as 250 to 300 ml of fluid collection.

The treatment depends on the clinical condition. If the hemothorax is small, serial chest x-ray films may be obtained for several days to ensure blood resorption, which is usually completed within 2 weeks. If blood appears to occupy one third or more of the hemithorax (500 to 2000 ml), a large-bore chest tube should be placed in the sixth intercostal space at the anterior axillary line. If bleeding is noted to continue at a rate of at least 300 ml/hour or if serial chest x-ray films show a worsening radiographic appearance, emergency thoracotomy is indicated.

MEDIASTINAL OR SUBCUTANEOUS EMPHYSEMA. Fractured ribs may result in the leakage of air into the mediastinum with spread into the subcutaneous soft tissues of the upper chest and neck. Clinically, subcutaneous emphysema is apparent by swelling of the neck and characteristic crepitation under the skin. On rare occasions, mediastinal air may be under sufficient pressure to force collapse of the great veins, which restricts blood return to the right side of the heart and consequently causes cardiac decompensation.

Subcutaneous emphysema typically resolves spontaneously. On occasion, however, the affected individual should be hospitalized for observation, and serial x-ray films taken to rule out progression of the condition.

CARDIAC INJURY

MYOCARDIAL CONTUSION. Blunt trauma to the chest wall may produce cardiac contusion. The most common mechanism of this injury is compression of the sternum against the steering wheel, as occurs in a rapid deceleration motor vehicle accident. Although cardiac contusion is not a common form of athletic trauma, participants in sports that involve great velocities and forces may sustain this injury.

The degree of myocardial injury ranges from localized contusion to complete myocardial rupture. Prompt recognition of even mild cardiac contusions is essential, since delayed ventricular rupture may occur for up to several months after the injury. On occasion, the coronary arteries may be damaged, resulting in thrombosis, which may lead to myocardial infarction. An additional potential complication of cardiac contusion is rupture of the intraventricular septum, with a resultant acute left-to-right shunt.

Cardiac contusion is diagnosed by maintaining suspicion based upon the mechanism of injury and by the characteristic electrocardiographic changes that are consistent with myocardial damage. The treatment of cardiac contusion is similar to that for acute myocardial infarction, including electrocardiographic monitoring in a hospital coronary care unit and cardiovascular support.

PERICARDIAL TAMPONADE. Acute hemorrhage into the pericardial cavity, or pericardial tamponade, is an uncommon athletic injury. Blunt trauma of a force sufficient to rupture the myocardium or lacerate a coronary artery may give rise to this often fatal injury. The most common mechanism of injury is a penetrating wound to the chest, such as that inflicted by a knife stab. This type of injury is not expected to occur in most sporting events, but it may transpire accidentally in sports that utilize high speed sharp objects or missiles carrying a risk of impalement. Examples include arrows in archery, the javelin in field events, and the epée in fencing.

Clinical features of a small cardiac tamponade include neck vein distention, shock, and cyanosis. Prompt recognition of the diagnosis, with confirmation by echocardiography if immediately available, should direct urgent pericardiocentesis. The definitive treatment is thoracotomy with pericardial decompression, and suture repair of the damaged myocardium. Massive cardiac tamponade almost always results in immediate death.

AORTA. Rupture of the aorta is a rare complication of blunt chest trauma in which the descending aorta undergoes torsion, and the aortic wall is disrupted at the ligamentum arteriosum. Occasionally, damage occurs to the ascending aorta at the root of the heart. Most victims of aortic rupture die immediately from massive exsanguination, but a few survive as a result of the formation of a "false aneurysm" between the periaortic tissues and the pleura. The diagnosis may be suspected on the basis of widening of the cardiac silhouette on chest radiograph. CT, MRI, or retrograde aortography is confirmatory. The treatment is immediate surgical repair.

ESOPHAGEAL INJURY

Most injuries to the esophagus are a result of penetrating trauma rather than blunt injury. Penetrating trauma, manifested by extreme chest pain, and the gradual onset of fever over several hours, may perforate the esophagus. Regurgitation of blood, hoarseness, dysphagia, and respiratory distress may also be present. The chest radiograph may show mediastinal air, widening, and a pleural effusion. The diagnosis is confirmed by water-soluble contrast radiography or esophagoscopy. The treatment is immediate surgical debridement, suture closure of damaged tissues, and drainage.

CONCLUSION

The abdominal cavity, by nature of its relative lack of bony protection, is quite susceptible to blunt trauma injury during athletics. The structures of the abdominal wall are often injured by direct compression forces, whereas the intra-abdominal organs are often damaged by compression against the spine. Injuries to the abdomen may become life-threatening, particularly if significant time passes without treatment. A major exsanguination from a ruptured blood vessel may rapidly progress to shock and death without prompt appropriate treatment.

Thoracic injuries are more likely to be life-threatening because of a disruption of the cardiopulmonary systems. Most serious intrathoracic injuries result from shearing forces of deceleration, which may disrupt vital structures. Penetrating trauma from objects such as a fractured, displaced rib, must also be considered as causes of thoracic injury. Injuries to the surface of the thorax typically manifest as muscle strains or ruptures, contusions, or bony fractures. The athletic health care professional must be well trained and knowledgeable in the early assessment, stabilization, and management of the various types of traumatic injuries that may involve the abdomen and chest.

REFERENCES

1. Bergqvist D, Hedelin H, Karlsson G, et al: Abdominal injury from sporting activities. Br J Sports Med 16:76–79, 1982.
2. Diamond DL: Sports-related abdominal trauma. *In* Ray RL (ed): Clinics in Sports Medicine — Emergency Treatment of the Injured Athlete. Philadelphia, WB Saunders, 1989, pp 91–99.
3. Taylor DC, Meyers WC, Moylan JA, et al: Abdominal musculature abnormalities as a cause of groin pain in athletes. Am J Sports Med 19:239–242, 1991.
4. deShazo WF: Hematoma of the rectus abdominis in football. Phys Sports Med 12:73–75, 1984.
5. US Department of Health, Education, and Welfare: National Health Survey of Hernias. Series B, No. 25, Dec 1960.
6. Nyhus LM, Bombeck CT: Hernias. *In* Sabiston DC (ed): Textbook of Surgery — The Biological Basis of Modern Surgical Practice, 13th ed. Philadelphia,WB Saunders, 1986, pp 1231–1252.
7. Haycock CE: How I manage hernias in the athlete. Phys Sports Med 11:77–79, 1983.
8. Douglas DM: The healing of aponeurotic incisions. Br J Surg 40:79, 1952.
9. Olsen WR: Abdominal trauma in the athlete. *In* Schneider RC, Kennedy JC, Plant ML (eds): Sports Injuries — Mechanisms, Prevention, and Treatment. Baltimore, Williams & Wilkins, 1985, pp 809–817.
10. Higgins GL: Penetrating trauma — Managing and preventing javelin wounds. Phys Sports Med 22:88–94, 1994.
11. Green GA: Gastrointestinal disorders in the athlete. Sports Med 1992; 11:453–470.
12. American College of Surgeons: Abdominal trauma. *In* Advanced Trauma Life Support Student Manual. Chicago, American College of Surgeons, 1989, pp 113–123.
13. Coant PN, Kornberg AE, Brody AS, Edwards-Holmes K: Markers for occult liver injury in cases of physical abuse in children. Pediatrics 89:274–278, 1992.
14. Affleck TP: Severe sports-related spleen injury. Phys Sports Med 20:109–123, 1992.
15. Buntain WL, Gould HR, Maull KI: Predictability of splenic salvage by computed tomography. J Trauma 28:24–34, 1988.
16. Maki DG, Reich RM: Infectious mononucleosis in the athlete: Diagnosis, complications, and management. Am J Sports Med 10:162–173, 1982.
17. Rutkow IM: Rupture of the spleen in infectious mononucleosis. Arch Surg 113:718–720, 1978.
18. Stricker PR, Hardin BH, Puffer JC: An unusual presentation of liver laceration in a 13-yr-old football player. Med Sci Sports Exerc 25:667–672, 1993.
19. Mustalich AC, Quash ET: Sports injuries to the chest and abdomen. *In* Scott WN, Nisonson B, Nicholas JA (eds): Principles of Sports Medicine. Baltimore, Williams & Wilkins, 1984, pp 236–240.
20. Hiatt JR, Harrier D, Koenig BV, Ransom KJ: Nonoperative management of major blunt liver injury with hemoperitoneum. Arch Surg 125:101–103, 1990.
21. Moon KL, Federele MP: CT in hepatic trauma. Am J Radiol 141:309–314, 1983.
22. Cywes S, Rode H: Blunt liver trauma in children — Non-operative management. J Pediatr Surg 20:14–18, 1985.
23. Henderson JM, Puffer JC: Abdominal pain in a football player. Phys Sports Med 17:47–52, 1989.
24. Murphy CP, Drez D: Jejunal rupture in a football player. Am J Sports Med 15:184–185, 1987.
25. Glenn JF, Harvard BM: The injured kidney. JAMA 173:1189, 1960.
26. Cianflocco AJ: Renal complications of exercise. Clin Sports Med 11:437–451, 1992.
27. Kulund DN: The Injured Athlete. Philadelphia, JB Lippincott, 1982, pp 332, 339.
28. Kenney P: Abdominal pain in athletes. Clin Sports Med 6:885–904, 1987.
29. Stricker PR, Puffer JC: Case report: Renal laceration — A skateboarder's symptoms are delayed. Phys Sports Med 21:59–68, 1993.
30. Siegel AJ, Hennekens CH, Soloman HS, Van Boeckel B: Exercise-related hematuria. JAMA 241:391–392, 1979.
31. Blalock NJ: Bladder trauma in long-distance runners. Am J Sports Med 7:239–241, 1979.
32. Hoover DL: How I manage testicular injury. Phys Sports Med 14:127–129, 1986.
33. DeLuca SA, Rhea JT, O'Malley T: Radiographic evaluation of rib fractures. Am J Radiol 138:91, 1982.

34. deLacey G: Clinical and economic aspects of the use of x-rays in accident and emergency departments. Proc R Soc Med 69:758, 1976.

35. Sullivan JA: *In* Grana WA, Kalenak A (eds): Clinical Sports Medicine. Philadelphia, WB Saunders, 1991, p 404.

36. Miller MD, Johnson DL, Fu FH: Rupture of the pectoralis major muscle in a collegiate football player: Use of magnetic resonance imaging in early diagnosis. Am J Sports Med 21:475–477, 1993.

37. Wolfe SW, Wickiewicz TL, Cavanaugh JT: Ruptures of the pectoralis major muscle. Am J Sports Med 20:587–593, 1992.

38. Zeman SC, Rosenfeld RT, Lipscomb PR: Tears of the pectoralis major muscle. Am J Sports Med 7:343–347, 1979.

39. McEntire JE, Hess WE, Coleman SS: Rupture of the pectoralis major muscle. J Bone Joint Surg 54A:1040–1046, 1972.

40. Lorentzen D, Lawson L: Selected sports bras: A biomechanical analysis of breast motion while jogging. Phys Sports Med 15:128–139, 1987.

41. Gehlsen G, Albohm M: Evaluation of sports bras. Phys Sports Med 8:89–98, 1980.

42. O'Donoghue DH: Treatment of Injuries to Athletes. Philadelphia, WB Saunders, 1984, p 337.

43. Orringer MB: Chest injuries in the athlete. *In* Schneider R, Kennedy JC, Plant ML (eds): Sports Injuries—Mechanisms, Prevention, and Treatment. Baltimore, Williams & Wilkins, 1985, pp 818–829.

CHAPTER 26

Shoulder Injuries

D A V I D   J.   M A G E E   *PhD, BPT, MSc, SPDIII, CAT(C)*
D A V I D   C.   R E I D   *MD, BPT, MCh(Orth), MCSP, MCPA, FRCS(C)*

A cursory glance at the shoulder belies the complexity of the proximal part of a kinematic chain that starts at the trunk and includes the scapula, glenohumeral joint, acromioclavicular joint, and sternoclavicular joint and ends at the hand and fingers.[1] Thus, it is always important to think in terms of the shoulder girdle as a whole, rather than any one articulation.[1] The human shoulder has evolved to allow an incredible range of motion for reaching and placing the human hand through a large functional arc. Elevation, depression, protraction, retraction, and rotation of the scapula, along with elevation and rotation of the clavicle, and, most importantly, forward flexion, extension, abduction, adduction, medial and lateral rotation, and circumduction of the glenohumeral joint allow an enormous peripheral arc of motion. Combined with flexion, extension, pronation, and supination of the elbow, these movements allow placement of the hand almost anywhere within this wide arc.[2] Unfortunately, every functional adaptation toward mobility demands sacrifice in terms of stability, a problem that is compounded by the large ranges of motion needed and high stress loads seen in sports involving the upper limb. Thus, the minimal bony support of the shoulder girdle has to be supplemented by strong ligaments and careful arrangement of muscle groups.[3,4] Even here, secure ligamentous structures would inhibit the arc of motion, and hence further emphasis has to be placed on the dynamic (muscular) support of the shoulder girdle complex.[5–8]

The anatomy of the shoulder complex makes it particularly vulnerable to certain injuries because stability has been sacrificed for mobility. The shoulder complex is made up of three bones: the scapula, the clavicle, and the humerus. These are linked together and to the body by four joints: the glenohumeral, acromioclavicular, sternoclavicular, and "scapulothoracic" joints. In the highly mobile situation, such as found in the shoulder, the bones and articular surfaces are positioned to contribute to stability. For example, the scapula faces 30 degrees anteriorly to the chest wall and is tilted upward 3 degrees to enable easier movement on the anterior frontal plane and movements above the shoulder, thus increasing forward reach.[9,10] The glenoid is tilted upward 5 degrees to help control inferior instability. Only about 25 to 30 percent of the humeral head covers the glenoid surface to allow significant movement at the glenohumeral joint.[11] To compensate, the glenoid labrum, which attaches tightly to the bottom half of the glenoid and loosely to the top half, increases the glenoid depth approximately two times, adding to glenohumeral stability.[9,12–14] Normally, when the humeral head is moved through its large ranges of motion, only a small amount of translation or excursion occurs between the humeral head and the glenoid. If the dynamic structures controlling this translation (primarily the rotator cuff) are injured, translation may increase, leading to increased wear on the glenoid labrum, failure of the static restraints (Table

TABLE 26–1
Restraints About the Glenohumeral Joint

Passive (Static)	Active (Dynamic)	
Capsule Labrum Coracohumeral ligament Superior glenohumeral ligament Middle glenohumeral ligament Inferior glenohumeral ligament Geometry of humeral articular surface Geometry of glenoid articular surface Coracoacromial ligament Articular cartilage compliance Joint cohesion	Supraspinatus Infraspinatus Subscapularis Teres minor	Humeral stabilizers
	Pectoralis major Latissimus dorsi Biceps (long head) Triceps Deltoid Teres major	Movers of glenohumeral joint
	Serratus anterior Latissimus dorsi Trapezius Rhomboids Levator scapulae Pectoralis minor	Movers of scapula

26–1), and eccentric overload of the dynamic restraints, resulting in instability and/or impingement.[15,16]

Many of the overuse problems of the shoulder complex result from problems under the acromial arch. The subacromial space under the arch and above the humeral head contains a bursa, soft tissue, and the rotator cuff tendons. Anything that narrows this space, including thickening of the coracoacromial ligament, swelling or thickening of the acromioclavicular joint, osteophytes, inflammation of the soft tissues or the anterior one third of the acromion (especially if the acromion is of the hooked variety), can precipitate impingement. The literature has reported three types of acromion: type I, flat (18 percent); type II, curved (41 percent); and type III, hooked (41 percent).[17]

The primary restraints about the glenohumeral joint are passive and active (Table 26–1); these work individually and in unison to provide stability where mobility is paramount. The static stabilizers include primarily the labrum, previously mentioned, and the glenohumeral ligaments (superior, middle, and inferior). These ligaments, which in reality are thickenings in the capsule, show a high degree of variability, especially the superior and middle glenohumeral ligaments. Of the three, the inferior glenohumeral ligament is the most important and shows the least variability. It acts as a hammock for the humeral head, preventing some inferior translation, with the anterior and posterior bands tightening on rotation (torsion) to limit anterior and posterior translation. This ligament takes on even greater importance with glenohumeral abduction. For example, at 0 degrees abduction, the subscapularis muscle alone prevents anterior dislocation, with the middle glenohumeral ligament acting as a secondary restraint. At 45 degrees abduction, the subscapularis muscle and the middle and inferior glenohumeral ligaments prevent anterior dislocation. At ≥ 90 degrees, which is the usual position of anterior dislocation, the anterior fibers of the inferior glenohumeral ligament are the primary restraints to anterior dislocation.[9,12,13,18] Secondarily, the bony head of the biceps tendon acts as a dynamic support to decrease stress anteriorly in the abducted and laterally rotated position.[19] Similarly, the posterior band of the inferior glenohumeral ligament prevents posterior translation above 90 degrees.[12] Thus, these passive restraints play a significant role in stabilization of the glenohumeral joint. Conversely, if they are hypomobile, they can restrict normal translation.[20]

The dynamic restraints about the shoulder (see Table 26–1) also play a significant role in shoulder stability. The rotator cuff muscles, acting as stabilizers, compress the humeral head into the glenoid, decreasing the amount of translation that occurs between the glenoid and humeral head.[12] Other dynamic restraints act as "movers" of the various bones of the shoulder complex. The scapular movers position the scapula so that the glenoid is stable for the humerus and may act isometrically, concentrically, or eccentrically depending on the movement desired and whether the movement is speeding up or slowing down. The humeral movers position the arm so that the hand can carry out its specific activities.[12,21]

Shoulder injuries in sports are primarily due to trauma (collision or noncollision) and overuse. Noncollision injuries include torsional injuries (e.g., a spiral fracture in pitching) and joint instability, often seen in pitching and swimming. The repetitive nature of some activities such as swimming, the power needed in weight lifting and football, the acceleration and velocities seen in throwing sports, and the impact produced by collisions and falls in hockey and skiing all serve to generate a significant number of injuries around the shoulder complex.

In the analysis of shoulder problems, there are several important concepts that must be considered:

1. Shoulder pain must always be distinguished from referred pain arising from the cervical spine.

Shoulder disorders may refer pain into the trapezius muscle proximally, sometimes into the root of the neck but more frequently to the insertion of the deltoid muscle. True shoulder pain rarely extends below the elbow.[22]

2. There is often coexisting cervical abnormality, especially in patients over the age of 50.[22]

3. Changes in posture and immobility of the thoracic spine and ribs can significantly influence the movement patterns of the shoulder complex, especially at the glenohumeral joint, as well as the dimensions of the subacromial space. Thus, a careful assessment of the cervical and thoracic spine's mobility is an important part of any shoulder assessment.

4. Stability of the shoulder complex begins with the periscapular muscle stabilizers and concludes with fine adjustment by the rotator cuff.[23] Most power movements and rapid accelerating motions begin with the lower limb and trunk musculature. If any of these muscles become weak or injured, muscular imbalance of synergic and prime mover muscles, often acting as a force couple, results in abnormal shear forces, which in turn can lead to instability (functional subluxation), impingement, and rotator cuff tears.[2,3,24]

Only by understanding these concepts and taking a holistic approach to the assessment and treatment of the shoulder will successful resolution of some of the more difficult sport-induced problems occur.[7,24]

SHOULDER ASSESSMENT

The key to clinical diagnosis of the spectrum of shoulder injuries in sports is recognition of the salient features in the history, identification of the precipitating or perpetuating factors, and careful palpation of the specific structures generating the pain. This allows an appropriate choice of further investigations and a logical approach to treatment.

According to Neer, impingement occurs against the anterior edge of the acromion, the coracoacromial ligament, and, at times, the acromioclavicular joint.[3] Structural narrowing of the subacromial space may be secondary to inferior acromial tilting, the so-called hooked (type III) acromion, an unfused acromial ossification center, or subacromial spurring.[25] In addition, acromioclavicular joint hypertrophy and marginal osteophytes may irritate the cuff.[5] Postural changes, particularly slouched, rounded shoulders and a poking chin, may also contribute to impingement. Magnetic resonance imaging (MRI) has demonstrated narrowing of the subacromial space as the shoulder girdle moves from a retracted to a protracted position.[26]

The function of the upper limb is to be able to put the versatile prehensile human hand through as large a functional range as possible. In this regard, the shoulder joint has to be considered particularly in relation to its role within the whole shoulder girdle. Thus, the sources of pain may be the nearby acromioclavicular articulation; the rotator cuff, whose job it is to fine-tune the large extrinsic muscles; the associated subacromial (subdeltoid) bursa; or the biceps tendon. In normal abduction, the ratio of glenohumeral motion to scapulothoracic motion is roughly 2:1, and it occurs with small variation in a steady flow throughout the range.[2] Pain can disrupt this smooth scapulohumeral rhythm. The embryologic derivation of the shoulder girdle from the cervical myotomes has resulted in a close relationship for specific innervation, as well as for referred pain. Thus, any complaint of shoulder girdle discomfort mandates a careful ruling out of cervical pathology.

HISTORY

Generally, shoulder abnormality is characterized by a feeling of instability, stiffness, or pain on use. These findings help to distinguish it from cervical pain, which is often present even at rest and is generally aggravated by chronic postural positions such as sitting, reading, or studying at a desk. Neck and shoulder pain may not be totally isolated, and in those 55 years of age and older, up to 20 percent of individuals may have some coexisting shoulder and cervical spine abnormality.[22] The clinical points that are most suggestive of pain of spinal origin include absence of shoulder tenderness, guarded cervical spine motion, decreased biceps strength and reflex, and a positive cervical compression test.[1] The most common pattern of cervical spine disease refers to the C5–C6 dermatome with pain and/or paresthesia over the shoulder, lateral arm, and even the forearm, as well as radiation to the well-known trigger points around the scapula (Table 26–2).

When the abnormality is in the shoulder, the most common pattern of pain radiation is to the deltoid insertion. Less commonly, pain radiates from the shoulder to the scapula, the base of the neck, or the elbow, in descending order of frequency. Infrequently, the pain is referred past the elbow but almost never into the hand.[22] Neck pain and dysesthesia radiating past the elbow normally implicate cervical spine disease, but

---

TABLE 26–2
Factors Suggesting Site of Origin of Shoulder Pain

Neck Pathology	Shoulder Pathology
Pain at rest	Pain with use
Pain with neck motion	Pain working overhead
Pain with overpressure on neck	Feeling of instability
Aggravated by postural positions	Local palpable tenderness
Pain past the shoulder	Painful arc of motion
Reflex changes	Pain into deltoid area
Altered peripheral sensation	Mainly dominant side
Guarded cervical spine motion	Relief with local injection

Note: Twenty percent of individuals over age 55 may have coexisting pathology.

nerve entrapment at the elbow or wrist or a local pathologic lesion within the hand must be considered.[1]

When the chief complaint is pain, it should be related to the athlete's age, occupation, recreational goals, and side dominance. Specifically, the examiner must ensure that the athlete is complaining of pain and not weakness or feeling of instability. The mode of onset is important, whether a single traumatic episode, which might signify a rotator cuff tear or subluxation, or repetitive in nature, related to the individual's occupation or pastime.

A family history of joint disease and the presence of other joint symptoms will help to identify the possibility of a generalized arthropathy. Inquiries regarding gastrointestinal problems or heart disease will distinguish referred pain from the viscera. In those age 45 and older, left shoulder pain related to activity must always raise the suspicion of cardiac symptoms and prompt further questions as to cessation with rest, associated chest and neck pain, and the presence of shortness of breath. Finally, if any meaningful treatment plan is to evolve, some knowledge of past therapy, response to the therapy, and compliance with these regimens, is required. In addition, with athletes, specific details of activities and their relation to pain and restriction of motion are required. For example, information on pain and weakness relative to the throwing motion, swimming stroke, or tennis stroke are necessary. Such information will enable informed modification of activity during treatment as well as assist in diagnosis.

PHYSICAL EXAMINATION

Adequate exposure of the athlete is necessary so that the initial examination can encompass the thorax, spine, and shoulder girdle. Viewing the athlete from behind allows an impression of wasting of the shoulder girdle muscles, specifically the supraspinatus, the trapezius, and the deltoid.[27] The presence and size of stretch marks or scars reflect poor quality collagen, and thus may be a clue to the possibility of generalized ligamentous laxity. Viewing from the side allows assessment of posture; specifically, a kyphotic thoracic spine and associated poking chin posture are suggestive of weakness, habit, or thoracic and cervical spine disease.[27]

General examination starts with a scanning examination of the cervical spine, especially if there is no history of trauma.[27] The object of the cervical scan is to exclude neurologic problems of the peripheral or central nervous system. Active motion of the cervical spine in all directions may be supplemented with specific overpressure in the four cervical quadrants to see if these positions trigger referred pain into the shoulder area.

Range of motion (ROM) of the shoulder girdle is done actively, which assesses the athlete's willingness to move and also the degree of pain, weakness, or impingement as seen by a painful arc, facial expression, or a reversed scapulohumeral rhythm. Abduction in both the frontal plane and scapular planes is assessed, watching for normal scapulohumeral rhythm. If the athlete is able to achieve 180 degrees of abduction actively, normal scapulohumeral rhythm is usually present. If 180 degrees of abduction cannot be achieved, the examiner must determine where and why movement is not occurring. For example, if clavicular rotation and elevation are restricted, abduction is limited to about 120 degrees. If there is no movement in the glenohumeral joint, abduction is limited to about 60 degrees. Furthermore, if lateral rotation at the glenohumeral joint does not occur during abduction, abduction is limited to about 120 degrees, 60 degrees of which occurs in the scapulothoracic joint and 60 degrees in the glenohumeral joint.[27] If there is any alteration in either of these active movements, along with active medial and lateral rotation, gentle passive range of motion is carried out to determine range of motion and end feel, followed by specific resisted isometric activity to test the individual muscles. Passive range of motion gives selective stressing primarily to the noncontractile elements, although the examiner should be aware that contractile tissue is being stretched at the extreme of the range of motion. If the entire capsule is involved, as with a frozen shoulder, infection, or capsulitis, a capsular pattern in which lateral rotation is most significantly affected, followed by abduction and medial rotation, is evident. The examiner should be aware, however, that an early capsular pattern may demonstrate only limitation of lateral rotation.[27]

Discrepancy between active and passive range of motion is usually secondary to pain, muscle weakness, nerve injury, or tendon or rotator cuff abnormality, or is purely volitional caused by some form of secondary financial gain. Active range-of-motion tests allow an observation of capsular or noncapsular patterns and give an overall impression of the amount of movement possible. Functional range of motion is most easily tested using the Apley scratch test (Fig. 26–1).

Testing for muscle strength is always done isometrically, in the position of most comfort. The examiner places the athlete's arm in the desired position and then asks the athlete to resist the movement with the instruction, "Don't let me move you." This isometric testing (Table 26–3) selectively stresses the contractile elements and, unless there is a considerable inflammatory response, allows isolation of the muscle and its associated tendon as the source of pain. It gives an overall impression of strength as well as inhibition of pain from the musculotendinous structures. Strength may be recorded according to the simple Oxford scale (1 to 5 scale) or by more sophisticated means such as isokinetic tests.

If a cervical lesion is suspected, a selection of muscles (myotomes) are chosen that help to identify the major nerve roots and nerves. Segments that test positive will be weak and pain free. Thus, the trapezius (neck side flexion and shoulder elevation) is examined to test C3–C4 cervical segments. Other specific cervical plexus levels are tested by abduction (deltoid, C5), flexion of the elbow (biceps, C6), extension of the elbow (C7), flexion of the wrist (C7), extension of the wrist (C6), thumb abduction (C8), and the intrinsics (T1) (Table 26–4).

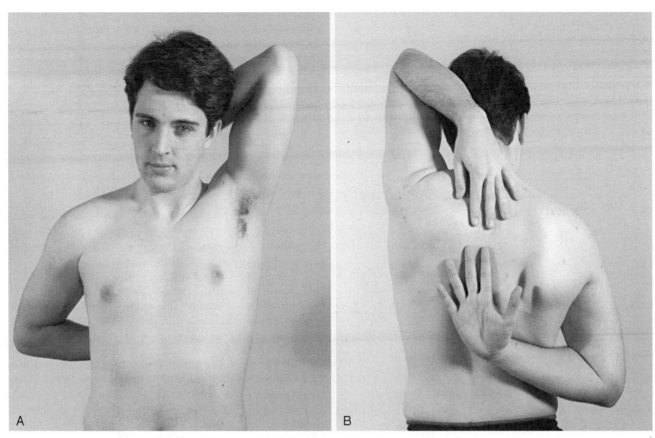

FIGURE 26–1. The Apley scratch test. *A*, Anterior view. *B*, Posterior view.

Shoulder impingement is associated with various degrees of inflammation and frequently occurs in athletes as a result of micro- or macrotrauma and functional instability. Impingement should have already been indicated as a source of the problem by the identification of a possible painful arc during attempted active abduction. Cross-flexion of the shoulder stresses primarily the acromioclavicular joint. It is considered a positive test only if the pain is carefully isolated to the acromioclavicular joint by the examiner's palpating fingers. The subacromial space is identified as a source of impingement by taking the arm passively into full abduction, followed by medial rotation (the Neer test). This test can be further supplemented by having the arm at 90 degrees of abduction and forward flexion, followed by forced medial rotation; this is the Hawkins test or sign (Fig. 26–2).[27] It may be enhanced by the athlete resisting a force applying downward pressure to the dorsum of the hand. Pink and Jobe state that the rotator cuff tendons are being impinged under the acromion with the Hawkins test, while the undersurface of the rotator cuff tendons is being impinged on the anterosuperior glenoid rim with the Neer test. They believed swimmers were more likely to have a positive Hawkins test than Neer test (see Chapter 16). The biceps is specifically examined by the classic Yergason test of flexion and supination with the arm in the neutral position and supplemented by the Speed's test in which the arm is held in the forward flexed (90-degree) position with the elbow extended, the athlete then attempts to resist extension of the shoulder, with the examiner giving eccentric resistance through the extension range. This test is usually more sensitive than the classic Yergason test because the tendon is moving through the bicipital groove.[27]

There has been a movement away from labeling specific structures in the diagnosis, and most of these painful shoulder abnormalities, including tendinitis and bursitis, are given the functional term *anterior impingement syndrome* to signify their close relationship to each other.[6,28] Where there is significant inflammation, impingement tests are often false positive, since all testing positions tend to be uncomfortable. Very inflamed tissues are uncomfortable even on passive stretch when put under tension by contraction of the associated muscle. Hence, by testing for pain in a nonimpingement position for each specific structure, it is sometimes possible to distinguish and isolate the inflammatory response of the tendon from a simple impingement. For example, a partial rupture of the biceps tendon within the joint may give positive impingement signs and may also be maximally painful when forearm supination and humeral flexion (the Yergason test) is resisted with the arm at the side and the elbow flexed to 90 degrees.

Diagnosis can be further confirmed by injecting approximately 3 ml of lidocaine (Xylocaine) directly around the most painful areas or 5 ml into the subacromial space and then waiting a suitable interval (usually a few minutes) before repeating the impingement test.[29] Relief of at least 50 percent of the athlete's

TABLE 26–3
Isometric Testing of Selected Muscles About the Shoulder

Muscle Tested	Test Position
Supraspinatus	Athlete's shoulder abducted to 90°, medially rotated and angled forward 30° so athlete's thumbs point toward floor ("empty can" position); pain on resistance Because of the synergistic role of supraspinatus in lateral rotation, rotator cuff tears (mainly supraspinatus) manifest as weakness in resisted lateral rotation with the arm by the side
Infraspinatus	Pain on isometric testing of lateral rotation, abduction, and horizontal abduction of arm
Teres minor	Pain on isometric testing of extension, lateral rotation, horizontal abduction, and abduction of arm
Subscapularis	Pain on isometric testing of medial rotation (arm by side) and abduction of arm
Biceps	Pain on resisted forward flexion of arm
Serratus anterior	Pain on resisted isometric elevation through abduction of arm
Trapezius (upper fibers)	Pain on resisted isometric shoulder girdle elevation
Trapezius (middle fibers)	Pain on resisted isometric shoulder retraction
Pectoralis major	Pain on resisted isometric adduction of arm

pain through the painful arc or the impingement positions is confirmatory of the source of the pain. Furthermore, where there is a suspicion of a tear of the rotator cuff, elimination of most of the pain allows a more specific examination of strength. The classic findings in a rotator cuff tear are difficulty in abduction in slight forward flexion and loss of lateral rotation power.

Shoulder instability due either to frank trauma or to functional instability is another common problem seen in athletes. A series of specific clinical tests will help unmask instability and its direction.[27] When the athlete is in the sitting position, the humeral head may be grasped through the bulk of the deltoid and attempts made to glide anteriorly and posteriorly (Fig. 26–3). Direct traction in the long axis of the arm may reveal a so-called sulcus sign as the humeral head subluxates inferiorly, indicating multidirectional instability.

Perhaps the easiest test to perform is the sitting or lying apprehension test for anterior instability. The abducted arm is firmly and carefully rotated laterally while anterior to posterior pressure is exerted on the proximal humerus (Fig. 26–4A). Ability to laterally rotate with a greater feeling of security with application of the anterior-to-posterior pressure is further evidence of instability as the cause of the initial apprehension (the relocation or Fowler test) (Fig. 26–4B). Direct posterior pressure with the arms slightly adducted and forward flexed to 90 degrees (the Norwood test) helps to determine posterior instability (Fig. 26–5).

The glenoid labrum grind, or "clunk," test is performed in an attempt to rule out internal derangement. Forward pressure is exerted over the humeral head as

TABLE 26–4
Screening Neurologic Levels in the Upper Limb*

Level Nerve	Sensory	Reflex	Motor	Method of Testing
C3, Spinal accessory	—	—	Trapezius	Neck side flexion
C4, Spinal accessory	—	—	Trapezius	Shoulder elevation
C5, Dorsal scapular	—	—	Rhomboids, deltoid	Hands on hips, push elbows back against resistance Shoulder abduction
C5–C7, Long thoracic	—	—	Serratus anterior	Patient pushed against wall; observe winging
C5, Circumflex	Lateral deltoid	Biceps jerk	Deltoid	Shoulder abduction
C6, Musculocutaneous	Dorsum of thumb	Biceps jerk Brachialis jerk	Biceps	Elbow flexion and wrist extension
C7, Radial	Dorsum of middle finger	Triceps jerk	Triceps	Elbow extension and wrist flexion
C8, Ulnar and median	Ulnar border hand	—	Thumb extension, finger flexors	Thumb extension and ulnar deviation
T1, Ulnar and median	Medial side of forearm and arm	—	Hand intrinsics	Finger abduction and adduction

*There are significant variations in individual anatomy and main testing areas and innervation given in various texts. When the screening test gives an indication of abnormality, more specific testing is required.
Data from Magee DJ: Orthopedic Physical Assessment. Philadelphia, WB Saunders, 1992.

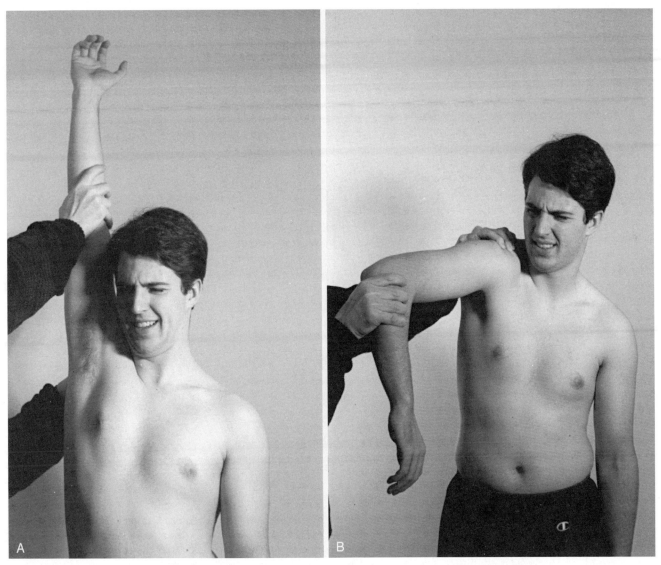

FIGURE 26–2. *A,* The Neer impingement test. *B,* The Hawkins-Kennedy impingement test.

the elbow is grasped, and the shoulder is circumducted or taken from flexion to extension (Fig. 26–6). During these maneuvers, the athlete may experience the apprehension of instability, or there may be a popping, grinding, or clunking sensation with or without pain, which may indicate the possibility of a glenoid labral lesion. Other tests of instability can be found elsewhere.[27]

Once the specific tests have been completed, the examiner can progress to testing sensation and reflexes, if appropriate. This testing is followed by joint play testing and palpation.

Palpation should be done very carefully with a visualization of the specific structures under the palpating fingers. If palpation is performed before the actual examination, the examiner must be cautious in assessing the pain and/or tenderness and must always be aware of the possibility of referred pain. Palpation should start at the sternoclavicular joint, move out along the clavicle and around the acromioclavicular articulation, followed by careful palpation around the anterior, lateral, and posterior margins of the acromion. The soft tissue triangles of the neck are palpated for abnormal nodes. The biceps tendon is gently probed, as is the supraspinatus tendon, the subdeltoid bursa, and, posteriorly, the insertion of the infraspinatus tendon. Palpation is completed by moving along the spine of the scapula and onto the muscle masses of the supra- and infraspinatus fossae, as well as the trapezius, in an attempt to identify trigger points. Palpation is most easily accomplished from behind, and the position of the athlete's arm should be changed during the examination to allow movement of the shoulder while palpating structures such as the biceps tendon, followed by movement of the arm into the medially rotated position with the forearm in the small of the back to uncover any rotator cuff abnormality, especially in the supraspinatus muscle.

Many techniques have been developed for radiologic examination about the shoulder. Regardless of which plane views the physician decides to use, the principle is to visualize the joint from at least two different angles

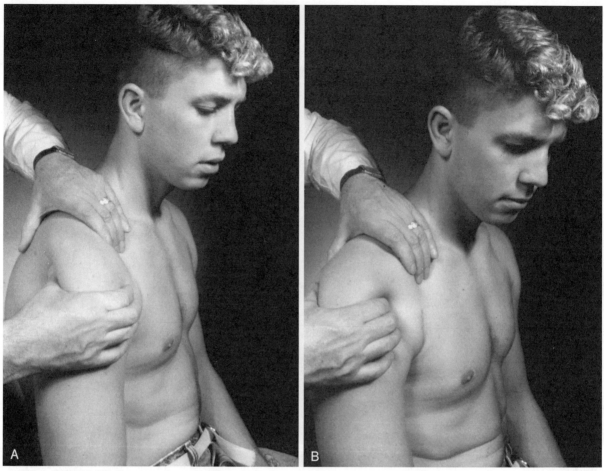

FIGURE 26–3. *A*, Anterior translation of humerus in sitting. *B*, Posterior translation of humerus in sitting.

to avoid a missed diagnosis. Normally, the anteroposterior and transscapular views are ordered.

The anteroposterior view is taken with the athlete's body turned 35 degrees medially to account for the normal shoulder anteversion of the glenoid (Fig. 26–7). The transscapular lateral view (the so-called Y view) is very useful, particularly after trauma, when it is difficult for the athlete to move the arm. In this particular view,

the athlete need not move the arm at all. The plate is held against the shoulder while the x-ray beam is pointed to show the body of the scapula in profile (Fig. 26–8). The glenoid is shown at the intersection of lines that form a Y.

Arthrograms, computed tomography (CT) scans, and MRI scans are also frequently used techniques, especially if the soft tissues are involved.[27]

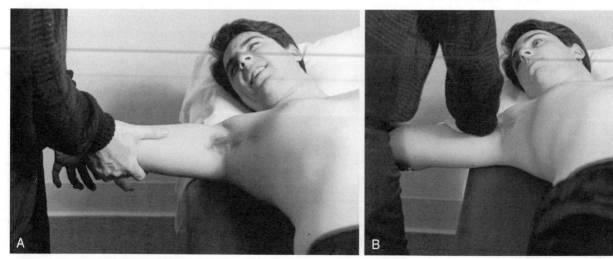

FIGURE 26–4. *A*, Anterior apprehension (crank) test for anterior instability. *B*, Relocation test.

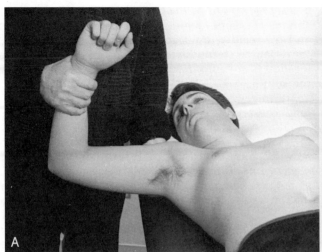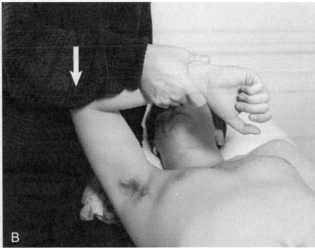

FIGURE 26–5. *A,* The Norwood test for posterior instability: position 1. The arm is taken into lateral rotation. *B,* The Norwood test for posterior instability: position 2.

DISLOCATIONS AND SUBLUXATIONS

Shoulder dislocations and subluxations can range in expression from a vague sense of shoulder dysfunction (atraumatic instability) to shoulder dysfunction due to repetitive microtrauma (functional instability) to frank dislocation caused by trauma. Thus, the practitioner must be aware that dislocations and subluxations, although most commonly caused by trauma in sports, may also be due to congenital joint laxity (hypermobility), congenital muscle weakness, and muscle weakness or atrophy after injury.

The signs and symptoms of any dislocation vary depending on the severity. As previously mentioned, the athlete may complain only of a vague sense of shoulder dysfunction, or pain may be one of the primary complaints, especially if the injury has been traumatic. Reduction of the dislocation or subluxation usually gives immediate relief of pain, although a dull ache may remain. Muscle spasm may make reduction difficult without the use of muscle relaxants, especially for the glenohumeral joint. Deformity, especially with dislocation, and loss of range of motion will be evident. Several days later bruising and ecchymosis will be seen.

If the joint is stressed after reduction, especially in the direction of dislocation, apprehension by the athlete will occur. If the athlete complains of paresthesia or numbness, the clinician must be aware of possible nerve injury.

STERNOCLAVICULAR JOINT

Dislocations of the sternoclavicular joint are quite rare, forming about 3 percent of all fractures and dislocations around the shoulder girdle.[30] The majority of these dislocations are anterior dislocations (with an anterior-to-posterior ratio approaching 20:1).[31] Nevertheless, when a posterior dislocation does occur, the complication rate is high, and thus it is important to recognize the injury and its potential life-threatening nature. The posterior dislocation may put pressure on the many vital structures lying between the sternum and the cervical spine, including the trachea, esophagus, and major vessels. It has been reported that

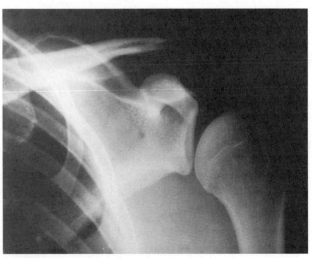

FIGURE 26–6. Clunk test for a glenoid labral lesion.

FIGURE 26–7. Anteroposterior radiograph of a normal shoulder.

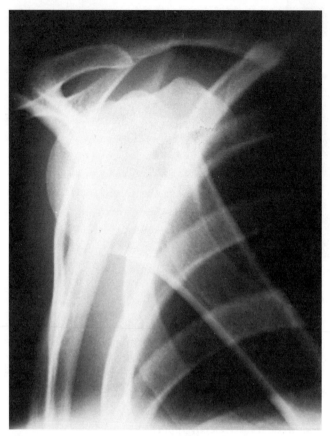

FIGURE 26—8. Transscapular lateral view (Y view) of a normal shoulder.

sporting activities are the second most common cause of these dislocations, which occur primarily as a result of direct or indirect trauma. Examples of direct sport trauma include a hockey player hitting the medial side of the clavicle on the goalpost or on another player's knee. With indirect injuries, the athlete is lying on his or her side, and the uppermost shoulder is compressed and rolled backward, resulting in an anterior sternoclavicular dislocation on the same side. If the shoulder rolls forward and is compressed, a posterior dislocation is more likely to occur.[31]

The sternoclavicular joint is stabilized primarily by strong ligaments. The anterior sternoclavicular ligament is a broad band supporting the anterior aspect of the joint, while the posterior sternoclavicular ligament is smaller and weaker, providing support to the posterior aspect of the joint. The costoclavicular ligament, shaped like an inverted cone, runs from the clavicle to the first rib and its adjacent cartilage. The interclavicular ligament, which provides minimal support to the joint, runs between the two sternoclavicular joints and also attaches to the manubrium sternum.

Sternoclavicular dislocations are classified in terms of degrees, and the classification is based more on injury to ligaments supporting the joint rather than the joint itself. A first-degree sternoclavicular dislocation classification results in minor tearing (1- or 2-degree sprain) of the sternoclavicular and costoclavicular ligaments with no true displacement of the joint. A complete tear (3-degree sprain) of the sternoclavicular ligaments and

a 2-degree sprain of the costoclavicular ligament constitute a second-degree sternoclavicular dislocation and, in reality, result in subluxation of the joint. A third-degree sternoclavicular dislocation is a true dislocation of the joint resulting from 3-degree sprains to the sternoclavicular and costoclavicular ligaments.

The injury is characterized by deformity; local pain or tenderness, especially on arm movement in which the shoulders are rolled forward; and subsequent ecchymosis. With a posterior dislocation or subluxation, there may be some shortness of breath or even venous congestion in the neck, with decreased circulation sometimes being evident in the arm. Radiologic confirmation requires a 40-degree cephalic tilt view. An axillary lateral view with the film aimed into the axilla and the plate above the shoulder is the best view for determining a sternoclavicular dislocation, but is sometimes difficult to obtain in athletes with acute injury.

The reduction of a posterior sternoclavicular dislocation is usually accomplished by extending the shoulders while using some form of roll or sandbag as a fulcrum along the spine. On most occasions reduction occurs easily, although some cases may require supplemental anesthesia. It may also be necessary to grasp the clavicle with the fingers or, where the anatomy is less defined, with some form of surgical instrument such as a towel clip. In the nonemergency situation, this grasping can be done under local or general anesthesia, but in the more urgent situation, where asphyxiation is imminent, it can be done without anesthesia.

If the main complaint after reduction is instability at the sternoclavicular joint, then treatment will frequently require sling support for anterior dislocation or a figure-of-eight bandage for posterior dislocation. The sling is worn for at least 2 to 3 weeks. Chronic instability may require surgical stabilization of the sternoclavicular joint, which is by no means uniformly successful. Chronic subluxation or damage to the intra-articular disc can produce long-term discomfort with repetitive or strong movements of the upper limb.

Complications of the anterior sternoclavicular dislocation include a cosmetic deformity, recurrent instability, and late osteoarthrosis, while complications of the posterior dislocation include the above plus pressure on or rupture of the trachea, pneumothorax, rupture of the esophagus, pressure on the subclavian artery or brachial plexus, voice change, and dysphagia. Although the incidence of one of these complications can be as high as 25 percent, only three deaths have been reported from the more serious complications associated with this injury.[31]

ACROMIOCLAVICULAR JOINT

The acromioclavicular (AC) joint is one of the most frequently injured joints in football, ice hockey, skiing, and rugby. These injuries, resulting in what is sometimes called a "separated" shoulder, account for 12 percent of the dislocations of the shoulder girdle.[30] The mechanism of injury is either a fall on the outstretched hand (FOOSH injury), a direct blow to the shoulder, or falling on the point of the shoulder.

There is considerable variation in the anatomy of this joint, with the articular surface orientation ranging from vertical to overriding at an angle of approximately 50 degrees.[31] There may be an intra-articular disc present in the joint that may be partial or complete. The disc can be damaged with an AC joint injury and may further degenerate with time; such discs may be implicated in some of the "clicking" that is heard and in some painful syndromes that occur in the joint post-traumatically. The major ligaments of the AC joint include the superior AC ligament, which reinforces the capsule superiorly, and the extrinsic bands of the conoid and trapezoid ligaments, which together make up the coracoacromial ligament or bundle. The dramatic variation in anatomy may account for the different vulnerability among individuals for separation. Indeed, it is not unusual to see veteran hockey players having subluxated both AC joints over a period of time.

During the abduction motion, there is up to 60 degrees of elevation and 50 degrees of rotation of the clavicle (scapulohumeral rhythm), and thus, in situations where there is degeneration and instability, there may be some degree of functional impairment, especially when the joint is placed under high loads.

Diagnosis is made by assessing the site of local tenderness, the degree of deformity, and the presence or absence of instability. Like the sternoclavicular joint, injury to the AC joint tends to cause very localized pain with minimal referral. Stressing the joint with cross-flexion will elicit pain in the injured AC joint. There may also be a palpable gap (step deformity) in the higher degrees of separation.

As in the sternoclavicular joint, AC joint injuries are classified according to ligamentous injury rather than injury to the joint itself (Table 26–5). There has been a suggestion that third-degree (type III) disruptions can be further divided according to the magnitude of displacement and the potential accompanying muscle and soft tissue stripping and tearing, as well as the direction of displacement of the distal clavicle.[1,31] For instance, displacement of the clavicle of more than 100 percent is often classified as a fourth-degree (type IV) injury. Type V injuries involve very severe deformity, because the distal end of the clavicle is displaced upward a significant degree toward the base of the neck. In addition, displacements may occur posteriorly through the trapezius or, on very rare occasions, inferiorly below the coracoid (type VI). The fourth-

TABLE 26–5
Classification of Acromioclavicular Joint Trauma

Classification	Salient Features	Management
1° (type I)	Minimal structural damage 1° sprain acromioclavicular ligament Local tenderness on palpation Full range of motion (may have pain at extreme) No structural strength loss Stress x-rays are normal	Re-establish full range of motion and strength
2° (type II)	Subluxation of acromioclavicular joint Tearing of acromioclavicular capsule 2°–3° sprain of acromioclavicular ligament 1°–2° sprain of coracoclavicular ligament Deltoid and trapezius muscles may be affected No significant increase in costoclavicular space on stress radiograph Slight widening of acromioclavicular joint on stress radiograph Definite structural weakness Detectable instability on stress Palpable gap or step deformity may be present Obvious swelling initially with later ecchymosis	Healing time is 6 weeks, although ligaments have good structural strength after approximately 3 weeks Limb support (sling) Modalities for pain relief (e.g., ice, TENS, interferential therapy) Ultrasound for collagen enhancement Strengthening and stability exercises Functional exercises (activities at functional speed with control)
3° (type III)	Dislocation of acromioclavicular joint Complete disruption of acromioclavicular capsule 3° sprain of acromioclavicular ligament 3° sprain of coracoclavicular ligament Deltoid and trapezius muscles torn from distal end of clavicle Step deformity obvious, often without stress Costoclavicular space increased on stress radiograph Widening of acromioclavicular joint on stress radiograph	May be treated surgically or conservatively If treated conservatively, deformity will remain but athlete will function remarkably well with only slight discomfort/instability at high loads Conservative treatment as above
Types IV, V, and VI	Modifications of type III (rare injuries) (see text)	Surgical repair required

TENS, Transcutaneous electrical nerve stimulation.

degree injuries are associated with considerable disruption of the deltoid and trapezius muscles, and although a third-degree separation may be treated nonoperatively,[32,33] there is a role for surgery in the treatment of fourth-, fifth-, and sixth-degree injuries because of the associated ligamentous disruption and because of cosmetic considerations in leaner individuals.

The ultimate function of the AC joint depends not so much on the amount of separation, but on the amount of pain that persists in the joint. Indeed, some first-degree dislocations and some of the more severe second-degree injuries are much more problematic in that they produce a great deal of pain in long-term follow-up.

Thus, early conservative treatment focuses on pain relief. Initially the athlete is placed in a sling, often accompanied by a swath, to remove the stress of the weight of the limb on the joint. As the pain decreases (within 5 to 7 days), range-of-motion and strengthening exercises, especially to the deltoid and trapezius muscles, are begun, with the athlete resuming activity 2 to 6 weeks after injury.[34]

For third-degree acromioclavicular joint injuries, complete reduction is not necessary for satisfactory function; in fact, in terms of strength, endurance, and function, nonsurgical and surgical treatment have been reported to be equally effective.[35–39] Depending on the preference of the surgeon, third-degree injuries may be treated surgically, but the results are seldom better than with conservative treatment, the recovery period is longer, and the complications of surgery must be considered. Some physicians advocate the use of a Kenny-Howard sling for 4 to 5 weeks. This sling pulls the arm superiorly while pushing the clavicle down, thus reducing the space between the acromion and clavicle. It has been reported that this reduction is often lost, even while the arm is still in the sling and the sling can lead to neurologic problems and skin breakdown.[39–41] Thus, the most common treatment for third-degree AC injuries in athletes is a swath and sling with treatment as pain allows, again stressing the deltoid and trapezius muscles. Immobilization is maintained for 7 to 10 days, and the athlete may return to activity within 2 weeks, although 6 weeks is more the norm.[42]

The complications of AC joint injury include a step deformity produced by the elevated distal end of the clavicle, early skin necrosis if the clavicle is widely displaced in a thin individual, osteoarthrosis, and continuing pain in the long term. In addition, for surgical procedures, complications include infection, wound dehiscence, pin migration, and recurrence of the instability, as well as the normal risks of general anesthesia.

GLENOHUMERAL DISLOCATIONS, SUBLUXATIONS, AND INSTABILITY

The glenohumeral joint is the most frequently dislocated major joint in the body, and in some series, glenohumeral dislocations are more common than all other joint dislocations combined.[43] Anterior dislocations of the shoulder account for between 80 and 95 percent of all shoulder girdle dislocations,[30,44,45] and recurrence is frequently the outcome of an initial traumatic dislocation. Classification is necessary to develop a logical treatment plan. Instabilities may vary from subtle subluxation to an obvious locked position in which the articular surfaces are no longer in contact (true dislocation). Recurrent transient subluxation results in a feeling of instability or loss of control due to positioning of the arm. An example of this would be forced hyperextension of the arm in elevation and/or lateral rotation, which may result in the "dead arm" syndrome seen in throwing athletes or tennis players when serving.[46,47]

Shoulder instability can range from a vague sense of shoulder dysfunction, resulting in atraumatic instability, to frank traumatic dislocation (Fig. 26–9). The basic classification of instabilities is traumatic and atraumatic. Neer added a third type, acquired.[48] The traumatic dislocation results from a single force that applies excessive overload to the soft tissues of the joint and often damages the glenoid labrum (Bankart lesion) along with disrupting the capsule. This type includes patients who present with *Traumatic Uni*directional instability with a *Bankart* lesion that responds well to *Surgery* (TUBS), as described by Matsen.[20] The atraumatic dislocation usually occurs in athletes with multiple joint laxities, who have frequently experienced episodes of subluxation before a relatively minor injury results in dislocation. These individuals often exhibit functional instability due to congenital hypermobility or congenital muscle weakness. This classification includes those patients who present with *Atraumatic Multidirectional* instability that is *Bilateral* and responds well to *Rehabilitation* (AMBRI).[20] If surgery is required, an *Inferior* capsular shift is best. Capsular laxity is common, and a frank

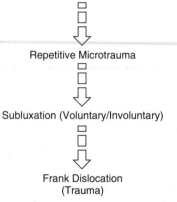

Vague Sense of Shoulder Dysfunction

(**A**traumatic **M**ultidirectional Instability in **B**oth shoulders that responds to Intensive **R**ehabilitation. If Surgery Necessary, **I**nferior Capsular Shift Used [**AMBRI**])

⬇

Repetitive Microtrauma

⬇

Subluxation (Voluntary/Involuntary)

⬇

Frank Dislocation (Trauma)

(**T**raumatic, **U**nidirectional Instability with **B**ankart Lesion Requiring **S**urgery [**TUBS**])

FIGURE 26–9. Shoulder instability spectrum.

Bankart lesion is not usually found in these individuals if surgery becomes necessary.[43] It must be remembered, however, that there are overlapping gradations of instability that cover the entire spectrum from TUBS to AMBRI.[15] Individuals with acquired instability are usually engaged in activities such as swimming, gymnastics, or baseball (i.e., pitching), where the repetitive microtrauma of ill-conceived stretching or rapid and large-range motion gradually contribute to capsular stretching. Although the shoulder becomes hypermobile, other joints may test in the normal ranges.[48] A traumatic episode may push the joint "over the edge" and produce the first frank dislocation, but this major episode is only a small component of the problem.[43]

Functional instability is becoming more and more frequently recognized as a pathologic entity that affects athletes, especially when the joint is put under high stress loads. The functional instability is due to large translation of the humeral head within the glenoid cavity as a result of overload and fatigue in the static and dynamic stabilizers of the shoulder.[16,49–54] Thus, the strong coordinated activity of the muscles and proper neuromuscular balance contribute significantly to a reduction in functional instability and the often associated impingement syndrome. The instability, which is due to asynchronous firing and fatigue of the humeral and scapular control muscles, can lead to subluxation and rotator cuff strains. Thus, movement control becomes the primary focus of the clinician when treating shoulder instability. Movement control focuses on strength, endurance, proprioception, and coordination. Burkhead and Rockwood[4] reported that 80 percent of patients with atraumatic subluxations had good or excellent results with conservative treatment using appropriate exercises. Thus, appropriate diagnosis and conservative treatment can lead to a successful outcome in the majority of athletes.

Although glenohumeral instability may occur in any direction, most acute locked dislocations are anterior, with posterior being the second most frequent. Although the functional instability is predominantly in one direction, testing in some individuals will reveal excessive motion anteriorly, posteriorly, and inferiorly, or in any combination of these directions, resulting in what is referred to as *multidirectional instability*.[55]

Voluntary instability is usually due to congenital hypermobility or laxity combined with the athlete using the shoulder muscles to purposely and spontaneously subluxate the joint.[43] There may be an element of secondary gain in these individuals, and treatment is difficult. *Involuntary instability* refers to a recurrent dislocation in individuals whose shoulders are so unstable they dislocate against their will.[5]

A dislocation may be acute or chronic. The acute frank dislocation is usually relatively easily reducible with adequate relaxation and, where appropriate, analgesia. Several methods have been advocated for reduction and may be found elsewhere.[31,56] Extreme care must be taken, however, to ensure that there is no damage to the axillary nerve during the reduction. For this reason, reduction by manipulation should be attempted only by experienced personnel. Occasionally the dislocation is irreducible and may require open reduction to extricate the structures barring reduction.

Chronic dislocation suggests that the humeral head has been out of contact with the glenoid cavity for a protracted period of time (i.e., days to years). Unreduced posterior dislocations are the most common because of the incidence of missed diagnosis. If the chronic nature of the dislocation is not recognized, attempts at closed reduction may produce a fracture.[57]

At the glenohumeral joint, there is a large humeral head with very little bony structural integrity, although the shallow glenoid cavity is deepened by the glenoid labrum.[9,12,14] The surface area of the head has been reported to be two to four times that of the glenoid.[58] However, the articular surfaces of the humeral head and glenoid are quite congruent, having radii within 3 mm. The area in contact tends to be greatest in mid-elevation rather than at the extremes.[58] The lax inferior capsule allows an adequate range of motion into elevation. Nevertheless, the surrounding soft tissue envelope is the primary contributor to stability in the normal glenohumeral joint.[59] The capsule is reinforced by the coracohumeral and glenohumeral ligaments, which act as checkreins, along with the dynamic muscle stabilizers, at the extremes of range of motion. There is a particularly weak area anteroinferiorly that leads into the subcoracoid recess. Nevertheless, translation of the humeral head on the glenoid is normally limited to a few millimeters in every direction.[60–63]

There are 120 degrees of glenohumeral motion, which is matched with 60 degrees of scapulothoracic motion, and unlike most movements at other joints, this large range of activity (scapulohumeral rhythm) is mainly brought about indirectly by muscles forming force couples generating rotary torques.[64] This lack of direct muscle action also contributes to the ease of dislocation and subsequent difficulty in protecting a lax joint simply with muscle hypertrophy.

The rotator cuff tendons and the long head of biceps have important dynamic roles in controlling glenohumeral translation and serve in a complementary function to adjust the tension in the capsuloligamentous system.[59] It is possible that stretch receptors within the capsular ligaments may be activated by tension to induce selective contraction of the surrounding musculature, thus protecting these structures at the extremes of motion (see Chapter 9).[65] Furthermore, contraction of these muscles compresses the humeral head into the glenoid cavity and increases the force needed to translate the head.[66] In addition, cadaveric experiments showed that simulated maximal contraction of the posterior rotator cuff muscles reduced anterior ligamentous strain, and posterior cuff contraction reduced anterior ligamentous strain.[67]

A second group of muscles affecting glenohumeral stability are the scapular control muscles (Table 26–6). These muscles position the glenoid beneath the humeral head, adjusting for the changing position of the arm. With periscapular dysfunction, there may be a failure to maintain a stable glenoid platform, an unlinking of scapulohumeral rhythm, and mild to severe winging of the scapula. It is these concepts that form the

TABLE 26–6
Scapular and Humeral Control Muscles

Scapular Control Muscles	Humeral Control Muscles
Trapezius	Deltoid
Serratus anterior	Pectoralis major
Levator scapulae	Latissimus dorsi
Rhomboids	Triceps
Latissimus dorsi	Rotator cuff
Pectoralis minor	Subscapularis
	Supraspinatus
	Infraspinatus
	Teres minor

basis for rehabilitation of the unstable shoulder and the emphasis on rehabilitation of the scapular control muscles, as well as the muscles controlling the humerus.[1]

Anterior dislocations probably account for about 95 percent of acute traumatic glenohumeral injuries.[31] They are most frequent in the young adult and are the result of excessive abduction and lateral rotation of the humerus. Pathologically, with the initial anterior dislocation, there may be rupture of the rotator cuff, detachment of the labrum, development of a subglenoid recess, and a redundant capsule or defect (Hill-Sachs lesion) in the humeral head. In cases in which no Bankart lesion is found, there may be disruption of the lateral capsule.[68] The capsule contains discrete thickenings (the glenohumeral ligaments) that come under tension when the joint is in the extremes of range, protecting against instability when all other mechanisms have been overwhelmed.[67] All ligaments of the shoulder work in an interconnected fashion. This is referred to as the *circle concept* (Fig. 26–10). In studies of posterior instability, damage occurs on both the anterior and posterior sides of the capsule.[68,69] Similarly, posterior laxity is a component of the pathomechanics of anterior instability.

The principles of diagnosing a dislocated or unstable shoulder have been outlined earlier in the chapter. Usually the diagnosis is self-evident from the history. On examination, if the shoulder is dislocated, there is usually a deformity or space under the tip of the acromion, resulting in prominence of the acromion, flattening of the deltoid muscle, pain, and loss of motion, with the arm tending to be supported in 30 degrees of abduction by the other arm. Full abduction is not possible. The humeral head may be palpable in the axilla. There may be paralysis or sensory loss based on injury to the axillary or, less frequently, the musculocutaneous nerve.

For dislocations of the shoulder, it is essential to take at least two views of the shoulder from two different angles to avoid a missed diagnosis, particularly a diagnosis of a posterior dislocation. Radiographs for an anterior dislocation should include a true anteroposterior view of the shoulder and a true lateral view of the scapula. A transscapular view is difficult to obtain in the acutely injured shoulder. In the chronic recurrent dislocation, a full medial rotation view may demonstrate a notch (Hill-Sachs lesion) in the humeral head.

In an anterior glenohumeral dislocation, the head of the humerus is driven or levered anteriorly (under the coracoid process), and thus it is sometimes referred to as a subcoracoid dislocation. The anterior capsule may be torn or the glenoid labrum may be stripped from the anterior aspect of the glenoid cavity, so the humeral head may be intracapsular or extracapsular. If the capsule alone is injured, the potential for healing is good. With greater damage and stripping of the glenoid labrum, the potential for recurrent dislocation is higher, because there is poorer potential for healing and spontaneous reattachment of the fibrocartilaginous labrum. The labral edge becomes atrophic and rounded, forming a poor anterior buttress to dislocation. Furthermore, the intact labrum is important in maintaining a vacuum suction–like effect that, although it is most important as a static stabilizer, does enhance dynamic support of the joint.[12,14] The glenohumeral joint is usually bathed in less than 1 ml of free synovial fluid.[67] This fluid aids in holding the articular surfaces together with viscous and intermolecular forces, which enhance the normal negative intra-articular pressure.[70,71]

There are several complications of anterior glenohumeral dislocations, of which recurrence is the most common. Others include fracture of the greater tuberosity of the humeral head and injury to the axillary, musculocutaneous, or median nerves. Subglenoid displacement of the humeral head into the quadrangular space damages the axillary nerve, causing paralysis of the deltoid muscle and loss of skin sensation in the region above the deltoid. More rarely, the musculocutaneous and median nerves and the brachial plexus may be involved.[72] Although clinically only about 20 percent of these dislocations show minimal signs and 5 percent significant evidence of neurologic involvement, Rockwood and Green have shown that there is electromyographic evidence of nerve injury in up to 80 percent of individuals.[31] This damage, however, is largely subclinical, with the athlete demonstrating no detectable weakness. Other complications include rotator cuff tears (the likelihood increases with increased age), tears of the glenoid labrum, damage to the humeral head (Hill-Sachs lesion), damage to the biceps tendon, and, on occasion, fractures and vascular injury must also be

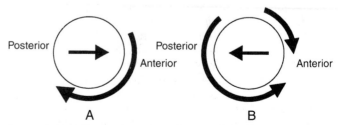

FIGURE 26–10. Circle concept of stability. Capsuloligamentous structures act together as a circular cuff. *A,* For anterior dislocation to occur, the capsular structures have to be disrupted as far as the 7 o'clock position posteriorly. *B,* For posterior dislocation to occur, a significant amount of anterior damage is necessary.

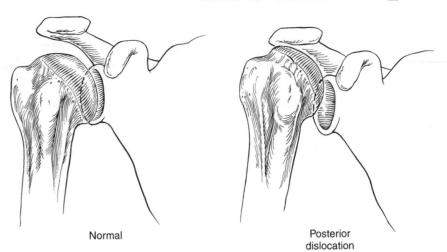

Normal

Posterior
dislocation

FIGURE 26–11. "Empty glenoid" sign of posterior dislocation on anteroposterior radiograph. Note how the head of the humerus fills the glenoid in the normal radiograph *(left)*. With a posterior dislocation, the glenoid is "empty," especially in its anterior portion *(right)*.

considered, as each will prolong the healing and treatment time.

Recurrent dislocations, sometimes referred to as "trick shoulders," tend to be anterior dislocations that are intracapsular.[45] They are due either to repeated traumatic dislocations, with each dislocation being easier to achieve, or to a congenital defect such as a lax capsule. In athletes under the age of 20, the recurrence rate has been reported to be as high as 80 percent, while nonathletes in the same age group demonstrated a recurrence rate of 30 percent. Between the ages of 20 and 30, the recurrence rate can be as high as 60 percent. The recurrence rate decreases with age, with very few recurrent dislocations occurring after age 40.[73,74] The majority (75 percent) of these dislocations occur within 2 years of the initial traumatic event.[47] Many of these dislocations are eventually treated surgically, since the anatomy of the labrocapsular complex has been disrupted. Nonoperative treatment is successful in some established recurrent dislocations, but for most individuals with multiple recurrent episodes, it is ineffective, due in part to the fact that the dynamic stabilizers (muscles) are in a poor position to control the humeral head with the arm abducted and laterally rotated. Furthermore, some of the power muscles, such as the pectoralis major and anterior deltoid, may dynamically contribute to pulling the humeral head out of joint if there is sufficient capsular laxity. Thus, surgical stabilization is appropriate for those with significant functional instability, and excellent success rates are usually achieved.[75] The choice of surgical technique will depend on the degree and direction of instability, the requirements for range of motion, and the preference of the surgeon.

Posterior or subspinous dislocations result from the arm being forced or thrust backward when it is forward flexed; these make up about 2 percent of glenohumeral dislocations. A posterior prominence (the humeral head) is often evident and rounding of the shoulder or deltoid is maintained, and so these dislocations are sometimes missed or misdiagnosed, especially in the heavier built individual. There may be some flattening of the anterior shoulder, and the coracoid process may be more prominent than on the uninjured side. The athlete will demonstrate limited lateral rotation (<0 degrees) and limited elevation (<90 degrees). In addition, medial rotation and cross-flexion will cause pain and apprehension. Posterior dislocations are recognized by the "empty glenoid" sign on the radiograph (Fig. 26–11). The anteroposterior (AP) view of the normal shoulder shows overlapping of the humeral head and glenoid shadows, which are absent or reduced with a posterior dislocation.

PRINCIPLES AND TREATMENT OF GLENOHUMERAL DISLOCATIONS

In the management of acute dislocations of the shoulder, an attempt must be made to characterize the injury. In fact, a major difficulty in developing a treatment plan from the older literature is the failure of the literature to adequately separate groups as to the underlying degree and direction of laxity.[76] Usually the glenohumeral joints are reduced by closed means with adequate anesthesia. It is important to recheck neural and vascular status both before and after reduction to ensure proper care.

Indications for surgery with open reduction include: irreducibility with closed reduction; the presence of a large flake of avulsed bone on the inferior glenoid margin, which will potentially contribute to future instability; a significantly displaced glenoid fracture involving a third or more of the articular surface; vascular impairment; and an associated tuberosity fracture. On occasion, a very athletic individual who, for social reasons, may desire a guarantee of stability in the shoulder may require early surgery.

For the anterior dislocation, after closed reduction, immobilization in the form of a swath and sling is used to prevent extension, abduction, and lateral rotation of the shoulder for 6 weeks in young adults. This promotes good capsular healing. It has been reported, however, that the period of immobilization has little relation to recurrence of dislocation.[77] Some authors[47,78] advocate a shorter period of immobilization (1 to 3 weeks). The duration of immobilization is dependent on the philosophy of the surgeon and type of reconstruction (if surgical repair was done).

The main point in acute anterior dislocation treatment is adequate early controlled immobilization. In the first 2 weeks after reduction, a program of strong isometric deltoid, shoulder abductor, adductor, and biceps work is instituted within the limits of pain tolerance. This minimizes muscle wasting as the edema and hemorrhage resolve and the shoulder becomes more comfortable. From 2 to 6 weeks after injury, the swath is removed for exercises several times each day. Small-range, gentle pendular exercises are begun. The emphasis is still on isometric activities, with shoulder medial and lateral rotator isometric exercises being added. In addition, concentric exercise through a limited range is permitted, bearing in mind that capsular healing is well under way at 3 weeks. The limits of range will be determined by pain and whether the athlete can comfortably control the movement. The controlled active movement will apply small amounts of stress to the joint structures to decrease the adverse effects of immobilization on the glenohumeral joint.[79–81] At no point during this time should abduction and forward flexion go beyond 90 degrees, nor should lateral rotation go past neutral. In older individuals, in whom the danger of stiffness from immobilization is greater than the risks of redislocation, the movement program is initiated sooner. Once immobilization has ended, the treatment protocol will follow the same principles indicated for postsurgery patients (see later discussion).

In all cases of dislocation, subluxation, or instability, a sincere, concerted effort at nonoperative treatment with well-planned and coordinated therapy must be attempted. The more lax the shoulder, the greater the collagen hyperelasticity, and the less trauma involved in the initial dislocation, the more important is this principle. Only when these methods have failed in the reduced or unstable shoulder should surgery be considered.

If surgery is elected, the spectrum of surgical approaches involves capsular plications of varying complexity (arthroscopic capsulorrhaphy; inferior, posterior, or anterior capsular shift; and subscapular muscle and capsule tightening in distinct layers [Putti-Platt] and as a single layer [Magnuson-Stack]). There are also bony procedures, including osteotomy and wedging of the glenoid (for posterior dislocation), humeral rotational procedures, osteotomies, and conjoint tendon transfer with the tip of the coracoid (Bristow procedure) (Table 26–7).[78,82–96]

Procedures that address the disrupted labrum and are plicated anteriorly (Bankart, Putti-Platt, and Magnuson-Stack procedures) are very effective but run the danger

TABLE 26–7
Common Surgical Procedures for Recurrent Anterior Dislocation

Type	Name	Procedure	Redislocation Rate*	Comment
Bone block	Eden-Hybbinette-Lange[83]	Bone block to increase anterior margin of glenoid	0–18%[82,84,95]; avg.: 6.0%	Decreases lateral rotation Late degenerative changes
Coracoid transfer	Bristow-Helfet[85]	Transfer of tip of coracoid process along with the conjoint tendon of biceps and coracobrachialis muscle	3–6%[82,85]; avg.: 1.9%[95]	A dynamic component Poor for throwing athletes 10% decrease in biceps power
Capsular repairs	duToit staple capsulorrhaphy[86]	Reattach anterior capsule to anterior glenoid margin	5–28%[87,94]; avg.: 8%[82,94]	Unacceptable redislocation and subluxation rates if not combined with other procedures
	Bankart procedure[88]	Reattach glenoid labrum and plicate anterior capsule	0–5%[78,89]; avg.: 3.3%[94]	Low dislocation rate May restrict lateral rotation
	Putti-Platt[90]	Reattach labrum and plicate capsule and subscapularis muscle separately	2–11%[89,91]; avg.: 2.8[94]	Good stability Addresses pathologic anatomy
	Magnuson-Stack[92]	Staple plication of entire anterior capsule and subscapularis muscle	2–17%[82,93]; avg.: 7.5%[95]	Problem with redislocation and biceps tendon

*Will vary with surgeon, patient population, length of follow-up, and numbers in series.

of restricting lateral rotation unduly in a percentage of individuals and may not be desirable for all athletes.[97] These procedures may be enhanced by resuturing any detached labral rim (Bankart repair). The Magnuson-Stack procedure is particularly difficult to adapt to the very active individual, since insufficient single-layer plication leads to an unacceptable redislocation rate, while overtightening gives inappropriate limitation of lateral rotation. The Bristow procedure works well for most athletes but results in some minor restriction of full abduction and of lateral rotation combined with abduction and extension. It is probably not the best choice for throwing athletes because of the need in these athletes for full lateral rotation in abduction, which may be limited by this procedure. However, it works well for football players, hockey players, and figure skaters, for example, because of the high degree of stability. Arthroscopic capsulorrhaphies, which involve plication of the capsule using arthroscopic stapling techniques, are appealing but have a high redislocation rate in the throwing athlete with very lax shoulders.[98]

For those requiring absolute full range of motion or who have any component of multidirectional instability, one of the inferior capsular shift procedures would be more appropriate.[99] The principle behind these repairs is to tighten the middle and inferior glenohumeral ligaments with due regard to the circle concept of instability (Fig. 26–10).

Following operative treatment, the traditional Putti-Platt procedure has a 1 to 5 percent incidence of recurrent dislocation; the Magnuson-Stack operation, 1 to 9 percent; and the Bristow repair, 1 to 6 percent.[95] Return to a high level of function is the rule with an appropriately selected and executed technique performed with due regard to the pathologic lesion and the activity goals of the athlete.

Initially, the aims of treatment postoperatively for the clinician are to stimulate circulation, decrease pain and inflammation, restore normal range of motion, increase strength, and restore proprioception. These aims can be accomplished by the use of ice, transcutaneous electrical nerve stimulation (TENS), interferential therapy, ultrasound, exercises, and mobilization depending on the stage of the lesion and presenting signs and symptoms.

Although many modalities can be and are used, the primary concern of the clinician is to restore the muscles by improving their strength, endurance, and proprioceptive control. In the early stages of rehabilitation, the stress is on scapular control and humeral head stabilization (see Table 26–6) and restoring the coordinated action of the force couples of the glenohumeral joint.[21,49,100] These force couples include the subscapular muscle, a primary stabilizer following anterior dislocation, counterbalanced by the infraspinatus and teres minor muscles, and the anterior deltoid, counterbalanced by the infraspinatus, teres minor, and subscapularis muscles.[18] By improving the strength and control of these force couples, the athlete will regain control of humeral head translation during dynamic movement.[49]

The basic rehabilitation plan will be modified depending on the type of surgery, surgical procedure used, precautions to treatment noted by the surgeon, individual surgeon's preference, the presence of pain, and the presence of restriction. In addition, the athlete's willingness to move and the quality of the athlete's movements will be of concern to the clinician. Thus, only broad guidelines are given for progression. However, the treatment principles remain constant: to relieve pain, observe for complications, regain muscle control, strengthen, regain range of motion safely, and retrain proprioceptive control. These aims are woven into an activity-specific protocol. Specificity plays a major role, with each program individualized to the athlete and his or her sport(s) and activities. With soft tissue operative techniques such as the Putti-Platt procedure, there must be sufficient time for capsular healing and with bony techniques such as the Bristow procedure, approximately 6 weeks are necessary to allow for union of the bone block before applying undue stress.

Initially, isometrics are instituted at several positions in the range of motion below shoulder level, with no lateral rotation beyond 0 degrees. The positioning and resistance will depend on the response of the athlete to pain and discomfort. The clinician must ensure that both scapular control and humeral muscle control receive attention (see Table 26–6).[21] Thus, the athlete is instructed to do proper isometrics into abduction, medial rotation, lateral rotation, extension, and a lower "empty can" position (below horizontal) for the supraspinatus, even with the athlete in a sling, as rhythmic stabilization exercises to the affected shoulder. If the athlete is complaining of pain in the shoulder, ice may also be used to give some relief. In addition, active exercise to the other joints of the arm and the rest of the body may be instituted. As the athlete improves (as evidenced by decreased pain and discomfort), isotonic exercises, especially flexion and extension, can be initiated (usually by the third or fourth day), again below shoulder level and with no lateral rotation beyond 0 degrees, within the pain-free and controllable range. By the fourth day, medial and lateral rotation to 0 degrees with the arm in the adducted position may be done very carefully. For the lateral rotators, only very careful isometrics should be performed to avoid excessive stress to the tissues. By the fifth day, the athlete may begin assisted abduction. By the sixth to eighth day, elevation through flexion may be begun, and by the end of the second week, the athlete should be able to attempt, very carefully, medial rotation and abduction. To achieve proper scapular and humeral control, exercises such as those shown in Table 26–8 are used when appropriate and when strength and pain allow.[101] Progression to free weights (5 lb [2.3 kg] or less for up to 30 repetitions) and tubing may be initiated, provided the athlete is able to control the movement.[102] This control is demonstrated by smooth, coordinated movement with minimal or no evidence of pain and discomfort.[103] Pappas et al.[102] found that weights heavier than 5 lb (2.3 kg) tended to precipitate loss of muscle balance in the shoulder. With further improvement, movement above shoulder height and into lateral rotation may begin. Again, it is essential that the athlete

TABLE 26–8
Scapular and Humeral Control Exercises

Scapular Control	Humeral Control
Bent-over rowing	Prone horizontal abduction
Pushups with a plus (maximum shoulder protraction)	"Scaption"* medial rotation ("thumbs down")
Press-ups	"Scaption"* lateral rotation ("thumbs up")
Forward punch-outs	Prone extension
Scapular squeezes	Side-lying medial and lateral rotation
	Prone 90°/90° (90° abduction, 90° elbow flexion) lateral rotation

Abduction in the plane of the scapula.

demonstrate control in terms of strength, endurance, and movement direction before being allowed to progress into these ranges of motion. At this stage, proprioceptive neuromuscular facilitation (PNF) techniques using rhythmic stabilization, slow reversals, and contract-relax techniques may be used. For example, the diagonal movement pattern into flexion, abduction, and lateral rotation with elbow flexion or extension is particularly effective for anterior shoulder dislocations, although movement into full range is discouraged, especially if the athlete demonstrates any signs of apprehension. With further improvement and control, PNF patterns may be performed with tubing, working toward functional speeds.

Treatment progression is aimed at further restoration of range of motion (the range necessary to do the activity, not necessarily hypermobility), continued strengthening of the appropriate muscle or muscle groups (isokinetic, concentric, eccentric, closed-chain, open-chain), increasing the speed of movement activity to functional levels, improving control of shoulder mechanics, increasing endurance, and continuing to restore proprioceptive control.[104] Active and resisted exercises may include progressive resisted exercises with minimal weight at the beginning, working up to heavier weights or using various exercise devices such as Nautilus or isokinetic machines. Isokinetic devices can be used to decrease reciprocal innervation time between the agonist and antagonists. They are also useful in providing accommodating resistance through the full range of motion and for eccentric training (in some isokinetic devices).[101] To improve control of the glenohumeral joint, the clinician can begin to stress the accelerators (concentric movement) and the decelerators (eccentric movement) (Table 26–9). Research has shown that eccentric control in throwing activities is more important than concentric control, and if eccentric fatigue occurs, injury is more likely.[105] Tubing may be used if the resistance and speed of contraction are carefully controlled. It is important that the shoulder not be overloaded, and the athlete must understand that the exercises can be done only at the speed at which

control (smooth, coordinated movement) is demonstrated. If range of motion is a problem, pullies or a broomstick or T bar routine may be used to assist in increasing the range of motion by adding a large, controlled lever force.[106,107]

As the athlete progresses, closed-chain proprioceptive activities such as pushups (progressing from a wall to a table to the floor), weight shifting, rhythmic stabilization, shifting from a quadriped to a tripod position, ball rolling to cause sudden alterations in joint position, sitting pushups, Profitter exercises using the hands, use of an upper body exerciser (UBE) or similar cycling devices for the upper limb, hand balancing or using a balance board, hand stair-climbing, and hand treadmill walking may be used.[18,106,108–111] All of these activities are excellent at improving strength, endurance, and proprioception, but the clinician must always watch for pain, discomfort, and fatigue, which will result in the loss of humeral and scapular control at the shoulder, causing compensation patterns while doing these activities.

Open-chain activities using devices such as the Body Blade and activities such as plyometrics and use of a medicine ball are helpful in later stages of rehabilitation to teach functional stabilization and control.

If the problem is one of atraumatic instability, the rehabilitation process follows a similar path, ensuring especially that the exercises demonstrate activation of the appropriate muscle or muscle groups and that proper functional control is achieved. Throughout the process, the principles of specificity apply (Table 26–10). Stabilization is best achieved by isometric exercises for static stabilization and eccentric exercises for dynamic stabilization. For strengthening, there should initially be low repetitions with high-intensity contractions. Eccentric exercises to the scapular control muscles, humeral control muscles, and brachialis muscle help improve their strength and endurance for decelerating the arm and for shock absorption.[18,112] Closed-chain shoulder activities, which should be encouraged when the athlete has attained suitable strength and control, include the activities previously mentioned. These activities also help to improve proprioception and maintain or restore dynamic muscle balance and flexibility.[111] Open-chain activities may be begun early with high-repetition low weights, as long as the athlete can control the movement. Activities such as deadlifts, military presses, and shrugs with weights in the hands should be avoided because of the long lever stress on

TABLE 26–9
Accelerators and Decelerators of the Glenohumeral Joint

Accelerators (Concentric Activity)	Decelerators (Eccentric Activity)
Pectoralis major	Supraspinatus
Pectoralis minor	Infraspinatus
Latissimus dorsi	Teres minor
Teres major	Posterior fibers of deltoid
Anterior fibers of deltoid	Triceps

TABLE 26–10
Principles of Specificity (Related to Sport and Rehabilitation)

Each athletic event makes specific demands in terms of its load (stress), rate, repetitions, duration, and neurophysiologic adjustments. When a new or modified task with a different demand in intensity, load, rate, repetition, duration, or neurophysiologic demand is instituted, an entirely new pattern of adjustment must be acquired. Thus, training and rehabilitation must be specific to the sport or activity in which the athlete hopes to take part. This principle applies to:

1. Cardiovascular fitness (aerobic/anaerobic activity)
2. Strength (isometric, isotonic [concentric/eccentric], isokinetic)
3. Open- and closed-chain activities
4. Motor skills/motor learning
5. Flexibility (static, dynamic)
6. Coordination
7. Proprioceptive control
8. Timing/reaction time/movement time
9. Progression
10. Biomechanical demands
11. Tissue healing and stress

To achieve a progression in the above areas, the clinician moves from:

1. General to specific
2. Simple to complex
3. Easy to difficult
4. Lesser to greater volume
5. Lesser to greater intensity
6. Lesser to greater frequency

the shoulder, which causes undesirable sheer forces and lack of control.[113] In addition, sleeping in a supine position with the hand under the pillow, fixing hair, reaching into the back of a car from the front seat, leaning back on arms while sitting for long periods, and putting on a backpack should be discouraged. Advanced exercises involving high speed and high energy and high-speed functional pattern exercises include isokinetic, tubing, PNF pattern, and medicine ball and plyometric activities. It is important when doing activities to stress functional diagonal patterns used in the sporting activity. This may be done using free weights or tubing exercises.

If inferior instability is present, the supraspinatus and deltoid muscles must be given special attention. As with other shoulder routines, the athlete must build up to full effort gradually, and it is important that the athlete always work within control. For multidirectional instability, the rehabilitation program should feature control training rather than pure strengthening. Strengthening of the scapular control muscles and supraspinatus, infraspinatus, and teres minor should be stressed, along with all three parts of the deltoid and biceps.[114–116] Biofeedback adapted to functional patterns is useful in this instance. Attention to scapular control, followed by periscapular strengthening and then rotator cuff control, is essential. Thus, the training and rehabilitation

program becomes much more functionally based, with all activities done at the speed at which the athlete has complete control and demonstrates proper coordinated movement. Only when the athlete can demonstrate this control should the speed of the activity be increased. Thus, control and endurance become primary factors along with strength.

While the athlete's shoulder is being rehabilitated, the clinician must keep in mind that the athlete will at some point be returning to activity. Thus, a program to maintain or restore cardiovascular fitness, being as specific to the sport as possible, should be instituted. It does little good to rehabilitate the initial trauma and have the athlete medically cleared to participate when he or she does not have the other necessary attributes (cardiovascular fitness, game-level fitness) to compete (see Chapters 11 and 13).

TENDINITIS AND IMPINGEMENT SYNDROMES

Shoulder pain due to impingement and bursitis would seem to be easily distinguishable from that due to post-traumatic instability. Nevertheless, one of the major changes in thinking with regard to shoulder problems is the realization that there is a spectrum of both injury and pathology with these conditions. At one end is the repetitive overuse situation, with gradual attrition and irritation of the tendons and bursae around the shoulder (the pure overuse injury); at the other extreme is the significant injury that dislocates the shoulder (the pure traumatic type), which frequently goes on to become a recurrent dislocating joint. Similarly, the spectrum of collagenous laxity ranges from extreme tightness to abnormally loose, and thus the trauma or overuse required to generate dislocation or subluxation varies. Between these two extremes can often be found the mildly unstable shoulder, which leads to impingement under the coracoacromial arch and pain, frequently seen in athletes such as swimmers. Also fitting into this spectrum is the aging process, which is frequently manifested more in the soft tissue cuff around the joint than at the joint surface itself. Furthermore, internal derangement in the form of labral tears and attrition to rotator cuff muscles and the biceps tendon have begun to be frequently diagnosed with the more prevalent use of the arthroscope and the increasing availability of MRI and CT scanning. Thus, the previously simple distinct diagnostic categories have become blurred into a spectrum of injuries.

Subacromial impingement is a condition that implies rotator cuff abnormality and actual mechanical abuttment of the rotator cuff and subacromial bursa against the coracoacromial ligament and acromion resulting from the force overload to the rotator cuff and bursitis occurring during the abduction, forward flexion, and medial rotation cycle of shoulder movement.[50,117] Such a movement is seen in swimmers who commonly swim up to 14,000 m per day (see Chapter 16). It has been reported that impingement may also occur when the arm is forward flexed, medially rotated, and adducted within the coracohumeral space. This "coracoid impingement syndrome" occurs when the lesser tuberosity of the humerus encroaches on the coracoid process and has been reported in tennis players and a weight lifter.[118] With force overload, the humeral and scapular control muscles become fatigued, leading to greater overload and muscle weakness and muscle imbalance in the humeral force couples.[50,117] Abnormal shear stresses, subluxation, and compression then lead to impingement.

In the early clinical stages (stages 1 through 3 [see Chapter 3, Table 3–5]), the athlete will complain of aching only after activity, and range of motion is normal. Seldom does the clinician see the athlete at this stage. Education can play a role, however. If the athlete believes the problem is starting to come on, there are different preventive measures that can be instituted. Athletes may modify the activity. For example, swimmers may use a different stroke (breaststroke), do only the leg portion of the stroke, or alter their stroke (e.g., different hand entry, altered body roll) during the workout, even if they want to use the impinging strokes in competition. The use of assistive devices should be kept to a minimum. For example, hand paddle use can increase the stress on the shoulder musculature, and use of a flutter board held in front of the head when doing kicking strokes leaves the arm in the vulnerable abducted and neutral or medially rotated position. The athlete should be instructed to apply ice, especially after a workout, and take the shoulders through a full range of motion, slowly and in a controlled fashion, before and after a workout. Ideally, muscle strength should be tested regularly to watch for weakness of the scapular or humeral control muscles.

In the next stage (stage 4), the athlete will complain of discomfort and even pain during and after the activity. On examination, a positive impingement sign will be elicited, and palpation may demonstrate acromioclavicular joint tenderness. Pathologically, changes consist of thickening and fibrosis of the tendon, involvement of the subacromial bursa, and residual adhesions.

In the final stages (stages 5 and 6), the athlete complains of continuous pain over the supraspinatus and biceps tendons and tenderness over the coracoacromial ligament. A painful arc in the "empty can" position is demonstrated, and range of motion is restricted. Radiographs may demonstrate infra-acromial and infraclavicular spurs, bony sclerosis near the supraspinatus insertion, and subacromial erosion. Factors that can contribute to the condition are shown in Table 26–11.

To properly treat impingement syndromes in athletes, time must be taken to explain the problem, and the athlete must understand that the outcome will depend on his or her compliance with the instructions of the clinician. Primarily, the physician will prescribe rest, anti-inflammatory medication, pain-relieving medication, and, in the odd case, surgery.

In the initial part of treatment, the clinician may prescribe ice before and after practice and teach the resting positions of the shoulder (e.g., pillow hugging) (Fig. 26–12) for relief while at home. Rest, if recom-

TABLE 26–11
Factors Contributing to Impingement Syndrome

- Functional instability
- Amount of overhead movement (e.g., number of swimming strokes/day)
- Clearance available under coracoacromial arch
- Thickness of supraspinatus and biceps tendon
- Flexibility of supraspinatus and biceps muscles
- Flexibility of coracoacromial ligaments
- Overstretching
- Use of training devices (e.g., hand paddles, tubing)
- Muscle strength, endurance, and control
- Shape of acromion (e.g., hooked type acromion most commonly associated with impingement)

mended, implies decreased distance, intensity, and/or frequency of activity. In other words, *relative* rest, not *total* rest, from the activity is recommended. Pendular exercises, such as Codman pendular arm swing exercises in which the athlete bends forward at the waist so the body is at a 45- to 90-degree angle to the hips and holds onto a table or chair for support, may be used initially, provided the exercises are pain free. The arm may then be horizontally swung in a variety of planes. These exercises are very useful in the early stages to maintain range of motion. Other Codman exercises include vertical arm swing exercises in which the athlete assumes the same position as previously described and swings the arm back and forth or in a circular fashion by drawing a circle approximately 6 to 10 inches in diameter in both clockwise and counterclockwise directions.

Short arc exercises with abduction and forward flexion up to 90 degrees (below horizontal plane) are usually prescribed, especially in the initial treatment phase. Exercises should be done in lateral rotation to facilitate clearance of the greater tuberosity under the coracoacromial ligament.[28] Stretching into abduction and medial rotation should be avoided, as this is the impingement position. Extreme care must be given

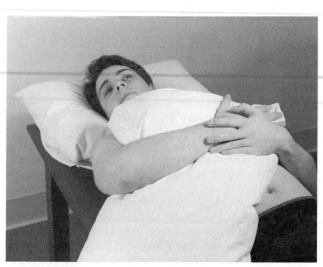

FIGURE 26–12. Pillow hugging: shoulder resting position.

when choosing the type of strengthening program to which the athlete is exposed, especially if the rotator cuff or biceps muscles are involved. Because the condition is an overuse one, further unsuitable exercises may aggravate the condition. If exercises are instituted, especially for the rotator cuff muscles, something should be taken out of the athlete's program to compensate. Tubing exercises, if done properly, are effective. In most cases, however, they should be kept to a minimum, because athletes do not do them correctly. To be performed correctly, tubing exercises should be done only at the speed at which the athlete has complete functional control of the activity. If functional control is lost, the stresses on the muscles, especially to the rotator cuff, may lead to increased irritation of the tendons.

In terms of strength about the shoulder, adduction should be the strongest, followed by extension, flexion, abduction, medial rotation, and lateral rotation. It is especially important to strengthen the medial humeral rotators (subscapularis, pectoralis major, latissimus dorsi, and scapular rotator muscles, especially the serratus anterior muscle), all of which show marked weakness when instability is demonstrated.[21] Thus, it is important to ensure scapular control and strength, if not before, then at least at the same time as humeral control exercises are being instituted (see Chapters 16 and 17).

Scapular control exercises are important, because these muscles maintain the normal relationship between the glenohumeral and scapulothoracic joints.[119] These muscles (see Table 26–6) provide a stable base for the arm, preserve deltoid fiber length so that acromiohumeral length is maintained, and lessen impingement of the rotator cuff.[18,49,64] Useful scapular control exercises include retraction and depression of the scapula, as well as elevation and protraction.[44,64] Scapular control exercises are given in Table 26–8.[101,120,121]

For the glenohumeral joint, humeral control exercises should be instituted for the rotator cuff and deltoid to prevent humeral head migration and to restore voluntary control of the humeral head through rotator cuff stabilization.[49] Humeral control exercises are shown in Table 26–8.[101,120,121] The humeral control strengthening exercises should initially concentrate on lateral rotation and the deltoid muscle, then move to the other humeral control muscles, and finally to medial rotation (subscapularis muscle). Controlled pullies or tubing may be used in the pain-free range of motion for forward flexion with the palm supinated, which causes lateral rotation of the humerus. Such movement in standing may provide gravity assistance to humeral depression.[122] Active assisted exercises using a T or an L bar are beneficial for range of motion.[44,123] Strengthening exercises will progress from isometric pain-free activity to isotonic pain-free activity. If the athlete has progressed sufficiently to be allowed to do weighted exercises, the weight should be strapped to the forearm, not held. If the weight is held, impingement is more likely to occur because of the additional muscle pull required to hang onto the weight. The weighted exercises that can be performed are shoulder shrugs to work the upper trapezius and pushups to work the serratus anterior,

provided it is not too irritable to the rotator cuff. As with shoulder instability, weights should be kept under 5 lb (2.3 kg).[102]

The clinician should keep in mind the specificity required by the athlete and include open and/or closed kinetic chain activities in the rehabilitation program. Closed-chain activities involve those activities in which the distal segment is fixed or holding on to an immovable object so fixation feedback is possible, thus providing better proprioception.[110] Chin-ups, dips, and many proprioceptive control activities (balance board) are considered closed-chain activities. Overuse injuries are less likely to occur during closed-chain activities. Closed-chain activities for the shoulder should be primarily eccentric to slow down the effects of gravity and inertia. These activities tend to compress the joint, increasing stability, and may be used in the reverse-origin insertion mode. For example, although the latissimus dorsi is viewed as an extensor and medial rotator of the shoulder, it may also be used as a trunk extensor. Open-chain activities simply refer to a moveable distal segment, as seen in grooming, eating, and swinging a racket or swimming. It is a concentric movement against gravity with no fixation feedback. Injury to the shoulder from overuse is most likely to occur during open-chain activities and is often the result of loss of functional control of the scapula and/or humerus.[110] Open-chain activities include free weight exercises and are often combined with proprioceptive activities (eyes open/closed) to teach free hand feedback.

Joint mobilization may be used, but the clinician must always keep in mind the possibility of hypermobility, which tends to be common in individuals with this complaint. If this is the case, the clinician must take time to determine which movements are hypomobile so that the joint play mobilization techniques to stretch the capsule can be much more effective.[123–127] Often, if the joint is hypermobile in one direction, it may be hypomobile in the opposite direction. For example, in throwing athletes, the posterior capsule tends to be tight and therefore requires mobilization, while the anterior capsule is hypermobile and requires protection. The clinician must also ensure that all joints of the shoulder complex have normal mobility. If there are signs of muscle hypomobility, the athlete may be encouraged to use muscle energy techniques, hold-relax techniques, or other types of muscle stretching. It is important to stress, however, that stretching should be done *only* in hypomobile directions. In most cases, the athletes tend to be hypermobile in most directions. Additional stretching techniques are not needed for these directions.

At the same time, the clinician, in conjunction with the coach, must work to correct mechanic faults in the athlete's technique. For example, in swimming, stroke modification aims to limit the extremes of abduction and medial rotation where the supraspinatus is most likely to impinge against the coracocromial ligament and the anterior leading edge of the acromion process. These stroke modifications should also limit the amount of time the arm spends in the adducted position to spare the wringing out of the "watershed" area of hypovascularity of the supraspinous tendon.[128] If the thumb or index finger enters the water first, there is greater medial rotation of the arm. Ideally, to prevent hypovascularity, at least during the rehabilitation process, the middle finger should enter the water first. Athletes should be taught that dropping the elbow during the recovery phase results in increased lateral rotation. As the arm comes out of the water, the athlete should attempt to get the hand in front of the elbow as soon as possible to lead with the hand. Ideally, athletes should be taught high elbow recovery leading with the hand, which again will decrease the period of hypovascularity to the rotator cuff muscles. Front crawl swimmers should be encouraged to shorten the stroke cadence by limiting follow-through. They should be taught to lean on the water-entering arm as so as to encourage body roll and keep the head up at arm entry. Breathing on alternate sides should be encouraged to increase roll. In some cases, a deltoid strap may be used.[129] The strap should fit as high up on the biceps as possible, close to the insertion of the deltoid muscle, and be snug enough to prevent slippage down the arm. It should feel tight only when the arm is in active use. Application of the band near the insertion of the tendons into the muscle may change the dynamics of the muscle orientation about the shoulder so that symptoms of impingement are mechanically decreased.

Because synchronization of the shoulder joints is important during normal athletic activities, the athlete must learn to work on neuromuscular functional control. Thus, any treatment program must show good muscle balance between the agonist and antagonist and also enable the athlete to work with properly controlled speed. It is important that this control be demonstrated at functional speed. Too often the clinician rehabilitates the athlete, only to the have the athlete return, complaining of problems when performing the activity in training or competition. Often the problem is due to lack of control at functional speeds. When referring to muscle balance in the humeral control muscles, there should be a good relationship between the medial and lateral rotators, between the flexors and extensors, and between the abductors and adductors. Isokinetic tests have shown that medial rotation–to–lateral rotation strength ratios should be approximately 3:2, extension-to-flexion strength ratios should be 5:4, and adduction-to-abduction strength ratios should be 2:1.[44,82,120]

PNF exercises for the upper limb are very good for teaching control and rhythmic stabilization in different parts of the range of motion through their diagonal patterns. The shoulder flexion, abduction, and lateral rotation pattern is especially useful for instability, although full range should not be attempted in those with an impingement syndrome.[44,49,113] The extension, adduction, and medial rotation pattern is good for abnormality occurring during the arm acceleration, arm deceleration, and follow-through phases of throwing by teaching control in these phases (see Chapter 17). Techniques such as slow reversals, contract-relax, rhythmic stabilization, and timing for emphasis are useful for treating instability by increasing awareness of

movement, stimulating appropriate irradiation from strong to weak muscles, and reinforcing weak patterns with strong patterns.[44,49,69] Tubing exercises using these patterns have also been found to be effective, provided they are done in a controlled fashion.

Plyometric programs for the upper limb are also useful in teaching functional control. Such programs should be designed to increase the excitability of the neurologic receptors and improve the reaction of the neuromuscular system.[49] It is important to teach the athlete to accept greater loads, remembering that, in this case, it is the rate of stretch rather than the length of stretch that is important.[130] Activities using a 2- to 4-lb ball (e.g., medicine ball or Plyoball), a bounce-back device (Plyoback) or a partner, or tubing (progressing from slow to fast sets) can be effective.[131]

ROTATOR CUFF INJURIES

Except for traumatic disruption, the rotator cuff muscles—supraspinatus, subscapularis, infraspinatus, and teres minor—are seldom the primary source of abnormality in the shoulder. These "caping" muscles are classified as humeral head movers acting in a short arc to maintain the position of the humeral head relative to the glenoid and to prevent excessive translation of the humeral head during shoulder movement.[114] Because of their location and function, however, they are prone to impingement, overuse, overload, and secondary weakness. In terms of muscle tearing itself (i.e., a 3-degree strain), the supraspinatus muscle is the most likely to be injured at the musculotendinous or the teno-osseous junction, not in the muscle belly itself.[132] Tears to the rotator cuff as a whole may be defined as partial-thickness tears and full-thickness tears from acute high-velocity trauma.[133] Aging can contribute significantly to these lesions because of intrinsic degenerative changes, such as osteophyte formation on the anteroinferior surface of the acromion, which lead to impingement syndromes; these changes may be associated with anterior dislocations in older individuals.[134] Generally, rotator cuff tears occur late in the shoulder deterioration process, after eccentric overload and secondary impingement, or in older individuals.[135] These injuries are being more frequently reported in younger throwing athletes (about 40 percent of those with shoulder abnormality); they rarely occur in normal healthy tissue, but they are sometimes associated with labial tears.[132,136–138] Microtrauma or repeated injury from the throwing motion can lead to decreased elasticity and tensile strength in the tendons of the rotator cuff, which may then be torn during the eccentric phase of throwing. Craven[132] called this phenomenon *athletically accelerated aging*. For this reason, the injury is sometimes referred to as *rotator cuff disease* and includes reversible tendon inflammation, irreversible tendon degeneration, partial- and full-thickness rotator cuff tears, and calcification.[133]

Rehabilitation will depend on the desired level of activity of the athlete and the athlete's motivation. Older patients tend to require more extensive rehabilitation. In addition, the size of the tear will influence the speed of recovery.[123] As treatment progresses, the clinician must ensure that the principles of specificity (see Table 26–10) are followed, as well as ensure proper technique and good endurance. It is important to remember that activation activity in the shoulder is a concentric movement, while stabilization is both static (isometric) and dynamic (primarily eccentric).[120]

Surgical repair of the rotator cuff may involve an open repair or a mini open repair using arthroscopy.[6,123] Arthroscopic debridement is possible for partial tears. Rehabilitation after an open repair is extensive. The athlete is given a sling for comfort, and isometric stabilization exercises are begun in the neutral position. These exercises may be accompanied by pain-relieving modalities. As with nonsurgical repair, activities can be progressed from assisted to active motion including such movements as elevation (to 90 degrees), lateral to medial rotation, T-bar activities (to assist movement and later to increase range of motion), and pendular exercises to the athlete's tolerance after 6 to 8 weeks. It may take up to 6 months before elevation above the horizontal is allowed. Once active movement has been accomplished with good coordinated movement, terminal stretching can be instituted, usually at about 3 months. Provided active movement is performed properly and the athlete demonstrates good coordinated control of the movement, resisted movements for humeral and scapular control can begin. The athlete must be warned that the rehabilitation process may take up to 2 years, and throwing can be instituted only when the athlete demonstrates good strength and mobility, a process that takes at least 12 months.[6,139]

The rehabilitation process after a mini repair follows the same process as for after open repair, but the time lines are shorter. Again, the clinician must spend a great deal of time ensuring that the athlete has good strength, endurance, coordination, and neuromuscular control of the scapular and humeral stabilizers.[123]

INJURIES TO THE SHOULDER IN THROWING

Several structures in the upper limb may be injured during the throwing motion (Table 26–12). In addition, there are several factors that contribute to shoulder injuries during the throwing motion. If the athlete opens up (i.e., rotates the body) too soon, it may lead to subacromial pain and bursal adhesions.[140] Opening up too rapidly or squaring the shoulders to the strike zone too soon causes the arm to lag behind the body, increasing the stress on the anterior shoulder and medial elbow. As the arm lags behind, the thrower rushes the arm forward to catch up; to do this, the elbow drops closer to the body, which is called "short-arming the ball" and places greater stress on the shoulder and elbow. The ball is then released early. Opening up too soon is caused by a short stride, the stride foot being too far to the opposite side of midline, the knee not being lifted high enough during windup, the pitcher trying to rush the delivery, or the pitcher starting to fatigue.[140,141]

If the pitcher opens up too late, it causes the arm to arrive at the release point before the shoulder. This is called "pitching with the arm" and also places too much stress on the shoulder. Opening up too late is due to foot stride being too far to the same side of midline, which results in the pelvis being unable to open up properly and so the body loses momentum.[140,141]

Other factors that may contribute to injuries in the shoulder are extending the glove arm, lifting the back leg from the ground too soon, and any anatomic abnormalities such as leg length discrepancy, scoliosis, or kyphosis.

Prior to beginning the pitching activity, the athlete must warm up, which may involve general stretching and massage activities. The warm-up should involve activities of stretching as well as neuromuscular activities to ensure timing and control. Exercises to improve mobility should be done without any throwing. The athlete should work up a sweat by using calisthenics before going to the pitching mound. The warm-up throws should begin at a distance shorter than that from the pitcher's mound to home plate, and the velocity of throws should begin with slow pitches, gradually increasing speed as the arm loosens up. Distance and speed are both increased gradually as the individual's arm warms up and good control is demonstrated. Curve balls and other specialty pitches should not be thrown until the arm has completely warmed up. An example of a pitching warm-up might be as follows: 30 balls at medium velocity, then ten fastballs, ten sliders, and ten curve balls, all of these with increasing speeds, for a maximum of about 80 pitches. Coleman et al.[142] developed a program for a simulated game to ensure the athlete is ready to go back to competition. They advocated a 15-minute warm-up throwing 50 to 80 pitches with increasing velocity. This is followed by five to eight sessions to simulate innings, interspersed with 9- to 10-minute rest periods throwing 12 to 18 pitches per session. The pitching selection is variable but should include six to ten fastballs per session. The clinician should remember that curve balls and sliders will add greater stress to the shoulder than fastballs. Brewster and Moynes Schwab[143] developed two programs: a seven-step program for pitchers and an eight-step program for catchers, infielders, and outfielders.

For any pitcher, the following principles should be followed: Ice should always be applied when the pitcher finishes throwing. The Specific Adaptation to Imposed Demand (SAID) technique should always be considered in any exercise routine the throwing athlete is given to do. The amount of force that the body or arm is subjected to should be increased gradually. It is important that the arm not be fatigued and that it be properly warmed up, including stretching, before beginning. Initially, the ball should only be tossed, not thrown. The athlete should be cautioned to ease off or stop if the arm becomes painful. It is important for the athlete to be able to differentiate between soreness and pain. If the soreness is in the muscle, one need not be as concerned as when the individual has pain in the tendons or in the joint areas, unless a muscle strain is

TABLE 26–12
Motion, Stress Site, and Injury Potential of Different Pitching Phases

Pitching Phase	Shoulder	Elbow	Forearm, Wrist, and Hand	Potential Injury Site
Windup/Stride	Flexion Lateral rotation	Flexion	Neutral	Rotator cuff Posterior capsule (shoulder) Biceps tendon Head of humerus Pectoralis major (insertion)
Arm cocking	Extension Lateral rotation Abduction	Flexion	Pronation	Medial rotators of shoulder Biceps tendon Triceps tendon Thoracic outlet syndrome (hyperabduction) Scapulothoracic bursa (inferior angle) Anterior capsule (shoulder) Medial epicondyle (elbow) Medial collateral ligament (elbow) Medial forearm compartment tendinitis Ulnar neuritis
Arm acceleration	Flexion	Extension	Supination	Anterior deltoid strain Pectoralis major strain Subscapularis strain (insertion) Latissimus dorsi strain (belly) Biceps tendinitis Biceps subluxation Rotator cuff impingement Humerus—spiral fracture Subacromial bursitis Medial collateral ligament (elbow) Elbow (medial epicondyle avulsion) Radiohumeral compression Forearm (flexor-pronator strain) Forearm (lateral compartment osteochondrosis)
Release and arm deceleration	Flexion Medial rotation Adduction	Extension	Pronation Wrist to neutral	Triceps tendinitis Rotator cuff Glenoid labrum Teres minor strain Glenohumeral subluxation (posterior) Triceps, ulna (traction spurs) Elbow (loose bodies) Fingertips (blisters)
Follow-through	Flexion Medial rotation Abduction	Extension	Pronation	Posterior capsule (shoulder) Triceps (insertion) Biceps strain Rotator cuff Glenoid labrum Scapulothoracic bursa (inferior angle) Brachialis strain Radiohumeral compression Olecranon process Pronator teres syndrome Forearm fascial compartment syndrome

suspected. The athlete must have full range of motion, or no throwing should be allowed. As the pitcher's development progresses, control should be the first thing that is developed. Once the athlete has control, then velocity can be considered, but the speed of throw should always be within the athlete's control ability. The athlete should progress from normal pitching to straight pitching to change-up, sinker, and cross-seam pitches. Breaking pitches (e.g., curves, sliders) should be the final types of pitches learned or attempted because of the increased stress they cause.

If the aim is to return the athlete to throwing sports after injury, the clinician must ensure that the throwing athlete has upper limb neuromuscular coordination strength and endurance, as well as normal range of motion and capsular flexibility. Thus, around the shoulder, the clinician must concentrate on the scapular and humeral control muscles. In addition, the clinician must ensure that all the joints work in a smooth, normal, coordinated movement and that they have been properly assessed. These include the glenohumeral, acromioclavicular, sternoclavicular, and scapulothoracic joints of the shoulder complex, as well as the spine, hips, knees, ankles, and feet.

FRACTURES OF THE SHOULDER GIRDLE AND HUMERUS

Fractures in the shoulder area are usually caused by a direct blow or FOOSH injury. To establish an accurate diagnosis and hence plan appropriate handling of fractures of the shoulder region, it is essential to have adequate radiologic films. The initial two films that should be ordered in this regard are an AP view of the shoulder region together with a transscapular lateral view (see Figs. 26–7 and 26–8). Depending on the location and visibility of the fracture lines, supplementary views of the scapula, clavicle, or shoulder may be taken. A CT scan is useful when the fracture is complex.

FRACTURES OF THE SCAPULA

The body of the scapula is heavily enclosed in muscles, which help control the shoulder and humerus, and thus is relatively protected from injury. Scapular fractures occur as a result of a direct blow or fall, and the important point with these fractures is to rule out underlying pulmonary injury (e.g., a collapsed lung, pneumothorax, or hemothorax) resulting from a possible accompanying rib fracture. Most scapular fractures heal with symptomatic treatment only and rarely give difficulty, as the bone fragments are well stabilized by the surrounding musculature.

Fractures in the region of the neck of the scapula and glenoid region, as well as fractures of the coracoid, are at some risk for injuring the neurovascular structures that pass in proximity through the thoracic outlet. The brachial plexus or associated nerve roots in particular may be injured with fractures to this region.

Rarely, the acromion or coracoid may be avulsed. If avulsion does occur, pinning or open reduction may be necessary to stabilize the fracture. In the younger athlete, the coracoid and acromial processes have secondary ossification centers that may be mistaken for fractures. Radiographs of the opposite side often help to solve this dilemma.

Intra-articular fractures of the glenoid may require open reduction if they involve enough of the joint to affect shoulder stability or mobility or if they are displaced sufficiently to increase the potential for degenerative changes in the joint. These fractures will also require more extensive therapy because of the potential for weakness and hypomobility resulting from the immobilization required after surgery, although the same principles apply as outlined in the section on dislocations and subluxations. Because hypomobility is of primary concern, the clinician should devote more time to joint play mobilization techniques.[124–127]

FRACTURES OF THE CLAVICLE

The clavicle is one of the most commonly fractured bones in children and adolescents; usually the mechanism of injury is a fall onto the shoulder, but occasionally these fractures may occur from a direct blow. The shoulder is driven downward, but the clavicle impinges on the underlying first rib and cannot continue its descent unless it fractures. The usual site of the fracture is between the medial two thirds and the lateral one third of the bone (80 percent of clavicular fractures).[31] Clavicular fractures may be classified into fractures of the proximal, middle, or distal portions of the bone. One must be aware that the brachial plexus lies not far away, and there is always the potential for injury to this structure. Open injuries may also occur, because the bone is very subcutaneous. Displacement of the clavicle often is minimal owing to the underlying subclavius muscle.

Fortunately, the clavicle demonstrates excellent healing properties, and the usual treatment is symptomatic support in a figure-of-eight bandage and/or sling and swath. Occasionally a simple supporting sling is sufficient if displacement has not occurred.

Open reduction of these fractures is very rarely indicated. Indications for open reduction include compound fracture, neurovascular compromise, or the occasional situation in which the proximal fragment becomes "buttonholed" in the trapezius or subcutaneous tissue.[31]

The clavicle usually heals with exuberant callus, and it is important to warn both the parents and the athlete that the healing may result in a very obvious bump because the bone lies subcutaneously. This bump tends to remodel to some degree over a period of years but may never completely disappear. Normal healing time varies from 6 weeks in young children to 8 weeks in adults. The area is tender and may need protection from heavy contact and stress for an additional 2 to 4 weeks.

Fractures at the extreme proximal end of the clavicle are often diagnosed as dislocations, but in the younger individual these may represent epiphyseal injuries. Thus, in growing individuals, epiphyseal fractures in this region should always be considered. The sternoclavicular epiphysis may remain open until the age of 25. Although these fractures may cause a prominent bump anteriorly, open reduction in this region is rather hazardous and is best avoided whenever possible.

PROXIMAL HUMERAL FRACTURES

The proximal humerus is a common site of injury in the young as well as in the elderly. In the skeletally immature athlete, the fracture frequently represents an epiphyseal fracture at the proximal humeral growth plate ("Little Leaguer's shoulder") and is most often associated with throwing sports. In the elderly, these fractures are usually through osteopenic bone and may occur with minimal trauma, or occasionally in association with dislocation.

There are many muscles in this region that can have a deforming force on the fracture, depending on where it has occurred. The rotator cuff muscles (supraspinatus, infraspinatus, and teres minor), which insert on the greater tuberosity, tend to abduct and laterally rotate the head fragment. Avulsion of the greater tuberosity by the supraspinatus is a common fracture in skiers of all ages. A fracture of the humeral head in which the fragment involves the lesser tuberosity but not the greater tuberosity will result in the subscapularis muscle tending to displace the fragment medially.

The clinician should again be reminded of how close the neurovascular structures are in this region and must always be aware of possible injury to the axillary artery or brachial plexus.

A useful system for classifying humeral head and neck fractures is Neer's four-part classification.[31,144] In this classification system, proximal humeral fractures are divided into displaced and nondisplaced. Neer defines displaced fractures as those in which there is more than 1 cm of displacement or more than 45 degrees of angulation. Nondisplaced fractures by these criteria may be termed one-part fractures, regardless of how many fracture lines are seen. A two-part fracture refers to displacement of the anatomic neck, surgical neck, lesser tuberosity, or greater tuberosity in relation to the remaining intact proximal humerus. Similarly, three- and four-part fractures refer to displacement of two or three fragments in relation to the main humeral fragment. Using this classification, the most common fracture in this region is a fracture involving the surgical neck, which may be displaced or nondisplaced (one-part or two-part fractures).[144] These injuries are particularly common in those over 60 years of age and occur as a result of either a fall on the outstretched hand or secondary to a lateral blow, such as a fall on the affected side.

With the fall on the outstretched arm, the shoulder and limb remain medially rotated. Normally, to accomplish full abduction, the humerus must laterally rotate. If lateral rotation is blocked, as in a fall, then the proximal humerus becomes impinged against the acromion. In young people, this impinging may result in a dislocation of the shoulder. In older people, a fracture of the proximal humerus is more common. If the fracture is displaced, there is a tendency for the shaft to migrate anteriorly and into an adducted position, secondary to the pull of the pectoralis major, while the head fragment becomes abducted, laterally rotated, and posterior to the shaft, secondary to the pull of the rotator cuff. Eighty percent of these fractures, however, are minimally displaced.

The most common medical treatment for these fractures is either a conventional sling or, preferably, a collar-and-cuff sling with the arm slightly adducted for comfort. The collar-and-cuff sling allows the weight of the arm to apply slight traction to the fracture. A swath about the chest may be used for stabilization and comfort, particularly for the first few weeks.

There is a tendency for the glenohumeral joint to stiffen very quickly after such injuries if the joint is not moved within the first 2 to 3 weeks of injury after the initial pain subsides. Good range of motion must be restored first, followed by active exercises and strengthening. It is essential with these fractures not to keep the limb immobilized for a prolonged period of time and to begin careful controlled motion (progressing from passive movement to active assisted to active movement), especially below shoulder height, as soon as possible. Carefully applied joint play mobilization techniques may also facilitate the return to full range of motion.[125–127]

With displaced fractures, traction is occasionally helpful in younger people, and open reduction and internal fixation may become necessary. The indications, however, are somewhat limited, as the shoulder has a wide range of motion, and thus a fair amount of angulation may be compatible with good function. Because most of these fractures tend to occur through osteoporotic bone in the elderly, there are many problems associated with internal fixation.

LITTLE LEAGUER'S SHOULDER

Little Leaguer's shoulder is an injury to the proximal growth plate of the humerus caused by a powerful medial rotation and adduction traction force on the proximal humeral epiphysis.[145] Such an injury occurs during the deceleration and follow-through phases of throwing or pitching (see Chapter 17). In addition, the rotational forces occurring during the arm-cocking and arm-acceleration phases can add to the problem. The result is a fatigue fracture, usually a Salter-Harris type I or II.[146] Radiologic signs, which may take up to 4 to 6 weeks to become evident, include widening of the epiphyseal plate, demineralization and rarefaction on the metaphyseal side of the physis, and metaphyseal bone separation. The athlete complains of acute shoulder pain when attempting to throw hard, which, if ignored, may result in an acute displacement of the weakened physis. Rest is the initial and primary treatment, and the bone may require up to 8 to 12 months to reossify and remodel. The athlete must have a full understanding of the problem and why absolute rest, at least initially, is essential. Therapy may include activities to improve strength, coordination, proprioception, endurance, and range of motion. The clinician should use the SAID principle when treating this condition and should ensure that although stress is applied to the injured area, the injury is never overloaded. Table 26–13 illustrates some of the preventive measures that may be used to decrease the chance of this injury occurring.

TABLE 26–13
Prevention of Little Leaguer's Shoulder

- Youngsters should be discouraged from pitching at home during and after the season
- Curve balls, sliders, and other breaking balls should be restricted or abolished
- Playing season should be shortened
- Pitchers should be restricted to 2 innings/game until the epiphysis closes
- Allow 3 to 4 days' rest between pitching days
- Ensure proper conditioning and warm-up
- Instruct pitcher in proper body mechanics
- Educate coaches and parents

FRACTURES OF THE GREATER TUBEROSITY

The majority of fractures of the greater tuberosity of the humerus are secondary to avulsions of the rotator cuff after glenohumeral dislocation. Displacement of the fragment by more than 1 cm implies an avulsion of the rotator cuff, and usually open reduction with internal fixation is recommended, not only to place the rotator cuff in a proper position for healing, but also to prevent later impingement.

FRACTURES OF THE LESSER TUBEROSITY

Fractures of the lesser tuberosity of the humerus are unusual injuries when seen in isolation. Normally they are seen after posterior dislocation of the glenohumeral joint, itself a rare injury in athletes, but they may also be associated with fractures of the neck of the humerus or occur after a seizure owing to muscle spasm. Again, this fracture represents an avulsion of the subscapular portion of the rotator cuff. Open reduction is necessary only if fragment displacement is severe. Only symptomatic treatment for pain and range of motion is necessary.

FRACTURES OF THE ANATOMIC NECK

Fractures of the anatomic neck of the humerus are rare injuries in isolation in athletics. The mechanism of injury is the same as for a dislocation (FOOSH injury), and in the young athlete, the ligaments and capsule tend to "give," resulting in a dislocation before the fracture occurs.[31] They are of great clinical importance, however, as there are no soft tissue attachments to the neck portion of the humerus. The blood supply to this region comes through the soft tissue attachments at the greater tuberosity and the lesser tuberosity. Thus, fractures in this location frequently develop late avascular necrosis, which may necessitate prosthetic replacement.

Neer's one- and two-part fractures around the proximal humerus have most often been described.[144] Three- and four-part fractures, in reality, represent permutations and combinations of these fractures and are seldom seen in sports except those involving very high impact forces (e.g., auto racing, skiing, equestrian events). Three-part fractures, particularly those involving the greater tuberosity, frequently require open reduction and internal fixation. Four-part fractures normally result in avascular necrosis of the humeral head, as all soft tissue attachments that supply blood to this region are stripped away from the head fragment. Early prosthetic replacement and mobilization are recommended for optimal results. These injuries, however, are severe, and because of the associated soft tissue problems in this region, a stiff shoulder frequently results, regardless of the treatment given.

In this region, fractures combined with dislocations may also occur. Thus, radiographs should always accompany dislocations to rule out the possibility of fractures. Patients with these severe injuries quite often develop complications, both early and late. Early complications include brachial plexus injury and/or vascular injury. Late complications include shoulder stiffness, malunion, nonunion, avascular necrosis, and myositis ossificans.

With any injury in the region of the humeral neck, transient lack of tone of the surrounding shoulder girdle musculature may occur. The initial radiographic appearance may then suggest an inferior dislocation or subluxation. If an axillary view or trans-scapular view is taken, however, it is obvious that the humeral head has remained in the joint. This transient inferior subluxation reverts to normal in a few weeks after the surrounding shoulder musculature returns to its normal tone.

HUMERAL SHAFT FRACTURES

The mechanisms of injury for humeral shaft fractures include direct forces (falls, crush injuries, projectiles), direct injuries (fall on the outstretched hand, twisting injuries, and stress fractures), and pathologic fractures. The shaft may be divided into proximal, mid- and distal portions. It is essential to always remember surrounding soft tissues, and a neurovascular examination should be performed with care to check for possible complications.

Most fractures of the humeral shaft can be handled by conservative means, the most common of which is the hanging cast. The ideal situation for a hanging cast is a displaced shortening fracture, either comminuted or oblique, in the mid- to distal humerus. The hanging cast is a lightweight plaster cast (no more than about two 4-inch rolls of plaster) that is applied from just above the fracture site down to the hand with the elbow at 90 degrees. A loop is placed at or just proximal to the wrist region, and its placement on either the dorsal or volar side of the wrist helps control varus and valgus angulation, while the height of the suspending collar and cuff helps control angulation in the anteroposterior plane. Basically, the system works by using gravity-assisted traction. However, it is essential that gravity be at work at all times; otherwise, deformity will occur. Thus, for the first few weeks until the fracture has some early consolidation, it is necessary for the individual to sleep in an upright position (i.e., in a recliner rocker). Until some early healing occurs, fracture position should be checked on a weekly basis. In the mid-shaft region, physicians will certainly accept shortening of up to nearly 1 inch, with 20 to 30 degrees of varus and approximately 20 degrees angulation in the anteroposterior plane.

A second method of handling fractures of the humeral shaft is with the use of a sugar-tong splint, which is essentially a plaster slab that runs from under the axilla down the medial aspect of the arm, under the elbow and up over the lateral aspect of the humerus, and over the top of the shoulder. As the plaster is setting, the arm is manipulated to reduce the fracture, and then a tensor bandage or gauze is wrapped around the arm to maintain reduction. This system has the advantage that the athlete can lie down with this particular type of a splint. However, adjustments are impossible to make once the cast is set, and thus if reduction is not adequate, the splint must be removed and reduction tried again.

Frequently open reduction is necessary for fractures of the humeral shaft. Indications for open reduction include compound injuries, irreducible injuries, pathologic fractures, vascular injury accompanying fracture of the shaft (occasionally with neurologic injuries), and multitrauma. The advantage of open reduction is early movement and mobilization of the upper limb. Internal fixation may be performed by means of either compression plating or intramedullary nail or rod. However, rotation is often hard to control with intramedullary devices.

While the fracture is healing, it is important to begin rehabilitation of the surrounding joints of the upper limb. The athlete should be instructed in pendular exercises for the shoulder, as well as range-of-motion exercises for the hand and elbow if possible; thus stiffness in all joints in the upper limb is minimized during healing.

Complications of humeral shaft fractures include neurologic injury, vascular injury, nonunion, pathologic fracture, and malunion. The most common neurologic complication is radial nerve palsy (10 to 20 percent).[147] This injury is usually secondary to a fracture in the distal one third of the humerus. Here the radial nerve is injured during the fracture or becomes entrapped in the fracture as it winds around the posterior aspect of the humerus along the radial groove of the humerus at mid-shaft and through the lateral intermuscular septum in the distal one third. Most of these injuries to the radial nerve are injuries of continuity (that is, contusion), and thus simple observation is in order. To assess neurologic injury, the clinician should test thumb opposition for normal function of the median nerve: holding the fingers, have the patient spread them against resistance to test the ulnar nerve; then have the patient extend the first metacarpophalangeal joint against resistance to test normal radial nerve function. Appropriate tests for the sensory distribution of each of these nerves should also be performed. Nerves tend to regenerate at about 1 mm/day (1 inch/month), and thus, the clinician can have some idea of how long it should take the nerve to recover by measuring the distance from the fracture to the next muscle innervated by that nerve. Electromyography (EMG) and nerve conduction studies are often performed, particularly 3 to 6 weeks after injury, and are useful for following progress with this problem. While awaiting the return of, for example, radial nerve function, it is important to maintain range of motion in the hand and wrist region. This area should also be dynamically splinted to prevent contracture and prolonged stretch of the extensor muscles.

Exploration of the radial nerve is recommended with compound fractures, as well as with failure of the nerve to show return of function after a reasonable length of time has passed. Exploration should also be done when radial nerve palsy appears after manipulation to reduce the fracture. In this particular situation, there is a high incidence of nerve entrapment in the fracture fragments.

Nonunion in the humeral shaft is usually secondary either to distraction of the fragments (i.e., overdistraction with a heavy cast) or to muscle interposition.

NERVE INJURIES

Most nerve injuries that occur in sport are transient in nature; these are termed *neurapraxia*. Nevertheless, several upper limb nerve injuries are indicative of a more serious injury, or *axonotmesis*. Transection of a nerve *(neurotmesis)* rarely occurs in athletics.

The etiology of most nerve injuries in sport is an acute episode of traction or a direct blow, crushing the nerve against underlying bony structures. More rarely, repetitive minor crushing, traction, or pressure results in dysesthesia or paralysis. For this reason, excellent functional recovery is usually anticipated in sports, and surgical exploration is rarely needed. However, the athlete must be advised that healing or full recovery will often take a long time. If an axonotmesis has occurred, degeneration will continue for 2 to 3 weeks, followed by slow regeneration. For an axonotmesis or neurotmesis, the best chance of recovery is 80 percent, but for a neurapraxia, 100 percent recovery can be expected. For information specific to the healing and resolution of nerve injuries, the reader is referred to Chapter 23.

THORACIC OUTLET SYNDROME

Thoracic outlet or inlet syndrome, also known as neurovascular compression syndrome , is a complex of signs and symptoms that result from compression of the neurovascular bundle as it emerges from the thorax and enters the upper limb. Depending on the site of compression and the structure involved, there are a variety of clinical manifestations. The presentation may be confusing, and the complaints and physical findings are often vague. Indeed, there is debate as to the existence of such a syndrome; and as a result, the attitude of the clinician dictates whether this syndrome is diagnosed with regularity or not at all.[148]

The narrow confines of the thoracic outlet may be considered the space (i.e., the costoclavicular space) between the relatively fixed immobile thorax, particularly the first rib and the clavicle (see Chapter 23). Traditionally, this space is extended to include the triangle between the anterior and middle scalene muscles, which border the nerve roots and trunks of the brachial plexus, en route to the upper limb, within the axillary sheath (anterior scalene syndrome and cervical rib syndrome) and where they pass beneath the lesser pectoral tendon and coracoid process (hyperabduction syndrome).[27]

During normal development of the human shoulder girdle, the scapula descends from a relatively high position at birth to a lower one during adolescence and maturation. These relationships are affected by hypertrophy or atrophy of muscles and chronic postural positions. Thus, as the configuration of this area changes throughout life, the possibility of a dynamic pathogenesis must be considered. Any factor that increases the angulation of the neurovascular structures can lead to symptoms. For example, abducting the arm to 180 degrees; pulling the shoulders down and back (e.g., wearing a heavy backpack); or muscle swelling from trauma, exercise, or hypertrophy may initiate the syndrome. Muscle weakness, trauma (e.g., fractured clavicle), arteriosclerosis, abnormal anatomy, and poor posture may all contribute as well.

Many problems in the thoracic outlet are congenital rather than acquired, but they occur within a dynamic state of changing relationships; thus, true thoracic outlet compression is rarely found before puberty. The scapula tends to descend more in females than males, which may partly explain the greater incidence of thoracic outlet syndrome in women. With increasing age and changing shoulder posture, particularly in association with excessive body weight and large breasts, the problem often becomes more manifest. It is worthwhile recalling that the suspension of the mobile scapula is entirely muscular in nature. The rhomboids and levator scapulae are particularly important to the possible pathogenesis of this problem, as well as when considering treatment. Direct and indirect trauma; a single blow; or repetitive, excessive use of the upper limb may trigger this syndrome. Furthermore, in the young athlete, it is often the particularly heavily muscled individual, with high trapezius and neck development, who runs the highest probability of developing this syndrome.

The first potential site of compression is within the interscalene interval (triangle) between the anterior scalene muscle anteriorly and the medial scalene posteriorly. Both muscles are attached to the first rib and serve as a framework for the brachial plexus. This triangle can be compromised by accessory muscles, hypertrophy of the existing muscles, the presence of a cervical rib, or fibrous bands. Accessory ribs are found in approximately 0.5 percent of the general population.[149]

The second major site of potential compression is between the mobile clavicle and the relatively fixed first rib. Fractures of the clavicle that produce large callus, congenitally bifid clavicles, a changing posture, a postfixed plexus, or a thickened, tight clavipectoral fascia may compromise this space by decreasing the area available for the neuromuscular bundle to pass through.

The third potential area of compression for the neurovascular structures is in the subcoracoid region adjacent to the pectoralis minor. Here the thickened clavipectoral fascia, often called the costocoracoid membrane, forms a dense line of fascia. With full circumduction of the arm, the coracoid process almost forms a fulcrum under which the subclavian vessels and the neurovascular structures must pass, increasing the path along which the bundle must move.

There are two major components to the syndrome, the first relating to problems with the major vessels and the second to pressure on the nerves. If thrombosis of the subclavian artery or vein is present, it is a clearly defined entity that is easily confirmed and usually presents with dramatic clinical signs (stiffness, especially in the hand; swelling in the hand; glossy appearance to the skin; coldness). There is usually no speculation regarding this problem. By contrast, the neural signs and symptoms (aching pain, pins-and-needles sensation, muscle atrophy) are more difficult to

pin down, even with sophisticated electrophysiologic tests, and are sometimes confused with cervical root problems.

Because of the various potential anatomic areas of compression and the variety of structures that can be involved, the clinical manifestations can be inconsistent in nature. The most common clear presenting symptom of thoracic outlet syndrome arises from compression of the lower trunk of the brachial plexus. The pain extends from the root of the neck to the shoulder and down the arm in a diffuse fashion. It may be accompanied by paresthesia involving the medial aspect of the hand, particularly the little finger and ring finger, or it may involve the entire medial aspect of the arm, particularly from the shoulder to the elbow. Less commonly, patients complain of weakness of the affected hand, and there may be detectable wasting.[1] Tennis or baseball players may experience difficulty gripping the racket or bat. Occasionally there is only painless intrinsic atrophy of the hand. Ultimately, the entire hand may be involved, but involvement usually starts on the ulnar side. Some athletes complain mainly of neck and shoulder pain, with vague discomfort extending into the trapezius and suboccipital region, which they may describe as a headache type sensation. During the history, it is important to determine whether the athlete relates the symptoms of upper limb motion in the arc in which the nerves are either stretched or compressed. Adopting the posture that either narrows the costoclavicular interval or allows compression of the underlying structures should reproduce the symptoms. Numbness and tingling in the hand with overhead movements must be distinguished from that occurring with shoulder instability, in which rapid movements are involved. Some athletes complain of nocturnal paresthesia, waking to find that they have slept with their arms in an overhead position.

Symptoms of arterial compression due to thoracic outlet syndrome are usually related to numbness of the entire arm, with rapid fatigue occurring during overhead exercises. These symptoms may be an isolated finding or may occur in association with some neural symptoms. When there is significant arterial compression, the hand may be obviously cool and pale compared with the contralateral side when both are held above the head. In addition, the radial pulse may disappear, only to return when the arm is replaced at the side. However, this phenomenon is frequently seen in the general population, and therefore, great care should be taken when drawing any conclusions from a weakening or a disappearing pulse with the arms above the level of the shoulder. Rarely, there are signs of acute arterial insufficiency with major vascular compromise to the hand or even the entire limb. Specific diagnostic tests for thoracic outlet should be performed. These include the Roos test, the Adson maneuver, and Halsted maneuver and are described in detail elsewhere.[27]

When venous compression in the thoracic outlet is the presenting problem, the athlete may present with a swollen, discolored limb several hours after a bout of intense exercise.[150] In the general population, unaccustomed activity, such as a project requiring overhead activity, may cause the problem, but with the athlete, it is usually a sudden change in exercise pattern, either different activity or an intense increase in volume of a specific overhead movement. Occasionally this obvious swelling and color change disappears over several hours so that by the time the athlete is examined by the clinician, there is little to see; thus, a careful history is important. When venous compromise is sufficiently severe or there is also occlusion of the subclavian vein, a visible venous collateral pattern may become evident across the athlete's shoulder, chest, and ipsilateral breast.

Inasmuch as the diagnosis of thoracic outlet compression is usually one of exclusion, an initial screening examination is mandatory, and differential diagnosis assumes significance. A detailed history is needed, and it is essential to evaluate the cervical spine, shoulder, elbow, and hand for evidence of neural compression. It is mandatory to differentiate this syndrome from the classic ulnar and median nerve compression syndromes and cervical radicular signs. Instability of the shoulder should be ruled out and the posture evaluated. A cervical spinal abnormality is the most common cause of paresthesia in the upper limb, and efforts should be made to distinguish radicular pain in the C8 and T1 distributions. Most disc diseases affect the C5–C6 level and, to a somewhat lesser extent, the C7 level. Thus, paresthesia in the ulnar side of the hand is more likely to be of distal origin. Any space occupying lesion within the thoracic outlet, particularly a Pancoast tumor at the apex of the lungs, can mimic the symptoms of thoracic outlet syndrome. Although the pursuit of health and fitness is not compatible with smoking, a large number of athletes smoke on a regular basis. The incidence of lung cancer parallels this habit, and so middle-aged and elderly athletes are not immune from lung tumors.

Peripheral entrapment of the ulnar nerve at the elbow and in the cubital tunnel, or in the hand in Guyon's canal, can produce typical dysesthesia in the ring and little fingers. Similarly, compression of the median nerve and the carpal tunnel may produce paresthesia in the distribution of that nerve, typically in the thumb and index and middle fingers, with wasting of the hyperthenar eminence. In a previously reported series of cervical rib resections for thoracic outlet syndrome, a large percentage of individuals subsequently required release of the ulnar or medial nerve peripherally.[1] It has been postulated that a double-crush syndrome, with irritation at a subclinical level at both sites, can combine to produce a significant clinical entity.[151,152] The clinician should remain pragmatic, however, and assume that in at least some of these instances, an incorrect diagnosis has been made.

Like thoracic outlet syndrome, reflex sympathetic dystrophy presents a constellation of peripheral symptoms, including dysesthesias, hypersensitivity, and muscle wasting. The key to diagnosing reflex sympathetic dystrophy is awareness of its possibility. A key feature is the disassociation among the sensations of touch, pressure, and pain. It is particularly difficult to distinguish the two syndromes if there is appreciable swelling within the hand. The presence of a "hot" bone scan, seen in reflex sympathetic dystrophy, helps to differentiate the two conditions.

Plain cervical spinal roentgenograms may help to rule out certain intrinsic conditions (e.g., cervical spondylosis, narrowed intervertebral discs, and osteophytic impingement). The presence of a cervical rib or long C7 transverse process may fit in with the findings of thoracic outlet compression. All athletes should undergo adequate studies of the apex of the lung on the affected side.

There is a discrepancy of opinion regarding the value of electrodiagnostic studies for this condition.[153] There is considerable difficulty in accurately determining the nerve conduction velocity through the thoracic outlet. In many ways, the biggest value of electrodiagnostic studies is to rule out peripheral entrapment (e.g., ulnar neuropathy at the elbow or hand or carpal tunnel syndrome of the median nerve at the wrist).

If there is significant evidence of arterial venous involvement suggesting thrombosis, aneurysm, or compression, it may be prudent to perform Doppler, angiographic, or venographic studies.

With the exception of athletes who present with an impending vascular catastrophe, the initial thrust of treatment for thoracic outlet syndrome should be nonoperative. Thorough assessment of muscle strength and posture leads to establishment of an adequate retraining program for the muscles of the scapula, shoulder girdle, and cervical spine. In females with large breasts, the purchase of an appropriate sporting bra is part of the treatment program. In situations where there has been a sudden change in activity pattern, treatment with anti-inflammatory medication, further corrected modification of activity, thorough investigation into past exercise habits, and a proposed direction of future training plans should be carefully determined.

When nonoperative treatment has failed and the diagnosis is firmly established, consideration of operative treatment is appropriate. The first rib resection is the usual, most effective treatment, as it deals with both the supraclavicular and the infraclavicular etiologic factors in this syndrome. The surgery may well be achieved through an axillary approach, as described by Roos in 1979, and allows fairly rapid resumption of physical activity.[154] Complications of this surgery include pneumothorax and occasional transient damage to the long thoracic nerve, with resulting winging of the scapula. Return to full activity should follow (1) an adequate rehabilitation program designed to provide full strengthening of the shoulder girdle muscles and re-establish the range of motion of the shoulder and (2) a plan of exercise progression for the ensuing season.

TUMORS

The proximal humerus is a relatively common site of bone tumors. Whenever a painful soft tissue lesion is not responding in the traditional fashion, repeat roentgenograms are advised, as many cases of bone tumor to the shoulder present as pain and are initially diagnosed as capsulitis, bursitis, or muscle injury.[1]

Simple bone cysts (a benign tumor) are common in the proximal humerus and probably represent an area of altered growth-plate activity. They are seen as a lytic lesion on plain films and are usually fluid-filled cysts (Fig. 26–13). Treatment depends on their size and the activity level of the patient. The decision to operate depends on the certainty of the diagnosis based on the classic appearance on the roentgenogram and the degree of potential mechanical weakening due to the size of the lesion. Stress fractures through these lesions are common.

Chondroblastomas are rare primary, usually benign, bone tumors of immature cartilage cell derivation (Fig. 26–14). Chondroblastomas comprise less than 1 percent of all primary bone tumors. Codman's description in 1931 pointed out the affinity of these tumors for the shoulder, and therefore this tumor has subsequently been referred to as a Codman tumor. However, the most frequent site is around the knee, followed by the pelvis, and then the shoulder region.[155] The peak age at onset is between 10 and 30 years. These lesions form within the epiphyseal area of long bones, with occasional metastatic expansion to adjacent areas. Radiographically, they appear as a more or less lytic, round or oval area of bone destruction. Histologically, they are locally aggressive. They tend to recur and, in rare cases, metastasize. The location of the lesion brings up a differential diagnosis of giant cell tumor and even aneurysmal bone cysts. Thus, biopsy is frequently mandatory.

The shoulder can be a site of malignant tumors such as an osteosarcoma or Ewing tumor, but by far the greatest number of malignant lesions are secondary, particularly from carcinoma of the breast. Thus, in the young and middle-aged female athlete presenting with a lytic lesion in the proximal humerus or shoulder, the possibility that it may be a secondary lesion must always be entertained, and even prior to biopsy, a search must be made for a primary source.

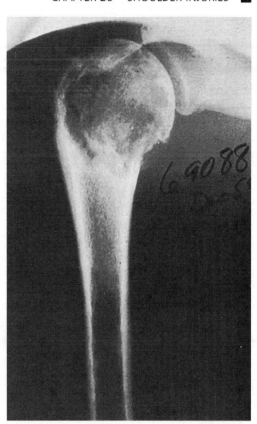

FIGURE 26–14. Chondroblastoma in the humerus. (From Bogumill GP, Schwamm HA: Orthopedic Pathology. Philadelphia, WB Saunders, 1984, p 445.)

CONCLUSION

The shoulder presents an interesting contrast of injuries, from relatively benign to life threatening. The majority of these injuries in athletics are due to overuse or trauma. Because of its relative proximity to the cervical spine, the clinician must always be aware of possible referral of symptoms. Because the shoulder is the proximal attachment of the arm, an extremity of great use in sport, the clinician must assess and treat carefully and ensure that the athlete is fully rehabilitated to return to full athletic activity.

REFERENCES

1. Reid DC: Sports Injury—Assessment and Rehabilitation. New York, Churchill Livingstone, 1992.
2. Reid DC: The shoulder girdle: Its structure and function as a unit in abduction. J Chart Soc Physiother 1969; 55:57–59.
3. Neer CS: Impingement lesions. Clin Orthop 1983; 173:70–77.
4. Burkhead W, Rockwood C: Treatment of instability of the shoulder with an exercise program. J Bone Joint Surg 1992; 70A:890–896.
5. Tehvanzadeh J, Ken R, Amster J: Magnetic resonance imaging of tendon and ligament abnormalities. Part I. Spine and upper extremities. Skeletal Radiol 1992; 21:1–5.
6. Kunkel SS, Hawkins RJ: Open repair of the rotator cuff. In Andrews JR, Wilk KE (eds): The Athlete's Shoulder. New York, Churchill Livingstone, 1994.

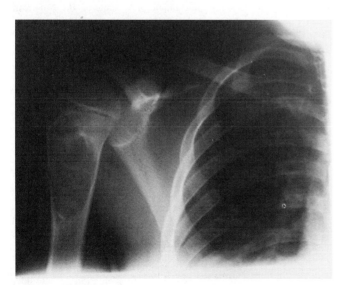

FIGURE 26–13. Simple bone cyst in the humerus. Note the pathologic fracture.

7. Jobe F, Kvitne R: Shoulder pain in the overhead athlete: The relationship of anterior instability and rotator cuff impingement. Orthop Rev 1989; 18:963–975.

8. Wickiewicz TL, Pagnani MJ, Kennedy K: Rehabilitation of the unstable shoulder. Sports Med Arthrosc Rev 1993; 1:227–235.

9. Warner JJ: The gross anatomy of the joint surfaces, ligaments, labrum and capsule. In Matsen FA, Fu FH, Hawkins RJ (eds): The Shoulder: A Balance of Mobility and Stability. Rosemont, IL, American Academy of Orthopedic Surgeons, 1993.

10. Mallon W, Brown H, Vogler J, Martinez S: Radiographic and geometric anatomy of the scapula. Clin Orthop 1992; 277: 142–154.

11. Howell SM, Kraft TA: The role of the supraspinatus and infraspinatus muscles in glenohumeral kinematics of anterior shoulder instability. Clin Orthop 1991; 263:128–134.

12. Bowen MK, Warren RF: Ligamentous control of shoulder stability based on selective cutting and static translation experiments. Clin Sports Med 1991; 10:757–782.

13. Lew WD, Lewis JL, Craig EV: Stabilization by capsule, ligaments and labrum: stability at the extremes of motion. In Matsen FA, Fu FH, Hawkins RJ (eds): The Shoulder: A Balance of Mobility and Stability. Rosemont, IL, American Academy of Orthopedic Surgeons, 1993.

14. Howell SM, Galinat BJ: The glenoid-labrum socket—a constrained articular surface. Clin Orthop 1989; 243:122–125.

15. Silliman JF, Hawkins RJ: Current concepts and recent advances in the athlete's shoulder. Clin Sports Med 1991; 10:693–705.

16. Pollock RG, Bigliani LU: Glenohumeral instability: Evaluation and treatment. J Am Acad Orthop Surg 1993; 1:24–32.

17. Bigliani LU, Ticker JB, Flatow EL, et al: The relationship of acromial architecture to rotator cuff disease. Clin Sports Med 1991; 10:823–838.

18. Speer KP, Garrett WE: Muscular control of motion and stability about the pectoral girdle. In Matsen FA, Fu FH, Hawkins RJ (eds): The Shoulder: A Balance of Mobility and Stability. Rosemont, IL, American Academy of Orthopedic Surgeons, 1993.

19. Rodowsky MW, Harner CD, Fu FH: The role of the long head of the biceps muscle and superior glenoid labrum in anterior stability of the shoulder. Am J Sports Med 1994; 22:121–130.

20. Matsen FA, Harryman DT, Sidles JA: Mechanics of glenohumeral instability. Clin Sports Med 1991; 10:783–788.

21. Bradley JP, Tibone JE: Electromyographic analysis of muscle action about the shoulder. Clin Sports Med 1991; 10:789–805.

22. Reid DC: Focusing the diagnosis of shoulder pain—pearl of practice. Phys Sports Med 1994; 22(6):28–45.

23. Neer CS: Anterior acromioplasty for chronic impingement syndrome in the shoulder: A preliminary report. J Bone Joint Surg 1972; 54A:41–50.

24. Reid DC: A practical approach to the painful shoulder. Can J Contin Med Educ 1991; 3(6):29–31.

25. Mudge MK, Wood VE, Frykman GK: Rotator cuff tears associated with os acromiale. J Bone Joint Surg 1984; 66A:427–429.

26. Solem-Bertoft E, Thuomas KA, and Westerberg CE: The influence of scapular retraction and protraction on the width of the subacromial space. An MRI study. Clin Orthop 1993; 296:99–103.

27. Magee DJ: Orthopedic Physical Assessment. Philadelphia, WB Saunders, 1992.

28. Ticker JB, Bigliani LU: Impingement pathology of the rotator cuff. In Andrews JR, Wilk KE (eds): The Athlete's Shoulder. New York, Churchill Livingstone, 1994.

29. O'Brien SJ, Pagnani MJ, Panariello RA, et al: Anterior instability of the shoulder. In Andrews JR, Wilk KE (eds): The Athlete's Shoulder. New York, Churchill Livingstone, 1994.

30. Cave EM: Fractures and Other Injuries. Chicago, Year Book, 1961.

31. Rockwood CA, Green DP: Fractures in Adults. Philadelphia, JB Lippincott, 1984.

32. Tibone J, Sellers R, Tonino P: Strength testing after third degree acromioclavicular dislocations. Am J Sports Med 1992; 20: 328–331.

33. Dias JJ, Gregg PJ: Acromioclavicular joint injuries in sport. Sports Med 1991; 11:125–132.

34. Glick JM, Milburn LJ, Haggerty JF, Nishimoto D: Dislocated acromioclavicular joint: Follow-up study of 35 unreduced acromioclavicular dislocation. Am J Sports Med 1977; 5:264–270.

35. Walsh WM, Peterson DA, Shelton G, Neuman RD: Shoulder strength following acromioclavicular injury. Am J Sports Med 1985; 13:153–158.

36. Wojtys EM, Nelson G: Conservative treatment of grade III acromioclavicular dislocations. Clin Orthop 1991; 268:112–119.

37. Bannister GC, Wallace WA, Stableforth PG, Hutson MA: The management of acute acromioclavicular dislocation—a randomized prospective controlled trial. J Bone Joint Surg 1989; 71B:848–850.

38. Dias JJ, Steingold RF, Richardson RA, et al: The conservative treatment of acromioclavicular dislocation—renew after 5 years. J Bone Joint Surg 1987; 69B:719–722.

39. Taft TM, Wilson FC, Oglesby JW: Dislocation of the acromioclavicular joint—an end-result study. J Bone Joint Surg 1987; 69A:1045–1051.

40. Allman FL: Fractures and ligamentous injuries of the clavicle and its articulation. J Bone Joint Surg 1967; 49A:774–784.

41. Bach BR, Van Fleet TA, Novak PJ: Acromioclavicular injuries—controversies in treatment. Phys Sports Med 1992; 20(12):87–101.

42. Dias JJ, Gregg PJ: Management of acromioclavicular joint injuries. Semin Orthop 1987; 2:239–245.

43. Higgs GB, Weinstein D, Flatlow EL: Evaluation and treatment of acute anterior glenohumeral dislocation. Sports Med Arthrosc Rev 1993; 1:190–201.

44. Loeb PE, Andrews JR, Wilk KE: Arthroscopic debridement of rotator cuff injuries. In Andrews JR, Wilk KE (eds): The Athlete's Shoulder. New York, Churchill Livingstone, 1994.

45. Mohtadi NG: Advances in the understanding of anterior instability of the shoulder. Clin Sports Med 1991; 10:863–870.

46. Rowe CR, Pierce DS, Clark JG: Voluntary dislocation of the shoulder: A preliminary report on a clinical, electromyographic, and psychiatric study of twenty-six patients. J Bone Joint Surg 1973; 55:445–460.

47. Rowe CR: Prognosis in dislocations of the shoulder. J Bone Joint Surg 1956; 38A:957–977.

48. Neer CS, Forster CR: Inferior capsular shifts for involuntary inferior and multi-directional instability of the shoulder. J Bone Joint Surg 1980; 62A:897–908.

49. Wilk KE: Current concepts in the rehabilitation of athletic shoulder injuries. In Andrews JR, Wilk KE (eds): The Athlete's Shoulder. New York, Churchill Livingstone, 1994.

50. Kvitne RS, Jobe FW: The diagnosis and treatment of anterior instability in the throwing athlete. Clin Orthop 1993; 291: 107–123.

51. Beynnon BD, Nichols CE, Pope MH: The kinematics of throws and strokes. In Matsen FA, Fu FH, Hawkins RJ (eds): The Shoulder: A Balance of Mobility and Stability. Rosemont, IL, American Academy of Orthopedic Surgeons, 1993.

52. Gowan ID, Jobe FW, Tibone JE, et al: A comparative electromyographic analysis of the shoulder during pitching: Professional vs amateur pitchers. Am J Sports Med 1987; 15:586–590.

53. O'Driscoll SW: Atraumatic instability: Pathology and pathogenesis. In Matsen FA, Fu FH, Hawkins RJ (eds): The Shoulder: A Balance of Mobility and Stability. Rosemont, IL, American Academy of Orthopedic Surgeons, 1993.

54. Glousman RE, Jobe FW: How to detect and manage the unstable shoulder. J Musculoskeletal Med 1989; 7:93–110.

55. Cooper RA, Brems JJ: The inferior capsular shift procedure for multidirectional instability of the shoulder. J Bone Joint Surg 1992; 74A:1516–1521.

56. Riebel GD, McCabe JB: Anterior shoulder dislocation: A review of reduction techniques. Am J Emerg Med 1991; 9:180–188.

57. Flatlow EL, Miller SR, Neer CS: Chronic anterior dislocation of the shoulder. J Shoulder Elbow Surg 1993; 2:2–10.

58. Soslowsky L, Flatlow E, Bigliani L, Mow VC: Articular geometry of the glenohumeral joint. Clin Orthop 1992; 285:181–190.

59. Pagnani MJ, Warren RF: The pathophysiology of anterior shoulder instability. Sports Med Arthrosc Rev 1993; 1:177–189.

60. Bowen M, Warren R: Ligamentous control of shoulder stability based on selective cutting and status translation experiments. Clin Sports Med 1991; 10:757–782.

61. Harryman D, Sidles J, Clark J, et al: Translation of the humeral head on the glenoid with passive glenohumeral motion. J Bone Joint Surg 1990; 72A:1334–1343.

62. Poppen N, Walker P: Normal and abnormal motion of the shoulder. J Bone Joint Surg 1976; 58A:195–201.

63. Hawkins RJ, Mohtadi NG: Clinical evaluation of shoulder instability. Clin J Sports Med 1991; 1:59–64.

64. Kibler WB: Evaluation of sports demands as a diagnostic tool in shoulder disorders. In Matsen FA, Fu FH, Hawkins RJ (eds): The

Shoulder: A Balance of Mobility. Rosemont, IL, American Academy of Orthopedic Surgeons, 1993.

65. Symeonides PP: The significance of the subscapularis muscle in the pathogenesis of recurrent dislocation of the shoulder. J Bone Joint Surg 1972; 54B:476–483.

66. Howell S, Galinat B, Renzi A, Morone P: Normal and abnormal mechanism of the glenohumeral joint in the horizontal plane. J Bone Joint Surg 1988; 70A:227–232.

67. Cain P, Mutschler T, Fu F: Anterior stability of the glenohumeral joint: A dynamic model. Am J Sports Med 1987; 15:144–148.

68. Neviaser R, Neviaser T, Neviaser J: Concurrent rupture of the rotator cuff and anterior dislocation of the older patient. J Bone Joint Surg 1988; 70A:1308–1311.

69. Engle RP: Proprioceptive neuromuscular facilitation for the shoulder. *In* Andrews JR, Wilk KE (eds): The Athlete's Shoulder. New York, Churchill Livingstone, 1994.

70. Browne A, Hoffmeyer P, An K, Morrey B: The influence of atmospheric pressure on shoulder stability. Orthop Trans 1990; 14:259–263.

71. Habermeyer P, Schmuller U, Wiedemann E: The intraarticular pressure of the shoulder: An experimental study on the role of the glenoid labrum in stabilizing the joint. Arthroscopy 1992; 8:166–172.

72. Travlos J, Goldberg I, Boome RS: Brachial plexus lesions associated with dislocated shoulders. J Bone Joint Surg 1990; 72B:68–71.

73. Simonet WT, Colfield RH: Prognosis in anterior shoulder dislocation. Presented at the Joint Meeting of the American Orthopaedic Society for Sports Medicine and the Japanese Orthopaedic Society for Sports Medicine, Maui, Hawaii, March 20–25, 1993.

74. Rowe CR: Recurrent transient anterior subluxation of the shoulder — the "dead arm" syndrome. Clin Orthop 1987; 223:11–19.

75. Zarins B, McMahon MS, Rowe CR: Diagnosis and treatment of traumatic anterior instability of the shoulder. Clin Orthop 1993; 291:75–84.

76. Higgs GB, Weinstein D, Flatow EL: Evaluation and treatment of acute anterior glenohumeral dislocations. Sports Med Arthrosc Rev 1993; 1:190–201.

77. Henry JH, Genung JA: Natural history of glenohumeral dislocation — revisited. Am J Sports Med 1982; 10:135–141.

78. Rowe CR, Patel D, Southmayd WW: The Bankart procedure — a long term end result study. J Bone Joint Surg 1978; 60A:1–16.

79. Akeson WH, Amiel D, Abel MF, et al: Effects of immobilization on joints. Clin Orthop 1987; 219:28–37.

80. Videman T: Connective tissue and immobilization — key factors in musculoskeletal degeneration? Clin Orthop 1987; 221:26–32.

81. Donatelli R, Owens-Burkhart H: Effects of immobilization on the extensibility of periarticular connective tissue. J Orthop Sports Phys Ther 1981; 3:67–72.

82. Reid DC, Saboe L, Burnham R: Current research of selected shoulder problems. *In* Donatelli R (ed): Physical Therapy of the Shoulder. New York, Churchill Livingstone, 1987.

83. Hovelius L, Akermark C, Albrektsson B, et al: Bristow-Latarjet procedure for recurrent anterior dislocation of the shoulder. Acta Orthop Scand 1983; 54:284–290.

84. Hehne HJ, Hubner H: Die Behandlung des Rezidivieremden Schulter Luxation nack Putti-Platt-Bankart und Eden-Hybinette-Lange. Orthop Prax 1980; 16:331–335.

85. Torg JS, Balduini FC, Bonci C, et al: A modified Bristow-Helfet-May procedure for recurrent dislocation and subluxation of the shoulder. Report of 212 cases. J Bone Joint Surg 1987; 69A:904–913.

86. Du Toit GT, Roux D: Recurrent dislocation of the shoulder. A 24 year study of the Johannesburg stapling operation. J Bone Joint Surg 1956; 38A:1–12.

87. Sisk TD, Boyd HB: Management of recurrent anterior dislocation of the shoulder. Du Toit type or staple capsulorrhaphy. Clin Orthop 1974; 103:150–154.

88. Bankart ASB: Recurrent or habitual dislocation of the shoulder. Br Med J 1923; 2:1132–1133.

89. Hovelius L, Thorling J, Fredin H: Recurrent anterior dislocations of the shoulder. Results after the Bankart and Putti-Platt operations. J Bone Joint Surg 1979; 61A:566–569.

90. Osmond-Clarke H: Habitual dislocation of the shoulder. The Putti-Platt operation. J Bone Joint Surg 1948; 30B:19–25.

91. Collins KA, Capito C, Cross M: The use of Putti-Platt procedure in the treatment of recurrent anterior dislocation with reference to the young athlete. Am J Sports Med 1986; 14(5):380–382.

92. Magnuson PB, Stack K: Recurrent dislocation of the shoulder. JAMA 1943; 123:889–892.

93. Karadimas J, Rentis G, Varouchas G: Repair of recurrent anterior dislocation of the shoulder using transfer of the subscapularis tendon. J Bone Joint Surg 1980; 62A:1147–1149.

94. Matsen FA, Tomas SC, Rockwood CA: Anterior glenohumeral instability. *In* Rockwood CA, Matsen FA (eds): The Shoulder, vol 1. Philadelphia, WB Saunders, 1990.

95. Rockwood CA: Subluxations and dislocations about the shoulder. *In* Rockwood CA, Green DP (eds): Fractures, vol 1. Philadelphia, JB Lippincott, 1975.

96. Banas MP, Dalldorf PG, DeHaven KE: The Allman modification of the Bristow procedure for recurrent anterior glenohumeral instability. Sports Med Arthrosc Rev 1993; 1:242–249.

97. Zarias B: Anterior shoulder stabilization using the Bankart procedure. Sports Med Arthrosc Rev 1993; 1:259–266.

98. Caspair RB, Beach WR: Arthroscopic anterior shoulder capsulorrhaphy. Sports Med Arthrosc Rev 1993; 1:237–242.

99. Warner JJP, Marks PH: Management of complications of surgery for anterior shoulder instability. Sports Med Arthrosc Rev 1993; 1:272–292.

100. Moseley JB, Jobe FW, Pink M, et al: EMG analysis of the scapular muscles during a shoulder rehabilitation program. Am J Sports Med 1992; 20:128–134.

101. Bonci DM, Sloane B, Middleton K: Nonsurgical/surgical rehabilitation of the unstable shoulder. J Sports Rehab 1992; 1:146–171.

102. Pappas AM, Zawacki RM, McCarthy CF: Rehabilitation of the pitching shoulder. Am J Sports Med 1985; 13:223–235.

103. Anderson TE: Rehabilitation of common shoulder injuries in athletics. J Musculoskeletal Med 1988; 5:15–26.

104. Wilk KE, Arrigo C: Current concepts in the rehabilitation of the athletic shoulder. J Orthop Sports Phys Ther 1993; 18:365–378.

105. Glousman R, Jobe FW, Tibone JE, et al: Dynamic electromyographic analysis of the throwing shoulder with glenohumeral instability. J Bone Joint Surg 1988; 70A:220–226.

106. Blackburn TA: Throwing injuries to the shoulder. *In* Donatelli R (ed): Physical Therapy to the Shoulder. New York, Churchill Livingstone, 1987.

107. Middleton K: Rehabilitation following shoulder arthroscopy. Sports Med Update 1989; 4:10–13.

108. Davies GJ, Dickoff-Hoffman S: Neuromuscular testing and rehabilitation of the shoulder complex. J Orthop Sports Phys Ther 1993; 18:449–458.

109. Borsa PA, Lephart SM, Kocher MS, Lephart SP: Functional assessment and rehabilitation of shoulder proprioception for glenohumeral instability. J Sports Rehab 1994; 3:84–104.

110. Cipriani D: Open and closed chain rehabilitation for the shoulder complex. *In* Andrews JR, Wilk KE (eds): The Athlete's Shoulder. New York, Churchill Livingstone, 1994.

111. Dickoff-Hoffman SA: Neuromuscular control exercises for shoulder instability. *In* Andrews JR, Wilk KE (eds): The Athlete's Shoulder. New York, Churchill Livingstone, 1994.

112. Bennett JG, Marous NA: The decelerator mechanism: Eccentric muscular contraction applications at the shoulder. *In* Andrews JR, Wilk KE (eds): The Athlete's Shoulder. New York, Churchill Livingstone, 1994.

113. Sutter JS: Conservative treatment of shoulder instability. *In* Andrews JR, Wilk KE (eds): The Athlete's Shoulder. New York, Churchill Livingstone, 1994.

114. Woo SL-Y, McMahon PJ, Debski RE, et al: Factors limiting and defining shoulder motion: What keeps it from going farther? *In* Matsen FA, Fu FH, Hawkins RJ (eds): The Shoulder: A Balance of Mobility and Stability. Rosemont, IL, American Academy of Orthopedic Surgeons, 1993.

115. McMahon MS, Zarins B: Multidirectional instability of the shoulder. *In* Andrews JR, Wilk KE (eds): The Athlete's Shoulder. New York, Churchill Livingstone, 1994.

116. Itoi E, Kuechle DK, Newman SR, et al: Stabilizing function of the biceps in stable and unstable shoulders. J Bone Joint Surg 1993; 75B:546–550.

117. Fu FH, Harner CD, Klein AH: Shoulder impingement syndrome — a critical review. Clin Orthop 1991; 269:162–173.

118. Dines DM, Warren RF, Inglis AE, Pavlov H: The coracoid impingement syndrome. J Bone Joint Surg 1990; 72B:314–316.

119. Paine RM, Voight M: The role of the scapula. J Orthop Sports Phys Ther 1993; 18:386–391.
120. Lephart SM, Kocker MS: The role of exercise in the prevention of shoulder disorders. *In* Matsen FA, Fu FH, Hawkins RJ (eds): The Shoulder: A Balance of Mobility. Rosemont, IL, American Academy of Orthopedic Surgeons, 1993.
121. Townsend H, Jobe FW, Pink M, Perry J: Electromyelographic analysis of the glenohumeral muscles during a baseball rehabilitation program. Am J Sports Med 1991; 19:264–272.
122. Keirns MA: Conservative management of shoulder impingement. *In* Andrews JR, Wilk KE (eds): The Athlete's Shoulder. New York, Churchill Livingstone, 1994.
123. Timmerman LA, Andrews JR, Wilk KE: Mini-open repair of the rotator cuff. *In* Andrews JR, Wilk KE (eds): The Athlete's Shoulder. New York, Churchill Livingstone, 1994.
124. Quillen WS, Halle JS, Rouillier LH: Manual therapy: Mobilization of the motion-restricted shoulder. J Sports Rehab 1992; 1:237–248.
125. Maitland GD: Peripheral Manipulation, 3rd ed. London, Butterworths, 1991.
126. Kaltenborn FM: Mobilization of the Extremity Joints: Examination and Basic Treatment Techniques. Oslo, Olaf Norles Bokhandel, 1980.
127. Lee D: A Workbook of Manual Therapy Techniques for the Upper Extremity. Delta, BC, DOPC Publishing, 1989.
128. Rathburn JB, MacNab I: The microvascular pattern of the rotator cuff. J Bone Joint Surg 1990; 52B:540–553.
129. Ciullo JV: Swimmer's shoulder. Clin Sport Med 1986; 5:115–137.
130. Wilk KE, Voight ML: Plyometrics for the shoulder complex. *In* Andrews JR, Wilk KE (eds): The Athlete's Shoulder. New York, Churchill Livingstone, 1994.
131. Gambetta V: Conditioning of the shoulder complex. *In* Andrews JR, Wilk KE (eds): The Athlete's Shoulder. New York, Churchill Livingstone, 1994.
132. Craven WM: Traumatic avulsion tears of the rotator cuff. *In* Andrews JR, Wilk KE (eds): The Athlete's Shoulder. New York, Churchill Livingstone, 1994.
133. Iannotti JP: Lesions of the rotator cuff: Pathology and pathogenesis. *In* Matsen FA, Fu FH, Hawkins RJ (eds): The Shoulder: A Balance of Mobility and Stability. Rosemont, IL, American Academy of Orthopedic Surgeons, 1993.
134. Neviaser RJ, Neviaser TJ, Neviaser JS: Anterior dislocation of the shoulder and rotator cuff rupture. Clin Orthop 1993; 291:103–106.
135. Abrams JS: Special shoulder problems in the throwing athlete: Pathology, diagnosis and nonoperative management. Clin Sports Med 1991; 10:839–861.
136. Andrews JR, Gidumal RH: Shoulder arthroscopy in the throwing athlete—perspectives and prognosis. Clin Sports Med 1987; 6:565–571.
137. Jobe FW, Giangarra CE, Kvitne RS, Glousman RE: Anterior capsulolabral reconstruction of the shoulder in athletes in overhand sports. Am J Sports Med 1991; 19:428–434.
138. Hurley JA, Anderson TE: Shoulder arthroscopy: Its role in evaluating shoulder disorders in the athlete. Am J Sports Med 1990; 18:480–483.
139. Hawkins RJ, Kunkel SS: Rotator cuff tears. *In* Torg JS, Welsh RP, Shepard RJ (eds): Current Therapy in Sports Medicine. Toronto, BC Decker, 1990.
140. Zarins B, Andrews JR, Carson WG: Injuries to the Throwing Arm. Philadelphia, WB Saunders, 1985.
141. Braatz JH, Gogia PP: The mechanics of pitching. J Orthop Sports Phys Ther 1987; 9:56–69.
142. Coleman AE, Axe MJ, Andrews JR: Performance profile–directed simulated game: An objective functional evaluation for baseball pitchers. J Orthop Sports Phys Ther 1987; 9:101–105.
143. Brewster C, Moynes Schwab DR: Rehabilitation of the shoulder following rotator cuff injury or surgery. J Orthop Sports Phys Ther 1993; 18:422–426.
144. Neer CS: Displaced proximal humeral fractures. I. Classification and evaluation. J Bone Joint Surg 1970; 52A:1077–1089.
145. Barnett LS: Little league shoulder syndrome: Proximal humeral epiphyseolysis in adolescent baseball pitchers—a case report. J Bone Joint Surg 1985; 67A:495–496.
146. Salter RB: Textbook of Disorders: Injuries of the Musculoskeletal System. Baltimore, Williams & Wilkins, 1983.
147. Connolly JF: DePalma's The Management of Fractures and Dislocations—An Atlas. Philadelphia, WB Saunders, 1981.
148. Howell JW: Evaluation and management of thoracic outlet syndrome. *In* Donatelli R (ed): Physical Therapy of the Shoulder. New York, Churchill Livingstone, 1987.
149. Grant JCB: Grant's Atlas of Anatomy, 5th ed. Baltimore, Williams & Wilkins, 1962.
150. Wright RS, Lipscomb B: Acute occlusion of the subclavian vein in an athlete: Diagnosis, etiology and surgical management. J Sports Med 1975; 2:343–347.
151. Nemoto R, Matsumoto N, Tazaki K, et al: An experimental study on the "double crush" hypothesis. J Hand Surg 1987; 12A:552–559.
152. Mackinnon SE: Double and multiple "crush" syndromes—double and multiple entrapment neuropathies. Hand Clin 1992; 8:369–390.
153. Caldwell JW, Crane CR, Krusen EM: Nerve conduction studies: An aid in the diagnosis of thoracic outlet syndrome. South Med J 1971; 64:210–213.
154. Roos DB: New concepts of thoracic outlet syndrome that explain etiology, symptoms, diagnosis and treatment. Vasc Surg 1979; 13:313–317.
155. Bateman JE: Tumors of the shoulder and neck. *In* The Shoulder and Neck. Philadelphia, WB Saunders, 1972.

CHAPTER 27

Elbow Injuries

JANET SOBEL *PT*
ROBERT P. NIRSCHL *MD*

The design of the human elbow is quite remarkable in its role as the link in the upper extremity kinetic chain, adjusting the length of the limb and position of the forearm while placing the hand in its most effective position. Extraordinary stability and joint alignment make it unusually resistant to arthritic overuse and dislocation. This design becomes compromised, however, when challenged by the demands of competitive sports. Elbow injuries are common in sports, occurring as a result of collision (direct blows and falls on the outstretched arm), as well as from cumulative overuse. As in injury to other areas, the factors involved in elbow injury include training intensity and frequency, general level of conditioning and sport preparedness, environmental stress and genetic factors, previous injuries, technique, external forces, and equipment. The elbow of the recreational athlete is often subject to a combination of repetitive submaximal stress induced by occupation,

daily activities, and sport, whereas that of the highly competitive athlete is subject to more constant repetitive microtrauma exceeding tissue ability to accommodate and repair itself. Types of injuries to the elbow are listed in Table 27–1.

In addition to previously mentioned factors, elbow injuries in young athletes may be caused by several other factors, such as strength imbalances during growth spurts or periods of accelerated bone growth, resulting in muscle–bone length imbalances, decreased flexibility, and impaired coordination. Factors concerning the epiphysis, a biomechanically weak link, must also be considered. Common adolescent elbow injuries such as osteochondritis dissecans of the capitellum and avulsion of the medial and olecranon apophysis are difficult additional problems not present in adults.

Although the normal elbow motion is 0 degrees to 150 degrees (extension to flexion) and approximately 85

TABLE 27–1
Injuries of the Elbow

- Osseous changes and articular changes
  - Bony hypertrophy
  - Traction spur formation
  - Osteochondral defects
  - Loose bodies
  - Joint degeneration
    - Chondromalacia
    - Osteophyte formation
  - Problems of skeletal immaturity
    - Epiphyseal
    - Apophyseal
    - Hypertrophy fragmentation and avulsion
  - Effects of fracture
  - Effects of dislocation
- Ligamentous changes
  - Stretching and tears
  - Contracture
  - Calcium deposition
- Soft tissue joint changes
  - Synovitis
  - Adhesive capsulitis
- Tendon alterations
  - Tendinosis/tendinitis
- Muscle alteration
  - Myositis, fibrosis, myositis ossificans
- Nerve alteration
  - Ulnar nerve entrapment in the cubital tunnel, ulnar nerve stretching and dislocation
  - Median nerve entrapment (pronator syndrome)
  - Radial nerve entrapment
  - Lateral antebrachial cutaneous nerve entrapment

degrees of pronation/supination, activities of daily living usually require only 15 degrees to 125 degrees of extension/flexion and approximately 50 degrees each of pronation and supination. Sports, however, which tend to create motion limitations, need the full range of motion for optimal performance and injury prevention.

Because the elbow is close to the end of the interconnected link in the kinetic chain, it often carries the burden of inadequacies and/or alterations elsewhere. As a result, elbow injuries are common in throwing and racket sports, as well as in gymnastics, boxing, wrestling, and certain field events such as javelin throwing. The kinetic chain injury potential also commonly involves the shoulder, as cited by several authors.[1–6] Priest et al.'s study of 2633 tennis players highlights this relationship: There was a 65 percent greater incidence of shoulder injury among tennis players with a history of tennis elbow than among those without a history of elbow problems.[5]

ANATOMIC AND BIOMECHANICAL CONSIDERATIONS

The elbow joint complex, which consists of the humeroulnar, radiohumeral, and radioulnar articulations, is inherently stable by skeletal design (Fig. 27–1). The exceedingly congruent humeroulnar joint acts as a

uniaxial hinge except in the extremes of flexion and extension. In flexion, there is 5 degrees of internal ulnar rotation, and at full extension, the ulna outwardly rotates 5 degrees.[7,8] This joint congruence keeps more of the medial olecranon surface in contact than at any other given point of flexion and extension and thus distributes the stresses of the cartilage. As a result, as suggested by Morrey and others,[8–10] degenerative changes rarely occur in the absence of a specific cause.

Additional stability is provided by the capsuloligamentous structure, as well as the kinetic relationships between the bony structure and their soft tissue attachments.[11] The ulnar collateral ligament (UCL), originating from the inferior surface of the medial epicondyle, consists of three parts: anterior oblique, posterior, and oblique. Because the UCL origin is posterior to the axis of joint flexion and extension, the ligamentous tension varies with elbow motion.[12] Throughout elbow flexion there is sequential tightening, so that some of the fibers of the anterior oblique ligament (AOL) are taut throughout elbow flexion. Through most of the motion (20 degrees to 120 degrees), the AOL provides the majority of functional contribution to the UCL. The AOL is the primary valgus stabilizer,[9] with the radiocapitellar joint offering secondary stability.[13,14] Fractures of the radiohumeral relationship and dislocations of the humeroulnar joint alter this stability.[15] In this circumstance, any compromise of the UCL will result in residual elbow instability except in full extension. Conversely, with a normal UCL, the radiohumeral joint does not appreciably contribute to the elbow valgus stability or axial rotation.

In the absence of the AOL of the UCL, there is moderate valgus laxity, even with a normal radiohumeral joint present. In this circumstance, the radiocapitellar joint is subject to compressive forces, with the resultant potential for loose bodies and fractures. Without the UCL, the radiohumeral joint and muscle activity offer resistance to valgus instability, but not to axial rotation.[12]

In full extension, valgus stability is equally divided among the UCL, the capsule, and the joint relationships.[13] The most anterior fibers of the UCL are the greatest constraints to valgus instability in flexion.[16] In studying 12 cadaver elbows, Sojbjerg et al. found elbow stability to be independent of the UCL beyond the last 20 degrees of extension. Sojbjerg also found that the annular ligament contributed to varus-valgus stability.[17] The posterior fibers of the UCL have negligible valgus stability effect, but they are linked in maximal flexion and are powerful constraints to elbow flexion beyond normal.[16]

The lateral collateral ligament (LCL) consists of the annular ligament, the poorly defined fan-shaped radial collateral ligament (RCL), the accessory collateral ligament (ACL), and the lateral ulnar collateral ligament (LUCL). The LCL is tense throughout the range of motion and is unaffected by elbow motion as the axis of rotation passes through its origin[12] (e.g., anatomic position is also the isometric position).

The RCL is taut throughout flexion.[18] The LUCL is taut only in extreme flexion (beyond 110 degrees) in the absence of load or valgus stress, but with varus load the LUCL is tense throughout the arc of motion.[18] O'Driscoll et al. describe the role of the LUCL as preventing posterolateral rotatory instability of the elbow.[19]

The interosseus membrane (IOM) acts to bind the radius and ulna together, thereby preventing displacement of the radius on the ulna.[20] The quadrate ligament, first described in 1854 by Denuce, is a fibrous band attached to the inferior border of the radial notch and the neck of the radius. It reinforces the inferior aspect of the joint capsule and is a stabilizer of the proximal radioulnar joint.[20] In full supination its anterior border tightens against the neck of the radius, drawing it against the proximal radioulnar notch. The quadrate ligament plays an important role in the reduction of radial head dislocations (e.g., Monteggia fractures, pulled elbows, and radiohumeral dislocations).[21]

The anterior capsule of the elbow joint complex (EJC) is characteristically thin and pliable, but the cruciate orientation of its fibers offers considerable strength.[22] It is exceedingly sensitive to injury, thereby thickening and predisposing the joint to flexion contractures. The anterior aspect of the joint is further susceptible to contracture and scarring because of the unique insertion of the brachialis muscle, which crosses the joint as a muscle instead of a tendon. Rehabilitative efforts to regain extension after brachialis muscle injury may lead to further complications, such as myositis ossificans or mechanical compression of the brachial artery and/or median nerve.[23]

Maximum capacity of the elbow joint occurs at approximately 80 degrees flexion (e.g., the intra-articular pressure is lowest).[13,24] Electromyographic (EMG) activity of all the major elbow muscles is minimal in this position as well.[24] For this reason, prolonged immobilization at 80 degrees invites maximum adhesions and is not recommended. Table 27–2 reviews the articular and ligamentous factors in elbow stability.

FUNCTIONAL ANATOMY

The muscles of the EJC affect movement throughout the upper extremity. The brachial, brachioradial, and biceps muscles are the primary muscles of elbow flexion, with the extensor carpi radialis longus (ECRL) and the pronator teres (PT) showing some accessory elbow flexor activity.[25]

The workhorse of the elbow joint, the brachial muscle, is unaffected by forearm rotation, because its line of pull remains unchanged.[26] Kapandji[20] describes the brachial muscle as one of the rare muscles of the body with only one function (i.e., elbow flexion), but

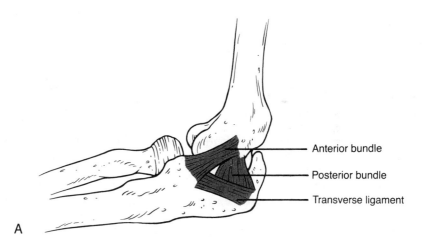

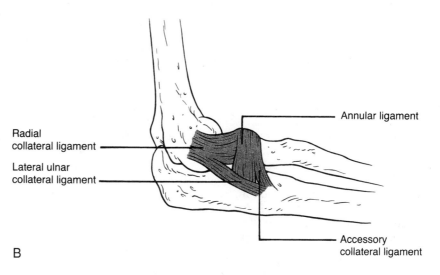

FIGURE 27–1. Elbow bones and ligaments. (From Richardson JK, Iglarsh ZA: Clinical Orthopaedic Physical Therapy. Philadelphia, WB Saunders, 1994, pp 222–223.)

TABLE 27–2
Articular and Ligamentous Contributions to Elbow Stability[7,8,11,12]

Stabilization	Elbow Extended	Elbow Flexed 90°
Valgus stability	Anterior capsule UCL and bony articular (proximal half of sigmoid notch) *equally divided*	UCL provides 55% 0% anterior capsule and bony articulation (proximal half of sigmoid notch)
Varus stability	Anterior capsule (32%) Joint articulation (55%) RCL (14%)	Joint articulation (75%) Anterior capsule (13%) RCL (9%)
Anterior displacement	Anterior oblique ligament Anterior joint capsule Trochlea-olecranon articulation (minimal)	
Posterior displacement	Anterior capsule Radial head against capitellum Coracoid against trochlea	
Distraction	Anterior capsule (85%) RCL (5%) UCL (5%) Triceps, biceps, brachial, brachioradial, forearm muscles	RCL 10% UCL 78% Capsule 8%

RCL, Radial collateral ligament, UCL, ulnar collateral ligament.

Cochran points out its action in joint compression.[7] The brachial muscle becomes more effective with the elbow flexed to 45 degrees and has maximum efficiency at 80 to 90 degrees.[7,20] Because its fibers are mostly muscular as it crosses the elbow joint (only 5 percent of its cross-section is tendinous at the joint), the brachial muscle carries a high risk for ectopic ossification about the elbow joint if rupture and intramuscular hemorrhage occurs.

The brachioradial muscle is relatively inactive in unloaded slow flexion except in the pronated forearm, where it shows slight activity. It is generally reserved for quick and powerful elbow flexion especially in the neutral or pronated forearm. It is maximally efficient at 100 to 110 degrees of flexion.[27] The brachioradial muscle also will cause forearm supination from full pronation and/or against resistance.[20,26]

The biceps long head, although it serves as an accessory for maintaining humeral head stability at the shoulder joint, also plays a role in elbow flexion, where overall it is more active than the short head.[20,26] The biceps is ineffective as a flexor in a pronated forearm, as the function of forearm supination becomes predominant in this position. Although it is a good flexor from 0 to 45 degrees, the biceps is strongest at 90 degrees.[7]

The best position for pure elbow flexion muscle activity is the neutral position, where all the flexors are active from 90 to 110 degrees flexion.[7,13,26–28] Only one third to one half of the maximal strength is generated in the first 30 degrees of motion, as these mechanical angles are less efficient.[13] The pronated forearm is the weakest position for elbow flexor power.[25,29]

The major elbow extensors are the triceps and anconeus. The anconeus is described as a dynamic stabilizer of the elbow joint in most positions,[13,27,30] but Pauly et al.[31] point out that it has less of a mechanical advantage at full extension. It is active throughout pronation and supination.[25,28,32]

The medial head of the triceps is the workhorse of extension, regardless of shoulder or forearm position.[31,32] The lateral and long heads are recruited against resistance.[28,31] Currier[33] studied EMG isometric activity of the triceps and anconeus in 41 normal males at 60, 90, and 120 degrees and found mean activity to be lowest at 60 degrees and highest at 90 to 120 degrees of elbow flexion. Kapandji[20] summarized the maximum efficiency of the upper extremity in his statement that the arms are best suited for climbing: maximum muscle efficiency occurs when the shoulder and elbow are simultaneously extending or flexing. The arm is weakest when the elbow is extending as the shoulder is flexing (i.e., pivoting forward). Funk et al.[25] studied five normal subjects and found the elbow muscles to be relatively quiet when valgus and varus stresses were applied at 90 degrees flexion, thus concluding that the static osteoligamentous constraints, not dynamic muscular forces, stabilize the elbow in this position (see Table 27–2).

The muscles of the common flexor origin, with the exception of the pronator teres, cross both the elbow and wrist joints.[23] The pronator teres is actually second to the pronator quadratus as a forearm pronator, but is unaffected by elbow position.[7,27,32] On the extensor side, the extensor carpi radialis brevis (ECRB) originates just anterior and distal to the lateral epicondyle, so that in elbow flexion and extension, it glides over the outer lateral capsule and over the bony lateral condyle. Thus, friction and tension forces are a potential source of pathologic ECRB changes at the elbow. The ECRB and its companion muscle, the ECRL, offer little in terms of elbow joint function.

The supinator, a flat muscle, essentially lacks any tendinous tissue.[22] Basmajian and Travill[27] described supination as elastic recoil initiated by pronation, continued by the supinator, and then augmented by the biceps when resistance was present. Kapandji,[20] in presenting the radius as a crank with three segments, explains that there are two mechanisms for moving the crank:

1. That of unwinding a cord coiled around an arm of the crank (accomplished by the short flat muscles, the supinator proximally and pronator quadratus distally).
2. That of pulling on the apex of one of the bends of the radius (accomplished by the biceps at the radial tuberosity attachment and by the supinator at the proximal one third of the radial attachment).

This relationship takes on great significance when the radius is fractured, as displacement and malunion can occur as a result of this dynamic muscle function.

NERVE FUNCTION ABOUT THE ELBOW

The act of pronation is innervated only by the median nerve, but pronation can be compensated for or intensified by shoulder abduction. The act of supination is innervated by the radial nerve to the supinator, as well as the musculocutaneous nerve to the biceps. The radial nerve is also the prime innervator of the triceps and is therefore the key to elbow extension. Elbow flexion has mixed innervation via the median nerve to the brachial muscle, the musculocutaneous nerve to the biceps, and the radial nerve to the brachioradial muscle. Nerve injury and entrapment are not uncommon about the elbow. The radial nerve is vulnerable to injury at the canal of Frohse as it enters into the proximal edge of the supinator. The median nerve is vulnerable at the antecubital fossa as it penetrates between the origins of the pronator teres (i.e., the pronator syndrome). The ulnar nerve is by far the most vulnerable to dysfunction and injury about the elbow. It is vulnerable to stretch or compression by entrapment by virtue of its location, the anatomic hereditary relationships, and elbow activity (i.e., flexion-extension arcs of motion). Nirschl[23] has defined three ulnar nerve zones about the elbow medial epicondylar groove (Table 27–3).

The ulnar nerve occasionally becomes entrapped in zone I by the arcade of Struthers or by a prominent medial intermuscular septum attachment to the proximal medial epicondyle. Zone II entrapments occur primarily due to joint disease (e.g., osteoarthritic spurs or rheumatoid synovitis compromising zone II space).

The most common etiology for nerve dysfunction is not tension, however, but compression in zone III, also known as the cubital tunnel or ulnar flexor arcade.

The more common etiologic factors related to ulnar nerve dysfunction are excessive traction due to a valgus elbow position (e.g., dynamic UCL instability in throwing sports or skeletal valgus resulting from fracture malunion). The most common tension etiology, however, is hereditary subluxation or dislocation of the nerve.

The nerve travels behind the medial epicondyle under the cubital tunnel, which extends from the medial epicondyle to the medial border of the olecranon process and serves as the tendinous origin of the flexor carpi ulnaris (FCU). As elbow flexion increases, the cubital retinaculum must stretch. Jobe and El Attrache[34] point out that the ulnar nerve essentially elongates in elbow flexion, and the medial head of the triceps can push it medially, so it is not normally a fixed structure unless trapped in zone III. Beyond the cubital tunnel, the nerve continues into the forearm between the two heads of the FCU, where entrapment can occur if the FCU muscles are hypertrophied, as in athletes participating in throwing sports. Mechanical errors in throwing exaggerate the potential of nerve dysfunction in these circumstances (e.g., "opening up" too late, dropping the elbow below the horizontal, and excessive numbers of one type of pitch) (see Chapter 17).

THE ADULT ELBOW IN THROWING

Because the elbow is close to the final link (or hand) in the kinetic chain of throwing, any alteration of the integrated movement may overstress it. Furthermore, the basic form, as well as the highly repetitive demands of throwing, are by their nature directly challenging to the integrity of the elbow. Jobe and El Attrache reported that the average angular velocity at the elbow during professional baseball throwing is 5000 degrees per second.[34] Others report it to be somewhere within the range of 1800 to 3000 degrees per second.[2,35,36] Whichever is correct, these velocities represent tremendous valgus forces at the medial elbow. As expected, especially in view of the rather meager stabilizing forces of the medial collateral ligament and common flexor origin, a high injury rate is the result. Tullos and King[37] in 1973 found that 50 percent of all professional baseball pitchers experienced performance-limiting shoulder or elbow pain during their careers. Adaptation of the arm to pitching commonly includes humeral hypertrophy (Gore et al.[38] report hypertrophy in 95 percent of all professional pitchers); hypertrophy of the pectorals, latissimus dorsi, and forearm flexors; elbow flexion contracture; and valgus deformity. King, Breslford, and Tullos[10] also reported an increased carrying angle in 30 percent of the pitchers they studied and elbow flexion contracture in the dominant arm in 50 percent.

TABLE 27–3
Nirschl Ulnar Nerve Zones at the Medial Epicondylar Groove

Zone I: Proximal to medial epicondyle
Zone II: At level of and posterior to medial epicondyle
Zone III: Distal to medial epicondyle

Although form may not play as critical a role in elbow injury potential in throwing sports compared with racket sports, some biomechanical factors are important. If the wind-up phase is rushed, less throwing energy is contributed from the legs and trunk.[39] Cochran[7] reports that body rotation accounts for more than half of the release velocity of the ball, and better throwers accelerate the ball over a shorter distance, releasing it from a position of greater spine extension.

Each phase of the pitching motion affects the elbow in a relatively characteristic fashion. The initial windup phase is one of low load to the arm, and elbow flexion is maintained by isometric contractions of the elbow flexors. During the stride of windup phase, the biceps contract to isometrically and eccentrically control the elbow angle, while the wrist and finger extensors concentrically move the wrist from slight flexion to hyperextension.[40] The massive valgus stresses to the elbow begin during the cocking phase, and the flexor pronator muscle mass must act to help dynamically stabilize the elbow against these forces. At this phase, the triceps acts isometrically to limit elbow flexion.

It is from late cocking phase through the acceleration phase that the elbow is subject to maximum valgus stresses as the body rotates ahead of the trailing arm.[41] The flexor-pronator group must apply varus force to the forearm and is easily subject to valgus overload to the medial elbow structures. Failure of these structures (UCL and common flexor origin) is followed by instability, lateral compression, and posterior injuries (olecranon fossa, chondromalacia, and chip fractures). During acceleration, an elbow flexed at 90 to 120 degrees is rapidly extended to approximately 25 degrees at ball release.[34] This movement places high shear forces on the articular cartilage and eccentric loading on the brachial and biceps muscles to resist uncontrolled extensions.[42]

Andrews[43] describes deceleration as the most violent phase in the throwing mechanism. The medial elbow stresses continue through deceleration as the common flexor and pronator muscles concentrically work to pronate and flex the wrist. The elbow flexors (biceps and brachial muscles) act eccentrically to decelerate the forearm. Failure of these groups with high elbow extension velocities can result in overextension injuries (compression posteriorly and stretch anteriorly). The pronator teres is very active in pronating the hand while the supinator acts eccentrically. Similarly, the wrist and finger flexors are very active concentrically and are opposed by the eccentrically acting extensors.

Multiple repetitions of all these forces on the elbow throughout the throwing motion create a high potential for injury to many anatomic areas of the joint (Fig. 27–2). The anterior compartment of the joint is least vulnerable to injury. Capsular sprains and chronic biceps tendinitis or brachial myositis may be additional

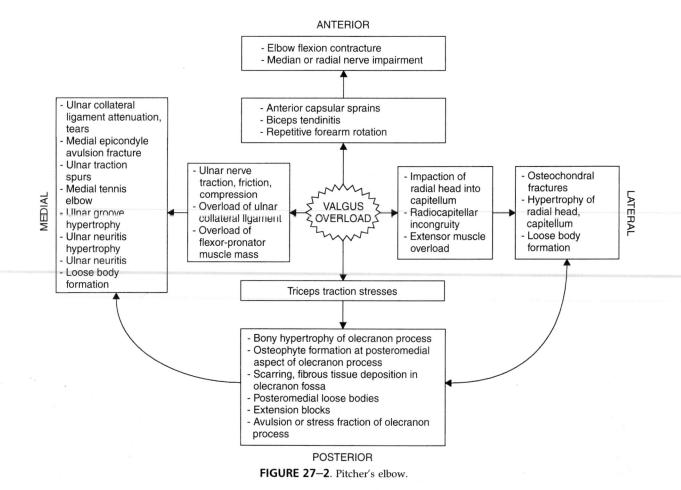

FIGURE 27–2. Pitcher's elbow.

factors leading to elbow flexion contracture. Repetitive rotational movements may result in radial nerve entrapments. Elbow flexion deformity, common in baseball players, is most likely the result of myositis and fibrosis of the common flexor origin but generally does not affect performance, as the range requirement for throwing is 20 to 120 degrees.[34] Posteriorly, repeated forced extension drives the olecranon into its fossa. This trauma may result in scarring and fibrous tissue deposition in the synovium of the olecranon fossa, osteophyte formation and/or chondromalacia at the posteromedial olecranon process, and loose body formation. Traction forces produced by triceps contraction may lead to avulsion fractures of the olecranon process, triceps tendinosis, or triceps avulsion off the olecranon.

All structures of the lateral aspect of the elbow are subject to injury from the throwing mechanism. The extensor muscles and tendons may be stretched and eccentrically overloaded in acceleration and follow-through, with resultant myositis and tendinosis/tendinitis. Valgus instability may lead to compressive forces at the radiocapitellar joint, resulting in synovitis, degenerative changes of the articular cartilage, loose body formation, radial head hypertrophy, and joint incongruity.

The medial elbow is commonly injured in the throwing sports. The violent forces from the late cocking phase through the acceleration phase are relatively continuous to the medial joint, where the anterior band of the medial collateral ligament (MCL) is the only significant stabilizer. Strains, myositis, and tears of the flexor muscle group commonly occur in throwing. Sprains, traction spurs, attenuation, and ruptures of the UCL also occur with some frequency, with resultant valgus instability.

Ulnar nerve impairment is common owing to zone II and zone III inflammatory changes, traction from the valgus instability, friction from recurrent subluxation, abrasion from osteophytes, and/or compression due to entrapment by the thickened or inflamed tissue in and about the cubital tunnel. Jobe and El Attrache[34] found both clinical and subclinical ulnar nerve dysfunction in 40 percent of competitive pitchers they studied.

Glousman et al.[44] performed EMG analysis during late cocking and acceleration in 19- to 30-year-old competitive pitchers, comparing muscular strength activity in injured versus noninjured elbows, as well as while throwing curve balls and while throwing fast balls. While flexor carpi radialis (FCR) and PT EMG activity did not increase to contribute dynamic stability to the UCL deficient elbows, the ECRL and ECRB, which oppose them, were more active in the injured arms. Thus, an asynchrony of muscular activity that leads to further problems is likely. Glousman et al. note that the FCR lies directly over the ACL and suggest that the lack of increased flexor activity may be the result of inhibition around the deficient UCL or it may be a predisposing preinjury pattern. In either case, emphasis on strengthening these muscles is essential. Only the biceps showed no difference between injured and noninjured elbows.

Elbow loose body formation is common in the pitching arm as a result of bony hypertrophy and exostosis, joint incongruity, and shear forces. Gore et al.[38] reported that 50 percent of loose bodies were in the posterior compartment, 31 percent were located medially, and 12 percent were located anteriorly and laterally in the elbows of pitchers who presented with the malady.

LITTLE LEAGUE ELBOW

In a study of 104 Little League baseball players, Pappas[45] found the elbow to be the most common site of complaint. The Houston study of 595 Little League pitchers found that 17 percent had elbow symptoms, and the Eugene study of 11- to 12-year-old pitchers found that 20 percent had structural changes at the elbow, 23 percent showed radiographic changes on the medial epicondyle[46]; 10 percent had limited extension, and 5 percent had lateral compartment changes. Young pitchers are subject to the same forces as adults, but the resulting injuries are to the weakest link on the adolescent kinetic chain, the epiphyseal plates.[47] These injuries are quite different from those in adults due to the lack of closure of the epiphysis and apophysis and the relative laxity of the medial elbow.[38] Although Little League rules impose limits on the frequency and duration of pitching, there are no limits imposed on practice frequency intensity or duration. Each young player is subject to variation in growth acceleration periods, neuromuscular coordination, and parent and peer influences. The medial elbow of the adolescent pitcher sees hypertrophy of the medial epicondylar apophysis, widening of the growth plate, and fracture and displacement of the epicondyle (Fig. 27–3).[42] Little League elbow was first identified in 1960 by Brogdon[47a] and Crow, and many studies have reported that its incidence usually peaks at approximately 13 years of age.[48]

In 1964 Adams[49] compared the elbows of 162 Little League pitchers with those of nonplayers. The stresses of acceleration and explosive forces placed on the medial elbow apophysis by the flexor pronator muscles create a mild separation of the medial epicondyle, resulting in hypertrophic fragmentation, irregularity, and sometimes avulsion of its ossification center. Tullos and King[50] reported this avulsion fracture through the medial elbow to be the most common injury in Little League pitchers. Gore et al.[38] found that Little League elbow was present in 33 percent of players. The lateral compression forces on the juvenile arm resulted in bony hypertrophy of the radial head and/or capitellum, as well as vascular insult to their ossific nuclei, which could lead to osteochondritis dissecans, osteochondral fractures, avascular necrosis of the radial head, and bony deformity of the radial head.[14,47,51]

Bassett and Breecher found changes in the lateral compartment of 10 percent of 13- to 14-year-old pitchers.[51] It is these lateral compression injuries that are most responsible for permanently disabling elbow injuries in young players.[38] Pappas[45] found osteochon-

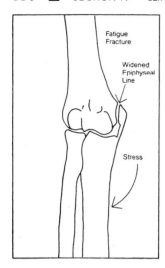
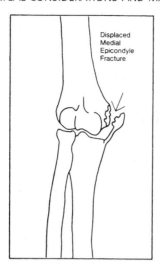
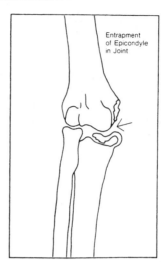

FIGURE 27–3. Little League elbow. (From Medich GF: Little League elbow, Sports Med Update 1989; 4:17.)

drosis in the younger players (<11 years old) and believed osteochondritis was more likely to occur in adolescents.

Posterior stresses may also result in apophysitis and avulsion fractures of the olecranon apophysis. Gore et al.[38] described a rare presentation of spiral fractures of the humeral shaft resulting from the inability of a young humerus to withstand the rotational torque imposed on it. The athlete with Little League elbow complains of progressive medial elbow pain and tenderness over the medical epicondyle; pain increases with pitching and is relieved with rest. Sometimes the athlete will have experienced a popping sensation, followed by pain, a decreased ability to throw, swelling, and ecchymosis. There is pain over the medial epicondyle and on passive extension and active flexion of the wrist and fingers. Elbow extension motion may be limited as well.

THE ELBOW IN TENNIS

The dominant arm of the elite tennis player has been found to undergo substantial adaptive changes because of the sport; these include humeral shaft hypertrophy, hypertrophy of the radius and ulna, and selected muscular hypertrophy.[5] Ellenbecker[3] has noted "that the repetition required for initial skill acquisition and subsequent practice and competition at all levels" may lead to overuse injuries about the elbow in tennis. The beginner and the recreational player are more likely to be injured as a result of poor form, while the advanced player has injuries resulting more from intensity and excessive demands. In either case, the incidence of elbow injury is extremely high among tennis players. A study by Hang and Peng[52] found a 37 percent incidence of lateral tennis elbow in 534 tennis players. Priest et al.[5] studied 2500 players and found a 45 percent incidence in world class players and a 47 percent incidence in average players. This is similar to Nirschl's[53] findings of a 50 percent incidence in 30+-year-old club players, as well as Cruchow and Pelletier's[54] report of a 39.7 percent incidence in recreational players. What is most outstanding in the statistics is the close relationship

between the incidence of tennis elbow and shoulder injuries among tennis players. In a survey by Priest and Nagel[55] of 84 world class players, 74 percent of the men and 60 percent of the women had a history of shoulder or elbow pain in the dominant arm that affected their play; 22 percent had both elbow and shoulder symptoms.

In 1980 Priest et al.[5] reported a 63 percent greater incidence of shoulder injury in tennis players who had a history of tennis elbow when compared with players with no tennis elbow history. These reports of the statistical relationship of elbow and shoulder pathoanatomy are similar to our observations and support our findings of muscle imbalances as predisposing factors to injury in the adjacent joint (shoulder or elbow). When testing 80 16- to 18-year-old nationally ranked tennis players, we found that 70 percent demonstrated significant shoulder muscle imbalances (USTA, unpublished data, 1988). In most cases, these young tennis players have no specific conditioning program to prepare their bodies for offsetting the musculoskeletal demands and imbalances imposed by the sport. It is common for these athletes to play 6 days a week for sessions of 2 or more hours. In addition, players who practice with ball machines or against a backboard are subjecting the arm to a greater number of balls per unit of time. Many of today's younger players are fashioning their form after the open-stance techniques demonstrated by the professionals, incognizant of the discernible subtleties. All ages of competitive players are also now using high-technology rackets fashioned to fit the needs and skill levels of the professional players. These rackets are capable of producing excessive torque and impact forces. Furthermore, they allow players to impart increased ball speeds without using good lower body mechanics for energy transfer. The basics of good tennis form involve transferring energy from the ground reaction to the lower body by using the legs, forward rotation weight transfer, and trunk and shoulder rotation for power. Poor form, in which the player fails to perform weight transfer and trunk rotation while leading with the elbow for power, predisposes to injury. As in all sports, injury potential is greater in players who bring genetic predisposition, avocational and occupational stresses, physical deficiencies, a history of previous uncorrected injury, and/or poor conditioning to the sport (Table 27–4).

Environmental factors, especially the court surface, also play a role. Consistent and unforgiving surfaces such as asphalt and concrete may result in late strokes. Inconsistent and unforgiving surfaces such as indoor carpet may lead to odd bounces, resulting in uncontrolled arm overload. This is also true of grass, where high ball velocity and ball bounce are commonplace. Clay is probably the most forgiving surface, but ball bounce consistency is dependent on its quality and upkeep.

An EMG analysis by Morris et al.[56] on nine professionals and college tennis players compared muscle activity in the serve and ground stroke. The muscles studied were the biceps and brachial muscles; the extensor muscles of the fingers; and the ECRL, ECRB, PT, and FCR. Morris et al. described the primary function of the elbow muscles in the ground stroke as one of forearm and wrist stabilization, allowing the arm to transfer energy from the trunk and shoulder to the racket. In the serve, the primary muscle function is to produce joint movement. Morris et al. found low muscle activity throughout the elbow in preparation and late follow-through. In all ground strokes with acceleration, there was marked activity of the wrist extensors, plus high biceps and brachial activity in the forehand stroke. These findings continued through the early follow-through phase.

Angular velocity in the tennis serve has been reported to reach 1700 degrees per second for elbow extension[35,57] and 315 degrees per second for wrist flexion.[58] In their EMG analysis, Morris et al.[56] found low muscle activity through the windup. There was high wrist extensor activity in the late cocking and acceleration phases, with additional high activity of the triceps when extending the elbow and of the PT when providing power and position to the forearm in acceleration. The biceps was the only muscle with significant activity in the follow-through, apparently acting as a decelerator.

Lateral tennis elbow, first described by Runge in 1873,[59] is reported to be far more common than medial tennis elbow in tennis. It is most commonly seen in 35- to 55-year-old players.[53,60] Because the origin of the ECRB is anterior to the elbow's flexion-extension axis of rotation, it is subject to a shearing stress in all movement of the forearms, especially where power is being imparted. Anterior rotation of the radial head against the tendon during pronation adds to the stresses. Thus, a vigorous grip with the hand ulnarly deviated and pronated can be excessively strenuous to the ECRB tendon.[61] Nirschl[62] likened the mechanical predisposition of the ECRB to a disadvantaged leverage system, in that the medially sloping lateral condyle creates a fulcrum effect via the prominent radial head.

Medial tennis elbow, although five times less common than lateral tennis elbow, is still a significant problem in tennis. The serve and overhead strokes subject the medial elbow and ulnar nerve to the same valgus stresses imposed by baseball pitching. Tennis ground strokes have been noted by Nirschl (Nirschl RP, personal observation, 1986) to subject the common flexor origin, primarily the PT and FCR, to tension overuse, resulting in medial tennis elbow.

THE ELBOW IN SWIMMING

Although the elbow is not a common site of complaint among recreational swimmers, the rigorous training demands of competitive swimming may magnify otherwise manageable stresses. Elbow injury can result from arm pull in the butterfly, the breast stroke, and, less frequently, the freestyle stroke, where an excessively high elbow position can result in medial tendon overload. Dropping the elbow results in a less effective angle with which to push the water back, which can also overload the extensor tendons.[63]

Johnson[64] describes the forces on the elbow that can lead to injury among the backstrokers. During the midportion of the pull-through, forces are maximized on the biceps and brachioradial muscles and the MCL,

TABLE 27–4
Stroke Factors in Tendinosis About the Elbow

Stroke	Recreational Player	Highly Skilled Player
Backhand	Poor weight transfer, front shoulder up, use of forearm extensors for power → lateral tennis elbow	Repeated concentrated contraction of wrist extensors for stabilization → lateral tennis elbow
Forehand	Late forehand with wrist snap to bring racket head to the ball → lateral tennis elbow or medial tennis elbow Faulty form of pronating over ball to impart topspin → medial tennis elbow	
Serve and overhead	Forceful extension → posterior tennis elbow	Valgus stress in cocking to acceleration → medial tennis elbow Forceful pronation and wrist snap on impact → lateral tennis elbow Forceful extension → posterior tennis elbow

which may result in overload injuries to these tissues. Triceps tendon strain or pinching of the synovium of the olecranon fossa can result from full elbow extension at the end of the pull-through.

THE ELBOW IN GYMNASTICS

Garrick and Regua[65] reported that although nearly one third of all gymnastics injuries occur in the upper extremity, only about 7 percent of these are likely to be elbow injuries. Snook[66] reported that of 66 major injuries, only four occurred at the elbow, and all of these were dislocations. Elbow injuries are far more common among female gymnasts than among males.[67,68] This is attributable to a variety of factors, including a tendency for girls to be most involved in the sport at a more vulnerable age (female maximum involvement occurs at 15 years of age; male maximum involvement occurs at 20 to 22 years of age).[68] Furthermore, competitive activities in female routines are more demanding to the elbow (e.g., the locked-out position for the women's floor exercises, vault, and beam). Finally, the increased valgus carrying angle of the female elbow may render it more vulnerable to medial instability problems.

In general, gymnastic elbow injuries are more likely to be due to a single traumatic event rather than overuse.[66] Priest and Wiese[69] studied 32 elbow injuries in 30 females, 28 of which were acute injuries (e.g., fractures, dislocations); two patients developed Panner disease. Elbow dislocation is the most common single-event gymnastic injury caused by an overwhelming hyperextension force. In a study by Priest[70] of fracture-dislocations of the elbow in 30 female gymnasts, the average age at injury was 13.6 years; all injuries were due to a fall on the outstretched hand (FOOSH), and 60 percent were due to a lack of adequate spotting and/or too thin a mat. Dislocation occurred most often on the uneven bars, followed by floor exercises, the balance beam, and, finally, vaulting.

Inability to regain full elbow extension can be devastating to the gymnast, as it is essential to sport performance. Osteochondritis, or Panner disease, may result from repeated use of the upper extremity as a weight-bearing structure with the elbow in the locked-out position. Finally, this demand on the elbow during the growing years, in combination with the natural valgus angle at the elbow, may result in stretching of the flexor muscle mass or the UCL, with resultant injury.

Certain issues are essential to prevent an upper extremity overuse injury in gymnastics. These include an effective upper body strengthening and flexibility program, cyclical training, and alternating swinging and support events in each workout. A lack of adequate spotters during practice and inadequate mat thickness have been implicated in the frequency of traumatic injuries. As Peter Korman, the Olympic medalist, noted, "All gymnasts work out and compete with ongoing problems in their upper extremities. These problems are only considered serious injuries when the gymnasts can no longer compete."[67]

BOXER'S ELBOW

Boxer's elbow has been described as an avulsion fracture of the olecranon process occurring as the olecranon impacts in the fossa when a forceful jab misses the target. Boxers in general do not have a high incidence of elbow injuries but can be subject to all of the maladies described in other sports.

TRAUMATIC ELBOW INJURIES

DISLOCATIONS

The elbow is second only to the shoulder as the most commonly dislocated joint. The sports of cycling, gymnastics, football, and wrestling contribute greatly to this statistic. In children under 10 years old, the elbow is the most dislocated joint. Dislocations of the elbow joint complex are classified by the displacement of the radius and ulna on the humerus. A posterior or posterolateral dislocation is by far the most common and is generally caused by a fall on the outstretched arm or by a violent hyperextension and abduction force.

Elbow hyperextension ruptures or avulses the UCL or fractures the medial epicondyle with the attached UCL. This allows the coronoid to disengage from the trochlea, and the olecranon levers posteriorly out of the fossa (Fig. 27–4). Additional injuries in posterior dislocations may include ruptures of the anterior capsule, LCL, the brachial muscle, and common forearm flexor and extensor origins, as well as radial head or radial neck fractures, tear of brachial artery, injury to nerves (ulnar, median or radial), and avulsion or entrapment and

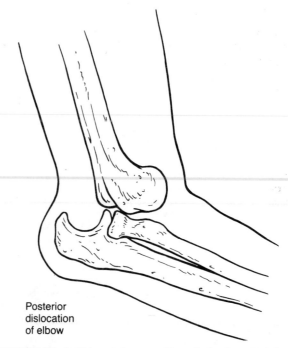

Posterior
dislocation
of elbow

FIGURE 27–4. Elbow dislocation. (From Richardson JK, Iglarsh ZA: Clinical Orthopaedic Physical Therapy. Philadelphia, WB Saunders, 1994, p 232.)

avulsion of the medial epicondylar apophysis. With a dislocation, the athlete generally presents with severe pain and swelling and the elbow held in 45 degrees of flexion, while the forearm appears shortened and the olecranon is prominent posteriorly.

Anterior dislocations are quite rare and are often the result of a direct blow to the olecranon posteriorly when the elbow is flexed. Generally, anterior traumatic elbow dislocation tends to occur as an isolated incident. Recurrence is not common unless ligament insufficiency exists.

Isolated dislocations of the radial head are not likely, although subluxation of the radial head in young children ("housemaid's elbow") occurs with some frequency.

FRACTURES

Fractures of the shaft of the humerus in sports may result from a direct blow, a fall on the outstretched arm, or an indirect rotary torque on a fixed arm (e.g., a spiral fracture in wrestling). These fractures present with a sudden, dramatic onset and intense pain. Diagnosis is easily confirmed by radiograph, and initial treatment falls under the immediate purview of an orthopaedic surgeon. Initial treatment options include closed reduction and cast bracing or open reduction and internal fixation. Complicating nerve injury (radial, median, or ulnar) may affect the treatment decision. The role of the physical therapist comes later, when the humerus is adequately stabilized.

A fall on the outstretched arm may result in a supracondylar fracture, with possible injury or compromise to the vascular supply to the forearm as a result of swelling of the fascial compartments or direct traumatic insult by bone fragments. If not considered and attended to immediately, an ischemic necrosis of these muscles (i.e., a Volkmann ischemic contracture) can be the tragic result. Complaints of coldness, numbness, and/or stiffness of the fingers in the presence or absence of a radial pulse call for immediate elevation of the arm, removal of all compressive bandages, and immediate orthopaedic surgical consultation.

Olecranon fractures usually occur from direct trauma (e.g., a fall from a bike). A fracture of this type is otherwise uncommon in athletic activity.

Acute valgus stress from a fall or a muscle contraction in throwing may lead to a fracture through the epiphyseal (apophyseal) plate of the medial epicondyle in young athletes. Salter type I fractures may occur in children with an open apophysis, wherein the entire apophysis is avulsed by the pull of the forearm flexors and the MCL progressing in quantification to the entire apophysis being either partially or totally avulsed by the pull of the common forearm flexors and the UCL. Type II fractures (avulsion through the apophysis with a fragment of bone) occur in adolescents with an essentially closed apophysis.[14,46]

Fractures of the radius and ulna are generally caused by direct blows. The critical issue in these fractures is to correct the angular displacement, restoring the normal anatomic skeletal bends (primarily in the radius) and the proper rotational alignment for pronation-supination.[71] If the radial fracture is in the proximal one third, each of the fragments is acted on by muscles with an agonistic effect (e.g., the supinators on the upper fragment and the pronators on the lower one), resulting in maximal displacement potential (e.g., the proximal fragment supinated and the distal fragment pronated). On the other hand, displacement is less marked in a radial fracture in the middle third of the shaft, because each fragment's displacement is checked (i.e., supination of the upper fragment is checked by the pronator, and only the pronator quadratus is pronating the lower fragment).[20] Distal one third fractures of the radius are relatively uncommon but may be difficult to immobilize because the extensors dynamically pull the distal fragment into dorsal displacement.

Isolated fractures of the ulna from a direct blow in contact sports (e.g., lacrosse, martial arts, hockey) are more likely to occur in the distal aspect.[72] The Monteggia fracture, in which there is dislocation (usually anterior) of the radial head with a displaced fracture of the ulna, is seen in cycling accidents and collision sports such as football. In any fracture or dislocation about the proximal radius, the posterior interosseous nerve may be insulted, resulting in dysfunction (usually temporary neurapraxia, which usually resolves with conservative treatment).[71]

Fractures of the coronoid process of the ulna, although rarely seen in isolation, occur in approximately 15 percent of athletes with posterior elbow dislocations.[73] The bone is avulsed by the brachial muscle when the elbow is hyperextended or by abutment of the trochlea during forcible posterior displacement of the proximal end of the ulna. There is some debate, dependent on the quantity of the fracture fragment, as to whether this displaced fragment results in recurrent dislocations.[14,73] Clinically, the elbow is swollen with marked limitation of motion (e.g., 50 to 90 degrees), and there is tenderness in the antecubital area, palpable crepitus, and anteroposterior instability.

CONTUSIONS

The humerus is subject to contusion from a fall or a direct blow in collision sports; such contusions may result in transitory loss of elbow motion, pain, and weakness of any involved muscles. Contusions occur most commonly at the bony projections. Contusions along the lateral epicondyle or posterolateral humerus may potentially injure the radial nerve. If so, the symptoms of pain into the forearm and wrist, numbness and tingling of the dorsal hand (usually the first dorsal web space), and wrist extensor weakness may exist.[72]

"Blocker's exostosis" describes a more serious contusion of the lateral humerus just distal to the deltoid insertion and lateral to the biceps muscles, with potential formation of a subperiosteal hematoma. Subsequent calcification within the hematoma may lead to myositis ossificans. A painful, firm mass is palpable just beyond the deltoid insertion.[72] Ice, a compression sling, or splint immobilization followed by gentle active range of motion and electrical stimulation are indicated. Passive stretching must be avoided so as not to further injure the muscle. Rarely, surgical removal when the injury process is completed (usually 1 year) may be appropriate.

A contusion along the medial epicondyle may result in ulnar nerve injury and possibly hemorrhage into the nerve fibers and sheath with permanent scarring and impaired nerve function. There are ulnar nerve symptoms of pain, numbness and tingling into the fourth and fifth fingers, weakness of the interossei, and tenderness along the zones of the medial epicondylar groove. A positive Tinel sign is usually present.

ACUTE MUSCLE–TENDON INJURIES

In general, injury may occur by tendon rupture from bone or at the musculotendinous junction or in the mid-muscle. Injury to the muscle–tendon units about the elbow generally results not from direct trauma, but from a violent eccentric tension load when the muscle–tendon unit is in concentric contraction (e.g., injury to the biceps or brachial muscle during forced elbow extension or to the triceps in forced elbow flexion). Injury prevention in these circumstances, other than developing contractile function, energy-absorbing capabilities, and flexibility that are superior to the tensile load, is virtually impossible. Peterson and Renstrom[74] found that after mid-muscle injury, although the active concentric force production capabilities of an injured muscle recover to 90 percent of the preinjury level by day 7, the tensile strength recovers to only 77 percent. Depending on the quantity of muscle injury, rehabilitation may take substantial time to restore full functional capabilities. Major hemorrhage into muscle also prolongs the rehabilitation time.

Rupture of the distal biceps tendon from the radial tuberosity is uncommon but not rare, occurring most commonly in middle-aged athletes. Because the biceps function (i.e., elbow flexion and forearm supination) is a backup to brachial and supinator function, surgical intervention may not be necessary to maintain activities of daily living. Baker and Bierwagen[75] studied 13 patients with biceps tendon rupture from the radius 15 months to 6 years after injury. The mechanism of injury in all was extrinsic violent extension against an actively flexing muscle (e.g., lifting a heavy object, as in a flexor curl, or spotting in gymnastics). Ten injuries were surgically repaired, followed by 4 weeks of postoperative immobilization, 4 weeks of active and passive motion, and then strengthening for 2 to 4 months. The three patients treated conservatively were in a sling for 3 weeks, followed by 5 weeks of range-of-motion exercises, and then strengthening for 4 months. Those who underwent surgery returned to normal strength and endurance of elbow flexion and supination (approximately 10 percent greater than in the nondominant arm), while those in the nonoperative group were significantly weaker in supination and elbow flexion with respect to the nondominant arm. The nonoperative group complained of movement restrictions out-

side of activities of daily living (e.g., inability to use a basketball, bat, or screwdriver). Bourne and Morrey[76] described a rare case of a partial rupture of the distal biceps, in which the tendon was partially avulsed from the radial tuberosity, then was surrounded by granulation and scar tissue that remained palpable. The patient would feel a pop, but swelling and bruising might or might not occur. The lacertus fibrosis, which assists in flexion but not supination, was intact and palpable. Elbow flexion and supination strength were somewhat compromised. For maximum result, Bourne and Morrey recommended surgical completion of the rupture, followed by reattachment. If less than normal function is acceptable to the patient (e.g., limited athletic aspirations), then 3 weeks of immobilization followed by progressive motion and strengthening may be considered.

Traumatic ligament sprains and ruptures to the UCL and LCL may result from a fall on the outstretched arm, a blow, or overwhelming force (e.g., in javelin throwers) or may accompany dislocation. Most commonly, however, ligament injuries occur as the result of repetitive overuse. In the dislocation group, healing may occur without surgery, but continuing evidence of instability indicates a need for surgical correction to achieve a stable elbow.[14]

REPETITIVE OVERUSE INJURIES

GENERAL CONCEPTS

Overuse injuries about the elbow often involve multiple pathoanatomic changes to different structures, including tendon, muscle, ligament, nerve, synovium, and articular surfaces. The changes are the products of a combination of intrinsic and extrinsic factors (i.e., multiple etiologies). Extrinsic factors include training errors, equipment, sport technique, and environmental conditions. Intrinsic factors include genetic and constitutional predisposition (e.g., malalignment, tissue quality), uncorrected sport-imposed deficiencies, muscular imbalance, and joint laxity. In the young athlete, these factors are compounded by the growth process, including periods of accelerated growth with relative soft tissue inflexibility and vulnerability of the apophysis to repeated overload.

ARTICULAR AND OSSEOUS OVERUSE INJURIES

A study by Gore et al.[38] on 29 symptomatic elbows in professional, amateur, and adolescent athletes in racket and throwing sports (javelin, football, tennis, baseball) revealed significant osseous changes in response to the stresses of these sports. Generalized bony hypertrophy (i.e., thickening of the humeral shaft cortex, medial elbow, olecranon, olecranon fossa, and ulnar groove) was present in 90 percent of adults. Diffuse stress (i.e., hypertrophy and hypermaturity of the open growth centers) was common among adolescents. Ninety-four percent of the professional baseball players and 55 percent of the adolescent baseball pitchers showed osseous abnormalities. Loose bodies were common in professional pitchers' elbows (posteriorly more so than medially, with the least number occurring in the anterior and lateral compartments). Seventy-five percent of professional pitchers had medial joint line (ulnar) traction spurs, and some avulsion of the medial epicondylar apophysis was present in 33 percent of adolescent baseball pitchers.

Goodfellow and Bullough[77] studied 28 necropsy subjects in an effort to determine why some cartilage undergoes degenerative changes and other cartilage does not. They found chondromalacia in the rim of the radial head (which normally lacks contact with an opposing surface), even in young subjects. In sharp contrast, the humeroulnar joint showed minimal changes (all surfaces of this joint contact the opposing cartilage at some point in their movement). Goodfellow and Bullough concluded that chondromalacia, or degeneration of the physical state of the articular cartilage, presents in those areas of cartilage that do not normally articulate with opposing cartilage. Their findings and conclusions are at variance with those of Nirschl, whose surgical observations on active athletes revealed significant chondromalacic changes in the olecranon fossa, posterolateral joint, capitellum, and center of the radial head. Interestingly, the rim of the radial head is usually spared of chondromalacic changes. Radiocapitellar chondromalacia likely results from valgus instability and repeated lateral compression stresses in a throwing elbow (a point perhaps not appreciated when dealing with elbows of nonathletes). Crepitus, catching, and tenderness to palpation are common chondromalacia symptoms.[78] Valgus extension overload and hyperextension overload syndrome, other effects of repeated hyperextension stress on an elbow with medial laxity, usually result in impingement of the posteromedial olecranon tip into its fossa, leading to osteophyte and loose body formation in this area.

Cox and Nirschl[79] have commonly noted combined anterior and posterior articular changes in racket and throwing sport athletes. The athlete complains of elbow pain that increases with stresses imposed by the sport. There may be catching, locking, crepitus, and loss of extension and flexion. The end points of motion feel hard and painful.

When bony blockade is present, the usual conservative efforts are generally unsuccessful. For posterior problems, Bryan[39] recommended surgical removal of the osteophytes. Rehabilitation starts with vigorous range-of-motion (ROM) exercise 2 days postoperatively, a return to light tossing at 6 weeks, and then full return to pitching at 10 weeks postoperatively. For combination problems, Cox and Nirschl[79] also recommend aggressive rehabilitation, starting at 2 days from the extended position; light throwing is usually started by 4 weeks. Because the combination problem includes surgical release of the anterior capsule, it is important to start from the extended position so as to eliminate recurrent anterior capsular scarring in a flexed position. A light extensor elbow immobilizer in the first 10 days postoperatively virtually eliminates the need for dynamic elbow splints and/or continuous passive motion (CPM) machines.

Triceps insertion problems may occur as a result of repeated traction on the proximal olecranon during the late ball release and sharp elbow extension phases of throwing or in the serve and overhead strokes of tennis. Injury can also occur to the olecranon apophysis at the triceps insertion. The young athlete (9 to 15 years old) will complain of pain at the insertion site (increased pain with extension), tenderness on palpation, and pain on a triceps provocative muscle test.[4,39] Olecranon stress fractures may occur in javelin throwers and baseball pitchers. Generally there is a long history of pain that recurs with throwing. Unless avulsion occurs, rest and gradual rehabilitation are effective treatment.

OSTEOCHONDRITIS DISSECANS AND PANNER DISEASE

Osteochondritis dissecans has been described by Harrelson[42] as the leading cause of permanent disability in the young pitching athlete. It usually presents in the capitellum of 12- to 15-year-olds as a result of vascular insufficiency from repetitive lateral compression at the radiocapitellar joint during the late cocking and acceleration phases in pitching or during the "back scratch" and acceleration phases of the tennis serve. Brown et al.[80] studied 18 athletes with osteochondritis dissecans and osteochondrosis (Panner disease), all participating in throwing and racket sports. They and Singer and Roy[81] described these two conditions as different stages of the same entity that are related to the age of the individual and the direction and level of activity. There is controversy, however, since Panner disease encompasses the entire capitellum and occurs at a younger age (i.e., 7 to 10 years). Loose body formation is much less likely to occur in Panner disease (Fig. 27–5). Pain is

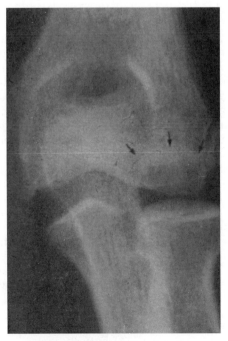

FIGURE 27–5. Panner disease.

present over the lateral and anterior elbow and is worsened by deep palpation or pronation-supination. Extension may be limited by 20 degrees or more secondary to a distortion of capitellar congruity and synovitis. Complete rest from the offending activity (i.e., compression loads) is indicated, combined with gentle stretching within the limited motion.

In those cases of osteochondritis dissecans that fail to respond to conservative treatment but in which loose bodies have not occurred, surgical drilling has been somewhat successful in restoring vascular supply. In those cases in which loose body formation results in grinding, catching, or extension block, surgical removal may be necessary. Return to racket and throwing sports is usually attainable, but return to a compression loading sport such as gymnastics is problematic.

BURSITIS

Of the superficial bursae about the elbow, the olecranon bursa is the most commonly injured in sports, usually from direct trauma, most often by falls (e.g., in wrestling, martial arts, football, roller blading). With chronic irritation, the bursal wall thickens, and inflammatory fluid fills the bursa. Infection may occur due to skin breakdown and poor blood supply in the area. If infection occurs, drainage plus antibiotic treatment is indicated.

Of the deep bursae, the bicipital radial bursae at the radial tuberosity may become inflamed. Symptoms include crepitus on pronation-supination. Treatment with anti-inflammatory medication, elimination of the offending activity, and gradual endurance and flexibility rehabilitation is generally successful.

MUSCLE–TENDON OVERUSE

LATERAL TENNIS ELBOW TENDINOSIS/LATERAL EPICONDYLITIS. The term *tennis elbow* was introduced in the 1880s by Major and Runge.[59] Prior to the 1970s, the offending pathoanatomy was thought to be inflammation about the lateral epicondyle or the extensor communis.[82] In 1979, Nirschl and Pettrone[83] described the surgical pathology as an alteration of the ECRB due to a degenerative process. Because no histologic evidence of inflammatory cells was present, the term *angiofibroblastic tendinosis* was coined as a histologically descriptive term. In lateral tennis elbow, this pathoanatomic change occurs primarily in the ECRB and secondarily at the extensor digitorum communis (EDC). Although the pathology was initially thought to be an inflammatory reparative process, as previously noted, no inflammatory cells were found in surgical specimens. Thus, Nirschl and Pettrone concluded that the term *tendinitis* is a misnomer. Although there is some discussion as to the exact order of progression, the theoretical progression is fatigue, infrastructure breakdown, and vascular compromise to the tissue, resulting in an altered nutritional state, oxygen deprivation, and, finally, angiofibroblastic tendinosis. In gross surgical examination, the tissue is easily identifiable and appears grayish, edematous, and friable.

In the lateral elbow, the ECRB is particularly vulnerable as it crosses the elbow and can be easily overloaded by excess eccentric contractions of the wrist extensors (commonly noted in the tennis backhand) to decelerate and/or absorb energy. The ECRB undergoes its greatest lengthening in an extended elbow with the forearm in pronation and the wrist flexed and ulnarly deviated (a common forced position in the tennis backhand).

The extensor muscles are subject to force overload by repetitive intrinsic concentric muscle contraction. The recreational athlete may subject the elbow to additional stress during his or her daily activities or occupation. Carpentry work, excessive computer keyboard time, weight lifting, needlework, cooking, gardening, playing the piano or video games, or any activity involving large amounts of wrist action or stabilization will contribute to tissue overload with compromised tissue reparability. Occupations at risk that may require surgical intervention include such diverse groups as construction workers, carpenters, musicians, journalists, politicians, and those in any occupation requiring repetitive forearm rotation and wrist extension.

In certain individuals lateral tennis elbow may also be associated with fibromyalgia in other areas. In 1969, Nirschl[84] described the mesenchymal syndrome. In about 15 percent of lateral elbow patients (women more so than men), systemic tendinosis occurred in which there were multiple sites of pain or tendon alteration. He theorized that the condition was due to a constitutional factor, most probably some form of tendon collagen distortion. Chop[85] suggested that cigarette smoking could be a factor, as nicotine decreases and distorts the peripheral circulation, thereby decreasing the oxygen and nutrition supply to the elbow. Notably, the use of steroid injections can contribute to other tendon changes, including tears, cellular death, and tissue distortion other than tendinosis.[86] These changes found at surgery are histologically distinguishable from tendinosis.

Clinically, pain is generally the primary complaint and is localized just anterior and distal to the lateral epicondyle. The pain is provoked by resisted wrist extension, as in lifting a coffee cup or shaking hands. Tenderness directly over the ECRB origin is the most common sign. Provocative resistance testing of the wrist extensors with the elbow extended is almost always positive. Cervical problems, particularly at C6–C7, should be ruled out. Other injuries to be considered in the differential diagnosis include posterior interosseus nerve entrapment, synovitis of the lateral compartment of the elbow, and osteophytes of the radiocapitellar joint.

The magnitude of lateral tennis elbow symptoms in large part reflects the volume of tendon alteration. Based on this observation, Nirschl has defined the stages of tendon overuse alteration (Table 27–5).

POSTERIOR INTEROSSEOUS NERVE ENTRAPMENT. In comparison with lateral tennis elbow tendinosis, posterior interosseous nerve entrapment is un-

TABLE 27-5
Nirschl Pathologic Stages of Tendon Overuse

Stage I:	Chemical inflammation
Stage II:	Tendinosis less than 50% of tendon origin or cross-sectional diameter.
Stage III:	Tendinosis greater than 50%
Stage IV:	Tendinosis with partial or complete tendon rupture

Note: Stages III and IV invariably result in surgical intervention.

common. The tenderness is more distal, and resisted supination is more painful than wrist extension. The nature of the pain is more of a vague, diffuse aching along the forearm and may be associated with numbness and tingling on the dorsum of the hand between the thumb and index finger if the superficial radial nerve (sensory branch) becomes entrapped. It is best to perform an EMG to validate the diagnosis. Werner[87] reported a cross-correlation in which 5 percent of his tennis elbow patients also had concurrent radial nerve entrapment. The differential diagnosis should also entertain the possibility of cervical osteoarthritis and radiculopathy.

SYNOVITIS OF THE POSTEROLATERAL COMPARTMENT OF THE ELBOW. Pain in the posterolateral gutter posterior to the lateral epicondyle may represent synovitis and/or chondromalacia. It has been our experience that this pain may be present after vigorous transverse friction massage to treat tennis elbow. In this instance, the symptoms will be fleeting. In the true synovitis presentation, the symptoms linger and often occur in combination with tennis elbow symptoms. The signs of synovitis include a palpable feeling of fullness in the gutter, often accompanied by crepitus. In the differential diagnosis, osteochondritis dissecans must also be considered.

MEDIAL TENNIS ELBOW TENDINOSIS (MEDIAL EPICONDYLITIS). Medial tennis elbow is similar to the lateral condition with respect to histologic pathoanatomy, but it occurs over the tip of the medial epicondyle, extending distally 1 to 2 inches along the common flexor origin (usually the PT and FCR). The racket and throwing sports, as well as the pull-through in swimming strokes, are common causes of overuse. Catching a divot in golf can also lead to the problem in the trailing arm.

The common signs include pain over the origin of the PT and FCR that increases with resisted provocative testing of wrist flexion and pronation with the elbow extended. Palpable tenderness is noted in the same areas on and about the medial epicondyle.

Neurapraxic symptoms of the ulnar nerve in zone III of the medial epicondylar groove, as it penetrates the FCU arcade, commonly accompany medial elbow tendinosis. Signs and symptoms include possible tenderness, a positive Tinel sign in zone III, possible motor dysfunction of the ulnar nerve–innervated muscles in the hand, and almost always sensory disturbance in the small and ring fingers.

A less common companion to medial tendinosis is UCL attrition and/or rupture at its attachment to the distal underside of the medial epicondyle. In this instance, tenderness will be at the distal underside of the medial epicondyle, and pain will be noted more so with valgus stress. With UCL rupture, valgus stress will also reveal instability.

POSTERIOR ELBOW TENDINOSIS. Posterior tennis elbow presents at the triceps insertion just proximal to the olecranon tip. Differential diagnosis includes olecranon bursitis, intra-articular (olecranon fossa) synovitis, chondromalacia, and loose bodies. The histology is similar to that in other tendinoses. Pain and tenderness are located at the triceps insertion. Provocative stress testing of resisted elbow extension and/or sitting press-ups magnifies the pain. Posterior tendinosis is most commonly seen in baseball pitchers and javelin throwers. The malady is commonly associated with olecranon compartment osseous changes.

TREATMENT OF ELBOW TENDINOSIS. The principles of tendinosis treatment are aimed at revitalization of the pathologic changes in the tendon. These changes have been described by Nirschl[53] as angiofibroblastic tendinosis with the histologic appearance of disorganized tendon, including young fibroblasts and vascular elements. Interestingly, there are no elements suggestive of an inflammatory etiology. The revitalization (i.e., treatment) process encourages revascularization with fibroblast and collagen production and, ultimately, collagen maturation. At the macro level, the rehabilitative process includes the enhancement of balanced muscular strength, endurance, and flexibility.

It should be noted that the pathologic elements may be focused in the tendons at the elbow, but strength loss is more global and often includes not only the forearm, but also the arm, shoulder, neck, and upper back muscle groups. The rehabilitation process must therefore include these areas as well.

The basic elements of the treatment protocol include the following:

- Control of pain
- Promotion of total healing
- Promotion of total body fitness with emphasis on total arm strengthening
- The control or elimination of abuse (i.e., injury-producing activity)
- Functional restoration of the arm through transitional exercise
- Surgical intervention as needed

LIGAMENT INJURIES

Jobe and Nuber[88] effectively summarize the stages of ligament change with injury. In the initial response, inflammation and edema occur with symptoms of acute pain with activity (such as throwing). Permanent changes, including scar formation, follow. Continued stress and bleeding may lead to calcification within the ligament. Pain plus loss of motion and joint crepitation often accompany these phases. Weakening of the ligament leads to the formation of ligament "stress risers" with increased vulnerability; these ultimately rupture (the final event may be minor stress). These phases are typical of attritional injury to the UCL in throwing athletes.

Injury to the LCL is less attritional and more likely to occur as a result of single-event macrotrauma, such as elbow dislocation or subluxation, or, as reported by Nirschl,[88a] from iatrogenic causes such as excessive surgical release of the common extensor tendon in older described techniques for lateral tennis elbow. Laxity or avulsion of the ulnar portion of the LCL may allow a rotatory subluxation of the ulnohumeral joint (possibly complete secondary dislocation). This has been described by O'Driscoll and Morrey[89] as posterolateral rotatory instability (PLRI) following single-event dislocating trauma. The ulnar portion of the LCL is lax or avulsed in this presentation, but the annular ligament is intact (i.e., the radioulnar joint remains intact). This rotatory subluxation occurs when the forearm supinates and the elbow extends, allowing both the radial head and the proximal ulna to slide posterolaterally below the capitellum. Symptoms include recurrent snapping and clicking or complete locking when subluxation of the elbow occurs during a supination and extension maneuver made either by the patient or by the examiner. The maneuver is essentially a lateral pivot shift test for PLRI that is best and most accurately done under anesthesia. If the test is positive, surgical reconstruction offers the best definitive treatment.[19,89]

PERIPHERAL NERVE DYSFUNCTION

The details of peripheral nerve anatomy, diagnosis, and treatment are addressed elsewhere in this text. Certain observations and concepts are presented by the physician author of this chapter concerning his experience in the area of the elbow.

ULNAR NERVE

The ulnar nerve is the most commonly injured or functionally altered nerve about the elbow. As previously noted, the medial epicondylar groove has been divided by Nirschl into three zones. Zone III (the area of the ulnar flexor arcade) is the most common offending area, with resultant compression neurapraxia symptoms secondary to impingement by a hypertrophied FCU muscle or a thickened retinaculum. In this situation, if conservative treatment fails, surgical decompression without ulnar nerve transfer has proven highly successful. Because the majority of ulnar nerve cases of this type are associated with medial tennis elbow, a combination tendon surgery and nerve decompression are performed.

Other compression etiologic factors concerning ulnar nerve dysfunction include the uncommon compression problems of zone II (joint synovitis or exostosis) and zone I (hypertrophied arcade of Struthers and medial intermuscular septum). Treatment of these compression neuropathies also consists of surgical decompression.

Ulnar nerve tension neuropathies are second in statistical importance to zone III compression neurapraxia. The most common of the tension group is congenital dislocation of the nerve (usually due to a shallow medial epicondylar groove). Other causes of tension neuropathy include elbow valgus instability (i.e., rupture of the UCL) and skeletal valgus deformity (either congenital or from a supracondylar fracture malunion [i.e., tardy ulnar palsy]). Ulnar nerve tension neuropathies are best addressed by anterior ulnar nerve transfer. If surgical intervention is undertaken, I recommend subcutaneous transfer utilizing a fascial buttress. Submuscular transfer should be avoided, as this technique is disruptive to the common flexor origin, increases postoperative morbidity, and has a high complication rate, including major scar formation about the transferred ulnar nerve.

I have noted occasional entrapment of the median nerve as it penetrates the PT arch (pronator syndrome) and the radial nerve as it enters the arcade of Froshe. These entrapments are highly uncommon, and the diagnosis must be confirmed by positive EMG findings.

The ulnar nerve is injured partly as a result of its superficial location, but most commonly because of intrinsic compressive and extrinsic tension forces. Although it is protected proximally and distally by musculature, it is unprotected in its medial epicondylar groove location. Of the three epicondylar zones, the cubital tunnel is most vulnerable (zone III). Several potential mechanisms of injury are possible and include the following:

- Single-event direct trauma (compression load)
- Tension. The nerve may become tethered by adhesions, but valgus stress is most common.
- Friction. Traction spurs, calcium deposits, or degenerative changes in the ulnar groove can compromise available space.
- Cumulative overload compression or entrapment with a thickened cubital tunnel retinaculum (the "Osborne lesion"). The arcuate ligament, which forms the roof of the tunnel, is increasingly taut beyond 90 degrees and may compress the nerve as elbow flexion increases. Hypertrophy of the FCU muscle may also cause compression of the nerve.
- Recurrent subluxation or dislocation out of the groove onto or over the tip of the medial epicondyle results in a combination of tension, compression, and friction. Childress[90] studied 2000 "normal" ulnar nerves in 1000 asymptomatic patients and found that in 16.2 percent of patients, the nerve displaced from its groove as the elbow flexed. Because none were symptomatic, he proposed that the probable cause is a congenital or developmental ligamentous laxity and the nerve remains asymptomatic until subjected to some form of trauma.
- Compression in zone I by the triceps medial head (often noted in weight lifters).
- Compression in zone II by medial joint line arthritic spurs or synovitis.

McGowan[91] defined three stages of ulnar neuropathy as follows:

- Stage I: paresthesias along digits 4 and 6, possibly from the hypothenar eminence.
- Stage II: weakness of the interossei.
- Stage III: atrophy of the interossei.

Likely symptoms include elbow pain about the medial epicondyle and in the ulnar nerve distribution, sensory radiation, and heaviness or clumsiness in the hand and fingers. The symptoms are worsened with activities involving valgus stresses or, in the occasion of nerve subluxation, by prolonged elbow flexion (e.g., during talking on the phone, sleeping with the elbow bent). In those with nerve dislocation, a painful snap or pop and sharp, radiating pain may accompany rapid elbow flexion and extension.

RADIAL NERVE

Mosher[92] describes the radial nerve as "almost totally a nerve of extensor function (except for the brachioradialis), which seems to have wandered astray by appearing in front of the elbow." To find its way back to the dorsal surface of the forearm, the motor branch (i.e., the posterior interosseus nerve [PIN]) passes through the radial tunnel, under the mobile wad of Henry (ECRB, ECRL, and brachioradial muscles) between the two heads of the supinator muscle. The proximal edge of the supinator forms an arch, the arcade of Frohse, under which it is most commonly entrapped. Other, less frequent compression sites include the fibrous band anterior to the radial head, under the fibrous borders of the ECRB, or, rarely, under the lateral head of the triceps.

Radial nerve entrapment is seen in throwers, swimmers, golfers, tennis players, and weight lifters. The symptoms of PIN compression differ somewhat from those of tennis elbow in that the complaint is a more diffuse, aching pain in the extensor muscles of the proximal forearm, possibly radiating into the dorsal aspect of the hand. Pain is increased by resisted supination of the extended elbow. Tenderness is experienced with palpation over the supinator muscle about four fingerbreadths distal to the lateral epicondyle. These symptoms, as well as possible night pain, distinguish PIN entrapment from lateral tennis elbow. Third finger extension should be tested in both problems, but for different reasons (i.e., to determine power loss in PIN entrapment and pain in tennis elbow).

MEDIAN NERVE

The median nerve is subject to compression under the ligament of Struthers, at the elbow, at the supracondylar process within the two heads of the PT, under the arch of the superficial head of the flexor digitorum superficialis, or under the lacertus fibrosis. Forced repetitions involving gripping and/or pronation of an extending forearm, as in weight lifting, gymnastics, and racket sports, may result in a vague, aching fatigue along the volar forearm, sometimes radiating distally to the hand. Electrodiagnostic testing of the sensory or motor distribution of the median nerve confirms the diagnosis.

Spinner and Linscheid[93] noted that an indentation of the flexor-pronator mass below the medial epicondyle may be a clinical sign suggesting that the lacertus fibrosis may be constricting the nerve in this location. Symptoms reproduced by resisting biceps contraction (i.e., supination and elbow flexion) will confirm this etiology. If the nerve is being compressed under the arch of the superficial flexor muscles of the fingers, resisted long finger flexion may reproduce symptoms. If the problem is at the PT, prolonged resisted pronation may reproduce the symptoms more so than direct pressure applied over the track of the PT (especially 4 cm distal to the antebrachial crease).

MUSCULOCUTANEOUS NERVE

Entrapment of the distal extension of the musculocutaneous nerve (i.e., lateral antebrachial cutaneous nerve) may occur over the lateral portion of the antecubital aponeurosis following repetitive and/or forceful pronation with elbow hypertension, compressing the nerve between the biceps tendon and the brachial fascia. A burning dysesthesia is experienced over the anterolateral forearm.

REHABILITATION

EVALUATION

The physical therapist's evaluation and treatment of acute single-event and overuse injuries of the elbow are guided by the athlete's subjective reports at the initiation of and throughout the rehabilitation process. Critical information needed from the outset is outlined in Tables 27–6 and 27–7.

PHYSICAL ASSESSMENT

INSPECTION

Hoppenfeld[94] described the normal carrying angle of the elbow (the angle between the long axis of the humerus and that of the ulna) as 5 to 10 degrees in males and 10 to 15 degrees in females; Morrey and An[13] reported the normal carrying angle to be 10 to 15 degrees in males and 15 to 20 degrees in females. Unilateral alterations in the carrying angle may result from a previous fracture. Valgus malunion often results in ulnar nerve dysfunction. Intra-articular fractures often result in carrying angle changes plus blockade of elbow motion.

Is joint swelling global or diffuse? With synovitis or effusion, the normal contour dimple of the lateral infracondylar recess may be obliterated. Local swelling suggests contusion. Olecranon bursa swelling is a classic sign of bursitis.

Reaction to cortisone injections may result in wasting of the subcuticular fat at the area of injection, usually

TABLE 27–6
Information Algorithm for Rehabilitation Protocol

1. Sport and activity
   a. Technique, training habits
   b. Recent changes in equipment (e.g., tennis racket head size, stringing tension, grip)
   c. Conditioning activities
2. Occupation
   a. Relevant daily activities (e.g., carpentry, musical instruments, needlework)
   b. Specific occupational activities
3. Onset of symptoms (acute vs. insidious)
   a. Date of onset
   b. Mechanism of injury (direct blows, hyperextension, hypertension, twisting, etc.)
   c. Any abnormal pops, sounds, or sensation? Any swelling?
4. Pain location
   a. Localized or diffuse, anterior-posterior, medial-lateral
   b. Anterior pain suggests biceps or capsule
   c. Posterior pain suggests olecranon bursitis, valgus extension overload syndrome (chondromalacia), triceps tendinosis
   d. Medial pain is often due to medial tendinosis, flexor/pronator mass strain, UCL injury (posterior to medial epicondyle), ulnar nerve compression
5. Quality of pain
   a. Aching, burning, or radiating may indicate nerve dysfunction
   b. Is the pain improving, worsening, or the same?
6. Is the pain affected by rest or activity or position of the elbow and/or forearm?
7. Pain intensity (see Table 27–7)
8. Additional symptoms (instability, snapping, catching or locking, loss of motion, or crepitus [may indicate articular changes, synovitis, loose bodies])
9. Prior injury history and surgeries
10. Symptoms in other body parts (shoulder, neck, back, legs, etc.)
    a. Neck and shoulder pathoanatomy may be associated problems
11. Medications
12. Current and prior treatment
    a. Results
    b. Unorthodox treatments (may need to question patient closely)

TABLE 27–7
Nirschl Classification of Tendinosis Phases of Pain

Phase I:	Mild pain after exercise activity, resolves within 24 hours
Phase II:	Pain after exercise activity, exceeds 48 hours, resolves with warm-up
Phase III:	Pain with exercise activity that does not alter activity
Phase IV:	Pain with exercise activity that alters activity
Phase V:	Pain caused by heavy activities of daily living
Phase VI:	Intermittent pain at rest that does not disturb sleep; pain caused by light activities of daily living
Phase VII:	Constant rest pain (dull aching) and pain that disturbs sleep

the end feel, the nature and location of the motion barrier, and the relationship of pain to the motion barrier should be noted. Normal elbow range of motion is 0 to 150 degrees flexion with 75 degrees pronation and 85 degrees supination.[95] Table 27–8 identifies normal factors limiting motion of the EJC. A 5-degree loss of terminal extension is considered a usual response to recurrent anterior capsular sprains and forearm flexor strains in throwing athletes and does not affect performance.[96] In gymnasts, on the other hand, such contractures will quite certainly affect performance and may result in having to end competitive participation. Hard end points and greater losses of motion may indicate arthritic and osseous etiologies and must be evaluated with radiographs and other means.

Loss of elbow flexion may be caused by osteophytic arthritis, intra-articular loose bodies, posterior capsule tightness, or possibly triceps tendinosis. Pronation and supination loss may occur as a result of osseous or soft tissue abnormality at the proximal or distal radioulnar joints. Bony synostosis or previous fracture must be considered in the differential evaluation.

STRENGTH

Although the data on elbow strength are relatively limited, some studies and clinical observations do provide basic guidelines, which will be discussed later in this chapter.[35,97–103] Initial manual muscle testing includes (Table 27–9) the following:

- Elbow flexed at 90 degrees with the forearm pronated, neutral, and supinated
- Elbow extended with forearm pronation, supination, and neutral
- Wrist flexion and extension and radial and ulnar deviation with the elbow straightened and flexed
- Finger abduction, flexion, and extension
- Dynamometer grip strength with the elbow flexed at 90 degrees and in full extension

Isokinetic testing may add valuable quantitative data. The ratio of pronation to supination and of wrist flexion to extension should be recorded. Pain (both location and intensity) on these tests is of great significance and

the lateral elbow. The atrophy is easily visible and sometimes occurs in conjunction with skin changes (i.e., thinning and loss of pigment). Hypersensitivity to touch or gentle percussion is often present.

It is essential to note alterations of muscular size, using the uninvolved arm for comparison. It is normal to see hypertrophy of the dominant forearm arm in athletes competing in racket and throwing sports. Circumferential forearm measurement using a tape measure is a simple and effective way to assess muscular size.

RANGE OF MOTION

Passive elbow flexion, extension, pronation, and supination should be evaluated. If restrictions are present, should also be recorded.[120] A review of the literature in isokinetic testing is presented in Tables 27–10 through 27–12.

SPECIAL TESTS FOR ASSESSMENT

LIGAMENTOUS INSTABILITY. Valgus and varus stress testing should be performed at approximately 20 degrees of extension, unlocking the olecranon from its fossa and relaxing the anterior capsule. Varus stress is applied with the humerus in relaxed internal rotation and the forearm in relaxed supination. Valgus testing is performed with the humerus in full external rotation and the forearm in relaxed supination. Posterolateral

stability testing is performed by axial loading as the elbow extends and the forearm supinates.

TINEL TEST FOR ULNAR NEUROPATHY. Tapping in the medial epicondylar groove will produce tingling (a positive result) along the ulnar nerve distribution. The clinician should accurately record the medial epicondylar zone in which the test is positive.

ELBOW FLEXION TEST FOR CUBITAL TUNNEL SYNDROME (ZONE III) COMPRESSION. Buehler and Thayer[104] reported a positive elbow flexion test in 13 patients with positive EMG results and clinical evidence of ulnar neuropathy. In this test the elbow is held in full flexion with the wrist extended for 3 minutes. All patients noted development of pain, numbness, and/or tingling along the ulnar nerve distribution. A positive test is usually reflective of entrapment in medial epicondylar zone III, but could also represent a nerve dislocation anteriorly over the medial epicondyle.

RADIOHUMERAL JOINT ASSESSMENT. Pain on provocative axial loading of the forearm with passive pronation and supination and with the elbow in extension suggests chondromalacia of the capitellum or radial head. Palpable pain and or crepitus anterolaterally or posterolaterally confirms the diagnosis of chondromalacia, synovitis, loose bodies, osteochondritis, or all of these.[105]

HUMEROULNAR JOINT. Pain on axial loading of the elbow while flexing and extending suggests chondromalacia of the humeral trochlea and ulnar articulation, as reported by Ferlic and Morrey.[105] Blockage of full flexion suggests scar tissue in the humeral coronoid fovea or bony exostosis of the ulnar coronoid process. Blockade of full extension is often the result of adhesions of the anterior capsule to the anterior humerus. Palpable crepitus of any fullness in the zone II area of the medial epicondylar groove (medial joint line) is often reflective of osteoarthritic exostosis and associated synovitis.

POSTERIOR OLECRANON COMPARTMENT. Palpable crepitus, fullness, or swelling is indicative of synovitis, chondromalacia, olecranon exostosis, loose body formation, or all of these. Associated bony blockade is particularly reflective of bony exostosis or olecranon fossa loose body formation.

LATERAL TENNIS ELBOW ASSESSMENT. Pain over the ECRB origin with the wrist extended (e.g., on lifting a coffee cup or using a computer keyboard), is a classic symptom of lateral tennis elbow. Anderson[106] described a test to stretch the extensor tendon by flexing the wrist while pronating and then supinating the forearm. Pain with resisted wrist and finger extension is a classic sign of the more common ECRB tendinosis. These provocative tests should be performed with the elbow first fully extended and then flexed at 90 degrees. If symptoms are reproduced with the elbow flexed, the degree of tendinosis is likely to be more significant (stage III or IV) and may indicate the need for surgical intervention. A test to differentiate lateral tennis elbow tendinosis from PIN entrapment is performed by resisted supination. Diffuse pain along the motor branches of the forearm muscles may indicate PIN entrapment. Palpable tenderness is less intense and more diffuse than the ECRB-focused tenderness of lateral tennis elbow ap-

---

TABLE 27–8
Normal Factors Limiting Motion of the Elbow Joint Complex

Motion	Active	Passive
Elbow flexion	Anterior muscle bulk of arm and forearm	RH against radial fossa of humerus, coronoid process against coronoid fossa, tension of triceps and posterior capsule
Elbow extension	Impact of olecranon in fossa, tautness of AOL of MCL, anterior capsule tension, biceps and brachial resistance	
Pronation	Passive resistance of the stretched antagonist quadrate ligament	Tissue impingement of FPL forced against FDP
Supination	Same as pronation	Same as pronation

AOL, Anterior oblique ligament; FDP, flexor digitorum profundus; FPL, flexor pollicis longus; MCL, medial collateral ligament; RH, radial head.

TABLE 27–9
Muscles Tested During Physical Examination

Elbow flexion: Biceps, brachial, brachioradial
Elbow extension: Triceps, anconeus
Forearm pronation: Pronator teres, pronator quadratus, brachioradial (full supination)
Forearm supination: Supinator, biceps, brachioradial (full pronation to neutral)
Wrist extension: ECLR, ECRB, ECU, EDC
Wrist flexion: FCR, FCU, FDS, PL

proximately 1 cm distal and anteromedial to the lateral epicondyle.

MEDIAL TENNIS ELBOW ASSESSMENT. Palpable tenderness over the tip of the medial epicondyle extending distally 1 to 2 inches along the track of the PT and FCR is the classic presentation. A positive provocative stress test elicits pain in the noted areas of palpable tenderness with resisted wrist flexion and forearm pronation. A positive test in 90 degrees of elbow flexion reflects a greater magnitude (stages III and IV) of tendinosis.

ULNAR COLLATERAL LIGAMENT ASSESSMENT. The mechanics of valgus stress testing has been discussed. A positive test (i.e., laxity that exceeds that in the opposite extremity) indicates a full-thickness tear of the ligament. Partial-thickness attritional tears may not demonstrate a positive valgus laxity, but may provoke pain. Evidence of palpable tenderness with provoked pain under and distal to the medial epicondyle should raise suspicions of partial damage to the UCL.

TREATMENT OF ELBOW INJURIES

The goal of any rehabilitation program is to return the injured area to its preinjured state, eradicate correctable injury-causing factors, and implement a maintenance fitness program to enhance performance and prevent reinjury. As part of the process, factors that predispose the elbow to injury must be considered (Table 27–13). Because the elbow is distal in the kinetic chain, any deficiency in the components of the chain, including the legs, must be corrected if injury recurrence is to be avoided.

Total upper quadrant assessment and conditioning are essential. General body conditioning (including the scapulothoracic, shoulder, arm, and hand muscle groups) can be initiated early on while still protecting the injured elbow. The importance of global rehabilitation was amplified by Priest et al.'s study,[5] which found twice as many shoulder injuries among tennis players with a history of tennis elbow. This has been our

TABLE 27–10
Elbow Isokinetic Results on Cybex Testing

Author	Population	Speed (deg/s)	Flexion/ Extension (%)	Approximate Peak Torque; Body Weight Flexion/ Extension (%)	Dominant vs. Nondominant (%)
Davies et al.[97]	U.S. cross-country ski team, 10 M, 10 F, dominant and nondominant averaged (female-male)	45 240 300	65–70 51–63 51–64	17–37/27–54 10–16/19–23 7–12/14–19	17–37/27–54
Wilk et al.[103]	Baseball pitchers	180 300	70–80 63–69		Flexors 10–20 Extensors 5–15
Schexneider et al.[99]	30 normal nonathletic males, dominant and nondominant aver-age	60 180 300		30/23 17 13	
Pawlowski & Perrin[98]	10 college baseball players, dominant and non-dominant averaged	60 240	10 100	23/23 Approx. 16	

TABLE 27–11
Forearm Isokinetic Results on Cybex Testing

Author	Population	Speed (deg/s)	Supination; Pronation Peak Torque (%)	Approximate Peak Torque; Body Weight Pronation/ Supination (%)
Sobel & Nirschl	70 normal tennis players (recreational and competitive), dominant arm	60	80°/s	
Ellenbecker[35]	22 highly skilled male tennis players	90 210 300	70 (work, 73) 73 (work, 73) 73 (work, 73)	7.8/5.5 (work, 8.5/6.3) 6.2/4.6 (work, 3.0/2.2) 5.2/3.8 (work, 1.6/1.2)

TABLE 27–12
Wrist Isokinetic Results on Cybex Testing

Author	Population	Speed (deg/s)	Wrist Extension/ Flexion Peak Torque (%)	Approximate Peak Torque; Body Weight Flexion/ Extension (%)	Dominant vs. Nondominant (%)
Van Swearingen[102]	32 normal nonathletes, 22–28 years old	60	62 (forearm neutral)		
Schexneider et al.[99]	30 normal, nonathletic males, dominant/ nondominant (averaged)	60 180 300	54 52 51	8/4.4 7/3.6 5/2.7	
Sobel & Nirschl*	70 normal recreational and competitive tennis players, male and female	60	60–70		10–20
Ellenbecker[35]	22 highly skilled tennis players, dominant	90 210 300	70 (work, 47) 64 (work, 45) 62 (work, 44)	8.4/59 (work, 10.3/4.9) 7.6/4.9 (work, 3.8/1.7) 6.7/4.2 (work, 2.1/0.91)	

*Unpublished Data; Virginia Sportsmedicine Institute, Arlington, VA, 1985.

observation as well.[4] Strizak et al.[101] studied isometric total arm strength in eight asymptomatic competitive tennis players and 12 nonplayers and compared the results to those in a population of symptomatic tennis elbow sufferers. The strength of the dominant arm was greater than that of the nondominant arm in all but the tennis elbow group. It has been our clinical experience that the great majority of athletes who present with tennis elbow have some, if not major, weakness of the scapulothoracic and rotator cuff muscle groups as noted by manual and isokinetic testing.

Although rehabilitation protocols are outlined in this section, attempting to fit each individual athlete's problems into a predetermined treatment protocol must be undertaken with caution. The success of a rehabilitation program is based on the ability of the program to be individualized to the magnitude of the pathologic lesion and to the athlete's lifestyle needs, goals, and rehabilitation progression. The progressive phases of injury rehabilitation are also based on the athlete's subjective and objective responses to treatment, as well as the clinician's knowledge of the stages of healing. In general, the phases are overlapping, and progression commonly vacillates throughout the rehabilitation period.

CONSERVATIVE TREATMENT

The basics of nonsurgical treatment for overuse injuries can be divided into two major stages: relief of pain and promotion of healing. The promotion of healing (stage II) consists of four phases: rehabilitative exercise, fitness exercise, advanced rehabilitation techniques, and control of abusive overload through activity modification, bracing, and proper equipment selection.

TABLE 27–13
Factors Predisposing to Elbow Injury

1. Genetic and constitutional factors
2. Sports and training factors
   a. Intensity, duration, and technique
3. Conditioning
   a. Strength, flexibility, and endurance
   b. Muscle imbalance
4. Previous injury with residual deficiency
   a. Correctable
   b. Not correctable

STAGE I: PAIN RELIEF AND INFLAMMATION CONTROLS

During this phase the injured area is protected against abusive overload while maintaining activity at as high a level as is possible or comfortable. Early exercise, therefore, to the noninjured adjacent areas, including overall fitness conditioning, is essential in the overall treatment process. Conditioning programs should include central aerobic exercise to enhance overall circulatory flow and oxygen diffusion. In most cases, this offers a great opportunity for the athlete to work on lower body and trunk agility drills, as well as plyometrics for improved sport performance.

Various modalities are used during this phase for their pain-relieving and anti-inflammatory effects. It has been our experience that each injury and each patient respond differently, and the therapist's best judgment should be combined with the patient's input in the choice of physical agents.

ICE. Ice is effective throughout the treatment program to slow the rate of cellular metabolic reaction, control histamine release, slow peripheral nerve conduction velocity, and promote vasoconstriction, thus lessening capillary bleeding and swelling.[61,107] Therefore, control of swelling is important not only for minimizing the harmful excesses of inflammatory exudation, but also for pain modulation.[108,109]

ULTRASOUND. Ultrasound is of questionable value in conservative approaches to soft tissue injuries about the elbow. It is contradicted with potential myositis ossification because of possible enhancement of osteoblastic proliferation. It is also contraindicated over open epiphyseal growth areas and thus is not to be used in children and adolescents.[110]

A number of studies on the use of ultrasound in tennis elbow revealed a significant placebo effect. Binder et al.[111] studied 76 tennis elbow patients, comparing ultrasound to a placebo. The subjects underwent 12 treatments over 4 to 6 weeks and were assessed based on pain and strength. Improvement was demonstrated in 63 percent of those treated with ultrasound and in 27 percent of the placebo group. Lundberg et al.[112] studied 99 patients age 21 to 63, comparing ultrasound, placebo, and rest. The ultrasound and placebo groups did equally well (36 percent and 30 percent, respectively, showed improvement), and both did better than the rest, 24 percent of whom improved. Straltford et al.[113] studied 40 patients, comparing phonophoresis to ultrasound placebo with transverse friction massage and to ultrasound placebo without massage. There was no difference among treatment groups, with all subjects demonstrating improvement. Similar findings were reported by Halle et al.[114] when they compared ultrasound with phonophoresis to transcutaneous nerve stimulation (TNS) and to injection. Leach and Miller[60] reported no noteworthy effect of ultrasound on tennis elbow.

It has been our experience that ultrasound is effective at the elbow only in the unusual case where there is a need to facilitate extensibility of scar tissue. Phonophoresis, in our opinion, has no role at the elbow, particularly in view of the known harmful effects of corticosteroids on tissue healing. It should be noted as well that many athletes present to physical therapy after having already received one or more cortisone injections. In our clinical experience, no patient has described a positive response to phonophoresis after ultrasound failed.

HIGH-VOLTAGE ELECTRICAL STIMULATION. High-voltage electrical stimulation may be useful in the early rehabilitation process to control pain and edema and enhance tissue vascularity. In postoperative cases or during periods of prolonged immobilization, it may be used for muscle contraction, thereby slowing muscular atrophy secondary to disuse, facilitating joint mobility, and minimizing the overall effects of immobility.[107,110] It has been our experience that it is useful in conjunction with moist heat to facilitate subsequent active rehabilitative exercise.

TRANSVERSE FRICTION MASSAGE. Transverse friction massage has been recommended by some therapists to minimize fibrous adhesions, promote revascularization of damaged tissue, and help in the maturation of collagen (healing tissue) into functional alignment.[107,115] Although no basic science studies have been presented to support these theories, this form of massage is widely used. Observation suggests that aggressive techniques are pain producing, and in some cases iatrogenically induced posterior lateral compartment synovitis has been noted. It is our opinion that transverse friction massage should be saved for situations in which scar adhesions are clinically present and healing alignment is likely to be resistant to molding by active exercise alone. This is most likely to occur in cases of chronic tissue damage. The athlete's subjective response to this treatment must be carefully monitored, as the induction of pain may compromise the long-range goals of rehabilitation.

CORTISONE INJECTIONS. Calvert et al.[116] reported that patient response to cortisone injection should occur with one or two shots and recommended minimal use of the arm in the week following injection. Warren[117] recommended avoiding cortisone shots initially and warned that the effects of cortisone will be only temporary unless an effective exercise program is performed. Sobel[6] has reported similar observations. Clark and Woodland[118] reported a 43 to 66 percent recurrence of tennis elbow after injections with two different types of steroid preparation. Kennedy and Willis[119] described evidence of collagen disorganization and weakening for up to 6 weeks following injections. In view of these reports, Nirschl[53] recommended cortisone injections only in those situations in which the pain is so severe as to preclude a meaningful rehabilitation exercise effort. It should be noted that the temporary comfort obtained with cortisone or any anti-inflammatory medication indicates only pain alteration, but does not imply that healing is occurring (e.g., revascularization; collagen production; or the enhancement of strength, endurance, or flexibility).

SUMMARY. The modalities discussed are effective in providing symptomatic relief early on in the rehabilitation program and can be discontinued once an effective exercise program is well tolerated. These modalities may again be useful from time to time if the pain or signs of chemical inflammation recur. Ice is an exception, in that it is indicated after exercise until the athlete has fully returned to his or her sport.

STAGE II: PROMOTION OF HEALING

Rehabilitative exercise to restore strength, endurance, and muscular balance; pain-relieving modalities; aerobics and general cardiovascular conditioning; and the absence of further abuse are necessary in the promotion of healing. The phases in stage II overlap considerably with those in stage I, but there is greater emphasis on rehabilitative exercise rather than symptomatic treatment.

PHASE I: REHABILITATIVE EXERCISE. Once exercise is initiated, progression to the next phase is based on the athlete's subjective symptoms (e.g., pain, stiffness, effect on daily function), as well as the therapist's objective findings (e.g., motion, swelling, strength, and ability to perform and handle specific performance criteria successfully). Early active motion is combined with passive mobilization as needed to restore normal range of motion, but in most cases, flexibility exercises per se are not stressed until reasonable strength has been restored (i.e., 75 percent of the opposite arm). (*Note:* It has been our experience that early stretching of inflamed tissue slows exercise tolerance. To minimize the potential for stretch overload of healing tissue, stretching should not be instituted until reasonable tensile strength is restored. Clinical observation suggests that 75 percent of uninvolved extremity strength is a workable practical starting point.)

If isometric exercises are used, multiangle isometrics as described by Davies[120] are recommended (beginning with symptom-limited submaximal contraction). Davies stresses the effectiveness of a gradient increase (i.e., a slow increase in intensity of contraction, then an isometric hold, and finally a gradual release). It should be noted that sudden contraction when joint effusion is present will cause painful capsular distention as a result of internal pressure buildup, whereas the gradient increase promotes accommodation.[1] Knott and Voss[121] described a similar effect when using proprioceptive neuromuscular facilitation (PNF) techniques.

Initial isotonic exercises are submaximal, avoiding any reproduction of symptoms. Daily exercise, two to three sets of 10 to 15 repetitions promotes muscle endurance while avoiding overload to the injured tissue.[1,6,103] We initially start with no weights and progress at 1- to 2-lb intervals once the athlete is able to tolerate the repetitions for two to three consecutive sessions (usually on a daily schedule). When a weight of 5 lb is reached, alternate-day isotonic strengthening with isokinetics and/or Isoflex rubber tubing is begun. Ellenbecker[122] studied 14 healthy students who used surgical tubing for wrist flexion and extension three times a week for 6 weeks (two sets of 15 repetitions). Comparison of the exercised wrist with the opposing control wrist during pre- and postisokinetic testing at 90 degrees and 300 degrees revealed no significant strength improvement. On the basis of this study, tubing alone should not be used as a substitute form of strengthening. All available forms of resistance exercise should be incorporated. Systematic progression of the rehabilitative exercise program continues, although the involved tissue is protected against abusive stresses as the level of involvement in daily activities is gradually increased.

Strength testing is indicated at this time in the rehabilitation program. Isometric (dynamometer grip) and isokinetic tests are most readily available. Conflicting results are reported in the literature, however, with respect to correlations between isometric and isokinetic muscular endurance and the testing protocols. Motzkin et al.[123] studied 32 healthy males and found no relationship between isometric and isokinetic endurance in the elbow flexors and extensors of either arm. They determined that isometric strength should last 60 to 80 seconds (flexion and extension, respectively) before dropping to 50 percent, while isokinetic strength drops 50 percent in 40 to 60 seconds (flexion and extension, respectively). Flexion isokinetic and nondominant arm efforts fatigued faster than extension

isometric and dominant arm efforts. These researchers concluded that there was a difference in the physiologic mechanism of endurance between the exercises that produce work and those that do not. Other studies comparing isometric and isokinetic peak torque outputs showed that a correlation does exist.[124,125] Van Swearingen[102] tested 32 normal students and found a high correlation between isometric torque and low-velocity (60 degrees per second) isokinetic torque in the wrist muscles in the neutral position. This correlation was higher in the pronated position. Tables 37–10 through 37–12 summarize the findings of isometric and isokinetic studies on the elbow, forearm, and wrist muscles.

Flexibility exercise should be initiated only after strengthening is well under way to minimize the potential for stretch overload of healing tissue. Static stretching with 10- to 20-second holds or using the contract-relax techniques of PNF are effective.[121,126]

PHASE II: FITNESS EXERCISE. Central aerobic and general fitness programs should be initiated as soon after injury as possible. The benefits of fitness are both physical and psychological. The sense of well-being that emanates from fitness is a powerful motivational tool as well.

Fitness exercise should include any of a wide variety of aerobic programs, as well as general strength and endurance training. Care must be taken to protect the injured elbow areas that are simultaneously going through the rehabilitation process.

PHASE III: ADVANCED TRANSITIONAL STRENGTHENING AND NEUROMUSCULAR CONTROL. Exercises to enhance neuromuscular control and muscular balance about the elbow (i.e., strength and flexibility and agonist/antagonist balance) are the focus of this phase. The goal is to promote effective high-speed function throughout the motion extremes that will be demanded by the sport. Plyometric activities are added to enhance explosive reactive movement for maximum sport performance. While the elbow functions primarily in open kinetic chain activities, closed kinetic chain exercise may be incorporated where dynamic stability of the proximal muscles need attention and/or for rehabilitation into sports such as gymnastics and football line play where the elbow must function in a closed kinetic chain fashion. The Profitter (Fig. 27–6) and Swedish ball (Fig. 27–7) offer the potential to individualize an exercise program tailored to the athlete's injury and sport demands.

PNF diagonals with dynamic stabilization and slow reversal hold are effective to enhance neuromuscular control of the elbow muscles and facilitate their role in the upper extremity kinetic chain.[121] Plyometric exercise with a medicine ball is invaluable to this phase of rehabilitation to help with proximal stabilization, to retrain effective synchrony of movements, and enhance effective explosive reactive movement. General upper body drills may include the following[103,108,126,127]:

- Medicine ball (2 to 4 pounds to start) techniques include throwing and catching side throws, soccer throws and chest passes, twists, and tosses. The athlete may be sitting, lying, kneeling, or standing.

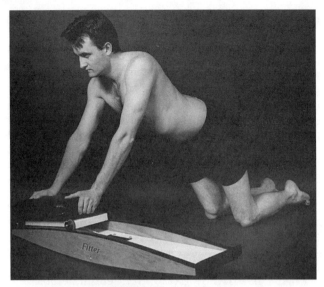

FIGURE 27–6. Profitter.

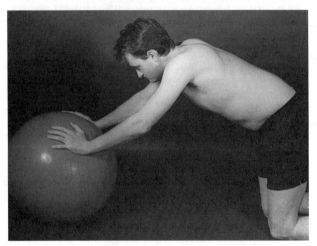

FIGURE 27–7. Swedish ball.

Any of these exercises performed against a mounted trampoline allow the athlete to work independently. Some authors recommend the use of up to 15-pound balls,[72,108,126] but in these cases careful monitoring is essential to avoid reinjury.

- Isoflex (surgical tubing) exercise throws and serves are initiated by holding the tube isometrically in full elbow flexion with the shoulder at 60 degrees flexion, followed by a release, allowing rapid, eccentric elbow extension and then quick reversal into flexion.
- Catching and throwing a weighted resistance (e.g., a punching bag or a car tire suspended by a rope).

PHASE IV: FORCE LOAD CONTROL AND RETURN TO SPORT. Once specific strength, muscular balance, flexibility, and endurance criteria are met, the athlete follows a methodical return-to-sport program. Appropriate sports equipment and bracing are addressed. The progression variables of intensity, duration, and frequency are systematically controlled, with attention to sport and training techniques. Emphasis is placed on adequate and appropriate warm-ups and cool-downs.

The athlete must fully understand the role of the warm-up in enhanced sport performance as well as injury prevention. A maintenance program for prevention of reinjury is designed in such a manner that the athlete will be willing and able to adhere to the program.

CONSERVATIVE TREATMENT OF TENNIS ELBOW

A number of studies on the treatment of tennis elbow show an inverse relationship between the duration of pain prior to treatment and the level of nonsurgical treatment success. The longer the duration of symptoms, the more difficult successful rehabilitation will be.[108,115,128] In addition, associated loss of wrist motion and decreased grip strength, indicative of a more chronic process and underlying changes in the muscle–tendon unit, are likely to impair the role of rehabilitation. Labelle et al.[129] surveyed all studies on tennis elbow and found a large placebo effect for all treatments, as well as poor quality of most of the studies.

Among the innumerable stage I treatments, the following are seen frequently in the literature:

- *Nonsteroidal anti-inflammatory medication.* It has been our experience that, when tolerated by the athlete, enhanced pain relief can facilitate early exercise and progression to stage II. Pain control may also be helpful later, during transition from one rehabilitation phase to the next phase. Initially, 2 to 3 weeks of medication should be all that is required. Leach and Miller[60] have reported a similar experience, using medication in conjunction with exercise.
- *Cock-up wrist splint.* The concept is to relieve tension on the wrist extensor tendons. This approach is recommended by some[108] in conjunction with pain-relieving modalities, stretching, and strengthening. In our experience, immobilization may achieve temporary comfort, but it tends to extend the rehabilitation time needed, as the side effects of immobility (atrophy, weakness, and decreased flexibility) must then be overcome.
- *Ultrasound and phonophoresis.* Ultrasound in and around the elbow epicondylar bony prominences has been ineffective and, on occasion, pain producing. The addition of cortisone cream (phonophoresis) has had no observed clinical benefit in our experience and has no support in the basic science literature. Ultrasound over the muscle mass may offer the usual benefits of deep heat application, but in relatively thin muscles, the advantage of a deep penetrating modality is questionable.
- *Electrical stimulation.* Four to six treatments of electrical stimulation focused over the ECRB origin and along the muscle belly over a 2- to 3-week period in conjunction with heat followed by early exercise is, in our experience, the most effective treatment for this condition in the majority of athletes. The achieved goals typically are pain and stiffness control in conjunction with muscle education. It is noteworthy that the occasional patient who notes exacerbated pain with the application of electrical stimulation

often presents subsequently for tennis elbow surgery. This pain response likely indicates more extensive tendinosis changes that are beyond the capabilities of conservative or nonsurgical care.

- *Steroid injections.* A number of authors recommend the use of steroid injections in patients whose pain is unresponsive to other treatment modalities and is interfering with progression in the exercise program.[60,62,110] These injections should never be considered curative and in our protocol must be accompanied by rehabilitative exercise for treatment success.
- *Transverse friction massage.* As discussed earlier, although commonly used, this technique offers no benefit and typically increases pain. Occasional onset of posterior lateral compartment synovitis has been noted after this treatment.
- *Forceful manipulation.* As described by Cyriax,[82] complete tearing of the ECRB has some proponents among physicians and therapists. In fact, however, no reported surgical observations are available to confirm exactly what forceful manipulation does. Speculation revolves about tearing of tendons, adhesions, synovium, the annular ligament, or other tissue. Failure to accurately identify pathoanatomy prior to the use of manipulation offers little in the treatment of elbow tendinosis.

COUNTERFORCE BRACING. Bracing is part of the healing process, as it controls abuse. The term *counterforce* was first introduced by Groppel and Nirschl.[62,130] The concept is to constrain the contractile expansion of muscle in a balanced and even manner, thereby decreasing the concentration of abusive forces to an injured area on the extremity (for tennis elbow, the lateral and medial elbow).

This type of bracing has proven extremely useful at the initiation of and throughout the rehabilitation cycle. Several studies support its use in this role. EMG and cinematographic studies by Groppel and Nirschl[130] found that muscle activity of the forearm extensors was lowered during the serve and backhand while wearing a specifically designed Count'R-Force brace (Medical Sports, Arlington, VA). Furthermore, the brace decreased the angular acceleration at the elbow in tennis ground strokes. Stonecipher and Catlin[131] isokinetically tested wrist extensor strength at 30 and 120 degrees per second in normal individuals with and without the brace and found no significant alteration in strength output. Wadsworth et al.[132] found increased grip and wrist extensor strength in symptomatic patients while utilizing the brace.

The brace generally enables the patient to initiate each phase of the exercise program, as well as return to sport with less or no pain. In most cases, the Count'R-Force brace should be utilized during rehabilitative exercise, in stressful daily activities, and on return to sport. The extent to which it is used is best determined by the athlete, but its use is not recommended at rest or with light activities of daily living (ADLs).

TOTAL ARM STRENGTHENING. Weakness of the entire extremity is common in tennis elbow, and total arm strengthening is of great importance in the overall treatment of tennis elbow. Immediate initiation of such exercise is recommended, especially for the shoulder and upper back. In addition to forearm extensor weakness, we have noted weakness of the scapular stabilizers, rotator cuff, hand, and forearm flexor muscles in patients with tennis elbow.

Strizak et al.[101] studied a composite total arm strength (TAS) factor (based on isometric testing of wrist flexion and extension, radial and ulnar deviation, pronation and supination, and finger flexion extension), comparing dominant to nondominant arms in healthy nonracket sport athletes, highly skilled tennis players, and those with a history of tennis elbow. He found statistically greater TAS-to–body weight (BW) ratios in the dominant arms of the control and tennis-playing groups, but not in the tennis elbow group.

A thorough evaluation of arm strength and appropriate exercise prescription to overcome imbalances are essential to tennis elbow rehabilitation. Throughout the rehabilitation phase, the injured tissue should be protected by avoiding aggravating ADLs and occupational activities, such as prolonged tight gripping; lifting with an outstretched arm; aggressive forearm pronation; extensive typing, writing, or use of a computer mouse; or extensive gardening, chopping, or plucking movements (e.g., playing musical instruments). Unavoidable activities should be protected by use of a Count'R-Force brace.

REHABILITATIVE EXERCISE (PHASE II). A study by Cruchow and Pelletier[54] in 1979 found that tennis players who did not undergo resistance training had increased recurrence of tennis elbow and those who continued maintenance exercise after an episode of tennis elbow had less incidence of recurrence (31 to 41 percent) than those who did not continue maintenance exercise.

Among the useful exercises to be incorporated into a tennis elbow program, the following are found frequently in the literature:

- UBE (Cybex Corp., Ronkonkoma, NY) for muscle endurance (utilizing the techniques of aerobic as well as anaerobic sprints).
- Grip strengthening using a foam ball or putty, with progression to a tennis ball.
- Broomstick curl-ups for the wrist extensors and flexors (equipment includes a weight suspended from the stick by a 3- to 4-foot cord curled over the stick).
- Isotonic resistance for all forearm muscle groups.
- Towel wringing, progressing from a bent elbow to full extension.
- The Powerstick (Power Pulleze Inc., Chester Heights, PA), an adjustable tension weighted bar resistance for forearm flexibility, strength and endurance conditioning.

ISOKINETIC EXERCISE. Ellenbecker[35] recommends starting with wrist flexion-extension before pronation-supination and beginning with the forearm supinated to allow gravity to assist the wrist extensors. He

TABLE 27–14
Medial Tennis Elbow Practice Schedule Return Guidelines (Progress If No Pain Increase)

	Day	Duration	Technique
Tournament Player	1	15 min	B only (2 handed); L (no late strokes)
	2	20 min	B (2 handed); L; Few F (2 handed)
	3	30 min	B; L; few F (no T); F; (no late strokes), (no topspin)
	4	35 min	B; L; BV; F (no T)
	5	40 min	B; L; BV; F (no T); Few O (to F court only)
	6	45 min	B; L; BV; F (no T); O (to F court only)
	7	1 hr	As day 6
	8	1 hr	B; L; BV; F (no T); FV; (no late strokes ever!)
	9	1 hr	All strokes easy
	10	1 hr (A.M.) 15 min (P.M.)	As day 9 B; L; F
	11	1 hr (A.M.) 30 min	B; 1; BV; F (no T); O; FV; S; (no T or AT) B; L; BV; F; (no T)
	12	1 hr (A.M.) 45 min (P.M.)	B; L; BV; F; O; FV; S; (no T or AT) B; L; BV; F; O
	13	1 hr (A.M.) 1 hr (P.M.)	Same as day 12 Same as A.M.
	14	1 hr (A.M.) 1 hr (P.M.)	B; L; BV; F As A.M.
	15		Resume normal practice/play schedule
Recreational Player*	1	15 min	L only
	2	20 min	L; B
	3	30 min	As day 2
	4	40 min	L; B; F; BV
	5	45 min	L; B; F; BV; few O
	6	1 hr	L; B; F; BV; O
	7	1 lu	L; B; BV; F; O; few S
	8	1 hr	L; B; F; BV; O; S; F; (no late strokes ever!)
	9		Resume normal practice/place schedule

*Progression for recreational player refers to actual playing days, not chronological days.
F, Forehand; FV, forehand volley; S, serve; U, underspin; B, backhand; SL, slice; BV, backhand volley; T, topspin; AT, American twist; L, lob; BL, backhand lob; FL, forehand lob; O, overhead.
Caution:
1. Use Medial Count'R-Force at all times.
2. Hit easily—hit through the ball.
3. Stay in balance.
4. Stay in hitting zone.
5. No late strokes.
6. Keep eye on ball.
7. Avoid frame shots.
8. Ice sore areas immediately after play.
From Nirschl RP, Sobel J: Arm Care: A Complete Guide to Prevention and Treatment of Tennis Elbow. Medical Sports Inc., Arlington, VA, 1995.

TABLE 27–15
Lateral Tennis Elbow Practice Schedule Return Guidelines (Progress If No Pain Increase)

	Day	Duration	Technique
Tournament Player	1	15 min	F only
	2	20 min	F; FL; few FV
	3	30 min	F; FL; FV; few O (to F court only)
	4	35 min	F; FL; FV; O; few S
	5	40 min	F; FL; FV; O; S (no SL, T or AT)
	6	45 min	As day 5
	7	1 hr	As day 6
	8	1 hr (A.M.)	F; FL; FV; O; S (no SL or AT); few B (2 handed)
	9	1 hr	F; FL; FV; O; S (no AT); B; (no BV)
	10	1 hr (A.M.) 15 min (P.M.)	F; FV; L; O; S; (no AT) B; (no U) F; FL; O
	11	1 hr (A.M.) 20 min (P.M.)	As day 10 As day 10
	12	1 hr (A.M.) 30 min (P.M.)	As day 11 F; FV; L; O
	13	1 hr (A.M.) 45 min (P.M.)	F; FV; L; O; S; B; few BV (no U) F; FV; L; O; S
	14	1 hr (A.M.) 1 hr (P.M.)	F; FV; L; O; S; B; BV As a.m.
	15		Resume normal practice/play schedule
Recreational Player*	1	15 min	F only
	2	30 min	F; FL; few FV
	3	35 min	F; FRL; FV; few O
	4	45 min	F; FL; FV; O
	5	1 hr	F; FL; O; S; few B (2 handed)
	6	1 hr	F; FV; FL; O; S; BV (2 handed); B
	7	1 hr	F; FV; L; O; S; B; BV (2 handed); B
	8	1 hr	F; FV; L; O; S; B
	9		Resume normal practice/play schedule

*Progression for recreational player refers to actual playing days, not chronological days.
F, Forehand; FV, forehand volley; S, serve; U, underspin; B, backhand; SL, slice; BV, backhand volley; T, topspin; AT, American twist; L, lob; BL, backhand lob; FL, forehand lob; O, overhead.
Caution:
1. Use lateral Count'R-Force at all times.
2. Hit easily—hit through the ball.
3. Stay in balance.
4. Stay in hitting zone.
5. No late strokes.
6. Keep eye on ball.
7. Two-handed backhand is protective.
8. Ice sore areas immediately after play.
From Nirschl RP, Sobel J: Arm Care: A Complete Guide to Prevention and Treatment of Tennis Elbow. Medical Sports, Inc., Arlington VA, 1995.

recommends starting with 30 to 50 submaximal repetitions at mid-speeds (60 to 180 degrees per second), progressing to maximal effort at 180 to 300 degrees per second, then full motion and with the elbow extended.

ISOFLEX EXERCISE. The term *isoflex* was introduced by Nirschl and Sobel.[100] The concept is that of tension cord resistance, which is now commonly used in the physical therapy community with surgical tubing or Theraband. It is our opinion that tension cord exercise is too important not to have an identifiable term equivalent to other forms of resistance exercise (e.g., isotonic, isometric, and isokinetic). It enables an emphasis on eccentric exercise, as well as stretching-shortening exercise, once these can be tolerated.

Isoflex exercise is more comfortable and effective when the tension cord is attached to a handle. This form of exercise is recommended for exercise of the cardinal six forearm muscle groups (i.e., wrist extension and flexion, pronation, supination, radial deviation, and ulnar deviation) after the athlete is capable of handling 3 lb of isotonic exercise (wrist extension) for 15 repetitions. In our treatment protocol, *Isoflex®* and isotonic exercise are alternated thereafter for three times each per week.

The tennis elbow exercise program that we have found to be most effective is outlined in the box below. The progression guidelines are based entirely on pain and any symptom exacerbation. Each exercise session is followed by application of ice. Medication, pain-relieving modalities, and counterforce bracing are employed as needed to allow a smooth efficient progression. A total arm strengthening program is incorporated, with emphasis on the scapular stabilizers and the rotator cuff to correct, most importantly, identified muscle imbalances of the entire arm.

Once full strength is achieved, exercises that include Powerstick, forearm flexibility, upper body plyometrics, and closed kinetic chain activities are added. The athlete may initiate full sport return, using the variables of strokes, duration, frequency, and, finally, competition. Counterforce bracing is often used as a protection. Initially a day off is recommended after each playing session. The backboard and ball machines are avoided in view of their increased repetitions and fast rebounds.

Davies and Ellenbecker[1] recommend starting with a foam ball to minimize impact stresses and using ground strokes only, followed by volleys mixed in with ground strokes, and finally serving with a foam ball at 40 to 60 percent velocity. Time on the court is then increased until finally match play is restarted. Nirschl has developed a specific return-to-play schedule as outlined in Tables 27–14 and 27–15.

Racket guidelines should be addressed during the rehabilitation program. Figure 27–8 demonstrates an accurate anthropometric measurement for determination of grip size. Chop[85] recommends that when the racket is gripped, the width of the index finger should fit between the tip of the ring finger and the base of the thumb. If the grip size is uncertain, it is probably best to go to a larger grip to minimize excessive wrist wobble and torque and the tendency to grip too tightly.[61,133,135] The multitude of available rackets, the changing tech-

---

TENNIS ELBOW PROGRAM

● Warm-up before exercise
● Counterforce bracing during exercise if recommended by the therapist or physician

PHASE IA: ISOTONIC EXERCISE TO 3 LB DAILY. Wrist flexion, extension, pronation, supination with elbow bent to 90 degrees, forearm supported. No weight to start, three sets of 15 to 20 repetitions. Once this is easily tolerated without symptom exacerbation for two to three consecutive sessions, add 1 lb, cut back to two sets of 15 repetitions. Progress to three sets of 20 repetitions. Go to 2 lb and repeat the process. Once this is easily tolerated, progress to 3 lb. Once at 3 lb, progress to phase II.

PHASE IB. Begin 50 to 100 repetitions throughout the day of squeezing a tennis ball and opening fingers against a rubber band. Elbow is bent to 90 degrees.

PHASE IIA: FUNCTIONAL PROGRESSION. Once patient is doing three sets of 20 repetitions with 3 lb, begin alternating strengthening with tubing (Isoflex) and/or isokinetic exercises as follows:

● 3×/week isotonics: two sets of ten repetitions; gradually work toward straightening the elbow. Once the elbow is almost straight, work up to two sets. When this is comfortable for three consecutive sessions, progress to 5 lb. Continue isotonic progress in this manner (usual end point is 5 lb for women and 8 lb for men).
● 3×/week Isoflex wrist flexion, extension, ulnar and radial deviation, pronation, supination; work up to 50 repetitions of each (usual end point).
● If the athlete has access to isokinetic equipment, the following progression is recommended:
  · 2×/week isotonics (elbow almost straight)
  · 2×/week Isoflex
  · 2×/week isokinetics. Midspeeds (120° to 180°/s) to start, 10 to 30 second bouts, then work into a velocity spectrum program (60°/s to 300°/s). Continue tennis ball and rubber band throughout the day, but with elbow just short of full extension.

PHASE III.

● Maintenance exercises
● Continue end point exercises for isotonic and Isoflex programs 3×/week

---

nology, and the paucity of information available for guiding tennis player choices make racket selection overwhelming to many. In general, medium-flex mid-size rackets (95 to 105 in² of hitting zone) are recommended.

Brody[134] recommends looser stringing, which increases the dwell time of the ball on the racket and thus decreases the shock that must be absorbed by the arm.

Further preventive measures in racket sports include the following:

· Players should use proper stroke mechanics. Proper strokes utilize trunk and shoulder rotation for power. Experienced players often overload by utilizing the relatively weak forearm muscles for power. Adequate instruction from a teaching tennis professional is recommended for all inexperienced players.

- In the athlete with lateral tennis elbow, consideration of a two-handed backhand is recommended.
- Players should play with players who hit the ball with a velocity that is comfortable for the player's game.
- Players should avoid tennis on wet or windy days.
- Slower, well-groomed playing surfaces (i.e., clay) offer some protection.
- Players should avoid solid-core or wet tennis balls.

Our approach to conservative treatment is summarized in Table 27–16.

SURGICAL CONSIDERATIONS IN ELBOW TENDINOSIS

Several overuse and traumatic injuries can contribute to elbow pain. The term *tennis elbow,* however, should be

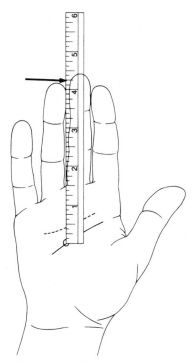

FIGURE 27–8. Measurement for racket grip. (From Nirschl RP: Elbow tendinosis/tennis elbow. Clin Sports Med 1992; 11(4):860.)

TABLE 27–16
Indications for Surgical Intervention in Tennis Elbow

1. Failure of a quality rehabilitation program
   a. Three or 4 months of supervised resistance exercise.
   b. Properly sequenced exercises
   c. Quality effort by the athlete
2. Presence of persistent pain (generally exceeding 1 year)
   a. Requiring sport or occupational activity change due to injury
   b. Pain at rest (*Note:* rule out other potential factors for rest pain, including malignancy)
3. Requirement of high activity level

---

reserved for those cases attributable to tendinosis of the forearm musculature. This tendinosis represents a degenerative change secondary to chronic repetitive activity (usually eccentric tension). Histologically, the changes appear as invasions of young vascular and fibroblastic tissue with collagen formation in an unorganized fashion. Such degenerative tissue has been termed *angiofibroblastic tendinosis.*[53] In the case of lateral tennis elbow, the ECRB is almost always involved, with involvement of the extensor communis being less common (30 percent in the Nirschl surgical series). In medial tennis elbow (golfer's elbow), degenerative changes are most commonly seen in the PT and FCR, to a lesser degree in the palmaris longus and FCU, and rarely in the superficial flexor muscles of the fingers.

Most cases of tennis elbow will respond favorably to an aggressive rehabilitation program incorporating the stages previously discussed in this chapter. A small percentage of cases, however, may not respond adequately to a quality rehabilitation program and may benefit from surgical management (see Table 27–16). Surgery should be considered for those athletes who continue to experience persistent pain and weakness with sports participation or daily activities. The final decision for surgery, however, is made by the athlete and should be based on the degree to which symptoms affect quality of life. It should be noted that it may take up to 3 to 4 months of daily rehabilitative exercise before a favorable result is experienced. Failure of comfort treatment (e.g., rest and medications, including cortisone injection) without adequate rehabilitation should not be considered a failure of conservative care.

Certain individuals have been identified who are at risk of experiencing a less favorable result with rehabilitative management alone and are therefore more likely to request surgery. These individuals include those who have received multiple cortisone injections (i.e., iatrogenic effects superimposed on original pathoanatomy), athletes who have experienced significant direct trauma to the lateral epicondyle, and patients with a history of mesenchymal syndrome (widespread tendinosis involving the shoulders, elbows, and wrists).[53,62]

SURGICAL PRINCIPLES

The surgical management of tennis elbow has undergone several developments. Early surgical technique focused on tension release of the common extensor (lateral) or flexor (medial) origins, as well as resection of the orbicular ligament. In 1979 Nirschl and Pettrone[83] introduced a new procedure for the surgical treatment of tennis elbow. The key to this technique is identification and removal of the pathologic tissue (angiofibroblastic tendinosis) (Fig. 27–9). In contrast to previous techniques, normal tendon origins are not released.

LATERAL TENNIS ELBOW SURGERY

The described technique (our preferred technique) and illustrations (Fig. 27–10) are for the classic case and

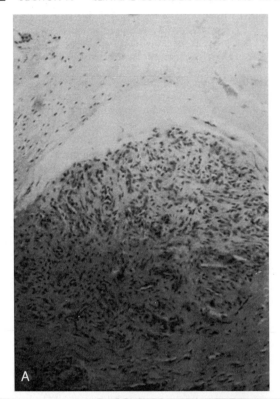

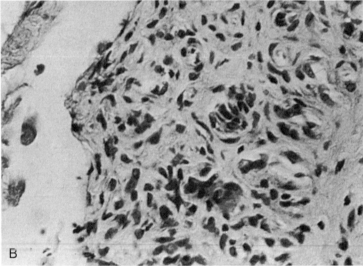

FIGURE 27–9. Fibroangiomatous hyperplasia. (From Nirschl RP: Elbow tendinosis/tennis elbow. Clin Sports Med 1992; 11(4):854.)

represent the majority of cases. The tissues most commonly involved laterally are the ECRB (100 percent) and the anterior edge of the extensor communis (30 percent). A bony exostosis of the lateral epicondyle is present in 20 percent of cases, and posterolateral synovitis is present in 5 percent. Such associated pathology is addressed at the time of surgery.

The incision extends from 1 inch proximal and just anterior to the lateral epicondyle to the level of the radial head. The interface between the extensor longus and extensor aponeurosis is identified, and a splitting incision is made. The extensor longus is then retracted anteromedially, bringing the extensor brevis origin into view. A common error surgeons often make is to penetrate too deeply with vertical dissection (i.e., beyond 2 to 3 mm), thereby failing to clearly identify the entire extensor brevis origin at its attachment points (the extensor aponeurosis and lateral epicondyle). The brevis origin normally attaches (1) to the underside anterior edge of the aponeurosis distal to the epicondyle at the anterior ridge of the epicondyle and (2) to the distal humeral ridge. In the properly selected case, the pathologic change of dull gray edematous tissue replacing normal glistening tendon will be noticed.

Tendinosis pathologic tissue often encompasses the entire origin of the extensor brevis to the level of the elbow joint. In approximately 35 percent of cases, pathologic tissue change will be noticed in the anterior underside of the extensor aponeurosis, and this is also removed. Calcific exostosis of the lateral epicondyle, if present, is removed after partially peeling away the anterior aspect of the extensor aponeurosis.

At the surgeon's discretion, a small longitudinal opening may be made in the synovium anterior to the radial collateral ligament for inspection of the lateral compartment. In the classic case, it is rare to have any lateral joint compartment, synovial fringe, or orbicular ligament changes.

The wounds are irrigated, and two or three drill holes are placed through the exposed cortical bone of the lateral condyle to cancellous depth to aid the healing process by enhancing vascular supply. It is unnecessary to suture the remaining areas of the extensor brevis, as some attachment at the level of the radial head remains. Minimal brevis retraction takes place, and the normal mechanical length is maintained. This concept is pertinent to regaining normal strength after healing has occurred.

MEDIAL TENNIS ELBOW SURGERY

The principles for medial elbow surgery (our preferred technique) are similar to those for the lateral elbow (Fig. 27–11). The goal again is to resect pathologic tissue without harm to normal tissue. Pathologic tissue is noted most often at the interface of the PT and the FCR (70 percent), often in both the PT and FCR (25 percent), and much less commonly in the FCR only (5 percent). Associated problems include ulnar nerve compression at zone III of the ulnar epicondylar groove (35 percent), congenital subluxation of the ulnar nerve (5 percent), medial collateral ligament laxity (5 percent), and olecranon fossa chondromalacia (5 percent).

For classic medial tennis elbow, a 3-inch incision is made longitudinally paralleling the medial epicondylar groove and starting approximately 1 inch proximal and just posterior to the medial epicondyle. Care is taken to avoid a sensory nerve branch (medial antebrachial cutaneous nerve) just distal and anterior to the epicondyle. Once the medial epicondylar area is exposed, a thin muscle layer may mask the pathologic changes underneath, so it is important to precisely locate the athlete's primary area of tenderness prior to administration of anesthesia, as the area of tenderness precisely indicates the area of pathologic change.

A longitudinal incision is made on the tendon origins, extending from the tip of the medial epicondyle distally for about 2 inches. The tendons are spread, and the lesion will come clearly into view if the surgical

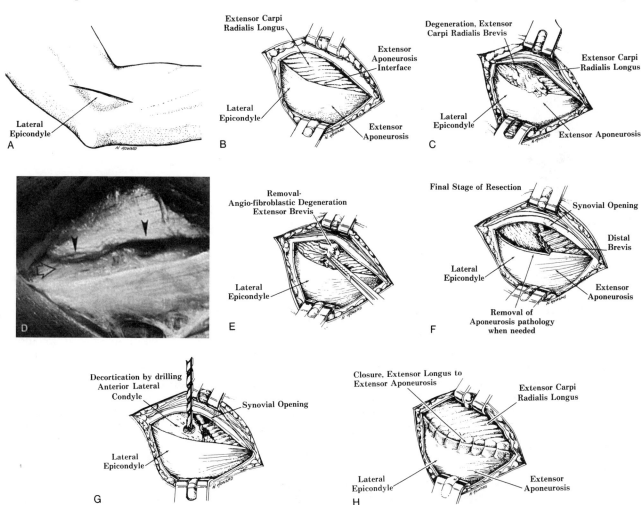

FIGURE 27–10. Lateral tennis elbow surgical sequence. (From Nirschl RP: Elbow tendinosis/tennis elbow. Clin Sports Med 1992; 11(4):862–863.)

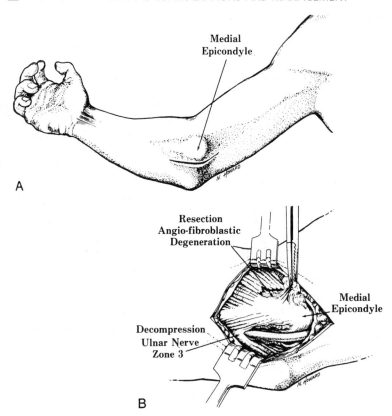

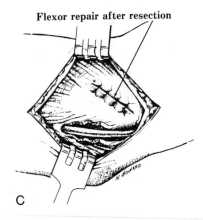

FIGURE 27–11. Medial tennis elbow surgical sequence. (From Nirschl RP: Elbow tendinosis/tennis elbow. Clin Sports Med 1992; 11(4):865.)

indications are correct. All excisions of pathologic tissue, including resection to the joint in the occasionally indicated case, are done longitudinally and elliptically. All normal tissue attachments to the medial epicondyle are left intact (e.g., the common flexor origin is a key medial stabilizer, and indiscriminate release of normal tendon attachment may lead to medial instability). After removal of tissue, the resulting elliptic space is closed with absorbable sutures (usually 0-0 or 0-1 in size).

ULNAR NERVE. As noted earlier in the chapter, the medial epicondylar groove is divided into three zones. The majority of ulnar nerve symptoms are the result of compression in zone III. Decompression of this zone by release of the ulnar flexor arcade will generally resolve the symptoms. Compression from osteophytic spurs, loose bodies, or rheumatoid synovitis can also occur in zone II, and compression in zone I may be caused by a

tight medial intermuscular septum or the retinaculum of Struthers.

Anterior transfer of the ulnar nerve is occasionally indicated, primarily when ulnar nerve symptoms are related to tension forces, including nerve subluxation or dislocation from the epicondylar groove, skeletal valgus (e.g., prior fracture malunion), dynamic valgus ligamentous instability, and surgical exposure to the medial elbow compartment. When ulnar nerve transfer is indicated, our preference is subcuticular, but with a fascial buttress from the common flexor origin.

POSTERIOR TENNIS ELBOW SURGERY

Triceps tendinosis most often occurs in combination with other posterior elbow problems, including extra-articular olecranon exostosis/bursitis and/or intra-articular olecranon fossa chondromalacia, exostosis, and loose fragments. The common etiologic factor is repetitive, aggressive elbow extension, which occurs in such varied sport activities as bowling, baseball pitching, football line play, track and field events (shot put, javelin), and heavy weight lifting.

Surgical intervention for a pure triceps tendinosis requires a longitudinal incision in the triceps tendon at or close to its olecranon attachment, followed by excision of any pathologically altered tissue. Associated problems are addressed as well and may include intra-articular arthrotomy or arthroscopy into the olecranon fossa. On occasion, we have encountered posterior involvement combined with either lateral or medial tennis elbow. All maladies are addressed during a single surgical procedure, through multiple incisions as needed.

POSTOPERATIVE PROTOCOL

The postoperative protocols for lateral, medial, and posterior tennis elbow are similar (see box below). The elbow is protected at 90 degrees for 1 week in a lightweight elbow immobilizer (Fig. 27–12). The immobilizer allows active use of the wrist, hand, and shoulder as the athlete's tolerance permits. The immobilizer is removed for active and active assisted range-of-motion exercise starting on postoperative day 3, but is worn at other times for up to 1 week. Most athletes tolerate normal activities of daily living (ADLs) by day 10. Rehabilitative exercises, as described previously, commence 3 weeks following surgery. A Count'R-Force elbow brace is worn during rehabilitative exercises, as well as during higher forearm activity (including ADLs and return to sport). Although full racket and throwing sport competitive activity is not recommended until full strength returns, modified sports technique patterns are often initiated 6 to 8 weeks after lateral elbow surgery and 10 to 12 weeks after medial or posterior elbow

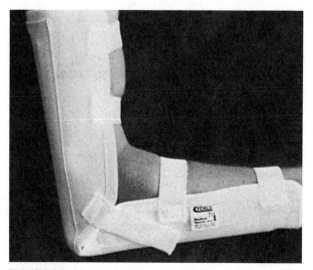

FIGURE 27–12. Elbow immobilizer. (From Nirschl RP: Elbow tendinosis/tennis elbow. Clin Sports Med 1992; 11(4):867.)

surgery. Full strength (and, thus, clearance for competitive play) is typically restored by 6 months, provided the athlete has adhered to a quality rehabilitative exercise program.

RESULTS OF SURGERY

Our experience with the described surgical techniques has been highly consistent and rewarding. Overall improvement to a level of activity that existed prior to the onset of symptoms has been observed in 90 percent of cases. Significant relief of pain in all activities has been observed in 97 percent of cases. However, a positive result depends on quality postoperative rehabilitation following surgery. A number of variables may play a role in individuals who experience unsuccessful results. These variables include the presence of pathologic involvement beyond tendinosis (e.g., associated nerve and ligament injury and osteoarthritis), emotional aspects of pain, and secondary gain issues (e.g., worker's compensation).

TREATMENT OF MEDIAL (ULNAR) COLLATERAL LIGAMENT INSUFFICIENCY

The conservative approach to attenuated lesions of the UCL should address stengthening the muscles that resist valgus forces while avoiding valgus stresses in daily activities and sports. An EMG study by Glousman et al.[44] compared muscle activity in throwing athletes with and without MCL insufficiency. Those with insufficiency demonstrated lower flexor and pronator activity and great wrist extensor activity in the muscles of the injured arm. Glousman et al. attributed this to the muscle's role in stabilizing and deceleration. It is conceivable that the lower muscle activity of the flexors and pronators is attributable, at least in part, to reflex inhibition. It is also likely that these muscle groups were already fatigued and overused in attempts to compensate for valgus instability.

In addition to strengthening the wrist extensors, it is essential to strengthen the wrist flexors, pronator teres, and biceps because of their role in resisting valgus forces. Pedegana et al.[136] isokinetically studied eight noninjured professional baseball players and found significantly greater dominant pronator strength at 60 and 180 degrees per second while no significant differences were found in supination, wrist flexion, or extension. They did find a statistically significant relationship between isokinetic wrist and elbow extensor strength and throwing velocity. It is likely that forearm muscle strength is necessary in throwing, as well as in resisting valgus stresses. Pawloski and Perrin,[98] on the other hand, found no statistically significant relationship between elbow extension or flexion strength and throwing velocity. Forearm strength likely is the more important factor.

Once normal motion, strength, endurance, resistance to fatigue, and muscle balance are fully restored, plyometric and sport-specific training can be initiated. The sequence is gradual over 6 to 8 weeks while

TENNIS ELBOW POSTOPERATIVE PROTOCOL

DAYS 1–7

2. Expect a good bit of soreness.
3. Keep elbow immobilized the majority of time.
4. Sleep on back if possible with arm on pillow on stomach.
5. Be sure to keep full shoulder motion and move shoulder fully several times each day.
6. Days 1–3: the elbow should stay bandaged and in the immobilizer at all times.
7. Starting about day 2: move fingers and wrist for 2 minutes, 3–5 times/day.
8. You may shower on the third day after surgery: remove bandages, and gently work the elbow in the shower. After showering, gently air or blow-dry the wound; cleanse gently with alcohol and apply antibiotic ointment and then cover the wound with adhesive bandages.
9. Days 3–6: wear the immobilizer most times except during showering, gentle limbering of the elbow, and mild ADLs.
10. Ice several times a day for 20–30 minutes at a time.
11. Medications: Use pain medications (such as acetaminophen [Tylenol] or mild codeine) or anti-inflammatory medications as prescribed by your physician. If you are taking no anti-inflammatory medicine, you may take aspirin. DO NOT TAKE ASPIRIN AND ANTI-INFLAMMATORY MEDICINE SIMULTANEOUSLY (the combination can cause stomach upset, ulcer, or excessive blood thinning).

EXPECT SOME DEEP ELBOW PAIN THROUGH THE NEXT WEEKS. THIS REFLECTS THE WORK DONE AND THE HEALING PROCESS!!!
RECHECK WITH YOUR DOCTOR IF:

- The wound looks "angry" (excessive swelling, redness, or dramatically increased pain that progressively worsens)
- Increased fever at wound or generalized throughout body

DAYS 7–17

1. Limber your elbow with bending and straightening motions; start in a warm shower.
2. By day 17, about 80% of elbow motion return is average.
3. Work on wrist, fingers, forearm pronation and supination (active motion).
4. Use arm for light activities.
5. Use immobilizer occasionally for protection only. Leave immobilizer off the majority of the time.

DAYS 17–21

1. Use counterforce brace with light tension when exercising.
2. Begin squeezing a Nerf ball.
3. Actively bend and straighten elbow through fullest possible range.
4. Do tennis elbow exercises as prescribed by your therapist or physician without any weight. Start with five repetitions, and work up to 15 repetitions of each.

3 WEEKS

1. Begin full tennis elbow program wearing counterforce brace.
2. Over the next 3 weeks, increase arm use in daily activities. Maintain or begin overall conditioning and aerobic program.
3. Relief of presurgery pain is usually noted in the 3- to 6-week period. If pain is increased, you may be overstressing the arm: ice 2–3 times/day, then decrease activities.
4. Full range of motion should be achieved by 6 weeks.
5. Perform upper quarter and total arm strengthening exercises.

6–10 WEEKS

1. Continue strengthening using tennis elbow program guidelines.
2. Advance total arm strengthening program with emphasis on scapular and shoulder muscles.

10 WEEKS TO 3 MONTHS

1. Achieve dominant arm strength 10% greater than nondominant arm on grip dynamometer and isokinetic testing.
2. Circumferential forearm measurement should demonstrate that the dominant arm is 1/4 to 1/2 inch greater than the nondominant arm (3/4 inch or more difference among elite athletes).
3. Begin sport-specific training (follow return protocols for tennis, Tables 27–14 and 27–15).
4. Arm should be comfortable, although phase III pain is occasionally noted.

3–4 MONTHS

1. Return to sport on gradual basis.
2. Continue conditioning and upper quarter strength programs.

6 MONTHS

1. Return to competitive play is usual (tennis, baseball, etc.).

monitoring symptoms with progression as indicated. Return-to-sport guidelines (e.g., ice and an interval throwing program) are essential. If the athlete is returning to a contact sport (such as football), then taping or bracing the elbow against the last 15 degrees of extension and against valgus stresses should be considered, especially after elbow dislocation.

Rehabilitation should include low back, hip, and abdominal strengthening (e.g., latissimus dorsi pulldowns, bent rows, pullovers, spinal twists, and PNF diagonals). A more global approach to conditioning is always in order, as the entire kinetic chain affects the elbow. Gamble[126] recommends tubing pulls that simulate the baseball swing and throw. Emphasis should be placed on eccentric exercises, as a high proportion of the loads in the throwing motion are eccentric in nature.[36,137]

The return-to-throwing program can begin by practicing the throwing motion in front of a mirror, with full attention to good throwing mechanics. Gentle, high-arc tosses, with minimal cocking and a smooth rainbow motion, are then initiated from level ground, increasing the distance from 90 feet to 180 feet. These allow the player to practice proper throwing mechanics and build endurance. Throwing high-arc tosses from the mound follows, then short tosses with less arc, and finally, practice in wind-up and cocking, with gradual progression, while throwing from the mound. Anderson and Ciolek[136a] recommend 2 to 3 days between workouts, working up to 40 to 45 throws at a low velocity before increasing to a higher velocity.

Specific interval training programs (ITPs) have been described in depth by several authors. A sample program may involve:

- warm-up, then stretching, then soft tosses at 10 to 90 feet
- long tosses emphasizing a good throwing form and follow-through for 5 minutes
- 30 short tosses at 1/4 to 1/2 intensity for 5 minutes
- repeat
- 120-foot toss with a 30-foot increase each few sessions to a maximum of 240 feet
- simultaneously, a 1/2-speed, 60-foot short toss is progressed to 3/4 speed, then breaking balls, then full activity.

Specific ITP protocols are described in depth in Wilk et al.[103] Davies and Ellenbecker,[1] and Blackburn.[137]

OPERATIVE INTERVENTION FOR UCL DEFICIENCY

In many instances, operative intervention for UCL deficiency may be unnecessary. Elbow dislocation in an otherwise non–valgus-stressed individual is typical of this category of patient. In those patients who subject their arms to valgus stress, however, surgical intervention may be required to restore preinjury function.

The diagnosis of instability and anatomic deficiency can be accurately made via clinical and magnetic resonance imaging (MRI) examination. With proper indications, the options are either to repair the existing ligament or to reconstruct the ligament with an autogenous tendon transplant. It is our experience that tendon transplant is best for the attritional rupture, as the quality of residual ligament is poor. In sudden single-event trauma through a previously normal (i.e., not attritionally injured and degenerated or calcified) ligament, primary repair may be successful.

The concept of reconstruction was initially reported by Jobe et al.,[138] and return to a high level of sports participation has been satisfying in greater than 50 percent of baseball pitchers. The original technique introduced by Jobe et al. (full release of common flexor origin and submuscular ulnar nerve transfer) has been amended by Nirschl and others[53,88a] to decrease morbidity, but the principle of autogenous tendon graft (usually the palmaris longus) through the medial epicondyle and to the proximal ulna has been retained.

POSTOPERATIVE REHABILITATION OF UCL RECONSTRUCTION. In an 8-year study of 16 javelin throwers and pitchers at 11 to 19 months after UCL reconstruction, Jobe et al. found that ten returned to their previous level of playing, one to a lower level, and five to professional sports.[138] Similarly good results have been reported by others.[103] The postoperative program after primary repair and reconstruction of a chronically insufficient ligament is quite similar, although range of motion should be delayed somewhat after repair. The congruency of the elbow joint allows for relatively early motion if done in a gradual, protected manner.

Table 27–17 outlines a postoperative protocol. Surgical considerations that may influence progression should be attended to, as well as the patient's pain and symptoms.

ULNAR NERVE TREATMENT

Ice, rest, medication, and alteration of throwing mechanics may be effective for ulnar nerve symptoms. Once ulnar nerve lesions become symptomatic and unresponsive to these modalities, surgical intervention is indicated.

The treatment of ulnar nerve dysfunction may vary widely depending on the magnitude of dysfunction and the etiology. The most common etiologic factors germane to an athletic population include compression neuropraxia in zone III of the medial epicondylar groove, often associated with medial tennis elbow tendinosis, tension overload secondary to valgus instability, and tension and compression overload secondary to a congenital dislocation of the nerve in association with repetitive elbow flexion-extension and valgus.

Conservative treatment in the form of elbow rehabilitation and anti-inflammatory medication may offer some opportunity for success in compression neuropraxia of zone III, but lingering symptoms almost always necessitate surgical intervention in the form of decompression (not unlike carpal tunnel syndrome).

Nerve dysfunction secondary to valgus instability and dislocation has no opportunity to resolve short of surgery unless a low activity level (i.e., no throwing or racket sports) is acceptable. Surgical intervention in this instance requires anterior nerve transfer. Our preference in this instance is subcuticular transfer with a fascial buttress formed from the common flexor origin. Although some authors recommend submuscular transfer, it is our opinion that the chance for complication and morbidity is much higher, without any significant benefit, than with the subcuticular technique.

POSTOPERATIVE REHABILITATION

The postoperative rehabilitation program (Table 27–18) is determined by the type of operative intervention.

TABLE 27–17
Protocol for Postoperative Rehabilitation of Ulnar
Collateral Ligament

Phase I: Postoperative days 1 to 10
Control inflammation, protect healing tissue
- Immobilize in 90° posterior splint or elbow
  immobilizer
- Wrist, hand, and shoulder mobility exercises
- Putty, grip exercises
- Wrist and hand isometrics, begin at 7 days
  postoperatively
- Modalities (electrical stimulation, ice) and
  medications as indicated

Phase II: Postoperative days 10 to 14
Early motion, promote healing
- Hinged brace to protect against valgus stresses, but
  allow flexion-extension motion
- Continue above exercises
- Sand and rice exercises for hand intrinsics
- Begin elbow motion 30° to 60°
- Biceps and triceps isometrics
- Modalities as needed

Phase III: Postoperative weeks 2 to 6
Progressive motion
- Hinged brace, progressively increase from 10° to 120°
  (off for active and active-assisted ROM)
- Progress to full elbow flexion by 6 weeks
  postoperatively
- Active elbow flexion, extension, pronation, and
  supination
- Wrist PRE program
- Shoulder PRE; avoid shoulder rotations until 6
  weeks
- Begin UBE
- Modalities as needed

Phase IV: Postoperative weeks 6 to 9
Early strengthening
- Isotonic concentric/eccentric elbow flexion-extension
  endurance and PRE program
- Full ROM at 6 weeks
- PNF diagonals with isotonic and manual resistance

Phase V: Postoperative months 2 to 4
Full strengthening
- Isoflex or surgical tubing
- Isokinetics at midspeed, progress to VSRP;
  emphasize biceps, triceps as needed

Phase VI: Postoperative months 4 to 6
Functional and sports-specific activities
- Isokinetic testing at 4 months postoperatively; adjust
  program to correct imbalance
- Plyometrics with tubing, medicine ball
- Begin ITP program once normal, pain-free motion,
  strength and endurance are demonstrated and sport-
  specific activities are under way without symptom
  exacerbation
- Ice throughout return program
- Return to sport at 6 months postoperatively (gradual
  program of throwing or tennis serve)

Note: Avoid valgus stresses until 4 months after surgery.
ITP, Interval training program; PNF, proprioceptive neuromuscular
facilitation; PRE, progressive resistive exercise; ROM, range of motion;
UBE, upper body ergometer; VSRP, Velocity Spectrum Rehabilitation
Program.

TABLE 27–18
Postoperative Rehabilitation of Ulnar Nerve Transfer

Phase I: Postoperative days 1 to 7
Control inflammation, retard atrophy, facilitate healing
- Posterior splint at 90° or elbow immobilizer at 90°
- Grip exercises, wrist and shoulder active motion
Phase II: Postoperative days 7 to 21
Early motion
- Remove splint for exercises
- Elbow 30° to 90° initially, progressing to 15° to full
  flexion
- Continue above exercises
- Shoulder, elbow, and wrist isometrics
- Sand and rice exercises for hand intrinsics
Phase III: Postoperative weeks 3 to 7
Early strengthening, normal motion
- Discontinue splint or immobilizer
- Work toward full elbow motion, emphasizing
  extension
- Begin strengthening elbow, forearm, wrist, hand
  exercises (isotonic, isokinetic, Isoflex)
- Shoulder conditioning
Phase IV: Postoperative weeks 7 to 9
Full strength, sport-specific activities
- Isokinetic strength testing (week 7)
- Emphasize eccentrics
- Initiate plyometric drills with medicine ball, tubing
- Once pain-free, normal strength, endurance, and
  flexibility are demonstrated, begin sport-specific
  training
Phase V: Postoperative weeks 9 to 16
- Interval training program (ITP)—weeks 9 to 12
- Progressive return to competition—weeks 12 to 16

Note: Total body conditioning throughout. For ulnar nerve decompression without nerve transfer, the protocol is accelerated.

In general, all the operative techniques involve soft
tissue without major ligament or tendon distortion. This
allows a rather rapid mobilization and strengthening
sequence.

In a pure decompression of the ulnar nerve in zone
III, range-of-motion exercises may be started within 24
hours and resistance strengthening of the forearm
muscle groups within 1 week. To illustrate the speed of
rehabilitation in this circumstance, Nirschl (personal
communication, 1977) reported on the return of a world
class tennis player, who won a U.S. National Championship just 59 days after surgery. In the more common
combination of nerve compression and medial tennis
elbow tendinosis, the rehabilitation sequence follows
that used for tendinosis.

In the anterior nerve transfer group, easy motion
exercises are started at 1 week after surgery, resistance
exercises at 3 weeks, and graduated return to throwing
sports at 3 months.

TREATMENT FOR LOSS OF ELBOW MOTION

Stiffness of the elbow is common after trauma and
immobilization because of the congruity of the joint, the
tightness of the capsule, and the tendency toward

scarring of the anterior capsule. The brachial muscle, which crosses the elbow, is also subject to excessive scarring and, on occasion, myositis ossificans in response to trauma.

Loss of motion at the elbow, especially loss of extension, is particularly challenging. High-intensity passive stretching can lead to greater motion loss and pain and can possibly stimulate myositis ossificans. The treatment specifics for loss of motion are dependent on the etiology of the motion loss. The basic etiologic categories include osseous problems (e.g., bony blockade from arthritic chondromalacia and synovitis, loose bodies, and bony exostosis) and soft tissue problems (e.g., adhesive capsulitis, usually in the anterior capsule, and fibrotic tendons, usually common flexor origin, triceps, or brachial muscle), or combinations thereof.

Conservative treatment for soft tissue problems includes early use of modalities to enhance circulation and collagen elasticity, followed by exercise. The UBE (Lumex Corp., Ronkonkoma, NY) is indicated to stimulate blood flow and disbursement of abnormal quantities of synovial fluid. Very low load, prolonged stretching may be employed, but the patient must be closely monitored for indications of reactive stiffening. Wilk et al.[103] described using a 2- to 4-lb hand-held weight with a towel roll placed behind the elbow to act as a fulcrum. The most effective techniques, however, are PNF techniques (contract–relax and hold–relax)[121] with active triceps extension and mobilization of the humeroulnar and radioulnar joints to enhance posterior glide of the ulna on the humerus.

Dynamic bracing has not been found to be generally effective in regaining the extremes of motion.

TREATMENT OF ELBOW DISLOCATIONS

Conservative treatment after reduction of an elbow dislocation involves brief immobilization followed by therapeutic exercise and return to sports. Some authors recommend prolonged immobilization, but the consequences of this can be devastating. Because of the joint congruity and low recurrence rate, immobilization beyond 1 week is not indicated.

Mehlhoff et al.[139] retrospectively studied the long-term effects of early mobilization. They found that prolonged immobilization after dislocation is strongly associated with a poor result (i.e., flexion contractures and pain). They recommended 2 weeks' maximum immobilization, with up to 4 weeks if some instability exists. This period is too long, in our opinion. In the occasional case of major instability, usually UCL and RCL surgical repair is indicated. Protzman[140] reported no recurrence of dislocation in 27 patients treated with active motion within 5 days of reduction.

Following reduction, the elbow is immobilized in a posterior splint or an elbow immobilizer at 90 degrees flexion for 3 to 4 days, during which time shoulder and wrist mobility exercises, as well as grip exercise, are performed. The elbow may then be removed from the immobilizer for active range of motion and isometrics (elbow flexion, easy extension, pronation, and supina-

tion) several times a day. Passive stretching is absolutely avoided because of the tendency toward scarring of the traumatized soft tissue and the possibility of recurrent posterior dislocation. The immobilizer may be discarded at 10 days, at which time exercise incorporating the entire arm is initiated. The elbow may then be supported in a hinged brace (set at 15 to 90 degrees) or a sling for several weeks, although this is usually unnecessary.

Once motion and strength are within 10 percent of normal, return to sports is initiated. For collision sports, a brace or taping to prevent elbow hyperextension and valgus forces may be used. Kulund[46] recommends taping the elbow in slight flexion or using a custom-made padded elbow sleeve around the arm and forearm to allow full flexion and avoid hyperextension.

Dislocations are rare, but loss of motion, joint stiffness, and heterotopic ossification are more likely complications. As with the discussions concerning elbow stiffness, the recently reported anterolateral approach to the elbow is ideal to correct recalcitrant postdislocation adhesive capsulitis. If postdislocation instability is a problem, primary repair or reconstruction with an autogenous tendon graft using either the UCL or the RCL is generally quite successful.

ARTHROSCOPIC REMOVAL OF LOOSE BODIES, DEBRIDEMENT OF OSTEOCHONDRITIS, EXOSTOSIS, AND ARTHROTOMY

Osteochondritis may be treated conservatively with rest, pain-relieving modalities, and gentle active exercise. However, a study by Tivon et al.[141] on surgical management of osteochondritis found the average increase in extension motion was approximately 20 degrees when compared with preoperative extension. Postoperative rehabilitation was initiated immediately in these cases.

The rehabilitation course after arthrotomy is the same as for arthroscopy except for a somewhat slower progression though each stage. After athroscopy, motion exercises begin immediately to avoid contracture and are limited only by pain and wound healing considerations. To allow for wound healing after arthrotomy, exercise should begin 5 to 7 days postoperatively. Occasionally, a CPM device may be indicated to nourish the articular cartilage, avoid edema and effusion, and minimize cross-linking of the scarring fibers.[23]

The prognosis for full return to most sports is excellent, although degenerative changes of the radio-capitellar joint may temper this prognosis, especially for gymnasts and pitchers. A study by Singer and Roy[81] of gymnasts with osteochondritis found that over a 3-year period, only 20 percent fully returned to the sport.

The overall goal of any elbow rehabilitation program, conservative or postoperative, is to restore the dynamic functional interplay of all aspects of the elbow joint complex. Any factors that affect this interplay must be addressed; thus, correction of total arm and upper quarter strength deficits and imbalances is important.

Improving the patient's commitment to a long-term rehabilitation program appropriate to his or her sport promises the best chance of minimizing further injuries. Effective education is the key to this commitment.

REHABILITATION

The most effective treatment for any overuse injury is its prevention. An overall program can be tailored to meet the identified demands and offset the deficits and imbalances of each sport. An effective program calls for ongoing interaction and communication among players (and parents of young players), coaches, and medical providers. Aspects of prehabilitation include the following:

- Vulnerable tissue should be sought out through fitness assessment, a thorough sport durability evaluation of the musculoskeletal system. In addition to musculoskeletal factors, this includes evaluations of the athlete's conditioning, training habits and equipment, and sport-specific performance.
- Activities independent of the sport, prior injury history (including treatments), and sports participation history are important considerations.
- Injury-producing overload in the sport must be controlled. This involves educating athletes and coaches on the importance of:

- Techniques of proper warm-up and cool-down and equipment selection guidelines,
- Good sport technique and knowledge of the effect of environmental conditions.
- Training programs to promote best sport performance and minimize injury potential. Periodization, which divides the annual training plan into segmented cycles, each with specific short-range goals, is designed to maximize the athlete's peak performance during the competitive season and to minimize the potential for overtraining by varying the exercise load, intensity, volume, and type. In sports such as tennis in which several major competitions occur each year, the cycles are modified accordingly.

- The athlete must take responsibility for listening to his or her body's warning signals.
- The athlete must be encouraged to report symptoms of injury to the coach early.
- Overtraining and its effects must be thoroughly understood by the athlete, coach, and (very important to the young athlete) parents. Effects and indications of fatigue and burnout are critical factors.
- The athlete should understand and know how to offset the effect of environmental conditions.
- Appropriate bracing should be used, if needed.
- A rehabilitative exercise program must be designed to address identified imbalances.
- The clinician should promote fitness exercise to overcome the inadequacies of the sport.
- The athlete should practice total arm strengthening throughout sport participation.

TABLE 27–19
Basic Upper Extremity Exercise Program

1. Shrugs
2. Scaption, progressing to "empty can"
3. Military press
4. PNF diagonal 2 (flexion-abduction–external rotation ↔ extension-adduction–internal rotation
5. Rows
6. Side-lying external rotation
7. Upper extremity "step-ups/down" (with involved arm on 4- to 8-inch step; the uninvolved arm "steps-down" to floor
   a. Involving elbow flexion/extension
   b. With elbow straight, involving scapular protraction/retracton
8. Biceps curls
9. Triceps extension
10. Forearm pronation/supination
11. Wrist extensor
12. Gripping (elbow flexed/extended)

PNF, Proprioceptive neuromuscular facilitation.

Table 27–19 outlines 12 basic exercises for the arm, an upper quarter foundation program that can be modified to meet individual need.

CONCLUSION

Enabling each athlete to maximize sport performance and minimize injury potential is the ongoing challenge of all involved with the athlete. Ongoing scientific research, with sensitivity to each patient's response to treatment approaches, provides the framework for improved future success.

We have reviewed pertinent functional anatomy and related it to the myriad of pathoanatomic alterations that commonly occur about the elbow. A clear understanding of the underlying pathoanatomy is critical to treatment success, defined as restoration to the patient's desired level of activity performance.

The key concept in treatment is the conservative pyramid: relief of pain, promotion of healing, adjunctive fitness programs of healing, adjunctive fitness programs, control of abusive activities, and transitional exercise in preparation of performance return (i.e., to sport, occupation, or performing arts). In those instances where conservative rehabilitation is inadequate, surgical intervention can be highly effective.

REFERENCES

1. Davies GJ, Ellenbecker TS: Total arm strength rehabilitation for shoulder and elbow overuse injuries. Orthopedic Physical Therapy Home Study Course 93-1. LaCrosse, WI, APTA Orthop Section, 1993, pp 1–22.
2. Dillman C: The upper extremity in tennis and throwing athletes. Presented at the US Tennis Association National Conference, Tucson, AZ, March 1991.
3. Ellenbecker TS: Shoulder injuries in tennis. In Wilk K, Andrews

J (eds): The Athlete's Shoulder. New York, Churchill Livingstone, 1994, pp 399–409.

4. Nirschl RP, Sobel J: Tennis. In Reider B (ed): Sports Medicine: The School-Age Athlete. Philadelphia, WB Saunders, 1991, pp 664–672.

5. Priest JD, Braden J, Gerberich JG: The elbow in tennis: Part 1. Phys Sports Med 1980; 8(4):80.

6. Sobel J: Shoulder rehabilitation — rotator cuff disease. In Pettrone FA (cd): Athletic Injuries of the Shoulder. New York, McGraw-Hill, 1995, pp 245–270.

7. Cochran VB: Biomechanics of the elbow-forearm complex. In Wadsworth TG (ed): The Elbow. New York, Churchill Livingstone, 1982, pp 31–47.

8. Morrey BF, Chao EY, Hui FC: Biomechanical study of the elbow following excision of the radial head. J Bone Joint Surg 1979; 61A(1):63–68.

9. Tullos HS, Bryan WJ: Functional anatomy of the elbow. In Zarins B, Andrews JR, Carson WD Jr (eds): Injuries to the Throwing Arm. Philadelphia, WB Saunders, 1985, pp 191–200.

10. King JW, Breslford HF, Tullos HS: Analysis of the pitching arm. Clin Orthop 1969; 67:116–123.

11. An Kai-Nan. Biomechanics: Basic relevant concepts. In Morrey BF (ed): The Elbow and Its Disorders, 2nd ed. Philadelphia, WB Saunders, 1993, pp 53–72.

12. Morrey BF, An Kai-Nan: Functional anatomy of the ligaments of the elbow. Clin Orthop 1985; 201:84–89.

13. An Kai-Nan, Morrey BF: Biomechanics of the elbow. In Morrey BF (ed): The Elbow and Its Disorders, 2nd ed. Philadelphia, WB Saunders, 1993, pp 53–72.

14. Bennett JB: Articular injuries in the athlete. In Morrey BF (ed): The Elbow and Its Disorders, 2nd ed. Philadelphia, WB Saunders, 1993, pp 581–595.

15. Hotchkiss RN, Weilan AJ: Valgus stability of the elbow. J Orthop Res 1987; 5:372–377.

16. Fuss FK: The ulnar collateral ligament of the human elbow joint. J Anat 1991; 175:203–212.

17. Sojbjerg JO, Oversen J, Nielsen S: Experimental elbow instability after transection of the medial collateral ligament. Clin Orthop 1987; 218:186–190.

18. Regan WD, Korinek SL, Morrey BF, et al: Biomechanical study of the ligaments around the elbow joint. Clin Orthop 1991; 271:170–179.

19. O'Driscoll SW, Bell DF, Morrey BF: Posterolateral rotatory instability of the elbow. J Bone Joint Surg 1991; 73A(3):440–446.

20. Kapandji IA: Physiology of the Joints: Vol 1, Upper Limb, 5th ed. Edinburgh, Churchill Livingstone, 1982.

21. Spinner M, Kaplan EB: The quadrate ligament of the elbow. Acta Orthop Scandinavia 1970; 41:632–637.

22. Morrey BF: Anatomy of the elbow joint. In Morrey BF (ed): The Elbow and Its Disorders, 2nd ed. Philadelphia, WB Saunders, 1993, pp 16–52.

23. Nirschl RP, Morrey BF: Rehabilitation. In Morrey BF (ed): The Elbow and its Disorders, 2nd ed. Philadelphia, WB Saunders, 1993, pp 173–180.

24. O'Driscoll SW, Morrey BF, An KN: Intraarticular pressure and capacity of the elbow: J Arthrosc Rel Surg 1990; 6(2):100–103.

25. Funk DA, An KN, Morrey BF, Daube JR: EMG analysis of the muscles across the elbow joint. J Orthop Res 1987; 5(4):529–538.

26. Basmajian JV, Latif MA: Integrated actions and functions of the chief flexors of the elbow. J Bone Joint Surg 1957; 39A(5):1106–1118.

27. Basmajian JV, Travill A: Electromyography of the pronator muscle of the forearm. Anat Rec 1961; 139:45–49.

28. An KN, Hui FC, Morrey BF, et al: Muscles across the elbow joint: A biomechanical analysis. J Biomech 1981; 14(10):659–669.

29. Rasch PJ: Effect of the position of the forearm on strength of elbow flexion. Res Q 1955; 27(3):333–337.

30. Morrey BF: Anatomy of the elbow joint. In Morrey BF (ed): The Elbow and Its Disorders, 2nd ed. Philadelphia, WB Saunders, 1993, pp 16–52.

31. Pauly JE, Rushing JL, Schering LE: An electromyographic study of some muscles crossing the elbow joint. Anat Rec 1967; 159:45–54.

32. Travill AA: Electromyographic study of the extensor apparatus of the forearm. Anat Rec 1962; 144:373–376.

33. Currier DP: Maximal isometric tension of the elbow extensors at varied positions. Phys Ther 1972; 52(12):1265–1276.

34. Jobe FW, El Attrache NS: Treatment of ulnar collateral ligament injuries in athletes. In Morrey BF (ed): The Elbow. New York, Raven Press, 1994, pp 566–577.

35. Ellenbecker TS: Elbow, forearm and wrist testing and rehabilitation. In Davies GJ (ed): A Compendium of Isokinetics in Clinical Usage, 4th ed. S&S Publishers, La Crosse, WI, 1992, pp 481–495.

36. Fleisig GS, Escamilla RF, Andrews JR: Biomechanics of throwing. In Zachazewski JE, Quillen WS, Magee DJ (eds): Athletic Injuries and Rehabilitation. Philadelphia, WB Saunders, 1996.

37. Tullos HS, King JW: Throwing mechanism in sports. Orthop Clin North Am 1973; 4:709–720.

38. Gore RM, Rogers LF, Bowerman J, et al: Osseus manifestations of elbow stress associated with sports. AJR 1980; 134:971–977.

39. Bryan W: Baseball in sports medicine. In Reider B (ed): Sports Medicine: The School-Age Athlete. Philadelphia, WB Saunders, 1991, pp 447–483.

40. DiGiovine NM, Jobe FW, Pink M, Perry J: An electromyographical analysis of the upper extremity in pitching. J Shoulder Elbow Surg 1992; 1:15–25.

41. Bowyer BL, Gooch JL, Geringer SR: Sports Medicine 2: Upper extremity injuries. Arch Phys Med Rehab 1993; 74(5):437.

42. Harrelson GL: Elbow rehabilitation. In Andrews J, Harrelson GL (eds): Physical Rehabilitation of the Injured Athlete. Philadelphia, WB Saunders, 1991, pp 443–472.

43. Andrews JR: Bony injuries about the elbow in the throwing athlete. In Pettrone FA (ed): AAOS Symposium on Upper Extremity Injuries in Athletes. St. Louis, CV Mosby, 1984, pp 221–232.

44. Glousman RE, Barron J, Jobe FW, et al: An electromyographical analysis of the elbow in normal and injured pitchers with MCL insufficiency. AMJS Med 1992; 20(3):311–317.

45. Pappas AM: Elbow problems associated with baseball during childhood and adolescence. Clin Orthop 1992; 164:30–41.

46. Kulund DN: The Elbow, Wrist, and Hand in The Injured Athlete, 2nd ed. Philadelphia, JB Lippincott, 1988, pp 360–372.

47. Hill JA, Polkow JJ, Brewster CE: Rehabilitation in baseball pitchers following surgery on the elbow. Contemp Orthop 1992; 24(4):445–449.

47a. Brogdon BG, Crow E: Little League elbow. Am J Roentgenol 1960; 83:671–675.

48. Hinz C: Little League elbow. Your Patients Fitness 1989; 2(4):5–8.

49. Adams JE: Injuries to the throwing arm: A study of traumatic changes in the elbow joint of boy baseball players. Cal Med 1964; 102:127–132.

50. Tullos HS, King JW: Lesions of the pitching arm in adolescents. JAMA 1972; 220(2):264–271.

51. Bassett RB, Breecher DB: Common Sports Injuries in Youngsters. Oradell, NJ, Medical Economics Books, 1987, pp 71–82.

52. Hang YS, Peng SM: An epidemiologic study of the upper extremity in tennis players with a particular reference to tennis elbow. J Formos Med Assoc 1984; 83:307–316.

53. Nirschl RP: Soft tissue injuries about the elbow. Clin Sports Med 1986; 5(4):637–652.

54. Cruchow HW, Pelletier D: An epidemiologic study of tennis elbow: Incidence, recurrence and effectiveness of prevention strategies. Am J Sports Med 1979; 7:234–238.

55. Priest JD, Nagel DA: Tennis shoulder. Am J Sports Med 1976; 4:28–42.

56. Morris M, Jobe FW, Perry J, et al: Electromyographic analysis of elbow function in tennis players. Am J Sports Med 1989; 17(2):241–247.

57. Dillman CJ: Presentation on the upper extremity in tennis and throwing athletes. US Tennis Association National Meeting, Tucson AZ, March 1991.

58. Van Gheluwe B, Hebbelinck M: The kinematics of the service movement in tennis: A 3-dimensional cinematographical approach. In Winter D, Normal R, Wells R, et al (eds): Biomechanics IX-B. Champaign, IL, Human Kinetics Publishing, 1983.

59. Runge R: ZurGenese & Behandllung des Schreibkrampfes. Klin Wochenschr 1873; 10:245.

60. Leach RE, Miller JK: Lateral and medial epicondylitis of the elbow. Clin Sports Med 1987; 6(2):259–272.

61. Kamien M: A rational management of tennis elbow. J Sports Med 1990; 9(3):173–191.

62. Nirschl RP: The etiology and treatment of tennis elbow. J Sports Med 1974; 2(6):308–323.

63. Fowler PJ, Webster-Bogaert MS: Swimming. In Reider B (ed): Sports Medicine: The School-Age Athlete. Philadelphia, WB Saunders, 1991, pp 429–446.

64. Johnson DC: The upper extremity in swimming. In Pettrone FA (ed): AAOS Symposium Upper Extremity Injuries in Athletes. St. Louis, CV Mosby, 1984, pp 36–46.

65. Garrick J, Regua R: Epidemiology of women's gymnastic injuries. Am J Sports Med 1980; 8(4):261.

66. Snook G: Injuries in women's gymnastics. Am J Sports Med 1979; 7(4):242.

67. Aronen JG: Problems of the upper extremity in gymnastics. Clin Sports Med 1985; 14(1):61–71.

68. Mandelbaum GR: Gymnastics. In Reider B (ed): Sports Medicine: The School-Age Athlete. Philadelphia, WB Saunders, 1991, pp 415–428.

69. Priest JD, Wiese DJ: Elbow injuries in women's gymnastics. Am J Sports Med 1981; 9:288–295.

70. Priest JD: Elbow injuries in gymnastics. Clin Sports Med 1985; 4(1):73–84.

71. Curtis RJ, Corley FG Jr: Fractures and dislocations of the forearm. Clin Sports Med 1986; 5(4):663–673.

72. The upper arm, elbow, and forearm. In Hunter LY (ed): AAOS Athletic Training and Sports Medicine, 2nd ed. Park Ridge, IL, 1991, pp 267–282.

73. Selesnick FH, Dolitsky B, Haskell SS: Fractures of the coronoid process requiring open reduction with internal fixation. J Bone Joint Surg 1984; 66A(8):1304–1308.

74. Peterson L, Renstrom P: Muscle injuries—strains. In Grana WA (ed): Sports Injuries: Their Prevention and Treatment. Chicago, Year Book Medical, 1986, p 465.

75. Baker B, Bierwagen D: Rupture of the distal tendon of the biceps brachii. J Bone Joint Surg 1985; 67A(30):414–417.

76. Bourne MH, Morrey BF: Partial rupture of the distal biceps tendon. Clin Orthop 1991; 271:143–148.

77. Goodfellow JW, Bullough P: The pattern of aging of the articular cartilage of the elbow joint. J Bone Joint Surg 1967; 49B(1):175–181.

78. Wilder R, Nirschl RP, Sobel J: Disorders of the elbow and forearm. In Bushbacher RM (ed): Musculoskeletal Disorders. Boston, Butterworth-Heineman, 1994, pp 153–169.

79. Cox WD, Nirschl RP: A modified lateral approach for release of post-traumatic elbow flexion contracture. Poster presentation at the American Academy of Orthopedic Surgeons Annual Meeting, Orlando, FL, February 19, 1995.

80. Brown R, Blazina ME, Kerlan K, et al: Osteochondritis of the capitellum. J Sports Med 1974; 2(1):27–46.

81. Singer KM, Roy SP: Osteochondrosis of the humeral capitellum. Am J Sports Med 1984; 12(5):351–360.

82. Cyriax J: Textbook of Orthopedic Medicine, Vol 1, 8th ed. London, Baillière Tindall, 1982, pp 168–181.

83. Nirschl RP, Pettrone FA: Tennis elbow: The surgical treatment of lateral epicondylitis. J Bone Joint Surg 1979; 61A:832.

84. Nirschl RP: Mesenchymal syndrome. Va Med Month 1969; 96:659.

85. Chop WM: Tennis elbow. Postgrad Med 1989; 86(5):301–308.

86. Chard M, Hazelman BL: Tennis elbow—a reappraisal. Br J Rheumatol 1990; 28(3):186–190.

87. Werner CO: A simple cure for chronic tennis elbow. Austr Fam Phys 1987; 16(7):953.

88. Jobe FW, Nuber G: Throwing injuries of the elbow. Clin Sports Med 1986; 5(4):621–636.

88a. Organ S, Nirschl RP: Salvage surgery to the lateral elbow. Presented at AOSSM Annual Meeting. Toronto, July 1995

89. Morrey BF, O'Driscoll SW: Lateral collateral ligament injury. In Morrey BF (ed): The Elbow and its Disorders, 2nd ed. Philadelphia, WB Saunders, 1993, pp 573–580.

90. Childress H: Recurrent ulnar nerve dislocation at the elbow. Clin Orthop 1975; 108:168–173.

91. McGowan AJ: The results of transposition of the ulnar nerve for traumatic ulnar neuritis. J Bone Joint Surg 1950; 32B:293–301.

92. Mosher JF: Peripheral nerve injuries and entrapments of the forearm and wrist. In Pettrone FA (ed): AAOS Symposium on Upper Extremity Injuries in Athletes. St. Louis, CV Mosby, 1984, pp 174–181.

93. Spinner M, Linscheid RC: Nerve entrapment syndromes. In Morrey BF (ed): The Elbow and Its Disorders, 2nd ed. Philadelphia, WB Saunders, 1993, pp 813–832.

94. Hoppenfeld S (ed): Physical examination of the elbow. In Physical Examination of the Spine and Extremities. Norwalk, CT, Appleton-Century-Crofts, 1976, pp 35–57.

95. Regan WD, Morrey BF: The physical examination of the elbow. In Morrey BF (ed): The Elbow and its Disorders, 2nd ed. Philadelphia, WB Saunders, 1993, pp 73–90.

96. Tullos HS, Bryan WJ: Examination of the throwing elbow. In Zarins B, Andrews JR, Carson WG Jr (eds): Injuries to the Throwing Arm. Philadelphia, WB Saunders, 1985, pp 201–211.

97. Davies GJ, Halbach JW, Carpenter MA: A descriptive muscular power analysis of the US cross country ski team. Med Sci Sports Exerc 1980; 12(2):441 (Abstract).

98. Pawlowski D, Perrin DH: Relationship between shoulder and elbow isokinetic peak torque, torque acceleration energy, average power and total work and throwing velocity in intercollegiate pitchers. Athletic Training 1989; 24(2):129–132.

99. Schexneider MA, Catlin PA, Davies GJ, Mattson PA: In isokinetic estimation of total arm strength. Isokinetics Exerc Sci 1991; 1(3):117–121.

100. Nirschl RP, Sobel J: Conservative treatment of tennis elbow. Phys Sports Med 1981; 9(6):43–54.

101. Strizak AM, Glenn GW, Spaega A, Nicholas JA: Hand and forearm strength and its relations to tennis. Am J Sports Med 1983; 11(1):234–239.

102. Van Swearingen JM: Measuring wrist muscle strength. J Orthop Sports Phys Ther 1983; 4(4):217–228.

103. Wilk KE, Arrigo C, Andrews JR: Rehabilitation of the elbow in the throwing athlete. J Orthop Phys Sports Ther 1993; 17(6):305–

104. Buehler MJ, Thayer DT: The elbow flexion test: A clinical test for cubital tunnel syndrome. Clin Orthop 1988; 233:213–216.

105. Ferlic DC, Morrey BF: Evaluation of the painful elbow: The problem elbow. In Morrey BF (ed): The Elbow and its Disorders, 2nd ed. Philadelphia, WB Saunders, 1993, pp 131–138.

106. Anderson T: Anatomy and physical examination of the elbow. In Nicholas JA, Hershman ER (eds): The Upper Extremity in Sports. St. Louis, CV Mosby, 1990, pp 273–288.

107. Cooper M: Use of modalities in rehabilitation. In Andrews J, Harrelson G (eds): Physical Rehabilitation of the Injured athlete. Philadelphia, WB Saunders, 1991, pp 85–140.

108. Harrelson GL: Introduction to rehabilitation. In Andrews J, Harrelson G (eds): Physical Rehabilitation of the Injured Athlete. Philadelphia, WB Saunders, 1991, pp 165–195.

109. Nirschl RP: Elbow tendinosis: Tennis elbow. Clin Sports Med 1992; 11(4):851–869.

110. Ernst E: Conservative treatment of tennis elbow. Br J Clin Pract 1992; 46(1):55–57.

111. Binder A, Hodge G, Greenwood AM, et al: Is therapeutic ultrasound effective in treatment of soft tissue lesions? Br Med J 1985; 290(10):512–514.

112. Lundberg T, Abrahamson P, Haker E: A comparative study of continuous ultrasound, placebo ultrasound and rest in epicondylalgia. Scand J Rehab Med 1988; 20:99–101.

113. Straltford PW, Levy DR, Gauldie S, et al: The evaluation of phonophoresis and friction massage as treatment for extensor carpi radialis tendinitis: A randomized controlled trial. Physiother Can 1989; 41:93–99.

114. Halle JS, Franklin RJ, Karaija BL: Comparison of four treatment approaches for lateral epicondylitis of the elbow. J Orthop Sports Phys Ther 1986; 8:62–69.

115. Galloway M, De Maio M, Mangine R: Rehabilitative techniques in the treatment of medial and lateral epicondylitis. Orthopedics 1992; 15(9):1089–1096.

116. Calvert PT, Allum RL, MacPherson IS, Bentley G: Simple lateral release in treatment of tennis elbow. J R Soc Med 1985; 78:912–915.

117. Warren RF: Tennis elbow (epicondylitis). In Pettrone FA (ed):

AAOS Symposium on Upper Extremity Injuries in Athletes. St. Louis, CV Mosby, 1984, pp 233–264.

118. Clark AK, Woodland J: Comparison of two steroid preparations used to treat tennis elbow. Rheumatol Rehab 1975; 14:47–49.

119. Kennedy JC, Willis RB: The effects of local steroid injection on tendons. Am J Sports Med 1976; 4:11.

120. Davies GJ: A Compendum of Isokinetics in Clinical Usage, 3rd ed. La Crosse, WI, S & S Publishers, 1987.

121. Knott M, Voss D: Proprioceptive Neuromuscular Facilitation. New York, Harper & Row, 1968.

122. Ellenbecker TA: Unpublished research, Health-South, Scottsdale, AZ, 1994.

123. Motzkin NG, Cahalan TD, Morrey BF, et al: Isometric and isokinetic endurance testing of the forearm complex. Am J Sports Med 1991; 19(2):107–111.

124. Knapik JJ, Ramos MV: Isokinetic and isometric torque relationships in the human body. Arch Phys Med Rehabil 1980; 61:64–67.

125. Otis JC, Gobold JH: Relationships of isokinetic torque to isometric torque. J Orthop 1983; 1:165–171.

126. Gamble JN: Strength and conditioning for the competitive athlete. *J Natl Strength Cond Assoc*, pp 111–147.

127. Chu D: Power Tennis Training. Champaign, IL, Human Kinetics Publishing, 1995.

128. Gerberich SG, Priest JD: Treatment of lateral epicondylitis. Br J Sports Med 1985; 19(4):224–227.

129. Labelle H, Gruber R, Joncas J, et al: Lack of scientific evidence for the treatment of lateral epicondylitis of the elbow. J Bone Joint Surg 1972; 74B(5):646–651.

130. Groppel J, Nirschl RP: A mechanical and electromyographical analysis of the effects of various joint counterforce braces on the tennis players. Am J Sports Med 1986; 14(3):195–200.

131. Stonecipher DR, Catlin PA: The effect of a forearm strap on wrist extensor strength. J Orthop Sports Phys Ther 1984; 6(3):184–189.

132. Wadsworth CT, Nielsen DH, Burns LT, et al: The effect of the counterforce armband on wrist extension and grip strength and pain in subjects with tennis elbow. J Orthop Sports Phys Ther 1989; 11:192.

133. Adelsberg S: An EMG analysis of selected muscles with racquets of increasing grip size. Am J Sports Med 1986; 14:139.

134. Brody H: Physics of the tennis racquet. Am J Physiol 1979; 6:482.

135. Groppel JL: Tennis for Advanced Players: And Those Who Would Like to Be. Champaign, IL, Human Kinetics, 1984.

136. Pedagana LR, Elsner RC, Roberts D, et al: The relationship of upper extremity strength to throwing speed. Am J Sports Med 1982; 10:352–352.

136a. Anderson TE, Ciolek J: Specific rehabilitation programs for the throwing athlete. Instr Course Lect 1989; 38:487–491.

137. Blackburn TA: Rehabilitation of the shoulder and elbow after arthroscopy. Clin Sports Med 1987; 6(3):587–606.

138. Jobe FW, Stark H, Lombardo SJ: Reconstruction of the UCL in athletes. J Bone Joint Surg 1986; 68A(8):1158–1163.

139. Melhoff TL, Noble PC, Bennett JB, Tullos HS: Simple dislocation of the elbow in the adult. J Bone Joint Surg 1988; 70A:244–249.

140. Protzman RR: Dislocation of the elbow joint. J Bone Joint Surg 1978; 60A:539–541.

141. Tivon MC, Anzel SH, Waugh TR: Surgical management of osteochondritis of the capitellum. Am J Sports Med 1976; 4(3):121–128.

CHAPTER 28

Hand and Wrist Injuries

FRANK C. McCUE III *MD*
OMAR D. HUSSAMY *MB, BChir, MD*
JOE H. GIECK *EdD, PT, ATC*

Injuries of the hand and wrist are common in athletics because the hand is characteristically in front of the athlete in most sports. Nevertheless, injuries to the hand and wrist are often ignored because frequently they do not prevent athletic participation. The key to proper care is early, accurate diagnosis and precise treatment, followed by an appropriate rehabilitation program. Conservative treatment is preferable for most injuries of the hand and wrist; most athletes can rapidly be returned to their normal activities.[1,2]

EXAMINATION OF JOINTS

Clinical examination of an injured joint requires knowledge of the functional and structural principles of anatomy. Observation is necessary to detect malrotation or angular deformities, both of which are accentuated when digits are actively flexed. Local tenderness and instability can be pinpointed through gentle examination. In determining joint laxity, an examination should always be made of the contralateral joint to compare variations in normal joint laxity. In some cases, a digital nerve block may be necessary to eliminate discomfort and allow the athlete to cooperate with the examination. Quality radiographs tailored to the specific joint may include posteroanterior, lateral, and oblique views for digital injuries. Stress radiographs are also helpful in assessing the degree of subluxation or ligamentous avulsion.

REHABILITATION PROGRAM

A rehabilitation program is based on the results of a thorough clinical examination and accurately documented measurements.[3] Initial examination includes the position of the hand at rest, evaluation of deformity, instability, active and passive motion, edema, and nerve and tendon functions.

Edema is best measured in the hand and wrist by circumferential measurements. These should be measured in centimeters and recorded in a consistent manner.

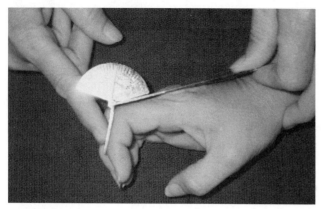

FIGURE 28–1. Goniometer suitable for measuring joint motion in the hand.

When active and passive motion is evaluated, standardized methods of measuring and recording should be used; a digital goniometer should be employed (Fig. 28–1). Active motion assesses the degree of motion that can be obtained in a joint by active muscle contraction. Passive motion determines the freedom that exists at a joint. Both active and passive motion should be measured and recorded; discrepancies between active and passive motion are a major factor in planning a successful rehabilitation program. Limitations in passive motion are indicative of problems with the joint itself or with its surrounding capsule. Limitations in active motion can be due to loss of tendon continuity, adherence of tendon to surrounding tissues, constriction of the tendon sheath, inflammation, subluxation, dislocation, or bowstringing of the tendon.

Manual muscle testing plays an important role in evaluating peripheral nerve lesions. To ensure consistency, a uniform system for recording muscle strength should be used. The numerical system 0 to 5, devised by Seddon, is a frequently used method. Jamar hydraulic dynamometers provide an accurate method of measuring grip strength. Several commercial pinch gauges are available. In acute and postoperative conditions, measuring grip and pinch strength is not appropriate. Resistive testing should not be started until motion is full and painless.

Edema is the hand's first reaction to injury. Acute edema is controlled with splints, compression dressings, icing, elevation, and active exercises. Edema responds well to Coban wrap, a means of providing constant pressure while allowing the freedom to exercise (Fig. 28–2).

Exercise is classified as active, active assisted, passive, or resisted. Active exercises should be initiated as soon as possible after injury, when adequate healing has occurred. Active exercises should be performed gently within pain tolerance to avoid tissue reaction, frequently to increase mobility, and through as complete a tendon excursion as possible to prevent tendon adherence.

Rehabilitation of hand injuries differs from that of other areas in that the hand is less forgiving in its response to overtreatment.[1] The hand responds to overexercise by developing increased pain, swelling, and stiffness. The effects of a poorly planned rehabilitation program can create a greater disability than that which was brought about by the initial injury.

After a comprehensive evaluation, the team physician must determine the course of action regarding treatment options. The main objective is to return the athlete to competition as quickly as possible while preventing permanent disability. The decision as to whether the player's injury can be safely protected to allow him to compete is totally that of the team physician.

FRACTURES AND DISLOCATIONS OF THE METACARPALS AND PHALANGES

Full restoration of hand function after skeletal disruption requires maximum range of motion with solid union of the fracture. Accurate diagnosis, fracture reduction, and an early rehabilitation program are essential to achieve these goals.[4]

Initial evaluation should include review of the mechanism of injury, and physical examination to evaluate swelling, pain, and limitations in motion or obvious deformities. Early management depends on the recognition of muscle and tendon forces on bone fragments that will result in residual deformity of the fragment. In certain types of avulsion fractures, the possibility of tendon rupture or injury to the interphalangeal

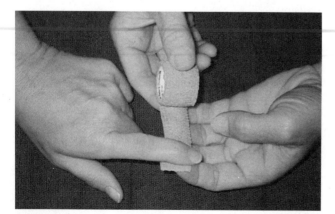

FIGURE 28–2. Coban wrapped in a single layer around a digit helps to control edema.

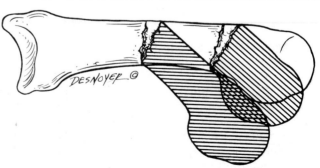

FIGURE 28–3. A boxer fracture occurs through the neck of the fifth metacarpal. Greater angulation is acceptable in the fourth and fifth metacarpals.

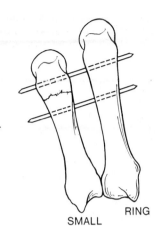
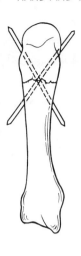
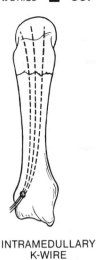

SMALL   RING

INTRAMEDULLARY
K-WIRE

FIGURE 28–4. Open reduction and internal fixation of an unstable metacarpal fracture. (From Hastings H II: Management of Extra-articular fractures of the phalanges and metacarpals. In Strickland JW, Rettig AC [eds]: Hand Injuries in Athletes. Philadelphia, WB Sanders, 1992.)

(IP) joints should be considered. Stress and comparison X-ray films of the opposite extremity are often needed to visualize subluxations or dislocations. A true lateral view of the digit is necessary to rule out injuries to the proximal and distal interphalangeal joints.[5]

Fractures are classified according to the direction of the fracture line with respect to the longitudinal axis of the bone. A transverse fracture line runs perpendicular to the long axis of the bone and extends throughout the entire bone. An oblique fracture line runs at an oblique angle to the long bone axis. A spiral fracture line rotates around and through the long bone axis causing both rotation and potential shortening. A comminuted fracture is one that is broken into more than two pieces. In an impacted fracture, the ends of the fragments are compressed together and may result in excessive shortening and angulation. The fracture line of an intra-articular fracture extends into the articular cartilage and may be displaced, creating an irregular joint surface and making anatomic reduction mandatory. An avulsion fracture is one in which a small fragment of bone pulls away from the large bone at the ligamentous or tendinous attachment.

Management of fractures is dependent on whether they are open or closed and stable or unstable. Closed injuries are usually more stable because soft tissue is not disrupted, whereas open fractures require special attention for wound care. Whether closed or open methods of treatment are used, immobilization or internal fixation must be sufficient to achieve adequate fracture stability; restore appropriate fracture alignment; and prevent excessive shortening, angulation, or rotation in order to allow early motion.[6]

METACARPAL FRACTURES

Metacarpal fractures are classified according to their location: head, neck, shaft, or base. Metacarpal (MC) fractures are more stable than phalangeal fractures because of the additional support provided by the adjacent bones and intrinsic muscles. Stable metacarpal fractures without a spiral component can be treated

with simple immobilization (Fig. 28–3). Fractures that are unstable or involve multiple metacarpals require internal fixation to allow early motion (Fig. 28–4). Edema is often present throughout the dorsal aspect of the hand because metacarpal fractures are often caused by dorsal crushing blows. Prolonged edema and direct trauma to the intrinsic muscles may result in intrinsic contracture. Proper immobilization followed by an early exercise program can help prevent an extension contracture. Metacarpophalangeal (MCP) joints should be immobilized in 60 to 70 degrees of flexion to prevent development of an extension contracture (Fig. 28–5). To counteract the effects of this splinting position, an early exercise program should be started to prevent intrinsic tightness. The MCP joints should be passively extended while flexing the interphalangeal joint.

The duration of immobilization required for healing of metacarpal fractures depends on the location of the fracture. Gentle active motion is not started for at least 3 weeks. Protective splinting then continues for an

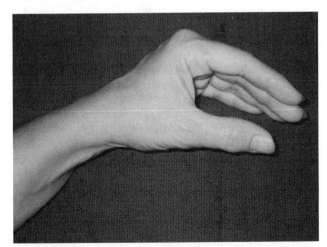

FIGURE 28–5. The intrinsic plus position with the metacarpophalangeal joints immobilized in at least 70 degrees of flexion and the interphalangeal joints fully extended. This prevents metacarpophalangeal extension contracture.

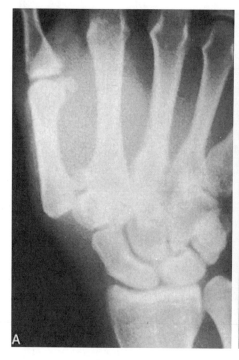
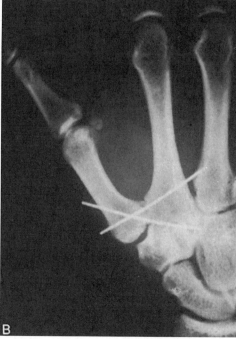

FIGURE 28–6. A radiograph demonstrating the Bennett fracture. (From McCue FC, Garroway RY: Sports injuries to the hand and wrist. *In* Schneider RC, Kennedy JC, Plant ML [eds]: Sports Injuries: Mechanisms, Prevention and Treatment. Baltimore, Williams & Wilkins, 1985.)

additional period as is deemed necessary by radiographic findings.[7]

THUMB METACARPAL FRACTURES

The usual mechanism of MC fractures of the thumb in athletes is axial compression. Thumb metacarpal fractures usually occur at the base and often involve the carpometacarpal joint. There are four types of fractures involving the base of the thumb metacarpal. There are two intra-articular types of fracture, Bennett and Rolando, as well as two extra-articular types. The Bennett fracture involves a small bony fragment that remains attached to the medial aspect of the volar ligament while the long abductor muscle of the thumb muscle pulls the metacarpal proximally (Fig. 28–6). The Rolando fracture involves a large dorsal fragment in addition to the volar lip fragment. The preferred method of treatment of both these fractures is closed reduction and K-wire percutaneous fixation. In cases in which there is soft tissue interposition, open reduction is required.

A rehabilitation program should be started at 3 to 4 weeks following initial treatment. To restore mobility to the thumb, the splint should be removed periodically to allow the athlete to perform active isolated and composite exercises. Wrist exercises should also be started to prevent stiffness. Protective splinting should continue for at least 6 weeks. When protective splinting is discontinued, exercises are upgraded from active to active assisted together with gentle stretching exercises. When medical clearance is given for the athlete to return to competition, it is the responsibility of the trainer or therapist to provide the athlete with adequate protection. Protection should be continued until motion has been fully restored and all pain has subsided.

REHABILITATION OF PROXIMAL INTERPHALANGEAL JOINT FRACTURES

Minimally displaced, stable fractures involving the proximal interphalangeal (PIP) joint should be immobilized for 3 weeks; gentle motion can then be initiated. Protective splinting continues for an additional 3 weeks, during which time it is removed for exercise.[2,8] Unstable or displaced fractures require open reduction to prevent angulation or rotation. After open reduction, immobilization should continue in the extended position for 2 weeks, after which gentle exercises are begun. Protective splinting should continue for an additional 3 weeks.[9,10] Early motion is necessary in rehabilitation of PIP joint injuries because it prevents tendon adherence to healing bone, torn periosteum, or scarred tendon sheath.[10]

ULNAR COLLATERAL LIGAMENT INJURIES

Abduction stress to the thumb while the metacarpophalangeal joint is near full extension can tear the ulnar collateral ligament. This injury has been described as an occupational feature of Scottish gamekeepers who dispatch rabbits by pulling forcibly on the neck; thus the term *gamekeeper's thumb*.[11] The injury is frequently seen in those who injure the ligament when the thumb is stressed by the ski pole strap during a fall.

In evaluating a suspected collateral ligament injury, it is essential to examine the uninjured thumb as well.[12] There is great variation in MP range of motion and stability. Laxity is best demonstrated by stressing the thumb in flexion to remove the stabilizing influence of the volar plate (Fig. 28–7). If the volar plate and accessory collateral ligaments have been injured as well, the thumb will demonstrate hyperextension laxity. Stress films are useful in documenting instability in abduction, and once again, they should be compared with the normal side. In addition, plain films may demonstrate a collateral ligament avulsion off the ulnar aspect of the proximal phalanx.[13]

Chronic laxity of the MCP joint is often seen following injury to the ulnar collateral ligament. Although the thumb adductor insertion is rarely injured concurrently, it alone cannot compensate for the loss of static stability.

A partially injured ligament will retain its normal anatomic relationship if properly immobilized in a thumb spica cast. The thumb is held in a slightly adducted position to reduce stress on the ligament. The thumb spica cast should be worn for 3 weeks, at which time it should be replaced by a volar splint. The splint is removed periodically throughout the day to allow the athlete to perform active isolated and composite exercises of the thumb and wrist. As stability of the thumb is necessary for functional use, splinting is continued until 6 weeks from the date of injury. Indications for surgical repair of acute ulnar collateral ligament injuries include gross clinical instability, interpositional soft tissue, and intra-articular displaced or rotated fractures.[14] Surgical repair of a chronic ulnar collateral ligament injury is only indicated to relieve pain and improve stability and to improve pinch strength. The results of surgical repair of chronic ligamentous injuries are not as good as those of acute injuries. The treatment goal is to re-establish or preserve stability of the thumb while returning the athlete to competition as quickly as possible without risking re-injury. The thumb is protected for a total of 3 months by either taping it to the index finger in adduction or by fabricating a silicone cast for participation in sports.

AVULSION OF THE FLEXOR DIGITORUM PROFUNDUS

Avulsion of the flexor digitorum profundus (FDP) is commonly referred to as a "jersey finger."[15] When an athlete grabs an opponent's jersey he feels a sudden pain in the distal phalanx, which is forcibly extended while it is actively flexed. This injury is most commonly seen in the ring finger. When the fingers are held in extension, there is no obvious deformity. Lack of active flexion of the distal interphalangeal (DIP) joint is often attributed to soft tissue swelling and tenderness. Examination of the injury should include testing of active flexion of the DIP joint. Radiographs should be obtained to rule out associated fracture; often a bony fragment from the distal phalanx is attached to the tendon.

Treatment should consist of primary repair with re-attachment of the deep tendon to the distal phalanx. However, if an athlete elects to undergo delayed repair, a therapeutic program of exercises should be performed to maintain mobility of all joints of the involved finger. Sufficient protection should be provided so as to prevent further injury to the digit during athletics.

Delayed surgical procedures are more extensive and may involve tendon grafting to restore mobility to the distal phalanx. Fusion of the DIP joint is an alternative mode of treatment.

The postoperative rehabilitation program for a jersey finger is similar to that for a flexor tendon repair. A dorsal splint is applied to hold the wrist in slight flexion. The MCP joints are immobilized in 60 to 70 degrees of flexion, and the PIPs and DIPs are held in relative extension. The splint is worn continuously for 3 weeks, at which time a hand therapy program is initiated. Active isolated and composite exercises are begun at this time as adequate soft tissue healing has occurred. Active exercises are performed gently within pain tolerance to increase mobility and through as complete an arc as possible to prevent tendon adherence. Exercises that are performed too vigorously or too often may result in a painful, swollen hand. Exercises should be performed periodically throughout the day with the use of a home program. During the third through fifth weeks postoperatively, the protective splint should be removed only to perform exercises. During this time the hand and wrist should be maintained in a protected position. To maintain the protected position, the wrist and fingers should not be simultaneously extended.

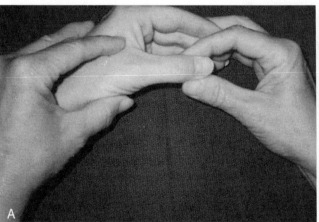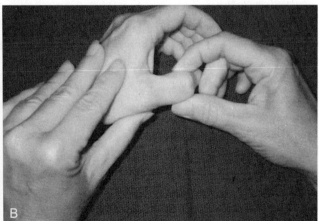

FIGURE 28–7. (A) The metacarpophalangeal joint is stressed in extensor *(A)* as well as flexion *(B)* to differentiate complete tears of the ulnar collateral ligament from partial tears.

When extending the fingers, the wrist should be flexed, and while extending the wrist, the fingers should be flexed. Care should be taken to avoid flexion contractures of the IP joints. If early contracture occurs, gently stretch the joint, using active assistive motion while supporting the wrist in flexion to maintain the protected position of the repaired tendon. Protective splinting is maintained for 5 weeks from the date of surgery. After splint use is discontinued, light functional use of the hand is allowed. Resisted exercises should not be performed until 8 weeks postoperatively. When the athlete is cleared by the team physician to participate, he or she should be provided with protection until full mobility has been restored.

BOUTONNIÈRE DEFORMITY

Boutonnière deformity is the second commonest closed tendon injury in athletes. The injury is caused by blunt trauma to the dorsal aspect of the PIP joint or acute flexion of the joint against resistance. A split in the dorsal covering of the PIP joint occurs where the central slip of the extensor tendon is avulsed from its insertion on the dorsal base of the middle phalanx. A bony fragment may or may not be attached. Early diagnosis can be difficult because deformity is not present acutely and develops later in digits that are untreated. Radiographs are usually negative. The classic boutonnière deformity consists of hyperextension at the MCP joint, flexion at the PIP joint, and hyperextension of the DIP joint.

After injury the PIP joint assumes a posture of 15 to 30 degrees of flexion. Point tenderness is present over the dorsal lip of the middle phalanx. The PIP joint is swollen and lacks full extension. The inability of the athlete to extend the PIP joint is often incorrectly attributed to pain and swelling. Often a digital block is necessary to allow for adequate examination. When an incorrect diagnosis is made, the finger is often splinted with the PIP joint held in slight flexion for comfort; splinting in this position will lead to further deformity.

Any digital injury that lacks more than 30 degrees of PIP extension along with dorsal tenderness over the base of the middle phalanx should be treated as an acute tendon rupture. The PIP joint should be splinted in full extension while the DIP joint should be left free to allow active flexion. This position of passive PIP extension and active DIP flexion serves to relocate the lateral bands to their original anatomic position on the dorsum of the PIP joint. The splint should be used for 6 to 8 weeks, at which time active exercises may be started. Open reduction and internal fixation is indicated only in acute injuries if an avulsion fracture of the middle phalanx constitutes one third of the articular surface.

In chronic injuries, when a fixed flexion contracture of the PIP joint has developed, either a safety pin splint or serial static splinting may be used to reduce the contracture gradually. If splinting is performed in a persistent manner, surgical intervention may not be needed in older neglected cases. Surgery is only indicated in cases that do not respond to splinting and hand therapy. Numerous surgical procedures have been developed to repair the chronic boutonnière deformity, but results are not uniformly predictable. The best result is obtained by early diagnosis and an adequate splinting program.

The athlete with an acute boutonnière deformity is allowed to participate in athletics wearing a splint. Protective splinting is continued until complete, painless motion has been restored.

PSEUDOBOUTONNIÈRE DEFORMITY

Damage to the proximal portion of the volar plate may produce the pseudoboutonnière deformity.[16,17] This resembles a classic boutonnière deformity, but the central slip remains intact. The pseudoboutonnière deformity is usually created by a twisting or hyperextension injury to the PIP joint.

The posture of a digit with a pseudoboutonnière deformity includes a flexion contracture of the PIP joint, slight hyperextension of the DIP joint, and radiologic evidence of calcification volar to the distal end of the proximal phalanx. In a pseudoboutonnière deformity, flexion contracture of the PIP joint is more resistant to passive extension than in the typical boutonnière deformity. In subacute cases, a safety pin splint can be used to reduce the pseudoboutonnière deformity. Even after correction, patients must be followed closely, since the deformity may recur. Night splinting should be performed to ensure that extension is maintained. Chronic pseudoboutonnière deformities are more resistant to splinting programs. If the deformity is fixed in greater than 40 degrees of flexion or is disabling to the athlete, surgical intervention is indicated.

Active exercises are begun at 6 to 8 weeks. The splint should be worn at all other times until the contracture has been reduced. It may then be removed during the day but worn at night to maintain extension. Protective splinting continues until complete, painless motion has been restored.

PROXIMAL INTERPHALANGEAL JOINT INJURIES

PIP joint dislocations are the commonest injuries in the hand. The spectrum of injuries to the PIP joint range from the athlete's jammed finger to irreducible fracture dislocations. An incomplete disruption can occur in which the ligament is either stretched or partially torn, resulting in pain and swelling but no instability of the joint. In other injuries, such as lateral dislocation and hyperextension injuries, there is complete rupture of the supporting ligaments. However, when the joint returns to normal alignment, the extent of disruption and exact site of injury are not apparent without specific testing. Clinical evaluation of the injured PIP joint requires testing of both active and passive stability of the joint.[18]

ACUTE DORSAL PROXIMAL INTERPHALANGEAL JOINT DISLOCATIONS

Dorsal displacement of the PIP joint is by far the commonest dislocation in the body. The mechanism of injury is usually hyperextension and longitudinal compression, such as that occurring in ball-handling athletes. The greater the longitudinal force involved, the greater the chance of producing a fracture-dislocation.

Treatment for dorsal dislocations that are unstable without an associated fracture is immobilization in 20 to 30 degrees of flexion. Treatment and rehabilitation are provided in two stages. During the first stage, the splint is worn for 3 weeks. While stabilizing the finger against the splint, blocking exercises are performed to isolate the deep and superficial flexor tendons. After the splint is removed, exercises to improve flexion continue, and extension exercises are begun. Once the splint is removed, a swan-neck splint may be worn to prevent hyperextension injury to the joint. The splint allows full flexion but blocks the last 10 to 15 degrees of PIP joint extension. Dynamic splints should not be instituted until 6 weeks from the time of injury.

In an unstable, displaced fracture in which multiple fragments are present, the fragments are excised and the volar plate advanced into the defect with a pull-out wire.[19] This volar plate advancement prevents dislocation from recurring.

The goals of rehabilitation are to prevent the development of contractures, restore mobility, and prevent attenuation of the volar plate. The digit is immobilized for 3 weeks. Active and passive resisted flexion exercises are started at this time with the digit protected in a dorsal extension block splint. Dynamic splints can be initiated after 3 to 5 weeks, but dynamic splints to improve flexion should not be used until after 5 to 7 weeks from the date of surgery.

PIP JOINT COLLATERAL LIGAMENT INJURIES

Incomplete tears of the radial and ulnar collateral ligaments of the PIP joints are termed *sprains*. Clinical examination shows the joint to be stable to both active and passive stability testing. The PIP joint is splinted for comfort, and after 1 week, gentle motion is begun. Protective splinting should continue for 3 to 4 weeks. Reduced motion places the joint at risk for reinjury and adequate, safe protection is mandatory if the athlete is allowed to participate in contact sports. Buddy taping does not allow adequate protection for acutely injured joints.

Completely ruptured collateral ligaments cannot resist passive stress but may be stable to the stresses of active motion. It is important to identify those ligamentous disruptions that are complete. Complete disruptions can result in joint instability such as a complex dislocation or subluxation, in which case early operative repair is necessary. Postoperative rehabilitation is critical to functional recovery. The rehabilitation of collateral ligament injuries requires a comprehensive program that includes the use of various modalities and the fabrication of appropriate splints that allow desired motion while protecting the joint from adverse lateral stresses. A protective splint allows the athlete to return to competition quickly without risking reinjury.

MALLET FINGER

This injury is common in athletes who are required to catch, as in basketball, and football. The injury occurs when a hard-thrown ball strikes the extended fingertip, forcing the DIP joint into flexion while the extensor mechanism is actively contracting. Tenderness is present over the dorsal aspect of the joint. The defect is created by a loss of continuity of the lateral bands at their insertion into the dorsum of the distal phalanx. The flexed position of the DIP joint may be created by the unopposed action of the flexor digitorum profundus tendon. The PIP joint may develop a position of hyperextension resulting from laxity of the volar plate and subsequent imbalance between the extensor and superficial tendons.

There are several distinct anatomic types of extensor mechanism injuries. The extensor tendon can be attenuated, ruptured, or avulsed from the base of the distal phalanx with or without a fragment of bone.

Forces that create the mallet finger deformity may also cause associated injury to the PIP joint. The PIP and DIP joints both must be examined clinically and radiographically; unrecognized and untreated joint injuries can result in serious residual disability.

Those injuries seen within 12 weeks following injury can usually be treated with the DIP joint splinted continuously in extension or slight hyperextension for 8 weeks. An additional 6 to 8 weeks of splinting should be employed during athletics. For daily use, the authors prefer a commercially available plastic splint (Fig. 28–8). The splint is available in eight sizes and will fit most patients. If commercially available splints do not fit, splints may be made from aluminum strips (Fig. 28–9). When applying splints, the position of hyperextension of the distal phalanx should be avoided, since excessive pressure created by such a position may result in skin breakdown. All patients should be evaluated at regular intervals to check skin condition. Splints may be

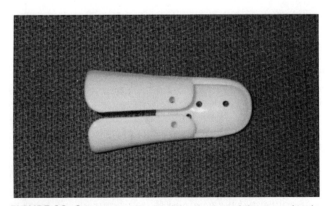

FIGURE 28–8. A stack splint used for the immobilization of mallet finger injuries.

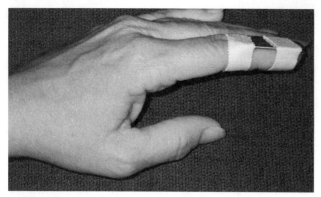

FIGURE 28–9. Dorsal aluminum splint used to protect a mallet finger.

removed for skin care, but it is important to instruct the patient not to allow the distal phalanx to drop into flexion during the early healing period.

Splints should be worn continuously for a minimum of 6 weeks. At the end of 6 weeks, the athlete is allowed to begin flexion exercises with the splint being worn at night for a further 2 weeks. If a loss of extension is noted at any time after splint removal, the splint is reapplied for another 2 weeks and the process repeated.

If compliance with a splinting program is not possible, a K-wire may be passed through the joint. Although use of a splint is still necessary postoperatively, the patient does not need to protect the distal phalanx from dropping into flexion while performing skin care. Those mallet fingers involving fractures of greater than 30 percent of the articular surface should be treated with open reduction and internal fixation.

WRIST INJURIES

Many wrist injuries that occur during athletics are often underestimated and passed off as sprains. The wrist functions to position the hand in space and transmit forces to the hand. Most wrist injuries in athletes are caused by falls on the outstretched hand or by repetitive stresses.[20,21]

SCAPHOID FRACTURES

Fracture of the scaphoid accounts for 70 percent of all carpal fractures. The usual mechanism of injury is a fall on the dorsiflexed wrist, and this is common in many sports.

Acute fractures of the scaphoid are often missed. After a fall, any athlete who has pain and tenderness over the radial aspect of the wrist should be treated as though the scaphoid is fractured. Radiographic examination should include six views: anteroposterior, lateral, right and left oblique, and clenched fist views with the wrist positioned in maximal radial and ulnar deviation. Immediately after an injury, the fracture may not be apparent on radiographic examination. Still, the scaphoid must be assumed to be fractured and treated by immobilization. All radiographs should be repeated

at 2 weeks postinjury. The fracture line usually becomes apparent, but if radiographs remain negative and the athlete remains symptomatic, a bone scan should be obtained.

A short arm-thumb spica cast is placed holding the wrist in slight flexion. In fractures that are unstable, a long arm-thumb spica cast should be used for 6 weeks followed by a short arm-thumb spica cast. The cast should fit snugly and should be changed every 4 weeks. Radiographs should be obtained to assess fracture healing every 3 to 4 weeks.

Most scaphoid fractures will heal in 3 to 4 months. After the fracture is healed as verified by radiographs, immobilization may be discontinued. A rehabilitation program of active exercises is begun to restore mobility to the wrist and thumb. Resistive exercises should not be allowed for at least 2 more months. Once adequate fracture healing has occurred, the athlete may return to competition, provided adequate wrist protection is used.

If a scaphoid fracture fails to unite after 6 months of continuous immobilization, it is unlikely to heal. Delayed union and nonunion can be due to inadequate immobilization, fracture displacement, carpal instability, and inadequate blood supply of the proximal fragment.[22] Bone grafting and internal fixation offer the best solution to this problem. Acute scaphoid fractures that are displaced should immediately be treated with open reduction and internal fixation.

FRACTURES OF THE HAMATE

Fractures of the hook of the hamate are frequently misdiagnosed as tendinitis or wrist sprains. The injury is suspected when an athlete complains of discomfort over the hook of the hamate. The fracture occurs when the bat or racquet strikes the hook of the hamate during a swing. Athletes may have few complaints when not participating in their sport.

The usual radiographic views do not detect this fracture. A carpal tunnel view is helpful in detecting a fracture line (Fig. 28–10) although a computed tomography (CT) scan is often necessary. Conservative treatment for an acute, nondisplaced fracture is possible, but the rate of nonunion is high. Most physicians choose to surgically excise the fragment acutely, since healing time is equal to that required for conservative treatment.

After the skin has healed, the athlete should be instructed in a program of modalities, whirlpool, or paraffin along with scar massage. Gripping exercises using the bat or racquet are begun as soon as this activity can be tolerated. Care should be taken not to progress to full activity until adequate soft tissue healing has occurred.

LUNATE DISLOCATION

Dislocation of the lunate bone arises when the athlete falls on the outstretched wrist. The chief complaint is pain in the wrist, although there may be numbness in the radial three-and-a-half digits of the hand resulting from compression of the median nerve in the carpal tunnel.

Simple anteroposterior and lateral radiographs detect this injury. The preferred treatment is open reduction of the lunate with pinning of the scaphoid to the lunate and capitate bones. The wrist is immobilized for 3 months, the pins being removed at 2 months. The athlete is then instructed in a range-of-motion program. There will be some permanent limi-

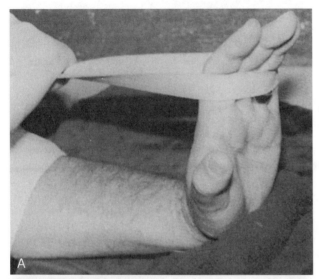

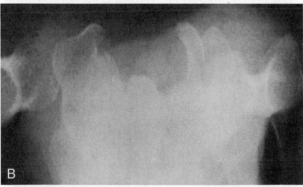

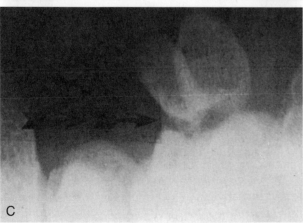

FIGURE 28–10. A carpal tunnel view is useful in the diagnosis of a hook of the hamate fracture. (From Zemel NP: Carpal fractures. *In* Strickland JW, Rettig AC [eds]: Hand Injuries in Athletes. Philadelphia, WB Saunders, 1992.)

tation of motion and grip strength in all individuals with this injury.[12]

KIENBÖCK DISEASE

Avascular necrosis of the lunate bone, which is also known as Kienböck disease, is thought to arise either because of repetitive trauma or an unrecognized fracture of the lunate. The athlete initially complains of pain and weakness of the wrist that is associated with use.

Early radiographs may be negative except for an ulnar minus variant. Ulnar variance refers to the relative lengths of the radius and ulna; these lengths may differ as measured on standard radiographs. Ulnar zero means the radius and ulna are of equal length, ulnar minus variance refers to the ulna being shorter than the radius and ulnar positive variance implies the ulna is longer than the radius. A high percentage of individuals with Kienböck disease have an ulnar minus variant of 2 mm or more. As the disease progresses, radiographic findings include loss of lunate height, fragmentation, proximal migration of the capitate, and degenerative changes in the wrist joint.

In cases of acute, nondisplaced fractures of the lunate, cast immobilization should be used. The cast is worn until radiographic healing is evident. A rehabilitation program for wrist mobilization is begun when adequate healing has occurred.

In the early stages, Kienböck disease can be treated with ulnar lengthening or radial shortening, since this discrepancy in bone length is thought to predispose the lunate to increased stress. In advanced cases of Kienböck disease, various surgical procedures have been employed, including prosthetic replacement, intercarpal fusion, proximal row carpectomy, or wrist fusion.

SOFT TISSUE OVERUSE INJURIES

Overuse injuries can affect a variety of sites. Tissue responds to injury by developing inflammation. In overuse injuries, the added effects of repetitive forces lead to microtrauma, which in turn triggers the inflammatory process as the tissue's ability to heal is overwhelmed. The musculotendinous unit is the tissue most commonly affected by overuse injuries.[23]

GANGLION CYSTS

After trauma to the wrist joint capsule, the synovium may herniate to form a ganglion cyst. This condition is most prevalent in female gymnasts. Wrist pain is greatest in extension but is occasionally present in flexion. Tenderness is present over the scapholunate interval, and a mass may be palpable.

Conservative treatment includes splinting, nonsteroidal anti-inflammatory drugs, taping, and a change in hand grip position during athletic activity. Recalcitrant cases may require surgical excision because aspiration is not productive. The possibility of recurrence always exists.

TENDINITIS

Tendinitis of the wrist is usually sports related. Symptoms include stiffness and an aching type of pain that is aggravated by activity and appears several hours after participation in sports. On clinical examination, tenderness is well localized over the involved tendons. Pain is increased by passive stretch of the affected tendon or by contraction of the associated muscle against resistance. Radiographs are usually normal, but occasionally calcification may be present within the tendon sheath.[24]

DE QUERVAIN DISEASE

Stenosing tenosynovitis of the first dorsal compartment of the wrist that houses the long abductor and short extensor of the thumb tendons is termed *De Quervain disease*. The athlete complains of pain localized to the radial side of the wrist, which is aggravated by movement of the thumb. Local tenderness and swelling over the first dorsal compartment are present. The Finkelstein test is positive. To perform the Finkelstein test, passively abduct and flex the first metacarpal while simultaneously flexing the metacarpophalangeal joint of the thumb to reproduce the pain if the test is positive (Fig. 28–11).

De Quervain disease is usually caused by overuse, but it can occur following a direct blow to the first dorsal compartment or as the result of an acute thumb sprain. Activities that require repetitive thumb abduction and extension combined with radial and ulnar deviation are thought to contribute to this condition. Conservative treatment should consist of splinting modalities and exercises. If symptoms do not subside, steroid injection can be helpful. In chronic situations, surgical intervention may be needed.

TENOSYNOVITIS OF OTHER DORSAL COMPARTMENTS

Tenosynovitis of the remaining five dorsal compartments of the wrist are much less common. The sixth dorsal compartment (extensor carpi ulnaris) of the wrist is the commonest site in this group. Inflammation of the second dorsal compartment (radial wrist extensors) is the next commonest form of dorsal tenosynovitis. It is associated with overuse and responds to conservative management.

Tenosynovitis that affects the fourth (extensor digitorum communis and extensor indicis proprius) or fifth (extensor digiti quinti) compartment is uncommon. If symptoms do not abate with conservative treatment, an anatomic abnormality should be suspected. Involvement of the third dorsal compartment (extensor pollicis

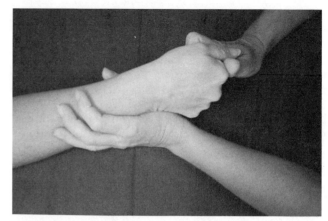

FIGURE 28–11. The Finkelstein test is helpful in the diagnosis of De Quervain disease.

longus) may occur as an isolated entity. Tenosynovitis of this compartment can result from degenerative changes at the Lister tubercle or from exostosis formation after a distal fracture. This puts the extensor pollicis longus at risk of rupture. As a preventive measure, careful radiographic evaluation of the distal radius is performed. In the presence of a bony abnormality, surgical intervention is indicated either to remove the exostosis or reroute the tendon to prevent rupture.[24]

RECURRENT SUBLUXATION OF THE EXTENSOR TENDON OF THE ULNAR WRIST

Recurrent subluxation of the extensor tendon of the ulnar wrist is characterized by a painful snapping over the ulnodorsal aspect of the wrist, especially on forearm rotation. Many of the cases are associated with a history of trauma involving athletic activity. The tendinous subluxation is caused by a disruption of the septum of the sixth dorsal compartment fibrosseous sheath. On supination and ulnar deviation of the wrist, the tendon displaces, and on pronation, the tendon relocates. Closed treatment by immobilizing the wrist in radial deviation and the forearm in pronation may be appropriate. If symptoms persist, surgical reconstruction is advisable.

FLEXOR TENDINITIS OF THE ULNAR WRIST

Flexor tendinitis of the ulnar wrist is associated with repetitive trauma and is quite common. The condition is characterized by tenderness over the tendon at the wrist. The pain is exacerbated by wrist flexion or ulnar deviation against resistance. Radiographs are usually negative, although calcific deposits may be seen in the area of the tendon.[25] Initial treatment includes avoidance of causative activity, immobilization, and nonsteroidal anti-inflammatory drugs. Steroid injection may be necessary. Occasionally, a recalcitrant case may require operative treatment to lyse peritendinous adhesions, excise the pisiform bone, or remove calcific deposits.

TRIGGER FINGER

Repeated trauma to the flexor tendon sheath can result in an inflammatory reaction with swelling that restricts the normal gliding of the flexor tendons within their sheath. This is especially true of the thickened portion of the sheath that forms the A1 pulley at the level of the distal metacarpal. A small nodule on the flexor tendon can impinge on the proximal or distal ends of the A1 pulley, creating a snapping sensation or locking the finger in the flexed position. Trigger finger is initially treated by splinting and steroid injection into the tendon sheath. If triggering persists, surgical release of the A1 pulley is required.

REHABILITATION OF OVERUSE INJURIES

Tendinitis and stenosing tendinitis can occur in any tendon of the hand and wrist. They are caused by repetitive overstretching or by the initiation of unaccustomed motion. All racquet sports create repetitive motions with sudden deceleration as the ball hits the racquet. Symptoms include a vague pain in the area of the affected tendon. Initial treatment to relieve inflammation includes splinting, therapeutic modalities, and avoiding the activity that creates the symptoms. Nonsteroidal anti-inflammatory drugs should be used judiciously.[26]

SPLINTING

Static splints are used for the protection of soft tissues inflamed by overuse. Resting splints should hold the hand and wrist in the functional position. Splinting should be combined with an individually tailored exercise program to prevent dysfunction from occurring. In some cases it may be necessary to allow structures to rest for several days prior to initiating an exercise program.[27]

MODALITIES

Therapeutic modalities are incorporated into the treatment protocol to relieve the symptoms caused by injured tissue.[28] The inflammatory response produces pain, heat, crepitus, erythema, swelling, loss of motion and eventual atrophy. Modalities help to decrease the inflammatory response and enhance tissue healing.

ICE. At the first sign of overuse, ice should be applied for 20 minutes each hour to relieve symptoms. Ice should be employed until a normal pain-free active arc of motion is present, swelling has subsided, and the involved site is no longer warm.

HEAT. As the acute symptoms subside, heat is applied to increase circulation and thus increase cellular metabolism. At this stage of the healing process, heat may be used prior to performing exercises, whereas icing is performed immediately afterwards. When switching to the use of heat, the involved area should be closely observed after each treatment for any signs of an increased inflammatory response. An overzealous ex-

ercise program may also exacerbate symptoms. If symptoms worsen, the exercise program should be downgraded and ice rather than heat should be used to allow for further healing.

ULTRASOUND. Therapeutic ultrasound uses high-frequency sound waves to produce thermal and nonthermal effects on the tissues. It is the treatment of choice when deep heat is required. The physiologic effects of therapeutic ultrasound include (1) increasing the extensibility of collagen tissue, thereby decreasing joint stiffness; (2) reducing pain and muscle spasm; (3) mobilizing edema; and (4) increasing blood flow and metabolism, thereby increasing motion and reducing inflammation.[15] Tendinitis of the hand and wrist responds well to ultrasound.

A conductive medium is required for the sound waves to penetrate to the affected tissue because ultrasound cannot be conducted through air. Although commercial gels, lotions, or mineral oil may be used, underwater ultrasound should be used to treat hands. When the submersion method is used, the sound head should be held 1 to 2 cm from the surface that is being treated. The intensity should be increased by 0.5 W/cm^2 to compensate for the energy that is dissipated into the water. Air bubbles that form on the sound head and on the area to be treated should be wiped away because air will impede the transmission of energy.

The sound head should be kept moving during the treatment at a rate of 2 to 4 cm/second. The head should be directed at a perpendicular angle to the surface being treated. A pulsed or continuous mode of ultrasound can be used, depending on whether heat is required. Pulsed ultrasound is used when treating scar tissue and for tissue healing, whereas the continuous mode is employed when deep heat is required. In areas such as the hand, which have little superficial soft tissue, higher-frequency ultrasound should be used. The depth of penetration is less with 3.0 MHz frequency and is better suited to treat areas such as the wrist, hand, and fingers. Some units do not offer variations in frequency and are usually set at 1.0 MHz. In these cases, intensities of less than 1.25 W/cm^2 should be used. The intensity should never exceed the pain threshold, and the athlete should not suffer excessive warmth during treatment.

Phonophoresis occurs when the energy of ultrasound is used to drive anti-inflammatory or analgesic medications directly into the tissues. This technique is an excellent analgesic with a resulting improvement in range of motion. Studies have shown that 10 percent hydrocortisone ointment is more effective than 1 percent cream.[29] The ointment should be massaged over the area prior to treatment to prevent air bubble formation that will impede transmission of the energy.

Several precautions must be observed to ensure that the use of therapeutic ultrasound is safe and effective. To avoid burns, ultrasound must be applied within pain-free limits. It should therefore not be used in areas with decreased sensation. Ultrasound is contraindicated with active infections and should be used with caution over open epiphyses. Ultrasound is not contraindicated over areas in which metal implants or hardware have been applied.

TRANSCUTANEOUS ELECTRICAL NERVE STIMULATION. Transcutaneous electrical nerve stimulation (TENS) is universally recognized as an acceptable method of treating acute and chronic pain.[30] Conventional TENS is best suited for treatment of overuse syndromes. The successful use of TENS depends on the correct placement of electrodes.[31,32] The area of application is dependent on the patient's description as well as the physical examination. As there is a strong correlation between trigger points, motor points, and acupuncture sites, the clinician should become familiar with their location in the upper extremity.

EXERCISE

Therapeutic modalities serve to reduce pain, swelling, and erythema so that exercise may be initiated. The objective of treatment of overuse syndromes is to allow the athlete to resume normal activity *as* healing occurs instead of rehabilitating him or her *after* healing has occurred. Strengthening and range-of-motion exercises are begun as soon as the inflammatory response is controlled, thus preventing the atrophy, dysfunction, and loss of motion that occurs as a result of disuse. Immobilization and rest may be necessary for several days before the initiation of exercises in acute overuse injuries.

After the application of the appropriate modality (heat, cold, or ultrasound), passive exercises are begun. A slow, steady stretch is held for 30 to 60 seconds and repeated three times. Isometric strengthening exercises are then initiated. Isometric exercises are most effective in the acute phase of treatment. An isometric exercise has a strength carry-over within a 20 degree range of motion. Initially, a patient exerts a force of 40 to 50 percent to gain strength. As symptoms subside, the athlete increases applied resistance isometrically. The exercises should be performed with the joint held in various positions for 6- to 8-second intervals.

The importance of isometric exercise in the strengthening program for overuse injuries cannot be overemphasized. Isokinetic exercises in the acute phase only serve to aggravate the injury. Three sets of ten repeti-

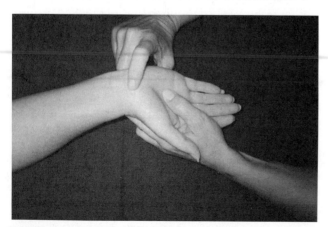

FIGURE 28–12. Percussion of the median nerve on the volar aspect of the wrist will elicit a Tinel sign in the presence of carpal tunnel syndrome.

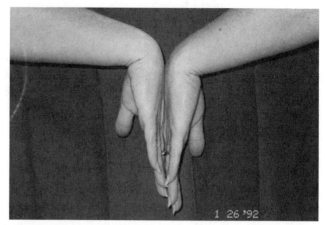

FIGURE 28–13. When the wrist is held in palmar flexion, the athlete experiences increased numbness and paresthesias in the radial three and one-half digits. This is termed a positive Phalen test.

tions of isotonically performed exercises with maximal pain-free resistance is an acceptable routine. Weight is progressively applied as soon as the exercises are tolerated through a full range of motion without evidence of tissue reaction. After eccentric muscle strength has been restored, isokinetic exercises may be initiated if necessary. Free weights are best used as they allow the most normal functional range of motion. Care should be taken not to overtrain when planning a wrist-strengthening program. As normal strength is regained, exercises to improve endurance may be added. This includes multiple sets and repetitions of exercises. The activity that contributed to the symptoms of overuse may be initiated at this time.

NERVE COMPRESSION SYNDROMES

MEDIAN NERVE COMPRESSION

Carpal tunnel syndrome is the most common compression neuropathy of the wrist. Any sports-related activity that involves repetitive wrist motion may be a causative factor. Clinical findings include paresthesias or dysesthesias of the radial three digits of the hand. Tinel sign (Fig. 28–12) over the median nerve and the Phalen test (Fig. 28–13) will be positive. Electromyography is an important diagnostic test in many cases.

Conservative treatment includes immobilization with the wrist in 10 degrees of dorsiflexion. Cessation of all activities that cause symptoms, steroid injection, and the use of nonsteroidal anti-inflammatory drugs may be helpful. Surgical treatment is indicated in cases resistant to conservative treatment.

ULNAR NERVE COMPRESSION

Compression of the ulnar nerve within Guyon's canal occurs less often than carpal tunnel syndrome. The condition is characterized by paresthesias of the ulnar one-and-a-half digits and weakness of the ulnar innervated muscles of the hand.

Treatment involves cessation of athletic activity that contributes to nerve compression. Splinting and nonsteroidal anti-inflammatory drugs may also be helpful. Surgical release of Guyon's canal and neurolysis is occasionally needed. Further discussion of peripheral nerve injuries may be found in Chapter 23.

REFERENCES

1. Bittinger S: The art of joint mobilization: The restoration of joint play. *In* Bowers WH (ed): The Interphalangeal Joints. New York, Churchill Livingstone, 1987, p 265.
2. Bittinger S: Sprains and joint injuries: Therapist's management. Hand Clin 2:99–106, 1986.
3. Beasley R: Rehabilitation of the Hand. *In* Hunter JM, Schneider LH, Mackin EJ, et al (eds): Rehabilitation of the Hand. St. Louis, CV Mosby, 1978.
4. Brunet ME, Haddad RJ: Fractures and dislocation of the metacarpals and phalanges. Clin Sports Med 5:773–781, 1986.
5. Hubbard LF: Metacarpophalangeal dislocations. Hand Clin 4:39–44, 1988.
6. Packer JW, Colditz JC: Bone injuries: Treatment and rehabilitation. Hand Clin 2:81–92, 1986.
7. McCue FC: How I manage fractured metacarpal in athletes. Phys Sports Med 13:83–87, 1985.
8. Bowers WH: Sprains and joint injuries in the hand. Hand Clin 2:93–98, 1986.
9. Mayer V, Gieck JH: Rehabilitation of hand injuries in athletes. Clin Sports Med 5:783–794, 1986.
10. Torkelson SH: Splinting the interphalangeal joints. *In* Bowers WH (ed): The Interphalangeal Joints. New York, Churchill Livingstone, 1987, pp 252–261.
11. McCue FC, Mayer V: Rehabilitation of common athletic injuries of the hand and wrist. Clin Sports Med 8:731–776.
12. Campbell CS: Gamekeeper's thumb. J Bone Joint Surg 37B:148–149, 1955.
13. McCue FC, Mayer V: Diagnosing and treating gamekeeper's thumb. J Musculoskel Med 5:53–63, 1988.
14. Cabrera JM, McCue FC: Nonosseous athletic injuries of the elbow, forearm and hand. Clin Sports Med 5:681–700, 1986.
15. Cooney WP: Sports injuries to the upper extremity. How to recognize and deal with some common problems. Postgrad Med 76:45–50, 1984.
16. Leddy JP, Packer JW: Avulsion of the profundus insertion in athletes. J Hand Surg 2:66, 1977.
17. McCue FC, Honner R, Gieck JH, et al: A pseudoboutonnière deformity. J Br Soc Surg Hand 7:166–170, 1975.
18. Redler MR, McCue FC: Injuries of the hand in athletes. VA Med 115:331–336, 1988.
19. McCue FC, Andrews JR, Hakala M, et al: The coach's finger. J Sports Med 2:270–275, 1974.
20. McCue FC, Honner R, Johnson M, et al: Athletic injuries of the proximal interphalangeal joint requiring surgical treatment. J Bone Joint Surg 52A:937, 1970.
21. Linsheid RL, Dobyns JH: Athletic injuries of the wrist. Clin Orthop 198:141–151, 1985.
22. Pettrone FA: Upper extremity injuries in athletes. St. Louis, CV Mosby, 1984.
23. Linscheid RL, Dobyns JH, Beabout JW: Traumatic instability of the wrist. J Bone Joint Surg 54:1612–1632, 1972.
24. Osterman AL, Moskow L, Dow DW: Soft tissue injuries of the hand and wrist in racquet sports. Clin Sports Med 7:329–347, 1988.
25. McCue FC, Garroway RY: Sports Injuries: Mechanisms, Prevention and Treatment. Baltimore, Williams & Wilkins, 1985.
26. Wood MB, Dobyns JH: Sports-related extra-articular wrist syndromes. Clin Orthop 202:93–102, 1986.
27. Gieck JH, Mayer V: Protective splinting of the hand and wrist. Clin Sports Med 5:795–807, 1986.
28. Gieck JH, Saliba EN: Application of modalities in overuse syndrome. Clin Sports Med 5:795–807, 1986.
29. Kleinkort JA, Wood F: Phonophoresis with 1% vs. 10% hydrocortisone. Phys Ther 55:1320–1324, 1975.
30. Bell AT, Horton PG: The use and abuse of hydrotherapy in athletics: A review. Athletic Train 22:115–119, 1987.
31. Mannheimer JS, Lampe GN: Transcutaneous Electrical Nerve Stimulation. Philadelphia, FA Davis, 1984.
32. Lampe GN: TENS Technology and Physiology. Codman & Shurtleff, 1984.

CHAPTER 29

Hip and Thigh Injuries

B A R B A R A   S A N D E R S   *PhD, PT, SCS*
W I L L I A M   C.   N E M E T H   *MD*

GENERAL CONSIDERATIONS

Although sports injuries to the knee, ankle, and shoulder are well documented and discussed, relatively little attention has been devoted to injuries of the pelvis, hip, and thigh. This is due in part to the relatively low incidence of problems related to this specific anatomic area and the infrequency of related career-threatening injuries. However, there are several important hip and thigh injuries with potentially dire consequences to function and a return to normal athletic activity if improperly managed. The purpose of this chapter is to discuss those entities in detail; dealing initially with the epidemiology of the injury; key factors involved in the differential diagnosis of the entity; treatment recommendations, including conservative and surgical care; and appropriate rehabilitation following medical treatment of the injury.

In the past 20 years, our knowledge of sports injury, its pathogenesis and appropriate treatment, has increased dramatically. This is due to increased athletic activity in our population with the myriad of running, new recreational and competitive sports, and fitness activities. Additionally, higher levels of performance have been sought and achieved in competitive sports as a result of appropriately applied scientific and physiologic principles. The ability to collect and analyze data using sophisticated computer systems has also increased our supply of information.

The incidence and distribution of injury to the pelvis, hip, and thigh varies significantly depending on the specific sporting activity involved. For example, contact sports—for example, like football, rugby, and soccer—have a relatively high incidence of injuries such as hip pointer, hematoma, and traumatic dislocations and fractures of the hip. In the endurance sports such as running and swimming, the overall incidence of traumatic injury is much lower and tends to be more specifically in the stress or overuse category. Serious injuries occur as a result of both types of activities. Specifically, stress fractures have an incidence ranging from as low as 4 percent of total sustained injuries in the casual exercise population to as high as more than 40 percent[1] in the more active population of military recruits. In the distribution of injuries to the lower extremity for all types of athletic activity, the knee, ankle, and foot are the most commonly involved, and behind that as a group are the injuries to the pelvis, hip, and thigh.

Sophisticated imaging techniques have been developed in the last 15 years, initially with computed tomography (CT) and more recently with magnetic resonance imaging (MRI). These techniques have allowed medical specialists to anatomically and pathophysiologically better understand sports injury patterns. Additionally, there has been significant progress made in rehabilitation. In contrast to immobilization in casts, rapid early mobilization following injury, when possible, is now the standard of care. This early mobilization alone has spurred on related research activities to improve even further the rapid return to sport that we are already experiencing.

EVALUATION OF HIP PAIN

No chapter on the pelvis, hip, and thigh would be complete without a discussion of the pathogenesis of hip pain. True hip joint pain is felt in the groin and thigh, not in the buttocks or over the trochanter. Most buttock pain derives from abnormalities of the back and lumbar spine rather than the hip joint itself, and consequently much confusion as to exact diagnosis can often exist.

It is important to acknowledge the possibility of the lumbar spine as a cause of certain patterns of pelvic and hip pain. There is a significant anatomic and biomechanical relationship between lumbar, pelvic, and proximal thigh structures that must be understood if clinicians are to appropriately treat these patients. The concept of referred pain must be kept in mind to make a concise diagnosis of hip and buttocks pain.

Pain in the upper sacroiliac joint area is often related to lumbar spine abnormalities such as lumbar strain, disc disease, and spondylolithesis (Fig. 29–1). This pain radiates from the lumbar area to the sacroiliac region and infrequently, below the area in a "sciatic" distribution. Primary sacroiliac pathology is rare, but seen occasionally in the systemic rheumatologic disorders. Occasionally, local soreness in the sacroalar area is due to sacroiliac bursitis. This manifests as a tender area of crepitus between the skin and the underlying sacroiliac joint.

Another pattern of posterior hip pain is the deep gluteal region over the piriformis muscle. This pain is generally due to lumbar pathology and is true referred pain. In some cases, because of congenital and developmental abnormalities, the piriformis and external rotator muscle group can become tight, causing secondary impingement of the sciatic nerve. This piriformis syndrome can result in "sciatic" pain as the nerve traverses from the sciatic notch underneath the piriformis down the leg. It is associated with local tenderness right over the piriformis muscle, decreased internal rotation of the hip (a result of external rotation contracture), and intermittent sciatica related to activity and overuse. It is seen especially in young gymnasts and dancers, and in older distance runners and ultra-athletes.

The third area of referred pain from the lumbar spine is in the lateral hip or trochanteric area. This type of pain is most often due to disc disease and strain patterns in the lumbar spine. It involves a more radiating type of pain often associated with some back symptoms and gluteal pain. There may or may not be associated tenderness along the trochanteric bursa; but the true

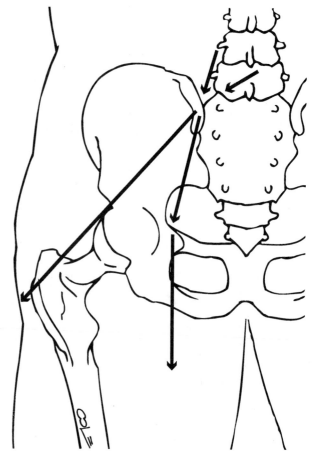

FIGURE 29–1. Pain patterns in lumbar pathology.

type of localized tenderness, swelling, and crepitus that is felt with trochanteric bursitis is not present if this is referred lumbar pain.

The fourth type of pain is due to radicular pathology. This pain pattern can be the most confusing of all because it can mimic true hip joint pathology and is also seen with retroperitoneal processes and intraabdominal and genitourinary abnormalities. Groin pain caused by lumbar pathology is rare, since most lumbar disease occurs in lower dermatomes. Consequently, the preponderance of pain in the groin or thigh is due to primary hip joint pathology or other local bone or muscle processes.

Thus, in the differential diagnosis of hip and thigh pain, one must always bear in mind that the lumbar spine is intrinsically involved in generating pain patterns in the sacroiliac, gluteal, lateral hip, and groin areas as well as the back. Additionally, an antalgic gait, which contributes to secondary lumbar strain patterns, can confound an exact diagnosis even more.

Furthermore, when a patient is queried as to the anatomic location of the hip, most will point to the posterior buttocks area, not the groin. It must be remembered that true hip joint pain occurs in the groin and thigh and to a much lesser extent in the lateral hip area. Most posterior and lateral pain is a symptom of lumbar pathology and much less often of sacroiliac or trochanteric bursitis.

FRACTURES AND DISLOCATIONS

Fractures and dislocations of the pelvis and femur can be divided into the following categories: stress fractures, traumatic fractures, avulsion fractures, and subluxations or dislocations.

STRESS FRACTURES

The signs and symptoms associated with stress fractures are often somewhat insidious. Initially, radiographs may not show any of the characteristic bony changes (lytic area surrounded by sclerotic bone) associated with stress fractures, since these can take 3 to 6 weeks to develop. Most of these athletes will report a gradual onset of pain related to activity, although occasionally the pain comes on suddenly. Important physical findings include the presence of tenderness and swelling in the area of stress fracture. Technetium bone scanning done at this point will show increased activity in the area of the stress fracture,[2] even though changes might not yet be apparent on x-ray film. Generally, if the fracture is subacute or chronic (greater than 4 weeks old), the fracture line or osteoblastic reparative "new" bone is visible on x-ray film.

The stress fracture is a metabolic event resulting from overuse. It occurs because the osteoclastic activity, in response to Wolff's law, antecedes the osteoblastic response of bone by 3 to 4 weeks (Fig. 29–2). Therefore, a great deal of osteolysis occurs prior to any notable effort by the bone to repair itself, and gross stress fractures develop as a result of the coalescence of these weakened areas.

For the diagnosis of stress fracture, MRI has proved extremely useful. Areas of decreased signal in the marrow of the involved bone at the site is compatible

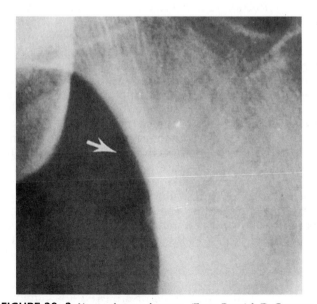

FIGURE 29–2. X-ray of stress fracture. (From Resnick D, Goergen TG, Niwayama G: Physical injury: Concepts and terminology. *In* Resnick D [ed]: Diagnosis of Bone and Joint Disorders, vol. 5. Philadelphia, WB Saunders, 1995.)

with the diagnosis of stress fracture if the appropriate history, bone scan, and x-ray findings are otherwise inconclusive.

STRESS FRACTURES OF THE PELVIS

Stress fractures of the pelvis are rare.[1] They are most often associated with running sports, although they have been reported in other activities that involve a great deal of conditioning and repetitive aerobic exercise. Most stress fractures of the pelvis involve the pubic rami. There are two recent reports, however, that involve a total of three cases of stress fracture of the sacrum, bringing the total number of reported cases in the literature to six.[3,4] Stress fractures of the pelvis are caused by patterns of overuse similar to those of other fractures but are infrequent compared with stress fractures in the legs. It is important in these cases to elicit an exact medical history in terms of alteration of training schedule, training methods, or recent participation in an event that has required excessive amounts of preparation. This is often the only way to separate these conditions from more serious bone tumors and infections, which can mimic stress fractures. This type of increased activity, leading to more rapid turnover of bone (osteoclysis), causes the stress fracture to occur.[5] There is no conclusive data as to particular risk factors involved in the evolution of stress fractures. Giladi reports only two variables that seem to correlate with a higher incidence of stress fracture in the lower extremities; retroversion of the hip and narrowing of the tibial shaft.[6,7]

In the pelvic area, stress fractures can become an extremely difficult diagnostic dilemma. Many serious bone tumors can resemble on x-ray film the changes that occur in stress fractures. Malignant bone neoplasms can occur proximally and involve the pelvis. Osteosarcomas, chondrosarcomas, and Ewing sarcoma of bone can all occur in the pelvis, and when they do, they have a poor prognosis. Appropriate early diagnosis and management is imperative. Additionally, other conditions in the pelvis can occur that resemble stress fractures. Some of these conditions include benign bone tumors such as osteoid osteoma, sacroiliac viral synovitis, retroperitoneal hematoma from trauma, osteomyelitis involving the pelvic bones, and other conditions involving either inflammation or irritation of the iliac apophysis or the pubic symphysis itself. Thus, the differential diagnosis of stress fracture involves sarcoma, benign bone tumors, infection, and certain cases of metabolic bone disease.

Stress fractures of the pubic rami generally occur on the inferior pubic rami adjacent to the symphysis pubis. They are seen largely in ultra-athletes, such as marathoners or triathletes who train and run excessive amounts. These injuries are more common in female than male runners, and the exact reason is unknown.[4,8,9] The pelvic stress fracture can be difficult to diagnose radiographically owing to the membranous nature of the bone, in which osseous changes are more difficult to detect than in other tubular bone involving more sclerotic diaphyseal structure.

Initial treatment for a stress fracture of the pelvis involves rest. Since the clinician is dealing with highly

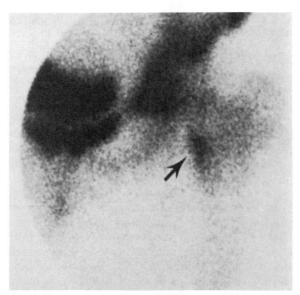

FIGURE 29–3. Stress fracture bone scan. (From Resnick D, Goergen TG, Niwayama G: Physical injury: Concepts and terminology. *In* Resnick D [ed]: Diagnosis of Bone and Joint Disorders, vol. 5. Philadelphia, WB Saunders, 1995.)

motivated athletes who may have difficulty with this type of treatment, passive-aggressive behavior such as noncompliance can result. The pelvic stress fracture takes anywhere from 6 to 8 weeks to heal, and initial treatment should involve absolute rest of the injured part until asymptomatic. Then gradual, incremental resumption of activities may occur, until an appropriate level of training and conditioning can be attained.

For pelvic stress fractures, there is no absolute contraindication to participation in sporting activities if the pain is not too severe (Fig. 29–3). However, if healing is to occur, a period of absolute rest is necessary to promote adequate reparative processes. In certain other stress fractures, it is absolutely imperative that the rest and other treatment regimens are carried out as prescribed lest further deterioration and major career-threatening complications arise.

STRESS FRACTURES OF THE FEMORAL NECK

Stress fractures of the proximal femur, including both the femoral neck and the femoral shaft itself, are relatively uncommon. They are seen in long-distance runners, triathletes, marathoners, and military recruits.[10–20] This lesion was first described by Wachsmuth in the 1930s, in a group of basic military recruits.[21] The incidence of femoral stress fractures in the entire lower extremity is less than 2 percent.[16,17] The exact cause of femoral stress fracture is unknown but definitely is related to overuse as evidenced by its frequent occurrence in long-distance runners. The incidence of these injuries is higher in women than men. The patient with femoral neck stress fracture complains of pain in the groin or thigh. This pain increases with activity. It may occur during running activity and persist for hours thereafter. There is generally, however, relief with rest.

Protracted periods of rest seem to relieve the symptoms. The pain can progress to the point at which it is fairly constant even without activity. This type of pain generally expresses itself in the groin, but it can also be in the anterior thigh or referred to the knee. Often, an antalgic gait is apparent. An abduction lurch is occasionally evident, and the Trendelenburg sign is positive. Range of motion can be limited secondary to pain. Early radiographs may not show any discernable lesion. A technetium bone scan is indicated in this particular situation, since it will be positive and determine the diagnosis.

The history is as important as the physical findings. The onset of pain some 3 to 4 weeks after increasing a training program, participating in strenuous competitive events, or altering the training regimen or equipment is almost always present in these individuals. The history is also important in terms of distinguishing this particular injury from other more serious types of osseous pathology that can manifest with radiographic changes that would be somewhat worrisome if taken out of context.

For most of these lesions, the initial treatment involves absolute rest and cessation of running. The treatment for stress fractures of the femoral neck depends on classification of the fracture. Devas initially described these fractures as either transverse, which usually occurred in older patients on the tension side of the femoral neck, or compression fractures, which occurred along the calcar on the medial side of the femoral neck.[10] The tension fractures have a poor prognosis and tend to go on to displace and cause further functional impairment. The fractures on the compression side seem to heal well if treated with conservative management. Further classification by Blickenstaff and Morris and a further management scheme by Fullerton and Snowdy support this approach.[14,17]

If the patient sustains a tension-type injury to the femoral neck, this fracture is treated aggressively with open reduction–internal fixation and only gradual resumption of activities following the surgical procedure. If the fracture is on the compressive side and is evident only on bone scan, not on radiograph, it is treated conservatively with rest and interruption of all running and traumatic activities to the extremity. In a compression femoral neck fracture, if there is a significant amount of fracture apparent on the x-ray film, the fracture is managed aggressively because it has a tendency to displace with associated complications. Return to athletic activity in these individuals should be allowed only once fracture healing and remodeling is complete, which can take up to 12 months. In these particular cases, internal fixation devices should be removed during the 12- to 18-month postsurgical period to allow full restoration of bone strength prior to engaging in excessive athletic conditioning and activity.

STRESS FRACTURES OF THE FEMUR

Stress fractures of the femur are even less common than those to the femoral neck.[22,23] This is due to the diminishing forces along the compressive side of the femur as one goes from hip joint to knee joint, decreasing the moment arm. Consequently, the forces across the bone on the compressive side are much lower, and stress injury in this area is much less common. When stress fractures do occur in the femur, they are treated with conservative management unless there is overt failure of cortical bone. If this occurs, generally, closed intramedullary rodding can be done, and the patient should be rehabilitated in an appropriate fashion and brought back rapidly to ambulatory status.

TRAUMATIC FRACTURES

TRAUMATIC PELVIC FRACTURES

Traumatic fractures of the pelvis do occur in sports, although they are rare. There are three different mechanisms involved in traumatic pelvic fractures: (1) avulsion or traction injury to the bony origin of or attachment of muscle, (2) direct compression with disruption of the pelvic osseous ring, and (3) direct blow to the pelvis itself. In the majority of cases, since the pelvis is a closed ring, an injury to one location in the pelvis will cause a contracoup fracture or sprain on the other side of the pelvic ring (Table 29–1).[24] For example, if superior and inferior pubic rami are fractured on the right side, there often will be sacroiliac disruption on the left side. When only one pelvic bone appears to be fractured as a result of compression or a disruptive injury to the pelvic ring, one should be aware that other structures may be involved, even though it may not be obvious on x-ray film. A solitary pelvic fracture can be sustained from a direct blow by a relatively sharp or circumscribed object. These injuries are seen largely in the iliac crest or pubic rami. Most pelvic fractures are sustained from severe high-velocity trauma such as a major fall or a collision in skiing, cycling, racing, or hang gliding.[25]

Pelvic fractures are generally treated conservatively, unless they are grossly displaced or unstable or they involve the hip joint. They are painful injuries. The diagnosis is made by eliciting pelvic pain by palpation or compression and verifying the fracture by pelvic

radiograph. If the bone around the hip is involved, Judet hip x-rays can be done to visualize possible acetabular involvement.[26] Additionally, CT and MRI scanning is useful. One test that can be done to help confirm the diagnosis of pelvic fracture is the pelvic "tap" test,[27] in which a stethoscope is placed over the pubic symphysis and the patella of each leg is tapped with a finger. The sound is transmitted up the femur to the pubic symphysis by osseous conduction. If the hip or pelvis is fractured, the tap is muffled on the involved side.

The stability of the pelvic ring is a consideration when deciding what type of treatment to employ. If there is significant pelvic asymmetry, sacroiliac disruption, or leg-length discrepancy, or if the pelvic ring itself is grossly disrupted, then open reduction and internal fixation or closed reduction with external fixation can be performed to provide improved anatomy and stability. Displaced fractures involving the acetabulum should be treated by open reduction if accurate coverage of the hip joint cannot be obtained by conservative means. The authors recommend treating these fractures conservatively unless there is significant anatomic or structural variation.

One associated factor involved in pelvic fractures is the significant amount of blood loss. The more severe pelvic fractures can cause hypovolemic shock if inadequate resuscitation and fluid replacement is not done. Fortunately, these injuries are rare in sporting activities.[25]

SACRAL AND COCCYGEAL FRACTURES

Fractures of the sacrum and coccyx are rarely seen in competitive athletics but can occur. They are caused by a direct blow onto the sacrococcygeal area. This can be seen in horseback riding or in any other type of activity in which a fall on the buttocks might occur. This is an extremely painful injury when it occurs.

X-ray film changes may be evident with angular deformity of the coccyx or lucent lines in the sacrum. Often fracture lines cannot be appreciated, although pain and deformity are evident. These fractures usually go on to heal without any functional impairment. In rare cases, coccygodynia, or persistent severe pain, can occur, which is very difficult to treat because of the rich complex of pain fibers (nociceptors) in this area. These fractures heal within 6 weeks and often show evidence of fibrous union although clinically healed.

Return to athletic activity should be restricted only if pain interferes with the activity. No further damage can be done by involvement in rigorous athletic activities if the pain is not impeding function.

FRACTURES OF THE HIP

Fractures of the hip are rare in the adolescent and young athletic population. They account for less than 2 percent of all hip fractures that occur.[28] A significant amount of sports trauma is usually involved in causing these injuries as opposed to the more common situation in which osteoporotic bone is the major factor contributing to the injury in the elderly population.

TABLE 29–1
The Tile Classification of Pelvic Disruption

Type	Characteristics
A	Stable
A1	Fractures of the pelvis not involving the ring
A2	Stable, minimally displaced fractures of the ring
B	Rotationally unstable, vertically stable
B1	Open book
B2	Lateral compression, ipsilateral
B3	Lateral compression, contralateral (bucket-handle)
C	Rotationally and vertically unstable
C1	Rotationally and vertically unstable
C2	Bilateral
C3	Associated with an acetabular fracture

From Tile M: Pelvic ring fractures: Should they be fixed? J Bone Joint Surg 1988; 70B:1–12.

TABLE 29–2
The Colonna Classification of Hip Fractures in Children

Type		Characteristics
I		Transepiphyseal fractures
	IA	Without dislocation
	IB	With dislocation of the femoral head from the acetabulum
II		Transcervical fractures
	IIA	Displaced
	IIB	Nondisplaced
III		Cervicotrochanteric fractures
	IIIA	Displaced
	IIIB	Nondisplaced
IV		Intertrochanteric fractures

From Colonna PC: Fracture of the neck of the femur in childhood. Ann Surg 1928; 88:902.

Even though these injuries are extremely rare in young athletes, they are important because of possible complications. The incidence of avascular necrosis is much higher in this particular age group[28] owing to the precarious nature of the blood supply to the subchondral region of the femoral head. This remains a problem until years after skeletal maturity, when collateral flow has developed.

These injuries do in fact occur more commonly in athletic children than they do in young skeletally mature adults, but, again, the injury is rare. The classification most commonly used for these particular types of fractures in children is that of Colonna (Table 29–2; Fig. 29–4).[29] In this particular classification, the fracture prognosis is dependent on the location of the injury and its interference with the blood flow to the femoral head. For type I fractures, the incidence of avascular necrosis approaches 100 percent. For types II and III fractures, the incidence of avascular necrosis varies from 30 to 50 percent. The recommended treatment for these fractures involves open-reduction internal fixation. These specific reductions are often difficult to obtain owing to the tight periosteal sleeve and excellent muscle tone in these children. Less than perfect anatomic reductions can result, further complicating these difficult fractures.

After surgery, most authors recommend immobilization in either a hinged brace or hip spica. The type IV, or intertrochanteric injury, usually has a much better prognosis. It is easier to reduce, heals better, and does not usually cause avascular necrosis of the femoral head.

These same injuries in athletic adults (i.e., femoral neck or subcapital hip fracture) also require exacting open reduction and internal fixation. These authors prefer to do this with smaller cannulated screws, at least three in number, to hold the head in anatomic position as healing occurs. The transcervical fracture in young adults has an incidence of avascular necrosis associated with it, but less than in children or the geriatric group. Intertrochanteric hip fractures, which vary in terms of degree of fragmentation and displacement, are treated surgically with open-reduction internal fixation. These require a moderate amount of time for healing, and the complications associated with this fracture, if anatomic reduction is accomplished and maintained, are minimal.

TRAUMATIC FEMORAL FRACTURES

Traumatic fractures of the femur are rarely seen in competitive athletics but can occur. Generally, the femoral bone is so strong compared with adjacent joints, especially the knee, that it seems to be spared in terms of traumatic injury. Fractures of the femur are seen in athletes in which high-velocity type mechanisms occur, such as football or rugby tackling, soccer, sports car driving, or hang gliding. Management of these fractures is aggressive with surgery offered to internally fix and stabilize the fracture when at all possible. This surgery can now be done without opening the fracture site, using small incisions and incurring minimal soft tissue damage. This form of stabilization allows for immediate mobilization of the hip and knee joints and shortens the hospital stay because it speeds recovery. Joint motion in both the hip and knee is desirable to maintain intra-articular cartilage nutrition and prevent joint stiffness and resultant weakness of the extremity.

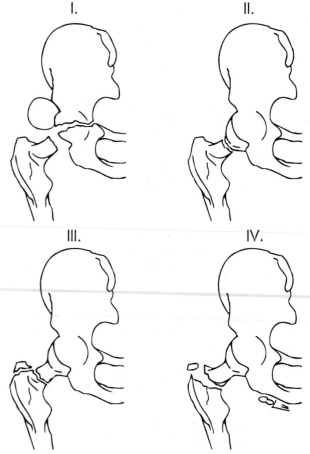

FIGURE 29–4. The Colonna classification of hip fractures in children. (From Colonna PC: Fracture of the neck of the femur in childhood. Ann Surg 1928; 88:902.)

AVULSION FRACTURES

The most common pelvic fractures involve avulsion injuries and are generally seen in the younger athlete with open epiphyses, or growth plates. These avulsion fractures of the apophyseal attachments of muscles to bone account for up to 15 percent of children's pelvic fractures.[28]

PELVIC AVULSION FRACTURES

In the pelvis, the most common site of avulsion fracture is the ischial tuberosity. This apophysis is torn loose, along with the medial hamstrings, as a result of violent hip flexion while the knee is extended. This injury is seen in sprinters, hurdlers, cheerleaders, and other jumpers as they engage in their specific athletic activities.

The injury is diagnosed radiographically by a displaced, usually crescenteric bony fragment in the area of the ischial tuberosity. By comparing the radiographic symmetry of one tuberosity to the other, the difference can be easily discerned (Fig. 29–5).[30] The patient gives a history of either a violent stretching or a jumping activity that caused acute pain in the tuberosity area. There is tenderness over the ischial tuberosity and pain on straight leg raising. The patient is unable to sprint or jump with any degree of freedom following this painful injury. These injuries can take months to heal. It is not uncommon to see patients with painful symptoms lasting up to 1 year.

The treatment for this particular problem involves rest and gentle stretching. Activities can be done if they are painless, and some level of conditioning can be maintained as it is desirable for healing (Table 29–3).

Another avulsion fracture in the pelvis involves the anterior inferior iliac spine, where the reflected head of the rectus femoris muscle takes its origin. This area is quite commonly avulsed. This injury usually occurs with an extension moment to the hip joint, again with the knee flexed, and it is commonly sustained in kicking sports. The treatment for this injury also is conservative. When healing does occur, it can be exuberant and involve considerable osteoblastic new bone formation and callus. Generally, this lesion heals more rapidly than its ischial tuberosity counterpart and has a better prognosis.

The anterior superior iliac spine can also be avulsed with vigorous contraction of the sartorius muscle. Tenderness is palpable directly over this anatomic landmark. This lesion tends to heal conservatively over a short period of time and does not have long-term disability associated with it. Additional injuries that involve avulsion of a portion of the iliac apophysis on either side can occur with sudden violent contractures of the external oblique abdominal muscle group. This is often seen in weight lifting and in contact sports that can lead to passive lengthening contractions of either the abdominal obliques, tensor, or gluteus muscles.

These particular traumatic avulsion injuries can be differentiated from apophysitis, based on their acute nature related to injury and their associated swelling and significant functional impairment. Apophysitis is generally characterized by a chronic low-grade inflammatory pain that comes on slowly and does not necessarily inhibit sports participation.

ILIOPSOAS AVULSION FRACTURE

Another type of avulsion fracture that occurs is avulsion of the lesser trochanter at the attachment of the iliopsoas tendon to the proximal femur. This is a result

TABLE 29–3
Management of Avulsion Injuries

Stage	Treatment
Acute (0–7 days)	Crutches, NWB; rest; ice
Subacute (7–14 days)	Gentle painfree ROM
	Assisted active ROM
	Protected gait
Rehabilitation (14 days on)	Progressive strengthening
	Gentle stretching
	Progressive return to functional activities and sport-specific activities
Return to sport	Progressive sport-specific activities

NWB = non–weight bearing; ROM = range of motion.

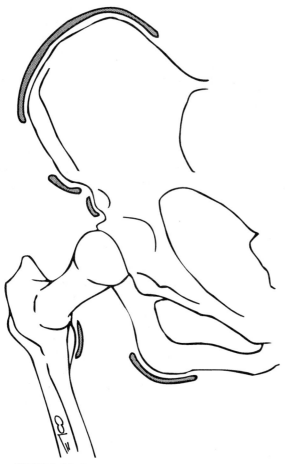

FIGURE 29–5. Diagram of pelvic avulsion fractures.

of a combination of forced hip flexion over an extended extremity. It is commonly seen in soccer when a player tries to kick a ball but finds the resistance of another foot or the ground in the way. These injuries are initially painful but usually heal over a period of 4 to 6 weeks. They are treated conservatively, and surgery is not indicated in this particular case.

TRAUMATIC SUBLUXATIONS AND DISLOCATIONS OF THE HIP

Traumatic subluxations and dislocations of the hip occur rarely in sports activities. However, when they do occur, they represent a true orthopedic and medical emergency. Much publicity has recently been given to this injury due to the visibility and notoriety of one athlete who sustained this particular injury.[31] These injuries actually account for a small number of the injuries that occur to the lower extremity as a result of sporting activity. The main concern that qualifies this injury as a medical emergency is the blood supply to the hip joint. With the hip subluxed or dislocated, the lateral femoral circumflex artery, from which the femoral head itself sustains most of its blood flow, can be compromised and circulation impaired. This can lead to avascular necrosis of the head if the condition is not rectified in a timely fashion. The consequences of developing avascular necrosis of the femoral head are severe in terms of the prognosis for both athletic participation and long-term joint function.

The vast majority of traumatic subluxations and dislocations to the hip are posterior. Less than 10 percent are anterior or inferior.[32] In the case of posterior subluxation, in which the hip is only transiently and partially dislocated, the mechanism of injury involves positioning of the extremity and an appropriate amount of muscle contraction to provide enough posterior movement to partially dislocate the hip. This, in fact, was the mechanism involved in the most notable recent hip subluxation involving a professional football player.[31]

The typical case of dislocation, however, involves an extreme posterior force to the flexed hip, leading to overt dislocation of the femoral head. Often this dislocation is associated with fracture fragmentation of the acetabulum, and this condition becomes a fracture-dislocation that may demand further surgical attention after the hip is reduced.

Again, the most important clinical feature of this injury is the grave prognosis even if managed properly. All efforts should be made to reduce a dislocated hip joint as rapidly as possible with the idea that this might improve the prognosis for survival of the head and ultimate hip joint function and integrity.

The fracture-dislocation classification of Epstein is useful in determining the type of care to render to the patient following injury (Table 29–4).[33] Open-reduction internal fixation is often recommended in a young athlete if the acetabulum is involved with a large posterior fragment. If significant comminution exists in the weight-bearing surface, then skeletal traction must be applied. Following reduction of a dislocated hip and appropriate reconstitution of joint surface, the treatment regimen is fairly exacting. The patient is initially kept off the hip until the pain has subsided. Once pain is alleviated, range-of-motion and strengthening activities are begun and gradual weight bearing is allowed as long as it can be accomplished without pain in the involved extremity. Crutches are used for whatever period of time necessary to provide adequate pain control. Current studies suggest that in a stable hip joint, enforcement of non–weight bearing has no long-term effect on the prognosis of the hip.[33] Curtailed activities are continued until normal range of motion has been obtained and strength is equal to the opposite side. At that point, it will be safe to return the patient to athletic activity if functional tasks have been mastered.

The ultimate prognosis following this injury cannot be determined until enough time has elapsed to allow the secondary changes of avascular necrosis to occur. This may take anywhere from 6 to 24 months. Generally within this period of time, avascular necrotic changes become apparent and management can be rendered based on the stage of the disease (Table 29–5).[34] The prognosis for subluxation and dislocation of the hip in a child is also guarded as evidenced by the Libri and Canale series in which up to 20 percent of their patients developed avascular necrotic changes of the hip.[28,35] Additional complications reported in children include loss of motion, ankylosis of the hip, and, occasionally, myositis ossificans. Overall, the prognosis for children with this injury is slightly better than adults but still significantly guarded.

In adults, the prognosis is poor. The incidence of avascular (aseptic) necrosis varies anywhere from 6 percent up to 40 percent.[36,37] Numerous other complications, including sciatic nerve injury, recurrent posterior dislocation, myositis ossificans, loss of motion of the hip, ankylosis, and post-traumatic arthritis have also been reported as a result of these injuries. From a prognostic point of view, the two most significant factors are the severity of injury and the length of time elapsing from injury until reduction of the dislocation. Anterior injuries are much less common and the degree of complications is less.

The authors' preferred method of treatment involves a rapid reduction of the dislocation. This often requires significant force, and many times a general anesthetic is desirable. The patient is hospitalized and managed at

TABLE 29–4
The Epstein Classification of Posterior Hip Dislocations

Type	Characteristics
I	With or without minor fracture
II	With a large single fracture of posterior acetabular rim
III	With comminution of the rim of the acetabulum and with or without a major fragment
IV	With fracture of the acetabular floor
V	With fracture of the femoral head

From Thompson VP, Epstein HC: Traumatic dislocation of the hip. J Bone Joint Surg 1951; 33A:746–778.

TABLE 29–5
Six Stages of Avascular Necrosis of the Femoral Head

Stage	Symptoms	Roentgenographic Changes
I	Asymptomatic	Subtle, mottled densities of femoral head
II	Asymptomatic	Infarct demarcated by increased density Sclerosis and/or cyst formation
III	Onset of mild, intermittent groin pain	Fine radiolucent fracture line 1–2 mm beneath subchondral plate (crescent sign) No flattening
IV	Sudden increase in pain with minor trauma/activity	Collapse Depression of fracture without joint narrowing or acetabular involvement
V	Pain with activity and rest	Severe degenerative arthritis of the hip Increased asymmetry of flattened femoral head with joint narrowing and/or acetabular changes
VI	Pain with activity and rest	Advance degenerative hip arthritis

From Marcus ND, Enneking WF, Massam RA: The silent hip in idiopathic aseptic necrosis. J Bone Joint Surg 1973; 55A:1351–1366.

bed rest or in skin traction for a day or two until comfortable. Following that, the patient is mobilized with progressive weight bearing on crutches until there are no symptoms with increased load. During this time frame, range of motion is obtained by both a continuous passive motion machine (CPM) and the intervention of a physical therapist with passive range-of-motion exercises to the extremity. Muscle stimulation to the hip flexors, extensors, abductors, and quadriceps and strengthening of those muscles can be accomplished as long as painless range of motion is present.

Return to activity can occur once adequate range of motion and strength are obtained. Again, whether or not a person goes back to athletic competition probably has very little to do with the ultimate prognosis for the hip joint. There is no research that supports persistent rest as a means of providing a better prognosis in these injuries; in fact, the opposite is true.

MUSCLE STRAINS

Muscle strains of the lower extremity are among the most common injuries in sports. Strains cause a significant amount of lost time from sports and are a common source of pain and reduced performance with return to competition.[38–40] A muscle strain is an indirect injury caused by excessive force or stress on the muscle rather than direct trauma to the muscle.[41] Injury often occurs when powerful contractions are combined with a forced lengthening of the muscle (eccentric contractions or lengthening contraction).[42] The injury is usually localized near the musculotendinous junction.[43]

O'Donoghue has described the spectrum of muscle injury quite well. He classifies muscle strain injuries in three categories, dependent upon the amount of damage that has occurred. The damage is dependent on the force placed on the muscle and the strength of the resistance. In first-degree strains, there is little tissue disruption. There is a low-grade inflammatory response to the injury. There is no loss of strength or range of motion. In second-degree strains, there is actual tissue damage with disruption of some fibers. Strength and range of motion are compromised and may result in any degree of involvement up to total loss of strength and function. The most severe category of injury, third-degree strains, indicates a complete disruption of the muscle-tendon unit (rupture) with grossly visible damage and will include complete loss of function of the unit.[44]

Muscles at the highest risk for muscle strain injury are usually the "two-joint" muscles, i.e., muscles whose length spans two joints and thus must stretch at more than one joint. For example, the hamstring muscles limit knee extension when the hip is flexed and limit hip flexion when the knee is extended. Joint motion at one of the joints can place increased passive tension on the muscle and make it more susceptible to injury. Another characteristic of frequently injured muscles is that they function in an eccentric contraction during participation in sports. The hamstrings function to decelerate knee extension in addition to flexing the knee. Similarly, the quadriceps limit knee flexion during knee extension following heelstrike.

Noonan and Garrett also state that the muscle with a relatively high percentage of type II (fast-twitch) fibers is more likely to be injured because of the implication of faster contraction of muscles.[43] Muscle strain injuries occur more often in sprinters or in athletes who perform activities with high speeds of acceleration. Therefore, muscle strain injuries are more common in sports such as track and field, football, basketball, soccer, and rugby.[45] In the lower extremity, the most common muscle strain injuries are to the adductor muscles of the thigh in horseback riders, calf muscles in tennis players, and hamstring muscles in runners.[46]

The initial treatment of acute muscle strain injuries has typically involved the universal pneumonic of RICE—rest, ice, compression, and elevation. Progressive treatment includes stretching to improve range of motion, reciprocal strengthening exercises, support bandaging, and medications. Medications usually include analgesics, nonsteroidal anti-inflammatories, and, occasionally, steroids. Surgical intervention is rare, even with complete ruptures of the muscle-tendon unit because these ruptures are difficult to repair owing to the nature of the muscle tissue itself. Treatment protocols are empirical, since there are few outcome studies addressing the effects of different treatments.

Prevention is a key element in managing muscle strain injuries. There are a number of factors that have been cited in the literature as relevant to the prevention of muscle injury. These include muscle strength, fatigue, warm-up muscle temperature, passive stretching, previous injury, and biomechanics of activity.

GLUTEUS MEDIUS STRAIN

Lloyd-Smith and colleagues reported on a series of 200 hip and pelvis injuries and indicated that gluteus medius strain and tendinitis were the most common soft tissue problems, accounting for 18 percent of total injuries.[47] Diagnosis is difficult because of the problem of differentiating between gluteus medius insertion tendinitis and trochanteric bursitis due to the proximity at the greater trochanter. Inflammation of the gluteus medius tendon causes tenderness just proximal to the greater trochanter and pain with resisted abduction. Pain over the lateral aspect of the trochanter and no pain with resisted hip abduction is thought to be trochanteric bursitis. Strains tend to be more acute and pain more constant compared with bursitis. Lloyd-Smith reported that the two conditions coexisted in about 10 percent of individuals, which may indicate the differentiation difficulty. Mechanism of injury is unclear but is most likely related to the seesaw tilt action of the pelvis when running. Significant leg-length discrepancy (>2.5 cm) tends to increase the stress involved in pelvic static and dynamic stabilization.[47]

Isolated strains of the tensor muscle of fascia lata muscle are rare. Because of its location, this muscle is frequently classified with the gluteal group. However, it also inserts into and helps form the anterior iliotibial tract to help flex the hip. It indirectly stabilizes the extended knee. With the lower extremity fixed, the tensor muscle of fascia lata helps with pelvic support. Strain of the tensor muscle of fascia lata is not always related to a tight iliotibial band, and therefore the Ober test may be negative. Diagnosis is made on the basis of pain over the muscle with palpation and discomfort with resisted activity. Treatment is consistent with that of other muscle strains—protected motion and local therapy, followed by progressive stretching, strengthening, and endurance activities as symptoms resolve.

ADDUCTOR STRAINS

Adductor strains ("pulled groin") are frequently seen in ice hockey, soccer, high jump, water skiing, swimming, and football—all activities requiring quick direc-tion changes or propulsion. Similarly, these injuries occur at the muscle-tendon junction and the adductor longus muscle is most frequently involved. Less severe injuries will occur in the muscle bellies. The usual mechanism of injury involves a sudden stretch caused by a forced external rotation of an abducted leg or by a stretching of the muscle group in a similar position without an adequate warm-up period.

An imbalance in strength between the abductor and adductor muscles may be the predisposing factor in these injuries. Two-joint muscles are also more susceptible to injury. Without sufficient rehabilitation, adductor injuries are similar to hamstring injuries in that individuals are susceptible to reinjury. Most injuries are first- and second-degree strains. Third-degree tears are rare and when they do occur are treated nonsurgically. Symptoms include pain with passive abduction and resisted active adduction and tenderness along the subcutaneous border of the pubic ramus.

Treatment for adductor strains is consistent with that for hamstrings and quadriceps injuries and includes rest, ice, and protection. Anti-inflammatory medication and treatment modalities are initiated after 24 to 48 hours. Stretching and range-of-motion exercise should begin as soon as possible in the pain-free range. Resistance exercises are included in the treatment regimen as pain subsides and motion improves.

A problem with adductor strains has been that they are usually ignored in strength-training workouts; therefore, emphasis should be placed on strength and endurance training activities. Stretching programs generally include the adductors. The saddle stretch, which is commonly used in warm-ups may be inadequate as a therapeutic approach. The saddle stretch is generally a simultaneous bilateral stretch, and as a rule stretching should be done unilaterally for maximum control and specificity. Alternative stretching exercises should be taught that require the athlete to stretch with the hip in neutral or in extension versus the flexed hip position.

HAMSTRING STRAINS

Hamstring muscle injuries are caused by either a vigorous stretch or a rapid contraction of the muscle. This muscle group is the most frequently strained muscle in the body.[48,49] The injury is commonly seen in activities such as running, sprinting, soccer, football, and rugby. Recurrence is common with hamstring injuries.

The hamstring muscles are composed of three separate muscles: semimembranosus, semitendinosus, and biceps femoris muscle of the thigh. The semimembranosus muscle originates on the ischial tuberosity and inserts on the posteromedial aspect of the tibia and knee joint. The semitendinosus muscle originates on the ischial tuberosity and inserts on the tibia with the gracilis and the sartorius muscles in the pes anserinus. The biceps femoris muscle of the thigh has two heads; the long head originates on the ischial tuberosity and the short head on the posterolateral femur. Both insert on the proximal fibula. The hamstring function is to extend the hip and flex the knee by synchronizing with other prime movers of the knee and hip. In addition, the biceps of the thigh rotates the flexed knee externally and the semimembranosis and semitendinosus muscles rotate it internally. As a two-joint (or biarthroidal) muscle, the hamstring works in closed kinetic chain activities or with co-contraction to direct the movement in a purposeful, coordinated motor pattern. Most of the hamstring activity is eccentric as a decelerator with walking or running activities.

In a review of the literature, Agre sites several studies of injuries to the hamstrings muscle group.[46] Brubaker and James found that hamstrings injuries accounted for 50 percent of injuries in sprinters and 20 percent of strain injuries in middle and distance runners.[48] Ekstrand and Gillquist reported that 47 percent of 36 strain injuries to soccer players were in the hamstrings.[50] They found that most injuries occurred during running and usually during warm-up or during the beginning of games. Dorman found that in 140 hamstring injuries, most occurred either early or late in practice or matches.[51] These reports support the importance of warm-up, flexibility, and endurance exercise prior to practice and competition.

Heiser and associates reported on hamstring injuries in intercollegiate football players.[52] They found a significant reduction in the number of hamstring injuries when muscle imbalances were evaluated and rehabilitated prior to practice and competition. These findings supported the theory that an imbalance in strength of the hamstrings bilaterally or in comparison with the quadriceps predisposes an athlete to hamstring injury. This finding is disputed by Worrell and co-workers and Paton and colleagues, who found no significant differences in hamstrings to quadriceps ratios in hamstring-injured and noninjured athletes.[53,54] Thus the relationship between hamstring muscles injury and muscle strength cannot clearly be defined.

A number of authors have investigated the relationship of hamstring flexibility with hamstring injury. Worrell and co-workers and Liemohn found that injured subjects were less flexible than noninjured subjects.[55,56] Other authors have reported no significant difference between groups. The ability to absorb force is somewhat related to resting length; therefore, the greater the resting length, the greater the ability to absorb force and avoid strain.

Worrell and colleagues have presented a theoretical hamstring-injury model—a multiple-factor model that identifies a relationship between strength, warm-up, fatigue, and flexibility.[55] This is useful in developing a model for the comprehensive approach of prevention and treatment and for evaluating causes of muscle strain injuries in a particular athlete.

Athletes should be evaluated before practice and competition, especially those athletes considered to be in high-risk activities, such as sprinting, jumping, and kicking. Evaluations should include flexibility and strength. In addition, the athlete should be well versed in stretching techniques and warm-up and cool-down activities.

Most injuries to the hamstrings are first- and second-degree strains, but there are a few third-degree strains, or complete ruptures of the muscle-tendon unit. The only third-degree strain in which surgery is occasionally indicated is when the tendon is avulsed at the tendon-bone interface. Injuries may occur in the tendon itself by avulsion at the ischium, or by tear in the muscle belly. These injuries are often devastating and prevent return to previous performance levels even with successful surgical repair and rehabilitation.

When assessing the injury, a good medical history of the injury from the athlete is of the most value. In the first-degree injury, athletes may not be consciously aware of injury until they have cooled down from practice or competition. Complaints will be of soreness over the hamstring muscles, but no obvious pain on palpation or swelling. Gait will be normal. Hip flexion range of motion will be normal with only a feeling of tightness reported. Resisted hip flexion and extension will elicit similar findings and will produce good strength.

In the second- or third-degree injury, the athlete may report having heard or felt a pop during activity. He will describe immediate pain. Swelling and severe pain will be present. Physical examination will reveal tenderness, limited passive straight-leg raising, and limited strength of the hamstrings secondary to pain. There may be a noticeable defect in the muscle belly as well, especially if assessed early. A few days following the injury, ecchymosis may be present over the muscle and with time descends down the back of the leg to the knee and even to the calf and ankle, based on dependence and gravity. The athlete with a third-degree injury probably needs crutches for ambulation. Gait is usually abnormal with no heelstrike and limited swing-through phase. The knee remains flexed. Palpation elicits moderate pain. Resisted knee flexion and hip extension causes moderate pain with second-degree injuries. With third-degree injuries, the pain is often less, the athlete complaining primarily of an aching type of pain. Resisted knee flexion and hip extension are weak. Passive hip flexion with knee extended is painful, and knee extension may be moderately limited with the hip flexed.

In first-degree strains, immediate treatment includes ice, compression, immobilization, and rest. As symptoms subside, these modalities are followed by stretching and strengthening and pain-free return to activity. Minor strains should not be treated lightly, because as many recurrent injuries or more severe injuries are preceded by minor injuries. Analgesics or nonsteroidal anti-inflammatory drugs (NSAIDs) may be given as necessary. The athlete should ambulate with full weight bearing only if gait is normal and pain free; if not, ambulation should be with crutches.

Second-degree injuries are handled similarly to first-degree injuries except for a longer treatment period. Controversy exists concerning treatment of third-degree injuries. Immobilization in extension is indicated for 48 hours. In addition, some physicians[57] have advocated the use of steroid injections into the site of the strain, although the benefit of this procedure has not been documented, and authors of this chapter do not recommend the procedure because steroids are detrimental to the healing of muscle tissue.

Exercises should include pain-free stretching and isometric contractions. Intensity should be gradually increased, keeping the activities in the pain-free level. Using this guideline will prevent further injury due to excessive rehabilitation. Once the athlete has achieved full pain-free range of motion and there is no residual soreness or tenderness, additional strengthening exercises can be included—closed-kinetic chain exercises, isokinetics, and isotonics. Ultrasound and gentle friction massage may be indicated in the resolution of adhesions within the muscle.

The athlete should be cleared for return to participation or competition when strength, endurance, flexibility, coordination, and athletic agility have been accomplished. The rehabilitation program should gradually build to include sports-specific drills, such as running, cutting, and jumping.

Chronic hamstring injuries usually occur as a result of insufficient rehabilitation or inappropriate progression of activities. Ekstrand and Gilquist found that many individuals sustain a re-injury within 2 months of returning to practice and competition.[50] Agre[46] found that many athletes had residual power and flexibility deficits resulting from inadequate rehabilitation of previous injuries (Table 29–6).

Ishikawa and associates reported on two rare cases of avulsion of the hamstring muscles from the ischial tuberosity without fracture of the ischium.[58] Only one of these cases involved an athletic injury and was sustained by a 22-year-old man thrown down during judo practice. The right hip was forcibly flexed and abducted with the athlete in single-leg stance. Surgical repair of complete avulsion of the long head of the biceps of the thigh, semitendinosus, and semimembranosus muscles was completed. After 53 months, the patient had returned to practicing judo with only occasional complaints of discomfort in the buttocks while running; range of motion and muscle strength were normal.

Blasier and Morawa reported on a complete rupture of the hamstring muscles at the ischial origin sustained as a result of a water skiing accident.[59] Surgical repair was successful, and 4 months after surgery the patient returned to recreational sports. Three years following injury he had full range of motion, and knee flexion strength was within normal limits.

Although hamstring injuries make up the largest percentage of muscle strain injuries to the thigh, the adductors and flexors are also susceptible to strain injuries. Loosli and Quick reported a 33 percent incidence of hip flexor adductor injury in high-level collegiate breaststroke swimmers.[60] Of 30 evaluated swimmers, 10 had a history of or presented with a significant flexor adductor injury. The majority of these athletes had primary adductor injuries (adductor magnus and adductor brevis). Loosli and Quick advocated prevention and treatment in order to minimize muscle strain injuries to swimmers. The program that they identified does not vary from the previously described approach. They emphasize stretching with warm-up and cool-down as well as endurance and strength training of all thigh musculature. Their recommendations also include a long warm-up of breaststroke kick prior to any high-intensity breaststroke workout.

QUADRICEPS STRAINS

Quadriceps strains are not common in sports. When seen, they are most frequent in soccer, weight lifting, football, rugby, and sprinting and usually involve the belly of the rectus femoris muscle of the thigh or the reflected head (which is diarthrodial). This type of injury can be disabling to the athlete because the quadriceps muscles are powerful extensors of the knee and work with the glutei and hamstrings for normal, coordinated walking, running, and jumping. Muscle tears usually occur with lengthening contractions of the involved muscle. Sudden or rapid deceleration from a sprint is a common event responsible for injury. The factors thought to contribute are tight quadriceps muscles, muscle imbalance between the two legs, leg-length discrepancy, inadequate cool-down, and insufficient warm-ups.

The rectus femoris muscle of the thigh is the most commonly injured muscle and usually tears in midsubstance. The vastus lateralis and vastus medialis are more rarely injured, but when injury does occur, it is in the mid- to upper third of the muscle belly. Despite persistence of muscle defects, third-degree injuries of the quadriceps muscle belly result in little or no functional disability, and surgical repair is not required.

In the first-degree quadriceps strain, the athlete may complain of tightness in the anterior thigh. Gait will be normal. There may be no swelling or discomfort with palpation. When asked to extend the knee from a flexed position, the athlete may not experience discomfort. If the hip is extended, there may be some discomfort, especially if the rectus muscle of the thigh is the involved muscle.

The athlete with a second-degree strain will experience more pain and some disruption of the normal gait

---

TABLE 29–6
Management of Muscle Strains*

Stage	Treatment
Acute (24–48 hours)	Ice Compression Crutches, possible immobilization Pain-free active ROM
Subacute (2–7 days)	Heat Electric stimulation Pain-free resisted ROM Pain-free stretching exercises NSAIDs
Rehabilitation	Discontinue crutches Progressive resistive exercises Swimming, cycling Jogging, running program
Return to sport	Progressive sport-specific activities

*Progression through management cycle depends on grade of injury. ROM = range of motion.

cycle. The knee may be kept in extension with protective maneuvers by the athlete. Interview of the athlete may indicate that a sudden twinge of pain down the length of the muscle was felt during activity. Swelling may be present, and palpation elicits pain. Resisted knee extension may produce pain. Active knee flexion range of motion is decreased. This is a good finding to classify the injury as a second or third degree.

Grade III strains are extremely painful, and ambulation is not possible without assistance of crutches. There may be an obvious defect in the muscle. Palpation indicates severe pain and may not be tolerated. Swelling is present. Resisted extension of the knee is not possible, and range of motion is severely limited. An isometric contraction is painful and may produce a muscle bulge or defect in the quadriceps muscles, especially the rectus muscle of the thigh. Treatment is similar to that described for the hamstring muscles strain, once again emphasizing pain-free range of motion and strengthening.

STRETCHING

An important aspect of the rehabilitation of any injury is stretching. However, this is a critical component in the rehabilitation of muscle strain injuries. For effective and safe performance, flexibility for specific demands is important. Flexibility refers not only to the range of motion available in a joint but includes the extensibility of the muscle-tendon unit. Rehabilitation and injury prevention programs should consider both dynamic and static flexibility.[61,62]

The three common techniques for stretching include (1) static stretching, (2) ballistic stretching, and (3) proprioceptive neuromuscular facilitation (PNF) techniques. Static stretching is the classic stationary stretch in which the limb is moved to position and stretched to a position of mild discomfort. These positions are generally quite simple, utilizing body weight or limb position, and no further resistance is required.

Ballistic stretching, although controversial, at times is a valuable addition to the development of dynamic flexibility. Ballistic stretching consists of moving the limb to position and adding quick bobbing movements at the end of the range instead of the long, slow stretch discussed previously. Ballistic stretching uses available range of motion and limb weight or muscle contraction to accomplish the increased flexibility. Although not widely accepted, it is an effective exercise when used properly and tailored to individual needs. All ballistic stretching should be preceded by static stretching and done only in small movements (using only 10 percent of range beyond that of static range), and movement should be progressive.

Proprioceptive neuromuscular techniques are used to place specific demands—promoting or hastening the response of tissues through the use of stimulation of the proprioceptors. PNF techniques include contract relax (CR), hold relax (HR), and contract relax antagonist contract (CRAC). CR techniques have the goal of relaxation of antagonistic pattern of movement. There is a static stretch at the end of range of motion with a gentle CR; as an assistant gently pushes for increased range, the part is moved passively into the agonistic pattern. The HR technique also achieves relaxation; however, the assistant provides maximal resistance to an isometric contraction at the end of range. CRAC uses the same approach as CR, but the antagonists contract and the assistant gently pushes the limb for increased range of motion.

There is no consensus on the best stretching technique.[63–68] Most studies[62] have shown that CRAC method of PNF stretching is the best but only slightly. Other studies have found that PNF techniques are better than static or ballistic techniques, and yet other studies[62,69] state that there is no difference. The choice of the technique depends on several factors—safety, ease of use, and the amount of assistance available.

Regardless of the techniques selected, it is widely accepted that stretching for 15 seconds may be as effective as stretching for 2 minutes and that individual responses to flexibility programs vary considerably. For increased flexibility to be maintained, it must be gained over a longer period of time. Zebas and Rivera[63] found that increases in flexibility were maintained after a 6-week stretching program and decreased with no exercise for 2 weeks, and that there was further gradual loss after 4 weeks of no exercise, but flexibility retained was greater than prior to the 6-week flexibility program. To maintain flexibility one should stretch at least once a week. To gain flexibility a program should be incorporated into the exercise routine three to five times per week.

Zachazewski[62] suggests the following flexibility routine: (1) general warm-up, (2) preparticipation stretching, (3) neuromuscular warm-up, (4) participation, and (5) postparticipation stretching. The general warm-up should consist of repetitive nonfatiguing exercise of muscle groups to be stretched for 10 to 15 minutes, allowing tissue temperatures to increase. Preparticipation stretching should include slow, static stretching followed by ballistic stretching, if appropriate. The key is caution and control of all stretching. During the neuromuscular warm-up, the athlete should simulate actual activity. The addition of PNF (therapist-assisted) stretching may be appropriate at this time. Following the participation in activity phase, the athlete should conclude with a postparticipation stretching program that includes slow stretching of specific muscle groups to further increase flexibility and to decrease or prevent muscle soreness as a result of strenuous activity during participation.

CONTUSIONS

A contusion is defined as an external blow to the muscle belly. This type of injury is associated with pain and swelling, decreased range of motion, and, occasionally, a palpable mass or hematoma.[70]

Contusions are classified in three grades or degrees. The first-degree contusion produces minimal discomfort for the athlete and should not restrict competition time. Grade II injuries are more painful and limit activity in extreme ranges of motion and strength.

Grade III contusions are associated with much more pain, swelling, and bleeding.

HIP POINTERS

Hip pointer is a nonspecific term and when used generally refers to an injury to the iliac crest as the result of a blow. The use of the term generally refers to contusions of the iliac crest over the tensor fascia lata muscle belly with associated hematoma but may also include tearing of the external oblique muscle from the iliac crest, periosteitis of the crest, and trochanteric contusions. Most injuries are due to violent contact with a piece of protective equipment such as a helmet or knee pad of another player in football and hockey; or in noncontact sports, when the player contacts the ground in a slide or dive. In volleyball, diving for the ball on hard courts produces significant bruising. The injury is most commonly seen in football but may occur in other contact sports such as rugby, soccer, wrestling, lacrosse, and ice hockey. Hip pads that are appropriate in design and properly fitted and work consistently can prevent or at least minimize the injury.

Muscles inserting on the iliac crest include the gluteus maximus and medius, tensor fascia lata, sartorius, quadratus lumborum, latissimus dorsi, external abdominal oblique, iliocostalis lumborum, and transversus abdominis muscles. When contracting, these muscles contribute to the discomfort and pain, as does any motion that causes rotation of the trunk or hip flexion. X-ray films may be indicated to rule out an iliac crest fracture or a displaced epiphyseal fracture (especially in younger athletes), which would require an extended healing period.

Symptoms are instantly disabling and painful. The trunk is flexed forward and toward the side of injury. The iliac crest is exquisitely tender to palpation and swelling is present. Abdominal muscle spasm may be present. Within 24 to 48 hours, the swelling is more diffuse, and an area of ecchymosis may become evident.

An athlete with a grade I hip pointer has a normal gait and normal posture and complains of slight pain with palpation with little or no swelling present. Full range of motion of the trunk may also be present. This level of injury should not prevent the athlete from competition. Grade II injuries are more painful and tender. There is noticeable swelling and an abnormal gait pattern. The athlete's posture may be slightly flexed to the side of the injury. Active trunk movement may be painful and range of motion limited, especially in side bending to the opposite side of the injury and in rotation both ways. The pain is quite debilitating and the athlete finds it almost impossible to return to competition. Return to activity takes at least 5 to 14 days. Athletes with grade III injuries complain of severe pain, swelling, and general bruising. Gait is slow and deliberate with short stride length and swing-through. Posture may present with a severe tilt to the side of injury. Range of motion of the trunk is limited in all directions. The athlete will be out of competition 14 to 21 days (Table 29–7).

TABLE 29–7 Management of Hip Pointers	
Stage	**Treatment**
Acute (24–48 hours)	Ice Rest Compression Crutches (if limp is present) Pain-free passive ROM Pain-free active ROM
Subacute (2–3 days)	Heat (when no swelling present) Pain-free active ROM Discontinue crutches (when no limp present) NSAIDs
Rehabilitation	Pain-free resisted ROM Cycling, jogging, running Sport-specific functional activities Custom padding
Return to sport	Progression of sport-specific activities

Initially, treatment of the classic hip pointer should include ice, rest, and compression. Crutches may be indicated if the hip is too painful for normal gait. Anti-inflammatory medications are indicated after 48 hours because they inhibit platelet function and promote hemorrhage. Later treatment should include ice coupled with ultrasound, heat, and transcutaneous electrical nerve stimulation (TENS). Pain-free range-of-motion exercises are essential to the recovery process. Active exercise should start as soon as possible, on the second day following injury, and helps to promote healing and decrease time for return to competition. As soon as pain-free active exercise can be accomplished, progressive resistive exercise may be performed and may include lower extremity and trunk strengthening. Compression garments can be worn during practice and competition.

In an uncomplicated hip-pointer contusion, pads should be used for protection from further injury in contact sports, and the athlete can return to activity in 3 to 7 days. Activity should increase as pain decreases. With grades II and III injuries, activity should be delayed until adequate healing occurs.

QUADRICEPS CONTUSIONS

Contusions of the anterior thigh and the quadriceps muscle groups are quite common. Blows occur by an accelerating knee or helmet or the edge of a thigh pad. Injuries of this nature are most often seen in sports such as football, rugby, soccer, basketball, and hockey. Contusions of the quadriceps are often accompanied by muscle strain injuries of that same muscle. A hematoma of some degree is usually present in a muscle contusion injury.

The most common contusions in the thigh are to the anterior and lateral thigh. The extent of the disability is dependent on the severity of the bleeding, the amount of muscle involved, and the treatment received by the athlete from the athletic trainer, physician, and/or physical therapist.

The athlete may complain of pain immediately following the injury, depending on the severity of the injury. If the pain is severe, the athlete may be unable to bear weight on that extremity. Treatment for the first 24 to 48 hours should follow the RICE protocol—rest, ice, compression, elevation. Further examination of the athlete indicates localized pain and loss of ability to fully flex and extend the knee. Knee flexion beyond 90 degrees is painful as is active extension against firm resistance. Loss of range of motion may be the best indicator of the severity of the injury. With a more severe injury, a palpable mass that is due to the hematoma may be present, and the athlete will be unable to establish a quadriceps contraction or a straight leg raise.

Further treatment following the immediate acute care should continue to provide compression and cooling to the entire area to minimize bleeding. The limb should remain in flexion and may be restrained with a wrap or support. To prevent further injury, this flexed position should not be forced but should be maintained for 48 hours. Re-evaluation may indicate continuation of the flexion, compression, icing program, for another 12 to 24 hours. Continued swelling despite this regimen may indicate continued hemorrhage. Further medical evaluation regarding bleeding is indicated in this case. The athlete should be put on crutches if he is unable to accomplish a pain-free gait; weight-bearing status should be non–weight bearing for 48 hours, then partial weight bearing in pain-free range.

During the subacute phase, range of motion is reassessed, and if full range of motion is not possible, non–weight bearing with crutches should be continued for 2 to 5 additional days with re-evaluation daily. During this phase, treatment should be directed toward restoration of motion. Goals of treatment should be to facilitate quadriceps action and eliminate quadriceps lag, increase range of motion to full active status, and start functional training. Ice or cool whirlpool can be continued. The use of physical agents such as pulsed ultrasound and high-voltage galvanic stimulation (HVGS) can be used to reduce edema. Assisted range of motion exercise and active flexion and extension exercises are encouraged. Quadriceps isometric exercises and hamstrings resistive exercises should be introduced.

Proprioceptive neuromuscular facilitation (PNF) exercise patterns may be used to strengthen, relax, or gain range of motion when there is spasm or reflex inhibition. Weight bearing as tolerated is allowed, and crutches can be discarded when there is greater than 90 degrees range of motion, no limp, and quadriceps control. There should be no forced stretching at this point. Quadriceps assisted stretching may be indicated but should be gentle and pain free. The goal is to maintain range of motion. Anti-inflammatory medications should also begin. Massage is not indicated at this time, and attempts to "rub it" or "work it out" should be discouraged because it will only increase trauma and hemorrhage. In more severe cases, gentle massage may be indicated after several days of rehabilitation and healing but should never be painful (Table 29–8).

Once the athlete has full range of motion, full weight-bearing gait should be resumed, and exercise program should progress to work on active range of motion and increased resistive quadriceps activity. The athlete may cycle with progression in a running program. Once the athlete has full, pain-free range of motion he or she can progress to sprinting, fast starts, and quick decelerations, and finally jumping or bounding. During the final phase of rehabilitation, the strengthening and conditioning exercise program should be more intensive and sport-specific as the athlete prepares to return to participation. Return to participation should not be allowed until the athlete has less than a 10 percent difference in strength between the injured and noninjured quadriceps and a hamstrings: quadriceps ratio of more than 60 percent.

Participants in contact sports should be evaluated for protective equipment. Prefabricated shells can be tried, or a custom protective shell of orthoplast, Plastizote, fiberglass, or similar materials can be made. Repeated injuries to the contusion increase the risk of myositis ossificans.

MYOSITIS OSSIFICANS

Myositis ossificans is the development of a lesion of heterotopic bone localized in the soft tissues adjacent to bone and associated with trauma, surgery, or disease such as paraplegia. It is a frequent complication of a combination of contusion with hematoma formation

TABLE 29–8
Management of Contusions

Stage	Treatment
Acute (24–48 hours)	Ice Rest Crutches, partial WB or NWB Pain-free passive ROM Pain-free active ROM
Subacute (2–5 days)	Pain-free resisted ROM Active ROM PNF relaxation patterns Partial WB Heat (when no swelling present) NSAIDs
Rehabilitation	Discontinue crutches (when no limp present) Active ROM Cycling, jogging, running Electrical stimulation Functional activities Consider equipment modification
Return to sport	Progression of sport-specific activities

NWB = non–weight bearing; NSAIDs = nonsteroidal anti-inflammatory drugs; ROM = range of motion; WB = weight bearing.

involving muscle. The importance of this condition rests in the fact that contusions are usually viewed as minor injuries by coaches and athletes and thus are not treated with much concern, although appropriate management of this initial injury can prevent or lessen the development of myositis ossificans.

The most common cause of myositis is trauma, and the lesion occurs primarily in contact sports such as football, rugby, and lacrosse.[71] The symptoms include a palpable, painful mass associated with progressive loss of knee motion. Treatment as described earlier for a quadriceps contusion should lead to an uneventful recovery for this athlete. There are several risk factors that should be avoided—continuing to play after injury, early massage of the injured area, and application of heat to the area. Other predisposing factors may be passive, forceful stretching, too rapid progression of rehabilitation, premature return to activity, re-injury of the same area, and innate predisposition to ectopic bone formation. Symptoms and findings may be confused with a femoral stress fracture or neoplasm. Other possible indicators of the development of myositis ossificans include increase in pain or decrease in range of motion following one or two treatment sessions, the persistence of warmth to palpation at the site of injury, or the palpation of increasing induration in the hematoma.

Roentgenographic signs of injury are present in the third to sixth week following injury. The initial appearance is that of fluffy calcification with indistinct margins lying in the soft tissue anterior to the femur. As the lesion matures, it enlarges, and margins become more distinct. It may coalesce with the anterior femur. Radionuclide bone scans may be employed to assess the maturity of the lesion. They can be confusing if done prior to typical radiographic changes. These lesions can be confused with malignant bone tumors both clinically and on histopathology; therefore, an extremely accurate history is mandated.

Early treatment of myositis ossificans consists of rest. Once the diagnosis is established, the athlete should begin a regimen of protected weight bearing with crutches. Rest and immobilization should continue until pain and inflammation subside. Following the acute period, there may be considerable loss of motion resulting from restricted muscle function. Early rehabilitation should be conservative and consist of active stretching and strengthening. Forceful passive stretching should be avoided for at least 4 months. Following treatment for a contusion and establishment of the diagnosis of myositis, there should be an immediate cessation of intensive exercises in rehabilitation programs; i.e., there should be no resisted strengthening or forced range-of-motion work, and treatment should be only passive. Anti-inflammatory agents are given, and all activities are reduced. The athlete should be re-evaluated frequently, initially after 10 days. If there has been no progression of the condition, once pain subsides, gentle range-of-motion and straight leg–raising exercises can be initiated. Progression of exercises should be slow and cautious.

If there is no improvement after 10 days, prednisone or a course of diphosphonates should be administered.

Activity progresses when the bone mass shows signs of stabilizing or maturing. The same criteria as discussed earlier should be applied for return to participation. In some cases, full range of motion may not be possible, and criteria may need to be modified. Even large ossific masses are compatible with full range of motion and good function.

Surgery is indicated only to reduce the mass effect of the ectopic bone and should never be done until a bone scan shows quiescence of activity. This is generally 9 to 12 months following injury. O'Donoghue states that early surgery usually results in recurrence and that an adequate incision should be made to fully visualize the entire mass.[44] When surgery is done, care must be taken in determining the pathologic diagnosis as osteogenic sarcoma and myositis ossificans look exactly like each other under a microscope; and of course, the treatments are radically different. An accurate medical history is often the only way to distinguish between the two lesions.

Wieder reported a case study of treatment of a 16-year-old boy with quadriceps femoris muscle myositis ossificans as a result of a springboard diving accident.[72] Treatment consisted of iontophoresis with 2 percent acetic acid solution followed by pulsed ultrasound. This regimen was followed for three times a week for 3 weeks. At the conclusion of treatment, radiography indicated a 98.9 percent decrease in the size of the ossified mass. Wieder suggested that this report demonstrated potential for a therapeutic program of acetic acid iontophoresis and ultrasound to eliminate myositis ossificans, but this treatment is thus far uncontrolled and the report anecdotal. Prevention of myositis ossificans is the best treatment. Trainers, coaches, therapists, physicians, and athletes should understand the seriousness of this injury and recognize the need for a careful and considerate progressive rehabilitation program (Fig. 29–6).

ACUTE COMPARTMENT SYNDROME

Most contusions resolve after a rather benign course of treatment, leaving the athlete with no residual symptoms. Complications may occur, however. One of these, although quite rare in the thigh, is development of a compartment syndrome. Compartment syndrome is defined as increased tissue pressure in a closed fascial compartment that compromises circulation to the nerves and muscles.[73,74] Diagnosis is based on pressure measurements, since the motor function of the femoral nerve is difficult to establish clinically when a large hematoma is present. Controversy exists over the actual pressures within a compartment that indicate surgical intervention is necessary. Suggested values above 40 mm Hg pressure are indicative. In this case, passive stretching into flexion is not diagnostic, since hematomas often cause intense pain with stretching. Rooser and colleagues reported on a series of eight cases of anterior thigh muscle contusion or rupture resulting in compartment syndrome.[75] All patients had an increased pressure in the quadriceps muscle ranging between 41 and 80 mm Hg. All cases were treated with a surgical

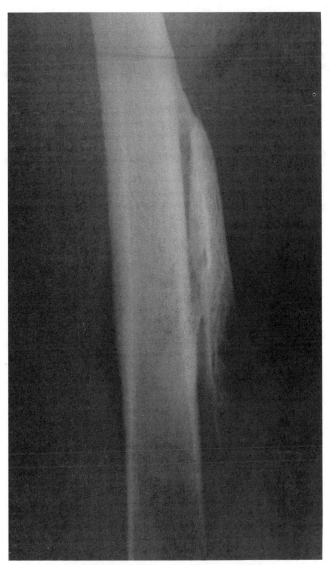

FIGURE 29–6. X-ray of myositis ossificans.

procedure consisting of an anterior or anterolateral skin incision, fasciotomy, and evacuation of hematomas. Rehabilitation was initiated within 2 days of surgery and within 4 weeks, all patients had normal function.

BURSITIS

The three major bursae around the hip that are susceptible to bursitis are the iliopsoas bursa (iliopectineal), the greater trochanteric bursa, and the ischial bursa. Bursitis is an inflammation of the bursas, which are fluid-filled sacs between bony prominences and the muscles or skin. Development of bursitis is a result of one or two mechanisms. The most common is inflammation secondary to excessive friction or shear forces as a result of overuse. Post-traumatic bursitis is the other mechanism, and it stems from direct blows and contusions that cause bleeding in the bursa with resultant inflammation.

Symptoms are usually benign and respond to symptomatic treatment such as rest, ice, and nonsteroidal anti-inflammatory (NSAIDs) medications. In the overuse form of bursitis, there is gradual onset of pain in the region, and this progresses proportional to activity. The pain can become severe enough that there is continuous pain even with rest.

Iliopsoas bursitis or iliopectineal bursitis are most often due to excessive activity. Osteoarthritis of the hip may also cause iliopectineal bursitis.[76] Differentiation between bursitis and iliopsoas muscle strain can be difficult. The pain is located in the inguinal area and radiates through the femoral triangle. It may also be associated with symptoms of a snapping hip. There is tenderness to palpation, which is most easily accomplished with the hip and knee flexed, leg externally rotated, and knee supported with muscle relaxation. Extremes of rotation in flexion and resisted hip flexion exercise may elicit discomfort. Meralgia paresthetica can cause radiation of pain into the front of the thigh and knee.

Treatment includes the use of NSAIDs and activity modification. Iliopsoas stretching is critical. The use of ultrasound or interferential current may also be indicated. Steroid injections and even surgical release of the iliopsoas tendon can be considered in chronic cases (Table 29–9).[77,78]

Trochanteric bursitis is often seen in runners, cross-country skiers, and ballet dancers. The greater trochanteric bursa lies between the gluteus maximus, tensor muscle of the fascia lata (TFL), and the surface of the greater trochanter. Trochanteric bursitis is characterized by a burning or deep aching sensation over or just posterior to the tip of the greater trochanter. It may be painful with walking during the early course. Pain is made worse by activity. The description usually is one of a dull ache in the hip with sharp pain as the hip moves from flexion to extension during weight bearing. Referral of pain down the lateral aspect of the thigh may be present. If there is a sudden sharp pain that occurs with certain movements, it could be secondary or related to a snapping hip problem.

Runners who do a great deal of road running will experience trochanteric bursitis in the "down side" leg. This is due to the functional leg-length discrepancy

TABLE 29–9 Management of Bursitis	
Stage	**Treatment**
Acute (24–48 hours)	Ice Compression Pain-free passive ROM NSAIDs
Rehabilitation	Heat Pain-free stretching and strengthening exercises Pain-free, progressive resisted ROM Gradual return to sport-specific and functional activities
Return to sport	Protective padding Progression of sport-specific activities

and is the source of friction between the greater trochanter and the iliotibial band during repetitive movements of the hip in flexion and extension. Overuse trochanteric bursitis is common in women runners who have an increased quadriceps (Q) angle and/or a possible leg-length discrepancy.[79] Lateral heel wear in running shoes may also cause excessive hip adduction leading indirectly to bursitis. Trochanteric bursitis can also occur in contact sports as a result of direct trauma. Football, soccer, and ice hockey players are susceptible to this injury. A blow can cause a huge, swollen, painful bursa over the area of the prominence of the trochanter.

Treatment is the same as for other sites of bursitis. However, in addition to rest and other measures, emphasis should be placed on stretching the iliotibial band and strengthening the gluteal muscles. Patients that do not respond may develop a chronically painful condition. After a series of local injections with anesthetics and cortisone, surgery may be considered. An orthotic evaluation should be performed to check for any biomechanical abnormalities of gait that could lead to dysfunction. Significant (>2 cm) leg-length discrepancies should be corrected.[80] Protective padding is indicated for participants in high-risk contact sports such as football.

Ischial bursitis is often due to a direct bruise or trauma after a fall and is uncommon. Since the ischial bursa lies between the ischial tuberosity and the greater gluteus muscle, the most important aspect of ischial bursitis is the differential diagnosis with a hamstring tear at the origin. When diagnosis is confirmed, treatment is the same as for other bursas. This problem usually responds well to treatment of measures of NSAIDs and rest and is resolved with no further need for treatment. Removal of ischial spurs for cases nonresponsive to the previously described treatment can be considered (Fig. 29–7).

SNAPPING OR CLICKING HIP

The snapping hip syndrome is a condition that develops secondary to a variety of intra-articular and extra-articular causes. Intra-articular causes include synovial chondromatosis, loose bodies, osteocartilaginous exostosis, and subluxation of the hip.[77] However, the most common cause is an extra-articular snapping of the iliotibial band over the greater trochanter, which can also result in trochanteric bursitis. Other extra-articular causes include snapping of the iliopsoas tendon over the iliopectineal eminence, the iliofemoral ligaments over the femoral head, and the long head of the biceps of the femur over the ischial tuberosity. Another possible cause of hip clicking is the suction phenomenon in the hip joint itself, which is due to negative pressure in the joint that exerts a "plunger" effect.

The clicking or snapping hip is common in athletes and most prominent in dancers and runners.[81–83] It is also commonly seen in cheerleaders and is much more common in females. Most complaints concern the sound or sensation of "clicking" rather than pain. This condition is generally painless and is present

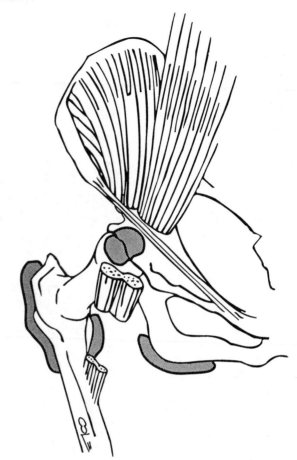

FIGURE 29–7. Anatomic diagram of bursa.

with specific flexion movements of the thigh such as sit-ups.

Once identification of contributing factors has been completed, treatment can be directed toward these factors—muscle tightness, muscle imbalance, poor training techniques, biomechanics of movement, which are at fault. Specific rehabilitation programs can be designed to reduce each of these factors. NSAIDs or injections with steroid preparations may help relieve symptoms while rehabilitation continues if trochanteric bursitis is an intermediate problem.

Zoltan and associates reported on seven patients with painful hip due to snapping of the iliotibial band over the greater trochanter and whose symptoms were nonresponsive to conservative treatment.[84] They describe a surgical procedure that includes excision of a portion of the iliotibial band over the greater trochanter and removal of the trochanteric bursa. They report this as an effective method to treat patients with a symptomatic snapping hip due to this condition.

OTHER CONDITIONS

APOPHYSITIS

Apophysitis is an inflammatory response to overuse in the growing child and is characterized by pain at the apophyseal growth attachment of muscle to bone.

It is generally insidious in onset without antecedent history of injury. Radiographic evaluation is required to rule out other abnormalities and look for pelvic asymmetry.

Clancy and Foltz first described a case of iliac crest tenderness to palpation and muscular spasm in a young long-distance runner.[85] There was a history of intensive training but no history of trauma. Therapy consisted of 4 to 6 weeks rest with an adjunct of ice application and NSAID medications. Apophysitis may be treated in the same manner as a hip pointer.

OSTEITIS PUBIS

Osteitis pubis is an inflammatory condition involving the pubic symphysis. Only recently has it been implicated as a significant sports injury.[86] It is most often encountered following suprapubic cystotomy and bladder surgery or as a degenerative process frequently associated with various metabolic conditions. As a sporting injury, the pain is characteristic because it is localized to the symphyseal area. It is exacerbated as a result of athletic activity. It is seen in severe form in long-distance runners, fencers, soccer players, and occasionally weight lifters, hockey, and football players. The pain is insidious and may radiate down into the groin or medial thigh. The characteristic finding is pain right over the pubic symphysis that is generally more prominent on one side. Associated abdominal muscle spasm may occur as a result of athletic activity. Eventually gait abnormalities can occur due to pain.

Early on, scant X-ray changes may be apparent, such as mild widening of the pubic symphysis, erosion along the cortical margins, and sclerotic reactive bone in the metaphyseal regions around the symphysis. In the chronic form, this area can appear moth-eaten on x-ray film. The precise cause of this particular problem is unknown, although it may be due to traction injuries at the origin of muscle from the pubic symphysis, where the adductor longus and brevis and gracilis muscles take their origin. This condition may also represent a type of overuse injury or stress fracture.[87] It is clear that in sports-related osteitis pubis, the pubic symphysis changes are more indolent and chronic and are due to overuse activities. Gross thinks that this lesion may be akin to shin splints and may involve periosteitis or tendinitis at the muscle attachments.

Treatment initially involves rest and use of NSAIDs. Holt reported excellent relief in resistant cases following the injection of corticosteroid into the involved area.[88] Occasionally, more aggressive treatment involving wedge resection of these lesions has been utilized.[89] This procedure has been used more for the nonathletic population.

TRANSIENT SYNOVITIS OF THE HIP

This infrequent condition occurs largely in children. Findings include a painful hip joint with an antalgic gait and limp. The exact cause of the transient synovitis is unknown, although it is thought that antecedent viral infection, allergic mechanism, or some type of microtrauma might be involved.

The diagnosis in this particular condition is made by exclusion because it is necessary to first rule out septic arthritis of the hip and other serious conditions. Consequently, once the patient is diagnosed as having primary hip pathology, an effort is made to eliminate bacterial synovitis as the primary cause. This is done with a good history and physical examination; blood work, including a CBC and sedimentation rate, and x-ray films of the hip. In the case of pyarthrosis, the joint may show capsular distention and osteomyelitis may also be apparent on the radiographs. Technetium bone scanning is also helpful; with bacterial infection, there is a much more intensely infected area. The sedimentation rate is generally much more elevated in bacterial than in viral infection. Hip aspiration must be done if pyarthrosis is strongly suspected.

The main reason that pyogenic hip arthrosis must be ruled out is the emergent surgery necessary to drain the septic joint to relieve pressure and preserve blood supply to the femoral head. Viral synovitis is treated conservatively without aggressive surgical treatment, and the prognosis is good. Other diseases of the hip that can mimic this particular transient synovitis include Legg-Calvé-Perthe disease, a type of avascular necrosis of the hip that occurs in children, juvenile rheumatoid disease manifesting in a monarticular fashion, and a slipped capital femoral epiphysis.

SLIPPED CAPITAL FEMORAL EPIPHYSIS

This particular disease is seen in children between the ages of 11 and 14 years. Males are affected more commonly than females, and black males are involved in a higher incidence.[90] The condition usually occurs in children who have delays of skeletal maturity and are obese. Occasionally, it is seen in aesthenic children, but it is generally not seen in children with normal development. Most of these slips occur around the time of puberty and can be related to some rather trivial injury that might have occurred during a sporting activity. Usually pain in the groin is the presenting complaint, which is occasionally referred down into the thigh or knee. Care must be taken to rule out this diagnosis in a child with a limp and knee pain.

Physical findings include loss of motion in the hip, especially internal rotation. Radiographs reveal a slip of the capital epiphysis compared with the other side. Acute slips are generally diagnosed within a period of 3 weeks following the onset of symptoms, chronic slips beyond that time. Slips are categorized based on the degree of slip that has occurred. Recommended treatment involves internal fixation of the slip in situ with threaded pins. Since the incidence of slip is high in the contralateral hip, prophylactic pinning should be considered.

The complications associated with slipped capital femoral epiphysis are severe. When manipulation is done, avascular necrosis increases dramatically. In black children, the prognosis is poor, with much higher incidence of avascular necrosis and chondrolysis; the exact reason is not yet known.

At any rate, these children need be managed with cautious optimism; the prognosis is guarded. They should probably be returned to athletic activity only as they reach skeletal maturity and the epiphyses fuse on both sides. Any other type of vigorous activity prior to that time is ill-advised.

MERALGIA PARESTHETICA

This condition is infrequent in athletes, but it can occur. The superficial branch of the femoral cutaneous nerve can be entrapped as it exits through the femoral canal in the groin. The wearing of skin-tight garments (such as a hip-pad girdle) or belts that compress this nerve at its exit from the inguinal canal is to be dis-

TABLE 29–10
Causes of Hip and Thigh Pain Other Than Traumatic Fracture

Location	Differential Diagnosis	Onset	Special Characteristics
Sacroiliac (SI) pain	1. Lumbar strain (LS) 2. Herniated nucleus pulposus (HNP) 3. Sacroiliac bursitis 4. Sacroiliac arthritis	1. Subacute/chronic 2. Subacute/chronic 3. Subacute/chronic 4. Subacute/chronic	1. Associated low back pain (LBP) 2. LBP and associated sciatica 3. Point-tender SI joint Crepitus; no change in radiographs 4. Point-tender SI joint with changes on x-ray films
Gluteal pain	1. LS/HNP (referred) 2. Pyriformis syndrome 3. Hamstrings strain (avulsion fracture) 4. Ischial bursitis	1. Subacute/chronic 2. Subacute/chronic 3. Acute 4. Subacute	1. See preceding 2. Tender over pyriformis; decreased external rotation of hip 3. Tender at injury point; history of injury 4. Tender over ischium; no injury
Trochanteric pain	1. LS/HNP (referred) 2. Trochanteric bursitis	1. Subacute/chronic 2. Subacute/chronic	1. See preceding 2. Exquisitely tender over trochanter; crepitus
Anterior hip and groin pain	1. LS/HNP (referred) 2. Hip pointer 3. Adductor strain 4. Stress fracture (femoral neck) 5. Hip pathology (synovitis, slipped capital femoral epiphysis, subluxation, snapping, avascular necrosis) 6. Inguinal hernia	1. Subacute/chronic 2. Acute 3. Acute 4. Subacute 5. Subacute 6. Acute/subacute/chronic	1. See preceding 2. Exquisitely tender over tensor fascia lata (TFL) muscle; history of direct blow 3. History of injury; tender in groin 4. History of injury; "Hot" bone scan ± changes on x-ray films 5. Painful range of motion; antalgic gait with abductor lurch 6. Hernia demonstrable with Valsalva maneuver on inguinal examination
Anterior thigh pain	1. Hip pathology (referred) 2. Contusion/strain 3. Compartment syndrome 4. Myositis 5. Stress fracture 6. Meralgia paresthetica	1. Subacute 2. Acute 3. Acute 4. Chronic 5. Subacute 6. Subacute	1. See preceding 2. History of injury; tender, swollen thigh; palpable muscle defect 3. Pain; swelling (tense); increased tissue pressure (>40 mm Hg) 4. Palpable mass; calcification seen on x-ray films 5. See the preceding 6. Dysesthetic thigh pain in superficial femoral nerve distribution
Posterior thigh pain	1. LS/HNP with sciatica 2. Hamstring strain	1. Subacute/chronic 2. Acute	1. See the preceding 2. History of injury; tenderness; palpable defect

couraged. An area of hyperesthesia, which can sometimes become dysesthetic and unpleasant, develops in the anterolateral thigh along the distribution of the superficial femoral nerve. Treatment is symptomatic. The condition generally improves over a period of time when the nerve impingement is removed.

CONCLUSION

Injuries to these pelvic and hip structures are less frequent than other parts of the leg but have potentially serious career-threatening consequences. Diagnosis is often problematic due to the prevalence of many confusing medical processes that can mimic these disorders (Table 29–10). An accurate medical history is imperative in reaching a specific diagnosis. Open-mindedness is also important in preventing inaccurate "shot-gun" diagnoses that can lead to improper management and poor programs for these conditions.

REFERENCES

1. Paty JG: Diagnosis and treatment of musculoskeletal running injuries. Semin Arthritis Rheum 1988; 18:48–60.
2. Harkess JW, Ramsey WC, Harkess JW: Principles of fractures and dislocations. In Rockwood CA Jr, Green DP, Bucholz RW (eds): Rockwood and Green's Fractures in Adults, vol 1, 3rd ed. Philadelphia, JB Lippincott Co, 1991, pp 1–180.
3. Peris P, Guañabens N, Pons F, et al: Clinical evolution of sacral stress fractures: Influence of additional pelvic fractures. Ann Rheum Dis 1993; 52:545–547.
4. Schils J, Hauzeur J: Stress fracture of the sacrum. Am J Sports Med 1992; 20(6): 769–770.
5. Wolff J: Das Gesetz der Transformation der Knochen. Berlin, A. Hirschwald, 1892, p 3.
6. Giladi M, Milgrom C, Simkin A, et al: Stress fractures. Am J Sports Med 1991; 19:647–652.
7. Giladi M, Milgrom C, Stein M, et al: External rotation of the hip. Clin Orthop 1987; 216:131–134.
8. Pavlov H: Roentgen examination of groin and hip pain in the athlete. Clin Sports Med 1987; 6(4):829–843.
9. Pavlov H, Nelson TL, Warren RF, et al: Stress fractures of the pubic ramus. J Bone Joint Surg 1982; 64-A:1020–1025.
10. Devas MB: Stress fractures of the femoral neck. J Bone Joint Surg 1965; 47-B:728–738.
11. Skinner HB, Cook SD: Fatigue failure stress of the femoral neck. Am J Sports Med 1982; 10:245–247.
12. Branch HE: March fractures of the femur. J Bone Joint Surg 1944; 26:387–391.
13. Sjølin SU, Eriksen C: Stress fracture of the femoral neck in military recruits. Injury 1989; 20(5):304–305.
14. Blickenstaff LD, Morris JM: Fatigue fracture of the femoral neck. J Bone Joint Surg 1966; 48A:1031–1047.
15. El-Khoury GY, Wehbe MA, Bonfiglio M, et al: Stress fractures of the femoral neck: A scintigraphic sign for early diagnosis. Skeletal Radiol 1981; 6:271–273.
16. Fullerton LR: Femoral neck stress fractures. Sports Med 1990; 9:192–197.
17. Fullerton LR, Snowdy HA: Femoral neck stress fractures. Am J Sports Med 1988; 16:365–377.
18. Johansson C, Ekenman I, Törnkvist H, et al: Stress fractures of the femoral neck in athletes. Am J Sports Med 1990; 18(5):524–528.
19. Lombardo SJ, Benson DW: Stress fractures of the femur in runners. Am J Sports Med 1982; 10:219–227.
20. Masters S, Fricker P, Purdam C: Stress fractures of the femoral shaft. Br J Sports Med 1986; 20:14–16.
21. Wachsmuth W: Atiologie der schleichenden frakturen. Chirung 16, 1937.
22. Butler JE, Eggert AW: Fracture of the iliac crest apophysis: An unusual hip pointer. J Sports Med 1975; 3:192–193.
23. Butler JE, Brown SL, McConnell BG: Subtrochanteric stress fractures in runners. Am J Sports Med 1982; 10:228–232.
24. Tile M: Pelvic ring fractures: Should they be fixed? J Bone Joint Surg 1988; 70-B:1–12.
25. Krissoff WB: Follow-up on hang gliding injuries in Colorado. Am J Sports Med 1976; 4:222–229.
26. Judet R, Judet J, Letournel E: Fractures of the acetabulum: classification and surgical approaches for open reduction. J Bone Joint Surg 1964; 46A:1615–1646.
27. Peltier L: Personal communication, 1974.
28. Canale ST, King RE: Pelvic and hip fractures. In Rockwood CA Jr, Wilkins KE, King RE (eds): Fractures in Children, vol 3, 3rd ed. Philadelphia, JB Lippincott, 1991, pp 992–1093.
29. Colonna PC: Fracture of the neck of the femur in childhood. Ann Surg 1928; 88:902.
30. Fernbach SK, Wilkinson RH: Avulsion injuries of the pelvis and proximal femur. Am J Roentgenol 1981; 137:581–584.
31. Stenger A: Bo's hip dislocates stellar athletic career. Phys Sports Med 1991; 19(5):17–18.
32. DeLee JC, Drez D Jr (eds): Orthopaedic Sports Medicine: Principles and Practice, vol 2. Philadelphia, WB Saunders, 1994.
33. Epstein HC: Traumatic dislocations of the hip. Clin Orthop 1973; 92:116–142.
34. Marcus ND, Enneking WF, Massam RA: The silent hip in idiopathic aseptic necrosis. J Bone Joint Surg 1973; 55A:1351–1366.
35. Libri R, Calderon JE, Capelli A, et al: Traumatic dislocation of the hip in children and adolescents. Ital J Orthop Traumatol 1986; 12:61–67.
36. Upadhyay SS, Moulton A: The long-term results of traumatic posterior dislocation of the hip. J Bone Joint Surg 1981; 63B: 548–551.
37. Stewart MJ, Milford LW: Fracture dislocation of the hip. J Bone Joint Surg 1954; 36A:315–342.
38. Speer KP, Lohnes H, Garrett WE: Radiographic imaging of muscle strain injury. Am J Sports Med 1993; 21:89–96.
39. Berson BL, Rolnick AM, Ramos CL, et al: An epidemiologic study of squash injuries. Am J Sports Med 1981; 9:103–106.
40. Glick JM: Muscle strains: Prevention and treatment. Phys Sports Med 1980; 8:73–77.
41. Garrett WE Jr: Muscle strain injuries: Clinical and basic aspects. Med Sci Sports Exerc 1990; 22:436–443.
42. Garrett WE Jr, Nikolaou PK, Ribbeck BM, et al: The effect of muscle architecture on the biomechanical failure properties of skeletal muscle under passive extension. Am J Sports Med 1988; 16:7–12.
43. Noonan TJ, Garrett WE: Injuries at the myotendinous junction. Clin Sports Med 1992; 11:783–806.
44. O'Donoghue DH (ed): Treatment of Injuries to Athletes, 4th ed. Philadelphia, WB Saunders, 1984.
45. Peterson L, Renstrom P: Muscle injuries-strains. In Grana WA (ed): Sports Injuries: Their Prevention and Treatment. Chicago, Year Book Medical Publishers, 1986, p 465.
46. Agre JC: Hamstring injuries: proposed etiological factors, prevention and treatment. Sports Med 1985; 2:21–33.
47. Lloyd-Smith, Clement DB, McKenzie DC, et al: A survey of overuse and traumatic hip and pelvic injuries in athletes. Phys Sports Med 1985; 13:131.
48. Brubaker CE, James SL: Injuries to runners. J Sports Med 1974; 2:189–198.
49. Garrett WE Jr, Califf JC, Bassett FH: Histochemical correlates of hamstring injuries. Am J Sports Med 1984; 98–103.
50. Eckstrand J, Gillquist J, Moller M, et al: Incidence of soccer injuries and their relation to training and team success. Am J Sports Med 1983; 11:63–69.
51. Dorman P: A report on 140 hamstring injuries. Aust J Sports Med 1981; 4:30–36.
52. Heiser T, Weber J, Sullivan G, et al: Prophylaxis and management of hamstring muscle injuries in intercollegiate football players. Am J Sports Med 1984; 12:368–370.
53. Worrell TW, Perrin DH, Gansnede, et al: Comparison of isokinetic strength and flexibility measures between hamstring injured and non-injured athletes. J Orthop Sports Phys Ther 1991; 13:118–125.
54. Paton RW, Grimshaw P, McGregor J, et al: Assessment of the effects of significant hamstring injury. J Biomed Eng 1989; 11:229–230.

55. Worrell TW, Perrin DH: Hamstring muscle injury: The influence of strength, flexibility, warm-up and fatigue. J Orthop Sports Phys Ther 1992; 16:12–18.

56. Liemohn W: Factors related to hamstring strains. J Sports Med 1978; 18:71–76.

57. McCue FW: Personal communication, 1978.

58. Ishikawa K, Kai K, Mizuta H: Avulsion of the hamstring muscles from the ischial tuberosity. Clin Orthop 1988; 232:153–155.

59. Blasier RB, Morawa LG: Complete rupture of the hamstring origin from a water skiing injury. Am J Sports Med 1990; 18:435–437.

60. Loosli AR, Quick J: Thigh strains in competitive breaststroke swimmers. J Sport Rehab 1992; 1:49–55.

61. Stanish WD: The use of flexibility exercises in preventing and treating sports injuries. In Leadbetter WB, Buckwalter JA, Gordon SL (eds): Sports-Induced Inflammation. Park Ridge, IL, American Academy of Orthopaedic Surgeons, 1990.

62. Zachazewski JE: Flexibility for sports. In Sanders BR (ed): Sports Physical Therapy, Appleton and Lange, 1991, pp 201–238.

63. Zebas CJ, Rivera ML: Retention of flexibility in selected joints after cessation of a stretching exercise program. In Dotson CO, Humphrey JH (eds): Exercise Physiology: Current Selected Research. New York, AMS Press, 1985.

64. Voss DE, Ionta MK, Myers BJ: Proprioceptive Neuromuscular Facilitation, Patterns and Techniques, 3rd ed. Philadelphia, Harper & Row, 1985.

65. Prentice WE: A comparison of static stretching and PNF stretching for improving hip joint flexibility. Athletic Train 1983; 18:56–59.

66. Markos PD: Ipsilateral and contralateral effects of proprioceptive neuromuscular facilitation techniques on hip motion and electromyographic activity. Phys Ther 1979; 59:1366–1373.

67. Sady SP, Wortman M, Blanke D: Flexibility training: Ballistic, static or proprioceptive neuromuscular facilitation? Arch Phys Med Rehab 1982; 63:261–263.

68. Tanigawa MC: Comparison of the hold-relax procedure and passive mobilization of increasing muscle length. Phys Ther 1972; 52:725–735.

69. de Vries HA: Electromyographic observations of the effects of static stretching on muscular distress. Res Q 1961; 32:468–479.

70. Ryan JB, Wheeler JH, Hopkinson WJ, et al: Quadriceps contusion: West Point update. Am J Sports Med 1991; 19:299–303.

71. Thorndike A: Myositis ossificans traumatica. J Bone Joint Surg 1940; 22:315–323.

72. Wieder DL: Treatment of traumatic myositis ossificans with acetic acid iontophoresis. Phys Ther 1992; 72:133–137.

73. Mubarak SJ, Owen CA, Hargens AR, et al: Acute compartment syndromes, diagnosis and treatment with the aid of the wick catheter. J Bone Joint Surg 1978; 60A:1091–1095.

74. Kahn JSG, Stanford R, McClellan T, et al: Acute bilateral compartment syndrome of the thigh induced by exercise. J Bone Joint Surg 1994; 76A:1068–1071.

75. Rooser B, Bengston S, Hagglund G: Acute compartment syndrome from anterior thigh muscle contusion: A report of eight cases. J Orthop Trauma 1991; 5:57 59.

76. Saudek CE: In Gould JA (ed): The hip. In Orthopaedic and Sports Physical Therapy, 2nd ed. St. Louis, CV Mosby, 1990, p 384.

77. Micheli LJ: Overuse injuries in children's sports: The growth factor. Orthop Clin North Am 1983; 14:337–361.

78. O'Neill DB, Micheli LJ: Overuse injuries in young athletes. Clin Sports Med 1988; 7:591–610.

79. Arnheim DD: Modern Principles of Athletic Training. St. Louis, CV Mosby, 1985.

80. De Palma B: Rehabilitation of hip and thigh injuries. In Prentice WE (ed): Rehabilitation Techniques in Sports Medicine. St. Louis, Times Mirror/Mosby College Publishing, 1990, pp 265–293.

81. Howse AJG: Orthopedist aid ballet. Clin Orthop 1972; 89:52.

82. Quirk R: Ballet injuries: The Australian experience. Clin Sports Med 1983; 2:507.

83. Schaberg JE, Harper MC, Allen WC: The snapping hip syndrome. Am J Sports Med 1984; 12:361–365.

84. Zoltan DJ, Clancy WG, Keene JS: A new operative approach to snapping hip and refractory trochanteric bursitis in athletes. Am J Sports Med 1986; 14:201–204.

85. Clancy WG Jr, Foltz AS: Iliac apophysitis and stress fractures in adolescent runners. Am J Sports Med 1976; 4:214–218.

86. Koch RA, Jackson DW: Pubic symphysitis in runners. Am J Sports Med 1981; 9:62–63.

87. Gross ML, Wolff A, Distefano M: Hip fractures in children. Orthop Grand Rounds 1986; 3:9.

88. Holt M: Personal communication, 1993.

89. Grace JN, Sim FH, Shives TC, et al: Wedge resection of the symphysis pubis for the treatment of osteitis pubis. J Bone Joint Surg 1989; 71A:358–364.

90. MacEwen GD, Bunnell WP, Ramsey PL: The hip. In Lovell WW, Winter RB (eds): Pediatric Orthopaedics, 2nd ed, vol 2. Philadelphia, JB Lippincott, 1986, pp 703–788.

BIBLIOGRAPHY

Abbate CC: Avulsion fracture of the ischial tuberosity: A case report. J Bone Joint Surg 1945; 27:716.

Adams RJ, Chandler FA: Osteitis pubis of traumatic etiology. J Bone Joint Surg 1953; 35A:685–696.

American Academy of Orthopaedic Surgeons (eds): Athletic Training and Sports Medicine. Chicago, American Academy of Orthopaedic Surgeons, 1984, pp 3, 223–234.

Antao NA: Myositis ossificans of the hip in a professional soccer player. Am J Sports Med 1988; 16:82–83.

Atwell EA, Jackson DW: Stress fractures of the sacrum in runners. Am J Sports Med 1991; 19:531–533.

Baker J, Frankel VH, Burstein A: Fatigue fractures: Biomechanical consideration. J Bone Joint Surg 1972; 54A:1345.

Berry JM: Fracture of the tuberosity of the ischium due to muscular action. JAMA 1992; 59:1450.

Blatz DJ: Bilateral femoral and tibial shaft stress fractures in a runner. Am J Sports Med 1981; 9:322–325.

Blecher A: Über den einfluss de parade-marches auf die enstehung der fuss geschwulst. Med Klin 1905; 1:305.

Bosacco SJ, Hollis SC, Berman AT: Insufficiency fracture of the sacrum. Orthopaedics 1990; 13(1):128–133.

Boyd AD, Sledge CB: Evaluation of the hip with pigmented villonodular synovitis. Clin Orthop 1992; 275:180–186.

Brunet ME, Hontas RB: The thigh. In DeLee JC, Drez D Jr (eds): Orthopaedic Sports Medicine: Principles and Practice, vol 2, Philadelphia, WB Saunders, 1994, pp 1086–1112.

Burgess AR, Tile M: Fractures of the pelvis. In Rockwood CA Jr, Green DP, Bucholz RW (eds): Rockwood and Green's Fractures in Adults, vol 2, 3rd ed. Philadelphia, JB Lippincott Co, 1991, pp 1399–1480.

Cady GW, White ES, LaPoint JM: Displaced fatigue fractures of the femoral neck. J Bone Joint Surg 1975; 57A:1022.

Ciullo JV: Lower extremity injuries. In Pearl AJ (ed): The Athletic Female, Human Kinetics. Champaign, IL, American Orthopaedic Society for Sports Medicine, 1993, pp 272–275.

Clement DB: Overuse running injuries. Phys Sports Med 1981; 9(5):47–58.

Colosimo AJ, Ireland MJ: Thigh compartment syndrome in a football athlete. Med Sci Sports Ex 1992; 958–963.

Cooper DE, Warren RF, Barnes R: Traumatic subluxation of the hip resulting in aseptic necrosis and chondrolysis in a professional football player. Am J Sports Med 1991; 19:322–324.

Daffner RH, Martinez S, Gehweiler JA: Stress fractures in runners. JAMA 1982; 247:1039–1041.

Del Beccaro MA, Champoux AN, Bockers T, et al: Septic arthritis versus transient synovitis of the hip. Ann Emerg Med 1992; 21:1418–1422.

Donald JG, Fitts WT: March fractures: A study with special reference to etiological factors. J Bone Joint Surg 1947; 29A:297–300.

Downing JF, Nicholas JA, Goldberg B: Four complex joint injuries. Phys Sports Med 1991; 19(10):81–95.

Ernst J: Stress fracture of the neck of the femur. J Trauma 1964; 4:71–83.

Frost A, Bauer M: Skier's hip—a new clinical entity? J Orthop Trauma 1991; 5(1):47–50.

Gamble JG, Simmons SC, Freedman M: The symphysis pubis. Clin Orthop 1986; 203:261–272.

Garrick JG, Webb DR: Sports Injuries: Diagnosis and Management. Philadelphia, WB Saunders, 1990.

Gibbens MW: March fractures of the neck of the femur. J Bone Joint Surg 1945; 27A:162–163.

Gleim GW, Nicholas JA, Webb JN: Isokinetic evaluation following leg injuries. Phys Sports Med 6(2):74–80.

Godshall RW, Hansen CA: Incomplete avulsion of a portion of the iliac epiphysis. J Bone Joint Surg 1973; 55A:1301–1302.

Harris NH, Murray RO: Lesions of the symphysis in athletes. BMJ 1974; 4:211–214.

Hasegawa Y, Ito H: Intracapsular pressure in hip synovitis in children. Acta Orthop Scand 1991; 62(4):333–336.

Hermel MB, Albert SM: Transient synovitis of the hip. Clin Orthop 1962; 22:21–26.

Herring SA, Nilson KL: Introduction to overuse injuries. Clin Sports Med 1987; 6:225–239.

Jackson DW: Low back pain in young athletes: Evaluation of stress reaction and discogenic problems. Am J Sports Med 1979; 7:364–366.

Jackson DW, Feagin JA: Quadriceps contusions in young athletes. J Bone Joint Surg 1973; 55A:95–105.

Jackson DW, Wiltse LL, Cirincoine RJ: Spondylolysis in the female gymnast. Clin Orthop 1976; 117:68–76.

Jacobs SJ, Berson BL: Injuries to runners: A study of entrants to a 10,000 meter race. Am J Sports Med 1986; 14:151–155.

James SL, Bates BT, Osternig LR: Injuries to runners. Am J Sports Med 1978; 6(2):40–50.

Kane WJ: Fractures of the pelvis. In Rockwood, CA Jr, Green DP (eds): Fractures, 2nd ed, vol 1. Philadelphia, JB Lippincott, 1984, pp 905–1011.

Krejci V, Koch P: Muscle and Tendon Injuries in Athletes. Chicago, Year Book Medical Publishers, 1979.

Kulund DN: The torso, hip, and thigh. In Kulund DN (ed): The Injured Athlete. Philadelphia, JB Lippincott, 1982, pp 350–360.

Kulund DN: The Injured Athlete. Philadelphia, JB Lippincott, 1988.

Lam SF: Fractures of the neck of the femur in children. J Bone Joint Surg 1971; 53A:1165–1179.

Langan P, Fontanetta AP: Reduction of dislocated hip with transepiphyseal fracture. Orthop Rev 1986; 15(9)586–589.

Latshaw RF, Kantner TR, Kalenak A, et al: A pelvic stress fracture in a female jogger. Am J Sports Med 1981; 9:54–56.

Lewinnek GE, Kelsey J, White AN, et al: The significance and comparison analysis of the epidemiology of hip fractures. Clin Orthop 152:35–43.

Lipscomb AB, Thomas ED, Johnston RK: Treatment of myositis ossificans traumatica in athletes. Am J Sports Med 1976; 4:111–120.

Lysholm J, Wiklander J: Injuries in runners. Am J Sports Med 1987; 15(2):168–171.

Maffulli N: Intensive training in young athletes. Sports Med 1990; 9(4):229–243.

Markey KL: Stress fractures. Clin Sports Med 1987; 6:405–425.

Martens MA, Hansen L, Mulier JC: Adductor tendinitis and musculus rectus abdominis tendopathy. Am J Sports Med 1987; 15:353–356.

Maydl K: Ueber subcutane muskel-und sehnenzerreissungen, sowie rissfracturen, mit berucksichtigung der analogen, durch directe gewalt enstandenen und offenen verletzungen. Deutsche Ztschr Chir 1882; 17:306–361 and 1883; 18:35–139.

McBryde AM Jr: Stress fractures in athletes. J Sports Med 1975; 3:2–217.

McBryde AM Jr: Stress fractures in runners. Clin Sports Med 1985; 4:737–752.

McCleod SB, Lewin P: Avulsion of the epiphysis of the tuberosity of the ischium. JAMA 1929; 92:1957.

McMaster PE: Tendon and muscle ruptures: Clinical and experimental studies on the causes and location of subcutaneous ruptures. J Bone Joint Surg 1933; 15:705–722.

McMaster WC, Walter M: Injuries in soccer. Am J Sports Med 1978; 6:354–357.

Mendez AA, Eyster RL: Displaced nonunion stress fracture of the femoral neck treated with internal fixation and bone graft. Am J Sports Med 1992; 20(2):230–233.

Merrifield HH, Cowan RFJ: Groin strain injuries in ice hockey. J Sports Med 1973; 1:41–42.

Metzmaker JN, Pappas AM: Avulsion fractures of the pelvis. Am J Sports Med 1985; 13:349–358.

Meurman KOA: Stress fracture of the pubic arch in military recruits. Br J Radiol 1980; 53:521–524.

Micheli L: Injuries to female athletes. Surg Rounds 1979; 2:44.

Milch H: Avulsion fracture of the tuberosity of the ischium. J Bone Joint Surg 1926; 8:832.

Muckle DS: Associated factors in recurrent groin and hamstring injuries. Br J Sports Med 1982; 1:37–39.

Murphy BJ, Hechtman KS, Uribe JW, et al: Iliotibial band friction syndrome: MR imaging findings. Musculoskel Radiol 1992; 185:569–571.

Nadkarni JB: Simultaneous anterior and posterior dislocation of hip. J Postgrad Med 1991; 37(2):117–118.

Noakes TD, Smith JA, Lindenberg G: Pelvic stress fractures in long distance runners. Am J Sports Med 1985; 13:120–123.

Noble CA: Iliotibial band friction syndrome in runners. Am J Sports Med 1980; 8:232–234.

Norman A, Dorfman HD: Juxtacortical circumscribed myositis ossificans: Evolution and radiographic features. Radiology 1970; 96:301–306.

O'Leary C, Doyle J, Fenelon G, et al: Traumatic dislocation of the hip in Rugby Union football. Irish Med J 1987; 80(10):291–292.

Orava S, Puranen J, Ala-Ketola L: Stress fractures caused by physical exercise. Acta Orthop Scand 1978; 49:19–27.

O'Toole ML: Prevention and treatment of injuries to runners. Med Sci Sports Exerc 1992; 24(9):S360–S363.

Pierson E Jr: Osteochondritis of the symphysis pubis. Surg Gynecol Obstet . 1929; 49:834–838.

Protzman RR, Griffis CG: Stress fractures in men and women undergoing military training. J Bone Joint Surg 1977; 59A:825.

Pruner RA, Johnston CE: Avulsion fracture of the ischial tuberosity. Pediatr Orthop 1990; 13(3):357–358.

Puffer JC, Zachazewski JE: Management of overuse injuries. Practical Ther 1988; 38:225–232.

Renne JW: Iliotibial band friction syndrome. J Bone Joint Surg 1975; 57A: 1109–1111.

Renner JB: Pelvic insufficiency fractures. Arthritis Rheum 1990; 33(3):426–430.

Robertson RC: Fracture of the anterior superior spine of the ilium. J Bone Joint Surg 1935; 17:1045.

Rogge EA, Romano RL: Avulsion of the ischial apophysis. J Bone Joint Surg 1956; 38A:442.

Rosenthal RE, Spickard WA, Markham RD, et al: Osteomyelitis of the symphysis pubis. J Bone Joint Surg 1982; 64A:123–128.

Rush LV, Rush HL: Avulsion of the anterior superior spine of the ilium. J Bone Joint Surg 1939; 21:206.

Safran MR, Garrett WE Jr, Seaber AV, et al: The role of warmup in muscular injury prevention. Am J Sports Med 1988; 16:123–129.

Schlickewei W, Elsässer B, Mullaji AB, et al: Hip dislocation without fracture. Injury 1993; 24(1):27–31.

Schlonsky J, Olix ML: Functional disability following avulsion fracture of the ischial epiphysis. J Bone Joint Surg 1972; 54A:641–644.

Schneider R, Kaye J, Ghelman B: Adductor avulsive injuries near the symphysis pubis. Radiology 1976; 120:567–569.

Scully TJ, Besterman G: Stress fracture—A preventable training injury. Milit Med 1982; 147:285–287.

Sim FH, Scott HG: Injuries of the pelvis and hip in athletes. In Nicholas JA, Hershmann EB (eds): The Lower Extremity and Spine in Sports Medicine. St. Louis, CV Mosby, 1986.

Solomonow M, D'Ambrosia R: Biomechanics of muscle overuse injuries: A theoretical approach. Clin Sports Med 1987; 2:241–257.

Stanish WD: Overuse injuries in athletes: A perspective. Med Sci Sports Exerc 1984; 16:1–7.

Stanish WD, Curwin S, Rubinovich M: Tendinitis: The analysis and treatment for running. Clin Sports Med 1985; 4:593–609; A:315–342.

Straehley DJ: A life-threatening femur fracture. Phys Sports Med 1991; 19(3):33–34.

Tachdjian MO: Pediatric Orthopedics. WB Saunders, Philadelphia, 1972.

Taylor DC, Meyers C, Moylan JA, et al: Abdominal musculature abnormalities as a cause of groin pain in athletes. Am J Sports Med 1991; 13:239–242.

Tsuno MM, Shu GJ: Myositis ossificans. J Manip Physiol Ther 1990; 13(6):340–342.

Walsh ZT, Micheli LJ: Hip dislocation in a high school football player. Phys Sports Med 1989; 17:112–114.

Walter NE, Wolf MD: Stress fractures in young athletes. Am J Sports Med 1977; 5:165–169.

Waters PM, Millis MB: Hip and pelvic injuries in the young athlete. Clin Sports Med 1988; 7:513–526.

White J: No more bump and grind. Phys Sports Med 1992; 20(3):223–228.

Wiley JJ: Traumatic osteitis pubis: The gracilis syndrome. Am J Sports Med 1983; 11:360–363.

Winternitz WA, Metheny JA, Wear LC: Acute compartment syndrome of the thigh in sports-related injuries not associated with femoral fractures. Am J Sports Med 1992; 20:476–477.

Yasuda T, Miyazaki K, Tada K, et al: Stress fracture of the right distal femur following bilateral fractures of the proximal fibulas. Am J Sports Med 1992; 20(6):771–774.

Yde J, Nielsen AB: Sports injuries in adolescents' ball games: Soccer, handball and basketball. Br J Sports Med 1990; 24:51–54.

Zarins B, Ciullo JV: Acute muscle and tendon injuries in athletes. Clin Sports Med 1983; 2:167–182.

CHAPTER 30

The Knee: Ligamentous and Meniscal Injuries

JAMES J. IRRGANG *MS, PT, ATC*
MARC R. SAFRAN *MD*
FREDDIE H. FU *MD*

FOUNDATION FOR SURGICAL AND NONSURGICAL MANAGEMENT OF KNEE LIGAMENT AND MENISCAL INJURIES

FUNCTIONAL ANATOMY AND BIOMECHANICS OF THE KNEE

Successful nonsurgical and surgical management of knee ligament and meniscal injuries requires knowledge of functional anatomy and biomechanics of the knee. The clinician must be able to integrate this information to evaluate the knee and to develop an appropriate treatment regimen.

The tibiofemoral joint is the articulation between the distal end of the femur and the tibial plateau. The femoral condyles are convex in the anterior-posterior and medial-lateral directions. They are separated by the intercondylar notch, which serves as the site of attachment for the anterior and posterior cruciate ligaments. The width of the intercondylar notch may be an important consideration for the risk of injury to the cruciate ligaments and for the development of loss of extension following anterior cruciate ligament reconstruction. The transverse anterior-to-posterior dimension of the lateral femoral condyle is greater than that of the medial femoral condyle[1] (Fig. 30–1). As a result, the lateral femoral condyle projects further anteriorly than does the medial femoral condyle and provides a bony buttress to minimize lateral displacement of the patella. The radius of curvature of the femoral condyles decreases from anterior to posterior and is shorter on the medial side than on the lateral side.[2] The anterior-to-posterior length of the articular surface of the medial femoral condyle is longer than that of the lateral femoral

623

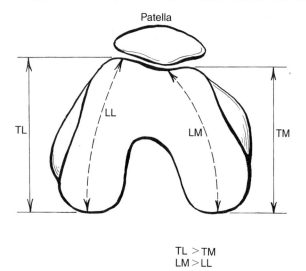

FIGURE 30–1. The transverse anterior posterior dimension of the lateral femoral condyle (TL) is greater than that of the medial femoral condyle (TM). The anterior-to-posterior length of the articular surface of the medial femoral condyle (LM) is longer than the anterior-to-posterior length of the articular surface of the lateral femoral condyle (LL). (From Cailliet R (ed.): 3rd ed. Knee Pain and Disability, Philadelphia, F.A. Davis, 1992.)

condyle[1] (Fig. 30–1). The longer articular surface of the medial femoral condyle facilitates external rotation of the tibia as the knee approaches terminal extension.

The medial tibial plateau is concave from anterior to posterior as well as from medial to lateral. The lateral tibial plateau is concave from medial to lateral, but it is convex from anterior to posterior (Fig. 30–2). The concavity of the tibial plateaus is increased by the presence of the menisci. The bony configuration of the knee lends little inherent stability. Stability of the knee depends on static and dynamic restraints. The static restraints include the joint capsule, ligaments, and menisci. Dynamic stability is provided by muscles that cross the knee and include the quadriceps, hamstrings, and gastrocnemius.

The ligamentous restraints of the knee include the collateral, cruciate, and capsular ligaments. The medial collateral ligament (MCL) is a broad band that runs from the medial epicondyle of the femur to insert on the tibia two to three finger widths below the medial joint line (Fig. 30–3). The MCL has been described as a thickening of the medial capsule and is divided into deep and superficial layers. The deep MCL is intimately attached to the medial meniscus and consists of the tibiomeniscal and femoromeniscal ligaments. The superficial band of the MCL runs from the medial epicondyle to insert distal to the tibial plateau. Because the superficial band of the MCL is further from the center of the knee, it is the first ligament injured when a valgus stress is applied. The MCL courses anteriorly as it runs from the femur to the tibia.

The lateral collateral ligament (LCL) is a cordlike structure that runs from the lateral epicondyle of the femur to the fibular head (see Fig. 30–3). The lateral collateral ligament courses somewhat posteriorly as it passes from the femur to the fibular head. It is separated from the lateral meniscus by the popliteus tendon, which in part explains the increased mobility of the lateral meniscus.

The anterior cruciate ligament (ACL) arises from the tibial plateau just anterior and medial to the tibial eminence. From the tibia, the ACL courses superiorly, laterally, and posteriorly to insert on the posterior

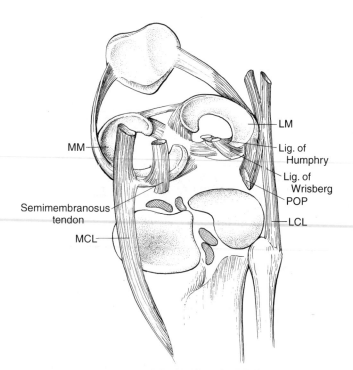

FIGURE 30–2. The medial tibial plateau is concave anterior to posterior, whereas the lateral tibial plateau is convex anterior to posterior. (From Kapandji IA: The Physiology of the Joints: Annotated Diagrams of the Mechanics of the Human Joints. Edinburgh, Churchill Livingstone, 1970.)

FIGURE 30–3. Ligamentous structures and menisci at the knee (MM, medial meniscus; LM, lateral meniscus; POP, popliteus tendon; MCL, medial collateral ligament; LCL, lateral collateral ligament). (From Girgis FG, Marshall JL, Monngem ARS: The cruciate ligaments of the knee joint; anatomical function and experimental analysis. Clin Orthop 1975; 106:218.)

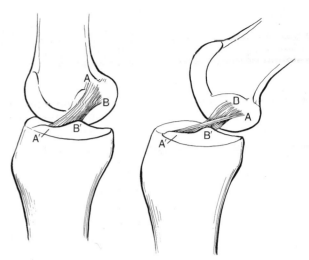

FIGURE 30–5. The anterior cruciate ligament is composed of two bundles. The anteromedial bundle (A-A') is taut in flexion. The posterolateral bundle (B-B') is taut in extension.

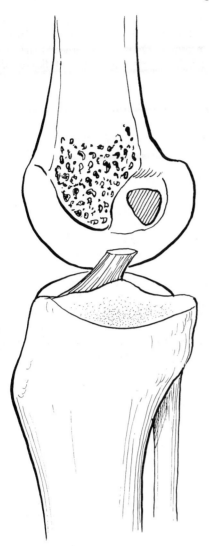

FIGURE 30–4. The anterior cruciate ligament arises from the tibial plateau anterior and medial to the tibial eminence and courses superiorly, laterally, and posteriorly to insert on the medial wall of the lateral femoral condyle.

margin of the medial wall of the lateral femoral condyle (Fig. 30–4). The ACL has been described as being composed of two bundles: the anteromedial bundle which is taut in flexion, and the posterolateral bundle, which is taut in extension (Fig. 30–5).

The posterior cruciate ligament (PCL) arises from the posterior margin of the tibia just inferior to the tibial plateau. From the tibia, the PCL courses superiorly, anteriorly, and medially to insert on the lateral wall of the medial femoral condyle (Fig. 30–6). The posterior cruciate ligament has been described as consisting of two bands, the anterolateral band, which is taut in flexion, and the posteromedial band, which is taut with the knee in extension. The anterior and posterior cruciate ligaments lie within the capsule of the knee, but they are considered to be extrasynovial.

The meniscofemoral ligaments course in a direction similar to that of the PCL. They arise from the posterior horn of the lateral meniscus and course superiorly and medially to insert on the lateral wall of the medial femoral condyle (see Fig. 30–3). The ligament of

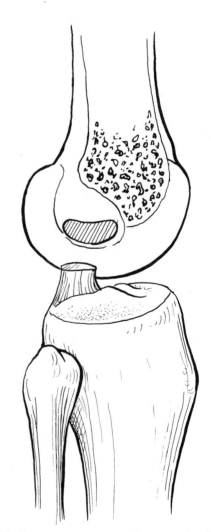

FIGURE 30–6. The posterior cruciate ligament arises from the posterior margin of the tibial plateau and courses superiorly, medially, and anteriorly to insert on the lateral wall of the medial femoral condyle.

Humphrey lies anterior to the PCL, whereas the ligament of Wrisberg lies posterior to the PCL. The meniscofemoral ligaments become taut with internal rotation of the tibia.

The posterior oblique ligament is a thickening of the posteromedial capsule. Fibers of the posterior oblique ligament course from the tibia superiorly and medially to the femur. The posterolateral corner of the knee is reinforced by the arcuate complex. The arcuate complex consists of the arcuate ligament, popliteus tendon, LCL, and posterior third of the lateral capsule.[3] The arcuate ligament arises from the fibular head and LCL to course superiorly and medially to insert along the popliteus tendon and lateral condyle of the femur.

The medial and lateral menisci lie between the tibial plateaus and femoral condyles (Fig. 30–3). The menisci improve stability of the knee by increasing concavity of the tibial plateaus. Additionally, the menisci function to absorb shock and distribute weight bearing over a greater surface area. Baratz and colleagues[4] demonstrated the effects of a partial or total meniscectomy on articular contact area and stress in the human knee. Total meniscectomy resulted in a concentration of high contact forces on a small area of the tibial plateau. Partial meniscectomy resulted in a smaller increase in contact stress. The increased tibiofemoral contact forces following meniscectomy may predispose individuals having undergone a total meniscectomy to long-term degenerative changes. As a result, partial meniscectomy is preferred to minimize the risk for long-term degenerative changes.

The outer third of the menisci is vascularized by the middle genicular artery and the inner third of the menisci is considered to be avascular. Therefore, peripheral tears of the menisci have the potential to heal and are often repaired surgically, but tears in the inner third (in the avascular zone) do not heal, and partial meniscectomy is often required. Partial meniscectomy is preferred over total meniscectomy to minimize the increase in contact forces, as noted by Baratz and associates.[4]

During flexion and extension of the knee, the menisci move posteriorly and anteriorly, respectively (Fig. 30–7). This movement is a result of the bony geometry of the tibiofemoral joint. Additionally, posterior movement of the medial meniscus during flexion is in part due to the insertion of a portion of the semimembranosus into the posterior horn of the medial meniscus. Similarly, fibers from the popliteus tendon

inserting on the posterior horn of the lateral meniscus pull the lateral meniscus posteriorly during flexion. Anterior movement of the menisci during extension is facilitated by fibers from the patellar tendon to the menisci. Anterior-posterior movement of the lateral meniscus is greater than that of the medial meniscus, which decreases susceptibility of the lateral meniscus to injury. During rotation of the knee, the menisci move relative to the tibial plateaus. During external rotation of the tibia, the medial meniscus moves posteriorly relative to the medial tibial plateau, whereas the lateral meniscus moves anteriorly relative to the lateral tibial plateau. During internal rotation of the tibia, movement of the menisci relative to the tibial plateaus is reversed.[2]

Flexion and extension of the knee combine rolling and gliding of the joint surfaces to maintain congruency of the joint surfaces. During flexion of the knee, the femur rolls posteriorly and glides anteriorly. During extension, the femur rolls anteriorly and glides posteriorly. The combined rolling and gliding of the joint surfaces maintains the femoral condyles on the tibial plateaus. Disruption of the normal arthrokinematics of the knee results in increased translation of the joint surfaces, which can lead to progressive degenerative changes of the articular surfaces.

The ACL and PCL have been described as a four-bar linkage system by Muller (1983) and serve to maintain normal arthrokinematics of the knee (Fig. 30–8A). Two bars of the four-bar linkage system consist of the ACL and PCL. The remaining two bars consist of the line connecting the femoral attachments of the ACL and PCL and the line connecting the tibial attachments of the ACL and PCL. The ACL and PCL are inelastic and maintain a constant length as the knee flexes and extends. As a result, the four-bar linkage system controls rolling and gliding of the joint surfaces as the knee moves. During flexion, the femur rolls posteriorly. This increases the distance between the tibial and femoral insertions of the ACL. Because the ACL cannot lengthen, it guides the femoral condyles anteriorly (Fig. 30–8B). Conversely, during extension of the knee, the femoral condyles roll anteriorly and the distance between the femoral and tibial insertions of the PCL increases. Because the PCL cannot lengthen, it pulls the femoral condyles posteriorly as the knee extends (Fig. 30–8C). Disruption of the ACL or PCL disrupts the four-bar linkage system and results in abnormal translation of the femoral condyles. Disruption of the normal arthokinematics of the knee may lead to repetitive injury of the menisci and joint surfaces and to the development of progressive degenerative changes over time.

LIGAMENTOUS RESTRAINTS OF THE KNEE

The primary restraint to anterior translation of the tibia is the ACL, which provides approximately 85 percent of the total restraining force to anterior translation of the tibia.[5,6] The remaining 15 percent of the restraining force to anterior displacement of the tibia is provided by the collateral ligaments, the middle portion of

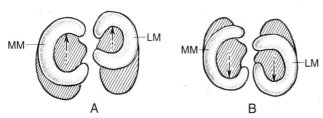

FIGURE 30–7. The menisci move anteriorly with extension *(A)* and posteriorly with flexion *(B)*. The right knee is shown (MM, medial meniscus; LM, lateral meniscus). (From Kapandji IA: The Physiology of the Joints: Annotated Diagrams of the Mechanics of the Human Joints. Edinburgh, Churchill Livingstone, 1970.)

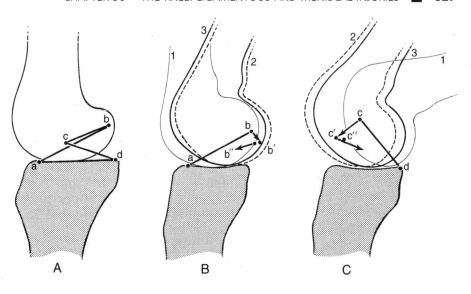

FIGURE 30–8. Four-bar linkage system. *A,* Four bars consist of the anterior cruciate ligament, ACL (line *ab*), posterior cruciate ligament, PCL (line *cd*), line connecting the femoral attachments of the ACL and PCL (line *cb*), and line connecting the tibial attachments of the ACL and PCL (line *ad*). *B,* During flexion, the femur rolls posteriorly. This increases the distance between the tibial and femoral insertions of the ACL. Because the ACL cannot lengthen, it guides the femoral condyles anteriorly. *C,* During extension of the knee, the femoral condyles roll anteriorly and the distance between the femoral and tibial insertions of the PCL increases. Because the PCL cannot lengthen, it pulls the femoral condyles posteriorly as the knee extends. (From Kapandji IA: The Physiology of The Joints: Annotated Diagrams of the Mechanics of the Human Joints. Edinburgh, Churchill Livingstone, 1970.)

the medial and lateral capsules, and the iliotibial band (Table 30–1).

The primary restraint to posterior displacement of the tibia is the PCL. The PCL provides approximately 85 to 95 percent of the total restraining force to posterior translation of the tibia.[5] The remaining 5 to 15 percent of the total restraining force to posterior displacement of the tibia is provided by the collateral ligaments, posterior portion of the medial and lateral capsules, and popliteus tendon. The ligaments of Humphrey and Wrisberg also provide restraint to posterior translation of the tibia, and their ability to do so increases with internal rotation of the tibia (Table 30–1).

The primary restraint to valgus rotation is the MCL. The anterior and posterior cruciate ligaments serve as secondary restraints to valgus rotation. When the knee is in full extension, the posterior capsule becomes a significant restraint to valgus rotation (Table 30–1). For varus rotation, the primary restraint is the LCL, and the anterior and posterior cruciate ligaments serve as secondary restraints. The restraining force provided by

the anterior and posterior cruciate ligaments, as well as the posterior capsule, increases when the knee is in full extension (Table 30–1).

External rotation of the tibia is restrained by the collateral ligaments, whereas internal rotation is restrained by the cruciate ligaments and the ligaments of Humphrey and Wrisberg (Table 30–1).

The quadriceps and hamstrings serve as dynamic stabilizers of the knee. In doing so, they assist the passive restraints in controlling kinematics of the knee. These muscles work synergistically with the cruciate ligaments to control motion of the knee dynamically. Unopposed contraction of the quadriceps is synergistic to the PCL and antagonistic to the ACL. Conversely, isolated contraction of the hamstrings is synergistic to the ACL and antagonistic to the PCL. It is theorized that activities that promote co-contraction of the hamstrings and quadriceps minimize tibial translation, and these have been advocated for rehabilitation of knee ligament injuries.[7] Dynamic stabilization of the knee to control abnormal motion depends on muscular strength and

	TABLE 30–1	
	Primary and Secondary Restraints of the Knee	
Tibial Motion	**Primary Restraint**	**Secondary Restraints**
Anterior translation	ACL	MCL, LCL; middle third of medial-lateral capsule; iliotibial band
Posterior translation	PCL	MCL, LCL; posterior third of medial and lateral capsule; popliteus tendon; anterior and posterior meniscofemoral ligaments
Valgus rotation	MCL	ACL, PCL; posterior capsule when knee fully extended
Varus rotation	LCL	ACL, PCL; posterior capsule when knee fully extended
External rotation	MCL, LCL	
Internal rotation	ACL, PCL	Anterior-posterior meniscofemoral ligaments

endurance as well as on development of appropriate neuromuscular control.

ROLE OF PROPRIOCEPTION

There has been an increased interest in the role of proprioception in the prevention and progression of injury to the knee.[8-11] Proprioception has been described as a variation in the sense of touch and includes the sense of joint motion (kinesthesia) and of joint position. It is mediated by sensory receptors located in the skin, musculotendinous unit, ligaments, and joint capsule. These sensory receptors transduce mechanical deformation to a neural signal, which modulates conscious and unconscious responses. It has been hypothesized that proprioception is important for providing smooth coordinated movement as well as for protecting and dynamically stabilizing the knee.[10,12-14]

It has been proposed that mechanoreceptors in the knee mediate protective reflexes. Solomonow and coworkers[10] described an ACL-hamstring reflex arc in anesthetized cats. High loading of the ACL resulted in increased electromyography (EMG) activity in the hamstrings, with electrical silence in the quadriceps. The increase in hamstring EMG activity was not evident when low to moderate loads were applied to the ACL. It was proposed that the ACL-hamstring reflex arc serves to protect the ACL during high loading conditions. It is doubtful, however, that this reflex arc can protect the ACL from injury if high loads are applied rapidly. Under rapid loading conditions, the ligament may be loaded and ruptured before sufficient muscle tension to protect the ligament can be generated.

Other proprioceptive reflexes originating from the joint capsule or musculotendinous unit probably exist. This was demonstrated by Solomonow and colleagues,[10] who reported increased hamstring EMG activity in a patient with an ACL-deficient knee during maximal slow speed isokinetic testing of the quadriceps. The increased hamstring EMG activity occurred simultaneously with anterior subluxation of the tibia at approximately 40 degrees of knee flexion and was associated with a sharp decrease in quadriceps torque and inhibition of quadriceps EMG activity. Because the ACL was ruptured, reflex contraction of the hamstrings could not have been mediated by receptors originating in the ACL. It was proposed that this reflex contraction is mediated by receptors in the joint capsule or hamstring muscles.

Several clinical studies have evaluated proprioception in terms of threshold to detection of passive motion and reproduction of passive joint position. Barrack and associates[9] demonstrated deficits in threshold to detection of passive motion in subjects with a unilateral ACL-deficient knee. Barett[13] demonstrated high correlations between measurements of proprioception and function ($r = .84$) and patient satisfaction ($r = .90$) in 45 patients who had undergone ACL reconstruction. Standard knee scores and clinical examination correlated poorly with the patient's own opinion and results of functional tests. Lephart and associates[11] studied threshold to detection of passive movement in patients who had undergone ACL reconstruction. Testing was performed at 15 and 45 degrees of flexion. Three trials were performed, moving into flexion and extension. The results indicated that threshold to detection of passive movement was less sensitive in the reconstructed knee compared with the noninvolved knee. Additionally, threshold to detection of passive motion was more sensitive in both the reconstructed and normal knees at 15 degrees of flexion compared with 45 degrees of flexion. Sensitivity to detection of passive motion was enhanced by the use of a Neoprene sleeve, which has implications for bracing following ACL injury and/or reconstruction.

Injury to the knee may result in abnormal sensory feedback and altered neuromuscular control, which may lead to recurrent injury. Proprioceptive training following knee injury and/or surgery should attempt to maximize the use of sensory information mediated by the ligaments, joint capsule, and/or musculotendinous unit to stabilize the joint dynamically. Proprioceptive training requires repetition to develop motor control of abnormal joint motion and may be enhanced with the use of EMG biofeedback. Initially, control of abnormal joint motion requires conscious effort. Through repetitive training, motor control of abnormal movement becomes automatic and occurs subconsciously. It should be noted, however, that the extent to which one can develop neuromuscular control of abnormal joint motion to stabilize the knee dynamically is currently unknown. Further research is required to determine the effectiveness of proprioceptive training to stabilize the knee dynamically.

OPEN VS. CLOSED KINETIC CHAIN EXERCISES

BIOMECHANICS

Open kinetic chain (OKC) exercise refers to exercise in which the distal segment is free to move, resulting in isolated movement at a given joint. At the knee, OKC exercise results in isolated flexion and extension. OKC knee extension is a result of isolated contraction of the quadriceps, and open chain knee flexion occurs as a result of isolated contraction of the hamstrings. Barratta and coworkers[14] and Draganich and colleagues[15] have demonstrated low levels of coactivation of the quadriceps and hamstrings during open chain knee extension. It is hypothesized that the hamstrings become active during the terminal range of extension to decelerate the knee and act as a synergist to the ACL to minimize anterior tibial translation produced by contraction of the quadriceps. During open chain knee extension, the flexion movement arm increases as the knee is extended from 90 degrees of flexion to full extension. This requires increasing quadriceps and patellar tendon tension, which can increase the load on the patellofemoral and tibiofemoral joints. During closed kinetic chain (CKC) exercises, the distal segment is relatively fixed, so that movement at one joint results in simultaneous movement of all other joints in the kinetic chain in a predictable manner. The lower extremity functions as a CKC as one squats over the fixed foot, resulting in simultaneous movement of the ankle, knee, and hip. CKC exercise for the lower extremity results in co-contraction of muscles throughout the lower extremity. For example, during squatting, the quadriceps contracts to control the flexion moment arm at the knee and the hamstrings contract to control the flexion moment arm of the hip. This resulting co-contraction of the quadriceps and hamstrings is thought to minimize translation and shearing forces at the knee. During CKC exercises for the lower extremity, the flexion moment arms at the knee and hip increase as one squats and require increased force of contraction of the quadriceps and hamstrings to control the knee and hip, respectively.

OKC and CKC exercises produce different effects on tibial translation and ligamentous strain and load. During active OKC knee extension, the shear component produced by unopposed contraction of the quadriceps depends on the angle of knee flexion (Fig. 30–9). Sawhney and associates[16] investigated the effects of isometric quadriceps contraction on tibial translation in subjects with an intact knee. Tibial translation was measured with the KT-1000 arthrometer (MedMetric, San Diego, Cal.) at 30, 45, 60, and 75 degrees of flexion. Open chain isometric quadriceps contraction against 10 lb of resistance applied to the distal aspect of the leg resulted in anterior tibial translation at 30 and 45 degrees of flexion. No significant tibial translation occurred at 60 or 75 degrees of flexion. It was determined that the quadriceps-neutral Q angle (i.e., the angle at which quadriceps contraction produces no anterior or posterior tibial translation) occurs between 60 and 75 degrees of flexion (Fig. 30–9A). OKC knee extension at angles less than the quadriceps-neutral position result in anterior translation of the tibia. This was demonstrated by Grood and coworkers[6] in intact cadaveric knees. Anterior translation of the tibia during OKC knee extension increased with loading of the quadriceps at angles less than 60 degrees of flexion. Sectioning of the ACL increased anterior translation during loaded and unloaded open chain knee extension. Anterior tibial translation produced by the quadriceps at knee flexion angles less than the quadriceps-neutral angle is a result of the anteriorly directed shear component of the patellar tendon force (Fig. 30–9B).

OKC knee extension at knee flexion angles greater than the quadriceps-neutral position results in posterior tibial translation. This is the result of a posteriorly directed shear component of the patellar tendon force at these angles of knee flexion (Fig. 30–9C).

OKC knee flexion is produced by isolated contraction of the hamstrings. It has been found that this results in posterior translation of the tibia and was demonstrated by Meglan and colleagues,[17] who found posterior tibial shear forces during isometric open chain knee flexion at 30, 60, and 90 degrees of knee flexion. The posterior shear force increased as flexion progressed from 30 to 90 degrees of flexion.

Several investigators have studied the in vivo and in vitro effects of OKC exercise on ACL and PCL strain.[18–21] During passive OKC movement in cadaveric knees, ACL strain decreases from full extension to a minimum value at 30 to 45 degrees of flexion.[18,21] Flexion beyond 45 degrees results in increased ACL strain, which reaches a maximum value between 105 and 120 degrees. Simulated open chain isometric and isotonic quadriceps activity in cadaveric knees significantly increased ACL strain relative to strain produced by passive motion at flexion angles from 0 to 45 degrees.[21] Quadriceps contraction at angles beyond 75 degrees of flexion reduced ACL strain relative to the strain produced by passive motion. This is probably due to the posteriorly directed shear component of the patellar tendon force, as described earlier. Similar results were found in vivo.[20] Simulated open chain hamstring activity in cadaveric knees significantly decreased ACL strain when compared with strain during passive motion at 75 to 105 degrees of flexion.[21] Kain and associates[22] demonstrated decreased strain on the ACL when the hamstring muscles contract before the quadriceps and simultaneous contraction of both is maintained.

Arms and coworkers[19] studied in vitro strain on the posterior and anterior fibers of the PCL during passive open chain knee flexion and extension. Strain on the posterior fibers of the PCL was reduced as the knee was passively flexed from 0 to 20 degrees. As flexion continued, strain on the posterior fibers increased. Maximum strain of the posterior fibers of the PCL was reached in full flexion. The anterior fibers of the PCL

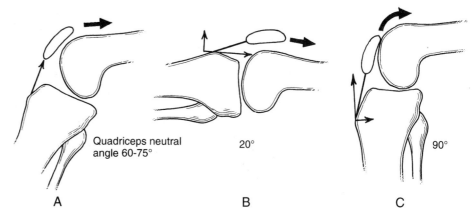

FIGURE 30–9. During open chain knee extension, tibial translation is a function of the shear force produced by the patellar tendon. *A,* Quadriceps neutral position. The patellar tendon force is perpendicular to the tibial plateaus and results in compression of the joint surfaces without shear force. *B,* At flexion angles less than the angle of the quadriceps neutral position, orientation of the patellar tendon produces anterior shear of the tibia. *C,* At angles greater than the angle of the quadriceps neutral position, patellar tendon force causes a posterior shear of the tibia. (From Daniel DM, Stone ML, Barnett P, Sachs R: Use of the quadriceps active test to diagnose posterior cruciate ligament disruption and measure posterior laxity of the knee. J Bone Joint Surg 1988A; 70:386–391.)

Quadriceps neutral angle 60-75°

20°

90°

A

B

C

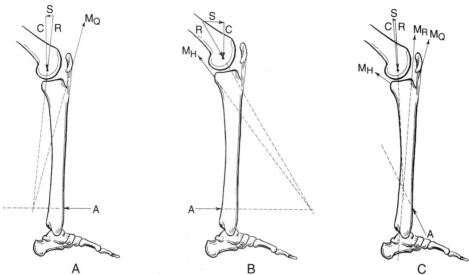

FIGURE 30–10. Free body diagram showing altered joint reaction forces during open chain knee extension, open chain knee flexion, and closed kinetic chain exercises for the lower extremity (R, resultant joint reaction force; C, compressive component of joint reaction force; S, shear-component of joint reaction force). A, Unopposed open chain quadriceps contraction. Force is applied perpendicular to the lower leg similar to open chain knee extension and results in posterior shear of the femur (M_Q; anterior shear of the tibia). B, Unopposed open chain hamstring contraction. Force is applied perpendicular to the lower leg similar to open chain knee flexion and results in anterior shear of the femur (M_H; posterior shear of the tibia). C, Closed kinetic chain leg press with co-contraction of quadriceps and hamstrings. Force is applied axially to the tibia similar to that provided by closed kinetic chain exercises for the lower extremity. The shear force (M_H, M_R, M_Q) that results from the axially applied load is reduced. (From Palmitier RA, An K-N, Scott SG, Chao EYS: Kinetic chain exercise in knee rehabilitation. Sports Med 1991; 11:402–413.)

were lax in full extension. Strain on the anterior fibers of the PCL rapidly increased, beginning at 10 degrees of knee flexion, and reached maximum strain in full flexion. The posterior fibers of the PCL were most lax between 15 and 30 degrees of flexion, whereas the anterior fibers of the PCL were most lax between 0 and 10 degrees. During simulated open chain isometric hamstring contraction against 40 kg, strain on the PCL was significantly increased over strain during passive knee flexion between 45 and 75 degrees of flexion.[19]

Although CKC exercises appear to decrease tibial translation and strain on the ACL, the effects on the PCL are unknown. Compression of the joint surfaces during weight bearing lends stability to the joint and reduces tibial translation. Additionally, during CKC exercises, there is co-contraction of the hamstrings and quadriceps. This occurs as the quadriceps contract to counteract the flexion moment arm at the knee and the hamstrings contract to counteract the flexion moment arm at the hip. It is proposed that co-contraction of the quadriceps and hamstrings minimizes anterior translation and reduces ACL strain. Ohkoshi and colleagues[23] reported increased hamstring activity during CKC exercises with increasing angles of trunk flexion. This resulted in increased posterior shear force at the knee with increased angles of trunk flexion.

Palmitier and associates[7] developed a biomechanical model that demonstrates reduced tibiofemoral shear forces when the line of force is applied more axially in relation to the tibia (Fig. 30–10). During open chain knee extension, resistance is applied perpendicularly to the distal aspect of the leg. The resultant force on the knee can be resolved to a compressive component, which is

perpendicular to the tibial plateaus, and a shear component, which is parallel to the joint surface. For open chain knee extension, posterior shear of the femur (i.e., anterior shear of the tibia) is produced (Fig. 30–10A). During open chain knee flexion with the force applied perpendicularly to the lower leg, anterior shear of the femur (i.e., posterior shear of the tibia) is produced (Fig. 30–10B). During CKC exercises with weight bearing through the extremities, the line of force is applied more axially in relation to the tibia. Resolving the resultant force on the knee into its shear and compressive components reveals a decreased shear compared with the open chain conditions (Fig. 30–10C).

Reduced shear with CKC exercises compared to open chain exercises was demonstrated in vivo by Lutz and coworkers,[17] who calculated shear forces during isometric OKC knee extension and flexion and CKC exercises at 30, 60, and 90 degrees of flexion. The results indicated less anterior shear forces at 30 and 60 degrees of knee flexion during the CKC condition compared with OKC knee extension. Additionally, there was significantly less posterior shear of the tibia during the CKC condition compared with open chain knee flexion at 60 and 90 degrees of flexion. The CKC condition produced a slight posterior shear force that remained constant at all angles of knee flexion. Voight and colleagues[24] used the KT-1000 to demonstrate decreased anterior tibial translation during maximal isometric CKC exercise compared with maximal isometric OKC knee extension at 30 degrees of flexion in normal and ACL-deficient subjects. Drez and associates[25] used a 4 degrees-of-freedom electrogoniometer to assess tibial translation in subjects with a unilateral ACL-deficient knee. The results revealed less anterior tibial translation with the leg press against 30 kg compared to leg extension against 4.5 kg. During the leg press exercise, there was only 0.1-mm side-to-side difference in tibial translation between the normal and ACL-deficient knee. The side-to-side difference in tibial translation during leg extension was 3.7 mm.

Based on these studies, it appears that CKC exercises minimize tibial translation and strain on the ACL and PCL. Two other studies, however, have indicated that CKC exercises may produce more load on the capsular and ligamentous structures about the knee than previously demonstrated. Meglan and coworkers[26] used EMG, motion analysis, and force plates to calculate net load on the knee and capsular and ligamentous structures during a variety of CKC exercises commonly used in weight training. Their results indicated that the net force on the knee is posteriorly directed throughout the range of motion. When a quadriceps-only model was used, they found an anterior shear load on the capsule and ligamentous structures between 20 and 40 degrees of knee flexion. When co-contraction of the quadriceps and hamstrings was used in the model, the anterior shear force increased in the range of 20 and 60 degrees of flexion. Meglan and colleagues[26] hypothesized that during CKC exercises the hamstrings contract to offset the flexion moment arm at the hip. Contraction of the hamstrings simultaneously increases the quadriceps force necessary to extend the knee. They hypothesized that contraction of the hamstrings was insufficient to negate the anteriorly directed shear force produced by the quadriceps. Bennyon and associates[27] arthroscopically implanted a Hall effect strain transducer on the anteromedial bundle of the ACL in subjects undergoing arthroscopic surgery. Following surgery, subjects performed squats with and without the use of a sport cord for resistance. The results indicated increased strain on the ACL during these exercises in the range of 0 to 60 degrees of flexion. The magnitude of the strain was about 4 to 6 percent above the strain on the ACL with the knee in full passive extension. These results appear to indicate that CKC exercises may not be as benign as previously thought for those undergoing rehabilitation following knee ligament injury or surgery.

At present, basic data on translation of the tibiofemoral joint and the strain and load on ligamentous structures imposed by open and closed kinetic chain exercises on the native or substitute ACL or PCL are incomplete. *Thus, developing a rehabilitation program following knee injury or surgery is an imprecise science.* Further research is required to develop a hierarchy of OKC and CKC exercises. This requires quantification of stresses and strains on the structures about the knee during a variety of exercises and functional activities. This has been attempted by Henning and coworkers,[28] who studied in vivo strain on the ACL in two subjects with a grade II ACL injury. The subjects performed a variety of exercises and activities, and the strain was reported relative to the strain produced by an 80-lb Lachman test. Less strain was produced with a one-legged squat compared to isometric quadriceps exercises with 20 lb, with the knee at 0, 22, and 45 degrees of flexion. Additionally, strain on the ACL increased as

activity progressed from crutch walking to cycling, walking, slow running, and fast running. These results must not be overinterpreted, because they represent only two subjects with a partial ACL tear. Further research to quantify the strain and load on various structures about the knee is necessary to validate current concepts for rehabilitation of the knee.

CKC exercises appear to be more functional than OKC exercises. During CKC exercises, simultaneous hip and knee extension occur when the subject rises from the flexed position. As a result of this movement, the rectus femoris lengthens across the hip while it shortens across the knee. Conversely, the hamstrings lengthen across the knee and shorten across the hip. The resultant concentric and eccentric contractions at opposite ends of the muscle produce a "pseudoisometric" contraction. Palmitier and colleagues[7] used the term *concurrent shift* to describe this phenomenon. This type of contraction is used during functional activities such as walking, stair climbing, running, and jumping, and cannot be reproduced by isolated OKC knee flexion and extension exercises.

Several studies have been conducted to describe EMG activity during controlled CKC exercises. Weiss[29] studied EMG activity in the quadriceps, hamstrings, and gastrocnemius using surface EMG during a minisquat from 0 to 60 degrees. EMG data were normalized as a percentage of maximum voluntary isometric contraction. The results indicated that the hamstrings and quadriceps are active throughout the range of motion. Quadriceps activity increased with increasing angles of knee flexion. There was greater muscle activity during the concentric phase as compared with the eccentric phase. The overall level of EMG activity for the quadriceps was approximately 4 to 6 percent of maximum voluntary isometric contraction and 2 to 4 percent of maximum voluntary isometric contraction for the hamstrings.

Ninos[30] conducted a similar study to determine the effects of hip position on muscle activity in the lower extremity. He studied patients squatting against 25 percent body weight with the hip in neutral rotation and with 30 degrees of external rotation. Surface EMG was used to sample electrical activity from the vastus medialis, vastus lateralis, semimembranosus-semitendinosus, and biceps femoris. The results indicated no significant difference in electrical activity with the hip in neutral or 30 degrees of external rotation. Quadriceps activity increased with increasing angles of knee flexion. Maximum quadriceps activity was about 20 to 30 percent maximum voluntary isometric contraction. Hamstring activity increased slightly as the angle of knee flexion increased. The maximum overall level of hamstring activity was 10 to 15 percent maximum voluntary isometric contraction. Greater activity of the quadriceps and hamstrings was found during the ascending phase as compared with the descending phase.

These studies indicate that, during CKC exercises, there is co-contraction of the quadriceps and hamstrings. As noted by Meglan and colleagues,[26] however, it is unknown whether this co-contraction is of sufficient magnitude to minimize stress on the ligamentous and capsular structures about the knee. Furthermore, this research was conducted on normal subjects. It is unknown whether similar muscle activity would be found in subjects with quadriceps weakness. It is our clinical impression that individuals can use substitute motor patterns in the presence of quadriceps weakness to perform closed chain exercises, which allows quadriceps weakness to persist. OKC knee extension exercises should be used to perform isolated strengthening for the quadriceps. Further research is needed to determine patterns of muscle activity during closed chain exercises in individuals with isolated muscle weakness.

Based on the above rationale, it is important to include both OKC and CKC exercises in rehabilitation programs following knee ligament injury or surgery. OKC exercises provide isolated exercise for the hamstrings and quadriceps. OKC knee extension from 75 degrees of flexion to full extension may stress the ACL, but should not produce significant stress on the PCL. Open chain knee extension from 90 to 75 degrees of knee flexion may produce increased stress on the PCL due to the posteriorly directed shear component of the force produced by the patellar tendon. Open chain knee extension between 60 and 90 degrees can be performed without jeopardizing the ACL and can be incorporated early in the rehabilitation program. Caution must be used to avoid undue stress on the ACL with OKC exercises, particularly between 0 and 45 degrees of flexion (Table 30–2). Additionally, caution must be used to avoid irritation to the patellofemoral joint with OKC knee extension exercises.

OKC knee flexion stresses the PCL, but results in reduced strain on the ACL. Following ACL injury and/or reconstruction, OKC knee flexion can be safely performed, but following PCL injury and/or reconstruction, OKC knee flexion should be avoided.

CKC exercises may be used to reduce tibial translation and minimize stress on the patellofemoral joint. Additionally, CKC exercises provide the specifity of training that is necessary to ensure restoration of function. A variety of CKC exercises can be incorporated into the rehabilitation program. CKC exercises must be performed properly to avoid use of substitute patterns of motion—improperly performed CKC exercises may allow weakness to persist. OKC exercises can be used to provide isolated training for the quadriceps and hamstrings to ensure complete rehabilitation.

TABLE 30–2
Summary of Open Kinetic Chain Extension of the Knee

Angle of Knee Flexion	Effect of Open Chain Extension
0–75°	Produced anterior tibial translation; antagonistic to ACL; synergistic to PCL
75°	Quadriceps-neutral angle
75–90°	Produced posterior tibial translation; synergistic to ACL; antagonistic to PCL

PATELLOFEMORAL CONSIDERATIONS

The effects of OKC versus CKC exercises on the patellofemoral joint must be considered when rehabilitating an individual following knee ligament injury and/or surgery. The patellofemoral joint consists of the articulation between the patella and the distal end of the femur. The patella is embedded in the knee extensor mechanism and is the largest sesamoid bone in the body. Proximally, the quadriceps inserts into the patella through the quadriceps tendon. Distally, the patella is connected to the tibia through the patellar tendon. The patella serves to protect the anterior aspect of the knee, increase the effective moment arm of the knee extensor mechanism, and centralize the divergent forces produced by the quadriceps. The tendency of the patella to sublux laterally produced by the Q angle, vastus lateralis, and lateral retinacular structures must be counterbalanced by the oblique fibers of the vastus medialis. Maintaining this balance is crucial to normal function of the knee extensor mechanism.

The patella is a triangular bone, with its base directed superiorly and its apex directed inferiorly. On the posterior aspect, the patella is described as having three facets. A central ridge that runs from superior to inferior divides the patella into medial and lateral facets. The odd facet lies on the medial border of the patella and engages the femur only during the extreme range of flexion. The posterior margin of the patella is covered by a thick layer of articular cartilage. This cartilage is thicker centrally than peripherally. This layer of articular cartilage is thicker than at any other joint in the body—perhaps up to 5 mm thick.[31] This layer of articular cartilage is important to reduce friction and aids in lubrication of the patellofemoral joint.

Stability of the patellofemoral joint depends on passive and dynamic restraints. Static restraints consist of the shape of the patellofemoral joint as well as on the medial and lateral patellofemoral ligaments. The lateral femoral condyle projects further anteriorly than the medial femoral condyle and serves as a buttress to minimize lateral displacement of the patella. Dynamic stability of the patellofemoral joint is provided by the quadriceps. The vastus medialis oblique (VMO) and medial retinaculum provide medial stabilization of the patella. The vastus lateralis, lateral retinaculum, and iliotibial band pull the patella laterally. The Q (quadriceps) angle is the angle formed by lines that connect the anterior superior iliac spine to the midpatella and the midpatella to the tibial tubercle. The Q angle results in lateral displacement of the patella when the quadriceps contracts. Lateral displacement of the patella is dynamically resisted by the VMO and medial retinaculum. Weakness of the VMO allows the patella to track laterally. Additionally, tightness of the lateral retinaculum and overpull from the vastus lateralis and iliotibial band can result in lateral displacement of the patella.

Prevention and/or treatment of patellofemoral symptoms following knee ligament injury or surgery must seek to maintain and/or restore balance of the medial and lateral stabilizers of the patellofemoral joint. This includes strengthening of the VMO and stretching of

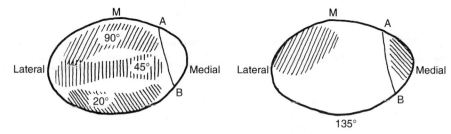

FIGURE 30–11. Patellofemoral contact pattern. Initial contact between the trochlear groove and inferior pole of the patella occurs at approximately 20 degrees of flexion. As flexion progresses, the area of contact migrates superiorly so that by 90 degrees of flexion, the entire articular surface of the patella except for the odd facet has articulated with the trochlear groove. At full flexion, the odd medial facet and lateral facet articulate with the intercondylar notch. (From Hungerford DS, Barry M: Biomechanics of the patellofemoral joint. Clin Orthop 1979; 144: 9–15.)

the lateral structures when they are tight. Strengthening of the VMO should include the use of both OKC and CKC exercises.

Hungerford and Barry[32] described the patellofemoral contact pattern as the knee moves through a full range of motion (Fig. 30–11). The patella initially makes contact with the femur in the trochlear groove at approximately 20 degrees of flexion. Initial contact is between the trochlear groove and inferior pole of the patella. As flexion progresses, the contact area on the patella progresses superiorly so that by 90 degrees of flexion, the entire articular surface of the patella, except for the odd medial facet, has articulated with the femur. As flexion continues beyond 90 degrees, the quadriceps tendon articulates with the trochlear groove and the patella moves into the intercondylar notch area of the femur. At full flexion, the odd medial facet and lateral facet of the patella articulate with the intercondylar notch. The odd medial facet articulates with the femur only at the end range of flexion. Knowledge of the patellofemoral contact pattern is useful to determine the limits of motion when performing OKC and CKC exercises in patients with patellofemoral symptoms. *Generally, exercises should be performed in the pain-free and crepitus-free range of motion.* It should also be noted that the patellofemoral contact area increases from 20 to 90 degrees of flexion. This increase helps distribute patellofemoral joint reaction forces over a larger area to reduce patellofemoral contact stress per unit of area.

Patellofemoral joint reaction force is a function of quadriceps and patellar tendon tension as well as of the angle formed between the quadriceps and patellar tendons (Fig. 30–12). This force compresses the patellofemoral joint, with increasing patellar and quadriceps tendon tension and increasing angle of knee flexion.

OKC and CKC exercises produce different effects on patellofemoral joint reaction force and contact stress per unit area. During open chain knee extension, the flexion moment arm for the knee increases as the knee is extended from 90 degrees of flexion to full extension, which results in increased quadriceps and patellar tendon tension and increasing patellofemoral joint reaction forces. Reilly and Martens[33] calculated peak patellofemoral joint reaction forces for knee extension against a 9-kg boot to be 120 kg at 36 degrees of flexion. At this angle of knee flexion, the patellofemoral joint reaction forces are concentrated on a relatively small contact area, resulting in large contact stresses per unit of area.

For CKC exercises, the flexion moment arm of the knee increases as the angle of knee flexion increases. Greater quadriceps and patellar tendon tension is required to counteract the increasing flexion moment arm, which results in increasing patellofemoral joint reaction force as the knee flexes. This force is distributed over a larger patellofemoral contact area, however, which minimizes the increase in contact stress per unit area.

Patellofemoral joint reaction forces during functional CKC activities were calculated by Reilly and Martens[33] and were found to be 0.5 times body weight during level walking, 3.3 times body weight on stairs, and 7.8 times body weight during a full squat. These results are consistent with activities that increase patellofemoral symptoms. Bandi[34] calculated patellofemoral joint reaction forces for squatting with the tibia perpendicular versus squatting when the center of gravity is allowed to shift forward. Squatting with the tibia perpendicular resulted in a patellofemoral joint reaction force equal to

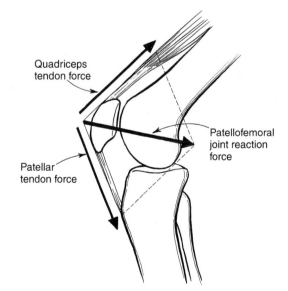

FIGURE 30–12. Patellofemoral joint reaction force. This is a function of patellar and quadriceps tendon tension as well as the angle formed between the quadriceps and patellar tendons. This force increases with increasing patellar and quadriceps tendon tension and increasing angle of knee flexion.

7.8 times body weight. Patellofemoral joint reaction force decreased to 3.9 times body weight when squatting with the center of gravity shifted forward. Shifting the body weight forward when squatting decreases the flexion moment arm at the knee and reduces quadriceps muscle force, resulting in decreased patellofemoral joint reaction forces.

Hungerford and Barry[32] compared OKC knee extension using a 9-kg wtd boot with squatting under body weight. Patellofemoral contact stress per unit area during open chain knee extension using a 9-kg boot exceeded that produced by squatting under body weight between full extension and 53 degrees of flexion. Between 53 and 90 degrees of flexion, patellofemoral contact stress per unit area produced by squatting under body weight exceeded that produced by open chain knee extension against a 9-kg boot.

Similar results were reported by Steinkamp and colleagues,[35] who compared patellofemoral joint biomechanics during leg press and leg extension exercises in 20 normal subjects. Resistance for the leg press was based on the amount of weight with which the subject could complete three sets of 10 repetitions on an inclined leg press. Resistance for the leg extension exercise was calculated by determining the amount of weight required for the leg extension exercise to produce a moment arm equivalent to the maximum moment arm obtained when the subject performed the leg press exercise. The results indicated that patellofemoral joint reaction force and patellofemoral contact stress per unit area are significantly greater during the leg extension exercise than during the leg press between 0 and 45 degrees of knee flexion. Between 50 and 90 degrees of knee flexion, patellofemoral joint reaction force and contact stress per unit of area were found to be significantly greater for the leg press exercise than for the leg extension exercise. The patellofemoral joint reaction stresses for leg press and leg extension exercises intersected at 48 degrees of knee flexion. These results are similar to those reported earlier by Hungerford and Barry.[32]

Following knee ligament injury and/or surgery, OKC and CKC exercises should be performed cautiously within the pain-free and crepitus-free range of motion to avoid the development of patellofemoral symptoms. Based on the biomechanics of the knee extensor mechanism, CKC exercises may be better tolerated by the patellofemoral joint than OKC knee extension exercises in the range from 0 to 45 degrees of flexion. In this range, CKC exercises can be used to develop lower extremity muscles in a functional manner. These exercises should be performed precisely, with the knee directly over the foot. CKC exercises may be initiated with isometric minisquats and progressed to active minisquats, step-ups, and leg press with resistance, as tolerated.

Based on the biomechanics of the knee extensor mechanism, OKC knee exercises may be better tolerated by the patellofemoral joint than CKC knee exercises in the range from 50 to 90 degrees of flexion. Formerly, short-arc quadriceps exercises in the range from 0 to 45 degrees of flexion were advocated for the management of patients with patellofemoral symptoms, but we have found that these exercises aggravate most patients. Performing OKC exercises between 90 and 45 degrees of flexion provides isolated exercise for the quadriceps and is usually tolerated well by the patient. If a patient is unable to perform resisted OKC knee extension exercises in this range of motion, then multiple angle isometrics can be used to improve isolated quadriceps muscle function. Focusing solely on CKC exercises to strengthen the quadriceps through a full range of motion for patients with patellofemoral symptoms may increase pain and allow isolated weakness of the quadriceps to persist.

EXAMINATION OF THE KNEE

SUBJECTIVE ASSESSMENT AND HISTORY

A thorough history and physical examination are essential for making the correct diagnosis and directing appropriate treatment. Often, these make most other studies unnecessary, except to confirm the clinical diagnosis.

One must be aware that athletes can have problems about the knee that affect the general population, and the problem may be intra-articular or extra-articular, mechanical or inflammatory. The history can help differentiate these. Furthermore, the patient may tell you the problem: "I felt a pop in my knee," or "My kneecap popped out of place." Knowing the patient's age or sport can provide clues about the type of injury to expect. The history can help direct questioning and allow the physical examination to focus on specific, subtle tests for meniscal, physeal, or ligamentous injury. Athletes may develop osteoarthritis (and associated degenerative meniscal tears), osteomyelitis, inflammatory arthritides, pigmented villonodular synovitis, osteochondritis dissecans, sarcomas (soft tissue and bony), vascular insufficiency, metabolic or hormonal conditions, neuromuscular diseases, and referred pain (lumbar spine disease).

The history can help determine the patient's activity level prior to injury and expectations following recovery. Also, it is important to determine the severity of the symptoms—are they disabling, or just a minor inconvenience? This can help in the planning and timing of treatment as well as in ensuring that patients have a realistic expectation of the outcome after the injury.

It must first be determined whether the injury is of traumatic origin. In traumatic injuries, the athlete should be queried about the mechanism of injury and location of the pain. This information provides the examiner with a clue about which anatomic structures are at risk. It should be determined whether the foot was planted, if it was a twisting injury, if the injury resulted from direct contact, and the direction of the forces involved. It is important to determine whether the athlete has injured the knee before, whether it is the same knee, and how it was treated. Was the athlete able to leave the scene unassisted, or was assistance required? This may indicate the severity of the injury. The athlete may be able to relate hearing or feeling a pop at the time of injury, so this may indicate a cruciate ligament tear or osteochondral fracture. Determining whether there was any deformity initially, which may have been reduced prior to being evaluated, is also helpful in diagnosing a patellar or tibiofemoral dislocation or periarticular fracture. It is also helpful to determine the time course of swelling of the knee after injury, because an acute effusion or hemarthrosis may indicate an intra-articular fracture or torn cruciate ligament.

The subacute or chronically dysfunctional knee requires the same history as above, because the injury may have been initiated by a traumatic event but never treated. The examiner must determine when the symptoms began in relation to a traumatic event. The athlete must relate whether the primary complaint is popping or clicking, giving way (instability), locking, pain, or swelling. The relationship between athletic activity and the patient's symptoms can also be helpful in determining the cause of the problem. Pain on takeoff (and, to a lesser extent, landing) in jumping is often due to extensor mechanism problems (patella, patellar tendon, quadriceps tendon), whereas instability on landing suggests ACL insufficiency or quadriceps weakness. A history of popping or clicking is frequently elicited and may be caused by a variety of conditions, both pathologic and normal.

Instability is often described as giving way, sliding, slipping out of socket, buckling, or the sensation that the knee may give out. When giving way exists, it is usually indicative of intra-articular pathology, including a displaced meniscal tear or cruciate ligament injury, resulting in a loose body or rotary instability. Impending giving way may be due to patellar subluxation or weakness of the extensor mechanism. Most patients with chronic rotatory instability can ambulate and perform activities of daily living without pain or instability. These patients complain of buckling during activities such as running, jumping, pivoting, or cutting. True locking is a mechanical block to full extension with uninhibited flexion and is usually indicative of a displaced meniscal tear. Other causes of locking include loose bodies, joint effusion, hamstring spasm, posterior capsulitis, and sometimes quadriceps mechanism disruption.

The complaint of pain needs to be clearly defined to be of benefit. The location, character, intensity, temporal variation, and activities that aggravate or alleviate pain must be determined. Aching pain associated with stiffness in the morning, rest, or after prolonged activity may indicate arthritic disease. Sharp pain associated with loading of the joint indicates a mechanical cause, such as a meniscal tear. The "theater sign," which is defined as knee pain with prolonged sitting with the knee bent, pain going down or up stairs or inclines, and retropatellar or diffuse anterior knee pain, all indicate of patellofemoral dysfunction. Although the location of pain may help limit the diagnosis, it is not always specific enough to give the exact diagnosis. An example of this is medial joint line pain, which is often associated with medial meniscal pathology. Patellar disorders,

MCL sprains, and medial unicompartmental arthritis, however, may also hurt in the same location. Lateral joint line pain may be associated with lateral meniscal tears, lateral unicompartmental arthritis, patellofemoral dysfunction, LCL sprain, or proximal tibiofibular instability. Pain after activity is characteristic of an inflammatory process, such as a plica or tendinitis. Bilateral knee pain may indicate an anatomic cause (such as patellofemoral malalignment syndrome) or systemic disease. Use of analgesic or anti-inflammatory medications may provide a clue about the severity of the symptoms. Constant pain may indicate an inflammatory process, tumor, or degenerative disease.

Obtaining a history of swelling is common following an injury, but the time from injury to its onset, the location, and amount should be determined, as well as its response to rest, activity, and medications. A large, acute hemarthrosis, occurring within 2 to 6 hours following injury, is secondary to an ACL rupture approximately 70 percent of the time,[36] although it may also be due to an intra-articular or osteochondral fracture. An acute hemarthrosis may also be due to patellar dislocation but, because the capsule is torn, the swelling is usually not as large as with a cruciate ligament disruption or fracture. An effusion developing 1 or more days after injury is usually a hydrarthrosis, secondary to a meniscal tear, synovitis, or sympathetic effusion. Chronic synovitis and its attendant effusion indicates intra-articular inflammation. In athletes, it is usually caused by a meniscal tear, advanced chondromalacia patella (patellar dysfunction—excessive lateral patellar compression syndrome), rotatory instability, or loose bodies. The differential diagnosis, however, must also include pigmented villonodular synovitis, osteochondritis dissecans, inflammatory and/or rheumatologic arthritis and other causes of synovitis.

A summary of the key questions included in the subjective assessment and history of individuals presenting with a knee injury is included in Figure 30–13. The patient intake should include questions related to onset of symptoms, onset date, history of previous injury, swelling associated with injury, and current chief complaint (Fig. 30–13A). The athlete should be questioned regarding the onset of symptoms (Fig. 30–13B). A gradual onset of symptoms is indicative of an overuse injury, such as tendinitis or patellofemoral pain. A rapid onset of symptoms without a history of an injury is indicative of an acute inflammatory condition, such as bursitis and tendinitis. A rapid onset injury, with or without contact, is indicative of sprains, subluxations, dislocations, or fractures. Knowledge of the location of the applied force during a contact injury may further elucidate the probable structures involved.

Athletes must be questioned to determine whether they have a history of a previous injury to the same knee (Fig. 30–13C). If the individual has a history of a prior injury, it should be determined whether this is the same injury as before. If the current injury is the same as the previous injury, it is important to determine how the injury resolved, what treatment was administered, and the effect of that treatment.

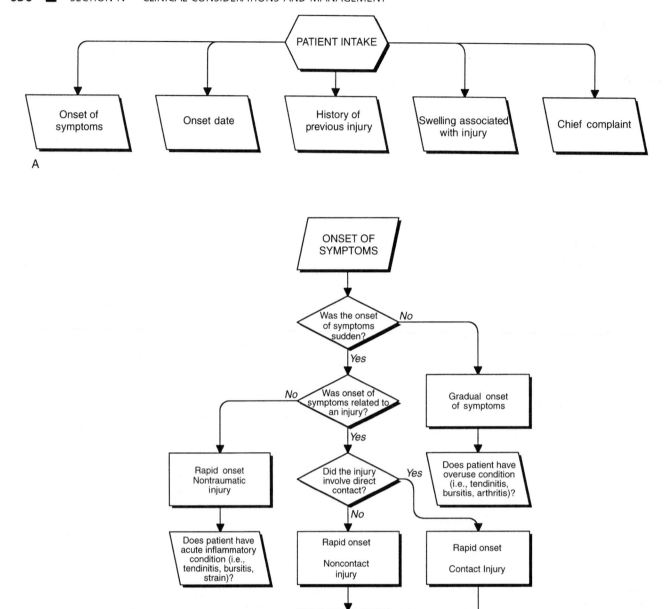

FIGURE 30–13. Clinical pathways for subjective assessment and history of individuals with knee injury. *A,* Patient intake. *B,* Assessment of symptoms.

A history of swelling associated with the injury is important to ascertain in (Fig. 30–13D). A history of rapid onset of swelling within 24 hours is indicative of a hemarthrosis and suggests injury to the anterior cruciate ligament, meniscus, and/or chondral surfaces. Swelling that occurs more than 24 hours after injury is indicative of reactive synovitis associated with an overuse injury.

Finally, the chief complaint must be determined (Fig. 30–13E). The complaint of pain must lead one to investigate the intensity, behavior, and location of that pain. Complaints of pain with forceful knee extension, catching, stiffness, and crepitus are indicative of patel-

lofemoral problems. Complaints of buckling and giving way are indicative of ligamentous and/or meniscal pathology.

Knowledge of the mechanisms of injury and signs and symptoms associated with different injuries can help guide the physician to the appropriate diagnosis, which can be confirmed by physical examination and ancillary studies. In practice, for the common problems, the same history is typically given by different individuals with only minor variations. Familiarity with the usual patterns also alerts the examiner when something does not fit. A discordant note, whether it is a sign or symptom that is out of the ordinary or unexpected, should alert the examiner and suggest a careful examination that may require a search for unusual causes.

PHYSICAL EXAMINATION

Complementing a good history is a thorough physical examination. Our general approach to examination of the knee is discussed first, followed by a discussion of specific tests and their rationale for diagnosing ligamentous instability and meniscal pathology. Tests for other problems are not discussed here because they are beyond the scope of this chapter.

Careful manual examination of the knee reveals most ligament disruptions. Some investigators suggest that up to 90 percent of all ligament disruptions can be diagnosed by clinical examination alone by an experienced clinician,[37,38] but the ability to diagnose meniscal injuries by physical examination alone is significantly less.[37,39–41] For multiple ligament injuries of the knee, the clinical examination is less accurate for determining all injuries.[37,42]

The motion resulting from a clinical test in a relaxed patient depends on the position of the limb at the start of the test, the point of application and direction of the force, and the ability of the examiner to detect displacement. In a normal patient, left-right, side-to-side difference is usually negligible, so an internal control often exists for most patients. For most knee ligament tests, pathologic motion during certain tests is associated with injury to a specific ligament or ligament complex. Pathologic motion exists with a test for a particular ligament if the ligament is partially or completely torn, but this motion may be even greater if other ligaments are disrupted (Table 30–1). For a specific motion, the structure that provides the greatest limitation is considered the primary restraint. When a primary restraint is disrupted, pathologic motion occurs, but its extent is limited by the remaining structures, called secondary restraints. Disruption of a secondary restraint does not result in pathologic motion if the primary restraint is intact, but disruption of the secondary restraint when the primary restraint is disrupted enhances pathologic motion. On all clinical laxity tests, the femur is held

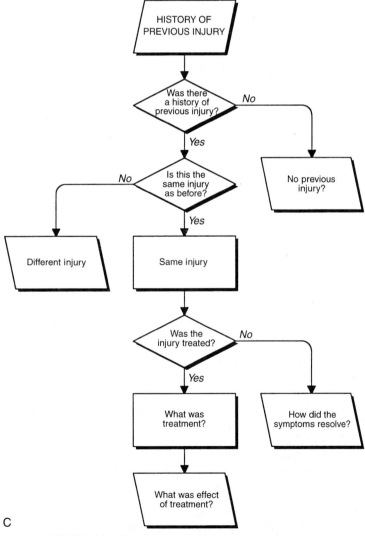

C

FIGURE 30–13. *Continued* C, History of previous injury.

Illustration continued on following page

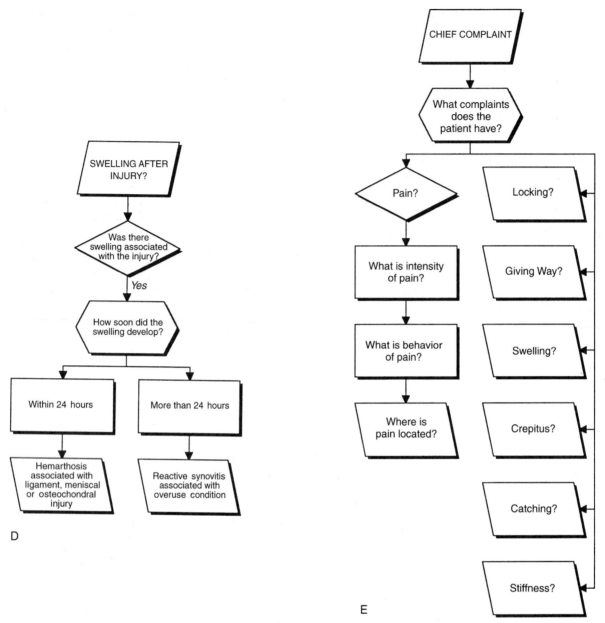

FIGURE 30–13. *Continued D,* Swelling after injury. *E,* Chief complaint.

steady and the tibial translation or rotation (joint space opening) is measured.

Meniscal injury, however, is more difficult to diagnose by clinical examination alone. No test is considered definitive and test reliability, although dependent on experience, is not as good as with ligamentous tests. The menisci are avascular in their inner 66 to 75 percent and, combined with a lack of pain fibers, meniscal injury can be present without pain or swelling.

A summary of the scheme to examine the knee is presented in Table 30–3. The patient is first examined standing in front of the examiner, and mechanical alignment of the lower extremities, symmetry, and foot type are assessed. The patient's gait is studied, noting the amount and time spent in stance phase, flexion and extension of the knee, medial or lateral thrust, and knee and foot progression angles. The patient also walks on the toes and heels to assess strength of the ankle dorsiflexors and plantarflexors and to rule out foot pathology as the source of any gait deviations. The patient may be asked to perform a "duck walk" (i.e., walk in the deep squat position) to rule out a meniscal tear (Childress' sign). Symptoms with squatting in the ascent or descent phase may be indicative of patellofemoral dysfunction, whereas pain with a deep knee bend may be indicative of meniscal pathology. The patient is also examined from behind to detect a popliteal cyst. The lower extremities are grossly evaluated for evidence of ecchymosis, such as that associated with contusions and muscle (hamstring and quadriceps) strains. Any obvious deformity is also noted.

Next, the patient is examined in the seated position with the knees flexed over the edge of the examining table. Alternatively, this part of the examination may be performed with the patient lying supine, with the knees bent to 90 degrees. The joint line is palpated for tenderness. As noted earlier, medial joint line pain may be indicative of a medial meniscal tear, patellofemoral problems, MCL sprain, or medial compartmental arthritis. Lateral joint line tenderness is most commonly associated with lateral meniscal tears, although patellofemoral dysfunction, lateral compartment degenerative arthritis, LCL sprain, or proximal tibiofibular arthritis may also present with lateral joint line tenderness. The patellar tendon is palpated from the patella to the tibial tubercle to determine that it is intact as well as to determine tenderness, consistency, and location. Patel-

---

TABLE 30–3
Physical Examination of the Knee

·Standing position
Mechanical alignment and symmetry of lower extremity
Foot type
Gait
Heel-and-toe walking
"Duck" walk
·Seated position
Palpation
   Medial joint line
   Lateral joint line
   Patellar tendon
   Tibial tubercle
   Proximal tibia (pes anserine bursa-Gerdy tubercle)
Sulcus tubercle angle (Q angle at 90°)
·Supine with knees extended
Palpation
   Warmth
   Swelling
   Patellar facets
   Quadriceps tendon
   LCL in figure-of-four position
Active and passive flexion and extension
Patellofemoral and tibiofemoral crepitus
Sag sign
Godfrey sign
Quadriceps active test
Anterior-posterior drawer
Lachman test
Varus-valgus stress test
O'Donoghue-McMurray test
Medial and lateral pivot shift
Reverse pivot shift
External rotation recurvatum test
Quadriceps atrophy
Hamstring and calf tightness
·Side-lying position
Ober test
·Prone position
Heel height difference (flexion contracture)
Apley compression/distraction test
External rotation of tibia at 30 and 90° of flexion
Reverse Lachman
Quadriceps flexibility

---

lar tendinitis is often tender at the inferior pole of the patellar or insertion to the tibial tubercle and may have a boggy consistency. With a patellar tendon disruption, the patient may still be able to extend the knee due to retinacular attachments, so the tendon must be palpated to ensure that it is not torn. The tibial tubercle is often tender in the adolescent with Osgood-Schlatter disease, an apophysitis of the tibial tubercle. In adulthood, the tibial tubercle is commonly asymptomatic. Palpation along the proximal tibia may reveal tenderness associated with pes anserinus bursitis or bursitis at Gerdy's tubercle. Stability of the proximal tibiofibular joint is assessed with the knee flexed beyond 80 degrees by pushing and pulling the fibular head in the anteroposterior plane. Finally, the sulcus tubercle angle (Q angle at 90 degrees of flexion) is measured to determine patellar malalignment.[43]

The patient is then positioned supine on the examining table, with the knees extended. The knee is inspected for gross deformity, including effusions. It is palpated for warmth and inspected for redness indicative of acute inflammation. Swelling about the knee must be assessed to determine its size and whether it is extra-articular, such as with prepatellar bursitis, or intra-articular. A large, tense effusion is often associated with an acute injury, such as a fracture or cruciate ligament injury, whereas a smaller effusion is associated with patellofemoral irritation. The patella is examined for facet tenderness, mobility, crepitus, and apprehension. Active and passive extension are then measured. Varus-valgus stability is examined with the knee in extension and 20 degrees flexion. If pain is elicited on this maneuver, it may be indicative of a meniscal tear (Bohler sign). A Lachman test is then performed with the knee in 20 degrees flexion to assess the integrity of the ACL. Both the amount of excursion and quality of the end point are noted. The knee is then actively and passively flexed and recorded and an O'Donoghue test is performed, followed by a true McMurray test. As the knee is brought into extension, one of the examiner's hands is maintained on the knee to palpate patellofemoral and tibiofemoral grinding and crepitation. Next, the knee is brought back to 90 degrees flexion, and the medial tibial plateau step-off is palpated while also looking for a posterior sag (indicative of a PCL tear). Anterior and posterior drawer tests are performed with the knee in 90 degrees flexion with the foot in neutral rotation as well as in internal and external rotation. The amount of translation and quality of end point for all these tests are recorded to assess for rotatory instability. A quadriceps active test can be performed if a posterior sag is identified.

The knee is then brought into a figure-of-four position to palpate the LCL and the medial joint line is palpated to test for pain associated with a medial meniscal tear (the Payr test). The flexed knee is then brought up to 90 degrees of knee and hip flexion to look for posterior sag (Godfrey sign). If a meniscal tear is suspected, the "bounce home" test can be performed at this point. The knee is then placed in extension and the thighs are measured for atrophy. If the examiner suspects a quadriceps tear, the suprapatellar insertion

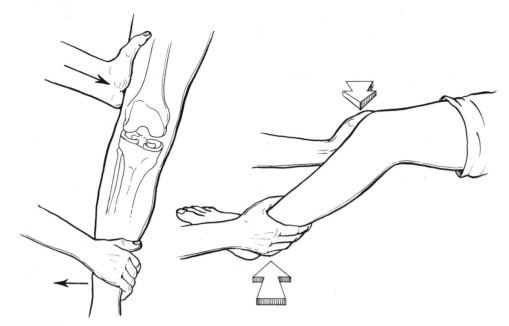

FIGURE 30–14. Valgus stress test in 30 degrees of flexion. The medial joint line gaps open when a valgus stress is applied across the knee. At 30 degrees of flexion, this test assesses the integrity of the medial collateral ligament.

of the quadriceps is palpated with the knee in extension. A pivot shift and reversed pivot shift are performed to confirm or rule out cruciate deficiency. When a PCL or multiple ligament injury is suspected, the external rotation recurvatum test is performed. Strength, sensation, and pedal and popliteal pulses are also assessed.

If lateral knee tenderness exists and the history is suggestive of iliotibial band syndrome, placing the patient in the lateral decubitus position to perform an Ober test is suggested. This assesses flexibility and relative tightness of the iliotibial band.

Finally, the patient is placed in the prone position. Inspection determines whether a flexion contracture exists by a difference in height between the patient's heels. Palpation reveals a popliteal cyst. With the knee flexed to 90 degrees, an Apley compression-distraction test can be performed to confirm or rule out meniscal tears. The feet are then externally rotated at 90 and 30 degrees to assess the integrity of the posterolateral corner when a PCL injury is suspected. With the knee flexed to 20 degrees, a reverse Lachman can be performed.

The lumbar spine should be examined in detail, including a careful neurologic examination to rule out referred pain from other locations. Additionally, the hip should be examined, because referred pain from the hip can often cause knee pain, especially in children, where a slipped capital femoral epiphysis often presents as knee pain.

SPECIFIC TESTS

MEDIAL COLLATERAL LIGAMENT

ABDUCTION (VALGUS STRESS) TEST. This test assesses the integrity of the MCL and medial instability in one plane only. The medial joint line gaps open when a valgus stress is applied across the knee while the patient is supine with the leg held in slight

external rotation (Fig. 30–14). The examiner's hand is placed on the lateral joint line to feel for opening of the medial joint line when valgus stress is applied from the lateral aspect of the knee. The knee is tested first in full extension and again in 20 to 30 degrees knee flexion. It is imperative to examine both knees, because some ligamentously lax individuals may have several millimeters of opening of the medial joint line, which may be normal for them. Depending on the amount of medial joint line opening in extension and slight flexion, the severity of injury to the MCL and associated structures can be determined. With the knee in full extension, capsular and other secondary restraints resist valgus stress, even when the MCL is disrupted. Flexion of the knee to approximately 20 degrees relaxes the secondary restraints for primary testing of the MCL.

If there is increased medial joint line opening of the affected knee with 20 to 30 degrees flexion, then the posterior oblique ligament and posteromedial capsule may be injured.

If there is excessive medial joint opening in full extension, a more severe injury to the secondary structures must be assumed. Medial joint line opening with the knee in full extension is indicative of injury to the MCL (superficial and deep fibers), posterior oblique ligament, ACL, PCL, posteromedial capsule, medial quadriceps expansion and retinaculum, and semimembranosus. With this more severe injury, one or more rotatory instability tests are also positive.

MCL injuries are graded as first, second, or third degree. A first-degree MCL injury is indicated by pain and tenderness along the ligament or at its insertion and the joint space opening is within 2 mm of the contralateral side, with a firm end point. For a second-degree injury, the end point is relatively firm and the joint space opens 3 to 5 mm more than the contralateral side in 20 degrees flexion and less than 2 mm more than the normal knee in full extension. A third-degree injury or a complete disruption of the MCL and associated structures is indicated by a soft end point, and the joint space opens more than 5 mm more than that of the normal knee in 20 degrees flexion and full extension.

LATERAL COLLATERAL LIGAMENT

ADDUCTION (VARUS STRESS) TEST. This test assesses the integrity of the LCL and thus lateral instability in one plane. The lateral joint line gaps open when a varus stress is applied to the knee while the patient is supine and the leg is held in slight external rotation (Fig. 30–15). External rotation of the leg uncoils the cruciate ligaments, requiring the collateral ligament to resist this stress. The examiner's hand is held on the medial joint line to feel for opening of the lateral joint line when varus stress is applied from the medial aspect of the knee. The knee is tested first in full extension and again in 20 to 30 degrees knee flexion. It is imperative to examine both knees, because some ligamentously lax individuals may have several millimeters of opening of the lateral joint line, which may be normal for them.

Depending on the amount of lateral joint line opening in extension and slight flexion, the severity of injury to the LCL and associated structures can be determined. With the knee in full extension, capsular and other secondary restraints such as the biceps femoris and popliteus resist varus stress, even when the LCL is disrupted. Flexion helps relax the secondary restraints for primary testing of the LCL.

If there is more lateral joint line opening of the affected knee with 20 to 30 degrees flexion, then the LCL, posterolateral capsule, arcuate-popliteus complex, iliotibial band, and biceps femoris tendon may have been injured.

If there is excessive lateral joint line opening in full extension, a more severe injury to the secondary structures must be assumed. Lateral joint space opening with the knee in full extension indicates some degree of injury to the LCL, posterolateral capsule, arcuate-popliteus complex, iliotibial band, biceps femoris tendon, ACL, PCL, and lateral head of the gastrocnemius. With this more severe injury, one or more rotatory instability tests are also positive.

Grading these injuries is the same as that for MCL injuries, by assessing the degree of opening of the lateral joint line.

PALPATION OF THE LCL. With the patient supine, the patient's hip is flexed to approximately 70 degrees, abducted maximally, and externally rotated with the knee flexed 70 to 90 degrees, so that the ipsilateral foot rests on the patient's contralateral leg (i.e., figure-of-four position). As the knee is allowed to relax passively, the examiner palpates the LCL from the fibular head to the femoral condyle. A firm, taut band, which is the LCL, should be easily palpated. If the patient's knee is not relaxed, the examiner may be fooled by the insertion of the biceps femoris. Both knees should be examined to compare the intact LCL with the injured one.

ANTERIOR CRUCIATE LIGAMENT

LACHMAN TEST. The Lachman test is the most sensitive clinical test for determining disruption of the ACL, particularly the posterolateral band.[38,44,45] This uniplanar test is for anterior instability or anterior translation of the tibia on the femur. Because the ACL is tight in full extension, the knee is examined in 20 to 30 degrees flexion, with the patient in the supine

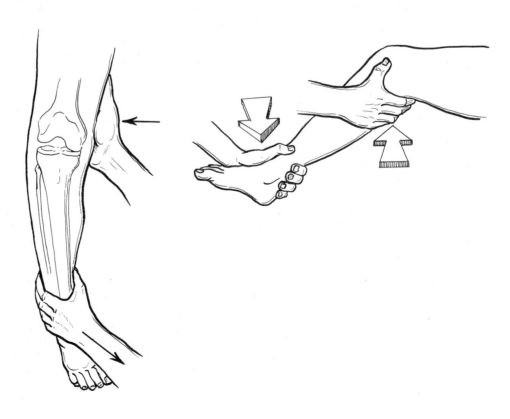

FIGURE 30–15. Varus stress test in 30 degrees of flexion. The lateral joint line gaps open when a varus stress is applied to the knee, indicating injury to the lateral collateral ligament.

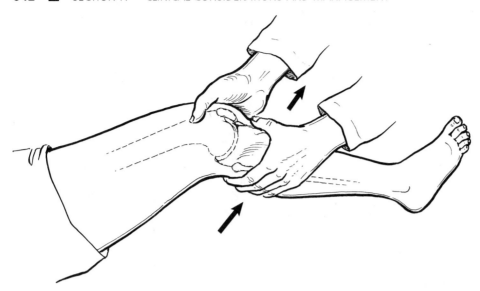

FIGURE 30–16. Lachman test. This is performed with the knee in 20 to 30 degrees of flexion. The distal femur is stabilized with one of the examiner's hands while the proximal tibia is pulled anteriorly with the other hand.

position. When testing the knee in slight flexion, the ACL is the primary restraining force that prevents anterior translation, because the secondary restraints are relaxed. The distal femur is stabilized with one of the examiner's hands while the proximal tibia is moved forward with the other hand (Fig. 30–16). A small support, such as a pillow, may be placed under the thigh to help support the thigh and provide the small amount of flexion necessary for this test. The amount of anterior translation and quality of the end point indicate injury to the ACL, posterior oblique ligament, and arcuate-popliteus complex. A soft or "mushy" end point, with excessive anterior translation as compared with the contralateral knee, is indicative of injury. The slope of the infrapatellar tendon also disappears.

The end point is graded as firm (normal), marginal, or soft. Anterior tibial translation is measured in millimeters. A left-right difference of greater than 3 mm is indicative of injury to the ACL.[46] If the end point and translation are normal, the Lachman test is negative. If the end point is soft and/or if there is increased anterior translation, however, then the Lachman test is positive. Care should be taken to ensure that the PCL is not torn, because this may give a false-positive Lachman test, allowing for more than a 3-mm increase in anteroposterior translation compared to the noninvolved side.

ANTERIOR DRAWER TEST. The drawer test is for determining anteroposterior uniplanar instability (Fig. 30–17). The difficulty with this test is determining the neutral starting position if the anterior or posterior cruciate ligament has been injured. The supine patient's ipsilateral hip is flexed to 45 degrees and the knee is flexed to 90 degrees. In this position, the ACL is nearly parallel to the tibial plateau. The examiner sits on the patient's forefoot to stabilize the leg. The examiner grasps the back of the proximal tibia with the index fingers and palpates the hamstring muscles to ensure they are relaxed. The examiner's thumbs are placed on the anterior medial and anterior lateral joint line to palpate anterior translation as the tibia is drawn forward on the femur. A step-off at the medial tibial plateau should be palpated to ensure the proper starting position (see PCL, later). The knee is tested with the foot in neutral rotation, external rotation, and then in internal rotation. The amount of translation and end point are compared with the contralateral (normal) knee. If excessive anterior translation is evident, the ACL (primarily anteromedial bundle), posterolateral capsule, posteromedial capsule, deep MCL, iliotibial band, posterior oblique ligament, and arcuate-popliteus complex may be injured.

Truly isolated acute ACL tears often produce only minimally increased anterior translation when the secondary stabilizers of the knee, including the posterior capsule and posteromedial and posterolateral capsular structures, are intact. False-negative results can also occur with a displaced ("bucket handle") meniscal tear, hamstring spasm, and hemarthrosis.

SLOCUM TEST. This test is similar to the anterior drawer test described earlier, with the tibia internally rotated 30 degrees.[47] If the majority of anterior translation occurs on the lateral side of the knee, and/or the amount of anterior translation increases or does not decrease, then anterolateral rotatory instability is indicated. With anterolateral instability, the ACL, postero-

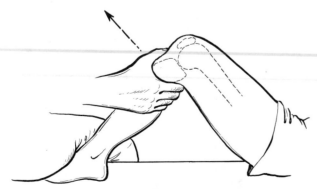

FIGURE 30–17. Anterior drawer test. This is performed with the knee in 90 degrees of flexion, with the examiner sitting on the patient's foot. The fingers should palpate the hamstring tendons to ensure that they are relaxed. The thumbs should be placed in the joint line medially and laterally to palpate anterior translation of the tibia during the test.

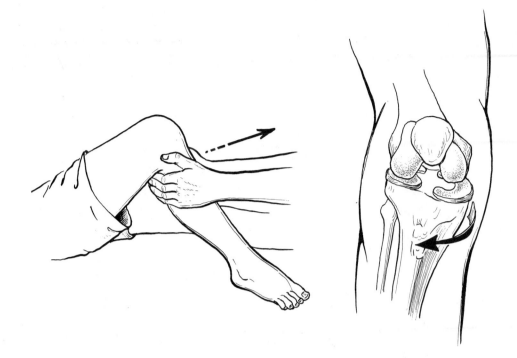

FIGURE 30–18. Slocum external rotation test. This anterior drawer test is performed with the leg externally rotated. Anteromedial rotatory instability is indicated if the majority of anterior translation occurs on the medial side and/or the amount of anterior translation remains the same or increases, indicating anteromedial instability compared to the anterior drawer test performed in neutral rotation.

lateral capsule, arcuate-popliteus complex, LCL, PCL, and iliotibial band (i.e., posterolateral corner) may be injured.

Next, the patient's foot is placed in 15 degrees external rotation as the examiner sits on the patient's forefoot. When the anterior drawer force is applied, the majority of anterior translation occurs on the medial side of the knee, and/or the amount of anterior translation is the same or increases, then anteromedial rotatory instability is present. This indicates injury to the MCL, posterior oblique ligament, posteromedial capsule, and the ACL (i.e., posteromedial corner) (Fig. 30–18).

Overrotating the foot can lead to a false-negative test, because this can tighten other secondary and tertiary restraints. Furthermore, tests for anteromedial rotatory instability are of less value when anterolateral rotatory instability is present.

PIVOT SHIFT TEST. This test is used to test for injury to the ACL as well as to assess anterolateral rotatory instability of the knee.[48–50] During this test, the tibia subluxates anterolaterally on the femur. This recreates the anterior subluxation-reduction phenomenon that occurs during functional activities when the ACL is torn. During the test, subluxation occurs in extension and reduction occurs between 20 and 40 degrees of flexion, which results in the patient feeling the sensation of instability that occurs when the knee buckles.

To perform this test, the patient lies supine, with the hip flexed to 30 degrees with no abduction. One of the examiner's hands holds the foot so that there is slight internal rotation (20 degrees) of the leg while the other hand is placed behind and lateral to the knee. The second hand is positioned so that the heel of the hand is behind the fibula, over the lateral head of the gastrocnemius, with the tibia internally rotated, which causes the lateral tibial plateau to sublux anteriorly as the knee is brought into extension. The examiner then

applies a valgus stress to the knee while maintaining an internal rotation torque on the tibia at the foot and ankle. As the knee is flexed to approximately 30 to 40 degrees, the tibia reduces or slides backward and the patient notes that the sensation is similar to that which occurs when the knee gives way (a positive test) (Fig. 30–19).

In extension, the secondary restraints of the knee, such as the hamstrings, lateral femoral condyle, lateral meniscus, and iliotibial band, are less efficient than in flexion to allow the lateral tibial plateau to sublux anteriorly. Reduction of the tibia on the femur during flexion is due to the iliotibial band tightening and moving from a position anterior to the axis of the knee to a position posterior to the axis of the knee, thus becoming a flexor of the knee and pulling the tibia back into its normal, reduced position. This test, then, has two phases—subluxation and reduction. The iliotibial band must be intact and under some tension (thus, no

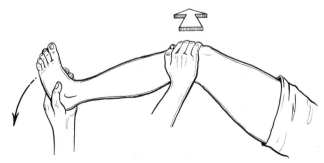

FIGURE 30–19. Lateral pivot shift test. This is performed with the patient supine. The heel of one hand is placed behind the head of the fibula, and the other hand is placed on the foot. Internal rotation and valgus force of the lower leg is produced with the knee in full extension to sublux the lateral tibial plateau anteriorly. The knee is then flexed to 20 to 30 degrees, which results in reduction of the lateral tibial plateau.

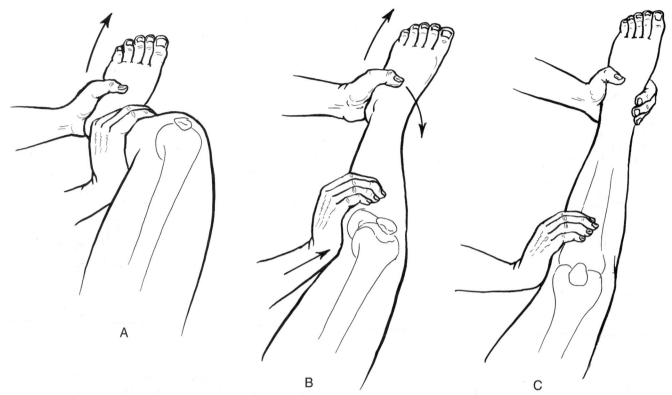

FIGURE 30–20. Jerk test of Hughston. *A,* The knee is flexed to 90 degrees, and the heel of one hand is placed behind the fibular head to produce internal rotation of the tibia. *B,* At 20 to 30 degrees, the lateral tibial plateau subluxes anteriorly. *C,* At full extension, the lateral tibial plateau is reduced.

hip abduction) for this test to work. Excessive hip adduction or abduction, a displaced meniscal tear, or torn MCL may give a false-negative result.

A positive test indicates injury to the ACL, posterolateral capsule, arcuate-popliteus complex, LCL, and iliotibial band. The reduction is graded by the examining clinician as 0 (absent), 1+ (slight slip), 2+ (moderate slip), or 3+ (momentary locking).[51]

LOSEE PIVOT SHIFT TEST. The Losee test is similar to the pivot shift test and is thought of by some clinicians as an extension pivot shift test.[52] The patient is placed supine on the examining table. The examiner then holds the patient's externally rotated ankle and foot between the forearm and abdomen. The patient's hip is flexed to approximately 30 degrees and the knee is flexed to 30 degrees to relax the hamstrings. In this position, the knee is in its reduced position. The examiner's other hand is placed so that the thumb is behind the fibular head and the fingers are over the anterior knee to produce an internal rotatory and valgus stress. The valgus force compresses the lateral structures of the knee, and the internal rotatory force produces anterior subluxation as the knee is extended. Just prior to full extension, a "clunk" is seen and felt as the tibia subluxes forward. A positive Losee pivot shift test is indicative of anterolateral rotatory instability and is associated with injury to the same structures injured with a positive pivot shift test.

JERK TEST OF HUGHSTON. This test is also similar to the pivot shift test and is often used, although it is not

as sensitive as the pivot shift test. The positioning is the same as with the pivot shift, but the patient's hip is flexed to 45 degrees and knee flexed to 90 degrees. The knee is extended while maintaining an internal rotation and a valgus force. At 20 to 30 degrees flexion, the tibia translates forward, causing subluxation of the lateral tibial plateau with a jerk if the test is positive. As the knee is extended further, the tibial plateau spontaneously reduces (Fig. 30–20).[53] This test indicates injury to the same structures as those listed for the pivot shift maneuver.

POSTERIOR CRUCIATE LIGAMENT

STEP-OFF TEST. This is a sensitive uniplanar test for determining posterior cruciate injury and posterior instability. Normally, the medial tibial plateau protrudes anteriorly 1 cm beyond the medial femoral condyle when the knee is flexed to 90 degrees (Fig. 30–21A).[54] This step-off is lost when there is a posterior sag of the tibia associated with injury to the PCL and other secondary restraints to posterior translation of the tibia (Fig. 30–21B). The patient is examined in the supine position with the knee flexed to 90 degrees. The examiner places the hands on either side of the proximal tibia at the joint line and palpates the hamstrings with the fingers to ensure that the patient is relaxed. The medial tibial plateau, which is easier to palpate than the lateral plateau, is felt in relation to the femoral condyle with the examiner's thumb. A 0.5-cm difference in the step-off between the involved and uninjured knees is considered a grade I laxity, whereas a 1-cm difference, in which the tibia and femoral condyles are flush, is considered a grade II laxity. If the anterior tibia lies posterior to the femoral condyle, indicating that there is more than a 1-cm difference between the involved and noninvolved knees a grade III laxity is considered to be present.[55,56]

POSTERIOR SAG TEST. This is a uniplanar passive test of PCL function and posterior instability. With the patient supine on the examining table, the hip flexed to 45 degrees, and the knee flexed to 90 degrees, viewing the knee from the lateral side reveals a loss of tibial tubercle prominence in a PCL-deficient knee (Fig. 30–22). If the PCL is torn, the tibia falls back or sags on the femur due to gravitational force. The posterior tibial displacement is more noticeable when the knee is flexed 90 to 110 degrees than when the knee is only slightly flexed. This test is less obvious when there is significant swelling of the knee. One must be aware of tibial tubercle enlargement (due to Osgood-Schlatter disease) or tibial plateau osteophytes, which can give a false-negative result. Different degrees of posterior sag represent varying degrees of injury to the PCL, arcuate-popliteus complex, posterior oblique ligament, and ACL.

QUADRICEPS ACTIVE DRAWER TEST. With the patient in the same position as for the posterior sag or

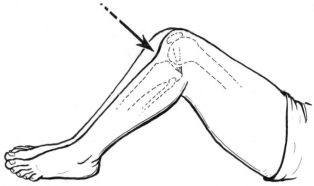

FIGURE 30–22. Posterior sag test. Viewing a posterior cruciate ligament-deficient knee at 90 degrees of flexion from the side reveals loss of prominence of the tibial tubercle.

posterior drawer test, the patient actively extends the knee by sliding the heel forward along the table. If the knee is posteriorly subluxed and the extensor mechanism is intact, the tibia translates forward and the knee reduces.[57] If this test is positive, the same structures are injured as with the posterior sag test.

GODFREY SIGN. This is a posterior sag test, with the supine patient's hips and knees flexed to 90 degrees (Fig. 30–23). The examiner holds the relaxed leg distally to prevent manual reduction of the tibia. The posterior sag of the proximal tibia may be accentuated by applying a posteriorly directed force to the proximal tibia. If this test is positive, the same structures may be injured as those listed for the posterior sag test.

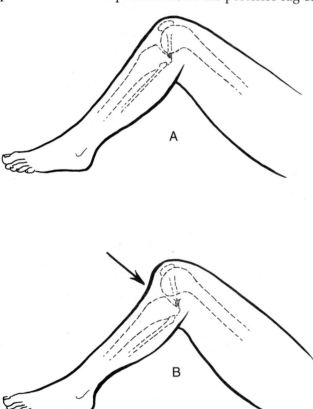

FIGURE 30–21. Step-off test. *A,* Normal relationship of the tibiofemoral joint. The medial tibial plateau protrudes anteriorly approximately 1 cm beyond the medial femoral condyle. *B,* With injury to the posterior cruciate ligament, the step-off is lost. The medial tibial plateau now lies either in line with or posterior to the medial femoral condyle.

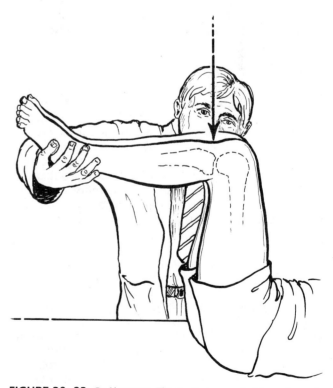

FIGURE 30–23. Godfrey test. This posterior sag test is performed with the patient's hips and knees flexed to 90 degrees. Disruption of the posterior cruciate ligament results in loss of prominence of the tibial tubercle.

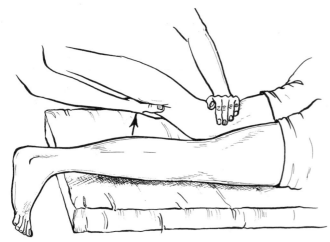

FIGURE 30–24. Reverse Lachman test. This test is performed with the individual lying prone and the knee flexed to 20 to 30 degrees. The distal thigh is stabilized by the examiner's proximal hand, and the distal hand is used to translate the proximal tibia posteriorly.

REVERSE LACHMAN TEST. This test for PCL insufficiency is performed with the patient lying prone, with the knee flexed to 20 to 30 degrees.[58] The examiner holds the distal femur to the examining table and grasps the proximal tibia anteriorly with the other hand. Using the hand on the femur to stabilize the thigh and to ensure that the hamstrings are relaxed, the examiner pushes the proximal tibia posteriorly (up), noting the amount of translation and quality of the end point (as with a regular Lachman test) (Fig. 30–24). A false-positive test may occur if the ACL is torn, allowing gravity to cause an anterior shift of the tibia. This test is not as sensitive for detecting a torn PCL, because the PCL functions more at 90 degrees of knee flexion.

POSTERIOR DRAWER TEST. As noted earlier, the drawer test is for anteroposterior uniplanar instability. The difficulty with this test is determining the neutral starting position if the ligaments have been injured. Nonetheless, this is the most useful test for diagnosing PCL injury. The supine patient's ipsilateral hip is flexed to 45 degrees and knee is flexed to 90 degrees. The examiner sits on the patient's forefoot to stabilize the leg. The examiner grasps the back of patient's proximal tibia with the index fingers, palpating the hamstring muscles to ensure that they are relaxed. The examiner's thumbs are placed on the anterior joint line to feel posterior translation as the tibia is drawn backward on the femur. The medial tibial plateau should be palpated as a 1-cm anterior step-off from the medial femoral condyle to ensure the proper starting position. The knee is tested with the foot in neutral position, external rotation, and then in internal rotation. The amount of translation and end point are again compared with the contralateral (normal) knee. If excessive posterior translation is evident, the PCL (primarily the anterolateral bundle), arcuate-popliteus complex, posterior oblique ligament, and ACL may be injured (Fig. 30–25).

Truly isolated acute PCL tears often produce only minimally increased posterior translation when the secondary restraints of the knee, particularly the posterior capsule and posteromedial and posterolateral structures, are intact. Some studies have suggested that the meniscofemoral ligaments are strong and may act as a secondary stabilizer to PCL function. A posterior drawer test with the leg in internal rotation is reduced if the posterolateral structures or, as some investigators have suggested, the meniscofemoral ligaments, are intact.[59] Some investigators believe that a posterior drawer cannot occur with an intact arcuate-popliteus complex, although laboratory studies have revealed that a posterior drawer of no greater than 10 mm as compared with the contralateral side can occur with an isolated PCL injury. False-negative results can occur with a displaced bucket handle meniscal tear, hamstring or quadriceps spasm, and hemarthrosis.

Grading of this test also requires comparison of the injured knee with the normal knee. Grade I injury occurs when the injured to noninjured side-to-side difference in posterior translation is less than 5 mm, which usually corresponds to posterior displacement of the tibial plateau to a position that is still anterior to the femoral condyles. A grade II PCL injury results in 5 to 10 mm more posterior tibial displacement on the involved side. This corresponds to posterior translation of the tibial plateau to the level of the femoral condyles. If the tibia can be posteriorly displaced 10 mm or more on the involved side compared with the noninvolved side, or posterior to the femoral condyles, then a grade III injury is present.[55,56] Although it is important also to assess the end point of the posterior drawer test, the end point may return to a normal, firm, feel in chronically PCL-deficient knees. Thus, the quality of the end point is not as sensitive as with the Lachman test.

HUGHSTON POSTEROMEDIAL AND POSTEROLATERAL DRAWER SIGNS. These tests for rotatory instability combined with PCL injury are analogous to the Slocum test for rotatory instability associated with ACL injury.[53] With the patient positioned for the posterior drawer test, the foot is internally rotated 30 degrees. Posteromedial rotatory instability is present if the majority of posterior translation occurs on the medial side of the knee and/or if the amount of posterior

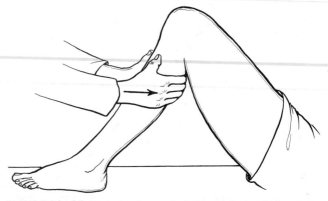

FIGURE 30–25. Posterior drawer test. The posterior drawer test is performed with the knee in 90 degrees of flexion. The fingers palpate the hamstrings posteriorly to ensure that they are relaxed, and the thumbs are placed in the anterior joint line to palpate posterior translation of the tibia when a posterior force is applied.

translation increases or does not change. Posteromedial rotatory instability is a result of varying degrees of injury to the PCL, posterior oblique ligament, MCL (deep and superficial), semimembranosus muscle, posteromedial capsule, and ACL (posteromedial corner).

Next, the patient's foot is placed in 15 degrees of external rotation as the examiner sits on the patient's forefoot. If the majority of posterior translation occurs on the lateral side of the knee, and/or if the amount of posterior translation increases or does not change, then posterolateral rotatory instability is present, indicating injury to the PCL, arcuate-popliteus complex, LCL, biceps femoris tendon, posterolateral capsule, and ACL (i.e., posterolateral corner). Overrotating the foot can lead to a false-negative test, because this can tighten other secondary and tertiary restraints.

REVERSE (JAKOB) PIVOT SHIFT TEST. This is the most sensitive test for posterolateral rotatory instability and is analogous to the pivot shift for ACL deficiency.[51,60] During this test, the posterolateral tibial plateau subluxes laterally and posteriorly on the femur. In this test, the knee starts in the subluxed position and the clunk associated with the test is that of the reduction phenomenon.

The patient lies supine, with the hip flexed and foot resting against the examiner's pelvis. The examiner uses one hand to support the lateral upper leg, with the palm on the fibular head. The ipsilateral knee is flexed to 70 to 80 degrees and the foot is externally rotated to sublux the lateral tibial plateau posteriorly. The examiner imparts a valgus stress to the knee while the knee is allowed to extend by gravity. As the knee approaches 20 degrees of flexion, the lateral tibia plateau shifts

forward, spontaneously reducing the subluxation (Fig. 30–26). The examiner must allow the foot to move back into neutral rotation as the knee is being extended to allow for reduction. When the knee is flexed again, the foot externally rotates and the lateral tibial plateau subluxes posteriorly.

This test evaluates the integrity of the structures listed for the posterolateral drawer test.

EXTERNAL ROTATION RECURVATUM TEST. This is another test for posterolateral rotatory instability and thus tests the same anatomic structures as listed earlier, with attention to the ACL, PCL, and posterolateral corner.[53] The patient is positioned supine on the examining table. The great toe of each foot is grasped and each foot is lifted off the table. While the extremities are elevated, the examiner observes for lateral rotation of the tibial tuberosity and hyperextension of the knee. The affected knee hyperextends to a greater degree than the noninvolved knee and appears to be in varus alignment (Fig. 30–27).

EXTERNAL ROTATION TEST AT 30 AND 90 DEGREES. This test helps determine the extent of injury to the PCL and posterolateral corner (LCL, arcuate-popliteus complex, posterolateral capsule, and biceps femoris).

With the patient lying prone, both knees are flexed to 90 degrees and an external rotation force is applied to both legs through the hindfeet (Fig. 30–28A). The amount of rotation of both extremities is observed. Then, the knees are extended to 30 degrees of flexion and both legs are externally rotated again (Fig. 30–28B). The amount of rotation is assessed. A difference of greater than 10 degrees external rotation between the

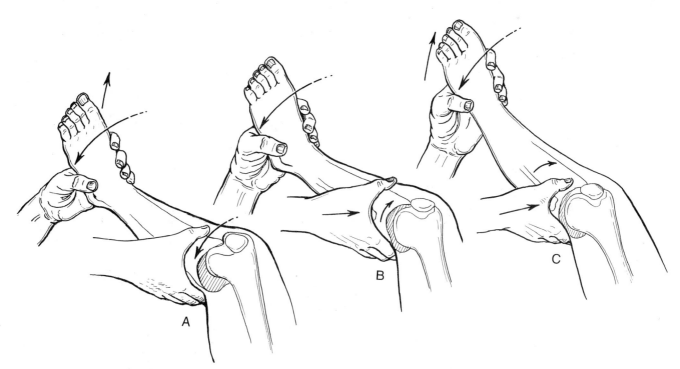

FIGURE 30–26. Reverse pivot shift test. *A,* The knee is flexed to 70 to 80 degrees. The proximal hand externally rotates the lower leg to sublux the lateral tibial plateau posteriorly. *B,* A valgus force is applied as the knee is passively extended. *C,* The lateral tibial plateau reduces as the knee approaches 20 degree of flexion.

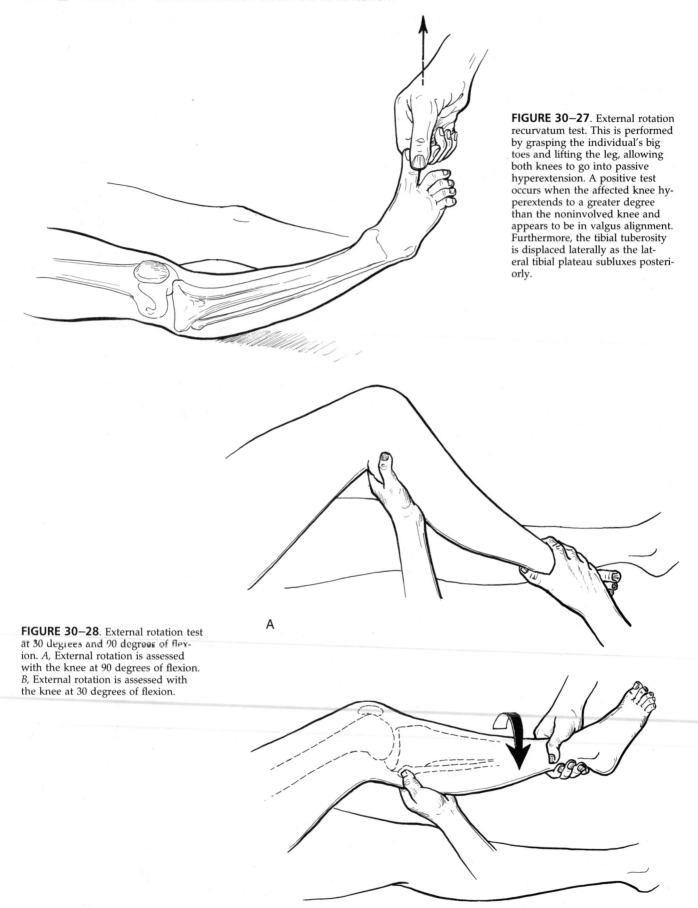

FIGURE 30–27. External rotation recurvatum test. This is performed by grasping the individual's big toes and lifting the leg, allowing both knees to go into passive hyperextension. A positive test occurs when the affected knee hyperextends to a greater degree than the noninvolved knee and appears to be in valgus alignment. Furthermore, the tibial tuberosity is displaced laterally as the lateral tibial plateau subluxes posteriorly.

A

FIGURE 30–28. External rotation test at 30 degrees and 90 degrees of flexion. A, External rotation is assessed with the knee at 90 degrees of flexion. B, External rotation is assessed with the knee at 30 degrees of flexion.

B

two knees is considered significant. If external rotation is greater in the affected knee at 30 and 90 degrees of flexion, then the PCL and posterolateral structures are injured. If the external rotation is increased only at 90 degrees, then the PCL is disrupted and the posterolateral corner is largely intact. If the external rotation is increased only at 30 degrees, the posterolateral corner is injured but the PCL is largely intact.[61]

POSTEROMEDIAL PIVOT SHIFT TEST. This new test has been introduced rather recently. When positive, it indicates injury to the PCL, MCL, and posterior oblique ligament.[62] All three structures must be injured for this test to be positive. The patient is positioned supine on the examining table and the knee is flexed greater than 45 degrees while applying a varus stress, combined with axial compression and internal rotation. If positive, this action results in the medial tibial plateau subluxing posterior to the medial femoral condyle. As the knee is brought into extension, the tibia reduces at approximately 20 to 40 degrees of knee flexion. Occasionally, the femur appears to internally rotate suddenly as the knee is extended.

MENISCUS

McMURRAY TEST. This is the classic and most specific test of meniscal injury.[63] The patient is positioned supine on the examining table with the knee completely flexed (heel to buttock). The examiner internally rotates the leg, applies a valgus force, and extends the knee while palpating the lateral joint line. This is repeated several times. Next, the leg is externally rotated and a varus stress is applied to the knee while palpating the medial joint line. A snap or click can be heard and felt along the joint line if a meniscal tear is present. A pop heard or felt in greater flexion is indicative of a more posterior tear.

JOINT LINE TENDERNESS TEST. This test is sensitive but not specific for meniscal pathology. The location of the tenderness should be noted as the anterior, middle, or posterior third on the medial or lateral joint line. Collateral ligament sprains, capsular irritation from nonmeniscal sources, or patellofemoral dysfunction may produce a false-positive finding.

BOUNCE HOME TEST. This is a nonspecific test for meniscal tears that block full extension. The patient is supine on the examination table and the knee is completely flexed so that the heel is at the buttocks. The examiner grabs the heel of the patient's foot. The knee is then passively extended to the end of the available range of motion. If full extension is not attained, or if there is a rubbery end feel ("springy block"), then something, most likely a displaced meniscus, is blocking extension.

O'DONOGHUE TEST. This test is a modification of the McMurray test, sometimes called a flexion McMurray or circumduction test. The patient is supine on the examining table. The knee is flexed to 90 degrees and rotated internally and externally and is then fully flexed and again rotated both ways. If the patient complains of pain with rotation in either direction, a meniscal tear or capsular irritation is present.

APLEY TEST. Another nonspecific test for meniscal injury is the compression-distraction test described by Apley.[64] The patient is positioned prone on the examining table, with the knee flexed to 90 degrees. The patient's thigh is steadied on the examination table with the examiner's hand or thigh. The examiner applies axial compression to the leg and rotates the tibia internally and externally. The test is then repeated with distraction of the knee while rotating the leg. If compression with rotation causes pain, the lesion is probably meniscal, whereas if distraction with rotation elicits pain, the lesion is possibly ligamentous.

PAYR TEST. This is a nonspecific test for medial meniscal injury.[58] The patient is positioned supine on the examination table and the extremity is placed in a figure-of-four position. If pain is elicited on the medial joint line, the test is considered positive for a middle or posterior medial meniscal lesion.

BOHLER SIGN. This is another nonspecific sign for meniscal injury. The patient lays supine on the examination table, and the examiner applies a varus or valgus stress to the knee. Pain along the joint line opposite to the stressed ligament is considered a positive test for meniscal injury. Pain is elicited due to compression of the injured meniscus between the tibia and femur. For example, valgus stress testing, which tests for MCL integrity, compresses the lateral compartment and may cause pain laterally if the lateral meniscus is injured.[58]

CHILDRESS' SIGN. This is also a nonspecific sign of meniscal pathology. The patient squats and performs a "duck walk." Pain, snapping, or a click is considered indicative of a posterior horn meniscal tear. Pain of patellofemoral origin may also produce symptoms with this test.

INSTRUMENTED TESTING OF THE KNEE

There are several knee ligament arthrometers commercially available for clinical use to quantify laxity of the knee. These include the Acufex Knee Signature System (Acufex Microsurgical, Inc., Norwood, MA), the Genucom Knee Analysis System (FaroMedical, Toronto, Canada), MedMetric KT-1000 Knee Ligament Arthrometer (MedMetric, San Diego, Cal.), and the Stryker Knee Laxity Tester (Stryker Corporation, Kalamazoo, Mich.). Of these, the MedMetric KT-1000 appears to be the most widely used.

The reliability and validity of these devices have been widely studied.[46,65–76] The Knee Signature System and Genucom appear to be less reliable than the MedMetric KT-1000.[71,72] Both these devices have higher 90% confidence limits than the KT-1000. Additionally, the Genucom tends to produce greater differences in displacement between the right and left knees of normal subjects.[73,74] The reliability of the Stryker Knee Laxity Tester has been questioned by King and Kumar,[70] who reported that more than 20 percent of normal knees showed more than a 2-mm variation between knees when tested by different examiners within the same day as well as when tested by the same examiner at a 3-week interval. Boniface and colleagues[77] reported that the Stryker Knee Laxity Tester is valid for detecting ACL injury. They reported that 89 percent of subjects with unilateral ACL injury had an increase of 2 mm or more compared with the uninjured side.

Intratester and intertester reliability for the Med-Metric KT-1000 have been reported to be high, both within and between days.[76] Wroble and associates[72] indicated that the 90 percent confidence limit for right-left difference with the KT-1000 measured at 89 newtons was ±1.6 mm and was ±1.5 mm when measured at 134 newtons. A confidence interval of this magnitude is within acceptable limits for the clinical diagnosis of ACL injuries. In vitro and in vivo research have demonstrated the KT-1000 to be a valid measure for the detection of ACL injury. The correlation between measurements made with the KT-1000 and those made with direct transducer readings in cadaveric knees was 0.97.[65] The mean anterior displacement in ACL-intact cadaveric knees was found to be 5.8 mm, which increased to 12.1 mm when the ACL was sectioned. In vivo studies demonstrated that 92 percent of normal subjects had a side-to-side difference in anterior displacement less than 2 mm, whereas 96 percent with confirmed unilateral disruption of the ACL had a side-to-side difference in anterior displacement greater than 2 mm.[65] Stratford and co-workers[66] and Highgenboten and colleagues[67] indicated that testing with the KT-1000 is more sensitive when performed with a 134-newton load or with manual maximum force. Highgenboten and associates[67] measured 68 patients with the KT-1000 at 15, 20, and 30 lb of force. Their results indicated that more patients demonstrate a side-to-side difference greater than 2 mm between the injured and noninjured legs at 30 lb of force than at 20 lb of force. It should be noted that, even with 30 lb of force, approximately 20 percent of patients with an ACL-deficient knee demonstrated a side-to-side difference less than 2 mm.

Based on this research, it appears that the KT-1000 is a clinically applicable instrument that can be used to assess anterior laxity in patients with an ACL-deficient knee. The KT-1000 measures anterior-posterior movement of the tibia relative to the femur. It includes patellar and tibial sensor pads (Fig. 30–29). The patellar sensor pad rests on the patella. When the patella is compressed against the femur, the patellar sensor pad indicates the position of the femur. The tibial reference pad rests in the area of the tibial tuberosity and provides a point of reference for the tibia. Relative motion between the patellar and tibial sensor pads is indicative of anterior and posterior translation of the tibia on the femur. The KT-1000 also includes a force-sensing handle that can be used to provide a 15-, 20-, and 30-lb anteriorly directed force as well as a 15- and 20-lb posteriorly directed force. Tibiofemoral motion is measured in millimeters as the relative motion between the patellar and tibial sensor pads and is displayed on a dial that can be zeroed to the neutral starting position.

Prior to using the KT-1000 to assess anterior-posterior laxity of the knee, it is necessary to screen for PCL injury. This is accomplished by observing for lack of a step-off between the medial femoral condyle and the medial tibial plateau. Additionally, the posterior sag test and/or active quadriceps drawer can be used to rule out injury to the PCL. Failure to detect a PCL-deficient knee prior to testing with the KT-1000 may result in a false-positive test for anterior laxity. With a PCL-deficient knee, gravity causes the tibia to sublux posteriorly. If this is undetected, then the reference position of the tibia is posterior to the true neutral position of the tibiofemoral joint. Performing a KT-1000 test from a starting position at which the tibia is posteriorly subluxed results in a false-positive increase in anterior translation. This occurs as the tibia is translated anteriorly from the posterior subluxed position to the neutral position. Failure to detect presence of a PCL injury when performing a KT-1000 test invalidates the results.

Once PCL injury has been ruled out, the patient's knees are placed in 20 to 30 degrees of flexion by placing a bolster under the distal aspect of the thighs. The bolster should be placed proximal to the knee to avoid restricting tibial translation. The angle of knee flexion

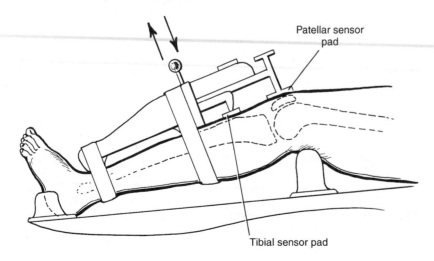

Patellar sensor pad

Tibial sensor pad

FIGURE 30–29. KT-1000 arthrometer for quantifying tibial translation. Relative movement of the tibiofemoral joint is measured as motion between the patellar and tibial sensor pads.

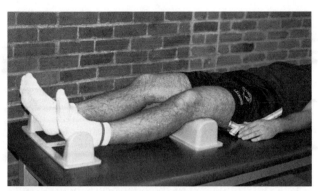

FIGURE 30−30. Position of the lower extremity for KT-1000 test. A Bolster is placed under the distal aspect of the thigh to flex the knee to 20 to 30 degrees. A foot rest is placed distal to the lateral malleolus to produce symmetric internal rotation of the tibia on the femur.

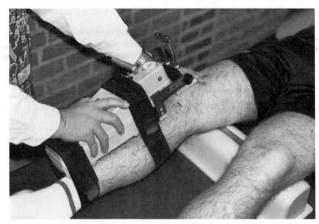

FIGURE 30−31. Proper alignment of the KT-1000 on the lower leg. The arrow on the arthrometer is aligned with the medial joint line and the arthrometer is slightly rotated onto the leg, so that compression of the patellar sensor pad directly compresses the patella against the femur without medial or lateral displacement. The height of the patellar sensor pad is adjusted so that the needle faces the 12 o'clock position on the dial. (MedMetric KT-1000 Knee Ligament Arthrometer, MedMetric, San Diego.)

should be recorded so that it can be repeated for future tests. A footrest is placed under the patient's feet just distal to the lateral malleoli to block external rotation of the leg, which produces relative internal rotation of the tibia in relation to the femur. Accurate placement of the footrest is important to obtain symmetric tibiofemoral rotation, which is necessary for an accurate test result (Fig. 30–30).

The KT-1000 is applied to the lower leg so that the arrow on the arthrometer is aligned with the tibiofemoral joint line. Additionally, the arthrometer should be slightly rotated on the leg so that compression of the patellar sensor pad against the patella causes the patella to compress directly against the femur, without medial or lateral displacement. The height of the patellar reference pad is adjusted so that the needle on the dial faces the 12-o'clock position. Once the arthrometer is accurately placed, it is secured to the leg by fastening two Velcro straps (Fig. 30–31).

The patient is encouraged to relax by oscillating the tibiofemoral joint. Several posterior pushes are performed to establish the neutral reference position prior to beginning the test. Once the neutral starting position of the tibiofemoral joint has been determined, the dial is rotated so that zero lies under the needle; this indicates the reference-neutral position for the test. Once the zero reference position has been set, the test is conducted by performing successive anterior pulls and posterior pushes through the force-sensing handle (Fig. 30–32). The amount of anterior displacement is recorded with the application of 15, 20, and 30 lb of force, as indicated by the force-sensing handle. Posterior displacement with the posterior push through the force-sensing handle is measured at 15 and 20 lb of force (Fig. 30–10). After each anterior-posterior cycle, the needle on the dial should return to the zero reference position. Failure to return to the zero reference point may indicate that the patient is not fully relaxed or that the arthrometer has moved from its initial starting position. Care should be taken when performing the test to avoid rotating or moving the arthrometer in a superior or inferior direction. The anterior drawer test is also performed with a maximum manual force, which is applied to the posterior aspect of the proximal calf.

The quadriceps active drawer test is performed by having the patient contract the quadriceps with sufficient force just to raise the heel off the table. Both the noninvolved and involved knees are tested.

Side-to-side differences are calculated for each level of force by subtracting translation of the involved side from the noninvolved side (noninvolved minus involved). Positive values are indicative of increased translation on the involved side. A side-to-side difference in anterior or posterior translation less 2 mm is considered normal. A side-to-side difference greater than or equal to 3 mm for anterior translation is considered to be diagnostic for injury to the ACL (Table 30–4).

The above procedure must be modified if the patient is suspected of having a torn PCL. Testing with the KT-1000 for a patient suspected of having injury to the PCL should be performed with the knee in the

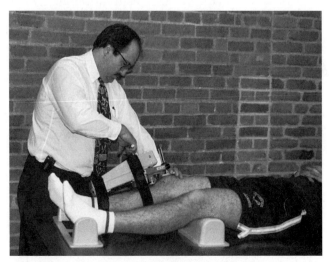

FIGURE 30−32. Anterior and posterior displacement are measured with the KT-1000 arthrometer. (MedMetric, San Diego.)

quadriceps-neutral position. The quadriceps-neutral position is defined as that angle of knee flexion at which contraction of the quadriceps does not result in anterior or posterior translation of the tibia. The quadriceps-neutral position is determined on the noninvolved knee by placing the knee in approximately 70 to 90 degrees of flexion. In this position, the patient is instructed to contract the quadriceps by sliding the heel along the table while translation of the tibia is palpated. The angle of knee flexion is adjusted until no tibial translation is felt to occur with isolated contraction of the quadriceps. Once the quadriceps-neutral angle has been determined, it is measured with a standard goniometer. Daniel and colleagues[57] found that the quadriceps-neutral angle averages 71 degrees.

Once the quadriceps-neutral angle is found, the KT-1000 arthrometer is placed on the leg so that the arrow on the arthrometer is in line with the tibiofemoral joint line. The arthrometer is held in place by securing the Velcro straps. When the arthrometer is secure and in place, the height of the patellar pad is adjusted so that the needle on the dial is directed toward the 12-o'clock position. The dial is adjusted to set the zero reference position for the knee. Anterior and posterior translation of the tibia are measured with 20 lb of force. Additionally, the patient is instructed to contract the quadriceps with the KT-1000 in place to determine the active quadriceps drawer displacement. Once measurements are completed on the noninvolved knee, the involved knee is placed at the same angle of knee flexion as the quadriceps-neutral angle found on the noninvolved knee. The KT-1000 arthrometer is applied to the leg, and anterior and posterior translation at 20 lb of force are measured. Additionally, the active quadriceps drawer is measured by having the patient contract the quadriceps muscle.

The active quadriceps drawer measurements are used to calculate corrected anterior and posterior translation for the noninvolved and involved knees. The corrected posterior drawer is calculated by adding the active quadriceps drawer to the measured posterior drawer. The corrected anterior drawer is calculated by subtracting the active quadriceps drawer from the measured anterior drawer (Fig. 30–33). Side to side differences for corrected anterior and posterior tibial translation are determined by subtracting the involved from the noninvolved knee. A positive value is indicative of more translation on the involved side. A noninvolved-to-

involved difference in corrected posterior translation greater than 3 mm is indicative of injury to the PCL.

Huber[78] found moderate test-retest reliability within and between novice and experienced testers. This was determined on 22 subjects who had a PCL-deficient knee or had undergone PCL reconstruction. Intraclass correlation coefficients (ICCs) for the novice tester were 0.67 for corrected posterior translation, 0.59 for corrected anterior translation, and 0.70 for determination of the quadriceps-neutral angle. For the experienced tester, ICC values were 0.79 for corrected posterior translation, 0.68 for corrected anterior translation, and 0.74 for determination of the quadriceps-neutral angle. Reliability between testers was 0.63 for corrected posterior translation and 0.64 for corrected anterior translation. Standard of error measurements were used to construct 95 percent confidence intervals. For the novice tester, the 95 percent confidence interval for corrected posterior translation was ±3.0 mm, whereas that for the experienced tester was ±1.2 mm. The 95 percent confidence interval between testers for corrected posterior translation was ±2.0 mm. These results indicate that the KT-1000 can be used with moderate reliability to measure anterior and posterior translation in a PCL-deficient knee. Furthermore, the experience of the tester is an important consideration when interpreting the results of the test.

SPECIAL DIAGNOSTIC STUDIES

ARTHROCENTESIS

The role of arthrocentesis following knee injury is to help determine whether an acute effusion is due to a fracture or cruciate ligament injury. Arthrocentesis may be helpful if radiographs are normal, or if a radiograph cannot be obtained, and the clinician's suspicion of fracture is high. In an acute injury, hemarthrosis is the result of a cruciate ligament injury approximately 70 percent of the time.[36] Because the diagnosis can readily be made based on the history, physical examination, and plane radiographs, arthrocentesis is rarely indicated. Aspiration of the fluid reveals nonclotting blood, indicating that it is truly an aspirate from the joint and not an inadvertent aspiration from a blood vessel. If fat globules are present in the aspirate, then the hemarthrosis is a result of an intra-articular fracture. Other sources of acute hemarthrosis include patellar dislocation, retinaculum tears, and peripheral meniscal tears.

Arthrocentesis is also indicated to provide relief of pain associated with large effusions. Performing an arthrocentesis to decompress the joint, followed by installation of 10 to 20 ml of 1 percent xylocaine, may relieve the patient's pain and allow the patient to relax, so that the knee may be thoroughly examined. If the diagnosis can be made by history and physical examination, and the patient is not in severe pain, arthrocentesis is not indicated. Basic research and clinical studies have shown that aspiration of the blood in a traumatically injured joint does not protect the cartilage or affect

TABLE 30–4 Interpretation of Side-to-Side Differences for KT-1000			
Test	Normal (mm)	Equivocal (mm)	Diagnostic (mm)
20-lb anterior drawer	<2	2–2.5	≥3.0
30-lb anterior drawer	<2	2–2.5	≥3.0
Maximum manual anterior drawer	<2	2–2.5	≥3.0

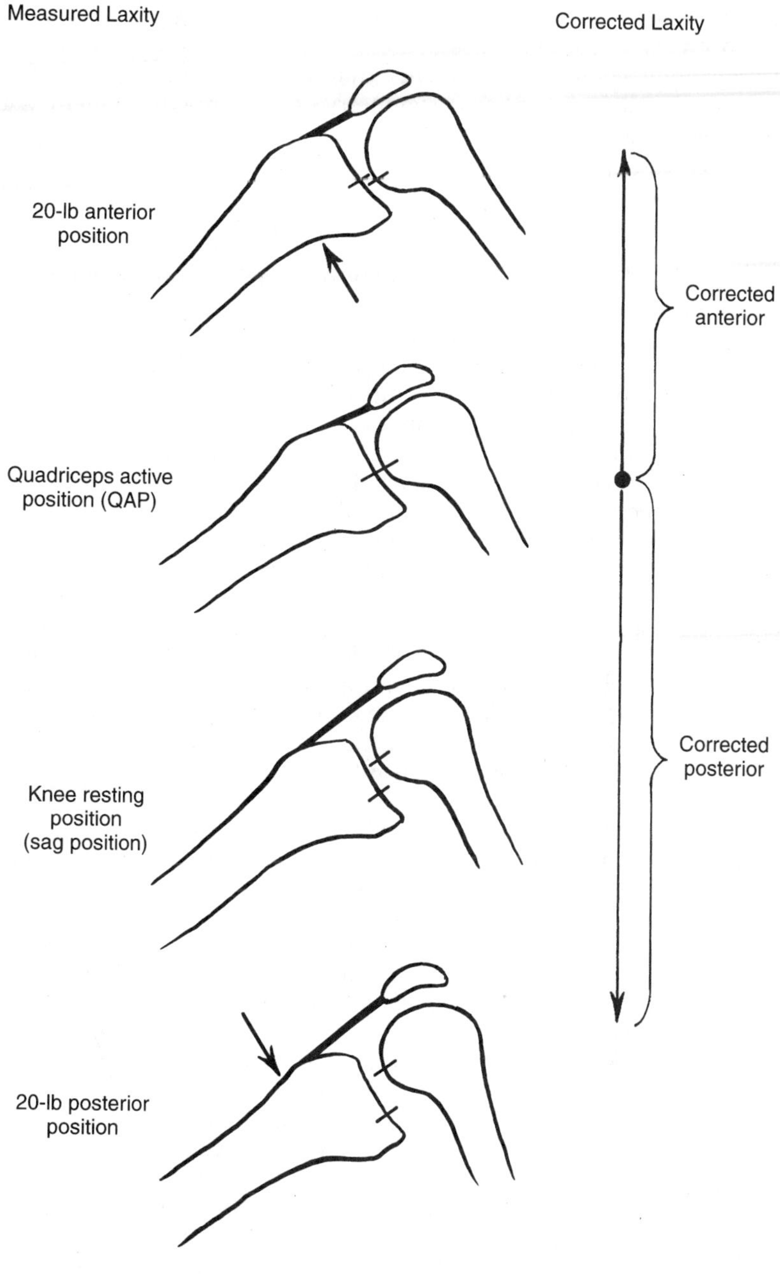

Measured Laxity

Corrected Laxity

20-lb anterior
position

Quadriceps active
position (QAP)

Knee resting
position
(sag position)

20-lb posterior
position

Corrected
anterior

Corrected
posterior

FIGURE 30–33. Use of quadriceps active drawer measurements to calculate corrected anterior and posterior translation in a posterior cruciate ligament (PCl)-deficient knee. The corrected posterior drawer is calculated by adding the active quadriceps drawer to the measured posterior drawer. The corrected anterior drawer is calculated by subtracting the active quadriceps drawer from the measured anterior drawer. (From Daniel DM, Stone ML, Barnett P, Sachs R: Use of the quadriceps active test to diagnose posterior cruciate ligament disruption and measure posterior laxity of the knee. J Bone Joint Surg 1988A; 70:386–391.)

joint stiffness.[79] Furthermore, this procedure is not without risk of introducing an infection to the knee joint.

In the chronic knee, arthrocentesis is indicated for nontraumatic or subacute injuries to rule out infection and inflammatory or crystalline arthropathy. In these cases, the fluid is evaluated for viscosity, color, cell count and differential, crystals, culture and sensitivity, and Gram stain.

RADIOGRAPHY

Radiographs of the knee should be obtained after any acute trauma. If the trauma is severe and the patient complains of pain when the knee is moved, radiographs should be obtained before physical examination begins. Fractures must be ruled out before the knee is manipulated because displacement of the fracture may cause

damage to other structures, including neurovascular structures.

Our standard radiographic series for the knee includes a flexion weight-bearing anteroposterior (AP) and lateral and skyline views. Because ligaments and menisci are radiolucent, radiography is used, for the most part, to exclude other causes of knee pain, swelling, deformity, and/or loss of function. Other radiographs obtained in special circumstances that may be beneficial include a long-cassette. AP weight-bearing, long-cassette radiograph to assess alignment, stress radiographs in cases of suspected ligamentous or physical injury, a cross-table lateral to look for hemarthrosis with a fat-fluid level, which is an indication of a fracture, and external and internal rotation views to look for loose bodies or oblique fracture lines. When viewing standard radiographs of the knee, the examiner should look for any obvious intra-articular or osteochondral fractures, calcification, joint space narrowing, epiphyseal damage, osteophytes or lipping, loose bodies, tumors, accessory ossification centers, alignment deformity (varus-valgus), patellar alta or baja, asymmetry of the femoral condyles, and dislocations. Secondary signs can be seen on plane radiographs to help diagnose ligamentous or meniscal injury.

Soft tissue swelling as seen on radiographs is helpful when those structures that are injured are surrounded by fat. An MCL injury may only reveal soft tissue swelling on the medial aspect of the knee. A bloody effusion, often associated with intra-articular ligament damage, is detected as a soft tissue density in the suprapatellar pouch on the lateral view. The presence of fat in the effusion or lipohemarthrosis suggests a fracture (osteochondral or intra-articular) and is identified as a fat-fluid level on a cross-table lateral projection. Although fat globules are occasionally seen in many other types of effusions, the accumulation of fat is much greater in cases of trauma.[80] Meniscal tears, although often associated with effusions, do not produce as large an effusion as a cruciate ligament disruption or intra-articular fracture. Furthermore, the timing of the radiograph to injury is important, because cruciate ligament injuries are associated with acute effusions, but meniscal tears usually do not produce a significant effusion for at least 12 hours.

Although extensive fractures about the knee are readily identified by standard radiographs, careful evaluation of the films may be required to detect avulsion injuries at the attachment sites of ligaments. This is particularly true of children, in whom cruciate ligament injuries frequently involve avulsion fractures. An avulsion of the ACL insertion may be seen on the flexion AP radiograph or on the lateral view by identifying the displaced fragment superior and anterior to the tibial spine.[81] The Segond fracture, also known as the lateral capsular sign, is an avulsion fracture of the lateral capsule posterior to the Gerdy tubercle on the proximal lateral tibia.[82] This fracture, seen on AP radiographs, is an indirect sign of ACL injury. The thin fragment of bone is vertically oriented and is located proximal and anterior to the fibular head and should not to be confused with a lateral ligamentous injury (see later). Avulsion of the tibial insertion of the PCL may be seen on lateral roentgenograms in the posterior intercondylar area. A PCL avulsion may be a small flake of bone or a large bony fragment. Lateral ligamentous injury may be identified on an AP or external rotation view as an avulsion of the biceps femoris or LCL insertion from the fibular head. Uncommonly, the MCL or LCL may avulse from the femoral condyle with a bony fragment. These injuries can be identified on AP radiographs.

Chronic knee injuries may also produce abnormal findings on radiographs. A chronic MCL injury may result in calcification at the site of injury. When this occurs at the femoral origin of the MCL, it is called Pelligrini-Stieda disease. Although the natural history of isolated cruciate ligament injuries is debated, most authors agree that, if untreated, the unstable knee develops degenerative osteoarthritic changes. Osteoarthritic change in the cruciate-deficient knee tends to occur first in the medial compartment, but the compartment with meniscal pathology often develops degenerative changes. This is best seen on 45 degrees flexion weight-bearing posteroanterior radiographs.[83] Degenerative changes identified on radiographs in a patient with a history of trivial trauma with signs of possible meniscal pathology may be suggestive of a degenerative meniscal tear.

Stress radiography has been advocated for knee ligament injuries, but this is difficult to carry out following acute trauma.[84] In chronic injury or in the anesthetized patient, these radiographs are more easily obtained and can be valuable. In children with varus or valgus instability, these films can differentiate between ligamentous disruption and a Salter I physeal fracture (fracture through the growth plate without displacement). Stress radiography is particularly popular in Europe to document knee instability in the sagittal and frontal planes,[85-89] but is not used as often in the United States. Using stress radiographs, the examiner can measure the anteroposterior displacement and medial and lateral joint space opening, including the relative position between the two compartments, to help diagnose knee ligament injuries.

ARTHROGRAPHY

Traditionally, single- and double-contrast arthrography was the "gold standard" for evaluating the menisci and plica and, to a lesser extent, the cruciate ligaments and articular surfaces.[40,90-95] This procedure is limited in that it is an uncomfortable, invasive procedure requiring a great deal of expertise to perform and interpret and exposes the patient to irradiation. Its use was prevalent prior to the advent of arthroscopy and magnetic resonance imaging (MRI). As a result, arthrography has largely been replaced by these two studies in most centers, but there are still specialized situations in which arthrography may be used to answer a specific question or in areas where the availability or quality of MRI is limited.

RADIONUCLIDE SCINTIGRAPHY

Radionuclide scintigraphy uses technetium-99 methylene diphosphonate (MDP) to screen for a variety of abnormalities. In general, the scintigram reflects the relative blood flow to an area as well as the degree of bone turnover (osteogenesis and osteolysis). The test is sensitive but nonspecific. It provides more information about osseous physiology than structural characteristics. The technique has traditionally been used to evaluate arthritic joints, stress fractures, tumors, osteonecrosis, infection, osteolysis, metabolic or metastatic bone disease, and reflex sympathetic dystrophy. Increased osseous metabolic activity as determined by scintigraphy has also been seen with knee disorders previously considered to involve only soft tissue failure, including symptomatic tears of the ACL.[96-103]

ULTRASONOGRAPHY

Ultrasonography has been used to evaluate various structures of the knee, including the menisci and the ligaments.[104] It is most useful in the evaluation of patellar tendinitis and partial patellar tendon tears. This technique is technician-dependent and, although inexpensive, has not been popularized for routine use for the evaluation of ligamentous and meniscal injuries. It is used in the United States primarily for evaluating patellar tendinitis and masses about the knee.

COMPUTED TOMOGRAPHY

Ever since the early application of computed tomography (CT) to the musculoskeletal system, this technique has been used to evaluate many disorders of the knee.[105-107] CT scanning, however, is best used for bony detail, because soft tissue detail is better with MRI or arthroscopy. Many conflicting descriptions have been reported with respect to the need for and type of intra-articular contrast material and patient positioning in the CT scanner. Thus, the clinical application of CT scanning following meniscal and ligamentous injury is currently not widely accepted.

MAGNETIC RESONANCE IMAGING

In the past, arthrography was frequently used to evaluate intra-articular structures of the knee, but now MRI has virtually replaced the arthrogram. MRI provides a sensitive, noninvasive, nonionizing radiation means for evaluating the structural integrity of the knee. This test is particularly helpful for visualizing soft tissue structures. Initially, MRI met some resistance because initial studies were less accurate than double-contrast arthrography, and the procedure was time-consuming and expensive.[108-111] Improvements in hardware and software, as well as increasing expertise in the interpretation of these studies, have overcome these problems, and MRI has become the procedure of choice for evaluating acute knee injuries.[112-117] Partial and complete tears of ligaments and menisci, as well as other pathologic changes, such as bone bruises and effusions, can be identified with MRI. Evaluation of the knee by MRI is reader-dependent, but its accuracy approaches 100 percent in diagnosing lesions of the PCL, ACL, medial meniscus, and lateral meniscus, with the lateral meniscus the least accurate.[113,115,117-120] Some clinicians believe that this technique is overused,[37] and in the future may be limited due to its expense. Nonetheless, MRI can help diagnose injuries when the patient cannot relax for an adequate examination and can provide a more complete evaluation of the knee than that limited to history, physical examination, and plane radiography. Use of the MRI has aided in identifying a new finding, bone "bruises" in patients with an ACL-deficient knee,[97] which may help play a role in understanding the natural history of this injury.

Our current medical indications for an MRI include the following: (1) an acutely injured knee in which an ACL tear is likely but it is unclear whether the patient has associated meniscal pathology, and the patient is considering nonoperative treatment for the torn ACL; (2) complete evaluation for preoperative planning of the multiple ligament-injured knee; (3) an unclear diagnosis based on history, physical examination, and plane radiography; (4) the patient who cannot relax or cooperate during physical examination; (5) a clinical course not commensurate with the clinical diagnosis; (6) a high-level athlete with an acute injury and in need of an immediate, thorough evaluation to determine the extent of injury and the need for surgical or nonoperative treatment; (7) evaluation for a discoid meniscus in a child with knee pain; (8) evaluation of an occult fracture; and (9) investigation of the cause of poor range of motion following ligament reconstruction surgery. Other uses of MRI include evaluation for soft tissue masses, tumors, osteonecrosis, osteochondritis dissecans, and extensor mechanism injuries, including tendinitis.

ARTHROSCOPY

Arthroscopy is currently the most commonly performed orthopaedic procedure in the United States. Arthroscopy allows for direct visualization of all intra-articular structures. It can be used to diagnose and surgically treat lesions of the knee. For many acute knee injuries, the best opportunity for complete recovery is with prompt and appropriate surgical treatment. Thus, the benefit to performing arthroscopy is that all pathology can be correctly identified and treated as needed. Arthroscopy uses smaller incisions than open surgery, allows better visualization with less morbidity, and can be performed without the use of a tourniquet. Partial tears of the ACL sometimes cannot be differentiated from complete tears, even with an examination under anesthesia. Using arthroscopy, the surgeon can determine whether the ACL is partially or completely torn. Furthermore, if the ligament is partially torn, the extent of injury can be ascertained and guide treatment. Arthroscopy can also be used to evaluate meniscal pathology and determine whether the lesion should be left alone, repaired, or excised. It has also been shown that complete isolated PCL disruptions may have a negative posterior drawer sign, even under anesthesia, but can be diagnosed with arthroscopy.[121]

Arthroscopy, although invasive, is a relatively low-risk procedure, with a complication rate less than 1 percent and an infection rate of approximately 0.1 percent.[122,123] Although there is also the risk of anesthesia, some authors have found local anesthesia to be effective and safe.[124-128] This is important, because several investigators are evaluating the efficacy of diagnostic and therapeutic office arthroscopy. Nonetheless, because some patients do not want surgery and that MRI is an effective, noninvasive, no-risk procedure, with a high level of sensitivity, specificity, and accuracy, diagnostic arthroscopy has been largely replaced by MRI.

EPIDEMIOLOGY, BIOMECHANICS, AND CLASSIFICATION OF KNEE LIGAMENT INJURIES

STRAIGHT PLANE VS. ROTATORY INSTABILITIES

There is much confusion regarding the terminology used to classify knee ligament injuries. This partially stems from the use of inappropriate terminology to describe and classify movement of the knee. Noyes and colleagues[129] defined terms that should be used to describe motion and position of the knee. Motion of the knee is accompanied by rotation and translation of the joint surfaces. Translation refers to movement that results when all points of an object move along paths parallel to each other. A fixed point on one surface engages successive points on the opposing surface, much like a tire sliding on an ice patch when the brakes are locked. In the knee, translation of the tibia is composed of three independent components known as translational degrees of freedom—medial-lateral translation, anterior-posterior translation, and proximal-distal translation. Translation of the tibia is commonly reported in millimeters of motion.

Rotation occurs when successive points on a given surface meet successive points on an adjacent surface. The surface appears to be going in circles about an axis of rotation. Rotation of the joint is similar to a tire rolling down a road. In the knee, there are three independent degrees of freedom for rotation. Flexion and extension rotation occurs in the sagittal plane about an axis located through the femur, which lies in the coronal plane. Abduction and adduction rotation occurs in the coronal plane through an axis located in the sagittal plane. Internal and external rotation of the knee occurs in the transverse plane around a vertical axis, which is located near the posterior cruciate ligament. Rotation of the knee is measured in degrees of motion.

Motion of the knee involves a complex combination of rotation and translation of the joint surfaces. According to the convex-concave rule, flexion of the knee is associated with posterior translation and rotation of the tibia. When the tibia is fixed, flexion of the knee occurs as posterior rotation and anterior translation of the femur. Extension of the knee involves anterior rotation and translation of the tibia. When the tibia is fixed, extension of the knee involves anterior rotation and posterior translation of the femur. This combination of rotation and translation is necessary to keep the femur centered over the tibial plateaus throughout the range of motion. As described earlier, rotation and translation of the joint surfaces during movement of the knee are controlled by the geometry of the joint surfaces as well as by tension in the ligamentous structures. Disruption of ligamentous structures alters the normal arthrokinematics of the knee and may lead to progressive degeneration of the joint surfaces.

The terms *laxity* and *instability* are often used interchangeably. The meaning of these terms must be clarified to improve communication among health care professionals when evaluating and treating knee ligament injuries. Laxity can be used to indicate slackness or lack of tension in a ligament or to describe looseness of a joint. Laxity is also used to indicate the amount of joint motion or play that results with the application of forces and moments. Laxity of a joint can be normal or abnormal. Therefore, the adjective *abnormal* should be used to indicate when laxity is pathologic. Additionally, laxity can refer to either translation or rotation, and this should be clearly specified. For example, anterior laxity of the knee can refer to either anterior translation or rotation of the tibia. If anterior laxity is used to describe translation of the tibia, it is preferable to use the more precise term *anterior translation.* The amount of laxity is often recorded as the difference between the involved and noninvolved knees and this should be clearly indicated. Owing to ambiguity in its use, Noyes and associates[129] recommend that laxity not be used to describe joint motion or displacement. They recommended using the term in a more general sense to indicate slackness or lack of tension in a ligament. When referring to motion of the knee, it is preferable to describe the specific motion as translation or rotation.

Noyes and coworkers[130] indicate that the term *instability* can be used to describe the symptom of giving way or the physical sign of increased mobility of the joint. To avoid ambiguity, they recommend avoiding use of instability to indicate an episode of giving way. They prefer to use it to indicate a physical sign that is characterized by an increase or excessive displacement of the tibia resulting from traumatic injury to the stabilizing structures.

Ligamentous injury to the knee results in varying degrees of abnormal laxity or instability, as described. Hughston[131] classified instability that arises as a result of a knee ligament injury as straight plane or rotatory instability.

A straight plane instability implies injury to the posterior cruciate ligament, allowing for equal translation of the medial and lateral tibial plateaus. According to Hughston, straight plane instabilities include posterior, anterior, medial, and lateral. Posterior instability occurs with injury to the posterior cruciate ligament combined with injury to the arcuate complex and posterior oblique ligament. This results in equal posterior translation of the medial and lateral tibia plateaus when a posterior drawer force is applied. Straight anterior instability occurs with a tear of the anterior and posterior cruciate ligaments along with the medial and lateral capsular ligaments. With a straight anterior instability, both tibial plateaus sublux anteriorly an equal amount when an anterior drawer test is performed. Straight medial instability occurs with a tear of the medial compartment ligaments as well as the posterior cruciate ligament. This results in a positive valgus stress test with the knee in full extension. Straight lateral instability occurs with a tear of the lateral compartment ligaments and the posterior cruciate ligament. This results in a positive varus stress test when the knee is in full extension.

A rotatory instability results when the posterior cruciate ligament is intact. With an intact posterior cruciate ligament, attempts to translate the tibia result in rotation of the tibia about the intact posterior cruciate ligament. As a result, rotatory instabilities involve unequal movement of the medial and lateral tibial plateaus. According to Hughston,[131] rotatory instabilities include anteromedial, anterolateral, and posterolateral. Anteromedial rotatory instability occurs when the medial compartment ligaments, including the posterior oblique ligament, are torn. Anteromedial rotatory instability may be accentuated by a tear of the anterior cruciate ligament. With anteromedial rotatory instability, valgus stress testing at 30 degrees of flexion is positive. Additionally, there is increased anterior translation of the medial tibial plateau when an anterior drawer test is performed with the tibia externally rotated, and the medial pivot shift test may be positive.

Anterolateral rotatory instability occurs with injury to the middle third of the lateral capsular ligaments and is accentuated by a tear of the anterior cruciate ligament. With anterolateral instability, an anterior drawer test results in increased anterior translation of the lateral tibial plateau. Additionally, the lateral pivot shift test is also positive.

Posterolateral rotatory instability implies greater posterior translation of the lateral tibial plateau compared with the medial tibial plateau when a posterior drawer force is applied. Posterolateral instability occurs with a tear of the arcuate complex, which results in a positive varus stress test at 30 degrees of flexion. Additionally, the external rotation recurvatum test is positive.

Combined rotatory instabilities, such as anteromedial and anterolateral rotatory instability, can also occur.

Butler and colleagues[5] developed the concept of primary and secondary ligamentous restraints. For each plane of motion of the knee, there is one ligamentous structure that serves as the primary restraint. This structure is responsible for restraining the majority of motion in a given direction. For example, the anterior cruciate ligament is the primary restraint for anterior translation of the tibia, providing approximately 85 percent of the restraining force.[5] Secondary restraints are those structures that take on a secondary role in restraining motion in a particular direction. For example, the secondary restraints for anterior tibial translation include the collateral ligaments, middle portion of the medial and lateral capsule, and iliotibial band. These are responsible for providing approximately 15 percent of the total restraining force to anterior translation of the tibia.[5]

The amount of ligamentous laxity or instability following injury to the ligamentous structures of the knee is dependent on the extent of injury and on the amount of force applied. Injury to the primary restraint with intact secondary restraints may result in a minimal increase in laxity during manual examination of the knee. If both the primary and secondary restraints are injured or stretched, however, clinical tests for laxity may demonstrate a large increase in motion compared with the noninvolved side. For example, isolated injury to the anterior cruciate ligament may result in only a slight increase in anterior tibial translation if the secondary restraints are intact. Over time, with repeated episodes of giving way, the secondary restraints may stretch out, resulting in increased anterior tibial translation. It is important to note that the secondary stabilizers are not as effective as the primary stabilizers in restraining motion in a particular direction. Therefore, over time, the secondary restraints tend to stretch out gradually when the primary restraint has been lost.

Another important consideration when performing and interpreting a clinical laxity test is the amount of force applied to the knee. Forces applied during a clinical laxity test are small, ranging from 20 to 40 lb. This is much less than the forces during in vivo activities, which may exceed 100 lb with strenuous exercise.[5] As a result, clinical laxity tests may not accurately describe stability of the knee when performing strenuous physical activities. The clinical laxity test may only demonstrate a slight degree of increased laxity. When performing more strenuous activities, higher loads are placed on the knee, which may result in greater laxity and in complaints of giving way.

ANTERIOR CRUCIATE LIGAMENT

The ACL is one of the most commonly injured ligaments in the knee. Some studies suggest that the ACL is the most commonly injured ligament in the general population.[132–134] Other investigators, however, believe that of all knee ligament injuries, including those that do not result in pathologic motion (grades I and II injuries), the MCL is the most commonly injured ligament.[132] The ACL is the primary stabilizer for resisting anterior translation of the tibia on the femur and serves to control hyperextension of the knee. The ACL also serves as a secondary stabilizer to resist internal and external rotation as well as varus and valgus stress. The ACL can be injured by contact or noncontact mechanisms of injury. Pathomechanics include a valgus force applied to a flexed, externally rotated knee with the foot planted, or hyperextension, often combined with internal rotation. Less common mechanisms of injury include hyperflexion or a direct valgus force. A direct valgus force may produce a tear of the MCL, ACL, and medial meniscus, which is known as the O'Donoghue triad.

Daniel and associates[135] reported that the incidence of acute anterior cruciate ligament injuries in a managed health care plan was 31 per 100,000 members annually. Ninety percent of anterior cruciate ligament injuries occurred in patients aged 15 to 45. The majority of ACL injuries occur as a result of sports activities, particularly those that place high demands on the knee (e.g., those involving jumping and hard cutting).

There is mounting evidence indicating that a narrow intercondylar notch width may place a patient at greater risk of injury. LaPraide and Burnett[136] reported a higher incidence of acute anterior cruciate ligament injuries in individuals with a narrow notch width index. The notch width index is defined as the ratio of the width of the anterior outlet of the intercondylar notch divided by the total condylar width at the level of the popliteal groove. Their prospective study involved 213 athletes at a Division I university, representing 415

ACL-intact knees.[136] Intercondylar notch stenosis was found in 40 knees (notch width index, less than 0.20), and 375 individuals had a normal notch width index. During the 2-year follow-up period, seven ACL injuries occurred, with six in knees with a narrow notch and one in a knee with a normal notch width. Souryal and Freyman[137] demonstrated similar results in 902 high school athletes followed prospectively. The overall rate of ACL injury during the 2-year follow-up was 3 percent. Athletes sustaining noncontact ACL tears had a statistically smaller notch width index. Of the 14 athletes with noncontact ACL injuries, 10 had a notch width index at least 1 SD below the mean.

At this time, no data support the premise that poor conditioning or increased physiologic laxity places an individual at greater risk for ACL injury, but women may be at higher risk for such an injury. Malone[138] reported that women participating in NCAA Division I basketball were eight times more likely than their male counterparts to sustain an ACL injury. Further research is needed to identify factors that may place women at higher risk for ACL injury.

Seventy-five percent of ACL ruptures occur in the midsubstance, whereas 20 percent are injuries involving the femoral attachment and 5 percent involve the tibial attachment.[139] Associated injuries include meniscal tears in 50 to 70 percent of acutely injured knees and up to 90 percent in chronic, ACL-deficient knees,[36,121,140] chondral injuries in 6 to 20 percent of ACL-injured knees,[36,121] collateral ligament injuries in 40 to 75 percent of ACL-injured knees,[140,141] and occasionally capsular injuries and knee dislocations.

The patient often relates an audible crack or pop at the time of initial injury. The patient also notes swelling within the first 2 to 6 hours and an inability to continue the activity.

Classification of knee ligament injuries is based on the extent of the tear and resulting degree of laxity. A grade I sprain involves a microscopic partial tear of the ligament, which overall remains intact. The ligament fibers are stretched, causing hemorrhage and microscopic disruption of the structure within the ligament. Examination of a grade I ACL sprain reveals no increased laxity compared with the contralateral knee, and the end point is firm. A second-degree sprain is also a partial tear, although the injury results in partial loss of function as determined by a slight increase in anterior translation with specific testing of the ligament (i.e., Lachman test or anterior drawer test), but a definite end point is noted, and the pivot shift is negative. A grade II ACL sprain may represent macroscopic or microscopic tearing, resulting in hemorrhage and stretching of the ligament, but it is still in continuity and functions to some degree. A third-degree sprain is a complete tear of the ligament. There is loss of ligament function, loss of joint stability, a 2+ to 3+ Lachman and anterior drawer, and a positive pivot shift test. Anterior translation of the tibia is excessive, and the end point is soft.

The natural history of an ACL-deficient knee is still unclear. The torn ACL does not heal.[142,143] ACL deficiency leads to rotatory instability in many patients and results in functional disability. This can occur with activities of daily living in some, with sports activities such as running (deceleration), cutting, and jumping in others, and with no functional instability in still another undetermined group. Repetitive episodes of instability may result in meniscal tears, which can result in arthritis. Debate exists as to whether isolated ACL tears, without meniscal pathology, result in degenerative changes within the knee joint.[49,133,135,140,142,144,145] ACL-deficient patients who undergo meniscectomy without ACL reconstruction, however, develop degenerative changes at a more rapid rate. A direct relationship exists between giving way (instability) and activity level, but many patients with an ACL-deficient knee can return to sports at a less stressful level of activity. Furthermore, functional instability may also be related to meniscal pathology. As discussed later, meniscal injury directly relates to the level of disability, pain, swelling, and frequency of reinjury.

POSTERIOR CRUCIATE LIGAMENT

Although the true incidence of PCL injuries remains unknown, injury to the PCL is thought to account for 3 to 20 percent of all knee injuries.[132,146,147] The PCL is the strongest ligament in the knee,[148] and as such, a significant force is required to rupture it. Most PCL injuries occur as a result of athletic, motor vehicle, or industrial accidents. The mechanism of most athletic PCL injuries is a fall on the flexed knee with the foot and ankle plantarflexed.[59,149] This imparts a posteriorly directed force on the proximal tibia, which ruptures the taut ligament that is parallel to the force vector, usually resulting in an isolated PCL injury.[150] Similarly, in a motor vehicle accident, the knee is flexed, and the tibia is forced posteriorly on impact with the dashboard. Another mechanism of injury to the PCL is a downwardly directed force applied to the thigh while the knee is hyperflexed, such as when landing from a jump.[151] Hyperflexion of the knee without a direct blow to the tibia can also result in an isolated PCL injury.[152]

Other mechanisms can result in injury to the PCL, but these usually also involve injury to other ligaments. Forced hyperextension can injure the PCL, but generally this also results in injury to the ACL.[146] A posteriorly directed force applied to the anteromedial tibia with the knee in hyperextension may also cause injury to the posterolateral corner,[146] and results in lateral and posterolateral instability. Significant varus or valgus stress injures the PCL only after rupture of the appropriate collateral ligament. Thus, when the PCL is torn, the integrity of the rest of the knee must be carefully evaluated as well.

Seventy percent of PCL disruptions occur on the tibial side, with or without an associated bony fragment, 15 percent occur on the femoral side, and 15 percent involve midsubstance tears.[139] Associated injuries with acute "isolated" PCL tears include chondral defects in 12 percent and meniscal tears in 27 percent, which occur more commonly in the lateral compartment.[153] As with chronic ACL tears, there is a greater incidence of meniscal and chondral lesions in the chronic PCL-deficient knee,[153] although in contrast to acute injuries, these more commonly involve the medial compartment.

The patient often relates an audible crack or pop at the time of the initial injury. The patient also notes mild to moderate swelling within the first 2 to 6 hours, but unlike ACL injuries, these individuals may return to activity and the injury is often thought to be a minor event.

As with the classification of ACL injuries, grading of PCL injuries depends on the extent of the tear and degree of resulting laxity. A grade I PCL sprain involves microscopic partial tearing of the ligament, which overall remains intact. The ligament fibers are stretched, causing hemorrhage and microscopic disruption of the ligament. Examination of a grade I PCL injury reveals no increased laxity compared with the contralateral knee, and the end point is firm. A second-degree sprain is also a partial tear, although the injury results in partial loss of function as determined by a slight increase in posterior translation during a posterior drawer, but a definite end point is noted, and the reverse pivot shift is negative. This may be a macroscopic or microscopic tear resulting in hemorrhage and stretching of the ligament, but it is still in continuity and functions to some degree. A third-degree sprain of the PCL is a complete tear of the ligament. There is loss of ligament function and loss of joint stability, with a 2+ to 3+ posterior drawer, and a positive posterior sag, Godfrey sign, quadriceps active drawer, and reverse pivot shift test. Posterior tibial translation is excessive, and the end point is soft.

The natural history of the PCL-deficient knee is controversial. Some patients experience almost no functional limitation and compete in high-level athletics, whereas others are severely limited during activities of daily living.[149,152,154–156] If adequate quadriceps strength can be obtained, Parolie and Bergfeld[149] suggests that most patients do well with nonoperative treatment. Dejour and coworkers[155] suggested that patients are symptomatic for the first 12 months, during which time they learn to adapt to the PCL injury. After this time, patients do well, with a high percentage returning to sports. They also reported[155] the development of degenerative changes involving the medial and anterior compartment in chronic PCL-deficient knees, but this finding has not been reported by others.[59,149,154] Laboratory studies confirm that PCL deficiency results in increased medial compartment and patellofemoral contact pressures that can result in arthritis of the knee.[157] It is unclear whether surgical reconstruction can alter the development of long-term degenerative changes. Furthermore, it appears that in some patients, the PCL may heal, although in a lengthened position.[158] This may explain the variable results of long-term studies of the PCL-deficient knee.

MEDIAL COLLATERAL LIGAMENT

As noted earlier, the MCL is the most commonly injured ligament in the knee.[132] The incidence of grade III injuries to the MCL, however, may be lower than those to the ACL.[132] The MCL is injured by a valgus stress to the knee that exceeds the strength of the MCL. This most commonly occurs from a blow to the lateral aspect of the knee during a sporting event. Uncommonly, a noncontact valgus injury to the knee, such as that which occurs in skiing, can produce an isolated tear of the MCL.

MCL injuries most commonly involve the femoral insertion site, which accounts for approximately 65 percent of all MCL sprains. Of all MCL sprains, 25 percent involve the tibial insertion. The remaining 10 percent of MCL injuries involve a deep portion of the MCL at the level of the joint line.[139] Associated tears of the medial meniscus occur in 2 to 4 percent of grades I and II MCL sprains, but medial meniscal tears do not occur with grade III MCL sprains.[159–161] This is most likely because compression of the medial compartment is required to tear the medial meniscus, whereas injury to the MCL requires tension that unloads the medial compartment.

The diagnosis of an MCL injury can be made from the history and physical examination alone and usually does not require MRI or arthroscopy. If the physical examination is difficult to perform, however, or damage to other intra-articular structures is suspected, an MRI can be helpful to determine the full extent of the injury. The patient often recalls being hit by another athlete while the foot was planted, feeling the impact on the lateral aspect of the knee and pain on the medial aspect of the knee. Rarely, patients may note a pop at the time of injury, but more commonly state that they felt a tearing or pulling on the medial aspect of the knee. Swelling occurs quickly at the site of injury, and ecchymosis may develop 1 to 3 days following injury. With a first- or second-degree sprain, the patient may be able to continue to play, but with a third-degree sprain the patient usually cannot continue to participate in sports. These patients usually walk with a limp and with the knee partially flexed, because extension stretches the ligament and causes further pain. Patients may not have an effusion if injury is isolated to the MCL.

Classification of MCL sprains depends on the extent of the tear and degree of laxity that results. A grade I sprain involves microscopic tearing of the ligament, which overall remains intact. The ligament fibers are stretched, causing hemorrhage and microscopic disruption of the ligament. Examination of the MCL by the aforementioned tests reveals no increase in laxity compared with the contralateral knee, and the end point is firm. There is, however, tenderness along the ligament. A second-degree sprain of the MCL is also a partial tear, but the injury results in partial loss of function, as determined by a slight degree of increased joint opening with valgus stress testing (3 to 5 mm) with the knee in 30 degrees of flexion, but a definite end point is noted. In full extension, the knee joint opens less than 2 mm more than the contralateral knee. A grade II sprain may represent macroscopic or microscopic tearing, resulting in hemorrhage and stretching of the ligament, but it is still in continuity and functions to some degree. An acute grade II MCL injury is tender to palpation and the patient notes pain with stress testing. A third-degree sprain is a complete tear of the ligament. There is loss of ligament function, with more than 5 mm of joint space opening compared with that of the noninvolved knee with valgus stress testing in 30 degrees of flexion and more than 3 mm of opening compared with the noninvolved knee in full extension. Furthermore, there is no definite end point with stress testing. Significant joint opening in full extension is indicative of medial capsular injury and also of possible injury to the cruciate ligaments. Severity of tenderness does not correlate with the extent of the injury. A third-degree sprain usually hurts less than a second- or first-degree injury.

The natural history of isolated MCL tears is for them to heal, regardless of the degree of injury.[160–166] Patients with proximal injuries involving the femoral insertion tend to have a higher incidence of stiffness. Additionally, proximal MCL injuries heal with less residual laxity as compared with injuries involving the tibial side.

LATERAL COLLATERAL LIGAMENT

Isolated injuries to the LCL of the knee are uncommon. In fact, they tend to be the least common injury to the knee, causing only 2 percent of all knee injuries that result in pathologic motion (grade III injuries).[132] The injury is usually the result of a direct varus stress to the knee, generally with the foot planted and the knee in extension.[167] Injury to the LCL tends to occur as a result of nonsports, high-energy activities,[132,167] because a direct blow to the medial aspect of the knee is an unusual occurrence in sports. Varus stress to the knee may also occur during the stance phase of gait, with sudden imbalance and shift of the center of gravity away from the side of injury resulting in tension on the lateral structures. This mechanism does not require an external force to the knee. Another cause of a varus stress to the knee is a sideswipe injury, in which one knee has a valgus stress and the other a varus stress. The varus injury often has a rotational component involved.

Straight varus injuries result in LCL disruptions. These tend to be tears from the fibular head, with or without avulsion in 75 percent of cases, from the femoral side in 20 percent, and midsubstance tears in 5 percent.[139] Associated peroneal nerve injuries are common (up to 24 percent); because the nerve is tethered as it courses around the fibular head.[167] These nerve palsies have a poor prognosis for complete recovery.[168]

Patients with injury to the LCL may hear or feel a pop in the knee and have lateral knee pain. An intra-articular effusion may represent a capsular injury or an associated meniscal or chondral lesion. Because the LCL is extra-articular, isolated LCL lesions do not commonly result in an effusion of the knee.

Often, LCL injuries occur in association with injury to other ligaments in the knee. A severe varus stress results in an LCL disruption, followed by disruption of the posterolateral capsule and PCL.

Classification of lateral collateral knee ligament sprains is dependent on the extent of the tear and the resulting degree of laxity. A grade I sprain involves microscopic partial tearing of the ligament, but the ligament overall remains intact. The ligament fibers are stretched, causing hemorrhage and microscopic disruption within the ligament. Varus stress testing reveals no increase in laxity compared with the contralateral knee, and the end point is firm, but there is tenderness along the ligament. A second-degree sprain is also a partial tear, but the injury results in partial loss of function as determined by a slight increase in joint opening with varus stress testing compared with the noninvolved knee (3 to 5 mm) with the knee in 30 degrees flexion, but a definite end point is noted. In full extension, the knee joint opens less than 2 mm more than the contralateral knee. A grade II LCL sprain may represent macroscopic or microscopic tearing, resulting in hemorrhage and stretching of the ligament, but it is still in continuity and functions to some degree. A grade II acutely injured LCL is tender to palpation, and the patient notes pain with stress testing. A third-degree sprain is a complete tear of the ligament. There is loss of ligament function, with more than 5 mm of joint space opening compared with the noninvolved knee with varus stress testing in 30 degrees of flexion and 3 mm or more than the non-involved knee in full extension. Furthermore, there is no definite end point with varus stress testing. Palpation of the ligament in the figure-of-four position reveals absence of tension in the ligament proximal to the fibular head.

The natural history of the untreated complete lateral collateral disruption has yet to be determined. Only a few studies with limited subjects have involved isolated LCL injuries. DeLee and colleagues[167] suggested that severe, straight lateral instability with more than 10 mm of joint opening compared with the contralateral knee usually implies that the ACL and/or PCL have been injured. From the few studies that have been reported, it appears that truly isolated LCL injuries do well with nonoperative treatment.[163,166,167]

KNEE DISLOCATIONS AND THE MULTIPLE LIGAMENT-INJURED KNEE

Knee dislocations and other less severe multiple ligamentous injuries make up approximately 20 percent of all grade III knee ligament injuries of the knee.[132] This diverse group of injuries is of variable severity and comorbidity. Other than combined ACL-MCL injuries, combined ligament injuries account for less than 2 percent of all knee ligament injuries.[132] Frequent combinations of two-ligament injury include the ACL-MCL (most common), PCL-MCL, ACL-LCL, and ACL-PCL.

To dislocate the knee, at least three ligaments must be torn.[169,170] Most often, both cruciate ligaments and one collateral ligament are torn to dislocate the knee.

Occasionally, fractures are associated with knee dislocations, but these fracture dislocations are considered a different entity from the dislocated knee and involve injury to only the ligaments. A person may dislocate the knee by simply stepping in a hole and hyperextending the knee (low energy). Dislocations can also result from a high-energy blow to the knee, such as that which with involvement in a motor vehicle accident. We have seen several athletes sustain low-energy knee dislocations during collisions in baseball, rugby, football, and soccer. Neurovascular injury is uncommon with knee injuries that involve only two ligaments. Dislocation of the knee does not occur when only two ligaments have been injured. Furthermore, injury to two ligaments does not result in enough translation of the joint to cause neurovascular injury. The exception to this is the LCL injury combined with a cruciate ligament injury, which results in enough lateral joint opening to produce injury to the peroneal nerve, as noted earlier.

Although the knee can dislocate in any direction, the most common direction is anterior or posterior.[171,172] Knee dislocations may involve damage to multiple structures within the knee, including the cruciate and collateral ligaments, capsular structures, menisci, articular surface, tendons, and neurovascular structures. The nerves and blood vessels in the popliteal space of the knee are easily stretched and torn during dislocation of the knee, and neurovascular injury must be ruled out in all cases. Associated injuries include vascular damage in 20 to 40 percent of all knee dislocations and nerve damage in 20 to 30 percent of knee dislocations. Some series of knee dislocations had an amputation rate of the involved extremity of up to 49 percent.[171,173,174] Posterior knee dislocations are associated with the highest incidence of popliteal artery injury,[171] and posterolateral rotatory dislocations have the highest incidence of nerve injury.[170] There is some evidence suggesting that low-velocity knee dislocations may uncommonly result in neurovascular injury.[175] Osteochondral and meniscal injuries are rare, particularly with low-velocity knee dislocations. This is most likely because a distraction force is required to dislocate the knee, whereas osteochondral and meniscal injuries result from compressive forces.[175]

The patient with a multiple ligament injury frequently gives a history of severe injury to the knee although, as noted earlier, the mechanism may be trivial. A pop is often noted by the patient. Swelling occurs within the first few hours, but it is not always large due to the associated capsular injury and extravasation of the hemarthrosis. The patient may note deformity of the knee if the knee dislocated and remained unreduced. The patient complains of instability and the inability to continue with sports and activities of daily living. Tibiofemoral dislocations are classified by the direction in which the tibia translates in relation to the femur. A knee can dislocate in any direction. For example, if the tibia lies anterior to the femur, the injury is called an anterior dislocation. Posterior, medial, and lateral dislocations of the knee can also occur. Rotatory dislocations occur when the knee dislocates in more than one direction; these include anteromedial, anterolateral, posteromedial, and posterolateral. Unfortunately, knee dislocations can spontaneously reduce, so this classification scheme is not useful. Furthermore, the amount of tibial displacement that occurs at the time of injury cannot be estimated from physical or radiographic findings. It is therefore helpful to describe the dislocated knee by the ligamentous structures that have been disrupted.

The natural history of knee dislocations and multiple ligament injuries is unknown. This is due to the uncommon nature of these injuries as well as to the many types of dislocations and mechanisms of injury (low velocity versus high velocity) that can occur. It is known, however, that vascular injury associated with knee dislocation, if left untreated or not repaired within 8 hours from the time of injury, results in an 86 percent amputation rate. If surgery to correct vascular injury is completed within 6 to 8 hours, the amputation rate is only 11 percent.[171] Associated nerve injury has a poor prognosis for recovery, regardless of the treatment.[176,177] The development of instability, loss of motion, and arthritis is unclear with nonoperative treatment. The level of function of patients with multiple ligament injuries is worse than those with an isolated knee ligament injury. Knee dislocations treated with immobilization and aggressive rehabilitation have surprisingly good results with regard to stability, absence of pain, and the range of knee flexion up to 90 degrees.[178] The incidence of arthritis following multiple ligament injuries has yet to be determined, but increased instability would be expected to result in a greater degree of arthritic changes.

TREATMENT OF KNEE LIGAMENT INJURIES

GUIDELINES FOR PROGRESSION OF REHABILITATION

Progression of the rehabilitation program following knee ligament injury and/or surgery should occur in a logical sequence. Generally, there is overlap in the phases of this progression. For example, muscle function may be addressed before full range of motion and flexibility have been restored. Progression of the patient through the sequence must be individualized and is dependent on the nature of the injury and/or surgery, principles of tissue healing, individual signs and symptoms, and response to treatment. Adequate time must be allowed for tissue healing and remodeling. During rehabilitation, care must be taken to avoid overaggressive treatment, which is indicated by a prolonged increase in pain following treatment and/or regression in the patient's progress.

The initial phase of the rehabilitation program should promote tissue healing and reduce pain and swelling. During this period, modalities such as cold and compression may be beneficial to decrease pain and swelling. There must be a balance between mobility and immobility. The healing tissues must not be overloaded. Overaggressive treatment during this period may disrupt the healing process, but prolonged immobilization may also have adverse effects. Prolonged immobilization is associated with decreased bone mass, changes in articular cartilage, synovial adhesions, and decreased strength and increased stiffness of ligaments and the joint capsule, which leads to joint contracture and loss of motion. Disuse results in atrophy and decreased oxidative capacity of muscle. It appears that immobilization may affect slow muscle fibers more than fast muscle fibers.[179,180]

The time required for soft tissue healing is variable. The response of soft tissue to injury is acute inflammation, which typically lasts for several days or until the noxious stimuli has been neutralized. During this period, cold and compression may be used to limit and control acute inflammation. Inflammation is followed by fibroplasia, which involves the proliferation of fibroblasts and the formation of collagen fibers and ground substance. Fibroplasia usually lasts for several weeks and results in the formation of granulation tissue, which is fragile, vascularized connective tissue. During this period, protected motion is encouraged, because it stimulates collagen formation and alignment. Excessive loading of the healing tissue during this period should be avoided, because it may result in disruption of the healing tissue and reinitiate the inflammatory process. Over time, granulation tissue matures and remodels and can withstand greater loads. This process is gradual and is dependent on stresses imposed on the tissue; Stresses should be gradually and progressively increased to allow the tissues to adapt to the functional demands placed on them.

Rehabilitation of the knee should ensure that full motion symmetric to the uninvolved knee is restored. Loss of motion following knee ligament injury and/or surgery adversely affect function. Loss of extension affects gait and results in patellofemoral symptoms. Loss of flexion interferes with activities such as stair climbing, squatting, and running. In the early phases of rehabilitation, passive, active assisted, and active range of motion exercises can be used to increase and/or maintain motion of the knee. In the latter stages of rehabilitation, active and passive stretching exercises can be used to restore motion. Stretching exercises should be sustained and use low force to maximize creep and relaxation of connective tissue to produce permanent elongation. Application of heat before and during the stretch and maintaining the stretch during cooling may also help produce permanent elongation.[181] Neurophysiologic stretching techniques such as contract-relax or contract relax-contract can help restore motion if the limitation is due to muscular tightness.

Mobilization of the patella also may be helpful in restoring motion. Inferior glide of the patella is necessary for flexion, and superior glide is necessary for normal functioning of the extensor mechanism. Decreased superior mobility of the patella interferes with the ability of the quadriceps to pull through the knee extensor mechanism and results in the development of a knee extensor lag. Medial glide and lateral tilt of the patella are necessary to stretch the lateral retinacular structures. The force used during patellar mobilization must be appropriate for the degree of inflammation present. Overly aggressive patellar mobilization aggravates pain and swelling, which can contribute to loss of motion. Mobilization of the tibiofemoral joint is rarely necessary but can help restore motion if the limitation of motion is due to hypomobility of the tibiofemoral joint.

Rehabilitation following knee ligament injury and/or surgery must restore function of the muscles that cross the knee as well as the muscles that influence segments proximal and distal to the knee. Following acute knee injury or in the immediate postoperative period, emphasis should be on regaining motor control. Often, acute pain and swelling result in inhibition of the quadriceps, and a knee extensor lag develops. During this period, quad sets, straight leg raises (SLR), and isometric hamstring exercises can be performed. Facilitation techniques such as vibration and tapping, as well as biofeedback and electrical stimulation, may be helpful in regaining motor control. Generally, it is more difficult to gain quadriceps control than control of the hamstrings.

Resistive exercises are initiated when the individual has regained full active motion of the knee. Initially, resistive exercises should be performed with light resistance for high repetitions to improve muscle endurance. This minimizes stress on healing structures about the knee and improves the aerobic capacity of slow twitch muscle fibers. OKC exercises can be used to provide isolated exercise for the hamstrings and quadriceps. Precautions must be taken to avoid overloading of healing tissues and development of patellofemoral symptoms. CKC exercises can be used to improve muscle function in functional patterns while minimizing patellofemoral stress. CKC exercises are progressed as tolerated and may include wall slides, minisquats, step-ups, and leg presses. Cycling is an excellent exercise for developing endurance of the lower extremity musculature while minimizing stress on the patellofemoral and tibiofemoral joints. The use of toe clips and pedaling with one leg can help increase hamstring activity. Other forms of endurance exercise for the lower extremity include the use of step machines, cross-country ski machines, and swimming.

In the later phases of rehabilitation, resistive exercises can be progressed to high-resistance, low-repetition exercises to develop muscle strength and power. High-resistance, low-repetition OKC exercises are used to improve isolated muscle strength, but care must be taken to avoid overloading the patellofemoral joint. High-resistance, low-repetition CKC exercises can be used to improve strength in functional patterns with less risk of developing patellofemoral symptoms. Exercises should incorporate both the concentric and eccentric phases of contraction. Concentric muscle function is necessary to accelerate the body while eccentric muscle function is necessary to decelerate the body. During a concentric contraction, the muscle shortens as it contracts, whereas during an eccentric contraction, the muscle elongates as it contracts. The force-velocity relationship is different for concentric and eccentric contractions. During a concentric contraction, muscle force decreases as the speed of shortening increases. During an eccentric contraction, muscle force increases as the speed of lengthening increases. Eccentric contractions produce higher levels of force due to lengthening of the series elastic component and facilitation of the stretch reflex. To ensure full restoration of function, rehabilitation should include concentric and eccentric exercises. Failure to incorporate eccentric exercise in the rehabilitation program results in the development of muscle soreness and an increased risk for reinjury with return to activity.

For athletes who require power to perform their sport, plyometric exercises should be incorporated into the final stages of the rehabilitation program. Plyometric exercises develop power and speed and incorporate lengthening of the muscle immediately before a powerful concentric contraction. These exercises include depth drops and jumps from 6- to 18-inch heights, bounding, hopping, and ricochets. The plyometric program must be carefully planned and implemented to avoid injury.

Once strength and endurance of the lower extremity musculature have been established, it is necessary to develop neuromuscular control to enhance dynamic stability of the knee. This requires learning how to recruit muscles with the proper force, timing, and sequence to prevent abnormal joint motion. Initially, this requires conscious effort, often with the help of biofeedback. Through practice and repetition, control of abnormal joint motion becomes automatic and occurs subconsciously.

Proprioceptive neuromuscular facilitation techniques such as rhythmic stabilization and timing for emphasis may be helpful for developing dynamic stability. A variety of functional activities can also be used to develop dynamic control of abnormal joint motion. These activities are generally progressed from slow to fast speed, from low to high force, and from controlled to uncontrolled activities. Emphasis should be on establishing proper movement patterns to enhance dynamic stability of the joint. Electromyographic biofeedback may be used to ensure that muscles are being recruited in the proper sequence to maintain joint stability. Activities for enhancing dynamic stability progress from walking, jogging-running, acceleration-deceleration, sprinting, jumping, cutting, pivoting, and twisting. Research is needed to determine the effectiveness of these techniques.

ACL INJURIES

Treatment of ACL injuries must be individualized and depends on the extent of pathology as well as on the level of disability experienced by the patient during sports and activities of daily living. As a result, decisions regarding the treatment of the ACL-deficient knee must be made in collaboration with the patient, physician, physical therapist, and athletic trainer. The type of treatment depends on many factors, including age, activity level, occupation, desire to continue sports, amount of functional instability, presence of associated injuries and arthritic changes, and amount of laxity. The willingness of the patient to modify activity to a level compatible with functional stability is the most important factor governing treatment options. Factors associated with a good outcome of nonoperative treatment include intact collateral ligaments, absence of meniscal injury and/or arthritis, and participation in low-demand sports that do not require running, jumping, or cutting.

Another factor mitigating against a surgical approach include a minimal increase in tibial translation with laxity testing. Surgical reconstruction of the ACL-deficient knee should be considered if instability of a knee prevents the patient from participating in sports and other activities. Additionally, surgery should be considered if there is associated collateral ligament damage or meniscal injury, or if there is a large increase in anterior tibial translation with laxity testing. Surgery should also be considered in most patients who have high expectations and plan to compete in sports that place high demands on the knee.

Partial tears of the ACL involving greater than 50 percent of the ligament are more likely to progress to complete tears if treated nonsurgically.[129] In general, however, there is little correlation between the percentage of the tear and clinical outcome.[129] ACL tears in skeletally immature individuals are more common than previously suspected. Initially, these patients are usually treated nonoperatively. If functional instability persists after rehabilitation, consideration must be given to reconstruction of the ACL. Skeletal immaturity is no longer an absolute contraindication to ACL reconstruction, but the patient must be followed closely to ensure that growth has not been arrested.

NONOPERATIVE TREATMENT. Nonoperative treatment following injury to the ACL may be indicated for those who had an isolated injury without damage to other structures and who are willing to modify their lifestyle to avoid activities that cause pain, swelling, and/or episodes of instability. Nonoperative treatment of ACL injuries does not mean that the injury is ignored. Treatment should actively involve the patient and includes exercise, functional training, bracing, and patient education.

Treatment following acute injury to the ACL should focus on resolving inflammation, restoring range of motion, regaining muscle control, and protecting the knee from further injury. Cold and compression can be used to decrease pain and swelling. Range of motion exercises should be performed to restore motion, which should improve as pain and swelling subside. Failure to regain motion, particularly extension, may indicate a torn meniscus and further diagnostic studies and/or surgery may be indicated. Isometric exercises for the quadriceps and hamstrings should be initiated to regain motor control and minimize atrophy. Assistive devices should be used for ambulation while the knee is still actively inflamed. The use of assistive devices can be discontinued once the patient has regained full extension without a quadriceps lag and can walk normally without gait deviations.

More aggressive rehabilitation can begin once inflammation has resolved and full range of motion has been restored. The emphasis at this time should be on improving strength and endurance of muscles that cross the knee. Particular emphasis should be placed on muscles that pull the tibia posteriorly (i.e., the hamstrings and gastrocnemius). The normal quadricep-to-hamstring ratio at a slow contractile velocity is approximately 3:2. It has been suggested that rehabilitation of an ACL-deficient knee should strive to develop a hamstring-dominant knee so that the hamstring-to-quadriceps ratio approaches 1:1. This seems to be a logical goal for rehabilitation of ACL injuries, but it should not be achieved at the expense of quadriceps weakness.

OKC and CKC exercises can be used to improve strength and endurance. OKC exercises can be used to provide isolated exercise for the hamstrings and quadriceps. Precautions must be taken to avoid the development of patellofemoral symptoms with OKC knee extension. Standing and seated calf raises can be used to develop the gastrocnemius and soleus, respectively. CKC exercises can be used to develop strength and endurance of the muscles of the lower extremity in functional patterns while minimizing patellofemoral stress. CKC exercises are progressed as tolerated.

Once strength and endurance of the lower extremity muscles have been established, it is necessary to develop neuromuscular control to enhance dynamic stability of the knee. Emphasis should be placed on learning to recruit the posterior muscles to minimize anterior subluxation of the tibia. The patient should be taught to "set" the hamstrings and gastrocnemius prior to foot strike.

Coactivation of the antagonist during contraction of the agonist has been proposed by Sherington.[182] Baratta and colleagues[14], and Draganich and associates[15] demonstrated coactivation of the hamstrings during resisted OKC knee extension. Antagonist-agonist coactivation probably originates from the motor cortex in the phenomenon known as direct common drive.[183] Activation of the muscle spindle can also facilitate contraction of the antagonist.[10] As the knee extends, muscle spindles lying within the hamstrings are activated and facilitate contraction. Training the hamstrings to stabilize the knee dynamically should capitalize on the phenomenon of coactivation.

A functional brace may be helpful as the patient returns to activity. It is unclear exactly how knee braces work, but many patients report improved function with the use of a knee brace. It is doubtful whether functional braces provide a physical restraint to abnormal joint motion. Several studies[184–187] have indicated that knee braces may restrain tibial translation at low force levels, but are ineffective in controlling abnormal joint motion at functional force levels. It has been proposed that knee braces function by improving proprioception. Lephart and coworkers[11] have demonstrated enhanced awareness of joint movement sense with the application of a neoprene sleeve. Application of a knee brace may stimulate cutaneous receptors and enhance proprioception. Additionally, knee braces may enhance conscious or subconscious awareness of the injury, allowing the individual to be protected from further injury.

Another important component of nonoperative management for ACL injuries is modification of lifestyle to avoid activities that are associated with pain, swelling, and episodes of instability. Repeated episodes of instability cause further injury to the joint, including stretching of secondary restraints and injury to the menisci and joint surfaces. Recurrent pain and swelling with activity indicate additional damage to the joint. Activities that are not tolerated by the joint should be eliminated to prevent irreversible degenerative changes. Activities that place high stress on the ACL-deficient knee include those that involve jumping, landing, cutting, pivoting, and rapid acceleration or deceleration on the involved extremity. Individuals who are unwilling or unable to modify their lifestyle to avoid activities that are associated with increased pain, swelling, and instability will likely fail nonoperative management and should consider surgical reconstruction.

SURGICAL TREATMENT. Surgical management of a torn ACL should be considered for those with associated injury to other structures as well as those who are unwilling or unable to modify their lifestyle to avoid activities that place high demands on the knee and are associated with episodes of instability. Surgical treatment of a torn ACL includes direct repair, repair with augmentation, and reconstruction with synthetic ligaments. Results of direct repair have been poor.[141,188,189] A few investigators, however, have been encouraged by repair with augmentation.[190,191] Reconstruction with synthetic ligaments to date has been poor, resulting in early failure and the development of wear particle debris that leads to reactive synovitis.[195–197] Reconstruction has been successful and remains the treatment of choice.[195–197] Reconstruction with augmentation does not appear to improve the results compared to reconstruction alone.[198–200] Additionally, the use of a ligament augmentation device may result in stress yielding of the graft, which may delay remodeling.

Currently, ACL reconstruction is most commonly performed using an arthroscopically assisted technique. Timing of surgery following acute injury is an important consideration to minimize the risk for postoperative loss of motion. Most authors recommend delaying surgery until inflammation has subsided and range of motion and muscle function have been restored.[201,202] It has been our experience that this usually occurs within 2 to 3 weeks following an acute injury. Several graft options exist, but the most commonly used is the central third bone-patellar tendon-bone autograft. Other grafts include the use of autogenous semitendinosus and gracilis as well as bone-patellar tendon-bone and/or Achilles tendon allografts. The graft is passed through tunnels drilled in the tibia and femur that replicate the anatomy and function of the native ACL. The graft is fixed within the tunnels with interference screws or to the bony cortex with spiked washers if bone-patellar tendon-bone is not used (Fig. 30–34). An adequate "notchplasty" must be performed to allow adequate space for the graft so that the knee can fully extend without impingement. This should be determined intraoperatively, and the notch should be enlarged if the graft impinges in the intercondylar area. With our current operative technique, patients generally return to sports within 6 to 9 months.

POSTOPERATIVE MANAGEMENT FOLLOWING ACL RECONSTRUCTION. Rehabilitation following ACL reconstruction must consider initial graft strength, fixation, and healing and maturation of the

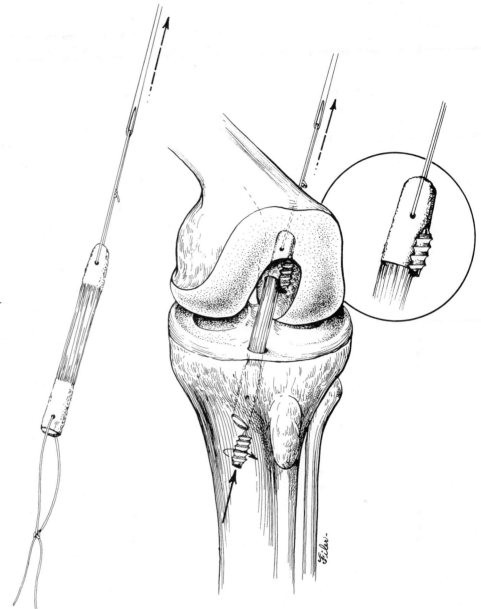

FIGURE 30–34. Anterior cruciate ligament reconstruction using a bone-patellar tendon-bone graft. Interference screw fixation is used to fix the graft within the tunnels.

graft. Initial graft strength depends on the quantity and quality of the material used, and has been investigated by Noyes and coworkers.[203] The central and medial thirds of the patellar tendon were found to be 186 percent and 159 percent of the strength of the native ACL, respectively. Weaker graft materials include the semitendinosus (70 percent), gracilis (49 percent), distal iliotibial track (44 percent), and fascia lata (36 percent). The use of stronger graft materials with solid fixation, such as that provided by an interference screw, allow more aggressive rehabilitation in the immediate postoperative period.

Graft strength is strongest at the time of reconstruction. Over time, the graft undergoes necrosis and remodeling. Healing and maturation of autogenous bone-patellar tendon-bone grafts in the animal model[204–209] and in humans[208,209] have been described. Others have described healing and maturation of allograft bone-patellar tendon-bone grafts in animal

models[207,210–212] and in humans.[213] Initially, the graft is avascular. By 6 weeks, the graft is enveloped in a synovial sheath. Revascularization begins 8 to 10 weeks postoperatively and is nearly complete by 16 weeks. Histologically, the graft shows signs of avascular necrosis 6 weeks after reconstruction. The graft is invaded by mesenchymal cells 8 to 10 weeks after reconstruction. These cells proliferate and form collagen by postoperative week 16. One year after reconstruction, the graft takes on the appearance of a ligament, with dense, oriented collagen bundles. Graft strength decreases during the period of necrosis and then increases as it remodels and matures, but it does not reach the original strength of the native ACL. Biomechanical studies have revealed that strength and stiffness of the graft is 30 to 50 percent of the native ACL 1 year after surgery.[206,211,213]

Even though the graft takes on the appearance of a normal ligament, it does not function the same as the native ACL. Evidence suggests that at 6 months after surgery, allografts demonstrate a greater decrease in their structural properties from the time of implantation, a slower rate of biologic incorporation, and prolonged presence of an inflammatory response as compared with autografts.[212] As a result, rehabilitation following allograft reconstruction may need to be less aggressive than that following autograft reconstruction. In spite of the research that has been done, little is known about the graft's ability to withstand loads and strain during healing and maturation. Thus, it is difficult to base rehabilitation following ACL reconstruction strictly on the time required for healing and maturation of the graft.

Postoperative rehabilitation following ACL reconstruction must minimize the adverse effects of immobility without overloading healing tissues. As discussed earlier, basic data on the strain and loads that the graft can withstand during healing and maturation are lacking. Additionally, studies on strain and loads imposed on the graft during exercise and activity are incomplete. Therefore, current trends in rehabilitation following ACL reconstruction are based on clinical experience.

Rehabilitation following ACL reconstruction has undergone significant changes over the last decade. In the 1970s and early 1980s, rehabilitation following ACL reconstruction was conservative. Paulos and colleagues[214] described a five-phase program that imposed time restraints thought to be necessary for graft healing and controlled forces that may have been deleterious to the healing process. In this program, range of motion was limited from 30 to 60 degrees in a cast brace and the patient was non–weight-bearing on crutches for 6 weeks. Toe touch weight bearing was initiated in the seventh week. The patient was allowed gradually to begin partial weight bearing on crutches at 12 weeks and was allowed to be in full weight bearing without assistive devices by postoperative week 16. Resisted exercises consisted of hamstring and limited arc quadriceps exercise, with light resistance for high repetitions. No mention was made of CKC exercises. Full return to activity was delayed for 9 to 12 months. There has been an interest in accelerated rehabilitation following ACL reconstruction, and was initially popularized by Shelbourne and Nitz.[215] The essential features of the program they proposed include early emphasis on restoration of full knee extension symmetric to the noninvolved side, immediate full weight bearing, use of CKC exercises to improve lower extremity muscle function, and return to full sports participation in 4 to 6 months. They compared the results of a group of patients who underwent an accelerated rehabilitation program with those of a group of patients who underwent a more traditional rehabilitation program that included immobilization in 10 degrees of flexion, delayed weight bearing, reliance on OKC exercises to improve quadriceps and hamstring function, and delayed return to full activity. Their results indicated that the accelerated rehabilitation program results in an earlier and more complete return of full extension and an earlier return to final flexion without adversely

affecting stability of the knee, as indicated by side-to-side differences in knee laxity scores. Additionally, isokinetic testing of the quadriceps revealed a higher mean percentage of involved-to-noninvolved scores from 4 to 10 months postoperatively. These differences in isokinetic scores, however, were eliminated 1 year following surgery. There were no differences in the patients' subjective assessment of their knee function. A second surgical procedure to recover loss of extension was required less often in patients who underwent the accelerated program. Based on these results, the use of an accelerated rehabilitation program following ACL reconstruction, was recommended because it resulted in earlier restoration of motion, strength, and function without compromising stability of the knee.

Loss of motion has been described as the most common complication following ACL reconstruction.[202,216–220] Sachs and associates[219] reported a 24 percent incidence of a knee flexion contraction greater than 5 degrees following ACL reconstruction. This was positively correlated with quadriceps weakness and patellofemoral pain. Harner and coworkers[202] reported an 11.1 percent incidence of loss of motion. In their study, loss of motion was defined as a knee flexion contracture greater than or equal to 10 degrees and/or knee flexion less than 125 degrees. All patients with loss of motion experienced loss of extension and two thirds also had loss of flexion. Factors significantly related to the development of loss of motion included reconstruction within 4 weeks of the initial injury, concomitant knee ligament surgery involving the medial capsule, and gender (male). There was a trend for patients with loss of motion to have had an autograft rather than an allograft and to be older but these trends did not reach statistical significance. Additionally, patients who developed loss of motion used a postoperative brace that limited full extension more often than patients who had normal motion following surgery. Loss of extension following ACL reconstruction leads to an abnormal gait, quadriceps weakness, and/or patellofemoral pain. Preoperative, intraoperative, and postoperative recommendations to minimize the risk for loss of motion were provided.

The goal for postoperative management following ACL reconstruction is to provide a stable knee that allows return to the highest level of function while at the same time minimizing the risk for loss of motion. To reduce the risk of loss of motion, postoperative management following ACL reconstruction should emphasize control of inflammation, restoration of full extension symmetric to the noninvolved knee, early range of motion and quadriceps exercises, and restoration of normal gait.

Cold and compression are used to reduce postoperative inflammation. These are applied immediately after surgery and used continuously for the first 7 days following surgery, or until the acute inflammatory reaction produced by surgery has subsided.

Goals for range of motion are to reach full extension symmetric to the noninvolved side within 2 to 3 weeks after surgery and full flexion within 8 weeks after surgery. These are achieved by immobilizing the knee

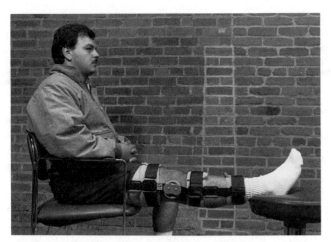

FIGURE 30–35. In the immediate postoperative period, the patient is encouraged to achieve full extension symmetrically to the noninvolved side. This is accomplished by sitting with the heel elevated and the knee unsupported.

in full extension in a postoperative rehabilitation brace or straight leg splint for the first week after surgery. This engages the graft in the intercondylar notch to reduce hemorrhage and intercondylar notch scarring. During the first postoperative week, the brace is unlocked several times daily for self-administered range-of-motion exercises. Additionally, the patient is encouraged to achieve full extension of the knee by lying prone with the lower leg unsupported or sitting with the leg elevated and the knee unsupported several times daily (Fig. 30–35). After the first postoperative week, the rehabilitation brace is left unlocked for all activities. When flexion improves beyond the range of the rehabilitation brace, use of the brace is discontinued. This typically occurs 3 to 6 weeks after surgery. Failure to progress and achieve the goals for range of motion should lead one to suspect development of loss of motion. Patients with suspected loss of motion should be evaluated carefully to determine the cause, which may be intercondylar scarring or capsulitis.[202] Appropriate management depends on the cause as well as on the length of time from reconstruction that the loss of motion is discovered.

One week following surgery the patient is instructed in self-mobilization of the patella. Inferior mobility of the patella is necessary for flexion. Superior mobility of the patella is necessary for normal function of the knee extensor mechanism. Decreased superior mobility of the patella interferes with the ability of the quadriceps to pull through the knee extensor mechanism and results in the development of a knee extensor lag. Medial glide and lateral tilting of the patella are necessary to maintain length of the lateral retinaculum. The force used during mobilization of the patella must be graded according to the degree of inflammation present to avoid aggravating pain and swelling.

Early quadriceps activity is encouraged. Beginning the day after surgery, quad sets are performed with the knee in full extension. It is believed that quadriceps exercises in this position primarily result in compression of the tibiofemoral joint, with little stress on the ACL. Quad sets are beneficial for regaining quadriceps control and also serve to maintain superior mobility at the patella. Straight leg raises are performed if the patient can do so with less than a 10 degree knee extensor lag. Additionally, isometric quadriceps exercises in the range of 60 to 90 degrees are performed, because it has been shown that they produce little or no active quadriceps anterior drawer.[16] These are initiated once the patient can flex the knee beyond 90 degrees. CKC exercises are initiated after the first postoperative week in preparation for weight bearing and to improve functional strength of the lower extremity. CKC exercises minimize patellofemoral stress and minimize anterior tibial displacement. CKC exercises are initiated in the form of bilateral isometric minisquats and are progressed as tolerated.

Initial ambulation after surgery is partial weight bearing with the brace locked in full extension. After the first postoperative week, the brace is unlocked to allow a normal heel-toe gait. Weight bearing is progressed as tolerated. The use of assistive devices is discontinued when the patient achieves full extension of the knee without a knee extensor lag and can demonstrate a normal gait pattern, which typically occurs 4 to 6 weeks after surgery.

The exercise program is progressed as tolerated by the patient, taking care to avoid activities that place high stress on the graft. OKC and CKC exercises as described earlier are used to increase strength and endurance of the lower extremity musculature. Proprioceptive activities are initiated to regain neuromuscular control of the knee. Functional exercises are emphasized throughout the rehabilitation program. Return to running is allowed when the patient is without inflammation, has full range of motion, and has recovered strength and endurance, as indicated by functional tests such as the one-legged hop and vertical jump tests. The patient must also be able to demonstrate a normal gait pattern while running. Return to running typically occurs 4 to 6 months after surgery. A gradual sports-specific functional progression allows return to sports within 6 to 9 months. A functional brace is recommended for the first 1 to 2 years after surgery.

A review of the results of 231 of our patients who underwent the above postoperative rehabilitation program revealed a 1.7 percent incidence of knee flexion contracture greater than 10 degrees 8 weeks following surgery.[221] This represents a marked reduction in loss of extension compared to that in our original study,[202] but the long-term functional outcome of this rehabilitation program is still to be determined. It appears that a more aggressive rehabilitation program following ACL reconstruction minimizes complications and maximizes restoration of function. Aggressive rehabilitation following ACL reconstruction, however, must be done in a manner that minimizes inflammation and its associated symptoms of pain and swelling, which predispose the patient to loss of motion. Complete disregard of sound basic scientific and rehabilitation principles to accelerate return to activity should be avoided. Additional research is necessary to document the long-term effects of accelerated rehabilitation following ACL reconstruction in terms of joint structure (i.e., stability, range of motion, strength, and degenerative changes) as well as the level of disability reported by the patient in terms of functional ability, symptoms, and return to activity.

PCL INJURIES

NONOPERATIVE MANAGEMENT. PCL injuries occur less frequently than ACL injuries. Isolated injury to the PCL does not produce the same degree of functional instability and disability that is seen with injury to the ACL. Many patients with an isolated injury to the PCL can return to their prior level of function with minimal symptoms. The level of function and patient satisfaction appear to be related to the ability of the quadriceps to stabilize the knee dynamically. Parolie and Bergfield[149] reported long-term results of 25 patients with PCL injuries who were managed nonoperatively. All patients who returned to their prior level of function and were satisfied with their results had involved side isokinetic quadriceps torque values greater than 100 percent of those of their noninvolved side. Conversely, those not satisfied with their knees had involved isokinetic torque values less than 100 percent of those of their noninvolved side. The level of function following PCL does not appear to be related to the degree of instability.[149,222] It should be noted however, that long-term follow-up of PCL injuries reveals the development of progressive pain and degeneration of the patellofemoral joint and medial compartment of the tibiofemoral joint.[155] This is likely due to altered arthrokinematics in the PCL-deficient knee.

Treatment following acute injury to the PCL is similar to that described for the management of acute ACL injuries. It should focus on resolution of inflammation, restoration of range of motion, and regaining motor control of the knee. Cold and compression are used to decrease pain and swelling. Range-of-motion exercises are performed to restore motion, which should improve as pain and swelling subside. Isometric exercises for the quadriceps, including quad sets and straight leg raises, (SLRs) are used to minimize quadriceps atrophy. Hamstring exercises are avoided at this time, because they contribute to increased posterior laxity. Also, the hamstrings do not appear to be as susceptible as the quadriceps to disuse atrophy. Assistive devices are used for ambulation while the knee is still actively inflamed. The use of assistive devices is discontinued when the patient has regained full extension without a quadriceps lag and can walk normally, without gait deviations.

More aggressive rehabilitation can begin once inflammation has resolved and full range of motion has been restored. The emphasis at this time is on improving endurance and strength of the quadriceps muscles. OKC knee extension exercises are used to provide isolated exercise for the quadriceps. Precautions must be taken to avoid the development of patellofemoral symptoms with OKC knee extension exercises. This is accomplished by performing these exercises with light resistance for high repetitions through a limited arc of motion. Heavy resistance OKC knee extension exercises through a range of 45 to 20 degrees of flexion should be avoided, because this results in the highest patellofemo-

ral joint reaction forces.[32,33] OKC knee extension exercises should be modified if the patient complains of pain or crepitus. CKC exercises are initiated and progressed as tolerated to improve endurance and strength of the muscles of the lower extremity in functional patterns.

OKC knee flexion exercises are to be avoided, because they contribute to increased posterior tibial translation. For patients with a PCL-deficient knee, the hamstrings are strengthened by performing open chain hip extension with the knee near terminal extension, which minimizes posterior tibial translation at the knee caused by the hamstrings. Additionally, CKC exercises can be performed to strengthen the hamstrings (Fig. 30–36). During CKC exercises, the hamstrings function to counteract the flexion moment arm at the hip. Their effect, of producing posterior tibial translation of the knee, is offset by simultaneous activity of the quadriceps. Proprioceptive training for the PCL-deficient knee should emphasize recruitment of the quadriceps to control posterior translation of the tibia dynamically. Individuals are progressed from walking to jogging-running, acceleration-deceleration, sprinting, jumping, cutting, pivoting, and twisting, as tolerated.

Generally, patients with a PCL-deficient knee do not complain of instability during physical activity, and the use of a functional brace is usually not necessary. If a patient with a PCL-deficient knee does require a functional knee brace, then one that is specifically designed for a PCL-deficient knee should be chosen. Most functional knee braces are designed for an ACL-deficient knee and do not benefit a patient with a PCL-deficient knee. When our PCL-deficient patients required use of a functional knee brace, the custom-fitted combined instabilities brace from DonJoy (Carlsbad, CA) has been used. Many patients with a PCL-deficient knee complain of patellofemoral symptoms and may benefit from the use of a neoprene patellar sleeve.

Because of the tendency for progressive deterioration of the anterior and medial compartments of the knee, patients with a PCL-deficient knee should be educated to avoid those activities that cause pain and swelling. Repetitive activities that involve high loading of the patellofemoral and tibiofemoral joints may accelerate this degenerative process and should be avoided.

SURGICAL MANAGEMENT. A number of important variables must be taken into account when deciding on how best to manage injury to the PCL. These include the type of injury, injury to associated structures, the patient's symptoms, activity level, goals, and expectations, as well as the acuity or chronicity of the injury. The goal of treatment is to restore stability and normal kinematics of the knee and to allow the patient to return to the preinjury level of activity. The best way to achieve this is still debatable. To serve as a guideline for management, we classify PCL injuries as avulsion injuries, isolated interstitial injuries, or combined ligament injuries. Isolated avulsion injuries to the PCL usually occur from the tibial insertion site. Tourisu[223] noted the posterior horn of the medial meniscus was also detached in 56% of the cases involving avulsion of PCL from its tibial insertion. Avulsion of the femoral

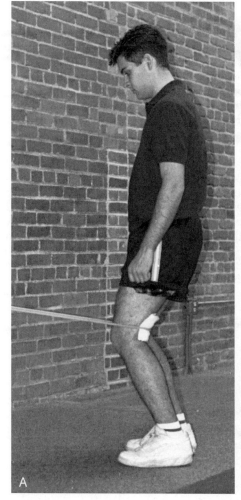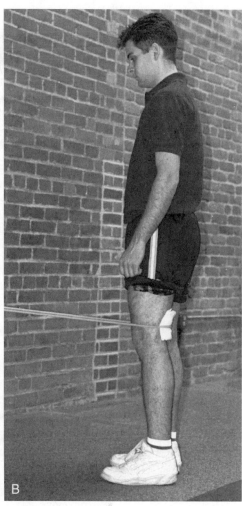

FIGURE 30–36. Closed chain knee extension exercises (A,B) are used to strengthen the hamstrings in the PCL-deficient knee. In this exercise, the individual performs terminal knee extension in the weight-bearing position. Resistance is applied posteriorly to the proximal thigh. Simultaneous contraction of the quadriceps counteracts the hamstrings' tendency to increase posterior tibial translation.

insertion site has also been reported.[150] The general consensus is that primary repair of avulsion injuries provides excellent stability and functional results if the fragment can be anatomically restored.[223–225] Tourisu[223] recommended open reduction and internal fixation of bony avulsion injuries if the bone fragment is greater than 3.1 cm and if it is separated more than 3 mm from its bed or displaced upward greater than 5 mm. Good results have also been reported for delayed unions and nonunions of bony avulsion injuries.[223,226] MRI or arthroscopy can be used to evaluate the nature of the bone fragment and the degree of displacement from the insertion site. Although the ligament may remain intact after an avulsion injury, plastic deformation can occur, making it nonfunctional.[223,226] In general, we recommend acute primary repair for bony avulsion injuries involving the PCL.

For interstitial tears of the PCL, the decision to perform surgery is based on the degree of resulting laxity as well as on injury to associated ligamentous structures. Grade I PCL injuries with less than 5 mm of increased posterior translation of the tibia are managed nonoperatively. Surgical reconstruction is recommended for isolated PCL disruptions that result in greater than 10 mm of increased posterior tibial translation compared with the noninvolved side or

when injury to the PCL is combined with injury to other ligamentous structures. It is important to note that a posterior drawer in excess of 15 mm is indicative of combined injury to the posterior cruciate ligament as well as posterolateral structures.[61] Controversy exists about whether to reconstruct a grade II PCL injury that results in 5 to 10 mm of increased tibial translation compared with the noninvolved knee. Isolated PCL tears can be reconstructed using an open or arthroscopic technique. Even though technically more demanding, we prefer to perform PCL reconstruction using an arthroscopically assisted technique because we believe it reduces operative morbidity and holds promise for improved clinical results. As with reconstruction of the ACL, PCL reconstruction has been performed using a variety of graft materials, including patellar and Achilles tendon allografts, patellar tendon, fascia lata, medial head of the gastrocnemius, semitendinosus-gracilis, and meniscus autografts, and synthetic replacements. Procedures involving use of the medial head of the gastrocnemius,[54,227–229] the semitendinosus gracilis,[228,229] the iliotibial band,[230] the meniscus,[231,232] Gore-Tex synthetic ligament,[233] and primary unaugmented repair[234–236] have all failed to produce consistent, objective results.

Our technique for PCL reconstruction consists of reproducing the anterolateral bundle of the ligament, because this is the largest and strongest band and it functions primarily with the knee in flexion. The procedure is performed by drilling the tibial tunnel so that it reproduces the distal-lateral portion of the tibial insertion site and drilling the femoral tunnel so that it reproduces the anterior portion of the femoral insertion site. An Achilles tendon allograft is passed through the femoral and tibial tunnels. We prefer to use an Achilles tendon allograft because of its length and strength, availability, lack of morbidity to the patient, and ease of passage, because it has one end without a bony block that can easily be passed through the acute angle required to go from the femoral to tibial tunnel. The femoral side, which includes the Achilles bone plug, is fixed with an interference screw, and the tibial side is fixed to the tibia with a screw and soft tissue spiked washer (Fig. 30–37). With our current techniques, patients who undergo arthroscopically assisted PCL reconstruction return to sports in approximately 9 to 12 months.

POSTOPERATIVE MANAGEMENT FOLLOWING PCL RECONSTRUCTION. The PCL is the primary restraint to posterior translation of the tibia on the femur.[5] Injury to the PCL leads to abnormal arthrokinematics of the tibiofemoral joint, which can result in degenerative changes of the patellofemoral joint and medial compartment of the tibiofemoral joint.[155] Reconstruction of the PCL has been proposed to delay and/or prevent these long-term degenerative changes.

The anatomy and function of the PCL have not been described as well as for the ACL. The PCL is described as having anterolateral and posteromedial components. The anterior portion becomes taut in flexion and is lax in extension, whereas the posterior portion is taut in extension and lax in flexion.[237–239] At our institution, it is the goal of the surgeon to reproduce the anterolateral portion of the PCL. It is believed that this portion of the PCL has a more important functional role in the kinematics and biomechanics of the knee. Arms and colleagues[19] demonstrated increased strain on the PCL

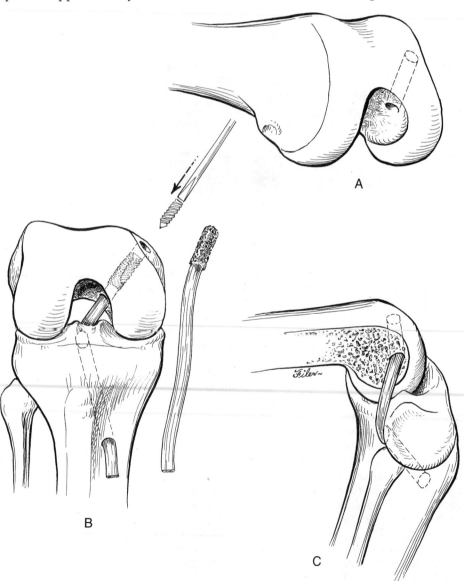

A

B

C

FIGURE 30–37. PCL reconstruction. *A,* PCL reconstruction is performed with an Achilles tendon allograft passed through the femoral and tibial tunnels. *B,* The femoral side is fixed with an interference screw. *C,* The tibial side is fixed with a soft tissue spiked washer and screw.

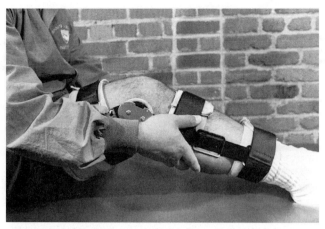

FIGURE 30–38. Passive range of motion following PCL reconstruction. This is done by lifting the proximal tibia to avoid posterior sagging of the tibia, which may jeopardize the graft in the immediate postoperative period.

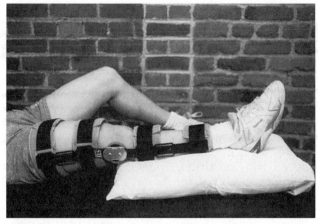

FIGURE 30–39. At rest, pillows are placed under the lower leg to prevent posterior sagging of the tibia in the immediate postoperative period following PCL reconstruction.

as the knee was flexed, reaching maximum strain at approximately 100 degrees of flexion. As a result, knee flexion in the immediate postoperative period is limited to avoid overloading the healing graft. This also minimizes the effects of gravity, which tend to create posterior sagging of the tibia.

Little is known about healing and maturation of the PCL graft. Bosch and associates[240] studied posterior cruciate graft fixation in sheep using a free patellar tendon graft and demonstrated good bone-to-bone incorporation at 6 weeks. In their study, postoperative management consisted of immediate partial weight bearing and range of motion beginning 2 weeks postoperatively. Clancy and coworkers[206] demonstrated revascularization of free patellar tendon grafts 8 weeks following surgery in rhesus monkeys. There have been no studies related to graft fixation and incorporation following PCL reconstruction in humans. Fixation of the Achilles tendon graft is vulnerable due to its distal soft tissue to bone fixation. This necessitates protection of the graft in the immediate postoperative period, until the graft has incorporated.

The maturation process of the PCL graft has not been definitively described, and the loads that it can withstand as it matures and remodels are unknown. Furthermore, the effect of loads imposed on the native or substitute PCL during exercise and functional activities is unknown. This lack of information makes it difficult to develop a scientifically based rehabilitation program following PCL reconstruction. OKC knee extension exercises in the range of 0 to 75 degrees produce anterior shear of the tibia relative to the femur. This should reduce strain on the PCL and can be incorporated early in the rehabilitation program to strengthen the quadriceps. OKC knee extension in the range from full flexion to 75 degrees produces posterior translation of the tibia and may increase PCL strain. OKC knee extension exercises in this range should be avoided in the early postoperative period. OKC knee flexion occurs as the result of unopposed contraction of the hamstrings and causes posterior translation of the tibia. Arms and colleagues[19] demonstrated increased

strain on the PCL with simulated contraction of the hamstrings. Following PCL reconstruction, OKC knee flexion should be avoided.

CKC exercises decrease tibial translation. This decrease is related to compression of the joint surfaces with weight bearing, co-contraction of the quadriceps and hamstrings, and a more axially aligned force in relation to the tibia. Lutz and associates[17] demonstrated posterior shear forces during CKC exercises, but the shear forces were less than those produced by OKC knee flexion. CKC exercises following PCL reconstruction are advocated to improve quadriceps and hamstring function while minimizing stress on the PCL and patellofemoral joint.

Rehabilitation in the immediate postoperative period following PCL reconstruction includes immobilization of the knee in a rehabilitation brace locked at 0 degrees extension. This is done to protect the distal soft tissue-to-bone fixation of the Achilles tendon graft. With the knee in full extension, tibiofemoral shear is minimized due to the small moment arm of the hamstrings when the knee is in this position. Additionally, the posterior capsule provides some restraint against posterior displacement of the tibia resulting from gravity. During the first postoperative week, the brace remains locked at all times. After the first postoperative week, the brace is unlocked for passive range-of-motion exercises and ambulation. Passive range of motion is performed by lifting the proximal tibia to protect against posterior sag (Fig. 30–38). At rest, pillows are placed distal to the knee to prevent posterior sagging of the tibia (Fig. 30–39). Exercises to regain motor control of the quadriceps are initiated and include quad sets and SLRs. Resistance for SLRs may be placed at the ankle if no quadriceps lag exists. During this period, open chain knee flexion and hip extension are avoided to minimize posterior tibial translation produced by the hamstrings. Resisted exercises for hip abduction and adduction are performed in the side-lying position, with the resistance applied proximal to the knee to avoid varus and valgus stress. Once good quadriceps control is demonstrated, OKC knee extension exercises may be performed in the seated position. During this exercise, the quadriceps functions concentrically and eccentrically to control knee flexion and minimize posterior translation of the tibia. In the immediate postoperative period, weight bearing is allowed.

The brace is unlocked for all activities 4 weeks after surgery. Use of the brace is discontinued after 6 weeks if range of motion permitted by the brace has been acquired by the patient (approximately 90 to 100 degrees of flexion). Patients continue to use assistive devices for gait until they can demonstrate full extension without a quadriceps lag and a normal gait without the use of the brace and assistive devices. During this period, CKC exercises in the range of 0 to 45 degrees of flexion are initiated. CKC exercises are progressed as tolerated. Hip extension is initiated with the knee in full extension. The patient may also begin resisted terminal knee extension in a CKC position, with resistance applied posteriorly to the proximal tibia (see Fig. 30–35). A stationary bicycle may be used to improve range of motion and lower extremity muscle function. Cycling is performed without toe clips to minimize hamstring activity. Balance and proprioception exercises are initiated once the patient is fully weight bearing.

Scientific justification for the end stages of rehabilitation following PCL reconstruction is not well developed at this time. Little is known about the effects of functional activities in vivo on the native or reconstructed PCL. Therefore, progression during this phase of the rehabilitation program is based on the patient's level of function and tolerance to the exercise program. Return to activity following PCL reconstruction is anticipated 9 to 12 months following surgery and requires sports-specific functional training.

MCL INJURIES

The philosophy for management of isolated MCL injuries has changed as a result of basic scientific and clinical studies. In the past, many of these injuries were treated with surgical repair followed by immobilization for 6 weeks. Studies in rabbits by Anderson and colleagues[74] and Weiss and associates[242] demonstrated that isolated MCL injuries heal when the ACL is intact. Similar findings were noted in clinical studies that demonstrated no difference in stability or function between patients with isolated MCL injuries who were treated nonoperatively versus operatively.[144,161,164,243] Isolated MCL tears heal well without surgery, regardless of the degree of injury, age of the patient, or activity level.[160–166] Usually, some residual valgus laxity can be elicited on physical examination after a grade II or III injury because the ligament may heal in a lengthened state, but this has little effect on knee function. Patients with combined MCL-ACL injuries, however, may require reconstruction of the ACL with or without repair of the MCL to restore stability and function to the knee. Reconstruction of the ACL alone for patients with a combined ACL-MCL injury may restore enough stability to the knee to allow the MCL to heal.

Acute treatment of isolated MCL injuries depends on the stability of the joint. Grades I and II MCL sprains that are stable with valgus stress testing are treated symptomatically without the use of a rehabilitation brace. Patients with isolated grade III MCL injuries that are unstable with valgus stress testing with a soft end point are treated with a hinged rehabilitation brace for 4 to 6 weeks. Typically, the brace is set to permit 0 to 90 degrees of motion. Use of a brace controls valgus stresses to allow the ligament to heal while allowing limited motion of the knee.

Treatment of acute MCL injuries should include the use of cold and compression to control pain and swelling. Early range of motion in the pain-free range is encouraged to facilitate healing and prevent development of a stiff knee. Transverse friction massage to the ligament may be beneficial to stimulate healing and orientation of the ligament fibers as well as to prevent the formation of adhesions. Isometric exercises for the quadriceps and hamstrings are initiated to minimize disuse atrophy. Assistive devices are used for ambulation until the patient demonstrates full extension of the knee without an extensor lag and can walk normally without gait deviations.

Once inflammation has resolved and range of motion has improved, the patient can begin OKC and CKC exercises to increase endurance and strength of the quadriceps and hamstring muscles. Exercises are progressed as tolerated, taking care to avoid the development of patellofemoral symptoms. As strength and endurance improve, the individual progresses through functional activities to enhance dynamic stability of the knee and to prepare for return to activity. Individuals returning to contact sports may use a functional knee brace to reduce the risk of reinjury. For MCL injuries, the brace should have good medial and lateral stays to control varus-valgus rotation.

LCL INJURIES

Treatment of acute isolated LCL injuries depends on the stability of the joint. Grades I and II LCL sprains that are stable with varus stress testing are treated symptomatically without the use of a rehabilitation brace. Patients with isolated grade III LCL injuries that are unstable with varus stress testing with a soft end point are treated with a hinged rehabilitation brace for 4 to 6 weeks. The brace is usually set to permit 0 to 90 degrees of motion. Use of the brace controls varus stresses to allow the ligament to heal while allowing limited motion of the knee.

Treatment of acute LCL injuries is similar to that described for MCL injuries. Cold and compression are used to control pain and swelling. Early range of motion in the pain-free range is encouraged to facilitate healing and prevent the development of a stiff knee. Isometric exercises for the quadriceps and hamstrings are initiated to minimize disuse atrophy. Assistive devices are used for ambulation until the patient demonstrates full extension of the knee without an extensor lag and can walk normally without gait deviations. Once inflammation has resolved and range of motion has improved, the patient can begin OKC and CKC exercises to increase endurance and strength of the quadriceps and hamstring muscles. As strength and endurance improve, the individual is progressed through functional activities to enhance dynamic stability of the knee and to prepare for return to activity. Individuals returning to contact sports may use a functional brace with good medial and lateral support to reduce the risk of reinjury.

Surgical management for isolated grade III LCL injuries is recommended for those patients who have chronic varus instability that affects their daily function or if they desire to continue sports activities. Additionally, surgery is recommended for those who have a bony avulsion that is displaced more than 3 mm. Reports on the results of LCL reconstruction are lacking. Reconstruction for the acute or chronic LCL injuries is usually reserved for multiple ligament-injured knees (see later).

Our technique for reconstruction of the chronically LCL-deficient knee depends on the acuity and severity of injury. For the acute LCL tear, the ligament can sometimes be reattached to its insertion using suture anchors or primary repair of the ligament can be performed. Often, however, the ligament is torn through its midsubstance and cannot hold sutures for repair. In these cases, as well as in the chronically LCL-deficient knee, we use an Achilles tendon allograft for reconstruction of the LCL. The bone plug of the Achilles tendon graft is placed in the fibular head and is fixed with an interference screw. The soft tissue end of the graft is fixed to the anatomic insertion of the LCL on the femoral epicondyle with suture anchors. Care must be taken that excessive stress is not placed on the graft as the knee is taken through a range of motion. Nonisometric placement of the graft can lead to stretching or tearing. The LCL remnants are sutured to the graft to provide added healing potential and possibly proprioceptive function.[244]

Following LCL reconstruction, patients are placed in a postoperative brace for 4 to 6 weeks to minimize varus stress. During this period, limited range-of-motion exercises from 0 to 90 degrees are performed. During the first postoperative week, isometric quadriceps and hamstrings exercises are initiated. A partial weight-bearing gait is used for 4 to 6 weeks following surgery to minimize stress on the graft. We have found that early, full weight bearing, particularly in the knee that demonstrates a varus thrust, leads to increased varus laxity. After 6 weeks, the patient is progressed to weight bearing as tolerated. Assistive devices are discontinued once the patient has full knee extension without a quadriceps lag and is able to demonstrate a normal gait pattern.

The rehabilitation brace is generally discontinued at 6 weeks postoperatively. At this time, emphasis is placed on regaining full range of motion as well as on developing muscle function for the lower extremity using OKC and CKC knee exercises. Proprioceptive activities are initiated to regain neuromuscular control of the knee. Gradual sports-specific functional progression allows return to sport within 6 to 9 months. A functional brace that provides varus stability is recommended for return to sports.

MULTIPLE LIGAMENT-INJURED KNEE

Immediate surgical intervention is necessary in the multiple ligament-injured knee that is associated with vascular injury or a compartment syndrome. Furthermore, the unreduceable knee dislocation, which is most often posterolateral, requires open reduction and an avulsed patellar tendon needs to be reattached to prevent a fixed posterior subluxation. These are the only absolute indications for surgical management of the multiple ligament-injured knee.

Based on the work of Taylor[178] on nonoperative versus operative treatment of knee dislocations, it is reasonable to conclude that nonoperative management could result in a functional knee depending on the patient's demands. Most authors, however, particularly in more recent reports, support open surgical techniques to restore stability and attempt to improve functional outcome.[172,201,245–247] Additionally, surgical management of the multiple ligament-injured knee may prevent or delay the onset of arthritis by improving joint stability. Functional deficiency that results from the multiple ligament-injured knee must be evaluated relative to the patient's age, occupation, recreational interests, and neurovascular status of the effected extremity before a decision is made to treat this problem surgically. When the authors opt for surgical management of this problem, they do so at least 5 days after initial injury if the clinical situation allows, but no longer than 3 weeks following injury. This allows the soft tissue inflammation to begin to recede and reduces interoperative bleeding. Also, the procedure may be able to be performed with arthroscopic assistance if it is done 10 to 14 days after injury. Waiting longer makes the repair more difficult due to scarring. We prefer to reconstruct both cruciate ligaments and repair the collateral ligaments and other structures as necessary, including the posterior lateral or posterior medial corner, arcuate complex, iliotibial band, and biceps femoris. Occasionally, the LCL cannot be repaired and requires reconstruction. We prefer reconstruction using allograft tissue to reduce surgical time and patient morbidity. Use of allograft tissue also ensures availability of graft tissue and minimizes difficulty with graft passage. The procedure is performed with arthroscopic assistance for the cruciate ligaments, particularly if the injury involves the ACL, PCL, LCL, and/or posterolateral corner with the ACL, PCL, or MCL avulsed off the tibial or femoral insertions. Otherwise, an open technique is used if the injury involves the ACL, MCL, PCL, and/or posteromedial corner, or if the patellar tendon must be reattached. In our experience, most patients are crutch-free and ambulating without a limp by 4 months.

MENISCAL INJURY

MECHANISM OF INJURY AND PATHOMECHANICS

A torn meniscus is the most common cause of mechanical symptoms in the knee. As such, arthroscopic meniscectomy is the most commonly performed arthroscopic procedure.[248] Turning or twisting on a loaded joint (weight bearing) may trap the meniscus between the joint surfaces and tear the meniscus. This may occur in combination with other injuries such as tears of the ACL that produce excessive tibial displacement on the loaded joint, causing the meniscus to displace and tear from its peripheral attachment. As a patient ages, the meniscus becomes less compliant and stiffer, subjecting it to injury with less force.[249,250] This fact, combined with the mucoid degeneration that comes with aging, results in older patients frequently developing meniscal tears that tend to be more complex in nature.

The menisci are not innervated by nocioceptors, and only the outer 10 to 33 percent is supplied by blood. The rest of the meniscus receives its nutrition from the synovial fluid and an interconnecting cistern and canal system from the fenestrated capillaries.[251,252] Meniscal tears are symptomatic because they render a portion of the meniscus abnormally mobile.[253] This mobile fragment causes pain, tenderness, and local synovitis by abnormally pulling on its remaining attachments. Furthermore, it can cause mechanical complaints such as catching and locking by dislodging and blocking joint motion. The patient may also note snapping and recurrent effusions. Isolated meniscal tears may result in joint swelling that develops more than 12 hours after the initial injury. The shape and location of a meniscus tear determine the symptoms and findings associated with a particular meniscal tear. Localized complaints of pain and joint line tenderness near the collateral ligament are probably the most characteristic findings. Anterior joint line pain rarely reflects meniscal pathology unless a bucket handle or ruptured bucket handle tear is present. Palpation for joint line tenderness reflects the capsular irritation resulting from the abnormal pull of a torn meniscus. Tears of the medial meniscus are more common than tears of the lateral meniscus.[254]

NATURAL HISTORY

Previously, it was suggested that a torn meniscus caused damage to the articular cartilage and thus resulted in the development of arthritis.[255] More recent studies, however, have found little evidence to suggest that meniscal tears cause osteoarthritis.[256] There is no observable change in the tibiofemoral pressure distribution pattern in the presence of a bucket handle tear, provided the torn segment maintains its normal anatomic position,[257] but displaced meniscal tears may result in abnormal wear of the articular cartilage and, in some situations, result in accelerated joint degeneration. This may be gleaned from studying the functions of the meniscus, which includes transmission of load across the tibiofemoral joint,[4,254,257–260] absorbing shock,[254,261,262] serving as a secondary restraint to tibiofemoral motion,[263–267] and aiding in joint lubrication.[268]

There are some meniscal lesions, even if associated with symptoms, that are best managed conservatively.

A diffusely degenerative meniscus or a pure cleavage tear without a large mobile fragment tends to cause mild symptoms that often respond to conservative treatment such as rest, nonsteroidal anti-inflammatory medications, and exercise. Furthermore, the meniscus in these situations most likely continues to serve its function and the patient does not benefit from its early removal.

Unless a tear is acute, peripheral, and stable (usually less than 7 mm in length), most meniscal injuries do not heal because of the lack of blood supply and high forces encountered by the meniscus. Some nonhealing tears, however, become asymptomatic with conservative treatment and, as noted earlier, do not require surgical intervention, but most meniscal lesions do require surgical management. This is particularly true of meniscal tears in the young athlete.

SURGICAL MANAGEMENT

If the knee is locked, or cannot be fully extended with a springy end point, the torn meniscal fragment is displaced. Meniscal pathology that results in blocked motion of the joint must be treated surgically. Furthermore, the patient who is an athlete may not be able to wait 4 to 6 weeks to determine whether conservative treatment is beneficial, and operative treatment should be instituted immediately.

MENISCECTOMY

Arthroscopic meniscectomy is the treatment of choice for a meniscal tear that is not appropriate for repair and causes significant symptoms that are unresponsive to conservative management. This may be related to the fact that total meniscectomy has been shown to result in premature degenerative arthritis of the knee.[269] Total meniscectomy has been shown to cause a 50 to 70 percent reduction in tibiofemoral contact area,[4,257] which results in a 235 percent increase in peak local contact pressure. Therefore, partial meniscectomy is preferred to total meniscectomy. Laboratory studies have shown that the reduced load transmission across the excised area is redistributed to the area between the remaining meniscus and articular cartilage. The degree of redistributed load transmission is dependent on the ratio of the amount of meniscus excised and the original load distribution.[4,257] Maintaining as much functioning meniscus as possible reduces the rate of development of arthritis as compared with total meniscectomy.

Meniscal surgery is performed arthroscopically to enhance visualization of the entire menisci, improve cosmesis, and reduce morbidity (compared with an arthrotomy). Arthroscopic partial meniscectomy should excise the mobile fragment and leave behind the residual meniscal rim that is stable, reasonably intact, and well contoured. Arthroscopic meniscectomy is done as an outpatient procedure and may be performed under local anesthesia.[124] Return to function following partial meniscectomy usually occurs within 2 to 6 weeks.

Rehabilitation following meniscectomy is dependent on the associated surgery that was performed and/or on underlying degenerative changes of the tibiofemoral and patellofemoral joints. Rehabilitation following meniscectomy without associated surgery or pre-existing degenerative changes includes controlling inflammation and restoring range of motion and muscle function, with an early return to activity expected. Associated surgery, such as concomitant ACL reconstruction, necessitates modification of the rehabilitation program and delays return to activity. Degenerative changes may slow the rehabilitation process and limit the level of activity to which the individual can return.

Rehabilitation following meniscectomy should begin immediately after surgery. Cold and compression are used to decrease pain and inflammation. Active assistive and active range-of-motion exercises are initiated to improve motion. Isometric quadriceps and hamstring exercises are used to regain motor control and minimize atrophy. Assistive devices are used for ambulation until the individual has regained full extension without a quadriceps lag and can demonstrate a normal gait pattern. Once range of motion is restored, OKC and CKC exercises are initiated to improve muscle endurance, strength, and power. Functional activities are initiated and progressed in a logical sequence to prepare the individual for return to activity.

For athletes who had no concomitant surgery or pre-existing degenerative changes of the joint, return to prior level of activity may occur in 2 to 3 weeks. Return to activity is delayed for individuals who had concomitant surgery. The length of time for return to activity following concomitant surgery is determined by the type of surgery that was performed and the expected rate of recovery. Pre-existing degenerative changes slow the rehabilitation process and delay restoration of motion and muscle function. Patients with degenerative joint changes do not tolerate exercises that cause high loads on the joint. Heavy resistance exercises should be avoided for these patients. Exercises that minimize impact loading of the joint, such as cycling, are better tolerated by these patients. Water exercises may be helpful, because the buoyant properties of water decrease the effects of weight bearing.

MENISCAL REPAIR

There has been great emphasis on meniscal repair as opposed to meniscectomy for the management of meniscal tears. As noted earlier, preservation of meniscal function may be important to prevent osteoarthritis. As a result, meniscal repair is indicated in situations in which successful healing is likely. Reparable tears, however, occur relatively infrequently. A current indication for a meniscal repair includes a single longitudinal tear at or near the periphery, where there is blood supply, in an otherwise normal meniscus.

At birth, the entire meniscus is vascular, but this is reduced to the peripheral third as a child. With aging, the blood supply of the meniscus is further reduced to less than 25 percent of the entire meniscus in the older adult.[270,271] Thus, reparable tears occur most commonly in the younger age group. Acute tears have a greater healing potential compared with chronic tears (i.e., those lasting longer than 2 months). The success of a meniscal repair in an ACL-deficient knee is not as high when the ACL is concurrently reconstructed.[272,273]

Techniques for meniscal repair have been modified to extend the indications for meniscal repair to regions where there is no blood supply. These include placing an autologous fibrin clot in the tear, rasping the synovial fringe to enhance synovial growth with its inherent blood supply, and creating vascular access channels.[274,275]

We prefer the arthroscopic "inside-out" technique to repair a torn meniscus.[275,276] After arthroscopic examination of the knee to confirm the presence of a reparable tear, a small skin incision is made on the side of the knee where the meniscus is torn to allow for visualization of the needles coming out of the joint.[275] The meniscal tear is rasped to clean the edges, which allows for adherence of blood and for coaptation of the torn edges. Sutures are placed through a cannula under arthroscopic visualization and are passed from the inside of the knee, through the meniscus, and out of the joint capsule under direct vision. The sutures are tied directly over the capsule (Fig. 30–40). Using this technique, the risk of injury to periarticular neurovascular structures is minimized, the repair is solid, and a high success rate is achieved.

Rehabilitation following meniscal repair includes a period of protected motion and weight bearing to allow the meniscus to heal. Motion is protected for 4 to 6 weeks in a rehabilitation brace that limits motion from 0 to 90 degrees. Motion beyond 90 degrees of flexion may jeopardize healing of the meniscus. During this period, the patient is encouraged to perform active assisted and active range-of-motion exercises within the protected range of motion. Additionally, isometric exercises are performed to maintain muscle tone. Protected weight bearing is continued for 4 to 6 weeks. After 4 to 6 weeks, the rehabilitation program is progressed as tolerated by the patient to restore range of motion and muscle function. Return to activity generally occurs within 3 months.

MENISCAL TRANSPLANTATION

Several investigators have begun to perform meniscal transplants for those patients who have had total or near-total meniscectomies.[277–281] Although early work is encouraging, it is too early to determine the ultimate success of this procedure. It appears, however, that once advanced arthritis is present, this technique is of no benefit.[278] Several methods have been utilized—allograft and prosthetic scaffolds are performed using arthroscopically assisted and open techniques, with and without bone plugs.[277–282] We prefer to perform an arthroscopically assisted technique using meniscal allografts. The bone plugs are maintained to allow for ingrowth of the meniscal insertions, and the periphery of the graft is sutured to the capsule (Fig. 30–41).

Following meniscal transplant, the patient is placed in a postoperative brace for 8 weeks. This brace is locked

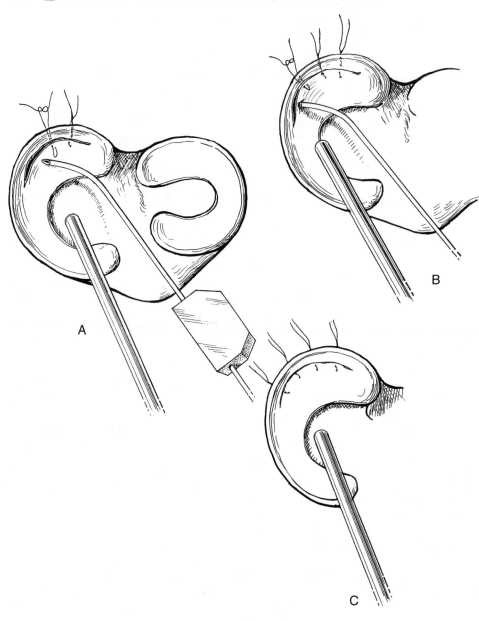

FIGURE 30–40. Meniscal repair is performed arthroscop-ically, passing the suture from in-side the knee *(A)* through the meniscus *(B)* to the outside of the joint capsule *(C)*, where the sutures can be tied under direct vision.

in full extension for the first 6 weeks to protect the meniscal transplant. During this period, the brace may be unlocked several times a day for passive range-of-motion exercises from 0 to 90 degrees as tolerated. Isometric exercises for the quadriceps, including quad sets and straight leg raises, are initiated immediately after surgery. Hamstring and weight-bearing CKC exercises are delayed for 6 to 8 weeks to protect the healing transplanted meniscus. For the first 6 weeks after surgery, the patient ambulates using a partial weight-bearing gait with the brace locked in full extension. At 6 weeks, weight bearing may be pro-gressed to weight bearing as tolerated and the brace may be unlocked for controlled gait training. The use of assistive devices may be discontinued 8 weeks follow-ing surgery provided there is full knee extension without a quadriceps lag, 90 to 100 degrees of flexion, and a normal gait pattern.

At approximately 8 weeks after surgery, the rehabili-tation program can be progressed to include CKC exercises for the lower extremity and OKC knee flexion exercises in the range from 0 to 60 degrees. The rehabilitation program should be progressed as toler-ated to restore full range of motion, muscle function, and proprioception. Return to sports activity is ex-pected 9 to 12 months after surgery.

ASSESSMENT OF FUNCTIONAL OUTCOME

Over the last 5 to 10 years, there have been many technologic advances in terms of diagnosis and treat-ment of knee ligament and meniscal injuries. Diag-nostic advances include the use of arthroscopy and magnetic resonance imaging. Arthroscopic procedures have been used to manage meniscal and ligamentous injuries surgically. Rehabilitation techniques have also changed, with emphasis on early restoration of motion and development of strength in functional patterns using closed kinetic chain exercises. The impact of these advances in diagnosis, treatment, and rehabilitation of knee injuries, on improved outcome, however, is unknown. There is a lack of clinical research to support the efficacy of current techniques for managing knee injuries. Almost all clinical studies to date are retrospective, with poorly defined end points. Well-designed clinical trials with clearly defined end points are needed to prove that advances in the management of knee ligament and meniscal injuries and their associated increased costs can lead to improved outcome.

Most definitions of outcome focus on physical impairments or the status of knee joint structure and function, including range of motion, strength, stability, and radiographic appearance. Little emphasis has been placed on assessing disability or the effect that impairment of the knee has on the patient's overall level of function.

In addition to documenting physical impairments, measurement of outcome following injury to the knee should focus on the resulting functional limitations and disability that a patient experiences. According to Nagi,[283] functional limitation is the limitation in performance at the level of the whole organism or person. Disability is defined as the limitation of performance of socially defined roles and tasks within a sociophysical environment. Following a knee ligament injury, a functional limitation may be the inability to perform activities that require cutting and pivoting. The resulting disability from this functional limitation may be the inability to participate in competitive sports, such as football or soccer, which require cutting and pivoting maneuvers. Outcome studies to document the effectiveness of advances in diagnosis and treatment of injuries should focus on the resulting functional limitations and disability that a patient experiences. Addi-

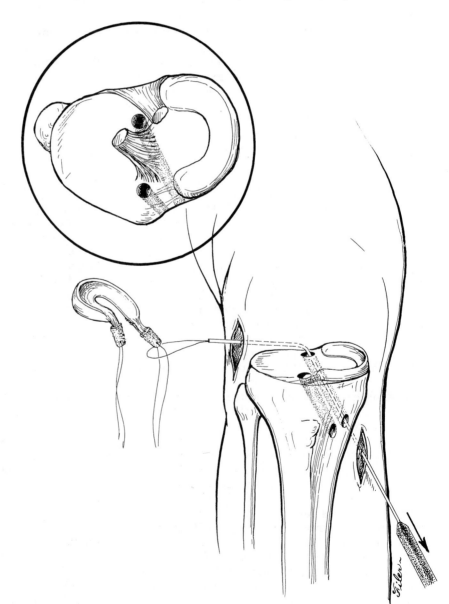

FIGURE 30–41. Arthroscopically assisted meniscal transplant. Bone plugs are maintained on the meniscal transplant to facilitate ingrowth of the meniscal insertions. *Inset,* The periphery of the graft is sutured to the capsule.

tionally, research is needed to establish the relationship between impairment of knee function and the resulting disability.

Outcome following knee injury must consider the patient's perspective of the impact of the injury on the level of function. Patients with residual knee laxity may be able to perform at their previous level of activity without symptoms and would consider themselves to have a good outcome. If outcome were determined on the basis of joint stability, however, these patients would be classified as having a poor outcome. Conversely, patients may have a good outcome in terms of joint stability but a poor outcome in terms of functional limitations and disability for various reasons, such as pain, apprehension, fear of reinjury, and lack of confidence. An instrument is needed to evaluate outcome that can measure the level of disability caused by a knee injury from the patient's perspective. This instrument must be tested to ensure its reliability and validity.

Although several instruments have been developed to assess outcome following knee injury, there is currently little agreement on how to report outcome following knee injury. This creates difficulty when comparing studies that report results for treatment of knee injuries. The International Knee Documentation Committee (IKDC)[284] has established guidelines for assessing outcome following knee ligament injury and/or surgery (Fig. 30–42). Overall rating of outcome is based on eight categories: (1) the patient's perception of their level of knee function; (2) symptoms including pain, swelling, and giving way; (3) range of motion; (4) laxity; (5) joint crepitus; (6) radiographic appearance of the joint; (7) graft site morbidity; and (8) functional strength. Each category is rated as normal, nearly normal, abnormal, or severely abnormal. The overall final rating is based on the worst rating for the categories of patient-reported function, symptoms, range of motion, and laxity. Over the last several years this instrument has been widely accepted in the orthopaedic community, but it has not been tested to ensure its reliability and validity. We have completed preliminary studies[285–287] indicating that this instrument may be overly critical in rating final outcome following knee ligament injury and/or surgery. Furthermore, outcome in terms of disability from the patient's perspective is only assessed with two items. Patients are asked to rate their level of satisfaction on a scale from 0 to 3 and to describe the function of their knee as normal, nearly normal, abnormal, or severely abnormal. The major focus of the IKDC guidelines is on rating impairment, and it is unknown how these relate to an individual's level of disability. Also, because the worst rating for any category determines the overall final rating, it is unlikely that this assessment battery is responsive to clinically significant differences over time. For example, if a patient's level of symptoms improves but the laxity remains unchanged, the overall final rating according to IKDC guidelines remains the same. This lack of responsiveness may fail to detect important changes in a patient over time. Further research is needed to establish the usefulness of reporting outcome following knee ligament injury and surgery according to IKDC guidelines.

Several other instruments have been developed to measure outcome from the patient's perspective following knee injury and/or surgery. The Lysholm Knee Scoring Scale has been widely used.[288–290] This instrument is a self-report completed by the patient and consists of a 100-point scale used to rate the patient's functional limitations in terms of walking with a limp, use of assistive devices, locking, giving way, pain, swelling, and ability to climb stairs and squat (Fig. 30–43). The intrapersonal coefficient of variation was determined to be 3 percent when the Lysholm Knee Scoring Scale was administered by the same orthopaedic surgeon at a 2-week interval.[289] Interpersonal coefficient of variation was found to be 4 percent when administered by an orthopaedic surgeon and a physical therapist on the same day. Test-retest correlation coefficients were 0.97 within testers and 0.90 between testers. The Lysholm Knee Scoring Scale was found to correlate significantly ($r = 0.78$) with the Marshall Scoring Scale. The disadvantage of the Lysholm Knee Scoring Scale is the questionable weighting scheme given to the categories, with 50 percent of the total score dependent on pain and swelling. No explanation of the weighting system was provided in the description of this instrument. Also, the Lysholm Knee Scoring Scale does not determine the individual's ability to perform running, cutting, and jumping maneuvers, making it likely to exhibit a ceiling effect when used with patients who place high demands on the knee.

The Cincinnati Knee Scale was originally presented by Noyes and colleagues.[291] It was a 50-point scale that rated activity level, pain, swelling, and giving way. This scale was subsequently expanded and described in greater detail[292] (Fig. 30–44). At that time, the Cincinnati Knee Scale consisted of two subscales, including symptoms and assessment of function. Symptoms accounted for 50 percent of the total score and included pain (20 points), swelling (10 points), and giving way (20 points). Assessment of function accounted for the remaining 50 percent of the total score and included overall activity level (20 points), walking (10 points), stairs (10 points), running (5 points), and jumping and twisting activities (5 points). The Cincinnati Knee Scale is a self-report completed by the patient, who is asked to rate symptoms and level of function for each knee separately.

Several authors have developed modified versions of the Cincinnati Knee Scale. Shelbourne and associates[215] described a 100-point modified Cincinnati Knee Scale that consisted of walking (20 points), stairs (10 points), running (10 points), jumping (5 points), cutting (5 points), pain (20 points), stability (20 points), and swelling (10 points). Olson and coworkers[293] also described a modified version of the Cincinnati Knee Scale that consisted of 100 points, including sports activity level (20 points), running (10 points), jumping and landing (10 points), cutting and pivoting (10 points), pain (10 points), swelling (10 points), partial giving way (10 points), and complete giving way (10 points). There have been no reports on reliability and validity for any versions of the Cincinnati Knee Scale described by these authors. The Cincinnati Knee Scale

Name: _____ First name: _____ DOB: ___/___/___ med. rec. #:_____
Examiner: _____ Date of examination: __/__/__ Date of injury/ies: __/__/__ ; __/__/__ Date of surgeries: __/__/__
Causes of injury: □ ADL*[2]   □ traff.   □ non-pivoting non-contact sports   □ pivoting non-contact sp.   □ contact sp. □ work
Time inj. to surg.: _____ (months)   □ acute (0-2 weeks)   □ subacute (2-8 weeks)   □ chronic (>8 weeks)
Knee involved: □ r. □ l.   opposite knee: □ norm.   □ injured   exam. under anesthes.:   □ yes   □ no
Postop. diagnosis: _____
Surgical proced.: _____
Status menisci: norm. □ med. □ lat.   1/3 removed: □ med. □ lat.   2/3 removed: □ med. □ lat.   compl. rem. □ med. □ lat.
Morphotype: □ lax   □ normal   □ tight   □ varus   □ valgus
Activ. level*[3]:   preinjury: □ I   □ II   □ III   □ IV   pretreatment: □ I   □ II   □ III   □ IV
                    present: □ I   □ II   □ III   □ IV   Eventual change knee-related: □ yes   □ no

GROUPS (PROBLEM AREA)	QUALIFICATION WITHIN GROUPS *[4]				GROUP QUALIFIC.			
	A: normal	B: nearly norm.	C: abnormal	D: sev. abnorm.	A	B	C	D*[4]
1. PATIENT SUBJECTIVE ASSESSMENT								
How does your knee function?	□ normally	□ nearly norm.	□ abnormally	□ sev. abnorm.				
On a scale of 0 to 3 how does your knee affect								
your activity level?	□ 0	□ 1	□ 2	□ 3	□	□	□	□
2. SYMPTOMS (absence of significant symptoms, at highest activity level known by patient) *[5]								
No pain at activity level *[3]	□ I	□ II	□ III	□ IV or worse				
No swelling at activity level *[3]	□ I	□ II	□ III	□ IV or worse				
No partial giving way at activity level *[3]	□ I	□ II	□ III	□ IV or worse				
No complete giving way at activity level *[3]	□ I	□ II	□ III	□ IV or worse	□	□	□	□
3. RANGE OF MOTION: Flex./ext.: documented side: __/__/__ opposite side: __/__/__ *[6]								
Lack of extension (from zero anatomic)	□ <3°	□ 3-5°	□ 6-10°	□ >10°				
△ *[7] lack of flexion	□ 0-5°	□ 6-15°	□ 16-25°	□ >25°	□	□	□	□
4. LIGAMENT EXAMINATION *[8]		3 to 5mm or	6 to 10mm					
△ *[7] Lachman (in 25°. flex.) *[9]	□ −1 to 2mm	□ −1 to −3mm[10]	□ or <−3mm	□ >10mm				
idem (alternative measurement, optional)	□ −1 to 2mm	□ 3-5/−1 to −3mm	□ 6-10/<−3mm	□ >10mm				
Endpoint: □ firm □ soft								
△ *[7] total a.p.transl. in 70° flex. *[9]	□ 0 to 2mm	□ 3 to 5mm	□ 6 to 10mm	□ >10mm				
idem (alternative measurement, optional)	□ 0 to 2mm	□ 3 to 5mm	□ 6 to 10mm	□ >10mm				
△ *[7] post. sag in 70° flex.	□ 0 to 2mm	□ 3 to 5mm	□ 6 to 10mm	□ >10mm				
△ *[7] med. joint opening (valgus rotation)	□ 0 to 2mm	□ 3 to 5mm	□ 6 to 10mm	□ >10mm				
△ *[7] lat. joint opening (varus rotation)	□ 0 to 2mm	□ 3 to 5mm	□ 6 to 10mm	□ >10mm				
Pivot shift *[11]	□ neg.	□ + (glide)	□ ++ (clunk)	□ +++ (gross)				
△ *[7] reversed pivot shift	□ equal (neg.)	□ slight	□ marked	□ gross				
	□ equal (pos.)				□	□	□	□
5. COMPARTMENTAL FINDINGS *[12]								
△ *[7] Crepitus patellofemoral	□ none/equal	□ moderate	□ painful	□ severe				
△ *[7] Crepitus medial compartment	□ none	□ moderate	□ painful	□ severe				
△ *[7] Crepitus lateral compartment	□ none	□ moderate	□ painful	□ severe				
6. HARVEST SITE PATHOLOGY *[13]								
Tenderness, irritation, numbness	□ none	□ slight	□ moderate	□ severe				
7. X-RAY FINDINGS (DEGENERATIVE JOINT DISEASE) *[14]								
Patellofemoral cartilage space	□ normal	□ >4mm	□ 2-4mm	□ <2mm				
Medial compartment cartilage space	□ normal	□ >4mm	□ 2-4mm	□ <2mm				
Lateral compartment cartilage space	□ normal	□ >4mm	□ 2-4mm	□ <2mm				
8. FUNCTIONAL TEST *[15]								
△ One leg hop (percent of opposite side)	□ 90-100%	□ 76-90%	□ 50-75%	□ <50%				
FINAL EVALUATION					□	□	□	□

FIGURE 30–42. International Knee Documentation Committee guidelines for evaluating outcome following knee ligament injury and/or surgery. (From Hefti F, Mullen W, Jakob RP, Staubli H-U: Evaluation of knee ligament injuries with the 1 KDC form. Knee Surg Sports Traumatol Arthrosc 1993; 1: 226–234.)

1. Please check the statement that best describes the way you walk.
   ___ I never walk with a limp.
   ___ I rarely walk with a limp or I walk with a slight limp.
   ___ I walk with a constant and severe limp.

2. Which of the following do you presently use as a support while you walk?
   ___ I can walk without crutches or a cane.
   ___ I can put some weight on my leg, but I need at least one crutch or a cane to walk.
   ___ I cannot put any weight on my leg when walking.

3. Do you experience LOCKING of your knee?
   ___ No, never.
   ___ My knee catches, but does not lock.
   ___ Yes, my knee locks occasionally.
   ___ Yes, my knee locks frequently.
   ___ Yes, my knee is locked all the time.

4. Do you experience slipping or giving way of your knee?
   ___ No, never.
   ___ Yes, rarely during sporting activities or other severe exertion.
   ___ Yes, frequently during sporting activities or other severe exertion.
   ___ Yes, occasionally during daily activities.
   ___ Yes, frequently during daily activities.
   ___ Yes, on every step.

5. Which of the following best describes your level of pain?
   ___ I have no pain in my knee.
   ___ I have occasional pain, which is slight and present only after severe exertion.
   ___ I have marked pain during severe exertion.
   ___ I have marked pain after walking more than 2 miles.
   ___ I have marked pain after walking less than 2 miles.
   ___ I have constant pain.

6. Which of the following best describes swelling in your knee?
   ___ I have no swelling.
   ___ I have swelling only after severe exertion.
   ___ I have swelling after ordinary exertion.
   ___ I have constant swelling.

7. Which of the following best describes your ability to climb stairs?
   ___ I have no problems on stairs.
   ___ I am only slightly impaired on stairs.
   ___ I can negotiate stairs, but only one at a time.
   ___ I cannot go up or down stairs.

8. Can you get into a full squat position?
   ___ Yes, no problems.
   ___ No, but I am only slightly impaired.
   ___ No, I cannot squat with my knee past 90 degrees.
   ___ No, I cannot squat at all.

THANK YOU FOR TAKING TIME TO COMPLETE THIS QUESTIONNAIRE.

FIGURE 30–43. Lysholm Knee Scoring Scale. (From Tegner Y, Lysholm J: Rating systems in the evaluation of knee ligament injuries. Clin Orthop 1985; 198: 43–49.)

also combines activities of daily living and sports activity, limiting its use for nonathletic subjects. Rating nonathletic subjects on a scale that is dependent on ability to perform sports results in an invalid score.

Bollen and Seedham[294] compared the Lysholm Knee Scoring Scale and Cincinnati Knee Scale in 41 subjects with documented unilateral ACL-deficient knees. They found a significant positive correlation ($r = 0.87$) between the two tests, but the median difference between the test scores was 13 points. The Lysholm Knee Scoring Scale consistently resulted in a higher overall rating than the Cincinnati Knee Scale. This has significant implications when trying to interpret results of clinical research related to treatment of the knee. Use of the Lysholm Knee Scoring Scale tends to overrate patients compared with use of the Cincinnati Knee Scale, perhaps because of the ceiling effect mentioned earlier.

To overcome the limitations identified for the Lysholm Knee Scoring Scale and the Cincinnati Knee Scoring Scale, we have begun to develop the Knee Outcome Survey, which consists of two separate scales to rate activities of daily living and sports activity. The Activities of Daily Living Scale (ADLS) of the Knee Outcome Survey includes items related to symptoms and functional disability during activities of daily living that are directly related to the patient's knee injury (Fig. 30–45). Symptoms on this scale include pain, crepitus, stiffness, swelling, instability, and weakness. Alternatives for each symptom are graduated in terms of the amount of disability that the symptom imposes on the patient during activities of daily living. Functional disabilities included on the scale are difficulty with walking, stairs, standing, kneeling, squatting, sitting, and rising from sitting. Alternatives for each functional activity are graduated, from no limitation to inability to perform the activity. The Sports Activity Scale of the Knee Outcome Survey includes items related to symptoms and functional disability during sports that are directly related to the individual's knee injury (Fig. 30–46). The same symptoms included on the ADLS are included on the Sports Activity Scale, but the alternatives for the items are graduated in terms of the amount of disability that the symptom imposes on the individual's ability to participate in sports. Functional disabilities on the scale include the ability to run straight ahead as well as the ability to jump and land, start and stop quickly, and cut and pivot on the involved knee. Alternatives range from being able to perform the activity without limitations to not being able to perform the activity.

Preliminary testing of the ADLS and Sports Activity Scale of the Knee Outcome Survey was accomplished by administering the survey to all patients presenting with a knee injury to the Center for Sports Medicine (University of Pittsburgh Medical Center) over a 3-month period. Patients concomitantly completed the Lysholm Knee Scoring Scale and the Modified Cincinnati Knee Rating Scale.[293] Additionally, patients provided an overall global subjective rating of their knee on a scale from 0 to 100, with 100 being their level of function prior to injury. The results indicated significant positive correlations between scores on the ADLS and the Lysholm Knee Scoring Scale ($r = 0.74$) and the ADLS score and the patients' self-rating ($r = 0.61$). There was also a significant positive relationship between the score on the Sports Activity Scale and the Cincinnati Knee Rating Scale ($r = 0.78$) and the Sports Activity Scale and the patient's self rating ($r = 0.51$).

In the same pilot study, the ADLS was readministered approximately 4 weeks after the initial survey was completed. At that time, patients were asked to state their change since initiation of treatment as greatly worse, somewhat worse, neither better nor worse, somewhat improved, or greatly improved. The mean

Symptoms: Please select the *HIGHEST* level of activity you can perform without significant pain, swelling or giving way. Exclude slight symptoms that do not cause you to limit or modify your activity.

Pain:

___ able to do strenuous sports activities that involve cutting, pivoting, and jumping (ex. basketball, football, gymnastics, soccer, etc.) without pain

___ able to do moderate sports activities that involve running, twisting, or turning (ex. tennis, hockey, skiing, wrestling, etc.) *or* heavy manual labor without pain

___ able to perform light sports activities that do not involve running, turning, or twisting (ex. cycling, swimming, golf, etc.) *or* light manual work without pain

___ able to perform sedentary activities (walking and other activities of daily living) without pain.

___ unable to perform activities of daily living without frequent or limiting pain

___ unable to perform activities of daily living without constant pain

Swelling:

___ able to do strenuous sports activities that involve cutting, pivoting, and jumping (ex. basketball, football, gymnastics, soccer, etc.) without swelling

___ able to do moderate sports activities that involve running, twisting, or turning (ex. tennis, hockey, skiing, wrestling, etc.) *or* heavy manual labor without swelling

___ able to perform light sports activities that do not involve running, turning, or twisting (ex. cycling, swimming, golf, etc.) *or* light manual work without swelling

___ able to perform sedentary activities (walking and other activities of daily living) without swelling

___ unable to perform activities of daily living without frequent or limiting swelling

___ unable to perform activities of daily living without constant swelling

Partial Giving Way (slipping of the knee, not resulting in a fall to the ground):

___ able to do strenuous sports activities that involve cutting, pivoting, and jumping (ex. basketball, football, gymnastics, soccer, etc.) without swelling

___ able to do moderate sports activities that involve running, twisting, or turning (ex. tennis, hockey, skiing, wrestling, etc.) *or* heavy manual labor without swelling

___ able to perform light sports activities that do not involve running, turning, or twisting (ex. cycling, swimming, golf etc.) *or* light manual work without swelling

___ able to perform sedentary activities (walking and other activities of daily living) without swelling

___ unable to perform activities of daily living without frequent or limiting swelling

___ unable to perform activities of daily living without constant swelling

Full Giving Way (buckling of the knee, resulting in a fall to the ground):

___ able to do strenuous sports activities that involve cutting, pivoting, and jumping (ex. basketball, football, gymnastics, soccer, etc.) without swelling

___ able to do moderate sports activities that involve running, twisting, or turning (ex. tennis, hockey, skiing, wrestling, etc.) *or* heavy manual labor without swelling

___ able to perform light sports activities that do not involve running, turning, or twisting (ex. cycling, swimming, golf, etc.) *or* light manual work without swelling

___ able to perform sedentary activities (walking and other activities of daily living) without swelling

___ unable to perform activities of daily living without frequent or limiting swelling

___ unable to perform activities of daily living without constant swelling

FIGURE 30–44. Cincinnati Knee Scoring Scale. (From Noyes FR, et al: Functional disability in the anterior cruciate insufficient knee syndrome. Sports Med 1984; 1:286–287.)

Illustration continued on following page

Functional Level: Please indicate your current level of function for each activity listed below. Check only the statement that describes your *highest* level of function.

Walking:

____ unable to walk
____ definite limitations
____ some limitations
____ no limitations walking

Stairs:

____ unable to climb stairs
____ definite limitations
____ some limitations
____ no limitations climbing stairs

Kneeling/Squatting:

____ unable to kneel or squat
____ definite limitations
____ some limitations
____ no limitations kneeling/squatting

Straight Running:

____ unable to run straight ahead
____ definite limitations
____ some limitations
____ no limitations running straight ahead

Jumping/Landing on Leg:

____ unable to jump or land on leg
____ definite limitations
____ some limitations
____ no limitations jumping or landing on leg

Hard Cutting, Pivoting, and Twisting:

____ unable to perform hard cutting, pivoting, or twisting
____ definite limitations
____ some limitations
____ no limitations performing hard cuts, pivots, or twists

FIGURE 30–44 *Continued*

gain scores for the ADLS (post-test minus pretest) for those that were greatly worse was –15.0, for those that were neither better nor worse, –9.8, for those that were somewhat improved, 11.0, and for those that were greatly improved, 23.7. These results appear to indicate that the ADLS can detect clinically significant changes over time in patients following injury or surgery of the knee. Further development and testing of the ADLS and Sports Activity Scale of the Knee Outcome Survey is warranted.

Most outcome studies related to treatment of knee ligament and meniscal injuries have focused on reporting physical impairment of the knee, including limitations in range of motion, strength, and stability. The relationship between physical impairment of the knee and functional limitations and disability experienced by the patient has been the subject of research. It has been hypothesized that deficits in range of motion, strength, and stability result in increased levels of functional limitations and disability. Snyder-Mackler and associ-

ates[295] demonstrated a significant relationship between isometric quadriceps peak torque and gait abnormalities. Decreased levels of isometric quadriceps peak torque were associated with an increased angle of knee flexion during gait. Wilk and coworkers[296] demonstrated a positive correlation between isokinetic knee extension peak torque at 180 and 300 degrees/sec and a Modified Cincinnati Knee Rating Score. Lephart and colleagues[11] failed to demonstrate a significant relationship between isokinetic peak torque and torque acceleration energy for the quadriceps and hamstrings at 60 and 270 degrees/sec to physical performance tests, including the shuttle run, carioca, and co-contraction semicircular run. Furthermore, there was no relationship between these isokinetic parameters and the Iowa Athletic Knee Rating Scale. Further research is needed to clarify the relationship between isometric and isokinetic strength of the quadriceps and hamstrings and functional limitations and disability experienced by the patient.

Instructions:

The following questionnaire is designed to determine the symptoms and limitations that you experience because of your knee while you perform your usual *daily activities.* Please answer each question by **checking the statement that best describes you over the last 1 to 2 days.** For a given question, more than one of the statements may describe you, but please mark ONLY the statement which best describes you during your usual daily activities.

Symptoms

1. To what degree does pain in your knee affect your daily activity level?
___ I never have pain in my knee.
___ I have pain in my knee but it does not affect my daily activity.
___ Pain affects my activity slightly.
___ Pain affects my activity moderately.
___ Pain affects my activity severely.
___ Pain in my knee prevents me from performing all daily activities.

2. To what degree does grinding or grating of your knee affect your daily activity level?
___ I never have grinding or grating in my knee.
___ I have grinding or grating in my knee, but it does not affect my daily activity.
___ Grinding or grating affects my activity slightly.
___ Grinding or grating affects my activity moderately.
___ Grinding or grating affects my activity severely.
___ Grinding or grating in my knee prevents me from performing all daily activities.

3. To what degree does stiffness in your knee affect your daily activity level?
___ I never have stiffness in my knee.
___ I have stiffness in my knee, but it does not affect my daily activity.
___ Stiffness affects my activity slightly.
___ Stiffness affects my activity moderately.
___ Stiffness affects my activity severely.
___ Stiffness in my knee prevents me from performing all daily activities.

4. To what degree does swelling in your knee affect your daily activity level?
___ I never have swelling in my knee.
___ I have swelling in my knee, but it does not affect my daily activity.
___ Swelling affects my activity slightly.
___ Swelling affects my activity moderately.
___ Swelling affects my activity severely.
___ Swelling in my knee prevents me from performing all daily activities.

5. To what degree does slipping of your knee affect your daily activity level?
___ I never have slipping of my knee.
___ I have slipping of my knee, but it does not affect my daily activity.
___ Slipping of my knee affects my activity slightly.
___ Slipping of my knee affects my activity moderately.
___ Slipping of my knee affects my activity severely.
___ Slipping of my knee prevents me from performing all daily activities.

6. To what degree does buckling of your knee affect your daily activity level?
___ I never have buckling of my knee.
___ I have buckling of my knee, but it does not affect my daily activity level.
___ Buckling of my knee affects my activity slightly.
___ Buckling of my knee affects my activity moderately.
___ Buckling of my knee affects my activity severely.
___ Buckling of my knee prevents me from performing all daily activities.

7. To what degree does weakness or lack of strength of your leg affect your daily activity level?
___ My leg never feels weak.
___ My leg feels weak, but it does not affect my daily activity.
___ Weakness affects my activity slightly.
___ Weakness affects my activity moderately.
___ Weakness affects my activity severely.
___ Weakness of my leg prevents me from performing all daily activities.

Functional Disability with Activities of Daily Living

8. How does your knee affect your ability to walk?
___ My knee does not affect my ability to walk.
___ I have pain in my knee when walking, but it does not limit my ability to walk.
___ My knee prevents me from walking more than 1 mile.
___ My knee prevents me from walking more than 1/2 mile.
___ My knee prevents me from walking more than 1 block.
___ My knee prevents me from walking.

9. Because of your knee, do you walk with crutches or a cane?
___ I can walk without crutches or a cane.
___ My knee causes me to walk with one crutch or a cane.
___ My knee causes me to walk with two crutches.
___ Because of my knee, I cannot walk, even with crutches.

10. Does your knee cause you to limp when you walk?
___ I can walk without a limp.
___ Sometimes my knee causes me to walk with a limp.
___ Because of my knee, I cannot walk without a limp.

11. How does your knee affect your ability to go up stairs?
___ My knee does not affect my ability to go up stairs.
___ I have pain in my knee when going up stairs, but it does not limit my ability to go up stairs.
___ I am able to go up stairs normally, but I need to rely on use of a railing.
___ I am able to go up stairs one step at a time with the use of a railing.
___ I have to use crutches or a cane to go up stairs.
___ I cannot go up stairs.

FIGURE 30–45. Activities of Daily Living Scale of the Knee Outcome Survey.

Illustration continued on following page

12. How does your knee affect your ability to go down stairs?

____ My knee does not affect my ability to go down stairs.

____ I have pain in my knee when going down stairs, but it does not limit my ability to go down stairs.

____ I am able to go down stairs normally, but I need to rely on use of a railing.

____ I am able to go down stairs one step at a time with the use of a railing.

____ I have to use crutches or a cane to go down stairs.

____ I cannot go down stairs.

13. How does your knee affect your ability to stand?

____ My knee does not affect my ability to stand. I can stand for unlimited amounts of time.

____ I have pain in my knee when standing, but it does not limit my ability to stand.

____ Because of my knee, I cannot stand for more than 1 hour.

____ Because of my knee, I cannot stand for more than 1/2 hour.

____ Because of my knee, I cannot stand for more than 10 minutes.

____ I cannot stand because of my knee.

14. How does your knee affect your ability to kneel on the front of your knee?

____ My knee does not affect my ability to kneel on the front of my knee. I can kneel for unlimited amounts of time.

____ I have pain when kneeling on the front of my knee, but it does not limit my ability to kneel.

____ I cannot kneel on the front of my knee for more than 1 hour.

____ I cannot kneel on the front of my knee for more than 1/2 hour.

____ I cannot kneel on the front of my knee for more than 10 minutes.

____ I cannot kneel on the front of my knee.

15. How does your knee affect your ability to squat?

____ My knee does not affect my ability to squat. I can squat all the way down.

____ I have pain when squatting, but I can still squat all the way down.

____ I cannot squat more than 3/4 of the way down.

____ I cannot squat more than halfway down.

____ I cannot squat more than 1/4 of the way down.

____ I cannot squat at all.

16. How does your knee affect your ability to sit with your knee bent?

____ My knee does not affect my ability to sit with my knee bent. I can sit for unlimited amounts of time.

____ I have pain when sitting with my knee bent, but it does not limit my ability to sit.

____ I cannot sit with my knee bent for more than 1 hour.

____ I cannot sit with my knee bent for more than 1/2 hour.

____ I cannot sit with my knee bent for more than 10 minutes.

____ I cannot sit with my knee bent.

17. How does your knee affect your ability to rise from a chair?

____ My knee does not affect my ability to rise from a chair.

____ I have pain when rising from the seated position, but it does not affect my ability to rise from the seated position.

____ Because of my knee, I can only rise from a chair if I use my hands and arms to assist.

____ Because of my knee, I cannot rise from a chair.

18. How would you rate your current level of knee function during your *usual daily activities* on a scale from 0 to 100, with 100 being your level of knee function prior to your injury?

_____

19. How would you rate the *overall function* of your knee during your *usual daily activities*?

_____ normal

_____ nearly normal

_____ abnormal

_____ severely abnormal

20. As a result of your knee injury, how would you rate your *current level of daily activity*?

_____ normal

_____ nearly normal

_____ abnormal

_____ severely abnormal

21. Since initiation of treatment for your knee, how would you describe your progress?

_____ greatly improved

_____ somewhat improved

_____ neither improved/worsened

_____ somewhat worse

_____ greatly worse

Changes in Daily Activity Level

Please use the following scale to answer questions A–C below.

1 = I was able to perform *unlimited physical work,* which included lifting and climbing.

2 = I was able to perform *limited physical work,* which included lifting and climbing.

3 = I was able to perform *unlimited light activities,* which included walking on level surfaces and stairs.

4 = I was able to perform *limited light activities,* which included walking on level surfaces and stairs.

5 = I was *unable to perform light activities,* which included walking on level surfaces and stairs.

A. ____ *Prior to your knee injury,* how would you describe your usual daily activity? Please indicate only the **HIGHEST** level of activity that described you before your knee injury.

B. ____ *Prior to surgery or treatment* of your knee, how would you describe your usual daily activity? Please indicate only the **HIGHEST** level of activity that described you prior to surgery or treatment to your knee.

C. ____ How would you describe your *current level* of daily activity? Please indicate only the **HIGHEST** level of activity that describes you over the last 1 to 2 days.

FIGURE 30–45 *Continued*

Instructions:

The following questionnaire is designed to determine the symptoms and limitations that you experience because of your knee while you participate in sports activities. Please answer each question by checking the statement that best describes you over the last 1 to 2 days. For a given question, more than one of the statements may describe you, but please mark ONLY the statement which best describes you when you participate in sports activities.

Symptoms

1. To what degree does pain in your knee affect your sports activity level?
   ___ I never have pain in my knee.
   ___ Knee pain does not affect my activity.
   ___ Slightly.
   ___ Moderately.
   ___ Severely.
   ___ Prevents me from performing all sports activities.

2. To what degree does grinding or grating of your knee affect your sports activity level?
   ___ I never have grinding or grating in my knee.
   ___ Grinding/grating does not affect my activity.
   ___ Slightly.
   ___ Moderately.
   ___ Severely.
   ___ Prevents me from performing all sports activities.

3. To what degree does stiffness in your knee affect your sports activity level?
   ___ I never have stiffness in my knee.
   ___ Knee stiffness does not affect my activity.
   ___ Slightly.
   ___ Moderately.
   ___ Severely.
   ___ Prevents me from performing all sports activities.

4. To what degree does swelling in your knee affect your sports activity level?
   ___ I never have swelling in my knee.
   ___ Knee swelling does not affect my activity.
   ___ Slightly.
   ___ Moderately.
   ___ Severely.
   ___ Prevents me from performing all sports activities.

5. To what degree does partial giving way or slipping of your knee affect your sports activity level?
   ___ I never have partial giving way or slipping of my knee.
   ___ Partial giving way does not affect my activity.
   ___ Slightly.
   ___ Moderately.
   ___ Severely.
   ___ Prevents me from performing all sports activities.

6. To what degree does complete giving way or buckling of your knee affect your sports activity level?
   ___ I never have complete giving way or buckling in my knee.
   ___ Knee buckling does not affect my activity.
   ___ Slightly.
   ___ Moderately.
   ___ Severely.
   ___ Prevents me from performing all sports activities.

Functional Disability with Sports Activities

1. How does your knee affect your ability to run straight ahead?
   ___ I am able to run straight ahead full speed without limitations.
   ___ I have pain in my knee but it does not affect my ability.
   ___ Slightly.
   ___ Moderately.
   ___ Severely.
   ___ Prevents me from running.

2. How does your knee affect your ability to jump and land on your involved leg?
   ___ I am able to jump and land on my involved leg without limitations.
   ___ I have pain in my knee but it does not affect my ability.
   ___ Slightly.
   ___ Moderately.
   ___ Severely.
   ___ Prevents me from jumping and landing.

3. How does your knee affect your ability to stop and start quickly?
   ___ I am able to start and stop quickly without limitations.
   ___ I have pain in my knee but it does not affect my ability.
   ___ Slightly.
   ___ Moderately.
   ___ Severely.
   ___ Prevents me from stopping and starting quickly.

4. How does your knee affect your ability to cut and pivot on your involved leg?
   ___ I am able to cut and pivot on my involved leg without limitations.
   ___ I have pain in my knee but it does not affect my ability.
   ___ Slightly.
   ___ Moderately.
   ___ Severely.
   ___ Prevents me from jumping and landing.

FIGURE 30—46. Sports Activity Scale of the Knee Outcome Survey.

Most outcome studies on knee ligament injuries report outcome in terms of knee joint stability. It is assumed that increased laxity, measured manually or with instruments such as the KT-1000, results in greater functional limitations and disability, but this has not always found to be the case. Lephart and associates[11] reported a nonsignificant relationship between the Iowa Athletic Knee Rating Scale Score and increased anterior translation of the tibia measured with the KT-1000. Over the last several years, we have collected outcome data on nearly 200 individuals undergoing knee ligament reconstruction. The average length of follow-up for these patients was 2.9 years. Laxity of the knee was assessed with the KT-1000 using a 30-lb and maximum manual anterior drawer and was reported as side-to-side differences between the involved and noninvolved knees. Manual laxity tests were also performed and were reported according to IKDC guidelines. Analysis of this data failed to demonstrate significant relationships between the involved and noninvolved side differences in the 30-lb and maximum manual KT-1000 scores for anterior tibial translation and the patient's perceived level of disability as indicated by the Modified Cincinnati Knee Score, or by the patient's self-rating on a scale from 0 to 100. A statistically significant relationship, however, was found between the pivot shift and the Cincinnati Knee Rating Scale ($r = -0.24$, $p = 0.002$) and the patient's self-rating on a scale from 0 to 100 ($r = -0.25$, $p = 0.001$). Additionally, significant relationships were found for the reverse pivot shift and the Cincinnati Knee Rating Scale ($r = -0.43$, $p < 0.001$) and self-rating on a scale from 0 to 100 ($r = -0.35$, $p < 0.001$). This indicates that increased laxity with the lateral pivot and reverse pivot shift tests results in greater functional limitations and disability as measured by the Cincinnati Knee Scale and self-rating on a scale from 0 to 100. Further research is needed to clarify the relationship between stability of the knee and functional limitations and disability experienced by the patient.

A variety of functional tests have been proposed to assess outcome following knee ligament injury and/or surgery. Tegner and colleagues[290] studied the one-legged hop, running in a figure-of-eight, running up and down a spiral staircase, and running up and down a slope in 26 individuals with an ACL-deficient knee and 66 uninjured soccer players. The results indicated significant performance deficits in individuals with an ACL-deficient knee compared with the uninjured soccer players. Barber and associates[297] evaluated the one-legged hop for distance, one-legged vertical jump, one-legged timed hop, shuttle run with no pivot, and shuttle run with pivot to predict lower extremity functional limitations in individuals with a ACL-deficient knee. Significant differences were found for ACL-deficient subjects compared to a normal group of subjects for all tests except the shuttle run with a pivot. The vertical jump and shuttle run tests were not capable of detecting functional limitations in the ACL-deficient subjects. For the one-legged hop tests, 50 percent of patients performed normally, but all reported giving way episodes during high-force activities, indicating a lack of sensitivity of such tests to identify functional limitations in these ACL-deficient patients. Lephart and coworkers[11] demonstrated a significant relationship between disability as defined by the Iowa Athletic Knee Rating Scale and performance time on the shuttle run, carioca, and semicircular co-contraction test. Also, those who were able to return to preinjury levels of activity demonstrated significantly better times on the functional performance tests than those who were unable to return to their prior level of activity. Wilk and colleagues[296] found weak positive correlations between the Modified Cincinnati Knee Score and one-legged hop for distance, one-legged hop for time, and one-legged cross-over test. Our data demonstrate a positive relationship between functional limitations and disability as measured with the Modified Cincinnati Knee Score and the patient's self-rating on a scale from 0 to 100 to the hop index and vertical jump index. The hop index is defined as the distance hopped on the

involved leg divided by the noninvolved leg multiplied by 100. The vertical jump index is calculated similarly.

It appears that functional performance tests may be better predictors of functional limitations and disability than measurements of physical impairment following knee ligament injury. It seems likely that deficits in functional performance tests would result in functional limitations and disability for an athlete. Functional performance tests that reproduce the stresses and strains on the knee that occur during athletic activities may be more likely to demonstrate functional limitations and disability. For example, carioca that involves a cross-cutting maneuver reproduces the pivot shift associated with anterolateral instability. It would be expected that this maneuver would be more stressful than a one-legged hop for distance in an individual with an ACL-deficient knee. Additional research is needed to identify functional performance tests that can predict functional limitations and disability following a knee ligament injury accurately.

Functional limitations and disability experienced by a patient following a knee ligament injury may have multifactorial causes. The disability experienced by a patient may be related to a combination of factors such as the type and extent of injury, symptoms, and physical impairment and to psychologic factors such as apprehension, lack of confidence, and fear of reinjury. A model that incorporates all these factors to predict outcome in terms of functional limitations and disability would be complex. We have analyzed data in our database in an attempt to develop a predictive model for disability following knee ligament surgery. The results indicate that outcome in terms of either the Modified Cincinnati Knee Rating Score or the individual's subjective self-rating on a scale from 0 to 100 is best predicted by the results of the reverse and lateral pivot shift tests and hop and vertical jump indices. These variables predict approximately 35 percent of the variance in the Cincinnati Knee Score and subjective self-rating. The amount of variability in the patient's subjective self-rating scale from 0 to 100 predicted by the model was increased to 69 percent by adding the patient's report of pain, swelling, and giving way during sports activities. This preliminary research demonstrates that a number of factors must be considered when attempting to determine outcome following knee ligament injury.

REFERENCES

1. Cailliet R: Knee Pain and Disability. Philadelphia, F.A. Davis, 1976.
2. Kapandji IA: The Physiology of the Joints. New York, Churchill Livington, 1970.
3. Blackburn TA, Craig E, et al: Knee anatomy: A brief review. Phys Ther 1980; 60:1556–1560.
4. Baratz ME, Fu FH, Mengato R: Meniscal tears: The effect of meniscectomy and of repair on intra-articular contact areas and stress in the human knee. Am J Sports Med 1986; 14:270–274.
4a. Muller W. The Knee: Form, Function and Ligament Reconstruction. New York, Springer-Verlag, 1990.
5. Butler DL, Noyes FR, Grood ES: Ligamentous restraints to

anterior-posterior drawer in the human knee. A biomechanical study. J Bone Joint Surg 1980; 62A:259–270.

6. Grood ES, Suntay WJ, Noyes FR, Butler DL: Biomechanics of the knee-extension exercise: Effect of cutting the anterior cruciate ligament. J Bone Joint Surg 1984; 66A:725–734.

7. Palmitier RA, An KN, Scott SG, Chao EYS: Kinetic chain exercises in knee rehabilitation. Sports Med 1991; 11:402–413.

8. Kennedy JC, Weinberg HW, Wilson AS: The anatomy and function of the anterior cruciate ligament as determined by clinical and morphological studies. J Bone Joint Surg 1974; 56A:223–235.

9. Barrack RL, Skinner HB, Buckley SL: Proprioception in the anterior cruciate ligament deficient knee. Am J Sports Med 1989; 17:1–6.

10. Solomonow M, Baratta R, Zhou BH, et al: The synergistic action of the anterior cruciate ligament and thigh muscles in maintaining joint stability. Am J Sports Med 1987; 15:207–213.

11. Lephart SM, Kocher MS, Fu FH, et al: Proprioception following anterior cruciate ligament reconstruction. J Sports Rehabil Med 1992; 1:188–196.

12. Walla DJ, Albright JP, McAuley E, et al: Hamstring control and the unstable anterior cruciate ligament–deficient knee. Am J Sports Med 1985; 13:34–39.

13. Barett DS: Proprioception and function after anterior cruciate ligament reconstruction. J Bone Joint Surg 1991; 73B:833–837.

14. Baratta R, Solomonow M, Zhou BH, et al: Muscular coactivation: The role of the antagonist musculature in maintaining knee stability. Am J Sports Med 1988; 16:113–122.

15. Draganich LF, Jaeger RJ, Krajl AR: Coactivation of the hamstrings and quadriceps during extension of the knee. J Bone Joint Surg 1989; 71A:1075–1081.

16. Sawhney R, Dearwater S, Irrgang JJ, Fu FH: Quadriceps exercise following anterior cruciate ligament reconstruction without anterior tibial displacement. Presented at the Annual Conference of the American Physical Therapy Association. Anaheim, June 1990.

17. Lutz GE, Palmetier RA, An KN, Chao EY: Comparison of tibiofemoral joint forces during open kinetic chain and closed kinetic chain exercises. J Bone Joint Surg 1993; 75A:732–739.

18. Arms SW, Pope MH, Johnson RJ, et al: The biomechanics of anterior cruciate ligament rehabilitation and reconstruction. Am J Sports Med 1984; 12:8–18.

19. Arms S, Johnson R, Pope M: Strain measurement of the hu-man posterior cruciate ligament. Trans Orthop Res Soc 1984; 9:355.

20. Bennyon B, Howe JG, Pope MH, et al: The measurement of anterior cruciate ligament strain in vivo. Int Orthop 1992; 16:1–12.

21. Renstrom P, Arms SW, Stanwyck TS, et al: Strain within the anterior cruciate ligament during hamstring and quadriceps activity. Am J Sports Med 1986; 14:83–87.

22. Kain CC, McCarthy JA, Arms S, et al: An in vivo analysis of the effect of transcutaneous electrical stimulation of the quadriceps and hamstrings on anterior cruciate ligament deformation. Am J Sports Med 1988; 16:147–152.

23. Ohkoshi Y, Yasuda K, Kaneda K, et al: Biomechanical analysis of rehabilitation in the standing position. Am J Sports Med 1991; 19:605–611.

24. Voight M, Bell S, Rhoades D: Instrumented testing of anterior tibial translation in open vs. closed chain activity. Phys Ther 1991; 71:S98.

25. Drez D, Paine R, Neuschwander DC: In vivo testing of closed vs. open kinetic chain exercises in patients with documented tears of the anterior cruciate ligament. Presented at the Annual Conference of the American Orthopaedic Society of Sports Medicine, Orlando, Fla, July 1991.

26. Meglan D, Lutz G, Stuart M: Effects of closed kinetic chain exercises for ACL rehabilitation upon the load in the capsular and ligamentous structures of the knee. Presented at the 39th Annual Meeting of the Orthopaedic Research Society, San Francisco, February 15–18, 1993.

27. Bennyon B, Horre JG, Pope MH, et al: The measurement of anterior cruciate ligament strain in vivo. Int Orthop 1992; 16:1–12.

28. Henning CE, Lynch MA, Glick KR: An in vivo strain gauge study of elongation of the anterior cruciate ligament. Am J Sports Med 1985; 13:1322–1326.

29. Weiss, JR: Electromyographic analysis of the minisquat exercise. Master's Thesis, University of Pittsburgh, 1990.

30. Ninos, JC: Electromyographic analysis of the squat performed in 0 and 30 degrees of lower extermity turn-out. Master's Thesis, University of Pittsburgh, 1993.

31. Williams PL, Warwick R: Functional Neuroanatomy of Man. Philadelphia, WB Saunders Company, 1975.

32. Hungerford DS, Barry M: Biomechanics of the patellofemoral joint. Clin Orthop 1979; 144:9–15.

33. Reilly DT, Martens M: Experimental analysis of the quadriceps muscle force and patello-femoral joint reaction force for various activities. Acta Orthop Scand 1972; 43:126–137.

34. Bandi W: Chondromalacia patellae and femoro-patellar arthrose. Helv Chir Acta 1972; 1 (Suppl):3.

35. Steinkamp LA, Dillingham MF, Markel MD, et al:, Biomechanical considerations in patellofemoral joint rehabilitation. Am J Sports Med 1993; 21:438–444.

36. Noyes FR, Bassett RW, Grood ES, Butler DL: Arthroscopy in acute traumatic hemarthroses of the knee. J Bone Joint Surg 1980; 62A:687–695.

37. Oberlander MA, Shalvoy RM, Hughston JC: The accuracy of the clinical knee examination documented by arthroscopy. A prospective study. 1993; Am J Sports Med 21:773–778.

38. Torg JS, Conrad W, Kalen V: Clinical diagnosis of ACL instability in the athlete. Am J Sports Med 1976; 4:84–93.

39. Anderson AF, Lipscomb AB: Clinical diagnosis of meniscal tears. Description of a new manipulative test. Am J Sports Med 1986; 14:291–293.

40. Gilles H, Seligson D: Precision in the diagnosis of meniscal lesion: A comparison of clinical evaluation, arthrography and arthroscopy. J Bone Joint Surg 1979; 61A:343–346.

41. Patel D: Arthroscopy of the plicae-synovial folds and their significance. Am J Sports Med 1978; 6:217–225.

42. DeHaven KE, Collins HR: Diagnosis of internal derangements of the knee. J Bone Joint Surg 1975; 57A:802–810.

43. Kolowich PA, Paulos LE, Rosenberg TD, Farnsworth S: Lateral release of the patella: Indications and contraindications. Am J Sports Med 1990; 18:359–365.

44. Jonsson T, Althoff B, Peterson L, Renstrom P: Clinical diagnosis of ruptures of the ACL: A comparative study of the Lachman test and anterior drawer sign. Am J Sports Med 1982; 10:100–102.

45. Katz JW, Fingeroth RJ: The diagnostic accuracy of ruptures of the ACL comparing the Lachman test, the anterior drawer sign, and the pivot shift test in acute and chronic knee injuries. Am J Sports Med 1988; 14:88–91.

46. Daniel DM, Stone ML, Sachs R, Malcom L: Instrumented measurement of anterior knee laxity in patients with acute anterior cruciate ligament disruption. Am J Sports Med 1985; 13:401–407.

47. Slocum DB, James SL, Larson RL, Singer KM: Clinical test for anterolateral rotatory instability of the knee. Clin Orthop 1976; 118:63–69.

48. Bach BR Jr, Warren RF, Wickiewicz TL: The pivot shift phenomenon: Results and description of a modified clinical test for ACL insufficiency. Am J Sports Med 1988; 16:571–576.

49. Fetto JF, Marshall JL: Injury to the ACL producing the pivot shift sign: An experimental study on cadaver specimens. J Bone Joint Surg 1979; 61A:710–714.

50. Galway HR, MacIntosh DL: The lateral pivot shift: A symptom and sign of ACL insufficiency. Clin Orthop 1980; 147:45–50.

51. Jakob RP, Staubli HU, Deland JT: Grading the pivot shift: Objective tests with implications for treatment. J Bone Joint Surg 1987; 69B:294–299.

52. Losee RE, Johnson TR, Southwick WO: Anterior subluxation of the lateral tibial plateau. A diagnostic test and operative repair. J Bone Joint Surg 1978; 60A:1015–1030.

53. Hughston JC, Norwood LA: The posterolateral drawer test and external rotational recurvatum test for posterolateral rotary instability of the knee. Clin Orthop 1980; 147:82–87.

54. Insall JN, Hood RW: Bone-block treatment of the medial head of the gastrocnemius for PCL insufficiency. J Bone Joint Surg 1982; 64A:691–699.

55. Harner CD: Posterior cruciate ligament. Presented at the Academy of Orthopaedic Surgeons, 61st Annual Meeting. New Orleans, February 1994.

56. Valtri DM, Warren RF: Isolated and combined PCL injuries. J Am Acad Orthop Surg 1993; 1:67–75.

57. Daniel DM, Stone ML, Barnett P, Sachs R: Use of the quadriceps active test to diagnose PCL disruption and measure posterior laxity of the knee. J Bone Joint Surg 1988; 70A:386–391.

58. Strobel M, Stedtfeld HW: Diagnostic Evaluation of the Knee. Berlin: Springer–Verlag, 1990.

59. Clancy WG Jr, Shelbourne KD, Zoellner GB, et al: Treatment of knee joint instability secondary to rupture of the PCL: Report of a new procedure. J Bone Joint Surg 1983; 65A:310–322.

60. Jakob RP: Observations on rotatory instability of the lateral compartment of the knee. Acta Orthop Scand 1981; 52(Suppl 191):1–32.

61. Gollehon DL, Torzilli PA, Warren RF: The role of the postero-lateral and cruciate ligaments in the stability of the human knee: A biomechanical study. J Bone Joint Surg 1987; 69A:233–242.

62. Owens TC: Posteromedial pivot shift of the knee: A new test for rupture of the PCL. A demonstration in six patients and a study of anatomical specimens. J Bone Joint Surg 1994; 76A:532–539.

63. McMurray TP: The semilunar cartilages. Br J Surg 1942; 29:407–414.

64. Apley AG: The diagnosis of meniscus injuries—some new clinical methods. J Bone Joint Surg 1947; 29B:78–84.

65. Daniel DM, Malcom LL, Losse G, et al: Instrumented measurement of anterior laxity of the knee. J Bone Joint Surg 1985; 67A:720–725.

66. Stratford PW, Miseferi D, Ogilvie R, et al: Assessing the responsiveness of five KT-1000 knee arthrometer measures used to evaluate anterior laxity at the knee joint. Clin J Sports Med 1991; 1:225–228.

67. Highgenboten CL, Jackson AW, Jansson KA, Meske NB: KT-1000 arthrometer: Conscious and unconscious test results using 15, 20, and 30 pounds of force. Am J Sports Med 1992; 20:450–454.

68. Wroble RR, Grood ES, Noyes FR, Schmitt DJ: Reproducibility of Genucom knee analysis system testing. Am J Sports Med 1990; 18:387–395.

69. Boniface RJ, Fu FH, Ilkhanipour K: Objective anterior cruciate ligament testing. Orthopaedics 1986; 9:391–393.

70. King JB, Kumar SJ: The Stryker knee arthrometer in clinical practice. Am J Sports Med 1989; 17:649–650.

71. Riederman R, Wroble RR, Grood ES, et al: Reproducibility of the knee signature system. Am J Sports Med 1991; 19:660–664.

72. Wroble RR, Van Ginkel LA, Grood ES, et al: Repeatability of the KT-1000 arthrometer in a normal population. Am J Sports Med 1990; 18:396–399.

73. Steiner ME, Brown C, Zarins B, et al: Measurement of anterior-posterior displacement of the knee. J Bone Joint Surg 1990; 72A:1307–1315.

74. Anderson AF, Snyder RB, Federspiel CF, Lipscomb AB: Instrumented evaluation of knee laxity: A comparison of five arthrometers. Am J Sports Med 1992; 20:135–140.

75. Highgenboten CL, Jackson A, Meske NB: Genucom, KT-1000, and Stryker knee laxity measuring device comparisons. Am J Sports Med 1989; 17:743–746.

76. Harten WP, Pace MB: Reliability of measuring anterior laxity of the knee joint using a knee ligament arthrometer. Phys Ther 1987; 67:357–359.

77. Boniface RJ, Fu FH, Ilkhanipour K: Objective anterior cruciate ligament testing. Orthopaedics 1986; 9:391–393.

78. Huber FE: Intratester and intertester reliability of the KT-1000 in the assessment of posterior laxity of the knee. Phys Ther 1994; 74:S52.

79. Safran MR, Johnston-Jones K, Kabo JM, Meals RA: The effect of experimental hemarthrosis on joint stiffness and synovial histology in a rabbit model. Clin Orthop 1994; 303:280–281.

80. Resnick D, Goergen TG, Niwayama G: Physical injury. In Resnick D, Niwayama G (eds): Diagnosis of Bone and Joint Disorders, 2nd ed. Philadelphia, WB Saunders, 1988, pp 2756–3008.

81. Pavlov H: The radiographic diagnosis of the anterior cruciate deficient knee. Clin Orthop 1983; 172:57–63.

82. Dietz GW, Wilcox DM, Montgomery JB: Segond tibial condyle fracture: Lateral capsular ligament avulsion. Radiology 1986; 159:467–469.

83. Rosenberg TD, Paulos LE, Parker RD, et al: The 45° posteroan-terior flexion weightbearing radiograph of the knee. J Bone Joint Surg 1988; 70A:1479–1483.

84. Warren RF: Acute ligament injuries. In Insall JN (ed): Surgery of the Knee. New York, Churchill Livingstone, 1984, pp 261–294.

85. Jacobsen K: Stress radiographical measurement of anteroposterior, medial, and lateral stability of the knee joint. Acta Orthop Scand 1976; 47:335–344.

86. Jacobsen K: Gonylaxometry. Stress radiographic measurement of passive stability in the knee joints of normal subjects and patients with ligament injuries. Accuracy and range of application. Acta Orthop Scand 1981; 52 (Suppl 194):1–263.

87. Kennedy JC, Fowler PJ: Medial and anterior instability of the knee. An anatomical and clinical study using stress machines. J Bone Joint Surg 1971; 53A:1257–1260.

88. Franklin JL, Rosenberg TD, Paulos LE, France EP: Radiographic assessment of instability of the knee due to rupture of the ACL. A quadriceps-contraction technique. J Bone Joint Surg 1991; 73A:365–372.

89. Torzilli PA, Greenberg RL, Insall JN: An in vivo biomechanical evaluation of anterior-posterior motion of the knee. Roentgenographic measurement technique, stress machine, and stable population. J Bone Joint Surg 1981; 63A:960–968.

90. Brown DW, Allman FL, Eaton SB: Knee arthrography: A comparison of radiographic and surgical findings in 295 cases. Am J Sports Med 1978; 6:165–172.

91. Crabtree SD, Bedford AF, Edgar MA: The value of arthrography and arthroscopy in association with a sports injury clinic: A prospective and comparative study of 182 patients. Injury 1981; 13:220–226.

92. Daniel DM, Daniels E, Aronson D: The diagnosis of meniscus pathology. Clin Orthop 1982; 163:218–224.

93. Dumas JM, Edde DJ: Meniscal abnormalities: Prospective correlation of double contrast arthrography and arthroscopy. Radiology 1986; 160:453–456.

94. Nicholas JA, Freiberger RH, Killoran PJ: Double contrast arthrography of the knee. Its value in the management of 225 knee derangements. J Bone Joint Surg 1970; 52A:203–220.

95. Thijn CJP: Accuracy of double contrast arthrography of the knee joint. Skel Radiol 1982; 8:187–192.

96. Dye SF, Andersen CT, Stowell MT: Unrecognized abnormal osseous metabolic activity about the knee with symptomatic ACL deficiency. Orthop Trans 1987; 11:492.

97. Marks PH, Goldenberg JA, Vezina WC, et al: Subchondral bone infractions in acute ligamentous knee injuries demonstrated on bone scintigraphy and magnetic resonance imaging. J Nucl Med 1992; 33:516–520.

98. Bauer KC, Persson PE, Nilsson OS: Tears of the medial meniscus associated with increased radionuclide activity of the proximal tibia. Report of three cases. Int Orthop 1989; 13:153–155.

99. Dye SF, McBride JT, Chew MH, et al: Unrecognized abnormal osseous metabolic activity in patients with documented meniscal pathology. Am J Sports Med 1989; 17:723–724.

100. Dye SF, Chew MH, McBride JT, Sostre G: Restoration of osseous homeostasis of the knee following meniscal surgery. Orthop Trans 1992; 16:725.

101. Lohmann M, Kanstrup IL, Gergvary I, Tollund C: Bone scintigraphy in patients suspected of having meniscus tears. Scand J Med Sci Sports 1991; 1:123–127.

102. Marymont JV, Lynch MA, Henning CE: Evaluation of meniscus tears of the knee by radionuclide imaging. Am J Sports Med 1983; 11:423–435.

103. Mooar P, Gregg J, Jacobstein J: Radionuclide imaging of internal derangements of the knee. Am J Sports Med 1987; 15:132–137.

104. Teitz CC: Ultrasonography in the knee. Radiol Clin North Am 1988; 26:55–62.

105. Passareillo R, Trecco F, Depaulis F, et al: Computed tomography of the knee joint: Technique of study and normal anatomy. J Comput Assist Tomogr 1983; 7:1035–1042.

106. Passareillo R, Trecco F, Depaulis F, et al: Computed tomography of the knee joint: Clinical results. J Comput Assist Tomogr 1983; 7:1043–1049.

107. Pavlov H, Hirschy JC, Torg JS: Computed tomography of the cruciate ligaments. Radiology 1979; 132:389–393.

108. Reicher MA, Bassett LW, Gold RH: High resolution magnetic

resonance imaging of the knee joint: Pathologic correlations. Am J Roentgenol 1985; 145:903–909.

109. Reicher MA, Rauschning W, Gold RH, et al: High resolution magnetic resonance imaging of the knee joint: Normal anatomy. Am J Roentgenol 1985; 145:895–902.

110. Reicher MA, Hartzman S, Duckwiler GR, et al: Meniscal injuries: Detection using MR imaging. Radiology 1986; 159:753–757.

111. Silva I, Silver DM: Tears of the meniscus as revealed by magnetic resonance imaging. J Bone Joint Surg 1988; 70A:199–202.

112. Polly DW, Callaghan JJ, Sikes RA, et al: The accuracy of selective magnetic resonance imaging compared with findings of arthroscopy of the knee. J Bone Joint Surg 1988; 70A:192–198.

113. Jackson DW, Jennings LD, Maywood RM, Berger PE: Magnetic resonance imaging of the knee. Am J Sports Med 1988; 16:29–38.

114. Crues JV III, Mink JH, Levy TL, et al: Meniscal tears of the knee: Accuracy of MR Imaging. Radiology 1987; 164:445–448.

115. Fischer SP, Fox JM, DelPizzo W, et al: Accuracy of diagnoses from magnetic resonance imaging of the knee. A multi-center analysis of one thousand and fourteen patients. J Bone Joint Surg 1991; 73A:2–10.

116. Raunest J, Oberle K, Loehnert J, Hoetzinger H: The clinical value of magnetic resonance imaging in the evaluation of meniscal disorders. J Bone Joint Surg 1991; 73A:11–16.

117. Gross ML, Grover JS, Bassett LW, et al: Magnetic resonance imaging of the PCL: Clinical use to improve diagnostic accuracy. Am J Sports Med 1992; 20:732–737.

118. Mandelbaum BR, Finerman GAM, Reicher MA, et al: Magnetic resonance imaging as a tool for evaluation of traumatic knee injuries. Am J Sports Med 1986; 14:361–370.

119. Mink JH, Levy T, Crues JV III: Tears of the ACL and menisci of the knee: MR imaging evaluation. Radiology 1988; 167:769–774.

120. Vellet AD, Marks P, Fowler P, Munro T: Accuracy of nonorthogonal magnetic resonance imaging in acute disruption of the ACL. Arthroscopy 1989; 5:287–293.

121. DeHaven KE: Diagnosis of acute knee injuries with hemarthrosis. Am J Sports Med 1980; 8:9.

122. DeLee JC: Complications of arthroscopy and arthroscopic surgery: Results of a national surgery. Arthroscopy 1985; 1:204–220.

123. McGinty JB: Complications of arthroscopy and arthroscopic surgery. In McGinty JB (ed): Operative Arthroscopy. New York, Raven Press, 1991, pp 47–54.

124. Shapiro MS, Safran MR, Crockett H, Finerman GAM: Local anesthesia for knee arthroscopy: Efficacy and cost benefits. Am J Sports Med 1994 23:50–54.

125. Besser MIB, Stahl S: Arthroscopic surgery performed under local anesthesia as an outpatient procedure. Arch Orthop Trauma Surg 1986; 105:296–297.

126. McGinty JB, Matza RA: Arthroscopy of the knee. Evaluation of an outpatient procedure under local anesthesia. J Bone Joint Surg 1978; 60A:787–789.

127. Minkoff J, Putterman E: The unheralded value of arthroscopy using local anesthesia for diagnostic specificity and intraoperative corroboration of therapeutic achievement. Clin Sports Med 1987; 6:471.

128. Wertheim SB, Klaus RM: Arthroscopic surgery of the knee using local anesthesia with minimal intravenous sedation. Am J Arthroscopy 1991; 1:7–10.

129. Noyes FR, Grood ES, Suntay WJ: Three-dimensional motion analysis of clinical stress tests for anterior knee subluxations. Acta Orthop Scand, 1989; 60:308–318.

130. Noyes FR, Mooar LA, Moorman CT III, McGinniss GH: Partial tears of the anterior cruciate ligament. Progression to complete ligament deficiency. J Bone Joint Surg 1989; 71B:825–833.

131. Hughston JC, Andrews JR, Cross MJ, et al. Classification of knee ligament instabilities: 1. The medial compartment and cruciate ligament. 2. The lateral compartment. J Bone Joint Surg 58A:159–179, 1976.

132. Miyasaka KC, Daniel DM, Stone ML, Hirschman P: The incidence of knee ligament injuries in the general population. Am J Knee Surg 1991; 4:3–8.

133. Johnson RJ: The ACL problem. Clin Orthop 1983; 172:14–18.

134. Pickett JC, Altizer TJ: Injuries of the ligaments of the knee: A study of the types of injury and treatment in 129 patients. Clin Orthop 1971; 76:27–32.

135. Daniel DM, Stone ML, Dobson BE, et al: Fate of the ACL injured patient: A prospective outcome study. Am J Sports Med 1994; 22:632–644.

136. LaPrade RF, Burnett QB: Femoral intercondylar notch stenosis and correlation to anterior cruciate ligament injuries: A prospective study. Am J Sports Med 1994; 2:198–202.

137. Souryal TO, Freeman TR, Evans JP: Intercondylar notch size and ACL injuries in athletes: A prospective study. Am J Sports Med 1993; 21:535–539.

138. Malone TR: Relationship of gender in anterior cruciate ligament (ACL) injuries of NCAA Division I basketball players. Presented at Specialty Day Meeting of the American Orthopedic Society for Sports Medicine, Washington, DC, February 23, 1992.

139. Tria AJ Jr, Klein KS: An Illustrated Guide to the Knee. New York, Churchill Livingstone, 1991.

140. Andersson C, Odensten M, Good L, et al: Surgical or non-surgical treatment of acute rupture of the ACL. A randomized study with long-term follow-up. J Bone Joint Surg 1989; 71A:965–974.

141. Sommerlath K, Lysholm J, Gillquist J: The long-term course after treatment of acute ACL ruptures. A 9 to 16 year follow-up. Am J Sports Med 1991; 19:156–162.

142. McDaniel WJ Jr, Dameron TB Jr: Untreated anterior ruptures of the cruciate ligament: A follow-up study. J Bone Joint Surg 1980; 62A:310–322.

143. Warren RF, Marshall JL: Injuries to the anterior cruciate and MCLs of the knee: A long-term follow-up of 86 cases — Part II. Clin Orthop 1978; 136:197–211.

144. Sandberg R, Balkfors B, Nilsson B, Westlin N: Operative versus non-operative treatment of recent injuries to the ligaments of the knee. J Bone Joint Surg 1987; 69A:1120–1126.

145. Wroble PR, Brand RA: Paradoxes in the history of the ACL. Clin Orthop 1990; 259:183–191.

146. Cooper DE, Warren RF, Warner JJP: The PCL and posterolateral structures of the knee: Anatomy, function and patterns of injury. Instr Course Lect 1991; 40:249–270.

147. Clendenin MB, DeLee JC, Heckman JD: Interstitial tears of the PCL of the knee. Orthopaedics 1980; 3:764–772.

148. Kennedy JC, Hawkins RJ, Willis RB: Tension studies of human knee ligaments: Yield point, ultimate failure and disruption of the cruciate and collateral ligaments. J Bone Joint Surg 1976; 58A:350–355.

149. Parolie JM, Bergfeld JA: Long-term results of non-operative treatment of isolated PCL injuries in the athlete. Am J Sports Med 1986; 14:35–38.

150. Trickey EL: Injuries to the PCL: Diagnosis and treatment of early injuries and reconstruction of late instability. Clin Orthop 1980; 147:76–81.

151. Insall JN, Hood RW: Bone block transfer of the medial head of the gastrocnemius for posterior cruciate insufficiency. J Bone Joint Surg 1982; 65A:691–699.

152. Fowler PJ, Messieh SS: Isolated PCL injuries in athletes. Am J Sports Med 1987; 15:553–557.

153. Geissler WB, Whipple TL: Intraarticular abnormalities in association with PCL injuries. Am J Sports Med 1993; 21:846–849.

154. Torg JS, Barton TM, Pavlov H, Stine R: Natural history of the PCL-deficient knee. Clin Orthop 1989; 246:208–216.

155. Dejour H, Walch G, Peyrot J, Eberhard P: The natural history of rupture of the PCL. Fr J Orthop Surg 1988; 2:112–120.

156. Keller PM, Shelbourne KD, McCarroll JR, Rettig AC: Nonoperatively treated isolated PCL injuries. Am J Sports Med 1993; 21:132–136.

157. Skyhar MJ, Warren RF, Ortiz GJ, et al: The effects of sectioning of the PCL and the posterolateral complex on the articular contact pressures within the knee. J Bone Joint Surg 1993; 75A:694–699.

158. Tewes DP, Fields MD, Fritts HM, et al: Longitudinal comparison of MRI findings in knees with PCL injuries. Presented at the Specialty Day Meeting of the American Orthopaedic Society for Sports Medicine, New Orleans, February 24, 1994.

159. Derscheid GL, Garrick JG: MCL injuries in football. Non-

operative management of grade I and II sprains. Am J Sports Med 1981; 9:365–368.

160. Holden DL, Eggert AW, Butler JE: The nonoperative treatment of grade I and II MCL injuries to the knee. Am J Sports Med 1983; 11:340–344.

161. Indelicato PA: Non-operative treatment of complete tears of the MCL of the knee. J Bone Joint Surg 1983; 65A:323–329.

162. Ballmer PM, Jakob RP: The nonoperative treatment of isolated complete tears of the MCL of the knee: A prospective study. Acta Orthop Trauma Surg 1988; 107:273–276.

163. Ellsasser JC, Reynolds FC, Omohundro JR: The non-operative treatment of collateral ligament injuries of the knee in professional football players. An analysis of seventy-four injuries treated non-operatively and twenty-four injuries treated surgically. J Bone Joint Surg 1974; 56A:1185–1190.

164. Fetto JF, Marshall JL: MCL injuries of the knee: A rationale for treatment. Clin Orthop 1978; 132:206–218.

165. Indelicato PA, Hermansdorfer J, Huegel M: Non-operative management of complete tears of the MCL of the knee in intercollegiate football players. Clin Orthop 1990; 256:174–177.

166. Jones RE, Henley MB, Francis P: Nonoperative management of isolated grade III collateral ligament injury in high school football players. Clin Orthop 1986; 213:137–140.

167. DeLee JC, Riley MB, Rockwood CA: Acute straight lateral instability of the knee. Am J Sports Med 1983; 11:404–411.

168. Terranova WA, McLaughlin RE, Morgan RF: An algorithm for the management of ligamentous injuries of the knee associated with common peroneal nerve palsy. Orthopaedics 1986; 9:1135–1140.

169. Cooper DE, Speer KP, Wickiewicz TL, Warren RF: Complete knee dislocation without PCL disruption, a report of four cases and review of the literature. Clin Orthop 1992; 284:228–233.

170. Shelbourne KD, Pritchard J, Rettig AC, et al: Knee dislocations with intact PCL. Orthop Rev 1992; 21:607–611.

171. Green N, Allen B: Vascular injuries associated with dislocation of the knee. J Bone Joint Surg 1977; 59A:236–239.

172. Roman PD, Hopson CN, Zenni EJ Jr: Traumatic dislocation of the knee: A report of 30 cases and literature review. Orthop Rev 1987; 12:917–924.

173. DeBakey M, Simeone F: Battle injuries in World War II: An analysis of 2,471 cases. Ann Surg 1946; 123:534–579.

174. Phifer T, Gerlock A, Vekovius W: Amputation risk factors in superficial femoral artery and vein injuries. Am Surg 1983; 199:241–243.

175. Shelbourne KD, Porter DA, Clingman JA, et al: Low-velocity knee dislocation. Orthop Rev 1991; 20:995–1004.

176. Towne LC, Blazina ME, Marmor L: Lateral compartment syndrome of the knee. Clin Orthop 1971; 76:160–168.

177. White J: The results of traction injury to the common peroneal nerve. J Bone Joint Surg 1968; 50B:346–350.

178. Taylor AR, Arden GP, Rainey HA: Traumatic dislocation of the knee: A report of 43 cases with special reference to conservative treatment. J Bone Joint Surg 1972; 54B:96–102.

179. Sargeant AJ, Davies CTM, Edwards RHT, et al: Functional and structural changes after disuse of human muscle. Clin Sci Mol Med 1977; 52:337–342.

180. Haggmark T, Jansson E, Erikson E: Fiber type, area metabolic potential of the thigh muscle in man after knee surgery and immobilization. Int J Sports Med 1981; 2:12–17.

181. Lehmann JF, Masock AJ, Warren CG, Koblanski JN: Effect of therapeutic temperatures on tendon extensibility. Arch Phys Med Rehab 1970; 51:481–487.

182. Sherington C: Reciprocal innervation of antagonist muscles: 14th note on double reciprocal innervation. Proc R Soc (London) 1909; B91:244–268.

183. Basmajian J, Deluca C: Muscles Alive, 5th ed. Baltimore, Williams & Wilkins, 1985.

184. Bassett GS, Fleming BW: The Lenox Hill brace in anterolateral rotatory instability. Am J Sports Med 1983; 11:345–348.

185. Beck C, Drez D, Young J, et al: Instrumented testing of functional knee braces. Am J Sports Med 1986; 14:253–256.

186. Colville MR, Lee CL, Ciullo JV: The Lenox Hill brace: An evaluation of effectiveness in treating knee instability. Am J Sports Med 1986; 14:257–261.

187. Wojtys EM, Loubert PV, Samson SY, Viviano DM: Use of a knee brace for control of tibial translation and rotation: A comparison,

188. Kaplan N, Wickiewicz TL, Warren RF: Primary surgical treatment of ACL ruptures. A long-term follow-up study. Am J Sports Med 1990; 18:354–358.

189. Andersson C, Gillquist J: Treatment of acute isolated and combined ruptures of the ACL. A long-term follow-up study. Am J Sports Med 1992; 20:7–12.

190. Sherman MF, Bonamo JR: Primary repair of the ACL. Clin Sports Med 1988; 7:739–750.

191. Sgaglione NA, Warren RF, Wickiewicz TL, et al: Primary repair with semitendinosus tendon augmentation of acute ACL injuries. Am J Sports Med 1990; 18:64–73.

192. Gillquist J, Odensten M: Reconstruction of old ACL tears with a Dacron prosthesis. A prospective study. Am J Sports Med 1993; 21:358–366.

193. Barrett GR, Line LL, Shelton WR, et al: The Dacron ligament prosthesis in ACL reconstruction. A four-year review. Am J Sports Med 1993; 21:367–373.

194. Paulos LE, Rosenberg TD, Grewe SR, et al: The Gore-Tex ACL prosthesis. A long-term follow up. Am J Sports Med 1992; 20:246–252.

195. Shelbourne KD, Whitaker HJ, McCarroll JR, et al: ACL injury: Evaluation of intra-articular reconstruction of acute tears without repair. Two to seven year follow-up in 155 athletes. Am J Sports Med 1990; 18:484–489.

196. O'Brien SJ, Warren RF, Pavlov H, et al: Reconstruction of the chronically insufficient ACL with the central third of the patellar ligament. J Bone Joint Surg 1991; 73A:278–286.

197. Buss DD, Warren RF, Wickiewicz TL, et al: Arthroscopically assisted reconstruction of the ACL with use of autogenous patellar-ligament grafts. Results after twenty-four to forty-two months. J Bone Joint Surg 1993; 75A:1346–1355.

198. Noyes FR, Barber SD: The effect of a ligament-augmentation device on allograft reconstructions for chronic ruptures of the ACL. J Bone Joint Surg 1992; 74A:960–973.

199. Moyen BJL, Jenny J-Y, Mandrino AH, Lerat J-L: Comparison of reconstruction of the ACL with and without a Kennedy ligament-augmentation device. A randomized, prospective study. J Bone Joint Surg 1992; 74A:1313–1319.

200. Clancy WG Jr, Nelson DA, Reider B, Narechania AG: ACL reconstruction using one-third of the patellar ligament, augmented by extra-articular tendon transfers. J Bone Joint Surg 1982; 64A:352–359.

201. Shelbourne KD, Wilckens JH, Mollabashy A, DeCarlo M: Arthrofibrosis in acute ACL reconstructions. The effect of timing of reconstruction and rehabilitation. Am J Sports Med 1991; 19:332–336.

202. Harner CD, Irrgang JJ, Paul JJ, et al: Loss of motion after ACL reconstruction. Am J Sports Med 1992; 20:499–506.

203. Noyes FR, Butler DL, Grood ES, et al: Biomechanical analysis of human ligament grafts used in knee ligament repairs and reconstructions. J Bone Joint Surg 1984; 66A:344–352.

204. Alm A, Stromberg B: Transposed medial third of patellar ligament in reconstruction of the anterior cruciate ligament. A surgical and morphological study in dogs. Acta Chir Scand 1974; 445:37–49.

205. Arnoczky SP, Warren RF, Ashlock MA: Replacement of the anterior cruciate ligament using a patellar tendon allograft. J Bone Joint Surg 1986; 68A:376–385.

206. Clancy WG, Narechania RG, Rosenberg TD, et al: Anterior and posterior cruciate ligament reconstruction in rhesus monkeys. J Bone Joint Surg 1981; 63A:1270–1284.

207. Shino K, Kawasaki T, Hirose H, et al: Replacement of the anterior cruciate ligament by an allogeneic tendon graft. J Bone Joint Surg 1984; 66B:672–681.

208. Alm A, Gillquist J, Stromberg B: The medial third of the patellar ligament in reconstruction of the anterior cruciate ligament. A clinical and histological study by means of arthroscopy or arthrotomy. Acta Chir Scand 1974; 445:5–14.

209. Yasuda K, Tomiyama Y, Ohkoshi Y, Kaneda K: Arthroscopic observations of autogenic quadriceps and patellar tendon grafts after anterior cruciate ligament reconstruction of the knee. Clin Orthop Rel Res 1989; 246:217–224.

210. Arnoczky SP, Tarvin GB, Marshall JL: Anterior cruciate ligament replacement using patellar tendon: An evaluation of graft

in cadaver, of available models. J Bone Joint Surg 1990; 72A:1323–1329.

revascularization in the dog. J Bone Joint Surg 1982; 64A:217–224.

211. Drez DJ, DeLee J, Holden JP, et al: Anterior cruciate ligament reconstruction using bone-patellar tendon-bone allografts: A biological and biomechanical evaluation in goats. Am J Sports Med 1991; 19:256–263.

212. Jackson DW, Grood ES, Goldstein JD, et al: A comparison of patellar tendon autograft and allograft used for anterior cruciate ligament reconstruction in the goat model. Am J Sports Med 1993; 21:176–185.

213. Shino K, Inque M, Horibe S, et al: Surface blood flow and histology of human anterior cruciate ligament allografts. J Arthrosc Rel Surg 1991; 7:171–176.

214. Paulos L, Noyes FR, Grood E, Butler DL: Knee rehabilitation after anterior cruciate ligament reconstruction and repair. Am J Sports Med 1981; 9:140–149.

215. Shelbourne KD, Nitz P: Accelerated rehabilitation after anterior cruciate ligament reconstruction. Am J Sports Med 1990; 18:292–299.

216. Mohtadi NGH, Webster-Bogaert S, Fowler PJ: Limitation of motion following anterior cruciate ligament reconstruction: A case control study. Am J Sports Med 1991; 19:620–625.

217. Noyes FR, Wojtys EM, Marshall MT: The early diagnosis and treatment of developmental patella infera syndrome. Clin Orthop Rel Res 1991; 265:241–252.

218. Paulos LE, Rosenberg TD, Drawbert J, et al: Intrapatellar contracture syndrome. Am J Sports Med 1987; 15:331–341.

219. Sachs RA, Daniel DM, Stone ML, Garfein RF: Patellofemoral problems after anterior cruciate ligament reconstruction. Am J Sports Med 1989; 17:760–765.

220. Strum GM, Friedman MJ, Fox JM, et al: Acute anterior cruciate ligament reconstruction: Analysis of complications. Clin Orthop 1990; 253:184–189.

221. Irrgang JJ, Harner CD, Fu FH, et al: Loss of motion following ACL reconstruction: A second look. Presented at the 12th Annual Meeting of the Arthroscopy Association of North America, Palm Desert, CA, April 4, 1993.

222. Dandy D, Pusey R: The long-term results of unrepaired tears of the posterior cruciate ligament. J Bone Joint Surg 1982; 64B:92–94.

223. Tourisu T: Isolated avulsion fracture of the tibial attachment PCL. J Bone Joint Surg 1977; 59A:58–72.

224. Burks RT, Schaffer JJ: A simplified approach to the tibial attachment of the PCL. Clin Orthop 1990; 254:216–219.

225. Drucker MM, Wynne GF: Avulsion of the PCL from its femoral attachment: An isolated ligamentous injury. J Trauma 1975; 15:616–617.

226. McMaster WC: Isolated PCL injury: Literature, review, and case reports. J Trauma 1975; 15:1025–1029.

227. Roth JH, Bray RC, Best TM, et al: PCL reconstruction by transfer of the medial gastrocnemius tendon. Am J Sports Med 1988; 16:21–28.

228. Wirth CJ, Jager M: Dynamic double tendon replacement of the PCL. Am J Sports Med 1984; 12:39–43.

229. Lipscomb AB, Anderson AF, Norwig ED, et al: Isolated PCL reconstruction. Long-term results. Am J Sports Med 1993; 21:490–496.

230. Ogata K: PCL reconstruction: A comparative study of two different methods. Bull Hosp Joint Dis 1991; 51:186–198.

231. Tillberg B: The late repair of torn cruciate ligaments using menisci. J Bone Joint Surg 1977; 59B:15–19.

232. Lindstrom N: Cruciate ligament plastics with meniscus. Acta Orthop Scand 1960; 29:150–152.

233. Jones RC, Richardson AB: Gore-Tex PCL replacement – preliminary clinical results. Orthop Trans 1990; 14:123–124.

234. Shirakura K, Kato K, Udagawa E: Characteristics of the isokinetic performance of patients with injured cruciate ligaments. Am J Sports Med 1992; 20:754–760.

235. Pournaras J, Symeonides PP: The results of surgical repair of acute tears of the PCL. Clin Orthop 1991;267:103–107.

236. Bianchi M: Acute tears of the PCL: Clinical study and results of operative treatment in 27 cases. Am J Sports Med 1983; 11:308–314.

237. Girgis F, Marshall J, Monajem A: The cruciate ligaments of the knee joint. Anatomical, functional and experimental analysis. Clin Orthop 1975; 106:216–231.

238. Kannus P, Bergfeld J, Jarvinen M, et al: Injuries to the posterior cruciate ligament of the knee. Sports Med 1991; 12:110–131.

239. Van Dommelen B, Fowler P: Anatomy of the posterior cruciate ligament. Am J Sports Med 1989; 17:24–29.

240. Bosch U, Kasperczyk W, Marx M, et al: Healing at graft fixation site under functional conditions in posterior cruciate ligament reconstruction. Arch Orthop Trauma Surg 1989; 108:154–158.

241. Anderson DR, Weiss JA, Takai S, et al: Healing of the medial collateral ligament following a triad injury: A biomechanical and histological study of the knee in rabbits. J Orthop Res 1992; 10:485–495.

242. Weiss JA, Woo SLY, Ohland KJ, et al: Evaluation of a new injury model to study medial collateral ligament healing: Primary repair versus nonoperative treatment. J Orthop Res 1991; 9:516–528.

243. Hastings DE: The non-operative management of collateral ligament injuries of the knee joint. Clin Orthop Rel Res 1980; 147:22–28.

244. Safran MR, Caldwell GL Jr, Fu FH: Proprioceptive considerations in surgery. J Sports Rehab 1994; 3:105–115.

245. Meyers MH, Harvey JP Jr: Traumatic dislocations of the knee joint. J Bone Joint Surg 1971; 53A:16–29.

246. Meyers MH, Moore TM, Harvey JP Jr: Follow-up notes on articles previously published in the journal. Traumatic dislocation of the knee joint. J Bone Joint Surg 1975; 57A:430–433.

247. Sisto DJ, Warren RF: Complete knee dislocation. Follow-up operative treatment. Clin Orthop 1985; 198:94–101.

248. Metcalf RW: Arthroscopic meniscal surgery. In McGinty JB (ed): Operative Arthroscopy. New York, Raven Press, 1991, pp 203–236.

249. Egner E: Knee joint meniscal degeneration as it relates to tissue fiber structure and mechanical resistance. Pathol Res Pract 1982; 173:310–324.

250. Hough AJ, Webber RJ: Pathology of the meniscus. Clin Orthop 1990; 252:32–40.

251. Bird MDT, Sweet MBE: A system of canals in semilunar menisci. Ann Rheum Dis 1987; 46:670–673.

252. Bird MDT, Sweet MBE: Canals in the semilunar meniscus: Brief report. J Bone Joint Surg 1988; 70B:839.

253. O'Connor RL: Arthroscopy. Philadelphia, JB Lippincott, 1977.

254. Arnoczky SP, Adams ME, DeHaven KE, et al: Meniscus. In Woo SLY, Buckwalter JA (eds): Injury and Repair of the Musculo-skeletal Soft Tissues. Park Ridge, IL, American Association of Orthopaedic Surgeons, 1988; pp 487–537.

255. Dandy DJ, Jackson RW: Meniscectomy and chondromalacia of the femoral condyle. J Bone Joint Surg 1975; 57A:1116–1119.

256. Fahmy NRM, Williams EA, Noble J: Meniscal pathology and osteoarthritis of the knee. J Bone Joint Surg 1983; 65B:24–28.

257. Ahmed AM: The load bearing role of the knee meniscus. In Mow VC, Arnoczky SP, Jackson DW (eds): Knee Meniscus: Basic and Clinical Foundations. New York, Raven Press, 1992, pp 59–73.

258. King D: The healing of the semilunar cartilages. J Bone Joint Surg 1936; 18:333–342.

259. King D: The function of the semilunar cartilages. J Bone Joint Surg 1936; 18:1069–1076.

260. Shrive NG, O'Connor JJ, Goodfellow JW: Load bearing in the knee joint. Clin Orthop 1978; 131:279–287.

261. Fithian DC, Kelley MA, Mow VC: Material properties and structure-function relationships in the menisci. Clin Orthop 1990; 252:19–31.

262. Voloshin AS, Wosk J: Shock absorption of meniscectomized and painful knees: A comparative in vivo study. J Biomed Eng 1983; 5:157–161.

263. Krause WR, Pope MH, Johnson RJ, Wilder DG: Mechanical changes in the knee after meniscectomy. J Bone Joint Surg 1976; 58A:599–604.

264. Levy IM, Torzilli PA, Warren RF: The effect of medial meniscectomy on anterior-posterior motion of the knee. J Bone Joint Surg 1982; 64A:883–888.

265. Markolf KL, Mensch JS, Amstutz HC: Stiffness and laxity of the knee: The contribution of the supporting structures. J Bone Joint Surg 1976; 58A:583–593.

266. Markolf KL, Bargar WL, Shoemaker SC, Amstutz HC: The role of joint load in knee stability. J Bone Joint Surg 1981; 63A:570–585.

267. Shoemaker SC, Markolf KL: The role of the meniscus in the

anterior-posterior stability of the loaded anterior cruciate deficient knee. J Bone Joint Surg 1986; 68A:71–79.

268. MacConaill MA: The functions of intra-articular fibro-cartilages with special reference to the knee and inferior radio-ulnar joints. J Anat 1932; 66:210–227.

269. Fairbank TJ: Knee joint changes after meniscectomy. J Bone Joint Surg 1948; 30B:664–670.

270. Clark CR, Ogden JA: Development of the menisci of the human knee joint. J Bone Joint Surg 1983; 65A:538–547.

271. Arnoczky SP, Warren RF: Microvasculature of the human meniscus. Am J Sports Med 1982; 10:90–95.

272. DeHaven KE, Black KP, Griffiths HJ: Open meniscus repair: Technique and 2 to 9 year results. Am J Sports Med 1989; 17:788–795.

273. Sommerlath K, Hamberg P: Healed meniscal tears in unstable knees: A long term follow-up of seven years. Am J Sports Med 1989; 17:161–163.

274. Arnoczky SP, Warren RF, Spivak J: Meniscal repair using an exogenous fibrin clot. J Bone Joint Surg 1988; 70A:1209–1217.

275. Scott GA, Jolly BL, Henning CE: Combined posterior incision and arthroscopic intra-articular repair of the meniscus. J Bone Joint Surg 1986; 68A:847–861.

276. Rosenberg TD, Scott SM, Coward DB, et al: Arthroscopic meniscal repair evaluated with repeat arthroscopy. Arthroscopy 1986; 2:14–20.

277. Swensen TM, Johnson DL, Aizawa H, et al: Human meniscal bony insertion sites: Gross, arthroscopic, and topographical anatomy as a basis for meniscal transplantation. Presented at the Sixty-First Annual Meeting of the American Academy of Orthopaedic Surgeons, New Orleans, February 1994.

278. Garrett JC: Meniscal transplantation: A review of forty-three cases with two to seven year follow-up. Presented at the Specialty Day Meeting of the American Orthopaedic Society for Sports Medicine, New Orleans, February 24, 1994.

279. Garrett JC, Stevensen RN: Meniscal transplantation in the human knee: A preliminary report. Arthroscopy 1991; 7:57–62.

280. Stone KR, Rosenberg T: Surgical technique of meniscal transplantation. Arthroscopy 1993; 9:234–237.

281. Stone KR, Rodkey WG, Webber RJ, et al: Development of a prosthetic meniscal replacement. *In* Mow VC, Arnoczky SP, Jackson DW (eds): Knee Meniscus: Basic and Clinical Foundations. New York, Raven Press, 1992, pp 165–173.

282. Arnoczky SP, Warren RF, McDevitt CA: Meniscal replacement using a cryopreserved allograft. An experimental study in the dog. Clin Orthop 1990; 252:121–128.

283. Nagi S: Disability concepts revisited: Implication for prevention. *In* Pope A, Tarlov A (eds): Disability in America: Toward a National Agenda for Prevention. Washington, DC, National Academy Press, 1991, pp 309–327.

284. Hefti F, Muller W, Jakob RP, Staubli H-U: Evaluation of knee ligament inuries with the IKDC. Knee Surg Sports Traumatol Arthrosc 1993; 1:225–234.

285. Harner CD, Irrgang JJ, Silverstein S, et al: Three to five year follow-up of allograft vs autograft ACL reconstruction. Presented at the Nineteenth Annual Meeting of the American Orthopaedic Society for Sports Medicine, Sun Valley, ID, July 12, 1993.

286. Harner CD, Irrgang JJ, Johnson D, et al: Three to five year results of allograft vs. autograft anterior cruciate ligament reconstruction: A matched pairs analysis. Presented at the Sixty-First Annual Meeting of the American Academy of Orthopaedic Surgeons, New Orleans, February 24, 1994.

287. Harner CD, Irrgang JJ, Allen A, et al: Outcome following isolated posterior cruciate ligament reconstruction. Presented at the Specialty Day Meeting of the American Orthopaedic Society for Sports Medicine, New Orleans, February 24, 1994.

288. Lysholm J, Gillquist J; Evaluation of knee ligament surgery results with special emphasis on use of a scoring score. Am J Sports Med 1982; 10:150–154.

289. Tegner Y, Lysholm J: Rating systems in the evaluation of knee ligament injuries. Clin Orthop Rel Res 1985; 198:43–49.

290. Tegner Y, Lysholm J, Lysholm M, Gillquist J: A performance test to monitor rehabilitation and evaluate anterior cruciate ligament injuries. Am J Sports Med 1986; 14:156–159.

291. Noyes FR, Matthews DS, Mooar PA, Grood ES: The symptomatic anterior cruciate-deficient knee. Part II: The results of rehabilitation and counseling on functional disability. J Bone Joint Surg 1983; 65A:193–194.

292. Noyes FR, McGinnis GH, Mooar LA: Functional disability in the anterior cruciate insufficient knee syndrome: Review of knee rating systems and projected risk factors in determining treatment. Sports Med 1984; 1:278–302.

293. Olson EJ, Harner CD, Fu FH, Silbey M: Clinical use of fresh frozen soft tissue allografts. Orthopedics 1992; 15:1225–1232.

294. Bollen S, Seedhom BB: A comparison of the Lyshom and Cincinnati knee scoring questionnaires. Am J Sports Med 1991; 19:189–190.

295. Synder-Macker L, DeLitto A, Bailey S, Stralka SW: Strength of the quadriceps femoris muscle and functional recovery after anterior cruciate ligament reconstruction: A prospective randomized clinical trial of electrical stimulation. J Bone Joint Surg 1995; 77A:1166–1173.

296. Wilk KE, Romaniello WT, Soscia SM, et al: The relationship between subjective knee scores, isokinetic testing, and functional testing in the ACL-reconstructed knee. JOSPT 1994; 20:60–73.

297. Barber SD, Noyes FR, Mangine RE, et al: Quantitative assessment of functional limitations in normal and anterior cruciate ligament-deficient knees. Clin Orthop 1990; 255:204–214.

BIBLIOGRAPHY

Bergfeld JA: Presented at the Sixty-First Annual Meeting of the American Academy of Orthopaedic Surgeons, New Orleans, February 24, 1994.

Collehon 1987, Bergfeld JA: Amer Orthop 1994, Presentation.

Deavila GA, O'Connor BL, Visco DM, Sisk TD: The mechanoreceptor innervation of the human fibular collateral ligament. J Anat 1989; 162:1–7.

Dye SF, Chew MH: The use of scintigraphy to detect increased osseous metabolic activity about the knee. J Bone Joint Surg 1993; 75A:1388–1406.

Katonis PG, Assimakopoulos AP, Agapitos MV, Exarchou EI: Mechanoreceptors in the posterior cruciate ligament. Histological study on cadaveric knees. Acta Orthop Scand 1991; 62:276–278.

Krenn V, Hofmann S, Engel A: First description of mechanoreceptors in the corpus adiposum infrapatellar. Man Acta Anat 1990; 137:187–188.

O'Connor BL, McConnaughey JS: The structure and innervation of cat knee menisci and their relation to a "sensory hypothesis" of meniscal function. Am J Anat 1978; 153:431–442.

Schultz RA, Miller DC, Kerr CS, Micheli L: Mechanoreceptors in human cruciate ligaments: A histological study. J Bone Joint Surg 1984; 66A:1072–1076.

Schutte MJ, Dabezies EJ, Zimny ML, Happel LT: Neural anatomy of the human anterior cruciate ligament. J Bone Joint Surg, 1987; 69A:243–247.

Tria AJ Jr, Hosea TM, Alicea JA: Clinical diagnosis and classification of ligament injuries. *In* Scott WN (ed): The Knee. St Louis, Mosby-Year Book, 1994, pp 657–672.

CHAPTER 31

The Knee: Patellofemoral and Soft Tissue Injuries

JENNY McCONNELL   *B App SCI (Phty), GDMT, M Biomed E*

JOHN FULKERSON   *MD*

Anterior knee pain is one of the most common conditions presenting to clinicians involved in the management of sports injuries.[1–5] The two most common causes of anterior knee pain in the athlete are patellofemoral pain syndrome, particularly in runners, cyclists, tennis players, and swimmers,[3,6–8] and patellar tendinitis, especially in those involved in jumping sports such as basketball, volleyball, and tennis.[5,8,9] Both these conditions are, in the athletic population, generally the result of overuse problems. Another major overuse injury adjacent to the patellofemoral region in runners is iliotibial friction syndrome.[1,3,10,11]

Overuse injuries abound in the patellofemoral region because the patellofemoral joint is essentially a "soft tissue" joint—that is, it is reliant on the soft tissue structures surrounding the patella to determine the position of the patella on the femur. The patella has been likened to a tent, with the surrounding soft tissue structures being the guy ropes.[2] Therefore, a thorough understanding of the anatomy and biomechanics of the region significantly enhances the clinician's approach to the assessment and management of patellofemoral problems.

This chapter therefore discusses the relevant anatomy and biomechanics of the patellofemoral joint, outlines the signs and symptoms of conditions of patellofemoral origin to assist in the differential diagnosis, and provides assessment procedures and intervention strategies for the clinician.

ANATOMY

SHAPE OF JOINT SURFACES

The patella is triangular in shape and slightly wider than high, with the base uppermost. It is divided into

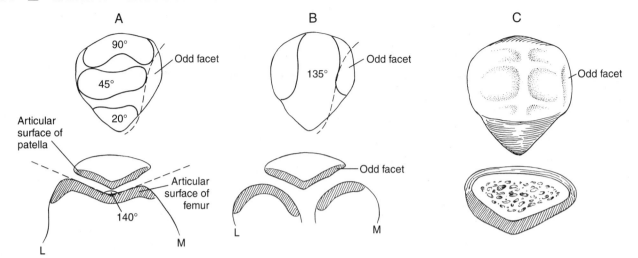

FIGURE 31–1. Articular surfaces of the patella and femur. Note the multiple ridges and surface areas of the retropatellar surface and the sulcus angle of the femoral trochlea (L, lateral; M, medial).

anterior and posterior surfaces and medial and lateral facets.[12]

The anterior surface of the patella is slightly convex in all directions and is divided into three parts. The rough superior third receives the deep fibers of the quadriceps tendon, the middle third contains numerous vascular orifices, and the inferior third, which is V-shaped, is enveloped by the patellar tendon. The posterior surface can be divided into superior and inferior portions. The inferior portion does not articulate with the femur and represents 25 percent of the patellar height but lies in close relationship to the infrapatellar fat pad.[2]

The articular cartilage of the central portion of the posterior surface is the thickest in the body, reaching 4 to 5 mm. Despite the amount of articular cartilage present, however, it may be susceptible to subsequent deterioration and failure because of poor load distribution. The distribution of load and patellofemoral compression have significant implications for the clinician. Treatment programs must consider this fact carefully. Attempts should be made to distribute a load as evenly as possible across as much surface area of the patella as possible during activities of daily living (ADL) function and rehabilitation.

The articular surface of the patella can be divided into as many as seven parts. The medial and lateral facets are separated by an obvious median ridge range. The lateral facet is longer than the medial. A smaller ridge divides the medial facet into the medial facet proper and the odd facet. The odd facet articulates with the medial femoral condyle only in extreme flexion. Two transverse ridges divide the articulating surface into superior, middle, and inferior thirds (Fig. 31–1).

The lateral facet is reported by Fujikawa and colleagues[13] as being almost flat and by Fulkerson and Hungerford[2] as being slightly concave in both the vertical and transverse planes. It lies at an angle of approximately 130 degrees to the medial facet and fits well with the lateral femoral condyle. It is usually longer and broader than the medial facet. The medial facet and the odd facet have a more complex geometry and are less congruent with the medial femoral condyle.[13] The odd facet has many variations in size and projection and may be concave or flat. It may also lie in the same plane as the medial facet or oblique to it by as much as 60 degrees. The medial facet also shows variation, but not as marked, and it is usually concave.[2]

Radiographic and cadaveric studies have allowed the patella to be classified into four types based on the size and shape of the medial and lateral facets.[14,15] These shapes are depicted in Figure 31–2 and summarized in Table 31–1. Type II is the most common patella shape, whereas type III is the least common. Both types III and IV tend to be unstable. It has not been firmly established whether patella type has any effect on symptoms or treatment outcome, but types III and IV have been

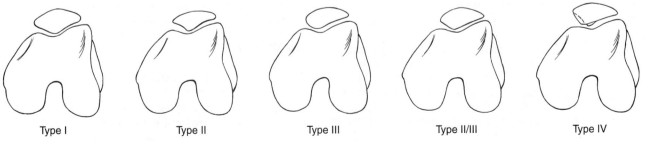

FIGURE 31–2. Patella shape—patellar configuration as determined by tangential roentgenographic views while the knee is flexed.

TABLE 31–1
Classification of Patella Types

Type	Facet Size	Facet Shape
I	Equal	Concave
II	Medial < lateral	Concave
III	Medial < lateral	Medial convex, lateral concave
IV	Medial < lateral	Medial flat or narrow

associated with a subluxing patella and are therefore more susceptible to articular cartilage damage.[16] The nonarticulating aspect of the posterior surface lies in close relationship to the infrapatellar fat pad.

TROCHLEAR SURFACE OF THE FEMUR

The trochlear surface of the femur is divided into medial and lateral facets that closely match the facets of the patella, particularly on the lateral side, and is convex in all directions. The lateral facet is higher and broader than the medial facet and extends more proximally.[2,17] The angle between the two facets is termed the *trochlear* or *sulcus angle* and is approximately 140 degrees.[17,18] The trochlear angle is usually slightly larger than the angle between the patellar facets (Fig. 31–1).[13]

Distally, the two facets form a trochlear groove, following the condyles posteriorly toward the tibiofemoral articular surface.[2,17] Proximally, the trochlear facets become the supratrochlear fossa. This fossa is filled by the prefemoral fat pad; hence, it is the fat pad, rather than the fossa, with which the patella articulates in full extension.

SOFT TISSUE STABILIZATION SYSTEM

The integrity and balance of the soft tissue structures are critical to the position and tracking of the patella. The position of the patella relative to the femur, especially in the first 20 degrees of knee flexion, is determined by the interaction of the surrounding soft tissue. After the first 20 degrees of knee flexion, as the patella begins to engage the trochlea, the bony architecture becomes increasingly responsible for joint stability. The lateral femoral condyle is more prominent anteriorly than the medial femoral condyle and provides a buttress against lateral patellar dislocation.[19] The patella, therefore, could be regarded as the point at which various converging anatomic elements — ligaments, muscles, aponeuroses, and capsule — intersect.[2] The patellar tendon and the medial and lateral retinacula comprise the passive elements of this soft tissue stabilization system. The four portions of the quadriceps provide the active elements of this system. These passive and active elements of the system, along with the bony confines of the trochlea, define the normal limits of patella excursion.

PASSIVE STRUCTURES

Anteriorly, the capsule is thin and loose to accommodate the large range of normal knee flexion. The capsule stretches medially to laterally across the anterior surface to contribute to the patellar retinaculum.[20] Proximal excursion of the patella from the tibia is limited inferiorly by tension in the patellar tendon. The peripatellar retinaculum interdigitates with the tendon medially and laterally.[2]

The lateral side of the knee is made up of various fibrous layers that form the superficial and deep lateral retinaculum. The anterior portion of the superficial layer of the lateral retinaculum consists of the fibrous expansion of vastus lateralis, running longitudinally along the lateral border of the patella and inserting into the patellar tendon.[20] Proceeding posteriorly, fibers from the iliotibial band interdigitate with fibers from the vastus lateralis and the patellar tendon to form the superficial oblique retinaculum (Fig. 31–3).

The deep layer, or deep transverse retinaculum, consists of three major components: (1) the epicondylopatellar band (lateral patellofemoral ligament), which provides superolateral static support for the patella; (2) the midportion, which is the primary support structure for the lateral patella, coursing directly from the iliotibial band to the patella; and (3) the patellotibial band, which provides inferolateral stability for the patella.[2] A large proportion of the lateral retinaculum arises from the iliotibial band. Because of this relationship, excessive lateral tracking, lateral patella tilt, and compression may result if the iliotibial band is tight. Lateral retinacular support is stronger than medial.

Medially, the capsule thickens to form a tough fibrous band, the medial patellofemoral ligament. This band inserts into the superior two thirds of the posterior part of the medial border of the patella. Medial patellar stability is further aided by the meniscopatellar ligament inferiorly. The meniscopatellar ligament inserts into the inferior third of the medial border of the patella, connecting the patella to the anterior portion of the medial meniscus.[2,17,20,21]

ACTIVE STABILIZERS

Most of the active stabilization of the patella is provided by the quadriceps muscle. The attachments of the individual heads of the quadriceps into the patella are considered structurally in three components — superficial, intermediate, and deep layers.

The superficial layer contains the rectus femoris (RF), which inserts into the superior pole and superior third of the anterior surface of the patella. The intermediate layer consists of the vastus lateralis (VL) and vastus medialis (VM), which unite to form a solid aponeurosis that inserts into the base of the patella just posterior to the RF insertion. The muscle fibers and fibrous insertion of the medial quadriceps descend further distally than the lateral quadriceps, attaching further distally on the medial condyle of the tibia.

The VM is divided functionally into two parts owing to the anatomic configuration of its fibers. Fibers of the

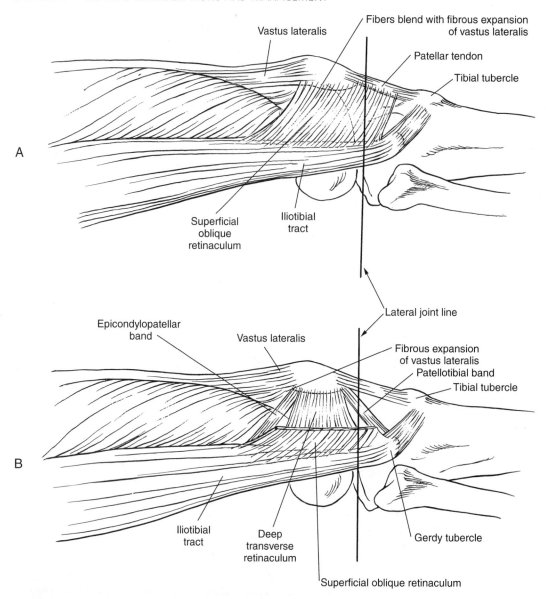

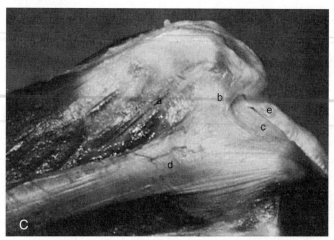

FIGURE 31–3. Anatomy of the lateral extensor mechanism and retinaculum. *A, B,* Lateral view of the extensor mechanism showing the orientation of the elements that make up the superficial and deep lateral retinaculum. *C,* Anatomic dissection of the intermediate layers of muscles and ligaments of the knee. *a,* Vastus lateralis obliquus; *b,* iliopatellar band; *c,* lateral patellotibial ligament; *d,* iliotibial tract; *e,* patellar tendon. (*A* and *B* from Fulkerson JP, Gossling HR: Anatomy of the knee joint lateral retinaculum. Clin Orthop 1990; 153:184.)

vastus medialis longus (VML) are oriented 15 to 18 degrees relative to the long axis of the femur in the frontal plane, whereas fibers of the vastus medialis obliquus (VMO) are oriented 50 to 55 degrees (Fig. 31–4).[24]

The VMO arises from the tendon of the adductor magnus[25] and is supplied in most cases by a separate branch of the femoral nerve.[24] The VML acts with the rest of the quadriceps to extend the knee. Although the VMO has no distinct function in extending the knee, it is active throughout knee extension, acting as the only dynamic medial stabilizer of the patellofemoral joint.[24] The VMO is responsible for keeping the patella centered in the trochlea of the femur. The centered position provided by the VMO enhances the efficiency of the VL during knee extension.[24]

Clinically, the VMO function of producing medialization of the patella has been verified in a study by Ingersoll and Knight.[26] After 3 weeks of electromyography (EMG) biofeedback training for the VMO, asymptomatic females were able to displace their patella medially during a quadriceps contraction as measured on a tangential x-ray. Bohannon[27] has also demonstrated that electrical stimulation of the VMO in a patient with chronically subluxing patellae prevented

dislocation of the patella while the electrical stimulation was being applied.

On the lateral side, fibers of the VL are oriented 12 to 15 degrees relative to the long axis of the femur in the frontal plane (Fig. 31–4). The distal fibers are more obliquely oriented than the proximal fibers. Hallisey and colleagues[23] noted that there is an anatomically distinct and oblique group of VL fibers (vastus lateralis obliquus, VLO) oriented 38 to 48 degrees relative to the long axis of the femur and separated from the main belly of the vastus lateralis by a thin layer of fat. The VLO interdigitates with the lateral intermuscular septum before inserting into the patella. Because of its interdigitation with the lateral intermuscular septum, these oblique fibers provide a direct lateral pull on the patella.

The remaining component, the deep plane, contains the vastus intermedius (VI), which inserts through a broad, thin tendon into the base of the patella, posterior to the other quadriceps insertions but anterior to the capsule. Additionally, it is attached to the lateral border of the patella and the lateral condyle of the tibia.[12] The direction of pull of the VI is along the line of the femur. The VI acting alone is the most efficient extensor. A 12 percent greater mean force is required by each of the other single long heads of the quadriceps compared with the VI to complete the same motion.[24]

The articularis genu (AG), usually distinct from the VI but occasionally blending with it, consists of several muscular bundles that arise from the anterior surface of the lower part of the shaft of the femur and attach to the upper part of the synovial membrane of the knee joint. Its function is to retract the synovial membrane of the knee joint proximally during extension of the leg, thereby preventing redundant folds of membrane between the patella and femur.[12]

If the attachment points of the VMO and VL are changed anatomically, the area of retropatellar surface contact can be dramatically changed.[28] This has significant implications for patients undergoing plication and realignment procedures for patellofemoral problems. It may explain why symptoms persist or recur in some of these patients. Symmetric displacement of the insertion points of the VMO and the VL tendons, either proximally or distally, results in greater changes at larger flexion angles (greater than 60 degrees). If the insertion points are shifted in an asymmetric manner, the distribution of pressure through the patella and femur is adversely affected at lower flexion angles (less than 60 degrees). At lower flexion angles, the effect of a lateral imbalance manifests itself as a rotation of the patella in the coronal plane, whereas at higher flexion angles the imbalance is more likely to produce a tilt of the patella in the sagittal plane. These may be critical factors for the therapist to consider in the rehabilitative management of patients who have undergone realignment procedures when designing therapeutic programs and exercise progressions.

The location and orientation of the pressure zone on the retropatellar surface are particularly sensitive to the magnitude and direction of tension in the VMO.[29] A 50

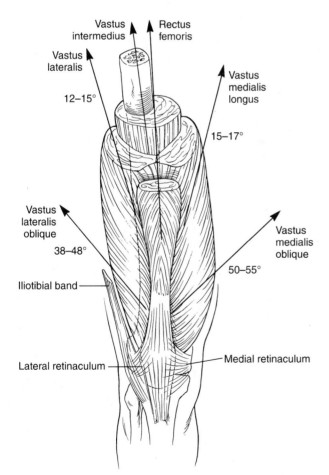

FIGURE 31–4. Components of the quadriceps femoris complex. Note the angle of insertion of the various components of the complex. The orientation of the muscle fibers dictates the line of action and pull on the patella.

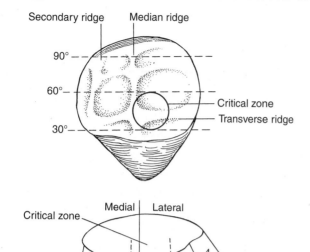

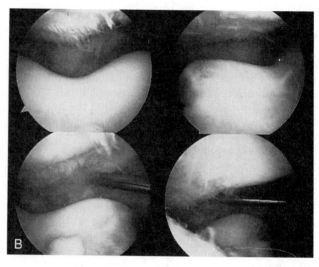

FIGURE 31–5. Zones of retropatellar pressure. *A,* The retropatellar surface must withstand contact pressure and joint reaction forces during activity. Chronic patellar malalignment may lead to lateral facet overload and deficient medial facet contact. This abnormal distribution of compressive forces may lead to articular cartilage degeneration on both the medial and lateral facets. The critical zone may be the first area to demonstrate abnormal responses to excessive compressive forces. *B,* Axial view arthrography showing smooth patellar cartilage joint line narrowing localized to the critical zone *(arrows).* (From Fulkerson JP, Hungerford DH: Disorders of the Patellofemoral Joint, 2nd ed. Baltimore, Williams & Wilkins, 1990, pp 105–108.)

percent decrease in tension in the VMO may result in a significant displacement of the patella laterally by up to 5 mm. VMO weakness or dysfunction relative to the VL may place patellofemoral compression almost entirely on the lateral patellar facet. Pressure on the lateral facet adversely affects the nutrition of the articular cartilage in the central and medial zones of the patella. Degenerative change occurs more readily in these areas. Therefore, one aim of the management of patellofemoral problems is to facilitate a balance between the medial and lateral structures. The purpose of this balance is to distribute pressure as evenly as possible over the largest area of the articular surfaces of the patella (Fig. 31–5).

FUNCTIONS OF THE PATELLA

The patella links the divergent quadriceps muscle to a common tendon. The major function of the patella is to increase the extensor moment of the quadriceps muscle. The patella also protects the tendon from compressive stress and minimizes the concentration of stress by transmitting forces evenly to the underlying bone.[2,30–33]

In the past, the patella was often considered to be a frictionless pulley, in which the force of the patellar tendon equals the force of the quadriceps tendon.[34] Other studies, however, have indicated that the patella acts more like a balance beam, adjusting the length,

direction, and force of each of its arms—the quadriceps tendon and the patella tendon—at different degrees of flexion (Fig. 31–6).[30,35–37] With increasing flexion, the patellofemoral contact area moves from distal to proximal on the patella surface. This change in contact area results in a change in the lever arm and mechanical advantage provided by the patella to the quadriceps.

PATELLAR EXCURSION

Movement of the patella over the femoral trochlea and condyles is controlled by the complex geometries of all the surfaces, muscles, and soft tissue structures. As the patella glides cephalad and caudad on the femur during flexion and extension of the knee, it rotates about three orthogonal axes.[13]

SAGITTAL PLANE MOVEMENT

The prime movement of the patella is in the sagittal plane, where the patella courses a proximal to distal path relative to the femoral condyles during flexion. The total excursion of the patella in this plane throughout the range of knee flexion is between 5 and 7 cm.[39] At full extension, the patella is not in contact with the femur but rests on the supratrochlear fat pad, so there is little compressive load (Fig. 31–7).[2,16] Between 0 and 10 degrees of flexion, the inferior third of the patella comes in contact with the trochlea, whereas the superior two thirds remains in the supratrochlear fossa (Fig. 31–7).[17] With increasing flexion, 10 to 20 degrees, the articular surface of the patella contacts the lateral femur on the inferior patellar surface.[13,38] In this position, the patellofemoral joint is still relatively unstable. From 30 to 60 degrees, the middle surface of the patella comes in contact with the middle third of the trochlea, with a broader band of contact, thus increasing the stability of the joint.[13,38] By 60 to 90 degrees, the upper third of the patella has a broad band of contact deep within the trochlea and is firmly in position by the trochlear facets.[13,17,38]

Beyond 90 degrees of flexion, the contact areas split into smaller areas medially and laterally on the upper patellar surface, corresponding to areas of contact on the medial and lateral condyles of the femur.[13,38] Although the patellofemoral contact area has diminished by this stage, there is extensive contact of the posterior surface of the quadriceps tendon with the trochlea.[38] It is not until 135 degrees of flexion that the odd facet of the patella makes contact with the medial femoral condyle (Fig. 31–7).[13,38] In degenerative patellae, the contact areas are on average 32 percent less than contact areas for normal patellae,[40] so there is less area to distribute the force. This increases patellofemoral contact pressures and may further accelerate the degenerative process.

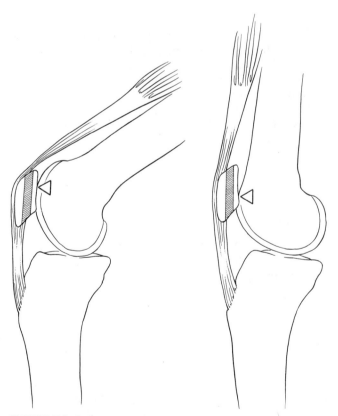

FIGURE 31–6. Patella as a balance beam. Patellofemoral contact pressure is identified by the arrow. Note the difference in the lever arm length as a function of knee flexion angle. Torque between the quadriceps and patellar tendons is balanced by the patella. (Reprinted From Huff U, Jones LC, Hungerford DS: Determination of forces transmitted through the patellofemoral joint. J Biomech 1988; 21:17, with kind permission from Elsevier Science, Ltd.)

FRONTAL PLANE MOVEMENT

In the frontal plane, the patella courses a path resembling a concave, lateral C-shaped curve. At full extension, the patella sits lateral to the trochlea and rests on the supratrochlear fat pad. The "screw home" mechanism of the tibiofemoral joint during terminal extension causes the tibia to rotate externally in relation to the femur, thus lateralizing the tibial tubercle.[2,38] When the knee is fully extended and the quadriceps are contracted, a valgus vector is produced as the patella is freed from the confines of the trochlea. Lateral forces acting on the patella are resisted by the medial retinaculum and the VMO. Passive medial displacement is approximately 20 percent greater than passive lateral displacement.[43]

During the first 20 degrees of flexion, the tibia derotates and the patella is drawn into the trochlear notch, as described earlier. The patella then remains in the trochlear notch until the knee has flexed to 90 degrees. Beyond 90 degrees, the patella moves laterally over the lateral condyle, so that at full flexion the lateral femoral condyle is completely covered by the patella and the medial condyle is, except for the lateral border, completely exposed. At this degree of flexion, the patella rotates around its vertical axis and shifts laterally as it slips into the intercondylar notch.[38]

Cadaveric studies have documented patella motion during knee extension. Moving from knee flexion toward extension between 120 to 30 degrees, there is a gradual medial glide of the patella in the frontal plane and a medial tilt in the sagittal plane. These patella motions reach a maximum at approximately 30 degrees.[36,45] Further knee extension between 30 and 0 degrees produces a lateral glide of the patella in the frontal plane and a lateral tilt in the sagittal plane. In the flexed position, slight changes in the rotation of the tibia have a significant effect on patellar rotation. The patella is confined to the trochlea and the patellotibial bands of the retinaculae are taut, so small changes distal to the retinaculae affect the patellar rotation.[45]

Another patellar movement of significance to the clinician is pitch, which occurs around a transverse axis. As the knee flexes, the contact area on the patella migrates proximally and the inferior pole of the patella rocks anteriorly in the sagittal plane.[13] As the knee extends, the inferior pole rocks posteriorly. Patients with a fat-pad irritation may exhibit symptoms due to pressure on the fat pad exerted by the inferior pole with full knee extension or hyperextension.

BIOMECHANICAL CONSIDERATIONS

Mathematical models have been used to describe forces acting on the patellofemoral joint in static equilibrium. This patellofemoral joint reaction force (PFJRF) as a result of knee flexion is depicted in Figure 31–8. The two forces acting on the patellofemoral joint are F_p and F_q, where F_p is the force in the patellar tendon and F_q is the force in the quadriceps tendon. Lever arms k and q are drawn in relation to the center

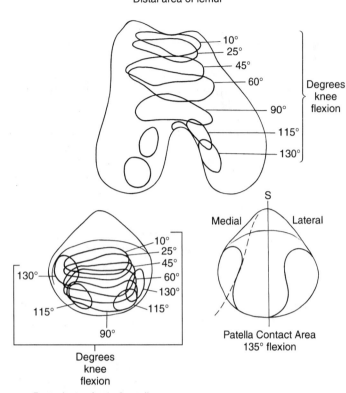

Patella Contact Area—Normal Tracking
Distal area of femur

FIGURE 31–7. Contact areas of the patellofemoral joint at different angles of knee flexion.

of the curvature of the contact area of the patellofemoral joint.

The resultant of these forces compresses the patella against the femur and can be calculated using the Maquet equation:

$$\text{Resultant } \sqrt{F} = Fp^2 + Fq^2 = 2FqFp * \cos \beta$$

where β is the angle between F_p and F_q.

The PFJRF is equal and opposite to this resultant force and acts perpendicular to the articular surfaces. It is the PFJRF that is most often referred to in discussing the compressive joint force. Figure 31–8 indicates that the resultant force increases with increasing flexion, because the angle between the patellar tendon and the quadriceps becomes more acute. As knee flexion increases, the effective lever arms q and k increase, requiring greater quadriceps force to resist the flexion moment of the body. An increase in PFJRF is the result in this squatting type of movement.

The PFJRF changes with various activities. During level walking, the PFJRF is half of body weight, during stair ascending and descending it is 3 to 4 times body weight, and during squatting it is 7 to 8 times body weight.[2,33,46] Ericsson and Nissell[47] demonstrated a PFJRF of 1.3 times body weight with ergonometric cycling, which further increased with increased work load and decreased seat height. This increase of PFJRF with flexion offers an explanation for the aggravation of patellofemoral symptoms experienced by individuals during flexed knee activities. Compressive force is also related to surface contact area. The PFJRF could increase even further with abnormal patella tracking and a decrease in articular contact surface area due to excessive lateral tilt or displacement. An increase in PFJRF is also the basis for the rationale of the management of patellofemoral pain, which emphasizes short arc quadriceps activity and straight leg raising maneuvers, thus avoiding weight-bearing and bent knee activities.

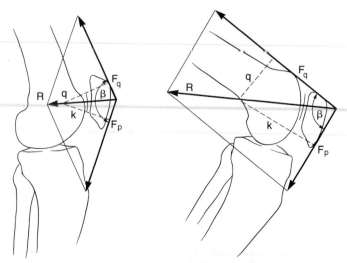

FIGURE 31–8. Effect of knee flexion on patellofemoral joint reaction force (PFJRF) (F_q, force of quadriceps tendon; F_p, force of patellar tendon; k, lever arm of patellar tendon; q, lever arm of quadriceps tendon; R, patellofemoral joint reaction force).

TABLE 31–2
Classification of Chondromalacia Patellae

Grade of Lesion	Appearance
1 — closed chondromalacia	Articular cartilage softening; appearance of a small blister; surface intact macroscopically; lesion may go unrecognized so the surface must be palpated with a blunt instrument
2 — open chondromalacia	Fibrillation of less than 0.5 inch in diameter
3 — open chondromalacia	Fibrillation of more than 0.5 inch in diameter
4 — open chondromalacia	Erosion to bone

Joints are, however, designed to handle compressive stress and they do this by maximizing the surface area of contact, with the resistance coming from the articular cartilage and subchondral bone.[48–51] The matrix of articular cartilage is a fiber-reinforced composite consisting of collagen and glycosaminoglycans that are linked to proteins to form proteoglycans. This composite resists both tension and compression. Thus, when load is applied to cartilage, it deforms gradually and reversibly, even though the pressure in the cartilage increases immediately.[48,50,52] The subchondral bone in high-stress areas has a high concentration of trabeculae. (Chapter 8 provides a more detailed explanation of this process.) The trabecular arrangement of the patella is greatest on the lateral surface and the midcrest regions, where the sheets are perpendicular to the articular surface. Medially, the sheets become more oblique, and in the central portion few sheets are found, so there is no well-characterized geometric organization.[53]

Articular cartilage adapts appropriately to the increased stresses imposed by strenuous physical exercise, particularly if the stress begins in adolescence.[54,56] On the other hand, it deteriorates if not loaded sufficiently. Because articular cartilage is avascular, it relies on the intermittent compression of the joint surfaces to be thoroughly nourished.[55] Cartilage softens and loses its shock-absorbing and load-distributing qualities, which explains the presence of nonprogressive surface fibrillation on the medial facet as an age-related change. Chondromalacia or softening of the articular cartilage in the patella is most common on the lateral facet, corresponding to the area of articulation in the 40 to 80 degree range of knee flexion (Table 31–2). This may be attributed to prolonged patellar tilt. Prolonged tilt results in the load being unevenly borne, which causes an alteration of the stiffness indices of the underlying bone. Because of this alteration in stiffness, a microfracture can result in the articular cartilage, and may also occur in the subchondral bone. Fortunately, the bone heals, but the articular cartilage, because it is avascular, does not. If excessive loading continues, as it may in someone with patella malalignment or maltracking, degeneration of the articular cartilage progresses until it affects the entire lateral facet.[53,57] (For a detailed description of the mechanical properties of bone and articular cartilage and how these structures dissipate forces, see Chapters 7 and 8.)

Degenerative changes in the patella can also cause increases in contact pressure. The involved cartilage exhibits a reduction in contact pressure due to decreased cartilage stiffness in the softened areas.[40,41] Macroscopically, normal cartilage around a chondromalacic lesion tends to demonstrate highly nonuniform pressure distributions, with the highest pressure being measured at regions directly bordering the chondromalacic cartilage.[40] Peak pressures are about twice as high as on the low-pressure zones of the same contact area. The change in the pressure differentials across the cartilage has been proposed as the mechanism for the spread of the lesion — that is, progressive degeneration.[40] Peak pressure areas can occur either medially or laterally and are not always located on one side of the lesion. If a chondroplasty or realignment procedure is to be performed, the surgeon needs to be aware of the highly nonuniform nature of the problem, because the macroscopically normal cartilage that is adjacent to mildly fibrillated or osteoarthritic cartilage may have inferior biomechanical properties and may not respond well to a traumatic insult or altered load bearing.[42]

FRONTAL PLANE MECHANICS

In the frontal plane, the Q angle has been used by many authors to estimate the angle of pull of the quadriceps muscle group.[2,58,59,60] The Q angle is formed by the bisection of a line from the anterior superior iliac spine (ASIS) to the midpole of the patella with a line from the tibial tubercle to the midpole of the patella. It forms a valgus vector, particularly in extension. The outer limit for the Q angle for males is 12 degrees and for females it is 15 degrees.[18,38,61] There is a higher Q angle in females because of the shape of the female pelvis. Several authors[2,17,62] have noted that the Q angle varies dynamically, decreasing with knee flexion and increasing with knee extension due to the external rotation of the tibia, which occurs during the screw home mechanism to allow full extension (Fig. 31–9).

FACTORS PREDISPOSING TO PATELLOFEMORAL PAIN

The 25 percent of the population (higher in the athletic population), who at some stage in their lives suffer from patellofemoral symptoms, demonstrate a failure of the intricate balance of the soft tissue structures. Anatomically, the lateral structures of the patellofemoral joint are much stronger than the medial, so any imbalance in forces usually causes the patella to drift laterally. Patellofemoral pain is a multifactorial problem. Table 31–3 summarizes the factors that may predispose an individual to patellofemoral pain.

There are many different causes of patellofemoral pain, from morphologic softening of the articular

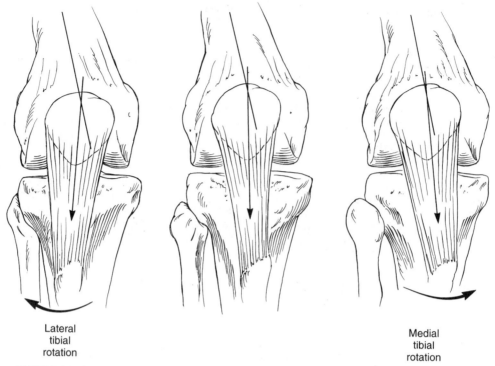

Lateral
tibial
rotation

Medial
tibial
rotation

FIGURE 31–9. Q angle as a function of knee flexion and tibial rotation. The Q angle increases with lateral tibial rotation and decreases with medial tibial rotation.

cartilage to a soft tissue retinacular problem. The mechanism of pain production due to chondromalacia is not fully understood. Articular cartilage is avascular and aneural, so it has been proposed that there are changes in energy absorption of the articular cartilage once degeneration has occurred in the middle and deep layers of the articular cartilage. This causes an increase in the intraosseous pressure of the subchondral bone and a transference of load from the articular cartilage to the richly innervated subchondral bone. When the degeneration progresses to the superficial layer of the cartilage, the byproducts of this degeneration irritate the synovium, causing synovitis and further pain.[2]

Cartilage damage can, however, occur without pain, and pain can occur without cartilage damage.[38,63] Therefore, for the therapist, the diagnosis of chondromalacia patellae is not particularly helpful. The diagnosis alone does not facilitate a useful management strategy. On the other hand, a useful management strategy could be to improve articular cartilage nutrition by optimizing the surface area of contact, which in turn decreases the load borne on a particular part of cartilage. Pressure is proportional to force and inversely proportional to surface contact area.

Soft tissue retinacular pain is common in patients with anterior knee pain. The source of the pain can often be located accurately if time is taken to palpate the periarticular soft tissues thoroughly. Patients whose patellae are chronically tilted laterally have adaptive shortening of the lateral retinaculum and often have evidence of small nerve injury in the lateral retinaculum.[2] The medial retinaculum can be recurrently stretched or abnormally stretched in some individuals in whom the soft tissue structures are not in balance.[63] Some patients present with inferior pain, which can indicate that there is an irritation or, in more severe cases, an impingement of the infrapatellar fat pad.[64,65] Areas of patellofemoral pain and the probable structures involved are summarized in Table 31–4.

TABLE 31–3
Predisposing Factors for Patellofemoral Pain

Factors	Cause
Abnormal biomechanics	Femoral anteversion; increased Q angle; patella alta, patella baja; excessive pronation; genu valgus, varus, recurvatum
Soft tissue tightness	Lateral retinaculum; iliotibial band; rectus femoris; hamstrings; gastrocnemius
Muscle imbalance	Vastus medialis obliquus; hip abductors, external rotators (gluteus medius posterior fibers)
Training	Sudden increase in mileage; increase in hillwork, stairs; change of training surface; change of footwear

TABLE 31–4
Relationship of Involved Structure to Pain Area

Pain Area	Involved Structure
Lateral	Small nerve injury, lateral retinaculum
Medial	Recurrent stretching, medial retinaculum
Inferior	Irritation of infrapatellar fat pad
Retropatellar	Probable articular cartilage damage
Superior	Quadriceps tendon (rarely, but must be considered)

BIOMECHANICAL FAULTS

Although a direct blow or a traumatic dislocation of the patella may precipitate patellofemoral pain, malalignment of the patella from biomechanical faults is increasingly believed to be the major contributory factor.[2,16,18,49,59,60,66,67] These faults may be structural or nonstructural. Structural causes of malalignment may be divided into intrinsic and extrinsic factors; extrinsic factors are more common and magnify the effect of the nonstructural faults.

STRUCTURAL FAULTS

INTRINSIC FACTORS. Intrinsic structural factors relate to dysplasia of the patella or femoral trochlea and to the position of the patella relative to the trochlea. Although uncommon, developmental abnormalities such as patellar dysplasia or hypoplasia create patellofemoral incongruence, with resultant instability of the patella.[66,68] A flattened femoral condyle (trochlear dysplasia) has a similar effect to patellar dysplasia.[66,68,69] Patella alta or patella baja may result in maltracking of the patella. Patella alta also results in a decrease in patellar stability.[68,70]

EXTRINSIC FACTORS. Extrinsic structural factors relate to the pull of the quadriceps on the patella relative to the relationship of the tibia and femur in the frontal and sagittal planes. These factors increase the possible lateral tracking and displacement of the patella.

An increase in the Q angle can be caused by increased femoral anteversion, external tibial torsion, or a lateral displacement of the tibial tubercle.[71,72] Often, individuals with an increased Q angle have "squinting" or infacing patellae and slight tibia varum, because knee flexion and extension are occurring about a medially rotated axis. These individuals usually present with an anteversion of the femur.[71] It has been suggested that the Q angle is a misleading sign of malalignment, because the Q angle is affected by several anatomic factors.[2,73] For example, the measurement of the Q angle, when a patella is laterally displaced, is often within normal limits, so a major contributory factor of patellofemoral pain may be dismissed because the Q angle is normal. It has also been shown that surgical intervention to decrease the Q angle in patients with patellofemoral pain does not alleviate the problem, but leads to different wear and pain patterns in the joint.[28,62]

Genu valgum causes an increase in the valgus vector force at the knee and hence increases the lateral tracking of the patella. In patients who exhibit genu recurvatum, the relationship of the patella within the trochlea is affected. The inferior pole of the patella is directed posteriorly into the infrapatellar fat pad.[65] This often irritates the fat pad and may be the source of the patient's symptoms. Genu recurvatum also affects the activation pattern of the quadriceps muscle; it does not perform well in a shortened range because of lack of use.[74]

NONSTRUCTURAL FAULTS

SOFT TISSUE TIGHTNESS. A decrease in the flexibility of the soft tissue structures that surround the patella is a significant contributory factor in the cause of patellofemoral pain. Soft tissue tightness is particularly prevalent during the adolescent growth spurt, when the long bones are growing faster than the surrounding soft tissues.[75] This not only leads to problems with lack of flexibility and alteration of stress through joints, but also to muscle control problems, in which the motor program can no longer control the limb appropriately. A decrease in the flexibility of the lateral retinaculum, hamstrings, rectus femoris, gastroc-soleus, or tensor fascia lata adversely affects the tracking of the patella. All the muscle groups affected are two-joint muscle groups.

As the knee begins to flex, a shortened lateral retinaculum comes under excessive stress as the patella is drawn into the trochlea. Tension is further increased as the iliotibial band (ITB) moves posterior to the epicondyle of the femur as flexion increases further. As a result, the ITB pulls posteriorly on the already shortened lateral retinaculum.[2,72] An increase in the lateral tracking and tilt of the patella is produced. Because of this lateral pull, weakness or laxity of the medial retinacula may result.[69]

A decrease in hamstring or gastroc-soleus flexibility may produce a cascade of events that results in an increase in the dynamic Q angle and patellofemoral compression. Tight hamstrings result in increased knee flexion at heel strike and during the stance phase of the gait or running cycle. This increase in knee flexion also requires an increase in dorsiflexion. If the full range of dorsiflexion has already occurred at the talocrural joint, further range is achieved by pronating the foot, particularly at the subtalar joint. This causes an increase in the valgus vector force and hence an increase in the dynamic Q angle.[77–79] These changes result in greater lateral patellar tracking and displacement and increase the PFJRF.

A shortened rectus femoris may not allow full excursion of the patella on the trochlea as the knee flexes, particularly when the hip is extended. Through its attachment into the iliotibial band, a tight tensor fasciae latae (TFL) promotes lateral tracking of the patella, particularly at 20 degrees of knee flexion when the band is at its shortest. These factors adversely alter patellofemoral contact areas and stress distribution.

MUSCLE IMBALANCE

Balanced activity of all portions of the quadriceps is critical for patellar control and normal tracking. Many factors may cause an alteration in this important balance, especially between the VMO and the VL.

The function of the VMO as the only dynamic medial stabilizer was mentioned earlier. The VMO is the most susceptible portion of the quadriceps to any type of joint effusion. The VMO may be inhibited by significantly less joint effusion compared with the VL and rectus femoris (20 and 60 ml, respectively).[80] This inhibition due to effusion may partly explain a selective atrophy of the VMO and the increased incidence of patellofemoral symptoms following other knee trauma or pathology in which a mild effusion was present, causing a maltracking of the patella during activity.

Many literature reports have demonstrated that individuals with patellofemoral pain may have an alteration in the amount of EMG activity of the VMO compared with the VL.[81–85] EMG recordings in normal subjects have demonstrated a 1:1 ratio of VMO:VL[81] and have shown that the VMO is tonically active.[82] EMG recordings in patients with patellofemoral pain have revealed that the ratio of VMO:VL activity is less than 1:1 and that the VMO is phasically active, reflecting a reduction in activity in the VMO rather than an increase in VL activity.[81,82] VMO and VL activity also differ according to the amount of knee flexion in symptomatic and asymptomatic individuals. In asymptomatic individuals, the VMO exhibits greater activity than the VL at 20 degrees of knee flexion than at 90 degrees, but subjects with patellofemoral pain show a reversal of EMG activity, with greater VMO than VL activity being present at 90 degrees and less at 20 degrees.[22] During functional weight-bearing activities such as walking, there may be less required of VMO and VL function as the body assumes a more upright position and the flexion moment of the knee is decreased.[83,84]

Voight and Wieder have also demonstrated changes in the reflex response time of the VMO in individuals with patellofemoral pain.[85] The VMO onset was significantly faster than the VL in normal subjects but, in patellofemoral pain syndrome subjects, there was a reversal of the normal onset of muscle activity, so that the VL fired significantly faster than the VMO.[85] Lateral displacement of the patella by as little as 5 mm (as might be caused by a tight lateral retinaculum or ITB) may result in up to a 50 percent decrease in maximum tension development of the VMO.[29] Findings from studies such as these emphasize the importance of patella position and a normal balance between the VMO and VL. The ability of the VMO to control the position of the patella is critical.

It remains unclear what mechanisms may be responsible for these neuromuscular changes. Most authors agree, however, that any neuromuscular imbalance

between the actions of the VMO and VL may be due to an initial mechanical disturbance that, over time, may lead particularly to depression of VMO neuromuscular activity.[81,86,87] Weh and colleagues[88] also suggested that muscle imbalance causing malalignment may be related to damage at the nerve root or anterior horn cell of the L3 and L4 segments.

Pelvic muscle imbalance and abnormal gait patterns may also contribute to patellofemoral dysfunction. Tightness in the iliotibial band results in overactivity in the TFL and diminished activity in both the VMO and gluteus medius posterior fibers. The faulty alignment pattern remains because the muscles in a shortened position (usually two-joint muscles, such as the TFL) are readily recruited and are strong, whereas muscles in an elongated position (usually postural muscles, such as the VMO) are difficult to recruit and are weak.[74] A subject with a short ITB demonstrates excessive medial rotation of the hip during the stance phase of gait, allowing the pelvis on the opposite side to drop and giving a Trendelenburg appearance.[74] This hip and pelvic movement increases the dynamic Q angle[89] and hence increases the potential for patella maltracking and patellofemoral pain.

Maintaining muscles in a clinically shortened or lengthened position alters their normal length tension properties.[92,93] Alteration in these length-tension properties may have small but profound effects on patellofemoral pain and tracking over time.

ALTERED FOOT BIOMECHANICS

Altered foot biomechanics such as excessive, prolonged, or late pronation alters the tibial rotation at varying times throughout the range, thus having an effect on patellofemoral joint mechanics.[77,79] In a series of 3500 injured runners, Lutter[3] found that only 10 percent of the extremities were judged to be normal biomechanically. He believed that, for the knee to function optimally, foot supination should begin when the center of gravity is at the midpoint of the knee, and that any rotational abnormality at the knee due to changes in the amount of pronation places increased stress on the joint. (See Chapter 18 for a detailed explanation of foot biomechanics.)

EXAMINATION

Clinically, a detailed history and physical examination are required to determine the causative factors of symptoms, correct diagnosis, and most appropriate method of management.

HISTORY

The clinician needs to elicit in the history the area of pain, the type of activity precipitating the pain, the history of the onset of the pain, the behavior of the pain, and any associated clicking, giving way, or swelling.[1]

The information obtained provides an indication of the structure(s) involved and the likely diagnosis. For example, if the type of activity that precipitated the patient's pain involved eccentric loading, such as jumping in basketball or increased hill work during running, patellar tendinitis is a likely diagnostic consideration.[1,5] On the other hand, if the athlete reports pain following tumble turning or vigorous kicking in the pool, the delivery of a fastball in cricket, or any other activity that involves fully loaded knee extension or hyperextension, an irritated fat pad might be suspected.[65] In both these conditions, the athlete complains of inferior patellar pain. Table 31–5 outlines the signs and symptoms of fat pad irritation and patellar tendinitis to aid in the differential diagnosis.[65] The patient with an irritated fat pad may often be aggravated by straight leg raise exercises, so it is essential for the therapist to recognize the condition and implement appropriate management to enhance rather than impede recovery. The clinical diagnosis of patellar tendinitis can be confirmed with diagnostic ultrasonography or magnetic resonance imaging (MRI). These investigations may show evidence of acute inflammation, with a thickened tendon and associated fluid, cyst formation within the tendon, or a partial tear within the substance of the tendon.[1] In conditions of extreme chronicity, degeneration of the tendon occurs with little inflammation—patellar tendinitis.

SYMPTOMS OF PATELLOFEMORAL PAIN

The patient usually complains of a diffuse ache in the anterior knee, which is exacerbated by stair ascent or descent.[1,2,4,7] For many, the knee aches when they are sitting for prolonged periods with the knee flexed. This is often called the "movie sign." Some patients may have crepitus, which is often a source of concern because they believe that the crepitus is indicative of "arthritis." The crepitus is mostly due to tight, deep, lateral retinacular structures, however, and can be improved with treatment. Abernathy and associates[95] examined the knees of 123 first-year medical students and found that asymptomatic patellofemoral crepitus was present in 62 percent.

Some patients may experience "giving way" or a buckling sensation of their knee. This occurs during walking or stair climbing (i.e., movements in a straight line) and is due to the reflex inhibition of the quadriceps muscle. It must be differentiated from the giving way experienced when turning, which may often be indicative of an anterior cruciate-deficient knee. Locking is another symptom that must be differentiated from intra-articular pathology. Patellofemoral locking is usually only a catching sensation in which the patient can actively unlock the knee; it is unlike loose body or meniscal locking, in which the patient is either unable to unlock or can only passively unlock the knee.[1,2,4,6] (See Chapter 30 for further information on anterior cruciate ligament and meniscal injuries.)

Mild swelling due to synovial irritation[2] may also occur with patellofemoral problems. Mild swelling causes an asymmetric wasting of the quadriceps muscle, whereby the VMO is inhibited before the VL and RF.[80,96,97] Therefore, an athlete who has primarily an intra-articular pathology, such as a meniscal or ligamentous injury, may have great difficulty resolving the subsequent secondary patellofemoral problem, particularly if the primary problem has not been identified.

When considering the possible differential diagnoses, the clinician must remember that the lumbar spine and hip can refer symptoms to the knee. For example, the prepubescent male with a slipped capital femoral epiphysis may present with a limp and anterior knee pain, and thus might initially be misdiagnosed as having patellofemoral pain.[1,2]

TABLE 31–5

Signs and Symptoms of Fat Pad Irritation and Patellar Tendinitis

	Fat Pad Irritation	Patellar Tendinitis
SYMPTOMS	"Tenderness" of inferior patella	"Tenderness" of inferior patella
	Complaints of "puffy" knees	Knees not "puffy"
	Pain exacerbated by prolonged standing, negotiating stairs	Pain exacerbated by jumping, mid to full squat
SIGNS	Hyperextended, locked-back knees	Nonsignificant Q angle: less than 15° in females and less than 12° in males
	In acute stage, pain ascending stairs as weight-bearing leg extends; pain down stairs in early range	Pain with three fourths to full squat
	Pain reproduced on extension overpressure	Pain with jumping
	Inferior pole painful to palpation	No pain on extension overpressure
	Posterior displacement of inferior pole passively and dynamically	Inferior pole painful to palpation
		No posterior displacement of inferior pole

Neural tissue may also be a source of symptoms around the patellofemoral joint. Lack of mobility of the L5 and S1 nerve roots and their derivatives can give rise to posterior or lateral thigh pain. Symptoms from neural tissue can be differentiated fairly easily from patellofemoral symptoms because the pain is exacerbated in sitting, particularly when the leg is straight, rather than in the classic movie sign position of a flexed knee. The slump sitting test quickly verifies the neural tissue as being a source of the symptoms.[98] Similarly, a peripheral nerve may scar down or become entrapped following arthroscopic surgery. The most common example is the infrapatellar branch of the saphenous nerve. Symptoms are sharp pain inferomedially, with or without slightly altered sensation laterally. They are reproduced on deep bending and jumping and are therefore frequently confused with patellar tendinitis symptoms because of the proximity to the tendon. Pain is reproduced with the patient prone, flexing the knee and externally rotating the tibia, to put the nerve on stretch.[99] Chapter 10 explains this mechanism in detail.

PATELLOFEMORAL INSTABILITY

Patellofemoral instability or recurrent patellofemoral subluxation is a variant of patellofemoral pain syndrome, in which there is actual subluxation of the patella. It is more common in females and tends to be associated with patella alta, a Q angle greater than 20 degrees, and dysplasia of the trochlea and patella.[1,68,100,101] Patients with patellofemoral instability complain of a sensation of giving way on certain movements. The giving way usually occurs when the femur rotates internally on a fixed, externally rotated tibia. When this happens acutely, there is usually swelling, which appears within 12 hours of the injury. If the fluid is aspirated, it is serosanguineous.[101] On the other hand, with an acute rupture of the anterior cruciate ligament, which is often injured with the same cutting action as described earlier for patellofemoral subluxation, the swelling occurs within the first few hours and a hemarthrosis is aspirated. It is important to x-ray all acute knee problems to ensure that there has been no disruption to the lateral femoral condyle during the subluxation.

Patients with patellofemoral instability have the same predisposing factors as those with patellofemoral pain syndrome (Table 31–3). They exhibit apprehension and sometimes pain on lateral movement of the patella. The apprehension sign confirms the diagnosis. Treatment is based on the same principles as those for patellofemoral pain management.

ILIOTIBIAL BAND FRICTION SYNDROME

The athlete, particularly the distance runner (and, to a lesser extent, the skier and the cyclist) who has increased the mileage, altered the terrain of the training, or changed footwear can complain of specific knee pain over the lateral femoral epicondyle, where the iliotibial band is being frictioned against the epicondyle of the femur.[1–3,102] In one report, iliotibial band friction syndrome accounted for 21 percent of knee injuries in runners.[3] These patients have a tight iliotibial band as confirmed on a modified Ober test, performed in the side-lying position with the pelvis in a stable position. The test consists of hip extension, adduction, slight external rotation, and knee flexion and extension; pain and sometimes a clicking is elicited.[102] Individuals with iliotibial friction syndrome may have faulty biomechanics (Table 31–3) that predisposes them to the condition, so correction of the faulty biomechanics as well as correction of any training errors must be addressed in treatment.

PLICA SYNDROME

Anterior knee pain, particularly along the medial edge of the patella, may be due to an inflamed synovial plica.[1,2,4,73,102] The synovial plica is a redundant fold in the synovial lining of the knee joint, extending from the fat pad medially under the quadriceps tendon and superiorly to the lateral retinaculum. The plica is an embryonic remnant.[4] Patients with an inflamed plica complain of pain in sustained flexed positions that progressively improves with increased activity. Some patients may be aware of a significant pop or snap as they flex and extend the knee. On examination, the plica is sometimes palpable as a thickened band, but should only be considered as the primary cause of symptoms if the patient fails to respond to appropriate management of the patellofemoral syndrome. An inflamed plica is usually only an indicator of a more complex problem involving abnormal patellofemoral mechanics.[1,2,103] It has been reported that as many as 60 percent of examined knees have a palpable plica, but the large majority are asymptomatic.[102,104] Arthroscopic resection of a thickened, inflamed plica in an athlete who has failed conservative management may sometimes be necessary.[105,106]

APOPHYSITIS IN THE ADOLESCENT

The tibial tubercle or inferior pole of the patella may be tender to palpation in the active, rapidly growing, usually male adolescent, indicating that there is excessive traction on the apophysis at the proximal or distal attachment of the patellar tendon.[107] If pain is elicited on palpation of the tibial tubercle, or the tibial tubercle appears elevated, a diagnosis of Osgood-Schlatter disease should be considered. Similar symptoms and physical findings at the inferior patellar pole of the adolescent athlete are known as the Sinding-Larsen-Johanssen syndrome. The diagnosis is a clinical diagnosis, so radiography is usually not necessary; it may be indicated to exclude bony tumor, in cases in which anterior knee pain is severe and there is a large amount of associated swelling. Bone tumors are rare but, in the 10- to 30-year-old age group, the knee is the site of osteogenic sarcoma.[1]

Both Osgood-Schlatter disease and Sinding-Larsen-Johanssen syndrome are regarded as self-limiting conditions—that is, the pain subsides at the time of bony fusion, which most clinicians suggest takes up to

2 years.[1,107] The traditional treatment approach is modified activity and, in extreme circumstances, rest from sport or other activities that cause symptoms.[1,107] This is difficult for active adolescents, because they are thoroughly enjoying their sport, and skill development and maturation can be lost through lack of participation and practice. The therapist, however, can be of much assistance for these individuals. Specific muscle training and stretching facilitating good flexibility of the quadriceps, hamstrings, ITB, and gastrocnemius-soleus are paramount. The use of a chopat strap or taping of the patella tendon may prove beneficial in decreasing the concentration of stress at the tibial tubercle (Fig. 31–10). All these treatment strategies are focused at decreasing the tension exerted on the apophysis during quadriceps contraction while allowing continued participation, provided the child is pain-free. Activities that cause pain and discomfort should be prohibited.

OSTEOCHONDRITIS DISSECANS IN THE ADOLESCENT

The adolescent patient with osteochondritis dissecans usually presents with intermittent pain and swelling of gradual onset. It must be differentiated from juvenile rheumatoid arthritis (Still disease) and a partial discoid meniscus. In the acute situation, the patient with osteochondritis dissecans may have an extremely painful, locked, and swollen knee. The swelling is a

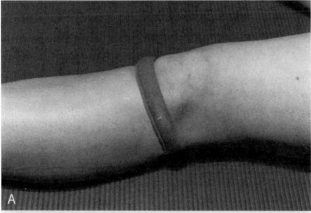

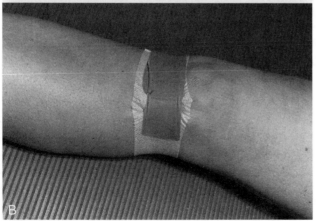

FIGURE 31–10. *A,* Chopat strap used for patellar tendinitis. *B,* Patellar taping procedure used for patellar tendinitis.

TABLE 31–6
Differential Diagnosis for Patellofemoral Pain

Symptoms	Possible Cause
Swelling	Intra-articular pathology; meniscus tear, effusion; ACL rupture, hemarthrosis; osteochondritis dissecans, effusion in the adolescent
	Bursa—localized pain, tender to touch; often hot
	Patellofemoral pain—small effusion
	Patellofemoral subluxation—large effusion
Giving way/buckle	ACL deficiency on turning or pivoting
	Patellofemoral instability with straight movements
Locking/catching	Meniscal or loose body pathology—difficult to "unlock" the knee
	Patellofemoral pain—easy to unlock
Movie sign	Patellofemoral pain—bent knee
	Compromise of S1 neural tissue—straight knee; sitting in slump position
Limp	Prepubescent individual—slipped femoral epiphysis
	Child—Perthes disease
	Patellofemoral pain
Crepitus—scraping, grinding, clicking	Osteoarthritis of the tibiofemoral or patellofemoral joints
	Patellofemoral pain
	Iliotibial friction syndrome
	Plica syndrome
Tenderness on palpation	Joint line—meniscal pathology
	Inferior pole—patellar tendinitis, fat pad irritation, adolescent (Sinding-Larsen-Johanssen syndrome)
	Tibial tubercle—Osgood-Schlatter disease

hemarthrosis, and the locking is due to a loose body from a defect at the lateral aspect of the medial femoral condyle.[1] This is confirmed on x-ray, and the patient requires an immediate orthopaedic referral for either fixation of the loosened fragment or removal of the detached fragment.[1,107]

The Table 31–6 summarizes the differential diagnoses for patellofemoral pain syndrome.

RADIOLOGIC EVALUATION OF THE PATELLOFEMORAL JOINT

To aid further in the diagnosis and management of patellofemoral pain, different radiologic procedures have been suggested. Formerly, however, wide variability in the radiographic findings of patients with patellofemoral dysfunction, and difficulty in demonstrating radiographic abnormalities consistent with clinical findings, contributed to confusion in the diagnosis and classification of those with patellofemoral pain disorders.[39,73,108] Despite this, numerous authors report that using certain techniques, malposition can be accurately and reliably evaluated radiologically.[18,108–112] One of the main disadvantages of radiologic examination is that the patient's knee is usually x-rayed when it is not weight bearing, with the quadriceps muscle relaxed, so the dynamic properties of patellar tracking are not considered.

Overall, there have been few studies using radiologic measurement of alignment as an evaluation of surgical or conservative treatment methods. Insall and coworkers[113] found that, after a proximal surgical realignment of the tibial tubercle, 52 of 57 subjects had congruence angles that were considered to be normal. Unfortunately, there were few preoperative measures for comparison. Möller[114] investigated patellar alignment in three groups (normal subjects, recurrent subluxers, and those with anterior knee pain) by measuring the congruence angle with and without the quadriceps contracted before and after 3 months of isometric quadriceps exercises. The congruence angle during a maximal quadriceps contraction became less positive for the recurrent subluxers after the exercise program. It did not change the angle for the other groups. Fulkerson and associates[115] have used computed tomography (CT) to assess patellofemoral alignment before and after surgical lateral release. The congruence angle and lateral patellofemoral angle were determined at 0, 10, 20 and 30 degrees preoperatively and postoperatively. The results demonstrated that lateral release significantly reduces abnormal patellar tilting. Reigler[116] had similar results when assessing the outcome of surgery.

In a study by Knight and Ingersoll,[26] it was demonstrated that 3 weeks of biofeedback training to the VMO was able to produce a significant ($p < 0.05$) decrease in the radiologic measurement of congruence angle, but 3 weeks of general quadriceps strengthening had no effect on the congruence angle.

Roberts[117] investigated the effect of patellofemoral taping on lateral patellar displacement, lateral patellofemoral angle, and congruence angle. The subjects were radiographed in standing, with the knee flexed to 30 degrees. It was demonstrated that, even though the changes were small, the patellofemoral angle and lateral patellar displacement improved significantly when taped ($p = 0.0003$ and 0.0002, respectively). The changes in congruence angle were not significant. Bockrath and associates[118] also found that there was no significant change in congruence angle with taping, but that patellar taping significantly reduced perceived pain levels during a 0.2-m (or 8-inch) step-down. They concluded that the reduction in pain was not associated with patellar position changes. McConnell, however, found[119] that when subjects performed maximal isometric contractions between 20 and 70 degrees while a lateral view of the patellofemoral joint was dynamically

imaged with video fluoroscopy, there was a change in the patellofemoral contact point (defined as the midpoint of the contact area) so that when the patella was taped the contact area was more distal than in the untaped situation. A corresponding increase in muscle torque was also found when the patella was taped.

BASIC METHODS

Using the anteroposterior view, the patella is evaluated for any fracture or bipartite configuration, as well as for gross positional changes such as dislocation or abnormalities of patellar height. Asymmetry of the femoral condyles may indicate abnormal femoral torsion or femoral neck anteversion.[39]

The lateral view in 30 degrees of knee flexion is used almost exclusively to determine patellar height. Various authors have proposed reliable methods for the assessment of patella alta and patella baja.[120,121] The lateral view may be a way of examining the position of the inferior pole of the patella relative to the femur to assess the problem of fat pad irritation, but this has not yet been considered in radiologic measurements.

The patellofemoral joint is best visualized on an axial or tangential view. The axial view describes the parallel relationship of the x-ray beam with respect to the axis of the anterior tibia, whereas the tangential view describes the perpendicular relationship of the x-ray beam to the joint surfaces.[111] Both these methods provide cross-sectional information about the relationship of the patella to the trochlear groove.[39]

A variety of methods and techniques have been described since the first tangential view was developed by Settegast in 1921. A number of modifications have been proposed, mainly in the variation of knee flexion angle and the angle of the x-ray beam. For reproducible tangential views, there are certain requirements. The x-ray beam and x-ray plate must be mutually perpendicular to avoid distortion.[111,122] Views with the knee flexed greater than 45 degrees are generally utilized.[39,111,123] The position of potential maximum instability is from 0 to 30 degrees, but this position is technically difficult to capture on an axial radiograph.[124–126] For the most reliable and reproducible results, 45 degrees seems to be the preferred position.[110] Some authors advocate that tangential projections throughout the range (i.e., 30, 60, and 90 degrees) are vital to the assessment of dynamic tracking of the patella.[124–126]

ADVANTAGES OF SPECIFIC PROCEDURES

COMPUTED TOMOGRAPHY. Computed tomography (CT) offers the advantage of a specific, definable plane. In general, CT is best performed using a midpatellar transverse image, including the posterior condyles of the femur. This enables the clinician to understand the relationship of the articulating midportion of the patella with its reciprocal portion of the trochlea at any degree of knee flexion. Midpatellar

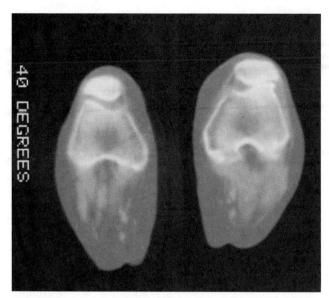

FIGURE 31–11. CT scan of lateral patellar tilt and displacement with the knee in 40 degrees flexion. Precise midpatella transverse tomographic images, using CT at 0, 15, 30, and 45 degrees knee flexion, give an accurate impression of patellar alignment.

transverse images through the posterior condyles with the knee flexed at 0, 15, 30, and 45 degrees provide an excellent depiction of how the patella enters the trochlea during flexion (Fig. 31–11). The images may be taken with the quadriceps contracted, as well as relaxed. On CT, the patella should be centered in the trochlea by 15 degrees of knee flexion, and the patella tilt angle should be 12 degrees or more for normal. The patellar tilt angle is determined by a line running along the lateral facet of the patella with respect to a line that runs across the posterior condyles of the femur. Flattening this angle suggests tilting of the patella.

MAGNETIC RESONANCE IMAGING. Early magnetic resonance imaging (MRI) had limited value in the evaluation of patients with patellofemoral pain. The use of MRI was prohibitive based on time and expense and on the quality and usefulness of the information obtained regarding patella position and tracking. More recently, however, CT and MRI have been used to image the patellofemoral (PF) joint during active or dynamic flexion and extension activities.[127–130] Kinematic and conventional MRI of the PF joint offer advantages over CT in not requiring ionizing radiation and in permitting the depiction of important passive and active soft issue PF joint stabilizers.[127–129] It has been suggested that dynamic MRI, which permits the assessment of the contribution of activated muscles and other soft tissue structures, is more sensitive than static imaging for demonstrating PF alignment and tracking abnormalities.[127–129] Statistically significant differences in patellar tracking patterns and imaging parameters (e.g., patellar tilt angle, bisect offset, lateral patellar displacement) between active and passive knee extension have been demonstrated by Brossmann and colleagues.[127] To date, constraints of acquiring images at 0.5 to 1.0 frames/sec have been encountered.[127–129] The use of echoplanar MRI in the future may allow a dramatic reduction of image acquisition time and greatly im-

proved resolution, allowing images of moving or changing structures to be acquired at near real-time rates of 10 to 16 frames/sec.[131]

BONE SCAN. A bone scan indicates whether there is true intra-osseous dysfunction and may localize the source of pain. A positive bone scan following knee trauma objectifies the problem and may even demonstrate whether there is more activity proximally or distally in the patella, as well as revealing a problem in the trochlea or elsewhere.

CLINICAL EXAMINATION

The clinical examination is important to establish the diagnosis and to determine the underlying causative factors of the patient's symptoms so that appropriate treatment can be implemented. The examination process is summarized in Table 31–7.

STANDING STATIC EXAMINATION

The patient is initially examined in the standing position to assess the alignment of the lower extremity. Biomechanical faults are noted so that the clinician has a reasonable indication of how the patient moves. The clinician looks at the femoral position, which is easier to see when the patient has the feet together. A position of internal rotation of the femur is a common finding in patients with patellofemoral pain. The term *internal femoral rotation* is preferred to femoral anteversion because the rotation applies not only to bony position but also to the soft tissue adaptation that occurs as a result of the femoral anteversion. Soft tissue changes are amenable to change by conservative management. Another reason to use rotation rather than anteversion is that these patients usually present without hip x-rays, so a true diagnosis of femoral anteversion should not be given without radiographic confirmation.

The internal femoral rotation often causes a squinting of the patellae, but if the lateral structures of the patellofemoral joint are tight, the patella may appear straight. The clinician is interested in the presence of an enlarged fat pad, which indicates that the patient may habitually stand in hyperextension or a "locked-back" position of the knees. The muscle bulk of the VMO is observed and compared with the other side. The VL and ITB are palpated to determine the resting tension. Presence of varus or valgus and/or torsion of the tibia is noted. The talus is palpated on the medial and lateral sides to check for symmetry of position. In relaxed standing, the patient should be in midstance position, so ideally the subtalar joint should be in midposition.[3,77] If the talus is more prominent medially, the patient's subtalar joint is pronated. The shape of the medial and lateral longitudinal arches are noted. If, for example, the medial longitudinal arch is flattened, the patient exhibits a prolonged amount of pronation during walking. The great toe and first metatarsal are examined for callus formation as well as for position. If the patient has callus on the medial aspect of the first metatarsal or

---

TABLE 31–7
Examination Checklist

STANDING-STATIC EVALUATION

Examine for biomechanical abnormalites by observing alignment from:

Front
- Normal standing
  - Position of the feet with respect to the legs
  - Q angle
  - Tibial valgum, varum
  - Tibial torsion
  - Talar dome position
  - Navicular position
  - Morton toe
  - Hallux valgus
- Feet together
  - Squinting patellae
  - VMO bulk
  - VL tension

Side
- Pelvic position—tilt
- Hyperextension of the knees

Behind
- PSIS position
- Gluteal bulk
- Gastrocnemius-soleus bulk
- Calcaneal position

STANDING DYNAMIC EVALUATION

Evaluate the effect of the bony alignment and soft tissue on dynamic activities:
- Walking, if no pain
- Steps, if no pain
- Squat, if no pain
- One-legged squat

SUPINE LYING

Determine causative factors of symptoms and formulate a diagnosis:
- Palpation of tibiofemoral joint line and soft tissue structures of patellofemoral joint
- Tibiofemoral tests
- Meniscal tests
- Ligament tests
- Thomas test—psoas, rectus femoris, tensor fascia lata
- Tests for hamstrings, gastrocnemius
- Slump test for dura length, particularly indicated if patient complains of lateral knee pain when sitting with legs out straight
- Hip tests (if applicable)
- Orientation of patella
  - Glide, dynamic glide
  - Lateral tilt, dynamic tilt
  - Anteroposterior tilt, dynamic AP tilt
  - Rotation

SIDE-LYING POSITION

Test for tightness of lateral structures:
- Medial glide—tests superficial lateral structures
- Medial tilt—tests deep lateral structures
- Ober test for iliotibial band tightness

PRONE POSITION
- Lumbar spin palpation (only applicable if dural test positive)
- Foot assessment
- Hip rotation
- Quadriceps flexibility
- Femoral nerve mobility

---

great toe, or has a hallux valgus, the therapist should expect the patient to have an unstable push-off in gait. When examined prone, this patient has one of the following forefoot deformities: a forefoot valgus deformity, a plantar flexed first ray deformity, or a Morton toe.

From the side, the clinician can observe pelvic position to determine whether there is an anterior tilt, posterior tilt, or sway-back posture.[132] The position of hyperextension or locked-back knees can be verified looking from the side. From behind, the level of the posterior superior iliac spine (PSIS) is checked, gluteal bulk is assessed, and the position of the calcaneum is observed. If the therapist finds that the calcaneum is in a relatively neutral or inverted position and that the talus is more prominent on the medial side, the patient probably has a stiff subtalar joint. Thus, from a person's static alignment, the clinician can have a reasonable idea of the dynamic picture, so it should be possible to anticipate how the patient will move. Deviations from the anticipated provide a great deal of information about the muscle control of the activity.

DYNAMIC EXAMINATION. The aim of the dynamic examination is not only to evaluate the effect of muscle action on the static mechanics, but also to reproduce the patient's pain or other associated symptoms. Reproduction of the patient's complaint of symptoms provides the clinician with an objective sign or activity by which to evaluate the effectiveness of the treatment. If treatment is effective, the symptoms produced during the initial examination should be abolished or decreased significantly on retesting.

The least stressful activity of walking is examined first. For example, individuals with patellofemoral pain who stand in hyperextension do not exhibit the necessary shock absorption at the knee at heel strike. Consequently, the femur rotates internally and the quadriceps does not function well in its shortened range due to lack of practice. If the patient's symptoms are not provoked in walking, evaluation of more stressful activities such as stair ascent or descent is performed. If symptoms are still not provoked, a double-leg or single-leg squat may be observed and used as a reassessment activity. For the athlete with subtle symptoms, the clinician often evaluates the control of the single-leg squat, because symptom production in the clinic may be difficult.

SUPINE LYING EXAMINATION

With the patient in the supine lying position, the clinician gains an appreciation of the soft tissue structures and begins to confirm the diagnosis. Gentle but careful palpation should be performed on the soft tissue structures around the patella.

1. The joint lines are palpated to exclude obvious intra-articular pathology.
2. Palpation of the retinacular tissues determines which parts of the retinaculum are under chronic recurrent stress because the chronically stressed areas are tight and, in many cases, tender.

3. Palpation of the quadriceps tendon assists in determining whether the patient has a quadriceps tendinitis.
4. If pain is elicited in the infrapatellar region on palpation, the clinician should shorten the fat pad by lifting it and the overlying soft tissues from the tibial tubercle toward the patella.

If the pain has gone on repeat palpation, the clinician can be relatively certain that the patient has a fat pad irritation. If the pain remains, however, the patient probably has a patellar tendonitis. The diagnosis is confirmed from the history and other examination procedures.

The hamstrings, iliopsoas, rectus femoris, tensor fascia lata (TFL), gastrocnemius, and soleus muscles are tested for length. Tightness of any of these muscles has an adverse effect on patellofemoral joint mechanics and must be addressed in treatment. The iliopsoas, rectus femoris, and TFL may be tested using the Thomas test. To perform the Thomas test, the patient stands with the ischia touching the end of the examination table. One leg is pulled to the chest to flatten the lumbar lordosis. The patient then lies down supine on the examination table, keeping the flexed leg close to the chest. The leg being tested should rest flat on the examination table with the hip in neutral position (at the same width as the pelvis) and the knee flexed to 90 degrees if the patient has appropriate iliopsoas, rectus femoris, and tensor fascia lata length. If the hip is in neutral position, but the knee cannot be flexed greater than 90 degrees, the rectus femoris may be considered tight. If the hip is flexed but lying in the plane of the body, the iliopsoas may be considered tight. If the hip remains abducted and flexed, the TFL may be considered tight. Lack of flexibility of the TFL may be further confirmed in the side-lying position by the Ober test. The Thomas test should be performed on both legs so that a bilateral comparison may be made. Hamstring flexibility may be examined by a passive straight leg raise once the lumbar spine is flattened on the examination table and the pelvis is stable. Between 80 and 85 degrees of hip flexion should be present with the knee extended and the lumbar spine flattened on the examination table for hamstring length to be considered adequate.

The knee should be passively flexed and extended, with overpressure applied, so that the clinician has an appreciation of the quality of the end feel. If any of these maneuvers reproduce pain, that maneuver can be used later in treatment and on subsequent visits as an objective method of testing the effect of the therapeutic intervention.[98] For example, the symptoms of fat pad irritation can often be produced with an extension overpressure maneuver. Change is monitored by evaluating the extension overpressure, with improvement being pain-free extension with overpressure and deterioration being when active extension causes pain.

One of the most essential parts of patellofemoral evaluation in the supine position is assessing the orientation of the patella relative to the femur. After patellar position has been assessed, the clinician aims to maximize the surface area of contact, so that for the

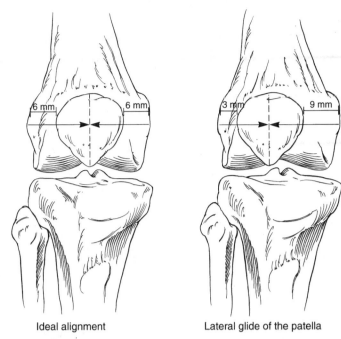

Ideal alignment   Lateral glide of the patella

FIGURE 31–12. Assessment of the glide component. Ideally, the patella should be centered on the superior portion of the femoral articular surface.

same amount of force there is less pressure being distributed through the overloaded part of the joint. To maximize the area of contact of the patella with the femur, the patellar position should be optimal before the patella enters the trochlea. The clinician needs to consider the patellar position not with respect to normal but with respect to optimal, because articular cartilage is nourished and maintained by evenly distributed, intermittent compression.[48,52,133]

An optimal patellar position is one in which the patella is parallel to the femur in the frontal and the sagittal planes and midway between the two condyles when the knee is flexed to 20 degrees.[136,137] The position of the patella is determined by examining four discrete components—glide, lateral tilt, anteroposterior tilt and rotation—in a static and dynamic manner. Determination of the glide component involves measuring the distance from the midpole of the patella to the medial and lateral femoral epicondyles. The patella should be sitting equidistant (± 5 mm) from each epicondyle when the knee is flexed approximately 20 degrees (Fig. 31–12). A 5-mm lateral displacement of the patella has been shown to cause a 50 percent decrease in VMO tension in vitro.[29] In some instances, the patella may sit equidistant to the condyles, but moves laterally, out of the line of the femur, when the quadriceps contracts, indicating a dynamic problem. The dynamic glide examines both the effect of quadriceps contraction on patellar position as well as the timing of the activity of the different heads of the quadriceps. The VMO and VL should be activated simultaneously, or even slightly earlier for the VMO.[85] In patients with PF pain, the VMO activity is often delayed.[85]

If the passive lateral structures are too tight, then the

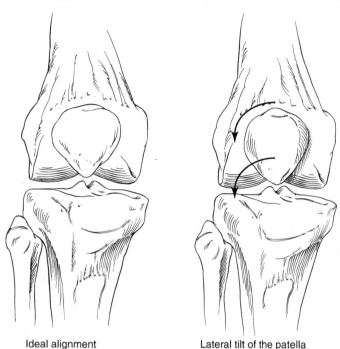

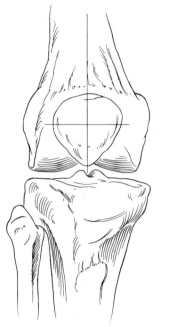

Ideal alignment   Lateral tilt of the patella

FIGURE 31–13. Assessment of the tilt component. Ideally, the patella should be parallel to the frontal plane of the knee. Commonly, in individuals with patella malalignment, there is an excessive lateral tilt.

patella tilts so that the medial border of the patella is higher than the lateral border and the posterior edge of the lateral border is difficult to palpate. This is a lateral tilt and, if severe, can lead to excessive lateral pressure syndrome.[2] The shaded area in Figure 31–13 represents the medial border of the patella, which is sitting away from the trochlea of the femur. When the patella is moved in a medial direction, it should initially remain

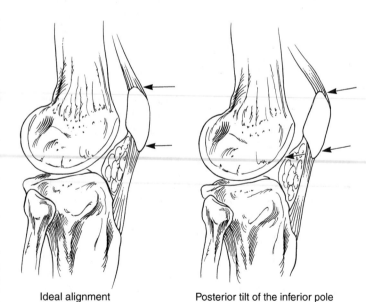

Ideal alignment   Posterior tilt of the inferior pole

FIGURE 31–14. Assessment of the anteroposterior component. Ideally, the superior and inferior poles of the patella should be parallel in the sagittal plane of the knee. Commonly, in individuals with patella malalignment, the inferior patellar pole pushes posteriorly into the infrapatellar fat pad. This may irritate the fat pad.

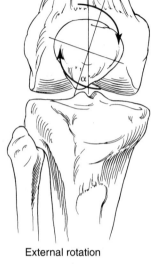

Ideal alignment   External rotation

FIGURE 31–15. Assessment of the rotation component. Ideally, the superior and inferior poles of the patella should be in line with the long axis of the femur. Commonly, in individuals with patella malalignment, there is an excessive lateral rotation of the inferior patellar pole.

parallel to the femur. If the medial border rides anteriorly, the patella has a dynamic tilt problem, which indicates that the deep lateral retinacular fibers are too tight, affecting the seating of the patella in the trochlea.

An optimal position also involves the patella being parallel to the femur in the sagittal plane. A common finding is a posterior displacement of the inferior pole of the patella, which results in fat pad irritation and often manifests as inferior patella pain that is exacerbated by extension maneuvers of the knee (Fig. 31–14).[65] A dynamic posterior tilt problem can be determined during an active contraction of the quadriceps muscle as the inferior pole is pulled posteriorly, particularly in patients who hyperextend.

To complete the ideal position, the long axis of the patella should be parallel to the long axis of the femur. In other words, a line drawn between the medial and lateral poles of the patella should be perpendicular to the long axis of the femur. If the inferior pole is sitting lateral to the long axis of the femur, the patient has an externally rotated patella (Fig. 31–15). If the inferior pole is sitting medial to the long axis of the femur, the patient has an internally rotated patella. The presence of a rotation component indicates that a particular part of the retinaculum is tight. Tightness in the retinacular tissue compromises the tissue[2] and can be a potent source of symptoms.*

---

*When reviewing the original biomechanics literature, the reader should be aware that many biomechanists describe patella rotation relative to the direction of movement of the *proximal* patellar pole. Therefore, the direction of rotation described here would be called "internal rotation" by many biomechanists.

SIDE-LYING

In the side-lying position, the retinacular tissue can be specifically tested for mobility. The patient's knee is flexed to 20 degrees, and the patella is moved in a medial direction. The therapist should be able to expose the lateral femoral condyle. The superficial retinacular fibers are implicated and considered to be tight if the lateral femoral condyle is not readily exposed (Fig. 31–16A). To test the deep fibers, the therapist places the hand on the middle of the patella, takes up the slack of the glide, and applies an anteroposterior (AP) pressure on the medial border of the patella (Fig. 31–16B). The lateral border should move freely away from the femur and, on palpation, the tension in the retinacular fibers should be similar. This test procedure can also be used as a treatment technique. The Ober test for iliotibial

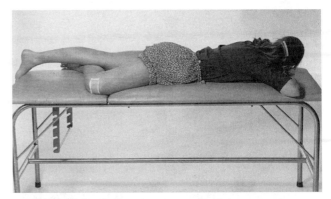

FIGURE 31–17. Figure-of-four stretch. This stretch is used to assess the flexibility of the anterior structures of the hip and the internal rotators. The distance from the anterior superior iliac spine (ASIS) to the examination table is measured.

band tightness may also be performed in the side-lying position to confirm the findings from the Thomas test in the supine position.

PRONE

In the prone position, the clinician may examine the foot to determine whether the patient has a primary foot deformity that is contributing to the patient's patellofemoral symptoms. The deformity needs to be addressed with orthotics or specific muscle training. (See Chapters 18 and 32 for more specific information on foot deformities.) With the patient in the prone position, the clinician can also evaluate the flexibility of the anterior hip structures by examining the patient in a figure-of-four position with the underneath foot at the level of the tibial tubercle (Fig. 31–17). This position tests the available extension and external rotation at the hip, which are often limited because of chronic adaptive shortening of the anterior structures as a result of the underlying femoral anteversion. The distance of the ASIS from the plinth is measured to provide the clinician with an objective measure of change. A modification of the test position can also be used as a treatment technique. The quadriceps may be tested for tightness in this position. It confirms the findings of the Thomas test for rectus femoris tightness. A lumbar spine palpation can be performed at this stage of the examination if the clinician believes that the knee symptoms have been referred from a primary pathology in the lumbar spine. The examination process is summarized in Table 31–7. Once the patellofemoral joint has been examined thoroughly, and the primary problems have been identified, the patient is ready for treatment.

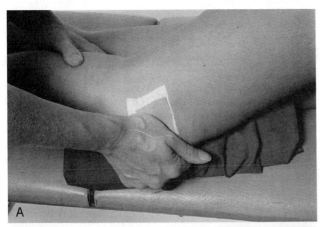
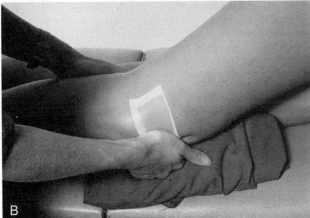

FIGURE 31–16. Assessing tension of the lateral retinaculum. A, Superficial retinaculum. The patient is placed in side-lying position. With the lower extremity supported, flexed approximately 20 degrees and in a relaxed position, the patella is cupped in the palm of the hand between the thenar and hypothenar eminences. A medial glide of the patella in the frontal plane is produced by the therapist. Excursion, resistance, and stiffness are assessed bilaterally. Symptoms, if present, are noted. B, Deep retinaculum. The patient is placed in a side-lying position, as described above. The thenar and hypothenar eminences are placed on the medial half of the patella. An anteroposterior force is directed against the medial half of the patella perpendicular to the femur to "gap" the lateral edge of the patella. Excursion, resistance, and stiffness are assessed bilaterally. Both techniques may be completed with the knee in varying degrees of flexion as assessment and treatment techniques.

CONSERVATIVE TREATMENT

The two primary aims of treatment are to optimize the patellar position to improve the lower limb mechanics which can significantly decrease the patient's symptoms.

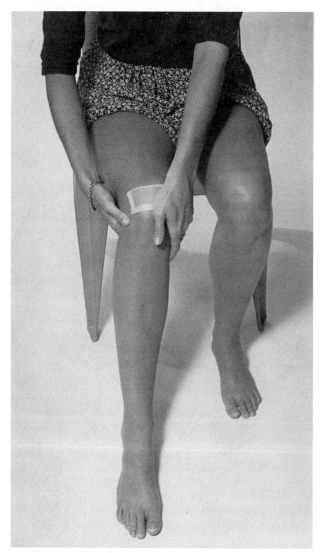

FIGURE 31–18. Self-mobilization of patella. With the knee in varying degrees of flexion and the foot on the floor, the patient exerts an anteroposterior force against the medial half of the patella to "gap" the lateral edge of the patella away from the femur in an effort to mobilize or stretch the lateral retinaculum. The pressure is maintained for 30 seconds and then released.

OPTIMIZATION OF THE PATELLAR POSITION

An optimal patellar position is achieved by stretching the tight lateral structures and by changing the activation pattern of the VMO. Stretching the tight lateral structures can be facilitated passively both by the therapist mobilizing the lateral retinaculum and the iliotibial band and by the patient performing a self-stretch on the retinacular tissue (Fig. 31–18). The most effective stretch to the adaptively shortened retinacular tissue, however, is obtained by a sustained low load, using tape, to facilitate a permanent elongation of the tissues. This uses the creep phenomenon, which occurs in viscoelastic material when a constant low load is applied. It has been widely documented that the length of soft tissues can be increased with sustained stretching.[138–142] The magnitude of the increase in displacement depends on the duration of the applied stretch — that is, if the stretch is applied for long periods, the increase in displacement is large (hence the term *time-dependent*).[141,142] Maintaining the tape for a prolonged period, plus training the VMO to change the patellar position actively, should have a significant effect on patellofemoral mechanics. Tape also unloads painful structures and provides a mechanical advantage to the quadriceps muscle.[117,143] Consequently, taping the patella facilitates recovery by enabling the patient to participate pain-free in activities while specifically training the VMO.

PATELLAR TAPING

Patellar taping is unique to each patient. Each component of the patellar position must be corrected. The order of correction and the tension of the tape are tailored for each individual based on the assessment of patellar position. The component that demonstrates the most significant amount of abnormality is always corrected first. The effect of each piece of tape on the patient's symptoms should be evaluated by reassessing the painful activity, which was determined during the examination. It may be necessary to correct more than one component. The tape should always improve a patient's symptoms immediately. If it does not, then the order in which the tape was applied or the components corrected should be re-examined. To protect the patient's skin, and to prevent irritation and possible breakdown, a light covering of hypoallergenic cloth tape is initially placed on the patellar area.

If a posterior tilt problem (posterior tilt of the inferior patellar pole) has been ascertained on assessment, it must be corrected first, because taping over the inferior pole of the patella aggravates the fat pad and exacerbates the patient's pain. The posterior component is corrected together with glide or lateral tilt, but the tape is placed on the superior aspect of the patella to lift the inferior pole out of the fat pad (Fig. 31–19A and B).

The lateral tilt component is corrected by placing a piece of tape firmly from the middle of the patella to the medial femoral condyle (Fig. 31–19C). The object is to lift the lateral border anteriorly so that the patella becomes parallel with the femur in the frontal plane. Again, the soft tissue on the medial aspect of the knee is lifted toward the patella.

Correction of the glide component involves placing a piece of nonstretch tape from the lateral patellar border and firmly pulling it to just past the medial femoral condyle (Fig. 31–20). At the same time, the soft tissue on the medial aspect of the knee is lifted toward the patella to create a tuck or fold in the skin superomedially. This provides a more effective correction of the glide component and also minimizes the friction rub (friction between the tape and the skin), which is relatively common in patients with extremely tight lateral structures.

External rotation (of the inferior pole of the patella relative to the long axis of the femur) is the most common rotation problem. To correct this, the tape is positioned at the inferior pole and pulled upward and medially toward the opposite shoulder while the superior pole is rotated laterally. Care must be taken so that the inferior pole is not displaced into the fat pad (Fig. 31–21). Internal rotation, on the other hand, is corrected by taping from the superior pole downward and medially.

After each piece of tape is applied, the symptom-producing activity should be reassessed. The clinician is

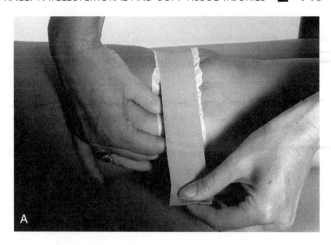

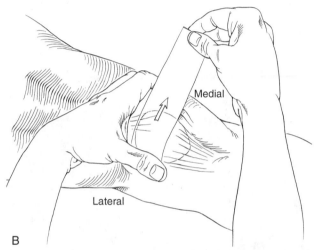

FIGURE 31–20. Correction of patellar glide. *A, B,* Tape is placed just lateral to the lateral border of the patella and is used to glide the patella medially on the femur. The thumb assists in gliding the patella medially, if necessary, while the fingers pull the skin toward the patella, creating a "wrinkle." Tape is anchored on the posteromedial aspect of the medial femoral condyle. Tape is *not* brought into the popliteal fossa, because this may irritate the skin in this area.

aiming for at least a 50 percent decrease in symptoms. If this is not achieved, further correction may be necessary, with ongoing evaluation of patellar position because correction of one component may change the other components. If the therapist cannot change the patient's symptoms with tape, one of the following must be considered:

1. The patient requires tape to unload the soft tissues, as well as the patellofemoral tape.
2. The tape was not well applied.
3. The assessment of patellar position was inadequate.
4. The patient has an intra-articular primary pathology that is inappropriate for taping.

UNLOADING SOFT TISSUE. The principle of unloading is based on the premise that inflamed soft tissue does not respond well to stretch. For example, if a patient presents with a sprained medial collateral ligament, applying a valgus stress to the knee aggra-

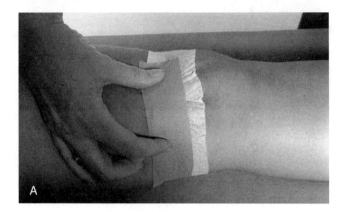

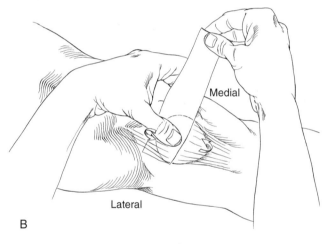

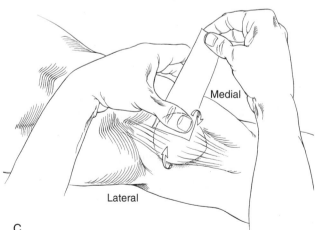

FIGURE 31–19. Correction of posterior and lateral tilt of patella. *A, B,* To correct an inferior tilt, tape is placed on the superior half of the patella. An anteroposterior force is exerted on the superior half of the patella to lift the inferior pole away from the femur and infrapatellar fat pad. *A, C,* To correct a lateral tilt, anteroposterior pressure is placed on the medial half of the patella to lift the lateral border away from the femur.

vates the condition, whereas a varus stress decreases the symptoms. The same principle applies for patients with an inflamed fat pad, an irritated iliotibial band, or a pes anserinus bursitis. The inflamed tissue needs to be shortened or unloaded. To unload the fat pad, the tape commences at the tibial tubercle and comes out in a wide V to the medial and lateral joint lines. As the tape is pulled toward the joint line, the skin is lifted toward the patella, thus shortening the fat pad. Figure 31–22 illustrates fat pad unloading. To unload the iliotibial band for the treatment of iliotibial friction syndrome, once the patellar position has been corrected, a V tape is applied above and below the lateral joint line to the middle of the femur and tibia, respectively. The soft tissue is lifted toward the patella.

PRINCIPLES OF USING TAPE TO CORRECT THE PATELLA. The tape is kept on all day, every day, until the patient has mastered how to activate the VMO during various functional exercises and activities. The tape is therefore similar to trainer wheels on a bicycle, which are discarded once the skill of riding a bicycle has been established. The tape is removed with care in the

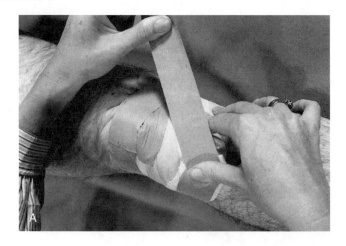

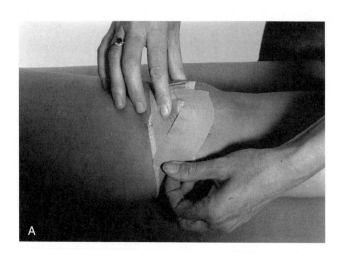

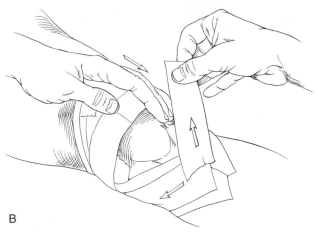

FIGURE 31–22. Fat pad taping. *A, B,* To "unload" the fat pad, tape is initiated at the tibial tubercle. Tape is pulled superiorly as the skin is pulled toward the patella, toward the joint line. Unloading strips are placed both medially and laterally.

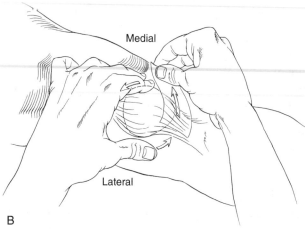

FIGURE 31–21. Correction of patella lateral-external rotation. *A, B,* Tape is initially placed at the inferior patella pole. The patella is grasped with the opposite hand and turned to decrease lateral-external rotation. Tape is anchored as depicted.

evening, allowing the skin time to recover. The tape can cause a breakdown in the skin, either through a friction rub or as a consequence of an allergic reaction. Table 31–8 summarizes the problems and solutions of skin irritation due to taping.

The patient should never train with or through pain or effusion, because it has been shown conclusively in the literature that effusion has an inhibitory effect on muscle activity.[80,96,97] If the patient experiences a return of the pain, the patient should readjust the tape. If the activity is still painful, the patient must cease the activity immediately. The tape loosens quickly if the lateral structures are extremely tight or if the patient's job or sport requires extreme amounts of knee flexion.

TRAINING THE VMO

If the VMO has no function in extending the knee, how can a therapist specifically facilitate a contraction? Emphasis on proper VMO function and on the specificity of training should be stressed during all exercise sessions. Biofeedback may be used to assist the patient in recruiting the VMO and to determine when the VMO is contracting during isolated activity and functional activities.

SPECIFICITY OF TRAINING. Before considering how to train the VMO, it should be noted that there is considerable evidence about the importance of specific training to facilitate skill improvement.[144,145] It is possible to identify at least four aspects of strength training specificity:

1. Strength training effects are largely muscle-specific, although they have been observed in the nonexercised contralateral limbs in subjects who have undergone unilateral exercise. The most likely explanation for contralateral strength changes is that the subjects learn muscle activation strategies so that they can lift heavier loads, and these activation strategies can be used by the contralateral limb.[144]

2. The training effect is joint angle-specific. If a muscle is trained isometrically at one angle or dynamically through a limited range, increases in strength occur where the training has taken place, with limited increases at other joint angles.[146,147]

3. The training response is specific to the type of contraction and the velocity of the contraction.[148] If muscles are trained at one velocity, they become stronger at that velocity and less so at other velocities. Rutherford and Jones demonstrated that after 12 weeks of concentric and eccentric training, subjects recorded a mean increase of 180 percent in isokinetic strength, but only a mean increase of 11 percent in isometric strength.[149]

4. Training is specific to limb position—that is, there is a postural specificity to training. One of the first studies on specificity of training demonstrated that after an 8-week isometric training program to the elbow flexors in standing, there was a significant increase in isometric elbow flexor torque but, when tested in supine lying, there was relatively little increase in the isometric elbow flexor torque.[150]

Thus, training causes changes within the nervous system to allow an individual to coordinate the activation of muscle groups better.

The findings from the literature therefore suggest that the effect of limb position and the relationship of the synergists should be considered if preferential activation of the VMO is desired. Pain-free weight-bearing activities should be commenced early in rehabilitation to improve the muscle activation for functional activities. A useful starting exercise is small range knee flexion and extension movements (the first 30 degrees) in walk stance position (Fig. 31–23). The patient should strive to maintain constant activity of the VMO. This functional activity should be pain-free. This position not only simulates the motion of the knee during the stance phase of walking, but is also the position where VMO recruitment is poor and the seating of the patella in the trochlea is critical.

If the patient is not pain-free in the walk stance position, small range flexion and extension movements could be commenced, with the weight either equally on both feet or partially through the symptomatic limb. For a patient who is having difficulty contracting the VMO, muscle stimulation or biofeedback should be used to facilitate the contraction.

The essential aspect of training for the therapist to remember is that in the early stages of rehabilitation, emphasis should be given to the timing and intensity of the VMO contraction relative to the VL. The VMO should come in slightly earlier than the VL but with the same intensity.[85] Biofeedback devices, particularly dual-channel devices, are extremely useful to facilitate this process because they give patients immediate feedback and reinforcement when the correct pattern is achieved.[90,91] EMG biofeedback training to the VMO has been shown to have a significant effect on the seating of the patella in the trochlea.[26] Biofeedback should be used whenever feasible to assist the patient in determining when the VMO is active relative to the VL

TABLE 31–8
Skin Problems Associated with Patellofemoral Taping

Problem	Description	Solution
Friction rub	Skin irritation due to pull of tape; occurs within 1 week; as skin "toughens," becomes less of a problem; common in 80% of patients to some extent; usually located on medial aspect of knee toward popliteal fossa	Lift skin over medial aspect of knee to a greater degree when taping. Take greater care when removing tape; remove skin from tape, not tape from skin. Use an adhesive tape remover. Condition and moisturize skin at night with skin lotion or skin cream. If skin breakdown occurs, discontinue taping until skin heals. If area of breakdown is small, cover with nonstick gauze or Bandaid prior to taping.
Allergic reaction	Raised, red, itchy rash all over the knee where tape has been placed; occurs within a day; rare, occurs in 5% of patients; patient usually has history of skin allergies	Discontinue taping. Ice may be helpful for itch and rash. Use topical cortisone cream, if needed. Use hypoallergenic tape only. Minimize time that tape is on.

in isolated strength training activities, as well as functional activities. Mirrors and self-monitoring by palpation should also be used as appropriate in the absence of suitable biofeedback equipment.

VMO recruitment may also be assisted through an isometric contraction of the adductor magnus. The adductors are rarely required to perform forcible adduction, but are essentially synergists in the complex patterns of gait activity.[12] The VMO arises from the tendon of the adductor magnus[25] and is usually supplied by a separate branch of the femoral nerve.[26] Because of this attachment and innervation, the therapist may also emphasize adduction of the thigh to the patient to facilitate a VMO contraction. When considering the use of resisted adduction to facilitate the VMO, the therapist must consider whether the patient is weight bearing and the position of the knee. Although not conclusive, activation of the adductor magnus has been demonstrated to improve the VMO contraction in a weight-bearing position and with the knee flexed, but not in a non–weight-bearing position with the knee straight.[151,153]

PROGRESSION OF TREATMENT. When attempting to strengthen the muscles used for a particular activity, the best training is the carefully monitored practice of the activity itself.[144] Because many patients experience pain during stair ascent and descent, one aim of

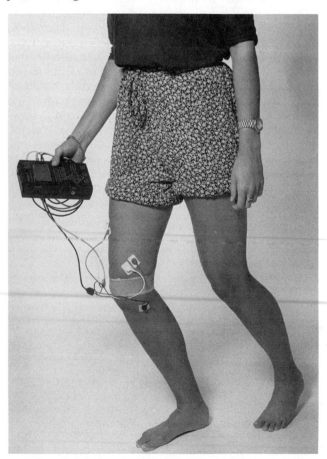

FIGURE 31–23. VMO training in walk stance with biofeedback. The patient demonstrates VMO training in walk stance position using dual-channel biofeedback. Appropriate mechanics at the foot, ankle, and hip must also be emphasized in this training activity.

treatment is to improve the patient's ability to negotiate stairs without reproducing symptoms. Patients need to practice stepping down over a progressive series of heights. At home, wooden or concrete blocks or bricks, a series of step stools, or a large telephone book may be used.

Initially, exercises should be performed using biofeedback in the clinic or a mirror so that the patient can observe changes in limb alignment and muscle activity. This progressive stepping activity needs to be performed slowly, so that deviations can be observed and corrected. Specific work on the hip musculature (to be discussed later) may be necessary to improve limb alignment. Some patients may only be able to do one repetition before the leg deviates or symptoms occur. This is sufficient to start with, because inappropriate practice can be detrimental to the condition or to developing sufficient motor control. The number of repetitions should be increased as the skill level and symptoms improve. Because the VMO is a stabilizing muscle,[82] endurance training is the initial goal. The emphasis of treatment at this stage should be on quality, not quantity. At first, a small number of exercises should be performed frequently throughout the day to achieve a carry-over from functional exercises to functional activities.

For further progression, patients can move progressively to larger step heights. The number of repetitions is initially decreased until the patient has control in this new range. Once control is achieved, the patient may slowly increase the number of repetitions again. As control improves, the patient can alter the speed of the stepping activity. Weights may be introduced in the hands or in a backpack to provide progressive resistance. As resistance increases, the number of repetitions and the speed of the movement should be decreased and built back up again. Training should be applicable to the patient's activities or sport. If the patient is a jumping athlete, jumping should be incorporated. Figure-of-eight running, bounding jumping off boxes, jumping and turning, and other pliometric routines are particularly appropriate for the high-performance athlete. The patient's VMO needs to be monitored at all times, however, for timing and level of contraction relative to the VL. The number of repetitions performed by the patient at a training session depends on the onset of muscle fatigue. The aim is to increase the number of repetitions before the onset of fatigue. Patients should be taught to recognize muscle fatigue or quivering, so that they do not train through the fatigue and risk exacerbating their symptoms. An overview of training progression is listed in Table 31–9.

When needed, patella taping should be used as a component of this functional training sequence on stair heights (Fig. 31–24). It was demonstrated in one study[154] that taping the patella into a medial glide significantly altered ($p < 0.05$) the onset of VMO activity in a group of asymptomatic subjects during stair ascent and descent. The onset of VMO activity was earlier during stair descent and later during stair ascent. Onset of VMO activity occurred as the knee was in a position of greater extension in both conditions. Based

TABLE 31–9 Overview of Treatment Progression*	
Initial treatment	Increase flexibility of anterior hip structures in figure-of-four position in prone Gluteus medius training in standing (15-second hold) Small range squats with gluteals contracted, dual-channel biofeedback on VMO and VL to monitor timing Specific VMO work in sitting Specific stretches—e.g., hamstrings, ITB, gastrocnemius, quadriceps
Subsequent training	Gluteus medius (20-second hold), build up to a 45-second hold Stepping from a small step (in front of mirror)—watch for deviation of hips and knees; start with small number until control has improved
Further progression	Gluteal work using Theraband around both ankles, extend and abduct the unaffected leg, gradually increase the number of repetitions Stepping from a larger step, maintaining control; changing speed of descent and ascent Deep lunge position, control alignment Jumping in the air, maintaining a gluteal contraction, watch alignment on landing Progress to hopping from a box and maintaining alignment as well as hopping and turning May incorporate weights Sport-specific activity, at slow speed to begin with and then faster activity Rapid change of direction, lunge to quick-stop drills If the athlete has good core stability and has not had pain during full training, may commence pliometric work; only for the high-level athlete

*This is intended as a guide only. Assessment is essential to evaluate progression.

on the position of the knee and the activity being performed, one could hypothesize that VMO activity under these conditions would assist in localization of the patella in the trochlea.[154]

IMPROVING LOWER LIMB MECHANICS

A stable pelvis minimizes unnecessary stress on the knee. Internal rotation of the hip increases the valgus vector force at the knee and can cause an increase in patellofemoral pain. If the gluteals, particularly the posterior fibers of the gluteus medius, are working well, there is less activity in the TFL. With less TFL activity, there is a decreased pull on the patella by the lateral retinacular fibers and therefore an enhancement of VMO activity, because the patella is not being displaced laterally.[29,74] It may be necessary to remind the patient of the location of the gluteus medius. This can be done effectively by asking the patient to stand side-on to a wall (Fig. 31–25). The asymptomatic leg closest to the wall is flexed at the knee so that the foot is off the ground and the hip is in a neutral position. The patient should have all the weight on the symptomatic (standing leg), which is flexed slightly (just off full extension).

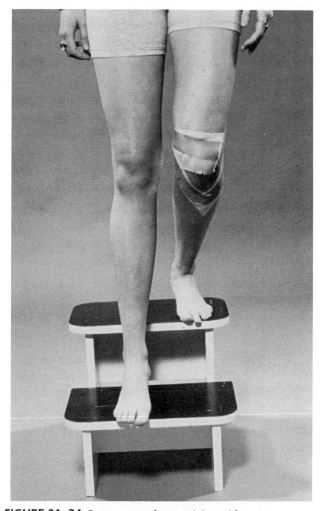

FIGURE 31–24. Step-up–step-down training with correct mechanics. Step-down activities should use progressive heights, which do not produce symptoms. Control and appropriate mechanics during the activity are emphasized. Emphasis is placed on having the toes forward, the knee progressing over the second metatarsal, not allowing the subtalar joint to go into excessive pronation, and maintaining a neutral hip (non–abducted/adducted) position as the individual works on controlled stair activity.

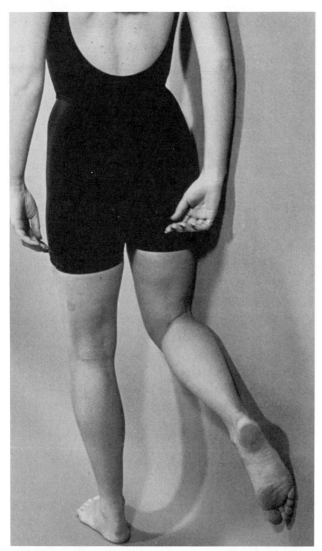

FIGURE 31–25. Gluteus medius training against wall in standing position. Emphasis is placed on maintaining a neutral hip position of the stance leg while the flexed knee is pushed into the wall. Correct mechanics at the ankle (no pronation) and knee (patella in line with the second metatarsal) are also emphasized.

The patient externally rotates the standing leg without moving the foot or the pelvis and at the same time pushes the other leg into the wall. If the patient is doing this exercise correctly, a burning in the gluteus medius is felt, especially if the contraction is sustained for at least 20 seconds. Common errors include the patient flexing too far forward with the hips so that the tension is felt in the ITB, the patient flexing the knee too much so that the quadriceps bears the brunt of the exercise, or the patient rotating the hips so that tension is felt in the back. Once patients have felt a strong contraction in the gluteal region, they are ready for further training.

Training may be progressed to standing on one leg. The pelvis is kept level and the lower abdominals and glutei are worked together while the other leg is swinging back and forward, simulating the activity of the stance phase of gait. An example of initial treatment is shown in Table 31–10 and a progression of treatment is presented in Table 31–11.

Some patients with marked internal femoral rotation may require a stretching of their anterior hip structures to increase their available external rotation and to assist gluteal work in the shortened range. This is done prone,

---

TABLE 31–10
Initial Treatment for Improving Lower Limb Mechanics

Case study: Male tennis player, aged 20 years, pain inferolateral, reproduced on a step-down. On examination, internally rotated femur, tight iliotibial band, tight hamstrings, poor gluteus medius posterior fibers, poor VMO. Patellar position—lateral tilt, posterior tilt, dynamic glide, neutral rotation.

- Tape patella—correct posterior and lateral tilt, correct dynamic glide, unload lateral retinaculum. Retest step, no pain.
- Stretch the tight lateral structures in side-lying with friction massage into retinaculum and release ITB, retest symptom producing activity. If pain has returned, tighten tape.
- Commence gluteal training against wall. Hold the contraction for 15 to 20 seconds. Repeat five times. This should not cause any pain.
- Place a biofeedback electrode on the patient's VMO and VL. The patient should be standing in front of a mirror. Ask the patient to squeeze the gluteals and do small bends of the knee, maintaining a constant VMO and gluteal contraction down and back up. The knees should be positioned over the feet. These small bends are performed in sets of ten. Perform five repetitions.
- The patient does another set of gluteal contracts against the wall.
- Stretch the anterior hip structures with the patient in prone, five repetitions with 4 seconds for each repetition.
- The therapist teaches the patient to tape the knee, the patient sits on the edge of a chair with the leg extended.
- The therapist teaches the patient to stretch the lateral structures by placing the heel of the hand in the middle of the patella, applying a posterior pressure on the medial border, and massaging the lateral retinaculum with the other hand.
- The therapist instructs the patient on the exercises to be done at home:
  Gluteal exercise against the wall, 5 times 20-second holds, 3 times per day.
  Anterior hip structures stretching, 3 times 4-second lift, pushing the pelvis into the ipsilateral hand. If can't achieve the lift, then just a push into the ipsilateral hand. This is performed once or twice a day.
  Small knee bends with gluteals squeezed, three or four repetitions, 20 times/day.
  Self-mobilizing of the lateral retinaculum, 30-second hold, 2–3 times/day.
  For tight hamstrings, a hamstrings stretch, performed in sitting, keeping the lumbar spine in lordosis.
- The patient may play tennis if the knee is taped and there is no pain while playing. If the pain returns, the tape should be readjusted. The patient must re-tape immediately after playing tennis because the tape has loosened and the supportive effect of the tape is lost.

TABLE 31–11
Progression of Treatment for Improving Lower Limb Mechanics

TREATMENT 2

- Check the squat.
- Check taping and examine skin.
- Check exercises.
- Increase time spent holding contraction in gluteal exercise to 30 seconds:
  Begin with phone book exercise in front of mirror. Watch pelvis. It should be level and the femur should not deviate. Therapist may have to remind patient to activate gluteus medius on standing leg and quadratus lumborum on non–weight-bearing leg to keep the pelvis level. Do in repetitions of five without stopping (down, hover, up, hover, down, hover, up, hover, etc.). This needs to be built up gradually to 10 repetitions and over the next few treatments increased to 10 times.

with the patient's hip of the symptomatic leg externally rotated, the foot underneath the extended asymptomatic leg, and the therapist's hands holding the pelvis down. The patient is instructed to lift the knee of the symptomatically externally rotated leg off the plinth.

MUSCLE STRETCHING

Appropriate flexibility exercises must be included in the treatment regimen. The involved muscles may include the hamstrings, gastrocnemius, rectus femoris, TFL, and ITB. The TFL and ITB are often difficult to stretch well and should be an area of concentration for proper flexibility, considering their attachment and influence on the lateral retinaculum.

To stretch the TFL, the patient should be taught the self-stretch illustrated in Figure 31–26. The patient initially lies on the side with the lower extremity that has the tight TFL uppermost. The heel is pulled to the buttock, and the hip is flexed so that the knee points forward (Fig. 31–26A). The hip is now circumducted and abducted to bring the thigh in line with the body in an abducted position. The heel is maintained in approximation to the buttock (Fig. 31–26B). The hip and thigh are then dropped back into extension and adduction (while the heel is kept in approximation with the buttock), and an initial stretch is placed on the TFL and ITB. Care must be taken to maintain control and not allow side bending at the waist (Fig. 31–26C). At this time, the opposite heel is placed on top of the knee, and the thigh is further adducted (Fig. 31–26D). A stretch should be felt in the area of the ITB at the patellofemoral joint.

The patient needs to be instructed precisely on how to perform the stretch and must be shown how to train the antagonist muscle in the new range gained immediately after the stretch.

CONSIDERATION OF FOOT PROBLEMS

Patients who exhibit prolonged pronation during midstance in gait should be shown how to train the supinators of their feet. Improved supinator function should improve the stability of the foot for push-off and decrease the increased valgus vector force created at the knee by the abnormal foot pronation. The position of training is midstance. The patient is instructed to "lift the arch" while keeping the great toe on the ground and pushing the first metatarsal and great toe into the ground. The rationale behind this exercise is that if the base of the first metatarsal is lifted using the tibialis posterior muscle, the line of action of the peroneus longus is improved. The peroneus longus can then efficiently act on the first metatarsal and improve the stability of the first ray in preparation for push-off.[77] If the patient is unable to keep the first metatarsophalangeal joint on the ground when the arch is lifted, the foot deformity is too extreme to correct with training alone, and orthotics is necessary to control the excessive pronation. (See Chapters 18 and 32 for further information about orthotic prescription.)

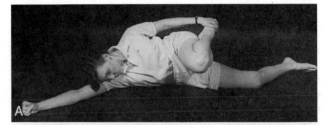
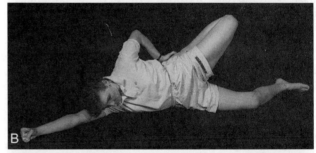
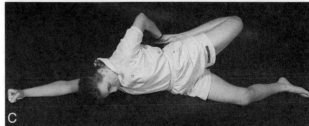
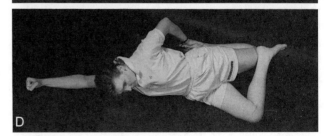

FIGURE 31–26. A–D, Stretch for the tensor fascia lata and the iliotibial band.

WEANING FROM TAPE

As stated earlier, the patient needs to wear the tape until the muscles have been endurance-trained. This may take a considerable amount of time for some. Functional tests should be performed to determine whether the patient is ready to be without the tape for daily activities. The following is a suggested functional test sequence that patients should be able to complete, with a 1- to 2-minute rest between each exercise and a 30-second rest between each set of step-downs:

1. Five sets of 10 continuous steps slowly, demonstrating good control.
2. One-minute quarter-squat against the wall.
3. One-minute half-squat against the wall.
4. Five sets of 10 continuous steps slowly, demonstrating good control.

The VMO and VL are monitored at all times. Deterioration in VMO activity relative to the VL indicates that the tape is not ready to come off. If the tape is ready to come off, the patient wears the tape on alternate days for 1 week. If there has been no recurrence of symptoms during that week, the patient may take the tape off for daily activities but should keep the tape on for sport. The patient should apply fresh tape after sport because the muscle will be fatigued and the old tape will be loose. When the VMO is fatigued, the patellofemoral joint is extremely vulnerable, and symptoms may recur. If the patient has been pain-free for a month and is not taped for daily activities, the tape may be removed for sport, provided the patient can carry out the functional test sequence described, being untaped and pain-free during the test.

The need for surgery may be minimal due to improved understanding of the cause of the patellofemoral pain, taping of the patella to reduce the symptoms, and specific training of the VMO and gluteals. Gerrard[155] demonstrated that 90.5 percent of patients were pain-free after seven treatments using taping and specific VMO training. Studies of other conservative therapies, in which treatment aimed at correcting the lateralization of the patella with exercises to strengthen the VMO (straight leg raise and inner range quadriceps exercises), did not demonstrate good long-term results.[58,71,156] Devereaux and Lachmann[156] found that only 28.6 percent were symptom-free after 13.1 months, whereas Gerrard found that 95 percent of respondents to a questionnaire had good to excellent results 1 year after the cessation of treatment, based on the approach described in this chapter. If the patient fails an appropriate conservative management program, however, surgery is indicated.

SURGICAL CONSIDERATIONS

Patients may fail nonoperative treatment for patellofemoral pain following even the best physical therapy, medical management, bracing, and modification of activity. In fact, there are some mechanical disorders of the knee extensor mechanism that are too severe to respond fully to nonoperative treatment. The following conditions may resist nonoperative treatment: (1) severe post-traumatic chondrosis-arthrosis; (2) persistent patellar tilt, with or without chondrosis or subluxation; (3) pathologic plica; (4) infrapatellar contracture; (5) postoperative neuroma or scar pain; and (6) recurrent dislocation. There has been a tendency to use certain operations, particularly lateral release, to treat any persistent anterior knee pain problem rather than to identify a specific procedure to correct the underlying abnormality.

CLINICAL EVALUATION

Prior to surgery, a complete history is imperative. The clinician should determine what caused the onset of pain or instability. Was there a history of trauma, and is there any suggestion of generalized arthritis, referred pain, underlying structural deformity, or secondary pain? One should also gain a feeling for the patient's personality. Those patients with dependent personalities are less likely to improve. If the onset of pain was spontaneous, it is more likely that the patient had an underlying structural malalignment. The clinician should establish if the primary problem is instability of the patella (subluxation or dislocation) or pain. If the problem is primarily pain, is it more intra-articular or periarticular?

The patient examination is similar to that of the patient being evaluated for nonoperative treatment, but greater emphasis is directed toward identifying the specific source(s) and mechanical origin(s) of pain, impairment and dysfunction that require surgical intervention and would not respond to conservative management.[157,158] The knee should be evaluated for evidence of patellar tilt, skin change, surgical scars, excessive varus or valgus, or contracture. The peripatellar retinaculum, patellar tendon, distal quadriceps, and infrapatellar area must be examined closely for evidence of neuroma, pain, or contracture. All surgical scars, including arthroscopy portals, should be palpated for induration and tenderness. A thumbnail run along the scar easily determines pain, which suggests scar neuroma. If the patient has had previous surgery, it should be determined whether there is a tender residual band of the lateral retinaculum. Patellar alignment should be evaluated actively and passively. The patella should be pressed on firmly to determine whether there is pain on compression that reproduces the patient's complaints of discomfort. Pain reproduced by compression is suggestive of articular cartilage breakdown. It should also be noted whether there is alteration of normal skin temperature, such as might occur in association with reflex sympathetic dystrophy. The examiner should note the degree of knee flexion pain or crepitation at which this occurs, because this helps localize a painful articular lesion (proximal lesions are painful in flexion past 75 to 80 degrees, whereas distal lesions are painful close to full extension). Any evidence of tilt or subluxation should be noted. In particular, the clinician must attempt to elevate the lateral patella away from the lateral trochlea to determine whether there is tethering of the patella laterally. The surgeon must take into consideration all radiologic studies to assist in determining the significance of tilt or subluxation.

CONDITIONS RESISTANT TO NONOPERATIVE MANAGEMENT

At the conclusion of the preoperative evaluation, the clinician should decide whether surgical treatment can offer a reasonable hope of improvement to the patient. There must be a specific, correctable problem that can be defined. Is it tilt? Is there arthrosis or chondrosis? If so, where is the lesion located? Is there a specific tender band of retinaculum or patellar tendon? Does the patella track laterally so that the extensor mechanism needs to be realigned (in addition to lateral release)? Is there any evidence of neuroma or scar pain from previous surgery? Is the pain related to malalignment, or is it post-traumatic?

LATERAL RELEASE

There are specific indications for lateral retinacular release, and there are many patients with resistant anterior knee pain who do not respond to lateral retinacular release but can benefit from other surgical procedures. A surgical release of the lateral retinaculum is used to decrease a pathologic patellar tilt (greater than 12 degrees) in the individual with a complaint of anterior knee pain and minimal evidence of articular degeneration or subluxation. Lateral release is not an appropriate procedure for treating many patients with significant instability (subluxation or dislocation) or the patella-extensor mechanism. Although lateral release has been (and occasionally still is) recommended to treat patellar subluxations, axial radiography, computed tomography, and laboratory studies using a cadaver knee model have clearly demonstrated that lateral release does not consistently relieve signs and symptoms of patellar subluxation.[2,159]

Lateral release is not generally effective in relieving pain related to patella articular degeneration.[160] Once the lateral facet of the patella has collapsed and degenerated,[161] releasing the lateral retinaculum does about as much to relieve contact stress on the degenerated cartilage as releasing the medial collateral ligament of a patient with medial compartment knee arthritis.

Finally, one must also recognize that a lateral release is unlikely to affect any meaningful change in a normally aligned patella that has been severely traumatized (e.g., fracture, dashboard injury), unless there is some secondary retinacular contracture and resulting patellar tilt needing release.

PERSISTENT PATELLAR TILT

Some patients with pathologic patellar tilt, with or without chondrosis or subluxation, do not respond to nonoperative treatment. In these patients, the surgical procedure selected is best determined after considering the extent and location of articular lesions, as well as evaluating the knee for evidence of subluxation associated with tilt. In short, tilt with minimal evidence of articular degeneration or subluxation usually responds well to lateral release alone.[2] One possible exception is the patient with chondral softening on the medial facet in whom greater contact pressure on soft cartilage may result after lateral release. Postoperative physical therapy is aimed at maintaining the mobility of the lateral structures by taping the patella as soon as the sutures from the arthroscopy site are removed and by training the VMO to keep the patella in the trochlea. Emphasis must also be given to the training of the gluteals to minimize any increase in tension in an overactive TFL and tight ITB.

When there is grade 3 or 4[162] articular breakdown on the lateral or distal medial facet in association with tilt, an anteromedial tibial tubercle transfer is more effective,[163,164] particularly if there is any associated lateral patellar subluxation (Fig. 31–27). In the absence of

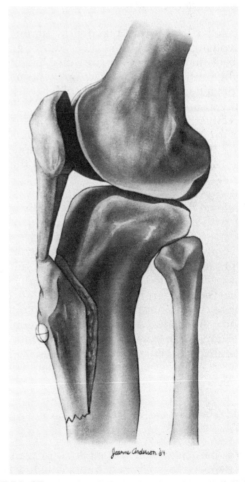

FIGURE 31–27. Transfer of tibial tubercle. Anteromedial tibial tubercle transfer reduces contact stress on the patella while realigning the extensor mechanism into a more medial orientation, thereby reducing or eliminating the likelihood of lateral patella subluxation or dislocation. (Redrawn from Fulkerson J, Hungerford D: Disorders of the Patellofemoral Joint, 2nd ed. Baltimore, Williams & Wilkins, 1990.)

articular disease, but when there is symptomatic sub-luxation associated with patellar tilt, a Trillat procedure may be most appropriate when all nonoperative measures to control the instability have failed to provide adequate relief.[165]

PATHOLOGIC PLICA

Some patients fail nonoperative treatment because of a persistent pathologic plica. Most significant pathologic plicae occur in the medial infrapatellar region and can be readily identified on clinical examination. To make this diagnosis, the clinician should be able to reproduce the patient's pain by palpating the plica. In most cases, the plica is a prominent band palpable by the examiner. In our experience, arthroscopic excision of a pathologic plica results in relief of pain in most patients. Broom, however, noted that pathologic plicae may sometimes be associated with patellar malalignment, so the examiner should be careful not to overlook other sources of pain related specifically to malalignment in patients with plicae.[166]

INFRAPATELLAR CONTRACTURE

Infrapatellar contracture may follow trauma or surgery involving the anterior knee. Although classic patella baja may occur, there are some patients with more subtle infrapatellar contractures who may have persistent pain with relatively little evidence of contracture. Only a careful and pointed physical examination can detect this. Such patients usually have rather diffuse retropatellar tendon pain, frequently aggravated by squeezing or palpating the infrapatellar tendon area. There is usually an associated tightness of the medial and lateral retinaculum.

In our experience, once physical therapy fails, one must evaluate this condition arthroscopically and then proceed with open release of the contracture, usually through a short lateral incision. In most cases, a lateral release is necessary, and one can then appreciate a dense tight infrapatellar fat pad. Release of the fat pad permits the surgeon to tilt the patella gradually up onto its medial edge, perpendicular to the trochlea. A complete release of infrapatellar scar, meticulous hemostasis, and immediate postoperative knee mobilization to full flexion are imperative in these patients. Results are generally excellent in properly selected patients when an adequate release and debridement have been carried out.

SEVERE POST-TRAUMATIC CHONDROSIS OR ARTHROSIS

Time is particularly important in the treatment of patients who have sustained trauma to the anterior knee. The clinician should remember that intraosseous homeostasis can take 18 months or more following injury.[166] One must carefully assess the degree of pain and whether the patient can reasonably tolerate a prolonged period of activity modification and supportive management to allow for spontaneous homeostasis.

It is impossible to know whether there will be relief of pain following such a long period, however, and patients with more severe pain cannot always tolerate this much time without treatment. Supportive measures including repeated ice applications, nonsteroidal anti-inflammatory medications, bracing, taping, and reassurance, but exercising, particularly resisted knee extension, is counterproductive in some of these patients.

Once the decision has been made to operate, the problem is whether the patella can be salvaged. Arthroscopic evaluation and debridement permit the surgeon to understand the extent of chondral injury once all soft tissue and retinacular problems have been solved. At the time of an initial arthroscopy, any post-traumatic neuroma, indurate (painful) retinaculum or tendon, and thickened plica or fibrillated articular cartilage should be excised. In the majority of patients, there is no need to release the lateral retinaculum unless there is significant tilt aggravating the problem. It is unusual to perform a patellectomy as an initial procedure, because many patients may benefit from soft tissue (retinacular) and articular debridement (chondroplasty) or patellar realignment. If an articular debridement has been performed, the therapist must initially avoid compression on the newly debrided area, and must communicate with the surgeon to determine where the chondroplasty has occurred.

The rehabilitation program follows the same principles as the nonoperative program. Emphasis is placed on specific VMO contractions in sitting and during other non–weight-bearing or minimal weight-bearing activities. Care is taken to avoid any compression on the area of chondroplasty. Taping may be used carefully to assist in controlling patellar position, provided no compression occurs on the newly debrided area. The therapist and patient must remember that rehabilitative progress from this type of surgery can be slow.

If arthroscopic treatment fails, a decision should be made as to whether there is sufficient articular cartilage to allow a transposition of the tibial tubercle (usually either medially, anteriorly, or both) to shift contact stress from damaged to healthy cartilage. In patients with extensive articular damage causing intractable pain, patellectomy or patella resurfacing may be the only viable options.

If there is healthy cartilage proximally on the patella, the tibial tubercle may be moved anteriorly. If the best remaining cartilage is proximal and medial, the patella should be moved anteromedially. If the proximal patellar cartilage is severely damaged (as it often is following dashboard injury), tibial tubercle anteriorization is less likely to be successful. In this case, patellectomy or resurfacing may need to be considered.

POSTOPERATIVE NEUROMA OR SCAR PAIN

The patient who has already had surgery and complains of persistent pain that is different than the original pain may have a postoperative neuroma or painful scar. This is a clinical diagnosis and is not usually difficult as long as one is looking for it. The thumbnail test (running the dorsum of the thumbnail over each scar) elicits the sharp pain of a neuroma in most cases. The clinician must be certain that this is not a diffuse sensitivity, suggesting reflex sympathetic dystrophy (RSD). Patients with RSD are not surgical candidates and may require pain management programs, sympathetic blocks, or surgical sympathectomy.

Sensitive scar or neuroma can be relieved transiently in the office using a local anesthetic injection, which confirms the diagnosis. Corticosteroids administered in conjunction with a local anesthetic do not usually provide lasting benefit to patients with a neuroma. In general, if a patient has failed nonoperative management and demonstrates a localized focus of pain in a scar, excision of this painful segment of tissue may be curative.

RECURRENT PATELLAR DISLOCATION

Recurrent patellar dislocation may be devastating to patellar articular cartilage and generally warrants early surgery if nonoperative treatment fails to restore stable tracking of the patella. Each patellar dislocation may result in a shearing off of articular cartilage from the medial patellar facet or lateral femoral trochlea. The cartilage may be stripped of bone so that it cannot be replaced. Consequently, restoration of stable patellar tracking is important, preferably before serious cartilage damage occurs.

Following an acute patellar dislocation, any fragment of articular cartilage with bone attached should be replaced anatomically, generally using an open lateral release incision and eversion of the patella to expose its medial facet for reconstruction. Very fine (8-0 or smaller) absorbable suture may help approximate the cartilage edges.

In our experience, it is best to restore patellar stability using lateral release and tibial tubercle transfer (as described by Trillat and reviewed by Cox[165]). Medial imbrication (overlapping of free edges) carries a substantial risk of increasing contact pressure on the medial patellar facet (because the medial retinaculum is oriented so that its imbrication pulls the medial patellar facet posteriorly as well as medially). When there is already damage to the medial patella following dislocation, anteromedial tibial tubercle transfer minimizes load increase on the medial patella while reorienting the extensor mechanism medially to minimize and hopefully eliminate the risk of lateral patellar dislocation.

In a skeletally immature patient, tibial tubercle transfer should not be done. Lateral release and careful medial imbrication may provide stability, or the surgeon may consider a semitendinosus tenodesis of the patella.[167,168]

SUMMARY

Surgical treatment can be extremely helpful in the management of patients with anterior knee pain resistant to nonoperative treatment. It is most important to direct surgical treatment specifically to the precise cause of the knee pain. Painful articular lesions should be debrided and unloaded, painful segments of the retinaculum or scar excised, alignment corrected, tilt relieved by lateral release, pathologic plicae excised, and contractures released. Surgery should not be initiated until there is a clear concept of what needs to be corrected in a patient who understands the risks involved as well as the potential benefits. The chosen surgical procedure requires appropriate postoperative management to optimize outcome.

REFERENCES

1. Brukner P, Khan K: Clinical Sports Medicine. Sydney, Australia, McGraw-Hill, 1993.
2. Fulkerson J, Hungerford D: Disorders of the Patellofemoral Joint, 2nd ed. Baltimore, Williams & Wilkins, 1990.
3. Lutter L: The knee and running. Clin Sports Med 1985; 4:685–698.
4. Jacobson K, Flandry F: Diagnosis of anterior knee pain. Clin Sports Med 1989; 8:179–195.
5. Molnar T, Fox J: Overuse injuries of the knee in basketball. Clin Sports Med 1993; 12:349–362.
6. Holmes J, Pruitt A, Whalen N: Lower extremity overuse in bicycling. Clin Sports Med 1994; 13:235–248.
7. Cox J: Patellofemoral problems in runners. Clin Sports Med 1985; 4:753–764.
8. Gecha S, Torg E: Knee injuries in tennis. Clin Sports Med 1988; 7:435–454.
9. Emerson R: Basketball knee injuries and the anterior cruciate ligament. Clin Sports Med 1993; 12:317–328.
10. Fox TA: Dysplasia of the quadriceps mechanism. Surg Clin North Am 1975; 55:199–225.
11. Apple D: End stage running problems. Clin Sports Med 1985; 4:657–670.
12. Williams P, Warwick R: Gray's Anatomy. London, Churchill Livingstone, 1980.
13. Fujikawa K, Seedholm B, Wright V: Biomechanics of the patellofemoral joint. Parts 1 and 2. Study of the patellofemoral compartment and movement of the patella. Eng Med 1983; 12:3–21.
14. Wiberg G: Studies of the femoropatellar joint. Acta Orthop Scand 1941; 12:319–410.
15. Baumgartl F: Das Kniegelenk. Berlin, Springer-Verlag, 1964.
16. Grana WA, Kriegshauser LA: Scientific basis of extensor mechanism disorders. Clin Sports Med 1985; 4:247–257.
17. Dahhan P, Delphine G, Larde D: The femoropatellar joint. Anat Clin 1981; 3:23–29.
18. Aglietti P, Insall J, Cerulli G: Patellar pain and incongruence. Clin Orthop Rel Res 1983; 176:217–224.
19. Wise HH, Fiebert IM, Kates JL: EMG feedback as a treatment for patellofemoral pain syndrome. J Orthop Sports Phys Ther 1984; 6:95–103.
20. Reider B, Marshall J, Koslin B, et al: The anterior aspect of the knee. J Bone Joint Surg 1981; 63A:351–356.
21. Fiske-Warren L, Marshall J: The supporting structures and layers on the medial side of the knee. J Bone Joint Surg 1979; 61A:61.
22. Petschnig R, Baron R, Engel A, et al: Objectivation of the effects of knee problems on vastus medialis and vastus lateralis with EMG and dynamometry. Arch Phys Med Rehab 1991; 2:50–54.
23. Hallisey M, Doughty N, Bennett W, Fulkerson J: Anatomy of the junction of the vastus lateralis tendon and the patella. J Bone Joint Surg 1987; 69A:545.
24. Lieb F, Perry J: Quadriceps function. J Bone Joint Surg 1968; 50A:1535–1548.
25. Bose K, Kanagasuntherum R, Osman M: Vastus medialis oblique: An anatomical and physiologic study. Orthopaedics 1980; 3:880–883.
26. Ingersoll C, Knight K: Patellar location changes following EMG biofeedback or progressive resistive exercises. Med Sci Sports Exercise 1991; 23:1122–1127.

27. Bohannon R: The effect of electrical stimulation to the vastus medialis muscle in a patient with chronically dislocating patella. Phys Ther 1983; 63:1445.

28. Ahmed AM, Burke DL, Yu A: In-vitro measurement of static pressure distribution in synovial joints—Part II: Retropatellar surface. J Biomed Eng 1983; 105:226–236.

29. Ahmed A, Shi S, Hyder A, Chan K: The effect of quadriceps tension characteristics on the patellar tracking pattern. *In* Transactions of the 34th Orthopaedic Research Society. Atlanta, 1988, p 280.

30. Buff H, Jones LC, Hungerford DS: Experimental determination of forces transmitted through the patellofemoral joint. J Biomech 1988; 21:17–23.

31. Hungerford DS, Barry M: Biomechanics of the patello-femoral joint. Clin Orthop Rel Res 1979; 144:9–15.

32. Kennedy JC, Alexander IJ, Hayes KC: Nerve supply of the human knee and its functional importance. Am J Sports Med 1982; 10:329–333.

33. Reilly D, Martens M: Experimental analyses of the quadriceps muscle force and patellofemoral joint reaction force for various activities. Acta Orthop Scand 1972; 43:126–137.

34. Ficat P, Hungerford D: Disorders of the patellofemoral joint. London, Williams & Wilkins, 1979.

35. van Eijden TMG, Kouwenhoven E, Verburg J, Weijs WA: A mathematical model of the patellofemoral joint. J Biomech 1986; 19:219–229.

36. Ahmed AM, Burke DL, Hyder A: Force analysis of the patellar mechanism. J Orthop Res 1987; 5:69–85.

37. Huberti HH, Hayes WC, Stone JL, Shybut GT: Force ratios in the quadriceps tendon and ligamentum patellae. J Orthop Res 1984; 2:49–54.

38. Goodfellow J, Hungerford D, Zindel M: Patellofemoral joint mechanics and pathology Parts 1 and 2. J Bone Joint Surg 1976; 3:287–299.

39. Carson W, James S, Larson R: Patello-femoral disorders—Parts I and II. Clin Orthop Rel Res 1984; 185:165–174.

40. Huberti HH, Hayes WC: Contact pressures in chondromalacia patellae and the effects of capsular reconstructive procedures. J Orthop Res 1988; 6:499–508.

41. Armstrong CG, Mow VC: Variations in the intrinsic mechanical properties of human articular cartilage with age degeneration and water content. J Bone Joint Surg 64A:88–94.

42. Akizuki S, Mow VC, Muller F: Tensile properties of human knee joint cartilage: I. Influence of ionic conditions, weight bearing and fibrillation on the tensile modulus. J Orthop Res 1986; 4:379–392.

43. Burgess R: Patellofemoral joint transverse displacement and tibial rotation. Unpublished project report, Graduate Diploma in Manipulative Therapy. Southern Australia Institute of Technology, Adelaide, South Australia, 1985.

44. Macquet P: Biomechanics of the Knee. New York, Springer Verlag, 1984.

45. van Kampen A, Huskies R: The three-dimensional tracking pattern of the human patella. J Orthop Res 1990; 8:372–381.

46. Matthews L, Sonstegard D, Henke J: Load-bearing characteristics of the patellofemoral joint. Acta Orthop Scand 1977; 48:511–516.

47. Ericsson M, Nissell R: Patellofemoral forces during ergometric cycling. Phys Ther 1987; 67:1365–1368.

48. Brandt K: Pathogenesis of osteoarthritis. *In* Kelley WN, Harris ED Jr, Ruddy S, Sledge CB (eds): Textbook of Rheumatology. Philadelphia, WB Saunders, 1981.

49. Radin E: A rational approach to treatment of patellofemoral pain. Clin Orthop Rel Res 1979; 144:107–109.

50. Minns KJ, Birnie A, Abernathy P: Stress analysis of the patella and how it relates to patellar articular cartilage lesions. J Biomech 1979; 12:699–711.

51. Björkstroöm S, Goldie I: Hardness of the subchondral bone of the patella in the normal state, in chondromalacia and in osteoarthrosis. Acta Orthop Scand 1982; 53:451–462.

52. Mow V, Eisenfeld J, Redler I: Some surface characteristics of articular cartilage—II. On the stability of articular surface and a possible biomechanical factor in aetiology of chondrodegeneration. J Biomech 1974; 7:457–467.

53. Raux P, Townsend P, Miegel R, et al: Trabecular architecture of the human patella. J Biomech 1975; 8:1–7.

54. Bland J, Stulberg SD: Osteoarthritis: Pathology and clinical

patterns. *In* Kelley WN, Harris ED Jr, Ruddy S, Sledge CB (eds): Textbook of Rheumatology. Philadelphia, WB Saunders, 1981.

55. Seedholm B, Takeda T, Tsubuku M, Wright S: Mechanical factors and patellofemoral osteoarthritis. Ann Rheum Dis 1979; 38:307–316.

56. Marar B, Pillay V: Chondromalacia of the patella in Chinese. J Bone Joint Surg 1975; 57A:342–345.

57. Townsend PR, Rose RM: The biomechanics of the human patella and its implications for chondromalacia. J Biomech 1977; 10:403–407.

58. Pevsner D, Johnson JR, Blazina MJ: The patellofemoral joint and its implications in the rehabilitation of the knee. Phys Ther 1979; 57:869–874.

59. Hvid I: The stability of the human patello-femoral joint. Eng Med, 12, (2), 55.

60. Lyon L, Benzl L, Johnson K: Q angle: A factor—peak torque occurrence in isokinetic knee extension. J Orthop Sports Phys Ther 1988; 9:250–253.

61. Draganich LF, Andriacchi TP, Andersson GBJ: Interaction between intrinsic knee mechanics and the knee extensor mechanism. J Orthop Res 1987; 5:539–547.

62. Huberti H, Hayes W: Patellofemoral contact pressures. J Bone Joint Surg 1984; 66A:715–724.

63. Fulkerson J, Gossling H: Anatomy of the knee joint retinaculum. Clin Orthop Rel Res 1980; 153:183.

64. Tsirbas A, Paterson R, Keene G: Fat pad impingement: a missed cause of patellofemoral pain. Aust J Sci Med Sport 1991; 23:24–26.

65. McConnell J: Fat pad irritation—a mistaken patellar tendinitis. Sport Health 1991; 9:7–9.

66. Kramer PG: Patella malalignment syndrome: Rationale to reduce excessive lateral pressure. J Orthop Sports Phys Ther 1986; 8:301–308.

67. McIntyre D, Wessel J: Knee muscle torque in the patellofemoral pain syndrome. Physiother Can 1988; 40:20–23.

68. Insall J: Chondromalacia patellae: Patellar malalignment syndrome. Orthop Clin North Am 1979; 10:117–125.

69. Kettlekamp DB: Current concepts review: Patellar malalignment. J Bone Joint Surg 1981; 63A:1344.

70. Micheli L, Slater J, Woods E, Gerbino P: Patella alta and the adolescent growth spurt. Clin Orthop Rel Res 1986; 213:159–162.

71. Malek M, Mangine R: Patellofemoral pain syndromes: A comprehensive and conservative approach. J Orthop Sports Phys Ther 1981; 2:108–116.

72. Fulkerson JP: Awareness of the retinaculum in evaluating patellofemoral pain. Am J Sports Med 1982; 10:147–149.

73. Minkoff J, Fein L: The role of radiography in the evaluation and treatment of common anarthrotic disorders of the patellofemoral joint. Clin Sports Med 1989; 8:203–260.

74. Sahrmann S: The movement system balance theory: Relationship to musculoskeletal pain syndromes. Phys Ther (in press).

75. Subotnik S: The foot and sports medicine. J Orthop Sports Phys Ther 1980; 2:53–54.

76. Buchbinder R, Naparo N, Bizzo E: The relationship of abnormal pronation to chondromalacia patellae in distance runners. J Am Podiatr Assoc 1979; 69:159–161.

77. Root M, Orien W, Weed J: Clinical Biomechanics, vol II. Los Angeles, Clinical Biomechanics Corporation, 1977.

78. Sagaki T, Yagi T: Subluxation of the patella: An investigation by computerized tomography. Int Orthop 1986; 10:115–120.

79. Tiberio D: The effect of excessive subtalar joint pronation on patellofemoral mechanics; a theoretical model. J Orthop Sports Phys Ther 1987; 9:160–165.

80. Spencer J, Hayes K, Alexander I: Knee joint effusion and quadriceps reflex inhibition in man. Arch Phys Med 1984; 65:171–177.

81. Mariani P, Caruso I: An electromyographic investigation of subluxation of the patella. J Bone Joint Surg 1979; 61:169–171.

82. Richardson CA, Bullock MI: Changes in muscle activity during fast alternating flexion and extension movements of the knee. Scand J Rehabil Med 1986; 18:51–58.

83. Reynolds L, Levin T, Medeiros J, et al: EMG activity of the vastus medialis oblique and vastus lateralis in their role in patellar alignment. Am J Phys Med 1983; 62:61–71.

84. Longhurst S: Variability of EMG during slow walking. *In* Proceedings of the Special Conference of the Canadian Society of Biomechanics. 1980.

85. Voight M, Wieder D: Comparative reflex response times of the vastus medialis and the vastus lateralis in normal subjects and subjects with extensor mechanism dysfunction. Am J Sports Med 1991; 10:131–137.

86. Boucher J, King M, Lefebvre R, Pepin A: Quadriceps femoris muscle activity in patellofemoral pain syndrome. Am J Sports Med 1992; 20:527–532.

87. Souza D, Gross M: Comparison of vastus medialis obliquus: vastus lateralis muscle integrated electromyographic ratios between healthy subjects and patients with patellofemoral pain. Phys Ther 1991; 71:310–320.

88. Weh L, Eickhoff W, Prahl R: Mediolaterale Quadrizepsdysbalance und Peripatellares Schmerzsyndrom. Z Orthop 1987; 125:48–53.

89. D'Amico JC, Rubin M: The influence of foot orthoses on the quadriceps angle. J Am Podiatr Assoc 1986; 76:337–339.

90. Wild J, Franklin T, Woods GW: Patellar pain and quadriceps rehabilitation—an EMG study. Am J Sports Med 1982; 10:12.

91. LeVeau B, Rogers C: Selective training of the vastus medialis muscle using EMG biofeedback. Phys Ther 1980; 60:1410–1415.

92. Williams PE, Goldspink G: Changes in sarcomere length and physiological properties in immobilised muscle. J Anat 1978; 127:459–468.

93. Gossman MR, Sahrmann SA, Rose SJ: Review of length-associated changes in muscle. Phys Ther 1982; 62:1799–1808.

94. McConnell J: An investigation of certain biomechanical variables predisposing an adolescent male to retropatellar pain. Unpublished thesis, Graduate Diploma in Manipulative Therapy, University of New South Wales, Sydney, Australia, 1983.

95. Abernathy PJ, Townsend P, Rose R, Radin E: Is chondromalacia a separate clinical entity? J Bone Joint Surg 1978; 60B:205–210.

96. Stokes M, Young A: Investigations of quadriceps inhibition: Implications for clinical practice. Physiotherapy 1984; 70:425–428.

97. de Andrade J, Grant C, Dixon A: Joint distension and reflex muscle inhibition in the knee. J Bone Joint Surg 1965; 47A:313.

98. Maitland GD: Vertebral Manipulation. London, Butterworths, 1986.

99. McConnell J: Promoting effective segmental alignment. In Crosbie J, McConnell J (eds): Key Issues in Musculoskeletal Physiotherapy. Oxford, Butterworth-Heinemann, 1993, pp 172–194.

100. Hughston J: Patellar subluxation: A recent history. Clin Sports Med 1989; 8:153–162.

101. Henry J: Conservative treatment of patellofemoral subluxation. Clin Sports Med 1989; 8:261–278.

102. Cross MJ, Crichton KJ: Clinical Examination of the Injured Knee. London, Harper & Row, 1987.

103. Meillon MB, Walsh WM, Shelton GL: The Team Physician's Handbook. Philadelphia, Hanley & Belfus, 1990.

104. Broom MJ, Fulkerson JP: The plica syndrome: A new perspective. Orthop Clin North Am 1986; 17:279–281.

105. Patel D: Plica as a cause of anterior knee pain. Orthop Clin North Am 1986; 17:273.

106. Jackson R, Marshall D, Fujisawa Y: The pathological medial shelf. Orthop Clin North Am 1982; 13:307.

107. O'Neill D, Micheli L: Overuse injuries in the young athlete. Clin Sports Med 1989; 7:591–610.

108. Schutzer SF, Ramsby GR, Fulkerson JP: The evaluation of patellofemoral pain using computerised tomography. Clin Orthop Rel Res 1986; 204:286–293.

109. Martinez S, Korobkin M, Fondren F, et al: Computed tomography of the normal patellofemoral joint. Invest Radiol 1983; 18:249–253.

110. Merchant AC, Mercer RL, Jacobsen RH, Cool CR: Roentgenographic analysis of patellofemoral congruence. J Bone Joint Surg 1974; 56A:1391–1396.

111. Laurin C, Levesque H, Dussault S, et al: The abnormal lateral patellofemoral angle. J Bone Joint Surg 1978; 60A:55.

112. Sagaki T, Yagi T: Subluxation of the patella: An investigation by computerized tomography. Int Orthop 1986; 10:115–120.

113. Insall J, Aglietti P, Tria AJ: Patellar pain and incongruence, II: Clinical application. Clin Orthop Rel Res 1983; 176:225–232.

114. Möller BN, Jurik AG, Tidemand-Dahl C, et al: The quadriceps function in patellofemoral disorders. Arch Orthop Trauma Surg 1987; 106:195–198.

115. Fulkerson JP, Schutzer SF, Ramsby GR, Bernstein RA: Computerized tomography of the patellofemoral joint before and after lateral release or realignment. Arthroscopy 1987; 3:19–24.

116. Reigler H: Recurrent patellar dislocation/subluxation. Clin Orthop Rel Res 1988; 27:201–209.

117. Roberts JM: The effect of taping on patellofemoral alignment—a radiological pilot study. In Jones M (ed): Proceedings of the Sixth Biennial Conference of the Manipulative Therapists Association of Australia, Manipulative Physiotherapists Association of Australia, Adelaide Australia, 1989; pp 146–151.

118. Bockrath K, Wooden C, Worrell T, et al: Effects of patella taping on patella position and perceived pain. Med Sci Sports Exercise 1993; 25:989–992.

119. McConnell JS: A mechanical investigation into the effect of taping the patella of patients with patellofemoral pain. Unpublished master's thesis, Biomedical Engineering, University of New South Wales, Sydney, Australia, 1992.

120. Insall J, Salvati E: Patella position in the normal knee. Radiology 1971; 101:101.

121. Insall J, Goldberg V, Salvati E: Recurrent dislocation and the high riding patella. Clin Orthop 1972; 88:67–69.

122. Laurin CA: Patellar position, patellar osteotomy—their relationship to chondromalacia: X-ray diagnosis of chondromalacia. In Chondromalacia of the Patella, vol 2. Baltimore/London. Williams & Wilkins, 1983, pp 11–23.

123. Bradley W, Ominsky S: Mountain view of the patella. Am J Radiology, 1981; 136:53–57.

124. Newberg AH, Seligson D: The patellofemoral joint: 30 degrees, 60 degrees, and 90 degrees. Radiology 1980; 137:57–61.

125. Imai N, Tomatsu T, Takeuchi H, Noguchi T: Clinical and roentgenological studies on malalignment of the patellofemoral joint. Part I: Classification of patellofemoral alignments using dynamic sky-line view arthrography with special consideration of the mechanism of the malalignment disorders. Nippon Scikeigeka Gakkai Zasshi J Orthop Assoc 1987; 61:1–15.

126. Imai N, Tomatsu T, Takeuchi H, Noguchi T: Clinical and roentgenological studies on malalignment of the patellofemoral joint. Part II: Relationship between predisposing factors and malalignment of the patellofemoral joint. J Jpn Orthop Assoc 1987; 61:1191–1202.

127. Brossmann J, Muhle C, Schorder C, et al: Patellar tracking patterns during active and passive knee extension: Evaluation with motion triggered cine MR imaging. Radiology 1993; 187:207–212.

128. Shellock FG, Mink JH, Deutsch AL, et al: Patellofemoral joint: Identification of abnormalities with active-movement "unloaded vs. loaded" kinematic MR imaging techniques. Radiology 1993; 188:575–578.

129. Shellock FG, Mink JH, Deutsch AL, et al: Kinematic MR imaging of the patellofemoral joint: Comparison of passive positioning and active movement techniques. Radiology 1992; 187:574–577.

130. Stanford W, Phelan J, Kathol MH, et al: Patellofemoral joint motion: Evaluation by ultrafast computed tomography. Skel Radiol 1988; 17:487–492.

131. Cohen MS: Rapid MR imaging: Techniques and performance characteristics. In Taveras JT, Ferrucci JT (eds): Radiology: Diagnosis/Imaging/Intervention, vol 1. Philadelphia, JB Lippincott, 1992; pp 1–19.

132. Kendall HD, Kendall FP, Boynton DA: Posture and Pain. Baltimore, Williams & Wilkins, 1952.

133. Helminen H, Kiviranta I, Tammi M, et al: Joint Loading. London, Butterworths, 1987.

134. Leveau BF: Basic biomechanics in sports and orthopaedic therapy. In Gould JA, Davies GJ (eds): Orthopaedic and Sports Physical Therapy. St. Louis, CV Mosby, 1985, pp 65–83.

135. Dumbleton JH, Black J: An Introduction to Orthopaedic Materials. Springfield, IL, Charles C Thomas, 1975.

136. McConnell J: The management of chondromalacia patellae—a long-term solution. Aust J Physiother 1986; 32:215–223.

137. McConnell J: Training the vastus medialis oblique in the management of patellofemoral pain. In Proceedings of Tenth Congress of the World Confederation for Physical Therapy, Sydney, Australia, May 1987.

138. Frankel VH, Nordin M: Basic Biomechanics of the Skeletal System, 2nd ed. Philadelphia, Lea & Febiger, 1980.

139. Herbert R: Preventing and treating stiff joints. In Crosbie J,

McConnell J (eds): Key Issues in Musculoskeletal Physiotherapy. Oxford, Butterworth-Heinemann, 1993; pp 114–141.

140. Hooley C, McCrum N, Cohen R: The visco-elastic deformation of the tendon. J Biomech 1980; 13:521.

141. Taylor D, Dalton J, Seaber A: Visco-elastic properties of muscle-tendon units. The biomechanical effect of stretching. Am J Sports Med 1990; 18:300.

142. Mckay-Lyons M: Low-load, prolonged stretch in treatment of elbow flexion contractures secondary to head trauma: A case report. Phys Ther 1989; 69:292.

143. Conway A, Malone T, Conway P: Patellar alignment/tracking alteration: Effect on force output and perceived pain. Isokinetics Exerc Sci 1992; 2:9–17.

144. Herbert R: Human strength adaptations—implications for therapy. In Crosbie J, McConnell J (eds): Key Issues in Musculoskeletal Physiotherapy. Oxford, Butterworth-Heinemann, 1993, pp 142–171.

145. Sale D, MacDougall D: Specificity of strength training: A review for coach and athlete. Can J Appl Sports Sci 1981; 6:87–92.

146. Sale D: Influence of exercise and training on motor unit activation. Exerc Sports Sci Rev 1987; 5:95–151.

147. Kitai T, Sale D: Specificity of joint angle in isometric training. Eur J Appl Physiol 1989; 64:1500.

148. Moffroid M, Whipple R: Specificity of speed of exercise. Phys Ther 50:1692–1700.

149. Rutherford O, Jones D: The role of learning and co-ordination in strength training. Eur J Appl Physiol 1986; 55:100.

150. Rasch PJ, Moorehouse LE: Effect of static and dynamic exercises on muscular strength and hypertrophy. J Appl Physiol 1957; 11:29.

151. Hodges P, Richardson C: An investigation into the effectiveness of hip adduction in the optimisation of the vastus medialis oblique contraction. Scand J Rehabil Med 1993; 25:57–62.

152. Hanten W, Schulthies SS: Exercise effect on electromyographic activity of the vastus medialis and the vastus lateralis muscles. Phys Ther 1990; 70:561–565.

153. Karst G, Jewett P: Electromyographic analysis of exercises proposed for differential activation of medial and lateral quadriceps femoris components. Phys Ther 1993; 73:286–295.

154. Parsons D: The effect of medial displacement of the patella on the onset of muscle activity in selected muscles of the quadriceps femoris in normal subjects. Unpublished honours thesis, Faculty of Health Sciences. Sidney, Australia, University of Sydney, 1993.

155. Gerrard B: The Patellofemoral pain syndrome: A clinical trial of the McConnell programme. Austr J of Physioth 1989; 35:70–80.

156. Devereaux MD, Lachmann SM: Patellofemoral arthralgia in athletes attending a sports injury clinic. Br J Sports Med 1984; 18:18–21.

157. Fulkerson J: Awareness of the retinaculum in evaluating patellofemoral pain. Am J Sports Med 1982; 10:147–151.

158. Fulkerson J: Evaluation of the peripatellar soft tissues and retinaculum in patients with patellofemoral pain. Clin Sports Med 1989; 8:197–202.

159. Post W, Fulkerson J: Distal realignment of the patellofemoral joint. Orthop Clin North Am 1992; 23:6–11.

160. Shea K, Fulkerson J: Pre-operative computed tomography scanning and arthroscopy in predicting outcome after lateral release. Arthroscopy 1992; 8:327–334.

161. Ficat P, Ficat C, Baileux A: Syndrome d'hyperpression externe de la rotule. Rev Chir Orthop 1975; 61:39–59.

162. Outerbridge R: Further studies on the etiology of chondromalacia patella. J Bone Joint Surg 1964; 46B:179–190.

163. Fulkerson J: Anteromedialization of the tibial tuberosity for patellofemoral malalignment. Clin Orthop Rel Res 1983; 177: 176–181.

164. Fulkerson J, Schutzer S: After failure of conservative treatment for painful patellofemoral malalignment: Lateral release or realignment?, Orthop Clin North Am 1986; 17:283–288.

165. Cox JS: Evaluation of the roux-Elmslie-Trillat procedure for knee extensor realignment. Am J Sports Med 1983; 10:300–310.

166. Broom M, Fulkerson J: The plica syndrome: A new perspective. Orthop Clin North Am 1986; 17:279–281.

167. Baker R, Carrol N, Dewar P, Hall J: Semitendinosis tenodesis for dislocation of the patella. J Bone Joint Surg 1972; 54B:1103–1109.

168. Hall J, Micheli L, McNamara G: Semitendinosis tenodesis for recurrent subluxation or dislocation of the patella. Clin Orthop Rel Res 1979; 144:31–39.

CHAPTER 32

Leg, Foot, and Ankle Injuries

JACK TAUNTON *MSc, MD, Dip. Sport Med. (CASM)*
CLYDE SMITH *BSc, DPT, SPD III*
DAVID J. MAGEE *PhD, BPT, CAT (C), SPD III*

The lower leg, ankle, and foot are the body's contact with the ground, providing both support and propulsion. Because of these roles, the area is highly susceptible to injury, either due to trauma or overuse (Table 32–1), because the forces experienced by the foot during activity are considerable. For example, a 150-lb man running a mile subjects each foot to a load of approximately 220 tons.[1] Thus, the lower leg, ankle, and foot must have the strength, endurance, and adaptability to withstand these loads.

The function of the lower limb is to propel and stabilize the body's center of gravity. This propulsion and stabilization occurs most often against gravity and ground reaction forces (see Chapter 13, Biomechanics of Running). The foot must be able to react to changes in surface (balance and proprioception), absorb shock, and at the same time provide acceleration and deceleration forces for movement of the body.[2] The ability of the body to perform these functions in an efficient and proficient manner involves strength, power, endurance, range of motion, and neurologic control. In addition, it is most important to remember that all body systems are involved in normal activity and, with injury, not only the area that is injured but also the body as a whole must be addressed during rehabilitation.

The function of the lower limb dictates that most of the injuries seen have to go through the same final stages of rehabilitation exercise and functional training before 100 percent return to activity. In many situations, the athlete has returned to complete participation before the tissues have progressed through the healing continuum (Fig. 32–1). In those cases, the athlete may need protective bracing, taping, or padding for a continued period of time until complete healing has taken place.

Breaking down the actions in the gait cycle is an important component of understanding the relationships and functional movements of the lower limb. (See Chapter 18, Biomechanics of Running, for more information on the running gait cycle.) Variations of changing direction, interaction of the foot within the shoe, and interaction of the shoe with even or uneven ground add multiple variables to the possible mechanisms of injury.

ASSESSMENT OF THE LOWER LEG, ANKLE, AND FOOT

Generally, lower leg, ankle, and foot pathology is characterized by a history of overuse or trauma. Thus, it becomes absolutely essential to determine the history of overuse or trauma, because these factors play a major role in what the clinician decides is necessary in terms of treatment, and return to activity, and the role of the athlete in this program.

Observation should include the shape of the foot and position of the foot and leg in the weight-bearing and non–weight-bearing positions. The height of the arches (longitudinal and metatarsal) should be noted, as

---

TABLE 32–1
Causes of Overuse Injuries to the Lower Limb

- Prolonged training season
- Impact force of activity
- Training or competing on hard surfaces
- Change of training surface
- Downhill running
- Lack of flexibility
- Individual muscle weakness or poor reciprocal muscle strength
- Overstriding
- Poor posture
- High mileage or sudden change in mileage
- Too much, too soon
- Overtraining
- Anatomic factors (e.g., malalignment)
- Wrong type of footwear
- Road and/or sidewalk camber

---

should any deformities or deviations, such as claw toes. A more detailed description of these deformities and deviations is found elsewhere.[3] The presence of calluses, blisters, and exostoses indicates pressure areas of the foot.

When assessing the lower leg, ankle, and foot, it is important to begin by considering the neutral position of the foot, which is defined as the midpoint of function of the foot where the talus and navicular are congruous.[4] This position must be established during both weight bearing and non–weight bearing to have a better understanding of how the athlete's foot is functioning normally.[5] In one case, the foot moves freely (non–weight bearing, or open kinetic chain), whereas in the other case, the foot is fixed and the body moves over it (weight bearing, or closed kinetic chain). The function of the lower limb is to provide contact with the ground and to move the body in the direction it wishes to go. Ideally, the clinician should view the foot during actual function (e.g., running, jumping), but this is difficult to do accurately unless high-priced equipment is available. If the foot is not found to be in neutral, especially on weight bearing, the clinician should note whether the foot is tending toward pronation (flat foot) or supination (cavus foot), because this is often a major determining factor in the corrective treatment to be given.

Range of motion of the foot and ankle should be observed including the athlete's willingness to move as well as the degree of pain, noting especially the amount of plantar flexion and dorsiflexion, inversion and eversion, and supination and pronation. These movements must be tested in weight bearing and non–weight bearing, and any differences noted. These same movements are tested passively to stress the noncontractile elements and to determine the end feels of motion.

Testing for muscle strength is done isometrically in the position of most comfort, which is usually the resting position. The athlete is appropriately positioned and is then asked to resist the movement by the instruction, "Don't let me move you." Testing in this fashion isolates the muscles and their associated ten-

dons as a source of pain. Usually, the strength is recorded according to the simple Oxford scale (1 to 5 scale), although isokinetic tests are sometimes used.

The most common special tests performed at the ankle are the anterior drawer sign and talar tilt. When doing the anterior drawer sign, the clinician must watch the movement of the foot as it is drawn forward in the ankle mortise. If excessive straight anterior movement occurs, it is indicative of both medial and lateral ligament insufficiencies at the ankle. If the foot moves anteriorly and medially when drawn forward (a more common case), it is indicative of injury to the anterior talofibular ligament and potentially the calcaneofibular ligament. The talar tilt test is performed to determine involvement of the calcaneofibular ligament. When the talus is adducted relative to the tibia and fibula, stress is placed on the ligament. If excessive movement or pain occurs, it is indicative of calcaneofibular ligament involvement. A more detailed description of these tests is given elsewhere.[3,6]

If injury to the Achilles tendon is suspected, the Thompson test is commonly performed.[7] The athlete lies prone, with the foot hanging over the end of the table. The clinician then gently grasps the soleus-gastrocnemius muscle belly and squeezes the muscle. If the foot plantar flexes, the tendon is intact. If the foot does not plantar flex, it is indicative of an Achilles tendon rupture (third-degree strain).

Because there is always the possibility of neurologic involvement following traumatic injury to the lower limb, ankle, and foot, the examiner should test sensation, being sure to differentiate among the various peripheral nerves.[8] This testing is followed by joint play testing and palpation.

Palpation should be a careful exercise, carried out in a systematic fashion by starting at the leg and working down over the ankle and into the foot. The clinician should try to visualize the structures under the palpating fingers. Any points of tenderness, pain, or deviations or deformities should be carefully noted.

Radiographic examination should complete the physical examination. Normally, anteroposterior and lateral views of the foot and ankle are taken, especially if a fracture is suspected. Consideration should be given to having these views taken in weight bearing and non–weight bearing. In some cases, if warranted by pathology, special techniques such as bone scans, computed tomography (CT) scans, and magnetic resonance imaging (MRI) may be requested.

SPECIFIC PROBLEMS AND TREATMENT

MUSCLE STRAINS

Muscle strains are seldom encountered in the lower leg, ankle, and foot except in the muscles of the lower leg, primarily the gastrocnemius and soleus. Gastrocnemius-soleus strains, sometimes referred to as tennis leg, are commonly seen in explosive sports such as court sports involving quick moves in all directions. The mechanism of forced dorsiflexion while the knee is extended or forced knee extension while the foot is dorsiflexed is the common cause. In addition, these strains occur in conjunction with muscular fatigue, particularly in the heat, with fluid-electrolyte depletion and muscle cramping followed by an actual tearing of the muscle fibers. Such injuries are sometimes seen in the final stages of a marathon or triathlon. These injuries occur primarily at the musculotendinous junction, between the muscles and the Achilles tendon, or in the medial head of the gastrocnemius muscle. The degree of pain, swelling, stiffness, and later ecchymosis, is a result of the muscle damage to the gastrocnemius or soleus. It was formerly believed that these injuries were strains of the plantaris muscle.

For grades I and II strains, treatment follows the principles of RICE (*r*est, *i*ce, *c*ompression, and *e*levation) and early weight bearing to tolerance during phase I of the healing continuum. At the time of initial injury, icing over a damp elastic wrap for compression with the leg elevated should be instituted. During the first 24 to 72 hours, one should continue to use cold with compression and to keep the limb in elevation. A normal gait pattern is encouraged, with a feathering or partial weight-bearing gait.

These strains need good external support and compression. The loss of the calf circulatory "muscle pump" mechanism often leads to soft tissue edema in the lower limb. The goals are to prevent further irritation of the damaged area and to aid venous and lymphatic fluid return by the use of pain-free movement. The limb should not be allowed to hang dependent any more than necessary, because this position only facilitates more swelling. These goals are met by crutches using a feathering gait (sole of foot just touching the ground for proprioception, not weight bearing), equal-thickness heel lifts (orthopedic felt) in both shoes (to prevent back and pelvic problems) so that in standing the entire sole of the foot can be in contact with the ground, not just the toes, and a compression tape technique to decrease stress on the muscle (Fig. 32–2). As dorsiflexion returns, the height of the heel lifts may be decreased to allow normal active movement during weight bearing.

Active foot and ankle movements can be carried out early within the pain-free range. Crutches should be used until normal gait can be achieved to prevent possible low back, knee, and circulation problems brought on by a faulty gait.

After the first day, ice massage and exercise are begun. The whole lower leg should be iced for 30 to 40 seconds, followed by active exercise for 2 to 5 minutes. The sequence is repeated for five to ten sets. Dorsiflexion against an elastic tube in elevation is used to facilitate relaxation of the gastrocnemius and soleus muscles and to aid in resolving swelling. Standing closed-chain exercises are then initiated. Partial weight-bearing squats and lunges may also be performed. During these movements, a 0.8- to 2-inch (2- to 5-cm) lift may be placed under both heels to keep the complete sole of the foot on the ground. Light plantar flexion exercises against elastic tubing are begun when the athlete is pain-free.

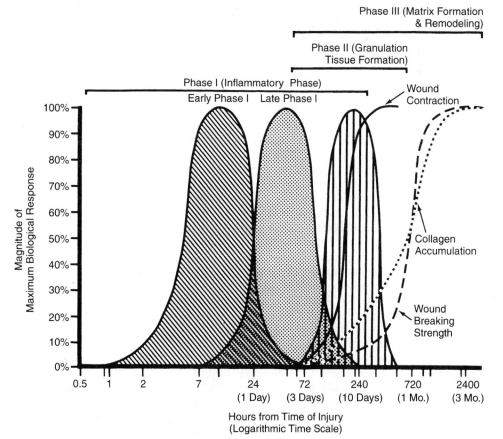

FIGURE 32–1. The three overlapping phases of wound repair. (From Daly TJ: The repair phase of wound healing, re-epithelialization and contraction. *In* Kloth CL, Mc-Culloch JM, Feedar JA (eds): Wound Healing: Alternatives in Management. Philadelphia, FA Davis, 1990, p 15.)

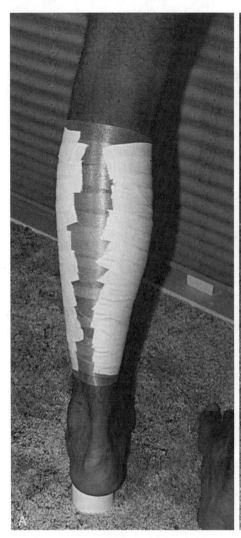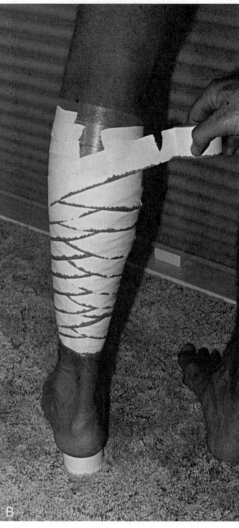

FIGURE 32–2. Calf compression taping technique. *A*, Step 1: Anterior leg taped as anchor. *B*, Step 2: Tape is crisscrossed over calf. Note that the heel is elevated during tape application.

Pulsed ultrasound is introduced after the first 24 hours to stimulate fibroblastic activity and collagen formation.[9] Ultrasound combined with muscle stimulation can be used to put mechanical strain through the tissue while providing a muscle pump for lymphatic and venous drainage.[10] The muscle stimulation frequency is set at 2 to 3 Hz to provide a muscle twitch, not tetanus (Table 32–2). High-voltage galvanic and interferential currents are frequently used to reduce inflammation, decrease pain, and provide some muscle pump action for venous and lymphatic drainage. Roy and Irvin[11] advocated the use of phonophoresis using a 10 percent hydrocortisone cream for the local application of anti-inflammatory medication. We have used other topical anti-inflammatory drugs, such as Myoflex or Flexall (both contain a salicylate), with ultrasound (phonophoresis).

Progression includes reduction in the height of the heel lifts as dorsiflexion range of motion returns, free stationary cycling, leg press, shuttle, heel raise, and eccentric drops (Table 32–3).[12] Massage techniques can be used to encourage the removal of interstitial fluid swelling and edema. We have found ice massage combined with active exercise (cryokinetics) to be of greater benefit than passive massage alone for the

reduction of swelling.[13,14] If the whole foot has been swollen, mobilization of the foot and ankle joints is usually required.[15–17]

Compression taping or elastic bandaging is usually required only for the first 2 to 14 days. In those athletes who begin treatment late—for example, 10 to 14 days after injury—or who are still non–weight bearing, with a dependent swollen limb, tape or tensor (Ace) bandage should be applied from the metatarsal heads to the top of the gastrocnemius muscle. The athlete must start moving the limb and get the sole of the foot on the ground with a partial weight-bearing gait as soon as possible. Ice massage and active exercise reduce the swelling. Resistance to dorsiflexion should be given, as well as unresisted exercise to the plantar flexors. The clinician should always be conscious of the possibility of deep venous thrombosis. If the athlete is fully weight bearing and limping, crutches should still be used to achieve a normal gait. As the initial inflammation and swelling are controlled, an appropriate rehabilitation program and drills may be instituted.

It is essential for the clinician to establish that the muscle-tendon unit is intact and has not been completely ruptured (third-degree strain). The Thompson test is used to determine whether the muscle-tendon unit is intact.[7] The clinician should also obtain the athlete's history. Classically, the athlete states that it felt like someone kicked the Achilles tendon; on further examination, the tendon is shown to be ruptured. For those with third-degree strains, surgical consultation is required. Surgical repair of the Achilles tendon may be open or closed, with open repair having a more predictable outcome.[18] Conservative nonsurgical treatment has been used in some cases but for the active individual, the technique is seldom used, because tendon strength is approximately 30 percent of normal and there is greater chance of rerupture in the nonsurgical group.[18] Postsurgery, the athlete is usually placed in a cast for 6 to 8 weeks, followed by an elevated heel in both shoes for about 1 month, or a functional orthosis is used.[18] Once the surgery is complete, the rehabilitation process follows a similar but delayed process to that seen for first- and second-degree strains. Special care has to be taken not to load stress on the repair too early in the rehabilitation process. Any stretching that is done should be gentle and "lazy." We use these terms to mean that only slight stress to the tissues is being felt by the athlete and the athlete is not pulling or pushing hard into the stretched position. Passive stretching to the healing tissue can be aggravating and should not be carried out until 4 to 6 weeks following severe injuries, and 10 to 14 days following minor strains, in the form of a prolonged (we advocate up to 2 minutes) static stretching.[19] The foot should be kept in a neutral position (no varus or valgus) during stretching, because

TABLE 32–2
Frequency and Clinical Use of Electrical Stimulation

Frequency	Muscle Response	Clinical Use
1–10 Hz	Light muscle twitch	Circulation, movement of both venous and lymphatic fluids; mechanical stress on tissues; education (sensory stimulation and stimulation of mechanoreceptors)
	Strong muscle twitch (almost painful)	Pain relief (acupuncture-like TENS)
30–50 Hz	Tetanus	Muscle education, strengthening and endurance
80–100+ Hz	Sensory*	Pain relief; stimulation of autonomic nervous system

*May also be tetanus but most frequencies in this range have short pulse width and are inefficient for muscle contraction.

TABLE 32–3
Five-Step Eccentric Program

1. *Warm-up:* a generalized exercise such as cycling or light jogging to increase body temperature and increase circulation. This exercise is not intended to load the tendon and should not be uncomfortable.
2. *Flexibility:* athlete performs at least two 30-sec static stretches of the affected muscle-tendon unit involved and its antagonist. More stretching can be done if hypomobility is felt to be a major factor in causing the athlete's symptoms.
3. *Specific exercise:* three sets are performed at the start with a brief rest and sometimes a stretch between each set. The athlete should feel a reproduction of the symptoms after 20 repetitions. If pain is felt earlier, the speed of movement is reduced or the load is decreased; if no pain is experienced, speed or load (not both) is increased. If this is the first exercise session and the initial level of loading is being determined, the intensity of exercise may be increased and the repetitions repeated until the appropriate level of intensity is reached.

   Begin with double heel raises (on both feet) on flat surface. Go up on two, down on one, 8 to 10 reps, three sets. Add 3 to 5 reps daily, working up to 30 reps in each set. Then do 40 doubles (on both feet) up on two, down on one, with 10 singles (on one foot), up and down on the affected side. Every third day, 3 to 10 doubles are taken away and 3 to 10 singles are added. When 50 singles are reached, add a 0.8- to 2-inch (2–5 cm) wedge under the forefoot to start increasing the range of motion. Start at half-reps and progress over a 10- to 14-day period to the previous reps. *Red flags are pain and/or stiffness.* If they occur, a rest day is taken and exercise is cut by 25 percent for the next workout.
4. *Repeat flexibility exercises.*
5. *Apply ice* 10 to 15 minutes to the affected (painful to palpation) area to prevent any inflammatory response provoked by microscopic damage to the tendon that might occur during the exercise.

Modified from Curwin SL: The aetiology and treatment of tendinitis. *In* Harries M, Williams C, Stanish WD, and Micheli LJ (eds): Oxford Textbook of Sports Medicine. New York, Oxford University Press, 1994. By permission of Oxford University Press.

this position keeps the Achilles tendon in a straight alignment and the foot out of overpronation while achieving dorsiflexion.

As range of motion at the ankle returns, strength drills using elastic resistance for all ranges are instituted. The elastic resistance provides easy control over the variables of range, load, type of contraction (concentric or eccentric), sets, and repetitions and allows control of speed and change of direction, which are hard to duplicate using other exercise modalities.

Friction massage followed by active exercise may do more to increase range of motion than passive stretching alone.[16] Deep tissue massage can be effective when combined with active exercise and icing but caution should be observed, because the actual area of injury must be allowed to stabilize before too aggressive a massage program is carried out.

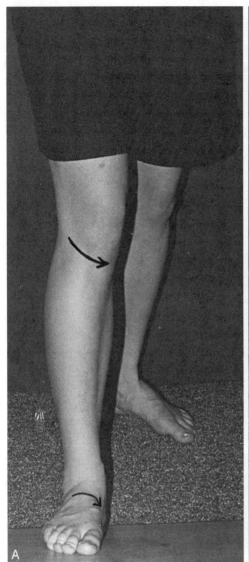
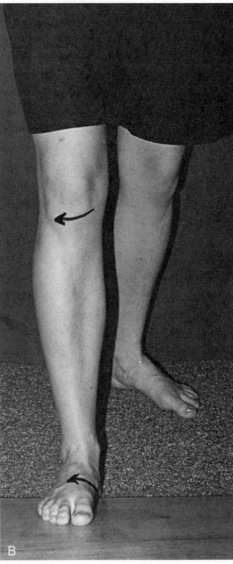

FIGURE 32–3. Foot exercise involving tibial rotation. *A,* Pronation and internal rotation of tibia. *B,* Supination and external rotation of tibia.

The basic premise to remember when rehabilitating the lower limb is that during most sporting activities, the foot functions on the ground (closed chain). The components of some sports (swimming, gymnastics, kick boxing) have elements during which the sole of the foot is not in contact with any surface (open chain). If possible, rehabilitation starts with the sole of the foot in contact with a surface, because better control is offered in closed-chain activities.[20]

The important principle of early closed-chain activities is to begin simply. One does not need a great deal of equipment to start the muscles contracting, to stimulate the circulation, or to retrain the nervous system. Movement at the knee and at all joints of the foot and ankle should be in a pain-free allowable range of motion. Bathroom scales can be used for weight bearing to educate the athlete to the amount of load desired and to achieve equality of weight distribution in standing, squatting, and lunging. Other early closed-chain activities include cycling with no resistance, walking in chest-deep water, and weight transfer while on parallel bars or on crutches. *No limping* should be seen or

allowed. Intrinsic foot exercises are important to control foot dynamics, which in turn controls some of the rotation forces transmitted up the leg (Fig. 32–3).

Proprioceptive training can be stressed early by the use of the BAPS system (Biomechanical Ankle Platform System) or balance board in sitting, supported standing, or free standing. All drills are in an environment that stresses control and progression of stress and strain on connective tissues during the early (inflammatory) phase I into the intermediate (proliferation) phase II, as described by Daly.[21] The effects of joint movement during healing were described as being beneficial, provided the forces are "not too great," and it was further stated that "the general concept at the present time is that very low cyclic loads on a ligament scar will promote scar proliferation and material 'remodeling'...."[21] It is the role of the clinician to control and progress this cyclic loading. Partial weight-bearing, proprioception, and balance exercises can be performed, progressing to full weight bearing with dynamic changes of speed, direction, stops, and starts. Free-standing drills can be done with the use of simple

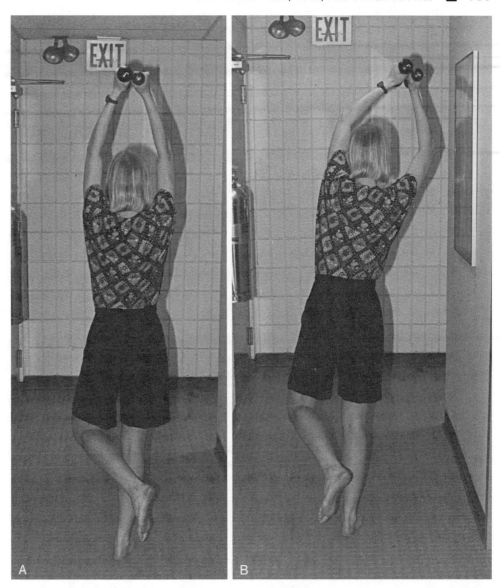

FIGURE 32–4. *A, B,* Using free weights to stress the ankle.

free weights to alter the center of gravity (Fig. 32–4). The weight can be lifted up and away from the body to change the relationship of the body's center of gravity to the base (the feet).

Early open-chain activities can start with active foot and ankle movements through a pain-free range of motion, being careful not to overstretch damaged tissues. The knee and hip may also be included in these movements. All movements can be done in elevation, on the level, or in a dependent position, but the dependent position should only be used with caution because of the adverse circulatory effects of this position. Water is a good medium in which to start early open chain activities. Water provides external support (the Pascal law: the deeper in the water, the greater the external support) and temperature control and allows good control of the speed of movement.[22]

As the athlete improves, more vigorous open and closed-chain activities can be instituted. These activities must be controlled so that the injured structures are not overloaded and chances of reinjury are kept to a minimum. Closed-chain activities include balance activities on a balance board, rebounder, or the BAPS system. Combined open- and closed-chain activities include skipping, hopping, jogging, retrorunning (backward running), and running drills (e.g., figure-eights, cutting drills).

The requirements of activities of daily living (ADL), training, and performance should be broken down to ensure specificity related to the athlete's sport. The rehabilitation program must be designed to progress through these requirements and the time continuum of healing. When the injury has specific limitations—for example, the use of a brace—the progression can be modified. Progression through the lower limb late stage rehabilitation program usually begins at about 6 to 8 weeks postinjury. In severe cases, it takes up to 12 weeks to fully rehabilitate.

If athletes are in a seasonal sport, they should be warned that before the next season they should prepare and train early to prevent recurrence of injury to the same side. In some cases, the opposite side is subse-

TABLE 32–4
Various Sports and Their Predominant Energy System(s)*

Sports and Sport Activity	ATP-PC and LA	LA-O₂	O₂
Baseball	80	20	—
Basketball	85	15	—
Fencing	90	10	—
Field hockey	60	20	20
Football	90	10	—
Golf	95	5	—
Gymnastics	90	10	—
Ice hockey			
Forward, defense	80	20	—
Goalie	95	5	—
Lacrosse			
Goalie, defense, attack men	80	20	—
Midfielder, man-down	60	20	20
Rowing	20	30	50
Skiing			
Slalom, jumping, downhill	80	20	—
Cross-country	—	5	95
Pleasure skiing	34	33	33
Soccer			
Goalie, wings, strikers	80	20	—
Halfbacks, or link men	60	20	20
Swimming and diving			
50 yards, diving	98	2	—
100 yards	80	15	5
200 yards	30	65	5
400, 500 yards	20	40	40
1500, 1650 yards	10	20	70
Tennis	70	20	10
Track and field			
100, 200 yards	98	2	—
Field events	90	10	—
440 yards	80	15	5
880 yards	30	65	5
1 mile	20	55	25
2 miles	20	40	40
3 miles	10	20	70
6 miles (cross-country)	5	15	80
Marathon	—	5	95
Volleyball	90	10	—
Wrestling	90	10	—

ATP, Adenosine triphosphate; PC, phosphocreatine; LA, lactic acid.
From Fox EL, Mathews DK: Interval Training. Toronto, WB Saunders, 1974, p 184.
*As a percentage.

quently injured. The authors have often seen the same athlete presenting with the same injury, in the same month, 1 year later.

The mix of power, strength, and endurance for athletes is dictated by their sport. Anaerobic and aerobic energy systems have to be stressed according to the requirements of the sport. Fox and Mathews[23] have broken sports down according to the energy system predominance required for each sport (Table 32–4). This table can be used as a guide for the mix of activities given in the final stage of rehabilitation.

Which tissues are damaged? What is required to protect them? What treatment facilitates healing and allows return to full function? The choices clinicians make to answer these questions must complement the time continuum of healing. This continuum (see Fig. 32–1) is broken into three phases, with each phase overlapping the other. There is no clear consensus as to when the third phase ends, but it may take up to 2 years.

TENDINITIS

Tendinitis in the lower leg is brought on by many common factors but treatment may differ due to the different anatomic causes of the problem. Most of the tendons in the lower limb have a synovial sheath surrounding the tendon. The Achilles tendon, however, has a peritendon sheath, which is not synovial. Common sites, causative factors, and signs and symptoms of tendinitis in the lower leg, ankle, and foot are summarized in Table 32–5. Poor-fitting footwear can often cause compression over the affected tendon. This is often the case in skaters, in whom the skate is fit so tight that the athlete usually has thickening and swelling over the extensor retinaculum. This injury is sometimes referred to as "skate bite."

Other tendinitis problems around the ankle are due to overuse, faulty foot mechanics, or trauma. The most likely cause is a combination of all these factors. In the case of tendinitis caused by overuse, the treatment consists of alteration of the athlete's training program and local treatment for inflammation. Poor foot mechanics require proper assessment and possibly the use of a foot orthosis.

Achilles tendon injuries are common in sports and are the most common tendinitis in the lower leg, ankle, and foot region. These injuries range from peritendinitis, tendinosis with degenerative changes, and insertional lesions often associated with bursitis to partial and complete ruptures. Achilles tendon inflammation is also seen with gout and some seronegative arthropathies (ankylosing spondylitis, ulcerative colitis, Crohn disease). The Achilles tendon, the common tendon of the gastrocnemius and soleus muscles, inserts into the calcaneus, adjacent to which are a superficial and retrocalcaneal bursa. The tendon itself has an area of relative avascularity about 0.8 inch (2 cm) above its insertion, which is the site of most torque on the tendon. This is the area of partial tears with secondary nodule formation and degenerative cysts seen in tendinosis.

Common symptoms of Achilles tendinitis include preactivity and morning stiffness, pain on stretch, pain under load such as going up onto the toes ("en pointe") with dancers, and pain with running. Clinical examination can reveal signs of local tenderness; muscle soreness and tenderness (often overlooked); crepitus; local nodules either within the tendon, which moves during dorsiflexion and plantar flexion, or within the peritendon, which does not move during these movements; limited dorsiflexion due to gastrocnemius-soleus spasm; or tendon adhesions. There is often limited power and, if chronic, there may be wasting of the calf muscles.

Investigation should include an x-ray for calcific tendon changes and insertional spurs, and ultrasonography for nodules or degenerative cysts. In persistent cases, arthritic blood screening should be carried out for rheumatologic conditions, possibly HLA-B27 for ankylosing spondylitis, and other seronegative arthropathies, if appropriate.

Treatment for the peritendinitis and bursitis with insertional injuries is conservative for the majority of cases. Some chronic adhesive peritendinitis may require tenolysis, which would remove the athlete from competition for 6 to 12 weeks. Conservative treatment in early conditions is best begun by taking a careful history and doing a lower leg examination to determine the cause, which may be overuse or a mechanical problem. If overuse is the cause, alterations in the training cycle to allow for rest and recovery are all the treatment required if the condition is caught early. If mechanical

problems do exist, they must be corrected before recovery can occur.

The clinician should check lower limb alignment, looking for a short leg or a pelvic rotation, which may be putting unequal stress through the Achilles tendons. This is often seen in feet in which one foot is in pronation and the opposite foot is in relative (or complete) supination. A similar relationship occurs when an athlete runs on roads or sidewalks with a camber.

It is important to check *all* footwear including everyday shoes that have been worn prior to the onset of symptoms (see later, Footwear Considerations). This can be informative and educational for the athlete about the reason for the problem. The clinician should watch for soft heel counters that do not provide adequate side wall support. An example is golf shoes, in which support is needed for side motion as well as for the constant change in terrain. Cleated shoes, because of their lack of heels, can allow the heel to drop lower than the forefoot on grass fields and put overstretch on the

---

TABLE 32–5
Tendinitis in the Lower Leg, Ankle, and Foot

Common Sites	Common Causative Factors	Signs and Symptoms

Achilles tendon just above its insertion into the calcaneus
Tibialis posterior just behind the medial malleolus
Tibialis anterior on the dorsum of the foot just under the extensor retinaculum
Peroneal tendon behind the lateral malleolus and at the insertion into the base of the fifth metatarsal
	Faulty foot mechanics producing friction and compression between the tendon, sheath, and underlying bony structure *or* causing compression of the tendon against the shoe
	Poor footwear that creates poor mechanics or is not fit properly (see Footwear Considerations)
	Training errors that include:
	  Intensity too high, with poor work:rest ratio
	  Muscle fatigue leading to mechanical breakdown of foot function
	  Poor training surface (dirty gym floor), sudden change from soft to hard or hard to soft (road camber change when running)
	  Sudden changes in program such as adding hills, sprints, or distance
	  Returning or progressing too quickly following an illness
	  Poor flexibility in the gastocnemius soleus muscles, which increases twist and whipping action of Achilles tendon because foot must increase pronation to increase dorsiflexion of the ankle joint in weight-bearing position; this in turn can produce chronic overstretching of Achilles tendon and result in microtears of tendon
	Trauma (direct blow)
	Infection from an overlying cut or a penetrating wound into the tendon
		Pain with active movement, aggravated in weight bearing
		Pain on passive stretching
		Localized tenderness
		Possible swelling and/or thickening in the tendon and peritendon tissues
		May have "snowball crepitus"
		Morning stiffness at site of lesion; this also occurs following any period of inactivity during the day when the part is not moved for 15–20 minutes or longer

gastrocnemius-soleus complex. When combined with poor side wall support, the Achilles muscle-tendon complex is put on stretch, with twisting of the tendon during weight bearing as the foot pronates. The increased pronation causes increased torque to the tendon. As the heels of shoes wear, they create a greater angle of calcaneal adduction at heel strike, which increases the forces needed to control the foot as it moves from heel strike to foot flat during the gait cycle (see Chapter 18, Biomechanics of Running). If the medial heel counter is not strong enough, the shoe breaks down and allows the foot to overpronate. It must be re-emphasized that all shoes worn need to be checked daily. If broken down, they do not allow the injured area to recover between activities. The everyday shoe can have the same poor qualities and structural breakdowns as athletic shoes, and thus cause low-grade repetitive stress on the Achilles tendon. Because of this, the tissues are never allowed to recover and usually enter the next exercise bout with a lower tolerance level.

The process of healing can be divided into three phases. Phase I is referred to as the inflammatory stage, phase II as the proliferation or fibroblastic stage, and phase III as the remodeling or maturation stage. Graded exercise in each of these stages is used to generate a different tissue response. The use of exercise as a strong stimulus in the healing of ligament and tendon is supported by Frank (Chapter 2) and Curwin (Chapter 3).

Early stage exercise is used to improve circulation and promote the removal of waste products, prevent disuse atrophy of surrounding musculature, maintain as much normal range of motion as possible without causing further damage, and stimulate fibroblastic activity.

Improving circulation includes both the vascular and the lymphatic systems for removing inflammatory exudate, providing nutrition, and aiding in fluid removal from the soft tissues. Removal of inflammatory byproducts assists in pain control. Controlling pain helps by preventing or minimizing the loss of motor control, coordination, and proprioception and allows the injured athlete to participate actively in early exercise rehabilitation and return to function sooner.

Phase I and early phase II exercises are not overly strenuous and are within pain tolerance. For lower limb injuries, they may be done in elevation to aid circulatory return. Early graded stress loads to the injured tissues help stimulate collagen fiber formation in functional planes. Rehabilitation exercises start with a combination of ice massage, active dorsiflexion using an elastic tube for resistance, gentle stretching of the calf, and eccentric calf exercise (Table 32–3). Appropriate temporary heel lifts made from high-density foam or orthopedic felt need to be added to both street and athletic shoes to decrease stress on the tendon. Their height can be reduced as pain-free range of motion improves.

During the intermediate phase II, exercises progress from gentle active range of motion in early phase II to muscle strengthening, power development, and cardiovascular, as well as muscle endurance, and more complicated neuromuscular control programs in the late stage of phase II. The dorsiflexion movements are done quickly to stimulate the anterior muscle groups working to control the foot and the eccentric activity of the dorsiflexors during that portion of the gait, from heel strike to midstance. The clinician must set all parameters for progression throughout phase II of healing. Range of motion should be controlled and limited to those ranges that allow free resisted movement without irritation to the damaged structures. Strengthening should be carried out, keeping in mind appropriate control of range, repetitions, sets, type of contraction, and speed of movement. Weight-bearing drills should be controlled by direction of movement, acceleration, and deceleration. The need for protective devices is usually required at this stage. Proprioceptive drills are important through all three phases of healing to ensure proper control of the joints during activity.

Phase III involves maturation of the collagen (scar) fibers. Progressive stress can be applied to the tissues so that the collagen tissue forms in the appropriate areas and along lines of stress.[24] The collagen strengthens and remodels as the weak hydrogen bonds that link collagen fibers in immature collagen become strong covalent bonds, linking the collagen fibers in mature scar.[25] Aggressive stretching and active resisted movements should not begin until pain and swelling have disappeared. Active movements within the pain-free range are encouraged. Heat may be used prior to exercise after the initial inflammation has resolved.

Cryotherapy techniques are widely used for all stages of rehabilitation. The most common response is to apply ice (cold) immediately after the injury to help control the hemorrhaging and thus control soft tissue swelling. This decreased swelling is thought to be brought on by the decrease in metabolic demands of the cooled tissues and the vasoconstriction of arterioles due to the cooling.[14] Application is recommended for 10 to 20 minutes, repeated every 2 hours for the first 72 hours. It is our experience that unless the venous and lymphatic systems are functioning near normal in the damaged tissues, it is best to stay with cooling modalities or a combination of heat and cold (contrast techniques) until the injury is well into the late stages of phase II. There is no evidence to demonstrate whether cold has a positive or negative effect on the healing of tissues, although it has been shown to decrease stress on tissue by decreasing swelling, decreasing pain, and lowering metabolism.[14] Cooling of nerve tissue has an analgesic effect and can be used to allow early pain control and thus early protected movement. Cold packs should be applied after exercise in phase I and early phase II of the healing continuum. Knight[14] has recommended 30 minutes of ice application after exercise. The use of cryokinetics (ice and exercise) as advocated by Knight[14] is also effective. We recommend this combination of ice and exercise as the most effective treatment modality during the rehabilitation stage. Ice massage can also be effective in the cooling of superficial sensory receptors and stimulation of circulation when combined with active exercise. We have found ice massage to be the most effective method to combine with exercise in chronic conditions. It is simple to use and the athlete can carry out the procedure at home with relative ease.

It should be kept in mind that it does not have to be ice but rather a cold medium that is applied. Cold water can often be just as effective as an ice bag. Nerve conduction decreases with cooling. Sensitivity of the skin receptors is decreased, so they are only one sixth as sensitive at 68° F (20°C) as they are at 95°F (35°C). At 41°F (5°C), they do not react to pressure and touch. Muscle spindles show an increased sensitivity to a slight lowering of temperature, but the sensitivity decreases as tissue temperature drops. At 80.6°F (27°C), some authors have reported a 50 percent decrease in reaction and a complete nerve block at 46 to 50° F (8 to 10°C).[26,27] These characteristics can be used to decrease pain and metabolic function in the early stages of an injury with the use of cool (77°F; 25°C) to cold (41°F; 5°C) water. Cold whirlpools can be an effective means of cold application. The water supports the tissues by displacement and also by compression (hydrostatic pressure) to offset some of the problems associated with a dependent limb. The deeper the submersion of the limb, the greater the hydrostatic pressure.[22] If there is concern about the possibility of increased swelling, the limb can be wrapped with a compression bandage before the limb is submerged in a cool whirlpool. The athlete can and should perform active movements within the pain-free range while the limb is suspended in the water.

Physical modalities can be used to reduce local inflammation and promote tissue healing. These include ultrasound, high-voltage galvanic currents, low-frequency electrical stimulation, interferential currents, and laser energy. Modalities that use electrical currents can be divided into those using direct currents and those using alternating currents.

Kloth and Feedar[28] summarized the use of electrical modalities and four waveform characteristics as needing controlled clinical research for the augmentation of soft tissue repair. The use of transcutaneous electrical nerve stimulation (TENS) for pain relief has been documented.[29] TENS should only be used in athletics in conjunction with an overall treatment approach. It is not to be used for the sole purpose of relieving pain and allowing the athlete to participate when tissues are not protected or healed.

The use of electrical muscle stimulation (EMS) for the production of muscle contraction is widely recommended and used in the field of sports therapy.[11,30,31] It is our opinion that it has a positive and useful clinical role in rehabilitation. It is used for re-education, to turn the muscle "on" following injury, to decrease soft tissue swelling, to strengthen, and to provide proprioceptive input, which are achieved by manipulation of the frequency (see Table 32–2). Dunlop[32] used MRI spectroscopy to demonstrate the use of EMS to produce intracellular changes similar to those found in voluntary muscle contractions. The clinical use of EMS tends to support these findings, but more research needs to be done.

Some studies have indicated an increase in fibroblastic activity with the use of ultrasound.[33,34] It is believed that the mechanical movement produced by the compression and rarefaction waveform stimulates collagen tissue synthesis and formation.

Curwin[12] and Dyson and colleagues[9] have reviewed ultrasound and its effects on tissue healing. They indicated that ultrasound used during the inflammatory phase and in the early proliferative phase can be beneficial. There is strong evidence to support that ultrasound can accelerate the resolution of inflammation and early advancement into the proliferation phase. Its use in the later phases of proliferation and the remodeling phase does not seem to be as beneficial.[9]

Low-energy laser irradiation is the newest of the modalities to be used by sports therapists. Early basic science and clinical trials indicate a positive response of healing tissues, especially for superficial wounds.[35,36] One of the authors has used both visible (HeNe) and infrared (GaAs) lasers clinically for 11 years and found them subjectively to be useful in pain relief, wound healing, and reduction of inflammation for ligament and tendon injuries.

Temporary relief of the pain often seen in tendinitis can sometimes be sustained by using adhesive felt strips lying in parallel with and adjacent to the tendons involved. The felt strips hold the footwear away from the tendon and transfer the forces over a larger area.

Topical anti-inflammatory drugs (5 percent ketoprofen, diclofenac, or indomethacin), transverse frictions followed by passive movements, and rest for 24 to 36 hours are also sometimes used to help break the inflammatory cycle.[21] Deep tissue massage to the gastrocnemius-soleus muscles relaxes the muscles and decreases stress to the Achilles tendon. Taping of the foot may also be used for protection.

Activities must be modified, and a time line of healing and expectations should be given to the athlete. For those rare individuals who see the clinician within days of the onset of symptoms, the condition can resolve in 10 to 14 days. For those athletes who show up after many months of symptoms, the same rehabilitation program is started but progress is slower. The tissue has thickened and organized and takes more time to remodel. Athletes presenting later can usually expect to take at least as long to recover as they have had the symptoms and, if there is tissue thickening around the tendon, it may take as long as 2 years for full resolution and recovery. These patients may also need a walking cast or Aircast to protect the Achilles tendon from the constant stresses applied during gait. The advantage of an Aircast is that it can be removed for exercise, icing, and local modalities. To maintain cardiovascular fitness, pool running is recommended. The same exercise program is followed but the time between progressions is longer and the slope of progression is gradual. It is important that attention be given to a total bilateral lower limb rehabilitation program. Proprioception is poor and the musculature of the upper leg and hip has wasted in some cases.

Similarly, tendinitis in athletes has also been seen in the peronei, tibialis posterior, and tibialis anterior, especially due to inequality of reciprocal muscle strength and in the presence of a cavus or planus foot or instability at the ankle.[37] Treatment of these tendon injuries follows a similar protocol as that used for Achilles tendinitis.

MEDIAL TIBIAL STRESS SYNDROME

Medial tibial stress syndrome (shin splints), a common overuse syndrome, is a periostitis that usually occurs at the posteromedial border of the tibia. The differentiation between this condition (Table 32–6) and a stress fracture is confirmed by a bone scan.[38,39] The mechanism of injury and the early symptoms are the same as those seen in tibial stress fractures. If the tibial stress syndrome is not treated early, it most likely will progress to a stress fracture. Periostitis is believed by many to be the result of traction of the deep medial compartment muscles or soleus on the fascial attachment to the medial tibial border.[40] There is a history of excessive weight bearing, such as jumping, running, or standing for prolonged periods, in combination with improper footwear for the athlete. There is often an associated varus alignment of the lower extremity, with excessive foot pronation. There is diffuse tenderness over the medial border of the tibia and often along the tendon of the tibialis posterior or soleus.[41]

Management should be aimed at reduction of local inflammation with icing and should include therapy modalities such as ultrasound, phonophoresis (lidocaine), iontophoresis (lidocaine), and anti-inflammatory medication.[42] Strength and flexibility exercises for the posterior and deep medial musculature are critical. Control of excessive pronation by motion control shoes (straight-lasted) and orthotics are impor-

tant. Curved lasted shoes with good shock-absorbing qualities are required for athletes with a more rigid foot (pes cavus) and excessive supination. As indicated earlier with stress fractures, an Aircast is often effective in reducing symptoms and controlling pain. The method by which this works is not clear. In chronic cases, surgical release of the fascia or periosteal stripping may be required.[40]

COMPARTMENT SYNDROMES

One should always be aware of a chronic compartment syndrome in the lower extremity in athletes, especially those in endurance sports. The lower leg is usually divided into four discrete compartments (anterior compartment, lateral or peroneal compartment, superficial calf compartment containing soleus and gastrocnemius, and deep calf compartment containing the flexors). Some authors add a fifth compartment containing the tibialis posterior muscle as an occasional separate unit within the deep calf compartment.[43,44] Each compartment contains muscles plus a neurovascular bundle. Compartment syndromes due to muscle hypertrophy have also been reported in the foot of active individuals.[45]

The most common form of compartment syndrome seen in athletics is the chronic rather than the acute syndrome. The acute syndrome with a fracture is seen

TABLE 32–6
Differential Diagnosis of Lower Leg Compartment Syndrome

	Compartment Syndrome	Shin Splints	Stress Fracture	Tumor
Pain (type)	Severe cramping, diffuse pain, and tightness	Diffuse along medial two thirds of tibial border	Deep, nagging, localized with minimal radiation	Deep, nagging (bone) with some radiation
Pain with rest	Decreases or disappears	Decreases or disappears	Present, especially night pain	Present, often night pain
Pain with activity	Increases	Increases	Present (may increase)	Present
Pain with warm-up	May increase or become present	May disappear	Unaltered	Unaltered
Range of motion	Limited in acute phase	Limited	Normal	Normal
Onset	Gradual to sudden	Gradual	Gradual	?
Altered sensation	Sometimes	No	No	Sometimes
Muscle weakness or paralysis	Maybe	No	No	Not usually
Stretching	Increases pain	Increases pain	Minimal pain alteration	No increase in pain
X-ray	Normal	Normal	Early, negative; late, positive (?)	Usually positive
Bone scan	Negative	Periosteal uptake	Positive	Positive
Pulse	Affected sometimes	Normal	Normal	Normal
Palpation	Tender, tight compartment	Diffuse tenderness	Point tenderness	Point or diffuse tenderness
Cause	Muscle expansion	Overuse	Overuse	?
Duration, recovery	None without surgery	None without rest	Up to 3 months	None without treatment

From Magee DJ: Sports Physiotherapy. Edmonton, Alberta, University of Alberta, 1988.

when a rapid compartment volume increase occurs due to the arterial bleeding associated with the fracture. In this situation, immediate fasciotomy is required. For the chronic type, the volume of the exercising muscle may increase by as much as 20 percent, which is the result of an increase in blood volume as well as an increase in transcapillary filtration of intravascular fluid.[46] Venous and lymphatic return is unable to keep up with the resultant increase in volume within the compartment space. Because the fascial sheath cannot stretch to accommodate this increase in volume, typical compartment signs and symptoms begin to occur. The athlete complains of compartment tightness, which occurs during or after exercise and is often more intense the next day (the "second day" phenomenon). There is associated swelling of the affected compartment and, rarely, a sensation of weakness of the compartment muscles. The anterior compartment is most commonly affected with paresthesia over the dorsum of the foot, classically the first web space (deep peroneal nerve), and weakness of the tibialis anterior, extensor digitorum longus, or extensor hallucis longus muscles.

The gradual onset of the compartment tightness with exercise is usually associated with a training error such as a sudden increase in training volume, intensity, or running downhill. In addition, there may have been a switch to running on harder surfaces or a change in footwear, especially in cases in which the heel is higher than the forefoot. Commonly, there may be an associated biomechanical foot abnormality such as pes planus with excessive pronation or, at the other extreme, a rigid pes cavus with tight gastrocnemius and soleus muscles.

The differential diagnosis (see Table 32–6) for a chronic compartment syndrome includes stress fractures, periostitis (shin splints), and tumors, particularly when considering the deep calf compartment syndrome. The clinician must also consider peripheral vascular disease or popliteal artery entrapment when assessing recurrent gastrocnemius-soleus tightness in the superficial calf compartment. Diagnosis of the chronic compartment syndrome involves measurement of the specific intracompartmental pressures during rest, exercise, and recovery, remembering that one or all of the compartments may be involved. Resting pressures are usually about 5 to 10 mm Hg. With exercise, pressures rise to between 20 and 30 mm Hg and remain high after exercise (20 mm Hg or greater after 5 minutes).[46,47] In some well-documented cases, typical signs and symptoms have occurred within what would be considered normal exercise pressures (i.e., under 30 mm Hg).[48,49]

Treatment for chronic compartment syndrome involves both operative and conservative measures. Fasciotomy is the most definitive operative treatment, but in some cases the condition resolves with a reduction in training volume or intensity, with a slow graduated return to training. In addition, icing, stretching (Fig. 32–5), and strengthening programs (e.g., tubing exercises or drills) are used, plus more appropriate footwear with orthotics or heel lifts to unload a tight gastrocnemius-soleus complex. Exercises for stretching and strengthening are more likely to succeed in those

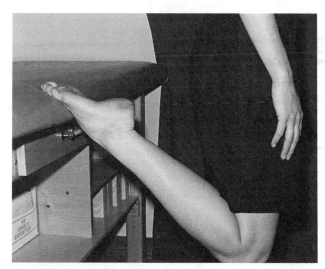

FIGURE 32–5. Stretching of the anterior compartment of the leg.

individuals who have had only one or two acute onsets due to poor conditioning. If the onset is slow and results from long periods of overtraining, the athlete must be encouraged to modify the training load. There must be increased emphasis on icing and stretching, combined with alteration of the training program. Training on softer surfaces with a graduated return to training on roads or synthetic surfaces is encouraged. If these conservative measures fail to resolve the compartment tightness, a fasciotomy is required. This surgery is now done as an outpatient procedure, with return to running in approximately 3 weeks. The results are usually good unless there have been ischemic changes and scarring of the muscles during a prolonged period of intense training with a chronic compartment syndrome. We have seen a few cases of recurrence with scarring over the fascia, but this was significantly reduced with early return to stretching exercises and early introduction of cycling and swimming during wound healing.

FRACTURES AND DISLOCATIONS

The tibia is the most common site for a stress fracture in the lower extremity. Matheson and coworkers[50] have shown that over 50 percent of stress fractures in athletes are in the leg and are usually seen in running and jumping athletes. Stress fractures are thought to represent an overuse failure of the bone along a continuum of failed adaptation, from accelerated osteoclastic remodeling to a complete fracture. Bone remodels in response to repetitive subthreshold stress, particularly in the face of muscle fatigue, which reduces the dampening effect of muscle activity to repetitive ground reactive forces in running or jumping. Stress fractures also occur at sites of repetitive muscle pull, such as at the insertion of the plantar fascia to the calcaneus or the soleus attachment to the medial border of the tibia, which initiates tibial periostitis and often leads to a stress fracture. Stress fractures are also seen in weakened bones, as in the female runner with secondary amenorrhea and resultant osteoporosis. The differential diagnosis for a stress fracture is included in Table 32–6. For the clinician, a red flag is raised by the athlete who complains of night pain or if a tender area is sensitive to ultrasound as the sound head is passed over it, which often causes a localized, acute, and sharp (spike) pain.

The history of a tibial stress fracture follows a usual pattern of pain. It occurs at first only after activity but, as the stress of weight-bearing activity continues, the pain is more intense after exercise and takes longer to resolve with rest periods. With repetitive stress, the pain then occurs during the activity and is only partially resolved with rest. Night pain along with pain at rest is most common. Eventually, the pain is always present and becomes intense with hopping or running. There is more and more local tenderness on palpation, often with local swelling, and eventually a callus can be felt. There is localized pain on hopping, with limited power to hop, and often disuse atrophy, with tibialis anterior or posterior weakness.

The diagnosis early in the history of development of the tibial stress injury is best done by bone scan with late callus formation and periosteal reaction seen with normal x-rays. Intense uptake on bone scan should be followed by CT scan or MRI to exclude the possibility of a complete fracture. This is particularly important with navicular stress fractures, femoral neck stress fractures, or anterior medial shaft tibial stress fractures.

Treatment for the uncomplicated stress fractures involves modified rest with non–weight bearing, pool running, swimming, or cycling until there is pain-free hopping. A graduated walk-run program is then initiated. The whole lower extremity needs to be retrained and rehabilitated due to the disuse atrophy that will have occurred. Appropriate footwear with better motion control and/or shock absorption needs to be considered. Tibial stress fractures are seen most commonly with excessive foot pronation and resultant internal tibial rotation (see Chapter 18). Orthotics may be required. Research has shown that early tibial stress injuries can be appropriately managed with an Aircast ankle brace.[51] Persistent cases can be resolved with electromagnetic bone stimulation.[52] The average tibial stress fracture resolves over an 8- to 12-week course.[50]

Matheson and associates[50] have shown that up to one third of stress fractures seen in runners occurs in the feet. The most significant of these involve the navicular, second or third metatarsal (March fracture), and the proximal shaft of the fifth metatarsal (Jones fracture).[53] These fractures are of concern, because they can lead to nonunion and complicated fractures and are difficult to protect and stabilize. Navicular stress fractures are commonly seen with excessive foot pronation, whereas fifth metatarsal stress fractures are seen with the more rigid pes cavus foot (Table 32–7).[54] Metatarsal stress fractures occur most frequently to the second and third metatarsals and are common in running and jumping sports. Common causative factors, as initially proposed by James and colleagues,[55] include training errors, changes in exposure to different surfaces, strength-flexibility dysfunction, poor

TABLE 32–7	
Common Injuries Associated with Foot Type	
Cavus (High Arch, Rigid) Foot	**Pes Planus (Flat Foot, Mobile)**
Plantar fasciitis	Tibialis posterior tendinitis
Metatarsalgia	Achilles tendinitis
Metatarsal and tarsal stress fractures	Plantar fasciitis
Peroneal tendinitis	Sesamoid disorders
Sesamoid disorders	Tibial stress syndrome
Iliotibial band friction syndrome	Patellofemoral pain

Modified from McKenzie DC, Clement DB, Taunton JE: Running shoes, orthotics and injuries. Sports Med 2:334–344, 1985.

shoes, and biomechanical variants such as excessive rearfoot and forefoot varus. Chrichton and associates[43] have noted that the second metatarsal is the most prone to stress fracture because the base of the second metatarsal extends proximally into the distal row of tarsal bones and is held rigid and stable by the bony architecture and ligament support. In addition, if the second metatarsal is longer than the first, as seen with the Morton-type foot, it is theoretically subject to greater bone stress. In addition, the second and third metatarsals are subjected to more stress in the hypermobile forefoot associated with excessive foot pronation. These stress fractures do well with modified rest and non–weight-bearing exercise (e.g., cycling, swimming, running in water) to maintain the athlete's cardiovascular fitness for 4 to 6 weeks and with a graduated return to running and jumping sports with supportive footwear and orthotics.

As with many stress fractures, the initial x-rays are often normal. A bone scan is frequently required for diagnosis. Stress fractures of the proximal shaft of the fifth metatarsal and the navicular often require more aggressive investigation and treatment. Because of their history of poor blood supply and delayed healing, CT scans are required to rule out a progression to a complete fracture. Both these fractures require aggressive treatment—not modified rest with non–weight-bearing exercise—but treatment in non–weight-bearing below-knee casts for 8 weeks for nondisplaced fractures. With cases of delayed union, nonunion, or especially displaced fractures, both the Jones and navicular fractures require internal fixation, with or without bone grafting. For delayed fractures, prior to surgery, we have found promising results with 6 to 8 weeks of electromagnetic bone stimulation. Again, as with other overuse foot injuries, appropriate sport shoes that match the foot type (Table 32–8), with adequate stability and shock absorption, are essential when returning the athlete to sport. Attention must also be given to foot control through the use of orthotics.

Rehabilitation efforts for stress fractures revolve around determining the cause and alleviating those that have led to the problem. Training errors such as overloading with inappropriate rest cycles, progression occurring too fast (often seen following an illness or break in the training cycle), and broken down or improper footwear are frequent causes.

A number of modalities are used for the local treatment of pain and inflammation, including high-voltage galvanic stimulation, interferential currents, laser, muscle stimulation, and ultrasound. There have been no good clinical trials to support the use of these modalities, but clinically, we have found that the use of visible red lasers and muscle stimulation (low-frequency twitch) for the reduction of pain are effective.

The main factor to control in stress fractures is weight bearing. Running and jumping activities should be substituted by cycling and pool running. Ice massage, stretching, and strengthening exercises for the foot and lower leg should be carried out in both open and closed chain positions. Low Dye taping of the foot during the early stage of rehabilitation helps support the strained tissues and serves as a clinical assessment to determine whether an orthotic can be of assistance.

Complete fractures of the tibia and fibula may also occur in sports because of the high torque and compression loads often placed on these bones. A typical example is the "boot top" fracture seen in skiing, in which a high torque load is placed on the lower leg. Because the foot and ankle are encased in a rigid boot, the fracture occurs at the top of the boot. The fracture is usually due to a rotation force and is often open because the tibia lies so close to the skin surface. The result is usually a spiral fracture. If the fibula is fractured above the level of the ankle joint, and was not caused by a direct blow to the fibula, it must be assumed that the tibiofibular ligaments have been torn and that the integrity and stability of the ankle mortise have been lost, until proven otherwise. This loss may require surgical correction and definitely prolongs the rehabilitation period.

Fractures of the ankle or malleoli of the tibia and fibula are also common in sports, and the clinician must always be wary of diagnosing an ankle sprain when it is actually a fracture. Immediate swelling is indicative of blood, and the examiner should be highly suspicious of a malleolar fracture. There are several ways these fractures can occur, and the mechanism of injury is similar to that seen for ankle sprains. With an inversion injury, if the talus does not "roll over" the medial malleolus, the malleolus fractures. Such a fracture is often accompanied by a sprain of the lateral ligaments of the ankle. Because the lateral malleolus extends as far as the distal aspect of the talus, a fracture of the lateral malleolus is often more likely to occur than a sprain if an eversion force is applied to the ankle. If the lateral malleolus fractures, however, there again may be an accompanying sprain to the deltoid ligaments. This is an important point for the clinician to consider because, when following the healing of the malleolus, it is often the injured ligaments that prolong the rehabilitation period. Rehabilitation following fracture to the lower leg, ankle, and foot follows the same format as for an ankle sprain.

Osteochondral fractures are sometimes seen in the talus. These fractures are also referred to as transchondral or dome fractures of the talus. They may be undisplaced (40 percent) or compressed (7 percent). These fractures should be managed with rest and protection until the fracture has healed. In about 25 percent of cases, there is a partial fragment, and this is cast to provide protection and rest. Displaced osteochondral fractures are seen in about 28 percent of cases, and surgery is required to remove the fragment. In other cases, if the fragment has not healed within a year, surgery may be considered to remove the fragment.[56]

Dislocations in the lower leg, ankle, and foot are rare due to the bony and ligamentous arrangements. When they occur, they are usually seen in conjunction with fractures. In some individuals, either due to trauma or weakness of the peroneal retinaculum, the peroneal tendons (brevis and longus) may sublux from their path behind the lateral malleolus, with associated stretching or tearing of the retinaculum.[37,57] In some individuals, appropriate rest restores the tendons to their usual location. In most athletes, however, surgical correction is recommended.[58]

ANKLE SPRAINS

Ankle sprains are one of the most common injuries seen in sports. Sprains to the ankle involve the lateral side more frequently than the medial side.[59] One should always be aware that because of the shape and structure of the ankle mortise, some lateral ligament sprains may have a fracture of some type associated with them. The opposite is true with eversion ankle injuries. It takes much more force to produce an eversion injury, and these sprains often have a fracture associated with them. A suspicion of a possible growth plate injury at the distal end of the fibula should always be considered in young children who sustain a lateral ankle injury. The ligaments in prepubescent children are stronger than the growth plate, so a growth plate fracture is likely to occur before the ligaments tear. In addition, the

TABLE 32–8 Features to Look for in a Running Shoe According to Foot Type	
Cavus (High Arch, Rigid) Foot	**Pes Planus (Flat Foot, Mobile)**
Curved last	Straight last
Slip last	Board last
Softer EVA	Motion control heel counter
Air sole	Additional medial support
Narrow flare	Wider flare
	Higher density EVA on medial side
Modifications	
Neoprene sole	Increased medial wedging on insole
Sorbothane insole	
Askton and Zekon insole	Soft orthotic
Soft orthotic	Semirigid orthotic

Modified from McKenzie DC, Clement DB, Taunton JE: Running shoes, orthotics and injuries. Sports Med 2:334–344, 1985.

clinician should always be aware that, although rare, forced inversion on the dorsiflexed or plantar flexed ankle may lead to talar dome fractures.[60]

Inversion and plantar flexion is the most frequent mechanism of injury and results in injury to the lateral ligaments of the ankle, usually the anterior talofibular and calcaneofibular ligaments. In some cases, the posterior talofibular ligament and peroneal tendons may also be injured.[61,62] If rotation occurs at the same time, the degree of injury is usually greater and includes the tibiofibular ligament. Disruption of the anterior talofibular ligament is the most frequent and most serious ligamentous injury because the ligament is a primary stabilizer of the ankle.[63] If a third-degree tear (complete rupture) to this ligament has occurred, anterior subluxation of the talus may occur.[64] These third-degree tears are seldom repaired surgically, but such a course may be considered for young, active athletes. If they are repaired surgically, the repair is usually done late rather than early, because most athletes function well without the surgery.[65] Because the inversion motion occurs at a high speed, the muscle cannot contract fast enough to take up the slack, and the ligament takes all the stress. When these lateral sprains occur, it has been reported that the common peroneal and/or posterior tibial nerve may be injured, especially with second- and third-degree sprains.[8] It is important for the clinician to check for this possibility, because it prolongs the rehabilitation period.

Nitz and associates,[8] in describing ankle sprains, referred to a different categorization scheme than is conventionally used. They defined a second-degree sprain as injury to the ligaments on the lateral aspect of the ankle as well as the deltoid ligament. They defined a third-degree sprain as tearing of the lateral ligaments, the deltoid ligaments, and the distal anterior tibiofibular ligament. Normally, damage to the ligaments is graded according to the cross-sectional tearing that takes place in the ligament. Instability of the ankle joint can occur when the anterior talofibular and/or the interosseous membrane are injured in the second- or third-degree classification. In fact, associated injury (strain, dislocation, rupture) to the peroneal tendons may lead to chronic lateral instability at the ankle. This is an important consideration for the clinician, because these tendon injuries often require surgical repair and need special emphasis during proprioceptive retraining.[6,61,66–69] Karlsson and Lansinger[65] reported that up to 20 percent of athletes may develop functional instability, even with suitable conservative care. They advocated ligament reconstruction rather than tenodesis (e.g., Evans repair), because both had good short-term results but tenodesis procedures had poorer long-term results. This type of injury involves the whole joint (intracapsular) and increases the healing time. Complete joint involvement is demonstrated by the swelling in the capsule, which shows up on both sides of the Achilles and posterior to the medial and lateral malleolus. For proper diagnosis, stress radiographs should be taken to determine the amount of instability and damage.[70,71]

As stated earlier, injury to the medial deltoid ligaments is much less common and is often accompanied by a fracture of the lateral malleolus. The mechanism of injury is usually abduction, eversion, and dorsiflexion. In some cases, there may be an accompanying avulsion fracture of the medial malleolus and the tibiofibular ligaments may be injured, affecting the stability of the ankle mortise. Syndesmosis sprains with injury to the anterior, posterior, and transverse tibiofibular ligaments and possibly the interosseous membrane may also lead to ankle instability and definitely prolong the rehabilitation period. The major complaints of the athletes is pain on push-off and stiffness in the ankle when these structures are involved.[72]

We have found that early partial weight bearing and immobilization with taping are effective. Taping and wrapping techniques for ankle sprains can be used for immediate care, protection, treatment, and evaluation. After an acute injury, taping and wrapping are used to provide compression and protection from unwanted movements, which may cause further injury. Wilkerson and Horn-Kingery[73] reported that focal compression with a U-shaped pad is most beneficial. These pads can be made of felt or in the form of commercially available, U-shaped, liquid-filled devices. Protective techniques allow normal movement patterns to occur but prevent abnormal or excessive movements. There remains controversy about the effectiveness of protective taping,[74] but many athletes find it to be desirable and effective in preventing recurrence of injury.[75,76] For some conditions, such as ankle sprains, it has become more efficient and cost-effective to use bracing,[77] although it has been reported that the brace's main positive effect may be due to proprioceptive feedback.[78,79] Braces, however, do offer the advantage that they are easier to readjust, thus restoring their effectiveness more quickly.[80] It has been reported that ankle braces limit motion relative to the unbraced ankle, but do not hinder performance.[81–85] Slight modifications of some techniques can be used as part of the overall treatment and management program, which allow normal movement and weight-bearing patterns to occur while at the same time protecting the area. Taping techniques can be used to evaluate some conditions by controlling specific movement(s) to see whether symptoms change. Commonly used taping and wrapping techniques are described elsewhere.[11,30]

We have used ice, compression, and weight bearing to tolerance to treat ankle sprains. Early active exercises, including dorsiflexion, squats, cycling, and BAPS drills, combined with icing (cryokinetics), are also effective.[86] Eiff and colleagues[87] have reported that early mobilization allows return to work and activity sooner. The athlete might be asked to perform active non–weight-bearing ankle activities in a cold whirlpool, ice water, or contrast bath. All these activities can be used to decrease swelling, thus decreasing pain resulting from pressure in the soft tissues. Laser and ultrasound treatments should be started during late phase I to help facilitate collagen formation.[9,36] Intermittent pressure devices such as a Jobst unit or Cryo/Cuff are effective in reducing swelling and can also be used with the limb in elevation. Surgical tubing is also effective and easy for the athlete to use.[88] No activity (passive or active) in any direction (late phase I, early phase II) that causes pain should be used at this stage. The drills should begin within the first 24 hours. "Relative rest" is used, meaning that no movement is performed that might overstretch the healing tissue. Range-of-motion exercise should be carried out in pain-free ranges only. The posterior calf muscles should be stretched to prevent spasm of these muscles. This stretching is easily accomplished within the pain-free range using osteopathic muscle energy techniques and stretching within the pain-free range of motion.[89]

The use of an Aircast brace should be started immediately, especially for lateral sprains.[79] Taping or an elastic bandage can be worn at the same time, so that compression can be maintained for the first 2 to 4 days following the injury. The Aircast is continuously worn for the first 2 to 4 weeks. The Aircast or Ankle Ligament Protector is then worn only during sporting activities for the next 5 to 6 months.[83,90]

During the fibroplasia phase of healing (phase III), the amount of collagen increases, as does its cross-linking. Because of the increasing tensile strength of the tissues, the treatment becomes more vigorous, evolving around stimulating the healing of the tissues as opposed to relieving pain or resolving inflammation. Exercise is used to facilitate tissue remodeling. Ice or cold baths following workouts are used to prevent problems that might arise from the tissues being irritated.

Transverse frictions (done with the ligament on stretch and at the extremes of range) can be used to mobilize ligamentous tissues and the forming collagen.[16] They are followed by active exercise to help maintain the newly acquired range of motion.

At this stage, if the athlete still has some limitation of range of motion in the talocrural, subtalar, or tarsal joints, appropriate mobilization techniques may be used to restore joint play. Corrigan and Maitland,[15,91] and Kaltenborn[17] have advocated several successful and easy techniques.

The most important overall principle to follow with ankle sprains is to rehabilitate the proprioceptive function of the muscles.[92,93] A common complaint is "I stepped on a small stone and went over on my ankle." In most of these situations, the athlete has regained full strength and range of motion but lacks the reflex control to contract the protective muscles fast enough when the ligaments are stretched.

Weight bearing is progressed from partial weight bearing to full weight bearing when the athlete can walk without a limp. Running in straight lines can be started when tolerated, progressing to more difficult drills with cutting, turning, and twisting.

Cardiovascular fitness is maintained with cycling, pool running, step machines, and ski and skate simulators, depending on the athlete's sport. When the athlete is ready to return to running, the method termed *three-thirds technique* may be effectively used. With this technique, the area in which the athlete runs in a straight line is divided into thirds (Fig. 32–6). This may be accomplished by dividing a basketball court or football field into thirds or any other suitable distance. The first third involves the athlete starting and building

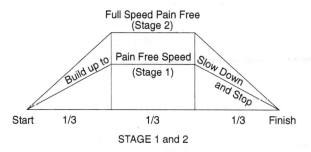

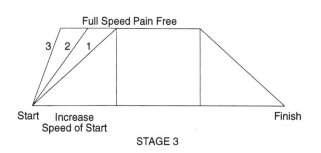

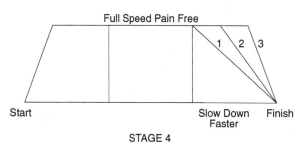

FIGURE 32–6. Three-thirds technique.

up speed to the pain-free speed to be attained in the middle sector. The middle third is the maximum speed the athlete can run in a pain-free fashion. The final third is the athlete running at the pain-free speed and slowing down to a stop. As the athlete continues to run and the injury improves, the speed of running in the middle third increases. When the athlete is running the middle third at full speed, the first third is increased in speed so that the athlete reaches full speed faster and faster. Once the athlete can start as quickly as possible, the "back" or last third is shortened so that the athlete slows down faster and faster. Basically, this means that the athlete runs from a stop position to a full-speed position faster and faster, until finally he or she can run as fast and as hard as possible from start to stop.

Functional activities such as those used for the knee may also be effective for ankle rehabilitation. These include the hop test, cross-over hop test, disco test, and leaning hop test.[94–96] The stages progress from interval running, backward running (retrorunning), side-to-side running, figure-of-eight running, cross-over, side-to-side shuffle, lazy s to sharp z running and cutting, jumping and skipping, and sport-specific patterns, including cutting on command.[2] These activities should be done so that the athlete is always in control but, when possible, the cardiovascular system is also stressed.

When the athlete can run forward and backward, hop, run, and cut, and run tight figure-of-eights at normal speed with no pain, he or she can return to stop-and-go sports. Running athletes (road racing and track) whose activity is in one direction may return to their sport much sooner than those requiring quick stops and change of direction. All athletes should continue to wear a protective ankle brace or support for the next 5 to 6 months of competition to prevent possible recurrence of injury.

MOBILE VERSUS RIGID FEET

Ideally, individuals taking part in sport have a relatively normal foot, with the foot in alignment with the leg and the talus acting as the key to the other tarsal bones and forefoot to maintain neutrality in the foot during static and dynamic activities. Thus, the foot has a normal medial longitudinal arch as well as a normal metatarsal arch, with the toes resting on the ground. In some individuals, this normal foot position is not present, resulting in either a pes planus (pronated foot) or a pes cavus (supinated foot). These deviations in themselves may not be a problem when normal stresses are applied. When abnormally high stresses or prolonged stresses such as those seen in sport are applied, however, problems can arise.

Pes planus, or a pronated foot, is a foot that has a tendency to be hypermobile due to lax ligaments and/or poor muscle support. Because the act of pronation of the foot enables the foot to dissipate shock on contact and allows it to adapt to uneven terrain, pronation is not usually a problem. Repeated excessive pronation, however, may put abnormal stress on the joints of the foot and may lead to increased valgus stress at the knee. In some individuals, the condition can lead to different pathology in the lower limb. If the condition is present and not causing any problems, it should be left alone but if it is causing problems, emphasis should be placed on improving reciprocal muscle strength and muscle proprioception in the foot and ankle. In addition, a control-type shoe may be used to help compensate for the overpronation (see Table 32–8).

Pes cavus or a supinated foot is usually more difficult to deal with because the foot is hypomobile, with an accentuated longitudinal arch, resulting in a decreased ability to absorb shock and a decreased ability to adapt to uneven surfaces. Because the foot cannot dissipate the force of contact, greater stress is placed on all the structures of the lower limb, with possible resulting pathology anywhere along the lower limb chain to the lumbar spine. Often accompanying the condition are loss of the metatarsal arch and clawing of the toes, which further affect locomotion and control. When individuals with a cavus foot are seen, there is little that can be done therapeutically except to relieve the symptoms. A cushion-type shoe is sometimes beneficial, and relative rest and modified activity may be of some help. Generally, the athlete has to be given a full understanding of the condition and the consequences of overloading the foot. It is important for the athlete to understand the necessity of cushioning the foot, and of wearing good shoes, and how quickly shoes can lose their shock absorption qualities. It has been shown that shoes lose up to 25 percent of their shock absorption capacity after being used to run 50 miles and lose up to 40 percent after running 250 to 500 miles.[97] Serious runners run 50 to 100 miles or more weekly, so proper, functional, cushioning shoes are of great importance.

TRACTION APOPHYSITIS

SEVER'S DISEASE

Calcaneal traction apophysitis, or Sever's disease, is seen in active preadolescents and adolescents (girls, 9 to 11 years; boys, 10 to 12 years). It is the calcaneal equivalent of Osgood-Schlatter disease of the tibial tubercle. It is commonly seen in running and jumping athletes who complain of heel stiffness and pain localized to the medial and lateral aspects of the calcaneal apophysis. Typically, the young athlete has excessive foot pronation and a tight gastrocnemius-soleus complex. Treatment is aimed at unloading the calcaneus, both with a heel lift and an orthotic. In addition, pre-exercise and postexercise stretching are beneficial. This is a self-limiting condition that resolves as the apophysis fuses, usually by age 13. During this period, activity modification may be required if pain-free running and jumping cannot be achieved with a heel lift (0.5 mm to start), orthotic, and stretching program. Cardiovascular fitness can be achieved with cycling, swimming, or pool running. Young soccer players are often helped with a switch to a multistudded boot rather than a boot with just two cleats under the heel. Young athletes with very tight heel cords may be helped by a night splint, commonly used in those with chronic resistant plantar fasciitis.

BASE OF THE FIFTH METATARSAL

This relatively common traction apophysitis is seen in the 11- to 13-year-old running and jumping athlete. It is commonly seen in athletes whose sports involve a great deal of lateral motion and frequent change of direction, such as soccer, field hockey, and basketball. It is also seen as a result of running on cambered or uneven surfaces, with traction stress of the peroneus brevis at its attachment to the base of the fifth metatarsal. Individuals with cavus feet and heel varus on static standing are at risk. There are localized swelling and tenderness, with pain on resisted foot eversion. Treatment is directed at inflammation control, activity modification, and motion control shoes with orthotic support.

Graduated strength, flexibility, and balance exercises for the foot and ankle are required. Ankle taping, bracing, or the use of an Aircast helps reduce ankle inversion and unload the traction stress caused by the peroneus brevis. Padding of the area is often helpful in restrictive boots such as those used for figure skating, skiing, and hiking. The boot can also be "punched out" or enlarged over this area.

NAVICULAR APOPHYSITIS

The adolescent 11- to 13-year-old athlete, particularly the one with excessive foot pronation, can develop traction stress at the insertion of the tibialis posterior into the navicular. Many, in fact, possess an accessory navicular that develops a traction irritation at the fibrous attachment to the main body of the navicular. This is seen in athletes in sports involving running, jumping, and change of direction. The differential diagnosis must always include a stress fracture, which can be determined by bone scan and CT scan. Treatment is again directed at inflammation control plus pronation control using orthotics with stable motion control shoes. The accessory navicular is much more prominent and may become irritated by direct pressure from ski boots and ice skates. As with the traction apophysitis at the base of the fifth metatarsal, boot modification and protective padding can be beneficial. Resistant cases of symptomatic accessory navicular irritation may require surgical resection with reattachment of the tibialis posterior tendon to the main body of the navicular.

OSTEOCHONDROSIS: KOHLER DISEASE

Kohler disease is a painful osteochondritis of the navicular seen in the very active young athlete (4 to 7 years old), more frequently in boys, who presents with a painful limp. There is swelling and local tenderness over the navicular. Beauchamp[98] described this condition as an "apparent" radiologic infarction of the navicular bone with the resultant wafer-shaped disc of sclerotic bone. Surprisingly, these young athletes do well with minimal long-term consequences, and there is a gradual development of a normal-appearing navicular bone. During the symptomatic period, the recommended treatment is 6 to 8 weeks of immobilization in a walking cast. Watson[99] stated that a walking cast followed by orthotic support may decrease the symptomatic period to 20 percent of that of the untreated athlete. We have been impressed with the use of a functional walking cast that can be removed for swimming or pool running for the serious age-class athlete.

FREIBERG DISEASE OR INFARCTION

This condition is a painful avascular necrosis of the second or, rarely, the third metatarsal head. It is seen in the 12- to 14-year-old active athlete who is often involved in running and jumping sports. Early x-rays may be normal, with later development of flattening of the involved metatarsal head. If seen early, deformity of the metatarsal head, which leads to early degenerative changes, can be prevented. Early treatment consists of exercise modification to eliminate excessive running and jumping plus orthotic foot support with a meta-

tarsal pad or bar to unload the involved metatarsal head. A rocker bar on the shoe may also be required. If pain persists and deformity develops with degenerative osteophytes, surgical consultation is appropriate. Surgical management involves either a cheilectomy, which is a cutting away of bony irregularities on the rim of the affected joint and capsular release or, with more extensive damage, a resection arthroplasty. Fortunately, most cases do not require surgery.

ANTERIOR METATARSAL AND MEDIAL LONGITUDINAL ARCH INJURIES

Both the medial longitudinal arch and the anterior metatarsal arch may be injured, often due to overuse, fatigue, or excessive activity on hard surfaces. The medial longitudinal arch is maintained by its bony arrangement, ligaments, and muscles. Because the ligaments become overloaded, a sprain results, often leading to the navicular bone being forced downward due to the weight of the body on the foot. This dropping of the navicular in turn leads to abnormal foot mechanics (e.g., pes planus), which can lead to injuries along the whole lower limb kinetic chain.

Injury to the anterior metatarsal arch or anterior metatarsalgia is usually the result of foot abnormalities (e.g., cavus foot), dysfunction of the intrinsic foot muscles, or poor-fitting shoes. Loss of this arch leads to calluses under and often bruising of the metatarsal heads. The condition is sometimes accompanied by clawing of the toes resulting from intrinsic insufficiency.

In both cases, the clinician should treat the symptoms and restore proper foot mechanics, which may involve electrical muscle stimulation, ultrasound, intrinsic foot exercises, proper fitting footwear, and orthotics.

PLANTAR FASCIITIS

Plantar fasciitis is an inflammatory stress syndrome of the plantar fascia or plantar aponeurosis. It is believed that this syndrome is related to the stress on the plantar fascia from the weight of an activity combined with weight transfer up onto the toes, which leads to metatarsophalangeal joint extension and causes a "windlass" effect on the plantar fascia.[100]

The plantar fascia is an important structure, stabilizing and locking the foot in supination prior to push-off in running. It usually is stressed with extensive foot pronation as the medial longitudinal arch collapses. Injury and stress usually occur at the medial calcaneal tubercle but may also occur within the midsubstance of the fascia. The periosteal reaction at its origin can result in hemorrhage and, ultimately, a heel spur. In many cases, heel spurs are asymptomatic, but are a sign of stress overload to the plantar fascia.

Typical symptoms include burning pain at the medial calcaneal tubercle, morning stiffness, and pain as the athlete walks on the toes, runs hills or stairs, pushes off from a dorsiflexed position (down lineman), or pushes off with internal rotation on the supporting limb (cutting motions in field sports). Signs include local tenderness (especially when the fascia is on stretch), pain on palpation, swelling, pain on passive toe extension with the foot in dorsiflexion, and some local swelling, although this is usually not evident. The condition is found in both rigid and mobile feet. It is important to check all footwear, which includes the everyday shoes that the athlete is wearing. Decreased flexibility in the gastrocnemius-soleus complex is commonly be found if the condition is seen in the pes cavus foot.

Biomechanical abnormalities of the foot may be significant contributing factors in the development of plantar fasciitis.[100] The foot goes through a precise series of movements during the running gait cycle (see Chapter 18). Overpronation and the resulting stretch and wringing of the plantar fascia during the stance phase can lead to straining of these tissues. If tight posterior muscles limit dorsiflexion, they may force the foot into pronation to achieve more range in dorsiflexion, which again increases stress on the plantar fascia. This mechanism is accentuated when running up even the smallest slope.

The differential diagnosis includes calcaneal stress fracture and plantar nerve entrapment, including tarsal tunnel syndrome, medial calcaneal nerve neuroma, subtalar joint arthritis, and insertional entothesis with seronegative arthropathies.[101]

Treatment is aimed at reduction of the inflammation, decrease of the tension on the plantar fascia, restoration of tissue strength and mobility, and controlling any biomechanical abnormality.

Inflammation can be controlled with ice, anti-inflammatory medication and, in recalcitrant cases, local corticosteroid injection.[102] A combination of Low Dye arch taping helps hold the foot in a neutral position and protects the plantar tissues from constant irritation during the early stages of rehabilitation.

Gastrocnemius-soleus stretching is important to increase dorsiflexion and to prevent the foot from going into increased pronation to compensate for the lack of dorsiflexion in the ankle. Heel lifts, heel cups, Low Dye or modified arch taping, low-frequency muscle stimulation, massage of the plantar fascia, intrinsic foot exercises, and assessment for proper footwear are all important in the therapy management of plantar fasciitis.[102] It is also important to assess and mobilize the joints of the ankle and foot. Of particular interest are the talocalcaneal joint, which often needs to be mobilized into adduction, and the talonavicular joint, which needs good translation of the navicular inferiorly on the talus. All other joints of the foot should be assessed and mobilization should be performed as needed.

Overall fitness is maintained through pool running, cycling, swimming for aerobic training and weight lifting for anaerobic systems. Running is restored through the use of a run-walk progression, with hopping, skipping, and jumping activities to follow.

If morning stiffness persists, the use of a night splint to maintain dorsiflexion of the plantar fascia may be useful. With the rare persistent case, surgical consultation is required. Surgery involves the release of the plantar fascia at its origin, heel spur removal, and exploration for nerve entrapment in scar tissue.

SESAMOIDITIS

Sesamoiditis involves trauma to the sesamoid bones in the tendons of the flexor hallucis brevis at its attachments to the base of the proximal phalanx of the hallux. This trauma can include a stress fracture, contusion, osteonecrosis, chondromalacia, or osteoarthritis of the sesamoid bones as they slide over and articulate with the head of the first metatarsal. Weight bearing on the toes increases the stress across the sesamoid bones. The condition is typically seen in jumping athletes, including volleyball and basketball players, gymnasts, and dancers.

The athlete complains of localized tenderness to the medial or lateral sesamoid with localized swelling and pain on weight bearing that increases with hopping. A triple-phase bone scan can be useful in differentiating a stress fracture from chondromalacia or local soft tissue inflammation. X-rays may show the common bipartite sesamoid. A "hot" bone scan indicates that this is an acute fracture process rather than an irritated previous bipartite sesamoid.

Treatment is aimed at reducing inflammation and unloading the inflamed sesamoid. Custom-made orthotics with appropriate padding or cut-out areas are usually successful. We have found that stress fractures of the sesamoid take 10 to 12 weeks to heal and functional casts, which can be removed for pool exercising, plus daily 8-hour electromagnetic therapy can often be useful.

The therapy modalities of ultrasound and laser for stimulation of healing and reduction of inflammation may prove useful.[36] Muscle stimulation to the plantar fascia using low-frequency (2 to 4 Hz) stimulation may help stimulate circulation and puts some mechanical stress through the tissues (see Table 32–2).[103] Ice massage combined with easy intrinsic foot exercises and calf stretching can be applied to the plantar aspect of the foot and the calf muscles.

For persistent pain that is not relieved by conservative means, surgical excision may be required. The major postoperative concern with the removal of the sesamoid is the development of significant hallux valgus, which may be prevented by the prescription of proper footwear and orthotics.

HALLUX VALGUS

Hallux valgus is usually seen in athletes with excessive foot pronation who use narrow footwear. Gould[104] has also attributed hallux valgus to the splayfoot syndrome associated with widening of the forefoot on weight bearing, resulting in increased laxity of the ligaments of the forefoot, particularly of the first and fifth metatarsal heads. The metatarsal angle with hallux valgus increases from 1 to 2 degrees to approximately 12 degrees with increased valgus deviation of the great toe toward the second toe. With this altered position, and with pronation and/or compression by footwear, the clinician can see the development of pinch calluses, exostosis, and a bursa thickening (bunion) at the first metatarsal head. Treatment is directed at controlled foot pronation using an orthotic and motion control footwear with adequate forefoot width. The callus can be trimmed, and icing and other modalities (e.g., ultrasound) can be used to decrease the bursitis.

With ongoing problems, surgical consultation is recommended. Gould[104] has suggested that surgical procedures be kept to a minimum in the active athlete and that osteotomy should be reserved until such time as the athlete switches to a more recreational sporting lifestyle. In the very active athlete, minimal surgical procedures, such as cheilectomy of the bunion, may be necessary.

HALLUX RIGIDUS AND TURF TOE

This disabling condition is associated with decreased range of motion at the first metatarsophalangeal joint and is accompanied by degenerative changes in the joint and "kissing osteophytes." Extension is usually reduced more than flexion, which makes running painful, especially uphill. Hallux rigidus is most frequently the result of repeated trauma but can also be seen following joint immobilization with a single traumatic episode or infection. In addition, it can be a result of "turf toe," when athletes stub their great toe. With turf toe, the toe is jammed or forced into hyperextension at the metatarsophalangeal joint when the boot grabs the artificial turf in sports such as soccer, football, baseball, or field hockey. This condition is also common in those in the performing arts, such as ballet. The condition progresses, with increasing restriction of joint motion. X-rays confirm the hypertrophic degenerative features, with joint space narrowing, often dorsal osteophytes, transverse joint space widening, and subchondral bone sclerosis. In late stages, as the metatarsophalangeal joint stiffens, hyperextension may be noted at the interphalangeal joint.

Treatment is aimed at the reduction of inflammation, protection, and restoration of normal range of motion. Treatment for inflammation may include icing, ultrasound, high-voltage galvanic currents, iontophoresis, or laser light energy.[36] Range-of-motion exercises are utilized in the early stages, with a requirement of 20 degrees of dorsiflexion for running sports and at least 10 degrees for walking and stair climbing. Range-of-motion exercises can be carried out in a cold whirlpool or contrast baths may be used during the inflammatory stage. Passive joint mobilizing techniques can be effective for pain relief, starting with accessory (joint play) movements and then moving into physiologic movement patterns when accessory movements are pain-free.[15] If stiffness persists, a warm whirlpool followed by icing is used. Sammarco[105] has outlined a non–weight-bearing exercise program for the rehabilitation of turf toe that involves stretching and strengthening, which is also useful for hallux rigidus. This program is combined with taping of the big toe to prevent hyperextension. If normal range of motion cannot be achieved, the use of an orthotic with a rocker bar or with a stiff-soled shoe with a rocker bar added can allow a pain-free gait. When the athlete returns to play, a properly fitted shoe with a stiffer sole should be used. The shoe can be combined with taping or a stiff insert to prevent hyperextension at the metatarsophalangeal joint.

With failure of an orthotic or shoe modification to provide relief, surgical consultation is needed. Surgical cheilectomy is the usual procedure; it does not sacrifice joint stability but improves range of motion.

MORTON NEUROMA

A Morton neuroma or interdigital neuritis is an injury of one of the common digital nerves as it passes between the metatarsal heads. The classic location is between the third and fourth metatarsal heads where the nerve is the thickest, receiving both branches from the medial and lateral plantar nerves. The digital nerves enter the forefoot between the superficial and deep transverse metatarsal ligaments in the interdigital space. Nerve irritation can then occur, with compression between the metatarsal heads when shoes are worn. In addition, Kopell and Thompson[106] have suggested that the nerve irritation occurs at the point where the nerve crosses the proximal edge of the transverse metatarsal ligament. Schamberger[107] has suggested that the irritation increases with the collapse of the transverse arch of the foot, putting the transverse metatarsal ligaments under stretch and thus compressing the common digital nerve and vessels. Excessive foot pronation can also be a predisposing factor, with more metatarsal shearing forces occurring with the prolonged forefoot abduction.[107]

The athlete complains of a burning paresthesia in the forefoot, often localized to the third web space and radiating to the toes. The symptoms are increased with hyperextension of the toes on weight bearing, as in squatting, stair climbing, or running. The symptoms are worse in shoes with a narrow toe box and higher heels. With ongoing nerve irritation and surrounding fibrous reaction or neuroma formation, the pain can become constant. On clinical examination, there is localized interdigital tenderness, possibly a positive Tinel sign, and often the well-described click with metatarsal head compression associated with a shoelike paresthesia. The presence of surrounding tenderness of the metatarsal heads requires a bone scan to rule out a metatarsal stress fracture.

Treatment is aimed at reducing inflammation and unloading the interspace between the bones. Cryotherapy, high-voltage galvanic currents, iontophoresis, laser, and ultrasound can all be used in an attempt to provide a local reduction of inflammation.[36,103] Local corticosteroid injections may be curative, along with an orthotic to prevent excessive pronation and with a metatarsal pad to reform the transverse arch and separate the metatarsal heads. Shoes with low heels and a wide toe box are essential. Failure of conservative management requires surgical excision, which is best done with a dorsal incision.

Other neurologic conditions such as anterior tarsal syndrome, medial calcaneal neuritis (jogger's foot), and tarsal tunnel syndrome are seen in the lower leg, ankle and foot. (See Chapter 23, for more information on these conditions.)

BLISTERS, CORNS, AND CALLUSES

The common areas for blisters are on the bottom of the foot under the metatarsal heads, over the insertion of the Achilles tendon, and on the side of and under the big toe. Shear and compression forces produced by poorly fitting shoes, wrinkled socks, tape, or repetitive action cause the dermal layers to separate and fill with fluid. Acute pain can result. If not treated properly, the athlete's performance can be affected, and improper management can lead to infection. If possible, the skin should not be removed from the blister, because this makes a sterile closed wound into an open wound. If the blister is large, it can be drained but only using a sterile technique. To protect hot spots, the "doughnut principle" should be used by cutting a hole in a sterile dressing or felt pad slightly larger than the damaged area. After applying the bandage over the area, the cut-out space can be filled with Skin Lube, which does not break down under body heat as easily as other petroleum-type lubricants. The area is then covered with a second dressing without the cut-out. If the blister has been drained, a topical antibiotic should be used to fill the space between the dressings. A second method is to apply Spenco Second Skin directly over the area and to cover with adhesive tape or a Bandaid to hold it in place. This method is better for blisters found on the bottom of the foot. If a blister is interfering with an athlete's performance, a topical analgesic to decrease the pain, followed by the application of Spenco Second Skin, which protects from further damage, may be used.

The same constant frictional forces that cause blisters acutely lead to the skin thickening and a callus forming in these areas due to chronic friction. As the callus thickens, it can add greater shearing stresses to the skin, and the separation of the callus from the underlying layers may result. If deep enough, small capillaries may rupture, forming a blood blister. Observation of callus formation on the bottom of the athlete's foot can be indicative of the type of foot function that is taking place. Callus formation always indicates that a poor-fitting shoe is being worn or abnormal stresses are being applied to the foot at some time. The stress may be applied not only by the training shoe but also by an everyday shoe.

Corns are found on the tops and between the toes and are usually classified as hard or soft. Those found between the toes are generally kept moist due to their location and are therefore soft. Immediate care requires the use of corn pads (doughnut principle) to distribute the forces away from the area. The soft corns require enough space in the toe box for the toes to remain dry and to provide air circulation between the toes. These conditions can be painful, and the underlying principle of treatment remains the same: relieve the stress, correct the foot mechanics, determine the foot and shoe interaction, and consider the surface on which the athlete is playing the sport.

Other dermatologic conditions such as athlete's foot, plantar warts, and subungual hematoma are discussed in Chapter 35, Dermatologic Considerations in Athletes.

FOOTWEAR CONSIDERATIONS

Proper shoe fit for both activity and everyday wear is poorly understood and certainly poorly done. This dilemma is as much the consumer's fault as it is the manufacturer's. When buying footwear, the following should be considered:

1. Determine length and width of the foot, and fit the forefoot width first. Both feet should be measured and the shoe fitted to the largest foot, because it is always easier to add parts to a shoe. Literature reports have noted that most people have one foot longer, with the left being the longest.[108] The length of the shoe should not be increased to improve the width. This is the most common error in fitting shoes, because it increases the length of the lever under the toes and contributes to hyperextension of the toes.

   Extra strain is placed on the longitudinal arches if the shoe is too narrow. The pressure over the heads of the first and fifth metatarsals creates bursitis, bunions, exostosis, hallux rigidus, hammertoes, and osteoarthritic changes. To test for proper width, the athlete should put full weight on the shoe (Fig. 32–7). The shoe upper should not overhang the sole of the shoe. On the other hand, if wrinkles appear across the top of the shoe, the shoe is probably too wide. Also, for a properly fitting upper, the lacing should be such that the eyelets are parallel from top to bottom. A shoe that is too narrow in the overpronating foot can force the first toe into valgus. The squeezing of the metatarsal heads can cause compression of the interdigital nerves between the metatarsal heads, sometimes resulting in a Morton neuroma. These problems are much greater in women. Frey and colleagues, as quoted by Quinn,[109] reported that 88 percent of women wear shoes between one and two sizes smaller in width than their feet. A shoe should never have to stretch to fit. Ice hockey players commonly wear skates that are one to two sizes too small to ensure a good snug fit, and they claim it gives them better control. Such action, however, increases the chances of foot problems and pathology.

2. The toe box (Fig. 32–8) should be wide enough and long enough to allow the toes to extend fully and to allow good alignment of the first toe on push-off. The toe box end of the shoe should be 0.5 inch (1 to 1.5 cm) from the end of the longest toe. If the toe box is too pointed, it pushes the first toe into a valgus position. The toe box should

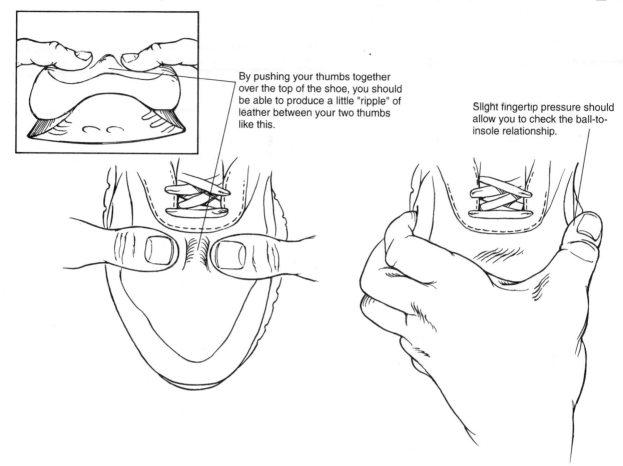

By pushing your thumbs together over the top of the shoe, you should be able to produce a little "ripple" of leather between your two thumbs like this.

Slight fingertip pressure should allow you to check the ball-to-insole relationship.

FIGURE 32–7. Checking shoes for proper width.

be rounded and not pointed. The condition of hallux valgus is not inherited, but the same foot type as one's parents is inherited. This, combined with poor fitting, often leads to the same foot problems.

3. The sole and instep of the foot must control the movement of the subtalar joint during midstance. The insole arch support should be properly positioned to provide support and cushioning. The outersole provides traction, durability, and cushioning. Ideally, this outersole should be a unit sole (no break in sole material) and vulcanized (fused) and stitched to the upper part of the shoe. This provides strength to the shoe. It is impossible to design a shoe that fits everyone—thus, the resulting use of orthotics. This portion of the shoe must be strong enough to hold the individual or an orthotic. Due to the force differences and the change in gait (see Chapter 18) a good running shoe may not make a good walking shoe. The running shoe needs to be stiffer, meaning that the forces of walking are not enough to make it function properly. Conversely, the walking shoe may not make a good running shoe. As the speed of gait increases, the forces to control motion have to increase as well.

4. The shoe should be designed to bend at the level of the metatarsophalageal joint. If it does not, ex-

cessive stress is placed on the foot and Achilles tendon. To test for this flexibility, the athlete should hold the heel of the shoe in one hand and attempt to push the toe of the shoe up with the index finger of the other hand. Similarly, one can hold the heel of the shoe and push the toe end down on a scale. The shoe should bend in the metatarsal area before the scale reads 10 lb (4.5 kg). If the shoe does not bend before 10 lb is reached, it is too stiff in the forefoot.

5. The heel has to be soft enough to absorb energy without overcollapsing during the gait cycle. Normally, the heel is 0.5 to 0.75 inch (1 to 2 cm) thicker than the sole of the forefoot to decrease stress on the Achilles tendon, especially in training shoes. This difference is not seen in racing flats. Cook and associates[97] pointed out that the shock attenuation properties of a shoe are lost according to the distance run. For example, 25 percent of shock absorption is lost after 50 miles, 33 percent lost after 100 to 150 miles and, between 250 and 500 miles, shoes retain less than 60 percent of their absorption capacity. The heels of the soles of shoes need to be kept in good repair, which may be accomplished with some type of rubberized shoe repair compound (e.g., Shoe Goo). When the heel wears down, it creates greater lever forces and leads to side wall and

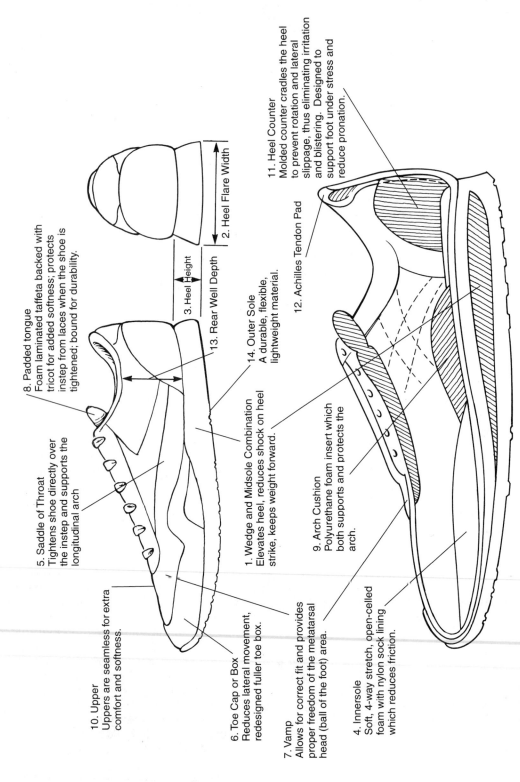

11. Heel Counter
Molded counter cradles the heel to prevent rotation and lateral slippage, thus eliminating irritation and blistering. Designed to support foot under stress and reduce pronation.

12. Achilles Tendon Pad

2. Heel Flare Width

3. Heel Height

13. Rear Well Depth

14. Outer Sole
A durable, flexible, lightweight material.

8. Padded tongue
Foam laminated taffeta backed with tricot for added softness; protects instep from laces when the shoe is tightened; bound for durability.

5. Saddle of Throat
Tightens shoe directly over the instep and supports the longitudinal arch

1. Wedge and Midsole Combination
Elevates heel, reduces shock on heel strike, keeps weight forward.

9. Arch Cushion
Polyurethane foam insert which both supports and protects the arch.

10. Upper
Uppers are seamless for extra comfort and softness.

6. Toe Cap or Box
Reduces lateral movement, redesigned fuller toe box.

7. Vamp
Allows for correct fit and provides proper freedom of the metatarsal head (ball of the foot) area.

4. Innersole
Soft, 4-way stretch, open-celled foam with nylon sock lining which reduces friction.

FIGURE 32–8. Anatomy of a running shoe.

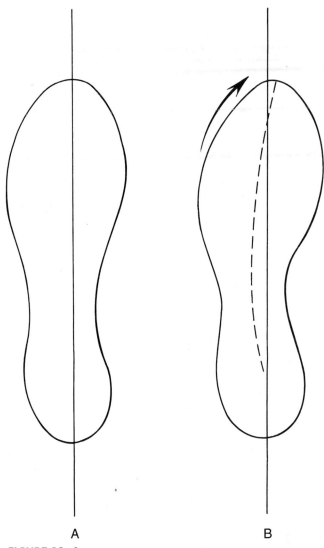

A   B

FIGURE 32–9. Straight *(A)* and curved *(B)* shoe lasts.

heel counter breakdown as the foot moves the shoe from supination at heel strike to pronation at midstance. This breakdown may not only be a problem in the athletic shoe but may also occur in the everyday shoe. By using this "favorite" pair of shoes, the athlete does not allow the tissues to rest and recover from the stress of training. Also, excessive flair to the heel may cause problems by causing an excessive "whip" of pronation at heel strike. The flair of the shoe's heel should never extend beyond the malleolus.

6. The shape of the shoe (lasting) is classified as straight, curved, or semi-curved (Fig. 32–9). Generally, individuals with a rigid type of foot (cavus foot) should wear a curved last shoe with sufficient cushioning. Those with a more mobile foot (pronated foot) need a shoe with more control. Straight-lasted shoes are usually more stable and designed for individuals with mobile (overpronating) feet. Thus, a straighter last and control shoe are required. This type of shoe needs good midfoot and heel counter control. It is our impression that most sport shoes have a last that

is too curved. If one looks down at the top of the shoe in weight bearing, and if it appears that the forefoot is sliding off the anterolateral border of the shoe, the last is too curved. In a shoe that has been worn for a while, this is easy to see as the shape the shoe has adapted to conform to the shape of the foot. When just sitting on a flat surface, the shoe should appear "balanced"—that is, it should not lean one way or the other. When viewed from behind, the heel cup should be straight and not lean in one direction or the other. If one takes a pencil and puts it against the inside back of the heel and pushes down, the shoe should come straight up and not deviate to either side. This indicates the proper balance of the shoe posteriorly.

7. The heel to forefoot height must be checked. In the athlete with a rigid or cavus foot, there should only be a slight difference in height, with good support under the subtalar joint. If the heel is too high in the rigid foot, too much weight is taken on the forefoot, which is not designed to absorb the extra energy. The lower heel allows energy to be taken through the full foot and reduces the force on the forefoot.

8. The width of the heel counter should allow for a snug fit of the heel in the shoe. This is the area that is often fitted first, resulting in some cases with the shoe not fitting in the forefoot. If the heel is too wide, it can be filled in by a piece of adhesive felt, heel cup, or something sewn in to fill in the space, which is more desirable than having a shoe too tight in the forefoot.

9. The following points should be remembered when fitting shoes[109]:
   a. The individual should shop for shoes at the end of the day when the feet are at their largest, or at least at the time of day when they plan to use the shoes. The socks that one plans to wear with the shoes should also be worn.
   b. Shoes should be fitted on weight-bearing feet and the athlete should at least "run" around the store in them to ensure a comfortable fit.
   c. Shoes should allow full extension of the toes.
   d. The feet should not bulge over the seams and should feel comfortable the moment they are put on.
   e. Defects of workmanship (e.g., crooked stitching) can occur in any pair of shoes. If they are present, ask for another pair of shoes.
   f. One should not believe that shoes will stretch to fit. This is especially true for nylon.
   g. Shoes that are designed for the activity should be bought.

10. Athletes should always watch for gimmicks in shoes. Flared heels, torsion bars, pumps, lights or air suspension may work for some but not for all. When one finds a shoe that fits properly, record the qualities of that shoe (e.g., straight-last, size [10 EEE], with stable heel counter and medium shock absorption) and look for the next

generation of shoe that has those qualities. Manufacturers bring out new models every 6 to 8 months to ensure a steady turnover of product.

REFERENCES

1. Mann RA: Biomechanics of running. *In* Mack RA (ed): Symposium on the Foot and Leg in Running Sports. St. Louis, CV Mosby, 1982, pp 1–29.
2. Jarvin JS, Ferkel RD: Ankle and foot injuries. *In* Fu FH, Stone DA (eds): Sports Injuries—Mechanism, Prevention, Treatment. Baltimore, Williams & Wilkins, 1994, pp 977–1000.
3. Magee DJ: Orthopedic Physical Assessment. Philadelphia, WB Saunders, 1992.
4. Bordelon RL: The form and function of the foot. Sports Med Update 1990; 5:3–7.
5. Lattanza L, Gray GW, Kantner RM: Closed versus open kinetic chain measurements of subtalar joint eversion: Implications for clinical practice. J Orthop Sports Phys Ther 1988; 9:310–314.
6. Feuerbach JW, Grabiner MD, Koh TJ, Weiker GG: Effect of an ankle orthosis and ankle ligament anesthesia on ankle joint proprioception. Am J Sports Med 1994; 22:223–229.
7. Thompson T, Doherty J: Spontaneous rupture of tendon of Achilles. A new clinical diagnostic test. Anat Res 1967; 158:126–129.
8. Nitz AJ, Dobner JJ, Kersey D: Nerve injury and grades II and III ankle sprains. Am J Sports Med 1985; 13:177–182.
9. Dyson M, Biol C, Biol MI: Role of ultrasound in wound healing. *In* Kloth CL, McCulloch JM, Feedar JA (eds): Wound Healing: Alternatives in Management. Philadelphia, FA Davis, 1990, pp 259–283.
10. Ebel A: Exercise in vascular diseases. *In* Licht S (ed): Therapeutic Exercise, 2nd ed. New Haven, E Licht, 1965, pp 851–867.
11. Roy S, Irvin R: Sports Medicine. Englewood Cliffs, NJ, Prentice-Hall, 1983.
12. Curwin SL: The aetiology and treatment of tendinitis. *In* Harries M, Williams C, Stanish WD, Micheli LJ (eds): Oxford Textbook of Sports Medicine. New York, Oxford University Press, 1994, pp 512–528.
13. Knight KL, Londeree BR: Comparison of blood flow in the ankle of uninjured subjects during therapeutic applications of heat, cold and exercise. Med Sci Sports Exerc 1980; 12:76–80.
14. Knight KL: Cryotherapy—Theory, Technique and Physiology. Chattanooga, TN, Chattanooga Corporation, 1985.
15. Maitland GD: Peripheral Manipulation, 2nd ed. London, Butterworth, 1977.
16. Cyriax JH: Clinical applications of massage. *In* Basmajian JV (ed): Manipulation, Traction and Massage, 3rd ed. Baltimore, Williams & Wilkins, 1981, pp 122–139.
17. Kaltenborn FM: Manual Therapy for the Extremity Joints, 2nd ed. Braddock, PA, Pittsburgh Regional Orthopedic Study Group, 1977.
18. Jones DC: Tendon disorders of the foot and ankle. J Am Acad Orthop Surg 1993; 1:87–94.
19. Sapega AA, Quedenfeld TC, Moyer RA, Butler RA: Biophysical factors in range of motion exercises. Phys Sports Med 1981; 9:57–65.
20. Grey GW: Rehabilitation of running injuries: Biomechanical and proprioceptive considerations. Topics Acute Care Trauma Rehabil 1986; 1:67–78.
21. Daly TJ: The repair phase of wound healing, re-epithelialization and contraction. *In* Kloth CL, McCulloch JM, Feedar JA (eds): Wound Healing: Alternatives in Management. Philadelphia, FA Davis, 1990, pp 14–24.
22. Bates C, Hanson N: The theories and principles of aquatic exercise therapy. Aquatic Exercise Therapy. Westbank, British Columbia, AET Consulting, 1992.
23. Fox EL, Mathews DK: Interval Training. Toronto, WB Saunders, 1974.
24. Longacre JJ: Scar tissue: Its use and abuse in light of recent biophysical and biochemical studies. *In* Longacre JJ (ed): The Ultrastructure of Collagen. Springfield, IL, Charles C Thomas, 1976, pp 511–524.
25. Price H: Connective tissue in wound healing. *In* Kloth CL, McCulloch JM, Feedar JA (eds): Wound Healing: Alternatives in Management. Philadelphia, FA Davis, 1990, pp 31–41.
26. Astrand P, Rodahl K: Temperature regulation. *In* Astraud P, Rodahl K (eds): Textbook of Work Physiology, 3rd ed. New York, McGraw-Hill, 1986, pp 583–645.
27. Barnes L: Cryotherapy—putting injury on ice. Phys Sports Med 1979; 7:130–136.
28. Kloth CL, Feedar JA: Electrical stimulation in tissue repair. *In* Kloth CL, McCulloch JM, Feedar JA (eds): Wound Healing: Alternatives in Management. Philadelphia, FA Davis, 1990, pp 221–257.
29. Kloth CL, Miller KH: Factors influencing wound healing. *In* Kloth CL, McCulloch JM, Feedar JA (eds): Wound Healing: Alternatives in Management. Philadelphia, FA Davis, 1990, pp 1–93.
30. Arnheim DD: Modern Principles of Athletic Training, 6th ed. St. Louis, CV Mosby, 1985.
31. Prentice WE, Henry CL: Therapeutic Modalities in Rehabilitation. *In* Prentice WE (ed): Rehabilitation Techniques in Sports Medicine. St. Louis, Times Mirror/Mosby College Publishing, 1990, pp 49–77.
32. Dunlop RJ: Electrical muscle stimulation protocols: Effects of force production and energy metabolism of the gastrocnemius muscle in humans. (thesis) Vancouver, BC, University of British Columbia, Faculty of Graduate Studies, 1991.
33. Harvey W, Dyson M, Pond JB, Grahame R: The stimulation of protein synthesis in human fibroblast by therapeutic ultrasound. Rheumatol Rehabil 1975; 14:237.
34. Povel JB, Woodward B, Dyson M: A microscopic viewing ultrasonic irradiation chamber. Phys Med Biol 1971; 18:521.
35. Cummings J: Role of light in wound healing. *In* Kloth CL, McCulloch JM, Feedar JA (eds): Wound Healing: Alternatives in Management. Philadelphia, FA Davis, 1990, pp 287–299.
36. Enwemeka CS: Laser biostimulation of healing wounds: Specific effects and mechanisms of action. J Orthop Sports Phys Ther 1988; 9:333–338.
37. Scheller AD, Kasser JR, Quigley TB: Tendon injuries about the ankle. Orthop Clin North Am 1980; 11:801–811.
38. Martire JR: Differentiating stress fracture from periostitis—the finer points of bone scans. Phys Sports Med 1994; 22:71–81.
39. Magee DJ: Sports Physiotherapy. Edmonton, Alberta, University of Alberta, 1988.
40. Detmer DE: Chronic shin splints: Classification and management of medial tibial stress syndrome. Sports Med 1986; 3:436–446.
41. Holder LE, Michael RH: The specific scintigraphic pattern of "shin splints in the lower leg": Concise communication. J Nucl Med 1984; 25:865–869.
42. Smith W, Wann F, Parette R: Comparative study using four modalities in shin splint treatments. J Orthop Sports Phys Ther 1986; 8:77–80.
43. Crichton PA, Fricker PA, Purdam CR, Watson AS: Injuries to the pelvis and lower limb. *In* Bloomfield J, Fricker PA, Fitch KD (eds): Textbook of Science and Medicine in Sport. Oxford, Blackwell Scientific, 1992, pp 381–418.
44. Davey JR, Rorabech CH, Fowler PJ: The tibialis posterior muscle compartment: An unrecognized cause of exertional compartment syndrome. Am J Sports Med 1984; 12:391–397.
45. Lokiec F, Sievner I, Pritsch M: Chronic compartment syndrome of both feet. J Bone Joint Surg 1991; 73B:178–179.
46. Wiley JP, Clement DB, Doyle DL, Taunton JE: A primary care perspective of chronic compartment syndrome of the leg. Phys Sports Med 1987; 15:111–120.
47. Pedowitz RA, Hargens AR, Mubarak SJ, Gershuni DH: Modified criteria for the objective diagnosis of chronic compartment syndrome of the leg. Am J Sports Med 1990; 18:35–40.
48. Beckham SG, Grana WA, Buckley P, et al: A comparison of anterior compartment pressures in competitive runners and cyclists. Am J Sports Med 1993; 21:36–48.
49. Logan JG, Rorabeck CH, Castle GS: The measurement of dynamic compartment pressure during exercise. Am J Sports Med 1983; 11:220–223.
50. Matheson GO, Clement DB, McKenzie DC, et al: Stress fractures in athletes. A study of 320 cases. Am J Sports Med 1987; 15:46–58.
51. Dickson TB, Kichline PD: Functional management of stress

fractures in female athletes using a pneumatic leg brace. Am J Sports Med 1987; 15:86–89.

52. Rettig AC, Shelbourne DK, McCarroll JR, et al: The natural history and treatment of delayed union stress fractures of the anterior cortex of the tibia. Am J Sports Med 1988; 16:250–255.

53. Eisele SA, Sammarco GJ: Fatigue fractures of the foot and ankle in the athlete. J Bone Joint Surg 1993; 75A:290–298.

54. McKenzie DC, Clement DB, Taunton JE: Running shoes, orthotics and injuries. Sports Med 1985; 2:334–344.

55. James SL, Bates BT, Ostering LR: Injuries to runners. Am J Sports Med 1978; 6:40–50.

56. Pettine KA, Morrey BF: Osteochondral fractures of the talus—a long-term follow-up. J Bone Joint Surg 1987; 69B:89–92.

57. Oden RR: Tendon injuries about the ankle resulting from skiing. Clin Orthop Rel Res 1987; 216:63–69.

58. Escalas F, Figueras JM, Merino JA: Dislocation of the peroneal tendons—long-term results of surgical treatment. J Bone Joint Surg 1980; 62A:451–453.

59. Kleiger B: Mechanisms of ankle injury. Orthop Clin North Am 1974; 5:127–146.

60. Shea MP, Manoli A: Recognizing talar dome lesions. Phys Sports Med 1993; 21:109–120.

61. Bassett FH, Speer KP: Longitudinal rupture of the peroneal tendons. Am J Sports Med 1993; 21:354–357.

62. Sobel M, Warren RF, Brourman S: Lateral ankle instability associated with dislocation of the peroneal tendons treated by the Chrisman-Snook procedure. Am J Sports Med 1990; 18:539–543.

63. Johnson EE, Markolf KL: The contribution of the anterior talofibular ligament to ankle laxity. J Bone Joint Surg 1983; 65A:81–88.

64. Wilkerson GB: Comparative biomechanical effects of the standard method of ankle taping and a taping method designed to enhance subtalar stability. Am J Sports Med 1991; 19:588–595.

65. Karlsson J, Lansinger O: Lateral instability of the ankle joint. Clin Orthop Rel Res 1992; 276:253–261.

66. Sobel M, Geppert MJ, Warren RF: Chronic ankle instability as a cause of peroneal tendon injury. Clin Orthop Rel Res 1993; 296:187–191.

67. Lentell GL, Latzman LL, Walters MR: The relationship between muscle function and ankle stability. J Orthop Sports Phys Ther 1990; 11:605–611.

68. Konradsen L, Ravn JB, Sorenson AI: Proprioception at the ankle: The effect of anesthetic blockage of ligament receptors. J Bone Joint Surg 1993; 75B:433–436.

69. Wilkerson GB, Nitz AJ: Dynamic ankle stability: Mechanical and neuromuscular interrelationships. J Sports Rehabil 1994; 3:43–57.

70. Rijke AM: Lateral ankle sprains—graded stress radiograph for accurate diagnosis. Phys Sports Med 1991; 19:107–118.

71. Glasgow M, Jackson A, Jamieson AM: Instability of the ankle after injury to the lateral ligament. J Bone Joint Surg 1980; 62B:196–200.

72. Taylor DC, Englehardt DL, Bassett FH: Syndemosis sprains of the ankle—the influence of heterotopic ossification. Am J Sports Med 1992; 20:146–150.

73. Wilkerson GB, Horn-Kingery HM: Treatment of the inversion ankle sprain: Comparison of different modes of compression and cryotherapy. J Orthop Sports Phys Ther 1993; 17:240–246.

74. Burks RT, Bean BG, Marcus R, Barker HB: Analysis of athletic performance with prophylactic ankle devices. Am J Sports Med 1991; 19:104–106.

75. Frankeny JR, Jewett DL, Hanks GA, Sebastianelli WJ: A comparison of ankle taping methods. Clin J Sports Med 1993; 3:20–25.

76. Scotece GG, Guthrie MR: Comparison of three treatment approaches for grade I and II ankle sprains in active duty soldiers. J Orthop Sports Phys Ther 1992; 15:19–22.

77. Gross MT, Bradshaw MK, Ventry LC, Weller KH: Comparison of support provided by ankle taping and semirigid orthosis. J Orthop Sports Phys Ther 1988; 9:33–39.

78. Carroll MJ, Rijke AM, Perrin DH: Effect of the Swede-O ankle brace on talar tilt in subjects with unstable ankles. J Sports Rehabil 1993; 2:261–267.

79. Feuerbach JW, Grabiner MD: Effect of the Aircast on unilateral postural control: Amplitude and frequency variables. J Orthop Sports Phys Ther 1993; 17:149–154.

80. Shapiro MS, Kabo JM, Mitchell PW, et al: Ankle sprain prophylaxis: An analysis of the stabilizing effects of braces and tape. Am J Sports Med 1994; 22:78–82.

81. Alves JW, Alday RV, Ketcham DL, Lentell GL: A comparison of the passive support provided by various ankle braces. J Orthop Sports Phys Ther 1992; 15:10–18.

82. Gross MT, Ballard CL, Mears HG, Watkins EJ: Comparison of Donjoy ankle ligament protector and Aircast sport-stirrup orthoses in restricting foot and ankle motion before and after exercise. J Orthop Sports Phys Ther 1992; 16:60–67.

83. Gross MT, Lapp AK, Davis JM: Comparison of Swede-O universal ankle support and Aircast sport-stirrup and ankle tape in restricting eversion-inversion before and after exercise. J Orthop Sports Phys Ther 1991; 13:11–19.

84. Bocchinfuso C, Sitler MR, Kimura IF: Effects of two semirigid prophylactic ankle stabilizers on speed, agility and vertical jump. J Sports Rehabil 1994; 3:125–134.

85. Gross MT, Everts JR, Roberson SE, et al: Effect of Donjoy ankle ligament protector and Aircast sport-stirrup orthosis on functional performance. J Orthop Sports Phys Ther 1994; 19:150–156.

86. Pincivero D, Gieck JH, Saliba EN: Rehabilitation of a lateral ankle sprain with cryokinetics and functional progressive exercise. J Sports Rehabil 1993; 2:200–207.

87. Eiff MP, Smith AT, Smith GE: Early mobilization versus immobilization in the treatment of lateral ankle sprains. Am J Sports Med 1994; 22:83–88.

88. McClushey GM, Blackburn TA, Lewis T: A treatment for ankle sprains. Am J Sports Med 1976; 4:158–161.

89. Case WS: Recovering from ankle sprains. Phys Sports Med 1993; 21:43–44.

90. Greene TA, Wight CR: A comparative support evaluation of three ankle orthoses before, during and after exercise. J Orthop Sports Phys Ther 1990; 11:453–466.

91. Corrigan B, Maitland GD: Practical Orthopedic Medicine. London, Butterworths, 1983.

92. Tropp H, Askling C, Gillquist J: Prevention of ankle sprains. Am J Sports Med 1985; 13:259–262.

93. DeCarlo MS, Talbot RW: Evaluation of ankle joint proprioception following injection of the anterior talofibular ligament. J Orthop Sports Phys Ther 1986; 8:70–76.

94. Losee RE: Diagnosis of chronic injury to the anterior cruciate ligament. Orthop Clin North Am 1985; 16:83–97.

95. Strobel M, Stedtfeld HW: Diagnostic Evaluation of the Knee. Berlin, Springer-Verlag, 1990.

96. Larson RL: Physical examination in the diagnosis of rotary instability. Clin Orthop Rel Res 1983; 172:38–44.

97. Cook SD, Kester MA, Brunet ME: Shock absorption characteristics of running shoes. Am J Sports Med 1985; 13:248–253.

98. Beauchamp R: Pediatric foot and ankle problems. Med Sport Sci 1987; 23:128–144.

99. Watson AS: Children in sport. In Bloomfield J, Fricker PA, Fitch KD (eds): Textbook of Science and Medicine in Sport. Oxford, Blackwell Scientific, 1992, pp 436–465.

100. Taunton JE, Clement DB: Evaluating heel pain in the recreational runner. Diagnosis 1988; 5:159–167.

101. Doxey GE: Calcaneal pain: A review of various disorders. J Orthop Sports Phys Ther 1988; 9:25–32.

102. Kosmahl EM, Kosmahl HE: Painful plantar heel, plantar fasciitis, and calcaneal spur: Etiology and treatment. J Orthop Sports Phys Ther 1988; 9:17–24.

103. Reid DC: Sports Injury Assessment and Rehabilitation. London, Churchill-Livingstone, 1992.

104. Gould N: Splay foot, hallux valgus and hallux rigidus. Med Sport Sci 1987; 23:121–127.

105. Sammarco JG: How I manage turf toe. Phys Sports Med 1988; 16:113–118.

106. Kopell HP, Thompson WAL: Peripheral entrapment neuropathies of the lower extremity. N Engl J Med 1960; 262:56–60.

107. Schamberger W: Nerve injuries around the foot and ankle. Med Sport Sci 1987; 23:105–120.

108. Cavanagh PR: The Running Shoe Book. Mountain View, CA, Anderson World, 1980.

109. Quinn M: If the shoe fits . . . surgery won't be necessary. Fam Pract 1994.

CHAPTER 33

Emergency Care of the Injured Athlete

BRUCE H. DICK MD
JEFFREY M. ANDERSON MD

The revolutionary changes occurring in all fields of medicine have afforded the health care professional an increased opportunity to salvage life and establish a framework for return to functional status. This opportunity is predicated on the ability of the clinician to understand signs, symptoms, and disease processes to deal with clinical problems intelligently. The acuity of this decision process is often magnified in the arena of sports medicine. Decisions regarding such issues as playing status, transport, and bracing are often made in the caldron of a sporting event with limited time, limited diagnostic capabilities, excessive crowd noise,

and pressure from coaches and players to return to competition.

The purpose of this chapter is to address the on-site management of acute athletic injuries. This goal is achieved by embracing the following:

- The historical and epidemiologic aspects of athletic injury, advanced trauma life support, advanced cardiac life support, and their application to sports medicine.
- The ethical and legal aspects of injury prevention, injury treatment, and athletic event coverage.

757

- The basic tenets of emergency medical care provision.

By incorporating these factors in decision making, the clinician can better understand the milieu of sports medicine.

HISTORICAL OVERVIEW

EPIDEMIOLOGIC BACKGROUND

The greatest amount of work done on sports-specific emergencies has been done in the area of neurologic injury,[1] specifically closed head trauma and cervical spine injuries. The sport in which most of the data have been gathered is football. The work of Schneider in the 1960s elucidated the risk of neurologic injury in football.[2] At that time, the predominance of neurologic morbidity and mortality occurred secondary to intracranial trauma, with cervical spine injury being less common. That was partly due to the design of and materials used in the football helmet during that era. Blocking and tackling techniques at that time involved using the shoulder as the primary sight of contact, with the player sliding the head to one side just prior to contact. By the early 1960s the football helmet was modernized, with improvements in the protective shell and the development of the modern face mask. In the late 1960s, the National Operating Committee on Standards for Athletic Equipment (NOCSAE) was established in the United States to develop and monitor safety standards for football helmets. By 1974, NOCSAE standards were being followed by all helmet makers. In 1978, it became mandatory at the collegiate level in the United States to use NOCSAE-approved helmets. High schools followed suit in 1980.

Another major development in the monitoring of catastrophic football injuries occurred in 1975 after 12 football players in New Jersey and Pennsylvania suffered severe cervical spine injuries.[3] The National Football Head and Neck Injury Registry was established, in response to this occurrence to track the occurrence of intracranial hemorrhage, fatal intracranial injuries, cervical spine fractures, subluxations, dislocations, and permanent quadriplegia resulting from cervical spine trauma on a national level. The initial action of the registry was to publish a retrospective review of neurologic trauma in football from 1971 to 1975.[4] This revealed a trend showing that intracranial injuries had diminished, associated with a striking increase in the occurrence of cervical spine trauma.[4] These changes were attributed to the improvement in helmet design, which lowered the intracranial injury rate but also allowed for techniques in which the head was used as the initial point of contact. These subsequently put the player's cervical spine at risk.

On presentation of these findings to the National Collegiate Athletic Association (NCAA) in 1976, rules 9-1-2N and 9-1-2-1 were adopted. These prohibited using the crown of the helmet as the initial site of impact ("spearing") and discouraged teaching such techniques. The National Federation of High School Athletic Associations (NFHSAA) adopted similar rules in the same year. Subsequent to these rule changes, there was yet another decrease in fatalities due to intracranial injuries and a significant decrease in cervical spine injuries.

Such a systematic application of sports-specific injury data has been and will be used to elucidate injury trends at such mass participation events as triathlons, road races, and auto races. In addition, the NCAA Injury Surveillance System (ISS), developed in 1982, provides data on injury trends to the NCAA Committee on Competitive Safeguards and Medical Aspects of Sports. Using this data, rule changes and protective equipment modification are implemented in an attempt to reduce injuries. Similar data banks are being constructed in other sports, such as boxing.

EMERGENCY MEDICAL CARE AND CARDIAC RESUSCITATION

In addition to the changes that have occurred in the prevention and incidence of neurologic injury, significant improvements have occurred in the care of the individual with cardiac arrest. In 1960, "closed-chest" compression was described.[5] Combined with mouth-to-mouth resuscitation, basic cardiopulmonary resuscitation (CPR) was developed to provide a form of artificial circulation and ventilation in the prehospital stage of patient care. The application and techniques of CPR have changed with time. In the United States, in 1966, the National Academy of Sciences-National Research Council (NA-NARC) recommended CPR training for all medical, allied health, and other professional personnel.[6] The standards were established by the American Heart Association (AHA), and the AHA became the primary overseeing body in the evolution of CPR and emergency cardiac care (ECC). Subsequent national meetings were held in 1973, 1979, 1983, 1985, and 1992.[7] The meetings addressed the standardization of curricula for basic life support (BLS), promotion of its teaching throughout the community, the development of protocols for advanced cardiac life support (ACLS), the development of standards for emergency cardiac care for children and infants, and re-evaluation of ECC standards in light of evolving medical knowledge.

ADVANCED TRAUMA LIFE SUPPORT (ATLS)

The principles of ECC provide guidelines for care in the case of cardiac arrest; in the athletic setting, however, the majority of scenarios encountered have a traumatic cause. Guidelines for the rapid assessment and therapy of trauma victims date to 1976, when the inadequate care received by a Nebraska surgeon following a traumatic incident prompted him to seek standardization of initial trauma care. The result of this situation was the development of the advanced trauma life support (ATLS) course, which was adopted by the

TABLE 33-1
Trimodal Trauma Mortality Distribution

Time After Injury	Injury Type	Salvage Potential
Seconds to minutes	Catastrophic; neurologic, cardiac	Minimal
Minutes to hours	Incracranial hemorrhage; visceral, thoracic	Good with proper intervention
Weeks	Organ failure, sepsis	Variable

American College of Surgeons Committee on Trauma in 1979.[8]

The principles of the course center around the trimodal distribution of trauma mortality (Table 33-1). The first peak in mortality occurs within seconds to minutes of injury. Death during this peak is usually secondary to catastrophic neurologic or cardiovascular injury, and it is unlikely that any of these patients can be saved. The second peak in mortality occurs within minutes to hours of injury. This is what is referred to as the "golden hour" in trauma management. Causes of mortality in these situations include various types of intracranial hemorrhage (ICH), thoracic injuries, such as tension pneumothorax or hemothorax, and visceral and skeletal injuries associated with a large amount of blood loss. The third peak in mortality occurs in days to weeks from injury and is usually the result of organ failure or sepsis. It is the second peak in the trimodal distribution of trauma mortality that is the focus of the ATLS course. It is believed that rapid and thorough assessment and resuscitation, performed immediately on contact with the trauma victim, reduce mortality. Prompt, organized, and complete evaluation and resuscitation at this time also limit complications that lead to mortality in the third trimodal peak.

The principles of ECC and ATLS emphasize a rapid, complete assessment of the injured or ill individual, with immediate institution of emergent therapy. By incorporating these principles into the evaluation and management of the injured athlete, the sports medicine practitioner is armed with a thorough, organized system upon which to rely in acute situations. Constant refocusing on the basic principles of airway, breathing, and circulatory management with continued respect for occult cervical spine injury, can prevent a myriad of oversights and errors that could occur in the emergent setting.

ADVANCE PREPARATION

The initial step in managing any athletic emergency occurs before an event takes place. Advance preparation is essential to the adequate management of any emergent situation. This involves individual preparation, provision of adequate facilities and supplies, appropriate personnel, coordination between event and health care personnel and facilities, previous rehearsal of common or serious situations, and periodic review and reassessment. Failure to prepare sufficiently places one at a disadvantage when a potential emergency does occur.

UNIVERSAL PRECAUTIONS AND IMMUNIZATION

The first step in the preparation for any athletic event should occur long before the first practice or game is even contemplated. A thorough review and update of universal precautions protocol and of the immunization status of each health care worker should be performed. Universal precautions in the prevention of disease due to bloodborne pathogens is the first line of defense in the prevention of these serious occupational risks to the health care provider.[9] Detailed guidelines exist for procedural protocols for the wide array of situations encountered on a daily basis by the health care provider in the routine and emergent administration of care to infirm or injured individuals. In addition to these protocols, immunization schedules for hepatitis B, tetanus, MMR (measles, mumps, and rubella) and influenza for health care workers have been issued.[9] Hepatitis B vaccine should be offered to all individuals on the sports medicine team. All adults should receive a tetanus-diphtheria booster at least once every 10 years. The complete series of combined tetanus-diphtheria toxoid should be given to patients who have not received the primary series. MMR vaccine should be administered to all individuals born after 1956 who lack evidence of immunity to measles. Also, although it carries no "universal" approval, it is our practice to offer influenza vaccine to all members of the sports medicine health care team.

FACILITIES

The facility at which an athletic event takes place needs to be inspected prior to every contest. Incumbent within this inspection is a thorough evaluation of field condition, weather conditions, where appropriate, and crowd composition. A detailed analysis of on-site medical capabilities and local and regional medical facilities must be reviewed prior to each game with all visiting team medical personnel. Also included is emergency vehicle route access, location and access to emergency equipment, location and training of emergency personnel, location and instruction on emergency communication devices, and any peculiarities in field layout and/or crowd contingencies.

The facilities hosting the athletic event must have communication available with a local hospital. The ideal situation is a direct phone line from the event site to the hospital emergency department, which should be unencumbered by other uses. The medical and surgical capabilities of the hospital must be fully addressed. If there are inadequate medical facilities locally, plans must be established for the transportation of the injured athlete to a more definitive care facility. Specifically, the medical coverage team must have access to a medical center with the neurosurgical capability to manage life-threatening focal and diffuse brain injuries, as well as spine injuries. Intensive care facilities should be sufficient to provide the level of care required for a critically injured patient, with immediate cardiac and orthopaedic care available.

There should be an established plan for transporting injured athletes both to the local facility and to a more distant facility if warranted by the situation. Emergency medical services (EMS) availability should be determined, addressing response time to the event site and the level of emergency medical services required on site, if any. Obviously, all sports do not require the same medical coverage. The degree of preparation and resources available depend on the nature of the sport, the size of the crowd attending the event, and state regulations. These facilities and plans need to be re-evaluated on a periodic basis to ensure their continued adequacy. There is no standardized schedule for this evaluation, but an annual reassessment of all emergency care provisions is recommended.

PERSONNEL

A designated team leader must be identified. Often, this is the team physician or head trainer. He or she is the person ultimately responsible for the immediate care of the injured athlete and serves to coordinate and direct the response of the medical care team. Baseline knowledge of CPR and basic life support is a must. For contact and collision sports, and sports where crowd size is an issue, ACLS and ATLS certification are mandatory. In addition, periodic proficiency testing with these protocols should be carried out to ensure the adequacy of the on-field responses of the team leader.

The medical personnel working with the team leader should all be certified in CPR and basic life support. In addition, they should have working knowledge and proficiency in the appropriate transport of the injured athlete.[10] The medical personnel working under the direction of the team leader should be a coherent, smoothly operating team. They should be well versed in the management of common scenarios. In addition, through a thorough knowledge of the epidemiology of sports-specific injury patterns, they should have the capability of managing any catastrophic injury that may occur.

EQUIPMENT

The equipment present at an event varies with the type of athletic occasion and should include the items listed in the box on the following page. A collision, "high-risk" sport such as football has different requirements than does a noncontact, "low-risk" sport such as tennis. Therefore, an accurate inventory of equipment suitable for all sports would be cumbersome. Preparedness, however, implies the availability of requisite supplies to manage common minor injuries, equipment necessary for basic and advanced cardiac life support, and supplies for spinal and extremity stabilization. If there is an ambulance at the event, much of this equipment can be found there. If not, it is incumbent on the physician or the institution to provide it.

ETHICAL AND LEGAL ASPECTS OF ATHLETIC EVENT COVERAGE

Sports medicine as a specialty is growing in popularity and practice. The advancement of preventive, surgical, and rehabilitative techniques has enhanced societal expectations. Because of this, when unexpected injury occurs, concern may be raised that some form of malpractice has occurred. Therefore, individuals providing medical care at athletic events must be cognizant of their role and function as caregivers. Caregivers may be spectators who volunteer their services for an injured player, volunteers who provide service for a school or institution, employees of the institution involved in the athletic event, or private contractors hired by the institution for episodic event coverage.[11] Although liability is present in any of these situations, the caregiver is held to different standards.

Liability occurs when a caregiver fails to exercise the knowledge, skill, and due care of a reasonably competent practitioner in the same class, acting in the same or similar circumstances. In addition, in circumstances in which caregivers are acting as a "Good Samaritan," they are not free from responsibility for their actions. Many states, however, have enacted Good Samaritan legislation that encourages medical and paramedical personnel to come to the aid of an injured or ill individual and, in those circumstances, the caregiver is not held to the same standard of care as with medical malpractice. Rather, the caregiver is held to the standard of avoiding gross negligence.[11]

Malpractice standards such as duty, breach of duty, standard of care, and negligence apply to sports medicine. There are some features of this relationship, however, that are unique to sports medicine. If the caregiver is the hired employee of an institution, there may be conflict between the caregiver's responsibilities to the athlete and those to the institution, creating an ethical and legal dilemma. It is important to note that from a legal standpoint the caregiver's duties are to the athlete, and not to the institution.[12] This is further emphasized in the American Medical Association's *Guide to Ethics*, which states that

> The professional responsibility of the physician who serves in a medical capacity at an athletic contest or sporting event is to protect the health and safety of the contestants. The desire of spectators, promoters of the event, or even the injured athlete that he or she should not be removed from the contest should not be controlling. The physician's judgment should be governed only by medical considerations.[13]

Athletes at different levels have differing abilities to participate in the decision making regarding their

EMERGENCY MEDICAL SUITE EQUIPMENT LIST

EQUIPMENT

Airway Management

Nasal airways—26, 28, 30 mm (two each)
Oral airways—3, 4, 5, 6 (two each)
Oxygen tank with mask and cannula
Bag valve mask
Endotracheal tubes—6, 5, 7.0, 7.5, 8.0 mm
Laryngoscope with blades and stylet
10-ml syringe
Bulb suction syringe
Surgilube, three packs

IV Fluid Management

IV catheters, 14 to 20 g (two each)
IV tubing set (two)
IV fluid, D5/lactated Ringer's (4 liters)

Spine Immobilization

Spine board
Stretcher
Cervical collar
Sand bags
Razor knife
Vacuum spine splint

Splinting and Bandaging

Splints
Slings
Crutches
Knee immobilizer
Ace bandages
Sterile gauze pads
Adhesive bandages
Adhesive tape, 1 inch wide
Kling

Surgical Equipment

Alcohol swabs
Betadine swabs
Hemostats
Suture kits, two-inch
Steristrips ¼-inch, ⅛-inch (six each)
Needles—18, 22, 25-gauge (six each)
Scalpels, disposable—10, 11 (two each)
Syringes—tuberculosis, 3, 5, 10, 50 ml

Examination Equipment

Stethoscope
Blood pressure cuff
Thermometer
Tongue blades
Tape measure
Reflex hammer
Otoscope, ophthalmoscope
Penlight
Eye chart

Miscellaneous

Scissors
Blankets
Ice
Q-tips
Ice bags

MEDICATIONS

Cardiac Medications

Atropine, 2-mg syringe
Epinephrine 1:1000, 2-mg syringe
Sublingual nitroglycerin (NTG), 0.4 mg
Lidocaine

Antiallergic Asthmatic Meds

Benadryl, 25-, 50-mg capsules
Epipen
Albuterol inhaler

Anti-Inflammatories

Ibuprofen, 600-mg tablets
Toradol, 30-, 60-mg injectable

Local Anesthetics

Lidocaine, 1%
Lidocaine, 1% with epinephrine
Marcaine, 0.5%

Pain Medications

Tylenol tablets
Morphine sulfate
Naloxone
Tylenol, no. 3 tablets
Demerol

---

return to play. Professional athletes may be given more latitude in sharing the risk regarding return to play. Therefore, their injuries may be treated less conservatively than a high school player with a similar injury. Implicit in this assumption is that the risk and benefit of return to play are clearly laid out for the athlete and no information is withheld. Failure to inform the athlete of potential long-term risks places the caregiver at significant malpractice risk.[12] The caregiver also remains responsible for the examination and assessment, even if athletes take the risk of competition on themselves.[11]

Conversely, athletes under the age of 18 require parental consent for medical care to be provided. It is essential that parental consent be obtained prior to the treatment of all but emergent injuries. The care provider for high school athletes must also realize that the athlete has less to gain by early return to competition than does the professional athlete, often has less ability to make medically appropriate decisions, and has less support should a permanent injury be sustained. It is the responsibility of the caregiver to treat underage athletes more conservatively and paternalistically.[12]

In summary, the legal and ethical responsibilities of medical personnel at athletic events vary with the situation. The overriding principles are *premum non cere* (first, do no harm) and a responsibility to the health and well-being of the athlete. The caregiver must develop field assessment competence, which requires the proper application of injury care and diagnostic principles to reduce morbidity and avoid unnecessary harm.

GUIDING PRINCIPLES IN EMERGENCY MANAGEMENT

Prioritization of assessment and subsequent management of the injured athlete is based on the extent and mechanism of injury. A rapid primary evaluation, followed by a more detailed secondary assessment, establishes treatment priorities and direct, definitive care. Distractions peculiar to the athletic setting, such as crowd noise, inclement weather, and interference from players and coaches, make it essential to follow established protocols. Assessment and treatment sequences are often carried out simultaneously.[8]

PRIMARY SURVEY

The primary survey can be broken down into five basic components represented by the mnemonic *ABCDE*:[8]

A, airway maintenance with cervical spine control

B, breathing and ventilation

C, circulation, hemorrhage control

D, disability, neurologic status

E, exposure

It is important to understand that the primary survey must be carried out with little or no movement of the injured athlete. Movement of the injured athlete prior to adequate cervical spine stabilization places the athlete at grave risk for catastrophic spinal cord damage.

The secondary survey logically follows the findings of the primary survey. In addition, the secondary survey is predicated on the clinical stability of the patient.

AIRWAY

The approach to the injured athlete is initiated by stabilizing the cervical spine of the injured athlete in the position found and asking "How are you?" The athlete's response provides important insight into airway patency and neurologic status. If the patient does not respond, one begins the assessment with an evaluation of the airway. The airway evaluation is initiated by looking, listening, and feeling for spontaneous respirations. Initial attempts to establish a patent airway include only the chin lift or jaw thrust maneuver.[8] If there are airway concerns in a prone athlete, the athlete should be logrolled to a face-up position. A team leader should stabilize the head and direct all move-

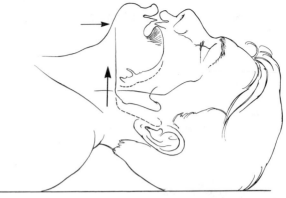

FIGURE 33–1. Chin lift procedure. The fingers are placed under the mandible (*small arrow*) and the jaw is lifted anteriorly (*large arrow*).

ments of the injured athlete. *An athlete with trauma to the clavicle or higher should be considered to have a cervical spine injury until proved otherwise.* In the airway management of an injured player with suspected cervical spine injury in sports such as hockey, lacrosse, and football, in which helmet and face mask use is required, the medical staff should avoid removing the helmet from the player, if at all possible. Proper management involves removing the face mask with a razor knife and instituting basic airway management protocols.

Basic airway management procedures include the chin lift and/or jaw thrust procedures. In the unconscious athlete, the tongue may prolapse backward and obstruct the hypopharynx. This simple obstruction can be corrected by the following maneuvers. The chin lift procedure is performed by placing the fingers of one hand under the mandible and gently lifting upward to bring the chin anterior (Fig. 33–1). The thumb of the same hand lightly depresses the lower lip to open the mouth. The thumb may also be placed behind the lower incisors. The chin lift maneuver should not hyperextend the neck. The jaw thrust maneuver is correctly performed by grasping the angles of the lower jaw, one hand on each side, and displacing the mandible forward (Fig. 33–2).

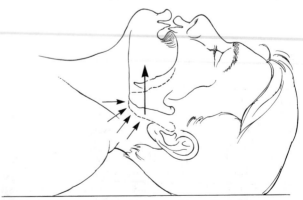

FIGURE 33–2. Jaw thrust procedure. The fingers are placed under the lower jaw (*small arrows*) and the jaw is displaced forward (*large arrow*).

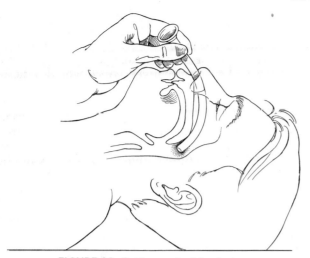

FIGURE 33–3. Nasotracheal intubation.

Advanced airway intervention techniques must be used with the understanding that the patient may have a cervical spine injury. Altered consciousness is the single most frequent indication for oral endotracheal intubation.[8] Trauma to the face, head, and neck, as well as anaphylaxis with actual compromise of the airway lumen, are other indications for advanced airway intervention. If there is immediate need for airway intervention and if the athlete is breathing, nasotracheal intubation should be attempted (Fig. 33–3). Oral endotracheal intubation (Fig. 33–4) should only be used in the unconscious patient because of the propensity to stimulate the gag reflex, causing vomiting and the risk of aspiration.[8]

Injuries that cause airway obstruction and subsequent disruption of normal anatomy are usually the result of high-velocity impact. Such maxillofacial injuries preclude the use of basic and/or advanced airway management techniques. Therefore, it is necessary to use surgical airway intervention in the emergent management of such injuries. Inability to intubate the trachea, however, is the only indication for creating a surgical airway. The least invasive surgical airway intervention is needle cricothyroidotomy, which is accomplished by palpating the cricothyroid membrane and puncturing the skin with a 14-gauge catheter over needle through the cricothyroid membrane, directed 45 degrees caudad. Aspiration of air signifies entry into the lumen. Surgical cricothyroidotomy is performed by making a skin incision over the cricothyroid membrane and extending through the membrane. A curved hemostat may be inserted to dilate the opening, and a small endotracheal tube or tracheostomy tube may be inserted. It is important to understand that the cricoid cartilage is the only circumferential support to the upper trachea.[8] In children under 12 years of age, this procedure is not recommended due to the risk of damaging this structure.

BREATHING

Once the athlete's airway is established, one must assess for spontaneous respiration. If there is no evidence of spontaneous respiration, assisted ventilation should be started, such as mouth to mouth, mouth to mask, or use of a bag valve device. During ventilation, the patient should always be assessed for adequate rise and fall of the chest with respiration and for bilaterality of breath sounds. In the intubated patient, the most common cause of unequal breath sounds is an endotracheal tube inserted into a mainstem bronchus (usually the right mainstem bronchus, because the angle of inclination from the trachea is less acute than the left). Three specific conditions that can compromise ventilation are tension pneumothorax, open pneumothorax, and large flail chest with pulmonary contusion. One must remember that assisted ventilation alone can predispose an individual to tension pneumothorax if excessive inspiratory pressures are used.

CIRCULATION

Evaluation of circulatory competency begins with the evaluation of state of consciousness, skin color, and pulse. If blood volume is reduced by 50 percent or more, cerebral perfusion may be critically impaired and unconsciousness results. Patients with pink skin, especially in the face and extremities, are rarely critically hypovolemic following injury. An ash-gray skin color of the face and extremities, however, usually indicates a blood loss of at least 30 percent.[8] Evaluation of the central pulse initially, and subsequently the femoral and carotid pulses, also yields valuable information about volemic status (Table 33–2). If there is a palpable carotid pulse, it indicates that the systolic blood pressure is at least 60 mm Hg. A femoral pulse becomes palpable at approximately 70 mm Hg. If the radial pulse is palpable, systolic pressure is at least 80 mm Hg. Femoral and/or

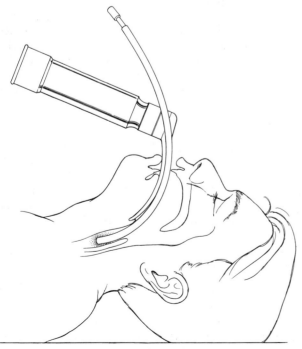

FIGURE 33–4. Oral endotracheal intubation.

TABLE 33–2
Pulse Points and Correlating Systolic Pressures

Pulse Point	Minimal Systolic Blood Pressure (mm Hg)
Radial	80
Femoral	70
Carotid	60

carotid pulses signify at least 50 percent of a residual blood volume. If a carotid pulse is absent, CPR should be initiated.

The quality of a palpable pulse is also valuable in the initial assessment. A rapid, weak, thready pulse is indicative of tenuous volume status. If time permits, evaluation of capillary refill in the nail beds is also of some assistance.

DISABILITY (NEUROLOGIC)

The next step in the primary survey is to make a rough, thorough assessment of the injured athlete's global neurologic status as quickly as possible (Table 33–3). Our preferred method when assessing level of responsiveness in the injured athlete is to use a modification of the AVPU scale. In this scale, *A* refers to alert, *V* indicates that the patient is responsive to verbal stimuli, *P* applies to the individual who is responsive only to painful stimuli, and *U* means the person is unresponsive. (The addition of *A* for the assessment of pupillary size and reactivity completes the modified scale.)

The neurologic evaluation during the primary survey is merely meant as a quick screen for gross assessment of the degree of central neurologic impairment. *An injured athlete who is only responsive to painful stimuli, has unequal pupils or pupils minimally responsive to light or accommodation, warrants immediate, appropriate transfer.* A thorough neurologic evaluation should be undertaken during the secondary survey. The primary neurologic survey serves the same purpose as the remainder of the primary survey—that is, to identify problems that are immediately life-threatening and to initiate therapy.

EXPOSURE

The final step of the primary survey is the most commonly overlooked. It involves full exposure of the injured athlete's body and a careful search for occult

TABLE 33–3
Modified AAVPU Scale

A—Alert
A—Assess Pupils
V—responsive to Verbal Stimuli
P—responsive to Painful Stimuli
U—Unresponsive

pathology. This is obviously most important in the unresponsive patient. It is also best performed off the playing surface. The examiner should have a high index of suspicion for subtle dermatologic, vascular, orthopaedic, and neurologic changes, which would indicate undetected pathology.

The overriding purpose of the on-field evaluation is to initiate emergent treatment and to establish transport protocols. Whereas treatment protocols are continuously re-evaluated and updated based on the clinical presentation of the injured athlete, the decision on the viability and method of transport is often based on information initially gained from the primary survey. It is necessary for the health care provider to ensure that the method of transport is appropriate for the current status of the injured athlete. In addition, although the entire primary and secondary survey can be more effectively performed away from the distractions that occur on the athletic field, it is not implied that emergent evaluation and resuscitations should wait until the patient is transferred into the training room. However, arrangements should be made early in the assessment to transfer the patient from the playing surface and, in the case of the seriously injured athlete, transfer to a hospital should be arranged as soon as possible.

Once the primary survey is completed and resuscitation of the patient is underway, the secondary survey takes place. This is a more deliberate evaluation of each body region or system. The various aspects of the secondary survey are discussed later.

NEUROLOGIC INJURIES

The specter of neurologic trauma should be anticipated in any sport. Although the frequency of severe central or peripheral nervous system injury is low, their varied presentation often makes these injuries the most difficult to evaluate and manage. Rapid and concise evaluation is the key to preventing neurologic morbidity from developing into mortality. It is incumbent on the health care team to provide for the proper care and transport of the neurologically injured athlete through meticulous prior planning.

INTRACRANIAL INJURIES

Intracranial injuries can be broken down into focal and diffuse brain injuries.[14] Focal injuries are thought of as causing a large amount of damage in a small area. Diffuse brain injuries are thought of as causing less damage but in a more widespread distribution.

FOCAL BRAIN INJURIES

Intracranial hemorrhage is the leading cause of death from head injuries in athletes.[16] There are four types of intracranial hemorrhage: epidural hematoma, subdural hematoma, intracerebral hematoma, and subarachnoid hemorrhage. The most dangerous of these expanding intracranial lesions is the epidural hematoma. Epidural hematomas are frequently caused by blows to the temporal region of the skull, causing laceration of the middle meningeal artery and rapid accumulation of blood in the epidural space. These lesions can be fatal within 30 to 60 minutes. A lucid interval (period of consciousness) is classically described with epidural hematomas, but need not occur. One third of patients with epidural hematomas presents with a lucid interval, one third does not experience unconsciousness until a period of time after the injury, and one third displays a persistent loss of consciousness from the moment of impact. Left untreated, the expanding epidural hematoma results in compression and shift of the brain, compression of the brainstem, coma, and death. Because there is theoretically no damage to the brain itself with the injury, rapid neurosurgical evacuation of the hematoma is lifesaving and curative.

Subdural hematomas most commonly result from acceleration or deceleration forces tearing the bridging veins and/or laceration of the small arteries within the subdural space.[16] Subdural hematomas commonly accumulate more slowly than epidural hematomas but, in the acute situation, symptoms produced are usually related to the region of the brain in which they occur.[17]

The fourth type of intracerebral bleed that can be encountered in the athlete is the subarachnoid hemorrhage in the subarachnoid space. It is commonly caused by hemorrhage of tiny surface vessels and is similar to a contusion. It can also be caused by rupture of an aneurysm or arteriovenous malformation.

DIFFUSE BRAIN INJURIES

The most common diffuse cerebral injury encountered is the concussion. Concussions vary in severity from a minor "ding" or "bell ringer," which frequently does not even come to medical attention,[18] to concussions that lead to coma and cardiorespiratory arrest. Different grading systems have been developed in an attempt to assess the severity of injury in athletes with concussion. Torg and colleagues have proposed a system with six grades of cerebral concussion based on clinical symptomatology (Table 33–4).[21] Grade I injuries are characterized by confusion and mild unsteadiness, but there is no aspect of antegrade or retrograde amnesia. Symptoms usually clear in 5 to 15 minutes, and

athletes can be permitted to return to competition, with close observation, once they are fully asymptomatic. Grade II concussions have confusion and antegrade amnesia, meaning amnesia pertaining to events since the injury without loss of consciousness. Grade II injuries and above are indications for removal from competition. Grade III concussions are characterized by retrograde amnesia without loss of consciousness. Grade IV concussions involve the player who has been knocked unconscious. Assuming that the patient is breathing spontaneously, the only immediate management is to immobilize the cervical spine and transport the patient from the field on a rigid backboard. Usually, the unconsciousness clears in a matter of a few seconds, but persistence of the unconscious state for several minutes or other signs of neurologic decompensation are grounds for immediate transfer to a hospital with neurosurgical services. Regardless of rapidity of return of consciousness, observation in the hospital should be strongly considered. Grade V concussions involve paralytic coma and possible cardiorespiratory arrest. Basic life support measures should be instituted immediately. Athletes with grade VI concussions are those who do not survive the cardiopulmonary arrest.

Of the six grades of concussions, the only grade that permits return to competition in a collision sport that day is the grade I concussion. In such a case, it is with careful observation, serial evaluation, and repeated questioning regarding the development of symptoms.

Cantu[20] has also described a grading scale for concussions that is based on the length of time of unconsciousness (Table 33–5). A grade I (mild) concussion is associated with no loss of consciousness and post-traumatic amnesia of less than 30 minutes. A grade 2 (moderate) concussion features either a loss of consciousness of less than 5 minutes or post-traumatic amnesia of more than 30 minutes. A grade 3 (severe) concussion is defined by loss of consciousness of greater than 5 minutes or post-traumatic amnesia of greater than 24 hours. Based on this grading scale, Cantu has developed a return to competition scale.[20]

FIELD EVALUATION AND MANAGEMENT OF CLOSED HEAD INJURIES

General concepts vital to the appropriate care of the individual with a closed head injury include adequate

TABLE 33–4
Torg Concussion Classification

Grade	Confusion	Amnesia	Loss of Consciousness	Return to Play
I	Yes	None	None	Asymptomatic
II	Yes	Antegrade	None	No
III	Yes	Antegrade, retrograde	None	No
IV	Yes	None	Transient	No
V	N/A	N/A	Coma	No
VI	N/A	N/A	Death	

From Torg JS (ed): Athletic Injuries to the Head, Neck and Face, 2nd ed. St. Louis, Mosby–Year Book, 1991, 225–231.

TABLE 33–5
Cantu Concussion Grading Scale

Grade	Loss of Consciousness	Post-Traumatic Amnesia
I	No	<30 min
II	<5 min	>30 min
III	>5 min	>24 hr

Return to Play*

	First Concussion	Second Concussion
I	Same game when asymptomatic	After 2 wk when asymptomatic × 1 wk
II	After asymptomatic, 1 wk	Minimum 1 month, asymptomatic 1 wk
III	Minimum 1 month, asymptomatic × 1 wk	Terminate season

From Stenger A: Keeping concussions from being fatal. Phys Sports Med 1992;20:54–55.
*A third concussion within one season, regardless of severity, is cause to terminate an athlete's season.

preparation (see earlier). There should be a team leader ultimately making decisions. There should be adequate equipment available to evaluate, immobilize, and transport the patient properly. There should be a treatment facility available that has neurosurgical and intensive care unit capabilities, and there should be rapid transportation readily available to this institution. Finally, the medical staff should be well rehearsed in anticipation of this type of catastrophic injury. *Because of the infrequent nature of this type of injury, general experience is insufficient preparation for the event, and rehearsal of the various situations is vital.* One must always remain cognizant of the ABCs in caring for these patients. Depending on the degree of injury, the athlete may be facing complete cardiorespiratory failure; therefore, *a*irway, *b*reathing, and *c*irculation need to be repeatedly assessed.

The initial on-field evaluation of a patient with a head injury involves assessing the level of responsiveness in a similar manner to that stated earlier (see Guiding Principles in Emergency Management). *Athletes who are unresponsive are considered to have a cervical spine injury.* They should have their cervical spine immobilized and be moved as stated earlier. With responsive athletes, questions about symptoms related to the cervical spine should be asked. If the athlete has no neck pain, numbness, weakness, or paresthesias in the extremities, one can move on to assessing cerebral function. Specifically, it is important to note the athlete's facial expression, orientation to time, place, and person, any evidence of amnesia, either antegrade or retrograde, and gait.[19] Once on the sideline, a complete neurologic assessment is performed involving full assessment of mental status, cranial nerve, motor, sensory, and deep tendon reflexes, and cerebellar function. Any focal signs elicited on neurologic testing, severe headaches, altered level of consciousness, or seizures should prompt

immediate transfer to a hospital with neurosurgical services for a computed tomography (CT) scan of the head.

If an athlete has persistent unconsciousness or rapidly deteriorating neurologic function, it may be incumbent on the supervising medical team to initiate therapy. With the realization that definitive therapy for mass lesions within the cranium is neurosurgical, steps are taken to decrease intracranial pressure. Ideally, the athlete should be intubated to assist in mild hyperventilation, but even if intubation supplies are unavailable, protection of the airway is vital. Adequate circulating volume should be maintained as much as possible, with blood pressure maintained within normal ranges. Situations that increase pressure in the head are to be avoided, including tight dressings around the neck and the Trendelenburg position. Hypotonic fluids increase cerebral edema and are to be avoided. Medications that can be used include furosemide, 20 to 40 mg IV, and mannitol, 50 to 100 g IV. These medications are used for their diuretic effect, with the intent of diminishing intracerebral water.[15]

CERVICAL SPINE INJURIES

Injuries to the cervical spine can result in a number of different spinal cord syndromes (Table 33–6). This is due in part to the isolated or combined involvement of bony, disc, ligamentous, and/or cord anatomic structures. Different causes have been postulated for the catastrophic neck injuries that can occur in athletes. Among these are hyperflexion, hyperextension, and rotational injuries.[21] It has been demonstrated, however, that axial loading is the predominant force that creates catastrophic spine injuries. With the neck flexed to approximately 30 degrees, cervical lordosis is lost, with the spine becoming a segmented column. When an axial load is applied with the neck in this position, the head is abruptly stopped on contact while the body continues. This compresses the cervical spine between the decelerating head and the body. The primary dissipation of force is through compression. With the spine's ability to dissipate the compressive force exceeded, it ultimately fails in the flexion mode.[21] Fracture, subluxation, or unilateral or bilateral facet dislocation can occur.

FIELD EVALUATION AND MANAGEMENT

The single most important evaluation and management point to remember is to suspect that a cervical spine injury exists. Therefore, the first procedure is to immobilize the head and neck immediately in a *neutral position* (see Chapter 21). At this time, airway breathing and circulation surveys can be rapidly performed. Subsequently, level of consciousness determinations can be made. *No attempt should be made to remove the helmet or chin strap of any injured athlete suspected of having a cervical spine injury.* At this time, the face mask can be rapidly removed by cutting through the plastic stays that hold it to the helmet. This procedure is preferred at this time, because it allows subsequent airway management if the athlete deteriorates. After initial assessment and stabilization of airway, breathing, and circulation, the neurologic status can be evaluated, including examination of the following: consciousness, withdrawal to pain, pupillary response, posturing, muscle tone, and/or weakness. If any significant abnormalities are found, the patient should be immediately transported.

If the athlete is found in the prone position, he or she must be logrolled to the face-up position and onto a spine board. This is a delicate procedure and should not be performed unless adequate, trained, coordinated personnel are present.

A medical support–athlete positioning team can be made up with as few as four to preferably six individuals. The team leader, positioned at the head, always gives commands and stabilizes the head and neck by applying slight traction. Three team members are positioned to roll the athlete toward themselves. One is positioned at the shoulder, one at the hip, and one at the knee. They must maintain the body in line with the head and spine during the roll. Another team member should be present with a razor knife to remove the face mask rapidly if this is indicated. In addition, this person should be familiar with intubation techniques if they are needed. The sixth team member is responsible for transporting medical supplies and assisting in transport of the athlete. Once the athlete has been moved or positioned in the face-up position, evaluation and management techniques are instituted.

PERIPHERAL NEUROLOGIC INJURIES

When an athlete presents during competition with neurologic symptoms, the health care practitioner must distinguish the minor blow from a potentially disastrous injury that would prohibit return to competition. The usual differential is between the common "burner" and the uncommon cervical spine injury. Certain findings are helpful in distinguishing the two. If the athlete has any bilaterality or involvement of the lower extremities with the symptoms, the extremities should be immobilized with the suspicion of an unstable cervical spine injury.[22] In the absence of such symptoms, the presence of significant neck pain or tenderness to palpation over the cervical spine indicates the need for immobilization. If the neck is nontender, a complete motor and sensory neurologic examination is performed. If a focal deficit is noted, the athlete is immobilized. In light of a normal neurologic examination, a full examination of the cervical spine is undertaken, testing active and resisted range of motion. If there is marked cervical spasm, loss of range of motion, or pain with examination, the athlete is immobilized. In their absence, the athlete can be permitted to move without restriction and should be re-examined every 5 minutes. Return to competition is prohibited until symptoms have completely resolved.

The most common peripheral nerve injury encountered in contact sports is the burner syndrome, so-named because of the circumferential burning sensation felt in one arm and hand (Table 33–6). Different causes for this syndrome have been proposed,[23] including traction on the brachial plexus, commonly occurring in a defensive football player who is shoulder tackling. In this situation, the tackler's shoulder is driven caudally and the neck is laterally bent away from the shoulder.[24] This places traction on the ipsilateral brachial plexus, especially the upper trunk. Another explanation is direct compression on the brachial plexus at Erb's point, thereby compressing the upper trunk and creating symptoms.

A nerve injury classification system has been developed that can be applied to brachial plexus injuries (Table 33–7).[23,25] The mildest nerve lesion is neuropraxia, which involves demyelination of the nerve without axonal injury. Conduction is blocked at the site of the lesion, but repair is rapid, usually within 3 weeks.

TABLE 33–6
Comparison of Spinal Cord Syndromes and Brachial Plexus Injuries

Syndrome	Pathology	Motor loss	Sensory loss	Prognosis
Central cord	Ischemia of central cord	Upper to lower	None	Good
Burning hands	Variant of central chord	None	Bilateral paresthesias	Good (transient changes)
Anterior cord	Anterior two thirds (distribution of anterior spinal artery)	Loss below lesion	Pain and temporary loss below lesion	Poor
Brown-Séquard	Hemitransection of cord	Ipsilateral	Contralateral pain and temporary loss	Poor
Posterior cord	Posterior third (distribution of posterior spinal artery—rare)	None	Dorsal column function	
Burner	Brachial plexus	Dependent on degree peripheral nerve damage	Unilateral, upper extremity only	Good (usually transient)

TABLE 33–7
Brachial Plexus Injury Classification

Grade				
Clancy	Seddon	Sunderland[25]	Pathology	Duration
I	Neuropraxia	I	Incomplete block, axon intact	Seconds to weeks
II	Axonotmesis	II	Distal axon degeneration, endo-neurium, perineurium, epineurium intact	Weeks to months
III	Neurotmesis	III	Distal axon degeneration, perineurium, epineurium intact	Months to years
		IV	Distal axon degeneration, epineurium intact	
		V	Nerve transection	

Axonotmesis is the next level of nerve injury; histologically, there is preservation of the epineurium. Wallerian degeneration occurs, and the entire distal axon degenerates. The intact epineurium, however, permits axonal regeneration, but the nerve is not functional until the entire axon is regenerated. The most severe nerve injury is neurotmesis, corresponding to complete nerve laceration or crush injury and resulting in disruption of the endoneurium. With complete disruption of the nerve and its sheath, nerve regeneration is rarely possible, with permanent loss of nerve function.

Clancy has developed a classification of burner injuries that corresponds with Seddon's nerve injury classification.[23] In addition, Sunderland has further expounded on the classification of burner syndromes and has associated those with the neurologic pathology that has occurred.[25] Clancy's grade I, II, and III injuries correlate with Seddon's neuropraxia, axonotmesis, and neurotmesis. Sunderland has further delineated the Clancy grade III-Seddon axonotomesis injuries into three further subdivisions of axonal injury. Grade I injuries show partial or complete conduction block. In addition, at the time of injury, there may be limited or no physiologic function. The axon and endoneurium are intact, and symptoms may last from several seconds up to 2 weeks. Grade II injuries exhibit motor and often sensory abnormalities persisting at 2 weeks. Electromyography (EMG) testing shows abnormalities at 3 to 4 weeks. Anatomically, the endoneurium, perineurium, and epineurium are intact. There is distal axonal and/or wallerian degeneration. Demyelination occurs secondarily to this. The duration of symptomatology can be weeks to months.

Clancy and Seddon have only one classification for neurotmesis, but Sunderland further subdivides these grade III injuries. According to Sunderland, grade III injuries all show axonal degeneration, but the perineurium and epineurium are intact. In Sunderland's grade IV injuries, only the epineurium is intact. In grade V injuries, there is complete nerve transection. Any grade III injury or higher has motor and sensory deficits at 1 year, with little or no evidence of improvement.

On-field examination of burners centers around their differentiation from cervical spine injuries. The motor examination is important, looking for weakness in any of the upper extremity muscles. Return to competition is prohibited as long as there are persistent sensory symptoms or abnormalities on neurologic examination.

One should always be aware of burning hands syndrome (see Table 33–7).[26] As the name implies, it is characterized by a burning sensation in both of the athlete's hands and is thought to be a variant of the central cord syndrome, selectively involving the fibers of the spinothalamic tract that supply pain and temperature to the upper limbs. Its bilaterality belies the lesion's location in the central cord—the more common burner or stinger is a peripheral lesion. Although the symptoms commonly resolve, they can be associated with both fractures and dislocations of the cervical spine, indicating a need to remove the athlete from competition and immobilize the cervical spine.

EYE, EAR, NOSE, AND THROAT

Injuries to the eyes, ears, nose, and throat (EENT) should be classified into soft tissue injuries, with or without involvement of the underlying bone or cartilage. Soft tissue injuries include injuries to the skin, subcutaneous tissue, muscle, nerves, and blood vessels. Each must therefore be considered when an injury is being evaluated.

OCULAR INJURIES

Ocular injuries are relatively frequent in sport, accounting for 1.5 percent of all sport injuries, but fortunately they are usually minor.[27] High-risk sports include those that involve high-speed balls or projectiles, or sticks or bats, or high levels of contact, such as baseball, racket sports, hockey, lacrosse, basketball, football, soccer, and volleyball. Extremely high-risk sports include combative sports such as boxing or martial arts.[28] The key to the successful outcome of an eye injury in sports is the performance of a thorough eye examination, followed by appropriate therapy or referral.

EXAMINATION

Although a complete eye examination requires equipment that cannot be kept on the field, a thorough on-field examination can screen out serious conditions that preclude return to competition and require further evaluation. The athlete's symptoms provide a significant amount of information regarding the severity of the injury. Loss or blurring of vision, boring or throbbing pain, photophobia, and diplopia are all disturbing symptoms. Their persistence should preclude return to play and trigger prompt, complete evaluation of the eye.

On-field examination of the eye begins with visual acuity testing. This is the single most important aspect of an eye examination. It can be done with any object—for example, finger, tongue blade, or penlight. Decreased visual acuity suggests pathology of the refractive apparatus, opacification of the ocular media, or injury to neurologic structures. Conjugate eye movement is determined by the symmetry of extraocular movements and the pupillary light reflex. Careful inspection of the eye is directed toward findings that suggest serious injury. Eyelids that are tensely swollen, ecchymotic, and preclude visualization of the eye may be indicative of severe injury. Eyelids that do not open spontaneously should not be forced open, risking further injury to the eye.[29] Extraocular movements should be fully assessed, and loss of movement in any direction is concerning. Loss of upward gaze is associated with orbital blowout fractures caused by entrapment of the inferior rectus or inferior oblique muscles.[30] Examination of the globe itself is done to look for evidence of forward displacement of the eye (exophthalmos) or posterior displacement of the eye (enophthalmos), as well as other evidence of significant trauma, such as lacerations or hemorrhages. Other ominous findings include irregularity or asymmetry of the pupils, blood in the anterior chamber (hyphema), or protrusion of uvea through the iris or sclera.[29] A funduscopic examination seeks evidence of papilledema or retinal abnormalities.

When faced with the question of whether the player can return to competition, several questions need to be answered. First, there should be none of the findings listed that would lead the examiner to be concerned about a potentially severe eye injury. Athletes must demonstrate that they do not have symptoms that can jeopardize their health while competing. Visual acuity should be normal. The athlete's symptoms of burning, itching, or tearing must not cause lapses in concentration or impairment of vision. The athlete should not be sent out into competition with topical anesthetic in the eyes, compromising the ability to clear away foreign material from the eye routinely. If all of these criteria are met, the athlete may return to competition with careful observation.

SPECIFIC OCULAR INJURIES

Abrasions to the surface of the cornea are common injuries and present with pain, tearing, injection, and photophobia. The diagnosis is made by fluorescein staining of the eye after topical anesthetic is applied. The abraded area appears as an area of green fluorescence. Treatment is with topical antibiotics and a pressure patch on the eye. The athlete cannot return to competition with this injury.

Foreign bodies can occur on the cornea or the conjunctiva. Symptoms include the sensation of a foreign body present, tearing (epiphora), pain, and photophobia. Magnification and/or fluorescein staining may be necessary to rule out the presence of a foreign body. Both the upper and lower conjunctival recesses need to be carefully examined. The upper eyelid should be everted. The examination is often facilitated with the use of a short-acting anesthetic. Superficial foreign bodies can often be irrigated or wiped off the surface of the eye with a sterile cotton swab. More deeply embedded foreign bodies may need to be removed under the magnification of a slit lamp with a sterile spud. After the foreign body is removed, the eye is treated with topical antibiotics and a pressure patch, just as with a corneal abrasion.

Discrete areas of hemorrhage over the sclera are subconjunctival hemorrhages. They can be caused either by minor trauma or barotrauma, as with scuba divers. No specific treatment is required, and the lesions resolve spontaneously in 10 to 14 days.[27] Any associated findings such as blurred vision, pain, photophobia, limitation of extraocular movements, lid swelling, or hyphema are associated with more severe injury to the eye. These need to be investigated, because they may be associated with facial fractures and injuries to the globe.

Traumatic iritis is inflammation of the iris and is most commonly caused by blunt trauma to the eye. The presentation includes pain, photophobia, and tearing. Examination may unveil injection of the conjunctiva in the perilimbal area and constriction of the pupil. A follow-up slit-lamp examination should show cells and flare in the anterior chamber. Treatment is with topical cycloplegics to limit the discomfort caused by the ciliary spasm and with topical steroids to diminish the inflammation.

Eyelid lacerations can be potentially serious due to the structures located in the lids and because of the cosmetic importance of the eyelids. Examination includes assessment of the anatomic relationship of the lid margins, the anterior surface of the globe, and opening and closing capabilities. Referral to an ophthalmologist is mandatory for repair of lacerations of the lid margins, for lacerations of the medial aspect of the lower lid (canalicular damage may be present) or the upper lid (potential damage to the levator palpebrae superioris muscle), or for any deep lacerations of either lid. Importantly, forces that can cause laceration of the soft tissues around the eye can also cause significant damage to the eye itself, and must be looked for.

A traumatic hyphema is a collection of blood in the anterior chamber of the eye that usually results from blunt trauma, with laceration of the globe. Hyphemas have a 25 to 35 percent association with other serious eye injuries, such as blowout fractures, iridodialysis (disinsertion of the iris from the ciliary body), vitreous hemorrhage, retinal detachments, and globe rupture.[27,29] If the quantity of blood in the anterior chamber is insufficient to obstruct the visual axis, no visual acuity deficits result. Therefore, this test is unreliable. Specific examination of the anterior chamber must be performed. For this reason, the athlete needs to be seen by an ophthalmologist promptly.

Fractures of the inferior orbital wall (roof of the maxillary sinus), or blowout fractures, are classically caused by blunt trauma to the eye, which increases intraorbital pressure and blows out the inferior orbital wall without damaging the orbital rim.[30] Classic presentation of this injury is with the triad of diplopia in upward and outward gaze, enophthalmos, and infraorbital nerve numbness. Visual acuity should be assessed, symmetry of extraocular movement documented, and the globe examined for retroinferior displacement, which causes a relative ptosis of the involved eye. Less commonly, the fracture can occur in the medial wall of the orbit and not present with the same classic findings. Because this fracture communicates with the ethmoid air cells, the only symptom may be subcutaneous emphysema, either spontaneously or only when the patient blows the nose. With blowout fractures, a thorough examination of the involved eye is also necessary due to the likelihood of direct eye trauma. Radiographic evaluation includes lateral, Waters, Caldwell, and optic canal views of the eye,[30] with positive findings including clouding of the maxillary or ethmoid sinuses resulting from prolapse of soft tissue from the orbit. Plain radiographs are often negative, and tomography or CT scan may be necessary for better visualization of the fracture. Initial management includes systemic antibiotics to attempt to prevent an orbital cellulitis. There has been a move to more conservative management of these fractures. Some surgeons still operate immediately on all fractures associated with herniation of the contents of the globe, whereas others wait 5 to 10 days to assess the spontaneous resolution of diplopia.[29,30]

Direct injury to the eye can also disrupt the integrity of the globe itself. Just as lacerations can occur in the soft tissues about the eye, they can occur to the eye itself. Corneal and scleral lacerations are caused by sharp, penetrating trauma to the eye. Superficial lacerations may not require surgical repair, but radiographs may be needed to rule out an opaque intraocular foreign body. Any laceration associated with prolapse of the intraocular contents or loss of the anterior chamber requires rapid surgical repair.[29]

Blunt trauma can also compromise the globe, with rupture occurring most commonly at the weakest point of the sclera, beneath the insertion of the rectus muscles. The important point is that these sites are not readily visible and are commonly overlooked. Symptoms include pain and decreased vision in the eye; signs include diminished intraocular pressure, blood in the anterior or posterior chambers, and a deepening of the anterior chamber angle. This particular physical examination feature is often subtle. Immediate management of any injury that compromises the integrity of the globe includes covering the eye with a rigid protective

shield. When applying the shield, it is vital to ensure that the pressure points rest on the orbital rims, not on the globe itself. Immediate referral should be made for surgery.

Retinal trauma can also be caused by athletic injuries. Damage can range from edema to detachment of the retina and is seen most commonly in sports that create a significant risk for blunt trauma to the eye, such as boxing and the martial arts. Symptoms of retinal damage depend on the area of the retina that is injured. If the pathology is peripheral, there may be minimal symptoms or defects in visual fields. If the injury involves the macula, there is a profound effect on central vision. Retinal breaks and detachments are commonly accompanied by flashing lights and the abrupt appearances of "floaters" in the field of vision. There may be visual field cuts on examination, and abnormalities may be seen on direct ophthalmoscopy, although binocular-indirect ophthalmoscopy is more effective for detecting retinal pathology. As with the other serious eye injuries, the findings of retinal breaks or detachment require immediate referral to an ophthalmologist for surgical therapy.

Many of the eye injuries discussed present at the time of injury, but injuries such as post-traumatic iritis, glaucoma, or cataract can arise later. Although they are not noted in the on-field evaluation, they are important sequelae of ocular trauma. The caregiver who has continuity of care with the athlete needs to be on the alert for changes that may herald the development of any of these conditions.

MAXILLOFACIAL, EAR, NOSE, AND THROAT INJURIES

In the initial evaluation and therapy of injuries in the area of the face and neck, there are several principles to be remembered. First, injuries in this area have a high association with serious injuries of the head and cervical spine.[31] There is also an increased risk of airway obstruction due to bleeding, emesis, or foreign bodies if there is significant injury in the mouth. As with any other injury, the appropriate sequence of events must be followed in the evaluation of these injuries. Infection is also a significant risk with injuries in this area because of potential contamination with oral, nasal, or sinus flora. There is also notable risk for chondritis in injuries involving the cartilage of the nose and ear.[32]

In the evaluation of these injuries, a basic knowledge of facial anatomy is necessary, especially of important soft tissue structures that can be injured, particularly the branches of the facial nerve and the parotid duct.[31] The facial nerve exits from within the parotid glands bilaterally, ramifying into its branches. The temporal branch courses upward within 1 cm of the lateral aspect of the eyebrow on its way to the frontalis muscle, and severing the nerve leads to loss of function in the muscle and noticeable facial asymmetry. The zygomatic and buccal branches share a significant amount of cross-innervation in their supply of the central muscles of the face. The marginal mandibular branch travels downward and anteriorly along the mandible and innervates the muscles at the angle of the mouth—the depressor anguli oris, in particular. Severing this nerve causes significant asymmetry in smiling. The cervical branch supplies the platysma and is of no great clinical importance if cut. The parotid duct runs in a course that can be approximated by drawing a line from the tragus of the ear to the angle of the mouth, and it can be transected by lacerations in this area.

Evaluation of facial injuries begins with observation, looking for evidence of ecchymosis, swelling, lacerations, puncture wounds, abrasions, and asymmetry. Particular attention needs to be paid to findings that indicate potentially serious head trauma. These include clear cerebrospinal (CSF) fluid draining from the nose or ear, raccoon eyes, the Battle sign (postauricular ecchymosis), and blood from the ear. Ecchymosis and swelling in the face can direct the examiner to potential underlying injuries. Linear lacerations, puncture wounds, and abrasions should be thoroughly cleaned and inspected for the presence of foreign material. This is all that is necessary for abrasions, but consideration needs to be given to closing lacerations. Care must be taken to assess for damage to underlying soft tissue structures before repairing lacerations.

Injuries to the ear generally include lacerations, avulsions, and auricular hematomas.[31,32] Lacerations of the ear require meticulous cleansing because of the risk of chondritis. Even so, systemic antibiotics are often given after repair of an ear laceration to act as prophylaxis against chondritis. Partial and complete avulsions should be kept moist with sterile saline while the patient is referred for definitive care.

Auricular hematomas present an interesting management problem. They form between the cartilage and the perichondrium of the ear due to blunt, shearing trauma, and are most common in wrestlers and boxers.[32] Their presence is important because the blood supply to the cartilage is through the perichondrium, so the vascular supply to the cartilage is disrupted as long as the hematoma is present.[32] Therefore, the hematoma should be aspirated with a sterile needle. After aspiration, a contoured pressure dressing is applied to the ear to prevent reaccumulation of the hematoma. Failure to aspirate the hematoma adequately can lead to necrosis of the cartilage and the cosmetic deformity known as "cauliflower ear."

Adequate evaluation of nasal injuries requires both external and internal inspection.[33] The most common injury to the nose is the nasal fracture, which can be detected without x-rays. Physical findings include epistaxis, nasal airway obstruction, asymmetry, crepitus to palpation, and periorbital ecchymosis. Hemorrhage control is accomplished through external pressure and/or internal packing. Intranasal examination is important to look for septal deviation and septal hematoma. Like an auricular hematoma, septal hematomas require prompt drainage to prevent necrosis of the nasal cartilage.[31,32] A small incision can be made in the nasal mucosa to permit drainage of the hematoma.[31,32] A small drain can be left in the area to make sure the hematoma is completely evacuated.[32] The affected side of the nose is also packed to prevent reaccumulation of the hematoma.

Maxillofacial fractures include Le Fort, sinus, and zygoma fractures. Le Fort fractures are maxillary fractures that are infrequently seen in sports because of the large amount of force required to create them. They are classified as types I, II and III by increasing order of severity. Physical findings include malocclusion, epistaxis, maxillary mobility, and nasal deformity, with flattening of the naso-orbital region. Le Fort I fractures occur just above the alveolar ridge, separating the palate from the rest of the face. Le Fort II fractures extend above the nasal pyramid. Le Fort III fractures completely separate the face from the rest of the cranium. The most important item to note on initial examination is dental occlusion. With normal occlusion, the maxillary and mandibular midlines should align, with the maxillary incisors slightly overhanging the mandibular incisors. The outer cusps of the upper molars should also be more lateral than those on the mandibular molars. Any significant deviation from this alignment or free motion of the palate is strongly suggestive of a fracture.[32] The patient should be closely observed for evidence of an intracranial injury and should be transported to the hospital for radiographic studies, which likely include CT scan to assess the fracture fully. Reduction and fixation of the fracture usually occur within a week.

Fractures of the walls of the sinuses can also occur with facial trauma. Uncomplicated maxillary fractures can be treated conservatively with antibiotics and observation. Frontal sinus fractures can be difficult to diagnose and to manage subsequently. Pain and swelling in the forehead are the most common symptoms associated with frontal sinus fractures, and local swelling can obscure cosmetic deformity. Frontal sinus fractures become particularly difficult to manage when the posterior wall is fractured, leading to communication with the anterior cranial fossa. In this situation, the athlete is kept upright to diminish CSF rhinorrhea and is observed closely for signs of meningitis. As with orbital blowout fractures, fractures of the ethmoid sinuses often present with subcutaneous emphysema and periorbital swelling. Antibiotics are important as prophylaxis against orbital cellulitis.

Zygoma fractures result from blunt trauma to the malar eminences and present with pain, swelling, and deformity in the area. Most of these fractures occur where the zygoma joins the temporal, frontal, and maxillary bones, and are therefore called tripod fractures.[32] The important local structure is the eye, and examination of the area should assess the eye for exophthalmos or enophthalmos and for full range of extraocular movements. The deformity of the tripod fracture is best seen by looking down from the top of the head, assessing the height of each cheekbone. Acute care of the injury is similar to that for other fractures of the face. Radiographs are obtained to assess the fracture, with the Waters and Caldwell views being the most sensitive. Antibiotics are given because the maxillary sinus fills with blood and is at risk for developing infection. Exploration of these injuries occurs if there is more than 1 cm of malar eminence depression, enophthalmos, or entrapment of extraocular muscles.[32]

Mandibular fractures are also relatively common in sports, occurring with a direct blow to the mandible. As much as any fracture in the face, mandibular fractures require special attention to maintaining an airway. Almost all mandibular fractures communicate with the inside of the mouth, creating a substantial amount of bleeding. Bleeding and potentially loose teeth can obstruct the airway. The tongue now has a mobile anterior attachment and may be more prone to falling back into the airway. A snug head dressing (Barton bandage) that wraps circumferentially from below the jaw and up over the top of the head can be used to hold the loose mandibular fragment in place. Plain mandibular films and Panorex views are obtained to evaluate the fracture. Because of the communication with the oral cavity, these fractures are treated as open fractures and treated with prophylactic antibiotics.[32]

Mandibular fractures can sometimes be confused with a mandibular dislocation, in which the mandibular condyles displace anteriorly after the mandible is rapidly depressed. Mandibular dislocations can be distinguished on physical examination by the inability to open the mouth more than 40 mm, inability to close, deviation to the side of injury, malocclusion (seen in both injuries), and joint popping or clicking. A mandibular dislocation should be reduced as soon as possible. This is usually done with the aid of systemic relaxants or sedatives and is performed with the physician's thumbs at the molars and the fingers extending back and under the angle of the mandible. A downward and posterior force is applied to the mandible, attempting to get the condyles to slip back into place.[32] This injury often results from a lateral blow to the jaw, making it more common in sports such as basketball and hockey, in which there is a higher rate of elbow trauma to the jaw.[33]

Soft tissue injuries of the neck are of particular importance. The initial concern is with the proximity of the cervical spine, with the worry being that a force that creates significant injury in the soft tissues may have injured the cervical spine. The other consideration is that there are many important structures in the neck, and injury to them must be carefully assessed. Laryngeal injuries are generally caused by blunt trauma to the larynx. The athlete suffering such an injury must be carefully assessed to rule out impingement of the airway and monitored closely for the development of hoarseness or stridor, two signs of swelling in the larynx. Early protection of the airway is important because if the swelling becomes critical, the airway may be unapproachable from above, necessitating a needle cricothyroidotomy to establish an airway.

Laceration of the neck requires great care because of the presence of large vascular structures, as well as the trachea and esophagus.[31] Surgical exploration may be necessary to rule out occult injury to deep structures. Gross laceration of the neck veins requires the application of an occlusive pressure dressing and immediate transport to the hospital. Laceration of the carotid artery may require clamping of the free ends and immediate transfer to the hospital. It is difficult to stop a carotid bleed with pressure alone.

Dental injuries include fractured, luxated, and avulsed teeth. In the acute setting, one should attempt to replace the avulsed tooth as rapidly as possible with minimal trauma.[33,34] If the tooth has been expelled from the mouth and is filthy from the external environment, it should be wiped gently before replacing it. The less trauma there is to the outside of the tooth, the greater the likelihood is that the tooth will "take" when reinserted. If the tooth cannot be replaced, it should be transported in a moist environment. An ideal location is under the tongue of the athlete. If that is not possible, submerging the tooth in milk or saline is optimal, but water can be used in their absence.[33,34]

THORACIC AND PULMONARY EMERGENCIES

There are many aspects of athletic competition that create risks for thoracic trauma. Most thoracic injury is blunt trauma experienced in collision sports, but some of the equipment used in sporting activity also has the potential to cause penetrating chest trauma. In addition to trauma to the chest, underlying pulmonary illness, such as asthma, may be exacerbated by exercise and the conditions and locations where athletes compete. Injuries to the chest and exacerbation of pulmonary disease can present emergencies that require rapid assessment and therapeutic measures. A thorough understanding of the physiology and mechanics of breathing and oxygen exchange underlies the treatment principle. Rapid intervention is the key.

THORACIC TRAUMA

TENSION PNEUMOTHORAX

The potential space that lies between the visceral and parietal pleurae within the chest cavity is a closed space. The generation of negative pressure within this potential space by expansion of the chest wall causes and maintains expansion of the underlying lung. Conversely, the development of positive pressure within this space leads to collapse of the lung. If the visceral pleural surface is disrupted and air is permitted to pass from within the lung to the pleural space, a closed pneumothorax is created. In some situations, the leak only occurs in one direction, as if there were effectively a one-way valve allowing air into the pleural space during inspiration but trapping it during expiration. As air progressively accumulates within the pleural space, it collapses the ipsilateral lung and begins to shift the mediastinum away as pressure accumulates. As the accumulation of air increases, intrathoracic pressure begins to increase markedly. Elevated intrathoracic pressure acts to decrease systemic venous return and, ultimately, cardiac output. This is the pathophysiology behind the development of tension pneumothorax.

Pneumothoraces can occur in athletes for various reasons. Blunt trauma such as that encountered in collision sports or penetrating trauma created by equipment can breach the visceral or parietal pleura. Many athletes also fit the description of the person most likely to suffer a primary spontaneous pneumothorax—a young, asthenic individual. Tension pneumothoraces are most commonly caused by blunt trauma to the chest, such as in a previously healthy individual who suffered a tension pneumothorax after falling while skiing and striking a mogul with the right anterior thorax.[35] Presenting symptoms are predominantly dyspnea and sharp chest pain. Findings on examination include diminished breath sounds on the side of the pneumothorax and hyperresonance on percussion over the involved lung. As the pathology progresses, the patient develops tracheal deviation away from the pneumothorax secondary to mediastinal shift, hypotension, and cardiopulmonary collapse.

Tension pneumothorax can be diagnosed radiographically, but in a severely symptomatic athlete with the above findings, emergent management must be undertaken without waiting for radiographic confirmation. Emergent management involves the placement of an 18-gauge needle in the second intercostal space in the midclavicular line. This releases the intrathoracic pressure and converts the tension pneumothorax to a simple pneumothorax. By reducing the intrathoracic pressure, the ipsilateral lung is allowed to expand somewhat, improving gas exchange but, more importantly, systemic venous return increases and cardiac output improves. Releasing the intrathoracic pressure allows time for placing a chest tube, the definitive therapy.

OPEN PNEUMOTHORAX

Penetrating chest trauma that creates a hole in the chest wall allows for communication between the pleural space and the external environment. This is an open pneumothorax or, as it is classically called, a "sucking chest wound."[36] Altered pulmonary biomechanics occurs because the relatively negative intrathoracic pressure is lost immediately as pressures equilibrate between the atmosphere and the pleural space. Laminar flow mechanics dictate that if the hole in the chest is two thirds the size of the trachea or greater, air preferentially enters the chest through the chest wall lesion, thereby impairing normal ventilation and resulting in hypoxia.[37]

Fortunately, treatment is relatively straightforward. The health care provider should cover the defect with a sterile occlusive dressing and tape it down on three sides. This effectively creates a one-way valve at the chest wall. With inspiration, the dressing is pulled against the chest, preventing the inflow of air through the wound. Expiration allows the passage of air out of the wound through the free edge, thereby preventing a tension pneumothorax.[37] Definitive treatment is by chest tube placement in the affected hemithorax, distant from the wound, and surgical closure of the wound.

FLAIL CHEST

Injury in which a section of the chest wall is discontinuous with the rest results in a flail chest; it is usually caused by multiple rib fractures. It destroys the bellows effect of the thorax and can significantly impair ventilation.[36] Importantly, this injury implies that a large force has been applied to the chest wall. It is more commonly seen in motor vehicle accidents than in athletic injuries, but must be suspected in an athlete with multiple rib fractures, especially when the fractures are both anterior and posterior. Its presence must also alert the health care provider to other possible injuries related to large forces delivered to the thorax, such as myocardial and pulmonary contusion.

The diagnosis of flail chest is often difficult because of the great amount of muscle splinting that occurs in the acute phase. Adequate clinical suspicion, however, should lead to serial examinations in a patient with multiple rib fractures. As muscular fatigue sets in, splinting diminishes, and an unstable segment becomes manifest.[37]

On-site management of flail chest involves respiratory support as required, vigilant observation for other injuries that could compromise cardiopulmonary performance, and transport of the athlete to a facility with an intensive care unit in case respiratory function deteriorates. Objective worsening in ventilatory function is an indication for endotracheal intubation and positive pressure ventilation.

HEMOTHORAX

Although a collection of blood in the pleural space can complicate both blunt and penetrating chest trauma, massive hemothorax often results from penetrating trauma to the chest.[36] The collection of a large amount of blood in one hemithorax significantly affects pulmonary mechanics as well as systemic hemodynamics. As blood accumulates, intrathoracic pressure increases, making lung expansion more difficult. The increasing pressure also causes mediastinal shift, ultimately elevating intrathoracic pressure in the contralateral hemithorax. This progression leads to critical hypoxia. Hemodynamically, the loss of a large volume of blood into the thoracic cavity obviously creates a serious loss of intravascular volume and may lead to shock.

Hemothorax should be considered in the athlete showing signs of shock. Characteristically, there is accompanying dyspnea with diminution of breath sounds and dullness to percussion on the side of the lesion. There may be mediastinal shift, creating tracheal deviation away from the involved side. Neck veins may be distended due to the increase in intrathoracic pressure or they may be flat because of volume loss.[37]

Initial therapy on site centers around the maintenance of the airway, attempts at ventilation with supplemental oxygen, and replacement of circulating volume. Two large-bore IV lines should be started as soon as possible, and rapid volume replacement with crystalloid should begin immediately. The athlete should be transferred immediately to the nearest trauma center.

TRACHEOBRONCHIAL AND PULMONARY EMERGENCIES

FOREIGN BODY ASPIRATION

Foreign body sources in athletes are numerous. They can include dental appliances, dental protective devices, gum, food, chewing tobacco or, in the case of upper airway trauma, teeth. Common symptoms include cough, wheezing, stridor, hoarseness, and dyspnea. The athlete may also have associated symptoms, such as retractions and accessory muscle recruitment. Unless there is a high level of suspicion, the symptoms can be confused with other respiratory problems, such as asthma.

If the athlete is not moving air, the Heimlich maneuver should be used in attempt to dislodge the foreign body. As long as the individuals can move air, their efforts at clearing the foreign body are more effective than those provided by the Heimlich maneuver. In this situation, the risks of abdominal trauma associated with the maneuver outweigh its benefit and preclude its usage. If the offending object is seen within the mouth, manual extraction can be attempted with a finger sweep.

If the object cannot be cleared from a totally occluded airway, a needle cricothyroidotomy (see earlier) may be necessary to establish an airway. Once the airway has been established, the athlete should be seen by an otolaryngologist for endoscopic extraction of the foreign body.

REACTIVE AIRWAYS DISEASE

Asthma and its variants are common, with the incidence of asthma estimated at 3 to 5 percent of the population.[38] The incidence of exercise-induced asthma in the American Olympic population has been reported to be 11 percent.[39] Whereas athletic participation was formerly precluded for individuals with asthma, improvements in the pharmacologic management of the disease have placed many of those with asthma on the playing fields and courts.

The pathophysiology of asthma is related to hyperreactivity of the airways that is triggered by mediators of inflammation, leading to inflammation and bronchospasm of the airways. Any number of different irritants may trigger an asthmatic attack, including airborne or ingested allergens, upper respiratory infection, atmospheric pollution, cold air, and emotional distress.

Symptoms experienced by individuals with an acute asthmatic attack include dyspnea, dry cough, and often a sensation of tightness in the chest, lack of energy, and being out of shape in comparison with their teammates. Findings on physical examination may include tachycardia, tachypnea with a prolonged expiratory phase, wheezing, and accessory muscle usage. The caregiver must be especially careful to assess air movement fully

TABLE 33–8
Banned Over-the-Counter Asthmatic Medications
• Phenylpropanolamine
• Pseudoephedrine
• Ephedrine
• Phenylephrine
• Systemic corticosteroids

on pulmonary auscultation. A severe exacerbation can present without wheezing because of inadequate air movement to produce the sound of a wheeze. In addition, ausculation during maximal forced expiration is necessary as this may elucidate subtle and expiratory wheezing.

Initial management of an exacerbation involves the use of a β_2-agonist metered dose inhaler (e.g., albuterol), which can be used every 20 minutes, if needed. It is helpful to document peak flow rates prior to each administration of the inhaler, which provides a semiobjective measure of pulmonary function. If the initial presentation is particularly severe or if the individual fails to get adequate relief after two administrations of the β_2-agonist inhaler, additional therapy at a definitive care facility must be instituted. This involves supplemental oxygen and IV medication. The asthmatic history can be helpful in deciding when to transport to the hospital. An athlete with a history of several admissions or intubation for the asthma should be transported to the hospital sooner than one whose previous asthma history included only occasional difficulty with exercise or cold exposure.

An athlete who has been treated for an acute asthmatic exacerbation with a respiratory rate of less than 20 bpm (beats per minute), heart rate of less than 100 bpm, no auscultatory evidence of wheezing, and symptomatic relief may return to competition under close observation. Any recurrence of symptoms or physical findings mandates removal from the athletic contest for definitive treatment. It is important to note that many over-the-counter medications for the treatment of asthma are banned by the United States Olympic Committee and NCAA (Table 33–8).

CARDIOVASCULAR EMERGENCIES

The initial evaluation and treatment of cardiovascular instability should have as its overriding goals the maintenance of vascular expansion, optimization of cardiac output, and enhancement of tissue oxygenation. Cardiogenic shock must be prevented through early identification of the potential cause and its reversal. General principles of cardiac resuscitation apply in the therapy of cardiovascular emergencies, but specific conditions require specific therapy.

Sudden cardiac death in an individual over the age of 35 is most commonly due to ischemic coronary artery disease. In an individual under the age of 35, it is more commonly related to inherited abnormalities of the heart.[44–47] Of the causes of sudden death in athletes younger than 35, the most common is hypertrophic cardiomyopathy,[46] a genetically transmitted condition characterized by asymmetric thickening of the interventricular septum with a nondilated left ventricle. Hypertrophic cardiomyopathy is followed in order of likelihood by idiopathic left ventricular hypertrophy (LVH), coronary artery anomalies, coronary heart disease, and ruptured aorta.[46] Ruptured aorta is most frequently due to cystic medial necrosis associated with Marfan syndrome, an inherited disorder of connective tissue.[48] With the exception of aortic rupture, the final common pathway in sudden death resulting from all these conditions is ventricular fibrillation, making it the most important arrhythmia to address when discussing emergency cardiac care of the athlete.

GENERAL MANAGEMENT PRINCIPLES

When a cardiac arrest is encountered, the overriding necessity is to provide ventilation and circulation for the individual. The basic ABCDEs of assessment and principles of CPR are easily forgotten when an unexpected emergency occurs. Initial reactions are to begin to use medications for the arrested individual, and a great deal of effort goes into memorizing the protocols in the ACLS course, but the failure to provide assisted ventilation and circulation for an arrested victim negates any value in regaining a viable cardiac rhythm.

It is also important to realize that regardless of how well prepared the health care staff may be, the site of an athletic event is not the optimal site to run a "code." Consideration must be given to immediate transportation of the athlete. How far one carries a code situation on site depends on a number of variables, such as equipment available on site, the physician's comfort and experience with handling cardiac arrests, transfer time to the hospital, and the type of personnel available to perform the transport, (e.g., emergency medical technicians, EMTs), versus paramedics. All these must be taken into consideration when deciding when to transport the athlete, so there are no set rules pertaining to time of transport. In general, however, "if you've reached the point at which one is pushing lidocaine, it's time to transport."

SPECIFIC CONDITIONS

MYOCARDIAL INFARCTION

Cardiac arrest caused by myocardial infarction is most commonly due to the development of ventricular fibrillation. This has important ramifications in treatment and is discussed in more detail later.

In the presence of an individual who is complaining of the symptoms of myocardial ischemia or infarction without cardiac arrest (e.g., chest pain, shortness of breath, diaphoresis, nausea, left arm pain, jaw pain), the hallmarks of care include ensuring adequate oxygenation, diminishing myocardial oxygen demand by the use of nitrates or morphine sulfate in athletes with adequate blood pressures, and rapidly arranging transport to a location where definitive care can be supplied.

Although the sports medicine practitioner most commonly cares for young, healthy individuals at low risk for coronary disease, athletic participation by older individuals continues to increase. Also, the public venues in which many athletic events occur place the health care provider in contact with the general public, in whom myocardial infarction is the most common cause of sudden death. The health care provider covering an athletic event may be called if a member of the audience suffers a cardiac arrest. It is also important to keep in mind that ischemic cardiac arrest can rarely occur in the younger individual. Contributing factors include a strong family history of coronary artery disease, familial hyperlipidemia, diabetes mellitus, or the recreational use of cocaine, which can cause coronary vasospasm and lead to ischemia and sudden death.

ARRHYTHMIAS

Ventricular fibrillation is the most common rhythm found in cardiac arrest. As noted earlier, it is the final common pathway in many arrest scenarios, whether the underlying abnormality is ischemic or structural in origin. When treating ventricular fibrillation, it is most important to remember that electricity heals. An unsynchronized dose of 200 to 300 joules (J) should be delivered to the athlete as soon as the rhythm is identified as ventricular fibrillation. If unsuccessful in converting the rhythm, defibrillation with 300 J should be repeated and then with 360 J, if necessary. CPR is held until all three defibrillations are attempted. After defibrillation is attempted, epinephrine is given at a dose of 1.0 mg IV, or approximately twice the dose diluted 1:10 with sterile saline or water through an endotracheal tube. Defibrillation is reattempted at 360 J after every dose of medication, and a quick check for a return of a viable cardiac rhythm and pulse is performed after each attempt at defibrillation. In the absence of defibrillatory capabilities, CPR is initiated. All medications are given with the intent to increase the effectiveness of the defibrillation. If defibrillation fails again after the administration of epinephrine, intravenous lidocaine is given in a bolus dose of 1 mg/kg, and defibrillation is reattempted. Refractory ventricular fibrillation can be treated with bretylium and repeated doses of epinephrine, each followed by attempts at defibrillation. With the exception of the times at which the athlete is being defibrillated, closed-chest cardiac massage and ventilation are performed.[7]

Asystole is the absence of a discernible cardiac rhythm. Apparent asystole on the monitor should be checked in more than one lead because fine ventricular fibrillation can resemble asystole in some chest leads, and therapy is markedly different for the two disorders. Therapy for asystole does not involve defibrillation, but consists of CPR and repeated doses of epinephrine, 1.0 mg IV or 2.0 mg diluted as above, administered by endotracheal tube. Atropine can also be given 1.0 mg IV and repeated once, with the hope of removing parasympathetic tone, which can inhibit cardiac activity.[7]

Pulseless electrical activity, or electromechanical dissociation (as it was formerly called) is evidence of cardiac activity on monitor without palpable pulses. Therapy for this rhythm, aside from CPR, is epinephrine in the same doses given earlier.[7] The key to managing this rhythm successfully, however, is the identification of the underlying abnormality causing the rhythm. Some of the more common causes of pulseless electrical activity are hypovolemia, pericardial tamponade, tension pneumothorax, pulmonary embolism, hypoxia, and metabolic acidosis.[7] Of these, only pulmonary embolism does not have the potential to be corrected readily by relatively simple means, so it is imperative to conduct a thorough search for the cause of pulseless electrical activity.

Supraventricular tachycardia (SVT) has been reported to lead to sudden cardiac death in athletes with underlying conduction system disorders, such as Wolff-Parkinson-White syndrome.[49] However, it is more commonly a cause of morbidity among otherwise healthy athletes. The most common supraventricular rhythm encountered in the athlete is sinus tachycardia, usually caused by volume depletion or pain. It is important to realize the frequency of resting sinus bradycardia in well-conditioned athletes. A heart rate of 90 may be of no concern in an average person, but in some athletes it is twice their resting rate of 45. Therapy is directed toward correction of the underlying problem. Paroxysmal supraventricular tachycardia can occur in some athletes, presenting with dyspnea and palpitations. In an otherwise stable individual, it usually responds well with observation and vagal maneuvers (Valsalva, carotid massage). Persistent or unstable SVT should be transferred to the hospital. The administration of adenosine, verapamil, or synchronized cardioversion would be highly inappropriate outside the controlled environment of the hospital, unless the athlete's instability dictated emergent synchronous cardioversion.

Atrial fibrillation and atrial flutter are unlikely in the athletic population. They are more likely to be encountered in the spectator population with underlying cardiac disease, usually ischemic. Therapy is dictated by symptoms. Diltiazem, β-blockers, verapamil, and digoxin are all used to control ventricular response.[7] Supplemental oxygen, intravenous access, and transport to the hospital are the rules of initial management.

Interpretation of the various bradycardias and heart blocks is difficult in the athletic population. Sinus bradycardia, sinus dysrhythmia, wandering atrial pacemaker, first-degree atrioventricular block, Mobitz type I atrioventricular block, and junctional rhythm have all been described as normal variants occurring more commonly in the athletic population.[50] Common sense dictates that if concerning signs and symptoms are present along with bradycardia or heart block, they should be treated. Concerning signs and symptoms include chest pain, shortness of breath, decreased level of consciousness, low blood pressure, shock, pulmonary congestion, congestive heart failure, and acute myocardial infarction.[7] On-site management includes the standard ABCDEs, supplemental oxygen, atropine, and transport to the hospital.

HYPOVOLEMIA

Hypovolemia is the diminution of circulating intravascular volume, potentially leading to tissue hypoperfusion or shock. In the athletic setting, it is often caused by processes leading to loss of body fluid such as vomiting, diarrhea, and excessive perspiration, with inadequate volume intake. It can also be caused by hemorrhage, which is the most common cause of massive loss of volume in an athlete.

Hemorrhage is defined as the acute loss of circulating blood. It is graded into four classes of increasing severity based on the volume of blood lost and associated signs and symptoms (Table 33–9). The categories were devised using studies in the general population. An athletic population can have different responses to the varying degrees of volume loss because of altered hemodynamics as well as the increased demand placed on the cardiovascular system with strenuous exercise. For example, as noted earlier, the athlete's heart may be slower to show tachycardia when using the strict criterion of heart rate greater than 100 because of the resting bradycardia seen in athletes. Also, smaller degrees of blood loss in the setting of strenuous activity may be more symptomatic, given the demands placed on the cardiovascular system and the ongoing loss of fluid due to perspiration. Basic management of hemorrhage is the maintenance of an airway, assisting breathing and oxygenation with supplemental oxygen, and replacing circulating volume.

	TABLE 33–9 Estimated Blood Loss Classification			
Class	I	II	III	IV
Blood loss (ml)	<750	750–1500	1500–2000	>2000
Blood loss (% blood volume)	<15	15–30	30–40	>40
Pulse (bpm)	<100	>100	>100	>100
Blood pressure	Normal	Normal	Decreased	Decreased

Class I hemorrhage is defined as the loss of up to 15 percent of total circulating blood volume (750 ml in a 70-kg male with a circulating volume of approximately 5 liters).[8] In the general population, there is minimal symptomatology with this amount of blood loss. There is a slight increase in the heart rate, but no changes are noted in blood pressure, pulse pressure, respiratory rate, or capillary refill. Treatment for this degree of blood loss is simply the replacement of lost fluid.

Class II hemorrhage is the loss of 15 to 30 percent of the circulating volume (750 to 1500 ml). Tachycardia is noted, as is tachypnea. There is also an increase in systemic sympathetic tone, leading to an increase in the diastolic blood pressure and a narrowing of the pulse pressure. An increase in capillary refill time may be noted, indicating a diminution of perfusion to the periphery. Also indicative of the decreased peripheral perfusion are subtle neurologic changes, such as anxiety, inattention, and hostility. There is no change in systolic blood pressure at this time, which is important because significant volume loss has occurred and there is clinical evidence of hypoperfusion without a drop in systolic pressure. Caregivers basing their care solely on the basis of a normal systolic blood pressure are dangerously undertreating this athlete. This degree of volume loss is managed on site with volume replacement using crystalloids. This method of volume replacement can be continued at the hospital and blood product use can be avoided if the blood loss can be controlled and the patient responds well to the crystalloid replacement.

Class III hemorrhage involves the loss of 30 to 40 percent of the circulating volume (1500 to 2000 ml). These injured athletes almost always exhibit the classic signs of hypovolemia, marked tachycardia, tachypnea, changes in mental status, and a measurable fall in systolic pressure. In a situation not complicated by other fluid loss, this is the smallest degree of blood that causes a drop in systolic blood pressure. This amount of blood loss almost always requires transfusion after initial fluid resuscitation with crystalloids. In the setting of other fluid losses, however, these same symptoms can be elicited with smaller amounts of blood loss, and it may be possible to avoid the use of blood products in such a scenario.

Class IV hemorrhage is characterized by the loss of more than 40 percent of the circulating volume (more than 2000 ml). This injured athlete is in grave danger and exhibits marked tachycardia, a marked drop in blood pressure, a very narrow pulse pressure or unobtainable diastolic blood pressure, negligible urine output, markedly depressed mental status, and cold, pale skin. Athletes with this degree of blood loss can be started with crystalloid fluid replacement, but transport to the nearest trauma center should not be delayed while attempting to start an intravenous line. They often require immediate transfusion and surgical intervention to control the bleeding. Loss of more than 50 percent of the circulating volume results in loss of consciousness, pulse, and blood pressure.

As always, it is the rapid, systematic initial assessment and definitive decision making that are vital for the athlete's well-being. If there is an obvious source of blood loss, it should be promptly addressed, but health care providers should never become so engrossed in a dramatic injury that they lose sight of the basic ABCDEs of care.

PERICARDIAL TAMPONADE

Pericardial tamponade is the compression of the chambers of the heart due to the accumulation of fluid, usually blood, in the pericardial space. The chambers are unable to dilate sufficiently and accept enough blood to provide adequate cardiac output and maintain metabolic function. Pericardial tamponade most commonly occurs due to penetrating trauma to the chest, but can also be seen with blunt trauma. Classic findings include muffled heart sounds, distended neck veins indicative of increased central venous pressure, and systemic hypotension (Beck triad). Due to the progression of the hemodynamic abnormalities, however, all these findings may be absent acutely. The heart sounds can be difficult to hear in a large athletic venue, regardless of the presence or absence of fluid in the pericardial space. Neck veins may not be distended because of hypovolemia.

In the setting of a deteriorating athlete with chest trauma who is not responding to regular ATLS protocols, the health care provider must seriously consider either a tension pneumothorax or pericardial tamponade, especially with evidence of diminished systemic blood pressure and elevated central venous pressure. Immediate therapy for pericardial tamponade is pericardiocentesis; this is best performed using the subxiphoid approach, entering the skin 2 cm below and 1 cm to the left of the xiphoid process. The needle is advanced until blood or fluid is returned from the pericardial space. An ECG lead can be attached to the needle to detect contact with the ventricle.

MYOCARDIAL CONTUSION

Cardiac concussion, or commotio cordis, is a functional, nonstructural injury to the myocardium that can result in ventricular dysrhythmia and cardiac arrest. Its occurrence has been reported in youth hockey and baseball players.[51,52] Fortunately, it is rare, but when it does occur, appropriate resuscitative techniques have had poor results. Commotio cordis is seen in the setting of direct blunt trauma with a missile, such as a hockey puck or baseball, to the anterior or left lateral chest wall. It seems to have an increased incidence in the pediatric and adolescent age groups, perhaps due to their increased chest compliance. Because of its dismal resuscitation rate, emphasis has been on prevention of the injury with adequate chest protection, but because of its uncommon occurrence, questions have been generated regarding the cost effectiveness of preventing the injury.

Cardiac contusion is a bruise to the myocardium resulting from blunt chest trauma. Criteria for diagnosis are highly variable, resulting in a range of incidence from 5 to 76 percent of patients sustaining blunt chest trauma.[53] As a clinical entity, it should be considered in a patient with significant blunt chest trauma.

Complications of myocardial contusion include arrhythmias, which are the most frequent complication. The arrhythmias range from isolated premature atrial contractions (PACs) and premature ventricular contractions (PVCs) to varying degrees of heart block, ventricular tachycardia, and ventricular fibrillation. Other severe complications include intramyocardial hematoma and local cellular necrosis, which can lead to late aneurysm formation or cardiac rupture. Its presentation can be vague and elusive. Many athletes complain of precordial chest pain similar to cardiac ischemia, but some are asymptomatic. *Chest pain that is not reproduced by palpation of the chest or movement of the anterior chest wall should be suspicious for myocardial contusion.* The most common clinical sign is sinus tachycardia. The electrocardiogram may show changes consistent with pericarditis or a typical myocardial infarction. Serum creatinine phosphokinase levels may be elevated, but this is a relatively insensitive test. Other tests involved in the diagnosis of myocardial contusion include two-dimensional echocardiography and radionuclide scans, but these are usually used when there is already concern about deterioration in cardiac function. There has also been some support in the literature for transesophageal echocardiography in the diagnosis of myocardial contusion,[54,55] but again, these reports involve already critically injured patients.

Because myocardial contusion can be so difficult to diagnose in its less symptomatic forms, and because it has potentially severe complications, it has provided many clinical dilemmas, and a need has arisen to identify a subset of patients at risk for myocardial contusion who are also at risk for cardiac complications. This has been attempted in the emergency room setting by Foil and associates.[56] They performed a retrospective review of 524 patients admitted over 33 months with a suspicion of myocardial contusion. Of these patients, 27 had cardiac-related complications. Of these 27, 23 had abnormalities on admission electrocardiograms, 3 had multiple other injuries requiring intensive care unit admission, and 1 experienced dysrhythmia 4 hours after admission, which led the authors to state that patients with isolated chest wall contusion, normal admission, 4-hour electrocardiograms, and no other major injuries need not be admitted.

This information is helpful in the emergency room setting, but still fails to answer fully the question of appropriate on-site management of the athlete with blunt chest trauma and no signs of cardiac decompensation. This remains a subjective call for the on-site health care provider. Proper management should be dictated by the severity of the athlete's chest discomfort, the magnitude of the force applied to the chest, and the presence or absence of other injuries.

ABDOMINAL AND PELVIC EMERGENCIES

Hemorrhage and peritoneal contamination due to rupture of an intra-abdominal organ or viscus and abdominal and/or pelvic organ contusion may present in a subacute manner. A high index of suspicion is necessary in the acute management of abdominal and pelvic trauma. A common mistake is often the failure to consider significant abdominal injury in an athlete suffering blunt trauma to the abdomen.[57] This section discusses the general approach to abdominal trauma in the athlete and then investigates specific abdominal and pelvic injuries.

INITIAL ASSESSMENT AND ON-FIELD MANAGEMENT

Abdominal visceral injury often has a subtle presentation. The most important determination to be made is the existence of an abdominal visceral injury, not the specific diagnosis. Hemorrhage is the hallmark of injury to the solid abdominal organs (liver, spleen, kidney), whereas peritonitis distinguishes injury to the hollow abdominal viscera. Knowledge of the mechanism of injury is helpful in beginning to assess an athlete suffering from an acute injury to the abdomen. The position of the athlete's body, as well as the specific site of the blow, are important in the evaluation. For example, renal injury is more common in an athlete whose body is extended and abdominal musculature relaxed, such as a receiver diving for a ball.[58] The location of the pain can also be helpful. Flank and back pain may indicate renal or ureteral injury. Left upper quadrant or lower thoracic pain could indicate splenic injury. Right upper quadrant or lower thoracic pain may signal hepatic injury. Associated symptoms can also be helpful. Splenic and hepatic injuries can cause ipsilateral shoulder pain due to referred pain from subdiaphragmatic irritation.

Physical assessment, once again, begins with the ABCDEs. Assessment of vital signs may show evidence of volume loss, which should immediately raise concern about intra-abdominal blood loss. Examination of the abdomen begins with inspection, specifically looking for flank ecchymosis (Turner sign) or periumbilical ecchymosis (Cullen sign). Either of these signs can indicate bleeding in the abdomen. The abdomen is auscultated, with concern caused by the absence of bowel sounds. The most important portion of the abdominal examination is palpation of the abdomen. Focal areas of tenderness, along with guarding and rebound tenderness, are worrisome. It is also important to examine the areas around the abdomen for injury. The lower rib cage is palpated for fractures that can lacerate the liver or the spleen. Flank tenderness or costovertebral angle tenderness can accompany renal trauma. The male genitalia are examined for evidence of testicular trauma, which can cause referred pain to the abdomen. Finally, a rectal examination is important. It is unlikely that blunt abdominal trauma can cause blood in the stool, but the examiner can also assess for a high-riding prostate, signifying marked pelvic trauma.

If the initial examination is negative, it does not exclude significant intra-abdominal trauma. In the setting of an injury with a high risk of intra-abdominal injury, the examiner should never be satisfied with one normal examination and, as long as there is any question regarding the presence or absence of injury, the player is held from competition.

SPECIFIC INJURIES

SPLENIC INJURIES

The spleen is the second most commonly injured abdominal organ after the kidneys. Up to 8 percent of all adult spleen injuries and 20 percent of all pediatric spleen injuries are sports-related, and spleen injuries account for approximately 10 percent of sports-related abdominal injuries.[61] Injury to the spleen should be considered in any athlete who has left upper quadrant pain, left lower chest trauma, or left shoulder pain. Physical examination can attempt to elicit the Kehr sign, in which left shoulder pain is elicited with the Trendelenburg position and palpation of the left upper quadrant. There is an increased frequency of traumatic splenic rupture associated with mononucleosis. Of all patients with mononucleosis, 0.09 to 0.2 percent sustain splenic ruptures, usually occurring between days 4 and 21 after trauma.[62]

With the realization of the spleen's important role in the reticuloendothelial system and the risk of postsplenectomy sepsis, there has been a shift in thinking about the management of acute splenic trauma. In an effort to determine which splenic trauma can be managed nonsurgically, a grading system, based on CT findings, has been established (Table 33–10). A class I injury exhibits a capsular avulsion, superficial laceration, or subcapsular hematoma smaller than 1 cm. Class II injuries have parenchymal laceration(s) 1 to 3 cm deep and central or subcapsular hematoma(s) smaller than 3 cm. Class III injuries are laceration(s) more than 3 cm deep, with central or subcapsular hematomas larger than 3 cm. Class IV injuries involve fragmentation into three or more pieces or a devascularized (nonenhancing) spleen.[63,64] In general, classes III and IV and most of class II injuries are treated surgically, whereas class I injuries are treated nonsurgically.

HEPATIC INJURIES

The liver is the third most commonly injured organ in sports-related trauma. Hepatic trauma should be considered in athletes with right upper quadrant pain, right lower rib fractures, or right shoulder pain. Like splenic injuries, the most likely injury in the liver is a laceration. As with the spleen, there have been attempts to manage hepatic trauma conservatively, with nonoperative management being successful in athletes who were hemodynamically stable.[65–67]

KIDNEY INJURIES

The kidney is the most frequently injured organ in sports-related abdominal trauma. Injuries that occur in the kidney due to athletic trauma include renal contusion, perinephric, subcapsular, and intrarenal hematomas, and laceration of the kidney. Renal pedicle injuries occur rarely.[58] Renal contusions are benign injuries that are handled conservatively with rest and fluid management, as are almost all small hematomas and lacerations. Even larger contusions and lacerations can be handled nonoperatively if there are no signs of bleeding.[58] The athlete with an acute renal injury usually presents with hematuria and significant flank pain. Hematuria, except in the case of a renal pedicle injury, is a sensitive sign, but not specific. Classically, evaluation of blunt renal trauma with hematuria has involved obtaining an intravenous pressure (IVP). Urologic literature, however, has stated that patients with hematuria, blunt renal trauma, without signs of shock do not require IVP evaluation due to the paucity of positive findings,[68–70] but athletes with penetrating injuries or with signs of shock do require imaging studies. One study has shown that contrast CT is more sensitive and specific when used for renal injuries.[68]

URETERAL AND BLADDER INJURY

Ureteral injuries are uncommon in athletes unless they are involved in motor sports. Both these injuries fall outside the realm of most sports, so are not discussed here. Bladder rupture occurs most commonly in relation to a significant pelvic injury, such as a fracture. In an athlete with a pelvic fracture, the presence of gross hematuria or an inability to void indicates a bladder or urethral injury. Retrograde cystography is the diagnostic procedure of choice.

TESTICULAR INJURY

Potential testicular injuries in the athlete include testicular torsion, testicular contusion, and testicular

TABLE 33–10
CT Classification of Splenic Injury

Class	Laceration	Hematoma	Fragmentation
I	<1 cm, superficial	<1 cm subcapsular	Negative
II	1–3 cm, parenchymal	<3 cm central	Negative
III	>3 cm, parenchymal	>3 cm central	Negative
IV	Devascularization		≥ Three fragments

rupture. Testicular torsion often presents atraumatically with an acutely swollen painful testis that is carried horizontally and higher in the scrotum than the opposite side. As the name implies, the pathology is related to the testis twisting on its suspensory ligaments, cutting off its blood supply. Rapid management is vital, given that the testis has a limited amount of time before it necroses. Diagnosis is with ultrasonography or radionuclide scan. A normal ultrasonogram effectively rules out testicular torsion.[71]

Testicular contusion and testicular rupture can be difficult to differentiate. The mechanism is blunt trauma, usually in contact sports. Symptoms of pain and swelling of the scrotum can be immediate. The most common injury or contusion is characterized by soft tissue swelling of the scrotum. Transillumination of the scrotal contents shows no gross accumulation of fluid. Treatment consists of ice, elevation, rest, oral analgesics, and support of the scrotum. Testicular rupture is more serious than the more common testicular contusion. It is characterized by disruption of the tunica albuginia covering of the vascular components of the testis. Scrotal bleeding is acute. Massive swelling is often associated. The physical examination should include transillumination, identifying significant fluid accumulation. Ultrasonography is helpful in the diagnosis. Rapid diagnosis is important in the setting of testicular rupture, because surgical repair of the damaged testis needs to be undertaken within 3 days to obtain a high rate of testicular salvage.[72] This has led to the practice of operating early on any significant testicular injury to obtain salvage where it matters.

MUSCULOSKELETAL EMERGENCIES

The overriding principle in the acute management of musculoskeletal emergencies is a thorough understanding of the neurologic, vascular, and anatomic structures of each affected region or joint. The prevention of morbidity and, in certain cases, mortality is based on this anatomic knowledge as well as on injury-specific complication rates. Although many of the emergencies that can complicate orthopaedic injuries are not initially encountered on the field, the initial assessment and care of an injured athlete have a profound effect on the development of complications. This section initially addresses on-field evaluation and management of orthopaedic injuries, with a later discussion of specific regional injuries and the attendant risks and potential complications.

INITIAL ON-FIELD ASSESSMENT AND MANAGEMENT

The initial assessment of an orthopaedic injury begins with visual inspection of the injured area. The examiner looks for obvious deformity, skin color changes, bruising, swelling, and open wounds. After visual inspection, the examiner gently palpates the injured area as well as the area proximal and distal to the injury. The examiner

feels for crepitus, tenderness, skin temperature, pulses (checking capillary refill), and sensation. Neurovascular evaluation is vital in the assessment of an orthopaedic injury. Many of the complications discussed in this section are related to disruption of the neurovascular supply to the extremity distal to the injury. Assessing motion and strength of an injured limb is also helpful. The athlete should be asked to move the extremity and the examiner should attempt to test muscle strength distal to the injury. The examiner should not passively move an extremity that the athlete refuses to move actively or that has an obvious fracture.[73] Often, in the setting of open fractures, the only valid motor examination of the injured extremity is done by the initial examiner due to pain and splinting secondary to muscle spasm.[74]

Initial management of musculoskeletal injuries centers around stabilization of the injury. Splinting is integral to the initial stabilization of injuries. Splinting helps prevent further soft tissue injury, aids in pain relief, may lower the incidence of fat embolism and shock, and facilitates patient transport.[75] Although splinting material should be part of the team physician's handbag, almost any rigid object padded with soft material can serve as a splint. Folded newspapers, magazines, and cardboard work well for the arm and forearm, and pillows bandaged around an injured lower leg or ankle are also effective.[75] Commercially available splints using vacuum or suction molding are also becoming popular. Splinting of open fractures does not differ from splinting of closed fractures, except that the open wound should be covered as soon as possible with a dry, sterile dressing to limit contamination. Probing of the wound outside the operating room is contraindicated and carries significant risk of contamination of the wound, further damage to underlying structures, and aggravation of hemorrhage.

The dilemma is whether to splint angulated fractures (i.e., to "splint them as they lie") or to attempt closed reduction of the fracture prior to transfer. Although the answer depends on the level of training of the initial examiner and on facility with managing the reduction of fractures, a safe guideline is to splint the fracture as it lies and arrange transport for radiographic studies. If the health care provider discovers a disruption of the vascular supply distal to a closed fracture, however, an attempt should be made at closed reduction by applying gentle traction to the fracture site. Frequently, this is adequate in reestablishing distal blood flow. One should not attempt reduction of open fractures because of the risk of soft tissue damage and contamination of the wound. In general, initial on-field examination and management should assess for possible life-threatening or limb-threatening injury, identify potential sites of injury, stabilize the injury, provide relief of discomfort, and avoid careless maneuvers that could increase the risk of further injury or complication.

Usually, the musculoskeletal assessment involves an injury of lesser magnitude, and the health care provider is faced with the question of whether the athlete can return to competition. This can be one of the most difficult decisions to make on the field. The decision making process involves several different components. Initially, assessment is directed toward ruling out any unstable injury that is at risk of worsening with further competition. This is done by assessment for possible fractures, ligamentous instability, or significant muscular dysfunction. The next level of assessment involves the determination of whether the present injury alters the athlete's performance and function, and should include an in-depth evaluation of whether the present injury is predisposed to further trauma and/or could lead to other associated injuries. This functional evaluation of the athlete indicates whether athletes can perform the tasks required by their position in a particular sport. A working knowledge of the sport being covered is essential. To be cleared to return to competition, athletes must demonstrate to the examiner that they can perform the specific tasks required in the sport, and are appraised and accepting of the inherent risks of continued participation. In general, athletes with lower extremity injuries need to demonstrate the ability to run, jump, and cut without significant dysfunction. Often, it is not the instability of an injury but the resultant dysfunction that precludes the athlete from returning to competition.

GENERAL COMPLICATIONS

As mentioned, musculoskeletal emergencies may not present at the time of injury but may manifest hours to days after the injury. In many cases, however, prudent on-site management can diminish the risk of these complications. It is important to be familiar with the presentations of these complications and their immediate therapy because they may require rapid, intervention at the time of presentation.

COMPARTMENT SYNDROME

Compartment syndromes have been described in the forearm and lower leg, but there have also been reports of compartment syndromes in the thigh secondary to contusions, fractures, and the application of military antishock trousers (MAST).[76,77] Some of the more common causes of compartment syndrome are open and closed fractures of the tibia, crush injuries of the lower leg, supracondylar fractures of the elbow, and fractures of the forearm. The underlying pathophysiology centers around the elevation of pressure within one of the fascial compartments of the involved extremity. The elevation in intracompartmental pressure produces compromise in the vascular supply, which leads to ischemia and soft tissue damage. As more soft tissue injury occurs, there is further pressure elevation within the compartment, and this vicious cycle propagates. It has been shown that muscular hypoxia and damage due to the combination of pressure and ischemia are greater than when caused by ischemia alone.[78,79] Not only does the ischemia affect the muscular components of the compartment, but the neural structures within

the compartment are also susceptible to ischemia. Deficits in neuromuscular function have been noted after the application of as little as 40 mm Hg of pressure for a period of 6 hours.[80] The ultimate outcome of compartment syndrome, if allowed to progress unchecked, is irreversible neuromuscular necrosis and sacrifice of the extremity.

To understand compartment syndrome in the lower leg, and its presentation and therapy, one must have a working knowledge of the anatomy involved. The lower leg is divided into four fascial compartments, the anterior, lateral, deep posterior, and superficial posterior compartments. The anterior compartment lies anterior to the interosseous membrane and contains the tibialis anterior, extensor digitorum longus, and extensor hallucis longus muscles. The innervation and blood supply in this compartment are supplied by the deep peroneal nerve and anterior tibial artery. This compartment is bounded medially by the tibia, anteriorly by the crural fascia, laterally by the anterior intermuscular septum, and posteriorly by the interosseous membrane. The lateral compartment is bounded anteromedially by the anterior intermuscular septum, anterolaterally by the crural fascia, posteriorly by the posterior intermuscular septum, and medially by the fibula. It contains the peroneal muscles, the longus and brevis, and the superficial peroneal nerve. The deep posterior compartment lies immediately behind the interosseous membrane, which separates it from the anterior compartment, and contains the tibialis posterior, flexor hallucis longus, and flexor digitorum longus muscles. Also within the compartment are the tibial nerve and posterior tibial vessels. Finally, the superficial compartment holds the gastrocnemius, soleus, and plantaris muscles.

Athletes with a compartment syndrome classically present with the complaint of pain out of proportion to their injury, as well as swelling and tightness of the affected limb.[81] Pain is exacerbated by passive stretching of the involved compartment. Although there may be signs of diminished perfusion, with decreased pulses and capillary refill, this is often a late finding, with significant intracompartmental damage occurring prior to this. The same can be said for motor and sensory changes in the limb. The five Ps apply—pain, pallor, pulselessness, paresthesias, and paralysis—and are classically discussed as findings suggestive of compartment syndrome. Diagnosis is confirmed by the measurement of intracompartmental pressures, with pressures of greater than 30 mm Hg as determined with the wick catheter.[76] Initial nonsurgical therapy for suspected compartment syndrome is the removal of all potentially constrictive materials from the involved extremity, including casts, cast padding, and compressive wraps.[81] Positioning the extremity is also important and, although it would seem that elevation is most beneficial, raising the extremity above the heart actually diminishes blood supply further, creating more ischemia. Therefore, the extremity should be positioned at the level of the chest.[81,82] Definitive therapy is surgical and involves fasciotomy with decompression of all the compartments.

CLOSTRIDIAL TETANUS

The development of clostridial infections in open wounds is another potential complication. Although there are two clostridial infections of clinical importance—clostridial myonecrosis, caused by *Clostridium perfringens,* and tetanus, caused by *C. tetani*—only tetanus is considered here.

Clostridial tetanus has the potential of invading any open wound, but it is preventable. Unimmunized individuals or those whose immunization has lapsed should be immunized against tetanus at the time of injury. Tetanus immune globulin can be administered to those with long lapses in their tetanus immunizations or with wounds particularly at risk for the development of tetanus. Three factors increase the risk of infection: deep wounds without exposure to air, ischemic wounds, and otherwise infected wounds.[83,84] The illness itself can be deadly, and the best treatment is prevention.

OPEN FRACTURES

Special mention should be made regarding the management of open fractures. An open fracture is an orthopaedic emergency because of the high incidence of complications.[85,86] Open fractures have been classified into three types, with the most severe classification of fractures being further divided into three subtypes (Table 33–11).[86] Type I fractures are the least severe. They encompass fractures associated with wounds smaller than 1 cm, minimal soft tissue damage, and no evidence of crush injury. There is generally little to no comminution of the fracture. Type II fractures have a wound that is greater than 1 cm. There is mild to moderate comminution of the fracture, with minimal to moderate degree of crush injury. These fractures are associated with a moderate degree of contamination. Type III fractures are the most severe and have been divided further into three different subtypes—IIIA, IIIB, and IIIC. Type III fractures feature extensive soft tissue damage and are often associated with high energy injuries. There is often extensive muscle devitalization, and the fracture is often significantly comminuted or displaced. These injuries are associated with a high degree of contamination. The following always make an open fracture a type III fracture: a shotgun wound, a high-velocity gunshot wound, a segmental fracture with displacement, a fracture with segmental loss in the diaphysis, a fracture associated with vascular injury that requires repair, a fracture that occurs in a highly contaminated area, such as a barnyard or stable, or a crush fracture caused by a high-velocity vehicle.[74] Type IIIA fractures, despite significant flaps, avulsions, or lacerations, have adequate soft tissue coverage of the fracture site. Type IIIB fractures are defined by periosteal striping of the exposed bone, with sufficient soft tissue loss so that local or free flaps are required for coverage. These fractures may also be associated with massive contamination or serious fracture comminution. Type IIIC fractures are characterized by arterial injury requiring repair.

The initial approach to these injuries is vital. *First, they must be recognized for the surgical emergencies that they are.* Rapid surgical debridement of devitalized tissues is vital to limit the incidence of wound sepsis.[87] These are not injuries that can be splinted overnight while waiting for the local x-ray facility to be open. Important on-field management is to limit contamination of the wound by covering it with a sterile dressing. Excessive cleansing and irrigation of the wound in the uncontrolled setting of the athletic venue is not recommended because of the potential risk of damage to exposed tissues, vessels, and nerves. Open fractures require surgical evaluation and debridement, and it is most beneficial to expedite this by getting the athlete to the hospital for definitive therapy. As stated earlier, splinting of open fractures is best done in the position in which the fracture is found. The wound should not be blindly probed on the field because of the risk of creating further bleeding, injury to soft tissues, or contamination of the wound. For these same reasons, bone fragments or portions of soft tissue should not be forced back into the wound.

FAT EMBOLISM SYNDROME

This syndrome is mentioned because of its relation to long bone fractures. Clinically, the most striking feature of the syndrome is marked respiratory distress that can progress to a full-blown adult respiratory distress syndrome (ARDS) picture. This is associated with marked tachypnea and tachycardia. Patients with fat embolism syndrome can also have marked changes in neurologic status characterized by restlessness, agitation, confusion, and even stupor and coma.[84] There is also a characteristic pattern of petechial development in the skin across the chest, around the neck, in the axillae, and in the conjunctivae that tends to develop 2 to 3 days after injury.[84] The pathophysiology of the syndrome has not been entirely elucidated. Historically, it has been

TABLE 33–11
Classification of Open Fractures

Type	Wound Size (cm)	Soft Tissue Injury	Bone Injury
I	<1	Negligible	Lack of comminution
II	>1	Muscle damage	Comminution
IIIA	>10	Severe, increasing	Severe comminution
IIIB	>10	Soft tissue damage	
IIIC	>10	Vascular injury	

TABLE 33–12
Acromioclavicular Separations

Type	Ligament Integrity*		Stability		PE
	AC	CC	A-P	Vertical	
I	+	+	+	+	Patient tender, without anatomic changes
II	–	+	–	+	+/– changes
III	–	–	–	–	Arm held adducted and supported
IV	–	–	–	–	Posterior inclination
V	–	–	–	–	Gross superior displacement with or without brachial plexus injury
VI	–	–	–	–	Inferior displacement

*AC, acromioclavicular; CC, coracoclavicular; AP, anteroposterior.

established that fat emboli have been found in the lungs and brain of individuals with a clinical scenario.[84] It is widely believed that these emboli come from the marrow of the fractured long bone, although the exact manner in which they cause the clinical picture has not been fully explained. The incidence of the syndrome has been estimated as 0.5 to 2.0 percent in long bone fractures and almost 10 percent in patients with multiple fractures.[88]

Sevitt[89] has reported that 25 percent of patients with fat embolism syndrome presented within 12 hours of injury, 75 percent presented before 36 hours after injury, and 85 percent presented before 48 hours after injury. The importance of mentioning this syndrome here is not because of its presentation on the field of play, but because of its occurrence shortly after the injury is sustained. The progression of symptoms to respiratory failure may be rapid, and it is important to consider this diagnosis when contacted by a patient with similar symptoms shortly after the fracture of a long bone.

REGIONAL APPROACH TO SPECIFIC INJURIES

This section examines particular anatomic regions and addresses the most common orthopaedic injuries in those areas or notes those injuries most fraught with complications. It is intended to be a practical guide to the management of those injuries, along with the recognition and management of their common complications that may present at the athletic venue.

SHOULDER GIRDLE AND SHOULDER

Acromioclavicular (AC) separation is a relatively common injury in collision sports. The most common mechanism of injury is a direct blow to the point of the shoulder.[90] AC separations are divided into six types (Table 33–12). A type I injury implies a sprain to the acromioclavicular ligaments, with no loss of stability. Type II injuries involve a tear of the acromioclavicular ligaments, without complete disruption of the conoid and trapezoid ligaments. Type III injuries are characterized by complete disruption of the acromioclavicular and coracoclavicular ligaments. Type IV injuries also have complete disruption of the acromioclavicular and coracoclavicular ligaments, along with detachment of the trapezius and deltoid muscles and posterior displacement, as noted in type V injuries. Type VI injuries occur when a superior force drives the distal end of the clavicle down into the subacromial or subcoracoid space, with complete disruption of the acromioclavicular and coracoclavicular ligaments.

Sideline evaluation of the athlete with a separation of the acromioclavicular joint involves close inspection of the area. An evaluation done shortly after the injury has the benefit of minimal soft tissue swelling obscuring the underlying anatomy. A distal neurovascular evaluation is also important because of the close proximity of underlying structures, such as the subclavian artery and vein and the brachial plexus. Type VI injuries, with their inferior displacement, have been associated with injury to the superior trunk of the brachial plexus, giving the athlete symptoms in the C5 and C6 distribution. Treatment of AC separations is immobilization of the arm adducted at the side, with the elbow flexed to 90 degrees. Inferior pressure is maintained on the clavicle while the sling suspends the arm. This maneuver generally provides significant pain relief and the athlete is then referred for x-ray.

Clavicular fractures can also occur from similar mechanisms. The vast majority of clavicular fractures occur in the middle third, followed in frequency by fractures to the distal third, and then the proximal third.[90] Athletes with clavicular fractures are usually relatively easy to identify. The affected arm is often held and supported by the opposite arm. There is usually significant pain and deformity. The fracture is generally palpable. Evidence of clavicular fracture obviously precludes return to play. Neurovascular examination of the upper extremity is important, because the subclavian vessels and brachial plexus are at risk of injury due to clavicular fractures. The medial cord lies closest to the clavicle and is the most frequently injured portion of the plexus.[90] There have also been reports of pneumothorax caused by clavicular fractures.[91,92] A complete pulmonary examination is therefore necessary to rule out the presence of pneumothorax.

Initial care for a fractured clavicle is a sling on the affected arm, along with the local application of ice. Figure-of-eight clavicle harnesses may be used, but they have not been shown to improve healing and are associated with a greater number of side effects.[93] Rarely is surgical intervention indicated with clavicular fractures, being reserved for a fraction of distal clavicular fractures, open fractures, or fractures associated with neurovascular injury.[90]

Traumatic anterior dislocation of the glenohumeral joint is also seen frequently in athletic competition, and studies have shown that approximately 90 percent of all shoulder dislocations occur anteriorly.[94] The classic mechanism of dislocation is abduction and external rotation of the arm, with a subcoracoid dislocation being the most common type of dislocation noted.[94] The athlete presents with marked pain and muscular spasm in the shoulder. Simple observation and palpation reveal a humeral head that is dislocated anteriorly and inferiorly. Complications associated with this injury include vascular damage to either the axillary artery or vein. Neural damage can also occur, with the most common injury being to the axillary nerve due to its close relationship to the proximal humerus as it passes through the quadrangular space.[94] The axillary nerve provides motor innervation to the deltoid muscle and sensory innervation to the lateral aspect of the proximal upper arm. The function of the axillary nerve should be assessed prior to and after any manipulation of the shoulder.

If the dislocated shoulder is acute, with no axillary nerve deficit noted, it can be reduced before marked muscle spasm sets in. This is generally attempted by applying longitudinal traction in the same plane that the arm is being held. The humerus is then gently flexed and abducted. A palpable, distinct clunk is noted. The basic principle is to be gentle. Forced humeral reductions have been associated with both glenoid and humeral shaft fractures.[94] The health care provider should be knowledgeable about both the reduction maneuver and its potential complications prior to reducing a suspected dislocated shoulder on the field.[94,95]

HUMERUS

Fractures of the humeral shaft can be associated with specific and immediate complications due to the anatomic relationships of the compartments and neurovascular structures about the humeral shaft. Fractures of the proximal humeral shaft involve one of four anatomic regions—the greater tuberosity, the lesser tuberosity, the anatomic neck, and the surgical neck. Greater tuberosity fractures are commonly associated with anterior shoulder dislocations. Frequently, when the shoulder is reduced, the greater tuberosity also anatomically reduces. Isolated lesser tuberosity fractures are rare and are generally associated with posterior dislocations. Anatomic and surgical neck fractures generally occur in an older population. Surgical neck fractures are more common. Fractures of the shaft of the humerus often reveal characteristic angulation. Proximal fractures assume an "apex medial" angulation due to the pull of the pectoralis major muscle on the proximal fragment. Midshaft fractures assume an "apex lateral" angulation due to the medially directed pull of the biceps, triceps, and coracobrachialis muscles on the distal fragment. In the absence of neurovascular compromise, all athletes with these injuries can be safely transported to the nearest health care facility in a supportive sling.

As in every fracture, distal neurovascular assessment is essential. The most common nerve injury occurring with midshaft humeral fractures is to the radial nerve.[90] Near the junction of the middle and distal thirds of the arm, the radial nerve lies in close apposition to the humerus, making it susceptible to injury with fractures at this site. The cause is commonly a stretching or contusion to the nerve that resolves spontaneously, although laceration of the nerve can occur. The motor and sensory components of all three nerves, however, must be assessed individually. Sensory function of the radial nerve is noted by testing sensation of the first dorsal web space, with the motor component being tested by assessing wrist and finger extension. The median nerve is tested in its sensory distribution over the palmar aspect of the index finger and its motor function noted in the thumb and distal interphalangeal index and middle finger flexors. Sensory evaluation of the ulnar nerve is tested on the palmar aspect of the little finger. Motor function is documented in the interosseous and lumbrical muscles of the hand. If a radial nerve palsy is detected on examination, immediate surgical exploration is not necessarily indicated. The vast majority of these injuries resolve spontaneously, and even those that do not can be repaired after some time has elapsed.

The brachial artery is also at risk for damage with a humeral shaft fracture. The identification of brachial artery disruption, through documentation of a pulseless distal upper extremity, is an orthopaedic emergency. Athletes with closed fractures should undergo arteriography to assess the degree of injury, and those with open fractures should proceed directly to open exploration and repair of the artery.

ELBOW

Elbow dislocations are the third most common joint dislocations in adults. The mechanism of injury is described as a fall on an outstretched hand, forcing the elbow into hyperextension.[83,95] The direction of the dislocation is therefore defined by the relationship of the radius and ulna to the distal humerus. The olecranon process becomes a fulcrum, with increasing degrees of hyperextension. The anterior location of the brachial artery and median and radial nerves subjects these structures to intimal damage and stretching with posterior dislocations. Elbow dislocation must therefore be treated as an orthopaedic emergency. Diagnosis is relatively straightforward. The elbow is held at approximately 45 degrees of flexion, the forearm is foreshortened, and the olecranon process is prominent. Treatment should be initiated after a thorough neurovascular examination, with specific attention being given to the integrity of the median and radial nerves and to the brachial artery distribution within the forearm. Reduction is accomplished by using longitudinal traction associated with an anteriorly directed force on the olecranon. The arm is then slowly flexed. A clunk is noted with reduction. The injured athlete should then be placed in a sling and arm swath for transport to the nearest health care facility for radiographic and possibly vascular workup.

Supracondylar elbow fractures, the most common type of pediatric elbow fracture, have been associated with compartment syndrome and with Volkmann ischemic contracture of the forearm.[81,83] This is secondary to damage of the brachial artery just above the elbow. Physical examination reveals a swollen, exquisitely tender elbow. The olecranon process is displaced posteriorly. The health care provider should be cognizant of the classic signs of pain and swelling in the forearm and significant pain with passive extension of the fingers of the involved extremity. If suspected, management of the possible compartment syndrome proceeds as described earlier (see Compartment syndromes). A volar compartment syndrome of the forearm has also been described in relation to a posterior dislocation of the elbow.[82]

FOREARM, WRIST, AND HAND

The hand and wrist are the most intricate articulations of the upper extremity. Morbidity associated with injuries of these anatomic structures is often significant. Evaluation of hand and wrist injuries is often confusing without a thorough knowledge of the structure and function of upper extremity anatomy.

Colles fracture is the most common wrist fracture seen in adults.[84] The fracture is commonly nonarticular, can be associated with a distal ulnar styloid fracture, and is dorsally angulated. Severe displacement can result in injury to the median nerve. A Smith fracture is a volarly angulated fracture of the distal radius, in contrast to the Colles fracture. Physical examination is similar in both in that the injured athlete presents with a swollen, painful wrist. Complete neurovascular examinations are necessary in both to rule out an associated nerve injury. Ulnar shaft or "nightstick" fractures can occur with blunt trauma to the forearm. A painful, swollen forearm with tenderness on palpation to the midshaft of the ulna is diagnostic. Fractures of both bones of the forearm are included secondary to the association with compartment syndrome. After complete neurovascular evaluation, all these fractures can be safely splinted and the athlete transported to an appropriate health care facility for fracture management.

The ulnar-collateral ligament of the first metacarpophalangeal (MCP) joint is vulnerable to injury. Two common names for this injury are "gamekeeper's thumb" and "skier's thumb." The mechanism of injury is that of a radially directed force applied to the thumb. Physical examination reveals swelling and tenderness at the ulnar aspect of the first MCP. In addition, laxity at both 0 and 20 degrees to radial stress is documented. Although athletes with this injury are routinely taped and allowed to continue playing, any athlete who presents with this injury should be splinted and referred for evaluation to an appropriate specialist.

Extensor tendon injuries are common athletic injuries. They usually occur over the MCP joint and are associated with penetration of the joint capsule. This is especially true if the injury is sustained in a fight. Flexor tendon injuries are mostly associated with hand wounds caused by sharp penetrating objects, although they can occasionally be caused by forced extension, such as occurs when a hand is caught in a jersey. Mallet finger, or "baseball finger," is a flexion deformity of the DIP joint of a digit. The mechanism of injury is forced flexion or jamming of the tip of the finger, which causes either a disruption of the extensor mechanism or a fracture at the dorsal base of the distal phalanx. Physical examination of the joint reveals pain, ecchymosis, and swelling about the DIP. In addition, the DIP is flexed, with the athlete unable to extend the joint actively. Radiographs are necessary to delineate the two types of injuries. Initial and longitudinal treatment is to splint the DIP in extension.

Fractures of the distal phalanx are common athletic injuries and are usually associated with crush injuries. The common association with a distal phalanx fracture is disruption of the nail matrix. By definition, these are considered open fractures and should be treated by repairing the lacerated nail bed, and by using antibiotics to prevent any infection. Physical examination is generally straightforward. Treatment involves splinting of the DIP joint only.

Fractures of the middle and proximal phalanges are also common athletic injuries. They are divided into articular and nonarticular categories. On the field, the physical examination is directed toward assessment of alignment and rotational deformities. The hand is splinted in the position of function, and the athlete is referred for radiographic documentation. Unlike distal phalanx fractures, middle and proximal phalanx fractures require immobilization of the whole hand.

Fractures of the metacarpals present with pain and swelling of the dorsum of the hand. The most common type of metacarpal fracture is the "boxer's fracture" of the fifth metacarpal. This injury occurs when an athlete strikes a hard surface with a closed fist. The concern with these fractures is the associated foreshortening and rotational abnormalities of the metacarpals. On physical examination, the digits should all point to the base of the scaphoid when flexed. Any deviation from this, as compared with the other side, is suggestive of a malrotation. Fractures of the second or third metacarpal are generally more stable due to the intrinsic tethering of these metacarpals, but anatomic reduction and maintenance become more important.

THIGH, HIP, AND PELVIS

Pelvic fractures are an orthopaedic emergency, with their severe complications of life-threatening hemorrhage and damage to internal structures. Fortunately, they are most commonly associated with high-velocity trauma and are rarely seen in athletes. In regard to the hip, its traumatic dislocation carries a significant risk of avascular necrosis.[96] Avascular necrosis has also been reported in an athlete who suffered a subluxation of the hip.[97] Because of the risk of avascular necrosis, management principles center around early reduction of the dislocation. Posterior dislocations can also be associated with acetabular fractures and are seen in automobile accidents. This injury carries a high rate of posttraumatic osteoarthritis, which can be diminished with open reduction and internal fixation of the fracture.

Several different injuries of the thigh carry the risk of complication. A simple thigh contusion can be associated with compartment syndrome of the thigh but, more commonly, it can significantly delay the athlete's return to play. An acute thigh contusion should be managed with a compressive wrap on the day of the injury. The area should be iced frequently. Local heat increases vascular flow to the area and thus should be avoided because of the risk of increasing bleeding in the area. The player should also either have the knee taped in flexion or be instructed to sleep with the knee flexed. The knee should never be forced into flexion, however. Without this measure, there is significant loss of flexion the next day, which can be difficult to restore. Actual fractures of the femur are rare in the athletic setting because of the large amount of force needed to create the injury, but they have occurred in collision sports. Therefore, a midshaft femur fracture should be considered when the pain or disability involving the thigh is severe. Midshaft femur fractures can also cause acute complications. They can lacerate the femoral artery, compromising blood supply distally, and can result in a large amount of blood loss into the thigh. As stated earlier with other injuries, a thorough distal neurovascular assessment is vital.

KNEE

Knee injuries are common in athletic participation. Although many knee injuries cause significant loss of playing time, few of them place the lower limb at acute risk. A notable exception to this is knee dislocation. Tibiofemoral dislocation carries a high risk of vascular injury. Because of its close anatomic proximity, the popliteal artery is placed at great risk with dislocation of the knee. Green and Allen[98] have reported a series of 245 knee dislocations in which there was a 32 percent incidence of injuries to the popliteal artery. Of the 33 limbs not undergoing vascular repair within 8 hours of the injury, 28 were amputated and 3 of the 5 salvaged limbs had severe ischemic injuries. This finding emphasizes the statement that knee dislocations should be considered a limb-threatening injury until proved otherwise. The presence of pulses on examination does not rule out a potentially devastating injury to the popliteal artery.[83] It also emphasizes the need for rapid vascular evaluation and repair to save the involved limb. Initial care of a dislocated knee involves gentle reduction and immobilization. One should avoid hyperextension of greater than 15 degrees and excessive varus stress, both of which can injure the peroneal nerve.[83]

Lateral dislocations of the patella usually occur in adolescents and are common athletic injuries. The mechanism of injury is a twisting type of injury to the lower extremity with the foot planted. This internally rotates the femur on the tibia, creates a laterally directed force on the patella with quadriceps contraction, and causes the patella to sublux or dislocate. Injured athletes often say that the knee "gave out" or "dislocated" or that they heard a "pop." Physical examination of the knee reveals prominent femoral condyles if the patella is dislocated. The knee is in a flexed position, and any attempt to move the joint is resisted. Reduction of a dislocated patella is obtained by slowly extending the affected knee while providing medial pressure to the patella. Although a dislocated patella is not an orthopaedic emergency, relocation provides almost instantaneous relief of pain. The health care provider should be aware that patella fractures have been associated with relocation maneuvers. The leg should be immobilized and the athlete transported to the appropriate health care facility for radiographic evaluation.

LEG

The tibia is the most commonly fractured long bone in the body. Its subcutaneous position frequently predisposes it to open-type fractures. Complications of tibial fractures have been shown to be related to the severity of injury.[99,100] One of the most common complications is the compartment syndrome (see earlier). Compartment syndromes are commonly described in the lower leg, so the caregiver must watch for the development of signs or symptoms. Another complication of tibial or fibular fractures is injury to the anterior tibial artery.[83] Identification of this injury can be difficult because if the injury occurs proximally, blood can be shunted through the peroneal artery to the dorsalis pedis artery, giving the patient both dorsalis pedis and posterior tibial pulses in the foot. Close observation is important for signs and symptoms of ischemia.

ANKLE AND FOOT

Emergent complications due to injuries to the ankle and foot are not common. The ankle is the most commonly injured joint of the lower extremity, however, so the health care provider must be aware of common complications or injuries. The "generic" lateral ankle sprain has been associated with peroneal nerve palsy as well as peroneus longus disruption.[101] An eversion sprain of the ankle, although not common, may be associated with syndesmosis disruption, interosseous hemorrhage, and fracture of the proximal fibula at or near the anatomic location of the common peroneal nerve. Therefore, a thorough mechanism of injury should accompany any routine ankle examination. A good habit to develop is to start by palpating the proximal fibula for tenderness. This is extended distally to include the distal fibula, anterior syndesmosis, and distal tibia. One should document sensation in the dorsal first web space and assess the integrity of the peroneal, extensor hallucis, tibialis anterior, and posterior tibialis muscles.

The calcaneus is the most commonly injured bone of the hindfoot. The mechanism of injury is usually a fall from a height, such as a pole vaulter missing the mat. There is an association in 25 percent of intra-articular calcaneal fractures with lumbar spine fractures.[83,102] Fractures of the talus and tarsal navicular are uncommon and are usually not associated with athletic encounters. An infrequent injury of the midtarsal region of the foot associated with those involved in the martial arts is the "locked cuboid."[103] Direct palpation of the cuboid along the peroneal groove elicits pain in this condition. Reduction should be reserved until radiographs confirm the absence of fracture. The athlete should be transferred splinted and non–weight bearing. Fractures of the metatarsals are not usually associated with emergent complications, but certain injury mechanisms should alert the health care provider to underlying pathology. Forced plantar flexion can fracture or dislocate the tarsometatarsal junction, the so-called Lisfranc fracture dislocation.[102] Although not an orthopaedic emergency, this particular injury carries a significant morbidity risk.

Achilles tendon rupture is most commonly seen in adults between the ages of 30 and 50 years. This injury can occur with no significant trauma. The mechanism of injury is a dorsiflexion force on the foot while the gastrocsoleus complex is contracting. Physical examination reveals a painful swollen calf, ecchymosis, a palpable deficit within the substance of the tendon, and weakness on plantar flexion against resistance of the foot. The Thompson squeeze test has also been described as a diagnostic entity, although its sensitivity is not a good reference. The injured athlete should be immobilized in 10 to 15 degrees of plantar flexion, made non–weight bearing, and transported to the nearest appropriate health care facility.

SUMMARY

The provision of care for the injured athlete is often a perplexing problem. Assessment, diagnostic, and transport procedures are routinely performed under circumstances of limited time, excessive crowd noise, inclement weather, unrealistic expectations of coaches and players, and the increasing specter of liability. The key to the proper assessment and management of the injured athlete is a thorough, systematic approach to game or event preparation, emergency medical service provisions, initial injury evaluation focusing on the ABCDEs, and appropriate, timely transport. Meticulous planning and preparation afford the competitive edge necessary to meet the challenge of the emergent care of the injured athlete.

REFERENCES

1. Clarke KS: An epidemiologic view. *In* Torg JS (ed): Athletic Injuries to the Head, Neck, and Face, 2nd ed. St. Louis, Mosby-Year Book, 1991, p 15.
2. Schneider RC: Serious and fatal neurosurgical football injuries. Clin Neurosurg 1966; 12:226.
3. Torg JS, Quedenfeld TC, Moyer RA, et al: Severe and catastrophic neck injuries resulting from tackle football. J Am Coll Health Assoc 1977; 25:224.
4. Torg JS, Quedenfeld TC, Burstein A, et al: National Football Head and Neck Injury Registry: Report on cervical quadriplegia 1971 to 1975. Am J Sports Med 1979; 7:127.
5. Kouwenhoven WB, Jude JR, Knickerbocker GC: Closed-chest cardiac massage. JAMA 1960; 173:1064.
6. Cardiopulmonary resuscitation: Statement by the Ad Hoc Committee on Cardiopulmonary Resuscitation of the Division of Medical Sciences, National Academy of Sciences-National Research Council. JAMA 1966; 198:372.
7. Guidelines for cardiopulmonary resuscitation and emergency cardiac care: Recommendations of the 1992 National Conference. JAMA 1992; 268:2171.
8. American College of Surgeons Committee on Trauma: Course overview, concept, and history. *In* Alexander RH, Proctor HJ (eds): The Advanced Trauma Life Support Course for Physicians Vol II: Student Manual. Chicago, American College of Surgeons, 1989, p 3.
9. Guide to Clinical Preventive Services: An assessment of the effectiveness of 169 interventions. *In* Report of the US Preventive Task Force. Baltimore, Williams & Wilkins, 1989.
10. Halpern BD: Down man on the field. Primary Care 1991; 18:833.
11. Walker EJ, Bianco EA, Hartmann PM: Legal aspects of sports medicine. *In* Birrer RB (ed): Sports Medicine for the Primary Care Physician. Norwalk, Appleton-Century-Crofts, 1984, p 326.
12. Richards EP III, Rathbun KC: Institutional practice: Teams, schools, and prisons. *In* Richards EP, Rathbun KC (eds): Law and the Physician: A Practical Guide. Boston, Little, Brown, 1993, p 451.
13. AMA Council on Ethical and Judicial Affairs: Code of Medical Ethics—Current Opinions. Chicago, American Medical Association, 1992.
14. Gennarelli TA: Head injury mechanisms. *In* Torg JS (ed): Athletic Injuries to the Head, Neck, and Face, 2nd ed. St. Louis, Mosby-Year Book, 1991, p 232.
15. Lehman LB, Ravich SJ: Closed head injuries in athletes. Clin Sports Med 1990; 9:247.
16. Cantu RC: Head and spine injuries in the young athlete. Clin Sports Med 1988; 17:459.
17. Seelig JM, Becker DP, Miller JD, et al: Traumatic acute subdural hematoma: Major mortality reduction in comatose patients treated within four hours. N Engl J Med 1981; 304:1511.
18. Yarnell PR, Lynch S: The "ding" amnestic states in football trauma. Neurology 1983; 23:196.
19. Vegso JJ, Lehman RC: Field evaluation and management of head and neck injuries. Clin Sports Med 1987; 6:1.
20. Cantu RC: Guidelines to return to contact sports after a cerebral concussion. Phys Sports Med 1986; 14:79.
21. Torg JS, Vegso JJ, O'Neill MJ, Sennett B: The epidemiologic, pathologic, biomechanical, and cinematographic analysis of football-induced cervical spine trauma. Am J Sports Med 1990; 18:50.
22. Bailes JE, Maroon JC: Management of cervical spine injuries in athletes. Clin Sports Med 1989; 8:43.
23. Clancy WG Jr: Brachial plexus and upper extremity peripheral nerve injuries. *In* Torg JS (ed): Athletic Injuries to the Head, Neck, and Face. Philadelphia, Lea & Febiger, 1982, p 215.
24. Hershman EB: Brachial plexus injuries. Clin Sports Med 1990; 9:311.
25. Sunderland S: Nerves and Nerve Injuries, 2nd ed. Edinburgh, Churchill Livingstone, 1978.
26. Maroon JC: "Burning hands" in football spinal cord injuries. JAMA 1977; 238:2049.
27. Zagelbaum BM: Sports-related eye trauma. Phys Sports Med 1993; 21:25.

28. Position statement from the International Federation of Sports Medicine on eye injuries and eye protection in sports. Br J Sports Med 1989; 23:59.

29. Brucker AJ, Kozart DM, Nichols CW, Raber IM: Diagnosis and management of injuries to the eye and orbit. In Torg JS (ed): Athletic Injuries to the Head, Neck, and Face, 2nd ed. St. Louis, Mosby-Year Book, 1991, p 650.

30. Forrest LA, Schuller DE, Strauss RH: Management of orbital blow-out fractures: Case reports and discussion. Am J Sports Med 1989; 17:217.

31. White MJ, Johnson PC, Heckler FR: Management of maxillofacial and neck soft-tissue injuries. Clin Sports Med 1989; 8:11.

32. Handler SD: Diagnosis and management of maxillofacial injuries. In Torg JS (ed): Athletic Injuries to the Head, Neck, and Face, 2nd ed. St. Louis, Mosby-Year Book, 1991, p 611.

33. Lephart SM, Fu FH: Emergency treatment of athletic injuries. Dent Clin North Am 1991; 35:707.

34. Bakland LK, Boyne PJ: Trauma to the oral cavity. Clin Sports Med 1989; 8:25.

35. Wilkinson DA, Moore EE, Wither PD, et al: A.T.L.S. on the ski slopes—a Steamboat experience. J Trauma 1992; 32:448.

36. Pate JW: Chest wall injuries. Surg Clin North Am 1989; 69:59.

37. Koster JK Jr, Sauders JH Jr, Stromberg RM: Thoracic injuries. In May HL (ed): Emergency Med, 2nd ed, vol 1. Boston, Little, Brown, 1992, p 705.

38. Fanta CH: Obstructive lung diseases. In May HL (ed): Emergency Medicine, 2nd ed, vol 1. Boston, Little, Brown & Company, 1992.

39. Risser WL: Exercise for children. Pediatr Rev 1988; 10:131.

40. Boxer MB, Greenberger PA, Patterson R: The impact of prednisone in life-threatening idiopathic anaphylaxis: Reduction in acute episodes and medical costs. Ann Allerg 1989; 62:201.

41. Stoloff R, Adams SL, Orfan N: Emergency medical recognition and management of idiopathic anaphylaxis. J Emerg Med 1992; 10:693.

42. Nichols AW: Exercise-induced anaphylaxis and urticaria. Clin Sports Med 1992; 11:303.

43. Adelman DC, Spector SL: Acute respiratory emergencies in emergency treatment of the injured athlete. Clin Sports Med 1989; 8:71.

44. Thompson PD, Funk EJ, Carleton RA, Sturner WQ: Incidence of death during jogging in Rhode Island from 1975 through 1980. JAMA 1982; 247:2535.

45. Waller BF, Roberts WC: Sudden death while running in conditioned runners aged 40 years or over. Am J Cardiol 1980; 45:1292.

46. Maron BJ, Epstein SE, Roberts WC: Causes of sudden death in competitive athletes. J Am Coll Cardiol 1986; 7:204.

47. Maron BJ, Roberts WC, McAllister HA: Sudden death in young athletes. Circulation 1980; 62:218.

48. Pyeritz RE, McKusick VA: The Marfan syndrome: Diagnosis and management. N Engl J Med 1979; 300:772.

49. Coslo FG, Benson DW Jr, Anderson RW, et al: Onset of atrial fibrillation during antidromic tachycardia: Association with sudden cardiac arrest and ventricular fibrillation in a patient with Wolff-Parkinson-White syndrome. Am J Cardiol 1982; 50:353.

50. Huston TP, Puffer JC, Rodney WM: The athletic heart syndrome. N Engl J Med 1985; 313:24.

51. Kaplan JA, Karofsky PS, Volturo GA: Commotio cordis in two amateur ice hockey players despite the use of commercial chest protectors: Case reports. J Trauma 1993; 34:151.

52. Abrunzo TJ: Commotio cordis: The single, most common cause of traumatic death in youth baseball. Am J Dis Child 1991; 145:1279.

53. Paone RF, Peacock JB, Smith DL: Diagnosis of myocardial contusion. South Med J 1993; 86:867.

54. Goldberg SP, Karalis DG, Ross JJ Jr: Severe right ventricular contusion mimicking cardiac tamponade: The value of transesophageal echocardiography in blunt chest trauma. Ann Emerg Med 1993; 22:745.

55. Orliaguet G, Jacquens Y, Riou B, et al: Combined severe myocardial and pulmonary contusion: Early diagnosis with transesophageal echocardiography and management with high-frequency jet ventilation: case report. J Trauma 1993; 34:455.

56. Foil MB, Mackersie RC, Furst SR, et al: The asymptomatic patient with suspected myocardial contusion. Am J Surg 1990; 160:638.

57. Colucciello SA, Plotka M: Abdominal trauma: Occult injury may be life-threatening. Phys Sports Med 1993; 21:33.

58. Kenney P: Abdominal pain in athletes. Clin Sports Med 1986; 6:885.

59. Knudson MM, McAninch JW, Gomez R, et al: Hematuria as a predictor of abdominal injury after blunt trauma. Am J Surg 1992; 164:482.

60. Powell DC, Bivens BA, Bell RM: Diagnostic peritoneal lavage. Surg Gynecol Obstet 1982; 155:257.

61. Haycock CE: How I manage abdominal injuries. Phys Sports Med 1986; 14:86.

62. Maki DG, Reich RM: Infectious mononucleosis in the athlete: Diagnosis, complications and management. Am J Sports Med 1982; 10:162.

63. Sugrue M, Knox A, Sarre R, et al: Management of splenic trauma: A new CT-guided splenic injury grading system. Aust NZ J Surg 1991; 61:349.

64. Mirvis SE, Whitley NO, Gens DR: Blunt splenic trauma in adults: CT-based classification and correlation with prognosis and treatment. Radiology 1989; 171:33.

65. Schweizer W, Tanner S, Baer HU, et al: Management of traumatic liver injuries. Br J Surg 1993; 80:86.

66. Delius RE, Frankel W, Coran AG: A comparison between operative and nonoperative management of blunt injuries to the liver and spleen in adult and pediatric patients. Surgery 1989; 106:788.

67. Galat JA, Grisoni ER, Gauderer MWL: Pediatric blunt liver injury: Establishment of criteria for appropriate management. J Pediatr Surg 1990; 25:1162.

68. Herschorn S, Radomski SB, Shoskes DA, et al: Evaluation and treatment of blunt renal trauma. J Urol 1991; 146:274.

69. Mee SL, McAninch JW, Robinson AL, et al: Radiographic assessment of renal trauma: A 10-year prospective study of patient selection. J Urol 141:1095.

70. Eastham JA, Wilson TG, Ahlering TE: Radiographic assessment of blunt renal trauma. J Trauma 1991; 31:1527.

71. Bird K, Rosenfeld AT, Taylor KJW: Ultrasonography in testicular torsion. Radiology 1983; 147:527.

72. Lupetin AR, King W III, Rich PJ, Lederman RB: The traumatized scrotum: Ultrasound evaluation. Radiology 1983; 148:203.

73. American College of Surgeons Committee on Trauma: Extremity trauma. In Alexander RH, Proctor RJ (eds): The Advanced Trauma Life Support Course for Physicians Vol II: Student Manual. Chicago, American College of Surgeons, 1989, p 181.

74. Chapman MW: Open fractures. In Rockwood CA, Green DP, Bucholz RW (eds): Fractures in Adults, 3rd ed, vol 1. Philadelphia, JB Lippincott Company, 1991, p 223.

75. Harkess JW, Ramsey WC, Harkess JW: Principles of fractures and dislocations. In Rockwood CA, Green DP, and Bucholz RW (eds): Fractures in Adults, 3rd ed, vol 1. Philadelphia, JB Lippincott, 1991.

76. Mubarak SJ, Owen CA, Hargens AR, et al: Acute compartment syndromes. Diagnosis and treatment with the aid of the wick catheter. J Bone Joint Surg 1978; 60A:1091.

77. Tarlow SD, Achterman CA, Hayhurst J, Ovadia DN: Acute compartment syndrome in the thigh complicating fracture of the femur. A report of three cases. J Bone Joint Surg 1986; 68A:1439.

78. Heppenstall RB, Scott R, Sapega A, et al: A comparative study of the tolerance of skeletal muscle to ischemia. J Bone Joint Surg 1986; 68A:620.

79. Sheridan GW, Matsen FA III: An animal model of the compartmental syndrome. Clin Orthop 1975; 113:36.

80. Sheridan GW, Matsen F, Krugmire R: Further investigations on the pathophysiology of compartment syndrome. Clin Orthop 1977; 123:266.

81. Rasul AT, Gustilo RB: Compartmental syndrome. In Gustilo RB, Kyle RF, Templeman D (eds): Fractures and Dislocations, vol 2. St. Louis, Mosby-Year Book, 1993, p 1251.

82. Matsen FA III, Winquist RA, Krugmire RB: Diagnosis and management of compartmental syndromes. J Bone Joint Surg 1980; 62A:286.

83. Wolin PM: Limb-threatening emergencies. In Cantu RC, Micheli LJ (eds): ACSM's Guidelines for the Team Physician. Philadelphia, Lea & Febiger, 1991, p 153.

84. Pellegrini VD Jr, Evarts CM: Complications. *In* Rockwood CA, Green DP, Bucholz RW (eds): Fractures in Adults, 3rd ed, vol 1. Philadelphia, JB Lippincott, 1991, p 335.
85. Werry DG, Meek RN: Clostridial gas gangrene complicating Colles' fracture. J Trauma 1986; 26:280.
86. Connolly JF: General problems. *In* Fracture Complications: Recognition, Prevention and Management. Chicago, Year Book Medical Publishers, 1988.
87. Gustilo RB: Open fractures. *In* Gustilo RB, Kyle RF, Templeman D (eds): Fractures and Dislocations, vol 1. St. Louis, Mosby-Year Book, 1993, p 169.
88. Gossling HR, Pellegrini VD Jr: Fat embolism syndrome: A review of the pathophysiology and physiological basis of treatment. Clin Orthop 1982; 165:68.
89. Sevitt S: The significance and classification of fat embolism. Lancet 1960; 2:825.
90. Chadwick R Jr, Kyle RF: Fractures and dislocations of the proximal humerus, scapula, sternoclavicular joint, acromioclavicular joint, and clavicle. *In* Gustilo RB, Kyle RF, Templeman D (eds): Fractures and Dislocations, vol 1. St. Louis, Mosby-Year Book, 1993, p 255.
91. Dugdale TW, Fulkerson JP: Pneumothorax complicating a closed fracture of the clavicle. Clin Orthop 1987; 221:212.
92. Meeks RJ, Riebel GD: Isolated clavicle fracture with associated pneumothorax: A case report. Am J Emerg Med 1991; 9:555.
93. Anderson K, Jensen PO, Lauritzen J: Treatment of clavicular fractures. Acta Orthop Scand 1987; 57:71.
94. Rockwood CA, Thomas SC, Masten FA III: Subluxations and dislocations about the glenohumeral joint. *In* Rockwood CA, Green DP, Bucholz RW (eds): Fractures in Adults, 3rd ed, vol 1. Philadelphia, JB Lippincott, 1991, p 1021.
95. Matsen FA III, Thomas SC, Rockwood CA Jr: Glenohumeral instability. *In* Rockwood CA Jr, Matsen FA III (eds): The Shoulder. Philadelphia, WB Saunders, 1990.
96. Cruess RL: Osteonecrosis of bone. Current concepts as to etiology and pathogenesis. Clin Orthop 1986; 208:30.
97. Cooper DE, Warren RF, Barnes R: Traumatic subluxation of the hip resulting in aseptic necrosis and chondrolysis in a professional football player. Am J Sports Med 1991; 19:322.
98. Green NE, Allen BL: Vascular injuries associated with dislocation of the knee. J Bone Joint Surg 1977; 59A:236.
99. Waddell JP, Reardon GP: Complications of tibial shaft fractures. Clin Orthop 1983; 178:173.
100. Blick SS, Brumback RJ, Poka A, et al: Compartment syndrome in open tibial fractures. J Bone Joint Surg 1986; 68A:1348.
101. Meals RA: Peroneal nerve palsy complicating ankle sprain. J Bone Joint Surg 1977; 59A:966.
102. Goossens M, DeStoop N: Lisfranc's fracture-dislocations: Etiology, radiology, and results of treatment. Clin Orthop 1983; 176:154.
103. Newell SG, Woodle A: Cuboid syndrome. Phys Sports Med 1982; 9:71.

CHAPTER 34

Psychology of the Injured Athlete

CAL BOTTERILL *PhD*
FRANCES A. FLINT *ATC, PhD*
LYDIA IEVLEVA *PhD*

The psychological dynamics in and around athletic injuries have become increasingly complex and significant. As the status, popularity, and payoffs of sport have escalated, so have the number and significance of injuries and their impact. The demands, challenges, and pressures of sport are greater, and increased visibility and scrutiny have heightened our awareness of powerful psychological and emotional dynamics.

Professionals engaged in sports medicine have witnessed cases of excruciating heartbreak and trauma, identity crisis and transition difficulty, and cases of miraculous recovery and growth. As careers and active lifestyles are jeopardized, the psychological and emotional impact approaches that of life-threatening challenges. On the other hand, highly motivated, fit, creative athletes and progressive sports medicine professionals have been on the leading edge of *pro-active* rehabilitation and health care possibilities.

All this has been occurring during an era of reawakening regarding the significance and potential of psychological and emotional factors in medical rehabilitation and health care.[1-3]

These forces have interacted to produce a powerful impact and some important implications for athletes, therapists, coaches, health care professionals, administrators, parents, and loved ones. This chapter summarizes key issues and aspects of the topic while sensitizing the reader to practical implications for the partners in the health and wellness challenge.

PSYCHOLOGICAL REACTIONS TO ATHLETIC INJURY

When an athletic injury occurs, and achievement goals and daily activities such as physical exertion and social interaction with teammates are affected, the injured athlete may experience severe psychological imbalance. It has been proposed that injured athletes experience psychological reactions similar to those following the death of a loved one.[4,5] Kübler-Ross,[6] in *On Death and Dying,* described the reactions to death as denial, anger, bargaining, depression, and finally, acceptance. These emotions and behaviors appear to be fairly common among injured athletes, and it may intuitively seem reasonable to expect some of these same feelings in injured athletes who are suffering from the loss of their normal (and loved) athletic lifestyles and, sometimes, the temporary loss of a meaningful identity. However, regardless of the severity of the injury, injured athletes should still consider themselves athletes and worthy human beings. In most cases, they have every intention of returning to sport once the rehabilitation process is complete. Thus, it may be unreasonable to extrapolate from the death and dying literature to the realm of injured athletes. In addition, to date, no empirical evidence exists to support the claims that injured athletes enter the death and dying paradigm.

What does occur psychologically when an athlete suffers from a major injury in which an extended hiatus from training and competition is experienced? When Drake Berehowski, a National Hockey League player, tore his anterior cruciate ligament and was out of competition for 9 months, he expressed the feeling of loss that the injury created. "You can't be with the guys anymore. You have to go back and do your therapy, and that's probably the hardest thing that I had to deal with, just being away from everyone, being away from the action, not being able to play."[7] When a first-year university level basketball player suffered a third-degree tear to her anterior cruciate ligament she stated, "At first, you might just think it's the end of the world; I did."[8] A senior in high school basketball who experienced the same injury agreed and commented, "I thought I had just twisted it . . . . When I came to the realization that I was going to be off for months at a time, that's when the fear set in and the discouragement."[9] Anecdotal testimony provides depth to the psychological experience and the beginning of empirically based foundation of knowledge on which to build psychological rehabilitation programs.

Current, ongoing research is beginning to contribute to knowledge relating to the psychophysiological reactions of athletes to injury. Both preinjury and postinjury data are being collected in the areas of affect, physical self-concept, and social support. Since this work is only in the preliminary stages, few generalizations can be made, but there are some emerging trends that can help

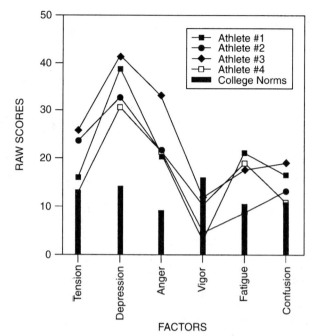

Male and female - In season Injury

FIGURE 34–2. Profile of mood states for four female and male athletes with second- or third-degree injuries sustained during the athletic season (Flint, October 1993).

us appreciate some of the psychological dynamics involved in athletic injuries. Over the course of a school year, baseline psychological data were collected on student/athletes at York University in Canada (Figs. 34–1 to 34–4). In addition, follow-up data were collected on any student athlete who sustained a 2nd degree (moderate) or 3rd degree (severe) injury during the course of varsity athletics. To date, the profile of mood states (POMS)[10] and a scale to determine feelings expressed after the injury[11] provide the most interesting insights. The POM scale was used to ascertain certain emotions both before and after injury and includes a college norm (nonathletes). Emotion or feelings reflected through the POMS included tension, depression, anger, vigor, fatigue, and confusion. As can be seen from Figures 34–1 and 34–2, reactions to the injury included marked increases in depression, anger, and tension and a decrease in the feeling of vigor compared with preinjury data. These profiles are the converse of the "iceberg" profile that has been used to describe healthy athletes.[12]

The second set of figures also shows an emotional reaction to the injury. Feeling of depression, frustration, and shock are extremely high and optimism reaches only a moderate level. Clearly, these injured athletes demonstrate that they are undergoing emotional trauma in conjunction with their physical injuries, loss of participation, or both.

Results obtained to date with an extremely small sample are supportive of the findings that athletes do undergo significant psychological and emotional stress related to injury. It is hoped that ongoing research will clarify the dynamics involved so that possible difficulties can be anticipated and preventive, therapeutic, and remedial guidelines can be suggested.

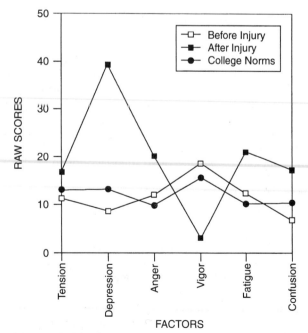

Male Population

FIGURE 34–1. Profile of mood state of a male athlete who suffered a fracture during the first game of the season. Pre- and postinjury POMS comparison (Flint, October 1993).

A review of research and literature by Vallerand[13] helps the health professional appreciate the spectrum of human emotions that are commonly experienced. Of the seven categories of emotion identified by Vallerand and listed here, it is interesting to note that as many as five might be identified as having "negative" dimensions: fear, anger, embarrassment, surprise, sadness, happiness, interest/excitement.

Even though it is desirable to operate as much as possible in the positive emotional domains, it clearly is important to learn to appreciate and respond to the functional dimensions of the other emotions. Injured athletes often experience the full spectrum of negative emotions, and those around them can often help by empathizing and helping them identify, accept, and respond constructively to the feelings involved.

Emotions, with the possible exception of sadness and grieving, tend to produce energy that when responded to or harnessed, can have functional payoff. Even sadness (feeling down, sorry for oneself or others) can eventually lead to a feeling of gratitude, but it can be the least functional and possibly the most dysfunctional emotion if one allows oneself to dwell in this domain.

Accepting and responding to the emotions one feels is a large part of what life is about. Learning to draw on and effectively use and respond to the full spectrum of emotions is part of what can be learned and worked on as a result of injury.

PSYCHOLOGICAL NEEDS DURING REHABILITATION

A review of the basic human psychological needs identified by Glasser[14] provides a valuable framework for anticipation and recognition of needs during injury

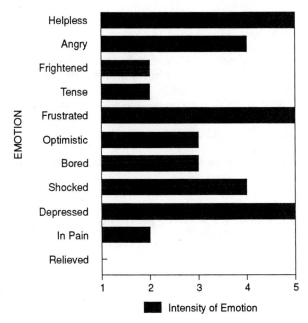

1 = Absolutely not
5 = Extremely so

FIGURE 34–3. Feelings after injury scale from a male athlete with a third-degree season-ending injury (Flint, October 1993).

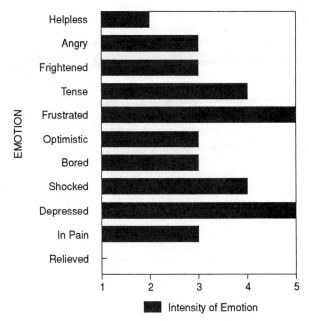

1 = Absolutely not
5 = Extremely so

FIGURE 34–4. Feelings after injury scale of a male athlete who suffered a season-ending second-degree injury (Flint, October 1993).

rehabilitation. As human beings we have basic needs for *acceptance, success, sensation, and control*. For many athletes, activity and feedback in sport provide a large part of their identity and meet many of their basic needs. On injury and during rehabilitation, these individuals' needs in such fundamental areas are likely to be heightened. They are likely to have a greater than normal need to be accepted, appreciated, and included. They are likely to have a greater than normal need to be considered worthy, capable, and important human beings. They may have heightened needs for sensation, enjoyment, and stimulation through other means when active sport outlets are not as available. And most important, the individuals involved are likely to have heightened needs for control, direction, and assurance.

Most elite athletes are strong-minded, assertive individuals with a high need for control who have learned to "take charge" of as much of their life as they can. It is extremely frustrating for them when a huge part of their destiny and prospects now seems beyond their control.

For these and other reasons, it is important that health care professionals help patients clarify what is beyond their control and what is reasonably within their control. It is critical to point out the important things that are within a patient's control in responding to an injury and rehabilitation, and the elements that need to be respected to optimize short-term and long-term health and welfare.

Elite athletes often have tremendous body awareness and a greater than normal need to know what is happening to and is possible with their bodies. In the absence of educational initiatives and strong advice and evidence, injured athletes may out of frustration try to "take charge" of their rehabilitation prescription and create their own diagnosis and prognosis, based on real or imagined personal needs.

Injury time can be a critical "teachable moment" in the lives of athletes. First, it can produce an awakening in terms of placing excelling in sport and one's own vulnerability in perspective. All too often, fairly irrational beliefs have crept into the lives of athletes. For example, (1) My *self-worth* is on the line in the next few moments; (2) I *must* perform for others; (3) I *must* be perfect; (4) The world *must* be fair.

Injuries sometimes sensitize athletes to the reality that there is life after sport and that even though sport is an exciting vehicle for development and accomplishment, it is best kept in perspective. Athletes who face life-threatening or career-threatening injury can end up being happy to be alive and better able to put perceived pressures into perspective.

Irrational beliefs and their created pressures can sometimes be corrected and relieved in responding to injury. If not, they may contribute to the individual's being prone to injury and vulnerable due to the inherent stress, pressure, distraction, and psycho-emotional "baggage" associated with an irrational perspective.

Second, injury time can provide the teachable moment to sensitize individuals to the critical dynamics of their psychophysiology. Glasser[14] has pointed out that at any given moment, human beings have four interactive components of total behavior: (1) doing, (2) thinking, (3) feeling, and (4) physiology.

Of the four components, feeling is probably the hardest to control directly but certainly is dynamically affected by behavior, thoughts, and physiology. Use of biofeedback equipment is sometimes the best way to demonstrate what a profound effect thoughts or behavior can have on feelings or physiology, or vice versa.

This highly dynamic model that we all influence and respond to everyday is the key to our health and welfare as well as our performance potential. Certainly, if we dwell on fears and negative thoughts, the tension produced can interfere with circulation and physiologic healing as well as performance.

Most elite athletes also recognize that if they don't look after their physiology (with proper exercise, diet, rest, and hydration) their ability to feel good, think positively, and behave effectively will eventually be influenced. When experiencing the frustration and stress of an injury, it is important to encourage therapeutic functional exercise with other body parts to the extent possible and to promote and monitor effective diet, rest, and hydration habits.

Finally, the cognitive and behavioral habits and focusing skills that can help optimize psychophysiology and performance can be taught and worked on as a result of the injury rehabilitation challenge.

For many athletes experiencing their first major injury there is little understanding of what the future holds. Since previous personal knowledge of injury and rehabilitation is usually not available, the athlete may feel lost and alone in unfamiliar territory.[15] To someone who strives for control of his or her own body and excels at domination in sport situations, this loss of control can create feelings of helplessness and frustration.

Of prime importance at this stage is a fear of the unknown. In this case, some of the unknown factors include a knowledge of the healing process, how much pain there will be, what rehabilitation involves, whether the athlete can return to preinjury skill levels, fear of disfigurement, and whether the athlete's status or place in the sport is assured.

The level of fear expressed by an injured athlete may be strongly influenced by the amount of his or her control over the future the injured athlete perceives.[16] If the injured athlete has an impression of control over the rehabilitation process and the return to competition, there may be a reduction in fear and a sense that the physical effects of the injury can be overcome. It appears that the best kind of information to give an injured athlete is a combination of sensory and procedural details that can help foster accurate expectations and assist in correct cognitive interpretations of sensations to be experienced.[17] Through this information, both procedural stress (immediate aspects such as rehabilitation) and outcome stress (long-term factors such as a return to competition) can be reduced.[18] Regardless of the specificity of the information, it is vital that open lines of communication exist so that the injured athlete can express his or her fears and gain input to help clarify the issues.[19,20] In the absence of accurate, honest, and optimistic information, complicating misperceptions and behaviors often develop.

When an athlete is injured and is told to "get" rehabilitation, the usual order of daily organization and workout scheduling is no longer in existence. This is particularly significant if the athlete has never been injured before and does not know what rehabilitation means. At this point, it is vital that the athlete regain a sense of order by being involved in planning the recovery.[21] This planning can give the athlete a feeling of being in control again and can provide the security of a structure in which the athlete can work to overcome the injury. One method of demonstrating to the injured athlete that control over the physical recovery process can be achieved is through the example of previously injured athletes.[22,23] Berehowski gained valuable information from formerly injured athletes on a return to competition after a major ligament reconstruction. "I did a lot of reading up on people who had been injured, and I realized that people have come back from this."[7] Since Berehowski did not know what to expect from his injury, he needed to gain a sense of control over the future, and previously injured athletes helped provide a basis for knowledge and understanding.

MODELING IN SPORTS INJURY REHABILITATION

How can therapists, physicians, and sports psychologists ensure that the injured athlete is receiving appropriate information about the recovery process? One of the best methods of communicating attitudes, behaviours, and skills is through observational learning, or modeling.[24] Modeling has long been considered an influential instructional tool in sports for the learning of motor skills and social behaviors.[25] The predominant theory of the modeling-behavior relationship comes from Bandura,[24,26,27] social-cognitive modeling theory being the most popular.

Bandura's[24] theory proposes that modeling, or observational learning, facilitates the transmission of socialization information and cognitive skills through behavioral and verbal cues provided by the model. As the model is watched by an observer, symbolic representation, or verbal coding, takes place, and these cues are stored in memory. Through this vicariously gained information, decision-making criteria are formed, and new behavioral patterns may be learned. Because we tend to compare our capabilities with those of others, seeing someone similar to ourselves complete a new task or demonstrate a particular behavior provides us with the information that we also have the capacity to re-create the action.[24] Examples of modeling effects are evident in sports, and teachers and coaches often rely on this teaching tool to enhance the learning of new physical skills.[25,28]

Observational learning has also had an impact in a medical context and has been used with cardiac patients,[29] children having surgery,[30] and endoscopy patients.[31] Within a sports rehabilitation setting, a videotaped modeling intervention has been found to be influential in aiding in recovery after anterior cruciate surgery in women basketball players.[15] The extension of this technique into the realm of sports injury management provides injury rehabilitation information, incentive, and behavioral cues for recovering athletes. Thus, athletes who have already recovered from injury and returned to competition are ideal models. Seeing someone similar to oneself successfully overcome the obstacle of an injury can help an injured athlete believe that recovery is possible.

Within the sports setting, there are numerous examples of the modeling effect with notable athletes such as Wayne Gretzky (hockey), Silken Laumann (rowing), Mike Foligno (hockey), and Kerrin Lee-Gartner (skiing), all of whom have recovered from major debilitating injury. In the case of Lee-Gartner, the 1992 Olympic winter games gold medal winner in women's downhill skiing, recovery from five knee surgeries and one broken ankle set the example for other Canadian skiers. The head coach of the Canadian ski team noted, "It will make us believe again. It will make injured skiers like Kate Pace and Lucie LaRoche say 'I can win again.' "[32] Indeed, Kerrin Lee-Gartner's example helped Kate Pace win a gold medal in 1993 in World Cup downhill competition while skiing with a fractured wrist. In this case, Pace herself has now become a model for other injured skiers.

In most cases, these sports modeling examples provide motivation and incentive to injured athletes, but very little information on the details of overcoming injury are conveyed. The observer generally sees the successful end-result of months of rehabilitation and is not exposed to the intricacies of the recovery process. Psychological strategies used to overcome obstacles, methods of maintaining motivation through the rehabilitation plateaus, and goal-setting techniques for re-entry into competition are not communicated. In this sense, then, the modeling experience is "informal" and may be of only motivational benefit. In order to ensure that pertinent details of the actual process of recovery are passed on to injured athletes, the modeling exposure should be formalized. "In formal modeling, a situation is created whereby one or more models presents specific verbal or visual cues that expose the observer to vicarious experiences, verbal persuasions, and emotional exhortations."[15] Thus, a model-observer situation is created to allow for optimal transmission of knowledge, behavior cues, and psychological strategies.

Kulik and Mahler[29] provide an example of formalized modeling within a medical setting. In this case, coping models were used to demonstrate the progression from the difficulties of immediate postsurgical conditions to self-sufficiency several days after surgery. Newly hospitalized cardiac patients were paired with postsurgical cardiac roommates and were thus exposed to postoperative sensations and events through this coping model. New patients learned what to expect immediately after the surgery, and their possible fears about the actual process were reduced by example in a formal modeling situation.

One way to ensure that the observer is provided with an optimal amount of information regarding the recovery from injury process and possible psychological strategies for handling problems is through the film or videotape medium.[15,30,33] Flint[15] used a coping model videotape as a psychological intervention with women basketball players. The videotape consisted of interviews with seven basketball players, all of whom had recovered from anterior cruciate ligament surgery. One player was followed from a few weeks postsurgery to 16 months after surgery and demonstrated the entire recovery process and return to competition. The other six players were all interviewed at various stages of recovery from surgery extending from 2 weeks to 7 years after surgery. All demonstrated a full and complete recovery from the injury and the surgery. Within the interviews, the models discussed the problems they encountered, how they overcame these obstacles, and how good it felt to return to competition. Each interview was culminated with scenes of the model's full physical function and capability to play basketball.

The modeling videotape was shown to women athletes who had just undergone reconstructive surgery for a torn anterior cruciate ligament. These recovering athletes viewed the videotape immediately after surgery, 2 months later, and 4 months postsurgery. Throughout this process, they were asked to identify anything or anyone in the videotape that caught their attention. One athlete noted, "A different part of each person caught my attention, either their determination or how quickly they recovered. I think it will [affect] my rehab progress, positively, of course."[8] In this case, an affinity between the models and the individual athlete helped provide motivation and incentive during the rehabilitation process. This athlete was encouraged throughout her rehabilitation by the thought that if they can do it, then so can I.

In another case, specific information about goal setting provided by one of the models was of particular relevance to an athlete. Bev Smith, a former All-American and a member of Canada's national basketball team was a model in the videotape, and her experiences of overcoming several knee surgeries gave her insight into the difficulties of rehabilitation. The athlete noticed Bev and commented, "She spoke of setting daily goals during rehab and trying to keep things in perspective. She also spoke of channeling energy into other things. This approach has certainly made my rehab time less frustrating."[8] Here we see that information has been provided on a specific psychological strategy for overcoming the frustration of long months of rehabilitation. While facing obstacles in the recovery process, this athlete was able to recall the words and actions of Bev Smith and use them to her advantage.

It was interesting to notice the characteristics, actions, or verbalizations of the models that were noted by the observers. In general, immediately after surgery, most of the models' comments identified by the observers related to the pain and emotional response to the surgery. There seemed to be a bond between some of the models and observers because of the shared experience of pain and emotional release. Two months later, the observers had moved from the emotion of the surgery and tended to notice specific aspects of the rehabilitation process. They identified with the model who progressed from one-legged bicycle pedaling to a complete bicycle workout. Finally, after 4 months of rehabilitation, the observers began noticing details such as which models wore a brace when returning to competition and the degree of dedication of the models throughout the rehabilitation process. Through the qualitative information gathered from recovering athletes, it was evident that they had identified with and paid attention to the examples set by the videotaped models.

The videotape format provides an opportunity to reconstruct the most desirable scenes and conditions that may be difficult or unrealistic to capture in a clinical setting.[34] By utilizing coping models, information needed by the injured athlete to promote the psychological aspects of recovery can be obtained. Seeing a similar individual struggle through rehabilitation, hearing a recovered athlete such as Bev Smith speak about setting daily goals for recovery and her commitment to the small details of rehabilitation, or hearing a similar athlete talk about the frustration of injury and the recovery process and the joy related to returning to competition can have a significant effect on recently injured athletes. For the athlete who has never experienced a major injury and does not know what to expect from rehabilitation, this may be particularly pertinent. The knowledge gained vicariously through coping models may provide the injured athlete with a sense of control over the situation. In this sense, the injured athlete gains an understanding of the task ahead and, more important, what strategies can be used to overcome any obstacles during the rehabilitation process.

What will ensure the strongest possible link between the injured observer and the model so that the observer will be encouraged to pay attention to the model? Bandura[27] and McCullagh and colleagues[25] have stressed the importance of model and observer characteristics. It is hoped that the observer will relate to the model and form a bond through identification of similarities and hence that the observer will have an incentive to pay attention to the actions or verbalizations of the model.[25] In sports injury rehabilitation, the most pertinent model and observer characteristics appear to be the similarity of injury or surgery, shared emotion (e.g., pain), feelings of frustration, dedication to recovery, and achievement of rehabilitation.[8]

Athletes who have sustained a major injury for the first time in their careers may not know if they have the capability to recover and return to competition. Since they do not have injury rehabilitation experience on which to rely, they may tend to judge their own prognosis on the basis of the experience of other athletes who have suffered from the same injury. Thus, the provision of models who have *successfully* recovered from injury can help furnish a strong psychological foundation on which to build confidence in the recovery process. The use of modeling, individually and in combination with other psychological intervention strategies, is a relatively new realm in sports rehabilitation.

EXCEPTIONAL PATIENTS

This section discusses the mental attributes and skills found to be associated with exceptional cases of sports injury recovery. Much of the information draws from extensive consulting experience, anecdotal information, plus the results of two comprehensive survey studies that examined a number of psychosocial factors related to sports injury rehabilitation of ankle and knee injuries.[35,36] Scores between those identified as either fast- or slow-healing subjects based on recovery time were compared. In the original study by Ievleva and Orlick,[35] the rate of recovery was found to be significantly related to the amount of practice of certain mental activities, most notably goal setting, healing mental imagery, and positive self-talk. The follow-up study by Loundagin and Fisher[36] revealed a similar pattern of results with the addition of focus of attention and stress reduction also being significantly related to recovery time.

COMMITMENT AND BELIEF

Just as commitment and belief are at the core of mental attributes and activities in pursuit of athletic excellence,[37] so, too, are they keys to achieving optimal recovery from injury. Patience and tenacity are necessary requisites when confronting any challenge and apply to the effort required to achieve full recovery from injury as well. Without faith and belief in one's own self-healing capacity and in the physician's, physical therapist's or trainer's skill or both, it is difficult to mobilize mental powers of healing to their fullest capacity. This difficulty can be especially pronounced in severe injury cases, in which great courage is required to commit the full effort toward an uncertain outcome. It sometimes takes a leap of faith to attempt to beat the odds, to overcome self-imposed or external limitations. The root meaning of the word *courage* draws from Latin *cor,* meaning *heart.* Therefore, to act with courage is to act with heart despite unknown consequences. Those who transcend the odds are never totally free from fear and doubt. What distinguishes exceptional athletes and healers is that they do not let the fears or doubts overshadow their heart's desire. They acknowledge the shadow, and press forward regardless, mobilizing positive efforts to achieve their goal.

SEEING THE OPPORTUNITIES AND POTENTIAL PAYOFFS

Seeing the opportunity for personal learning and growth is conducive to enhancing the process of recovering from an injury. Although the injury may pose a crisis in an athlete's life, it can be approached in two ways. Just as the word for *crisis* in Chinese has two meanings, *danger* and *opportunity*—rather than viewing an injury as a major obstacle and a disruption that destroys the chances for athletic success, one may instead view it as a challenge to overcome, a learning and growth opportunity, or a strengthener.

Injuries often produce unplanned but sometimes beneficial "time outs" from competitive demands. The break from competitive and training demands can result in a more rested, clearer-minded performer with a better focus and perspective. In addition to the break from competitive stress, the athlete is often able to adjust priorities and return refreshed with better perspective, increased sense of mission, and decreased pressures and expectations. In some cases, building stress, fatigue, pressures, and a questionable perspective may have contributed to injury proneness.

Just as a broken bone heals stronger than before following proper rehabilitation, patients should be reassured that they can come back mentally tougher and stronger from injury setbacks. Exceptional patients use the injury rehabilitation challenge as an opportunity to apply and develop the attitudes, mental skills, and behaviors that can make a difference in rehabilitation and in the rest of their lives.

When asked in the Ievleva and Orlick[35] study whether the time out provided by the injury resulted in any valuable lessons, or perspectives that contributed to later achievement, subjects in the fast-healing group reported deriving enhanced insight and enjoyment from their sport, whereas those in the slow-healing group could find no benefits whatsoever. Those athletes who accepted the injury as a challenge and opportunity and drew lessons from the experience demonstrated much shorter recovery times. These athletes showed greater determination to see the positives than the negatives. These findings are supported by the Loundagin and Fisher study,[36] in which athletes in the fast-healing group reported feeling more positive about the time out and recognized greater benefit from the

opportunity, whereas the slow-healing group viewed the experience as completely negative. This is consistent with observations of world class athletes who have made remarkable recoveries from serious and potentially career-ending injuries in which there was always some form of gain in terms of insight or approach to training that substantially improved the athlete's subsequent training, performance, or both.

According to Ievleva and Orlick, "To enhance the recovery process, exceptional athletes accept the injury, and do everything in their power to initiate a positive and complete recovery. They also take advantage of what can be learned from the experience (e.g., about oneself and the relationship to one's sport)."[20]

Caregivers and others in an injured athlete's support network are in an excellent position to assist this process of exploration and growth, which may ultimately take the athlete to a higher level later than he or she might have achieved without the injury experience.

MENTAL SKILLS

Mental skills or activities associated with successful athletic preparation and performance may likewise be applied to exceptional recovery from injury. Some of the key skills include goal setting, positive self-talk, relaxation, and mental imagery.

GOAL SETTING

Goal setting and visualization of goals being achieved are the first step toward applying mental training skills, whether goals are performance- or recovery-oriented. The results from injury studies by Ievleva and Orlick[35] and Loundagin and Fisher[36] indicated that the fast healers practiced much more goal setting than the slower healers. This was especially the case with daily goal setting.[35,36] It is recommended that specific and objectively measurable goals related to rehabilitation be set for every physical therapy session and every day, week, or month.

Having set goals, the practice of mental imagery may be applied to deepen and promote the conviction of the desired end. Goal setting is an indirect link to the practice of end result or affirmation imagery (discussed following). Setting a goal is a statement of expectation, hence a conceptualization of success. Inherent in goal setting is the periodic contemplation, or imagining of, achievement of that goal. The act of goal setting alone conjures up an image of success, control, or those activities in which one can engage that are consistent with achieving that goal. Those goals that are most immediately attainable are also most easily conceived and seen in the imagination. This is consistent with the findings from the Ievleva & Orlick[35] study, in which both daily goal setting and healing imagery were more closely related to recovery time than other categories of goal setting and imagery practiced.

Orlick,[38] however, has identified several kinds of goals that can be beneficial in developing motivation, focus, and perspective in the patient or performer.

Although they need to be combined with realistic short-term goals, *dream* goals can often have tremendous motivational and focusing value. The challenge of matching or exceeding a best-ever rehabilitation or postinjury performance can sometimes produce tremendous energy, conviction, and persistence. A continuum of target possibilities from *exceptional* through *typical* to *complicated* helps the patient respect and appreciate the spectrum of possibilities but often triggers dream goals and high aspirations.

Probably the most important goal is that of the daily *process*—making improvement in focus, attitude, rehabilitation exercises, and relationships. Some athletes even take advantage of injury opportunities to develop new attributes (e.g., lower-body flexibility or upper-body strength). In addition to improved mental skills athletes can emerge from rehabilitation with new physical capacities.

Goals in school, outside interests, time and relationship management can also be important during rehabilitation. Orlick[38] also encourages goals of *self-acceptance* and *self-appreciation* in the event that some dreams are temporarily delayed or not possible. This helps people separate their self-worth from their goals and frees them to strive unburdened.

POSITIVE SELF-TALK AND ATTITUDE

Thinking in positive ways contributes to personal well-being and enhanced health. A positive outlook indicates adjustment to the new condition and an orientation toward improvement. In contrast, a negative outlook indicates preoccupation with the implication of the injury, which can lead to reduced effort toward improvement.

Internal dialogue is a reflection of one's attitude and outlook. As such, the degree to which this self-talk is positive may be the degree to which healing is enhanced. This was confirmed in an injury study demonstrating that those whose self-talk was positive, self-encouraging, and determined healed much more rapidly than those whose self-talk tended to be totally negative, self-deprecatory, and unforgiving.[35] In addition, the Loundagin and Fisher[36] study reportedly found the greatest incidence of self-talk control occurred during exercise. See Table 34–1 for representative examples.

It is generally accepted that success in any endeavor depends on the extent to which one has a positive attitude. This may be particularly challenging in lengthier rehabilitations, in which the road may seem endless. The quality of recovery, however, depends on maintaining a positive perspective to permit the physiological healing processes to flow unobstructed. Although one cannot control the fact of the injury and may be facing a long rehabilitation, thinking about it can be directed and controlled. Rather than focusing on all that has gone wrong, and dwelling on the negative, it is more effective to focus on the positive possibilities—those within personal control—and what can be done to enhance the situation and recovery. In his book *Full Catastrophe Living,* Kabat-Zinn[39] discusses his work with

TABLE 34–1
Examples of Positive Self-Talk from the Fast-Healing Group and of Negative Self-Talk from the Slow-Healing Group[20]

Positive Self-Talk

- How can I make the most out of what I can do now?
- I can beat this thing.
- I can do anything.
- I can do it. I can beat the odds and recover sooner than normal.
- I want to go spring skiing. I'll be totally healed by then.
- I have to work to get my leg as strong as the other one.
- It's feeling pretty good.
- It's getting better all the time.

Negative Self-Talk

- It's probably going to take forever to get better.
- I'll never make up for the lost time.
- What a stupid thing to do—dumb mistake.
- What a useless body.
- It will never be as strong again.
- Stupid fool! Stupid injury. Stupid leg.
- I talked to myself about how frustrated I was. There is nothing good about this, and there is nothing I can do about it.
- Why me?

Adapted from Ievleva L, Orlick T: Mental paths to enhanced recovery from a sports injury. *In* Pargman D (ed): Psychological Bases of Sport Injuries. Morganton, WV, Fitness Information Technology, Inc., 1993. Reproduced with permission.

severely physically impaired patients who come to his stress reduction clinic as a final resort after exhausting the resources of the medical system. During the course of his 8-week class in mindfulness meditation, he counsels the participants to recognize that there is often much more *right* with one's body than there is ever *wrong*. Thus, it is much more conducive to healing to appreciate what is going well than to focus on what is not.

Positive thinking can influence belief and perspective, and belief is often translated into action through positive self-talk. Monitoring internal dialogue can be effective in taking control, guiding positive thoughts, and reducing negative thoughts. This is done by first planning to think in positive terms and second, by responding to any negative thoughts that may still occur, using them as cues to switch to positive thoughts. Injured athletes invariably have moments when they make disparaging remarks to their injured body part (e.g., "Stupid, useless knee"). Ask them to reflect on how they would feel and respond if spoken to in such terms, and then invite them to consider speaking positively, kindly, and lovingly to the injured part, much as one might speak to an injured child (e.g., "It's ok, knee. I'm going to take care of you; you're going to take care of me; you're getting stronger all the time. Together we're going to make you as good as new.").[20]

RELAXATION

Relaxation practice in any of its various forms—for example, physical relaxation, meditation, progressive relaxation, breath control, or yoga—plays an integral role in behavioral medicine and stress reduction programs. The health and wellness benefits accrued from engaging in relaxation on a regular basis have been well documented. Numerous studies have established the following list of relaxation effects that are the specific means by which the health benefits take place:

- Decreased heart rate
- Reduced respiration
- Enhanced oxygen consumption
- Reduced muscle tension
- Decreased galvanic skin response
- Redistribution of blood flow
- Reduced blood pressure and hypertension
- Reduction in lactate
- Reduction in cholesterol
- Enhanced reactivity to stress
- Reduced cortisol
- Enhanced immune system

Stress tends to reverse the effects for each of those items.

Relaxation helps open the mind-body channels that regulate the body. Through relaxation practice, awareness of and connection to the body can be increased, thereby enabling inner control over the body. Using relaxation in combination with imagery, it is also possible to initiate physical and behavioral change.[40–43]

It is common for tension level to increase, especially in the injured area, owing to the stress of being injured.[44,45] Regularly practicing a relaxation routine can be effective in relaxing the area and relieving the tension. Staying loose and relaxed facilitates recovery. When the body is more relaxed, blood circulation is enhanced. The greater the blood flow, the faster injured tissues are repaired.[20,46–48]

Also, the fact that cortisol levels rise with stress[49,50] and inhibit muscle fiber repair[51] further suggests the need for stress reduction in the form of relaxation becomes more evident because relaxation has been shown to reduce cortisol levels.[52–58]

The fast-healing group in the Loundagin and Fisher[36] study used relaxation techniques to manage stress level to a greater extent than the slow-healing group.

MENTAL IMAGERY

It is important to recognize that the body's healing powers are continually in progress, whether or not one chooses to exercise conscious control over healing. Employing positive images of healing and images of being fully recovered, however, are useful in enhancing belief and mobilizing one's own healing powers to maximize the healing potential already existing within an individual.

Four basic kinds of imagery may be applied during injury rehabilitation; they are

1. Recovery or affirmation imagery: imagining one's recovery goals being achieved or imagining oneself with the capacity to achieve all goals
2. Healing imagery: envisioning and feeling healing taking place
3. Treatment imagery: imagining the physical therapy treatment promoting quick and efficient recovery
4. Performance imagery: mentally rehearsing performance skills

Both of the injury studies mentioned here found a significant relationship between the practice of imagery and recovery time. In the Ievleva and Orlick[35] study, healing imagery was most closely related with fast recovery, whereas in the Loundagin and Fisher[36] study, both healing and recovery imagery were equally related to fast recovery. In addition, negative imagery, or images reliving the initial injury, tended to cancel out the benefits of positive healing imagery.[20,35]

END RESULT OR AFFIRMATION IMAGERY. The following is a model for recovery imagery adapted by Ievleva & Orlick[20] for sports injury derived from the application for cancer treatment found in *Getting Well Again* by Simonton and colleagues:[59]

1. Select a goal.
2. Relax.
3. See yourself with goal already met.
4. Imagine, with as many details as possible, your feelings, having reached your goal.
5. See the response of others close to you regarding your achievement.
6. Go over the steps it took to reach your goal and experience satisfaction at each level.
7. Allow yourself to feel happy about reaching your goal.
8. Gradually come back to the present.
9. Then open your eyes and commence action on that first step.

> For those who have difficulty seeing or feeling their goals being achieved, or who get negative images, it is suggested they stop and acknowledge their doubts and fears, and then make a list of all the positive attributes that will enable reaching the goal (e.g., talent, treatment, tenacity, etc.). This is done to help them believe or to recognize that they have the tools necessary to meet the goals and are in control.[20]

HEALING IMAGERY. Currently, the value of imagery for healing is gaining increasing acceptance in modern medicine. There are many clinical reports of therapeutic benefits resulting from imagery. Whereas most are anecdotal in nature, there is increasing documentation of cases to support the healing benefits of engaging in healing imagery.[1,60–64]

In the groundbreaking work of Simonton and colleagues,[59] positive results were reported as a result of implementing a relaxation and imagery program with cancer patients diagnosed as medically incurable. A total of 41 percent showed improvement, of whom 22.2 percent experienced complete remission and 19.1 percent, tumor regression. This was subsequently followed up and supported in a study by Hall.[65]

It is most effective to elicit relaxation before commencing with imagery practice. A state of calm and quiet allows for greater receptivity and flexibility of the mind with which to direct and control imagery. In fact, a state of mental and bodily relaxation is generally considered a prerequisite for all work with therapeutic guided imagery. Common forms of relaxation include focus on diaphragmatic breathing, meditation, or some form of the progressive relaxation technique.

"Imagining the healing process can be enhanced by knowing precisely what it looks like physiologically. It is not essential that it be realistic, but it must symbolize positive change."[20,59,66,67]

What precisely is to be imagined is determined individually. An image that works for one person may not be as effective for someone else. For example, among the Simontons' cancer patients, one patient saw her white cells as "killer sharks" attacking the cancer cells, whereas another saw the white cells as white knights.[59] The important feature is to see one's own bodily resources as being powerful and effective.[20] An athlete recovering from a fracture might imagine the blood flow to the injured area and "feel" the healing, strengthening effects.

TREATMENT IMAGERY. Suggestions that chemotherapy or radiation treatment are effective are incorporated in the Simonton guided imagery program. The emphasis, however, is on the body's own resources leading the battle against cancer. This principle can be applied to the physical therapy setting as well—for example, " . . . seeing and feeling the treatment, minimizing scar tissue, increasing blood flow, or strengthening the muscle or tissue. Athletes should be clearly informed about what the treatment is designed to do so that they can imagine those effects taking place."[20]

Progressive sports medicine practitioners Arnheim[68] and Swearingen[69] point out the importance of the patient being educated about the goals and process of healing and treatment so that meaningful detailed imagery can be facilitated. The athlete then can play a much more active role in optimizing rehabilitation responses and can increase feelings of control and influence.

PERFORMANCE IMAGERY. Because injured athletes are unable to practice physically, mental practice becomes that much more important if they are to maintain a certain skill level. Performance imagery can be a powerful tool in this respect. Not only does it provide a medium in which to rehearse sport skills, it helps prepare for situations that are infrequently encountered in physical practice or competition. Imagery practice can be effective in preparing injured athletes for any number of competitive or practice situations and thus helps them to retain confidence in their ability and to dissipate any lingering fears they may have of re-injury on return to competition.[20] Progressive desensitization using imagery and simulation may be necessary to help eliminate fears and doubts that could lead to injury proneness.[70]

Every effort should be made before a return to competition to have the athlete feel as if he or she is a physically, psychologically, and emotionally recovered as opposed to a recovering performer. Evidence from physical tests, biofeedback, imagery, and practice reports can all assist in accomplishing this belief.

When approaching a return to training and competition, it is important to incorporate in the performance

---

TABLE 34-2
Summary of Imagery Application During Rehabilitation

1. Visualizing healing taking place in the injured area
2. Imagining treatment being optimally effective
3. Imagining moving freely and efficiently through the specific motions and situations that put the most demand on the injured area
4. Re-experiencing or imagining individual skills required for best performance—to stay sharp and mentally connected with one's sport
5. Calling up the emotional and physical feelings that characterize best performances
6. Visualizing returning to competition and performing at one's best again
7. Imagining feeling positive, enthusiastic, and confident about returning to training and competition

Adapted from Ievleva L, Orlick T: Mental paths to enhanced recovery from a sports injury. *In* Pargman D (ed): Psychological Bases of Sport Injuries. Morganton, WV, Fitness Information Technology, Inc., 1993. Reproduced with permission.

---

imagery details of the use of such protective devices as taping or braces as are required for actual activity. An omission of such detail in the imagery may result in the kind of pain, soreness, or discomfort that would typically occur if physically performing the activity without the protective device. This circumstance occurred with a university basketball player with whom the authors worked who habitually taped his previously injured ankles before every practice and game to avoid soreness. He had, however, inadvertently neglected to do so in his imagery. Once the taping was included in subsequent imagery, the soreness did not recur.

Timing is an important consideration in the athlete's readiness to practice certain forms of imagery. For example, it may be advisable to focus solely on relaxation and pain management immediately following knee reconstruction surgery before commencing with healing imagery. It may not be feasible to practice performance imagery until enough healing has taken place for the athlete to feel ready to contemplate being active and performing again. In some cases, the injury may have been so dramatic or traumatic that if there has not been enough opportunity for rest, it would be unreasonable to expect the athlete to have sufficiently recovered psychologically, not to mention physically, to apply the mental energy required to implement self-directed healing (Table 34-2).

STAYING ACTIVE

Exceptional patients are those who are extraordinarily active within the limitations of their injury. If they have an injury of the lower body, they use upper-body exercisers. As soon as possible, they start working out with the nonaffected and affected limbs. Some even look to new mediums (such as swimming pools) to remain as active as possible. Not only does this help prevent loss of fitness and atrophy, it is extremely therapeutic. The therapeutic effects of regular exercise on biochemistry and psychophysiology has been well documented.[71] These effects can be reversed if athletes are kept inactive for long, and inactivity can make them more prone than normal to depression, tension, and frustration.

Athletes experiencing injury are especially appreciative of being able to stay active and work through some of their frustrations through physical exercise. Benefits of dissipation of excess energy, maintenance of a sense of control, reduction of stress, and retention of self-image have been identified.[71–75]

CHARACTERISTICS OF PEAK PERFORMERS

Exceptional injury rehabilitations like that of Silken Laumann (a Canadian rower) who made a miraculous comeback from a serious rowing accident in time to achieve a silver medal in the 1992 Barcelona Olympics are reminders of the qualities of peak performers. The attributes initially identified by Garfield[76] are recognized in top performers in many fields[77] and provide a framework for optimizing human potential in demanding circumstances. These individuals are

1. *Motivated by "mission."* Top performers not only have dreams and goals, they *passionately* invest in seeing, feeling, and realizing them. Their sense of "mission" inspires focus and energy.
2. *Action-oriented.* Peak performers have a strong *work ethic.* They stay assertive, enjoy "going for it," and epitomize the slogan "Just do it."
3. *Self-mastery.* People who get to the top and stay are always working on personal and situational *excellence.* They want to see "how good they can be" and enjoy working on technical, tactical, physical, and mental development goals.
4. *Flexible and in control.* Peak performers are creative and can see solutions and maintain perspective when others cannot. They also are mentally "tough" and can *focus* effectively and *refocus* when necessary. This flexibility and control is usually due to superior *preparation*—physical, mental, and emotional.
5. *Challenged by change.* Top performers prepare not only for the expected but also the unexpected. They see demanding or changing conditions as the ultimate challenge and *opportunity* to test and develop themselves. They enjoy positive rivalries and being tested, and they believe in the slogan, "Tough times don't last, tough people do."
6. *Team-oriented.* Peak performers are "team" people. They *care* enough to encourage, challenge, and support teammates when necessary. They remain respectful and appreciative of the many roles of players and of the attributes necessary to create and maintain an effective team.

These attributes and the skills involved epitomize attitudes of the best patients and top health care professionals. Exceptional patients are not exactly "patient." They respect medical knowledge and physiology but are pro-active in their pursuit of an optimal response. They serve as inspirational models to other patients and to health care professionals.

Health care professionals who show these attributes often have a profound effect on the patients and professionals around them. Their enthusiasm, professionalism, and caring nature have a powerful influence on belief, trust, and motivation. It is important to nurture these peak performer attributes in patients and to model them whenever possible.

OPTIMIZING REHABILITATION CONDITIONS AND SERVICES

As a result of progressive sports medicine research, Gordon[78] has identified important skill areas and procedures for trainers, therapists, and health care professionals. Training in these areas can help equip professionals to optimize patient responses to injury.

SKILLS

1. Effective communication and active listening skills are required by practitioners and are often undermined by overloaded treatment schedules in busy clinics.
2. Cognitive restructuring skills such as self-instruction training and stopping thoughts could be taught to therapists for use by athletes in combating negative reasoning and/or promoting rehabilitation performance.
3. Shaping behavior through schedules of positive reinforcement can combat dysfunctional behaviors such as moaning, arguing, lack of attention, and nonadherence. Dealing with behavior problems in general enhances the effectiveness of therapists, whose professional conduct is often reflected in their characteristic reactions to these problems.
4. Relaxation and visualization techniques can promote internal healing and oppose pain. Relaxation in general also helps conserve vital energy required to fight lengthy periods of discomfort.
5. Goal setting is used by most athletes and can readily be applied to the recovery process by trainers or therapists.

PROCEDURES

1. Peer modeling is a form of group therapy in rehabilitation that is known to promote performance, particularly in cases in which motivation and enthusiasm are lacking.
2. Knowledge about and explanations related to the cause of injury, the extent of damage, and what has to happen internally for healing to occur is an important part of the therapist's role. Athletes should be encouraged to ask questions about their injury.
3. Provision of sensory information in a specific and clear (comprehensible) manner is very much ap-

preciated by athletes. This information, for example, regarding what the athlete will feel and for how long, reduces feelings of helplessness and lack of personal control during treatment.

4. Finally, all types of social support identified in the literature could be provided by therapists. These include active listening, emotional support, emotional challenge, shared social reality, technical application, and technical challenge. With only a little effort, therapists could contribute meaningfully to all types of support without compromising their function of helping athletes recover as opposed to "looking after" them.

Creative, caring, dedicated health care professionals and support people can have a tremendous effect in optimizing psychological, emotional, and physical recovery and growth.

The absence of these skills and procedures has probably complicated and limited many rehabilitations in the past. In reacting to health care professionals who evasively said they didn't want to give "false hope," an outstanding athlete/patient from Sweden, Egon Oosteren, suggested, "The opposite of hope is hopelessness, and that is totally unacceptable."

Clearly, those facing health challenges want honesty, optimism, and caring. Those in a position to help should not let their schedules, fears, or backgrounds prevent them from providing what patients really need.

INJURY-PRONENESS AND PREVENTION

The study of the psychophysiological dynamics during injury rehabilitation sensitizes one to the importance of these factors in injury prevention.

Confidence, preparation, focus, and development all can play a role in injury prevention. Knowing one has the physical, technical, tactical, and mental resources to face the demands in competitive sport can help prevent stress, tension, and injury proneness (Fig. 34–5). There is no substitute for thorough preparation and development of athletes in the technical, tactical, physical, and mental areas. As the demands of sports grow, it is important to do an increasingly better job of athlete development and preparation.

However, if the perceived demands in a situation begin to exceed the perceived resources, it is fairly easy to appreciate how the *physical* or *psychological* effects of stress might interfere with performance and contribute to escalating stress and injury proneness. An adaptation of Nideffer's model (see Fig. 34–5)[79] demonstrates how stress can physically or psychologically interfere with effective functioning.

Injury-proneness can be related to fitness, genetics, technique, tactics, equipment, or psychological factors such as stress, confidence, and focus. Even subconscious needs, doubts, or fears about readiness to perform can produce the physical and psychological effects outlined in Figure 34–5 that can make an athlete injury-prone.

Athletes sometimes progress through their careers virtually injury-free and carefree in their approach to sport and suddenly face a frustrating and complicated "injury year" in which they have one injury after another. The initial injury sometimes triggers a complex emotional and psychological reaction that involves heightened sensitivity to injury risk and personal fallibility. Athletes then often begin to overanalyze the demands they face and any potential limitations in the resources they bring to competition. In the process, they lose the clear-minded, confident focus that helps optimize performance and minimize injury risk.

Every effort must be made to ensure that athletes are not injury-prone when they return to action. Complete injury rehabilitation involves psychological as well as physical, technical, tactical, and equipment considerations. Systematic progressive simulations and performance drills can play a critical role in the athlete's regaining confidence and focus. Evidence of improved strength, flexibility, speed, co-ordination, or stamina can be a powerful force in breaking through from the perception of recovering to that of recovered athlete. Coaches, trainers, doctors, and therapists should take advantage of every opportunity to provide confidence-building progression and feedback.

The athlete's personal work on the relaxation, imagery, focusing, self-talk, and rehearsal skills described earlier in the chapter helps facilitate psychological as well as physical rehabilitation. The confidence and control that comes from progressively applying these mental skills can play a large role in preventing or overcoming injury-proneness.

Reinforcement, positive rational thinking, and a sense of humor from those around the athlete can also assist in the progressive desensitization of fears, doubts, and overanalysis to an optimistic, task-relevant focus and mindset.

If there are concerns an athlete may still be injury-prone, simple biofeedback measures during real or imagined simulations can help detect complicating psychophysiological responses. Further progressive training, desensitization, and re-sensitization to an optimistic task-relevant focus may be necessary.

If it is suspected that subconscious fears, doubts, needs, or guilt feelings might be contributing to injury-

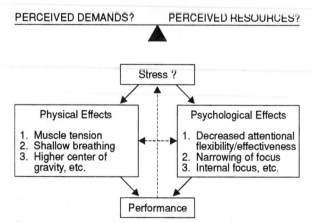

FIGURE 34–5. Adapted from Nideffer R: Prevention and treatment of injury. *In* Nideffer R (ed): The Ethics and Practice of Applied Sport Psychology. Ithaca, NY, Mouvement Publications, 1981.

proneness, every effort should be made to enlist the help of someone trained in clinical psychology, psychiatry, or hypnosis.

This same model can then be valuable in helping assess if the athlete is ready to return to competition following injury. It is important that the athlete feel technically, tactically, physically, and mentally ready to take on the demands of competition.

Fitness is an important element in injury prevention. Stamina, flexibility, and strength all help increase confidence, reduce injuries, and increase capabilities. It is also important to remember that fitness is a state as well as a set of capabilities, and rest, diet, and hydration are equally important in optimizing potential and minimizing injury-proneness. Mental fitness is also a state as well as a set of capabilities—mental and focusing capacities—that can be influenced by both a state of fitness and psychological overload or stress.

Although mental skills are sometimes the last area to be appreciated after fitness, skill development, and strategies, they can play a critical role in finalizing preparation and accomplishing a clear-minded, confident focus.

Mental skills, together with a rational perspective, can help athletes "park," or set aside excessive demands and pressures created by others. Coaches and athletes are wise to deliberately reduce demands and expectations if irrationally escalated and exaggerated by others. This is especially important when an athlete is returning after injury and is complemented by a primary focus on one's game plan and personal and situational excellence and execution.

MALINGERING AND SECONDARY GAINS

For most highly motivated, take-charge athletes, malingering is never a problem. More often, ambitious athletes need to be held back a bit to prevent their pushing themselves too much too soon and complicating the rehabilitation process.

However, as the pressures and demands of sport have increased, secondary gains from being injured may subtly and subconsciously become factors in an athlete's response. Heil[21] has identified increased attentions from significant others, sympathy and social support, release from day-to-day responsibilities, escape from stressful situations, and medication use as potential secondary gains for injured athletes.

Rotella and associates[80] have identified a list of potential reasons for malingering in sport (Table 34–3).

For the most part the key to preventing malingering in sport would seem to be maintaining enthusiasm for the primary payoffs and potential of effective rehabilitation and return to action. A crisp, enthusiastic, professional environment around the clinic, rehabilitation and practices can help ensure primary motives and pro-active behavior maintain precedence over any competing secondary or subconscious motives. Establishing and reviewing long-term, short-term, and situational goals can help prevent malingering tendencies.

TABLE 34–3
Reasons for Malingering in Sport

- Using an insignificant injury to rationalize loss of starting status, reduction in playing time, and poor competitive performance
- Using an injury-related disability to prevent loss of athletic scholarship
- Using injury to account for apparent decrease or change in motivation for participation
- Using injury to offset the personal realization of insufficient ability (talent) to compete successfully
- Using injury to attract needed or desired attention from others that has not been forthcoming elsewhere
- Using injury to demonstrate personal courage by "playing hurt."
- Using injury to offset expectations of coaches, teammates, and parents
- Using injury as a reason to desist from performing, thereby not contributing skill, talent, and ability to the team's effort, and thus expressing hostility or anger toward coaches, teammates, or parents
- Using injury to avoid the rigors of practice but still be able to compete since the coach may need the athlete's services on game day (athlete does not wish to "waste" his or her body)
- Using minor injury to avoid play in order to save the body for intercollegiate or professional competition, in which the material rewards are greater than those at the present level
- Using injury as a way of disengaging from a dimension of life that has proved to be undesirable but also unavoidable (all males in the family traditionally play football)

Adapted from Rotella R, Ogilvie B, Perrin D: The malingering athlete: psychological consideration. *In* Pargman D (ed): Psychological Bases of Sport Injuries. Morgantown, WV, Fitness Information Technology, Inc., 1993. Reproduced with permission.

Good rehabilitation environments involve a healthy mix of empathy, support, and challenge to maximize rehabilitation potential. Behavioral expectations for optimizing rehabilitation are made clear and every effort is made to maintain a high level of trust, respect, and optimism. "Tough love" and professionalism are sometimes necessary to help people through difficult phases in their lives. A mix of empathy, support, belief, and challenge can often help people go past feeling sorry for themselves and continue with effective responses.

Honesty and openness about possible psychosomatic influences that could be complicating rehabilitation and return to form may be necessary. At the same time, respect for athletes' abilities to know their bodies must be maintained together with a trust that those involved really want to do what is right.

REBUILDING CONFIDENCE

The components of confidence identified by Gill[71] provide an excellent framework for efforts to rebuild it:

(1) past experiences, (2) vicarious experiences, (3) verbal persuasion, (4) emotional state.

In order to rebuild confidence, athletes can review past successful experiences to counteract temporary doubts and can work hard in practice on activities they do confidently. They can also empathize with or vicariously experience great performances by others and see and feel greatness as they mentally rehearse and use creative imagery. Being positive and supportive of others often leads to reciprocal support and confidence, and every effort should be made for athletes in need of confidence to hang around energizing, confident believers. Self-talk can also be made more positive, convincing, and persuasive if it has slipped. Finally, becoming emotional, energized, or aroused often leads to increased feelings of confidence. Most emotions other than sadness produce energy; thus, if one becomes passionate and engages in energizing activities or thoughts, confidence can be increased and intensity channeled into a positive primary focus.

In summary, confidence is most related to *quality preparation*. A quick review of past highlights and future prospects is best followed by a total focus on the here and now—the current game plan. A quick review of future opponents' capabilities should be followed by a comprehensive rehearsal of the athlete's own game plan in the key situations that will be encountered. A final phase in quality preparation is to rehearse maintaining focus in some of the key contrasting conditions that may occur in the competition (e.g., contrasting crowd conditions, scores, opponent behavior, and officials calls).

SUMMARY

The psychological dynamics involved in preventing injuries and helping athletes work through injury rehabilitation are often complex and extremely significant.

The mind-body relationship is highly interactive and two-way, influencing every element of readiness for challenges and responsiveness to situations. Injury or physical threat to health and capability has a profound effect on emotions and thoughts, and there is now little doubt that thoughts and feelings can have a profound influence on ability to perform or recover.

Informed health care professionals can be invaluable in sensitizing athletes, coaches, parents, and administrators to this powerful psychophysiology and its many *practical* implications. The empathy of a parent, the interest of a coach or teammate, the caring of an administrator together with the skills of health care professionals can make huge differences in the lives affected. It is too important not to take seriously.

REFERENCES

1. Achterberg J: Mind and medicine: The role of imagery in healing. J Am Soc Psychic Res 1989; 83(2):93–100.
2. Justice B: Who Gets Sick. Los Angeles, J.P. Tarcher, 1987.
3. Moyers B: Healing and the Mind. New York, Doubleday, 1993.
4. Pedersen P: The grief response and injury: A special challenge for athletes and athletic trainers. Athletic Training 1986; 21:312–314.
5. Rotella RJ, Heyman SR: Stress, injury and the psychological rehabilitation of athletes. In Williams JM (ed): Applied Sport Psychology: Personal Growth to Peak Performance. Palo Alto, Mayfield, 1986, pp 343–364.
6. Kübler-Ross E: On Death and Dying. New York, MacMillan, 1969.
7. Berehowski D: Personal interview with F. Flint, September 1993.
8. Flint FA: The psychological effects of modeling in athletic injury rehabilitation. Doctoral dissertation, University of Oregon, 1991. Microform Publications No. BF 357.
9. Townsend L: Personal interview with F. Flint, August 1993.
10. McNair DN, Lorr M, Droppleman LF: Profile of Mood States. San Diego, Educational and Industrial Testing Services, 1971.
11. Smith AM, Scott SG, O'Fallon W, Young ML: The emotional responses of athletes to injury. Mayo Clin Proc 1990; 65:38–50.
12. LeUnes AD, Hayward SA, Daiss S: Annotated bibliography of the profile of mood states in sport. J Sport Behav 1988; 11:213–291.
13. Vallerand R: Emotion in sport. In Straub W, Williams J (eds): Cognitive Sport Psychology. Lansing, NY, Sport Science Associates, 1984.
14. Glasser W: Control Theory. New York, Harper & Row, 1984.
15. Flint FA: Seeing helps believing: modeling in injury rehabilitation. In Pargman D (ed): Psychological Bases of Sport Injuries. Morgantown, WV, Fitness Information Technology, 1993, pp 183–198.
16. Johnson M: Dimensions of recovery from surgery. Int Rev Appl Psychol 1984; 33:505–520.
17. Anderson KO, Masur FT: Psychological preparation for invasive medical and dental procedures. J Behav Med 1983; 6:1–40.
18. Weinman J, Johnston M: Stressful medical procedures: An analysis of the effects of psychological interventions and of the stressfulness of the procedures. In Maes S, Spielberger CD, Defares PB, Sarason IG (eds): Topics in Health Psychology. New York, Wiley & Sons, 1988, pp 205–217.
19. Fisher AC, Hoisington LL: Injured athletes' attitudes and judgements toward rehabilitation adherence. Athletic Training, 1993; 28:48–53.
20. Ievleva L, Orlick T: Mental paths to enhanced recovery from a sports injury. In Pargman D (ed): Psychological Bases of Sport Injuries. Morgantown, WV, Fitness Information Technology, 1993, pp 219–245.
21. Heil J: A comprehensive approach to injury management. In Heil J (ed): Psychology of Sport Injury. Champaign, IL, Human Kinetics, 1993, 137–149.
22. Hardy CJ, Crace RK: The dimensions of social support when dealing with sport injuries. In Pargman D (ed): Psychological Bases of Sport Injuries. Morgantown, WV, Fitness Information Technology, 1993, pp 121–144.
23. Wiese DM, Weiss MR: Psychological rehabilitation and physical injury: The role of the sports medicine team. Sport Psychologist 1:318–330.
24. Bandura A: Social Foundations of Thought and Action: A Social Cognitive Theory. Englewood Cliffs, NJ, Prentice-Hall, 1986.
25. McCullagh P, Weiss MR, Ross D: Modeling considerations in motor skill acquisition and performance: An integrated approach. In Pandolf KB (ed): Exercise and Sport Sciences Reviews, vol 17. Baltimore, Williams & Wilkins, 1989, pp 475–513.
26. Bandura A: Principles of Behavior Modification. New York, Holt, Rinehart & Winston, 1969.
27. Bandura A: Self-efficacy: Toward a unifying theory of behavioral change. Psychol Rev 84:191–215.
28. Weiss MR, Klint KA: "Show and tell" in the gymnasium: An investigation of developmental differences in modeling and verbal rehearsal of motor skills. Res Q Exerc Sport 1987; 58:234–241.
29. Kulik JA, Mahler HI: Effects of preoperative roommate assignment on postoperative anxiety and recovery from coronary-bypass surgery. Health Psychology 1987; 6:525–543.
30. Melamed BG, Siegel LJ: Reduction of anxiety in children facing hospitalization and surgery by use of filmed modeling. J Consult Clin Psychol 1975; 43:511–521.
31. Shipley RH, Butt JH, Horwitz B, Farbry JE: Preparation for a stressful medical procedure: Effect of amount of stimulus pre-exposure and coping style. J Consult Clin Psychol 1978; 46:499–507.

32. Byers J: Canadian ski gold an inspiration to others. The Toronto Star, Feb 16, 1992, p E18.

33. Thelen MH, Fry RA, Fehrenbach PA, Frautschi NM: Therapeutic videotape and film modeling: A review. Psychol Bull 1979; 86:701–720.

34. Anderson LA, DeVellis BM, DeVellis RF: Effects of modeling on patient communication, satisfaction, and knowledge. Med Care 1987; 25:1044–1056.

35. Ievleva L, Orlick T: Mental links to enhanced healing: An exploratory study. Sport Psychologist, 1991; 5(1):25–40.

36. Loundagin C, Fisher L: The relationship between mental skills and enhanced injury rehabilitation. Poster presentation at Annual Meeting of AAASP, Montreal, 1993.

37. Orlick T: The psychology of human excellence. Contemp Thought Sport Psychol Hum Perform 1992; 1(1):112–127.

38. Orlick T: Psyching For Sport. Champaign, IL, Human Kinetics, 1986.

39. Kabat-Zinn J: Full Catastrophe Living: Using the Wisdom of Your Body and Mind to Face Stress, Pain, and Illness. New York, Delacorte, 1990.

40. Green EE, Green AM, Walters ED: Biofeedback for mind/body self-regulation: Healing and creativity. In Peper E, Ancoli S, Quinn M (eds): Mind/Body Integration: Essential Readings in Biofeedback. New York, Plenum, 1979, pp 125–140.

41. Patterson DM: Progressive relaxation training: Overview, procedure and implication for self-regulation. In Peper E, Ancoli S, Quinn M (eds): Mind/Body Integration: Essential Readings in Biofeedback. New York, Plenum, 1979, pp 187–200.

42. Rossman ML: Imagine health! Imagery in medical self-care. In Sheikh A (ed): Imagination and Healing. Farmingdale, NY, Berkley Books, 1984, pp 231–258.

43. Korn ER, Johnson K: Visualization: The Uses of Imagery in the Health Professions. Homewood, IL, Dow Jones–Irwin, 1983.

44. Brewer B, Raalte J, Linder D: Role of the sport psychologist in treating injured athletes: A survey of sport medicine providers. J Appl Sport Psychol 1991; 3:183–190.

45. Yukelson D: Psychology of sports and the injured athlete. In Bernhardt D (ed): Sports Physical Therapy. New York, Churchill Livingstone, 1986, pp 173–195.

46. Benson H: The Relaxation Response. New York, William Morrow, 1975.

47. Bresler DE: Conditioned relaxation: The pause that refreshes. In Gordon JS, Jaffe DT, Bresler DE (eds): Mind, Body, and Health: Toward an Integral Medicine. New York, Human Sciences, 1984, pp 19–36.

48. Bresler DE: Mind-controlled analgesia: The inner way to pain control. In Sheikh AA (ed): Imagination and Healing. Farmingdale, NY, Berkley Books, 1984, pp 211–230.

49. Selye H: Stress Without Distress. New York, Harper & Row, 1974.

50. Borysenko M, Borysenko J: Stress, behavior and immunity. Gen Hosp Psychiatry 1982; 4:59–67.

51. Perna F, McDowell S: The association of life-stress and cognitive coping strategy with symptoms, immunosuppression and injury among Olympic athletes. Lecture presentation at Annual Meeting of AAASP, Montreal, 1993.

52. Bevan AJ: Endocrine changes in transcendental meditation. Clin Exp Pharmacol Physiol 1980; 7(1):75–76.

53. DeGood DE, Redgate ES: Interrelationship of plasma cortisol and other activation indices during EMG biofeedback training. J Behav Med 1982; 5(2):213–223.

54. Green RG, Green ML: Relaxation increases salivary immunoglobin A. Psychol Rep 1987; 61:623–629.

55. McGrady A, Woerner M, Bernal GAA, Higgins JT: Effect of biofeedback-assisted relaxation on blood pressure and cortisol levels in normotensives and hypertensives. J Behav Med 1987; 10(3):301–310.

56. McGrady A, Turner JW, Fine TH, Higgins JT: Effects of biobehaviorally-assisted relaxation training on blood pressure, plasma renin, cortisol, and aldosterone levels in borderline essential hypertension. Clin Biofeedback Health 1987; 10(1):16–25.

57. Holden-Lund C: Effects of relaxation with guided imagery on surgical stress and wound healing. Res Nurs Health 1988; 11:235–244.

58. Jin P: Changes in heart rate, noradrenaline, cortisol and mood during Tai Chi. J Psychosom Res 33(2), 197–206.

59. Simonton OC, Matthews-Simonton S, Creighton JL: Getting Well Again. New York, Bantam Books, 1978.

60. Cousins N: Head First: The Biology of Hope and the Healing Power of the Human Spirit. New York, Penguin Books, 1989.

61. Cousins N: Belief becomes biology. Advances 1989; 6(3):20–29.

62. Epstein G: The image in medicine: Notes of a clinician. Advances 1986; 3(1):22–31.

63. Epstein G: Healing Visualizations: Creating Health Through Imagery. New York, Bantam Books, 1989.

64. Krippner S: The role of imagery in health and healing: A review. Saybrook Rev 1985; 5(1):32–41.

65. Hall HR: Hypnosis and the immune system: A review with implications for cancer and the psychology of healing. Am J Clin Hypn 1983; 25(3):92–103.

66. Green EE, Green AM: Beyond Biofeedback. New York, Delacorte/Seymour Lawrence, 1977.

67. Jaffe DT, Bresler DE: Guided imagery. In Gordon JS, Jaffe DT, Bresler DE (eds): Mind Body, and Health: Toward an Integral Medicine. New York, Human Sciences, 1984, pp 56–69.

68. Arnheim DD: Modern Principles of Athletic Training. St. Louis, Times Mirror/Mosby College Publishing, 1985.

69. Swearingen RL: The physician as the basic instrument. In Gordon JS, Jaffe DT, Bresler DE (eds): Mind, Body, and Health: Toward an Integral Medicine. New York, Human Sciences, 1984, pp 101–106.

70. Rotella RJ, Campbell MS: Systematic desensitization: Psychological rehabilitation of injured athletes. Athletic Train 1983; 18(2): 140–142.

71. Gill D: Psychological Dynamics in Sport. Champaign, IL, Human Kinetics, 1985.

72. Crossman J: Psychological and Sociological Factors Supporting Athletic Injury. Coach Rev 1986; May/June: 54–58.

73. Salisbury N: The comeback trail. New Body 1984; 3(6):56–58.

74. Steadman JR: Rehabilitation of skiing injuries. Clin Sports Med 1982; 1(2):289–294.

75. Willis H: Some psychological effects of athletic injuries. Physiother Sport 1983; 5(3):16–17.

76. Garfield C: Peak Performers. New York, Avon Books, 1986.

77. Botterill C, Friesen R: Peak Performer Attributes. Paper presented at Canadian Association of Sport Sciences, Saskatoon, Canada, 1992.

78. Gordon S: Sport psychology and the professional training of health care professionals. Assoc Advanc Appl Sport Psychol Newsletter, Summer 1991.

79. Nideffer R: Injury prevention and rehabilitation. In Nideffer R (ed): The Ethics and Practice of Applied Sport Psychology. Ithaca, NY, Mouvement Publications, 1981.

80. Rotella RJ, Ogilvie B, Perrin D: The malingering athlete. In Pargman D (ed): Psychological Bases of Sport Injuries. Morgantown, WV, Fitness Information Technology, 1993.

CHAPTER 35

Dermatologic Considerations in Athletics

D O N   G R O O T   *MD, FRCP(C), FACP*
P A T R I C I A   J O H N S T O N   *MClSc, MBA*

THE SKIN

The skin is not simply a sack in which the organs, bones, and muscles of the body are housed. It is in itself a vital organ that teems with nerves, blood vessels, pigment cells, and glands. The skin is the largest organ of the body and is highly visible and vulnerable. In its protective role, the skin is often the first and only part of the body to be injured in athletic activity.

The skin protects the body from harmful external factors such as trauma, ionizing radiation, ultraviolet light, and toxic fumes and chemicals. Through dilation or contraction of blood vessels and excretion from the sweat glands the skin monitors and manages temperature fluctuations that could disrupt the functioning of the internal organs. It also signals many internal diseases, providing early warning signs for such conditions as hormonal imbalance, internal cancer, diabetes, and the AIDS virus.

Although the skin is unique, varying from individual to individual and from race to race as well as from one area of the body to the next, its basic structure is the same in all individuals. The skin is divided into three layers: the epidermis, the dermis, and fat (Fig. 35–1).

The epidermis is the top layer of the skin. It extends along the surface, dipping into the dermis to surround hair follicles and oil glands. At a molecular level the epidermis is very effective at blocking the entry of foreign materials to the deeper layers of the skin and the internal organs.

The epidermis is made up of two types of cells: keratinocytes and dendritic cells. The clear appearance of the dendritic cells differentiates them from the keratinocyte cells, which contain cytoplasm and are connected by intracellular bridges. The keratinocytes are arranged in layers, whereas the dendritic cells are distributed throughout the epidermis. The basal cell layer of the keratinocytes is a single layer of elongated cells that borders the dermis. The many-sided squamous cells form the next layer. The thickness varies from five to ten cells laid down in a meshlike fashion. At its interface with the next layer of granular cells, the squamous cells flatten. The granular cell layer varies in thickness with the horny layer. Where the horny layer is thin, such as the skin of the back, the granular layer

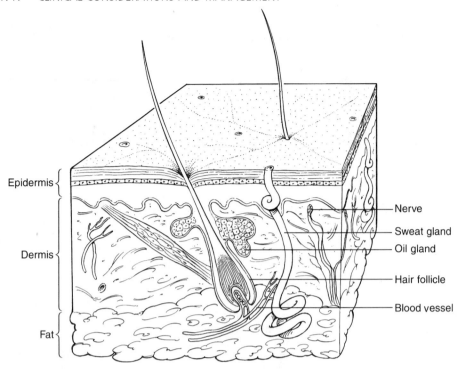

FIGURE 35–1. Elements of the skin.

is only one to three cells deep. Where the horny layer is thick, such as on the palm of the hand or sole of the foot, the granular layer may be ten cells thick. The granular cells are characterized by their diamond shape. Their cytoplasm contains keratohyaline granules, which contain tonofibrils that keep the skin flexible. This is in contrast to the keratin granules of the nails and hair, which are hard because they are devoid of tonofibrils. The fourth horny layer of the epidermis is highly keratinized. As new skin cells, produced in the deeper layers of the epidermis, push upward, the dead cells of the superficial horny layer, known as the stratum corneum, are sloughed. This turnover takes 3 weeks on average.[1]

The mucosa of the mouth differs from other skin surfaces in that the epidermis does not contain a granular or horny layer except on the hard palate and dorsum of the tongue.[1]

Three types of dendritic cells are present in the epidermis: melanocytes, Langerhans cells, and indeterminate dendritic cells. The last-named are thought to be related to the Langerhans cells, which are part of the immunologic system. These epidermal Langerhans cells provide a first-response reaction to foreign antigens that come in contact with the skin. The melanocytes produce melanin, which is transferred to and stored in the basal cell layer of the epidermis, providing the skin with its color.[1]

The nails of the fingers and toes originate from the epidermis of the nail matrix, which is the moon-shaped structure at the proximal end of the nail (Fig. 35–2). The cells of the nail plate are not vital and consist of keratinized cells.[1]

The dermis is the second layer of the skin. Divided into two layers, the papillary dermis and the reticular

dermis, it contains the building blocks of the skin. Collagen, a fibrous protein, is the most abundant fibroblast of the dermal connective tissue. Collagen provides strength and structure to the skin; it is most abundant in the deeper reticular layer of the dermis but is also found in the papillary dermis. Elastins, also a major component of the reticular dermis, are elastic proteins that give the skin tone and suppleness, so that it will snap back into place when stretched. The breakdown of fibrous and elastic proteins is responsible for many of the signs of aging, such as sagging skin and wrinkles.

The papillary dermis contains blood vessels that deliver essential nutrients to and remove wastes from the skin. The complex system of nerves in the papillary dermis makes the skin one of the most sensitive organs of the body.

The glands of the skin are found in the papillary dermis, although they extend into the basal layer of the epidermis. Sebaceous glands secrete lipids to lubricate the skin; eccrine glands release sweat to regulate fluctuations of body temperature; and apocrine gland secretions are responsible for body odor. These glands

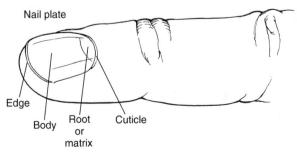

FIGURE 35–2. Elements of the nail.

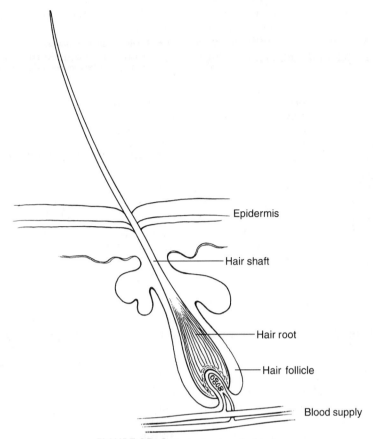

Epidermis

Hair shaft

Hair root

Hair follicle

Blood supply

FIGURE 35–3. A single strand of hair.

vary in their location, size, and distribution. For example, eccrine glands are most abundant in the palms of the hands and soles of the feet and are nonexistent along the vermilion borders of the lips.

Although the hair follicle is an appendage of the epidermis, it extends into the papillary dermis, where it receives its blood supply and surrounding network of nerves (Fig. 35–3). The hair follicle is alive and grows at an average rate of 1/2 to 1 inch per month. The shaft or visible portion of the hair consists of dead, keratinized cells.[2]

A layer of fat underlies the dermis. It plays an important role in providing a protective pad between the skin and the underlying skeletal and muscular structures. Subcutaneous fat is also responsible for giving the skin a full, healthy look.[2]

In its role as an interface between the body and an often hostile environment, the skin is subject to frequent and often damaging abuse. This is particularly the case with athletes. In mild cases, sports-related skin injuries may simply be annoying, yet in severe cases may impede an athlete's ability to perform.

Frequently, a direct causal relationship can be established between the athletic activity and a skin condition. Blisters are an obvious example. In other circumstances, a pre-existing skin condition is aggravated by the athletic activity. Acne under protective padding, known as acne mechanica, is an example.

Age also affects the way in which the skin responds to trauma. As time passes, the skin breaks down with repetitive trauma. Blisters and bruises are more likely to occur, and the skin does not heal as well, increasing the likelihood of unacceptable scarring. The passage of time also affects the efficiency with which the sebaceous glands produce the natural lubricating oils of the skin, creating dry skin problems, especially with exposure to environmental factors such as wind and chlorine in pools.

The most common dermatologic problems in athletes are caused by trauma, equipment, heat/sweat, communal contact, and environmental exposure.[3]

CONDITIONS CAUSED BY TRAUMA

It is difficult to participate in any sport without experiencing some form of trauma to the skin. Lacerations and bruising are typical, but other traumatically induced skin problems may result in irritating discomfort.

LACERATIONS AND ABRASIONS

Lacerations are categorized according to the depth of the wound. A superficial laceration or abrasion involves the epidermis and possibly a small superficial portion of the dermis. A partial-thickness wound extends into the dermis but does not sever it entirely, whereas a full-thickness wound involves the entire dermis.

Superficial and partial-thickness wounds will generally re-epithelialize without direct intervention. The wound should be cleansed with water and any dirt gently removed. A medicated (antibiotic) dressing, such as mupirocin (Bactroban) ointment under a semiocclusive (e.g., Mepore) bandage, may be applied to stanch any bleeding and to protect the wound from infection. After an initial 24-hour period when re-epithelialization has begun, the dressing is changed.

Full-thickness wounds, which sever the dermis, take longer to heal. If the skin is cut so that two opposing edges can be brought together, suturing is the treatment of choice. If, on the other hand, a piece of the skin has been removed, suturing is not possible. A major loss of skin may require direct intervention with grafting. However, in many instances the wound can be left to heal on its own after it has been thoroughly cleansed.

The removal of dirt and debris from a wound is important for proper healing. If debris is left behind, permanent discoloration in the form of a dirt tattoo may result. Running water through the wound may be adequate; however, if the wound is dirty a more aggressive approach is required. Under local anesthetic, the wound is scrubbed with a disposable, sterile, surgical brush that contains an antiseptic cleansing solution. Any foreign material, such as glass or gravel, is carefully removed and necrosed tissue debrided.

Once the wound is properly prepared, healing can take place. Some areas of the body, such as the face, heal faster and better than others, such as the leg, depending largely on the blood supply to the region. The body lays down a base of granulation tissue with a circular pattern of collagen fibers to fill in the missing dermis. This process causes the wound to contract, drawing the epidermal edges closer together. The skin loses its ability to retain water in the damaged area, contributing to the formation of a scab from the inflammatory deposits. Although the scab plays an important role in the control of infection, it can also slow the healing process. To encourage more rapid epithelialization it is best to keep a wound moist with an appropriate dressing. A topical antibiotic, such as Bactroban ointment under a semiocclusive (e.g., Mepore) dressing, will reduce the risk of infection.

In cases in which the skin is cut (either ragged or linear) and two opposing edges can be brought together, sutures or adhesives may be used to encourage rapid repair and to minimize a cosmetically unsatisfactory result. Once again the wound must be properly cleansed, in the same manner that was discussed previously.

Sutures will be required for extensive full-thickness wounds. Absorbable sutures are used to repair the deep dermal and subcutaneous layers. This is important to strengthen the closure. The epidermal layers are generally brought together with nonabsorbable sutures that are removed after an average of 5 to 14 days, depending on the location of the wound. Care must be taken to avoid tension at the epidermal margins, as this contributes to tissue necrosis and the subsequent formation of weak scar tissue. If there is poor blood supply to the wound or infection, the healing process will be compromised.

Adhesive materials, such as Histoacryl, are becoming popular alternatives to superficial sutures for joining the epidermal borders of wounds. They offer the advantage of avoiding the risk of cross-hatching when excess tension is placed on the sutures; also, there are no sutures to be removed.

Steri-strip and Butterfly bandages are effective in cases of superficial and partial-thickness lacerations in which the two opposing epidermal edges can be brought together easily and held in place by the tape.

Scarring is inevitable with full-thickness wounds. The cosmetic result may vary according to intrinsic and extrinsic factors. Intrinsic factors include a hereditary predisposition for scar formation or poor nutrition; extrinsic factors include poor surgical technique, infection, compromised blood supply, use of topical or systemic steroids, and foreign materials in the wound. Scars may be categorized as normal, hypertrophic, keloid, or atrophic. A normal scar, although never regaining the strength of untraumatized tissue, is flat and similar in color to the surrounding skin. Hypertrophic and keloid scars are both overgrown, the difference lying in the mass of scar tissue deposited and the tendency for recurrence. Keloid scars tend to be extensively overgrown and have a high rate of recurrence despite numerous interventional therapies. Atrophic scars are deficient in collagen and tend to be weak and depressed.

An unacceptable scar may be excised and resutured, although the likelihood of recurrence is high, especially in the case of genetic predisposition to scar formation. A more successful approach combines several therapeutic techniques.

To be successful, scar revision requires an observant eye and a creative multidimensional approach. Component analysis of the scar is the first step. A scar may be raised, uneven, vascular, or devoid of color (hypopigmented). Pressure dressings, application of silicone sheets, and cortisone-impregnated tape applied to the wound during the healing process will help control the formation of a raised or hypertrophic scar. Once the scar has formed, cortisone injected directly into a scar with a Ligmaject pressure syringe will flatten it. Resurfacing with a vaporizing laser, such as the CO_2 or KTP laser, will smooth out a lumpy scar and blend the edges into the adjacent normal tissue. Red discoloration due to vascularity can be removed with one of the target-specific lasers, such as the flash pump dye or KTP laser. Hypopigmentation may be solved by meticulous injection of flesh-colored pigment into the scar using a microimplantation technique.[2]

PURPURA (BRUISING) AND HEMATOMAS

Purpura, the term given to bruising, is derived from the Greek name for a mollusk, porphyra, from which a deep purple dye can be obtained. Bruising occurs when blood escapes into the skin or the mucous membranes; it is characterized by a purplish red discoloration of the skin resulting from red cell extravasation.[3]

Although the cause of red cell extravasation varies, in sports, bruising is largely the result of blunt trauma. The

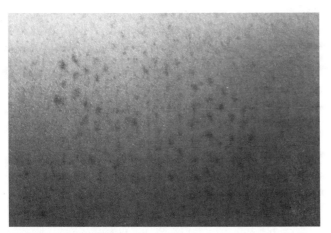

FIGURE 35—4. Patterned petechiae ("boarded" hockey player).

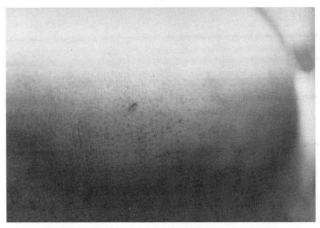

FIGURE 35—5. Dirt tattoo (cyclist fall on asphalt).

two types of bruises most commonly seen in athletes are petechiae and ecchymoses. Petechiae are purpuric lesions, which are less than 3 mm in diameter, and often occur in groups.[4] An example of petechiae may be seen in a hockey player who has been checked into the boards. His garment may leave a pattern of tiny vascular eruptions that match the weave of the cloth.[3] This is known as jersey bruise or patterned petechiae (Fig. 35–4). Ecchymosis is a bruise larger than 3 mm in diameter.

An ice pack applied with pressure immediately after the trauma will help stanch the bleeding and control swelling. With time, the macrophage cells of the body will clear away the blood cell particles, and the bruise will gradually fade from a deep purple or red discoloration to a green or yellow tone and finally disappear.

A unique type of bruising or petechiae found only in athletes, adolescents in particular, is referred to as black heel or black palm. It is characterized by a grouping of bluish black specks on the back of the heel or the padded portion of the palm. It is due to the rupturing of the papillary capillaries in the skin. Athletes who participate in high-impact sports that involve jumping, twisting, and sudden shearing movements or stops, such as basketball, football, lacrosse, tennis, and squash, are candidates for a black heel. Black palm has been reported in athletes participating in sports involving friction and pressure to the palm of the hand, such as weight lifting, tennis, mountain climbing, and golf.[5,6] No intervention is required for this condition, as there is no associated pain or functional disruption of the foot or hand. Reassurance that these black skin lesions do not represent mole cancer is often sought by the athlete. Once the sport is stopped for the season, the condition spontaneously disappears.

Another type of ecchymotic condition unique to athletes is known as runner's rump. Postecchymotic hyperpigmentation occurs in the cleft of the buttocks owing to the constant repetitive contact between the cheeks of the buttocks. The condition is asymptomatic and subsides with a decrease in running.[6]

Hematomas may occur when the blood does not seep into the skin or mucous membranes but becomes trapped and pools in a confined space, such as under the fingernail or toenail (subungual hematoma). They may have to be drained, especially in circumstances in which the pressure from the trapped blood is very painful, as is the case with subungual hematomas. A needle into the collection of blood may aspirate enough blood to relieve the pressure. Massage assists absorption of the loculated serous blood components of clear hematomas (seromas) that may be trapped in skeletal soft tissue.

DIRT TATTOOS

Dirt tattoos occur when dirt or other debris is embedded in the skin from a traumatic injury, such as a fall on an asphalt surface while cycling or running. This is sometimes referred to as road rash (Fig. 35–5).

If a wound is properly cleansed after an injury, dirt tattoos are usually prevented. In instances in which the debris has been incorporated into the skin during the healing process, no amount of cleansing will remove the resulting discoloration.

The advent of laser technology has made it possible to remove dirt tattoos with a minimal risk of scarring. The type of laser selected for the surgery is important. Lasers that target the pigment in the skin, leaving the remaining tissue relatively untouched, ensure the best results. Several lasers have the color-specific selectivity to remove blue/black/brown discolorations in the skin, including the Q-switched ruby, the KTP, and the double-frequency YAG lasers.

The selective affinity of the laser light for certain discolorations allows the laser surgeon to remove pigment from the skin with minimal disruption to the surrounding tissue. The energy emitted by the laser light when it hits the targeted pigment causes a microscopic fragmentation of the pigment particles. The macrophage cells of the immune system then carry the minuscule waste particles away.[2]

The methods of tattoo removal used in the past generally left unsightly scars. Resurfacing techniques such as salabrasion (salt scraping), dermabrasion (mechanical scraping), lasabrasion (laser vaporization), and chemical peels as well as surgical techniques such as skin grafting were the only available options for the

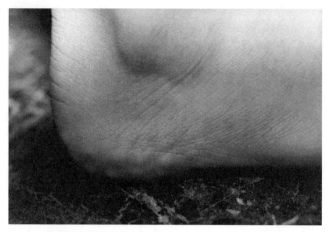

FIGURE 35–6. Piezogenic papules (squash player).

removal of tattoos. The new target-specific lasers have driven these techniques into obsolescence.

Decorative tattoos are popular among some athletes. The trend is to tattoo a team logo or insignia into the skin. These tattoos may be removed in a similar fashion to dirt tattoos, although red and yellow pigments are more resistant to laser therapy.[7]

PIEZOGENIC PAPULES

Piezogenic papules have been reported in athletes participating in prolonged endurance events such as marathons and triathlons (Fig. 35–6).[6] These skin-colored bumps most commonly occur on the medial and lateral aspects of the heel and are due to a herniation of the subcutaneous fat into the dermis.[4]

The athlete may experience pain only when the foot is bearing weight. However, the pain can be such that it will prevent the athlete from continuing with the sport. These papules have been reported, with no associated pain, in the general population. Therefore, there is some speculation as to why some individuals with this condition are prone to pain. Such factors as faulty weight bearing, bony spurs, and secondary inflammatory changes to the deep dermis have been discussed.[5]

Intralesional injections of the cortisone triamcinolone acetonide (Kenalog) will shrink the fat, providing relief to the individual who suffers pain. If there is no associated pain, intervention is not indicated except for cosmetic reasons.[8] Orthotic support to the heel has been of benefit to some sufferers.[6]

LEG VEINS

Repetitious high-impact sports, such as running and aerobic dancing, can dilate and weaken the walls of the small superficial veins of the legs, leaving spider-like venous patterns on the skin. This condition is four times more common in women than in men.[9] Although harmless, many individuals find this condition cosmetically disturbing.

If the veins are blushlike and indistinct, treatment with a vascular laser, such as the flash lamp pulse dye laser, will suffice. The light from this laser passes harmlessly through the epidermis and is selectively absorbed by the targeted vessels. Upon contact a microscopic fragmentation of the blood vessels occurs, resulting in a localized bruise. The macrophage cells remove the debris, leaving normal intact skin behind.[2]

Sclerotherapy is still the treatment of choice for well-defined vessels. An irritating solution, such as salt, sugar, and alcohol in various concentrations, is injected into the small spider-like veins using a fine needle. The solution inflames the walls of the vein, causing them to adhere to one another, preventing the influx of blood. Eventually the vein shrinks and disappears. Larger varicose veins are sometimes treated with sclerosants; however, in cases in which they are too large they need to be surgically ligated.

HERPES ZOSTER

Herpes zoster is a virus that lies dormant in the nervous system. A traumatic blow to the spine or exhaustion can stimulate the virus to run down a nerve root with a linear distribution on the surface of the skin, resulting in the condition commonly known as shingles. It is believed that herpes zoster results when a latent form of the chickenpox virus (varicella) is activated. Unlike chickenpox, the herpes zoster rash is not contagious and is localized to an area innervated by a single nerve. It occurs on only one side of the body.[10]

The rash is characterized initially by painful red bumps (papules) that fill with a clear fluid, giving a blister-like appearance (vesicles). The vesicles then become infected (pustules). As the pustules dry up, a crust is formed that falls off in the final stages of healing.[11] Scars may result. The initial stages of the virus may be accompanied by a high fever, headache, and general malaise. The entire cycle may take 3 to 4 weeks.

When the initial signs of the virus are noted, oral acyclovir (Zovirax) has been found to be the most effective agent for aborting the disease cycle. It should be administered immediately. Once the virus has taken hold, the medication loses its effect. The usual dose is 800 mg, five times a day for 7 days. Since the drug is of little value once the rash reaches the vesicular stage, early diagnosis is crucial.

APHTHOUS ULCER (CANKER SORE)

Aphthous ulcers, superficial erosions of the mucous membrane lining of the mouth, are sometimes caused by blunt trauma to the face. The ulcers can be very painful and may interfere with eating. Bacterial infections may exacerbate the discomfort and contribute to further deterioration of the tissue. Tantum Oral Rinse, a mild topical analgesic, may be used to control inflammation and alleviate the discomfort. In more severe cases, cortisone injections have provided some relief. Vaporization of the ulcer with the CO_2 laser has been helpful in promoting the healing process.[12]

Mouth guards protect the teeth from fractures in contact sports, and the smooth outer surface may also help prevent ulcers from resulting when the mucosal lining is forced against the teeth from a blow to the face.

PYOGENIC GRANULOMA

Pyogenic granulomas are benign vascular tumors that may occur after traumatic injury. Their color range is bright red to reddish brown. The size, shape, and texture of these lesions tend to vary. They frequently form crusts and ulcerate, although some show a transition from vascular tissue to vascular and fibrous tissue, forming a hemangioma. Continuous trauma to the same area contributes to ongoing necrosis and bleeding of the tumor. Surgical excision or laser vaporization is generally the treatment of choice.

SURFER'S NODULES

Surfer's nodules are small, benign, fibrotic growths that occur in the dermis and subcutaneous tissue of the skin on the top of the feet of dedicated surfers. They result from continuous localized trauma and hemorrhaging. Over time the lesion may calcify, contributing to bone deformities in the area. However, in most cases the condition is nonsymptomatic. Surfers rarely seek treatment, as the nodules tend to have symbolic meaning for them.[6]

CONDITIONS CAUSED BY EQUIPMENT

Equipment-related skin problems are more common in some sports, such as hockey and football, than in others. Occlusive material, chemicals in the cloth, and friction or pressure from the garments contribute to a wide variety of skin conditions. Prevention plays an important role in the management of equipment-related skin problems.

ACNE MECHANICA

A combination of friction, pressure and heat from occlusive clothing and equipment may cause swelling of the pore openings of an athlete's skin, preventing the oil glands from draining properly. The trapped oil ferments, causing the gland to become irritated, inflamed, and in some cases infected, resulting in acne (Fig. 35–7). The problem is common in the regions of the back, neck, shoulders, and face because of the high concentration of oil glands in these areas. It is particularly troublesome in sports that require heavy padding and protective equipment, such as hockey and football, and in which taut synthetic garments are worn. Other sports in which there appears to be a relatively high incidence of acne mechanica include cross-country

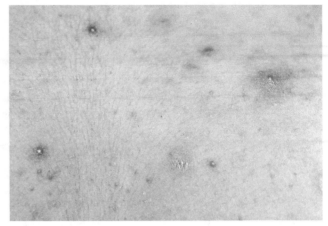

FIGURE 35–7. Acne mechanica (football shoulder pad).

skiing, speed skating, competitive cycling, and aerobic dancing. Golfers, hikers, and mountain climbers may experience acne mechanica along the strap lines of the equipment that they carry on their back and over their shoulders. Weight lifters may notice that the problem is particularly troublesome on their back because of contact with plastic-covered weight benches.[6]

Undergarments made of absorbant material specially designed to wick moisture away from the skin, such as Coolmax, Supplex, and Drylette, will help keep the skin dry and control the irritating friction caused by garments that do not absorb moisture and breathe, such as nylon. Proper cleansing of the skin immediately after an activity is important. Using a mild soap, the involved areas should be gently scrubbed with lukewarm water and a rough washcloth. Aggressive cleansing, particularly with abrasive soaps, may cause further swelling of the pore openings, compounding the problem.

Generally, over-the-counter preparations for the treatment of acne mechanica have little effect, although preparations containing benzoyl peroxide may be helpful in drying up some lesions.

Application of a sulfur mixture, such as Sulfacet lotion, may help open the pores to encourage better drainage of the oil from the glands and decrease inflammation from bacterial overgrowth. Sulfur lotions may be very drying, so they should be used sparingly. To further control inflammation, 1 percent hydrocortisone powder may be added to the lotion.

Medications for acne are categorized as topical or systemic. Tretinoin, a member of the retinoid (vitamin A) family, is a topical antibacterial and pore-opening agent that has proved effective in controlling milder forms of acne mechanica. Unfortunately, the antibacterial drugs that are taken systemically for other forms of acne, such as tetracycline, erythromycin, and minocycline, are not as effective for acne mechanica. However, they may help prevent a milder form of acne from becoming infected and cystic. Isotretinoin (Accutane), which is the best medication currently available for pustulocystic acne, controls the secretions of the sebaceous glands, preventing the buildup of thick oils in the pores. Unfortunately, it can wreak havoc with athletes, as the side effects may interfere with their performance.

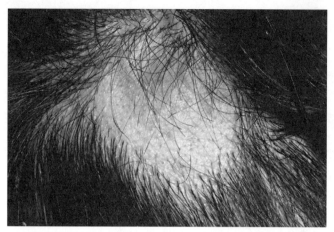

FIGURE 35–8. Traction alopecia (hockey helmet induced).

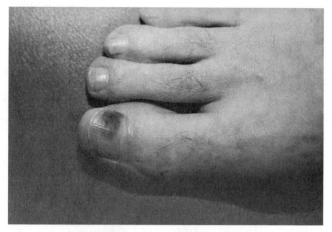

FIGURE 35–9. Jogger's toe (marathoner).

Aching muscles and joints, lack of energy, general lethargy, and dehydration are among the expected side effects when isotretinoin is prescribed.

FOLLICULITIS

Folliculitis, inflammation and infection of the hair follicles, is a problem for some athletes, particularly on the scalp, when helmets are required to protect the head from injury. It may also occur in padded areas of athletes who are particularly hairy, such as on the thighs or back and shoulders. Contributing factors are occlusion, heat, pressure, and friction. Folliculitis is characterized by raised red bumps around the hair follicles. When scar tissue forms, it is referred to as folliculitis keloidalis. This condition is more common in black athletes because the pressure from the athletic equipment pushes the ends of the tightly curled hair back into the skin, which reacts to the embedded keratin of the hair shaft. Keloid refers to a dense overgrowth of fibrous tissue forming a large, raised scar. These scars tend to be cosmetically unacceptable, especially when they occur on the forehead and cheeks. Prevention in some individuals may be as simple avoiding short haircuts.

Medical intervention is generally not required with folliculitis unless bacterial infection is involved. Then a topical antibacterial agent, such as clindamycin, may be recommended or in some cases a systemic antibiotic, such as minocyline. The formation of keloid scars may require injections of cortisone, which flatten the scar. Resurfacing with a vaporization laser smoothes out the lumpy fibrous tissue and blends the edges to the normal surrounding tissue. This approach often helps to cosmetically improve the appearance of the scar. Excision is generally not recommended, because the scar tissue will usually recur.

ALOPECIA

Alopecia refers to loss of hair, which can occur in athletes as a result of friction from equipment causing the hair shaft to fracture (Fig. 35–8). A snug-fitting helmet may help prevent this problem. Hair styling to camouflage the problem will improve the appearance of a bald patch. Once the offending equipment is no longer required, the hair usually grows back. If permanent damage to the hair follicle results, replacement surgery may be required. In this case, a patch of normal hair from another area of the head is used to replace the bald spot, using grafting techniques.

SUBUNGUAL HEMORRHAGES

Chronic, repetitive contact of the edge of the toenail plate with athletic footwear will cause hemorrhaging under the nails. The condition is characterized by a blue-black discoloration under the nails and a tenderness on palpation. Subungual hemorrhaging of the toes has been referred to as skier's toe,[13] tennis toe,[14] and jogger's toe (Fig. 35–9).[15] The condition can occur in any sport in which the toenail and the athletic footwear are in repetitive, abrupt contact. In some cases the nail matrix is damaged, impeding the growth of the nail and resulting in a permanently disfigured nail plate.

If the hemorrhaging is significant, the blood may need to be drained in order to relieve the pain caused by the built-up pressure under the nail. The finger or toe is frozen with a ring block, which numbs the nerves of the digit. Using an extremely hot paper clip, nail drill, or twirling scalpel, a small hole is created in the nail plate through which the blood can drain. Electrocautery or a vaporization laser (CO_2) will serve the same purpose but obviously requires more sophisticated equipment. Relief from pain is immediate once the digit regains normal sensation as the local anesthetic wears off.

Properly fitting footwear is essential to prevent chronic hemorrhaging. One should avoid footwear that is too short or does not allow adequate room for unrestricted vertical movement of the toes. Keeping the toenails trimmed to the margin where the skin and nail come in contact will also help to control the problem.

INGROWN TOENAILS

Another condition of the toenail that can be particularly troublesome to the athlete is referred to as ingrown nails. Rather than the nail plate growing in an anterior direction, it tends to grow peripherally, cutting deep into the skin. When this occurs, the spicules of nail need to be removed to prevent acute pain and infection. Alternatively, the edge of the nail may be elevated with a piece of tape, paper, or pledget of cotton wool to encourage the nail to grow above and beyond the inflamed skin.

The first step in prevention is to ensure properly fitting footwear that has adequate anterior and vertical movement in the toe box. Trimming the nails straight across with V-shaped grooves notched into the nail edge will encourage anterior, inward growth of the nail. Rubbing a glass slide across the middle of the nail will also stimulate the nail to grow toward the center rather than peripherally into the soft tissue of the skin.[3]

BLISTERS

Repetitive friction will cause a separation within the epidermis or between the epidermis and the dermis. The resulting gap fills with fluid exudate and, in some cases, blood, resulting in what is commonly referred to as a blister.

Footwear that fits properly is the first step in preventing blisters. Absorbent socks are also important, as the tropical environment of athletic footwear also contributes to the formation of blisters. Foot powders such as Zeasorb cellulose powder are helpful in keeping the feet dry. Talcum is less effective because it is essentially a powdered rock that can be abrasive and is not effective in absorbing moisture. In areas particularly prone to blister formation, a protective dressing such as Spenco 2nd Skin may be applied prophylactically or, once the blister has formed, to protect the area from further trauma and to relieve discomfort. In those sports in which blisters may occur on the hands, such as cycling and gymnastics, protective gloves should be worn.

The management of blisters is fairly straightforward. Under sterile conditions, the blister should be drained; otherwise, pressure in the area can cause further peripheral separation and a more extensive blister. Draining will also help relieve the pain. The epidermal covering should be left intact until underlying healing takes place, at which time the covering will dry up and slough on its own. This helps prevent infection and promote rapid re-epithelialization. To drain the blister, a sterile needle should be used to puncture the epidermal covering. The excess fluid is aspirated or allowed to drain into a dressing. This procedure is repeated several times over a 24-hour period, if necessary, to release fluid buildup. A protective dressing is applied to discourage further friction to the involved area.[3]

CALLUSES AND CORNS

Calluses and corns are medically referred to as conditions of hyperkeratosis, which is an excessive overgrowth of the superficial layer of keratin on the surface of the epidermis. Hyperkeratosis occurs in areas of chronic friction. The friction may be mild in areas of structural abnormality or bony prominence, or it may be excessive in areas where the underlying structure is normal but the tissue is subjected to repeated stress (hands of a gymnast, heels of a runner). Architectural imbalance of the foot, poor walking or running habits, and poorly fitting footwear may all contribute to the formation of calluses and corns.[16]

Calluses commonly occur on the feet but may appear on any part of the body that is subject to repeated external pressure and friction, as may be the case with athletic equipment or padding. For example, calluses commonly occur on the hands of cyclists, oarsmen, gymnasts, golfers, and individuals who play racket sports.[6]

Padded, well-ventilated gloves help prevent calluses of the hands, and properly fitting footwear is the first step to the management of calluses on the feet. Further intervention may or may not be indicated. Some individuals view their calluses as a natural protection from blisters. Others find that calluses tend to contribute to the formation of blisters or eventually interfere functionally with performance. Soaking the feet in warm water will soften the callus such that it is easy to pare down with an abrasive material such as pumice stone or a scalpel in cases of very thick keratin. Regular application of salicylic acid plasters, which gradually eat away at the keratin, has also proved effective. Generally, once the offending source of friction has been removed, the skin will return to normal without intervention.[6]

Corns are distinguished from calluses by a deep central core of keratin. They tend to be exclusive to the feet and occur over the bony prominence of the toes and lateral edge of the metatarsals. Neuroclavi and keratomas are terms commonly used for cornlike formations on the bottom of the feet. Owing to the tenderness of corns and neuroclavi, they are particularly annoying to athletes.

Warts (verrucae) underlying calluses may sometimes be misdiagnosed as corns. A simple test helps distinguish the two. A corn is more painful under direct pressure than a wart, whereas a wart is more painful when pinched.[5]

Correction of poorly fitting footwear and orthotics for architectural imbalances that contribute to the formation of hyperkeratosis are important to the prevention of repetitive formation of corns after treatment. To remove the core, cantharidin (an extract from the blister beetle) is applied to the lesion and kept under a salicylic acid plaster for 3 days. A blister forms under the keratosis, separating it from the underlying dermis. The resulting blister may be quite tender. It does, however, make the removal of the core and the surrounding keratosis easier. Recurrence is common.[6]

LICHEN SIMPLEX CHRONICUS

Thickening of the skin due to chronic rubbing or scratching is referred to as lichen simplex chronicus. Individuals who develop lichen simplex chronicus in areas where the buttocks are continually rubbing against the metal seat of a rowing machine are said to have rower's rump.[6] The condition is relatively asymptomatic and will self-resolve with cessation of the activity.

CHAFING

Chafing occurs in areas of prolonged friction and usually involves a coarse, sweaty garment. Unprotected nipples are particularly vulnerable. The inner upper thigh is also a common place of irritation as skin rubs against the hem of a pair of shorts or skin rubs against skin. The former condition is frequently referred to as jogger's nipples,[17] and the latter is termed chafing.

Erosion of the skin of the areolae and nipples is particularly troublesome to male long-distance runners wearing loose-fitting T-shirts. The nipple may bleed and is very tender because of the chafing. A popular solution is the application of petroleum jelly to the nipple. Although helpful, it is not always effective. To avoid the problem, several options are available: close-fitting, nonocclusive, absorbent undergarments; no shirt at all; or a piece of circular, flesh-colored adhesive tape applied over the nipple.[6] Women are less prone to the problem because of the soft exercise brassieres that are now available. The nipple will be very sensitive for several days after injury and may need to be protected from further chafing by regular clothing.

Chafing between the upper thighs is characterized by inflamed, tender skin, sometimes accompanied by a burning sensation. To prevent the problem, long, close-fitting shorts (cycling shorts) or tights made of nonocclusive, absorbent material should be worn. Loose-fitting shorts and pants should be avoided.

A mild cortisone cream, such as Westcort cream, applied two to three times a day to chafed nipples or skin will provide rapid relief and encourage healing in the area.

PSEUDOBURSITIS

Pseudobursitis is characterized by swelling, inflammation, and tenderness in an area of chronic friction, causing a subcutaneous pocket to form in which serous fluid gathers. Hence the name pseudobursitis or false bursitis, because the fluid does not gather in an established bursa but in a friction-induced sac.

This condition is common to hockey defensemen, in whom the extra padding at the front of the skate rubs under the pressure of the laces (Fig. 35–10). Pseudobursitis among hockey players is often referred to as skate bite, reflecting the painful nature of the condition.

At one time surgical removal of the lesion was the treatment of choice. Today, however, potent topical cortisone salves, such as Dermovate or Temovate ointment, applied regularly to the area, controls the inflammation and decreases the discomfort. Once the offending equipment is no longer worn or proper protection is provided, the condition resolves on its own, and the cortisone treatments are no longer necessary.

DERMATITIS

Dermatitis and eczema are used synonymously to describe conditions in which the skin is inflamed. The causes are many and varied, but characteristically the skin is red, itchy, and scaly, and accompanied by vesicular papules. Laymen's terms abound for this condition and generally are sport specific. For example, hockey players refer to dermatitis as "gunk," a term not found in any medical dictionary.

A common cause of dermatitis and allergic reactions in athletes is the chemicals in garments. Formaldehyde, which is used in cloth to prevent mildew and wrinkling and to preserve color, is very irritating to the skin when leached out with sweat (Fig. 35–11).

Some individuals are hereditarily predisposed to irritable skin, a condition referred to as atopic dermatitis. Athletes with this condition are particularly susceptible to equipment-related irritation of the skin as well as environmental factors such as chemicals in swimming pools.

Cortisone salves applied frequently may be used to relieve the dermatitis, once present. However, prevention is important in controlling the condition. Careful washing of clothing will help prevent contact dermatitis. Detergent should be used sparingly in the wash, as detergents and softeners are a source of skin irritation in themselves. Bleach should be avoided, as it may activate rubber elastic, making it more allergenic. A cup of powdered milk added to the second rinse cycle will remove the formaldehyde in new clothing. The formaldehyde molecules bind with milk caseins and are flushed away with the rinse water (Table 35–1).[8]

CONDITIONS CAUSED BY HEAT/SWEAT

The skin of the athlete is often immersed in a tropical type environment because of the rise in body temperature through exertion and the body's natural cooling mechanism, sweating. Infectious organisms such as bacteria, viruses, and fungi thrive in this type of environment, and skin problems may result.

The stratum corneum, or superficial layer of the epidermis, plays an important role in preventing the invasion of infective microorganisms. To serve this purpose well, the stratum corneum must be dry and intact. The macerating effect of heat and moisture on the skin lowers its defenses, making it vulnerable to infection.

HERPES SIMPLEX (FEVER BLISTERS, COLD SORES)

Herpes simplex, one of the most common viruses (Fig. 35–12), has two classifications. Type 1 generally occurs on the face but may occur in the genital region. Type 2 is more often a genital condition, although orogenital contact has somewhat changed the distinction of type 1 and type 2 herpes by location. Type 2 herpes generally

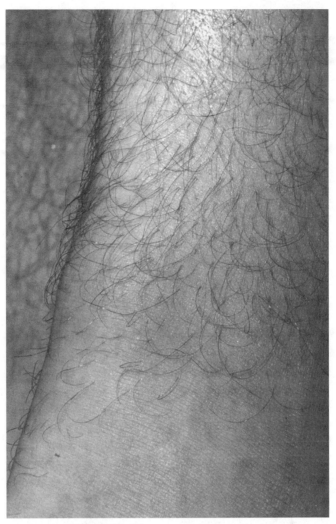

FIGURE 35–10. Pseudobursitis (skate bite).

occurs after puberty, whereas type 1 herpes may occur at any age.

Herpes simplex is passed through skin-to-skin contact and can be aggravated by an increase in body temperature, exposure to sunlight, menstruation, ingestion of certain spicy foods, and a depression in the immune system due to illness. Blunt trauma may also activate the virus owing to an increase in the body temperature and local immune deficiency at the site of the injury. Herpes may also result from exposure to infected saliva.

The primary herpes infection is characterized by painful, raised, erythematous lesions of the skin, known as vesicles. The vesicles contain intra- or intercellular fluid, giving the lesion a blister-like appearance. Erosion of the skin and the mucous membrane in the area of the lesion is common and may be quite extensive. The infection may last from 2 to 6 weeks before healing spontaneously. Recurrence of the infection tends to be less traumatic. The lesions are smaller, less painful and last on average 1 week.[11] Avoiding contact with an individual with an active herpesvirus infection is the best means of prevention.

Acyclovir (Zovirax) is the systemic treatment of choice for herpes simplex. It is most effective when taken in the very early stages of the infection. A sensation of tingling at the site of a previous infection is an indication of a recurring episode. Treatment with acyclovir should be initiated immediately, using a recommended course of 200 mg five times a day for 5 days or more.[11] If the drug has not been taken early enough to abort the lesion, the area must be kept clean and dry. Some physicians recommend the use of a topical antibiotic to prevent secondary bacterial infection in the area. Other topical agents for the treatment of herpes have not proved to be effective. However, it has been shown that the use of topical acyclovir (Zovirax ointment) reduces the contagious nature of the herpes. Once the infection takes hold, it generally runs its course.

INTERTRIGO

Intertrigo is a condition in which the skin becomes inflamed because of moisture and constant friction in skin folds. It differs from chafing in that chafing is

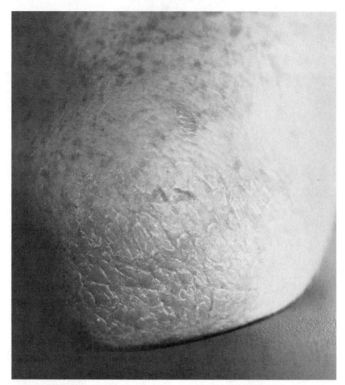

FIGURE 35–11. Contact dermatitis (elbow pad formaldehyde eczema).

caused by friction between two skin surfaces or the skin and a garment, whereas intertrigo is caused by the maceration of the stratum corneum in areas where moisture has difficulty escaping, such as skin folds. In athletes this commonly occurs in the groin or axillary regions. The symptoms include burning, itching, and redness of the skin. Secondary bacterial (candidiasis) or fungal (tinea) infections may accompany intertrigo. In severe cases, the skin becomes eroded and weeping. Blockage of the sweat pores in these areas causes small sweat gland cysts known as miliaria.

Loose, absorbent, cotton underclothing is the first step in drawing moisture away from the skin. The area should be cleansed frequently and when thoroughly dry, a fine absorbent dusting powder, such as Zeasorb cellulose powder, applied. Talcum powders should be avoided, as they can be abrasive and do not absorb moisture well. Underarm deodorants can be irritating to the skin and should be avoided as long as the condition persists. Emollients, such as silicone-based creams (Prevex), may help reduce friction in more severe cases. If antibacterial, antifungal, and mild cortisone preparations are prescribed, the emollient should be applied on top of these to maximize the absorption of the active therapeutic agent into the skin. In cases in which the skin is actually eroded, wet medicated compresses, such as Burosol, may help in the healing process.

MILIARIA

Miliaria refers to damage to the sweat gland, and, depending on the extent of damage, it may be classified as crystallina, rubra, or profunda.

Miliaria crystallina refers to a superficial obstruction of the sweat duct. It is found in individuals who sweat profusely and is characterized by multiple groupings of thin, clear-walled vesicles.[18]

Miliaria rubra, sometimes referred to as prickly heat rash, is caused by increased body temperature with associated profuse sweating (Fig. 35–13). It is commonly seen in individuals who wear occlusive exercise garments or who exercise in hot, humid environments. Crops of erythematous papules cause a very uncomfortable prickly sensation in the skin. Because the sweat cannot escape through the blocked pores, it leaks into the epidermis, resulting in a crop of irritated, itchy papules and vesicles.[18]

Miliaria profunda is the result of chronic miliaria rubra and involves more extensive damage to the sweat duct. This condition is relatively uncommon except in the tropics; it is characterized by asymptomatic pale, hard papules under the surface of the skin and may cause discomfort.[18]

Generally speaking, there is no effective treatment for miliaria. It is best managed by avoiding those circumstances that promote the condition by causing an increase in body temperature and profuse sweating. Unfortunately, for the athlete this is more easily said than done. Occlusive clothing that does not breathe, or excessive clothing in the case of out-of-door sports, should be avoided. Frequent changes to clean absorbent cotton or silk clothing that draws moisture away from the skin are important. Molecularly fine dusting powder, such as Zeasorb cellulose powder, may be helpful. Cool showers or baths will offer some relief, followed by an application of calamine lotion. As calamine lotion can be drying to the skin, a moisturizer applied over it may

TABLE 35–1
Prophylactic Measures for Skin Conditions

Measure	Rationale
Wear full or partial underclothing of soft 100% cotton.	Prevents dermatitis due to sweat gland leaching of chemicals and dyes. Draws moisture away from the skin, preventing maceration of the stratum corneum and avoiding the development of a breeding ground for bacterial and fungal infections.
Use a minimal amount of detergent (1/4 cup) when washing clothing. Avoid bleach. Add powdered milk to the second rinse cycle to wash away formaldehyde in new garments.	Detergents, bleach, and softeners are sources of irritation. Bleach can activate rubber and elastic, making them more allergenic. Formaldehyde in new clothing will bind to caseins in the powdered milk. These will be flushed away with the rinse water.
Use protective dressings such as Spenco 2nd Skin on skin surfaces exposed to trauma or friction.	Provides a buffer against trauma and friction and protects blisters from further injury.
Use a moisturizer immediately after showering.	Controls dryness and reduces the likelihood of asteatotic eczema. This is particularly important in cool, dry climates. Scaly, cracked skin is more susceptible to contact dermatitis and infections.
Use a protective wrap such as Pro-Wrap Foam under adhesive tape.	Adhesive tape can irritate the skin when next to the skin or when being removed.
Wear properly fitting equipment, especially footwear.	Reduces friction. For example, individually casted skates and water molding of skate boots will immobilize the foot, reducing friction.
Wear protective clothing.	Layer clothing in various ambient temperatures to allow for adjustment to changes in body heat. Wet/dry suits, underwater boots and gloves, and bathing caps provide protection in the water. Wide-brim hats, tightly woven cloth, and sunglasses protect against the sun's rays.
Wear protective creams.	A broad-spectrum sunscreen with an SPF of 15 or more will protect against UVA and UVB wavelengths of light. Apply when the skin is cool and dry. Oil-based ointments, such as vaseline, should be used on the lips and around the nostrils to protect them from dehydration due to cold and wind conditions.
Postpone shaving and washing exposed skin surfaces when participating in sports in cold temperatures.	The natural oils of the skin provide insulation from the wind and cold.

Adapted from Groot DW, Johnston PJ: A review of sports-related skin problems. Can J CME 1990;2:19–27.

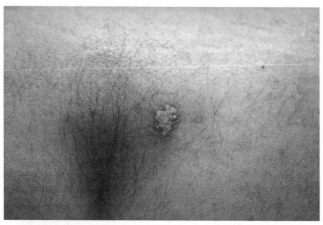

FIGURE 35–12. Herpes simplex (recurrent viral infection).

FIGURE 35–13. Miliaria rubra (prickly heat rash).

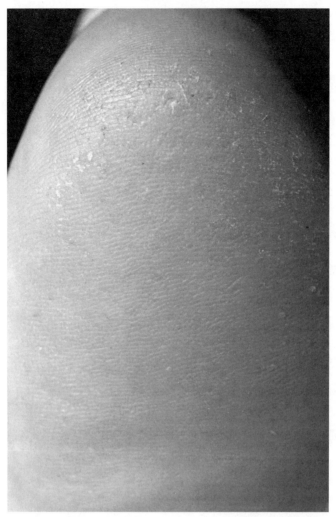

FIGURE 35–14. Pitted keratolysis (bacteria induced).

be required. However, moisturizers in themselves can create problems by plugging the sweat pores and aggravating the condition. As a last resort, acetaminophen (Tylenol or Tempra) taken to lower the body temperature may be helpful.

ACROCHORDONS

Acrochordons are frequently referred to as skin tags. They are small benign polyps that are characteristically soft, pedunculated, and pigmented. Acrochordons generally appear in regions of chronic friction, such as the neck, the armpits, the groin creases, and under the breasts. Skin, like muscle and bone, tends to grow in the direction of physical stress and friction. In these areas the skin is confused with the multiplicity of movements and simply grows outward. Combined with sweat and heat these lesions may become irritated and itchy.

Although acrochordons are benign, most individuals seek treatment for cosmetic purposes. Several effective techniques are used to remove these lesions. Small ones may be clipped with surgical scissors, while cryotherapy, electrocauterization, tying off with stitches, and laser vaporization are effective techniques for removal of larger lesions. Touch-up treatments are usually required, as there is a tendency for recurrence.[2]

PITTED KERATOLYSIS

Maceration of the skin under conditions of sweat and heat create the ideal environment for a condition known as pitted keratolysis. A bacterial microorganism infiltrates the horny layer of the skin, causing a superficial infection on the soles and undersurfaces of the feet. These circular, pitted lesions may blend to produce large irregular margins. As the condition is largely asymptomatic, individuals may be unaware that they have it, although repetitive trauma, such as running, may cause tenderness. The lesions may take on a green or brown discoloration and may be responsible for a foul odor of the feet (Fig. 35–14).

Application of a topical antibiotic, such as Fucidin cream or Bactroban ointment, twice daily for 10 days will rapidly resolve this problem in most cases. Soaking the soles of the feet in an aluminum pie plate for 10 minutes in a mixture of 1 tbs of formalin and 18 tbs of water will help reduce sweat production and odor.

CONDITIONS OF COMMUNAL CONTACT

The interactive nature of sports places most athletes in an environment of communal contact. Even the cleanest facilities afford an opportunity for the transfer of bacteria, fungi, and viruses. Although any part of the body is susceptible, the feet are most commonly involved.

DERMATOPHYTES

Dermatophyte is the medical term for ringworm, a fungus that causes keratin breakdown and inflammation of the skin. The moist, hot conditions created when an individual sweats during an athletic activity cause maceration of the stratum corneum, creating an ideal environment for fungal growth.

There are many different species and strains of dermatophytes, and the clinical features of the skin changes will vary somewhat depending on the type and size of the dermatophyte that is causing the problem. Variations in skin response are also dependent on the area of the body that has been infected and the immune response of the individual.[18]

Common areas of the body for dermatophyte infection, particularly among athletes, include the feet, the fingernails and toenails, the axillae, and the groin. Tinea pedis, an infection of the feet, is commonly referred to as athlete's foot. If the nail plates of the feet or hands are involved, the condition is called onychomycosis or tinea unguium. Jock itch is the lay term for tinea cruris or fungal infection of the groin. Ringworm may also be found in other areas of the body: Tinea corporis involves the entire body; tinea capitis, the scalp; tinea barbae, the beard; tinea faciei, the face; and tinea manuum, the hands.

TINEA PEDIS

Tinea pedis (athlete's foot) generally begins in the toe clefts but may spread to other areas of the foot, particularly the sole. Scaling, peeling, and fissuring of the skin are clinical features of tinea pedis. Itchiness and an unpleasant foot odor are common. The condition may be aggravated by secondary bacterial infection (Fig. 35–15).

Walking barefoot in communal areas such as locker rooms, showers, and along the sides of swimming pools is one of the most common means of dermatophyte transfer. Wearing protective footwear, such as thongs, in these areas is recommended. Keeping the foot dry, particularly between the toes, to prevent maceration of the skin so that it does not become a breeding ground for infection is important. Towel drying after cleansing followed by blow drying with cool air from a hair dryer is helpful. Absorbent socks and foot powders, such as Zeasorb cellulose powder, are recommended.

TINEA UNGUIUM

Onychomycosis refers to fungal infection of the nail plate, while tinea unguium refers more specifically to

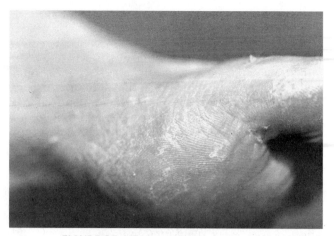

FIGURE 35–15. Tinea pedis (athlete's foot).

the ringworm dermatophytes. In either case, fungal invasion of the nail plate presents a major therapeutic challenge. The nails of athletes play an important protective role in sports requiring either the hands or the feet. Yet trauma and the environmental conditions to which athletes are exposed—heat, sweat, occlusion, and communal exposure—make the nails of the athlete more susceptible to fungal infections.

Fungal infection of the nail plate usually begins with a single digit. The typical early warning sign is a small area of discoloration, white or yellow, at the lateral free edge of the nail plate. It is at this point that treatment should be instigated to prevent damage to the nail plate and involvement of the other digits. As the fungus spreads inward and to the base of the nail, the discoloration may become darker and the nail plate becomes thicker. Subungual hyperkeratosis (thick scale under the nail) will cause the nail plate to lift and crack. Discomfort may accompany gross involvement of the nail plate.

Avoiding communal exposure by wearing protective footwear in sports facilities is the first step in prevention. The sharing of sports equipment such as gloves and footwear should also be avoided. Absorbent cotton socks, glove linings, and powders will help control the conditions that support the growth of fungi.

TINEA CRURIS

Tinea cruris (jock itch) is more common among men than women. This is probably due to the fact that men perspire more than women. Further, the skin is more occluded in the groin area of men because of the scrotum's being in contact with the skin of the thighs and because of the type of undergarments that men wear.[18] It is an interesting aside that jock itch usually appears in the left groin crease first because the left testicle descends lower than the right. Raised erythematous (red) plaques with distinct margins characterize tinea cruris. These plaques appear in the groin, extending down the thigh and onto the scrotum, giving a butterfly-like appearance. The condition is very itchy.

The fungus may be transferred from the feet to the groin, particularly when toweling off. Sharing of sports equipment, clothing, or towels contributes to the transfer of dermatophytes from one individual to the next.

To prevent the spread of tinea cruris, sports equipment, including towels, should not be shared (even after towels have been laundered). Also, individuals with athlete's foot should be cautioned to dry the body before drying the feet in order to avoid autoinfection of other areas, particularly the groin. Loose-fitting, absorbent undergarments are essential to the control of this condition, as dermatophytes thrive in occlusive, tropical environments.

The treatment of tinea pedis, tinea unguium, and tinea cruris is very similar. A topical antifungal cream, such as Lamisil, Micatin, Nizoral, or Canesten, is applied, after thorough cleansing and drying of the affected area, twice daily for 2 to 6 weeks. In resistant cases, systemic medication, such as Nizoral, Fulvicin, or Lamisil, taken orally may be required.

WARTS

Verucca is the medical term for wart. It is a virus that infiltrates the epidermal layer of the skin and susceptible mucosal membranes. Because the virus is made of DNA, it mimics the body's genetic makeup. This confuses the immune system, rendering the virus resistant to the body's natural defense mechanisms.

Athletes are particularly susceptible to the wart virus because of exposure through communal facilities and the role that trauma plays in the inoculation of the virus into the epidermal cells. Autoinfection, whereby the virus is transferred from one part of the body to another, is common. For example, warts may be transferred from the hands to the shaft of the penis or from the feet to the hands. Skin-to-skin contact with an individual with warts will also spread the infection. Verrucae may appear on any part of the body but are most common on the hands and feet. Common verrucae are characterized by raised, firm papules that tend to be paler than the surrounding tissue and have a rough, horny surface.[11]

Plantar warts commonly occur at pressure points on the bottom of the foot (Fig 35–16). They are characteristically flat or slightly raised, firm, circular lesions. A rough, kerototic surface is surrounded by a smooth, horny border. Plantar warts may vary from pale, flesh tones to yellowish gray lesions. These warts may be painful for some individuals.[11]

Warts may spontaneously regress after a few weeks or may last for years. One school of thought is to leave the wart to follow its natural course. Owing to the contagious nature of warts and the social stigma attached to them, however, the authors advise seeking treatment as soon as possible.

Various topical agents are available for the treatment of warts. These include preparations of salicylic acid and lactic acid, formalin in water, glutaraldehyde in aqueous ethanol, and podophyllin. These preparations are generally applied daily to the wart under an occlusive dressing. Patience and determination are required.

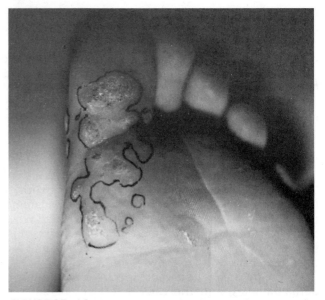

FIGURE 35–16. Plantar warts (outlined prior to laser removal).

If the warts are recalcitrant, more aggressive measures may be necessary to get rid of them. Cryotherapy, laser vaporization, and surgical removal are common strategies. Cryotherapy utilizes liquid nitrogen, which causes a localized frostbite that kills the virus. Alternatively, the liquid nitrogen may be applied less aggressively at 3-week intervals to stimulate the immune system to eradicate the wart. The flash pump dye laser and KTP laser may be used to selectively compromise the supply of nutrients from the blood vessels and thereby cut off the wart's lifeblood. Another technique utilizes a vaporizing laser, such as the CO_2 laser, to heat the individual cells of the wart to 100° C or 212° F, causing the lesion to disappear in a plume of steam and tissue particles.[1] The advantage of laser vaporization over surgical removal is that the laser light seals the blood vessels, creating a better visual field for distinguishing the root of the wart from normal tissue. In this manner, the surgeon can be more certain that the entire wart has been removed with minimal disturbance of the surrounding tissue. This decreases the time required for healing, minimizes the amount of scar tissue formation, and reduces the likelihood of recurrence. Surgical removal involves an excision of the wart with a scalpel. This technique is rarely used today because of the formation of scar tissue and a high rate of recurrence.

PSEUDOMONAS

Many athletes find the tropical waters of a hot tub therapeutic. However, if the pH and chemicals of the water are not properly monitored, hot tubs become breeding grounds for the ubiquitous bacterium *Pseudomonas*.[13] A diffuse rash occurs on areas of exposed skin. The rash may be tender and itchy and is characterized by red, raised papules. Of interest, these microorganisms often give off a distinct fruity odor. Open sores may become infected, complicating the healing process. In the worst-case scenario, the bacterium may penetrate the internal organs, causing a systemic infection that may require hospitalization.

It is important to meticulously clean the hot tub with bleach and to find the proper chemical balance for the water to prevent further bacterial invasion. If the source of infection is a public facility, the maintenance staff should be informed and the facility should be avoided until it is properly cleaned.

Systemic medication with antibiotics such as Cipro will clear up the infection. If the nail plate is involved, soaking the nails in vinegar twice daily helps kill the bacteria. When the infection involves the hair follicles, causing a "hot tub folliculitis," topical agents such Burosol compresses and Garamycin ointment are recommended in combination with systemic antibiotics.

CONDITIONS OF ENVIRONMENTAL EXPOSURE

The skin is one's protective covering from the harsh realities of the environment, yet it cannot stand alone or it will break down under the volley of destructive forces. The onus is on the athlete to take the necessary preventive measures to protect the skin from ultraviolet light, chemicals, and temperature fluctuations in the environment.

PHOTO INJURY

The sun is like a double-edged sword. It provides individuals with light and warmth. It stimulates the production of essential nutrients to sustain life on earth. It stimulates the metabolism of vitamin D, which is necessary for the development of a strong skeletal structure. It has the capacity to heal. Yet, excess amounts of sun exposure can at the very least contribute to aging of the skin; at most, through invasive skin cancers, sun exposure can kill. The sun emits three types of radiation: visible, infrared, and ultraviolet. It is overexposure to ultraviolet light that can be harmful to the skin. Ultraviolet light consists of three basic wavelengths: ultraviolet A (longest), ultraviolet B (midrange), and ultraviolet C (shortest).

The impact of ultraviolet C (UVC) rays is controlled by the ozone layer in the atmosphere, where these rays are absorbed. The epidermis is able to provide a protective barrier from the small amount of UVC light that may filter through the atmosphere. However, if larger doses reach individuals as a result of deterioration of the ozone layer, the UVC rays will be a major contributing factor in the formation of skin cancers.

Ultraviolet B (UVB) was at one time thought to be the major cause of sun damage to the skin because its impact is visible in the form of a sunburn. However, it is now known that ultraviolet A (UVA) rays are absorbed into the epidermis and the dermis more efficiently and in much greater amounts than UVB rays, posing an even greater threat to the health of the skin. This is particularly important given that tanning parlors claim that the ultraviolet A light that they use is safe. UVA and UVB rays may also damage the eyes and the immune system. Damage to the lens and retina of the eye may cause cataracts and visual acuity problems. Ultraviolet light may also interfere with the functioning of the Langerhans cells of the skin. These cells play an important role in recognizing infections and setting the defense mechanism of the immune system in motion. Therefore, damage to these cells reduces the effectiveness of the immune system, increasing susceptibility to viral and other diseases.[2]

UVA and UVB rays stimulate a change in the normally well-organized cells of the epidermis, resulting in skin cancers. There are three basic types of skin cancers: squamous cell, basal cell, and malignant melanomas. The name reflects the level of cell involvement.

Basal cell and squamous cell carcinomas generally arise in individuals over the age of 40 years who have experienced long-term exposure to ultraviolet light. Common areas of the body for these tumors to appear include the face, the outer rim of the ears, the lower lip, the neck, the upper chest, the forearms, and the back of the hands.

Clinically, a basal cell carcinoma begins as a small red, brown, or light flesh tone spot on the skin. It has a distinct pearly appearance and raised borders. Basal cell carcinomas enlarge steadily at one site but tend not to spread to other areas of the skin or metastasize to internal tissue. Without early intervention, the tumor will continue its slow, insidious growth. As the lesion grows larger, it may become scaly and may bleed and crust in a repetitive fashion.[20] Surgical removal is the treatment of choice. Early intervention is recommended, as the small tumor can generally be scooped out with a curette, leaving a cup-shaped lesion that heals with little or no residual scar tissue. Although a recurrence after removal is rare (less than 4 percent), this technique allows a recurring cancer to surface rather than being trapped under scar tissue. The larger the lesion, the more invasive the surgery becomes, increasing the risk of a cosmetically unacceptable scar.

Squamous cell carcinomas pose a greater threat than basal cell carcinomas because they grow quickly, spread rapidly, and are more likely to metastasize. Initially, a squamous cell carcinoma may appear as a raised, red or white, scaly sore on the skin that tends not to heal. It may bleed and may rapidly evolve into a large, ulcerated tumor.[20] Early diagnosis is important in nipping this potentially dangerous cancer in the bud, and surgical removal is the treatment of choice. An early warning sign of the potential development of squamous cell carcinomas is the appearance of actinic keratoses or sunspots. Although it is rare that these red, scaly spots change into squamous cell carcinomas, they indicate the extent to which the skin has been damaged by solar radiation and suggest that regular examination of the skin for more sinister lesions be performed.

Melanomas are the most dangerous type of skin cancer. Five and one-half percent of persons with melanomas die from the condition, and it is alarming to note that the incidence of melanomas has increased by 100 percent over the past 15 years.[20] These cancers develop in and around moles and are less likely to be associated with sun exposure. They are commonly found on the trunks of men and the legs of women. The highest incidence is seen between the ages of 25 and 50 years, although in 2 percent of cases, melanoma develops in individuals under the age of 20 years.

Persons with a family history of melanoma, numerous moles on their body, excessively large moles, or moles that are unusual in color, texture, or shape are at greater risk for the development of the disease. If a mole or pigment spot suddenly appears on the skin or an existing mole shows signs of change in shape, color, size, or surface texture, it should be checked for malignancy. Variations of color within the mole and seepage of color beyond the border of a mole also serve as important indicators of malignancy. Itching and bleeding moles are cause for concern. Melanomas may go through a period of slow growth prior to entering a rapid growth phase during which they quickly metastasize to underlying tissue and spread throughout the body. Early intervention is absolutely essential for a successful outcome. In fact, the most significant breakthrough in the treatment of melanomas has been the identification and removal of nonmalignant moles known as dysplastic nevi. Research has demonstrated that 20 to 35 percent of malignant melanomas developed from nonmalignant dysplastic nevi; it has been suggested that these figures are an underestimate, because many melanomas overgrow the pigmented lesion to which they attach.[20] In comparison with normal nevi, a dysplastic nevus tends to be variable and asymmetric in color. It is also likely to be much larger (1 to 2 cm) than a normal nevus and to have irregular margins. Over time, normal nevi stop growing outward and become raised, soft, and devoid of pigment; dysplastic nevi, on the other hand, continue to spread out from the center, remain pigmented, and are flat. It is not uncommon for people to have more than one lesion. The removal of dysplastic nevi significantly reduces the risk of developing a malignant melanoma in the future.[21]

If the threat of skin cancer is not enough to encourage an athlete to use protective measures, it may help to be aware that exposure to ultraviolet light contributes significantly to the aging of the skin. Photo-aging is characterized by wrinkles and dilated blood vessels as well as by pigment and texture changes. Although much can be done to rejuvenate the skin through medicated creams, chemical peels, and lasabrasions, it is far easier and less costly to prevent the problem from occurring in the first place.

Staying out of the sun is probably the best protective measure, however unrealistic for most athletes. Therefore, the next best alternative for preventing sun damage is the liberal and frequent use of a broad-spectrum sunscreen as well as wearing protective clothing. In the event that adequate precautionary measures have not been taken and a sunburn occurs, steps should be taken to minimize the damage to the skin. In the early stages of a burn, the body releases the chemical prostaglandin into the skin. This chemical is responsible for the red, irritated tenderness of a burn. Acetylsalicylic acid (aspirin) is an antiprostaglandin.

SUN PROTECTION

1. Minimize the amount of sun exposure that you receive, particularly in the middle of the day, when ultraviolet radiation is most intense. Be aware that a light cloud cover does not protect against the damaging rays of the sun and that reflective surfaces such as water, snow, sand, and concrete are sources of ultraviolet radiation, as they will reflect up to 85 percent of the sun's rays.
2. Apply a broad-spectrum sunscreen, which protects against UVA and UVB wavelengths, daily to sun-exposed areas of the skin. The sun protection factor (SPF) should be 15 or more. Sun protection factor refers to the time greater than normal that it takes for ultraviolet light from the sun's rays to burn the skin. For example, if the unprotected skin burns in 1 minute, an SPF 15 sunscreen would allow 15 minutes of sun exposure before a sunburn will occur. Ombrelle 15, Ombrelle 30 Extreme, PreSun 30 and Photoplex are examples of broad-based sunscreens.
3. Apply adequate amounts of sunscreen, 1 ounce for one body for one application, and be thorough in covering the exposed areas of the skin.
4. Apply sunscreen to a cool body, 1/2 hour before sun exposure, so that it will bind more effectively to the skin.
5. Wear sunscreen under loosely woven clothing or wet clothing. The ultraviolet radiation can penetrate through cloth.
6. Reapply sunscreen throughout the day according to the amount of sun exposure. Water and sweat will wash away the sunscreen, so reapplication every hour is important. Sunscreen should be applied to dry skin 20 minutes before exposure to more moisture.
7. Wear protective clothing: tightly woven cloth, sun hats, and sunglasses.
8. Avoid tanning salons. Fifteen minutes of exposure to UVA light from a tanning bed is equivalent to 3 days of sitting in the sun. The UVA rays penetrate deep into the skin, so that superficial burning does not occur unless the skin is exposed for long periods of time.[1]

Therefore, if taken in high doses prior to the onset of inflammation and redness, acetylsalicylic acid will inhibit prostaglandin release. Two adult aspirin three times daily for 2 days will suffice, if the individual's digestive system can take it. Enteric-coated aspirin is less irritating to the stomach. Acetaminophen (Tylenol or Tempra) is effective in reducing the discomfort of the sunburn, but it does not have the beneficial effect of inhibiting prostaglandin release, which will prevent the sunburn from occurring.

Photo injury is a major factor in the aging of the skin. Many individuals seek help after the damage has been done. There are many alternatives available to rejuvenate the skin. Medicated creams, containing tretinoin or alpha hydroxy acid, applied daily to the skin will even out the color and reduce the fine wrinkles by realigning the collagen in the dermis. Hydroquinone will bleach the brown discolorations known as age spots.

Pigment changes, such as age spots, may also be removed with a target-specific laser, such as the Q-switched ruby or KTP laser. The laser light has a selective affinity for dark pigment in the skin. On contact the energy of the light is emitted, causing the pigment cells to break into tiny particles that are carried away by the immune system. Another commonly used technique is cryotherapy, although this carries a greater risk of scarring. A localized frostbite to the age spot is created with the application of liquid nitrogen, causing the pigmented lesion to split away from the normal skin. In the same fashion that age spots can be removed with a target-specific laser, fine superficial veins can be removed with a laser such as the flash lamp pulse dye laser or the KTP laser. These veins often appear on the face and neck after years of excessive sun damage.

Resurfacing techniques, such as chemical peels and lasabrasions, work at a deeper level to realign the collagen and elastins of the dermis, remove unwanted pigment, smooth out fine to moderately deep wrinkles, and even out the texture changes.

Implant therapies are helpful when deep furrows appear in the skin. These follow natural muscle pull lines. Sterile substances such as bovine collagen (Zyderm and Zyplast) or Gortex, in some select cases, are implanted into the deep furrow to fill the depression.

If gravity begins to pull on skin weakened by excessive sun exposure, surgical redraping techniques such as eyelid lifts, brow lifts, and face lifts will help correct the problem.

It is important to reiterate that many of the signs of aging can be prevented or certainly minimized by protecting the skin from sun exposure. The therapeutic alternatives discussed above are not magical, and they have inherent risks. They also do not eliminate the need to take protective measures against the sun.[2]

COLD TEMPERATURE CUTANEOUS INJURY

With exposure to extremely cold environmental conditions, severe tissue damage will ensue. Skiers, skaters, bobsledders, snowmobilers, rock and ice climbers, horseback riders, and sailors are some of the sports-minded individuals who are susceptible to skin injury due to cold weather conditions.

COLD URTICARIA

Urticaria is synonymous with hives, which is an edematous swelling of the dermis or subcutaneous tissue in response to stimuli such as drugs, foods, food additives, inhalants, infections, heat, sweat, and cold, to name a few. Cholinergic (sweat-induced), cold, and mechanical urticaria are common among athletes. Accurate diagnosis is crucial to therapeutic success. Cholinergic urticaria is best treated with agents that reduce production of the chemical mediator acetylcholine. People who have a high level of cold proteins in their blood, which may be a reflection of systemic disease such as lupus erythematosus or a viral illness, are more prone to develop hives when exposed to a cold

environment. In these cases, the underlying cause must be addressed therapeutically. Otherwise, avoidance of cold exposure is the best prophylaxis. Antihistamines may be helpful when cold conditions are unavoidable. Mechanical urticaria is best treated by avoiding direct pressure to the skin, as in the case of properly fitting equipment.

CHILBLAINS

Chilblains or perniones develop when conditions are cold and damp. To preserve heat, vasoconstriction is the body's defense against the cold. However, this defensive action may compromise the tissue of the skin, making it a pawn in the battle against the cold. Chilblains appear on protruding extremities such as the fingers, toes, nose, and ears. The heels of the feet, the lower legs, and the thighs may also be involved. The skin and subcutaneous tissue swell, becoming itchy and red. Blistering may occur and, in more severe cases, ulceration.[22]

Chilblains are self-limiting. Once the humid, cold conditions disappear, so do the chilblains. Keeping the extremities warm and dry, even when indoors, is the first step to management of this problem. Vasoconstriction can be controlled by wearing properly fitting footwear and gloves. If treatment is required, topical corticosteroids may be prescribed to control the inflammation, and systemic vasodilators may be necessary to monitor the vasoconstriction.[13]

FROSTBITE

Frostbite is a paramount concern of winter sports athletes. Extremely cold conditions, especially at high altitudes or combined with a severe wind chill, will cause the tissue of the skin to freeze. In the initial stages, the individual experiences a very painful burning sensation. At this point individuals should remove themselves from the cold conditions, because once the pain subsides, freezing of the tissue has begun. As the temperature of the skin drops to $-2°C$ metabolism at the cellular level stops, causing destruction of enzymes and proteins.[22] Ice crystals begin to form inside and outside the cell.

A white patch on the skin is the first sign of freezing. The patch will spread as more tissue becomes involved and will remain devoid of color until removed from the cold. In mild cases, the skin may simply be red and inflamed for several hours. In more severe cases, blistering may occur. Frostbite may extend beyond the skin to involve the muscles, nerves, vascular structures, and bones. Extensive loss of tissue (gangrene) may result. In cases in which loss of tissue does not occur, the involved areas may be numb and hypersensitive to cold for several months owing to the damage to blood vessels and nerves.[22] Once removed from the cold, the affected body part should be rapidly rewarmed by immersing it in circulating water of 38° to 44°C (100° to 110°F),[23] and further exposure to extreme cold should be avoided.

Ensuring that all exposed skin is properly covered

prior to venturing into the cold is the first step in prevention. The face is generally of greatest concern; facemasks help. By not shaving, men can take advantage of the natural protection offered by their beards. Not washing prior to taking part in outdoor activities will allow the natural oils of the skin to provide a protective film against the cold. The use of sunscreens will provide double protection against two environmental hazards.[6]

Avoiding restrictive clothing prevents vasoconstriction. Wearing layers of lightweight clothing helps monitor temperature fluctuations. Inner garments should be such that they draw moisture away from the skin.[24] Preserving and managing changes in body heat and moisture will help protect against the dangers of chilblains, frostbite, and hypothermia.

EXOSTOSIS

Chronic wet and cold conditions, such as those experienced by surfers, may lead to the growth of bony spurs in the ear canal known as exostosis. Some serious surfers consider these lesions to be a kind of status symbol. These lesions may be removed surgically;

however, they are generally considered to be asymptomatic.

CHEMICAL DAMAGE

Pigmentary changes in the hair may result from long-term exposure to chemically treated waters. It is not the chlorine or bromine but the copper in chemically treated pools that is responsible for the change in hair color. When the copper ions of a chemically treated pool become integrated into the hair matrix, the hair takes on a greenish coloration that is very disturbing to most people. A bathing cap should be worn in chemically treated waters to prevent the problem. Another alternative is to wet the hair and apply a moisturizing conditioner before entering the pool, although most public facilities frown on this practice. Specialized shampoos and conditioners, such as Ultra-Swim chlorine combatting shampoo and conditioner and Le Remouver shampoo, are available to help remove some of the green discoloration from the hair.

Chemicals in swimming pools also contribute to hair

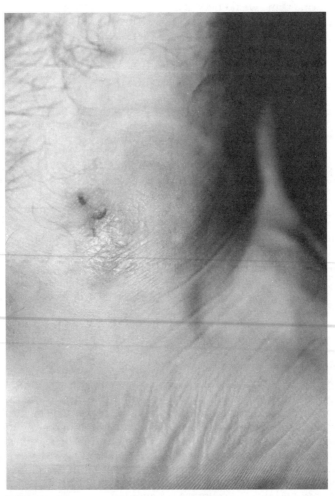

FIGURE 35–17. Asteatotic eczema (long-distance chlorine pool swimmer).

shaft fragility, resulting in split ends and hair breakage. Thorough rinsing of the hair after shampooing helps control the problem. Conditioners contain proteins that help to temporarily mend damaged hair by binding hair shaft cells. Oils in conditioners also replenish the natural oils that have been stripped from the hair by exposure to chemicals and shampooing. They also contain quaternary compounds that help to control "fly-away" hair, a common problem in dry, cold climates and air-conditioned rooms.[1] In the case of severe damage, the only alternative is to cut the hair. To prevent the problem, a bathing cap should be worn.

ASTEATOTIC ECZEMA

When dryness due to lipid depletion results in irritated, inflamed skin, the condition is referred to as asteatotic eczema (Fig. 35–17). This is a particularly common condition in athletes who are exposed to environmental conditions that strip the skin of its natural oils. Such environmental factors may include wind, chemicals in swimming pools, and deodorant soaps.

The skin is dry, itchy, scaly, and irritated. This can be particularly annoying to the athlete. The best treatment option for eczema is prevention. A soap that contains a high concentration of fat (animal, glycerin or resin) should be used when bathing or washing the face. A deodorant or antiperspirant should be used separately. In severe cases, Cetaphil lotion is a good soap substitute. Be sure that the skin is thoroughly rinsed, pat dry, leaving the skin slightly moist, and apply a moisturizer. Moisturizers with perfumes should be avoided, as they irritate the skin. The moisturizer does not replenish the natural oils but prevents the oil and moisture in the skin from escaping. Chemically enhanced moisturizers contain agents such as urea, glycolic acid, and lactic acid that improve the entrapment of the skin's natural oils, for example, Uremol 10 and Lac-Hydrin lotions. Calmurid cream is particularly useful for cracked and fissured heels. Apply the cream before going to bed, wrap the feet in a plastic (SARAN) wrap, and cover them with socks in order to maximize effectiveness.[2]

In severe cases, topical cortisone may be required or a course of treatment with controlled ultraviolet light.

CONCLUSION

Throughout this chapter the authors have touched on some of the common skin problems encountered by the athlete. The protective role the skin plays in maintaining one's health cannot be overemphasized. As in any other area of medicine some simple yet effective precautions may prevent skin diseases which can interfere with training and performance.

REFERENCES

1. Lever WF, Schaumburg-Lever G: Histopathology of the Skin. Philadelphia, JB Lippincott, 1983.
2. Groot DW, Johnston PA: Young As You Look. Edmonton, Canada, InForum, 1993.
3. Groot DW, Johnston PA, Miller P, Sather G: Skin problems of a professional hockey club: a season in review. Cont Derm 1988; 2:13–22.
4. Lynch PJ, Boyer JT: Clotting disorders in the skin (purpura). In Fitzpatrick TB, Eisen AZ, Wolff K, et al (eds): Dermatology in General Medicine. New York, McGraw-Hill, 1971, pp 1168–1171.
5. Wilkinson DS: Cutaneous reactions to mechanical and thermal injury. In Rook A, Wilkinson DS, Ebling FJ, et al (eds): Textbook of Dermatology, vol 1. Oxford, Blackwell Scientific, 1986, pp 587–622.
6. Basler RSW: Skin injuries in sports medicine. J Am Acad Dermatol 1989; 21:1257–1262.
7. Johnston PA, Groot DW: Tattoos: art or injury. Pulse 1993; 7(2):14–15.
8. Groot DW, Johnston PJ: A review of sports-related skin problems. Can J CME 1990; 2:19–27.
9. Ryan TJ, Wilkinson DS: Diseases of the veins and arteries—leg ulcers. In Rook A, Wilkinson DS, Ebling FJ, et al (eds): Textbook of Dermatology, vol 2. Oxford, Blackwell Scientific, 1986, pp 1187–1227.
10. Oxman MN: Varicella and herpes zoster. In Fitzpatrick TB, Eisen AZ, Wolff K, et al (eds): Dermatology in General Medicine. New York, McGraw-Hill, 1971, pp 1600–1616.
11. Nagington J, Rook A, Highet AS: Virus and related infections. In Rook A, Wilkinson DS, Ebling FJ, et al (eds): Textbook of Dermatology, vol 1. Oxford, Blackwell Scientific, 1986, pp 657–720.
12. Evans JG: Recurrent aphthous stomatitis: management of a patient. Oral Health 1993; 8:27.
13. Basler RSW: Skin problems in winter sports. In Casey MJ, Foster C, Hixson EG (eds): Winter Sports Medicine. Philadelphia, FA Davis, 1989.
14. Resnick SS, Lewis LA, Cohen BH: The athlete's foot. Cutis 1977; 20:351–355.
15. Sher RK: Jogger's toe. Int J Dermatol 1978; 17:719–720.
16. Gibbs RC, Boxer MC: Abnormal biomechanics of feet and their cause of hyperkeratosis. J Am Acad Dermatol 1982; 6:1061–1069.
17. Levit P: Jogger's nipples. N Engl J Med 1977; 297:1127.
18. Champion RH: Disorders of the sweat glands. In Rook A, Wilkinson DS, Ebling FJ, et al (eds): Textbook of Dermatology, vol 3. Oxford, Blackwell Scientific, 1986, pp 1891–1893.
19. Roberts SOB, Mackenzie DWR: Mycology. In Rook A, Wilkinson DS, Ebling FJ, et al (eds): Textbook of Dermatology, vol 2. Oxford, Blackwell Scientific, 1986, pp 921–923.
20. Sun Facts. Kingston, The Canadian Dermatology Association, 1993.
21. McLean D: Dysplastic nevus: precursor to melanoma. Med North Am 1986; 32:4460–4462.
22. Champion RH: Cutaneous reaction to cold. In Rook A, Wilkinson DS, Ebling FJ, et al (eds): Textbook of Dermatology, vol 3. Oxford, Blackwell Scientific, 1986, pp 623–635.
23. D'Ambrosia RD: Cold injuries encountered in winter sport. Cutis 1977; 20:365–368.
24. Washburn B: Frostbite. N Engl J Med 1962; 266:974–989.
25. Mikelionis J: Mountains, snow and skin. Cutis 1977; 20:346–347.

CHAPTER 36

Medical Problems in Athletes

J A M E S   C.   P U F F E R   MD

Many consider the discipline of sports medicine to be primarily concerned with athletic trauma. Although musculoskeletal injury is commonly seen by the physician who cares for athletes, the recognition and management of medical problems that may occur as a result of athletic participation are also critically important, as is the comprehensive management of athletes with pre-existing medical disease. Appropriate care for these problems affords the opportunity for the athlete to participate optimally in his or her chosen sport. In fact, a University of Arizona study has demonstrated that the management of medical problems accounts for the highest incidence of visits to the team physician by a large population of men and women athletes at the intercollegiate level.[1]

SUDDEN CARDIAC DEATH

The relationship of exercise and sudden death has been a topic of considerable interest since the well-publicized deaths of runner Jim Fixx, Olympic volleyball player Flo Heyman, and basketball star Reggie Lewis. Athletes who succumb to sudden cardiac death can be separated into two distinct groups. Deaths that occur in young athletes are frequently the result of inherited cardiac disorders, whereas deaths of middle-aged athletes are, for the most part, caused by atherosclerotic coronary artery disease.

A seminal study has described the autopsy findings in 29 young athletes who died suddenly.[2] Twenty-two of these athletes died of unequivocal cardiovascular disease, of which 14 cases were attributed to familial hypertrophic cardiomyopathy. This disorder, which is genetically transmitted, has been characterized by marked asymmetric hypertrophy of the interventricular septum in relationship to the posterior ventricular wall. This results in almost complete obliteration of the left ventricular cavity and, in approximately 20 to 25 percent of those affected, obstruction of the left ventricular outflow track. Left heart catheterization studies in patients with the obstructive form of hypertrophic cardiomyopathy demonstrate significant left ventricular outflow obstruction and obliteration of the left ventricular cavity during systole with extremely high ejection fractions.

Since most individuals with this form of cardiomyopathy die suddenly before the age of 35 years, athletes who are affected by this disorder may give a positive family history for sudden death at an early age. Any history of syncope, dizziness, associated shortness of breath, palpitations, or chest pain during exercise must be viewed with serious concern and the possibility of hypertrophic cardiomyopathy seriously considered. Physical examination may be unrevealing but, when remarkable, will usually reveal a displaced left ventricular impulse and a harsh systolic ejection murmur that is accentuated by the Valsalva maneuver in those with the obstructive form of this disorder. Although the electrocardiogram is typically abnormal, it is important to note that it may be normal in as many as 10 percent of patients with hypertrophic cardiomyopathy.

Hypertrophic cardiomyopathy should not be confused with the normal physiologic changes that occur in the athlete's heart in response to chronic exercise, the so-called athletic heart syndrome. These changes have been well described[3] and, in endurance athletes, are characterized by initial dilatation of the left ventricular cavity with subsequent concentric thickening of the left ventricular wall to normalize wall tension. In athletes who perform primarily isometric activity, hypertrophy is seen without dilatation. Distinction between these two entities can be made echocardiographically. Athletes with obstructive hypertrophic cardiomyopathy will demonstrate a left ventricular free wall that exceeds 15 mm and a septal:free wall ratio greater than 1:3. Systolic anterior motion of the septal leaflet of the mitral valve can be demonstrated as well. Conversely, athletes with the athletic heart syndrome will have a left ventricular free wall that is less than 15 mm in thickness and a septal:free wall ratio of less than 1:3. Occasionally, septal:free wall ratios greater than 1:3 are seen in athletes, but these are probably normal in the absence of absolute left ventricular hypertrophy. In athletes in whom there is a question with respect to this issue, cessation of activity will result in regression of the normal physiologic changes described above, whereas cardiac dimensions will not change in the athlete with hypertrophic cardiomyopathy.

Recent work has demonstrated that there may be wide variation in the expression of this disorder. In fact, both lethal and nonlethal forms of obstructive hypertrophic cardiomyopathy may exist.[4] However, until further refinement of genetic screening, all athletes with this condition should be precluded from vigorous athletic participation.

Marfan's syndrome is also a cause of sudden death in young athletes. This occurs as a result of cystic medial necrosis of the intima of the aorta, which predisposes to aortic dissection and rupture. These athletes can be recognized by their tall stature; their relatively long arms, legs, and fingers; and the presence of anterior chest deformities, thoracic kyphosis, or scoliosis. Common cardiac findings include evidence of mitral valve prolapse, mitral regurgitation, or aortic regurgitation. Subluxation of the lens is also a common finding in these individuals, who will typically have marked myopia.

This disorder is genetically transmitted, and, therefore, a positive family history for this disorder coupled with any of the findings noted above should lead the physician to perform a careful screening examination to exclude this disease. This should include noninvasive cardiovascular evaluation with echocardiography in an effort to demonstrate dilatation of the ascending aorta as well as slit-lamp examination to detect subluxation of the lens. Those athletes found to have this disorder should be precluded from participating in activities that increase mean arterial pressure and thereby increase the risk of aortic dilatation and subsequent aortic rupture.

Coronary artery abnormalities are the second most common cause of exercise-associated death in young patients. The most commonly reported coronary artery abnormality in the young athlete at autopsy is an anomalous left coronary artery that originates from the right sinus of Valsalva and then makes an abrupt turn to course between the pulmonary artery and the aorta.[2] Anomalous right coronary arteries and single coronary arteries have been reported as well. Although it is impossible to screen for these anomalies on routine preparticipation examination, any athlete who presents with symptoms of syncope, near-syncope, or chest pain requires thorough evaluation to rule out the possibility of anomalous coronary arteries.

In the older athlete, atherosclerotic coronary artery disease is almost always the cause of sudden death. The incidence of sudden death for joggers between the ages of 30 and 64 years was found to be approximately one sudden death per year for every 7620 joggers in the state of Rhode Island.[5] This equated to approximately one death for every 396,800 hours of jogging. Although the absolute number of jogging deaths was extremely low in this study, there was an approximate seven times greater chance of dying suddenly while exercising than when sedentary. In the middle-aged athlete, therefore, it is critically important to assess whether risk factors for coronary artery disease exist. If so, consideration should be given to noninvasive screening to rule out coronary artery disease with stress testing.

HYPERTENSION

Athletes can develop hypertension just as any other individual can. However, treatment of the athlete with hypertension presents an interesting challenge to the clinician, since one would like to optimize blood pressure control without a deleterious effect on performance. In understanding the management of hypertension in athletes, it is important to appreciate some hemodynamic considerations that will influence therapy.

Blood pressure, in the hemodynamic sense, can be conceptualized as a product of both cardiac output and peripheral vascular resistance.[6] In young athletes, hypertensive changes in blood pressure are most commonly the result of a significant increase in cardiac output with minimal changes in peripheral vascular resistance. Heart rate, renal blood flow, plasma renin activity, and catecholamines are all elevated in the young hypertensive athlete, and cardiac output is increased 10 to 20 percent over that seen in normal subjects. The hypertension of young athletes, therefore, has been characterized as a hyperadrenergic or hyperdynamic hypertension. On the other hand, in middle-aged or older athletes, hypertensive blood pressure change is most likely a reflection of significant increases in peripheral vascular resistance with no change or a decrease in cardiac output.

These differences are important when management is considered. Since there is no critical level of blood pressure that identifies excess risk, the definition of hypertension obviously remains arbitrary. By convention, most would define hypertension as a blood pressure that exceeds 140/90.

The work-up of the hypertensive athlete should include a careful history taking. This should ascertain whether there is a family history of hypertension, diabetes, or cardiovascular disease; the known duration of blood pressure elevation; the results of previous treatment; and whether symptoms of secondary hypertension exist. Other important features of the history include questions about the use of anabolic steroids or oral contraceptives and abuse of alcohol or tobacco, all of which may contribute to blood pressure elevation.

The physical examination should be complete and thorough, but special attention should be paid to an accurate blood pressure measurement, which usually will require the use of an appropriate-size blood pressure cuff for larger athletes. Careful attention also should be given to the optic fundi, the cardiovascular system, the peripheral pulses, and the presence of abdominal murmurs. Considerable debate exists over the appropriate laboratory studies to obtain in the athlete who is hypertensive, but a reasonable work-up might include a routine urinalysis; complete blood count (CBC); and serum potassium, creatinine, cholesterol, and uric acid levels as well as a fasting blood glucose value and electrocardiogram, since these tests would most cost-effectively screen for secondary causes of hypertension.

Pharmacologic management of those athletes who require medication for control of their blood pressure should be targeted to the specific underlying hemodynamic derangement, as discussed above. The ideal antihypertensive agent for use in competitive athletes should meet the following criteria: (1) It should be free of any depressant effect on the myocardium; (2) it should have no arrhythmogenic potential; (3) it should preserve the redistribution of blood flow to exercising muscle; and (4) it should not interfere with efficient substrate utilization for energy demands.[7] In the young athlete, the agents that meet all these criteria are the angiotensin converting enzyme (ACE) inhibitors. The use of beta-blockers should be discouraged because of their known ability to impair left ventricular function, their unfavorable effect on serum lipids, and their negative influence on the mobilization of lipids during prolonged submaximal exercise. Likewise, diuretics are unsuitable first-line agents for the athlete because of their unfavorable effect on serum lipids, their potential to cause hypokalemia and hypomagnesemia, and their negative influence on volume status. For the older patient, appropriate first-line agents include the calcium channel blockers and the ACE inhibitors. A combination of both these agents may be beneficial in treating the older athlete whose blood pressure is resistant to treatment with either agent used singly. The hypertensive black athlete deserves special mention because of the volume-dependent nature of the hypertension. He or she may respond to very small doses of diuretic such as hydrochlorothiazide, 12.5 mg daily. Other options for this population include antiadrenergic agents as well as the calcium channel blockers. For the athlete participating in events at which drug testing will be done, special consideration must be given to the choice of therapeutic agents, since beta-blockers (in some events) and diuretics are banned by both the International Olympic Committee (IOC) and the National Collegiate Athletic Association (NCAA) testing protocols.

EXERCISE-INDUCED BRONCHOSPASM

Exercise-induced bronchospasm is a disorder that has been reported in approximately 8 to 12 percent of athletes. It occurs in 40 percent of individuals with known allergic rhinitis and in 90 to 95 percent of those with known asthma. It has been reported in 6 to 8 percent of athletes with no history of either of these disorders. A survey of 597 Olympic athletes revealed that 67 of them had exercised-induced bronchospasm, for a prevalence of 11.2 percent.[8] This group won a total of 41 medals in 14 different sports during the 1984 Summer Olympic Games, demonstrating that with proper treatment athletes with this disorder can compete at the highest levels of sport.

By definition, exercise-induced bronchospasm is the 15 percent reduction in either peak expiratory flow rate or forced expiratory volume in 1 second, which typically occurs 6 to 8 minutes after vigorous exercise. This reduction in pulmonary function can last as long as 60 minutes after the termination of exercise. Recent work suggests that bronchospasm occurs as a result of airway cooling with increased minute ventilation during exercise and rapid rewarming when ventilation diminishes.[9] Evaporative water loss leads to changes in epithelial cell osmolarity and temperature change secondary to airway cooling. The release of chemical mediators, including histamine, neutrophil chemotactic factor, eosinophil chemotactic factor, and the leukotrienes, can mediate both early and late reactions to exercise.

Exercise-induced bronchospasm may go undetected in as many as 30 percent of athletes,[10] and, therefore, screening is critically important. The diagnosis of exercise-induced bronchospasm can be made by eliciting a history of cough, shortness of breath, or wheezing associated with exercise. Past medical history of asthma or allergic rhinitis should heighten suspicion of exercise-induced bronchospasm in individuals with exercise-related complaints. If necessary, validation of the clinical impression can be made with an exercise test in which the athlete exercises at 85 to 90 percent of maximal predicted heart rate for a period of 5 minutes with postexercise spirometry. These tests can be done in a controlled laboratory situation using either a treadmill or a bicycle ergometer; however, a simple field test using a hand-held spirometer may be the most sensitive in identifying athletes with suspected exercise-induced bronchospasm.

Treatment should consist of the prophylactic use of an inhaled beta-agonist or cromolyn sodium prior to exercise. The beta-agonist albuterol should be considered as the initial agent, given its rapid onset and longer duration of action compared with other beta-agonist preparations. This agent should typically be given in inhaled form 15 to 20 minutes prior to exercise and may be repeated if symptoms occur once exercise begins. In those patients not responsive to albuterol, a trial of cromolyn sodium may be used. A combination of both agents may provide considerable synergism in the difficult-to-control patient.[11] In athletes with known asthma, an inhaled corticosteroid preparation should be used on a daily basis to treat the underlying airway inflammation that is the hallmark of this disorder. An inhaled beta-agonist then can be used in conjunction with this treatment prior to exercise. All these medications can be utilized by athletes who will be competing under circumstances in which drug testing may take place as long as they are appropriately declared.

Prevention is vitally important in minimizing the impact of exercise-induced bronchospasm on performance. This includes not only the regular use of the medications described above but also careful attention to appropriate warm-up; the use of a mask or muffler to warm inspired air in cold, dry climates; and the avoidance of exercise when environmental pollutants are present at elevated levels.

ANEMIA

Exercise-related anemia has been a well-recognized disorder in athletes for some time. Reduction in both red blood cell mass and hemoglobin concentrations in long-distance runners over the course of a 20-day run have been demonstrated[12] as well as the chronic changes in blood parameters in endurance athletes of all types. Several possible explanations for anemia in athletes have been advanced. With chronic endurance exercise, a significant increase in plasma volume is noted. This disproportionate increase without a concomitant increase in red blood cell mass has been likened to the "pseudoanemia" seen during the second trimester of pregnancy. This has been viewed as an adaptive mechanism that attempts to maximize cardiac output and oxygen transport. Considerable attention has also been focused on the mechanical destruction of red blood cells as a plausible explanation for this phenomenon.

True anemia in the athlete increases in likelihood as hemoglobin values drop below 11.5 g/dl in women and 13.5 g/dl in men, although lower thresholds may be tolerated for elite athletes. Nutrition may play just as critical a role in the development of true anemia in athletes as it does in nonathletes. In fact, it is well known that iron deficiency anemia is more common in female athletes than in their male counterparts; nutritional surveys conducted on elite athletes have demonstrated that as many as 90 percent of women may have inadequate intake of dietary iron.[13] Evaluation of the athlete who is anemic should include a very careful review of dietary intake as well as a CBC and examination of the peripheral blood smear. In the athlete with a low hemoglobin suggestive of true anemia, a serum ferritin level is helpful, as this is the most sensitive indicator of iron deficiency (a value below 15 ng/ml strongly suggests iron deficiency). Completion of the work-up with determination of folate and vitamin B_{12} levels as well as an appropriate hemolytic study can be performed if indicated in patients without evidence of iron deficiency. Those athletes found to have iron deficiency anemia should have further evaluation to determine the source of their blood loss or inadequate iron intake or both.

The effect of iron deficiency anemia on performance is well understood; for that reason, athletes who are found to have this disorder should receive appropriate iron supplementation in the form of ferrous sulfate, 325 mg orally three times daily. In athletes in whom the hemoglobin is at low-normal levels with a low serum ferritin value, a therapeutic trial of iron can be instituted; a concomitant rise in serum hemoglobin indicates the presence of iron deficiency anemia. The issue of whether nonanemic iron deficiency should be treated has received considerable attention. A frequently cited study, in which athletes donated 2 units of blood and were subsequently reinfused with the washed red blood cell components to restore their hematocrit while still iron deficient, demonstrated no reduction in performance from baseline and the iron-deficient, nonanemic state.[14] For this reason, therapeutic iron therapy is not indicated in this population, but an effort should be made to ensure adequate intake of dietary iron.

SICKLE CELL TRAIT

Approximately 6 to 10 percent of the black population carries the sickle cell trait. The incidence of sickle cell trait in 579 football players in the National Football League has been found to be 6.7 percent.[15] Although there have been isolated reports of deaths in athletes with sickle cell trait secondary to sickling crises, current evidence suggests that the remote chance of a sickling crisis should not justify a policy of unnecessary restrictions on the athlete with sickle cell trait. All black athletes should be offered the opportunity to have sickle cell testing performed and should be advised of the results. They should also be informed of the early symptoms of a sickling crisis (bone pain, abdominal pain, and arthralgia) and should seek immediate medical attention if these are experienced. Since dehydration and high altitude have been implicated in the precipitation of sickle cell crises in individuals with sickle cell trait, exercise at altitudes should be avoided and appropriate hydration should be guaranteed during vigorous physical activity.

DIABETES MELLITUS

The athlete who is diabetic deserves special attention. It is well known that diabetes alters the metabolic response to exercise. In well-controlled type I diabetics (insulin dependent) as well as in type II diabetics (non–insulin dependent, usually with adult onset), excessive insulin availability results in increased muscle glucose uptake and diminished liver glucose production. This will produce a drop in blood glucose. On the other hand, the poorly controlled type I diabetic has diminished muscle glucose uptake and increased liver glucose production owing to an excessive rise in counterregulatory hormones and inadequate insulin availability.[16] This results in increased blood glucose. Therefore, it should be obvious that the exercising diabetic must follow several precautions to avoid untoward reactions during exercise. These precautions include ingestion of carbohydrate before exercise, avoidance of exercise at the time of peak insulin action, and avoidance of injecting insulin into large muscle groups that will be exercised most actively.

The athlete should always exercise with a companion who is aware of the potential problems of this disorder and who knows what to do in an emergency. The athlete who is hypoglycemic (excessive insulin present) will usually experience the sudden onset of weakness, lethargy, and headache, possibly accompanied by pale, moist skin and drooling. These individuals will quickly respond to the administration of concentrated carbohydrate, which they should always have readily available for use under these circumstances. On the other hand, the athlete who is hyperglycemic (insufficient insulin present) usually develops symptoms of irritability and abdominal pain associated with exaggerated breathing, a fruity odor on the breath, low blood pressure, and a rapid, weak pulse over the course of days. These athletes should be immediately transported to an emergency facility for definitive care.

Regularity of exercise is extremely important to minimize glucose instability.[17] This provides an opportunity for appropriate adjustment of insulin dosages in the type I diabetic. If hypoglycemia occurs repeatedly during regularly scheduled exercise, the appropriate insulin component should be reduced as necessary. The type I diabetic who is exercising regularly may require as much as a 10 to 20 unit reduction in daily dose. The athlete should keep a careful daily diary of insulin dosage and exercise intensity, duration, and frequency that can be monitored by both the athlete and the physician at regular intervals. Fluid replacement is essential for all athletes but is particularly important for the diabetic in order to avoid dehydration secondary to osmotic diuresis. The diabetic athlete should be encouraged to drink plenty of fluid before, during, and after exercise. Appropriate equipment is also essential, with particular attention paid to the shoes to avoid unnecessary foot problems that may occur secondary to peripheral neuropathy.

PROTEINURIA

Functional proteinuria may be seen in athletes after vigorous exercise[18] and may be detected on routine urinalysis during preparticipation examinations. Proteinuria in the athlete, which has been termed pseudonephritis,[19] usually is idiopathic and benign, but more serious causes must be excluded. The usual cause of proteinuria in young athletes, other than exercise per se, is orthostatic proteinuria. This diagnosis can be confirmed by home urine sampling methods.[20] The athlete is instructed to void completely before retiring. Upon first arising in the morning, the athlete voids into a sample container, which is appropriately labeled. At some point later in the day, the athlete collects a second sample. This is repeated on 3 separate days, and then the samples are analyzed. The absence of protein in the first voided specimens in the morning and subsequent demonstration of protein in the specimens obtained later in the day confirm the diagnosis. Orthostatic proteinuria has an excellent prognosis if the 24-hour collection yields less than 750 mg of protein, if there is no evidence of hypertension, and if the patient is able to demonstrate a consistently negative protein dipstick on recumbency.

HEMATURIA

Gross hematuria in the athlete is usually secondary to mechanical trauma in the bladder and can be confirmed by cystoscopy.[21] Cystoscopic examination will reveal contusions of the posterior wall of the bladder and the trigone. This "kissing" lesion is believed to be caused by the flaccid posterior wall of the bladder striking the base of the bladder during impact.[22]

Microscopic hematuria has also been described in athletes. Glomerular filtration and renal blood flow diminish as exercise intensity increases. This causes a subsequent increase in glomerular permeability secondary to hypoxia with excretion of erythrocytes into the urine. Microscopic hematuria has been shown to reverse within 24 hours of exercise in long-distance runners who participated in a 100 km race.[23] Hematuria, whether microscopic or macroscopic, should never be ascribed mistakenly to exercise, however, and always deserves a careful and thorough evaluation to rule out more serious causes of genitourinary bleeding.

CHRONIC FATIGUE/OVERTRAINING

Perhaps no greater diagnostic challenge exists than the evaluation of an athlete who presents with either chronic fatigue or depression. The dynamic interplay between psychologic, physiologic, and sociologic factors provides a unique set of variables that the physician must assess and evaluate. Depression and fatigue are symptoms that frequently can be used interchangeably by the athlete. In fact, it is important to differentiate between these two entities. This is perhaps most easily done by viewing fatigue as a physical phenomenon, whereas depression is more psychologic.

The highly motivated athlete, who is frequently possessed with the will to win and to perform well, will be frustrated by poor performance that may be due to unrecognized fatigue. This will lead to increased effort to improve performance, by increasing either practice time or the intensity devoted to a specific endeavor, resulting in increasing fatigue and worsening performance. This cycle results in deterioration of not only the athlete's performance but also his or her mental well-being. As the athlete becomes increasingly exhausted and frustrated with worsening performance, depression may begin to manifest itself through altered mood state, sleep disturbance, and vegetative behavior. While it is important to note that depression, either endogenous or reactive, may occur as a primary disorder in the absence of physiologic fatigue, the most common syndrome seen in the competitive athlete is the coupled chronic fatigue/depression syndrome.[24] This typically occurs as a result of overtraining.

Significant increases in training volume and intensity

can lead to a vicious circle that can manifest clinically in the form of chronic fatigue and depression. The inability of the athlete to adapt to increasing training volume or intensities has been described as a phenomenon of overtraining that can lead to the state known as staleness. Clinically, staleness can be recognized by symptoms of fatigue, irritability, and depression. This phenomenon has been studied in 12 male swimmers in whom psychologic, physiologic, and performance changes were measured following a sudden increase in training load.[25] Psychologic assessments were done before, during, and after 10 days of increased training. Daily training distance was increased from 4000 to 9000 M per day, and intensity was maintained at 94 percent of maximum oxygen consumption. There was a significant increase in the reported ratings of pressure, anger, fatigue, and mood disturbance, with a reduction in the general sense of well-being. There was also a significant increase in complaints of muscle soreness and exercise intensity, and when psychologic assessments were compared with physiologic data compiled on each swimmer, there was close agreement between the psychologic and physiologic assessments.

Muscle glycogen was an important physiologic parameter assessed in this study.[26] Muscle biopsies demonstrated clear evidence of depletion of muscle glycogen stores in those athletes with the greatest number of psychologic complaints. These athletes were not adequately replenishing the muscle glycogen stores that had been depleted by the increased intensity and quantity of training. An interesting corollary of this work was the ability to classify athletes as responders or nonresponders to increased training load based upon their psychologic and physiologic assessments. A blinded author was able to accurately predict all the responders as well as five of the six nonresponders based upon evaluation of their psychologic assessment.

These data underscore the importance of recognizing the symptoms of fatigue and depression as manifestations of overtraining. Additionally, the monitoring of psychologic parameters by the clinician may be useful in predicting those individuals at greatest risk for the development of staleness and the chronic fatigue/depression syndrome. Finally, there is a high correlation between inadequate muscle glycogen stores and the subsequent manifestations of overtraining.

Primary prevention of this syndrome is important. The diet of any athlete performing at intense levels of exercise for prolonged periods should consist of a high percentage of carbohydrate. The typical American diet of 46 percent carbohydrate does not supply sufficient carbohydrate to replenish glycogen stores. A high-performance athlete requires a diet containing 60 to 70 percent carbohydrate to optimize glycogen repletion. This is equivalent to approximately 8 g of carbohydrate per kg of body weight daily. Since only 5 percent of the muscle glycogen that is utilized during exercise is resynthesized each hour following exercise, at least 20 hours are required for complete repletion of glycogen after exhausting exercise if 8 g of carbohydrate are consumed. After intense training sessions, muscle is perhaps most receptive to glycogen replenishment, and

the athlete should attempt to consume 2 g of carbohydrate per kg within 15 to 30 minutes after finishing exercise. This is most easily accomplished by using one of the high-carbohydrate sports drinks.

Once an athlete has developed signs and symptoms of fatigue and depression associated with overtraining, the therapeutic interventions necessary to reverse them are clear. The first step is for the clinician to recommend to the coach a dramatic reduction in training volume and intensity. The duration and amount of this reduction are determined by the severity of symptoms but almost always involve several days of complete rest. Second, a high-carbohydrate diet needs to be instituted immediately. This should consist of approximately 600 g of carbohydrate daily. Additionally, the clinician needs to provide appropriate support and assurance during the recovery phase, as these athletes may experience significant mood disturbance. After resolution of symptoms, the clinician, athlete, and coach may carefully develop a graduated return to activity with careful monitoring of both mood and performance.

INFECTIOUS MONONUCLEOSIS

Infectious mononucleosis is a self-limited disease caused by the Epstein-Barr virus (EBV). Approximately 3 percent of college-aged students contract this illness annually.[27] Athletes typically present with fever, sore throat, fatigue, malaise, and enlarged lymph nodes. Physical signs typically peak at about the fourteenth day of illness and are characterized by lymphadenopathy, splenic enlargement, tonsillar hypertrophy with or without exudate, a red pinpoint enanthema of the palate, and mild periorbital swelling. Laboratory assessment, if performed, will reveal a normal to mildly elevated white count with a left shift, atypical lymphocytes on a peripheral smear, elevated liver function tests, and positive serology. Complications, which occur in less than 1 percent of patients, can include splenic rupture, encephalitis, aseptic meningitis, pneumonitis, and hemolytic anemia.

Most college athletes are not terribly incapacitated by this illness, usually suffering a loss of only 1 week of classes. The more critical issue is that of return to play. Athletes may resume athletic activity when they are afebrile, when their spleens have returned to normal size, and when laboratory tests (CBC, liver functions tests), if they were obtained, have normalized.[28] In most instances, this will require about 1 month. Premature return risks the possibility of a ruptured spleen, although this can occur while at rest and without contact.

The other potential catastrophe that can occur with premature return to play is head injury. Torg and coworkers have reported three cases of serious head injury in football players suffering from mononucleosis after relatively minor contact.[29] Potentially life-threatening intracranial injury can occur under these circumstances as a result of altered compliance of cerebral vasculature and predisposition to the second-impact phenomenon.

The treatment of infectious mononucleosis is expectant and supportive. Corticosteroids have no role in the routine management of this illness and should be reserved for those with serious complications. "Chronic" infection with EBV has been argued by some to be responsible for the chronic fatigue syndrome; however, recent work has convincingly demonstrated that this is not the case.[30]

HUMAN IMMUNODEFICIENCY VIRUS INFECTION

The human immunodeficiency virus (HIV) is a ball-shaped retrovirus that has been causally linked to the acquired immunodeficiency syndrome (AIDS). Because this virus can be transmitted from one person to another via blood, significant concern has been voiced about the potential for transmission of HIV during athletic competition. To date, not one case of HIV transmission during athletic participation has been reported that has been scientifically verified; this is remarkable, given that approximately 3 in every 1000 people are infected with HIV and that we are at least 10 years into the epidemic of HIV infection.

HIV could potentially be transmitted on the athletic field only by the exposure of one athlete to the HIV-infected blood of another. HIV transmission has not been demonstrated for saliva or tears, and HIV has never been grown or isolated from sweat. Given this, it is important to note that to date health care workers with intact skin exposed to HIV-infected blood have never become infected, and only 3 in 1000 have become infected after being stuck with a needle contaminated with HIV-infected blood.[31] Using known prevalence and exposure rates and assuming that conversion rates similar to those for health care workers, Brown and Drotman showed that the risk of being infected by HIV in the National Football League was well below 1 infection in 1,000,000 games.[32]

In view of the extremely low risk for HIV infection during athletic competition, primary concern must be focused on minimizing and preventing the spread of HIV through more common routes. Athlete education in this regard is extremely important as is the employment of universal precautions within the training room.

UPPER RESPIRATORY INFECTION

Upper respiratory infection (URI) occurs commonly in athletes, as it does in the nonathletic population, and is usually viral. Care for these athletes is supportive. More critical is the question of whether athletes who suffer from URI should be allowed to exercise, given the potential for the development of viral myocarditis. Although the potential for this is exceedingly low, experimental data exist to suggest that strenuous exercise increases the severity of viral myocarditis in laboratory mice.[33] In general, the athlete who is febrile and has systemic signs of viremia (myalgia, fatigue, and malaise) should refrain from exercising.

Are athletes more prone to URI? While moderate exercise may enhance immune function, intense, fatiguing exercise can alter T-cell number and function[34] and decrease natural killer (NK) cell function.[35] Given that NK cells are the first line of defense against certain viruses, it is not difficult to surmise that intense exercise may lead to increased risk of infection from certain viruses. In fact, runners have been shown to be at increased risk of URI after running a marathon.[36]

OTHER COMMON INFECTIONS

While acute pharyngitis is usually viral in origin and is a common complaint in URI, it can result from infection by the streptococcus. Differentiation of viral from bacterial pharyngitis is important, because appropriate treatment with antibiotics can hasten recovery and reduce the likelihood of transmission of this disease to others. A throat culture has been long recognized as the gold standard for making the correct diagnosis, although the development of rapid antigen tests has simplified the quick diagnosis of streptococcal pharyngitis in the training room setting. Although these tests lack the sensitivity and specificity of a throat culture, they are nevertheless useful when combined with other clinical information gathered in the diagnosis of streptococcal pharyngitis.

Conjunctivitis can be caused by chemical irritation (such as in swimmers), bacteria, or viruses. A careful history and clinical examination can usually quickly sort out the most likely cause, and appropriate treatment can be instituted. The use of antibiotic solutions or ointments is indicated only when bacterial infection is likely. Infection with the herpes virus can be particularly worrisome, and these patients should be referred to an ophthalmologist for definitive care. Conjunctival injection and eye pain can also present as a result of eye trauma (usually a finger in the eye) and subsequent corneal abrasion. The use of fluorescein instilled in the eye and a cobalt blue light will reveal the characteristic fluorescent stain on the cornea that confirms this diagnosis. The eye should then be patched and the athlete carefully followed by the physician until this heals (usually within 24 hours).

Otitis externa is a common infection of the external ear canal typically seen in aquatic athletes. It is a polymicrobial infection that is best treated with an otic antibiotic solution after meticulous debridement of squamous debris and cerumen from the external canal.

GASTROINTESTINAL PROBLEMS

Gastrointestinal problems in the athlete are usually a result of the effect of exercise on the motility of the gastrointestinal (GI) tract. However, functional symptoms are frequently seen in athletes prior to competition. These are usually caused by stress and anticipation, which can directly affect the sensitive gut of some athletes. Symptoms, which may be present in either the upper or the lower GI tract, can be managed in the same manner as the physiologic syndromes that are the direct result of exercise and are described below.

Heartburn, nausea, and vomiting have been reported during exercise in athletes, and it appears that the severity of symptoms is directly related to the intensity of exercise.[37] High-intensity exercise reduces gastric emptying, and therefore the athlete suffering from symptoms referable to the upper GI tract should avoid fatty, high-calorie meals, eating easily digested food prior to competing. Low osmolar, cold liquids should be consumed during exercise to facilitate rapid gastric emptying and absorption by the proximal gut. The use of H_2 blockers should be reserved for those with reflux that is not amenable to the simple measures described above.

Cramping, the urge to defecate, and diarrhea are common symptoms referable to the lower GI tract. Their severity is also directly related to the intensity of exercise.[37] When evaluating these symptoms in athletes, it is critical to rule out underlying causes that may not be attributable to exercise. Indeed, attributing GI symptoms to exercise should be done only after excluding other, potentially serious causes. When symptoms are found to be related to exercise, treatment can be directed at avoiding exacerbating food and ingesting a low-residue meal prior to activity. Caffeine should be avoided because of direct stimulatory effects on the GI tract. Since fluid status may influence the severity and frequency of symptoms,[38] hydration before and during activity is critical. Medication should be reserved for significant symptoms that are not amenable to the simple measures described above; the agent used should have no effect on the central nervous system and should not inhibit sweating. Loperamide in low doses may be an excellent choice.

Rectal bleeding can occur after strenuous exercise, and it has been shown that whether the source is in the upper or lower GI tract, it is secondary to relative ischemia.[39] Despite this fact, a full and careful evaluation of the athlete who presents with rectal bleeding after strenuous exercise is always indicated to rule out structural (e.g., hemorrhoids) or pathologic causes of bleeding. For those in whom serious disease has been excluded, a trial with an H_2 blocker may ameliorate symptoms if bleeding originates in the upper GI tract.

Acute gastroenteritis may occur in athletes. This illness is usually self-limited and resolves with supportive care. Although this illness is viral in most instances, pathologic bacteria and parasites can cause diarrhea and need to be excluded in the patient with fever, severe diarrhea, and protracted symptoms.

SUMMARY

Medical problems occurring in athletes may be directly related to the specific type of activity in which they participate. Awareness and familiarity with these exercise-related syndromes are helpful in the clinical evaluation of those who present with these problems but should never replace a careful and thoughtful search for more serious underlying conditions. Only

after excluding more serious illness can we comfortably ascribe an athlete's symptoms to exercise or activity alone.

REFERENCES

1. Hirsh FJ: The generalist as team physician. Phys Sports Med 1979;7:89–95.
2. Maron BJ, Roberts WC, McAllister HA, et al: Sudden death in young athletes. Circulation 1980;62:218–229.
3. Huston TP, Puffer JC, Rodney WM: The athletic heart syndrome. N Engl J Med 1985;313:24–32.
4. Watkins H, Rosenzweig A, Dwang DS, et al: Characteristics and prognostic implications of myosin missense mutations in familial hypertrophic cardiomyopathy. N Engl J Med 1992; 326:1108–1114.
5. Thompson DD, Funk EJ, Carleton RA, Sturner WQ: Incidence of death during jogging in Rhode Island from 1975 through 1980. JAMA 1982;247:2535–2538.
6. Messerli FH, Garavaglia GE: Cardiodynamics of hypertension: a guide to selection of therapy. J Clin Hypertens 1986;3:100S–108S.
7. Chick TW, Halperin AK, Gacek EM: The effect of antihypertensive medications on exercise performance: a review. Med Sci Sports Exerc 1988;20(5):447–454.
8. Pierson WE, Voy RO: Exercise-induced bronchospasm in the XXIII Summer Olympic Games. Acta Paediatr Jpn 1987;29:695–700.
9. Gilbert IA, McFadden ER Jr: Heat and water flux in the intrathoracic airways and exercise induced asthma. J Clin Invest 1992; 90:699–704.
10. Rupp NT, Guill MF, Bruduno S: Unrecognized exercise-induced bronchospasm in adolescent athletes. Am J Dis Child 1992;146: 941–944.
11. Woolley M, Anderson SO, Quigley BM: Duration of protective effect of terbutaline sulfate and cromolyn sodium alone and in combination on exercise-induced asthma. Chest 1990;97:39–45.
12. Dressendorfer RH, Wade CE, Amsterdam EA: Development of pseudo-anemia in marathon runners during a 20-day road race. JAMA 1981;246:1215–1218.
13. Clements TB, Asmundson RC: Nutritional intake and hematological parameters in endurance runners. Phys Sports Med 1982;10(3):37–43.
14. Celsing F, Blomstrand E, Werner B, et al: Effects of iron deficiency on endurance on muscle enzyme activity in man. Med Sci Sports Exerc 1986;18:156–161.
15. Murphy JR: Sickle cell hemoglobin (Hb AS) in black football players. JAMA 1973;225:981–982.
16. Jensen MD, Miles JM: The roles of diet and exercise in the management of patients with insulin dependent diabetes mellitus. Mayo Clin Proc 1986;61:813–819.
17. Landry GL, Allen DB: Diabetes mellitus and exercise. Clin Sports Med 1992; 11(2):403–418.
18. Poortmans JR: Postexercise proteinuria in humans—facts and mechanisms. JAMA 1985;253:236–240.
19. Gardner KD: Athletic pseudonephritis: alteration of urine sediment by athletic competition. JAMA 1956;151:1613–1617.
20. Stewart DW, Gordon JA, Schoolwarth AC: Evaluation of proteinuria. Am Fam Physician 1985;29(4):218–225.
21. Blacklock NG: Bladder trauma in the long distance runner: ten thousand meters hematuria. Br J Urol 1979;49:129.
22. Abaranel J, Benet A, Lash D, et al: Sports hematuria. J Urol 1990; 143:887–890.
23. Alvarez C, Mir J, Obaya S, Fragoso M: Hematuria and microalbuminuria after a 100 kilometer race. Am J Sports Med 1987;15(6): 609–611.
24. Puffer JC, McShane JM: Depression and chronic fatigue in athletes. Clin Sports Med 1992;11(2):327–338.
25. Morgan WP, Costill DL, Flynn MG, et al: Mood disturbance following increased training in swimmers. Med Sci Sports Exerc 1988;20:408–414.
26. Costill DL, Flynn MG, Kirwang P, et al: Effects of repeated days of intensified training on muscle glycogen and swimming performance. Med Sci Sports Exerc 1988;20:249–254.
27. Ryan AJ, Evans AS, Hoogland RJ, Seifert M: Infectious mononucleosis in athletes. Phys Sports Med 1978;6:41–56.

28. deShazo WF: Returning athletic activity after infectious mononucleosis. Phys Sports Med 1980;8:71–72.
29. Torg JS, Beer C, Bruno LA, Vegso J: Head trauma in football players with infectious mononucleosis. Phys Sports Med 1980;8:107–110.
30. Gold D, Bowden R, Sixbey J, et al: Chronic fatigue: a prospective clinical and virologic study. JAMA 1990; 264:48–53.
31. Henderson DK, Fahey B, Wily M, et al: Risk for occupational transmission of human immunodeficiency virus type I (HIV-I) associated with clinical exposures. Ann Intern Med 1990;113:740–746.
32. Brown LS, Drotman P: What is the risk of HIV infection in athletic competition? 9th International Conference on AIDS. Berlin, June 1993.
33. Ilback NG, Fohlman J, Friman G: Excercise in coxsackie B3 myocarditis: effects on heart lymphocyte subpopulations and the inflammatory reaction. Am Heart J 1989;117(6):1298–1302.
34. Deuster PA: Excercise-induced changes in populations of peripheral blood mononuclear cells. Med Sci Sports Exerc 1988;20:276.
35. Mackinnon LT: Excercise and natural killer cells. What is the relationship? Sports Med 1993; 7:141.
36. Nieman DC, Johanssen LM, Lee JW, et al: Infectious episodes in runners before and after the Los Angeles Marathon. J Sports Med Phys Fit 1990; 30:316–328.
37. Riddoch C, Trinick T: Gastrointestinal disturbances in marathon runners. J Sports Med 1988; 22:71–74.
38. Rehrer NJ, Janssen ME, et al: Fluid intake and gastrointestinal problems in runners competing in a 25 km race marathon. Int J Sports Med 1989; 19(Suppl.):22–25.
39. Schwartz AE, Vanagunas A, Kamel PL: Endoscopy to evaluate gastrointestinal bleeding in marathon runners. Ann Intern Med 1990;113:632–634.

Special Topic Areas

CHAPTER 37

The Female Athlete

A U R E L I A N A T T I V *MD*
E L I Z A B E T H A. A R E N D T *MD*
R I C H R I E H L *ATC*

Through the centuries there has been a dramatic change in attitudes toward women's participation in sports and athletic competition. In ancient Greece, women were not allowed to participate in or even observe the sacred Olympic events. In fact, the punishment for a woman observing the events was to be hurled off a cliff! Even in the modern Olympic games, founded by Pierre de Coubertin in 1902, women were excluded from participation because women's sports were thought to be "against the laws of nature."

Despite the exclusion of females from organized activities in many sports, females partook in individual and community-based activities in great numbers, proving the critics wrong with many of these ill-founded fears. This was particularly true with endurance running, with the thrust of early activity occurring outside of organized, higher level competition. It was not until the 1984 Summer Olympic Games that the International Olympic Committee allowed women to participate in the marathon run, an event previously believed to be too stressful for women.[1]

In the United States, the adoption of Title IX to the Education Amendments Act in 1972 was a pivotal point in the history of girl's and women's participation in sports and exercise.[1,2] The Title IX rule stated that, "No person in the United States shall, on the basis of sex, be excluded from participation in, be denied the benefits of, or be subject to discrimination under any educational program of action receiving federal financial assistance."[1] This ruling resulted in a dramatic increase in female sports participation, with a 600 percent increase in girls' participation in high school sports witnessed shortly thereafter, compared to only a 20 percent increase in boys' sports participation during this same time period.[1]

Thus, since the 1970s there has been much more acceptance of and appreciation for women's roles in sports and athletics. Despite these positive steps toward increasing participation in sports for girls and women, societal and cultural factors still exist that disproportionally affect the opportunities to participate in sports, especially for young girls.[2] Health professionals and educators must increase their awareness of the benefits of sports and exercise for women, as well as the potential risks, so that widespread involvement in sports and exercise will continue to be encouraged in the safest possible way.

EXERCISE TRAINING AND PHYSIOLOGY: GENDER DIFFERENCES

PRE- AND POSTPUBERTAL DIFFERENCES

Gender differences in strength, aerobic capacity (Vo2max), and endurance performance are much more subtle before puberty.[3–5] Prepubertal boys and girls have similar strength. Boys have somewhat higher Vo2max throughout childhood, but when corrected for lean body mass, this difference disappears. Similarly, endurance performance is slightly better in boys before puberty. Gender differences in performance may be due to social rather than biologic constraints,[3] including psychologic barriers, lack of appropriate role models for girls, and fewer opportunities, among other reasons.

At puberty these gender-related performance discrepancies become exaggerated, primarily as a result of hormonal changes (i.e., increased estrogen in girls and increased testosterone in boys). At puberty, girls show a relative increase in body fat and boys, a relative increase in muscle mass. This inequality of muscle mass after puberty is reflected in decreased muscle strength, power, and speed in women compared with men.[3–5]

MUSCLE STRENGTH

Absolute upper extremity muscle strength in women averages 40 to 75 percent that of men, whereas absolute lower extremity strength averages 60 to 80 percent that of men. These differences are primarily due to muscle mass size differences between men and women.[6] Women, however, have the same capacity for strength gains as men (controlling for body composition and size). Strength gains are the result of both muscle hypertrophy and neuromuscular recruitment. Women do not experience the same degree of increased muscle hypertrophy as men, mostly because of lower levels of testosterone.[6]

AEROBIC CAPACITY (Vo2max)

Women have a lower maximal level of aerobic capacity (Vo2max) by about 10 to 30 percent (relative to body weight) compared with men. The physiologic reasons for this difference include a lower oxygen carrying capacity in women, as well as lower blood volume, fewer red blood cells, lower hemoglobin content, smaller hearts, lower stroke volume, higher percentage of body fat, and smaller muscle fiber area.[4–6] There is a strong genetic component to the Vo2max differences. Training programs (interval and continu-

ous) produce similar increases in aerobic capacity in women and men.

ENDURANCE PERFORMANCE

Women trail men by about 6 to 15 percent in most endurance events. Differences in body size and body composition most likely explain these sex differences in endurance performance. Although muscle fiber composition is similar in men and women, both fast- and slow-twitch muscle fibers tend to be larger in men. Training programs, both interval and continuous, produce similar improvements in endurance performance in men and women.[5]

MENSTRUAL CYCLE AND ORAL CONTRACEPTIVES: EFFECT ON PERFORMANCE

Although studies are limited, it appears as though there is no significant difference in athletic performance during menstruation compared with other phases of the menstrual cycle. With regard to oral contraceptives, a few studies suggest a small decrease in Vo2max, as well as a decrease in strength, on low-dose oral contraceptives, but other studies contradict these conclusions. Unfortunately, the studies to date are limited and complicated by the variety of preparations on the market. More research will have to be performed before conclusions are made regarding effects of oral contraceptives on athletic performance.[5,7]

MUSCULOSKELETAL CONSIDERATIONS IN THE FEMALE ATHLETE

Much has been written concerning the anatomic differences between the sexes that may form the basis for differences in athletic performance, athletic potential, and musculoskeletal injuries. It is important to establish that there are significant variations in characteristics between the sexes. With the exception of injuries that involve female or male sexual organs and/or hormonal makeup, the injuries sustained by men and women are similar.

INJURY RATES

There are few data to support the notion that women and girls are injured more frequently than men and boys.[8] Early studies of the first female cadets in military institutions concluded that significant differences in performance variables and injury rates were heavily influenced by traditional sex bias. Young women were not conditioned to specific skill preparation for a given activity, which resulted in more injuries in the female athletes. Equipment differences, specifically footwear, were also a very large contributory factor. When the footwear was corrected and the female cadets were given a proper conditioning program, the injury rates were reduced.

Much of the current literature supports the fact that injury patterns are more sport-specific than sex-specific or gender based. Sprains and strains are the most common type of injury, with contact sports displaying more injury patterns than noncontact sports.[8] However, there are several types of injuries that seem to be more prevalent among female athletes than male athletes. There is increasing concern that women have a greater risk of anterior cruciate ligament (ACL) injury, particularly in sports that involve jumping and pivoting, such as basketball and soccer.[8–11] This concern is supported by an increasing body of epidemiologic data that points to a greater incidence of severe knee injuries, specifically injury to the ACL, in women than men.[8–11]

Other injuries that are prevalent among female athletes include patellofemoral pain syndrome (PFPS),[5,8] patellar subluxations/dislocations,[5,8] low back problems (spondylolysis and spondylolisthesis),[5,8,12,13] bunions, and stress fractures.[5,8]

Injuries, regardless of the athlete's gender, occur for many reasons. Both intrinsic and extrinsic factors may contribute to an injury. Intrinsic factors are those that come from within the person, such as strength, flexibility, biomechanical malalignment, and psychologic stamina. Extrinsic factors are those that are related to an outside force being applied to the person. These include the playing surface, equipment, environmental conditions, training errors, and coaching errors. How these various contributory factors may relate to the specific injury patterns among female athletes will be discussed.

ANTERIOR CRUCIATE LIGAMENT INJURIES

Much has been theorized concerning the increased rate of ACL injuries in the female athlete, with no conclusive evidence to date. Research studies have identified specific sports that are considered to carry a higher risk of ACL injuries. When both sexes are considered, gymnastics, soccer, basketball, football, and lacrosse, respectively, are the sports with the highest ACL injury rates, according to the 1991–1992 NCAA Injury Surveillance Survey. When comparing gender-related injury patterns, the rate of ACL injury is greater in female athletes in gymnastics, soccer, and basketball (Fig. 37–1).[8–11]

What are the factors, both intrinsic and extrinsic, that are responsible for this difference in ACL injury rates? Intrinsic factors may include ligament size, inherent ligament laxity, intracondylar notch width, muscular weakness, and biomechanical alignment. Extrinsic factors may include level of skill, level of playing experience, shoe-surface friction interface, type of activity, and gender-specific avoidance patterns.[8–11] The etiologies for an increase in ACL injury patterns are most likely multifactorial. Further research is required before one can be conclusive regarding this gender-specific injury pattern and its etiology.

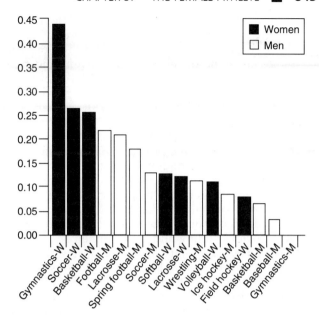

All data are shown per 1000 athletic exposures

FIGURE 37–1. ACL injury rate by sport. All data are shown per 1000 athletic exposures. M, Men; W, women. (From NCAA Injury Surveillance System, NCAA, Overland Park, KS.)

PATELLOFEMORAL PAIN SYNDROME

PFPS is more common in female than male athletes. It typically affects young women from adolescents through 30 years of age and is manifested most commonly as anterior knee pain exacerbated by prolonged knee flexion ("theater sign") and stair climbing (especially going down the stairs). A number of biomechanical factors have been proffered to explain the etiology of PFPS; it is believed that these biomechanical factors add to increased stress on the soft tissues around the patellofemoral joint and/or a subtle malalignment of the patella as it tracks in the trochlear groove. These include an increased Q angle, excessive pronation of the foot, internal rotation of the tibia, increased femoral anteversion, and genu valgum at the knee. These biomechanical features, alone or in combination, have been referred to as the *miserable malalignment syndrome.* Women are reported to have miserable malalignment syndrome with greater frequency than men, although few population studies have analyzed this critically. Other intrinsic factors may include muscular imbalances, specifically weakness of the vastus medialis with overpowering of the laterally directed muscles, patella alta, and limb length discrepancies.[8]

Extrinsic factors can also contribute to PFPS. Poor training techniques, hill running, improper seat height while cycling (exaggerating knee flexion), and improper footwear are some of the extrinsic factors leading to abnormal patellar mechanics.

In the treatment of PFPS, it is imperative that the underlying factors be identified, whether they be intrinsic, extrinsic, or a combination of the two. Education with regard to proper training techniques, running on nonrigid surfaces, cross-training, selecting proper footwear, correcting biomechanical malalignments, avoiding excessive camber in the road, and avoiding excessive incline or decline running (hill or stair running), are some of the ways to prevent and treat PFPS.[8] The majority of patients with PFPS, if properly evaluated and treated, are able to improve their function and reduce their pain with conservative treatment.

If intrinsic factors are the cause, they must be addressed to alleviate the problem. Muscular strengthening and flexibility programs are often of benefit to address muscular imbalances. Orthotic devices and proper shoe selection may help in correcting biomechanical malalignment. Patellar taping, as described by McConnell,[14] has shown to be of assistance in relieving excessive patellar tilting and malalignment.

PFPS is an overuse injury, and there are few satisfying surgical solutions. Current surgical solutions are directed at attempts to better align the patella, based on the theory that the pain is secondary to subtle malalignment. Arthroscopic debridement is frequently used as a surgical solution, with generalized debridement of the underneath surface of the patella. Although subjectively patients frequently report improvement, there are few studies that examine the efficacy of arthroscopic debridement of the patella for pain reduction or functional improvement.[8]

PATELLAR DISLOCATIONS AND SUBLUXATIONS

Patellar dislocation and subluxation are also fairly common in the female athlete.[8] Many of the predisposing factors for patellar dislocations also contribute to PFPS. In fact, these disorders are thought to lie on a continuum. An important distinction is that patellar dislocations are acute injuries, whereas PFPS is an overuse injury.

Treatment for an acute dislocation of the patella can follow a conservative or aggressive course. Most patellar dislocations and subluxations are treated conservatively with stabilization of the patella (in a knee sleeve or immobilizer), combined with an extensive rehabilitation program emphasizing the medial dynamic stabilizers. Although conservative treatment is the preferred treatment choice for first-time dislocations, surgery is indicated in the acute phase if loose body formation is noted on radiographs. If conservative treatment fails, surgery may be indicated to help stabilize the patella in those athletes experiencing chronic dislocations.

LOW BACK INJURIES

Certain types of low back injuries have been found to be more common in the female athlete, especially in the female gymnast.[8,12,13] These injuries include spondylolysis or fracture of the pars interarticularis, as well as spondylolisthesis, in which forward slippage of one vertebra on an adjacent vertebra occurs. The etiology of spondylolysis and spondylolisthesis is multifactorial,

and whether the injury is acute or chronic may have important implications in treatment.

Spondylolisthesis is most common in female athletes 9 to 13 years old. Because this is a time of rapid growth and development, the slippage may increase in severity, and significant disability can arise if the condition is not prevented and treated early on.[8,12,13] Any young female athlete with persistent low back pain should be evaluated carefully to assess the specific cause of her pain. Radiographs of the lumbosacral spine should include oblique views to look for the pars interarticularis defect. If the radiograph is normal but clinical findings suggest a pars defect, a bone scan is indicated.

Treatment of an athlete with a pars interarticularis defect is controversial.[8,12,13] A positive bone scan indicates recent trauma to that area. Although treatment remains controversial, most physicians favor immobilization in a brace for a minimum of 3 months in an attempt to heal the affected area. Whether the defect heals with bony or fibrous union is debatable; however, there is convincing evidence that brace treatment is helpful in those with a positive bone scan.

If the patient has positive radiographic signs and a negative bone scan, conservative treatment is the method of choice. This consists of a rehabilitation program emphasizing stretching of the lumbodorsal fascia and hamstrings, as well as abdominal strengthening. Brace treatment can be tried as an adjunctive measure if muscle strengthening and a period of rest are unsuccessful in relieving pain. However, brace treatment in this regard is meant to reduce the tension and inflammation in the surrounding tissue. It is not used to imply that there can be any bony healing with this method of treatment. Surgery, including fusion, is occasionally performed in some cases of spondylolisthesis that are recalcitrant to conservative treatment.

BUNIONS

Bunions are more common in women than in men and may be due to genetic factors, to athletic shoes that are inappropriately fit, or to frequent use of high-heeled shoes, as well as other factors. Bunions can be seen in women participating in all sports and can be a significant deterrent to exercise. Stress placed on the feet and toes is often accentuated by the type of footwear worn by female athletes, not only during sports activity, but also in activities of daily living. Shoes with narrow toe boxes can be causative factors, especially when accompanied by high heels. Treatment and prevention involve footwear that is properly fitted, usually shoes with a wide forefoot and narrow enough heel to prevent the foot from sliding forward in the shoe.[8]

In addition to appropriate footwear, conservative treatment includes the use of protective pads to reduce pressure on the metatarsal head. In a pronated foot with a bunion deformity, treatment with a medial arch support may help to reduce some medial-side bunion discomfort. Anti-inflammatory agents are also of benefit. Surgery may be indicated in cases that are refractory to conservative treatment.

STRESS FRACTURES

Special considerations must be given to the developing and maturing woman when considering stress fractures and stress reactions of bone. Menstrual irregularities have been associated with an increased incidence of stress fractures.[15–17] Such fractures are largely seen in long bones, even though few studies have shown a decrease in bone mineral density in the long bones of amenorrheic women. However, this is due in part to limitations in the techniques available to measure bone density in earlier studies.

Menstrual dysfunction in athletes may lead to premature bone loss.[18–21] It is the hypoestrogenic state that is thought to lead to loss of bone mineral density, whether it be in the postmenopausal woman who is not on estrogen replacement or in the premenopausal athlete with amenorrhea or oligomenorrhea.[18–21] Low progesterone has been proposed as an underlying factor that may lead to osteoporosis, although studies are limited.[22] Thus, the exact relationship among menstrual dysfunction, low bone mineral density, and stress fractures is not clearly defined. Normal menstrual function does not preclude the development of a stress fracture. Confounding variables, including diet, body composition, training errors, and biomechanical limb considerations, play a role in the increased development of stress fractures in female athletes.

A complete menstrual history is essential for the complete evaluation of any stress fracture in a woman. A decrease in the frequency of the menstrual cycle associated with increased training should be a cause for concern. A nutritional history should be obtained and the possibility of disordered eating patterns evaluated. If a problem is identified, the woman should be directed to a physician adept in the evaluation and treatment of these problems as quickly as possible.

MENSTRUAL DYSFUNCTION AND BONE CONCERNS

DEFINITION OF TERMS

A variety of menstrual irregularities may occur in the woman involved in sports and exercise. These menstrual irregularities may have significant health consequences for women, including an impact on bone health.[15–24] Common terms used in describing menstrual dysfunction include *eumenorrhea, oligomenorrhea,* and *amenorrhea*. These terms reflect normal menstrual cycles (eumenorrhea), irregular menstrual cycle length of 35 to 90 days (oligomenorrhea), and the absence of menstrual bleeding (amenorrhea). Amenorrhea is further classified into *primary amenorrhea,* referring to a woman who has never had a menstrual period (menarche > 16 years of age), and *secondary amenorrhea,* the absence of menstrual periods in a woman who has had established menstrual cycles. There is no consensus on a standard definition for secondary amenorrhea, but absence of menstrual periods for 3 to 6 consecutive months or more is commonly used.

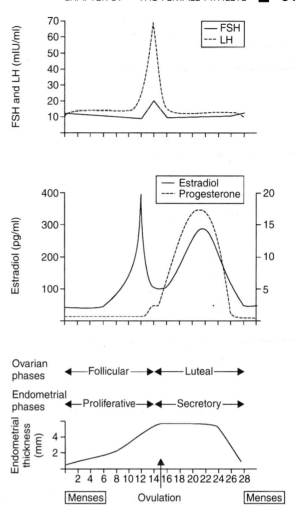

FIGURE 37–2. Hormonal events during the menstrual cycle, phases of the ovarian and endometrial cycles, and endometrial height throughout the menstrual cycle (From Shangold M, Mirkin G: Women and Exercise: Physiology and Sports Medicine, 2nd ed. Philadelphia, FA Davis, 1994.)

The above definitions describe menstrual dysfunction by the presence or absence of menstrual bleeding. There is also a spectrum of menstrual dysfunction defined by hormonal levels that change according to follicular and luteal development. The normal menstrual cycle encompasses two phases: the follicular phase and the luteal phase (Fig. 37–2). In luteal phase dysfunction, there is a shortened luteal phase and insufficient progesterone production. The athlete may or may not present with irregular menses. Research shows that this type of menstrual dysfunction may be very prevalent in the female athlete.[5,23,24] Another type of dysfunction is that of chronic anovulation and unopposed estrogen. Estrogen is produced, but there is no basal body rise, and progesterone levels are lower. The athlete may present with short or long cycles (oligomenorrhea). The most widely studied and frequently observed type of menstrual dysfunction in athletes is hypoestrogenic amenorrhea. It is this type of amenorrhea that is thought to have the most detrimental effects on bone health, as well as other potential complications.[18–21,23,24]

PREVALENCE OF MENSTRUAL DYSFUNCTION IN THE FEMALE ATHLETE

There is an increased prevalence of oligomenorrhea and amenorrhea among athletes. Reported prevalence in the female athlete varies from 3.4 to 66 percent, compared with 2 to 5 percent in the general population.[5,23,24] Athletes competing in performance sports (such as gymnastics, figure skating, dance) or endurance sports (such as distance running), appear to be at an increased risk for menstrual dysfunction. The reasons for this are multifactorial, but most likely revolve around inadequate nutrition and caloric intake to meet energy demands, as well as the training intensity of the exercise, stress, and changes in body composition, along with other factors.[23,24]

The actual prevalence of luteal phase dysfunction, chronic anovulation, and hypoestrogenic amenorrhea in female athletes is not known. Menstrual dysfunction in this group may represent spectrum of menstrual disease, with hypoestrogenic amenorrhea at the extreme. Athletes may present with different hormonal patterns in a given period of time, depending on environmental and other factors.

POTENTIAL COMPLICATIONS OF MENSTRUAL DYSFUNCTION IN ATHLETES

A most disconcerting potential complication in the female athlete with menstrual dysfunction is skeletal demineralization (premature osteoporosis). The prevalence of premature osteoporosis among female athletes is not entirely certain. What is certain, however, is that bone loss in an amenorrheic athlete is rapid and may not be entirely reversible.[18-21]

Another potential complication of menstrual dysfunction in athletes includes infertility. Infertility, however, is thought to be reversible if exercise related. There is no evidence to date that future fertility is altered in those women with a history of exercise-associated menstrual dysfunction.

Theoretical complications of hypoestrogenic amenorrhea in the female athlete not on hormone replacement therapy include an increase in cardiovascular disease, as seen in the postmenopausal woman not on estrogen replacement. Another potential theoretic complication includes endometrial hyperplasia and an increased risk of adenocarcinoma of the uterus in the female athlete with unopposed estrogen, such as seen in women with chronic anovulation.[5,23,24] Much more research will have to be done to see if these potential complications exist in the female athlete.

CONTRIBUTORY VARIABLES ASSOCIATED WITH MENSTRUAL DYSFUNCTION IN ATHLETES

The etiology and pathophysiology of menstrual dysfunction in athletes is not entirely certain and is probably multifactorial.[23,24] Certain contributory vari-

ables, however, have been associated with menstrual dysfunction. These variables include a history of delayed menarche, as well as nulliparity, increased exercise intensity, poor nutritional habits and low caloric intake, disordered eating patterns, low body fat and/or weight loss, stress, and certain "high-risk" sports, as mentioned previously. In many female athletes, one or more of these variables may coexist.

PROPOSED MECHANISMS OF MENSTRUAL DYSFUNCTION IN ATHLETES

Two popular theories exist regarding the specific mechanisms leading to exercise-associated menstrual dysfunction.[25] One is that of inhibition of the hypothalamic gonadotropin-releasing hormone (GnRH) pulsatile secretion, which decreases luteinizing hormone (LH) and follicular stimulating hormone (FSH) by activation of the adrenal axis in strenuous and endurance exercise. The other is that of an "energy drain." This energy drain is the result of insufficient caloric intake to meet the demands of energy expenditure during exercise. The body responds with a decrease in basal metabolic rate at the expense of follicular development.

CLINICAL EVALUATION OF MENSTRUAL DYSFUNCTION IN ATHLETES

Evaluation of menstrual dysfunction is recommended if there is an absence of menstrual cycles for 3 months or more or a recurrent pattern of irregular menstrual periods and oligomenorrhea. In the young woman with delayed menarche, an evaluation is recommended if there is no menstrual period by age 16.[24]

Exercise-associated amenorrhea is a diagnosis of exclusion. Thorough workup is indicated to rule out other potential causes of menstrual dysfunction in the active and athletic woman.

When taking the history, the current and past menstrual patterns should be assessed, including the age at menarche.[24,26] A sexual history, pregnancy history, and history of oral contraceptive use should be obtained. A physical activity level, nutritional history, and history of weight fluctuations and disordered eating should also be obtained.

Stressors, medications, associated symptoms (such as hirsutism, acne, galactorrhea), and family history (such as thyroid disease, menstrual irregularity, osteoporosis) should be discussed. A complete physical and pelvic examination is important to rule out other types of menstrual dysfunction.[5,24] Recommended laboratory tests include a urine pregnancy test to rule out pregnancy (the most common reason of amenorrhea in a young woman), a highly sensitive thyroid stimulating hormone (TSH) test to look for underlying thyroid disease, an FSH test to assess hormonal status, and a prolactin test to look for a pituitary adenoma. A progesterone challenge test can be used in the amenorrheic woman to assess the estrogen state. No vaginal bleeding following a 7 to 10-day trial of oral medroxy-progesterone suggests a hypoestrogenic state.

TREATMENT AND PREVENTION OF MENSTRUAL DYSFUNCTION IN ATHLETES

The treatment of menstrual dysfunction is important to avoid the potential complications discussed earlier.[5,24] Treatment varies depending on the type of menstrual dysfunction. Luteal phase dysfunction requires no specific treatment in the female athlete unless pregnancy is desired. Optimal nutrition, however, and appropriate calcium intake are important to maximize bone health.

Women with chronic anovulation and a normal estrogen state may be treated with monthly progestin to protect the endometrium or with oral contraceptives if sexually active. Calcium intake of 1200 mg/day is recommended, ideally through diet. However, calcium supplementation is recommended if dietary intake is insufficient.

The hypoestrogenic amenorrheic woman causes the most concern and presents the greatest challenge. Treatment is recommended as soon as possible, as bone loss is rapid and may not be reversible.

Oral contraceptive pills or cyclic estrogen/progestin is indicated after other causes of amenorrhea have been ruled out.[5,24] Other variables, however, must be looked at in the prevention of this abnormal endocrine state. The athlete should be encouraged to consider decreasing exercise intensity, if excessive. Nutrition and caloric intake should be optimized, with a calcium intake of 1500 mg/day recommended. Disordered eating patterns, if present, should be treated utilizing psychological and nutritional counseling, and stress reduction techniques should be used if indicated. Bone density testing may be beneficial, especially in an athlete with 6 or more months of amenorrhea. The importance of education, counseling, and the multidisciplinary team approach cannot be overemphasized in these women.

DISORDERED EATING

MAGNITUDE OF THE PROBLEM

The term *disordered eating* is preferred to the term *eating disorder* because of its emphasis on the spectrum of pathologic patterns of eating. At the extremes, this term refers to frank eating disorders as defined by the strict *Diagnostic and Statistical Manual (DSM-IV)* criteria of anorexia nervosa (Table 37–1) and bulimia nervosa (Table 37–2),[27] with poor nutritional habits at the other end of the spectrum. Although many athletes may not fit the *DSM-IV* criteria, they are still at risk for developing serious endocrine, skeletal, and psychiatric disorders.[28–33] The mortality rate from anorexia nervosa (treated anorectic patients) ranges from 10 to 18 percent.[34] In addition to the serious psychiatric consequences and high rate of suicide, multiorgan problems, including serious cardiac arrythmias and gastrointesti-

nal problems, as well as effects on growth and development, can occur.

Disordered eating patterns often develop in the young female athlete driven to excel in her sport.[28–30,32,33] The focus on achieving or maintaining an "ideal" weight or body image or percentage of body fat may put the athlete at risk for the development of disordered patterns of eating. This in turn may lead to menstrual dysfunction and subsequent premature osteoporosis. Because this triad of disorders is often seen together, especially in the young female athlete, it has been referred to as the *female athlete triad* (Fig. 37–3).[29,30]

PREVALENCE OF DISORDERED EATING IN FEMALE ATHLETES

The prevalence of disordered eating in female athletes, based on a series of small studies, ranges from 15 to 62 percent.[33,35–38] A higher prevalence is seen in certain sports in which subjective judging and aesthetics are important (gymnastics, dance, figure skating, diving, synchronized swimming), as well as in sports in which peak performance is associated with low body fat (distance running).

The prevalence of anorexia and bulimia in the general female population is estimated at 3 to 5 percent for bulimia and 1 to 3 percent for anorexia.[27,28] Disordered eating is much more prevalent in women than men (9:1

TABLE 37–1
Diagnostic Criteria for Anorexia Nervosa

1. Refusal to maintain body weight at or above a minimally normal weight for age and height (e.g., weight loss leading to maintenance of body weight less than 85% of that expected; or failure to make expected weight gain during period of growth, leading to body weight less than 85% of that expected).
2. Intense fear of gaining weight or becoming fat, even when underweight.
3. Disturbance in the way one's body weight or shape is perceived; undue influence of body weight or shape on self-evaluation, or denial of the seriousness of the current low body weight.
4. In postmenarchal females, amenorrhea (that is, the absence of at least three consecutive menstrual cycles). (A woman is considered to have amenorrhea if her periods occur only following hormone, e.g., estrogen, administration.)

Specify type:
Restricting types of anorexics do not regularly engage in binge eating or purging behavior (self-induced vomiting or the misuse of laxatives or diuretics) during episodes of anorexia nervosa.

Binge eating and purging types regularly engage in binge eating or purging behavior (self-induced vomiting or the misuse of laxatives or diuretics) during episodes of anorexia nervosa.

Data from American Psychiatric Association, Task Force on DSM-IV: DSM-IV Draft Criteria. Washington, DC, APA, 1993, pp 1–2.

TABLE 37–2
Diagnostic Criteria for Bulimia Nervosa

1. Recurrent episodes of binge eating. An episode of binge eating is characterized by both of the following:
   a. Eating in a discrete period (e.g., within any 2-hour period) an amount of food that is definitely larger than most people would eat during a similar period of time and under similar circumstances, and
   b. A sense of lack of control over eating during the episode (e.g., a feeling that one cannot stop eating or control what or how much one is eating)
2. Recurrent, inappropriate compensatory behavior to prevent weight gain, such as self-induced vomiting, misuse of laxatives, diuretics, or other medications, fasting, or excessive exercise
3. The binge eating and inappropriate compensatory behaviors both occur, on average, at least twice a week for 3 months
4. Self-evaluation is unduly influenced by body shape and weight
5. The disturbance does not occur exclusively during episodes of anorexia nervosa

Specify type:
Purging type: the person regularly engages in self-induced vomiting or the misuse of laxatives or diuretics.

Nonpurging types: the person uses other inappropriate compensatory behaviors, such as fasting or excessive exercise, but does not regularly engage in self-induced vomiting or the misuse of laxatives or diuretics.

Data from American Psychiatric Association, Task Force on DSM-IV: DSM-IV Draft Criteria. Washington, DC, APA, 1993, pp 1–2.

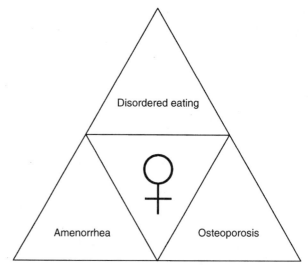

FIGURE 37–3. Picture of some young female triathletes. (Reprinted with permission of American College of Sports Medicine 1992, The Female Athlete Triad slide presentation.)

ratio), although it is often seen in certain men's sports such as wrestling.

CONTRIBUTORY FACTORS

The pressure to excel; the desire to achieve an "ideal" body weight; weight standards; unrealistic expectations; and pressure from coaches, parents, schools, organizations, society, and oneself all may contribute to the development of disordered eating.[28–30,39] Frequently, athletes' motivation for engaging in disordered eating behavior is the belief that weight loss will result in enhanced performance. A low self-esteem, poor body image, and a family history of disordered eating are often contributing factors. There is also thought to be a time-sensitive period, a "window of vulnerability," especially during adolescence and young adulthood, in which disordered eating patterns may develop.[28–30,39]

CLINICAL EVALUATION OF DISORDERED EATING IN THE FEMALE ATHLETE

The physician caring for female athletes should keep a high index of suspicion regarding the presence of disordered eating. Because of the secretive nature of disordered eating, as well as the presence of denial,

an athlete will usually not bring up the subject. The preparticipation physical examination presents an ideal opportunity to screen athletes for disordered eating.[26,29,39]

When taking a history, questions regarding abnormal menstrual function should be asked, including specific questions regarding the presence of anorexia, bulimia, specific pathogenic weight control behaviors (such as use of laxatives, diet pills, diuretics, self-induced vomiting, and overexercise), fears of becoming fat, weight fluctuations, dissatisfaction with appearance, and pressures from the coach to lose weight.[39]

The athlete with disordered eating patterns should be referred to a primary care physician familiar with treating disordered eating in athletes for a more extensive physical as well as pelvic examination, if menstrual dysfunction is present. Laboratory testing should include a complete blood cell (CBC) count, chemistry panel, electrolyte and thyroid function tests, and a urinalysis. An electrocardiogram is often indicated, depending on the severity of the disorder.[39]

TREATMENT AND PREVENTION OF DISORDERED EATING IN ATHLETES

The multidisciplinary team of primary care physician, psychologist, and nutritionist must work closely together in treating these athletes.[39] In some cases the athlete will have to be on medication (e.g., antidepressant medication), and in more serious cases hospitalization may be necessary. Removal of the at-risk athlete from competition may be indicated. Discussions regarding redefining athletic goals may also be necessary for the athlete with significant problems with disordered eating. Treatment ultimately lies in prevention of the problem and the potential health consequences that may occur.[28–30,39]

NUTRITIONAL CONCERNS IN THE FEMALE ATHLETE

NUTRIENT REQUIREMENTS

The female athlete has similar nutrient requirements as male athletes, with the exception of calcium and iron.[5,28,40]

CALCIUM

Calcium recommendations depend on the menstrual status of the female athlete. If she is amenorrheic (hypoestrogenic amenorrhea), then 1500 mg/day of calcium are recommended to maintain calcium balance. If she has normal estrogen levels and normal menstruation, 1200 mg/day of calcium are indicated. Dietary calcium is preferred to supplementation, but because many female athletes have low caloric intakes, supplementation is often indicated. If the athlete does supplement, it is best to divide the total dose of calcium supplementation to two or three doses a day to enhance absorption.

IRON

Iron deficiency is common in women (prevalence, 20 to 30 percent). Whether it is more common in female athletes than in women in general is controversial.[41,42] It is important to differentiate iron deficiency anemia from iron deficiency without anemia, as well as pseudoanemia (also called *sports anemia* or *runner's anemia*). Pseudoanemia is a dilutional anemia commonly seen in runners, especially endurance runners. It is a normal physiologic adaptation to running in which the plasma volume expands, with a resultant drop in hematocrit secondary to this increase in plasma volume.[41,42]

The most common sources of iron loss in women include menstruation and iron-poor diets. Research suggests that vegetarian athletes are at higher risk for iron deficiency owing to less bioavailability of the iron from nonmeat sources. Other sources of iron loss include gastrointestinal bleeding (seen in runners and other endurance athletes) and (less commonly) sweat, urine, or "footstrike hemolysis."[41,42]

It is probably not cost effective to screen all female athletes for iron deficiency. High-risk athletes may be screened; these include endurance athletes, those who might have disordered eating, and/or those who complain of fatigue and decreased performance. Serum ferritin is the most sensitive screening test for iron deficiency (< 12 mg/dl is diagnostic). A decreased serum iron and increased total iron binding capacity (TIBC) can also be seen with iron deficiency. A CBC count should be obtained to assess whether iron deficiency with anemia is present.

The effect of iron deficiency on athletic performance is controversial.[41,42] Most studies conclude that iron deficiency with anemia decreases performance, and low ferritin without anemia does not.[41,42] However, athletes with low ferritin alone are at higher risk for the development of iron deficiency anemia and should be followed.

Treatment of iron deficiency anemia includes iron supplementation in varying amounts depending on the severity of the anemia. Iron supplementation may be indicated for more than 6 months to replenish iron stores. Dietary counseling is important to assist in the prevention of further iron deficiency. The recommended dietary allowance (RDA) for women is at least 15 mg/day. Dietary recommendations include (1) eating more lean red meat or dark meat poultry, alone or in combination with iron-rich foods from vegetable sources (enhances absorption); (2) including vitamin C–rich foods with meals to increase iron absorption; (3) avoiding coffee or tea with meals (decreases iron absorption); and (4) cooking with cast iron skillets and pans.[5,41,42]

Those athletes with iron deficiency without anemia may or may not need iron supplements. An increase in dietary iron is helpful, as well as close follow-up for development of anemia.

Those athletes with normal iron stores do not need iron supplementation. The possibility of other mineral deficiencies may occur with iron supplementation. Prevention of iron deficiency should be discussed through dietary measures for all female athletes.

STRESS URINARY INCONTINENCE

A number of female athletes complain of stress urinary incontinence, or involuntary loss of urine, during physical exertion.[5,43,44] Physical activity involving a Valsalva maneuver increases intra-abdominal pressure, which may lead to an increase in intravesical pressure that exceeds the maximum urethral pressure, with resultant urine leakage during exercise. Female athletes in sports such as gymnastics, as well as in other sports involving running and jumping, may complain of this problem during exercise. Exercise-induced increases in intra-abdominal pressure are transient and should not produce chronic pressure alterations at rest or anatomic abnormalities.

Women who have had one or more vaginal deliveries have a higher prevalence of urinary incontinence with exercise. However, many nulliparous women may also experience stress incontinence with exercise. Women may not mention this problem because of embarrassment and may stop exercising because of frustration and inconvenience.

The sports medicine physician may recommend that the female athlete avoid excessive fluid ingestion for 2 to 3 hours prior to exercising and urinate before practice or competition. This recommendation must be tailored to the sport and weather conditions, however, to avoid dehydration, especially in a prolonged endurance event. Fluids should be encouraged after events to ensure adequate hydration. A mini-pad can be worn during exercise to minimize discomfort and embarrassment.

Kegel exercises (pelvic muscle exercises) may also be beneficial in preventing urine leakage.[5,43,44] These can be done at any time, but especially during urination to stop the urine stream. A daily or twice-daily regimen is recommended with increasing repetitions until 10 minutes' duration or fatigue. The anatomy of the pelvic and urogenital structures should be reviewed to increase the woman's awareness and assist in the success of the treatment.

The woman's menstrual status should be ascertained, as a hypoestrogenic state may contribute to problems of pelvic floor dysfunction, and benefit may be seen after hormone replacement.

Many women athletes who experience stress urinary incontinence will have normal anatomy. Some, however, may have a pre-existing anatomic defect in the posterior urethrovesical angle and may need surgical correction if the above treatments do not help. Physicians working with female athletes should be aware of problems of stress urinary incontinence and discuss appropriate management when indicated.

CONCLUSION

Despite the historical struggles, women in the 1990s are participating successfully in sports and exercise more than ever before. There are some potentially devastating medical and orthopaedic problems, however, that have serious health consequences for the female athlete. The physician providing health care to the female athlete must have a knowledge of the many special concerns that may arise during training and competition. Most of the problems discussed are preventable and can be avoided with careful screening, education, and counseling during the preparticipation examination or other encounters with the athlete. The multidisciplinary team approach to the health care of the female athlete is the most effective way of ensuring safe and healthy sports participation as well as optimal enjoyment from sports.

REFERENCES

1. Squire DL: Female athletes. Pediatr Rev 1987; 9(6):183–190.
2. Lutter JM: History of women in sports. Clin Sports Med 1994; 13(2):263–279.
3. Rowland TW: Exercise and Children's Health. Champaigne, IL, Human Kinetics Books, 1990.
4. Sanborn CF, Jankowski CM: Physiological considerations for women in sport. Clin Sports Med 1994; 13(2):263–279.
5. Shangold M, Mirkin G: Women and Exercise—Physiology and Sports Medicine, 2nd ed. Philadelphia, FA Davis, 1994.
6. Wilmore JH: Practice of Pediatrics. Philadelphia, Harper & Row, 1984.
7. Lebrun CM: The effect of the phase of the menstrual cycle and the birth control pill on athletic performance. Clin Sports Med 1994; 13(2):419–441.
8. Arendt E: Orthopedic issues for active and athletic women. Clin Sports Med 1994; 13(2):483–505.
9. Arendt E, Dick R: Gender specific knee injury pattern in basketball and soccer. Presented at the American Orthopedic Society for Sports Medicine Conference, Sun Valley, Idaho, 1993.
10. Ireland ML: Female athlete at risk: ACL injuries in females. Presented at the American Orthopedic Society for Sports Medicine Conference, Sun Valley, Idaho, 1993.
11. Ireland ML, Wall C: Epidemiology and comparison of knee injuries in elite male and female United States basketball athletes. Med Sci Sports Exer 1990; 22:14.
12. Mandelbaum BR: Gymnastics. In Reider B (ed): Sports Medicine: The School-Age Athlete. Philadelphia, WB Saunders, 1991, pp 415–428.
13. Micheli L: Back injuries in gymnastics. Clin Sports Med 1985; 4:85–95.
14. McConnell J: The management of chondromalacia patella: A long term solution. Aust J Physiother 1986; 32(4):215–223.
15. Barrow EW, Sasha S: Menstrual irregularity and stress fractures in collegiate female distance runners. Am J Sports Med 1988; 16:209–216.
16. Lloyd T, Triantafyllou SJ, Baker ER, et al: Women athletes with menstrual irregularity have increased musculoskeletal injuries. Med Sci Sports Exerc 1986; 18:374–379.
17. Myburgh KH, Hutchins J, Fataar AB, et al: Low bone density is an etiologic factor for stress fractures in athletes. Ann Intern Med 1990; 113(10):754–759.
18. Cann CE, Martin MC, Genant HK: Decreased spinal mineral content in amenorrheic women. JAMA 1984; 251:626–629.
19. Drinkwater BL, Bruemner B, Chestnut CH: Menstrual history as a determinant of current bone density in young athletes. JAMA 1990; 263(4):545–548.
20. Drinkwater BL, Nilson K, Chestnut CH, et al: Bone mineral content of amenorrheic and eumenorrheic athletes. N Engl J Med 1984; 311(5):277–281.
21. Myburgh KH, Bachrach LK, Lewis B: Bone mineral density at axial and appendicular sites in amenorrheic athletes. Med Sci Sports Exerc 1993; 25(11):1197–1202.
22. Prior JC, Vigna YM, Schechter MT, et al: Spinal bone loss and ovulatory disturbances. N Engl J Med 1990; 323(18): 1221–1227.
23. Loucks AB, Horvath SM: Athletic amenorrhea: A review. Med Sci Sports Exerc 1985; 17(1):56–72.
24. Otis CL: Exercise-associated amenorrhea. Clin Sports Med 1992; 11(2):351–362.
25. Loucks AB: Effects of exercise training on the menstrual cycle: Existence and mechanisms. Med Sci Sports Exerc 1990; 22:275.
26. Johnson MD: Tailoring the preparticipation exam to female athletes. Phys Sports Med 1992; 20(7):61–72.
27. American Psychiatric Association. Diagnostic and Statistical Manual of Mental Disorders: IV, 4th ed. Washington, DC, APA, 1994.
28. Brownell KD, Rodin J, Wilmore JH: Eating, Body Weight and Performance in Athletes: Disorders of Modern Society. Philadelphia, Lea & Febiger, 1992.
29. Nattiv A, Agostini R, Drinkwater BL, et al: The female athlete triad: The inter-relatedness of disordered eating, amenorrhea and osteoporosis. Clin Sports Med 1994; 13(2):405–418.
30. Yeager K, Agostini R, Nattiv A: The female athlete triad: Disordered eating, amenorrhea, and osteoporosis. Med Sci Sports Exerc 1993; 25(7):775–777.
31. Palla B, Litt IF: Medical complications of eating disorders in adolescents. Pediatrics 1988; 81:613.
32. Mansfield MJ, Emans SJ: Anorexia nervosa, athletics, and amenorrhea. Pediatr Clin North Am 1989; 36:533–549.
33. Rosen LW, McKeag D, Hough KO, et al: Pathogenic weight control behavior in female college athletes. Phys Sports Med 1986; 14:79–86.
34. Ratnasuriya RH, Eisler I, Szmukler GI, et al: Anorexia nervosa: Outcome and prognostic factors after 20 years. Br J Psychiatry 1991; 158:495.
35. Dummer GM, Rosen W, Heusner WW: Pathogenic weight-control behavior of young competitive swimmers. Phys Sports Med 1987; 15:75.
36. Rosen LW, Hough BJ: Pathogenic weight control behaviors of female college gymnasts. Phys Sports Med 1988; 16(9):141.
37. Sundgot-Borgen J: Prevalence of eating disorders in elite female athletes. Int J Sport Nutr 1993; 3:29.
38. Warren BJ, Stanton AL, Blessing DL: Disordered eating patterns in competitive female athletes. Int J Eat Disord 1990; 9:565.

39. Johnson MD: Disordered eating in active and athletic women. Clin Sports Med 1994; 13(2):355–369.

40. Steinbaugh N: Nutritional needs of female athletes. Clin Sports Med 1984; 3(3):649–670.

41. Eichner E: The anemias of athletes. Phys Sports Med 1986; 14(9):122–130.

42. Eichner E: Sports anemia, iron supplements, and blood doping. Med Sci Sports Exerc 1992; 24(9):S315–S318.

43. Nygaard I, Delancey JO, Arnsdorf L, et al: Exercise and incontinence. Obstet Gynecol 1990; 75:848–851.

44. Wallace K: Female pelvic floor functions, dysfunctions, and behavioral approaches to treatment. Clin Sports Med 1994; 13(2):459–481.

CHAPTER 38

Preparticipation Sports Physicals

BRIAN HALPERN *MD*
TAB BLACKBURN *MEd, PT, ATC*
BRIAN INCREMONA *MD*
STEVE WEINTRAUB *DO, BS*

The preparticipation evaluation (PPE) is frequently viewed by the athlete in a negative light. It is a common misconception that the process is designed solely to seek out abnormalities that will disqualify the individual from participation. This is inaccurate and does not reflect the spirit with which the PPE is designed or performed. In addition to obtaining "negative information," which would prohibit participation, the PPE should uncover "positive information," which, when addressed appropriately, may enhance performance and prevent injury. While negative information may be obtained from 1 to 5 percent of the time, the likelihood of obtaining positive information has been reported to be as high as 86 percent.[1] The primary purpose of the PPE is to ensure the safety and maintain the health of the athlete.[2] Both are accomplished by seeking negative and positive information relative to athletic participation, providing an avenue for access to counseling and otherwise neglected health care issues, assessing adequate physical development in the adolescent, and assuring that legal and insurance requirements designed to protect the athlete are adequately fulfilled (Table 38–1).[3]

Information obtained during the history or physical examination may prompt a diagnostic workup for an underlying condition that is potentially injurious or life-threatening. Although this negative information may prohibit or limit the athlete's participation in certain activities, the benefits cannot be ignored. In addition, after appropriate evaluation, the athlete may either return to the sport or be encouraged to partici-

pate in alternative and more acceptable activities. For example, an athlete with a history of exercise-induced syncope or a heart murmur consistent with hypertrophic cardiomyopathy requires a thorough cardiac evaluation. Although the presence of such a disorder would prohibit participation in sports such as basketball or wrestling, the athlete could be directed toward a less vigorous activity such as golf or bowling, depending upon the recommendations of the cardiologist. An epileptic who is poorly controlled despite optimal medical therapy is best directed away from swimming but may be well suited for tennis.[2,3]

Positive information, such as untreated previous injury or inadequate muscular strengthening and flexibility, indicates the need for evaluation, proper treatment, or appropriate rehabilitation to reduce the risk of injury, thus bringing the athlete to the optimal level of performance prior to the season onset.[1–3] The PPE is not intended to replace the annual physical examination but is meant as a screening process to detect conditions requiring further evaluation or referral before sporting activities are allowed.[1–3] At times, however, this examination represents the only opportunity to identify issues relevant to the athlete's general health. For example, detection of a testicular mass enables early treatment and cure of a potential malignancy that might have gone unnoticed until advanced and incurable.

Time permitting, and particularly if performed one to one, the PPE provides an excellent opportunity to establish a database, discuss health-related issues such

TABLE 38–1
Objectives of the PPE

Primary Objectives	Secondary Objectives
Detect conditions that may limit participation	Determine general health
	Counsel on health-related issues
Detect conditions that may predispose to injury	Assess maturity
	Assess fitness level and performance
Meet legal and insurance requirements	

From Bergfeld J, Lombardo J, Nelson M: Pre-Participation Physical Examination. A joint publication by the American Academy of Family Physicians, the American Academy of Pediatrics, the American Medical Society for Sports Medicine, the American Orthopaedic Society for Sports Medicine, and the Osteopathic Academy of Sports Medicine. Chicago, 1992.

as immunizations, and offer counseling. Nutrition, obesity, tobacco and drug use, and safe sex practices are among the issues that can be effectively addressed by the health care professional.[2–4] For some athletes, the PPE may be the only annual health assessment performed, making it an essential contact with a physician of record. Most importantly, this is an excellent opportunity for the primary care or team physician to establish rapport with the athlete.

Physical maturity assessed by Tanner staging may be of benefit in detecting those adolescent athletes who are less fully developed and may therefore be at increased risk for physical and emotional injury if allowed to compete in contact sports with athletes who are fully developed (Fig. 38–1).[3] This is a controversial subject not well documented in the literature. Nonetheless, physical maturity provides, at least theoretically, an objective measure of preventable injury risk.

Finally, the PPE must satisfy legal and insurance requirements. These may be dictated by the particular state or province, school district, or insurance carrier. One study revealed that while 35 of 45 states surveyed required yearly examinations, three states required examinations to be performed every 3 years, and six states had no specific requirements.[5] Furthermore, there is a marked disparity among the states regarding both the quality and the content of the evaluation. While 36 states furnished a PPE form, 11 did not include a section to screen medical history, and 8 did not specify which organ systems required examination. Only 38 of the states required that the physician perform the evaluation.[5] It is obvious, therefore, that the health team not only must be familiar with the specific requirements of their district but also must assume the responsibility for providing a thorough evaluation tailored to the individual athlete. A fine example of a PPE form is presented in Figure 38–2.[3]

With these objectives in mind, we will offer specific guidelines for preparticipation evaluation of the athlete and discuss the rationale for particular components. In addition, laboratory testing will be addressed as well as guidelines for clearance of the athlete for participation.

THE EVALUATION

The optimal time to perform the PPE is approximately 6 weeks prior to the start of practice sessions for the season. This early assessment will allow ample time for evaluation or correction of detected abnormalities without interfering with the adequate preparation of the athlete and team for the season. PPE for fall sports may be performed during the spring provided there is a mechanism for reporting and evaluating illness and injuries incurred during the summer.[2–4]

The ideal frequency for performing the PPE is unknown. Although the complete yearly evaluation is popular, it is probably unnecessary and inefficient unless there is a change in the evaluating physician or if records are unavailable.[2] A joint publication prepared by the American Academy of Family Physicians, the American Academy of Pediatrics, the American Medical Society for Sports Medicine, the American Orthopaedic Society for Sports Medicine, and the American Osteopathic Academy of Sports Medicine (hereafter referred to as the joint publication) recommended that an entry-level complete evaluation be performed, followed by a limited annual re-evaluation. The entry-level history and physical examination are discussed in detail below. The re-evaluation should concentrate on the medical history (the same history form used in the entry-level evaluation) and a limited physical examination, including height, weight, blood pressure, pulse, visual acuity, cardiac auscultation, and examination of the skin.[2,3]

The format for the evaluation depends upon the community, the availability of personnel and facilities, the number of athletes requiring screening, and the personal preference of the evaluator. The evaluation may be part of the annual health examination done by the athlete's private physician. Although this offers the benefits of privacy and a greater familiarity with the athlete's family history and provides an optimal setting for counseling, the cost is higher and the time commitment on the part of the physician is significant.[4] It also assumes that the physician is sufficiently interested in, and knowledgeable about, the aspects of medicine relevant to safe participation in sports, without being unreasonably conservative.[3]

The group/station format permits more rapid assessment of a higher volume of athletes at a lower cost. Ancillary personnel such as physical therapists, trainers, nurses, and coaches may be utilized to facilitate the process and to expand on the type of information obtained (for example, having trainers and coaches assess flexibility, strength, and endurance). To be successful, however, this format requires excellent coordination among personnel. It is also more impersonal, allowing little opportunity to address issues of personal concern to the athlete.[3,4]

MEDICAL HISTORY

The medical history is undoubtedly the most important tool in the PPE. Considering that between 36 and

74 percent of all problems detected in athletes are revealed in the medical history, it is surprising that several states do not specifically require its use.[4] The joint publication proposes a medical history form that is relatively complete, yet efficient.

Obtaining information regarding past hospitalizations and surgery may be useful in identifying medical illness and in establishing control of chronic disease. An athlete who may not list asthma under the heading of medical problems if it is currently inactive may be more apt to recall an episode requiring hospitalization. This signals a serious form of the disease. Multiple or recent admissions suggest a poorly controlled chronic condition in an athlete with asthma, diabetes, or a seizure disorder.[3] Obtaining a surgical history ensures that adequate time has been allowed for healing prior to return to sports activity[2,3] and documents surgical procedures after which participation is inadvisable. For

example, an athlete who has undergone evacuation of a subdural hematoma would not be permitted to participate in collision/contact sports, while a history of myotomy for hypertrophic cardiomyopathy would preclude participation in most sports.

Proper documentation of medications taken by the athlete is important, for a variety of reasons. It may offer insight into the presence, severity, and control of chronic disorders such as diabetes mellitus, asthma, dysrhythmias, hypertrophic cardiomyopathy, seizure disorders, and hyperlipidemia. Such documentation also allows the team physician to be prepared in the event of a medical emergency. For example, glucagon and insulin as well as a glucose-measuring instrument should be available for the use of a diabetic athlete.[2] Chronic use of over-the-counter medications such as antihistamines may predispose to heat injury or lead to decreased alertness. Questions about the use of oral

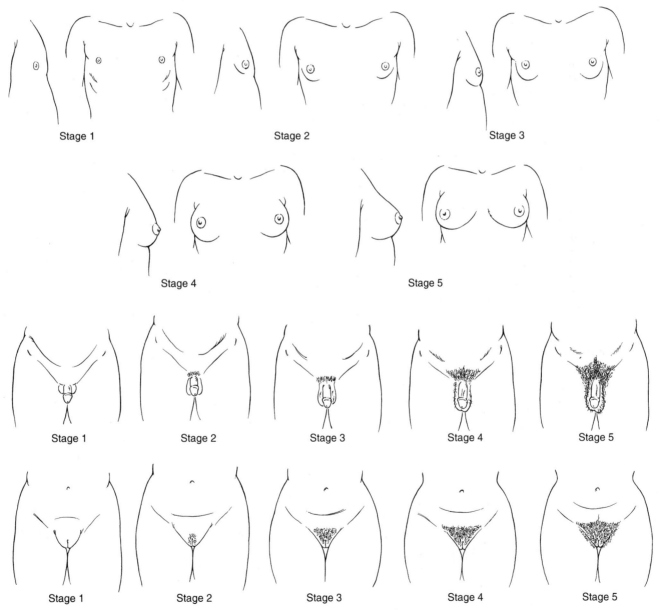

FIGURE 38–1. Tanner stage examination.

Preparticipation Physical Evaluation

History

Date _____

Name _____ Sex _____ Age _____ Date of birth _____

Grade _____ Sport _____ _____ _____

Personal physician _____

Address _____   Physician's phone _____

Explain "Yes" answers below:

		Yes	No
1.	Have you ever been hospitalized?	☐	☐
	Have you ever had surgery?	☐	☐
2.	Are you currently taking any medications or pills?	☐	☐
3.	Do you have any allergies (medicine, bees or other stinging insects)?	☐	☐
4.	Have you ever passed out during or after exercise?	☐	☐
	Have you ever been dizzy during or after exercise?	☐	☐
	Have you ever had chest pain during or after exercise?	☐	☐
	Do you tire more quickly than your friends during exercise?	☐	☐
	Have you ever had high blood pressure?	☐	☐
	Have you ever been told that you have a heart murmur?	☐	☐
	Have you ever had racing of your heart or skipped heartbeats?	☐	☐
	Has anyone in your family died of heart problems or a sudden death before age 50?	☐	☐
5.	Do you have any skin problems (itching, rashes, acne)?	☐	☐
6.	Have you ever had a head injury?	☐	☐
	Have you ever been knocked out or unconscious?	☐	☐
	Have you ever had a seizure?	☐	☐
	Have you ever had a stinger, burner or pinched nerve?	☐	☐
7.	Have you ever had heat or muscle cramps?	☐	☐
	Have you ever been dizzy or passed out in the heat?	☐	☐
8.	Do you have trouble breathing or do you cough during or after activity?	☐	☐
9.	Do you use any special equipment (pads, braces, neck rolls, mouth guard, eye guards, etc.)?	☐	☐
10.	Have you had any problems with your eyes or vision?	☐	☐
11.	Have you ever sprained/strained, dislocated, fractured, broken or had repeated swelling or other injuries of any bones or joints?	☐	☐

☐ Head ☐ Shoulder ☐ Thigh ☐ Neck ☐ Elbow ☐ Chest
☐ Forearm ☐ Shin/calf ☐ Back ☐ Wrist ☐ Ankle ☐ Hand ☐ Foot

		Yes	No
12.	Have you had any other medical problems (infectious mononucleosis, diabetes, etc.)?	☐	☐
13.	Have you had a medical problem or injury since your last evaluation?	☐	☐

14. When was your last tetanus shot? _____

When was your last measles immunization? _____

15. When was your first menstrual period? _____

When was your last menstrual period? _____

What was the longest time between your periods last year? _____

Explain "Yes" answers:

_____

_____

_____

I hereby state that, to the best of my knowledge, my answers to the above questions are correct.

Date _____

Signature of athlete _____

Signature of parent/guardian _____

FIGURE 38–2. Preparticipation physical examination form. (From Bergfeld J, Lombardo J, Nelson M: Pre-Participation Physical Examination. A joint publication by the American Academy of Family Physicians, the American Academy of Pediatrics, the American Medical Society for Sports Medicine, and the Osteopathic Academy of Sports Medicine. Chicago, 1992.)

Preparticipation Physical Evaluation *continued*

Physical Examination   Date _____

Name _____   Age _____   Date of birth _____

		Height _____ Weight _____ BP _____ / _____ Pulse _____					
		Vision R 20/ _____ L 20/ _____ Corrected Y N Pupils _____					

			Normal	Abnormal findings				Initials
COMPLETE	**LIMITED**	Cardiopulmonary						
		Pulses						
		Heart						
		Lungs						
		Tanner stage	1	2	3	4	5	
		Skin						
		Abdominal						
		Genitalia						
		Musculoskeletal						
		Neck						
		Shoulder						
		Elbow						
		Wrist						
		Hand						
		Back						
		Knee						
		Ankle						
		Foot						
		Other						

Clearance:

    A. Cleared

    B. Cleared after completing evaluation/rehabilitation for: _____

    C. Not cleared for: ☐ Collision

                   ☐ Contact

                   ☐ Noncontact   _____ Strenuous   _____ Moderately strenuous   _____ Nonstrenuous

                   Due to: _____

Recommendation: _____

_____

Name of physician _____   Date _____

Address _____   Phone _____

Signature of physician _____

FIGURE 38–2. *Continued*

birth control are needed to obtain an adequate menstrual history and promote discussion of safe sexual practices, sexually transmitted diseases, and pregnancy. Finally, the abuse of potentially dangerous ergogenic substances, such as anabolic steroids, human growth hormone, and cocaine, should be uncovered through direct inquiry.[2,3]

A history of allergy to medications or environmental substances is useful and will prevent the inadvertent administration of harmful pharmacologic agents. The need for injection of epinephrine in the past may signal the presence of allergy to *Hymenoptera* venom, exercise-induced anaphylaxis, or severe environmental allergies. Thus alerted, the team physician should ensure that his medical bag includes epinephrine in case of a recurrence.[2,3]

When evaluating the cardiovascular system it is imperative to elicit from the athlete a history of loss of consciousness, dizziness, and chest pain during or after exercise as well as sudden death occurring in a family member under 50 years of age. Syncope or near-syncope should raise strong suspicion of underlying cardiovascular abnormalities, including hypertrophic cardiomyopathy, aberrant origin of the left coronary artery, underlying dysrhythmia, and valvular disease.[6] Additionally, a history of heart murmur palpitations is useful information when compiling a differential diagnosis. Sudden death in the athlete under 30 years of age nearly always has a cardiovascular cause and is commonly the result of one of three conditions. Chest pain during exercise in the athlete over 30 years of age, and in younger athletes with congenital hyperlipidemia, should always prompt evaluation for atherosclerotic cardiovascular disease, which is the most common cause of sudden death in these individuals. Although chest pain in the young athlete rarely indicates significant cardiovascular pathology, it should not be ignored. Potentially dangerous causes include anomalous origin of the coronary artery, hypertrophic cardiomyopathy, mitral valve prolapse, and congenital aortic stenosis.[6] A history of sudden death in a family member 50 years of age or younger may suggest a predisposition to hypertrophic cardiomyopathy, Marfan syndrome, mitral valve prolapse, or a prolonged QT syndrome.[2,3,7]

A previous history of elevated resting blood pressure may be revealing. If positive, one must pay careful attention not only to the present blood pressure but also to historical and physical findings that suggest a cause of secondary hypertension. For example, paroxysmal tachycardia and anxiety may indicate pheochromocytoma, whereas diminished femoral pulses may indicate coarctation of the aorta. The physician should also inquire into the use of illicit drugs such as anabolic steroids, amphetamines, and cocaine, all of which have pharmacologic properties that may induce hypertension.

The history should uncover skin infections that could be transmitted to other players during contact sports, such as wrestling, or to a common medium, such as swimming pool water or shower floors. Such infections include herpes simplex, impetigo, tinea corporis and tinea pedis, molluscum contagiosum, scabies, and pubic lice.[3] If the athlete has a history of acne, it is important to be aware of prescribed medications that may induce sun sensitivity or other organ toxicity. Acne is commonly exacerbated by sweating, abrasion, and restrictive clothing, creating a nuisance for the athlete involved in contact sports. Counseling regarding methods of prevention and control is often helpful in alleviating self-consciousness and discomfort in the athlete.

The neurologic history should include previous head injury, noting the occurrence of loss of consciousness or amnesia. Seizures and episodes of neurapraxia should be recorded. It is essential to know the number, severity, and approximate date of previous injuries to the head when determining the athlete's ability to participate in contact/collision sports. It is likewise helpful to be aware of recommendations from other physicians advising restriction from participation. This issue will be discussed later in greater detail.

Neurapraxias, more commonly known as burners, stingers, or pinched nerves, result from a stretching or compression injury to the cervical nerve root or brachial plexus; cervical spinal cord injuries may cause transient quadriplegia or generalized limb dysesthesias. Although these conditions are usually self-limiting, a history of recurrent burners or transient quadriplegias warrants cervical spine radiographs, a detailed examination of the neurologic system, and careful consideration of appropriate athletic participation.[2,3] A history of seizures requires a detailed inquiry regarding previous treatment, frequency of recurrence, and whether adequate control has been achieved with medications. A poorly controlled seizure disorder obviously places limitations on participation.

A history of heat-related injury should be elicited, including cramping, syncope, exhaustion, and heat stroke. Athletes who are particularly predisposed are those with previous heat-related injury and those ingesting medications that impair the body's ability to release heat (i.e., antihistamines). It is prudent to compile a list of athletes with this predisposition in order that health personnel trainers and coaches can ensure aggressive hydration before, during, and after practice or events.

A history of coughing spells or dyspnea during or after exercise should raise the suspicion of exercise-induced bronchospasm. This disorder, although easily diagnosed and treated, often goes undetected, which may lead to the frustrating and unfortunate situation in which the athlete experiences difficulty with conditioning or is viewed by coaches as unmotivated.[2,8] Particular attention should be paid to the athlete with environmental allergies or seasonal rhinitis; up to 40 percent of these individuals will experience exercise-induced bronchospasm. Up to 80 percent of asthmatics will be similarly affected.[3] Although exercise-induced bronchospasm is the most common cause of respiratory complaints in the athlete, one must also be alert to the possibility of congenital heart defects, cardiomyopathy, or valvular dysfunction.

By asking the athlete to report any special equipment worn for sports participation, the examiner may be alerted to injuries or conditions that would otherwise have gone unnoticed. For example, use of a tennis elbow brace may indicate persistence of an unresolved epicondylitis. In this case, proper treatment and rehabilitation may be offered in order to prevent progression of the process and unnecessary down time for the athlete. Likewise, use of a neck roll will alert the examiner to inquire about previous neurapraxia and carefully search for persistent neurologic impairment.

Questions relating to disorders of vision are designed to identify the athlete with significantly impaired vision in one eye, for example, a history of trauma that led to loss of an eye or retinal detachment. Of greatest concern are those athletes with best corrected vision poorer than 20/50.[3] These athletes as well as those who have suffered the loss of one eye require protective eye gear and counseling regarding the risks involved in their particular sport. It is important to be familiar with the type of corrective lenses that an athlete uses to facilitate a back-up pair of lenses in case of loss or damage. Protective eyewear, as in polycarbonate goggles, offers good protection for the normal and abnormal eye.

A complete musculoskeletal history should include previous fractures, sprains, strains, tendinitis, dislocations, subluxations, and symptoms suggesting arthritis. Follow-up inquiries should focus on the nature of the injury, the specifics and duration of treatment and rehabilitation, and the need for surgical intervention. The residual effects of the injury and its effect on the athlete's participation should be noted. Symptoms suggesting arthritis require a detailed diagnostic workup at a later date or appropriate referral.

The presence of other medical problems and conditions should be established. Disorders such as diabetes mellitus, asthma, seizures, and chronic inflammatory processes require careful evaluation in order to ascertain the severity of the condition, the level of control, and the medications necessary for treatment. Consultation and frequent communication with a subspecialist during the season may be advisable for optimal management and, in certain difficult cases, to allow the athlete's continued participation. Special attention should be paid to problems that have occurred since the last evaluation, as they are the most likely to affect the athlete's ability to participate.

Given the risk of open wound injury inherent in many sports, it is advisable to have on record the date of the most recent tetanus booster administration. Being able to refer to medical records for an accurate date rather than relying upon recall will avoid the cost of unnecessary immunizations while protecting against a tetanus infection.

For female athletes, the menstrual history should include age of menarche, date of the last menstrual period, longest time between periods, and regularity or irregularity of the cycle.[2,3] The age of menarche is a clue to the athlete with primary amenorrhea and helpful in assessing physical maturity. Oligomenorrhea and amenorrhea require further evaluation or counseling, as even oligomenorrhea has been associated with an increased risk of poor bone mineralization, stress fractures, and potential osteoporosis. The theoretical risk of endometrial hyperplasia and neoplasia has not yet been proved but is also of concern.[9,10] It is important to discuss eating habits and nutrition to help identify those with eating disorders (i.e., anorexia nervosa, bulimia nervosa).

Since studies have shown that less than 50 percent of information reported by athletes is corroborated by their parents, it is recommended that the prepubescent and adolescent athlete's history be reviewed and signed by the parents prior to the preparticipation evaluation.[2,3] In addition, a careful review of the history with the athlete by the physician prior to the examination is essential in order to clarify and expand upon areas of concern.

THE PHYSICAL EXAMINATION

The physical examination performed during the preparticipation evaluation is not intended to be complete but rather should focus on the systems that are of most concern to the athlete and the sport or activity of choice. Particular attention should be given to problem areas detected during review of the history. The format proposed in the joint publication is reproduced in Table 38–2[3] and will be discussed in detail below. Height and weight should be recorded and compared with standardized growth charts when abnormality is suspected. Extremely thin individuals should be questioned about weight loss, eating patterns, body image, and, in the case of females, menstrual dysfunction. Appropriate referral is indicated when an eating disorder such as anorexia nervosa or bulimia is suspected.

OPHTHALMIC EXAMINATION

Examination of the eye should include visual acuity testing using the standard Snellen eye chart. Vision corrected to poorer than 20/50 or the absence of one eye warrants a discussion with the athlete and possibly the parents about the potential dangers of contact sports. At the very least, protective eyewear should be required. Documentation of "physiologic anisocoria" (pupils of unequal size) is useful. Although many normal persons have a slight difference in pupil size, awareness of this baseline anisocoria is important if the athlete is later evaluated for a head injury.[3]

CARDIOVASCULAR EXAMINATION

Blood pressure should be measured and recorded with particular attention given to adequate cuff size. A too-small cuff on a large athlete who requires a thigh cuff could cause a falsely elevated reading. If the initial reading is elevated, the test should be repeated after 20 minutes' rest in the supine position. Classifications of hypertension in adults and children have been published and should be available for comparison (Table 38–3).[3]

The pulse should be counted and assessed for regularity of rhythm. Frequent premature beats, pauses,

TABLE 38–2
Components of the Physical Examination

Height
Weight

Eye Examination
- Visual acuity (Snellen chart)
- Legal blindness in one eye
- Protective eyewear
- Glasses or contact lenses
- Equal pupil size (anisocoria)

Cardiovascular Examination
- Blood pressure
- Pulses (radial, femoral)
- Heart (size, rate, rhythm, murmurs, arrhythmias)

Pulmonary Examination
- Symmetric diaphragmatic excursion
- Clear breath sounds
- Asthma; other chronic lung disease

Abdominal Examination
- Masses
- Organomegaly
- Kidney (abnormal)

Skin
- Acne
- Impetigo rash
- Furuncle, carbuncle
- Herpes
- Scabies
- Lice
- Molluscum contagiosum
- Suspicious nevi or lesions

Musculoskeletal Examination
- Genitalia (male)
- Single or undescended testicle
- Testicular mass
- Hernia

Maturity (Tanner staging)

From Bergfeld J, Lombardo J, Nelson M: Pre-Participation Physical Examination. A joint publication by the American Academy of Family Physicians, the American Academy of Pediatrics, the American Medical Society for Sports Medicine, the American Orthopaedic Society for Sports Medicine, and the Osteopathic Academy of Sports Medicine. Chicago, 1992.

or irregularities, although common in the athlete and probably benign, may be evaluated further by electrocardiogram (ECG) or stress ECG. Simultaneous palpation of the radial and femoral arteries is a useful screening method for aortic coarctation.[2,3]

Auscultation of the heart should be performed with the patient in the standing and supine positions, as abnormalities are not uncommonly transient and positional. The regularity of the rhythm should again be established, and the quality of the heart tone should be noted. The second heart sound (S_2) may be hyperdynamic in hypertrophic cardiomyopathy and diminished in congenital aortic stenosis, whereas a fixed splitting of S_2 suggests the presence of atrial septal defect (ASD). The first heart sound (S_1) may be diminished if significant mitral insufficiency exists. Extra sounds should be soft. Although a third heart sound (S_3) is usually physiologic in young people, a fourth heart sound (S_4) may indicate hypertrophic cardiomyopathy or aortic stenosis. A midsystolic ejection click at the apex of the heart is a frequent finding in mitral valve prolapse, whereas one that is heard early in systole and is loudest at the base may be indicative of aortic or pulmonary stenosis.

Finally, murmurs should be carefully evaluated. Physiologic murmurs, common in the athletic heart, can usually be distinguished from more ominous murmurs by simple techniques such as the Valsalva and squat-stand maneuvers. These maneuvers reduce the volume of blood that returns to the left side of the heart. For example, when one goes from a lying to a standing position, blood will pool in the lower extremities and the physiologic murmur will become softer.[4] Physiologic murmurs are typically low in intensity. They are appreciated best along the left sternal border and do not radiate to the neck or axilla. They are crescendo-decrescendo midsystolic murmurs. In contrast, hypertrophic cardiomyopathy produces a midsystolic, harsh-sounding, diamond-shaped murmur that is loudest at the left lower sternal border and apex. This murmur is typically augmented by maneuvers that reduce the left ventricular end-diastolic volume as explained previously (i.e., phase 2 of the Valsalva maneuver and standing from the squatting position).[6,12]

The murmur of mitral valve prolapse usually follows a midsystolic click. It occurs late in systole, is crescendo in configuration, is appreciated best at the apex, and is augmented by the same maneuvers as for hypertrophic cardiomyopathy. It often radiates to the axilla. The findings may be transient or positional—thus the need for auscultation in both the standing and the supine positions.[6]

The murmur of aortic stenosis is loudest at the base, with radiation to the neck. It is crescendo-decrescendo and begins in early systole, shortly after S_1. The intensity is decreased with phase 2 of the Valsalva maneuver, as is true with physiologic murmurs. Therefore, it is important to note the accompanying features in order to distinguish between the two (i.e., displaced point of maximal intensity [PMI], diminished S_2, radiation, and ejection clicks are present in aortic stenosis and not in the physiologic murmur). Detection of any murmur not clearly consistent with a physiologic murmur requires referral to a cardiologist with a recommendation for echocardiography.

The presence of certain musculoskeletal abnormalities may forewarn of cardiovascular abnormalities. For example, kyphoscoliosis, pectus excavatum or carinatum, hypertelorism, or arachnodactyly should raise suspicion of Marfan syndrome as should ectopia lentis, striae distensae, and abnormal cardiac findings. If clinical suspicion is high, a thorough cardiovascular evaluation, including echocardiogram, may be warranted to rule out a dilated aortic root, which predisposes the athlete to sudden death.[12]

Although the athlete with endocarditis or pericarditis would rarely escape detection in an appropriate referral setting, the athlete with mild carditis might be asymptomatic. More likely, however, the athlete would manifest one or more of the following: fatigue, dyspnea or diminished exercise tolerance, palpitations, precordial discomfort, myalgias, fever with disproportionate tachycardia, and dysrhythmias and conduction disturbances on ECG. Most feared is the progression to congestive cardiomyopathy or sudden death from dysrhythmia, which can be caused by Coxsackie B virus and echovirus, bacterial infection with diphtheria, and connective tissue diseases such as lupus.[15]

The evaluating physician should be familiar with normal cardiovascular variations that might be mistaken for a pathologic condition, resulting in unnecessary restriction of activity. Components of the "athletic heart syndrome" may be bradycardia, S_3 and S_4 gallops, and functional heart murmurs on examination. Normal variant ECG findings in this syndrome include sinus bradycardia, sinus arrhythmia, first-degree and second-degree type I atrioventricular (AV) block, right or left atrial enlargement, augmented QRS voltage, early repolarization with T-wave inversion in leads V1–V4, and abnormal ST- and T-wave segment depression with exercise stress testing. Finally, enlargement of all four chambers detected by echocardiogram is not uncommon in the well trained athlete.[7]

PULMONARY EXAMINATION

On pulmonary examination the examiner should auscultate for normal breath sounds in all fields. Wheezes, rhonchi, rubs, or rales should prompt referral to the athlete's personal physician before clearance is granted.[3] A prolonged expiratory phase, particularly in an athlete with a history of asthma or allergic rhinitis, should raise suspicion of bronchospasm. These athletes require referral and careful observation for exercise-induced asthma.

GASTROINTESTINAL EXAMINATION

The abdomen should be examined carefully for masses, tenderness, hepatomegaly, and splenomegaly with the athlete supine and exposed from the lower ribs to the anterior superior iliac spine.[2,3]

SKIN EXAMINATION

Examination of the skin should be performed throughout the evaluation, observing for lesions consistent with herpes, impetigo, molluscum contagiosum, tinea capitis or corporis, and secondary syphilis. Detection of these entities can preclude participation in sports. In contrast, lesions consistent with atopic dermatitis, contact dermatitis, psoriasis, seborrhea, and nevi suspect for malignancy require further evaluation but not necessarily restriction from participation.

GENITOURINARY EXAMINATION

The genitourinary (GU) examination of the male athlete should note the absent or undescended testicle and assess for testicular irregularity or mass. Examination for inguinal and femoral hernias should be performed as well. Any evidence of sexually transmitted disease should prompt counseling and immediate referral for treatment. The Tanner stage should be determined during examination of the genitals and counseling provided in the event of inappropriate development (see Fig. 38–1). The general examination provides an excellent opportunity to discuss safe sex practices and instruct the athlete in self-examination for testicular cancer, the leading cause of cancer death in young men.

The GU examination of the female is best deferred to the athlete's private physician; actually, this is not a requirement for female athletes, although it may be warranted based on the athlete's medical history.[2] It is

---

TABLE 38–3
Categories of Hypertension — Diastolic (mm Hg)

Diastolic Blood Pressure	Adults*	Children†		
		10–12 Years Old	*13–15 Years Old*	*16–18 Years Old*
120 + 115–119	Severe (≥115)	Severe (≥90)	Severe (≥92)	Severe (≥98)
110–114 105–109	Moderate (105–114)			
100–104 95–99 90–94	Mild (90–104)		Significant (86–91)	Significant (92–97)
85–89 80–84		Significant (82–89)		

*The 1988 Report of the Joint National Committee on Detection, Evaluation and Treatment of High Blood Pressure. Arch Intern Med 1988; 148(5):1023–1038.
†Report of the Second Task Force on Blood Pressure Control in Children—1987. Pediatrics 1987; 79(1):1–25.

prudent to suggest a pelvic examination and Papanicolaou smear for sexually active athletes as well as those whose history is positive for dysfunctional uterine bleeding or amenorrhea. The Tanner stage is probably best determined by having the athlete self-rate her pubic hair pattern and breast development.[3] This has been shown to correlate well with the objective observations of the physician (see Fig. 38–1).[2,3]

DENTAL EXAMINATION

A dental evaluation will add useful information to the PPE, and the involvement of dentists will ensure proper evaluation during the screening. Tooth and gum disease may cause significant time away from practice or games, and pain and infections of teeth and gums will also keep an athlete from performing at peak efficiency. The evaluation of the teeth should include gum condition and the presence of cavities. Follow-up with the athlete's family dentist is encouraged as soon as possible when problems are found. The importance of using mouthguards or masks to protect the athlete's mouth and teeth can be stressed during this part of the examination. The need is, of course, sport specific.

NEUROLOGIC EXAMINATION

The neurologic examination in the PPE need not be too complicated. Assessing pupillary reactivity to light, evaluating cranial nerves, doing a brief motor-sensory examination of the upper and lower extremities, and testing deep tendon reflexes may be the extent of the examination.

Most important to focus on is a history of head or spinal trauma, peripheral nerve injuries, and seizure disorder. This history will direct the neurologic examination and also guide the physician's decision as to whether to clear an athlete for competition.

MUSCULOSKELETAL EXAMINATION

The musculoskeletal (MS) examination may vary according to the history of the individual and the preference of the examiner. A 13-point MS screening examination is proposed in the joint publication[3]; it is a minimum screening that should be adequate to detect most important MS abnormalities in athletes. It may be expanded to a more complete evaluation of a particular problem area identified during history taking or on physical examination. A complete knee, ankle, or shoulder evaluation is frequently necessary.[3] The purpose of the examination is to identify injuries requiring further assessment and rehabilitation as well as abnormalities in flexibility and strength that may predispose the athlete to injury. In one study, an effective evaluation was reported to have reduced the number of significant injuries by 75 percent.[3] In this study, 63

percent of the 196 athletes screened were determined to have problems needing rehabilitation. The complete evaluation need be performed only at entry level unless a specific injury or symptom detected on a yearly follow-up questionnaire prompts a limited re-examination.

The components of the 13-point musculoskeletal screening are as follows:

1. Assessment of symmetry of the bony structures of the trunk, pelvis, and upper and lower extremities, noting in particular symmetry of the pelvis and shoulders, enlargement of the acromioclavicular and sternoclavicular joints, and swelling of the points of extremities.
2. Evaluation of the cervical range of motion in flexion, extension, lateral bend, and lateral rotation.
3. Resisted shoulder shrug to assess trapezius strength.
4. Resisted shoulder abduction in the neutral position and in 30 degrees of forward flexion (plane of the scapula) with internal rotation, in order to assess deltoid and supraspinatus strength, respectively.
5. Evaluation of shoulder range of motion for the degree of internal and external rotation.
6. Evaluation of elbow range of motion for the degree of flexion and extension.
7. Evaluation of wrist range of motion for the degree of pronation, supination, flexion, and extension.
8. Evaluation of the hand and finger range of motion with the fingers in a fist and then spread wide.
9. Assessment of symmetry of the trunk, pelvis, and upper and lower extremities from behind. Particular attention should be paid to scapular asymmetry, pelvic tilting, and hamstring and calf atrophy.
10. Observation of the back and spine with the athlete in the forward flexed/knees extended position to detect scoliosis and assess hamstring flexibility.
11. Observation of the lower extremities from the front, which allows evaluation of quadriceps symmetry during contraction and relaxation, genu valgus or varus, and excessively pronated or supinated feet.
12. Observation during squatting and duck walking, which allows a gross functional assessment of the hip, knee, and ankle.
13. Observation of the lower extremities during heel standing and toe standing to evaluate strength and range of motion in dorsiflexion and plantar flexion, respectively.[3]

Additionally, some practitioners recommend the anterior apprehension test as a screen for anterior shoulder instability; the patellar grind and Lachman tests to evaluate for patellofemoral syndrome and anterior cruciate ligament (ACL) integrity, respectively; and the anterior drawer and talar tilt test to evaluate stability of the ankle.[13]

PHYSICAL FITNESS PROFILE

Specialized fitness evaluations performed by coaches or athletic trainers may be of aid in detecting deficits in strength and flexibility that may predispose to injury. Testing may include a detailed evaluation of total body flexibility, including goniometric measurements of hamstring, quadriceps, gastrocnemius, shoulder, and low back range of motion. Strength may be assessed by manual muscle testing, grip strength, pushups, sit-ups, and isotonic lifts.[1] Power may be measured by vertical jump and reach, stair climbing, and various weight machines. Speed can be assessed by timed sprints, while endurance is tested by a timed 12-minute run.[4] These are usually not necessary in order to clear an athlete for participation but are helpful in establishing a baseline and identifying deficiencies early in the season. In this way, there will be adequate time to bring the athlete to an optimal level of performance prior to the start of competition.[1] The Physical Fitness Profile should be considered an essential part of the preseason examination.

Body composition should be measured in athletes who must meet weight standards in order to compete (i.e., wrestlers and boxers) as well as those who require a slender body habitus to perform effectively (i.e., gymnasts and dancers).[4] Although underwater weighing is the gold standard for determining body composition, it is expensive and impractical. A study comparing various methods for determining the minimum weight allowable for a specific body fat percentage revealed that the most accurate method was skinfold measurement utilized in the modified Loman equation.[3] Body fat percentage and minimum allowable weight should be determined several weeks before the season. Athletes should not be permitted to participate at levels less than 7 percent body fat. Females may require 12 to 15 percent body fat in order to maintain regular menses.[11] In addition, athletes should be required to participate in the same weight class at the beginning and end of each session to avoid rapid weight gain and loss and to prevent achieving less than their minimum allowable body fat percentage.[3]

LABORATORY ASSESSMENT

The use of laboratory testing during the PPE is controversial. Perhaps the most frequently utilized screening test has been the urine dipstick analysis for protein, glucose, and blood. Although limited data are available on the subject, urine testing has proved ineffective in detecting renal disease in children.[2,3] Given the low incidence of true renal pathology in the population, the relatively high incidence of benign intermittent proteinuria and hematuria among athletes, and the cost of testing, urine dipstick analysis cannot be recommended as a routine component of the PPE. Similarly, there is no evidence to support the routine use of blood work such as hemoglobin and hematocrit, complete blood count, and blood chemistries. It should be noted, however, that a few states require particular laboratory tests as a component of a PPE, and that

physicians are obliged to comply with such laws.[5] Should historical or physical findings suggest a need for laboratory investigation, the appropriate referral should be arranged and, if necessary, clearance delayed until the issue is resolved.

Although a few clinicians recommend routine ECG and echocardiogram screening, this would increase the cost of the evaluation and the time required to a prohibitive degree not justified by the number of cases that would be detected. It is generally accepted that these tests be reserved for athletes with suggestive positive historical or clinical findings.[3,12]

DETERMINING CLEARANCE

When determining whether an abnormality will rule out participation in a particular sport, the following questions proposed by Smith and Lombardo should be asked: (1) Does this abnormality increase the risk of injury to the athlete or to other participants? (2) Can participation be enabled by medication, rehabilitation, or protective bracing or padding? If so, can limited participation be allowed in the interim? (3) Finally, if clearance is disallowed for a particular sport, are there other sports or activities in which the athlete can safely participate?[2,3]

Most experts base their clearance decisions upon the recommendations of the American Academy of Pediatrics Committee on Sports Medicine guidelines, which break down a relatively comprehensive list of sports into various categories according to the level of contact and intensity (Table 38–4).[2] Commonly encountered abnormalities are listed along with these suggested guidelines for allowance or disallowance of participation in the various categories of sports (Table 38–5). The interpretation of these guidelines depends upon the clinical judgment of the physician in concert with a well-informed athlete and family.

The athlete may be "cleared without restriction," "cleared after completing evaluation/rehabilitation for" a specific abnormality, or "not cleared for" a specific category of sports.[3] Any restriction should be discussed in detail with the athlete, family, and training and coaching staff in order to eliminate unnecessary confusion and anxiety. Special emphasis should be placed upon the recommendation of alternative acceptable activities. The abnormalities included by the American Academy of Pediatrics Committee on Sports Medicine are addressed in the following discussion.

The athlete with an acute illness requires individual assessment by a qualified physician. Participation of the febrile athlete should be deferred until the infection has been controlled and the temperature lowered. This will minimize the risk of dehydration and heat injury as well as the risk of contamination of other athletes.

Carditis is the first of the listed subcategories of cardiovascular abnormalities. Although uncommon, it deserves mention as a potential cause of sudden death. An athlete suspected of having myocarditis should obviously be restricted from participation and referred to a cardiologist for evaluation.

TABLE 38–4
Classification of Sports

Classification by Contact			Classification by Strenuousness		
Contact/Collision	**Limited Contact**	**Noncontact**	**High to Moderate Intensity**		
Basketball	Baseball	Archery		**High to Moderate**	**High to Moderate**
Boxing*	Bicycling	Badminton	**High to Moderate**	**Dynamic and Low**	**Static and**
Diving	Cheerleading	Body building	**Dynamic and Static**	**Static**	**Low Dynamic**
Field hockey	Canoeing/kayaking	Bowling	**Demands**	**Demands**	**Demands**
Football	(white water)	Canoeing/kayaking	Boxing*	Badminton	Archery
Flag	Fencing	(flat water)	Crew/rowing	Baseball	Auto racing
Tackle	Field	Crew/rowing	Cross-country	Basketball	Diving
Ice hockey	High jump	Curling	skiing	Field hockey	Equestrian
Lacrosse	Pole vault	Dancing	Cycling	Lacrosse	Field events
Martial arts	Floor hockey	Field	Downhill skiing	Orienteering	(jumping)
Rodeo	Gymnastics	Discus	Fencing	Ping-pong	Field events
Rugby	Handball	Javelin	Football	Race walking	(throwing)
Ski jumping	Horseback riding	Shot put	Ice hockey	Racquetball	Gymnastics
Soccer	Racquetball	Golf	Rugby	Soccer	Karate or judo
Team handball	Skating	Orienteering	Running (sprint)	Squash	Motorcycling
Water polo	Ice	Power lifting	Speed skating	Swimming	Rodeoing
Wrestling	Inline	Race walking	Water polo	Tennis	Sailing
	Roller	Riflery	Wrestling	Volleyball	Ski jumping
	Skiing	Rope jumping			Water skiing
	Cross-country	Running			Weight lifting
	Downhill	Sailing			
	Water	Scuba diving	**Low Intensity (Low Dynamic and Low Static Demands)**		
	Softball	Strength training			
	Squash	Swimming		Bowling	
	Ultimate Frisbee	Table tennis		Cricket	
	Volleyball	Tennis		Curling	
	Windsurfing/	Track		Golf	
	surfing	Weight lifting		Riflery	

*Participation not recommended.
Used with permission of American Academy of Pediatrics Committee on Sports Medicine, 1994 Policy Statement. "Medical Conditions Affecting Sports Participation."

It is generally accepted that athletes with hypertension in the mild range may participate safely in competitive sports, provided their private physician is aware of the problem and that secondary causes of hypertension have been investigated. The vast majority of affected athletes have mild hypertension and will probably benefit from an exercise program of moderate intensity, measured by a maximum predicted heart rate of 50 to 70 percent during exercise. Exercise has been shown to decrease exertional and resting diastolic blood pressure. This beneficial effect on resting diastolic blood pressure may be lost with exercise intensity above 70 percent of the maximum predicted heart rate and strenuous exercise has been demonstrated to produce elevations in diastolic blood pressure.[16] For this reason it is probably unwise to allow athletes with more than mild elevation in blood pressure to participate until adequate control of hypertension has been achieved.

Athletes with mild forms of congenital cardiac abnormalities who are asymptomatic and have a normal chest x-ray and ECG are generally acceptable candidates for participation in all competitive athletics. Examples include the presence of mild pulmonic stenosis, aortic stenosis, mitral valve prolapse, and patent ductus arteriosus. A small atrial septal defect or ventricular septal defect is acceptable provided that pulmonary artery pressure is normal.[6,17,18] Owing to the inherent increased risk of sudden death, athletes in whom the

family history, medical history, response to cardiopulmonary questions, or findings on examination lead to the diagnosis of the following disorders should generally be restricted from participation in vigorous exercise: hypertrophic cardiomyopathy, Marfan syndrome with evidence of aortic root dilatation, coronary artery disease, congenital anomalies of the coronary arteries, high-grade ventricular arrhythmia not resolving with exercise, coarctation of the aorta, myocarditis, dilated cardiomyopathy, prolonged QT syndrome, valvular heart disease, cyanotic congenital heart disease, and pulmonary hypertension.[7] Idiopathic concentric left ventricular hypertrophy with left ventricular wall thickness greater than 16 mm has also been associated with sudden death in athletes and warrants restriction from vigorous activity.[19]

Mitral valve prolapse is common among the general population and does not warrant concern unless associated with syncope, significant arrhythmia, significant mitral insufficiency, chest pain, or a family history of sudden death associated with mitral valve prolapse.[3,18] Athletes in whom Marfan syndrome is clinically suspected should undergo echocardiographic evaluation to detect aortic root dilatation.

Although various dysrhythmias have been reported in the asymptomatic athlete without organic heart disease, the athlete with symptoms suggestive of dysrhythmia (i.e., palpitation, presyncope, syncope)

TABLE 38–5
Disqualifying Conditions for Sports Participation

Conditions	Collision*	Contact†	Noncontact‡	Other§
General				
Acute infections: Respiratory, genitourinary, infectious mononucleosis, hepatitis, active rheumatic fever, active tuberculosis	X	X	X	X
Obvious physical immaturity in comparison with other competitors	X	X		
Hemorrhagic disease: Hemophilia, purpura, and other serious bleeding tendencies	X	X	X	
Diabetes, inadequately controlled	X	X	X	X
Diabetes, controlled	††	††	††	††
Jaundice	X	X	X	X
Eyes				
Absence or loss of function of one eye	X	X		
Respiratory				
Tuberculosis (active or symptomatic)	X	X	X	X
Severe pulmonary insufficiency	X	X	X	X
Cardiovascular				
Mitral stenosis, aortic stenosis, aortic insufficiency, coarctation of aorta cyanotic heart disease, recent carditis of any etiology	X	X	X	X
Hypertension on organic basis	X	X	X	X
Previous heart surgery for congenital or acquired heart disease	‖	‖	‖	‖
Liver, enlarged	X	X		
Skin				
Boils, impetigo, and herpes simplex gladiatorum	X	X		
Spleen, enlarged			X	X
Hernia				
Inguinal or femoral hernia	X	X	X	
Musculoskeletal				
Symptomatic abnormalities of inflammations	X	X	X	X
Functional inadequacy of the musculoskeletal system, congenital or acquired, incompatible with the contact or skill demands of the sport	X	X	X	
Neurologic				
History of symptoms of previous serious head trauma or repeated concussions	X			
Controlled convulsive disorder	¶	¶	¶	¶
Convulsive disorder not moderately well controlled by medication	X			
Previous surgery on head	X	X		
Renal				
Absence of one kidney	X	X		
Renal disease	X	X	X	X
Genitalia				
Absence of one testicle	**	**	**	**
Undescended testicle	**	**	**	**

*Football, rugby, hockey, lacrosse, and so forth
†Baseball, soccer, basketball, wrestling, and so forth.
‡Cross country, track, tennis, crew, swimming, and so forth
††No exclusions
‖Each patient should be judged on an individual basis in conjunction with his cardiologist and surgeon.
¶Each patient should be judged on an individual basis. All things being equal, it is probably better to encourage a young boy or girl to participate in a noncontact sport rather than a contact sport. However, if a patient has a desire to play a contact sport and this is deemed a major ameliorating factor in his or her adjustment to school, associates, and the seizure disorder, serious consideration should be given to letting him or her participate if the seizures are moderately well controlled or the patient is under good medical management.
**The Committee approves the concept of contact sports participation for youths with only one testicle or with an undescended testicle (s), except in specific instance such as an inguinal canal undescended testicle(s), following appropriate medical evaluation to rule out unusual injury risk. However, the athlete, parents, and school authorities should be fully informed that participation in contact sports for youths with only one testicle carries a slight injury risk to the remaining healthy testicle. Fertility may be adversely affected following an injury. But the chances of an injury to a descended testicle are rare, and the injury risk can be further substantially minimized with an athletic supporter and protective device.
From Smith NJ (ed): Sports Medicine: Health Care for Young Athletes. Chicago, American Academy of Pediatrics, 1983.

should be carefully evaluated before being cleared for participation. Helpful diagnostic tests include ECG, echocardiogram, exercise stress testing, and ambulatory ECG monitoring. Each case must be reviewed individually with consideration given to the particular dysrhythmia detected, the hemodynamic state of the athlete during the dysrhythmia, the presence or absence of structural heart disease, and the particular sport for which clearance is being sought. Detailed recommendations were proposed by the American College of Cardiology at the 16th Bethesda Conference of 1985. These should be consulted when there is doubt; however, some general recommendations can be made. The following lists dysrhythmias that do not preclude participation for athletes without symptoms or structural heart disease:

- Sinus node dysfunction
  - Tachycardia
  - Bradycardia
  - Sinus arrhythmias and pause
  - Sinus exit block
  - Wandering pacemaker
- Junctional escape beats or rhythms
- Premature junctional complexes
- Premature ventricular complexes (resolve or show no increase with exercise)
- First- or second-degree AV block that does not worsen during exercise
- Right bundle branch block

More significant dysrhythmias probably warrant consultation with a cardiologist.[18]

Clearance of the athlete with impaired vision includes those whose best corrected vision is less than 20/50 in one eye. These athletes should be prohibited from boxing, martial arts, and wrestling, for which adequate protection would not be available. High-risk sports, including football and racquetball, can be permitted with two provisos: (1) that protective goggles be worn, and (2) that a discussion regarding potential risks and liabilities be held with the athlete, his or her family, and any involved administrative personnel.[3]

An athlete with a solitary kidney should consider taking no part in full contact/collision sports, as this will avoid the risk of injury and the possible resultant need for dialysis or transplantation. If the solitary kidney is in any way abnormal or is positioned such that the risk of trauma is high (i.e., pelvic, iliac), even limited contact/collision activity should be avoided.[3] Organomegaly should always prompt a search for an underlying infection, malignancy, or metabolic abnormality. These athletes should be barred from all contact/collision sports until resolution has occurred. Probably the most frequently encountered dilemma is the return to contact/collision sports for the athlete recovering from acute infectious mononucleosis with persistent splenomegaly. The incidence of splenic rupture is highest during the second and third weeks of illness, when the spleen usually achieves its maximum size, then regresses over the next 7 to 10 days.[20] Although the precise recovery time has not been established, it is probably wise to prohibit the athlete from contact/collision sports until 4 weeks from the onset of illness, or until the left upper quadrant tenderness and palpable spleen tip are no longer appreciated on examination.

It would be difficult to propose comprehensive guidelines for clearance of all musculoskeletal injuries. Areas of previous injury, including sprains, strains, overuse injuries, and apophyses detected during the PPE, should be examined for functional stability, range of motion, strength, persistent swelling, and inflammation. In each case an individual assessment must be made regarding the athlete's ability to perform in a particular sport without an increased risk of injury. If these parameters are significantly abnormal, clearance should be deferred until appropriate rehabilitation or orthopaedic evaluation has been completed. If an athlete has undergone a recent surgical procedure or reconstruction, a letter of clearance from the involved surgeon should be obtained.

Participants in contact/collision sports have a relatively high risk of sustaining cerebral concussion. A 10 and 20 percent risk per season has been reported in high school football and hockey players, respectively.[21] There are conflicting criteria in the literature regarding severity grading and recommendations for return to play following concussion. In addition, there is little objective evidence to support these recommendations, which are based primarily upon clinical experience and intuition. While the most critical evaluation is that done on the field at the time of injury, the decision to return to play will be affected by a history of previous concussion. It is, therefore, essential to elicit a thorough history during the PPE so that the physician on the field will be able to make an informed and safe decision regarding return to play. Also, if more than one concussion occurred during a previous season, depending on the severity, the athlete may be unable to take part in another contact/collision sport until the appropriate observation period has elapsed. Athletes with a history of head injury requiring surgery should be referred for evaluation and clearance by a neurosurgeon prior to participation[3]; contact/collision sports are inadvisable in this situation.

Injury to the cervical roots or brachial plexus resulting in neurapraxia (burners, stingers) should not prohibit participation provided that the athlete is asymptomatic with a normal neuromuscular examination. A history of transient quadriplegia secondary to spinal injury should prompt evaluation by a neurosurgeon prior to clearance. If evaluation by magnetic resonance imaging (MRI) suggests a functional spinal stenosis, many authors advise against participation in contact/collision sports.[22] Of note, roentgenographic evaluation of the cervical spine has been shown to be unreliable in the evaluation of possible spinal stenosis. The vertebral canal:vertebral body ratio method described by Torg has been demonstrated to yield a positive predicted value of only 12 percent.[20] MRI, therefore, appears to be the study of choice in determining the presence of spinal stenosis.[22]

Although a well-controlled seizure disorder does not preclude participation in contact/collision sports, it is recommended in the joint publication that affected individuals be advised against participation in the following: skiing, scuba diving, rope and rock climbing, gymnastics on a high apparatus (high bar, rings, parallel bars, uneven bars, balance beam), parachuting, hang gliding, and high diving.[3] Athletes with poorly controlled seizures should be referred to a neurologist prior to clearance. If seizures remain poorly controlled, participation should be prohibited from the aforementioned activities, in addition to swimming, weight lifting, archery, riflery, and javelin toss.[23]

A history of spontaneous pneumothorax in the asymptomatic athlete with a normal examination should not mean exclusion from sports participation except for scuba diving. It occurs most commonly in otherwise healthy young adults and is clearly unrelated to exertion.[24] Clearance assumes, however, that an adequate evaluation including chest x-ray and pulmonary function testing has been performed to rule out underlying pulmonary disease. This type of evaluation is particularly important in the older athlete.

Infectious dermatologic disorders including herpes simplex infection; impetigo; furuncles; carbuncles; tinea corporis, capitis, or barbae; scabies; louse infestation; and molluscum contagiosum necessitate treatment and resolution before clearance can be granted for wrestling, boxing, martial arts, swimming, sports requiring shared use of mats or headgear (gymnastics and baseball), or other close contact sports.

Athletes with a single functional testicle should be advised against participation in contact/collision sports. Those choosing to participate should be strongly advised to wear a protective cup.[3]

The athlete with a direct or indirect inguinal hernia who has signs and symptoms of incarceration or strangulation should be referred immediately for surgical consultation and repair. In the absence of a symptomatic hernia, most cases can be managed with elective surgical repair at the end of the season. Owing to the higher incidence of incarceration, strangulation, and recurrence, however, femoral hernias should be referred for immediate surgical repair.[25]

The disorders discussed in this chapter represent only those most commonly encountered by the primary care physician and therapist during the PPE. When uncertainty exists regarding the athlete's ability to participate safely in a particular sport, clearance should be deferred until a consultation with the appropriate medical specialist has been obtained.

CONCLUSION

The PPE is important for yielding both negative and positive information. The rarely detected negative information, although necessitating restrictions from certain activities, will theoretically prevent the potential fatality associated with a serious underlying medical condition. The more commonly detected positive information will aid in the prevention of injury and will facilitate the return of the athlete to optimal form prior to participation. The history and physical evaluation should be brief and efficient, addressing the issues relative to safe participation in sports. Although not a substitute for the annual health evaluation, the PPE should serve to detect serious conditions that may otherwise go unnoticed. It may also afford a setting to provide counseling on relevant health-related issues. While clearance should be based upon the recommendations outlined earlier, the final decision is based on the clinical judgment of the physician in conjunction with a well-informed athlete and his or her family.

REFERENCES

1. Kubler WB, Chandler TJ, Maddus RE: A musculoskeletal approach to the pre-participation physical examination: Preventing injury and improving performance. Am J Sports Med 1989; 17(4):1–7.
2. Smith DM, Lombardo JA, Robinson JB: The pre-participation evaluation. Prim Care 1991; 18(4):777–807.
3. Bergfeld J, Lombardo J, Nelson M: Pre-Participation Physical Examination. A joint publication by the American Academy of Family Physicians, the American Academy of Pediatrics, the American Medical Society for Sports Medicine, the American Orthopaedic Society for Sports Medicine, and the American Osteopathic Academy of Sports Medicine. Chicago, 1992.
4. Henderson JM, et al (eds): Sports Medicine I. Monograph, Edition No. 160, Home Study Self-Assessment Program. Kansas City, MO, American Academy of Family Physicians, 1992.
5. Feinstein RA, Soileau EJ, Daniel WA: A national survey of pre-participation physical examination requirements. Phys Sports Med 1988; 16(5):51–59.
6. Strong WB, Steed D: Cardiovascular evaluation of the young athlete. Pediatr Clin North Am 1982; 29(6):1325–1339.
7. Van Camp SP: Sudden death. Clin Sports Med 1992; 11(2):291–302.
8. Kyle JM, Walker RB, Hanshaw SL: Exercise-induced bronchospasm in the young athlete: Guidelines for routine screening and initial management. Med Sci Sports Exerc 1992; 24:856–859.
9. Shangold M, Rebar RW, Wentz AL: Evaluation and management of menstrual dysfunction in athletes. JAMA 1990; 263(12):1665–1669.
10. Barrow GW, Saha S: Menstrual irregularity and stress fracture in collegiate female distance runners. Am J Sports Med 1988; 16(3):209–215.
11. Clark RR, Kuta JM, Sullivan JC: A comparison of methods to predict minimal weight in high school wrestlers. Med Sci Sports Exerc 1993; 25(1):151–158.
12. Braden DS, Strong WB: Pre-participation screening for sudden cardiac death in high school and college athletes. Phys Sports Med 1988; 16(10):128–140.
13. Cherney SB: The preseason orthopaedic screening examination. Sports Med Clin 1984; 1(2):1–7.
14. Fields KB, Kelaney M: Focusing the pre-participation sports examination. J Family Pract 1990; 30:304–312.
15. Wenger NJ, Abelmann WH, Roberts WC: Myocarditis. *In* Hurst JW (ed): The Heart, 7th ed. New York, McGraw-Hill, 1990, pp 1256–1277.
16. Tanji JL: Exercise and the hypertensive athlete. Clin Sports Med 1992; 11(2):291–302.
17. Braden DS, Strong WB: Pre-participation screening for sudden cardiac death in high school and college athletes. Phys Sports Med 1988; 16(10):128–139.
18. Mitchell JH, Maron BJ, Epstein SE: 16th Bethesda Conference: Cardiovascular abnormalities in the athlete: Recommendations regarding eligibility for competition. J Am Coll Cardiol 1985; 6(6):1186–1232.
19. Pelliccia A, Maron BJ, Spataro A: The upper limit of physiologic cardiac hypertrophy in highly trained elite athletes. N Engl J Med 1991; 324(5):293–301.

20. Schooley RT, Dolin R: Epstein-Barr virus. *In* Mandell GL (ed): The Principles And Practice Of Infectious Disease, 3rd ed. New York, Churchill Livingstone, 1990, pp 1172–1181.

21. Roberts WO: Managing concussions on the sidelines. Phys Sports Med 1992; 20(6):66–72.

22. Cantu RC: Functional cervical spine stenosis: A contraindication to participation in contact sports. Med Sci Sports Exerc 1993; 25(3):316–317.

23. American Academy Of Pediatrics: Committee On Sports Medicine. Recommendations for participation in competitive sports. Pediatrics 1988; 81(5):737–739.

24. Fraser RG, Paré JA, Paré PD: Pneumothorax. *In* (eds) Diagnosis of Diseases of the Chest, 3rd ed. Philadelphia, WB Saunders, 1991, pp 2741–2744.

25. Rich BS, Hough DO, Monroe JS: Inguinal mass in a college football player: A case study. Med Sci Sports Exerc 1993; 25(3):318–320.

CHAPTER 39

Nutritional Concerns in Athletes

SUSAN CUMMINGS *MS, RD*
MARY JANE REWINSKI *BS, RD*

Athletic performance can be optimized by adequate nutrition. Thus, there are nutritional concerns specific to athletes. For this reason, the athlete is particularly vulnerable to health claims that may or may not be accurate. Misleading nutritional information may make it difficult for the athlete to make appropriate decisions regarding nutritional intake. It seems that new claims are made as often as old ones are disproved. The objective of this chapter is to provide nutritional information based on current scientific findings and to provide a guide for assessing an athlete's intake and developing a nutritionally adequate sports diet. By beginning with the assessment, the health professional can determine an individual's current nutritional excesses, deficiencies, or both and can develop an individualized plan.

THE NUTRITIONAL ASSESSMENT

In order to prescribe a dietary regimen, a thorough assessment to determine the athlete's health and nutritional status is an important first step. The initial assessment should include an interview to determine dietary intake, eating behaviors, and dietary patterns. A physical examination by a primary care physician is also recommended to determine current health status. The initial information obtained in the physical examination should also include laboratory data (for example, a complete blood count) providing objective information that may substantiate physical findings and dietary deficiencies or excesses noted in the dietary intake analysis. Anthropometric data such as height, weight, height to weight ratio, and body composition should also be documented at baseline; these can be used as a standard to measure body composition changes and to determine training strategies for the athlete.

ENERGY NEEDS

The longer and more effectively an athlete trains, the more efficient the body becomes at burning calories and using oxygen. Efficiency of energy burned refers to the quantity of energy required to perform a particular task in relation to the actual work accomplished.[1] Factors that determine energy requirements for athletes are (1) body composition, which determines basal metabolic rate (BMR); lean body mass accounts for approximately 75 percent of all calories burned, and since athletes generally have higher lean body mass, they have 5 percent higher BMR than nonathletic individuals; (2) sex; females generally have a 5 to 10 percent lower BMR than males; (3) energy expenditure for training, competition, and daily activities; and (4) whether an athlete is gaining or losing body weight.

Highly trained endurance athletes burn energy more efficiently than less well trained athletes. They also burn a large number of calories simply because of the extended time spent in training. Studies of elite endurance athletes show that these athletes report consuming on average about 55 kcal per kg body weight per day versus an average recommended intake of about 35 kcal per kg per day for nonathletes.[2] Table 39–1 lists caloric expenditure for various physical activities.

DETERMINING NUTRIENT INTAKE

Using any combination of the following dietary methodologies, the health professional can estimate calories and nutrients consumed by the athlete.

THE 24-HOUR RECALL

This method requires the athlete to report what he or she has eaten in a 24-hour period, beginning with the first thing in the morning and continuing throughout the day, including beverages and snacks. Record time, food, and amount eaten. Since the 24-hour recall relies on memory and may not be representative of a typical or average intake, combining it with questions regarding food frequency will provide a more complete overview of the athlete's usual intake. For example, how many times in a week do you eat this for breakfast? If you didn't have this, what would you have? How many times a week do you skip breakfast?

THE FOOD FREQUENCY QUESTIONNAIRE

A food frequency questionnaire is designed to obtain both qualitative and semiquantitative descriptive information about usual food intake.[3] This is accomplished by assessing the frequency with which foods are eaten during a specified time (daily, weekly, or monthly). The advantages of a food frequency questionnaire are that it is relatively inexpensive and can be administered by nonprofessionals or can be self-administered. A disadvantage to its use is that it is time consuming, and accuracy depends on either a trained person sitting with the individual defining portions sizes and quantities or the individual understanding the usually very lengthy questionnaires and accurately self-assessing portions and frequency.

A shortened version of the food frequency questionnaire would be to go through the food groups—starches, fruits, vegetables, protein, dairy, and fats (Fig. 39–1)—and question how often and in what quantity the athlete eats these foods, including what foods and beverages the athlete consumes prior to and just after exercise, training, and an event; what typical snack foods; and what if any nutritional supplements the athlete takes.

THE FOOD RECORD

A food record is a record maintained by an individual and consists of the exact quantity of food eaten within a specified period of time, usually 3 to 7 days. The accuracy depends on the individual's diligence and integrity. Over a specific period of time, the method provides a fairly accurate estimate of food consumption.

By keeping a food record for 7 days, total caloric intake can be found and compared with weight changes to determine the level of exercise and caloric intake that produces weight maintenance, weight loss, or weight gain.

EVALUATION OF NUTRIENT INTAKE

COMPUTER PROGRAMS

When purchasing a software system for computerized dietary analysis, an accurate nutrient data base is essential. The source of the database, its completeness in terms of the range of foods listed, and the availability of nutrient values for individual foods must be determined. The validity of the computer program for calculating nutrient intakes must also be assessed. The food is entered in the database after it is coded, usually manually. The nutrient intake is then calculated by the software package. The software package should provide total nutrients per meal, total nutrients for each day, average daily nutrient intake per major food group and subgroups, and average frequency of consumption of major food groups and subgroups.

STANDARD TABLES OF RECOMMENDED INTAKE

Most methods of evaluating intake involve comparisons with tables of recommended nutrient intake. The Recommended Dietary Allowances[4] (RDAs) are listed in Table 39–2. The RDAs are recommended intakes, not requirements. They were designed for the evaluation of groups, not individuals, and were set to meet the nutrient needs for healthy people. If a healthy individual consumes two thirds of the RDA, he or she is considered to be meeting the nutrient requirement, since the RDA is set on the high side to meet population needs. The nutrient needs of an athlete are discussed later in this chapter.

The evaluation of nutrient intake is an estimate that depends on the accuracy of the methods used for dietary assessment and analysis. To identify specific nutrient deficiencies, biochemical and clinical assessments should be done along with the dietary assessment.

THE DIETARY INTERVIEW

In addition to collecting information regarding actual dietary intake, the dietary interview is used to develop a rapport with the individual athlete and to assess general eating patterns. Questions should address where most meals are eaten; who prepares the food; any foods the athlete avoids; snacking patterns and choices; the athlete's ethnic or cultural practices; what, if any, vitamins, minerals, or other nutritional supplements are used; and what is individual's perception of good nutrition: "In your opinion, what constitutes a poor eating day?" "What constitutes a good eating day?" "How often does each occur?" "What are your most difficult challenges in eating a 'healthy' diet?"

The dietary interview should also include questions regarding training and competition practices. It is important to know the amount of time spent in training as well as the intensity and duration of the individual's activity in order to calculate caloric needs. Specific questions regarding eating and drinking patterns before, during, and after an event are also important.

MOTIVATION AND READINESS FOR BEHAVIORAL CHANGE

The step after evaluating an athlete's intake and determining needs, is to make recommendations for change. One of the most common errors made by health professionals advocating behavior change is to tell the individual what to do and expect that a behavior change will occur. Attention should be given to whether the individual is ready, motivated, and willing to make the change or changes. Experts in the area of health promotion are suggesting that a shift from an action to a stage paradigm is occurring. The stage paradigm is a proactive and interactive model for behavior change and can be used to assess an individual's readiness in regards to making changes; it also provides guidelines for professional intervention.[5] The stages of change are shown in Table 39–3. During the assessment, it would be useful to determine the athlete's stage in order to determine an appropriate intervention strategy. An example would be the athlete who has no idea that his or her diet is nutritionally inadequate and therefore may not be ready to take action and start goal setting. Information regarding nutrition and exercise is first needed to move her or him to the next stage, contemplation. Once the athlete has contemplated making the dietary changes, it is time to clarify any preconceived notions and provide additional information regarding the benefits of the change. The athlete may then be ready to move to the preparation stage. During this stage, he or she is able to identify a motivation for taking action and begins to investigate strategies for change. In the box is a list of action strategies for the athlete ready to implement changes. Learning where the individual is regarding readiness to make changes requires good listening skills on the part of the interviewer. The interviewer can learn what motivates the athlete and where to start in the process of making behavior changes.

NUTRIENT RECOMMENDATIONS

The body requires at least 40 nutrients, which are classified into six groups: the macronutrients protein, carbohydrate, and fat; the micronutrients vitamins, minerals, and water. These nutrients are classified as essential because they cannot be made in the body and must therefore be supplied from the diet.

MACRONUTRIENTS

There are three categories of macronutrients: protein, carbohydrate, and fat; and two categories of micronutrients: vitamins and minerals. The macronutrients, in addition to alcohol, provide energy in the form of calories (Table 39–4); vitamins, minerals, and water have no calories and therefore are not a source of energy.

PROTEIN

Requirements for protein are actually requirements for amino acids, the building blocks of protein. Protein can be compared to a chain-link fence, the links representing amino acids. (There are nine amino acids not stored by the body, termed essential amino acids, and therefore need to be supplied by the diet.) Protein is the component of many hormones, is a constituent of antibodies for the body's immune system, and is a part of every enzyme in the body. About 45 percent of the human body is protein; second to water, it makes up the largest percentage of material in the human body. Although carbohydrate is the body's most used source of energy, in aerobic sports, amino acids may supply up to 15% of the total energy used.[6]

Evaluation of protein needs should consider the energy content of the diet. Although protein requirements are based on degree and intensity of training, energy intake is the most important factor affecting protein requirements. When energy intake is less than that required by the body, protein breakdown occurs to provide the energy needed. Therefore, sports that require specific body weight such as wrestling, dancing, and gymnastics may lead to insufficient energy intake, and protein needs may exceed the RDA.

An athlete's protein requirement is dependent on energy intake and the degree and intensity of training. The effect of training on protein needs is transient. Initially, protein losses increase with training but after a period of 5 to 14 days, return to normal.[7] Protein may actually be more efficiently utilized in a well-trained individual;[8] therefore, well-trained athletes may need less protein than those beginning an exercise program. There is some discrepency in data, which may be due to the study designs, regarding the effect of intensity of exercise on protein requirement.[9] The rate of amino acid use appears to depend on glycogen stores. Lemon and Mullin found that the rate of amino acid utilization during exercise in individuals with depleted glycogen stores increased with exercise.[10] The implication is that muscle glycogen stores may have a protein-sparing effect.

BRANCHED-CHAIN AMINO ACIDS. Three amino acids, leucine, valine, and isoleucine, are branched-chain amino acids. These amino acids are predominantly oxidized during exercise and are essential amino acids. Increased utilization of branched-chain amino

TABLE 39–1
Caloric Expenditure for Various Physical Activities

Body Weight
($kcal \cdot min^{-1} \cdot kg^{-1}$)

Kg Pounds	45 100	48 105	50 110	52 115	55 120	57 125	59 130	61 135	64 140	66 145
Sedentary Activities										
Lying quietly	.99	1.0	1.1	1.1	1.2	1.3	1.3	1.4	1.4	1.5
Sitting and writing, card playing, etc.	1.2	1.3	1.4	1.5	1.5	1.6	1.7	1.7	1.8	1.8
Standing with light work, cleaning, etc.	2.7	2.9	3.0	3.1	3.3	3.4	3.5	3.7	3.8	3.9
Physical Activities										
Archery	3.1	3.3	3.5	3.6	3.8	4.0	4.1	4.3	4.5	4.6
Badminton										
Recreational singles	3.6	3.8	4.0	4.2	4.4	4.6	4.7	4.9	5.1	5.3
Social doubles	2.7	2.9	3.0	3.1	3.3	3.4	3.5	3.7	3.8	3.9
Competitive	5.9	6.1	6.4	6.7	7.0	7.3	7.6	7.9	8.2	8.5
Baseball										
Player	3.1	3.3	3.4	3.6	3.8	4.0	4.1	4.3	4.4	4.5
Pitcher	3.9	4.1	4.3	4.5	4.7	4.9	5.1	5.3	5.5	5.7
Basketball										
Half court	3.0	3.1	3.3	3.5	3.6	3.8	3.9	4.1	4.2	4.4
Recreational	4.9	5.2	5.5	5.7	6.0	6.2	6.5	6.7	7.0	7.2
Vigorous competition	6.5	6.8	7.2	7.5	7.8	8.2	8.5	8.8	9.2	9.5
Bicycling, level										
(mph) (min/mile)										
5 12:00	1.9	2.0	2.1	2.2	2.3	2.4	2.5	2.6	2.7	2.8
6 10:00	2.7	2.8	3.0	3.1	3.2	3.4	3.5	3.6	3.8	3.9
8 7:30	3.4	3.6	3.8	4.0	4.1	4.3	4.5	4.7	4.8	5.0
10 6:00	4.2	4.4	4.6	4.8	5.1	5.3	5.5	5.7	5.9	6.1
11 5:28	5.0	5.2	5.5	5.7	6.0	6.2	6.5	6.7	7.0	7.2
12 5:00	5.7	6.0	6.3	6.6	6.9	7.2	7.5	7.8	8.1	8.4
13 4:37	6.8	7.1	7.5	7.8	8.2	8.5	8.8	9.2	9.5	9.9
Bowling	2.7	2.8	3.0	3.1	3.3	3.4	3.5	3.7	3.8	3.9
Calisthenics										
Light type	3.4	3.6	3.8	4.0	4.1	4.3	4.5	4.7	4.8	5.0
Timed vigorous	9.7	10.1	10.6	11.1	11.6	12.1	12.6	13.1	13.6	14.1
Canoeing										
(mph) (min/mile)										
2.5 24	1.9	2.0	2.1	2.2	2.3	2.4	2.5	2.6	2.7	2.8
4.0 15	4.4	4.6	4.9	5.1	5.3	5.5	5.8	6.0	6.2	6.4
5.0 12	5.7	6.0	6.3	6.6	6.9	7.2	7.5	7.8	8.1	8.4
Dancing										
Moderate (waltz)	3.1	3.3	3.5	3.6	3.8	4.0	4.1	4.3	4.5	4.6
Active (square, disco)	4.5	4.7	5.0	5.2	5.4	5.6	5.9	6.1	6.3	6.6
Aerobic (vigorous)	6.0	6.3	6.7	7.0	7.3	7.6	7.9	8.2	8.5	8.8
Fencing										
Moderate	3.3	3.5	3.6	3.8	4.0	4.1	4.3	4.5	4.6	4.8
Vigorous	6.6	7.0	7.3	7.7	8.0	8.3	8.7	9.0	9.4	9.7
Field hockey	5.0	6.3	6.7	7.0	7.3	7.6	7.9	8.2	8.5	8.8
Football										
Moderate	3.3	3.5	3.6	3.8	4.0	4.1	4.3	4.5	4.6	4.8
Touch, vigorous	5.5	5.8	6.1	6.4	6.6	6.9	7.2	7.5	7.8	8.0
Golf										
Twosome (carry clubs)	3.6	3.8	4.0	4.2	4.4	4.6	4.7	4.9	5.1	5.3
Foursome (carry clubs)	2.7	2.9	3.0	3.1	3.3	3.4	3.5	3.7	3.8	3.9
Power cart	1.9	2.0	2.1	2.2	2.3	2.4	2.5	2.6	2.7	2.8
Handball										
Moderate	6.5	6.8	7.2	7.5	7.8	8.2	8.5	8.8	9.2	9.5
Competitive	7.7	8.0	8.4	8.8	9.2	9.6	10.0	10.4	10.8	11.1
Hiking, pack (3 mph)	4.5	4.7	5.0	5.2	5.4	5.6	5.9	6.1	6.3	6.6

From Williams MH: Nutrition for Fitness and Sport, 2nd ed. Copyright 1988 Davenport, IA, William C. Brown Communications, Inc. 1988. All rights reserved. Reprinted by permission.

68 150	70 155	73 160	75 165	77 170	80 175	82 180	84 185	86 190	89 195	91 200	93 205	95 210	98 215	100 220
1.5	1.5	1.6	1.6	1.7	1.7	1.8	1.8	1.9	1.9	2.0	2.0	2.1	2.1	2.2
1.9	2.0	2.0	2.1	2.2	2.2	2.3	2.4	2.4	2.5	2.5	2.6	2.7	2.7	2.8
4.1	4.2	4.4	4.5	4.6	4.8	4.9	5.0	5.2	5.3	5.4	5.6	5.7	5.9	6.0
4.8	4.9	5.1	5.3	5.4	5.6	5.7	5.9	6.0	6.2	6.4	6.5	6.7	6.9	7.0
5.4	5.6	5.8	6.0	6.2	6.4	6.6	6.7	6.9	7.1	7.3	7.4	7.6	7.8	8.0
4.1	4.2	4.4	4.5	4.6	4.8	4.9	5.0	5.2	5.3	5.4	5.6	5.7	5.9	6.0
8.8	9.1	9.4	9.7	10.0	10.3	10.6	10.9	11.2	11.5	11.8	12.1	12.4	12.7	13.0
4.7	4.8	5.0	5.2	5.3	5.5	5.6	5.8	5.9	6.1	6.3	6.4	6.6	6.8	6.9
5.9	6.0	6.3	6.5	6.7	6.9	7.1	7.3	7.4	7.7	7.9	8.0	8.2	8.5	8.6
4.5	4.7	4.8	5.0	5.1	5.3	5.4	5.6	5.7	5.9	6.0	6.2	6.4	6.5	6.7
7.5	7.7	8.0	8.2	8.5	8.7	9.0	9.2	9.5	9.7	10.0	10.2	10.5	10.7	11.0
9.9	10.2	10.5	10.9	11.2	11.5	11.9	12.2	12.5	12.9	13.2	13.5	13.8	14.2	14.5
2.9	3.0	3.1	3.2	3.3	3.4	3.5	3.6	3.7	3.8	3.9	4.0	4.1	4.2	4.3
4.0	4.2	4.3	4.4	4.6	4.7	4.9	5.0	5.1	5.3	5.4	5.5	5.7	5.8	6.0
5.2	5.4	5.5	5.7	5.9	6.1	6.3	6.4	6.6	6.8	6.9	7.1	7.3	7.5	7.7
6.4	6.6	6.8	7.0	7.2	7.4	7.6	7.9	8.1	8.3	8.5	8.7	8.9	9.1	9.4
7.5	7.8	8.0	8.3	8.5	8.8	9.0	9.3	9.5	9.8	10.0	10.3	10.6	10.8	11.1
8.7	9.0	9.3	9.5	9.8	10.1	10.4	10.7	11.0	11.3	11.6	11.9	12.2	12.5	12.8
10.2	10.6	10.9	11.3	11.6	12.0	12.3	12.6	13.0	13.3	13.7	14.0	14.4	14.7	15.0
4.1	4.2	4.4	4.5	4.6	4.8	4.9	5.0	5.2	5.3	5.5	5.6	5.7	5.9	6.0
5.2	5.4	5.5	5.7	5.9	6.1	6.3	6.4	6.6	6.8	7.0	7.1	7.3	7.5	7.7
14.6	15.1	15.6	16.1	16.6	17.1	17.6	18.1	18.6	19.1	19.6	20.0	20.5	21.0	21.5
2.9	3.0	3.1	3.2	3.3	3.4	3.5	3.6	3.7	3.8	3.9	4.0	4.1	4.2	4.3
6.7	6.9	7.1	7.4	7.6	7.8	8.0	8.2	8.5	8.7	8.9	9.1	9.4	9.6	9.8
8.7	9.0	9.3	9.5	9.8	10.1	10.4	10.7	11.0	11.3	11.6	11.9	12.2	12.5	12.8
4.8	4.9	5.1	5.3	5.4	5.6	5.7	5.9	6.0	6.2	6.4	6.5	6.7	6.9	7.0
6.8	7.0	7.3	7.5	7.7	7.9	8.2	8.4	8.6	8.9	9.1	9.3	9.5	9.8	10.0
9.1	9.4	9.7	10.0	10.3	10.6	10.9	11.2	11.5	11.8	12.1	12.4	12.7	13.0	13.3
5.0	5.2	5.3	5.5	5.7	5.8	6.0	6.2	6.3	6.5	6.7	6.8	7.0	7.1	7.3
10.0	10.4	10.7	11.0	11.4	11.7	12.1	12.4	12.7	13.1	13.4	13.8	14.1	14.4	14.8
9.1	9.4	9.7	10.0	10.3	10.6	10.9	11.2	11.5	11.8	12.1	12.4	12.7	13.0	13.3
5.0	5.2	5.3	5.5	5.7	5.8	6.0	6.2	6.3	6.5	6.7	6.8	7.0	7.1	7.3
8.3	8.6	8.9	9.2	9.4	9.7	10.0	10.3	10.6	10.8	11.1	11.4	11.7	12.0	12.2
5.4	5.6	5.8	6.0	6.2	6.4	6.6	6.7	6.9	7.1	7.3	7.4	7.6	7.8	8.0
4.1	4.2	4.4	4.5	4.6	4.8	4.9	5.0	5.2	5.3	5.4	5.6	5.7	5.9	6.0
2.9	·3.0	3.1	3.2	3.3	3.4	3.5	3.6	3.7	3.8	3.9	4.0	4.1	4.2	4.3
9.9	10.2	10.5	10.9	11.2	11.5	11.9	12.2	12.5	12.9	13.2	13.5	13.8	14.2	14.5
11.5	11.9	12.3	12.7	13.1	13.5	13.9	14.3	14.7	15.0	15.4	15.8	16.2	16.6	17.0
6.8	7.0	7.3	7.5	7.7	7.9	8.2	8.4	8.6	8.9	9.1	9.3	9.5	9.8	10.0

Table continued on following page

TABLE 39–1 *Continued*
Caloric Expenditure for Various Physical Activities

Body Weight (Continued)

Kg Pounds	45 100	48 105	50 110	52 115	55 120	57 125	59 130	61 135	64 140	66 145
Hockey, ice	6.6	7.0	7.3	7.7	8.0	8.3	8.7	9.0	9.4	9.7
Horseback riding										
Walk	1.9	2.0	2.1	2.2	2.3	2.4	2.5	2.6	2.7	2.8
Sitting to trot	2.7	2.9	3.0	3.1	3.3	3.4	3.5	3.7	3.8	3.9
Posting to trot	4.2	4.4	4.6	4.8	5.1	5.3	5.5	5.7	5.9	6.1
Gallop	5.7	6.0	6.3	6.6	6.9	7.2	7.5	7.8	8.1	8.4
Horseshoes	2.5	2.6	2.8	2.9	3.0	3.1	3.3	3.4	3.5	3.7
Jogging (see running)										
Judo	8.5	8.9	9.3	9.8	10.2	10.6	11.0	11.5	11.9	12.3
Karate	8.5	8.9	9.3	9.8	10.2	10.6	11.0	11.5	11.9	12.3
Mountain climbing	6.5	6.8	7.2	7.5	7.8	8.2	8.5	8.8	9.2	9.5
Paddle ball	5.7	6.0	6.3	6.6	6.9	7.2	7.5	7.8	8.1	8.4
Pool (billiards)	1.5	1.6	1.6	1.7	1.8	1.9	1.9	2.0	2.1	2.2
Racquetball	6.5	6.8	7.1	7.5	7.8	8.1	8.4	8.8	9.1	9.4
Roller skating (9 mph)	4.2	4.4	4.6	4.8	5.1	5.3	5.5	5.7	5.9	6.1
Running (steady state)										
(mph) (min/mile)										
5.0 12:00	6.0	6.3	6.6	7.0	7.3	7.6	7.9	8.2	8.5	8.8
5.5 10:55	6.7	7.0	7.3	7.7	8.0	8.4	8.7	9.0	9.4	9.7
6.0 10:00	7.2	7.6	8.0	8.4	8.7	9.1	9.5	9.8	10.2	10.6
7.0 8:35	8.5	8.9	9.3	9.0	10.2	10.6	11.0	11.5	11.9	12.3
8.0 7:30	9.7	10.2	10.7	11.2	11.6	12.1	12.6	13.1	13.6	14.1
9.0 6:40	10.8	11.3	11.9	12.4	12.9	13.5	14.0	14.6	15.1	15.7
10.0 6:00	12.1	12.7	13.3	13.9	14.5	15.1	15.7	16.4	17.0	17.6
11.0 5:28	13.3	14.0	14.6	15.3	16.0	16.7	17.3	18.0	18.7	19.4
12.0 5:00	14.5	15.2	16.0	16.7	17.4	18.2	18.9	19.7	20.4	21.1
Sailing, small boat	2.7	2.9	3.0	3.1	3.3	3.4	3.5	3.7	3.8	3.9
Skating, ice (9 mph)	4.2	4.4	4.6	4.8	5.1	5.2	5.5	5.7	5.9	6.1
Skiing, cross-country										
(mph) (min/mile)										
2.5 24:00	5.0	5.2	5.5	5.7	6.0	6.2	6.5	6.7	7.0	7.2
4.0 15:00	6.5	6.8	7.2	7.5	7.8	8.2	8.5	8.8	9.2	9.5
5.0 12:00	7.7	8.0	8.4	8.8	9.2	9.6	10.0	10.4	10.8	11.1
Skiing, downhill	6.5	6.8	7.2	7.5	7.8	8.2	8.5	8.8	9.2	9.5
Soccer	5.9	6.2	6.6	6.9	7.2	7.5	7.8	8.1	8.4	8.7
Squash										
Normal	6.7	7.0	7.3	7.7	8.0	8.4	8.7	9.1	9.5	9.8
Competition	7.7	8.0	8.4	8.8	9.2	9.6	10.0	10.4	10.8	11.1
Swimming (yards/min)										
Backstroke										
25	2.5	2.6	2.8	2.9	3.0	3.1	3.3	3.4	3.5	3.7
30	3.5	3.7	3.9	4.1	4.2	4.4	4.6	4.8	4.9	5.1
35	4.5	4.7	5.0	5.2	5.4	5.6	5.9	6.1	6.3	6.6
40	5.5	5.8	6.1	6.4	6.6	6.9	7.2	7.5	7.8	8.0
Breaststroke										
20	3.1	3.3	3.5	3.6	3.8	4.0	4.1	4.3	4.5	4.6
30	4.7	5.0	5.2	5.4	5.7	5.9	6.2	6.4	6.7	6.9
40	6.3	6.7	7.0	7.3	7.6	8.0	8.3	8.6	8.9	9.3
Front crawl										
20	3.1	3.3	3.5	3.6	3.8	4.0	4.1	4.3	4.5	4.6
25	4.0	4.2	4.4	4.6	4.8	5.0	5.2	5.4	5.6	5.8
35	4.8	5.1	5.4	5.6	5.9	6.1	6.4	6.6	6.8	7.0
45	5.7	6.0	6.3	6.6	6.9	7.2	7.5	7.8	8.1	8.4
50	7.0	7.4	7.7	8.1	8.5	8.8	9.2	9.5	9.9	10.3

68 150	70 155	73 160	75 165	77 170	80 175	82 180	84 185	86 190	89 195	91 200	93 205	95 210	98 215	100 220
10.0	10.4	10.7	11.0	11.4	11.7	12.1	12.4	12.7	13.1	13.4	13.8	14.1	14.4	14.8
2.9	3.0	3.1	3.2	3.3	3.4	3.5	3.6	3.7	3.8	3.9	4.0	4.1	4.2	4.3
4.1	4.2	4.4	4.5	4.6	4.8	4.9	5.0	5.2	5.3	5.4	5.6	5.7	5.9	6.0
6.4	6.6	6.8	7.0	7.2	7.4	7.6	7.9	8.1	8.3	8.5	8.7	8.9	9.1	9.4
8.7	9.0	9.3	9.5	9.8	10.1	10.4	10.7	11.0	11.3	11.6	11.9	12.2	12.5	12.8
3.8	3.9	4.0	4.2	4.3	4.4	4.5	4.7	4.8	4.9	5.2	5.2	5.3	5.4	5.6
12.8	13.2	13.6	14.1	14.5	14.9	15.4	15.8	16.2	16.6	17.1	17.5	17.9	18.4	18.8
12.8	13.2	13.6	14.1	14.5	14.9	15.4	15.8	16.2	16.6	17.1	17.5	17.9	18.4	18.8
9.8	10.2	10.5	10.8	11.2	11.5	11.8	12.1	12.5	12.8	13.1	13.5	13.8	14.1	14.5
8.7	9.0	9.3	9.5	9.8	10.1	10.4	10.7	11.0	11.2	11.6	11.9	12.2	12.5	12.8
2.2	2.3	2.4	2.5	2.6	2.6	2.7	2.8	2.9	2.9	3.0	3.1	3.2	3.2	3.3
9.8	10.1	10.4	10.7	11.1	11.4	11.7	12.0	12.4	12.7	13.0	13.4	13.7	14.0	14.4
6.4	6.6	6.8	7.0	7.2	7.4	7.6	7.9	8.1	8.3	8.5	8.7	8.9	9.1	9.4
9.1	9.4	9.7	10.0	10.3	10.6	10.9	11.2	11.6	11.9	12.2	12.5	12.8	13.1	13.4
10.0	10.4	10.7	11.1	11.4	11.7	12.1	12.4	12.8	13.1	13.4	13.8	14.1	14.5	14.8
10.9	11.3	11.7	12.0	12.4	12.8	13.1	13.5	13.8	14.3	14.6	15.0	15.4	15.7	16.1
12.8	13.2	13.6	14.1	14.5	14.9	15.4	15.8	16.2	16.6	17.1	17.5	17.9	18.4	18.8
14.6	15.1	15.6	16.1	16.6	17.1	17.6	18.1	18.5	19.0	18.5	20.0	20.5	21.0	21.5
16.2	16.8	17.3	17.9	18.4	19.0	19.5	20.1	20.6	21.2	21.7	22.2	22.8	23.3	23.9
18.2	18.8	19.4	20.0	20.7	21.3	21.9	22.5	23.1	23.7	24.2	24.8	25.4	26.0	26.7
20.0	20.7	21.4	22.1	22.7	23.4	24.1	24.8	25.4	26.1	26.8	27.5	28.1	28.8	29.5
21.9	22.6	23.3	24.1	24.8	25.6	26.3	27.0	27.8	28.5	29.2	30.0	30.7	31.5	32.2
4.1	4.2	4.4	4.5	4.6	4.8	4.9	5.0	5.2	5.3	5.4	5.6	5.7	5.9	6.0
6.4	6.6	6.8	7.0	7.2	7.4	7.6	7.9	8.1	8.3	8.5	8.7	8.9	9.1	9.4
7.5	7.8	8.0	8.3	8.5	8.8	9.0	9.3	9.5	9.8	10.0	10.3	10.6	10.8	11.1
9.9	10.2	10.5	10.9	11.2	11.5	11.9	12.2	12.5	12.9	13.2	13.5	13.8	14.2	14.5
11.5	11.9	12.3	12.7	13.1	13.5	13.9	14.3	13.7	15.0	15.4	15.8	16.2	16.6	17.0
9.9	10.2	10.5	10.9	11.2	11.5	11.9	12.2	12.5	12.9	13.2	13.5	13.8	14.2	14.5
9.0	9.3	9.6	9.9	10.2	10.5	10.8	11.1	11.4	11.7	12.0	12.3	12.6	12.9	13.2
10.1	10.5	10.8	11.2	11.5	11.8	12.2	12.5	12.9	13.2	13.5	13.9	14.2	14.6	14.9
11.5	11.9	12.3	12.7	13.1	13.5	13.9	14.3	14.7	15.0	15.4	15.8	16.2	16.6	17.0
3.8	3.9	4.0	4.2	4.3	4.4	4.5	4.7	4.8	4.9	5.1	5.2	5.3	5.4	5.6
5.3	5.5	5.6	5.8	6.0	6.2	6.4	6.5	6.7	6.9	7.1	7.2	7.4	7.6	7.8
6.8	7.0	7.3	7.5	7.7	7.9	8.2	8.4	8.6	8.9	9.1	9.3	9.5	9.8	10.0
8.3	8.6	8.9	9.2	9.4	9.7	10.0	10.3	10.6	10.8	11.1	11.4	11.7	12.0	12.2
4.8	4.9	5.1	5.3	5.4	5.6	5.7	5.9	6.0	6.2	6.4	6.5	6.7	6.9	7.0
7.1	7.4	7.6	7.9	8.1	8.3	8.6	8.8	9.1	9.3	9.5	9.8	10.0	10.3	10.5
9.6	9.9	10.2	10.5	10.9	11.2	11.5	11.9	12.2	12.5	12.8	13.1	13.5	13.8	14.1
4.8	4.9	5.1	5.3	5.4	5.6	5.7	5.9	6.0	6.2	6.4	6.5	6.7	6.9	7.0
6.0	6.2	6.4	6.6	6.8	7.0	7.2	7.4	7.6	7.8	8.0	8.2	8.4	8.6	8.8
7.3	7.5	7.8	8.0	8.3	8.5	8.8	9.0	9.2	9.4	9.7	9.9	10.2	10.4	10.7
8.7	9.0	9.3	9.5	9.8	10.1	10.4	10.7	11.0	11.3	11.6	11.9	12.2	12.5	12.8
10.6	11.0	11.3	11.7	12.0	12.4	12.8	13.1	13.5	13.8	14.2	14.5	14.9	15.2	15.6

Table continued on following page

TABLE 39–1 *Continued*
Caloric Expenditure for Various Physical Activities

Body Weight (Continued)

Kg Pounds	45 100	48 105	50 110	52 115	55 120	57 125	59 130	61 135	64 140	66 145
Table tennis	3.4	3.6	3.8	4.0	4.1	4.3	4.5	4.7	4.8	5.0
Tennis										
Singles, recreational	5.0	5.2	5.5	5.7	6.0	6.2	6.5	6.7	7.0	7.2
Doubles, recreational	3.4	3.6	3.8	4.0	4.1	4.3	4.5	4.7	4.8	5.0
Competition	6.4	6.7	7.1	7.4	7.7	8.1	8.4	8.7	9.1	9.4
Volleyball										
Moderate, recreational	2.9	3.0	3.2	3.3	3.5	3.6	3.8	3.9	4.1	4.2
Vigorous, competition	6.5	6.8	7.1	7.5	7.8	8.1	8.4	8.8	9.1	9.4
Walking										
(mph) (min/mile)										
1.0 60:00	1.5	1.6	1.7	1.8	1.8	1.9	2.0	2.1	2.2	2.2
2.0 30:00	2.1	2.2	2.3	2.4	2.5	2.6	2.8	2.9	3.0	3.1
2.3 26:00	2.3	2.4	2.5	2.7	2.8	2.9	3.0	3.1	3.2	3.4
3.0 20:00	2.7	2.9	3.0	3.1	3.3	3.4	3.5	3.7	3.8	3.9
3.2 18:45	3.1	3.3	3.4	3.6	3.8	4.0	4.1	4.3	4.4	4.5
3.5 17:10	3.3	3.5	3.7	3.9	4.0	4.2	4.4	4.6	4.7	4.9
4.0 15:00	4.2	4.4	4.6	4.8	5.1	5.3	5.5	5.7	5.9	6.1
4.5 13:20	4.7	5.0	5.2	5.4	5.7	5.9	6.2	6.4	6.7	6.9
5.0 12:00	5.4	5.7	6.0	6.3	6.5	6.8	7.1	7.4	7.7	7.9
5.4 11:10	6.2	6.6	6.9	7.2	7.5	7.9	8.2	8.5	8.8	9.2
5.8 10:20	7.7	8.0	8.4	8.8	9.2	9.6	10.0	10.4	10.8	11.1
Water skiing	5.0	5.2	5.5	5.7	6.0	6.2	6.5	6.7	7.0	7.2
Weight training	5.2	5.4	5.7	6.0	6.2	6.5	6.8	7.0	7.3	7.6
Wrestling	8.5	8.9	9.3	9.8	10.2	10.6	11.0	11.5	11.9	12.3

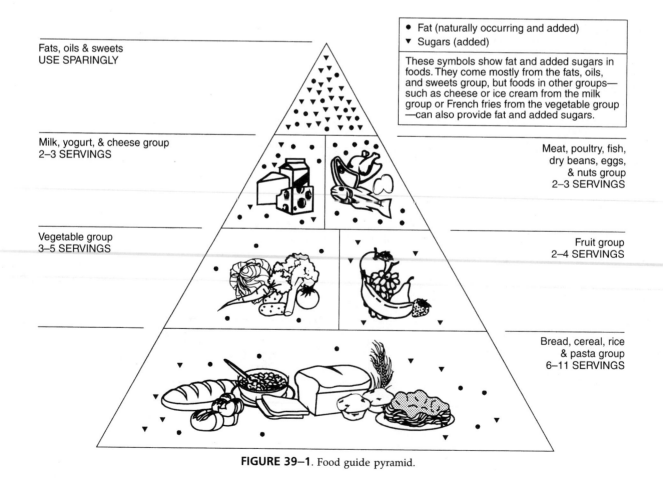

FIGURE 39–1. Food guide pyramid.

68 150	70 155	73 160	75 165	77 170	80 175	82 180	84 185	86 190	89 195	91 200	93 205	95 210	98 215	100 220
5.2	5.4	5.5	5.7	5.9	6.1	6.3	6.4	6.6	6.8	7.0	7.1	7.3	7.5	7.7
7.5	7.8	8.0	8.3	8.5	8.8	9.0	9.3	9.5	9.8	10.0	10.3	10.6	10.8	11.1
5.2	5.4	5.5	5.7	5.9	6.1	6.3	6.4	6.6	6.8	7.0	7.1	7.3	7.5	7.7
9.8	10.1	10.4	10.8	11.1	11.4	11.8	12.1	12.4	12.8	13.1	13.4	13.7	14.1	14.4
4.4	4.5	4.7	4.8	5.0	5.1	5.3	5.4	5.6	5.7	5.9	6.0	6.1	6.3	6.4
9.8	10.1	10.4	10.7	11.1	11.4	11.7	12.0	12.4	12.7	13.0	13.4	13.7	14.0	14.4
2.3	2.4	2.4	2.5	2.6	2.7	2.8	2.9	2.9	3.0	3.1	3.2	3.2	3.3	3.4
3.2	3.3	3.4	3.5	3.6	3.7	3.9	4.0	4.1	4.2	4.3	4.4	4.5	4.6	4.7
3.5	3.6	3.7	3.8	4.0	4.1	4.2	4.3	4.4	4.5	4.7	4.8	4.9	5.0	5.1
4.1	4.2	4.4	4.5	4.6	4.8	4.9	5.0	5.2	5.3	5.4	5.6	5.7	5.9	6.0
4.7	4.8	5.0	5.2	5.3	5.5	5.6	5.8	5.9	6.1	6.3	6.4	6.6	6.8	6.9
5.1	5.3	5.4	5.6	5.8	6.0	6.2	6.3	6.5	6.7	6.9	7.0	7.2	7.4	7.6
6.4	6.6	6.8	7.0	7.2	7.4	7.6	7.9	8.1	8.3	8.5	8.7	8.9	9.1	9.4
7.1	7.4	7.6	7.9	8.1	8.3	8.6	8.8	9.1	9.3	9.5	9.8	10.0	10.3	10.5
8.2	8.4	8.7	9.0	9.2	9.5	9.8	10.1	10.4	10.6	10.9	11.2	11.5	11.8	12.0
9.5	9.8	10.1	10.4	10.8	11.1	11.4	11.8	12.1	12.4	12.7	13.0	13.4	13.7	14.0
11.5	11.9	12.3	12.7	13.1	13.5	13.9	14.3	14.7	15.0	15.4	15.8	16.2	16.6	17.0
7.5	7.8	8.0	8.3	8.5	8.8	9.0	9.3	9.5	9.8	10.0	10.3	10.6	10.8	11.1
7.8	8.1	8.3	8.6	8.9	9.1	9.4	9.7	9.9	10.2	10.5	10.7	11.0	11.2	11.5
12.8	13.2	13.6	14.1	14.5	14.9	15.4	15.8	16.2	16.6	17.1	17.5	17.9	18.4	18.8

acids and increased breakdown of protein are two factors contributing to the increased protein requirement in endurance athletes.[11] Protein intakes for endurance athletes range from 1.0 to 1.5 g/kg of body weight.[11,12] Some research indicates that an intake of 2 g/kg of body weight/day may be required by some endurance athletes. These recommended levels of protein intake are based on an energy intake that is equal to energy expenditure and can be obtained readily in a well-balanced diet.[13]

Laritcheva et al.[14] demonstrate that protein intake less than 2 g/kg/d in some champion weightlifters was associated with a negative nitrogen balance during intensive training. This intake was adequate, however, when the athletes were not training intensively.

It is unlikely that amino-acid oxidation plays an important role in providing energy for strength training because, although it may be intense, each bout is brief. Also, weight training may actually improve the efficiency of protein utilization.[8] Carbohydrate in the form of glycogen is the major fuel for strength activities.

Most research on the actual protein intake of athletes in developed countries reveals that the average athlete consumes protein in the highest recommended range.[15] Those at highest risk of consuming inadequate protein are individuals who already have elevated protein requirements for reasons other than sports; those who consume inadequate calories; and those who participate in multiple daily training sessions. Protein needs can be calculated both as a percentage of total energy and on a per kilogram body weight basis. For athletes with exceptionally high energy intakes, providing 12 to 15 percent of total energy from protein may be excessive. When energy intake is low, as may be observed for many young women or in low–body weight athletes, protein needs calculated as a percentage of energy may be inadequate. In both of these cases, 1.0 to 1.5 g protein per kilogram body weight may be a more appropriate guide for intake than protein as a percentage of total energy.[16]

Table 39–5 lists dietary sources of proteins. To add 1 lb of muscle per week, an additional 100 g of protein would be needed in the diet.[17] One hundred g of protein in a week is 14 g protein per day, which is obtained in 2 oz of high biologic value protein such as meat, poultry, fish, cheese, or 2 cups of milk or yogurt. Extra protein is not preferentially laid down as muscle mass. Extra protein is used as an energy source if calories and carbohydrate are inadequate, stored as fat if the protein is in excess of calorie needs, or used for its primary and structural roles (formation of tissues, hormones and antibodies; maintenance of water and acid-based balance; and control of blood-clotting processes). For discussion on the use of amino acid supplementation, see Chapter 15.

SPECIAL CONSIDERATIONS. In females, one potential problem with consuming excessive protein is research has shown that increasing dietary protein leads to elevated calcium excretion.[18,19] A high-protein diet combined with a low intake of calcium can, over time, lead to osteoporosis. Most studies have been done

TABLE 39–2
Recommended Dietary Allowances,[a] Revised 1989

Category	Age (years), or Condition	Weight[b] (kg)	(lb)	Height[b] (cm)	(in)	Protein (g)	Fat-Soluble Vitamins Vitamin A (μg RE)[c]	Vitamin D (μg)[d]	Vitamin E (mg α-TE)[e]	Vitamin K (μg)
Infants	0.0–0.5	6	13	60	24	13	375	7.5	3	5
	0.5–1.0	9	20	71	28	14	375	10	4	10
Children	1–3	13	29	90	35	16	400	10	6	15
	4–6	20	44	112	44	24	500	10	7	20
	7–10	28	62	132	52	28	700	10	7	30
Males	11–14	45	99	157	62	45	1,000	10	10	45
	15–18	66	145	176	69	59	1,000	10	10	65
	19–24	72	160	177	70	58	1,000	10	10	70
	25–50	79	174	176	70	63	1,000	5	10	80
	51+	77	170	173	68	63	1,000	5	10	80
Females	11–14	46	101	157	62	46	800	10	8	45
	15–18	55	120	163	64	44	800	10	8	55
	19–24	58	128	164	65	46	800	10	8	60
	25–50	63	138	163	64	50	800	5	8	65
	51+	65	143	160	63	50	800	5	8	65
Pregnant						60	800	10	10	65
Lactating	1st 6 months					65	1,300	10	12	65
	2nd 6 months					62	1,200	10	11	65

[a]The allowances, expressed as average daily intakes over time, are intended to provide for individual variations among most normal persons as they live in the United States under usual environmental stresses. Diets should be based on a variety of common foods in order to provide other nutrients for which human requirements have been less well defined. See text for detailed discussion of allowances and of nutrients not tabulated.

[b]Weights and heights of Reference Adults are actual medians for the U.S. population of the designated age, as reported by NHANES II. The median weights and heights of those under 19 years of age were taken from Hammill et al. (1979) (see pages 16–17). The use of these figures does not imply that the height-to-weight ratios are ideal.

[c]Retinol equivalents. 1 retinol equivalent = 1 μg retinol or 6 μg β-carotene. See text for calculation of vitamin A activity of diets and retinol equivalents.

on sedentary females, and more research is needed on athletes to determine the role of exercise, dietary protein, and calcium in the development and prevention of osteoporosis in athletes.

The metabolism of protein requires more water than carbohydrate or fat metabolism. As dietary protein increases, increased water intake is recommended to minimize dehydration.

VEGETARIAN DIETS AND PROTEIN. Vegetarian diets are divided into four categories: vegan, or only plant products; lacto, plant products and dairy products but no eggs; lacto-ovo, plant and dairy products and eggs; and partial vegetarian, including all of the preceding plus poultry and fish but no other animal products. Table 39–6 lists vegetarian food sources for important nutrients.

Plant sources of protein alone can provide adequate amounts of essential amino acids. Whole grains, legumes, vegetables, seeds and nuts all contain essential amino acids. It was once thought that vegetarian sources of protein needed to be consciously combined in order for the vegetarian to meet his or her protein needs. For example, legumes that are low in the amino acid methionine but high in the amino acid lysine need to be eaten with grains high in the amino acid methionine but low in lysine, but most vegetarian diets provide adequate protein without conscious food combining.[20] Athletes who are striving for a high-carbohydrate (60–70 percent), low-fat, and moderate protein diet can benefit from a well-planned vegetarian diet. Table 39–7 provides a daily food guide for planning a vegetarian diet, and Figure 39–2 is a sample lacto-vegetarian menu.

CARBOHYDRATES

Carbohydrates are the body's preferred source of energy and are used to spare protein for body growth and repair. The body has limited ability to store carbohydrates. The predominant method of storage is in the form of glycogen, an intracellular polysaccharide. Glycogen is stored in the liver and muscle. The liver's glycogen storage is used to maintain blood glucose levels, whereas muscle glycogen is used by the muscle for energy. An athlete's performance—greater endurance and delayed fatigue—can be maximized by ensuring greater energy reserve in the form of muscle glycogen for endurance and strength activities. Muscle glycogen is the preferred carbohydrate fuel for endurance activities such as marathon running, cross-country skiing, distance cycling, and swimming, which require greater than 65 percent VO$_2$ max.[21,22] Muscle glycogen

Water-Soluble Vitamins							Minerals						
Vita-min C (mg)	Thia-min (mg)	Ribo-flavin (mg)	Niacin (mg NE)	Vita-min B_6 (mg)	Folate (μg)	Vita-min B_{12} (μg)	Cal-cium (mg)	Phos-phorus (mg)	Magne-sium (mg)	Iron (mg)	Zinc (mg)	Iodine (μg)	Sele-nium (μg)
30	0.3	0.4	5	0.3	25	0.3	400	300	40	6	5	40	10
35	0.4	0.5	6	0.6	35	0.5	600	500	60	10	5	50	15
40	0.7	0.8	9	1.0	50	0.7	800	800	80	10	10	70	20
45	0.9	1.1	12	1.1	75	1.0	800	800	120	10	10	90	20
45	1.0	1.2	13	1.4	100	1.4	800	800	170	10	10	120	30
50	1.3	1.5	17	1.7	150	2.0	1,200	1,200	270	12	15	150	40
60	1.5	1.8	20	2.0	200	2.0	1,200	1,200	400	12	15	150	50
60	1.5	1.7	19	2.0	200	2.0	1,200	1,200	350	10	15	150	70
60	1.5	1.7	19	2.0	200	2.0	800	800	350	10	15	150	70
60	1.2	1.4	15	2.0	200	2.0	800	800	350	10	15	150	70
50	1.1	1.3	15	1.4	150	2.0	1,200	1,200	280	15	12	150	45
60	1.1	1.3	15	1.5	180	2.0	1,200	1,200	300	15	12	150	50
60	1.1	1.3	15	1.6	180	2.0	1,200	1,200	280	15	12	150	55
60	1.1	1.3	15	1.6	180	2.0	800	800	280	15	12	150	55
60	1.0	1.2	13	1.6	180	2.0	800	800	280	10	12	150	55
70	1.5	1.6	17	2.2	400	2.2	1,200	1,200	300	30	15	175	65
95	1.6	1.8	20	2.1	280	2.6	1,200	1,200	355	15	19	200	75
90	1.6	1.7	20	2.1	260	2.6	1,200	1,200	340	15	16	200	75

[d]As cholecalciferol. 10 μg cholecalciferol = 400 ɪᴜ of vitamin D.

[e]α-Tocopherol equivalents. 1 mg *d*-α-tocopherol = 1 α-ᴛᴇ. See text for variation in allowances and calculation of vitamin E activity of the diet as α-tocopherol equivalents.

[f]1 ɴᴇ (niacin equivalent) is equal to 1 mg of niacin or 60 mg of dietary tryptophan.

Reprinted with permission from Recommended Dietary Allowances: 10th edition. Copyright 1959 by the National Academy of Sciences. Courtesy of the National Academy Press, Washington, D.C.

stores represent about 1500 kcal of carbohydrate, whereas liver stores represent about 320 kcal of carbohydrate, and a smaller amount of carbohydrate in the form of glucose is found in the blood.

High-intensity, short-duration exercise (sprinting) relies on the anaerobic pathway for the production energy. Only glucose derived primarily from the breakdown of muscle glycogen can be used as fuel. Muscle glycogen is used about 18 times faster when glucose is broken down anaerobically than when glucose is broken down aerobically. During high-intensity exercise (more than 70 percent of aerobic capacity) and in extended mixed anaerobic and aerobic sports (such as soccer, basketball, football drills, and interval running or swimming) the anaerobic pathway is also used. A more rapid rate of muscle glycogen breakdown occurs in these events.

Exercise of low-to-moderate intensity is fueled almost entirely aerobically. Increased epinephrine, norepinephrine, and growth hormone and decreased insulin promote the release of fatty acids from the adipose tissue into the bloodstream. Half of the energy is supplied by these fatty acids, while muscle glycogen and blood glucose supply the rest for this type of event. However, muscle glycogen is the predominant fuel for most types of exercise.

It is extremely important that endurance athletes (triathletes, cyclists, marathon runners) consume a high-carbohydrate diet since one of the limiting factors in prolonged performance is glycogen depletion. Trained muscles have a large capacity to store glycogen. The recommended "sports diet" contains 60 to 70 percent of total calories as carbohydrate and should be consistently maintained. An athlete needs 3 to 5 g of carbohydrate per pound of body weight, depending whether he or she is moderately or extremely active.[23] Therefore, a 150 lb person would need between 450 and 600 g of carbohydrate per day.

The training and diet regimen termed *modified carbohydrate loading* is used to maximize glycogen storage and has been accepted since the 1980s, when it was recognized that the original carbohydrate-loading scheme, which involved a carbohydrate-depletion phase, resulted in a diminished ability to train before the competitive event and introduced potential health risks. Athletes who train exhaustively on successive days or who compete in prolonged endurance events (90 minutes or longer) should consume a diet that provides 65 to 70 percent of total Calories as carbohydrate. The athlete should include at least 3 days of intake that includes 800 g of carbohydrate per day (or 6 to 10 g of carbohydrate per kilogram of body weight

TABLE 39–3
Stages of Change

Stage	Description	Intervention at This Stage
Precontemplation	Athlete unaware of, denies, or minimizes the problem or need to make a change	Provide personalized information, allow athlete to express emotions or feelings
Contemplation	Aware of the problem but weighing costs/benefits of change	Encourage support networks; give positive feedback about athlete's abilities to make the change; clarify notions, misconceptions, i.e., carbohydrates are *not* fattening; emphasize expected benefits
Preparation/motivation	Decision to make change, plans to do so within the next month	Encourage athlete to set specific, achievable goals; reinforce small changes that athlete may have already achieved
Action	Plan is in progress, attitudinal/behavioral changes have begun	Refer to an education program for behavioral skill training and to learn tools and techniques to implement goals; set, implement, and evaluate goals
Maintenance/relapse	Action plan maintained over 6 consecutive months; high rate of relapse before 6 months	Encourage athlete to anticipate and plan for potential difficulties; if a lapse or relapse occurs, go back to previous stage(s); do not assume that initial action means permanent change; do not be discouraged or judgmental about a lapse or relapse

ACTION STRATEGIES

COMMON PROFILE OF MANY ATHLETES

1. Skipping meals, most commonly the preworkout meal
2. Consuming 50–70% of total calories in the evening
3. Consuming greater than 30% of calories from fat

GUIDELINES

1. REDISTRIBUTING CALORIES THROUGHOUT THE DAY:
   To keep blood glucose even and prevent hypoglycemia, which results in fatigue, shakiness, or irritability the athlete should eat small, frequent meals or snacks every 3–4 hours. If this is not possible, fruit, fruit juice, or a 6–8% carbohydrate solution should be consumed during workout to avoid hypoglycemia.

EXAMPLE

Breakfast	7:00 am
Snack	10:30 am
Lunch	1:00 pm
Snack	4:00 pm
Dinner	7:00 pm
Snack	Optional

MORNING WORKOUT

- Encourage small snack (examples: fruit or yogurt, foods that do not cause discomfort) during the workout or of fruit juice if the athlete prefers workout on an empty stomach

AFTERNOON WORKOUT

- Encourage consumption of full breakfast which includes a protein source, a low-fat, low protein lunch, a carbohydrate mid-afternoon snack and after working out, a high carbohydrate dinner with moderate protein.

EVENING WORKOUT (AFTER 7:00 PM)

- Lunch should be the main meal of the day, providing daily protein, carbohydrate and fat. A high carbohydrate, no or low-fat dinner should be consumed about 2 hours before working out.

2. SELF-MONITORING
   Eating is often subjective and is regulated by external forces such as time of day, mood, stress, social activities, workout schedule, etc. Maintenance of a food diary will assist athletes in observation of their habits to assess the value of their food intake. From the diary, actions can be planned, goals set, and changes implemented. The diary may then be used by a dietitian for analysis of food intake.

DATE	TIME	FOOD	AMOUNT	FAT	CARBOHYDRATE	PROTEIN	BEVERAGE	WORKOUT

TABLE 39–4
Balancing the Sports Diet*

Nutrient	Calories†	Sports Diet (%)
Carbohydrate	4 calories	60–70
Protein	4 calories	15–20
Fat	9 calories	15–20

*Recommended distribution of macronutrients for an athlete.
†Calories per gram of nutrient.

per day) and a week of tapered workouts that ends in complete rest the day before competition.[16] Training is altered as follows:[23]

Day 3 (before the event)	Exercise 20 minutes only
Day 2 (before)	Exercise 20 minutes only
Day 1 (day before)	Rest
Event Day	

This dietary protocol maintains high glycogen stores and may be followed numerous times throughout the year without health risk.[16] If an athlete adheres to a high-carbohydrate diet but does not train to develop muscle strength and endurance, there will be a limited capacity to store glycogen. However, reducing exercise 2 days before the event and resting the day before allows the muscles the opportunity to replace depleted glycogen stores. Rest is an essential part of carbohydrate loading.

FAT

Dietary fat provides essential fatty acids and is necessary for absorption of fat-soluble vitamins. It is an energy source that provides flavor and meal satiety. Fat in food converts more efficiently to body fat than other macronutrients.

The degree to which fats are used as fuel during exercise is determined by exercise intensity and duration, diet, endurance training history, and altered metabolic state.[24] Fatty acid metabolism requires more oxygen than carbohydrate metabolism. Low-intensity exercise ($<50\%$ VO_2 max) may rely extensively on free fatty acids for fuel. As exercise intensity increases, there is a greater requirement for glucose as fuel. Blood glucose and muscle and liver glycogen are the primary fuels when energy is needed rapidly.

Aerobic training increases the cell's mitochondria and enzymes involved in fatty acid oxidation, thereby enhancing the athlete's ability to burn fat as fuel efficiently. This increased ability is demonstrated in four distinct ways:[24] a more efficient use of oxygen; more oxygen can be used at a given work load; less glycogen and more fat used to meet energy needs; and lower lactate production, representing more complete oxidation—improved oxygen use of energy substrates. Training increases the rate of fat utilization by changing the oxidative potential of the muscle.

The body's need for dietary fat is only about 3 to 10 g per day (<10 percent of total calories). Americans, however, consume 34 to 37 percent of total calories as fat. Most healthy people have sufficient stores of body fat. The average 150-lb person with 10 to 20 percent

TABLE 39–5
Protein Sources*

Type	Nutritional Breakdown	Food Sources
Lean sources, serving size 1 oz	55 cal, 0 g CHO, 7 g protein, 3 g fat	Lean beef and pork Fish Poultry without skin
Medium-fat sources, serving size 1 oz (or otherwise noted)	75 cal, 0 g CHO, 7 g protein, 5 g fat	Ground beef Skim/part skim mozzarella, ricotta 4 oz tofu 1 egg
High-fat sources, serving size 1 oz (or otherwise noted)	100 cal, 0 g CHO, 7 g protein, 8 g fat	Corned beef, spare ribs, cheese (cheddar, Swiss), cold cuts 1 hot dog 1 Tbsp peanut butter
Dairy, non-fat	90–150 cal, 12 g CHO, 8 g protein, 0 g fat	8 oz skim milk Non-fat yogurt
Dairy, low-fat, 1–2%	90–150 cal, 12 g CHO, 8 g protein, 3–5 g fat	8 oz 1–2% milk Plain low-fat yogurt, 1–2%
Dairy, high-fat	90–150 cal, 12 g CHO, 8 g protein, 8 g fat	8 oz whole milk
Vegetables Fruits and fat contain no protein	25 cal, 5 g CHO, 2 g protein, 0 g fat	1/2 c cooked or 1 c raw

Adapted from the American Dietetic Association exchange list.
Cal = calories; CHO = carbohydrate; c = cup; g = gram; oz = ounce; tbsp = tablespoon.

TABLE 39–6
Vegetarian Nutrition: Food Sources of Important Nutrients

Nutrient	Rationale	Food Sources	
		Animal	Plant
Protein: amino acids	In 1988 the American Dietetic Association stated that although plant foods contain less of the essential amino acids than equivalent quantities of animal food, a vegetarian diet provides adequate amounts of amino acids when a variety of foods are eaten over the course of the day, not necessarily within each given meal. Mixtures of proteins from grains, vegetables, legumes, seeds, and nuts eaten over the course of the day compliment one another in their amino acid profiles without the necessity of precise planning and complimentation of proteins within each meal.	Meat Poultry Fish Eggs Low-fat dairy products	Dried beans, peas, lentils Grains Tofu/Tempeh Soy milk Nuts & seeds Whole grain breads & cereals Starchy vegetables
Vitamin B_{12}	This vitamin is found primarily in animal products. Plants do not produce or contain B_{12}, so vegetarians who do not eat eggs or dairy products could develop a deficiency. Since the human body has several years' store of B_{12}, and actual requirements of B_{12} are so miniscule, the vitamin deficiency is rare among vegetarians. It is recommended that strict vegetarians who regularly avoid dairy products, eggs, or fortified foods take a non–animal derived supplement at least 3 times a week, since a vitamin B_{12} deficiency can lead to serious neurological damage.	Meat Poultry Fish Eggs Low-fat dairy products	B-12 Fortified breakfast cereals Bread & pasta B_{12} fortified soy milk Some brands of nutritional yeast (e.g., Red Star T-6635)
Calcium	Major dietary source is milk and milk products. Since lacto-ovo vegetarians include dairy products in their diet, they are easily able to meet their nutrient requirements. For strict vegetarians, it can be more difficult to fulfill their requirement. However, with proper planning and variety, calcium needs can be adequately met. Because vegetarians consume less protein than non-vegetarians, they absorb more calcium, since an excess intake of protein causes the body to excrete calcium through the urine. Vegetarians may consider taking a supplement to ensure they are getting enough calcium.	Low-fat dairy products Salmon & sardines with bones	Cooked, dark leafy greens Firm tofu/tempeh Calcium-fortified soy milk Cooked broccoli; cooked white beans Rhubarb Figs
Iron	Plant foods contain less iron than does meat and the iron in plants is not as easily absorbed by the body. Calcium can interfere with the absorption of iron by the body. Save calcium supplements for between meals or bedtime. Tea and coffee hamper absorption of iron. Limit caffeine for 1 hour before or after meals. Vegetarians can dramatically increase their absorption of iron by adding vitamin C–rich foods or beverages to their meals (e.g., citrus fruit or juices, tomatoes, broccoli). Cooking food in iron cookware also adds to iron intake.	Organ meats Meat Poultry Fish Shellfish Egg yolk	Firm tofu Dried beans Dark, leafy greens Whole grain & enriched breads, cereals, pasta Bulgur Black strap molasses Prune juice Dried fruits
Riboflavin	Major dietary source is dairy products. Include a variety of foods containing riboflavin. The more restrictive diets should include products fortified with riboflavin.	Low-fat dairy products Red meat Eggs	Whole grains Fortified cereals Broccoli Dark leafy greens Winter squash Fresh mushrooms
Zinc	There are a variety of plant sources of zinc. Choosing a variety of zinc-containing foods helps ensure adequate intake.	Oysters Meat Eggs Poultry Seafood	Wheat germ Firm tofu Legumes Cooked spinach; cooked broccoli Whole grain breads & cereals
Vitamin D	Major dietary source is dairy products. The more restrictive diets should include products fortified with vitamin D, such as soy milk.	Low-fat, fortified milk products Fish oils Eggs	Low-fat, fortified soy milk Vitamin D-fortified margarines Sunlight

From the Massachusetts General Hospital Department of Dietetics.

TABLE 39–7
An Introduction to Vegetarian Food Groups: Daily Food Guide for Vegetarian Diets

Food Group	Number of Servings/Day	One Serving Equivalent
Bread, grains, cereal, pasta, & starchy vegetables	6–11 servings/day Include whole grain products for trace minerals and fiber	1 slice whole grain bread 1/2 bagel, corn tortilla (6"), bread sticks (2) 1/2 cup cooked whole grains (hot cereal, rice, bulgur, couscous, kasha, quinoa, barley, pasta) 1 oz ready-to-eat cereal 1/2 cup starchy vegetables (corn, peas, lima beans, potatoes, winter squash) 3 cups air-popped popcorn 4–6 crackers, whole grain, low fat 1 oz pretzels, whole grain 1 oz tortilla chips, no oil
Dried beans, tofu, eggs, nuts, seeds	3–5 servings/day dried beans, tofu, tempeh Limit egg yolks to 2–3 per week Peanut butter, nuts, seeds—use sparingly owing to high fat content	1/2 cup cooked beans (black, garbanzo, pinto, kidney, Great Northern) 1/2 cup cooked split peas, lentils, black-eyed peas 4 oz tofu/tempeh 1 whole egg, 2 egg whites 2 Tbsp. peanut butter 1/4 cup nuts, seeds (almonds, walnuts, sunflower, pumpkin)
Fruits, vegetables	5–9 servings/day Include one good source of vitamin C at each meal (e.g, citrus, tomatoes, red peppers). Include at least one good source of betacarotene daily—deep green and dark orange fruits and vegetables (e.g., carrots, apricots, dark green leafy vegetables, spinach)	1/2 cup cooked vegetables 1 cup raw vegetables 1/2 cup chopped, cooked or canned fruit 1 medium whole fruit 1/2 cup fruit juice 3/4 cup vegetable juice
Milk, yogurt, cheese	2–3 servings/day	1 cup milk, buttermilk, skim or 1% fat 1 cup yogurt, low fat or nonfat 1 oz cheese, low fat or fat-free 1/2 cup cottage cheese, 1% low fat or fat-free
Fats, oils, sweets	As appropriate for additional calories and essential fatty acids	1 tsp. oil, butter, margarine, mayonnaise 1 Tbsp. diet margarine, reduced calorie mayonnaise, salad dressing (oil based) 2 Tbsp. reduced calorie salad dressing 1 Tbsp. jam, jelly, all-fruit spread

The key to all well-balanced vegetarian diets is planning and variety. The daily food guide preceding can be the basis for planning a nutritionally adequate vegetarian diet. The daily food guide is based on a lacto- or lacto-ovo vegetarian diet. A vegan or total vegetarian diet excludes milk, yogurt, cheese and eggs, and includes additional servings from each of the other groups with the inclusion of nutritional yeast or B_{12}-fortified products to ensure an adequate intake of vitamin B_{12}.
From Massachusetts General Hospital Department of Dietetics.

body fat stores has between 63,000 and 126,000 potential kcals as fat.[6] A high-fat diet limits the amount of carbohydrates stored, and since carbohydrates are necessary for the complete oxidation of fats, a high-fat diet may in fact reduce endurance.

Dietary sources of fat include added fats and hidden sources of fat. Examples of added fats are butter, margarine, oils, mayonnaise, and salad dressings. Fat found in meat, skin of poultry, nuts, seeds, and baked products are examples of hidden fats. Since fat consumed in amounts in excess of body needs is most likely to be stored in the form of adipose tissue, reducing total fat intake is one way to reduce total calories. Alcohol promotes fat storage;[25] therefore, it may be beneficial to count alcohol calories as part of the athlete's total fat allowance. Sources of dietary fat and calories from fat are listed in the box.

ALCOHOL

Although alcohol has a high caloric content (7 kcals/g), it has limited food value. Alcohol acts on the brain by depressing its ability to reason and make judgments. Information-related processes are slowed; fine-motor skills are decreased; reaction time is reduced; coordination, balance, and visual perception are altered; and muscular reflexes are impaired. Athletes involved in sports such as tennis and racquetball, which demand the athlete's rapid reflex response, are most affected.[26]

Alcohol can weaken the heart's pumping force[27] and diminish sprinting, middle-distance,[28] and endurance performance.[29] One of the most harmful effects of alcohol in an athletic event is evident in prolonged endurance contests. The liver is the primary organ for the detoxification of alcohol. Once alcohol is present in the blood, the metabolism of alcohol takes priority over other liver functions. An elevated level of blood alcohol may block the biochemical pathway that supplies extra glucose to the body. A drop in blood glucose during an endurance event could lead to early fatigue.

Peak concentration of alcohol in the blood occurs within 1 hour of consumption, depending on whether or not food is in the stomach. Since the absorbed alcohol is distributed within the water compartments of cells, it can disturb the water balance in muscle cells and consequently alter the cellular enzymatic activity producing ATP, the substrate that provides fuel for muscle contraction, active transport, and biosynthesis within the body.[26] Body size and composition alter dose/response; a small, lean athlete is likely to experience fatigue sooner than a larger person with more body fat.

MICRONUTRIENTS

The micronutrients are vitamins (Table 39–8) and minerals. Vitamins are complex organic compounds and exist in very small quantities in foods. The role of vitamins is in the action of several hundred enzymes that serve as catalysts to body function such as muscle contraction, digestion, absorption, and metabolism. The

A SAMPLE MENU	YOUR SAMPLE MENU
Breakfast 4 oz. orange juice 1 cup hot cereal 1 piece fresh fruit 1 tsp. margarine 4 oz. low-fat milk	**Breakfast**
Lunch 4 oz. apple juice 1 cup vegetarian chili 1 cup tossed salad 1 tbsp. Italian dressing 1 slice whole-grain bread 1 tsp. margarine	**Lunch**
Snack 1 piece fresh fruit	**Snack**
Dinner 1 cup pasta entree with vegetables (with 1 tbsp. oil) 4 oz. sauteed tofu **or** 1 cup bean soup 1 slice whole-grain bread 8 oz. low-fat milk	**Dinner**
Snack 1 sesame roll 1 tbsp. peanut butter 4 oz. low-fat milk	**Snack**

FIGURE 39–2. Sample lactovegetarian menu. (From the Massachusetts General Hospital Department of Dietetics.)

D I E T A R Y   F A T

A diet that consists of 20% of total calories from fat includes the following grams of total fat—for example:

$$1200 \text{ kcals} \times 0.20 = 240 \text{ kcals from fat}$$

$$240 \text{ kcals from fat}/9 \text{ kcals per gram*} = 27 \text{ g of fat}$$

CALORIES	GRAMS OF FAT
1500	33
1800	40
2000	44
2500	55

Since hypercholesterolemia is a risk factor for coronary artery disease, it is recommended that dietary sources of fat that increase serum cholesterol be limited in those persons who have hypercholesterolemia or are at risk of developing coronary artery disease. Saturated fats in the diet raise serum cholesterol, particularly low-density lipoprotein (LDL), which is associated with plaque buildup. Polyunsaturated fats lower both LDL and high-density lipoprotein (HDL), which is known to provide protection from plaque buildup. Monounsaturated fats lower LDL but do not lower HDL and therefore are the dietary fat of choice.

DIETARY SOURCES OF FAT

*SATURATED: animal fats, cocoa butter, palm and coconut oils, hydrogenated oils.

*POLYUNSATURATED: vegetable oils.

*MONOUNSATURATED: canola oil, olive oil

*(*All fats contain 9 kcals per gram.)*

---

findings of studies evaluating the effectiveness of high-level vitamin or mineral supplementation on athletic performance lead to the conclusion that large therapeutic doses of vitamins and/or minerals are not useful in improving athletic performance.[30] Focusing on the quality of the athlete's caloric intake to ensure that the vitamins and minerals necessary for optimal functioning of energy metabolic process are present is of primary importance. Physical activity increases the need for some vitamins and minerals; however, the increased need can be met by a diet that provides a variety of foods and is high in complex carbohydrates, moderate in protein, and low in fat. Individuals who consume a low-calorie diet are at risk for low vitamin and mineral intake.

WATER-SOLUBLE VITAMINS

Water-soluble vitamins are vitamin C and the B complex vitamins. These vitamins act as coenzymes or cofactors in metabolic reactions involved in the oxidation of food and the production of energy. Water-soluble vitamins are not stored and therefore need to be consumed on a daily basis. The B complex vitamins, thiamin, riboflavin, niacin, pyridoxine, cyanocobalamin (B_{12}), pantothenic acid, folacin, and biotin, work together to ensure proper digestion, muscle contraction, and energy release.

There has been speculation about whether supplementation of the B complex vitamins enhances energy release and as a result leads to improved physical performance.[30] However, since there have been reports of toxic effects of pyridoxine (vitamin B_6) and niacin, supplementation in large doses is not recommended. Table 39–8 lists food sources for these vitamins.

Vitamin C is used in the synthesis of collagen, epinephrine, and anti-inflammatory corticoids of the adrenal gland. It aids in healing, facilitates iron absorption, and may serve as an antioxidant. Supplementing vitamin C is popular among athletes, possibly as a result of its role in the healing process and the expectation that high doses of vitamin C will improve physical performance, which appears to be unfounded.[31] Well-controlled studies have reported no benefits of vitamin C supplementation on strength, maximum oxygen consumption, or aerobic capacity.[32–36]

FAT-SOLUBLE VITAMINS

The fat-soluble vitamins are A, D, E, and K, which are stored by the body in fat. Since these vitamins are stored in the body, excess intake can lead to toxicity. There are few studies on the relation of vitamins A, D, and K regarding physical performance. Vitamin E, an antioxidant, has not been shown to maximize oxygen consumption, strength, power, or muscular endurance.[37,38] More research is needed on vitamin E and athletic performance. Table 39–8 lists food sources of fat-soluble vitamins.

MINERALS

For young athletes and women of all ages, the intake of two minerals are of concern; these are iron and calcium.

IRON. Iron is a component of hemoglobin and myoglobin and is essential for oxidative metabolism to occur. Problematic factors associated with exercise are hemolysis of erythrocytes, alterations in iron metabolism, hematuria, increase in erythrocyte osmotic fragility resulting in decreased red blood cell survival time, and a possible shift in the oxygen dissociation curve.[39]

Athletes, especially endurance athletes, tend to have lower hemoglobin concentrations than nonathletes. This has been known as sports anemia and is a misnomer because the most common cause of a low hemoglobin concentration in an endurance athlete is a false anemia.[40] Sports anemia may occur in athletes owing to an increase in plasma volume associated with the initiation of training. Causes of sports anemia are thought to be hemodilution and physiologic adaptation.[41,42] Regular aerobic exercise expands the baseline plasma volume, diluting the red blood cells and thus the hemoglobin concentration. True sports anemia will not respond to supplementation. No treatment is required as the condition is self-correcting.[39,42]

TABLE 39–8
Vitamins: Charting Your Course

Vitamin	Major Food Sources	Adult RDA*	What It Does	Potential Benefits	Supplementation
A	Milk, egg, liver, cheese, fish oil. Plus fruits and vegetables that contain beta carotene. (You need not consume preformed vitamin A if you eat foods rich in beta carotene.)	800 RE (8,000 IU), women; 1,000 RE (10,000 IU), men *1 cup = 140 RE*	Promotes good vision; helps form and maintain skin, teeth, bones, and mucous membranes. Deficiency can increase susceptibility to infectious disease.	May inhibit the development of certain tumors; may increase resistance to infection in children.	Not recommended, since toxic in high doses.
Beta carotene (not a vitamin, but converted to vitamin A in the body)	Carrots, sweet potatoes, cantaloupe, leafy greens, tomatoes, apricots, winter squash, red bell peppers, pink grapefruit, broccoli, mangos, peaches.	No RDA; experts recommend 5–6 mg (milligrams) *1 medium carrot = 12 mg* *1 sweet potato = 15 mg*	Converted into vitamin A in the intestinal wall. As an antioxidant, it combats the adverse effects of free radicals in the body. Best known of a family of substances called carotenoids.	May reduce the risk of certain cancers as well as coronary artery disease.	6–15 mg (equal to 10,000–25,000 IU of vitamin A) a day for anyone not consuming several carotene-rich fruits or vegetables daily. Nontoxic.
C (ascorbic acid)	Citrus fruits and juices, strawberries, tomatoes, peppers (especially red), broccoli, potatoes, kale, cauliflower, cantaloupe, Brussels sprouts.	60 mg *1 orange = 70 mg* *1 cup fresh O.J. = 120 mg* *1 cup broccoli = 115 mg*	Helps promote healthy gums and teeth; aids in iron absorption; maintains normal connective tissue; helps in healing of wounds. As an antioxidant, it combats the adverse effects of free radicals.	May reduce the risk of certain cancers, as well as coronary artery disease; may prevent or delay cataracts.	250–500 mg a day for anyone not consuming several fruits or vegetables rich in C daily and for smokers. Larger doses may cause diarrhea.
D	Milk, fish oil, fortified margarine also produced by the body in response to sunlight.	5 mcg (micrograms), or 200 IU; 10 mcg, or 400 IU, before age 25 *1 cup milk = 100 IU*	Promotes strong bones and teeth by aiding the absorption of calcium. Helps maintain blood levels of calcium and phosphorus.	May reduce the risk of osteoporosis.	400 IU for people who do not drink milk or get sun exposure, especially strict vegetarians and elderly. Toxic in high doses.
E	Vegetable oil, nuts, margarine, wheat germ, leafy greens, seeds, almonds, olives, asparagus.	8 mg, women; 10 mg, men (12–15 IU) *1 Tbsp canola oil = 9 mg* *1 Tbsp margarine = 2 mg* *1 oz peanuts = 2 mg* *1 cup kale = 6 mg*	Helps in the formation of red blood cells and the utilization of vitamin K. As an antioxidant, it combats the adverse effects of free radicals.	May reduce the risk of certain cancers, as well as coronary artery disease; may prevent or delay cataracts; may improve immune function in the elderly.	200 to 800 IU advised for everybody; you can't get that much from food, especially on a low-fat diet. No serious side effects at that level, though diarrhea and headaches have been reported.
K	Intestinal bacteria produce most of the K needed by the body. The rest is supplied by leafy greens, cauliflower, broccoli, cabbage, milk, soybeans, eggs.	60–65 mcg, women; 70–80 mcg, men *1 cup broccoli = 175 mcg* *1 cup milk = 10 mcg*	Essential for normal blood clotting.	May help maintain strong bones in the elderly.	Not necessary, not recommended.
Thiamin (B₁)	Whole grains, enriched grain products, beans, meats, liver, wheat germ, nuts, fish, brewer's yeast.	1–1.1 mg, women; 1.2–1.5 mg, men *1 pkt oatmeal = 0.5 mg*	Helps cells convert carbohydrates into energy. Necessary for healthy brain, nerve cells, and heart function.	Unknown.	Not necessary, not recommended.
Riboflavin (B₂)	Dairy products, liver, meat, chicken, fish, enriched grain products, leafy greens, beans, nuts, eggs, almonds.	1.2–1.3 mg, women; 1.4–1.7 mg, men *1 cup milk = 0.4 mg* *3 oz chicken = 0.2 mg*	Helps cells convert carbohydrates into energy. Essential for growth, production of red blood cells, and health of skin and eyes.	Unknown.	Not necessary, not recommended.

Vitamin	Food Sources	RDA	Function	Possible Benefits	Cautions
Niacin (B₃)	Nuts, meat, fish, chicken, liver, enriched grain products, dairy products, peanut butter, brewer's yeast.	13–19 mg 3 oz chicken = 12 mg 1 slice enriched bread = 1 mg	Aids in release of energy from foods. Helps maintain healthy skin, nerves, and digestive system.	Large doses lower elevated blood cholesterol.	Megadoses may be prescribed by doctor to lower blood cholesterol. May cause flushing, liver damage, and irregular heart beat.
B₆ (pyroxidine)	Whole grains, bananas, meat, beans, nuts, wheat germ, brewer's yeast, chicken, fish, liver.	1.6 mg, women; 2 mg, men 1 banana = 0.7 mg 1 cup lima beans = 0.3 mg	Vital in chemical reactions of proteins and amino acids. Helps maintain brain function and form red blood cells.	May boost immunity in the elderly.	Megadoses can cause numbness and other neurological disorders.
B₁₂	Liver, beef, pork, poultry, eggs, milk, cheese, yogurt, shellfish, fortified cereals, fortified soy products.	2 mcg 1 cup milk = 0.9 mcg 3 oz beef = 2 mcg	Necessary for development of red blood cells. Maintains normal functioning of nervous system.	Unknown.	Strict vegetarians may need supplements. Despite claims, no benefits from megadoses.
Folacin (a B vitamin; also called folate or folic acid)	Leafy greens, wheat germ, liver, beans, whole grains, broccoli, asparagus, citrus fruit and juices.	180 mcg, women; 200 mcg, men 1 cup raw spinach = 110 mcg 1 pkt oatmeal = 150 mcg 1 cup asparagus = 180 mcg	Important in the synthesis of DNA, in normal growth, and in protein metabolism. Adequate intake reduces the risk of certain birth defects, notably spina bifida.	May reduce the risk of cervical cancer.	400 mcg, from food or pills, for all women who may become pregnant, in order to help prevent birth defects.
Biotin (a B vitamin)	Eggs, milk, liver, brewer's yeast, mushrooms, bananas, tomatoes, whole grains.	No RDA; experts recommend 30–100 mcg	Important in metabolism of protein, carbohydrates, and fats.	Unknown.	Not necessary, not recommended.
Pantothenic acid (B₅)	Whole grains, beans, milk, eggs, liver.	No RDA; experts recommend 4–7 mg	Vital for metabolism of food and production of essential body chemicals.	Unknown.	Not necessary, not recommended. May cause diarrhea.

*These figures are not applicable to pregnant women, who need additional vitamins and should seek professional advice.

What is a vitamin?

Among the achievements for which this century will surely be remembered is the discovery of vitamins, a scientific advance truly beneficial to humanity. For hundreds of years, of course, people had noticed that certain foods seemed to prevent diseases – most famously, the limes or lemons that British sailors ate to ward off scurvy – but the first vitamin was isolated in the lab only in 1911. That was thiamin, a B vitamin. Now 13 vitamins are known. In the past, vitamins were discussed in terms of preventing deficiency diseases (beriberi, caused by a lack of thiamin, for instance, or scurvy, by a lack of vitamin C). The RDAs (Recommended Dietary Allowances), devised by scientists in the U.S. and revised and updated over the years, were designed partly to prevent such deficiency diseases and partly to meet the needs, as they were understood, of healthy people.
But we still have much to learn about the functions of these powerful chemicals. Indeed, in the last decade alone, hundreds of scientific studies have found that vitamins play a much larger role in health than was dreamed of even 20 years ago.

Vitamins are organic substances required to regulate the functioning of cells. They are essential to life. They take part in myriad biological processes, among them promoting good vision, forming normal blood cells, creating strong bones and teeth, and ensuring the proper function of the heart and nervous system. While vitamins supply no energy, they do aid in the conversion of foods into energy. The 13 vitamins fall into two categories: fat-soluble (A and its precursor beta carotene, D, E, and K) and water-soluble (the B vitamins and C). This distinction is important because the body stores fat-soluble vitamins in the liver and fatty tissue for relatively long periods (many months), but it stores the water-soluble vitamins for only a short time (up to a few weeks). In general, you have to consume vitamins: the body cannot manufacture them (though it does synthesize some vitamin K, D, and B₁₂ and convert beta carotene into vitamin A). For a description of the specific functions of each vitamin, consult the chart.

Who needs supplements?

If you follow the government's dietary recommendations, you may not need supplements to meet the RDAs. Still, we think it's wise for adults to consume extra amounts of the antioxidants (vitamins E and C and beta carotene), and for premenopausal women to eat a folacin-rich diet or take supplements (see chart for recommended amounts).
Most people do *not* need a daily multivitamin and mineral supplement, although millions of Americans take one. It can't be said too often that a pill a day won't turn a poor diet into a healthy one. However, elderly people, especially those who may have reduced their food intakes for any reason, may benefit from a daily multivitamin. So may frequent aspirin takers, heavy drinkers, smokers, and those with impaired immune systems. Pregnant women have special needs and should follow professional advice.
Taking huge doses of most vitamins is not wise. Some vitamins – A and D, specifically – are toxic in large doses. Others, like niacin, have serious side effects in large doses. Excess amounts of the water-soluble vitamins, in particular, will simply be eliminated by the body. In planning your diet and in taking supplements, we urge you to stick with the amounts recommended on the chart.

Reprinted with permission of the University of California at Berkeley Wellness Letter. © Health Letter Associates, 1994.

The most common cause of true anemia in athletes is iron deficiency anemia, which may not stem from the athleticism.[43] Many reports of iron deficiency anemia in athletes, especially women endurance athletes, imply that a large percentage of women athletes are iron-deficient, that women athletes are uniquely prone to iron deficiency anemia, and that a low serum ferritin level causes fatigue and harms athletic performance even in the absence of anemia. These implications may be unwarranted.[44] Low serum ferritin values may be common to elite women athletes and yet do not represent iron deficiency, since plasma volume expansion could dilute a serum ferritin level. When 100 women college athletes were compared with nonathletic coeds, differences in iron balance were minor. In a review of many studies of iron balance in athletes, Clarkson[45] concluded that athletes are not iron-depleted any more so than the general population.

There is evidence that in the absence of anemia, a low serum ferritin does not curtail athletic performance. When mild iron deficiency anemia was induced by venesection of healthy runners, and the anemia (not the iron deficiency) was obviated by transfusion, the subjects' exercise capacity was unchanged from baseline.[46] It may be difficult to distinguish mild iron deficiency anemia from dilutional pseudoanemia. When this occurs, an empiric trial of iron therapy, ferrous sulfate, 325 mg, taken three times a day for 2 months, is prudent. A rise in hemoglobin level of at least $1g/dl^{-1}$ proves that the anemia was due at least in part to iron deficiency.[46]

Table 39–9 lists dietary sources of iron. As stated in Chapter 15, it is not necessary for all female athletes to ingest iron supplements. However, if an athlete is supplementing iron based on a physician's recommendation, is taking a daily multiple vitamin with iron to meet the RDA for iron, or is consuming dietary sources of iron, the following are recommendations to enhance absorption: (1) include a source of vitamin C at the same time (see Table 39–9) and (2) do not consume iron within 1 hour of having coffee or tea, since these interfere with iron absorption.

A discussion on blood doping can be found in Chapter 15.

TABLE 39–9
Dietary Sources of Iron

Nonvegetarian Sources of Iron	Vegetarian Sources of Iron
>5 mg/Serving	**4–9 mg/Serving**
Liver (high in cholesterol) 3 oz	Fortified cooked cereal, 3/4 c
Oysters 1/2 c	Fortified dry cereal, 1 oz
3–5 mg/Serving	**6–7 mg/Serving**
Most beef, lean	1/2 cup tofu
1–3 mg/Serving	**3–4 mg/Serving**
Fish; chicken	Soybeans, 1/2 c
	Lentils, 1/2 c
	Pumpkin/squash seeds, 1 oz

TABLE 39–10
Dietary Sources of Calcium

Calcium-enriched bread, 2 slices	580 mg
8 oz Lactose-free calcium-fortified nonfat milk	500 mg
8 oz yogurt, plain, nonfat	452 mg
8 oz yogurt, low fat	415 mg
8 oz milk, skim	352 mg
8 oz yogurt, fruit	314 mg
Minute Maid calcium-enriched orange juice, 8 oz	293 mg
Swiss cheese, 1 oz	272 mg
Dry cereal, 3/4 cup (variable amount)	250 mg
Cheddar cheese, 1 oz	204 mg
Sardines, canned in water with bones, 2 oz	185 mg*
Mozzarella, 1 oz	183 mg
Tofu with calcium sulfate, 3 oz	150 mg†
Almonds, 1/4 c	94 mg
Broccoli, turnip greens, 1/2 c	36 mg

*Average of major brands.
†Estimates of brands.
Supplements: calcium carbonate (example, Tums) is better absorbed with meals; calcium citrate (examples, enriched orange juice, tablets) is better absorbed on an empty stomach.

CALCIUM. Many athletes having low body weight do not consume enough calories or choose low nutritional quality foods and do not therefore consume adequate calcium. Calcium is necessary for the contractile ability of muscles, the maintenance of healthy bones and teeth, blood clotting, and nerve transmission. Since bone formation and dissolution is a continuous process, calcium must be supplied to the cells on demand. When dietary calcium is low, the body draws from its own reserves in bone, which reduces bone density and can lead to stress fractures. Women are at higher risk because they have thinner bones and as they mature, lose bone density at a faster rate. Amenorrhea, found in many female athletes, is also associated with decreased spinal bone mass.[47]

Osteoporosis is a major health concern for women. Calcium intake; estrogen level; alcohol, caffeine, and protein intake, family history; and the type and amount of physical activity are all related to the development of osteoporosis. Ninety-nine percent of dietary calcium is deposited in the bone. Increased physical activity improves the efficiency of calcium utilization and is important for the maintenance of optimal bone mass and strength.

The RDA for calcium is listed in Table 39–2. Female athletes who become amenorrheic may need additional calcium—as much as 1500 mg/day. Table 39–10 lists dietary and supplemental sources of calcium.

SODIUM. Sodium (Na) is an essential mineral needed to regulate water balance in the cells and to maintain blood volume and normal nerve and muscle activity. Sodium increases the absorption of fluids in the small intestine. Sodium also helps maintain the osmotic drive for drinking and reduces water clearance associated with reduced serum electrolyte concentration that results from electrolyte losses during exercise. In athletes who train daily at high intensity or in high temperatures, a prolonged state of hypohydration can occur. Rehydration occurs when a dilute solution of sodium rather than plain water is consumed under these conditions.[48]

Sodium makes up as much as 40 percent of common table salt (chloride constitutes the remaining approximately 60 percent). Requirements for sodium vary with age, environmental conditions, and level of activity. However, it is recommended that a healthy sedentary adult consume 500 to 2400 mg per day, which can be achieved by consuming a typical American diet. During prolonged exercise in hot weather, sodium losses in sweat and urine may exceed 10 g per day. The sodium concentration of sweat is approximately 50 mEq/L; the average daily urine sodium loss is 120 mEq/L.[49] Therefore, an athlete working out 4 hours per day and losing sweat at a moderate rate of 1.5 L per hour, may benefit from a dilute sodium mixture (80 to 120 mg Na/8 oz water) or a slightly more liberal use of sodium with meals. Concentrated salt tablets are generally not recommended and may actually be harmful. Acclimatization to heat or exercise can compensate for some but not all sodium loss.[50] Heat-acclimated subjects lose considerably less salt at a given sweat rate than their unacclimated counterparts. The amount of sodium lost increases as sweat rate increases. During exercise bouts lasting more than 3 hours, sodium losses can result in hyponatremia, a plasma sodium content of less than 130 mEq sodium/L, a potentially fatal condition that can be prevented.[48]

FLUIDS

To prevent dehydration, fluids should never be restricted; they need to be taken before, during, and after exercise. Dehydration adversely affects muscle strength, endurance, and coordination. It also increases the risk of cramps, heat exhaustion, and life-threatening heat stroke.[51,52] During exercise, heat produced within working skeletal muscle is carried by the convective flow of blood to the body core, elevating its temperature and stimulating warm receptors located in the anterior hypothalamus. In response to the rise in temperature, sweating is initiated. The loss of sweat means the loss of vital body fluids, which can result in circulatory and thermal impairments if these fluids are not replaced. Fluid, electrolyte, and energy supplementation are desirable during exercise to support circulatory, metabolic, and thermoregulatory functions and to maintain plasma volume.

To monitor fluid lost during training and exercise sessions, the athlete should weigh before and after each session. For each pound lost (0.45 kg), 16 oz of fluid should be consumed. Sufficient fluids should ideally be consumed during exercise so that weight remains constant before and after activity. It is important to drink fluids before becoming thirsty. Work capacity can be reduced by 10 to 15 percent with a 2 percent loss of body fluids.

The process of rehydration depends on both gastric emptying and intestinal absorption. For exercise longer than 60 to 90 minutes, using a 6 to 8 percent carbohydrate solution (for example, diluted fruit juice, Gatorade, Exceed) during the event optimizes stamina and endurance, since the carbohydrate helps to maintain normal blood glucose levels and to provide energy for muscle.[53] Highly concentrated sweets (greater than 8 percent) tend to empty more slowly from the stomach than diluted fluids and impair fluid absorption. Therefore, they are not recommended during the event.[54] Cold fluids help cool core body temperature and leave the stomach more rapidly than warm fluids.

Once the gastric contents empty into the small intestine, this solution must be absorbed before any benefit of hydration is realized. Absorption from the small intestine is accelerated by the combination of glucose and sodium.[55] It has been reported that the most effective glucose to sodium ratio promoting water absorption is 2:1.[56,48] Fluid replacement recommendations and symptoms of dehydration are boxed on the following page. (See Chapter 14 for further details.)

CAFFEINE. Some research has shown that caffeine may facilitate the use of fats stored in the muscle as an energy source during exercise. However, most investigators suggest that caffeine's effect is an enhanced psychologic function leading to greater work output and/or increased tolerance to fatigue. Response to the effect of caffeine is variable. In some athletes, performance is hindered because of adverse effects such as anxiety, nervousness, and upset stomach. In addition, caffeine is a diuretic, and consumption before or during an event can lead to dehydration. It also increases basal metabolic rate and heat production.[57] Caffeine is considered a banned substance by the International Olympic Committee and United States Olympic Committee in some situations and sports because of its metabolic effects.

Urinary caffeine levels above 12 μg per milliliter may be considered a sign of caffeine doping. This level would be reached by consuming 6 to 8 cups of coffee in one sitting followed by the test within 2 to 3 hours.[58] A dose of 5 mg/kg of body weight would provide a stimulant effect and would not be considered doping. For additional discussion on the use of caffeine in athletics, see Chapter 15.

FOOD INTAKE BEFORE, DURING, AND AFTER EXERCISE

Before exercise, it is most important that the athlete have adequate carbohydrate and fluid intake. Foods eaten prior to an event should be familiar and comforting. Depending on individual preference, the pre-event meal should be consumed 2 to 6 hours before activity and provide 85 to 200 g of carbohydrate.[59] The meal should be low in fat and protein and high in complex carbohydrate. Five to 10 minutes before exercise or competition, a 5 to 6 percent carbohydrate solution may be consumed to maintain blood glucose levels. For endurance sports, it has been recommended that food eaten 1 hour before exercise supply 0.5 to 0.9 g of carbohydrate per pound of body weight.[60] Table 39–11

TABLE 39–11
Carbohydrate Content of Food and Beverages

Food	CHO (grams)	Beverage	CHO (grams/ 8 oz)
Apple	21	Gatorade	36
Banana, large	40	Apple juice	30
Baked potato, large	51	Exceed High	58
Yogurt, fruited (1 c)	40	Carbohydrate source	58
Bread, whole wheat, 2 slices	22	Carboplex	54
Bagel, medium	50	Exceed	17
Raisins, 2/3 c	79	Cranapple juice	43
Rice, 1 c	50		
Spaghetti, w/sauce, 1 c	37		
Tortilla, flour	15		
Waffles, buttermilk, 2	29		

CHO = carbohydrates.

lists the carbohydrate content of various food and beverages. Pre-exercise meal guidelines and a list of liquid meals are boxed on the next page. Liquid meals can be consumed closer to exercise time because of shorter gastric emptying time; they produce low stool residue, keeping weight gain after a meal to a minimum; and they provide an alternative to solid meals for day-long competitions and multiple events.

Many high school and college coaches try to set guidelines for an entire team regarding safe pre-exercise eating. Because each athlete is unique, this is not effective. Each individual must discover the best pre-exercise foods for his or her own body. This is based on trial and error.

Adverse gut reactions occur in 30 to 50 percent of endurance athletes. Complaints include stomach and upper gastrointestinal problems such as heartburn, vomiting, bloating, and stomach pain and lower gastrointestinal problems such as gas, intestinal cramping, urge to defecate, loose stools, and diarrhea. Sports performed in a relatively stable position such as cycling, swimming, and cross-country skiing seem to cause fewer gastrointestinal problems compared with sports that jostle the intestines such as track events, running, football, and basketball.

Untrained individuals just beginning an exercise program report more gastrointestinal problems than do well-trained individuals who may have gradually built up tolerance to exercise and who have discovered their tried and true pre-exercise foods. Gastrointestinal problems also occur more frequently in younger athletes who may have less nutrition knowledge and experience with precompetition foods. Women may experience more problems than men, particularly during menstruation. Hormonal shifts at this time may contribute to looser bowel movements. During easy and moderately high exercise, the body can simultaneously digest food

and comfortably exercise. During intense exercise, the shift of blood flow from the stomach to the working muscles may cause gastrointestinal problems. High-fat foods eaten shortly before exercise can cause problems. Low-fat, high-carbohydrate foods that are tried and true favorites are recommended pre-exercise.

During endurance exercise of more than 1 hour, consuming approximately 25 g of carbohydrate every 30 minutes has been reported to delay fatigue.[61] Since gastric emptying and absorption time is faster with carbohydrate-containing sports beverages they are often better tolerated by athletes during activity. These also have the added advantage of replacing fluids. Consuming highly concentrated sugar drinks such as fruit juice and soda during exercise may cause stomach distress; therefore a 6 to 8 percent carbohydrate solution is recommended during exercise (see Fluid Guidelines box).

The fastest glycogen replacement occurs within the first 2 hours following exercise. Blood glucose, insulin, and glycogen synthetase levels remain high to promote glycogen synthesis and replete muscle reserves.[62] Muscle will replete glycogen to a higher degree when as much as 600 g of easily digestible carbohydrate is consumed within the first 1 to 3 hours following exercise. Within the first hour postexercise, it is recommended that 0.75 g of carbohydrate per pound of body weight be consumed, followed by a second dose 1 to 3 hours later.[23] Many athletes are not ready to eat within an hour postevent; therefore high-carbohydrate juices immediately after are an excellent way to restore glycogen, followed by a high-carbohydrate meal 1 to 3 hours later. High-carbohydrate drinks such as soda, which also replace glycogen stores, are void of addi-

F L U I D G U I D E L I N E S

EVENT	CUPS (8-OZ)
2 hours before	2–3
15 min before	1–2
Every 15–20 min during	1
Afterward	Until urine is pale

Symptoms of Dehydration

Dark urine
Small volume of urine
Elevated heart rate
Headache

Fluid Weight Loss in Pounds	Effect
1.5	Increased body temperature
4.5	Impaired performance
7.5	Gastrointestinal problems, heat exhaustion
10.5	Hallucinations
15.0	Circulatory collapse

Fluid	Carbohydrate (%)
Gatorade	6
Exceed	7
Cola	11
Apple juice	10

PRE-EXERCISE MEAL GUIDELINES

During exercise, athletes rely primarily on their pre-existing glycogen and fat stores.

Effects of a pre-exercise meal should be tested during training, not before an event.

Carbohydrate feedings before exercise can help restore suboptimal liver glycogen stores.

HOW MUCH CARBOHYDRATE PRE-EXERCISE: 1–4 g/kg body weight consumed 1–4 hours before exercise. Guidelines: high carbohydrate, low fat, moderate protein, extra fluid, appropriate portions.

Large meal: 4–6 hours prior
Lighter meal: 2–3 hours prior
Snack: 0.5–1.0 hour prior

Timing varies with duration and intensity of exercise and personal preference.

Caution: simple sugar pre-exercise may cause hypoglycemia, lightheadedness.

Liquid Meals:

Nutrament (12 oz)	360 kcal	16 g PRO*	52 g CHO*	10 g fat
Exceed (8 oz)	360 kcal	14 g PRO	54 g CHO	9.5 g fat
GatorPro (8 oz)	360 kcal	16 g PRO	58 g CHO	7 g fat

*CHO = carbohydrate; PRO = protein.

tional nutrients such as vitamin C. Alcohol is not recommended as either a fluid or glycogen replacement for all of the reasons already discussed in this chapter and because it is low in carbohydrate and has a diuretic effect.

WEIGHT MANAGEMENT

The diet industry is a 31 billion dollars a year business. This business encompasses commercial diet programs, sales of books, weight-loss products and low-fat diet foods and drinks. Fad diets are popular because of the promise of quick and easy weight loss. Fad diets may be particularly attractive to athletes because of claims to alter body composition. The truth of the matter is that if it sounds too good to be true, it is. Ketogenic diets are not appropriate for athletes because of problems with secondary dehydration and hyponatremia (low serum sodium). Most fad diets are nutritionally inadequate, and because hypocaloric diets cannot meet the energy needs of athletes in training, they may promote depletion of glycogen stores and loss of lean body mass.

An appropriate weight-loss program begins with a complete assessment[63] of the athlete, discussed in the beginning of this chapter. The assessment would include anthropometries: height, weight, and body composition; weight and diet history; 24-hour recall and food frequency assessment; and information re-

garding activity, including duration and intensity; stage of change should also be assessed.

Basal metabolic rate can be estimated using height, weight, and age (see Table 39–15 later in this chapter for the Harris-Benedict formula). To estimate caloric needs for maintaining current weight, add an activity factor of 1.3 for normal activities of daily living and 1.5 for the very active individual, then add any additional calories burned during exercise (listed in Table 39–1). Decreasing the maintenance calories by 500 kcals per day would promote a weight loss of approximately 1 lb a week; doing additional exercise to utilize an additional 500 kcal, would promote a 2-lb per week weight loss. A weight loss of 1 to 2 lb per week is a realistic, appropriate goal. With well-trained athletes, measuring body composition using skin calipers, underwater weighing, or bioelectrical impedance for an analysis of body composition is a better determinant of fat loss than using the scale. The scale weighs water, muscles, and fat and, therefore, does not distinguish whether fat was lost or muscle (which is heavier than fat) was gained. The goal is to decrease body fat and preserve lean body mass.

The athlete should be referred to a registered dietitian, who will develop an individualized meal plan based on the athlete's likes, dislikes, lifestyle, ethnic food practices, and socioeconomic factors. The diet should be a high-carbohydrate sports diet, limiting fats to 20 percent of total calories. The Action Strategies box early in this chapter lists guidelines for recommending behavioral changes to accomplish the weight-loss goal.

Weight goals should be appropriate and based on both genetic and environmental factors affecting the athlete's weight status. Emphasis should be placed on realistic goals, long-term weight maintenance, and a healthy lifestyle, which includes healthful eating and physical activity. Behavioral-cognitive therapy is an important adjunct to any diet program. Factors associated with successful weight loss are self-monitoring (food records), goal setting, social support, and length of treatment. Factors associated with successful maintenance are physical activity, self-monitoring, and continued contact with the weight management therapist or counselor. Those factors associated with weight regain are restrictive dieting, life stresses, negative coping style, and emotional or binge eating patterns.[64] It is extremely important to assess the presence or potential risk of eating disorders, particularly in sports in which thinness is stressed.

EATING DISORDERS AND THE ATHLETE

Concern is escalating about the eating disturbances and harmful practices of weight control in the athlete. These practices range over a wide spectrum of behaviors that include severe dieting; binge eating; fasting; the abuse of laxatives, diuretics, and diet pills; and use of ipecac and self-induced vomiting. It is an irony that the athlete striving for low body weight by any of these methods ultimately compromises health and athletic performance.

TABLE 39–12
Diagnostic Criteria

Anorexia Nervosa

1. Refusal to maintain body weight at or above a minimally normal weight for age and height (e.g., weight loss leading to maintenance of body weight less than 85% of that expected; or failure to make expected weight gain during periods of growth, leading to body weight less than 85% of that expected).
2. Intense fear of gaining weight or becoming fat, even when underweight.
3. Disturbance in the way one's body weight or shape is perceived; undue influence of body weight or shape on self-evaluation, or denial of the seriousness of the current low weight.
4. In postmenarchal females, amenorrhea, that is, the absence of at least three consecutive menstrual cycles. (A woman is considered to have amenorrhea if her periods occur only after hormone, such as estrogen administration)

Specific types:
Restricting does not regularly engage in binge eating or purging behavior (self-induced vomiting or the misuse of laxatives or diuretics) during episodes of anorexia nervosa.
Binge eating and purging type regularly engages in binge eating or purging behavior (self-induced vomiting or the misuse of laxatives or diuretics) during episodes of anorexia nervosa.

Bulimia Nervosa

1. Recurrent episodes of binge eating. An episode of binge eating is characterized by both of the following:
   a. Eating in a discrete period (e.g., within any 2-hour period) an amount of food that is definitely larger than most people would eat during a similar period of time and under similar circumstances.
   b. A sense of lack of control over eating during the episode (e.g., a feeling that one cannot stop eating or control what or how much one is eating).
2. Recurrent, inappropriate compensatory behavior to prevent weight gain such as self-induced vomiting; misuse of laxatives, diuretics, or other medications; fasting; or excessive exercise.
3. The binge eating and inappropriate compensatory behaviors both occur, on average, at least twice a week for 3 months.
4. Self-evaluation is unduly influenced by body shape and weight.
5. The disturbance does not occur exclusively during episodes of anorexia nervosa.

Specific types:
Purging regularly engages in self-induced vomiting or the misuse of laxatives or diuretics.
Nonpurging uses other inappropriate compensatory behaviors, such as fasting or excessive exercise, but does not regularly engage in self-induced vomiting or the misuse of laxatives or diuretics.

From the Diagnostic and Statistical Manual of Mental Disorders, 4th ed. Washington, DC, American Psychiatric Association, 1994.

The prevalence of eating disorders in the general population appears to be increasing and is estimated to occur in 1 to 4 percent of adolescent and young women, predominantly white upper- and middle-class students. However, increasing numbers of eating disorders are also being reported in males, minorities, and women of all age groups. At present 90 to 95 percent of all cases occur in females.[65]

The prevalence of eating disorders in athletes is unknown. Drummers and co-workers reported that in a survey of 9- to 18-year-old swimmers, 15.4 percent of the girls and 3.6 percent of the boys used pathogenic weight-loss techniques.[66] Rosen and associates reported that 32 percent of the female athletes from ten varsity level sports engaged in at least one pathogenic weight-control practice: 25 percent used diet pills, 16 percent used laxatives, 14 percent used self-induced vomiting, and 5 percent used diuretics.[67] In a survey of male high school and college wrestlers, 63 percent of college and 43 percent of high school wrestlers were preoccupied with food during the season, 41 percent of college and 29 percent of high school wrestlers reported eating out of control between matches; and 52 percent of college and 26 percent of high school wrestlers fasted at least once a week.[68] A survey of female college gymnasts reported all 42 gymnasts were dieting (50 percent for appearance, 50 percent for performance) and 62 percent used at least one pathogenic weight-control practice. In addition, 66 percent were told by coaches that they were too heavy.[69]

Seemingly, sports that emphasize thinness and low body weight for appearance or optimal performance such as gymnastics, dance, diving, figure skating, long-distance running, swimming, and cross-country skiing or that utilize weight classification such as wrestling, crew, weight lifting, and body building place the athlete at increased risk for developing an eating disorder. Athletes in sports such as basketball or football that do not focus on leanness may be at a lower risk.[65]

DIAGNOSTIC CRITERIA FOR EATING DISORDERS

Eating disorders are defined according to diagnostic criteria for anorexia nervosa and bulimia nervosa. For a diagnosis of either anorexia nervosa or bulima nervosa, all criteria must be met. Table 39–12 lists these diagnostic criteria. However, it is important to consider the wide spectrum of disordered eating patterns and pathogenic weight-control practices that fall in the gray areas outside the diagnostic criteria. In the case of either frank eating disorders or disordered eating behaviors, there is equal concern about the serious medical consequences if these are left untreated.

EFFECT OF EATING DISORDERS ON ATHLETIC PERFORMANCE

When viewed in the context of the medical complications that occur as a consequence of eating disorders, impaired athletic performance and increased risk of injury seem inevitable. Reduced calories and, therefore, reduced nutrients and fluid, along with electrolyte imbalances, often lead to a decline in endurance, strength, reaction time, speed, and the ability to concentrate.[70] The athlete with anorexia nervosa or with restricted eating leading to semistarvation will demonstrate reduced oxygen consumption; reduced energy expenditure; maximal heart rate; maximal exercise capacity; and a decrease in muscular strength, speed and coordination.[71,72] These changes were all observed by Rosen and colleagues in female athletes following 6 months of semistarvation.[71] The alteration in body composition led to a 28 percent reduction of oxygen consumption during a standard task of moderate intensity. Energy expenditure per minute during work decreased by 23 percent. This was similar to the decrease in body weight (24 percent) during semistarvation. Changes in muscular strength, speed, and coordination were also noted. Grip and back dynamometric strength decreased by 28 and 38 percent, respectively. Manual speed and tapping speed declined by approximately 5 percent and coordination by 17 percent.

There is also evidence of increased risk of delayed wound healing, shin splints, and stress fractures related to restricted calories and nutrients, specifically calcium, which is required for bone health. In women, a deficiency of estrogen resulting in irregular menses or amenorrhea leads to a lower bone mineral density.[73]

For the athlete with bulimia nervosa or one using a pathogenic weight-control method, the electrolyte and fluid abnormalities can result in dehydration or edema, muscular fatigue, leg cramps, dizziness, lightheadedness, and weakness.[65] Since restricted eating and pathogenic weight-control methods often coexist, the athlete may show physical impairment common to both anorexia and bulimia nervosa. Because of the body's capacity to adapt to deficiencies in nutrition or to the insult of pathogenic weight-control methods, a decline in athletic performance due to disordered eating may not be seen for some time.[70]

SYMPTOMATOLOGY

Because features of anorexia and bulimia nervosa can coexist, a blend of signs and symptoms may be observed. The athlete with anorexia nervosa or very low body weight often has a dramatic physical presentation specific to the starvation syndrome. This may include significant weight loss; edema; excessive bruising; fine downy (lanugo) hair, which is notable on the face, shoulders and back; dry skin that may have a yellow cast; hair loss; and cyanosis of extremities.[74] The individual often wears multiple layers of clothes in part to conceal a low body weight, but also as a result of increased cold intolerance. The athlete may complain of fatigue or overabundant energy, headaches, and abdominal pain and may voice fear of being fat or becoming fat in the face of ongoing weight loss or maintenance of low body weight. Often the individual exceeds the training regimen and engages in aimless physical activity.[75–77] Anxious or agitated behavior, obsessionality, mood lability, social isolation, bizarre eating behavior, sleep disturbances, intense preoccupation with food, depressed affect, impaired concentration, or indecisiveness are all common events that may be observed.[78]

The athlete with bulimia nervosa engaging in purging behaviors may be more difficult to identify as he or she is often normal weight, appears healthy, and is secretive in behavior.[75] The primary concern is this population is the electrolyte and fluid abnormalities that can lead to cardiac arrhythmias, specifically hypokalemia.[75,77] Signs of chronic, self-induced vomiting include Rossel's sign, or scarring on the dorsum of the hand used to stimulate a gag reflex, bilateral parotid gland enlargement, and erosion of dental enamel. If ipecac is being used to induce vomiting, the athlete must be warned of cardiac toxicity and irreversible cardiac myopathy.[75]

If laxatives and diuretics are being used, the athlete should be informed that weight change is caused by dehydration and that weight will return to normal or be followed by reflex peripheral edema.[75,77] Laxatives do not significantly alter calorie absorption. Laxatives act predominantly on the colon to cause water secretion and rapid evacuation of feces with minimal effect on the small intestine, the primary site of calorie absorption. In a study by Bo-Linn and associates, a decrease in calorie absorption of only 12 percent occurred when the laxative Correctol was administered during a controlled meal.[79]

The physical signs that are suggestive of bulimia nervosa include frequent fluctuations in weight or limited weight loss; variable athletic performance; dental erosion; bruises on the neck or knuckles; enlarged parotid glands, which appear as chipmunk-like pouches under the angle of the jaw; and bloodshot eyes. The athlete may complain of weakness, dizziness, aches, pains, leg cramps, sore throat, and abdominal pain.[75]

Unlike the individual with anorexia nervosa, the athlete with bulimic patterns can appear extroverted or anxious and depressed. It is not uncommon for other impulsive behaviors to surface. Frequently, this involves drugs or alcohol. He or she may resort to stealing money for binge food, laxatives, diet pills, or diuretics or steal the items directly.[74] Although the athlete with anorexia may avoid eating or eat extremely small amounts of food, those with bulimia may be observed to consume large amounts of food not consistent with their weight, which may be followed by immediate trips to the bathroom. They may also engage in erratic pattern of restricted eating preceding or following these occasions of large food intake. As with anorexics they, too, may voice concerns about their weight or express fear of being or becoming fat.[77]

INTERVENTION

Recovery from disordered eating patterns, anorexia, or bulimia nervosa can be slow and arduous with an uneven course over a period of months or years. It is not uncommon for athletes to continue to struggle with concerns about weight and eating after their athletic careers are over. Treatment requries a multidisciplinary team that includes medical monitoring, psychological intervention, and nutritional counseling.[80] The nutritionist must be a registered dietitian knowledgeable in eating disorders and sports nutrition.

Hospitalization may be required if weight loss is 30 percent of desirable body weight; cardiac function is compromised; or for hypotension, dehydration, or electrolyte abnormalities. Hospitalization may also be indicated if outpatient treatent fails to improve symptoms or a worsening of symptoms occurs after 3 months of outpatient treatment.[70]

There are no published data on prognosis for recovery from eating disorders in athletes. The prognosis for nonathletes treated for eating disorders has been reported as follows: 50 percent of patients do well; 30 percent have some improvement but continue to struggle with weight, body image, and relapses, and 20 percent do poorly.[70]

The nutritionist working with an athlete on an outpatient basis has a dual role as nutrition educator and nutritional therapist. Nutritional counseling occurs in ongoing collaboration with the physician and psychotherapist. Progress takes place over a variable length of time and can occur only with the willing participation of the person. Small, progressive goals are established, focusing on nutritional restoration and normalization of eating and weight.

The following issues are typically addressed:

1. Nutrition requirements for health and athletic performance
2. Appropriate body fat and weight range
3. Normal and abnormal eating and hunger patterns
4. Normal metabolic rate and aberrations associated with abnormal eating
5. Symptomatology and medical complications common to eating disorders
6. Predicting refeeding symptoms

NUTRITIONAL REQUIREMENTS FOR HEALTH AND ATHLETIC PERFORMANCE

The nutritional requirements to promote health and ensure optimal athletic performance are presented at the beginning of this chapter. These guidelines provide a critical foundation for the athlete to begin to identify goals for change in food intake and eating patterns. To cover micronutrient deficiencies caused by inadequate food intake, a multivitamin with minerals containing 100 percent of RDA is recommended.[75,78] An additional daily calcium supplement of 1000 to 1500 mg is usually suggested for the amenorrheic female.

BODY FAT AND WEIGHT RANGES

In a given sport, body fat, not body weight is the most important factor influencing performance. Although it is generally true that the leaner the athlete, the better

the performance, it is also extremely important for the athlete to recognize that driving body weight too low can have major repercussions.[81] Table 39–13 provides a reference of values of relative body fat for, in most cases, elite athletes in selected sports. There are two important concerns regarding body fat recommendations.[81] First, there are inherent errors in existing techniques for measuring body composition that must be considered. Second, individual variability is a factor. Some athletes are able to achieve slightly lower values and improve performance, whereas other find it impossible or undesirable.

When athletes are educated about body composition and body fat percentages for their sport, they may be willing to increase food intake and allow for some weight gain. Ranges of body fat and body weight are important to allow for individual variability and normal fluctuations. In the event that a lower body fat is desirable and reasonable, the athlete with an eating disorder must first work toward normalizing eating and metabolism and must be carefully guided by the nutritionist.

TABLE 39–13
Ranges of Relative Body Fat for Men and Women Athletes

Sport	Men	Women
Baseball, softball	8–14	12–18
Basketball	6–12	10–16
Body building	5–8	6–12
Canoeing and kayaking	6–12	10–16
Cycling	5–11	8–15
Fencing	8–12	10–16
Football	6–18	—
Golf	10–16	12–20
Gymnastics	5–12	8–16
Horse racing	6–12	10–16
Ice and field hockey	8–16	12–18
Orienteering	5–12	8–16
Pentathlon	—	8–15
Racketball	6–14	10–18
Rowing	6–14	8–16
Rugby	6–16	—
Skating	5–12	8–16
Skiing	7–15	10–18
Ski jumping	7–15	10–18
Soccer	6–14	10–18
Swimming	6–12	10–18
Synchronized swimming	—	10–18
Tennis	6–14	10–20
Track and field		
Running events	5–12	8–15
Field events	8–18	12–20
Triathlon	5–12	8–15
Volleyball	7–15	10–18
Weight lifting	5–12	10–18
Wrestling	5–16	—

From Wilmore JH: Body weight standards and athletic performance. *In* Brownell KD, Rodin J, Wilmore JH (eds): Eating, Body Weight and Performance in Athletes: Disorders of Modern Society. Philadelphia, Lea & Febiger, 1992, p 326.

NORMAL AND ABNORMAL EATING AND HUNGER PATTERNS

A normal hunger pattern is a cyclical, predictable fluctuation in the intensity of hunger that is experienced throughout the day. It is unique to every person and varies according to nutrient and caloric intake, regularity of food intake, sleep patterns, biological function, and activity.[80] Abnormal hunger and eating patterns develop when an individual develops a set of arbitrary rules about food and eating that disregards body signals.[80]

For the individual with an eating disorder, hunger is experienced in various ways. The anorexic experiences hunger and low body wieght as an accomplishment based on a self-defined system to foster control, safety, and security. The anorexic usually denies feeling hungry. For the bulimic, hunger is a frightening omen of an impending binge and loss of control. The purge is usually a corrective measure to prevent weight gain.

TABLE 39–14
Abnormal Eating Patterns in Anorexia Nervosa and Bulimia Nervosa[75,78,80]

Anorexia Nervosa

1. Food intake is restricted and constant in content from day-to-day.
2. Hunger is controlled by high-bulk, low-calorie, calorie-free, and/or strongly flavored food (lemon juice, vinegar, pepper, mustard).
3. Large amounts of caffeine or carbonated beverages, chewing gum, or hard candy may be consumed to control hunger.
4. Fat-containing food is stringently avoided.
5. Food may be prepared and eaten in a ritualistic manner that may appear bizarre.
6. Claims to be vegetarian may be a guise to avoid fat-containing animal protein.
7. There is often a complex interplay between calories consumed, amount of hunger-suppressing foods eaten, amount of exercise performed, and the amount of strongly flavored foods eaten.

Bulimia Nervosa

1. May have regular pattern, albeit restricted, of food intake and regular binging and purging patterns.
2. Food intake, binging, and purging patterns may be chaotic.
3. Often relies on similar hunger suppressing foods and substances as in anorexia nervosa.
4. Late afternoon and evening are common time frames for extreme hunger to override control and result in binging and purging.
5. Binging can last for minutes to hours before purging, or there can be several binges and purges in succession.
6. Binges are highly variable in caloric content; 1200 to 11,500 kcals per episode have been reported.
7. Fat-containing food is stringently avoided, and as in anorexia nervosa, the individual may claim to be vegetarian to avoid fat-containing animal protein.

During nutrition counseling, the role of normal hunger is continuously reinforced. The body is relentless in its eforts to maintain homeostasis and aggressively pursues an adequate daily caloric intake, the intake of calories on a regular cyclic basis throughout the day, and the intake of sufficient protein.[81] Helping the athlete establish a consistent eating pattern of a minimum of three meals per day with the inclusion of protein and carbohydrate is fundamental. Establishing meal consistency and nutritional adequacy occurs in a slow, stepwise manner based on small, concrete goals that the individual feels he or she can successfully accomplish (Table 39–14).

NORMAL METABOLISM AND ABERRATIONS ASSOCIATED WITH ABNORMAL EATING

Since most poeple with an eating disorder spend significant time, energy, and thought pursuing a low body weight, it is crucial to establish understanding of the metabolic adaptations to restricted eating and low body weight. By learning about the factors that determine weight regulation and normal metabolism, the athlete can begin to understand that how he or she eats ultimately interferes with weight control and athletic performance and explains many of the physical symptoms experienced (Table 39–15).

SYMPTOMATOLOGY AND MEDICAL COMPLICATIONS OF EATING DISORDERS

The athlete needs to connect the physical complaints and changes in health, well being, or athletic performance with the eating disorder. A review of medical complications can have a powerful influence on the athlete who is often quite simply feeling "sick and tired" and may also be worried about health and performance. Table 39–16 lists various symptoms and medical complications of eating disorders.

PREDICTING REFEEDING SYMPTOMS

The greatest challenge for the individual with an eating disorder is coping with weight fluctuations. As the athlete increases food and fluid intake and decreases or ceases purging behaviors, he or she must be prepared to see weight changes. There is a tendency to automatically assume weight shifts are caused by increases in fat or muscle mass. Weight increases are usually due to replacement of fluid, substrate, and electrolyte store.[75,78,80]

Significant increases in carbohydrate following a period of prolonged restriction can lead to a 1- to 5-lb weight gain. Decrease in or cessation of purging behaviors such as use of laxatives, diuretics, or self-induced vomiting can result in a 5- to 10-lb weight gain from rebound edema. This fluid retention can last up to 2 months as the body normalizes hydration.[55]

The dietitian has an important role as a member of the eating disorder treatment team and as a resource for all athletes. Access to accurate nutrition information, healthy weight-management techniques, and nutri-

TABLE 39–15
Explanation of Normal Metabolism and Consequences of Abnormal Eating[75,78,80]

1. Define metabolism and regulation of body weight
2. Estimate caloric requirements at normal metabolic rate

    Calculate Harris-Benedict equation[82] to predict normal resting energy expenditure
    Women: 655 + (4.4 × weight in pounds) + (4.3 × height in inches) − (6.8 × age in years)
    Men: 66 + (6.2 × weight in pounds) + (12.7 × height in inches) − (6.8 × age in years)

    Multiply the resting energy expenditure × 1.3 for sedentary activity
    Add caloric requirements for exercise or sports event
3. Estimate current caloric and nutrient intake from a 24-hour recall
4. Describe compensatory mechanism of decreased metabolic rate to conserve muscle and fat stores in response to restricted food intake[80]
    For anorexia nervosa, a 20 to 40% decrease from normal metabolic rate can be expected
    For bulimia nervosa, 0 to 15% decrease from normal metabolic rate can be expected (depends on severity of purging and restricted eating patterns)
5. Relate the connection between abnormal eating and obsessional thinking about food, weight, and hunger
6. Discuss steps in normalizing metabolic rate
    For anorexia nervosa, increase calories from current level by approximately 250 to 300 calories to promote slow, steady weight gain.
    For bulimia nervosa, maintain or slowly increase calories, if appropriate, while primarily focusing on stabilizing eating patterns to decrease binges and purges

tional requirements for health and athletic performance is essential to curb the rise in eating disorders in the athletic world.

SUMMARY

In order to determine an athlete's nutrtional needs and whether they are being met, a complete assessment is necessary. The assessment consists of subjective data: what the athlete has to say about his or her nutritional status; objective data, including anthropometric indices (height, weight, body composition); laboratory data (complete blood count, lipid profile), caloric vitamin, and mineral intake; and percentage of total calories contributed by carbohydrate, fat, and protein. An interview is an important component of the assessment and a good time for the practitioner to build a rapport with the athlete, learn about his or her eating and training practices and determine the athlete's motivation and readiness to make dietary changes.

The recommended sports diet consists of 60 to 70 percent carbohydrates, 10 to 15 percent protein, and 20 percent fat. Most nutritional requirements can be met

with a balanced diet. Protein needs are best met through dietary sources. Complex carbohydrates are the body's most efficient source of energy and an abundant source of vitamins and minerals. Dietary fats are the most energy-dense of the macronutrients and are needed in limited amounts in the diet. Since individual needs for calories, and nutrients may vary, individual needs should be assessed.

Water-soluble vitamins are the vitamin B complex and vitamin C. Based on their use in the body, these vitamins may play a role in athletic performance. All of these are readily available in the diet, primarily from grains, fruits, and vegetables. The role of fat-soluble vitamins and athletic performance is not well studied, and their role in athletic performance is unclear.

The timing of meals and snacks may have a great impact on an athlete's level of energy and physical status. Consumption of pre-exercise and competition foods should be based on the duration and intensity of the activity and the athlete's individual preferences. Precompetition foods should be tried and true favorites. With activities lasting 90 minutes or longer, a diluted carbohydrate drink, about 6 to 8 percent carbohydrate, helps to prevent dehydration and provides energy to maintain blood sugar levels. After an event, high-carbohydrate intake is recommended because glycogen replacement is most efficient immediately following the exercise.

Athletes may be particularly susceptible to the marketing of fad diets and gimmicks. Weight-loss goals

TABLE 39–16
Medical Complications of Eating Disorders

- For women irregular periods, cessation of periods (amenorrhea), reproductive complications
- Lowered metabolism
- Fatigue
- Weakness
- Cold intolerance
- Muscle wasting (including heart tissue)
- Anemia
- Dehydration
- Electrolyte abnormalities: dizziness, lightheadedness, weakness
- Fluid retention
- Delayed gastric emptying: bloating, early fullness, indigestion
- Constipation
- Diarrhea
- Hypoglycemia
- Stomach pain
- Esophageal tears
- Sore throat
- Dental erosion
- Parotid gland enlargement
- Rectal bleeding
- Frequent bruising
- Slow wound-healing
- Night blindness
- Dry skin and lips
- Dry, dull hair or significant hair loss

The following nonprofit organizations offer a variety of services to individuals with eating disorders, their families, and health care professionals:

American Anorexia/Bulimia Association, Inc.
418 East 76th Street
New York, NY 10021
(212) 734–1114

Anorexia Nervosa and Related Eating Disorders (ANRED)
P.O. Box 5102
Eugene, OR 97405
(503) 344–1144

National Anorexic Aid Society (NAAS)
5796 Karl Road
Columbus, OH 43229
(614) 436–1112

National Association of Anorexia Nervosa and Associated Disorders (ANAD)
P.O. Box 271
Highland Park, IL 60035
(708) 831–3438

NCAA Videotapes on Eating Disorders/Karol Media
350 N. Pennsylvania Avenue, Box 7600
Wilkes-Barre, PA 18773-7600
(800) 526–4663

should be realistic and achievable. Athletes trying to meet weight requirements or who are working to improve their fat to lean body mass ratio, should be individually assessed, and a program of exercise and diet should be developed based on the assessment. Concern has been escalating about eating disorders in athletes and health professionals; coaches and trainers working with athletes should be able to recognize the signs and symptoms of anorexia nervosa and bulimia. Early detection and intervention may increase the chances of successful intervention.

As technology improves and research expands, the science of nutrition provides us with information that, if implemented, will increase quality of life and optimize the athlete's performance. Since it is a science of interest to our population in general, the popular press will continue to sensationalize information regarding nutrition. The diet and supplement industry are not strictly regulated in this country; therefore athletes need to seek out nutritional experts for accurate nutrition information and to develop individualized plans to optimize performance.

REFERENCES

1. McArdle WD, Katch FI, Katch UL: Exercise Physiology: Energy, Nutrition and Human Perforamnce, 2nd ed. Philadelphia, Lea & Febiger, 1986.
2. Klaas R, Saris WH: Limits of energy turnover in relation to physical performance: Achievement of energy balance on a daily basis. J Sports Sci 1991; 9:1–15.
3. Willett W, Sampson L, Stampfer MJ, et al: Reproducibility and validity of a semiquantitative food frequency questionnaire. Am J Epidemiol 1985; 122:51–65.
4. National Research Council: Recommended Dietary Allowances, 10th ed. Washington, DC: National Academy of Sciences; 1989.
5. Prochaskas J, DiClemente C, Norcross J: In search of how people change: Applications to addictive behaviors. Am Psychol 1992; 47(9):1102–1114.
6. Berning J, McKibben G, Benardot D, Fike S: Fuel supplies for exercise. In Bernardot D (ed): Sports Nutrition: A Guide for the Professional Working with Active People, 2nd ed. The American Dietetic Association, Chicago, 1992; pp 11–19.
7. Gontzea I, Sutzescu R, Dumitrach S: The influence of adaptation to physical effort on nitrogen balance in man. Nutr Rep Int 1975; 11:231–236.
8. Marable NL, Hickson JF, et al: Urinary nitrogen excretion as influenced by a muscle-building exercise program and protein intake variation. Nutr Rep Int 1979; 19:795–805.
9. Butterfield GE. Whole-body protein utilization in humans. Med Sci Sports Exerc. 1987; 19:S157–S167.
10. Lemon PWR, Mullin JP: Effect of initial muscle glycogen levels on protein catabolism during exercise. J Appl Pysiol 1980; 48:624–629.
11. Tarnopolsky M, MacDougall D, Atkinson S: Influence of protein intake and training status on nitrogen balance and lean body mass. J Appl Physiol 1988; 64:187–193.
12. Dohm GL, Williams RT, Kaspereck GJ, et al. Increased secretion of urea and N-methylhistidine by rats and humans after a bout of exercise. J Appl Physiol, 1982;52:27–33.
13. Houtkooper L: Food selection for endurance sports. Med Sci Sports Exerc 1992; 24(Suppl 9)S349–S359.
14. Laritcheva KA, Alovaya NI, Shubin VI, Smirnov PV. Study of energy expenditure and protein needs of top weight lifters. In Parizkova J, Rogozkin VA (eds): Nutrition, Physical Fitness and Health. Baltimore, University Park, Press, 1978, p 155.
15. Burke L, Read R: Diet patterns of elite Australian male triathletes. Phys Sports Med 1987; 15:140–145.
16. Position of the American Dietetic Association and the Canadian Dietetic Association: Nutrition for physical fitness and athletic performance for adults. J Am Diet Assoc 1993; 93(6):691–696.
17. Williams MH: The role of protein in physical activity. In Williams MH (ed): Nutritional Aspects of Human Physical and Athletic Performance. Springfield, IL Charles C Thomas, 1985.
18. Heaney RP: Protein intake and the calcium economy. J Am Diet Assoc 1993; 93:1261–1262.
19. Nordin BEC, Need AG, Morris HA, Horowitz M: Sodium, calcium and osteoporosis. In Burckhardt P, Heane RP (eds): Nutritional Aspects of Osteoporosis. New York, Raven Press, 1991; pp 85:279–295.
20. Position of the American Dietetic Association: Vegetarian diets. J Am Diet Assoc 1993; 93(11):1317–1319.
21. Sherman WM, Lamb DR: Nutrition and prolonged exercise. In Lamb DR, Murray R (eds): Perspectives in Exercise Science and Sports Medicine: Prolonged Exercise. Indianapolis, Benchmark Press, 1988, pp 213–280.
22. Roberts KM, Noble EG, Hayden DB, Taylor AW: Simple and complex carbohydrate – rich diets and muscle glycogen content of marathon runners. J Appl Physio 1988; 57:70–74.
23. Clark N: Nanc Clark's Sports Nutrition Guidebook. Champaign, IL, Leisure Press, 1990.
24. Wright ED, Paige DM: Lipid metabolism and exercise. J Clin Nutr 1988; 7:28–32.
25. Berg, FM: Alcohol promotes fat storage. Obesity Health, Nov/Dec 1993;107–108.
26. Berning J, McKibben G, Benardot D, Fike S: Fuel supplies for exercise in sports nutrition. In Benardot D (ed): Sports Nutrition: A Guide for the Professional Working with Active People, American Dietetic Association Chicago, 2nd ed. 1992, p 18.
27. Lange RM, Borrow KM, Neumann A, Feldman T: Adverse cardiac effects of alcohol ingesting in young adults. Ann Intern Med 1985; 102:742–747.
28. McNaughton L, Preece D: Alcohol and its effects on sprint and middle distance running. Br J Sports Med 1986; 20:56–59.
29. Houmard JA, Langenfeld ME, Wiley RL, Seifert J: Effects of the acute ingestion of small amounts of alcohol on 5-mile run times. J Sports Med 1987; 27:253–257.
30. Keith RE: Vitamins in sport and exercise. In Wolinsky I, Hickson JF (eds): Nutrition, Exercise and Sport. Boca Raton, FL, CRC Press, 1989, p 34.
31. Gerster H: The role of vitamin C in athletic performance. J Am Coll Nutr 1989; 8:636–643.

32. Baily D, Carron AV, Teece RD: Effect of vitamin C supplementation upon the physiological response to exercise in trained and untrained runners. Int Z Vitaminforsch 1979; 40:435–441.

33. Henschel A, Taylor H, Brozek J, et al: Vitamin C and ability to work in hot environments. Am J Trop Med Hyg 1944; 24:259–265.

34. Howald H, Segesser B: Ascorbic acid and athletic performance. Ann Ny Acad Sci 1975; 258:458–464.

35. Keren G: The effect of high dosage vitamin C intake on aerobic and anaerobic capacity. J Sports Med Phys Fitness 1980; 20:145–148.

36. Rasch P, Arnheim D, Klafs C: Effects of vitamin C supplementation on cross-country runners. Sportsartzliche Prax 1962; 5:10–13.

37. Sharman IM: The effects of vitamin E and training on physiological function and athletic performance in adolescent swimmers. Br J Nutr 1971; 26:265–276.

38. Lawrence JD, Bower RC, Riehl WP, Smith JC: Effects of alpha-tocopherol acetate on the swimming endurance of trained swimmers. Am J Clin Nutr 1975; 28:205–208.

39. Clement DB, Sawchuk LL: Iron status and sports performance. Sports Med 1984; 1:65.

40. Eichner ER: Sports anemia: Poor terminology for a real phenomenom. Gatorade Sports Sci Exchange 1988; vol 1(6).

41. Sherman AR, Krammer B: Iron, nutrition and exercise. In Wolinsky I, Hickson JF (eds): Nutrition in Exercise and Sport. Boca Raton, FL, CRC Press, 1989, pp 291–300.

42. Eichner E: Sports anemia, iron supplements and blood doping. Med Sci Sports Exerc 1992; 24:S315–S318.

43. Eichner E. The anemias of athletes. Phys Sports Med 1986; 14:122–125, 129–130.

44. Eichner ER: Facts and myths about anemia in active women. Your Patient Fitness 1990; 5(1):12–16.

45. Clarkson PM: Vitamins and trace minerals. In Lamb DR, Williams MH (eds): Perspectives in Exercise Science and Sports Medicine, vol 4, Ergogenics. Indianapolis, Brown and Benchmark, 1991, pp 123–182.

46. Celsing FJ, Svedenhag J, Pihlstedt P, Ekblom B: Effects of anemia and stepwise-induced polycythemia on aerobic power in individuals with high and low hemoglobin concentrations. Acta Physiol Scand 1987; 129:47–57.

47. Drinkwater BL, Nilson K, Chesnut CH, et al: Bone mineral content of amenorrheic and eumenorrheic athletes. N Engl J Med 1984; 311:277–281.

48. Gisolfi CV, Duchman SM: Guidelines for optimal replacement beverages for different athletic events. Med Sci Sports Exerc 1992; 24(6):679–687.

49. Hiller WDB: Dehydration and hyponatremia during triathlons. Med Sci Sports Exerc 1989; 21:S219–S221.

50. Morimoto T, Miki K, Nose H, et al: Changes in body fluid and its composition during heavy sweating and effect of fluid and electrolyte replacement. Jpn J Biometeorol 1981; 18:31–39.

51. Nadel ER: Limits imposed on exercise in a hot environment. Sports Sci Exchange 1990; 3:27.

52. Sawka MN, Pandolf KB: Effects of body water loss on physiological function and exercise performance. In Gisolfi CV, Lamb DR (eds): Perspectives in Exercise Science and Sports Medicine, vol 3, Fluid Homeostasis During Exercise. Indianapolis, Benchmark Press, 1990, pp 1–38.

53. Coggan AR, Coyle EF: Carbohydrate ingestion during prolonged exercise: Effects on metabolism and performance. Exerc Sports Sci Rev 1991; 19:1–40.

54. Coyle EF, Montain SJ: Benefits of fluid replacement with carbohydrate during exercise. Med Sci Sports Exerc 1992; 24(Supplement 9):S324–S330.

55. Leiper JB, Maughan RJ: Comparison of absorption rates from two hypotonic and two isotonic rehydration solutions in the intact human jejunum. Clin Sci 1988; 75(Supplement 19):22P.

56. Lifshitz F, Wapnir RA: Oral hydration solutions: Experimental optimization of water and sodium absorption. J Pediatr 1984; 106:383–389.

57. Williams MH: Beyond Training: How Athletes Enhance Performance Legally and Illegally. Champaign, IL, Leisure Press; 1989.

58. US Olympic Committee: Drug Control Program. Committee on Substance Abuse Research and Education, 1986.

59. Sherman WM: Carbohydrate feedings before and after exercise. In Lamb DR, Williams MH (eds): Perspectives in Exercise Science and Sports Medicine, vol 4, Ergonomics: Enhancement of Performance in Exercise and Sport. Indianapolis, Benchmark, 1991, pp 1–34.

60. Sherman WM, Lamb DR: Nutrition and prolonged exercise. In Lamb DR, Murray R (eds): Perspectives in Exercise Science and Sports Medicine, Vol 1, Prolonged Exercise. Indianapolis, Benchmark Press, 1988, pp 213–280.

61. Sherman WM, Maglischo EW: Minimizing chronic athlete fatigue among swimmers: Special emphasis on nutrition. Sports Sci Exchange Nov 1991; 4(35).

62. Coyle EF: Carbohydrates and athletic performance. Sports Sci Exchange Oct 1988; 1(7).

63. Cummings S: Obesity management. In Carlson KM, Eisenstat S (eds): Primary Care of Women. Chicago, Mosby Year Book (in press).

64. Foreyt JP, Goodrick GK: Factors common to successful therapy for the obese patient. Med Sci Sports Exerc 1991; 23:292–297.

65. Brownell KD, Rodin J: Prevalence of eating disorders in athletes. In Brownell KD, Rodin J, Wilmore JH (eds): Eating, Body Weight and Performance in Athletes: Disorders of Modern Society. Philadelphia, Lea & Febiger, 1992.

66. Drummer G, Rosen L, Heusener W, et al: Pathogenic weight-control behaviors of young competitive swimmers. Phys Sports Med 1987; 15:75–84.

67. Rosen L, McKeag D, Hough D, Curley V: Pathogenic weight-control behavior in female athletes. Phys Sports Med 1986; 14:79–86.

68. Steen SN, Brownell KD: Current patterns of weight loss and regain in wrestlers: Has the tradition changed? Med Sci Sports Exerc 1990; 22:776.

69. Rosen L, Hough D: Pathogenic weight-control behaviors of female college gymnasts. Phys Sports Med 1988; 16:141–145.

70. Johnson MD, Disordered eating in active and athletic women. Clin Sports Med 1994; 13:335–369.

71. Malina RM: Physique and body composition: Effects on performance and effects of training, semistarvation and overtraining. In Brownell KD, Rodin J, Wilmore JH (eds): Eating, Body Weight and Performance in Athletes: Disorders of Modern Society. Philadelphia, Lea & Febiger, 1992.

72. Eichner ER: General health issues of low body weight and undereating in athletes. In Brownell KD, Rodin J, Wilmore JH (eds): Eating, Body Weight and Performance in Athletes: Disorders of Modern Society. Philadelphia, Lea & Febiger; 1992.

73. Snow-Harter SM: Bone health and prevention of osteoporosis in active and athletic women. Clin Sports Med 1994; 13:389–404.

74. Herzog DB, Copeland PM: Eating disorders. N Engl J Med 1985; 313:295–303.

75. Luder E, Schebenach J: Nutrition management of eating disorders. Top Clin Nutr 1993; 8:48–63.

76. MsSherry J: The diagnostic challenge of anorexia nervosa. Am Fam Physician 1984; 29:139–145.

77. Eating disorders in young athletes. Phys Sports Med 1985; 13(11):89.

78. Rock CL, Yager J: Nutrition and eating disorders: A primer for clinicians. Int J Eat Disord 1987; 6:267–280.

79. Bo-Linn GW, Santa Ana CA, Morawski SG, Fordtran S: Purging and calorie absorption in bulimic patients and normal women. Ann Intern Med 1983; 99:14–17.

80. Reiff DW, Rieff KKL: Eating Disorders: Nutrition Therapy in the Recovery Process. Gaithersberg, MD, Aspen, 1992.

81. Wilmore JH: Body weight standards and athletic performance. In Brownell KD, Rodin J, Wilmore JH (eds): Eating, Body Weight and Performance in Athletes: Disorders of Modern Society. Philadelphia, Lea & Febiger, 1992.

82. American Psychiatric Association: Diagnostic and Statistical Manual of Mental Disorders, 4th ed. Washington, DC, American Psychiatric Association, 1994.

CHAPTER 40

Protective Equipment Considerations

ETHAN SALIBA *PhD, ATC, PT, SCS*
SUSAN FOREMAN *MEd, MPT, ATC*
RICHARD T. ABADIE, JR. *BA, EMC*

In 1968, there were 32 fatalities due to participation in organized football and 4 additional fatalities in sandlot play.[1] Although the incidence of fatalities was above average that year, severe injuries in organized sports have been greatly reduced by efforts to improve protective equipment. Injury prevention is a major role of sports medicine professionals. When used properly, athletic equipment can contribute significantly to injury prevention. Equipment has evolved as a result of research and testing of materials as well as from the examination of mechanisms of injury. Football has the greatest incidence on injury, therefore, the focus has been on protective football gear. Other sports have benefited from the research and development of football equipment, however. This chapter covers the common materials used in protective padding and presents an overview of some of the protective equipment used in athletic competition.

The purpose of athletic equipment is to prevent injury or to protect an existing injury. Protective equipment attempts to restrict the motion of a certain body part, reduce friction between surfaces that come into contact, or absorb energy of a direct blow. The selected materials should allow the force to be dispersed over a large area so that the force at any one place is minimized.[2] Athletic equipment is not effective unless the proper fit is maintained and the use of the equipment is thoroughly explained.[3] Equipment cannot eliminate injuries, but it can help prevent them and reduce their severity.

There is debate as to whether protective equipment can increase the incidence of injury by allowing some athletes to participate with reckless abandon. The football player's "armor" can allow higher-velocity impacts because the shock is well absorbed by the protective padding. These high-speed collisions can result in a greater incidence of joint injury because equipment cannot protect the athlete adequately from indirect forces. As a result, the sport of rugby does not allow any protective equipment—pads, wraps, helmets,

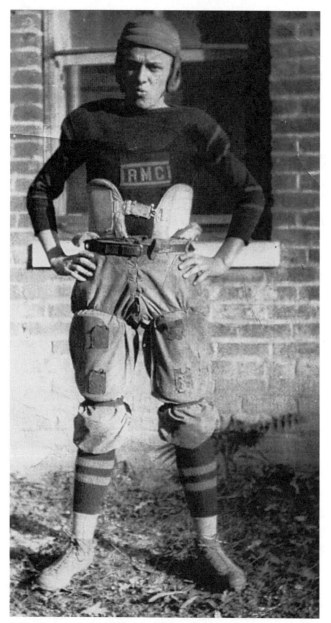

FIGURE 40–1. Football equipment from the 1930s: Leather helmet, no facemask, rib protector, thick canvas football pants with pads sewed or strapped into place.

or braces—even to prevent reinjury. Many women's sports organizations, such as lacrosse, believe that protective equipment will change the nature of the game to one with more physical contact.[4] Women's lacrosse, however, does permit the use of padding or bracing to prevent reinjuries and to allow earlier return to participation after injury.

Modern protective equipment utilizes technological advances in plastics for energy absorption and impact deflection. For example, football shoulder pads were originally fabricated out of leather by saddlemakers to disperse forces and reduce shock. Pants were made of thick leather with layers of cotton to provide hip, knee, and thigh protection. Helmets were also originally fabricated from leather (Fig. 40–1). Football facemasks were not added until 1954, after helmets were made

from plastic shells.[4] Modern equipment is produced from strong but lightweight plastics, covering a variety of shock-absorbing material.

Protective equipment has been developed and has subsequently become required for some sports to help reduce the incidence of specific injuries. This equipment can have varying styles to accommodate the different functional needs of the various sports. Additionally, there are subtle differences in equipment even between positions within the same sport. For example, lineman shoulder pads typically allow less movement and provide more protection compared with shoulder pads for a receiver, which are lighter and allow greater mobility.

Protective equipment is also available to protect a previously injured area. Once functional criteria have been met to allow an athlete's return to activity, added protection should be considered to help prevent reinjury. Commercial protective equipment for specific injuries can be purchased or can be fabricated by athletic trainers or therapists. The availability of materials and creativity are the only restricting factors in fabricating such protective equipment.

Any modifications of the athlete's equipment should be done according to the manufacturer's specification and should not alter the fit of the original equipment. Care should be taken not to cause stress or cracking of the original material on impact, such as might result from drilling holes.[5] To do so may also void the manufacturer's warranty. Specialized pads such as flank pads, arm extensions, or rib protectors are also commercially available to protect specific areas (Fig. 40–2). Most commercially produced special pads fit well with standard pads and can be secured with the existing brackets or Velcro. However, many times the smaller and less costly adaptations will perform just as well. For example, foam donuts with or without a hard orthoplast or plastic covering can be taped or wrapped into place. Spray adherent may prevent slippage of custom-made pads during competition, or the device can be sewn into existing pads (Fig. 40–3).

LIABILITY AND STANDARDS

The legal issues associated with athletic equipment have become a concern, since catastrophic injuries can occur with improperly fitted or maintained equipment or if the device is used incorrectly. The equipment manager or other designated personnel should regularly inspect athletic equipment for defects, be knowledgeable about proper fit, and be able to instruct and warn the athlete about proper use of equipment.[6]

Because injuries of varying degrees of severity happen in sports, equipment manufacturers have attempted to protect themselves from litigation by developing standards of quality to ensure that the equipment does not fail under normal athletic circumstances and that the equipment does not contribute to injury. The National Operating Committee on Standards for Athletic Equipment (NOCSAE) was established in 1969 to

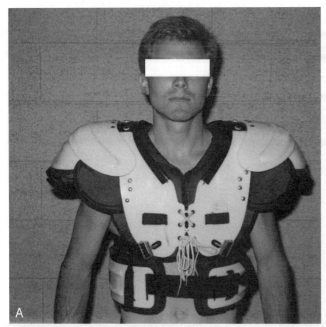

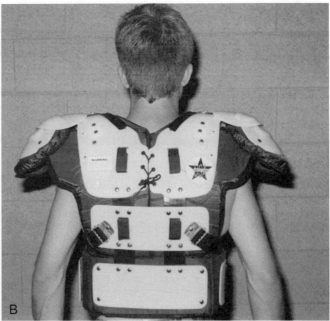

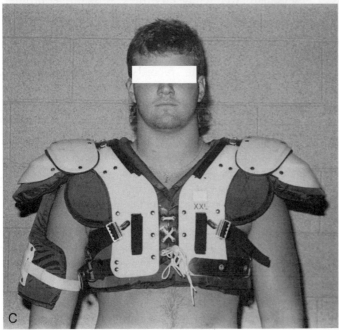

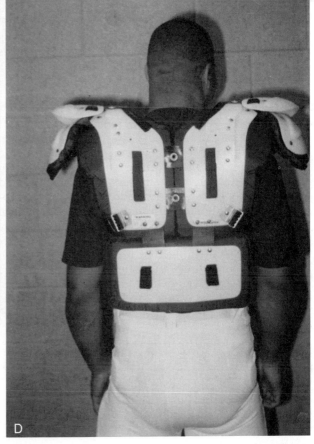

FIGURE 40–2. Standard extensions to football shoulder pads: *A,* Rib combination often used with football quarterbacks; *B,* posterior aspect of rib combination; *C,* lateral arm protector, deltoid extension; *D,* back extension "kick plate."

develop safety standards for football helmets, and the results of its extensive testing were published in 1973.[7] Currently, baseball, softball, and lacrosse helmets and facemasks are also NOCSAE certified; standards were developed for these helmets in 1983 and 1987, respectively.[1]

Other testing agencies have provided standards for equipment used in various sports not covered by

NOCSAE, such as ice hockey and bicycling. The Canadian Standards Association (CSA) and American Society for Testing and Materials (ASTM) also provide standards and testing for athletic equipment. These companies describe the material standards of equipment such as hockey helmets and facemasks so that injuries to the face and head can be consistently prevented or minimized.[8]

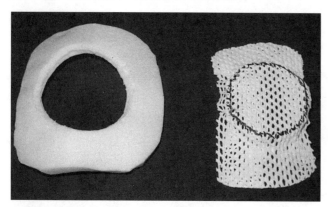

FIGURE 40–3. A custom-fabricated pad: A donut pad is cut from Thermoplast, and firmer Hexalite is molded and attached to the donut to give better protection. This pad is used to protect the acromioclavicular joint.

TABLE 40–1
Factors to Consider in Equipment Testing
• Limitations of size, weight, shape, materials, and durability of the device, with respect to the athletic performance, injury to other players, aesthetics, and cost
• Injury mechanisms—compression, tension, shearing
• Single or multiple impact protection
• Mechanisms of injury and the ability of tissues to withstand that injury at the protected location
• Equipment reassessment for weakness

Testing of equipment is performed under realistic conditions, and in some cases, physical models of the body part and impact surface are created. Football helmets are tested with blunt impact, whereas baseball helmets are tested by focal area impacts such as high-velocity baseballs and swinging bats to simulate potential injury. Torsional stresses may also be imposed, but it is difficult to determine exactly how the body will react in slightly different circumstances. As a result, models cannot be used accurately in all situations (Table 40–1).

WARNING THE ATHLETES

It should be understood that no equipment can prevent all injury. Standards are developed to provide guidelines in the manufacture and maintenance of materials and equipment. Players should be warned about the proper use and limitations of athletic equipment. Athletes should be informed of the dangers of sports participation repeatedly in a manner that they understand. They should never be told that the equipment can do something that it cannot do. NOCSAE warnings are required and must be placed on the exterior of all approved helmets and emphasize that no helmet can protect a player's neck (see box below). This

fact should be reiterated to athletes so that they understand the risks involved in playing sports.[1]

RESPONSIBILITIES OF THE EQUIPMENT MANAGER

Equipment managers or other appropriate personnel must ensure that teams buy the best-quality equipment possible and that used or worn-out equipment is discarded rather than passed down to younger or less skilled athletes. The person responsible for the equipment of a large group such as a football team should maintain appropriate records about guarantees or warranties, any repair or reconditioning requirements, and the age of the equipment.[5] This information may be necessary to demonstrate testing or standards of equipment, and it may be essential if the equipment is implicated in a serious injury. Intercollegiate and professional athletic teams typically hire certified equipment managers to organize, maintain, purchase, and dispense equipment. The Athletic Equipment Manager's Association serves as the certifying agency for this profession.

The inadequate use or improper selection or fit of equipment, or missing equipment, is an act of negligence. Beyond that, all personnel affiliated with a sports team are responsible for ensuring that athletes properly use the required equipment. The individual who is responsible for the fitting and maintenance of athletic equipment is one of the most important members of the athletic support staff. He or she should be aware of the specific purpose of each piece of equipment, the fitting criteria, and the sport-specific mandates and legalities.

NOCSAE WARNING TO BE PLACED ON THE EXTERIOR OF ALL FOOTBALL HELMETS
Do not strike an opponent with any part of this helmet or facemask. This is a violation of football rules and may cause you to suffer severe brain or neck injury, including paralysis or death. Severe brain or neck injury may also occur accidentally while playing football. **No helmet can prevent all such injuries.** **You use this helmet at your own risk.**

MATERIALS USED

Numerous materials are used in the manufacture of modern protective athletic equipment. Every material of a given density, thickness, and temperature has certain properties that help define that material's use.[8] Soft materials usually have a lower density and are lightweight because of air incorporated into the material. Soft materials protect optimally at low levels of impact intensity. Open-cell foams are low-density materials in which the cells are connected to allow air passage from cell to cell. Similar to a sponge, these materials have the capacity to absorb fluids and are commonly used to pad bony prominences or hard edges of protective equipment and custom fabricated pads. Open-cell foams generally do not have good shock-absorbing qualities because they deform quickly under stress.

Firmer, higher-density materials of the same thickness offer less cushioning at low levels of impact, but they absorb more energy by deformation at higher levels of impact.[4] Closed-cell foam is used primarily for protection because air cannot pass from one cell to another. Ensolite (Uniroyal Co., Mahawka, IN) is an example of a closed-cell shock-absorbing material sold in a variety of thicknesses and used commonly in hip pads, thigh pads, and knee pads.

Air management pads are a relatively new type of protective padding and are often used when maximal shock absorption is required in lightweight gear. These pads are constructed of various open- and closed-cell foam pads encased in polyurethane or a nylon material.[9] This encasement is airtight, which prevents quick deformation of the foam so that the energy is dissipated over a broad area. Air pads are frequently used in football shoulder pads, and various companies incorporate different designs of foam placement within the nylon encasement. These pads are more expensive than traditional equipment, and the linings must be replaced or patched if the nylon is torn because this allows too much air to escape on impact. Nylon prevents fluids from entering the pads, which helps avoid adding significant weight to the equipment. Body fluids such as sweat and blood are easily cleaned from the nylon material with a weak bleach solution. Sanitation of traditional padding is more difficult because even closed-cell foam absorbs some fluids.

Resilience or memory is another property of materials used in protective equipment. Resilience is the ability of a material to regain its shape quickly after impact. Highly resilient materials are used when protection from repeated impacts is required.[8] Nonresilient materials can be used when one-time or occasional impact is made, although the protective equipment may be ruined by that impact. These materials must be checked to ensure that the athlete does not continue to use the equipment if the material is crushed or compacted by repeated impacts. For example, the Styrofoam inside bicycle helmets is lightweight and will crush on impact to protect the skull. When the material has been altered due to impact, it no longer offers adequate protection and should be replaced. Nonresilient materials are tested by an independent company to determine whether deformation and energy absorption occurs below levels that would cause injury.

Silicone, fiberglass, Plastazote, thermoplastic materials (Orthoplast, Aquaplast), neoprene, moleskin, felt, and adhesive foams are among the materials used in fabricating customized splints or equipment.[10] Each has a unique protective ability to conform to the body, deflect impact, absorb shock, or immobilize a body structure. Lightweight plastics and foams can be combined to optimize the products' ability to absorb or deflect an impact. Most equipment companies combine

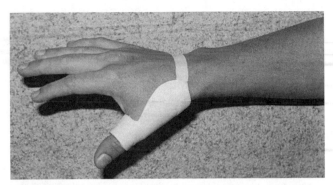

FIGURE 40–4. A thermoplastic splint. Depending on the league and sport, this splint may be used in a game to help stabilize the thumb. Athletic tape is often used to hold the device in place.

materials, depending on the function of the particular piece of gear. This provides comfort and cushion close to the body, and firmer, nonyielding materials are placed on the outside to transfer the stresses over a broad area.[11] Sports medicine clinicians should be familiar with various materials and how they react on impact so that combinations of materials can be used effectively to prevent injury or reinjury.

THERMOPLASTIC MATERIALS

There are various thermoplastic materials that can be used for splint or custom pad fabrication (Fig. 40–4). Thermoplastics, which were developed in the 1960s, become moldable when heated.[12] When hardened, the material gives rigid support to help restrict motion at a joint, such as on the hand. The material can also be used to relieve impact at an area when used in conjunction with a softer, more shock-absorbing material such as foam. The number of companies producing thermoplastics has substantially increased, and the types of materials vary considerably. Different thermoplastic materials have unique characteristics such as moldability, durability, and thickness, which may make one material more suitable for a problem than another. Several of the available materials are identical in composition but are offered by various distributors under different names.

Thermoplastics can be divided into two basic categories: plastic and rubber. Subclassifications, which include plastic/rubber-like and rubber-like, exhibit characteristics of both groups.[12] The plastic group uses a polycaprolactone base with varying amounts of inorganic filler, resins, and elastomers. These agents act as modifiers that affect the memory, stiffness, and durability of the material. The base of the rubber group is composed principally of polyisoprene, which also has varying amounts of fillers and therefore demonstrates different characteristics.

The plastic category tends to be more conforming than the rubber-type materials. Therefore, plastic is more appropriate for small splints such as on the hand. Plastics include materials such as Aquaplast Bluestripe (WFR/Aquaplast), Orfit (North Coast Medical), Multiform I and II (Alimed), and Orthoplast II (Johnson &

Johnson). Rubber-like materials include Ultraform Traditions (Sammons) Orthoplast (Johnson & Johnson), Aquaplast Greenstripe (WFR/Aquaplast), and Synergy (Roylan).

The working temperatures of these materials range from 150° F to 180° F. Most thermoplastics should be heated for about 1 minute with the material flat to minimize distortion or stretching. Most can then be manipulated for 3 to 4 minutes before resuming their hardened form. Some changes can be made with a heat gun, but this should not be done while the splint is on the athlete.

Thermoplastic materials come in varying thicknesses and degrees of perforation. Perforation allows for ventilation in the material but can compromise the durability, especially when subjected to the forces associated with athletic competition.[13] Table 40–2 summarizes the various qualities associated with some of the thermoplastic materials. Shelf life also affects the quality of these materials.

There are also high-temperature thermoplastics that become malleable at temperatures of 325° F to 350° F (163° C to 177° C). These can be vacuum molded or shaped over plaster models. Heat guns can be used to make modifications. These materials can be transparent and are useful, for instance, if a full-contact facemask is desired to allow protection of a facial injury (e.g., W-Clear [Smith Nephew Rolyan]).

SOFT MATERIALS

Other materials frequently used in splint or protective equipment customization include felts and foams. These materials are available in various thicknesses and may have adhesive backing, allowing easy application. Moleskin and orthopaedic felts are frequently used in the athletic environment. Moleskin is a soft, 1/16-inch-thick cotton backcloth with self-adhesive backing. It is used to protect the athlete from abrasive forces in high-stress areas or to cover edges of splints. Orthopaedic felt is made of polyester, polypropylene, and viscose and has numerous applications, including bridging equipment around injured sites or as temporary orthotic materials.

Foam padding is used to help absorb shock and can be used alone in custom padding or in conjunction with thermoplastic materials, depending on the amount of impact resistance needed.[11] Plastazote (Apex Foot Products, South Hackensack, NJ) is heat-activated, lightweight, closed-cell foam that is heated for 5 to 10 minutes in a convection oven at 285° F (140° C). This polyethylene material can be formed to the part to be protected and provides lightweight padding and support.[4] Sorbothane (Sorbothane, Inc., Kent, OH) is a self-adhesive viscoelastic polymer padding that dissipates and absorbs impact forces. This material is available in sheets or in prefabricated pads that can be placed in ball gloves, shoes, or splints. PPT (Professional Protective Technologies, Inc., Division of Langer Biomedical Group, Deer Park, NY) is a nylon-coated, open-cell padding material that absorbs shock. It is a durable material frequently used in supporting devices such as thigh and elbow sleeves to add protection in impact areas. PPT is also used over tender or sensitive areas, especially in footwear.

SEMIRIGID MATERIAL

Scotchcast fiberglass/polyurethane splints soften at room temperature (70° F to 75° F) and provide a one-step, easily moldable splint that sets in 3 to 4 minutes. Functional strength in the material is attained in 20 minutes. Scotchwrap has 25 percent of the fiberglass resin of Scotchcast, which causes it to be less rigid when dry. This could be an alternative to RTV 11 rubber in high school athletes, since it is easier to apply. However, a referee may require the material to be covered with soft padding during participation to avoid injury to other players.

Hexcelite or X-Lite (Smith Nephew Rolyan) is a low-temperature thermoplastic with an open-weave design that allows fabrication of lightweight, highly ventilated splints. This material becomes malleable with warm tap water and is self-bonding, so multiple layers can be used to increase the rigidity of the device.

Silicone elastomer has been popular in fabricating soft splints. This material is used when a more rigid material is considered illegal in sporting competition. Silicone elastomer casting is appropriate with certain types of hand or wrist injuries or when a fracture has reached a healing state that would not be compromised with less rigid protection. The liquid-style elastomer is reinforced with layers of gauze bandaging when used for casting. The set-up time is controlled by a separate catalyst that is added to the silicone when the cast is made. Because the silicone cast is nonporous in its finished form, it is typically worn only during competition. Skin maceration can occur if the cast is worn for too long. The athlete should wear a bivalved cast or splint at all other times until the injury has healed.

RULES FOR INDIVIDUALIZED PROTECTIVE EQUIPMENT

Rules regarding legal equipment in high school football are established by the National Federation of State High School Association. The previous rule regarding the use of splinting materials stated that hard substances in their final forms such as leather, rubber, plastic, plaster, or fiberglass constitute illegal equipment when worn on the elbow, forearm, wrist, or hand, even when covered with soft padding. This rule was meant to protect an injured athlete from further harming himself or herself, but it often resulted in the athlete compromising needed protection by substituting softer, legal materials.[14] Intercollegiate and professional athletes are allowed to wear hard and unyielding substances (e.g., casts) below the elbow if they are covered with one-half-inch closed-cell foam.

The rule was changed based on injury data from the National Collegiate Athletic Association (NCAA) and

TABLE 40–2
Comparison of Thermoplastics

	Working Temperature (° F)	Rigidity	Shrink-age	Stretch	Drap-ability	Mold-ability	Bond	Mem-ory	Comments
Plastic									
NCM Clinic (Precision Splint/RS 3000) North Coast/Polymed	160–170	3	1	3	3	3	3	2	Easy to work and contour
Polyform/Kay Splint—Rolyan/Sammons	150–160	2	1	2+	3	3	3	1	Easy to mold; do not overheat
Ultraform (Sammons)	160	2	2	2	3	2	2	1	Nice feel/texture
Aquaplast, Bluestripe (WFR/Aquaplast)	160–180	2	2	3+	3	3	3	2	Better cut pattern when translucent; highly moldable
Orthoplast II (Johnson & Johnson)	150–170	2	1	3	2	2	3	1	Looks, behaves like Multiform
Multiform I & II (AliMed)	150–180	3	2	3	3	2	3	1	Inexpensive; easy to mold and work
Plastic and rubber-like									
NCM Preferred/Custom Splint/JU1000 North Coast/Polymed	160–170	3	1	2	3	2	2	1	Versatile; skin rash with perspiration
Ultraform 294 (Sammons)	160	3	1	1	1	1	2	2	Difficult to form
Polyflex II/Kay Splint, Isoprene Rolyan/Sammons	160	2	1	3	3	3	2	1	Good for small/large orthoses; scraps recyclable
Aquaplast (WFR/Aquaplast)	160–180	2	3	3	3	3	3	3	Needs work with edges—for experienced splint makers
Orfit Soft (North Coast)	160–180	2	2	3	3	3	3	3	Similar to Aquaplast—shrinks less when allowed to cool on patient
Rubber-like									
NCM Spectrum/Ultrasplint/MR 2000 North Coast/Polymed	170	2	1	1	1	2	2	1	Reshapes and edges roll easily
Ezeform/Kay Splint III Rolyan/Sammons	170	3	1	1	1	2	3	1	Good for large othoses; easy trim edge
Aquaplast (Aquaplast)	160–180	2	2	2	2	3	3	3	Great colors; contours nicely, easy to work
Aquaplast Greenstripe (WFR Aquaplast)	160–180	2	2	2	1	2	2	3	Less conforming but more rigid for larger othoses
Orfit Stif (North Coast)	135	3	2	2	1	2	3	3	Increased thickness good for large orthoses
Synergy (Rolyan)	160	1	1	1	1	2	1	2	Attractive/nice feel; takes effort to contour
Rubber									
Orthoplast (Johnson & Johnson)	160	1	1	1	1	3	2	1	Good edges, worse contour
Ultraform Traditions (Sammons)	160	2	2						Not tested

Range of scores is 1 (least) to 3 (most).
From Breger-Lee DE, Buford WL: Propertes of thermoplastic splinting materials. J Hand Ther 1992; 4:202–211.

TABLE 40–3
Legality of Hard Casts in High School Football

- The cast or splint must be constructed of approved material (no metal or plaster)
- The cast or splint must be covered by a minimum of ½-inch closed-cell foam
- A written authorization form must be signed and available to the officials at the beginning of the competition that indicates that the athlete may participate in football with the cast or splint
- The officials should check and approve the paperwork and the padded cast or splint prior to the game
- The referee has the authority to eject a player if he or she is using the cast or splint as a weapon

from a pilot program in six states. The National Federation of State High School Association will now allow "hard, abrasive or unyielding substances on the hand, wrist, forearm, or elbow if the substance is covered on all exterior surfaces with no less than one-half inch thick, high density, closed-cell polyurethane, or a material of the same minimum thickness and similar physical properties." In addition, "a licensed medical physician must approve in writing any playing cast or splint, and the document must be available for the contest officials to verify that the hard material is properly padded according to new guidelines."[14] In the case of a fracture, it would have to be considered by a physician to be stable or "healed," but that additional protection or immobilization is advisable.

Materials approved in the current ruling would allow fiberglass, Scotchguard soft cast, thermoplastics, and rubber materials but would prohibit plaster and metal. Soft materials do not require additional padding but must be determined to be "soft" by the attending game official (Table 40–3).

HELMETS

The advent of the football helmet and, more specifically, the plastic shell with the facemask dramatically increased the number of injuries in sports. The number of head and facial injuries was reduced but the increased protection allowed the head to become a "weapon," therefore increasing the risk of cervical spine injuries.[3] This increase in injuries generated a heightened interest in the proper maintenance and fitting of helmets. No helmet design can completely prevent head injury but it can reduce the magnitude of a blow by dispersing or deflecting forces.

Currently, catastrophic head injuries are relatively uncommon in organized sports if protective equipment is used properly. Head injuries can occur from direct or indirect contact when the head strikes another surface and when there is motion of the brain within the skull. Additionally, scalp injuries such as lacerations can occur with direct impact. Injury to the scalp and skull from blunt trauma can be greatly minimized or eliminated with properly fitted helmets. However, contrecoup injuries caused by motion of the brain within the cranial cavity and shearing of the brain tissue are much more difficult to predict, prevent, and test.[8]

Many sports require protective head gear because of an increased potential for head injury (Table 40–4). Standards for helmets and head gear are defined in the rules and regulations of each particular sport.

HELMET LININGS

Helmet linings have changed over the decades. Initially, leather linings were the only means of force absorption in head gear. The lining has since progressed from suspension webbing, to using water or air cells, to the contemporary closed-cell padding with air bladders (Fig. 40–5). The air bladders, used to absorb shock as well as to maintain proper fit, should be inspected daily by the players to ensure that adequate inflation is maintained.

HELMET SHELLS

The manufacturers of football helmets have slightly different helmet reconditioning and retirement requirements, although they each use similar materials. Generally, all helmets should be reconditioned every 2 years. The polycarbonate alloy shell has a 5-year warranty, and the ABS plastic shell has a 2-year warranty. The AHI (Athletic Helmets, Inc.) helmet should be retired after 6 years. Riddell recommends retiring its helmet after 10 years, based on data collected from tests performed on helmets as they were reconditioned. Additionally, independent laboratory analysis of resin base characteristics of the plastic shell under environmental stresses showed significant changes in the material qualities over time.

A rubber liner was devised to fit on the outer surface of the plastic shell in the 1980s. This was proposed to provide an additional shock-absorbing quality. However, the frictional forces that this external liner added created significant concern among equipment professionals. The company that produces this product states that the safety issue regarding additional frictional forces has been appropriately addressed through impact research.[15] It concludes that the rubber liner is an effective and safe addition to the standard football helmet. This outer padding device is currently used on an individual basis.

TABLE 40–4
Sports Requiring Helmets

- Football
- Ice hockey
- Mens' lacrosse
- Baseball
- Softball
- Whitewater sports (kayaking)
- Amateur boxing
- Bicycling

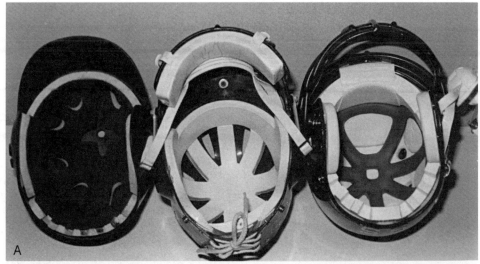

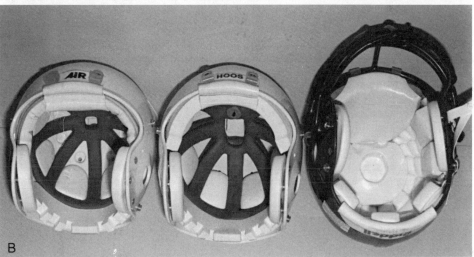

FIGURE 40–5. Helmet linings: *A*, Baseball, lacrosse, and football air helmets *(left to right)*. *B*, Various types of air helmets; AHI single-bladder, AHI double-bladder, and Riddell air helmets *(left to right)*.

HELMET SAFETY

Several factors must be considered when using protective head gear. Most important, instruction in proper technique should prevent the intentional use of the head as an initial point of contact. Players should be taught to keep the head up when tackling. Additionally, motion of the head with respect to the body should be limited by protective equipment to the greatest degree tolerable. In football, this is done by the combined use of helmets and shoulder pads to reduce the range of motion of the cervical spine.

In material design, helmets and attachments should be as slippery and as conforming to the shell as possible to minimize rotational acceleration of the head. When the surface of the helmet is abraded or dirty, the helmet can essentially "grab" onto other surfaces, allowing friction-generating forces to be directed to the athlete rather than being deflected. Helmets must meet the appropriate standards, and they must be routinely inspected so that good condition can be maintained (Tables 40–5 and 40–6).

TABLE 40–5
Suggested Daily Helmet Inspection Checklist by NOCSAE

Each player should inspect his helmet before each usage, as follows:
1. Check foam padding for proper placement and any deterioration.
2. Check for cracks in vinyl or rubber covering of air, foam, or liquid padded helmets.
3. Check that protective system or foam padding has not been altered or removed.
4. Check for proper amount of inflation in air-padded helmets. Follow manufacturer's recommendations for adjusting air pressure at the valves.
5. Check all rivets, screws, Velcro, and snaps to ensure that they are properly fastened and holding protective parts.

If any of the above inspections indicates a need for repair and/or replacement, notify your equipment manager. This is your responsibility
NEVER WEAR A DAMAGED HELMET.

TABLE 40–6
Suggested Weekly Helmet Inspection Checklist by NOCSAE

These steps should be completed by qualified personnel:
1. Check helmet fit using manufacturer's instruction procedures.
2. Examine shell for cracks, particularly noting any cracks around holes (where most cracks start) and replace any that have cracked. *Do not use a helmet with a cracked shell.*
3. Examine all mounting rivets, screws, Velcro, and snaps for breakage, distortion, and/or looseness. *Repair as necessary.*
4. Replace face guards if bare metal is showing, there is a broken weld, or the guard is grossly misshapen.
5. Examine for helmet completeness and replace any parts that have become damaged, such as sweatbands, nose snubbers, and chinstraps.
6. Replace jaw pads when damaged. Check for proper installation and fit.
7. Examine chinstrap for proper adjustment and inspect to see if it is broken or stretched out of shape; also inspect the hardware to see if it needs replacement.
8. Read instructions provided by manufacturer regarding care and maintenance procedures. Always follow these procedures.

Caution: Only paints, waxes, decals, or cleaning agents approved by the manufacturer are to be used on any helmet. It is possible to get a severe or delayed reaction from using unauthorized materials, which could permanently damage the helmet shell and affect its safety performance.

Currently, AHI and Riddell are the only two manufacturers that produce football helmets.[5] Litigation and high insurance premiums have prohibited many athletic equipment makers from producing football helmets. The companies that still manufacture helmets have been forced to increase the cost drastically because of the high insurance fees. This cost is still negligible, considering the extensive consequences of a head injury.

All football, batting, and lacrosse helmets should bear the NOCSAE seal of approval to ensure that the established standards have been met. Other sports utilize other testing organizations. Helmets that are no longer under warranty should be reconditioned or discarded.

HELMET FITTING

Proper fit of helmets is essential to protect the athlete from injury. The athlete should be comfortable and confident with his or her equipment. Lack of confidence can impair performance and possibly lead to injury. "Firm but comfortable" should be the guideline.

To prevent injury to the face from helmet slippage, however, the helmet must be snug and stay in place at impact. Additionally, if the helmet provides adequate pressure on all contact points, the forces will be dispersed throughout a larger area. The exact fitting techniques can vary slightly among different helmet models and between manufacturers, and the person in charge of equipment should stay current with any variations. Each manufacturer has published fitting instructions based on the unique characteristics of its product (see Helmet-Fitting Guidelines box).[5] These guidelines should be incorporated in the fitting considerations (Fig. 40–6).

Thickness of padding can also be varied to ensure proper fit. Changing the padding does not void a warranty as long as pads are not interchanged between the different brands of helmets. Always follow the manufacturer's guidelines for fitting to avoid potential litigation. The order of checking the fit should be height, chinstrap, neck, back, front, sides, jaw pads, facemask. The goal is to obtain a proper initial fit and to maintain a proper fit throughout the season.

PROTECTIVE EQUIPMENT FOR THE FACE

FACEMASKS

Most facemasks for football are made of heavy-gauge plastic-coated steel. NOCSAE has developed standards for strength and durability at high school and college levels so that an adequate amount of space is maintained between the faceguard and the face on impact.

The two companies that currently manufacture football helmets also produce facemasks. Both companies use a NOCSAE-approved steel that is coated with different materials. One company also produces a plastic-type facemask called Kra-Lite (Riddell, Chicago, IL), which is also NOCSAE-approved. The Kra-lite is used extensively by high schools because it is lighter in weight than the steel-coated mask and offers similar protection. However, the plastic must be inspected frequently; any damage can seriously weaken the structure. Cold temperatures can make the plastic more brittle, and equipment should be inspected weekly for any defects.

Manufacturers of football helmets offer similar styles of steel-coated facemasks, although there may be a unique design feature specific to each brand. The available styles provide a range of protection for the jaw, mouth, nose, and eyes, allowing an equipment manager to choose the facemask that will give each player adequate protection and optimal visibility (Fig. 40–7). For example, a visual obstacle has been added by using a facemask with greater nose protection. Variations of standard facemask styles include a double-wire configuration that is available for reinforcement and a "U-bar" that helps keep hands and feet away from the eyes. The position the athlete plays typically determines the style he or she uses, unless there is a unique need or preference (Table 40–7).

Custom facemasks can be made by each company to accommodate for injuries such as a broken jaw. All modifications and extensions should be made by the manufacturer.

Some athletes who want added protection without a visual restriction can use a polycarbonate shield with the facemask. Players who wear contact lenses often

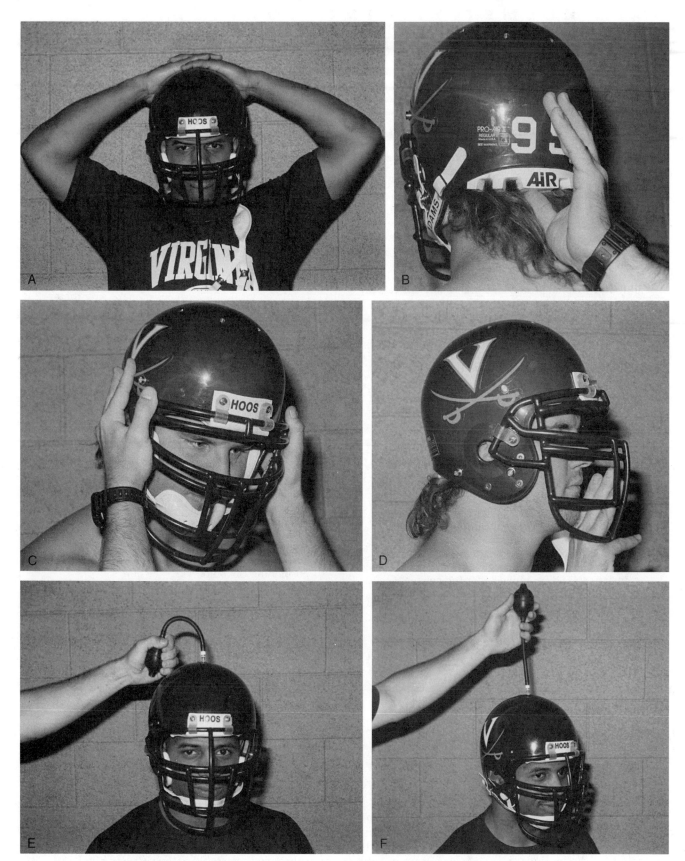

FIGURE 40–6. Fitting a football helmet. (See Helmet-Fitting Guidelines box for explanation.

HELMET-FITTING GUIDELINES

All helmets should be visually inspected for any defects before fitting. In addition to checking the outer shell, the inside support system should be inspected to ensure that the padding has adequate resiliency and that air liners are intact. Padding should be replaced with respective manufacturers' parts. Warranty should be checked before issuing a helmet.

1. Medical history—concussions, maxillofacial injuries, or sensitivity to any material.
2. Previous experience—success or problems with previous use of specific helmets may be useful information.
3. Hair length—short hair is advisable when fitting helmets and during the season; hair should be wet during fitting to simulate the sweaty state typically present during activity.
4. Size determination—circumferential or caliper measurements may be used to establish a general size category (e.g., small, medium, or large). These measurements run from the forehead, 1 inch above the eyebrows, and extend to the occipital prominence. Make sure the ears are not included in the tape measurements.
5. Helmet fitting (follow manufacturers' recommended guidelines)—

HEIGHT:

The front rim of the helmet should be 1 inch (one to two finger widths) above the eyebrows. Have the athlete interlock his fingers on top of the helmet and pull downward to ensure that the helmet stays at the desired height (Fig. 40–6A). Pressure should be placed at the center of the helmet. Adjustments can be made by modifying the top pads. If adequate height cannot be achieved, try a different type of helmet.

CHINSTRAPS:

Usually the four-point chinstrap is used, which helps prevent the helmet from pivoting when contact is made. The two-point chinstrap may be used occasionally by professional quarterbacks or kickers but is illegal in college or high school leagues. The chinstrap should be applied after the helmet height has been determined to maintain proper position while the other pads are checked and adjusted. The cup should fit squarely on the chin. The front straps are applied first, followed by the back straps. The tension should be equal, and the straps should be aligned equally.

NECK:

The padding at the posterior rim of the helmet should be firm but comfortable. The base of the skull should be covered. This area is important because it keeps the helmet from shifting forward, which can cause the helmet to hit the nose. There should be no gaps in the pads. When pressure is applied to the helmet (not the facemask) in a rotational motion and in anterior/posterior directions, the skin on the forehead should move, indicating an appropriate amount of contact (Fig. 40–6B).

BACK TO FRONT:

The front should be inspected by rotating the shell from side to side while looking to see if the skin moves with the helmet (Fig. 40–6C). Pull with one hand on the back of the helmet. There should be no gapping between the forehead and front. Finally, when the helmet is removed, the skin on the forehead should not be blanched from too much pressure.

SIDES:

The earholes should align with the external ear canals. The cheek pads should be in firm but comfortable contact with the cheeks. A finger can be placed inside the earholes to make sure there is firm pressure on the sides.

FACEMASK:

The playing position is an important consideration as to the type of facemask that is appropriate. Manufacturer's instructions should be followed when applying the mask. There should be two to three finger widths between the mask and the player's nose (Fig. 40–6D). The athlete's vision should not be impaired.

ADJUSTMENTS:

The air bladders can be adjusted most easily, but the inflating device is frequently used improperly. To inflate the bladder, the bulb should be held with an arch in the hose and bulb (Fig. 40–6E); to deflate, the bulb is in a straight position (Fig. 40–6F). Untrained individuals often have good intentions of inflating the bladder, but they may inadvertently be releasing the air by improperly positioning the bulb.

FINAL INSPECTION:

Check the fit without the chinstrap in place. (A) Attempt to rotate the helmet down on the nose of the player. Rotational forces should be exerted from the sides of the helmet, rather than from the facemask. (B) Side-to-side rotation should result in movement of the soft tissue of the forehead, rather than movement of the helmet. The jaw pads can be adjusted if necessary. (C) The player places his hands on the top of the helmet and pulls down. Pressure should be felt at the top of the head if proper seating has been attained. (D) A general guideline should be *firm but comfortable*.

---

prefer the shield because there is less chance that a finger or hand can hit the eye. The shield can also be tinted to reduce glare from the sun. Some players, however, think that the polycarbonate shield prevents adequate heat dissipation, and they can fog up in cold weather. The shields can become scratched when transported in equipment bags.

All football facemasks are secured to the helmet with plastic binders that can easily be cut with scissors if the athletic trainer needs access to the player's airway in an emergency. The helmet and chinstraps should be left in place because they stabilize the player's head and neck, but the facemask can be removed with little movement or jarring.[16]

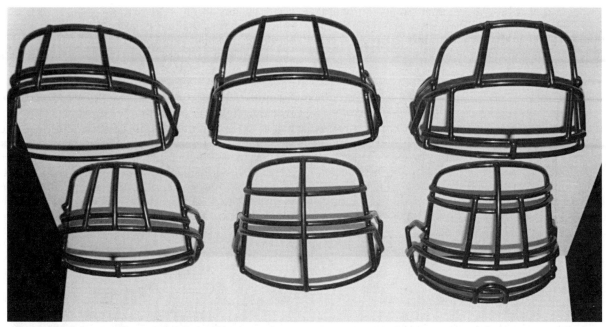

FIGURE 40–7. Different facemask configurations.

Ice hockey helmets often protect the face, although this is not required at the professional level. The facemask or plastic protector must meet either CSA or ASTM standards (which are similar). Standards require mesh in the steel wire masks to be small enough to prevent penetration of a blade simulator in testing.[8] Because the play of hockey is more upright than that of football, the facemask can rest against the chin, making it less likely to catch on other surfaces. Most professional hockey players prefer polycarbonate eye protectors because they offer greater field of vision. The plastic is cut high at the mouth and just below the nose so that the plastic does not fog when the athlete warms up.[17]

Lacrosse facemasks protect the face from impact of either the stick or the ball. Men's lacrosse rules mandate helmets and facemasks with a NOCSAE standard. The strength of the steel wire is intermediate compared with that required in football and ice hockey. The facemask is well off the face, but padding around the chin area protects the athlete if the facemask is driven backward in a collision.[17] Four-point chinstraps are used on all helmets (Fig. 40–8A).

Facemasks are now available that protect the jaw area and can be attached to baseball and softball batting helmets. These devices can also be used on players in the field. ASTM standards have been developed, and progress is being made to require facemasks on batters in Little League baseball. The prototypes are wire cage or a clear plastic guard that is attached to the batting helmet and shields the mouth and jaw area, with an opening at the mouth to prevent fogging. The eyes are not covered but are well protected from impact because the ball will not fit between the helmet's visor and the jaw protector (Fig. 40–8B).

CHINSTRAPS

Chinstraps help secure a helmet on the head. Certain sports such as bicycling and kayaking use a single strap that is hooked under the chin. A single strap allows some rotation of the helmet but is usually adequate in maintaining the appropriate position of the helmet on the top of the head. Football and lacrosse use four-point chinstraps to prevent rotation of the helmet.

Chinstraps are connected to the helmet with metal grommets that must be replaced occasionally. There are many companies that produce similar chinstraps. Different styles include the hard shell lined with a vinyl-dipped foam or a soft cup made of leather or vinyl. The hard cup gives the athlete added padding on the chin, and the soft cup primarily functions to hold the helmet in place. Some chinstraps are available in different cup sizes.

In football, the four-point chinstraps are secured by either the high-hookup or the low-hookup (Fig. 40–9). The Riddell helmets are drilled for low-hookup, and the AHI helmets are drilled for high-hookup. Either helmet can be modified by punching through a marked area on

TABLE 40–7 Facemask Type by Position Played	
Facemask	**Playing Position**
Oral protection only	Quarterback, running backs, defensive backs, kickers, wide receivers
Nose and oral protection	Fullbacks, linebackers, tight ends
Jaw and oral protection (with or without nose protection)	Quarterbacks, linebackers, linemen

the helmet and attaching a grommet. Some equipment managers have found that the decreased angle of the low-hookup means that there is less chance of the chinstrap rotating off the chin.

EYE PROTECTION

Eye injuries in sports are frequent, but many professionals believe that the severity of eye injuries can be minimized or prevented with proper protective gear.[18–21] (See Types of Eye Protectors on next page.) There are more than 100,000 sports-related eye injuries yearly, with more than 25 percent resulting in serious complications or blindness.[18] Sports have been catego-

rized as low, high, and extremely high risk for eye injury, and rule changes have made protective eyewear required in some instances.

Low-risk sports are those that do not involve a thrown or hit ball, use of a stick or bat, or close aggressive play with body contact. Low-risk sports include track and field, swimming, gymnastics, and rowing. High-risk sports involve the use of a high-speed ball or puck, the use of a bat or stick, and close aggressive play with body contact. These sports include hockey, basketball, football, racquet sports, lacrosse, baseball, handball, soccer, and volleyball. Extremely high-risk sports are the combat sports, including boxing or full-contact karate. The incidence of eye injury in racquet sports has been found to be greater in higher-

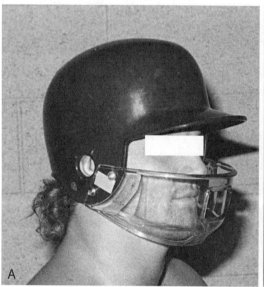
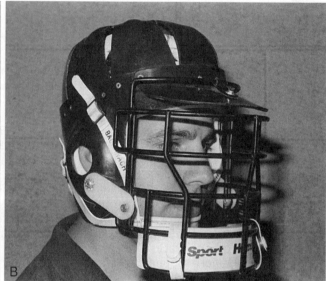

FIGURE 40–8. Facemasks used in other sports: *A,* plastic facemask used on batting helmets. *B,* Lacrosse facemask.

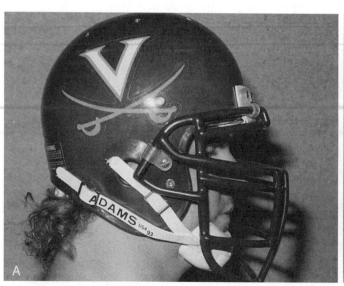
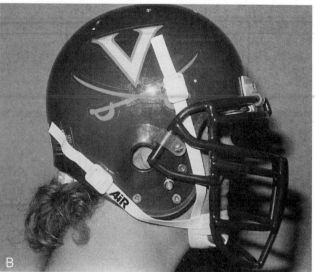

FIGURE 40–9. Chinstraps: *A,* Low-hookup chinstrap (hard-cup); *B,* high-hookup chinstrap (soft cup).

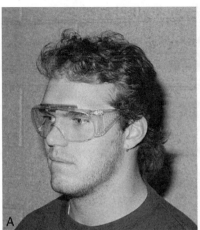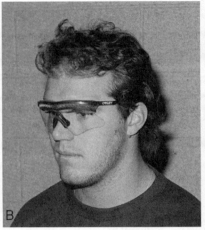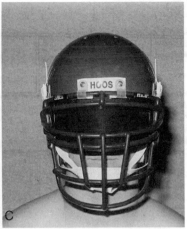

FIGURE 40–10. Examples of eye protectors: *A,* Plastic and lens are all one piece; *B,* separate plastic lens; *C,* polycarbonate shield attached to football facemask.

skilled, more experienced players, despite the initial impression that novice athletes seem to be more at risk. This finding was attributed to the faster, more aggressive nature of the skilled participant, along with the tendency to "keep the eye on the ball."[19]

The rapid rise in interest in racquet sports in the 1970s and 1980s resulted in a substantial increase in the incidence of eye injuries. Racquetball speeds have been measured to exceed 130 miles per hour.[22] Eye guard standards were established initially by the CSA in 1982 and by the ASTM in 1986. Several of the early eye pro-

tectors, including the open eye guards (class III), were found to be ineffective in dissipating the forces generated during racquet sport competition or in stopping the ball from entering the eye guard opening.[19,22]

Lens materials in approved eye protectors are composed of plastic or polycarbonate material, both of which can be incorporated with prescription lenses. CR 39 plastic lenses with an industrial thickness of 3.0 mm may be used, but they scratch rather easily and are not impact resistant. CR 39 lenses are generally less expensive but are often thicker and heavier than polycarbonate lenses. Polycarbonate, with more than seven times the impact resistance of CR 39 plastic, has the greatest impact resistance of the clear materials developed.[19]

EYEGLASSES VS. CONTACT LENSES

Properly constructed eyeglasses provide some inherent protection, although they have several disadvantages compared with contact lenses during sports participation. The disadvantages include difficulty in keeping them in place, perspiration or dirt that may distort vision, fogging, decreased peripheral vision, and difficulty fitting under head protection. Everyday eyeglasses are not safe in racquet or contact sports because glass or hardened plastic lenses may shatter on contact, resulting in serious eye injuries. Eye protectors with shatterproof polycarbonate or CR 39 prescription lenses give good protection during sports activities. Some prescriptions, however, are unavailable in the plastic.

Contact lenses do not provide protection from contact with an object or another player, but they are less cumbersome, do not fog, and do not decrease peripheral vision. Soft contacts are generally preferred over hard contacts because there is less chance of them breaking, and soft contacts have a higher survival rate when they fall out of the eye.

"ONE-EYED" ATHLETES

An athlete is considered to be "one-eyed" if the corrected vision is 20/200 or less in one eye.[18] These individuals should wear appropriate eye protectors at

---

TYPES OF EYE PROTECTORS

Total head protector. A helmet or face protection used in high-energy sports (football, lacrosse, hockey) that shields the entire face and head.

Full face protector. Used in sports that threaten the face but not the brain, such as fencing, catching, or umpiring. Additional eye protection can also be worn with this type of protector.

Helmet with separate eye protector. The eye protector is attached to the helmet in many cases. This type of protection is used in ski racing, auto racing, cycling, and horseback riding.

Helmet only. These provide partial eye protection, such as in boxing.

Sports eye protectors. These are available in different designs and provide protection to the eyes only. These are recommended for sports that do not use other head gear, such as baseball or softball (fielders), soccer, and cross-country skiing. Participants in racquet sports should always wear some form of protective eye gear. The different classifications of these protectors are:

- Class I—a molded single-unit lens and frame (Fig. 40–10*A*)
- Class II—lens mounted in a separate frame (Fig. 40–10*B*)
- Class III—protector that contains no lens that is used alone or over eyeglasses

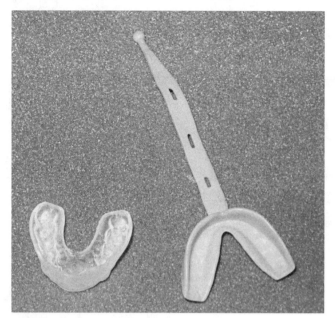

FIGURE 40–11. Examples of mouthguards: custom (*left*) and heat-molded (*right*).

all times to ensure protection of the good eye. One-eyed athletes should not participate in extremely high-risk sports (boxing) and should be hesitant to engage in collision or contact sports because of the possibility of eye injury even with proper protection. The decision to play is up to the athlete, the athlete's parents if he or she is a minor, and the physician. Legal counsel may be necessary if handicap discrimination is an issue. A signed waiver may be indicated, stating the necessity of using protective eyewear and the possibility of injury to the good eye. Class I or II sports eye protectors should be worn at all times during athletic endeavors, with an additional face shield if there is a significant potential for injury.

MOUTHGUARDS

Mouthguards were introduced to high school football players in 1955 and became mandatory pieces of equipment in 1962.[23] College football players, however, were not required to wear mouthguards until 1973. Mouthguards have effectively reduced the incidence of split lips, broken teeth, and temporomandibular joint injury. In addition, they have helped decrease the severity of concussions due to their shock-absorption qualities. Many sports medicine practitioners and dentists recommend mouthguards for all athletes in both recreational and competitive sports whenever contact is possible.[24] Currently, mouthguards are required in football, field hockey, ice hockey, and men's and women's lacrosse. To help enforcement of the rule, the NCAA adopted an addendum in 1990 that required mouthguards to be a high-visibility color such as yellow or orange so that referees could easily identify unprotected players.

There are two effective types of mouthguards available: custom made and mouth formed (Fig. 40–11).[24] Custom-made mouthguards are produced from molds

made of the athlete's teeth. These devices are preferred by athletes because they make it easier to breathe and talk during play and generally feel more comfortable. However, cost may inhibit the use of custom mouthguards, since mouth-formed models provide similar injury prevention. Mouth-formed guards are made from pliable plastic that is moldable when heated. The athlete dips the mouthguard into hot water to soften the plastic and then gently bites into the plastic to mold the device to the teeth. This activity should be supervised to prevent burns to the mouth. Various sizes are available, and the athlete should cut down the excess only if the device extends beyond the posterior molars. Some athletes attempt to cut the device to a size that covers only the four front teeth. This practice voids the product's injury prevention warranty and could result in an airway obstruction. The effectiveness of the mouthguard in absorbing shock in the bite and thus preventing concussions is limited when the mouthguard is cut too small.[23]

The mouthguard is often attached by a strap to the facemask in football and lacrosse to keep the athlete from losing it. This strap should be designed so that excessive force will tear it away from the mouthguard to prevent the stress from being transferred to the athlete's teeth.

EAR PROTECTORS

The ears are protected from shearing forces and contusions by most helmets. Even though helmets are not used in boxing, wrestling, and water polo, ear protection is required because of the high incidence of ear injury. "Cauliflower ear," a hematoma in the outer ear, may occur without the use of appropriate equipment. This hematoma often requires aspiration, and a splint is applied to prevent the hematoma from returning. If adequate pressure is not maintained, the blood

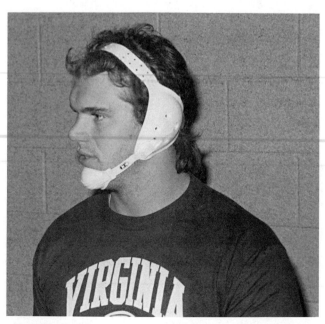

FIGURE 40–12. Example of ear protector: wrestling headgear.

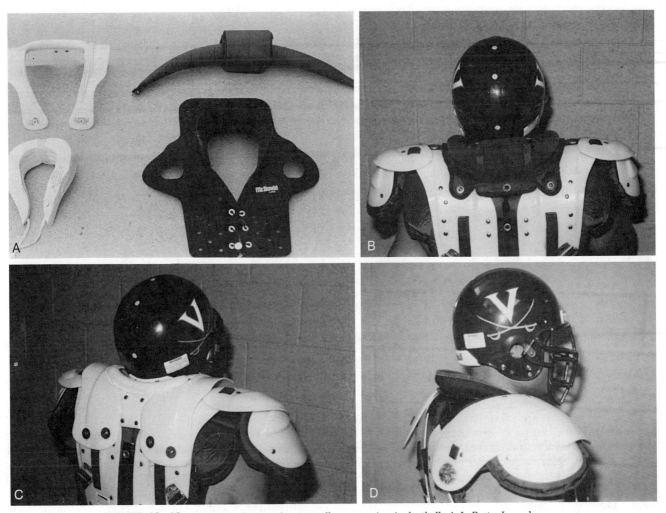

FIGURE 40–13. Examples of cervical spine collar protection in football: *A,* LaPorta, Long horn, neck roll, and Cowboy collars. *B,* Long horn neck roll. *C,* LaPorta attached to shoulder pads. *D,* Cowboy collar.

and exudate collect between the skin and cartilage and may solidify, causing a permanent deformity. This type of injury is preventable with appropriate ear protection (Fig. 40–12).[10]

NECK PROTECTION

Training is the single best protector against cervical spine injury in sports. The athlete should be taught to make impact with the head up to prevent compressive loading of the cervical spine, which is the most common mechanism for spinal cord injury.[16] Any impact made to the top of the head increases the chance of serious cervical spine injury.

There are combinations of helmet and shoulder pads that can prevent certain injuries of the neck by restricting motion. The brachial plexus can be injured in sports with a forceful lateral flexion of the neck or shoulder depression.[2] This injury varies in its severity and is commonly called a "burner" or "stinger" because of the sharp radiating pain along the affected upper extremity (see Chapter 23). Fit of the shoulder pads is perhaps the most important aspect of preventing

brachial plexus injuries.[16] If such an injury occurs, the shoulder pads should be modified when the athlete is cleared to play so that extremes of cervical motion are limited. A molded collar around the neck may be used, but it must be snug and limit the motion that causes the pain. Commercial products or collars can be added to the shoulder pads to further restrict problematic motions. These include the Cowboy collar (McDavid, Chicago, IL), Long Horn neck roll, LaPorta collar, and numerous others of similar design (Fig. 40–13).

The conventional neck collar made of closed-cell foam is frequently used in high school football. This type of collar restricts motion by engaging the bottom of the helmet. The Long Horn, Cowboy, and LaPorta collars restrict motion by making contact with the sides and back of the helmet. The Long Horn collar is larger in diameter than the conventional foam collar, which limits cervical motion by restricting helmet movement. Motion restriction can be further isolated by putting auxiliary pads over the Long Horn collar at specific sites. The Cowboy collar is a closed-cell polyethylene foam that fits underneath any shoulder pad. This collar can be further reinforced by adding a plastic back plate along the posterior aspect of the support. The LaPorta

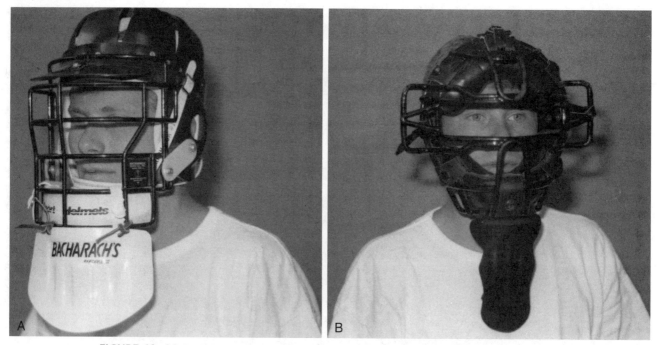

FIGURE 40–14. Examples of throat protection: *A*, Throat protector in lacrosse goalie's equipment. *B*, Larynx extension for baseball catcher.

collar is a more rigid plastic shell that is secured directly to the shoulder pad arch. The helmet wedges into the collar, limiting the degree of cervical excursion.

The anterior neck or larynx is protected in sports that utilize a high-velocity projectile such as a baseball, hockey puck, or lacrosse ball. Goalies and catchers are especially susceptible to injuries in this area and should wear hanging plastic shields from their facemasks (Fig. 40–14).

SHOULDER PADS

Football shoulder pads are generally made of a lightweight yet hard plastic on the exterior that can effectively deflect a blow. The inner lining of the shoulder pads is composed of closed-cell or open-cell padding that absorbs the shock and distributes it over a broad area. Football pads provide the ultimate protection for the shoulder, clavicle, sternum, and scapula. Attachments can be added to the equipment to provide protection to the cervical spine, upper extremity, abdomen, ribs, flank, and back (Fig. 40–15). Ice hockey and men's lacrosse also utilize shoulder pads, but they are not as extensive or as protective as the football pads (Fig. 40–16).

There are two main types of football shoulder pads: cantilever and flat pads.[4,5] The channel system has been incorporated into both the cantilever and the flat pads. The channel system utilizes a series of long, thinner pads that are attached by Velcro into the shoulder pads. The pads are fitted to the athlete so that there is air space at the acromioclavicular joint.[9] The pressure is placed entirely on the anterior and posterior aspect of the shoulder. Many think that this system provides maxi-

mal protection when the pads are properly fitted and the inner pads are aligned to the individual (Fig. 40–17).

Cantilever pads are so named because of the hard plastic bridge they make over the superior aspect of the shoulder to protect the acromioclavicular joint. They are now built to be lightweight, allow maximum range of motion, and distribute the force and pressure of a blow throughout the entire shoulder, chest, and back. Cantilever pads come in three types: inside, outside, and double cantilever. The inside cantilever fits under the arch of the shoulder pads and rests against the shoulder. It is more common because it is less bulky than the outside cantilever. The outside cantilever sits on top of the pad, outside of the arch. It provides a larger blocking surface and affords more protection to those who are in constant contact, such as linemen. The double cantilever, which is a combination of both the inside and the outside cantilever, affords a player the greatest amount of protection but is not feasible for all positions due to its bulk (Fig. 40–18).

Flat pads do not use the cantilever struts and generally allow greater mobility. These pads are different from the earlier generation of flat pads because they use the "air management" system. The air management system is a combination of both open- and closed-cell foam pads encased in nylon, which is placed under the protective hard plastic. When contact is made with the shoulder, air is distributed throughout the padding to create an "air pocket" between the athlete and the shoulder pads. Flat pads are generally used for receivers and quarterbacks because they are lightweight and less restricting. However, they are becoming more popular for offensive linemen who principally use their hands to block. The flat pads must use the belt buckle strapping to create an archlike effect in the pads and to minimize

ANTERIOR VIEW

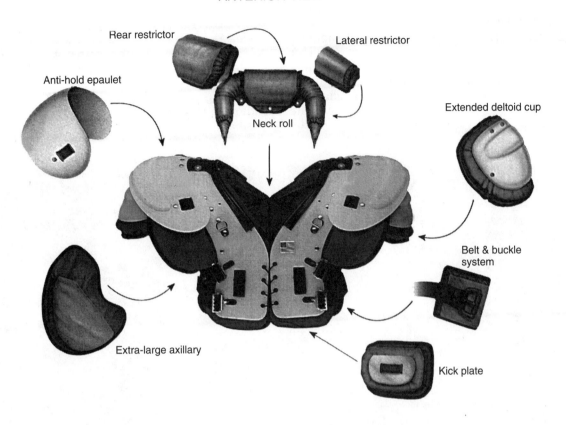

POSTERIOR VIEW

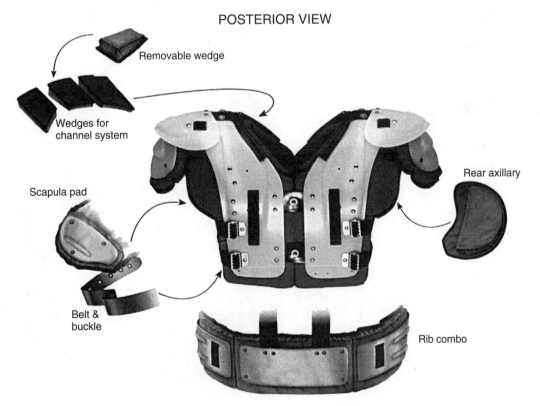

FIGURE 40–15. Shoulder pad components and common attachments.

pad displacement. The elastic webbing straps typically used in shoulder pads are inadequate for proper stabilization of flat pads.[5]

In addition to the cantilever, the football shoulder pads consist of an arch, two sets of epaulets, shoulder cups, and anterior and posterior pads. The arch around the cantilever is shaped to fit the contour of the upper body. The shoulder flaps, also called epaulets, extend from the edge of the arch over the shoulder caps. These further protect the top of the

entire shoulder area. The shoulder cups also attach to the arch and are located just below the epaulets and should cover the deltoid. The posterior pads cover the trapezius and other posterior muscles in addition to covering the scapula and spine. The anterior pads cover the pectoral muscles as well as the sternum and clavicle. Anterior pads may be slanted forward or even built up in pads made for linebackers and others who routinely receive blows anteriorly or from an upright position.

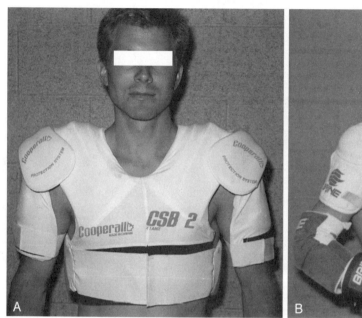
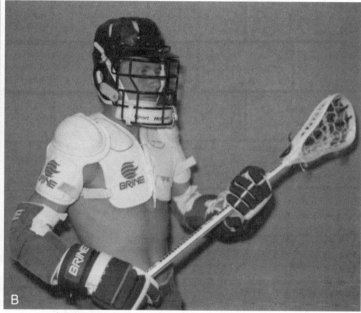

FIGURE 40–16. Examples of hockey and lacrosse shoulder pads: *A*, Ice hockey shoulder pads; *B*, lacrosse shoulder pads.

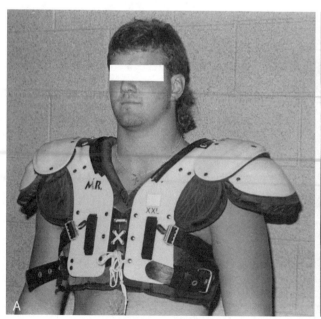
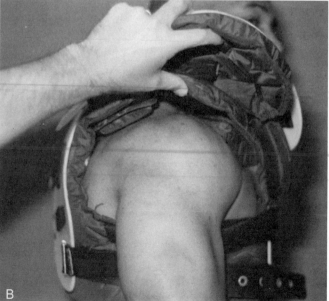

FIGURE 40–17. Examples of flat pads: *A*, Flat pad with belt attachment to help maintain an "air" pocket at the top of the shoulder on impact. *B*, Channel system features wedges of Velcro on the inside of pads to protect the acromioclavicular joint.

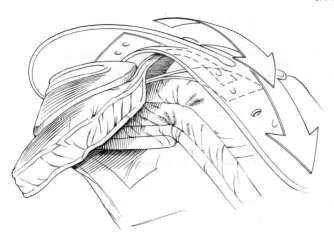

FIGURE 40–18. Schematic of cantilever pads.

TABLE 40–8
Shoulder Pad Categorization by Position

- Quarterbacks
- Wide receivers
- Kickers
- Offensive linemen
- Defensive linemen
- Running backs
- Defensive backs
- Fullbacks
- Linebackers

Pads should be selected based on the athlete's position, body type, and history of injury.[3,5] Playing position often determines what style of shoulder pad is used (Table 40–8). For example, anterior and posterior padding extends lower in order to protect the sternum and ribs of linemen, linebackers, and fullbacks, whereas defensive ends require the greater protection of larger cups and flaps for tackling. Offensive backs and receivers require smaller shoulder cups and flaps to allow them greater mobility when passing and catching. Cantilevers also come in different sizes so that quarterbacks and receivers who need more glenohumeral movement are not restricted. Linemen, who require little glenohumeral movement but need more protection against constant contact, use larger cantilevers. The shoulder pad can be customized by the equipment manager in many ways to give greater protection from injury or to make the pads lighter and more mobile. For example, a drop-back passer may not need as much padding as a running quarter-back. A speed receiver who does not catch balls in the middle of the field would require less padding than a receiver who blocks or catches in the middle of the field. A fullback would need enhanced protection because of his constant hitting with or without the ball.

Shoulder pads must be correctly fitted and be in good condition to provide optimal protection for an athlete.[3,5] Each athlete must be fitted with quality equipment by knowledgeable personnel. Many injuries are caused by improper fit of the equipment rather than design flaws. Consultation with an athletic trainer or sports physical

---

FITTING PROTOCOL FOR FOOTBALL SHOULDER PADS

1. Check pads for possible damage.
2. Review personal and medical history (history of AC joint sprains, burners).
3. Fit without a T-shirt to allow visualization of body parts.
4. Use the chest girth measured at the nipple line or measure the distance between shoulder tips to determine size. Body weight is used by some manufacturers to determine initial size.
5. Select pads for player's position.
6. Place the shoulder pads on the player and tighten all straps and laces. The lacers should be pulled together until touching. Tension on straps should be equal on both sides and as tight as functionally tolerable to ensure proper force distribution of the pads. Check to see that the clavicle is covered completely and that the neck opening is large enough for comfort but not too large, as this will allow exposure of the clavicles when the arms are raised. There should be enough room on either side of the neck roll to allow comfort when the arms are raised fully (Fig. 40–19A).
7. Anterior view: Make sure the laces are centered over the sternum and that there is no gap between the two-halves. There should be full coverage of the acromio-clavicular joint, clavicles, pectoral muscles, and trapezius muscles. Caps should cover the deltoid muscles. The medial aspects of the clavicles should

not be exposed. Ifthe clavicles can be palpated without moving the pads, refit with a smaller pad. The inner padding (under the deltoid caps) should align with the tips of the shoulders. This fit can be confirmed by placing a ruler vertically on the lateral aspect of the deltoid muscle. The pads should align with the vertical ruler within half an inch (Fig. 40–19B).
8. Lateral view: The acromioclavicular joint is protected by the channel or cantilever system. Raise the deltoid cap and visualize if the channel or air space is in the proper location. This can be assessed by running a hand along the clavicle. The deltoid should be adequately covered by the deltoid cap (Fig. 40–19C).
9. Posterior view: There should be full coverage of the scapulae and rhomboid muscles. The latissimus should be adequately covered. The lacers should be pulled together slightly and should be centered over the spine.
10. The axillary straps or belts should be secured so that the pads do not shift. The straps should be tight enough to allow only two fingers to be inserted under the strap. The strap is not tight enough if the hand can be slid under the straps or pad.
11. Final inspection: check the shoulder pads with the helmet and jersey in place to determine the final fit. Have the athlete raise his arms to ensure comfort and no impingement in the cervical region.

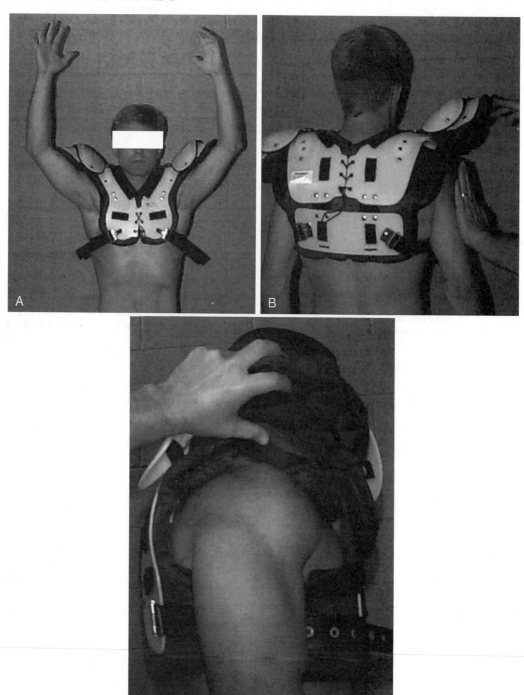

FIGURE 40–19. Fitting of shoulder pads.

therapist may be necessary to address unique medical conditions and whether additional padding may be necessary.

RIB AND FLANK PADS

Flak Jacket (American Pneumatics Co., Houston, TX) is a combination fiber and air-filled bladder that provides protection for rib or low back contusions (Fig. 40–20A). The device fits with most standard shoulder pads and can be used to prevent injury in athletes who frequently get hit from behind—such as running backs. Quarterbacks often receive blows while their arms are abducted, making the anterior ribs and abdomen vulnerable to injury. Special combinations of shoulder and rib pads are manufactured by some companies to give quarterbacks flexibility and range in the shoulder and added protection to the flank.

Body suits made of mesh with pockets to hold rib and hip pads can be used to add protection to the sides and back (Fig. 40–20*B*). Although these suits are manufactured for football, they are easily adapted to other sports when additional protection is needed to prevent reinjury.

CHEST PROTECTION

Hockey and lacrosse goalies and baseball catchers wear flexible, resilient chest protectors that are made of a dense, energy-absorbing material (Fig. 40–21). These chest protectors provide protection to the ribs, sternum, and underlying tissues. It has been suggested that young baseball and softball players (younger than 12 years) should wear chest protectors in the infield because their rib cages are less rigid, leaving the heart at risk from direct impact. A focal impact to the chest in preadolescents increases the risk of ventricular fibrillation and death. Rutherford and associates[25] reported more deaths from impacts to the chest than to the head

in baseball and softball injuries in this younger age group.

BRAS

Sports bras are designed to restrict excessive movement of the breasts during exercise, which can cause bruising and stretching of the suspensory ligaments. The bra should have wide elastic straps to prevent friction or binding, and all metal should be covered. There should be no seams in the cup area. Sports bras should be constructed of a firm compressive material and should allow for absorption of perspiration.

HIP PADS

Hip pads are required in football and ice hockey. Hip pads are usually composed of hard polyethylene

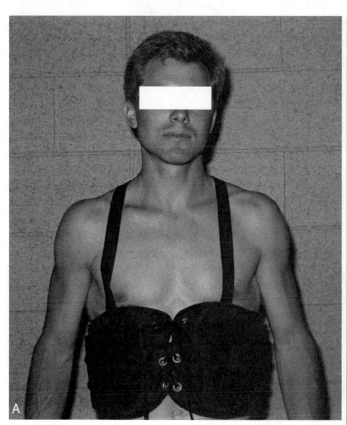

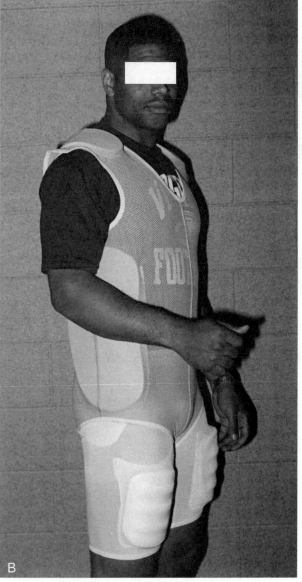

FIGURE 40–20. *A*, Example of rib protector. *B*, Body suit worn under the pants and shoulder pads to give protection to the ribs and flanks.

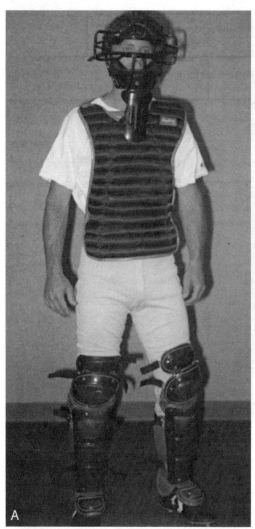

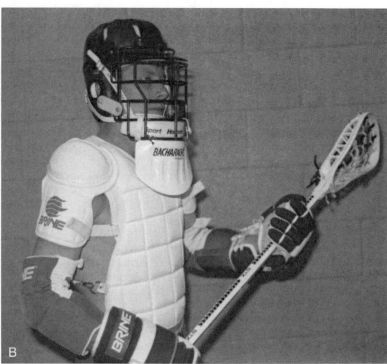

FIGURE 40–21. Examples of chest protectors: *A*, Chest protector for baseball catcher; *B*, chest protector for lacrosse goalies.

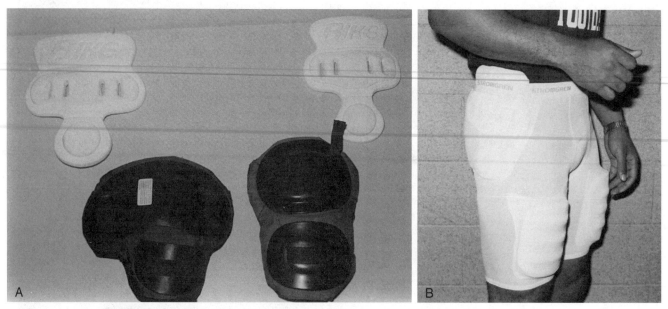

FIGURE 40–22. Examples of hip pads: *A*, Various types and sizes of hip pads for football. *B*, Girdle with pockets to hold hip and thigh pads can be used in many sports such as basketball to protect an injury.

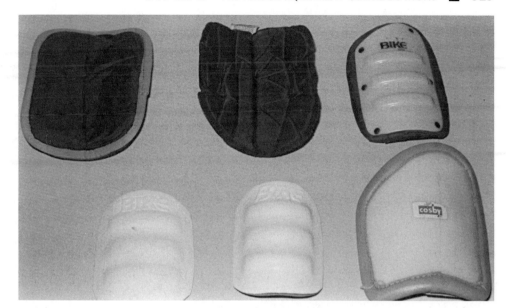

FIGURE 40–23. Examples of sizes and types of thigh pads.

covered with layers of Ensolite. These pads are designed to protect the iliac crest, greater trochanter, and coccyx.[26] The NCAA requires that all football players wear hip and tail pads and that these pads cannot be altered (Fig. 40–22A).

A girdle with pockets can hold the pads in place, although the iliac crest pad may slip (Fig. 40–22B).[3] A belt can better secure the iliac crest pads in place to prevent hip pointers. Air management pads can also be used to protect the iliac crest. These afford maximal protection but are usually not used unless there is an existing injury, because they are larger than standard hip pads.

JOCKS

Sports that utilize a high-velocity projectile such as a baseball, lacrosse ball, or hockey puck require protection of the genitalia for male participants.[10] A hard plastic shell fits into an opening in the athletic supporter to deflect forces.

THIGH PADS

Thigh pads protect the anterior thigh from contusions. Most thigh pads are made of polyethylene encased in Ensolite, but there are numerous commercially produced thigh pads of all sizes and shock absorbency to provide thorough protection of the anterior and lateral thigh (Fig. 40–23). Some football players believe that speed is hindered by large thigh pads. These players attempt to cut their thigh pads and remove the hard plastic center.[4] This practice should be discouraged because of the high risk of contusions to this area.

Properly fitting football pants are essential in maintaining proper placement of thigh and knee pads. Thigh pads should be centered over the quadriceps muscle group approximately 6 to 7 inches above the kneecap. When using asymmetrical thigh pads, the larger flare

should be placed on the lateral aspect of the thigh to avoid injury to the genitalia.

Deep quadriceps contusions are common in all contact sports, although only football and hockey require thigh pads. Athletes in other sports may benefit from wearing football thigh pads in a girdle to protect a healing contusion. Some athletic trainers suggest that basketball players, especially those who frequently drive the lane, wear thigh pads in practice. Stromgren has produced a girdle with thigh pads sewn in place; these are easily used with the equipment of any other sport.

KNEE PROTECTION

PADS

Football knee pads help prevent contusions from impact with other players or the turf. Many football players in skill positions opt to cut their football pants at the knee to allow greater mobility in running.

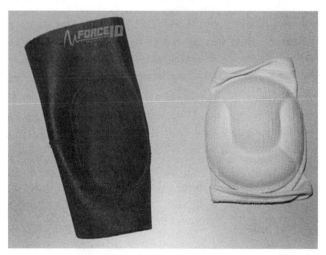

FIGURE 40–24. Examples of knee pads to protect the knees from impact.

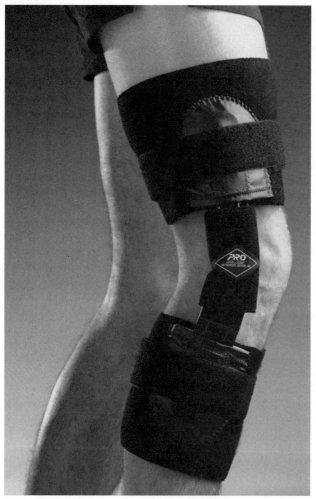

FIGURE 40–25. Example of prophylactic knee brace. (Courtesy of PRO Orthopedic Devices, Inc., Tucson, AZ.)

Unfortunately, this does not allow proper pad stabilization of the anterior knee. Thus, players should not be permitted to alter their pants. Legally, the NCAA requires that the pad cover the knee.

Other sports may use knee pads to reduce the impact of the patella on a hard surface such as a gym floor. Volleyball players often use elastic knee pads with soft fiber filling to protect the knee. Wrestlers may also use knee pads or neoprene sleeves because of the potential for impact on the mat (Fig. 40–24).

BRACES

Braces are often used in sports to protect the knee from both compression forces and torsional stress. Knee braces are categorized according to their function: prophylactic, functional, or rehabilitative.[27] A prophylactic brace is used to reduce the incidence or severity of injury to uninjured normal anatomy or to a fully rehabilitated injury. A functional brace provides protection against reinjury following rehabilitation and/or surgical reconstruction of an injured knee. A rehabilitative brace provides protection of healing structures by limiting mobility following injury or surgery.

The proper selection of a brace depends on the goal of the brace, the athlete's sport and position played, the cost, and the player's acceptance of the device.

Prophylactic knee braces are commonly seen as hinged braces on the lateral aspect of knees of football linemen (Fig. 40–25). Some programs require interior linemen to wear the braces because of the high forces that can be imparted to the knee. Some studies have shown a reduction in the number of knee injuries and fewer surgical interventions when athletes wear these braces.[28] However, other investigators have shown an increase in knee injuries in a Division I college football team during a period when players were required to wear lateral knee braces.[29]

There are various factors that make these epidemiologic studies inconclusive. For example, there have been seven rule changes in college football since 1981, when these and other studies were conducted. The rule changes include penalties for blocking below the waist, chop blocking below the knee, running into the kicker, and executing crackback blocks. A crackback block is a play in which a receiver runs downfield and comes back to block behind the defensive secondary in a running play. These rule changes were designed specifically to reduce the incidence of knee injuries.[28] In addition to the rule changes, there were inconsistencies in the approach toward medial collateral ligament (MCL) injury management. Some physicians prefer conservative management rather than surgical intervention for grade III MCL injuries. Therefore, the number of knee injuries requiring surgery may not be consistent among testers.

The American Academy of Orthopaedic Surgeons presented a position statement on prophylactic knee braces in 1987 that reiterated the lack of conclusive evidence that knee braces reduce the incidence or severity of knee injury.[10] Prophylactic knee braces should not be required equipment. The decision to wear braces should be made on an individual basis, and lateral knee stabilizers should be available if they make the athlete feel more confident.

Functional knee braces are designed to restore functional stability to the knee after an athlete has suffered a ligamentous disruption.[30] Most functional braces on the market today are made for persons who are anterior cruciate ligament (ACL) deficient. The Lenox Hill derotation brace was the first functional knee brace. It was designed in 1972 for Joe Namath, a professional football player with an anteromedial rotatory instability. Currently, there are numerous functional knee braces available, both "off the shelf" and custom fit (Fig. 40–26).

There are two basic styles of ACL braces: hinge-post-strap and the hinge-post-shell. There are numerous companies that produce each type of brace. The Don Joy Defiance (Smith & Nephew, Carlsbad, CA) and the Lenox Hill Precision Fit (Lenox Hill Brace Co., Long Island City, NY) are examples of the hinge-post-strap; the CTi (Innovation Sports, Upper Marlboro, MD) is an example of the hinge-post-shell. Both types attempt to control forward translation of the tibia on the femur or a functional pivot shift of the affected knee. Factors to consider when ordering a functional knee

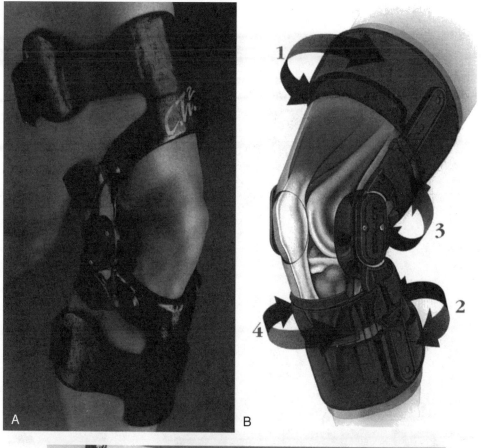

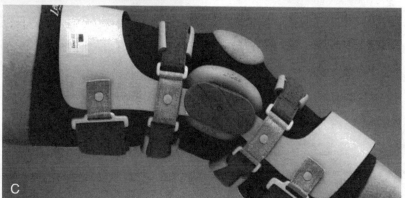

FIGURE 40–26. Examples of functional knee braces: *A*, CTi 2 brace; *B*, Don Joy Defiance 4-point brace; *C*, Lennox Hill precision-fit brace. Courtesy of PRO (Orthopedic Devices, Inc., Tucson, AZ.)

brace include fit, cost, migration or slipping with activity, and weight. The Don Joy Defiance and the Lenox Hill Precision Fit each weighs approximately 17 oz. Range of motion blocks are offered in most functional braces to help control hyperextension and hyperflexion. Functional knee braces can be used during rehabilitation to give an athlete added security and stability with early activity. *No athlete should be allowed to participate fully in contact sports unless he or she has been fully rehabilitated and can demonstrate functional activity both with and without the brace.* It should be reiterated to the athlete that the brace can help control stability, but it does not replace strengthening of the limb, and the brace cannot prevent all injury.

The disadvantages of knee bracing during competition include cost, weight, difficulty in sizing, and breakdown of Velcro fasteners, buckles, and elastic straps. Migration of the brace during vigorous activities severely affects its ability to stabilize the knee. Additionally, psychologic dependency may adversely affect an athlete in competition. Braces should not create a threat to other players and should be well padded on all metal surfaces. Many braces are now fabricated so that no metal is exposed, eliminating the need for additional padding.

Rehabilitative knee braces have three functions: to provide rigid immobilization at a selected angle, to permit controlled range of motion through predeter-

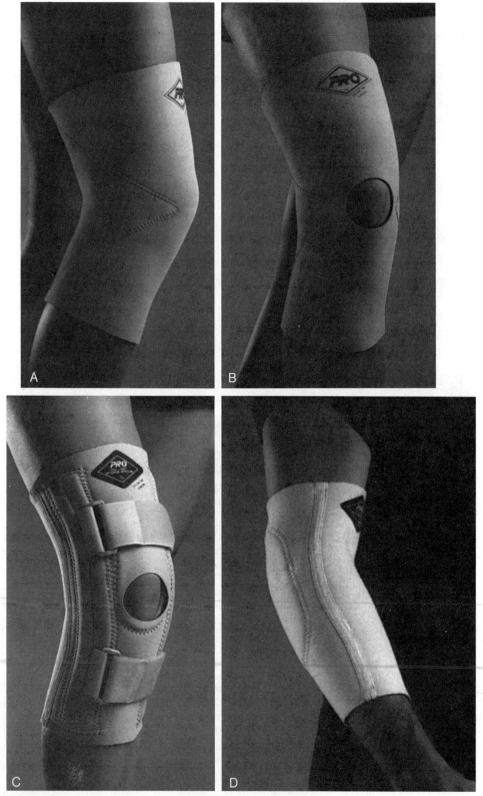

FIGURE 40–27. Neoprene braces: *A*, Neoprene knee sleeve; *B*, knee sleeve with opening at the patella; *C*, knee sleeve with patella stabilizers and felt buttresses sewed inside; *D*, neoprene elbow sleeve with extra padding at the olecranon. (Courtesy of Pro Orthopedic Devices, Tucson, AZ.)

mined arcs, and to provide protection from accidental loading in non-weight-bearing patients.[30] When choosing a rehabilitative knee brace, accurate control of range of motion, limited migration, and edema control should be considered. The brace should be able to conform to various leg sizes and shapes. This is important, because muscular atrophy usually occurs postoperatively.

PATELLAR BRACES

Patellofemoral problems are common, and the use of patellar braces may give some athletes relief. Patellar braces act primarily to dissipate forces, maintain patellar alignment, and improve patellar tracking.[31] Some braces attempt to minimize lateral displacement of the patella with a felt buttress or strap to hold the patella in a more medial position. Other braces are sleeves with a hole cut out for the patella, contributing to stabilization of the patella and minimizing compressive forces. The brace should be comfortable so that the athlete is more likely to wear it, and it should be part of an overall program to reduce patellofemoral stresses.

NEOPRENE BRACES

Neoprene is the nylon-coated rubber material used in wet suits. One or both sides of the material can be covered with nylon, which allows better absorption of sweat and less skin breakdown. Neoprene gives firm compression and retains body heat, which may increase local circulation. Its application in protective equipment ranges from padding of vulnerable areas such as the elbow, to muscular compression such as in a hamstring injury, to minimal stabilization of a joint such as a knee (Fig. 40–27). Neoprene sleeves and wraps are comfortable, allow full mobility, and provide the athlete with proprioceptive feedback in the affected area. Adaptations such as hinges or straps can be made to neoprene sleeves to enhance their joint-stabilizing properties. When choosing a neoprene device, one should consider fit, purpose, and appropriate modifications to allow for joint mobility. Seams should be secure and not cause additional pressure on the skin. Proper care and cleansing as recommended by the manufacturer should minimize any dermatologic problems.

SHIN GUARDS

Soccer, ice hockey, and field hockey players as well as baseball catchers are required to wear shin guards in intercollegiate play (Fig. 40–28). Most shin guards are constructed of a hard, deflective outer layer and an inner layer of thin foam. Other shin guards are constructed with plastic stays sewn into a felt material.

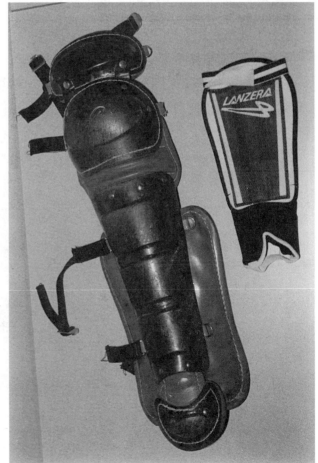

FIGURE 40–28. Shin guards: Baseball catcher's shin guard (also incorporates a knee guard *(left);* soccer or field hockey shin guard *(right).*

This design gives the athlete a more comfortable fit, since it conforms easily to the leg. Velcro straps and stirrups help stabilize the device inside the sock. Shin guards can also incorporate padding or plastic shells over the ankle malleoli, which is also a site for contusions.

ANKLE BRACES

Ankle braces attempt to stabilize the ankle to reduce the incidence of sprains (Fig. 40–29). Ankle braces can be used as a preventive or a postinjury supportive device. The purpose of an ankle brace is to minimize the amount of inversion and plantar flexion at the ankle. Ankle braces are used prophylactically in sports with close contact such as basketball, where there is a high likelihood of landing on another player's foot and spraining the ankle. There are numerous brands and designs of ankle braces available, giving athletes or sports medicine professionals choices when considering the degree of protection needed, comfort, and fit inside the shoe.

Several studies have been conducted that examine the benefit of ankle bracing over ankle taping. Bunch and associates[32] claim that tape initially restricts greater range of motion than braces but provides equal support after 20 minutes of exercise. However, tape has been shown to provide residual restriction in inversion-neutral and inversion-plantar flexion after a 3-hour football practice.[33] Other authors found that ankle braces provided a greater restriction in range of motion[34] and that injury rates were lower with bracing.[35] Several commercial brands were used in the research, and many of the investigations incorporated the use of numerous types of braces within each study.

Ankle braces and athletic tape are often compared for comfort and for effectiveness in preventing or minimizing ankle injuries. Bracing can be a cost-effective means of restricting ankle mobility and takes less time to use. However, many athletes prefer the comfort and stability offered by properly applied athletic tape.

ELBOW, FOREARM, WRIST, AND HAND PADS

Injuries to the hands or fingers are among the most common injuries in sports—and the most neglected. These injuries often cause minimal functional disability, and adequate protection with splinting materials may disqualify the athlete. In collegiate and professional football, no rigid material can be worn at the elbow or below unless it is adequately padded with closed-cell foam. Rules vary about the legality of protective equipment on the hand, depending on the sport and league. Clinicians should consult an authority about specific rules for individual cases before making custom-fabricated pads or splints to be used below the elbow.

To prevent injury to the hand, gloves are often worn in addition to many types of foam or neoprene pads for the distal aspect of the upper extremity. Gloves with silicone gel or foam padding are used in football, baseball, hockey, and lacrosse (Fig. 40–30).

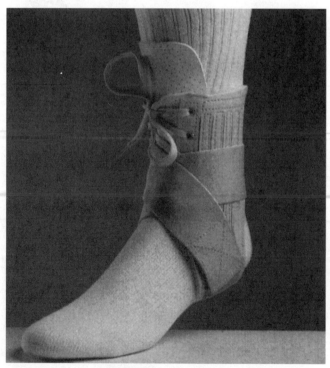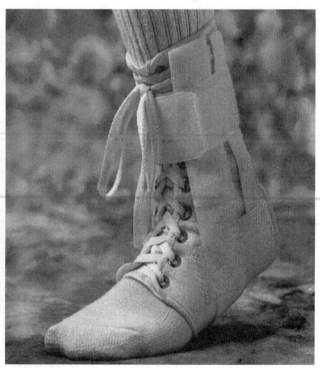

FIGURE 40–29. Ankle braces to prevent lateral ankle sprains: Pro ankle brace *(left)*; Rocketsoc by Don Joy *(right)*. (Courtesy of PRO Orthopedic Devices, Inc., Tuscon, AZ.)

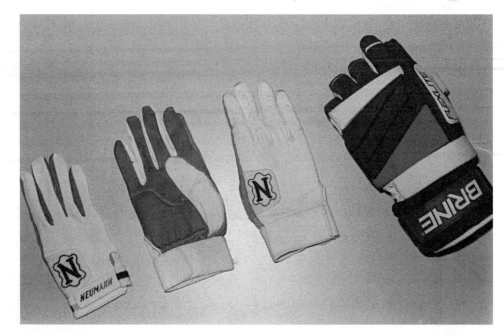

FIGURE 40–30. Examples of gloves for football and lacrosse. Varying amounts of dorsal and palmar padding are used, depending on the amount of contact.

R U N N I N G   S H O E   S E L E C T I O N

For runners, the most important piece of protective equipment is the running shoe. A key to remember when considering a new purchase is that if you have a shoe that is working well for you, do not change models. Changing to the latest model or a different brand is frequently a factor in running injuries.

1. Comfort. There should be no pressure spots on any part of the foot. The athlete should not assume that the shoe will stretch out.
2. Toe clearance. There should be a thumb's breadth (1/2 inch) between the longest toe and the end of the shoe. The toes should be able to fully extend. Make sure that the longer foot is used to determine the size. One foot is longer than the other in 75 percent of the population.
3. Shoe width. Eyelets should be at least 1 inch apart with normal lacing. The forefoot is typically the widest part of the foot and usually increases with activity. Shoes should give firm support at the heel and should not allow heel slippage.
4. Heel height. The running shoe should position the heel at least 1/2 inch above the outsole to minimize stretch on the Achilles tendon. Heel height is varied by the use of a wedge placed between the midsole and the heel counter of the shoe.
5. Forefoot cushioning. This area should be firm and well cushioned, as most of the vertical force occurs just behind the metatarsal heads.
6. Arch support. This provides support along the medial aspect of the shoe. This area should resist compression as the foot progresses through the footflat phase when pronation occurs. The arch support is typically provided by the insole or molded sock liners. The upper of the shoe can provide some support if adequate reinforcement is part of the design of the shoe.
7. Sole. The midfoot region should have moderate support but should not be rigid. Soles that are too rigid can transmit too much stress to the heel and leg, but if the sole is too flexible, forefoot and midfoot injury can result. If the shoe bends easily into a U shape, it is considered too flexible. Typically, the sole tread of running shoes comes in the horizontal bar or waffle design. The horizontal bar is generally considered appropriate for asphalt or concrete, and the waffle tread is more appropriate for off-road work, where traction is more important.
8. Midsole. This region provides shock absorption and motion control. The midsole is composed of ethylene vinyl acetate (EVA), polyurethane, or a combination of the two. The firmness of EVA can vary and is recognized as having good cushioning qualities, but it will break down over time. Polyurethane has minimal compressibility and therefore has good durability and stabilizing qualities. The use of a combination of these materials allows the shoe to provide good stability and motion control from the polyurethane and good shock absorption from the EVA.
9. Heel counter. This part of the shoe is considered critical in controlling rearfoot motion. Thermoplastic or fiberboard materials are used, the latter being found in lower-priced shoes. Thermoplastics are preferred, as they maintain their shape much longer, especially in adverse weather conditions. The heel counter should be firm, not collapsing when compressed. A heel counter stabilizer helps prevent heel counter breakdown.

FOOTWEAR

Appropriate footwear is one of the most important and often intimidating pieces of athletic equipment. There are numerous shoe manufacturers producing hundreds of models. The principal concern for clinicians is the possibility of an injury resulting from an improper selection. The shoes should be comfortable, prevent injury, and not deter performance (see Chapter 32).

It is not necessary to have a sport-specific shoe for all activities. Individuals may benefit from wearing shoes specific to their activities if they perform their sports more than three times a week.[36] Sport-specific shoes attempt to provide extra protection for stresses particular to that activity or to accommodate conditions unique to the surface on which the sport is played (Fig. 40–31A). Running shoes generally have extra flexibility in the forefoot region to accommodate the necessity for toe-off. Walking shoes have a more rigid forefoot to

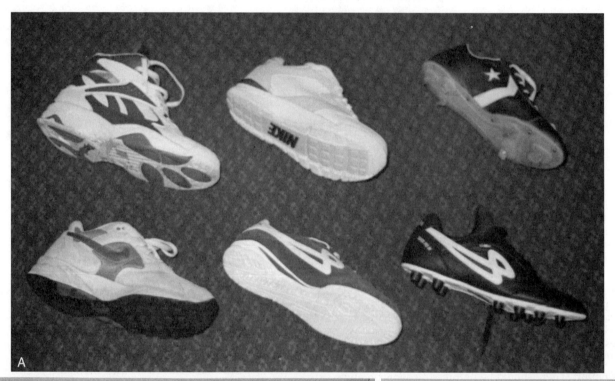

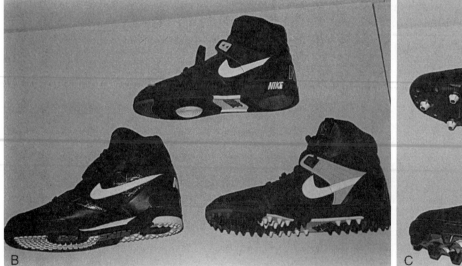

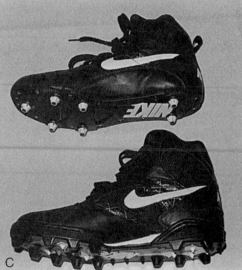

FIGURE 40–31. Various types of shoes. *A, (left to right):* Basketball shoes; low-top court shoes; metal cleats for baseball; running shoes; flat soccer shoes; molded rubber cleats on soccer shoes. *B,* Dry-weather football shoes: flat and "turf." *C,* Football shoes for grass: seven screw-in studs for optimal traction *(top);* molded cleats on outer sole *(bottom).*

prevent the bending stress placed through the forefoot and toes. Court shoes such as those for tennis, racquetball, and basketball provide extra lateral support to protect the ankle from excess side-to-side motion. Cross-trainer shoes attempt to combine flexibility and lateral stability but are not advisable for extensive running. Cleats are produced for various field sports and are designed for different surfaces and field conditions, including artificial turf, natural grass, and wet conditions.

There are numerous manufacturers of football shoes that have similar features. The shoe may be a low-top or a high-top with different soles, depending on the type of playing surface. Low-top shoes are typically used on the running-intensive positions (e.g., running backs, defensive backs, or quarterbacks). The use of low-top shoes is often discouraged because of the loss of additional ankle support that high-top shoes provide. The use of athletic tape over the shoe (spatting) to provide additional support is discouraged because of the difficulty in accessing the foot or ankle should an injury occur. The types of soles available for different playing surfaces include:

ARTIFICIAL SURFACES (Fig. 40–31*B*)

Basketball sole. Flat bottom sole with small grooves to enhance traction. Football players, especially linemen, wear this type of shoe on dry artificial surfaces.

Multicleated. 150 molded cleats or "turf shoes" for dry-weather activity.

Molded cleats. Molded sole with cone-shaped cleats of varying heights for increased traction in wet weather.

GRASS (Fig. 40–31*C*)

Seven-studded. Seven removable, or "screw-in," cleats on the bottom sole. Gives best traction on wet surfaces. These shoes are poorly tolerated for everyday use because they have little foot support.

Molded cleats. Molded sole with large cleats on the perimeter of the shoe and smaller cleats located centrally. This shoe cradles the foot, therefore providing adequate support and comfort.

It is difficult to stay current with the numerous brands and models of shoes available. Finding an athletic shoe store that employs serious recreational athletes can be helpful in selecting appropriate shoes. This selection process should include knowlege of certain orthopaedic concerns, such as over- or underpronation and bunions, as well as an athlete's physical characteristics and activity goals.

When selecting the size of the shoe, do not rely on sizing to be standardized. Sizes can vary considerably among manufacturers, and even within the same model and company. The last of the shoe can affect sizing, as can what factory a particular shoe was constructed in. Women with wide feet may consider a boy's or man's shoe for a better fit. Women's sizes run 1.5 sizes larger than men's sizes (e.g., a 9.5 woman's size is equal to a man's 8.0).

ORTHOTICS

Orthotic devices such as shoe inserts can be used to accommodate for or help correct certain lower extremity postural malalignments (Fig. 40–32). Small modifications in the subtalar joint position can affect the stresses placed throughout the kinetic chain, such as at the ankle, knee, hip, or vertebra. Orthotic devices attempt to balance the foot in a subtalar neutral position to help the foot and ankle complex undergo normal pronation and supination at the appropriate phases of gait. Orthotics can be used to help control excessive motion of the foot or allow for limitations in range of motion. Various types of orthotics can be used as part of the total management of stress fractures, arch pain, plantar fasciitis, bunions, shin splints, and patellofemoral problems.

Temporary orthotics can be fabricated by sports medicine clinicians by cutting pads from orthopaedic felt or closed-cell foam and placing the pad inside the shoe. Some manufacturers produce prefabricated pads such as arch supports and heel lifts that are easily added to the sock liner of the shoe. Custom orthotics are made from a cast or impression of the athlete's feet in a neutral position. The shoe insert is fabricated from a positive of this mold, and variations are made, depending on the postural malalignments of the lower extremity or the symptoms. Posts or wedges are secured to the insert. The sock liner of the shoe is removed before positioning the custom orthotic. The athlete should be encouraged to "break in" the new orthotic as he or she would break in a new pair of shoes.

CONCLUSION

The fabrication, fitting, and use of protective equipment to prevent or treat injuries should be coupled with

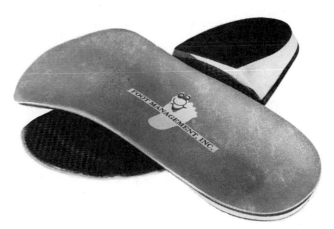

FIGURE 40–32. Examples of orthotic devices for shoe insertion. (Courtesy of Foot Management, Inc., Salisbury, MD.)

education. Athletes and coaches should be informed that although equipment is used to decrease the risk of injury or reinjury, prevention of injury and reinjury cannot be guaranteed. The athlete should be shown how the equipment should be worn and used. He or she should be told to inspect the equipment each day and to replace any damage to the pads, straps, or braces. Additionally, the athlete should be asked whether the device fits comfortably and should be told to report any discomfort the device causes. Any injury or reinjury must be reported to the athletic trainer or team physician. Educating the athlete also includes reinforcing the importance of conditioning or rehabilitation. If the coaches, sports medicine personnel, and equipment managers all exhibit a positive attitude toward a piece of protective equipment, with emphasis on protection rather than using the device as a weapon, injuries surely can be prevented.

REFERENCES

1. NOCSAE Manual. Overland Park, KS, 1993.
2. Roy S, Irvin R: Sports Medicine: Prevention, Evaluation, Management and Rehabilitation. Englewood Cliffs, NJ, Prentice-Hall, 1983, pp 45–51.
3. Gieck J, McCue FC: Fitting of protective football equipment. Am J Sports Med 1980; 8:192–196.
4. Gieck J: Protective equipment for sport. In Ryan AJ, Allman FL (eds): Sports Medicine. New York, Academic Press, 1989, pp 211–242.
5. American Equipment Manager's Certification Manual. Health Care Forum, Inc. Athletic Equipment Managers Association, 1992.
6. Nygaard G, Boone TH: Coaches Guide to Sport Law (publication for the American Coaching Effectiveness Program). Champaign, IL, Human Kinetics, 1985.
7. Hodgson VR, Thomas LM: Biomechanical study of football head impacts using a head model-condenser version. Final report prepared for National Operating Committee on Standards for Athletic Equipment (NOCSAE), 1973.
8. Hodgson VR: Athletic equipment and injury prevention. In Mueller FO, Ryan AJ (eds): Prevention of Athletic Injuries: The Role of the Sports Medicine Team. Philadelphia, FA Davis, 1991, pp 48–63.
9. Miller R: Presentation on protective padding. NATA National Convention and Symposium, Columbus, OH, 1987.
10. Arnheim DD: Modern Principles of Athletic Training. St. Louis, Times Mirror/Mosby College Publishing, 1989, pp 734–775.
11. Rovere GD, Curl WW, Brownig DC: Bracing and taping in an office sports medicine practice. Clin Sports Med 1989; 8:497–515.
12. Breger-Lee DE, Buford WL: Properties of thermoplastic splinting materials. J Hand Ther 1992; 4:202–211.
13. Mayer V, Gieck J: Rehabilitation of hand injuries in athletics. Clin Sports Med 1986; 5:783–793.
14. Almquist J: Presentation on the high school cast rule for football as governed by the National Federation of High School Associations. Virginia Beach, 1994.
15. Procap product testing. Pennsylvania State University Biomechanics Laboratory, 1991.
16. Watkins RG: Neck injuries in football players. Clin Sports Med 1986; 5:215–246.
17. American Society for Testing and Materials: Philadelphia, 1994.
18. American Academy of Ophthalmology: The Athlete's Eye. San Francisco, American Academy of Ophthalmology, 1982.
19. Easterbrook M: Eye protection in racket sports: an update. Phys Sports Med 1987; 15:180–192.
20. Orlando RG: Soccer-related eye injuries in children and adolescents. Phys Sports Med 1988; 16:103–106.
21. Labelle P, Mercier M, Podtetenev M, Trudeau F: Eye injuries in sports: results of a five year study. Phys Sports Med 1988; 16:126–138.
22. Easterbrook M: Eye injuries in squash and racquetball players: an update. Phys Sports Med 1982; 10:47–56.
23. Heintz WD: Mouth protection in sports. Phys Sports Med 1979; 7:45–46.
24. Kulund D: The Injured Athlete. Philadelphia, JB Lippincott, 1988.
25. Rutherford GW, Kennedy J, McGhee L: Baseball and softball related injuries to children 5–14 years of age. Washington, DC, US Consumer Product Safety Commission, Epidemiology, Division of Hazard Analysis, 1984.
26. Deitsch MA, Fashover T: Football hip pad protection for hip pointers and AC sprains on ice hockey players. Athletic Training 1981; 16:2.
27. Hald RD, Fandel D: Taping and bracing. In Mellion MB (ed): Office Management of Sports Injuries and Athletic Problems. Philadelphia, Hanley & Belfus, 1988.
28. Hansen BY, Ward JC, Diehl RC: The preventive use of the Anderson knee stabler in football. Phys Sports Med 1985; 13:75–81.
29. Rovere GD, Haupt HA, Yates CS: Prophylactic knee bracing in college football. Am J Sports Med 1987; 15:111–116.
30. Cawley PW: Postoperative knee bracing. Clin Sports Med 1990; 9:763–769.
31. Cawley PW, France P, Paulos LE: Comparison of rehabilitative knee braces: a biomechanical investigation. Am J Sports Med 1989; 17:141–146.
32. Bunch RP, Bednarski K, Holland D, Macinati R: Ankle joint support: a comparison of reuseable lace-on braces with taping and wrapping. Phys Sports Med 1985; 13:59–62.
33. Fumich RM, Ellison AE, Guerin GJ, Grace PD: The measured effect of taping on combined foot and ankle motion before and after exercise. Am J Sports Med 1981; 9:165–170.
34. Alves JW, Alday RV, Ketcham DL, Lentell GL: A comparison of the passive support provided by various ankle braces. J Ortho Sports Phys Ther 1992; 15:10–18.
35. Rovere GD, Clarke TJ, Yates CS, Burley K: Retrospective comparison of taping and ankle stabilizers in preventing ankle injuries. Am J Sports Med 1988; 16:228–233.
36. Wichmann S, Martin DR: Athletic shoes: finding the right fit. Phys Sports Med 1993; 21:204–211.

CHAPTER 41

The Child and Adolescent Athlete

LORI A. THEIN MS, PT, SCS, ATC

Organized sports participation by young athletes is increasing and is gradually replacing time that was spent in free play. Many young children are involved in multiple sports, and parents find themselves busy keeping track of their children's soccer, softball, gymnastics, dancing, and swimming events. Approximately 7 million students, nearly half of all males and one quarter of all females between the ages of 8 and 16 years, are involved in some organized sporting activity.[1] High schools in the United States offer as many as 32 competitive sports for boys and 27 for girls.

The participation of children and adolescents in sports poses a unique set of problems for the sports medicine professional. Although children spend plenty of time participating in free-play activities, organized training and sports place different stresses on the young athlete. These stresses are above and beyond those encountered in activities of daily living, and questions arise concerning physical and psychological issues related to participation. The push for recognition of elite athletes at the international level has spawned a grass roots effort to start children training at an earlier age in hopes of fine-tuning high-level skills as they approach adulthood. However, as witnessed by high-visibility sports such as gymnastics and figure skating, children are entering the elite class at much younger ages. This produces a series of issues open to debate within the medical and coaching communities. The questions related to physical, physiological, and psychological

development and sports participation by the adolescent and child athlete are addressed in this chapter.

EPIDEMIOLOGY OF INJURY

Participation of children and adolescents in organized sports and training has received a great deal of attention in the last two decades. Beginning in the early 1960s with the advent of the President's Council on Physical Fitness and Sports, focus on the physical condition of children has increased. Decreasing fitness levels in children has prompted growth in organized training for this age group. However, despite the health benefits known to occur with exercise, the young athlete's participation in organized sports has been questioned because of the possible risks of injury. The mode, frequency, duration, and intensity of exercise and the level of organization have been questioned. This has prompted studies to determine the incidence and rate of injuries in pediatric and adolescent athletes.[1-7] An estimated 91,667 hospitalizations and 2,564,558 emergency room visits occurred in 1985 as a result of sports injuries in children aged from 0 to 19 years.[6] Emergency room visits resulting from sports injuries occurred four times more often than emergency room visits for motor vehicle occupant injuries.[6] The indirect cost of childhood sports injuries in 1982 was estimated at 13.2 million dollars, and the direct costs were estimated to be

933

567.6 million dollars.[6] In the youthful athlete, injuries are often contusions, sprains, and simple fractures. The sports resulting in the most injuries per participant hour in a 1979 study were football, basketball, gymnastics, soccer, and baseball, in the order named.[8] Other studies have found the injury rates to be the highest in football, wrestling, and girls' and boys' gymnastics.[9,10] When evaluating injury statistics in the literature, one must keep in mind differences in methodology and definitions of terms, which may lead to errors in data interpretation.[11]

In 1978, DeHaven[12] reported on 161 athletic injuries to children aged 15 years and younger over the course of 18 months. The number of injuries to boys exceeded those to girls 124 to 37, and most injuries occurred in the older adolescents. Nearly 80 percent of the injuries involved the knee and included sprains, strains, fractures, and meniscal injuries. Sports producing the most injuries were football for boys and gymnastics for girls.[12] A higher incidence of injuries occurred in boys than in girls.[13] Unsupervised sports produced 40 percent of the injuries, followed by physical education classes at 38 percent, and organized sports accounted for 15 percent of injuries. However, one must bear in mind the changing face of sport in today's society with girls representing a larger proportion of the sports population. Additionally, evaluation, documentation, and follow-up procedures have improved, providing more specific injury information.

In 1982, Backx and colleagues[14] collected epidemiologic data on 7,468 children aged 8 to 17 years in a 6-week period. They found an incidence of 10.6 injuries per 100 participants, 31 percent of whom required medical consultation.[14] The lower extremity was involved in 75 percent of the injuries, the ankle accounting for 26.5 percent and the knee 21.9 percent of all injuries. When evaluating the injury setting, 62 percent of all injuries occurred in organized sports, 21 percent in physical education classes, and 17 percent in unsupervised sports activities. Unlike the previous studies, no significant differences were noted between the boys and the girls. These authors thought that the choice of sport was a more important determinant of the injury pattern than gender. Another large study looked at injuries over the course of an entire year and found an incidence of 39.3 per 100 athletes, of whom 40 percent were referred to a physician. When analyzing days of participation missed, 29 percent missed only 1 day, and 70 percent missed 5 days or less.[15]

More recent studies have concurred with some aspects of earlier epidemiologic data. A consistent finding is that injury incidence increases with age when comparing children with adolescents.[3,13,16] For example, the injury rate for junior high students is about one third that of high school students' injuries.[16] A study of injuries at two large wrestling tournaments involving 1742 participants aged 6 to 16 years found an overall injury rate of 12.7 percent. An increasing incidence of injury was correlated with increasing age and weight.[17] There is still some question concerning different injury rates in boys compared with girls and incidence differences related to type of sport. A large retrospective

study of adolescents between the ages of 8 and 19 years seen at one facility from 1980 to 1990 reported 724 cases of tendinitis and apophysitis, 88 occurring in the upper extremity and 636 in the lower extremity. A total of 253 girls and 192 boys were evaluated and treated. Conservative management was effective in most cases.[18] It is difficult to draw any conclusions from the many studies because of variations in data collection procedures, definition of injury, and presentation in the literature.[11,19]

Finally, when studying serious injuries such as acute fractures and dislocations of the cervical spine in children and adolescents, McGrory and associates[20] found that the older children (aged 11 to 15 years) were more likely to sustain injuries during sports and recreational activities, compared with younger children, who were injured as a result of falls. Their injuries demonstrated a pattern similar to that of adults, and there was a higher male-to-female ratio than in the younger years. The age- and sex-adjusted incidence of cervical spine fractures and dislocations was 7.41 per 100,000 participants per year. The sports producing these injuries were primarily diving, gymnastics, football, and wrestling.[20]

The constantly changing face of sport in society today results in continuous fluctuation of the epidemiologic literature. The passage of Title IX in 1972 spawned an expansion of girls' sports, resulting in an increase in their injuries; and the development of new equipment such as in-line skates and snowboards has resulted in new injury categories. The sports medicine professional must keep abreast of the changing nature of youths' sports to provide guidance to athletes, parents, and coaches regarding participation.

PHYSICAL DEVELOPMENT AND CHARACTERISTICS

GROWTH AND MUSCULOSKELETAL DEVELOPMENT

Musculoskeletal injuries in the pediatric and adolescent athlete are of great concern to parents, coaches, and the health care community. A thorough understanding of the normal developmental characteristics of the child helps the sports medicine professional to recognize injuries specific to this population. An awareness of the potential risks and benefits of participation in sports allows adults to direct children to age- and skill-appropriate activities. This will enable the sports medicine professional to guide coaches and parents in appropriate activity choices for their child athlete and will provide a sound basis for realistic expectations for all involved.

Boys and girls grow at similar rates in height and weight throughout childhood. The most rapid growth occurs shortly before birth and subsequently slows and remains relatively steady until adolescence.[21] The infant has a relatively large head, long trunk, and short limbs. By adulthood, the head will have doubled in size, whereas the trunk will have tripled. The upper extremi-

TABLE 41–1
Comparisons of Various Musculoskeletal Development Characteristics Between Boys and Girls

Landmark	Boys	Girls
Onset of puberty (yrs)	12.5	10.5
Peak height velocity (yrs)	14.10 ± 0.92	12.14 ± 0.88
Height added during spurt (cm)	7–12	6–11
Age reaching adult stature (yrs)	18–21	17–18
Percentage of adult height at 2 yrs	49.4%	52.7%
Percentage of adult height at 5 yrs	62.0%	66.4%
Percentage of adult height at 10 yrs	77.6%	84.5%
Percentage of adult height at 15 yrs	95.4%	99.1%

Compiled from Smith,[21] Porter,[22] Lowrey,[23] and Tanner.[24]

ties increase in size by a factor of four and the lower extremities by a factor of five. Between ages 2 and 3 years, children may add as much as 10.2 cm to their height, and continue to add approximately 5.1 to 7.6 cm/year until adolescence. In the preadolescent years, the rate of growth is disproportionate throughout the body. There is a greater increase in the length of the limbs relative to the trunk, and the center of gravity moves caudally.[22]

The onset of puberty occurs at approximately 10.5 years for girls and 12.5 years for boys (Table 41–1). Disproportionate growth of various body parts during this developmental phase is the rule, resulting in changes in body shape and proportion. The peak velocity of growth in height for girls in the United States is generally during the 12th year (peak 12.14 ± 0.88 years), and the average girl will add from 6 to 11 cm at this time. This same landmark generally occurs during the 14th year for boys (peak 14.06 ± 0.92 years), whose growth will range from 7 to 12 cm during this growth spurt.[21] Most girls reach their adult stature at age 17 to 18 years, whereas boys reach their adult height at age 18 to 21 years.[22]

Tanner noted that adult height could be predicted based on the child's height. A 2-year-old *boy* is generally at 49.4 percent of his adult height, a 5-year-old at 62 percent, a 10-year-old at 77.6 percent, and a 15-year-old at 95.4 percent. He found height at the age of 3 years to be the best predictor of adult height of any early age.[24] Progression of girls' height follows the same pattern, although some differences are noted during adolescence. A 2-year-old *girl* averages 52.7 percent of adult height; a 5-year-old, 66.4 percent; a 10-year-old, 84.5 percent; and a 15-year-old is at approximately 99.1 percent of her adult height.[24] Girls and boys are generally the same height during childhood, and girls are taller than most boys at ages 12 to 13 years. However, when boys enter puberty approximately 2 years later, this situation reverses.[21] When anthropometric measures are used to determine skeletal maturity, height

demonstrates the strongest correlation, followed by weight, width, and circumference.[25]

Like height, weight increases steadily throughout childhood and adolescence. Weight gains of approximately 2 kg/year are normal for the preschool years, and a youngster will have doubled his/her 1-year weight by age 5 years.[22] Weight gain during the preschool years is around 2.0 kg/year with steady gains of roughly 2.7 kg/year from ages 6 to 9 years. By age 10, the child's weight is generally ten times the birth weight.[22] Peak weight velocity follows peak height velocity by 0.25 years in boys and 0.63 years in girls.[26] A study of children throughout puberty noted an average 113 percent increase in boys' and a 76 percent increase in girls' total body weight during puberty.[27] Variance in adolescent growth spurts can result in dramatic physical differences between two children of the same chronological age. At the start of puberty in boys, there can be differences of as much as 100 lb and 5 years in bone age between two boys of the same chronological age.[21] For this reason, criteria other than chronological age should be considered in the organization of collision sports such as football. Two children of the same chronological age may be extremely unevenly matched physically, resulting in unfair and unsafe competition.

Measurements of muscle mass and strength demonstrate increases proportional to weight gain during childhood. Although muscle mass and strength are related, they are not equivalent. Strength measurements include a neurologic component (recruitment, motor control, etc.) that simple muscle mass measurements do not consider. At birth, skeletal *muscle mass* accounts for approximately 25 percent of total body weight, and this increases to 35 percent at age 5 years and to 40 percent at maturity. When evaluated by sex, girls' percentage of muscle mass increases to 40 to 45 percent by age 13 years and then decreases after this age. In contrast, boys' muscle mass increases from approximately 42 to 54 percent.[28] Two accelerations in this proportion occur, the first between ages 1.5 and 5 years and the second during adolescence.[21] A boy's muscle mass will double between the ages of 11 and 17 years, and the peak muscle growth occurs simultaneously with peak height velocity. Overall, a girl's muscle mass increases four times and a boy's five times between the ages of 5 and 18 years. Girls reach the maximum muscle growth during their 12th year, whereas boys reach their maximum on average during their 14th year.[22]

After birth, gains in *strength* are due to hypertrophy of the existing muscle fibers.[28,29] By age 6 years, the distribution of types I, IIA, and IIB fibers is nearly the same as in the adult.[29] Prior to puberty, minimal differences exist between boys and girls in upper- and lower-extremity strength, boys on average demonstrating slightly greater strength than girls at all ages.[28,30] Girls' muscle mass doubles between the ages of 9 and 15 years, and they reach peak muscle growth approximately 6 months after peak height velocity. Increases in muscle strength closely follow increases in muscle mass in both sexes (approximately 9 to 12 months after peak

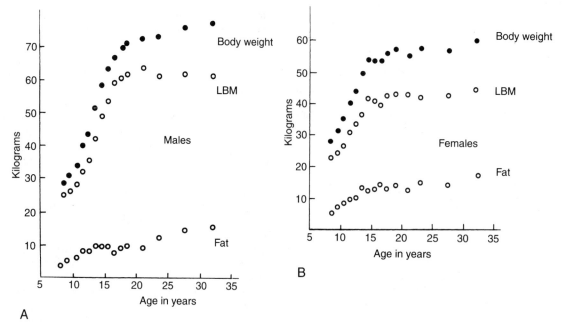

FIGURE 41–1. Changes in body composition in males *(A)* and females *(B)* between the ages of 10 and 35 years. (From Falkner F, Tanner JM (eds): Human Growth: A Comprehensive Treatise, 2nd ed., vol 2. New York, Plenum Press, 1985.)

height and weight gain).[22] Muscle mass and size are closely related to skeletal maturity during puberty but are weakly correlated in childhood.[25] However, although attainment of peak strength development is a good indicator of maturity in adolescent boys, it is not in girls.

Evaluation of motor skill acquisition during the school-age years demonstrates an increase in gross motor skills such as running, jumping, and throwing. The child should develop the adult forms of these skills somewhere between the ages of 6 and 10 years. Sex differences can be noted in motor skills, even at a young age. Boys generally outperform girls in a variety of gross motor tasks such as running, jumping, and throwing throughout childhood, whereas girls are generally better than boys at fine motor tasks at ages 5 to 6 years. Boys continue to improve in motor skills until at least 17 to 18 years, whereas girls' development drops off at 14 years.[22] It is unclear to what extent this reflects differences in socialization. The adolescent with poor motor abilities should have specific drills and activities to improve the skills related to his or her sport, and to reduce the likelihood of injury.

BODY COMPOSITION

The relative proportion of lean body mass and adipose tissue is important to most athletes and receives a tremendous amount of emphasis in society as a whole. From age 8 years until adolescence, boys and girls add a steady amount of adipose yearly, and boys and girls appear to have similar distributions of fatty tissue.[27] At adolescence, girls begin to slow the addition of adipose to a rate that is lower than before or after

adolescence. Boys, in contrast, demonstrate a net loss of adipose tissue at adolescence, gaining lean body mass at a greater rate (Fig. 41–1).

Buckler found a steady decline in appendicular skinfolds and increases in axial skinfolds in boys during puberty, suggesting a change in the distribution of body fat.[27] The girls demonstrated increases at all sites. Training can affect body composition even in children. Trained children have demonstrated increases in lean body mass and decreases in percentage of body fat when compared with untrained children.[31]

BONE DEVELOPMENT

Skeletal maturity is often used as the measure of physical maturity in the young adult and is a more accurate reflection of his or her maturity than chronological age. According to Roche, bone maturation is the process whereby the tissue undergoes alterations in each of its parts as it progresses from the embryonic rudiment of a bone to the adult form.[32] The increased size of the bone occurs as a result of a combination of hyperplasia, hypertrophy, and the storage of organic or nonorganic materials in and around the cells.[32] Bone growth occurs either with an intermediate cartilage structure that is eventually replaced by bone (endochondral) or without a cartilage model (intramembranous).[33] Most bones are formed with a cartilage model first (endochondral), with the exception of the skull, carpal and tarsal bones, and part of the clavicle, which are formed intramembranously. The long bones increase in length by endochondral ossification and increase in width by a second process involving intramembranous ossification. Growth takes place at the pressure physis, or epiphyseal growth plate. This is in distinction to a traction physis, which is the site of a tendinous attachment. A traction physis does not contribute to the longitudinal growth of the bone and is more commonly referred to as an apophysis.[34] The epiphyseal plate is weaker than the surrounding bone, thus making it susceptible to injury.

After birth, ossification begins to take place in the cartilaginous ends of the long bones. These epiphyses develop separately from the long shaft of the bone, and may contain several "secondary" ossification centers (Fig. 41–2).[32] For example, the primary ossification center of the femur is the shaft, and secondary centers exist at the proximal and distal epiphyseal plates. Ossification continues at the epiphysis throughout early childhood until only the epiphyseal plate remains between the shaft and the ossified epiphysis. Once the epiphysis has ossified, continued longitudinal growth

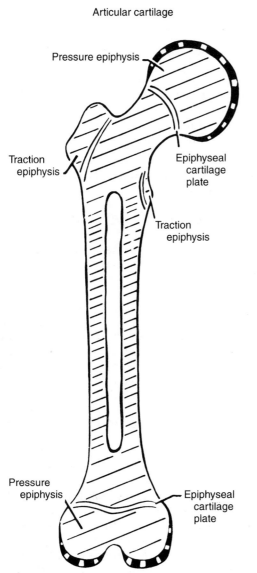

Articular cartilage

Pressure epiphysis

Traction epiphysis

Epiphyseal cartilage plate

Traction epiphysis

Pressure epiphysis

Epiphyseal cartilage plate

FIGURE 41–2. Drawing of a young femur bone demonstrating the types of epiphyses. The epiphyseal cartilage provides for the longitudinal growth of the bone. (From Moore KL: Clinically Oriented Anatomy, 3rd ed. Baltimore, Williams & Wilkins, 1993.)

occurs on the diaphyseal side of the epiphyseal plate. It is this plate that is responsible for the continued longitudinal growth of the bone. Growth in the length of the bone is a result of growth in the length of the metaphysis and diaphysis. The diaphysis is the elongated, cylindrical portion of the bone, and the metaphysis is the wider portion at the end of the shaft, adjacent to the epiphyseal growth plate. Despite the amount of longitudinal growth that occurs at the epiphyseal plate, its thickness does not change. This is because of a balance between the interstitial growth of the plate's cartilage cells (making it thicker), and calcification, death, and replacement of cartilage by bone on the metaphyseal side. This results in the epiphysis moving farther away from the metaphysis.[34]

The shape and orientation of the epiphyseal plate is a result of tension and compression forces. Salter[34] has identified four zones of the epiphyseal plate (moving from epiphysis to metaphysis): (1) zone of resting cartilage, which anchors the epiphyseal plate to the epiphysis; (2) zone of proliferating cartilage, which is the most active site of interstitial cartilage cell growth; (3) zone of maturing cartilage, containing progressively enlarging and maturing cartilage cells; and (4) zone of calcifying cartilage, which is the weakest zone of the epiphyseal plate (Fig. 41–3). Matrix is abundant in the first two layers, which are therefore strong. The matrix is thin in the fourth layer, making this layer the most vulnerable. The blood supply to the epiphyseal plate is from the epiphyseal side, and any disruption may therefore result in epiphyseal plate necrosis and cessation of growth. As the child approaches maturity, the epiphyseal plate begins to fuse to the shaft, and longitudinal growth slows and eventually ceases (Fig. 41–4).[34]

A similar growth process occurs at the traction physis, or apophysis, although there is no change in bone length. Recent studies have however noted significant histologic differences between these two types of physes, especially at the tibial tubercle.[35] Specific structural adaptations, including a zone of endochondral bone formation, a zone of membranous bone formation through fibrocartilaginous tissue, and a zone of membranous bone formation through fibrous tissue, accommodate the specific tensile stresses from the quadriceps.[36] The apophysis may be susceptible to injury owing to constant tension via the muscle-tendon attachment. These attachments can put an excessive load on the weaker cartilage zones, causing changes in the normal response. These changes might include localized soft tissue swelling and rarefaction or fragmentation at the muscular attachment.

One important issue in adolescence is the association between chronological age and bone age. Numerous scales and grading systems of maturity exist, thereby confounding published information on bone age and maturity. Additionally, bones vary in the chronological age at which they reach adult maturity levels.[32] Before puberty, chronological age correlates well with bone age as the child increases in both height and weight. However, during puberty, bone age can be expected to accelerate as height accelerates. Thus, bone age in this

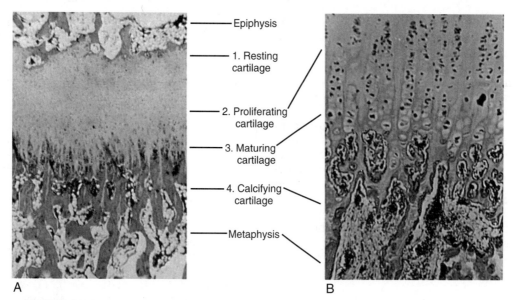

FIGURE 41–3. Histology of an epiphyseal plate (from the upper end of the tibia of a child). *A,* Low power; *B,* high power. (From Salter RB: Textbook of Disorders and Injuries of the Musculoskeletal System, 2nd ed. Baltimore, Williams & Wilkins, 1983.)

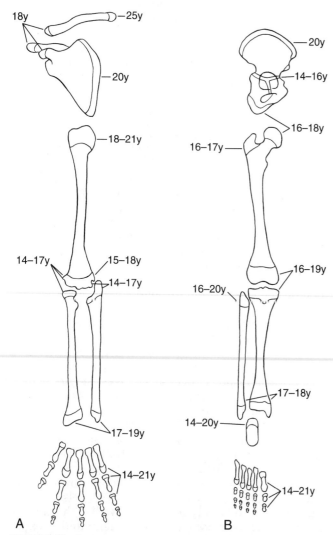

FIGURE 41–4. Schematic of ages of physeal closure in the major long bones of the arm *(A)* and leg *(B)*. (From Ogden JA: Skeletal Injury in the Child. Philadelphia, WB Saunders, 1990.)

population is more closely related to the timing of puberty than to actual chronological age. Buckler found the age at which 95 percent of adult height was reached and the age of menarche to be more closely related to bone age than to chronological age.[27]

PHYSIOLOGIC DEVELOPMENT AND CHARACTERISTICS

CARDIORESPIRATORY DEVELOPMENT

The heart and lungs in the child are proportional to his or her body size. The size of the heart increases from about 2/3 oz at birth to 7 oz at age 15 to 16 years, whereas the rate of contraction decreases from 120 to 70 to 80 beats per minute at age 16 years. This decrease is due in part to an increase in stroke volume and cardiac output with growth. The heart is oriented more horizontally in the child than in the adult, and as the child grows, the heart becomes more vertical. Blood pressure remains steady from years 2 to 5, after which it rises gradually until it reaches adult values during puberty.[22] The hemoglobin concentration, hematocrit, and red blood cell count are all lower in the child than in the adult, reaching adult values during adolescence.

Pulmonary diffusing capacity is lower in children than adults, since the rate of gas diffusion is dependent on the surface area of the alveolar membrane.[29] Respiration is accomplished primarily by the diaphragm until age 5 to 7 years, when the transition to the thoracic muscles for respiration occurs. Respiration efficiency is similar in boys and girls throughout childhood until adolescence, when boys become more efficient than girls.[37] Maximum pulmonary ventilation is about the same in children, adolescents, and adults when expressed per kilogram of body weight. However, submaximal ventilation per kilogram of body weight is higher in the child, suggesting a lower ventilatory reserve.[31]

Maximal oxygen uptake is the standard measure that assesses aerobic fitness. As boys and girls grow, their maximal oxygen uptake increases at the same rate until approximately age 12 years. Thereafter, the boys continue to demonstrate increases until about 18 years, whereas girls do not progress much in their maximal oxygen uptake beyond 14 years (Fig. 41–5).[31] This is generally the result of increases in muscle mass because maximal aerobic power is strongly related to lean body mass. In boys, absolute Vo_2max increases from approximately 1.0 L/min^{-1} at age 6 to 3.2 L/min^{-1} at age 16 years. When expressed relative to body weight, the boys' value remains constant from ages 6 to 16 years at about 53 ml/kg/min^{-1}. Girls' values approximate boys' between the ages of 6 and 12 years, but the girls achieve a maximum of about 2.0 L/min^{-1} at age 14 years, which then declines. When described relative to body weight, the girls' Vo_2max decreases with age from 52 L/kg/min^{-1} at age 6 years to about 40.5 L/kg/min^{-1} at age 16 years. This decrease likely is due to an increase in adipose tissue, which thereby increases total body weight, and a decreasing proportion of lean body mass.[38] The maximal increase in Vo_2max appears to occur in the same year as peak height velocity. At age 14 years, the difference in maximal oxygen uptake between boys and girls is about 25 percent, and this number increases to about 50 percent by age 16 years.

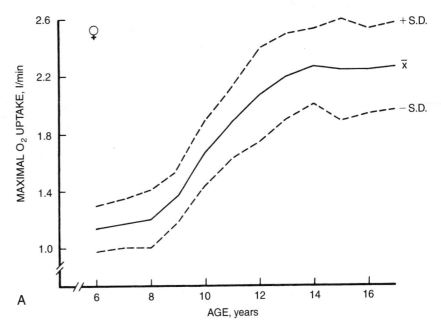

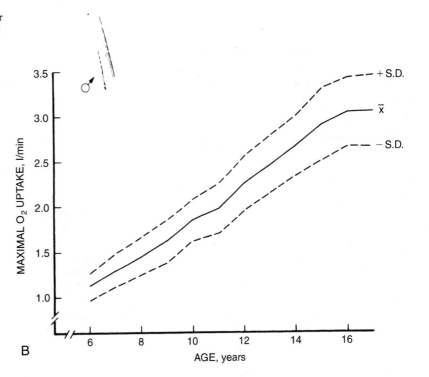

FIGURE 41–5. Maximal O_2 uptake in children and adolescents. Data from 179 girls (A) and 178 boys (B) who performed an all-out progressive-continuous protocol on a treadmill. (From Bar-Or O: Pediatric Sports Medicine for the Practitioner: From Physiologic Principles to Clinical Applications. New York, Springer-Verlag, 1983.)

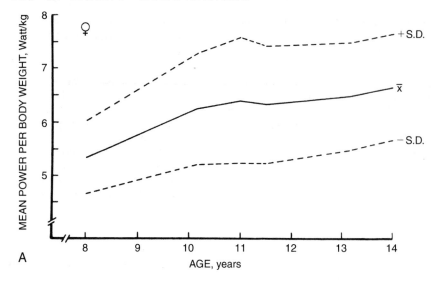

A

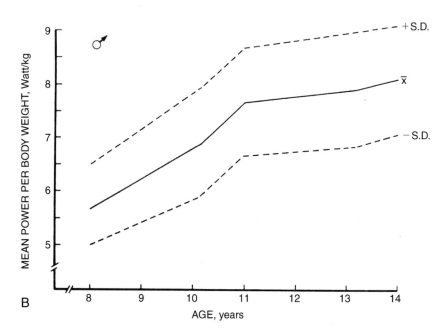

B

FIGURE 41–6. Anaerobic capacity per kilogram of body weight in children and adolescents: 144 girls (A) and 145 boys (B). Mean power during a Wingate anaerobic test. (From Bar-Or O: Pediatric Sports Medicine for the Practitioner: From Physiologic Principles to Clinical Applications. New York, Springer-Verlag, 1983.)

Oxygen uptake appears to be primarily determined by stroke volume in circumpubertal boys. Stroke volume reflects oxygen uptake throughout puberty with the exception of the period of most rapid growth. Arteriovenous oxygen difference also increases during the period of most rapid growth with little change in any other stage.[39]

The capability of children to perform maximal anaerobic activities is much lower than that of the adolescent or the adult (Fig. 41–6).[31] Performance on the Wingate anaerobic test is positively correlated with age, the 8-year-old boy producing approximately 70 percent of the power of an 11-year-old boy, even when results are normalized for body weight.[31] The same holds true for peak power performance, or the explosivity of the muscle contraction. Differences in anaerobic performance appear to be unrelated to age or muscle mass, and the differences between children and adults may be due to the glycogen utilization rate.[40]

The maximal heart rate of children ranges between 195 and 215 beats per minute, and the submaximal heart rate declines during the growth years, but the maximal heart rate does not decline until after maturity. Girls demonstrate a higher heart rate than boys, on the average of 10 to 20 beats per minute. It is possible that this is related to a lower stroke volume seen in girls.[31] Boys also demonstrate a faster decline in postexercise heart rate than girls.

RESPONSES TO ACUTE EXERCISE

When a child begins to exercise, heart rate and cardiac output increase as the work intensity increases. However, when compared with the adult, the child's heart rate is higher and the stroke volume is lower. Children are also much less mechanically efficient than adults, using more energy than the adult for the same activity and intensity. One study found an 8-year-old child running at 180 m/min to be operating at approximately 90 percent of Vo_2max, whereas a 16-year-old operated at only 75 percent of his Vo_2max.[41] Additionally, children demonstrate a greater arteriovenous oxygen difference and increased blood flow to the exercising muscle than adults. This would suggest an improved oxygen delivery system in the child that may compensate for a decreased cardiac output (Table 41–2).[29] During exercise, the rise in systolic blood pressure is proportional to the exercise intensity, but the same small child demonstrates lower systolic and diastolic blood pressures than the adolescent. This may be due to the lower stroke volume and cardiac output or it may be due to a decreased peripheral resistance. Boys have higher peak systolic blood pressure than age-matched girls, and black children have higher arterial blood pressure than white children.[42]

When exercising at a maximal or submaximal level, the child has a higher respiration rate, and tidal volume generally is the same or lower when compared with the exercising adult (Table 41–3).[31] The ventilatory breaking point, or the point at about 60 percent Vo_2max when pulmonary ventilation accelerates, occurs earlier in children. Increasing blood lactate levels are thought to be the trigger for this increase, which is often concomitant with anaerobic threshold. This results in a relative tachypnea and shallower breathing in the child when compared with the exercising adolescent or adult. A decrease in ventilatory equivalent (increased efficiency) with age also supports this finding. No sex-related differences in ventilatory equivalent are noted.[29]

THERMOREGULATION AND EXERCISE

An area of concern with children and sports is their relative inability to dissipate heat during exercise. The

TABLE 41–3
Respiratory Function During Exercise in Children Compared with Adults

Function	Child's Response Compared with Adult's
Ventilation/kg body weight, maximal	Same
Ventilation/kg body weight, submaximal	Higher
Ventilatory "breaking point"	Earlier
Respiratory rate, submaximal and maximal	Higher
Tidal volume, vital capacity, maximal	Lower
Tidal volume, vital capacity, submaximal	Same or lower
Ventilatory equivalent, submaximal and maximal	Higher
Dead space, tidal volume	Same
Partial pressure of arterial Co_2	Somewhat lower

From Bar-Or O: Pediatric Sports Medicine for the Practitioner: From Physiologic Principles to Clinical Applications. New York, Springer-Verlag, 1983, p 31.

primary cooling mechanism in the exercising individual is evaporation, which is dependent upon body surface area. The child has a smaller absolute surface area than the adult, although relative to mass, surface area in the child is 36 percent greater than the adult's.[31] This allows a greater heat transfer to or from the body surface in the child. The child generates more metabolic heat per unit body size than the adult and has a lower cardiac output at a given metabolic rate. Additionally, lower sweating rates and initiation of sweating at a higher core temperature have been documented in the child.[43] This is true both absolutely and when normalized for body surface area. Sweat glands are fully developed in the child by 3 years of age; however, the adult's sweat glands excrete 2.5 times as much sweat as the child's at rest and during exercise.[31] This may help the child to conserve water but may also lead to increases in core temperature and forms the basis for the child's relative intolerance to exercise in the heat. However, children appear to tolerate exercise in neutral or moderately warm environments as well as adults.[44–46] Anaerobic performance (30 seconds duration) in children has not been found to be adversely affected by temperature. Children are capable of acclimating to warm environments although at a slower rate than adults.

The decreased sweating response may be related to the relatively low plasma pool found in prepubertal children.[29] Voluntary hypohydration may exacerbate the heat intolerance seen in this population. Plasma volume generally drops 10 to 15 percent in the early stages of exercise, and this fluid must be replaced.[31] Voluntary hypohydration has been documented in children who were exercising in the heat but were not forced to drink.[47] Voluntary fluid intake was 66 percent of the intake necessary to replenish fluid losses, and

TABLE 41–2
Central and Peripheral Hemodynamic Responses to Exercise in Children Compared with Adults

Function	Child's Response Compared with Adult's
Heart rate (submaximal)	Higher, especially first decade
Heart rate (maximal)	Higher
Stroke volume (submaximal and maximal)	Lower
Cardiac output (submaximal)	Somewhat lower
Arterio-mixed venous O_2 difference (submaximal)	Somewhat higher
Blood flow to active muscle	Higher
Systolic and diastolic blood pressure (submaximal and maximal)	Lower

From Bar-Or O: Pediatric Sports Medicine for the Practitioner: From Physiologic Principles to Clinical Applications. New York, Springer-Verlag, 1983, p 19.

urinary output decreased in response. Final values were fluid loss of 1 to 2 percent of initial body weight, and each 1 percent weight loss was correlated with a 0.28°C rise in core temperature. At equal levels of percentage weight loss, children demonstrated a greater rectal temperature rise than adults.[47]

ADAPTATIONS TO TRAINING

There is evidence that cardiac hypertrophy results from endurance training in children.[31] Increases are also noted in total hemoglobin (but not hemoglobin concentration), plasma volume, and blood volume with endurance training.[29] These chronic responses to aerobic training mirror responses seen in adults. Stroke volume increases with training in pubescent children, although no change is seen prior to puberty. The submaximal heart rate decreases, and submaximal cardiac output is unchanged or slightly decreased, whereas maximum cardiac output increases with training in this population.[29] However, there is no change in arteriovenous oxygen difference, suggesting no change in extraction. No changes are noted in systolic or diastolic blood pressure or in total peripheral resistance.[48]

Pulmonary adaptations to training in children include increases in tidal volume, respiratory rate, and ventilation during maximal exercise. Decreases are seen in submaximal minute ventilation and respiratory rate, whereas no change is seen in vital capacity.[27]

It is currently unclear whether the aerobic system in the child will adapt with training. It is difficult to distinguish the effects of growth and maturation from those of training in the child. At the core of this question is the validity of testing the aerobic power in children in the same way it is tested in adults. Most activities are performed at a submaximal level, and training may result in changes at the submaximal level that are not evident with maximal testing.[41] Some studies have found maximal aerobic capacity to improve with training in preadolescent children and have concluded that children respond to training the same way as adults. Others have found the improvements to be in line with normal growth and developmental changes.[41] In a slightly older population, children ages 10 to 15 years and girls ages 8 to 13 years were found to increase their oxygen consumption by 2 to 16 percent and 18 to 26 percent, respectively, with endurance training.[39,49] As with adults, most of the changes occurred in the first 6 weeks of training.

Training seems to have less of an effect on children under the age of 10 years. However, improvements in performance with training are noted with children. Bar-Or suggests that these improvements may be due to (1) increased mechanical efficiency, (2) improved anaerobic capacity, (3) poor sensitivity in measurement tools, or (4) training effects of free play confusing results.[31]

Increases in muscle strength do occur in children following a training stimulus. A study of boys and girls ages 10 to 11 years participating in a 3-week resistive training program showed strength increases of greater than 40 percent.[50] Blimkie and colleagues studied strength training in prepubescent boys and also found strength increases that were independent of changes in muscle size. The authors speculated that strength increases were due to neurologic changes not measured in the study.[51]

MUSCULOSKELETAL PROBLEMS

Children are susceptible to the same acute and overuse injuries as adults. Children who overtrain are just as likely to develop an overuse syndrome as adults. In addition, there are several musculoskeletal problems specific to the child or adolescent. These problems are not necessarily *caused* by sports participation but may first be detected by the sports professional treating young athletes. It is imperative to recognize a growth-related injury early to assure prompt and appropriate medical intervention.

OSTEOCHONDROSES

Injuries involving avascular necrosis and its sequelae are considered osteochondroses. There is a great deal of confusion surrounding the terminology in this body of literature. Osteochondrosis, osteochondritis, osteochondritis dissecans, Panner disease, little leaguer elbow, and similar terms are often used interchangeably. In general, osteochondrosis is a disease of the growth center (see following) in children characterized as a degeneration or necrosis followed by regeneration or recalcification, whereas osteochondritis is an inflammation of both bone and cartilage.[52] Osteochondritis dissecans is a type of osteochondrosis that results in pieces of articular cartilage breaking off into the joint.[52] These processes at various joints have acquired specific names, usually labeled by the person first describing the entity in the literature.

Osteochondroses usually involve the epiphyseal center at the end of a long bone entirely covered by articular cartilage. The pressure epiphysis has a precarious blood supply, which puts it at greater risk than the epiphyseal center of a small bone. Osteochondroses are more common in children aged 3 to 10 years, affect boys more often than girls, and affect lower extremities more often than upper extremities.[34] The most commonly affected areas are the lateral aspect of the medial femoral condyle, the femoral head, the talus, and the capitellum.[19]

The etiology of osteochondroses is currently unknown, although theories have been proposed. Some suggest a genetic factor in the vascular configuration of the epiphysis.[19] This causes an infarction resulting from an embolism of small blood vessels in the area. Others have supported a trauma theory, particularly in light of the increased incidence noted in the lower extremities and in boys.[34,53] Finally, some believe that the fragment represents a separate ossification center that has become detached.[19,34,53]

Pathologic changes seen throughout the course of the disorder correlate well with the radiographic changes seen. Salter has outlined four phases of the pathologic process that may range in duration from 2 to 8 years.[34] The first phase is the early phase of necrosis, in which the osteocytes and bone marrow cells in the epiphysis die from avascularity but no change is noted in the bone. This phase may last a year or longer while the articular cartilage continues to grow, and the child usually remains asymptomatic. The second phase is the phase of revascularization with bone deposition and resorption, in which the surrounding tissues respond to the dead bone. The body attempts to revascularize the dead epiphysis, resulting in radiographic changes, including ossification of the cartilage around the rim of the epiphysis. Continued bone deposition and resorption results in fragmentation of the epiphysis. This phase can last from 1 to 4 years. The third phase is that of bone healing, when bone resorption ceases and the fibrous and granulation tissue is replaced by bone. This bone is still plastic and can respond to loading according to the Wolff law. The final phase is that of residual deformity. When bony healing is complete and remodeling has ceased, the remaining deformity will persist.[34]

The basic principles of treatment focus on preventing the debilitating deformity that remains after remodeling. Generally, the patient does not present until the second phase, at which time the process cannot be reversed.[34] The condition is self-limiting, and the patient's primary need is guidance regarding weight-bearing and activity modifications. The goal is to prevent any secondary morbidity as the patient progresses through the phases and to prevent significant residual deformity as the bone remodels. Participation in sports and recreational activities depends on the site and extent of osteochondrosis. Those with significant involvement of large portions of a weight-bearing surface need to be treated more conservatively than those with small areas of involvement on non–weight-bearing surfaces. Maintenance of normal articular surface and joint congruity is essential in the prevention of degenerative joint disease as the young athlete ages.

LEGG-CALVÉ-PERTHES DISEASE

Legg-Calvé-Perthes disease is an idiopathic avascular necrosis of the femoral head occurring in children between the ages of 3 and 12 years. Boys are seen much more frequently with this problem (80 percent) than girls, and unilateral involvement (85 percent) is much more common than bilateral.[55] There is approximately an 8 to 12 percent familial predisposition.[56] Children presenting with Legg-Calvé-Perthes disease are more likely to live in an urban area, to have delayed bone age, and to be 1 inch (boys) to 3 inches (girls) shorter than their peers, suggesting some correlation with a constitutional delay in growth.[56,57]

As implied by the term *idiopathic*, the cause of Legg-Calvé-Perthes disease is not well understood. A vascular cause has been suggested, with damage to the blood vessels from trauma or disease causing an avascular necrosis of the femoral head. Excessive fluid pressure from a synovial effusion in the hip joint has also been suggested to explain disruption of the femoral head blood supply, but only approximately 1 percent of cases have a history of transient synovitis.[56] Epidemiologic studies support a systemic disorder involving the epiphyseal cartilage, with manifestation at the femoral head. Histologic studies demonstrate a thickening and disorganization of the epiphyseal plate and cartilage that could prevent penetration of vessels into the growth plate, resulting in avascular necrosis.[56]

The pathology of Legg-Calvé-Perthes disease is a progressive necrosis of the bone and marrow of the epiphysis of the femoral head, involving either the entire epiphysis or only part of it. If the epiphyseal plate becomes involved, growth disturbances will occur, likely resulting in a short, broad femoral neck. A study of 80 patients found that 90 percent had interference with physeal growth, 25 percent demonstrating premature physeal closing.[57] During the revascularization phase, the child is at risk for subluxation from abnormal forces, flattening of the femoral head as a result of head collapse, or both. Over the course of 2 to 3 years, new bone will gradually form, replacing the necrotic bone. Late degenerative joint disease can result from residual deformity and incongruity of the joint surfaces. Several classification systems exist, classifying either chronologically or by the extent of the disease. In addition to the classification system discussed previously, another system categorizes the process into four stages: initial, fragmentation, reossification, and healed.[57]

Clinically, the child with Legg-Calvé-Perthes rarely presents in the first phase, which is often termed the "quiet" phase owing to a lack of symptoms. Approximately 17 percent provide a history of trauma.[57] Presentation is generally in one of the later phases, owing to hip or referred knee pain. Pain may also be referred to the inner thigh, and the child may present with a limp. Pain is generally activity-related, which often contributes to delayed presentation and recognition. In the later stages, there is likely a motion loss, particularly in hip abduction and internal rotation. Radiographs confirm the diagnosis, with changes in bone density, bone resorption, and fragmentation noted (Fig. 41–7). Differential diagnosis includes rheumatoid arthritis, slipped capital femoral epiphysis, congenital dysplasia of the hip, and congenital coxa vara.[55]

Treatment depends on the radiographic classification of the disease and the philosophy of the treating physician. Nonoperative treatment has been divided into several categories, including therapy to improve hip range of motion, non–weight bearing in a brace, weight bearing in a brace that limits hip movement, and weight bearing in a brace that permits free movement.[56] Some children with less than half of the femoral head involved and no evidence of subluxation may require observation only. For those requiring treatment, the key principle is containment of the femoral head (to prevent subluxation and motion) and protected weight bearing.[34] This philosophy attempts to equalize pressure on the femoral head to assist with remodeling by containing it within the acetabulum. An abduction brace can

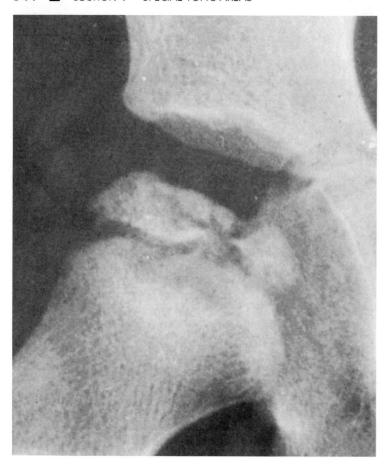

FIGURE 41–7. Legg-Perthes disease in the late phase of revascularization, with bone deposition and bone resorption going on simultaneously in different areas of the head. (From Salter RB: Textbook of Disorders and Injuries of the Musculoskeletal System, 2nd ed. Baltimore, Williams & Wilkins, 1983.)

prevent subluxation and help maintain the normal contour of the femoral head.

The prognosis varies with age and severity of the disease. Long-term follow-up studies show that 70 to 90 percent of patients with Legg-Calvé-Perthes disease will be active and pain-free 20 to 40 years later. However, at 48-year follow-up, 50 percent had disabling arthritis and pain.[57] In general, children under 5 years do well, whereas the prognosis for children from ages 5 to 7 years is fair, and children over the age of 7 years have a poor prognosis.[34] The age of 8 years appears to be a watershed, older children having a much poorer prognosis.[57] The prognosis is formed during the revascularization and early bone healing stages. Those demonstrating involvement of the entire head, subluxation, or significant deformity are more likely to develop secondary degenerative changes.

When making decisions about sports participation for the child or the adult with a history of Legg-Calvé-Perthes disease, the extent of damage to the hip and the prognosis will determine appropriate activities. Any instability, deformity, or significant degenerative joint disease precludes involvement in sports or exercises requiring extensive running, cutting, or jumping. If the joint is unstable, it may be necessary to limit the range of motion during exercises. Pool exercise may be an ideal medium for this population, owing to the minimized weight bearing. No contact sports should be allowed until the subchondral bone of the epiphysis is formed.

OSTEOCHONDRITIS DISSECANS

The convex surface of some joints may be susceptible to avascular necrosis of a small portion of subchondral bone, which can eventually become detached. This condition is most commonly found in the knee but can also affect the capitellum, patella, femoral head, and talus. Osteochondritis dissecans, a type of osteochondrosis, is the most common cause of loose bodies in the young child. Boys are affected nearly twice as often as girls, with the majority of patients ranging between ages 10 and 20 years. The most common site at the knee is the medial femoral condyle (Fig. 41–8).[58]

The etiology of osteochondritis dissecans is unknown, some theorizing trauma and vascular insufficiency, which leads to bone infarction. Again, there is some familial predisposition for this problem. However, Cahill states that the etiology is likely multifactorial, including some predisposing condition and unrecognized trauma or an accessory ossification center and torsional impaction.[59] Cyclical loading of the bone produces a type of subchondral stress fracture.

The pathology of osteochondritis dissecans includes an area of avascular necrosis on the epiphysis generally no larger than 2 cm and often smaller.[34] The osteocytes in the area die, although the overlying articular cartilage remains intact. A space is created between the living and dead bone by the ingrowth of fibrous tissue, separating the necrotic area. As with all osteochondroses, a process of deposition and resorption occurs, resulting in plasticity of the area. As this occurs, the normally convex surface may flatten. Eventually, healing takes place unless the fragment is displaced by trauma or other cause.

The extent of clinical signs and symptoms is related to stability of the fragment. If the fragment is maintained in position by the overlying articular cartilage, symptoms may be very mild. Symptoms are generally those of pain, giving way, swelling, catching, and, occasionally, locking. True locking is a symptom of a loose body and may indicate displacement of the osteochondral fragment. Diagnosis is confirmed by radiographs or magnetic resonance imaging.

The treatment depends on the size of the lesion, location (weight bearing surface), and stability. If the lesion is still intact, with healthy overlying cartilage, the goal is to prevent detachment of the fragment. Above all, it is important to maintain the integrity of the articular surface. If there is a large lesion on a weight-bearing surface, surgery may be indicated to fixate the fragment. Detached or partially detached fragments with interruption of the overlying articular cartilage should be removed, unless they are very large, in which case they should be fixated.[34] Cahill has outlined four surgical precepts in the case of osteochondritis dissecans: (1) when possible, restore the joint surface, (2) enhance the blood supply of the fragment, (3) use rigid fixation in the case of instability, and (4) begin joint motion as soon as possible postoperatively.[59]

As with treatment, prognosis varies depending upon the size, location, and stability of the fragment. Clearly, a fragment that heals in place has a very good prognosis. A large fragment on a weight-bearing surface generally has a poor prognosis, likely progressing to early degenerative joint disease. Cahill notes that if juvenile osteochondritis dissecans does not heal by

bony union prior to closure of the distal femoral epiphyseal plate, then adult osteochondritis dissecans will result. This has a much poorer prognosis than the juvenile form.[59] These same factors influence decisions about sports participation. Participation in running, jumping, and cutting sports is certainly acceptable after a thorough rehabilitation program. Those at risk for early degenerative joint disease may benefit by limiting their participation in vigorous weight-bearing sports.

PANNER DISEASE

Osteochondrosis of the capitellum was first described by Panner in 1929.[60] True osteochondrosis occurs in children between the ages of 3 and 11, and like Legg-Calvé-Perthes disease, goes on to bone healing. The whole capitellum is involved, and the bone goes through the phases characteristic of other osteochondroses. The prognosis is good, and deformity is unlikely.

Osteochondritis dissecans of the capitellum is often considered to be a separate entity from osteochondrosis but may actually represent different stages of the same disease. If an osteochondral fragment becomes detached and loose within the joint, it is considered to be osteochondritis dissecans. Although the term *osteochondritis* is used, there is often no evidence of inflammation. The prognosis is dependent on the age of the patient, type and level of activities, and the severity of the original lesion.[61] Those participating in highly competitive throwing sports, throwing more advanced pitches, or having a greater volume of activity may present a treatment challenge. As with other osteochondral lesions, the etiology is suspected to be traumatic or vascular. The throwing athlete appears to be particularly susceptible, owing to the compressive forces on the lateral elbow, which reinforces a trauma theory. Singer and Roy note that despite the number of theories regarding etiology, some type of disordered endochondral ossification occurs and is associated with trauma or vascular impairment.[61]

As stated previously, the cause of osteochondrosis is unknown, with theories of vascular insufficiency or trauma. Local avascular necrosis of the capitellum leads to loss of subchondral bone, articular depression, loss of normal joint congruency and deformity of the capitellum. Fragments may become displaced, resulting in loose bodies at the radiohumeral joint. Once the pathology has progressed to include the lateral elbow, the prognosis for return to throwing, particularly at a competitive level, is guarded. For this reason, education of parents, children, and coaches to facilitate early detection and intervention is critical. The adults charged with the adolescent's care should be capable of recognizing the early signs and symptoms of Panner disease and of referring the youth to the appropriate medical professional.

Three stages of the disease have been described, group I involving children up to age 13 years.[62] This group likely represents Panner's original classification. The lesion rarely displaces, and the epiphysis progresses through the stages outlined previously.

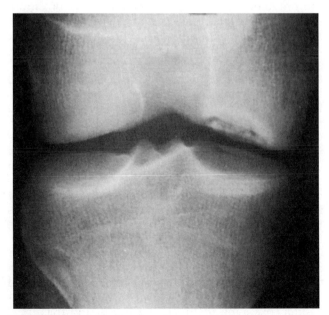

FIGURE 41–8. Osteochondritis dissecans of the medial femoral condyle. (From Insall JN: (ed) Surgery of the Knee. New York, Churchill Livingstone, 1984.)

Because the elbow is not a weight-bearing joint, symptoms may be minimal, and the child may never present for evaluation. Those presenting are likely to complain of pain and motion loss, and rarely their disease progresses to surgery.

Group II patients range from 13 years to adulthood and have a history of chronic repetitive stresses to the elbow. Onset of symptoms may be insidious. They may demonstrate a loss of motion at the elbow in addition to localized pain. Treatment includes activity modification and possibly surgery to stabilize a loose fragment or to remove loose bodies.[62]

Group III patients generally present in the second decade of life with complaints of pain, loss of motion, catching, locking, and swelling. Symptoms may have been intermittent for several years but have worsened recently, possibly owing to detachment of one or more fragments. Treatment is frequently surgical to fixate loose fragments and remove loose bodies. The prognosis is poor in this group.

Diagnosis of Panner disease is generally confirmed by radiographs demonstrating cystic changes in the capitellum and blunting of the capitellum with enlargement of the radial head.[62] Pappas notes that variations in the size and density of the ossific nucleus with apparent fragmentation is associated with osteochondrosis. This may represent an alteration of the normal vascular development and ossification pattern.[63] If the epiphyseal plate is involved, growth alterations can occur.

Participation in sports and recreational activities are generally self-limited in the adolescent. Treatment and participation in sports and activities by the adolescent vary, depending upon the extent of involvement, the phase of presentation, and whether or not surgery has been performed. Generally, the athlete may return to sports after full mobility, strength, and function have returned to the arm.

SLIPPED CAPITAL FEMORAL EPIPHYSIS (ADOLESCENT COXA VARA)

A slipped capital femoral epiphysis is seen most often in adolescents from ages 10 to 16 years and occurs most commonly in boys. Its prevalence is approximately 0.71 to 3.41 per 100,000 children.[64] The condition is bilateral in approximately 25 to 30 percent of cases. A recent study of 224 children diagnosed with slipped capital femoral epiphysis found a 37 percent occurrence of bilaterality. The mean age at diagnosis was 13 ± 1.7 years with the duration of symptoms 5 ± 5.0 months.[65,66] Those who had a sequential bilateral slip were younger at initial presentation than those who did not develop a subsequent second slip. The common somatotype presenting with a slipped capital femoral epiphysis is an overweight adolescent with underdeveloped sexual characteristics and, occasionally, the tall, thin child.

The etiology of femoral epiphysis slipping is currently unknown, but some theories exist. Some speculate that slippage is the result of a period of rapid growth in combination with the obliquity of this epiphyseal plate and minor traumas. Although slippage can occur during physical activity, no causal relationship has been found between sports and slipped capital femoral epiphysis. The specific body type associated with this condition has resulted in speculation about an underlying endocrine disorder contributing to the slippage. Although this has yet to be proved, one study of adolescents with slipped capital femoral epiphysis showed 25 percent to have decreased active thyroid levels, 76 percent to have decreased testosterone levels, and 87 percent to have decreased growth hormone levels.[67] An imbalance between growth hormone and sex hormones may result in weakening of the epiphyseal plate.[34]

In a slipped capital femoral epiphysis, the femoral head slips at the epiphyseal plate and displaces inferiorly and posteriorly relative to the neck (Fig. 41-9). The periosteal attachment remains intact posteriorly with secondary remodeling of the femoral neck resulting in a progressive coxa vara deformity. A subsequent acute injury or failure to recognize the early stages of slipping may result in further slip and complete separation of the epiphysis from the neck. This may disrupt the precarious blood supply to the femoral head, resulting in avascular necrosis. The condition is divided into three grades of severity: mild, less than 30 degrees of slippage of the epiphysis on the metaphysis; moderate, 30 to 60 degrees; and severe, greater than 60 degrees of slippage.[68] Traditionally, slipped capital femoral epiphysis has been categorized as acute, chronic, and acute-on-chronic. There is a suggestion that this system is cumbersome and may be misleading and that slips should simply be classified as stable or unstable.[66]

The early clinical signs and symptoms may go undetected owing to mild symptoms at the hip and referred pain to the ipsilateral knee. Fleisher found that 29 percent of slipped capital femoral epiphysis diagnoses were missed on the first evaluation.[69] Frequently, the only complaint on presentation is that of diffuse knee pain. The knee examination will be unremarkable; however, if the sports medicine professional assesses one joint proximal and one joint distal to the knee, subtle signs leading to the diagnosis of slipped capital femoral epiphysis may be detected. There is often no history of trauma and if present, it is often mild. Limping may be noted, and a progressive external rotation of the hip may result in a waddling type gait. Clinical suspicion should be high in the young athlete with the aforementioned body type, history of mild trauma, unremarkable knee examination, and mild hip symptoms, including loss of motion and palpable tenderness. Loss of motion is usually in the directions of internal rotation and abduction, and as the hip is passively flexed, it will roll into external rotation. The hallmark clinical sign is a loss of hip internal rotation. Diagnosis is confirmed by radiographs and is best seen in the lateral "frog position" projection with the hip in flexion, abduction, and external rotation. Differential diagnosis includes Legg-Calvé-Perthes disease, congenital coxa vara, rheumatoid arthritis, and fracture.[55]

The primary treating principle is the protection of the blood supply to the femoral head. In the early stages,

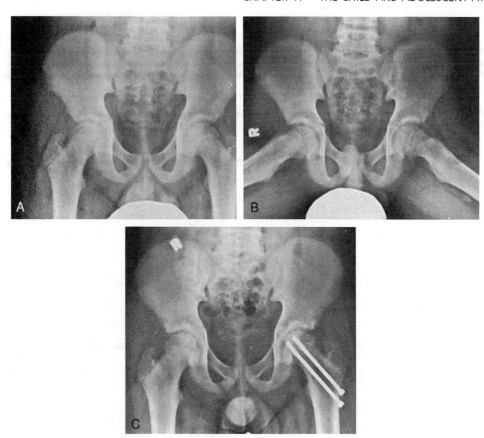

FIGURE 41–9. Radiographs of a 13-year-old 200-pound basketball player who developed left anterior thigh pain. *A* and *B*, Anteroposterior roentgenogram is essentially normal, but the frog-leg lateral view demonstrates an early slipped capital femoral epiphysis. *C,* An in situ pinning was performed. (From Nicholas JA, Hershman EG (eds): The Lower Extremity and Spine in Sports Medicine. St. Louis, CV Mosby, 1986.)

this means avoiding further slippage and maintaining the reduced position until the epiphyseal plate has closed. The child presenting with the signs and symptoms of a slipped capital femoral epiphysis should be placed non–weight bearing on crutches and should be directed to a physician immediately. If the slip is minimal (< 1 cm), it should be surgically stabilized to prevent any further slippage. A complete slip should be reduced and then surgically stabilized. Follow-up care must continue until the physes have closed because of a 30 percent chance that the opposite side will slip. Treatment by hip spica casting has proved unfavorable, with a high incidence of avascular necrosis and chondrolysis.[70,71] A single screw appears to reduce the chances of these complications when compared with single or multiple pinning or spica casting.[72,73]

The prognosis following a slipped capital femoral epiphysis depends on the degree of slippage and the status of the blood supply to the femoral head. Cases detected early with minimal slipping have a good prognosis, whereas those with more severe slips are likely to have residual deformity and progressive disability. Duration of symptoms in mild slips has been shown to be approximately 13 weeks; moderate slips, 24 weeks; and severe slips, 40 weeks. There is evidence that these hips will develop radiographic evidence of degenerative joint disease at intermediate-range follow-up.[64] This factor, along with the amount of deformity, determines the quantities and types of sports that are safe for the adolescent with a slipped capital femoral epiphysis. Impact and cutting sports, which place a great demand on the hip, may need to be limited for the long-term health of the hip.

OSGOOD-SCHLATTER DISEASE

Osgood-Schlatter disease was first described by Osgood and Schlatter in 1903 and is considered an apophysitis of the tibial tubercle.[74] Athletes generally present with symptoms between the ages of 8 and 13 years in girls and 10 and 15 years in boys, at the beginning of their growth spurt. The symptoms are frequently bilateral.

Although Osgood-Schlatter disease is considered by many to be an apophysitis, there is some question as to whether or not an inflammatory process is involved. Maffulli describes an apophysitis as a chronic inflammation and avulsion of cartilage and bone from the developing ossification center, whereas Singer and Henry state that there is no inflammatory process present.[19,75] The physis beneath the tibial tuberosity is composed of fibrocartilage and has a different histologic appearance from other physes.[75] Ossification of this apophysis occurs by membranous ossification from a cartilaginous tongue-shaped downward continuation of the upper tibial epiphysis.[34] The essential lesion appears to be an avulsion of small portions of the tibial tuberosity's ossification center with callus formation causing an elevation of the anterior portion of the tibial tuberosity.[54] The adaptive change in the tibial tubercle shows a direct correlation between the amount of fibrous tissue and the level of traction exerted on the tibial tubercle.[35]

The athlete presenting with Osgood-Schlatter disease complains of pain in the anterior aspect of his or her knee in the region of the tibial tubercle. An enlargement of the tibial tubercle commonly accompanies symptoms and is often exquisitely tender. There is rarely an acute injury but rather a history of repetitive running, jumping, or both that precipitates symptoms. Occasionally, a fall or a blow directly on the tibial tubercle can initiate symptoms. Pain with resisted quadriceps contraction and passive quadriceps stretching may exacerbate symptoms. Radiographs may demonstrate soft tissue swelling in the area of the patellar tendon insertion with or without fragmentation of the tibial tuberosity. In some cases, irregular, multiple areas of ossification may be seen, and in some, ossification may be completely absent.[54] Ossification within the patellar tendon itself is not consistent with Osgood-Schlatter disease but represents a different pathologic process. A study of Osgood-Schlatter disease in 82 patients with high-resolution ultrasonography found four different ultrasonographic results, all with the same clinical diagnosis. These results included (1) a normal ossification center with swelling noted in the cartilage and subcutaneous tissues displaced forward, (2) additional fragmentation of the nucleus, (3) primary patellar tendinitis with or without ossification center involvement, and (4) infrapatellar bursitis with or without ossification center involvement.[76] Because radiographic findings are often inconsistent, Osgood-Schlatter disease is often a clinical diagnosis.[11]

Treatment for this condition in the past was quite drastic. Immobilization in long leg casts or splints was not uncommon. Currently, treatment of the mild forms of Osgood-Schlatter disease is symptomatic. Guidance should be provided to the young athlete and his or her parents and coaches to help determine an appropriate type and level of activity at various stages of symptoms. When the athlete is experiencing anterior knee pain with activity and the tibial tuberosity is palpably tender, activities involving running and jumping should be limited. When the athlete is asymptomatic, activity is unrestricted. Rehabilitative exercises should be incorporated to promote appropriate strength and flexibility in the surrounding musculature, including quadriceps, hamstrings, iliotibial band, and gastrocnemius. The time frame until complete resolution of symptoms may be as long as 12 to 18 months or until the apophysis is fully ossified. Avulsion fracture of the tibial apophysis is a rare phenomenon and requires urgent surgical fixation.

Some athletes may experience Osgood-Schlatter type symptoms into adulthood. This is usually the result of ossicles in the patellar tendon or failure of the proximal

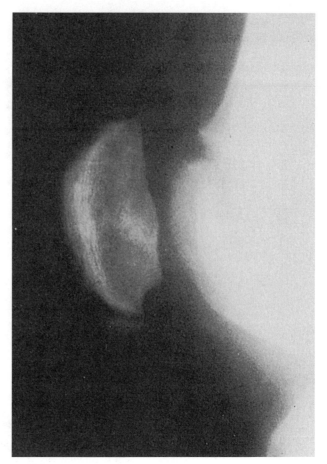

FIGURE 41–10. Sinding-Larsen-Johansson syndrome in a young patient. (From Singer KM, Henry J: Knee problems in children and adolescents. Clin Sports Med 1985; 4(2):388.)

fragment to unite. Those individuals failing to improve with appropriate conservative measures may undergo surgical fixation or removal of ossicles.[54]

Athletes with Osgood-Schlatter disease can usually continue to participate in sports and activities. Participation in running and jumping sports is often self-limited when symptoms are increased. Return to full activity is usually within a few days to a few weeks of an exacerbation of symptoms. Maintenance of good flexibility in the quadriceps, hamstrings, and iliotibial band may prevent or decrease the severity of exacerbations.

SINDING-LARSEN-JOHANSSON SYNDROME

Sinding-Larsen-Johansson syndrome is an apophysitis of the distal pole of the patella and usually occurs in children ages 8 to 13 years. Like other apophysitides, the onset is frequently gradual and is often seen in children involved in running and jumping sports. The primary complaint is that of anterior knee pain localized to the distal pole of the patella. There may be a prominence at the distal pole and irregularity and fragmentation seen in this area on radiographs (Fig. 41–10).[75] Micheli and Fehlandt found four cases in their study of apophysis injuries, all of which resolved with conservative management, including strengthening and flexibility of the lower extremity musculature.[18]

Treatment of Sinding-Larsen-Johansson syndrome is symptomatic, with activity modifications when the knee is sore along with appropriate stretching and other rehabilitative measures to decrease pain and inflammation. Symptoms generally resolve quickly, and no indications of an increased susceptibility for the development of patellar tendinitis have been reported.[75] Rarely, athletes continue to present with symptoms and may require surgical excision of fragments. Return to full sports activity after thorough rehabilitation (mobility, strength, flexibility, function) is reasonable with or without surgery. Differential diagnoses include patellar tendinitis, infrapatellar bursitis, Osgood-Schlatter disease, patellofemoral pain, fat pad impingement, and patellar instability.

DISCOID MENISCUS

Overall, meniscal problems in children and adolescents are uncommon. However, a congenital discoid meniscus can be a cause of lateral knee pain and meniscal symptoms in this population. One study found a discoid meniscus to be present in 7 percent of their cases, and it was bilateral in 4.5 percent.[77] A discoid meniscus is the result of a developmental anomaly in which the meniscus remains disc-shaped rather than developing into the normal semilunar shape. This is rarely found in the medial meniscus, and a familial pattern has been noted. The discoid meniscus is generally thicker than normal and lacks the normal posterior attachments.[34] Some speculate that the abnormal attachments of the ligaments of Wrisberg and Humphry are responsible for the resulting shape of the discoid meniscus.[53]

The child with a discoid meniscus presents with symptoms of clicking or clunking. This is the result of the lateral femoral condyle riding over the posterior margin of the meniscus, causing a clicking or a visible shift at the tibiofemoral joint. The lack of mobility of the discoid meniscus and its constant trauma by the lateral femoral condyle makes it susceptible to tearing.

Diagnosis of a discoid lateral meniscus is made by subjective history and clinical examination consistent with a meniscal injury. There may or may not be a history of acute trauma. Aching pain, lateral joint line pain, or both are likely to be present, and the catching or locking may be reproducible with clinical examination procedures. Suspicion of a discoid meniscus may be supported by routine radiographs demonstrating a widening of the lateral joint space owing to the increased thickness of the lateral meniscus.[53] A lateral cyst may also be present, and the clinical diagnosis can be confirmed by magnetic resonance imaging, arthrography, or arthroscopy.

Treatment is generally surgical and varies with the area of damage and the specific anomaly found. The overall goal is to normalize the meniscus, converting it from a flat disc shape to an O shape.

TARSAL COALITION

A tarsal coalition is a congenital union between two or more tarsal bones. The fusion may be complete or incomplete and usually involves the talus, calcaneus,

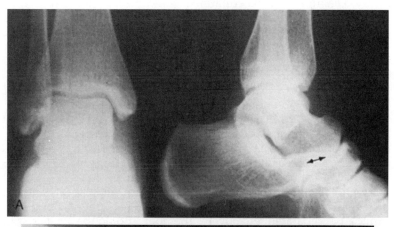

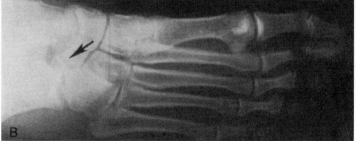

FIGURE 41–11. Tarsal coalition in a patient diagnosed with chronic lateral ankle sprains. *A,* Anteroposterior and lateral views of the ankle are normal. A calcaneonavicular bar was suspected from the lateral view of the foot. *B,* Oblique view of the foot clearly demonstrates a calcaneonavicular bar. (From Nicholas JA, Hershman EG (eds): The Lower Extremity and Spine in Sports Medicine. St. Louis, CV Mosby, 1986.)

navicular, cuboid, or cuneiforms. The fusion between two or more bones begins as cartilaginous bars that may calcify to become osseous or may remain fibrous or cartilaginous. Calcification generally occurs during adolescence, at which time symptoms may appear. Coalitions are most commonly found at the calcaneonavicular, followed by those at the talocalcaneal site. The etiology of tarsal coalition is unknown, although there appears to be a strong hereditary component.[78] Many cases go undiagnosed until noted following an ankle sprain (Fig. 41–11).[79]

The presence of a tarsal coalition restricts motion in the tarsal bones, leading to a progressive decrease in subtalar motion. Fusion can occur at the anterior, middle, or posterior facets, and limited calcaneal mobility may be difficult to detect, owing to midtarsal movement.[78] The foot assumes a flatfooted position owing to the forcing of the calcaneus into a position of valgus to compensate for the decreased mobility of the subtalar joint. In contrast to the flatfooted appearance usually associated with hypermobility, the foot with tarsal coalition is actually rigid. This problem has been termed *rigid valgus foot* and *peroneal spastic flatfoot* as a result of associated peroneal spasm and contracture.[34,79]

Tarsal coalition frequently goes undetected until adolescence, when the cartilaginous bars begin to ossify. The athlete generally presents with a chief complaint of pain and peroneal spasm. An injury may cause a previously asymptomatic coalition to become symptomatic. Diagnosis of a tarsal coalition is suspected in the case of an adolescent athlete with a flat foot but decreased talocalcaneonavicular mobility. This decreased mobility can increase stress at the ankle joint, and coalition should be suspected in cases of peroneal spasm that lingers longer than usual following an ankle injury. Diagnosis can be confirmed with anteroposterior, lateral, oblique, and posterior subtalar (Harris) view radiographs, tomograms, or computed tomography.[79] A coalition may be missed on routine radiographs following an ankle sprain.

Treatment options include resecting the bar or performing a triple arthrodesis, depending upon the presence or absence of secondary degenerative changes. Triple arthrodesis involves both the subtalar and midtarsal joints. If the coalition is discovered before degenerative changes occur, surgical excision of the coalition has good results. Surgery attempts to restore normal talocalcaneonavicular mobility and to prevent attritional changes. If secondary degenerative disease has occurred and the bones cannot be separated effectively, the foot should be realigned and fused with the heel in slight valgus and the forefoot plantigrade.[78] This surgery should be performed only after skeletal maturity has been attained.

Athletes may return to participation in sports and recreational activities following surgery and an appropriate rehabilitation program to restore motion, strength, and function in the ankle. Pain may limit participation in impact activities in a joint that has developed secondary degenerative changes.

SEVER DISEASE

Sever disease at the calcaneus is similar to Osgood-Schlatter disease at the tibia. The calcaneus provides attachments for the Achilles tendon, plantar fascia, and the intrinsic muscles of the foot. It is the most common cause of heel pain in the child and adolescent athlete and specifically affects the Achilles tendon insertion into the posterior calcaneus. Sever disease is most often seen in boys between the ages of 8 and 15 years. Like Osgood-Schlatter disease, the etiology of Sever disease is unknown. It likely represents a similar traction injury or even partial avulsion of the calcaneal apophysis. Micheli and Fehlandt treated 64 cases in boys and 28 cases in girls with stretching, strengthening, and anti-inflammatory drugs with good results.[18] Tight heel cords were noted in all cases, and other foot malalignments were noted in many.

The athlete with Sever disease presents complaining of localized pain over the attachment of the Achilles tendon, but localized swelling is rare. An early heel rise on initial swing of gait in an attempt to decrease the pull of the Achilles may be noticeable. Enlargement of the attachment site is indicative of the repetitive stress at the ossification center. The os calcis apophysis ossifies from multiple centers and normally appears dense in lateral radiographs in both symptomatic and asymptomatic individuals, making radiographic diagnosis difficult.[34] For this reason, diagnosis is generally made by physical examination.

This condition is typically self-limiting and resolves within a year. A heel lift may decrease symptoms by effectively shortening the Achilles tendon. Athletes with significant foot malalignment may benefit from other orthotic treatment. Additionally, treatment should include frequent gentle stretching to prevent shortening of the musculotendinous complex. Participation in sports is limited only by pain. When symptoms are increased, activities producing symptoms should be minimized.

MISCELLANEOUS APOPHYSEAL PROBLEMS

Although the most common sites for apophyseal problems in children and adolescents are the calcaneus and tibial tuberosities, the young athlete can develop problems at many tendinous attachments. Other sites include the ischial tuberosity at the attachment of the hamstring muscles, the anterior inferior iliac spine at the origin of the rectus femoris, and the anterior superior iliac spine at the attachment of the sartorius. Avulsions at the ischial tuberosity and anterior superior iliac spine with forceful kicking have been reported.

Apophysitis of the iliac crest at the attachment of the abdominal oblique muscles has been seen in adolescents, most commonly in distance runners. Micheli and Fehlandt reported 22 cases in girls and 10 cases in boys in their large retrospective study.[18] This problem was most commonly seen in runners; and in girls, it was next most common in dancers. They reported tightness in the hip musculature, including positive Ober, Thomas, and Ely testing. The hallmark finding was palpable tenderness along the anterior third of the iliac crest.

LITTLE LEAGUER ELBOW

Little Leaguer elbow was first described by Brogdon and Crow in 1960 in reference to an avulsion of the ossification center of the medial epicondyle of the humerus in adolescents as a result of the repetitive stresses of throwing.[80] Since that time, the term has come to include a number of conditions ranging from the initially described lesion to flexor muscle tendinitis, osteochondral fractures of the capitellum, and loose bodies and degenerative joint changes in the lateral compartment. Because of its ambiguity, the term *Little Leaguer elbow* should be abandoned in favor of a more specific diagnosis describing the particular pathology found. The elbow is a most common site of complaints among young throwers, especially baseball pitchers.[81] Although the problem is most frequently associated with baseball, the same set of problems can be found in other throwing sports, including water polo, javelin tossing, and tennis. Studies of the incidence of elbow pain in Little League players find approximately 20 percent of athletes reporting elbow pain, although few missed any days of participation. Pathology in the elbow appears to be rare, with reported prevalence of degenerative disease in the lateral compartment of about 1 in 10,000.[82] However, radiographic changes, including evidence of accelerated growth, separation, and fragmentation at the medial epicondylar epiphysis have been found in 95 percent of 80 pitchers aged 9 to 14 years.[83] These same changes were present in only 15 percent of 47 nonpitching little league players and in 8 percent of age-matched active children.[83]

The growth plate and associated soft tissue structures such as ligaments and tendinous attachments are at risk for injury until fusion is complete. The ossification center of the capitellum fuses at approximately age 14.5 years in boys and 13 years in girls, whereas the ossification center of the radial head fuses at roughly 16 years in boys and 14 years in girls. Fusion of the ossification center in the medial humeral epicondyle is not complete until approximately age 17 years in boys and 14 years in girls.[63] Elbow pain in a young thrower likely represents a continuum of problems ranging from tendinitis to osteochondritis dissecans of the capitellum. The throwing motion places a great deal of valgus stress on the medial elbow, particularly during the cocking phase. A significant distraction force on the medial side is countered by a compressive force on the lateral side and a translatory force across the olecranon. These forces are reduced during the acceleration phase, but forces associated with elbow extension and forearm pronation during release and deceleration combine to produce compression and shearing of the radial head on the capitellum. The forces across the elbow vary, depending on the type of pitch thrown, and are significant when throwing a fastball, sidearm, or straight overhead.

A number of problems can result from the forces at the adolescent's elbow. The anterior oblique portion of the medial collateral ligament is critical for stability in the throwing elbow. Because of its close attachment to the epiphyseal plate at the distal humerus, excessive traction can produce changes at the growth center, including delayed closure of this growth plate, traction apophysitis at the origin of the common flexor tendon, osteophyte development, ulnar nerve traction injuries, and fragmentation and widening of the medial epicondylar apophysis. An acute avulsion fracture of the medial epicondylar apophysis can also occur. The continued medial distraction forces and resultant medial instability can progress to changes on the lateral aspect of the elbow caused by compression forces. Changes in the lateral elbow are less common and are more frequently seen in the older adolescent (ages 14 to 15 years). These are likely to manifest as osteochondrosis of the capitellum.

Treatment of throwers with elbow pain depends on the stage of the pathology. Pappas outlines four grades of functional severity and makes treatment recommendations based on the specific phase.[63] Athletes presenting in phase I generally complain of aching during performance with no limitation of performance and no residual pain. There are no physical examination findings and no radiographic changes. Athletes in this phase often respond after a brief period of rest, rehabilitative exercises, and activity modification. Exercises generally include strengthening exercises for the arm and forearm musculature and stretching if there is any muscular tightness noted on examination. Activity modification includes decreasing the number and frequency of aggravating throws. Phase II severity includes symptoms of aching, pain, or both during performance and a mild limitation of performance and mild postexercise achiness. Some localized tenderness may be elicited, and early radiographic changes such as separation and fragmentation of the epiphysis may be observed on comparison views. These athletes require a longer period of rest and rehabilitation, including a progressive throwing program before full return to competition. Athletes presenting in phase III complain of pain during performance and note a change in their performance owing to pain. Physical findings include localized tenderness, occasional loss of extension, increased valgus laxity compared with the contralateral side, and clear radiographic changes such as separation and fragmentation of the medial epicondylar epihysis. Treatment includes a longer course of rest and rehabilitative strengthening until the athlete is symptom-free and continued follow-up until the physes have ossified. Phase IV findings include a significant alteration of performance owing to pain, localized swelling, decreased motion, and advanced radiographic changes such as radiocapitellar loose bodies. Surgery may be considered, depending on the athlete's age and the extent of changes.[63]

The key to the prevention and treatment of elbow pain is the recognition of the underlying overuse problem and appropriate intervention. The primary issue in prevention is limiting the total number of throws. Little League rules have been constructed to prevent excessive throwing in the growing athlete by limiting the number of innings pitched and games played per week. However, many young athletes continue to throw on off days at home and with friends and family, thereby continuing to overload the elbow. Overzealous parents, peers, and coaches can place excessive pressure on the young athlete to spend spare time practicing in addition to scheduled practices and games. A second issue is the type of pitches thrown by the young athlete. The young pitcher should be encouraged to spend his or her time working on proper form and technique, attempting to control the pitch placement within the batting zone. Off-speed pitches and breaking balls such as the curveball, slider, and changeup should be reserved for postadolescence.

LITTLE LEAGUE SHOULDER

Injury to the proximal humeral epiphyseal plate in young throwers has been called Little League shoulder. Like Little Leaguer elbow, the term *Little League shoulder* implies an overuse injury but does not signify a specific diagnosis. Hence, this term should be abandoned in favor of a specific diagnosis. The extent of injury can vary anywhere from widening of the epiphyseal plate, to a stress fracture, to an occult fracture. The injury can occur in any thrower but is most often found in pitchers.[84] The most common presentation is of a boy between the ages of 12 and 15 years who is a baseball player. The rotational torques during the acceleration phase and the traction forces during deceleration are likely to be the underlying mechanism of injury. The strength of the joint capsule relative to the epiphyseal plate (five times stronger) predisposes the growth plate to injury.[34]

The athlete with a proximal humeral epiphyseal plate injury complains of pain in the shoulder. There may or may not be a history of a specific episode precipitating the symptoms. Palpation deep within the axilla may detect tenderness. Radiographs may demonstrate early changes, including widening of the epiphyseal plate with demineralization and rarefaction on the metaphyseal side.[84] More severe injury to the growth plate can occur with a forceful exertion, resulting in a Salter type II fracture.

If displacement of the fracture is minimal, a sling may be used to rest the shoulder for approximately 3 weeks. If there is significant displacement, closed reduction may be attempted, after which the shoulder is immobilized for 3 weeks.[34] Return to activity should follow a course of rehabilitation and functional progression once the athlete has been cleared to begin throwing.

FRACTURES IN THE YOUNG ATHLETE

EPIPHYSEAL PLATE INJURIES

One of the common issues that arises when considering the young athlete's participation in sports is the risk of epiphyseal plate injuries, including fractures. Damage to the epiphyseal plate can result in arrested growth, and those arguing against children's participation in activities such as weight training focus on this risk. A radiographic study of 60 competitive gymnasts supports this concern. Assessment of the distal radius growth plate demonstrated a significant delay in maturation for girls.[85]

The epiphyseal plate is most vulnerable at the zone of calcifying cartilage on the metaphyseal side. It is weaker than the surrounding bone, joint capsule, and ligaments but still accounts for only 15 percent of all fractures in childhood.[34] This is because of the firm attachment of the epiphysis to the metaphysis peripherally. The blood supply to the epiphyseal plate is derived from the epiphyseal surface and if disrupted can result in necrosis of the epiphysis and epiphyseal plate. Areas of risk are the proximal femoral epiphysis and the proximal radial epiphysis because of a blood supply that courses around the femoral neck. In the lower limb, more longitudinal growth occurs at the epiphyseal plate about the knee than at the ankle or hip. In contrast, the upper extremity grows more in length from the shoulder and wrist than from the elbow.[34] The prognosis following an epiphyseal plate fracture varies, depending on the type of fracture, status of the blood supply, and age of the athlete. If the blood supply is disrupted, the growth plate severely damaged, or both, the resultant deformity will depend on the amount of growth expected from that growth plate. Clearly, the younger the child, the more the deformity that will result if growth is disturbed.

The mechanism of injury causing an epiphyseal plate fracture is the same mechanism that is likely to cause a ligament sprain or dislocation in the adult. Varus and valgus stresses in the lower extremity and elbow and excessive torsional stresses can result in trauma to the epiphyseal plate.

Epiphyseal plate fractures have been placed in five categories by Salter and Harris, in order of increasing risk of disruption of physeal blood supply and growth arrest (Fig. 41–12). Other classifications of physeal fractures exist, but the Salter-Harris classification remains the most practical and most easily remembered system. In a type I fracture, there is complete separation of the epiphysis without any fracture through the bone, and it is usually caused by a shearing force. The prognosis following this type of fracture is good provided the blood supply is intact.

A type II fracture is the most common and involves the plate and a triangular segment of the metaphysis. This type is usually caused by a combination of shearing and bending forces, and the periosteum is torn on the convex side but intact on the concave side of the angulation, resulting in an intact periosteal hinge on the metaphyseal fragment side.[34] Treatment is generally with closed reduction, and the prognosis is good provided the blood supply is intact.

A type III epiphyseal plate injury extends into the joint, passing through the articular cartilage at the joint. This intra-articular fracture extends from the articular surface through the epiphysis to the epiphyseal plate and then transverses the plate to the periphery. This

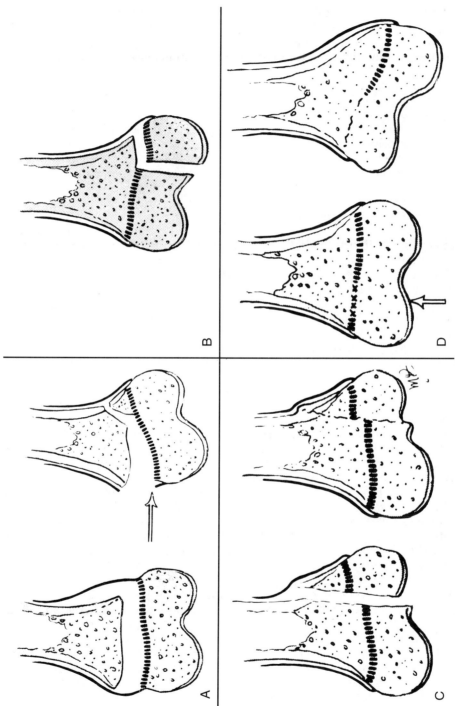

FIGURE 41–12. Salter–Harris classification of epiphyseal plate injuries. *A,* Type I injury, separation of epiphysis *(left)*; type II injury, fracture-separation of epiphysis *(right)*; *B,* Type III injury, fracture of part of the epiphysis. *C* Type IV injury, fracture of epiphysis and epiphyseal plate *(left)*; bony union will cause premature closure of the plate *(right)*. *D,* Type V injury, crushing of the epiphyseal plate *(left)*; premature closure of the plate on one side with a resultant angular deformity *(right)*. (From Salter RB: Textbook of Disorders and Injuries of the Musculoskeletal System, 2nd ed. Baltimore, Williams & Wilkins, 1983.)

type of fracture is also caused by a shearing force and is most often seen at the distal tibial epiphysis.[34] A type III fracture generally requires open reduction to restore the joint surface. Failure to do so will result in an unequal distribution of loads across the joint surface. The prognosis following this relatively uncommon fracture is good provided the blood supply is intact.

A type IV is like a type III injury in that it is intra-articular and extends through the epiphysis to the epiphyseal plate. Rather than transversing the plate to the periphery, however, it continues along the same course through the metaphysis. The most common site of the type IV epiphyseal plate fracture is the lateral condyle of the humerus (supracondylar fracture). The supracondylar humeral fracture is associated with a high incidence of malunion and the risk of Volkmann ischemia. Like a type III injury, open reduction is necessary to restore the joint surface and approximate the fractured growth plate. The prognosis with this type of injury is poor because of the difficulty in reducing and maintaining a perfect alignment at the epiphyseal plate.[34]

Finally, a type V fracture is a crush injury to the epiphyseal plate, a relatively uncommon injury. It is usually seen at the knee and ankle and is often missed because the epiphysis is frequently not displaced. Salter recommends avoidance of weight bearing for at least 3 weeks to prevent further compression of the plate.[34] The prognosis following a type V epiphyseal plate fracture is poor owing to the significant trauma to the growth plate and its blood supply.

OTHER FRACTURE TYPES

The young athlete is more at risk for a fracture than a ligamentous injury owing to the relative strength of the soft tissue as compared with the bone. Children have a stronger and more active periosteum that allows for significant remodeling after a fracture. The high osteogenic activity also allows healing to take place much faster in the child than in the adult. The child can correct and remodel for what appears to be significant deformities and shortening. Residual angulations can correct spontaneously if the plane of deformity is in the same plane as the motion at the nearest joint. For example, a varus or valgus angulation at a humeral supracondylar fracture will not correct because motion at the elbow is in the sagittal plane. Additionally, the body does not correct well for rotations. This becomes important in fractures in the hand when one segment of the fracture becomes rotated on another. Any residual rotational deformity can result in an inability to clench the fingers into a fist. In children under 12 years of age, 1.0 to 1.5 cm of shortening can be made up in the remodeling phase.

Some fracture types are specific to children. The greenstick fracture is an incomplete fracture in which the angulation force bends the cortex on the compression side and breaks it on the distraction side.[55] A greenstick fracture results from bending forces at both ends of the bone, causing tension at the diaphysis.

There is an obvious deformity, and maintenance of the reduction is difficult because of the fracture's tendency to return to its original position.[5] A torus, or "buckle," fracture is the result of a longitudinal compressive force along the shaft of the bone. This results in a remodeling of the metaphysis, causing it to bulge. This bulge makes the metaphysis look like the base of a column, and the name is derived from *torus,* the Latin word meaning *protuberance.*[5] Because the cortex is still intact, the prognosis is excellent.

SPECIAL ISSUES

WEIGHT TRAINING FOR CHILDREN

The increase in sports participation by children of all ages has prompted questions regarding the risks and benefits of weight training for this population. Weight, or strength, training should be distinguished from weight, or power, lifting. Weight training uses weight machines or free weights to increase muscular strength, power, or endurance. In contrast, weight lifting is a competitive category in which the athlete attempts to lift a maximum amount of free weight at one time.[85] There are questions regarding the benefit of weight training in children owing to their lack of circulating androgens. Before puberty, serum testosterone levels are insufficient to produce significant muscular hypertrophy as a result of strength training. Concerns about the possibility of epiphyseal plate injuries discourage some from recommending weight training for the young athlete.

Several studies have been done to assess the results of strength training in children and adolescents. In a classic study, Rutherford and Jones found that strength increases were not correlated with actual changes in the muscle. This led the authors to conclude that neurologic changes occur to improve the coordination and activation of the muscles tested.[87] These same findings were supported by Blimkie and coworkers in a study of 26 boys aged 9 to 11 years.[51] Sewell and Micheli looked at strength training in boys and girls aged 10 to 11 years and found significant increases in strength compared to a control group.[50] Studies of prepubescent, pubescent, and postpubescent boys found significant increases in strength in all groups following a strength training program.[88] In 1985, the National Strength and Conditioning Association reported that prepubescent children could improve their strength and motor performance as a result of strength training.[89] Other benefits of appropriate strength training programs in this population include a decrease in serum lipid levels and a decrease in blood pressure in hypertensive adolescents.[90,91]

The question of possible epiphyseal plate damage and other injuries as a result of weight training has received some attention in the literature, although the information is scanty, often relying on athlete recall for data collections.[92] One study found no injuries during a 9-week training session of 10- to 11-year-old children, whereas another found 43 cases of injuries having a direct relationship to weight training.[50,93] However, many of the injuries observed were in poorly supervised settings, when young athletes were lifting maximal weight through full range of motion with poor control.[89] In contrast, weight-training programs with proper supervision and guidance for young athletes have a very low incidence of injury. The US Consumer Product Safety Commission reported 8543 weight-lifting injuries in athletes presenting to the emergency room who were children between ages 0 and 14 years. Nearly 40 percent of those injuries occurred in unsupervised settings in the home.[92]

In general, children participating in strength-training programs can increase their strength despite the lack of circulating androgens. Recommendations for weight training in this age group include proper warm-up and cool-down, with use of body weight as resistance before progressing to free weights. The focus in this group should be on proper technique, with appropriate supervision and coaching. Repetitions should be high and the resistance should be kept low, and maximal or Olympic-type lifts should be avoided until maturity. Strength training in this population can be an adjunct to the child's participation in other sports, improve body image, and prepare his or her techniques for postadolescent strength training.

LONG-DISTANCE RUNNING AND CHILDREN

As the number of adults participating in endurance activities such as long-distance running increased in the last two decades, so did the number of young athletes. The health care community found itself in the midst of a dilemma, realizing the importance of supporting lifetime activities such as long-distance running but voicing concern over the possibility of injuries in the young athlete. Participation beginning at an early age is essential in developing lifelong habits of exercise, but issues such as distance, intensity, and total mileage were unclear.

The prepubertal child demonstrates similar adaptations to training as the adult. In fact, children are quite well suited for endurance activities. There is no evidence at this time that supports an increased incidence of injury with distance running in children. The American Academy of Pediatrics Committee on Sports Medicine issued a statement on the risks of distance running in children.[94] They recommended that children be allowed to participate in such events as long as the child enjoys the activity and is asymptomatic.[94] However, their relative lack of heat tolerance makes young distance runners more susceptible to heat illness. Extra precautions should be taken to limit training and encourage extra fluids in a warm environment.

One must remember, however, that children and adolescents are susceptible to the same overuse injuries as are adults. Therefore, both the physical and psychological signs of overtraining should be monitored. George Sheehan said, "No horse ran itself to death until there was a rider on its back, and similarly, no child did anything repetitive enough to cause overuse injury, whether it was throwing a baseball, swimming the breaststroke, or running on a street for 10 miles, before there was some structured aspect to the activity."[95] The purpose and goal of long-distance running should be addressed and discussed with the child, and training should be kept in an appropriate balance with other activities.

SOCIOLOGIC ISSUES

The positives and negatives of increased organized sports participation by today's youth are the subject of much debate. The changing social structure in society now encourages youth to participate in an ever-increasing menu of organized sporting activities provided by school programs and outside agencies. How does one counsel the child-athlete regarding the number of choices available? Pressure from peers and coaches plays an important role in the decision-making process in the older child, and parental support or discouragement significantly influences choices made by the younger athlete.

Most adults and children can recall being encouraged to participate in youth sports. It is a traditional belief that these activities "build character" and will affect development throughout the child's entire life. However, these theories have not been consistently supported by research.[96] This does not mean that these beliefs are necessarily untrue. However, they may be true for some children but not for others. Consider the child who perceives that a failure in the sport is his or her own fault, the child who witnesses and models unsportsmanlike behavior, or the child who receives constant criticism from coaches, parents, or peers. In each of these cases, sports will likely have a negative influence. It is difficult to reach any conclusion about the risks and benefits of participation in youth sports, and it is unlikely that research will provide us with any definitive answers because of the great variability among sports experiences. Coakley believes that the outcomes of participation are a result of the conditions under which participation occurs.[96] The sports experience is more likely to contribute to the child's overall development if the sport fits the child's age and stage of development.[96] For example, children aged 2 to 7 years need to focus on the mastery of physical control and performance, whereas children aged 7 to 10 years must learn how to cope with authority figures other than parents. Children aged 10 to 13 years need to develop close friendships and share everyday experiences with friends.[96] Understanding the relationship between these developmental needs and sports can help the parent and coach guide the young athlete into appropriate sports.

In addition to questions about choosing a particular sport, there are also questions about the level of sports participation, from organized and highly structured, to unorganized or "free play." There are some significant differences between free play and organized sports. As the game starts, the spontaneous play group spends the most time on organizational problems, whereas the competitive team has most of these details preset by adults.[97] Some argue that organized sport, with its rules and adult intervention, eliminates the opportunity for children to set their own standards and resolve discrepancies. Rules are made and modified as needed by the free-play group. Some players are given special privileges or handicaps based on the judgment of the group. For example, some players may be forced to bat with their nondominant arm, and others are given a 5-second lead after hitting the ball. Under the coaches' direction in organized play, orders are given, and the players respond in a routine and predictable manner. The emphasis in this setting is on the development of sports skill, whereas the emphasis in unstructured sports is on the development of interpersonal skills. Coakley suggests that children in organized teams learn obedience, but children in free play learn discipline.[97] For the pick-up game, the experience of play is an end in itself; in contrast, the game is a means to an end in the organized team.[97]

The quantity of time spent in organized play can impact on the time spent in unorganized games in several ways. It has been found that children participating in Little League have little time for free play as a result of the team's schedule. Participation in organized sports has demonstrated that children spend more time in fewer sports and abandon games 2 to 3 years earlier than before the introduction of organized sport.[97]

Parental involvement in a child's sport can have a positive or negative effect on the child. When parents become involved in children's sport, they have a tendency to place unreasonable demands on the young athlete, with excessive focus on winning. Many parents are participating as volunteer coaches and officials with little or no training. This can have significant impact on the young athlete who fears losing at sport will result in parental rejection. A potentially dangerous situation exists when a child believes that parental affection is based on his or her athletic performance. Additionally, excessive parental involvement may interfere with the child's opportunity to develop self-discipline and a sense of responsibility.[98]

The psychological impact of intensive training in the young athlete is yet another question being studied. Many sports medicine professionals can relate cases of child athletes presenting to the clinic with vague complaints and minimal findings. At this point, the question of who is driving the athlete to participate becomes important. The child athlete's physical symptoms may be due to excessive psychological stress and should be treated for this problem simultaneously with treatment for the physical problems. Rowley focused on six issues related to intensive training in youth athletes. These included gender, peer relationships, anorexia syndromes, injury, educational attainment, and emotional problems.[99] The emotional stress of sports has been shown to produce psychosomatic complaints, while the belief that participants in school sports perform better academically has not been supported.[99]

Of particular importance, it was noted that young athletes who experienced significant life events such as parental illness, separation, divorce, or death were more likely to sustain a significant injury.[99]

CONCLUSION

Young athletes pose a set of issues specific to their age, physical maturity, and sociologic development. The sports medicine professional must be well versed in the potential problems unique to this population. Their relative heat intolerance, growth-plate weakness, and apophyseal problems are all possible factors predisposing to injury. Additionally, children are susceptible to the same injuries as adults. Weight training appears to be a safe activity for preadolescents as long as it is well supervised and the focus remains on technique and not on heavy lifting. Long-distance running can be a safe activity as long as the environmental and psychological concerns are addressed. The motivation behind the young athlete's participation in organized sports and training (including long-distance running) must be critically evaluated both by the sports medicine professional dealing with that athlete and by society as a whole.

REFERENCES

1. Stanitski CL: Common injuries in preadolescent and adolescent athletes: Recommendations for prevention. Sports Med 1989; 7:32–41.
2. Nilsson S, Roaas A: Soccer injuries in adolescents. Am J Sports Med 1978; 6(6):358–361.
3. Schmidt-Olsen S, Jorgensen S, Kaalund U, et al: Injuries among young soccer players. Am J Sports Med 1991; 19(3):273–275.
4. Shively RA, Grana WA, Ellis D: High school sports injuries. Phys Sports Med 1981; 9:46–50.
5. Wilkins KE: The uniqueness of the young athlete: Musculoskeletal injuries. Am J Sports Med 1980; 8(5):377–382.
6. Guyer B, Ellers B: Childhood injuries in the United States. Am J Disease Child 1990; 144:649–652.
7. Busch MT: Sports medicine in children and adolescents. In Morrissy RT (ed): Pediatric Orthopaedics, 3rd ed. Philadelphia, JB Lippincott, 1990.
8. Chambers RB: Orthopaedic injuries in athletes (ages 6–17). Am J Sports Med 1979, 7.195.
9. Garrick JG, Requa RK: Injuries in high school sports. Pediatrics 1978; 61:465–469.
10. McClain LG, Reynolds S: Sports injuries in a high school. Pediatrics 1989; 84:446–450.
11. Landry GL: Sports injuries in childhood. Pediatr Ann 1992; 21(3):165–168.
12. DeHaven KE: Athletic injuries in adolescents. Pediatr Ann 1978; 7(10):96–119.
13. Zaricznyj B, Shattuck LJ, Mast TS, et al: Sports-related injuries in school-aged children. Am J Sports Med 1980; 8(5):318–323.
14. Backx FJ, Erich WB, Kemper AB, et al: Sports injuries in school-aged children: An epidemiologic study. Am J Sports Med 1989; 17(2):234–240.
15. Garrick JG, Requa RK: Injuries in high school sports. Pediatrics 1978; 61:465–469.
16. Apple DF: Adolescent runners. Clin Sports Med 1985; 4(4): 641–655.
17. Lorish TR, Rizzo TD, Ilstrup DM, et al: Injuries in adolescent and preadolescent boys at two large wrestling tournaments. Am J Sports Med 1992; 20(2):199–202.

18. Micheli LJ, Fehlandt AF: Overuse injuries to tendons and apophyses in children and adolescents. Clin Sports Med 1992; 11(4):713–726.

19. Maffulli N: Intensive training in young athletes: The orthopaedic surgeon's viewpoint. Sports Med 1990; 9(4):229–243.

20. McGrory BJ, Klassen RA, Chao EY, et al: Acute fractures and dislocations of the cervical spine in children and adolescents. J Bonc Joint Surg 1993; 75A:988–995.

21. Smith NJ: Children and parents: Growth, development and sports. In Strauss RH (ed): Sports Medicine. Philadelphia, WB Saunders, 1984.

22. Porter RE: Normal development of movement and function: Child and adolescent. In Scully RM, Barnes MR (eds): Physical Therapy. Philadelphia, JB Lippincott, 1989.

23. Lowrey GH: Growth and Development of Children, 8th ed. Chicago, Year Book Medical Publishers, 1986.

24. Tanner JM: Foetus into Man: Physical Growth from Conception to Maturity. Cambridge, MA, Harvard University Press, 1978.

25. Beunen G: Biological age in pediatric exercise research. In Bar-Or O (ed): Advances in Pediatric Sport Sciences. Champaign, IL, Human Kinetics, 1989.

26. Tanner JM: Standards from birth to maturity for height, weight, height velocity, and weight velocity: British children. Arch Dis Child 1966; 41:454.

27. Buckler J: A Longitudinal Study of Adolescent Growth. New York, Springer-Verlag, 1990.

28. Malina RM: Growth of muscle tissue and muscle mass. In Falkner F, Tanner JM (eds): Human Growth: A Comprehensive Treatise, 2nd ed, vol 2. New York, Plenum, 1985.

29. Zauner CW, Maksud MG, Melichna J: Physiological considerations in training young athletes. Sports Med 1989; 8(1):15–31.

30. Blanksby BA, Bloomfield J, Elliot BC, et al: The anatomical and physiological characteristics of pre-adolescent males and females. Aust Paediatr J 1986; 22:177–180.

31. Bar-Or O: Pediatric Sports Medicine for the Practitioner: From Physiologic Principles to Clinical Applications. New York, Springer-Verlag, 1983.

32. Roche AF: Bone growth and maturation. In Falkner F, Tanner JM (eds): Human Growth: A Comprehensive Treatise, 2nd ed, vol 2. New York, Plenum, 1985.

33. Riegger CL: Mechanical properties of bone. In Gould JA, Davies GJ (eds): Orthopaedic and Sports Physical Therapy. St. Louis, CV Mosby, 1985.

34. Salter RB: Textbook of Disorders and Injuries of the Musculo-skeletal System, 2nd ed. Baltimore, Williams & Wilkins, 1983.

35. Ogden JA: Development and maturation of the neuromusculo-skeletal system. In Morrissy TR (ed): Pediatric Orthopaedics, 3rd ed. Philadelphia, JB Lippincott, 1990.

36. Ogden JA, Hempton RF, Southwick WO: Development of the tibial tuberosity. Anat Rec 1975; 182:431–456.

37. Valadian I, Porter D: Physical Growth and Development: From Conception to Maturity. St. Louis, CV Mosby, 1980.

38. Beunen G, Malina R: Growth and physical performance relative to the timing of the adolescent spurt. Exerc Sport Sci Rev 1988; 16:503–540.

39. Cunningham DA, Paterson DH, Blimkie CJR, et al: Development of cardiorespiratory function in circumpubertal boys: A longitudinal study. J Appl Physiol 1984; 56(2):302–307.

40. Inbar O, Oded B: Anaerobic characteristics in male children and adolescents. Med Sci Sports Exerc 1986; 18:264–269.

41. Bailey DA, Malina RM, Mirwald RL: Physical activity and the growth of the child. In Falkner F, Tanner JM (eds): Human Growth: A Comprehensive Treatise, 2nd ed, vol 2. New York, Plenum, 1985.

42. Alpert BS, Flood NL, Strong WB, et al: Responses to ergometer exercise in a healthy biracial population of children. J Pediatr 1982; 101(4):538–545.

43. Bar-Or O: Climate and the exercising child: A review. Int J Sports Med 1980; 1:53–56.

44. Drinkwater BL, Kupprat IC, Denton JE, et al: Response of prepubertal girls and college women to work in the heat. J Appl Physiol 1977; 43:1046–1053.

45. Haymes EM, Buskirk ER, Hodgson JL, et al: Heat tolerance of exercising lean and heavy prepubertal girls. J Appl Physiol 1974; 36:566–571.

46. Haymes EM, McCormick RJ, Buskirk ER: Heat tolerance of exercising lean and obese prepubertal boys. J Appl Physiol 1975; 39:457–461.

47. Bar-Or O, Dotan R, Inbar O, et al: Voluntary hypohydration in 10- to 12-year-old boys. J Appl Physiol 1980; 48(1):104–108.

48. Eriksson BO, Koch G: Effect of physical training on hemodynamic response during submaximal and maximal exercise in 11–13 year old boys. Acta Physiol Scand 1973; 87:27–39.

49. Brown CH, Harrower JR, Deeter MF: The effects of cross-country running on preadolescent girls. Med Sci Sports Exerc 1972; 4(1):1–5.

50. Sewell L, Micheli LJ: Strength training for children. J Pediatr Orthop 1986; 6:143–146.

51. Blimkie CJR, Smith K, Garner K, et al: Strength training effects in prepubescent boys. Med Sci Sports Exerc 1990; 22(5):605–614.

52. Dorland's Medical Dictionary, 26th ed. Philadelphia, WB Saunders, 1981.

53. Insall JN: Surgery of the Knee. New York, Churchill Livingstone, 1984.

54. Strizak AM, Stroberg AJ: Knee injuries in the skeletally immature athlete. In Nicholas JA, Hershman EG (eds): The Lower Extremity and Spine in Sports Medicine. St. Louis, CV Mosby, 1986.

55. Brashear HR, Raney RB: Shands' Handbook of Orthopaedic Surgery, 9th ed. St. Louis, CV Mosby, 1978.

56. Wenger DR, Ward WT, Herring JA: Current concepts review: Legg-Calvé-Perthes disease. J Bone Joint Surg 1991; 73A:778–788.

57. Weinstein SL: Legg-Calvé-Perthes disease. In Morrissy RT (ed): Pediatric Orthopaedics, 3rd ed. Philadelphia, JB Lippincott, 1990.

58. Aichroth P: Osteochondritis dissecans of the knee. In Insall JN (ed): Surgery of the Knee. New York, Churchill Livingstone, 1984.

59. Cahill B: Treatment of juvenile osteochondritis dissecans and osteochondritis dissecans of the knee. Clin Sports Med 1985; 4(2):367–384.

60. Panner HJ: A peculiar affection of the capitulum humeri resembling Calvé-Perthes disease of the hip. Acta Radiol 1929; 10:234.

61. Singer KM, Roy SP: Osteochondrosis of the humeral capitellum. Am J Sports Med 1984; 12(5):351–360.

62. Jobe FW, Nuber G: Throwing injuries of the elbow. Clin Sports Med 1986; 5(4):621–636.

63. Pappas AM: Elbow problems associated with baseball during childhood and adolescence. Clin Orthop Rel Res 1982; 164:30–42.

64. Morrissy RT: Slipped capital femoral epiphysis. In Morrissy RT (ed): Pediatric Orthopaedics, 3rd ed. Philadelphia, JB Lippincott, 1990.

65. Loder RT, Aronson DD, Greenfield ML: The epidemiology of bilateral slipped capital femoral epiphysis. J Bone Joint Surg 1993; 75A(8):1141–1147.

66. Loder RT, Richards BS, Shapiro PS, et al: Acute slipped capital femoral epiphysis: The importance of physeal stability. J Bone Joint Surg 1993; 75A(8):1134–1140.

67. Wilcox P, Weiner D, Leighley B: Maturation factors in slipped capital femoral epiphysis. J Pediatr Orthop 1988; 8:196–200.

68. Schoenecker PL: Slipped capital femoral epiphysis. Orthop Rev 1985; 5:71–76.

69. Fleisher GR: Slipped capital femoral epiphysis without hip pain leads to missed diagnosis. Pediatrics 1992; 89:660–662.

70. Carney BT, Weinstein SL, Noble J: Long-term follow-up of slipped capital femoral epiphysis. J Bone Joint Surg 1991; 73A(5):667–674.

71. Meier MC, Meyer LC, Ferguson RL: Treatment of slipped capital femoral epiphysis with a spica cast. J Bone Joint Surg 1992; 74A(10):1522–1529.

72. Aronson DD, Carlson WE: Slipped capital femoral epiphysis: A prospective study with a single screw. J Bone Joint Surg 1992; 74A(6):810–819.

73. Ward WT, Stefko J, Wood KB, et al: Fixation with a single screw for slipped capital femoral epiphysis. J Bone Joint Surg 1992; 74A(6):799–809.

74. Osgood RB: Lesions of the tibial tubercle occurring during adolescence. Boston Med Surg J 1903; 148:114.

75. Singer KM, Henry J: Knee problems in children and adolescents. Clin Sports Med 1985; 4(2):385–398.

76. DeFlaviis L, Nessi R, Scaglione P, et al: Ultrasonic diagnosis of Osgood-Schlatter and Sinding-Larsen-Johansson diseases of the knee. Skel Radiol 1989; 18:193–197.

77. Bullough PG, Vosburgh F, Arnoczky SP, et al: The menisci of the knee. *In* Insall JN (ed): Surgery of the Knee. New York, Churchill Livingstone, 1984.

78. Donatelli RA: The Biomechanics of the Foot and Ankle. Philadelphia, FA Davis, 1990.

79. Turco VJ, Spinella AJ: Injuries to the foot and ankle in the skeletally immature athlete. *In* Nicholas JA, Hershman EG (eds): The Lower Extremity and Spine in Sports Medicine. St. Louis, CV Mosby, 1986.

80. Brogdon BG, Crow NE: Little leaguer's elbow. Am J Roentgenol 1960; 83:671–675.

81. Jenkins W, Kegerreis S: Throwing injuries. *In* Sanders B (ed): Sports Physical Therapy. Norwalk, CT, Appleton & Lange, 1990.

82. Hunter SC: Little leaguer's elbow. *In* Zarins B, Andrews JR, Carson WG (eds): Injuries to the Throwing Arm. Philadelphia, WB Saunders, 1985.

83. Adams JE: Injury of the throwing arm: A study of traumatic changes in the elbow joints of boy baseball players. Calif Med 1965; 102:127.

84. Kulund DN: The Injured Athlete. Philadelphia, JB Lippincott, 1982.

85. Caine D, Roy S, Singer KM, et al: Stress changes of the distal radial growth plate. Am J Sports Med 1992; 20(3):290–298.

86. Risser WL: Musculoskeletal injuries caused by weight training. Clin Pediatr 1990; 29(6):305–310.

87. Rutherford OM, Jones DA: The role of learning and coordination in strength training. Eur J Appl Physiol 1986; 55:100–105.

88. Pfeiffer RD, Francis RS: Effects of strength training on muscle development in prepubescent, pubescent and postpubescent males. Phys Sports Med 1986; 14(9):134–143.

89. Weltman A: Weight training in prepubertal children: Physiologic benefit and potential damage. *In* Bar-Or O (ed): Advances in Pediatric Sport Sciences. Champaign, IL, Human Kinetics, 1989.

90. Hagberg JM, Ehsani AA, Goldring D, et al: Effect of weight training on blood pressure and hemodynamics in hypertensive adolescents. J Pediatr 1984; 104:147–151.

91. Weltman A, Janney C, Rians CB, et al: The effects of hydraulic-resistance strength training on serum lipid levels in prepubertal boys. Am J Dis Child 1987; 141:777–780.

92. Blimkie CJR: Resistance training during preadolescence. Sports Med 1993; 15(6):389–407.

93. Brady TA, Cahill BR, Bodnar LM: Weight training–related injuries in the high school athlete. Am J Sports Med 1982; 10(1):1–5.

94. American Academy of Pediatrics Committee on Sports Medicine: Risks in distance running for children. Pediatrics 1990; 86(5):799–800.

95. Micheli LJ: Sports in childhood: A round table. Phys Sports Med 1982; 10(8):52–60.

96. Coakley JJ: Social dimensions of intensive training and participation in youth sports. *In* Cahill BR, Pearl AJ (eds): Intensive Participation in Children's Sports. Champaign, IL, Human Kinetics, 1993.

97. Coakley JJ: Sport in Society: Issues and Controversies. St. Louis, CV Mosby, 1978.

98. Vaughan LK: Psychological impact of organized sports on children. *In* Micheli LJ (ed): Pediatric and Adolescent Sports Medicine. Boston, Little, Brown, 1984.

99. Rowley S: Psychological effects of intensive training in young athletes. J Child Psychol Psychiatry 1987; 28:371–377.

CHAPTER 42

The Athlete with a Disability

KATHLEEN A. CURTIS *PhD, PT*
ROBERT S. GAILEY JR. *MSEd, PT*

Fifteen or twenty years ago, on any given afternoon, a local charity organization would host a track meet for the "handicapped" where an indiscriminate number of events would be offered. Participants would often compete in their street clothes and everyday wheelchairs, prostheses, or braces. Many competitors had never practiced or even attempted some of the events before the day of competition. However, everyone would have a day of fun and excitement.

Today, for the accomplished athlete with a disability, athletics is a world of aerodynamic wheelchairs and high-tech equipment costing thousands of dollars; scientific performance analysis; and year-round training for regional, national, and international competitions. The grassroots infrastructure of disabled athletics is still firmly in place, with charity groups, public schools, and local disabled sports organizations hosting improved, structured weekend competitions for novice and intermediate-level competitors. Additionally, the poten-

tial vertical growth of competition has flourished within disabled athletics for gifted and serious competitors.

Over the past decade, disabled athletics has matured into a finely structured group of organizations dedicated to providing athletes of all disabilities with an equitable playing field for competition, while allowing individual athletes the opportunity to rise through the ranks of competition, depending on their athletic ability. Thanks to the relentless efforts of a persistent few, disabled competitors are beginning to enjoy the satisfaction of training, competing, and receiving the recognition so richly deserved yet frequently bestowed only on able-bodied athletes. Only recently have a few disabled athletes found themselves featured in the sports section of newspapers, magazines, and television. Unfortunately, the majority of the media still regards these talented athletes as "human interest" stories. This chapter provides a comprehensive overview of the complexities and challenges of disabled ath-

TABLE 42–1
Competitive Sports and Recreation Activities Offered by U.S. Disabled Sports Organizations

Sport	1	2	3	4	5	6	7	8
Alpine skiing	x		x		x			x
Archery			x	x		x		
Basketball	x	x	x					x
Boccie						x	x	
Bowling	x					x		x
Canoeing			x					x
Cross country	x					x		x
Cycling	x		x		x	x		x
Diving	x							
Equestrian						x		x
Figure skating								x
Floor hockey								x
Goal ball					x			
Gymnastics					x			x
Handball	x							
Ice hockey	x							
Judo					x			
Nordic skiing	x		x		x			x
Poly hockey								x
Powerlifting		x	x	x	x	x	x	x
Racquetball			x					
Road racing	x		x	x				x
Roller skating								x
Shooting	x	x	x	x		x	x	
Slalom				x		x	x	x
Soccer	x					x		x
Softball	x	x						x
Speed skating	x				x			x
Swimming	x	x	x	x	x	x	x	x
Table tennis	x	x	x	x		x	x	x
Team handball						x	x	x
Tennis	x		x	x				x
Track and field	x	x	x	x	x	x	x	x
Volleyball	x		x					x
Weight lifting			x	x				
Wrestling	x				x			

Key:
1. AAAD: American Athletic Association of the Deaf
2. DAAA: Dwarf Athletic Association of America
3. DSUSA: Disabled Sports USA (amputees)
4. WSUSA: Wheelchair Sports USA
5. USABA: United States Association of Blind Athletes
6. USCPAA: United States Cerebral Palsy Athletic Association
7. USLASA: United States Les Autres Sports Association (other disabilities)
8. SOI: Special Olympics International (developmentally disabled)
Adapted from Paciorek MI, Jones JA: Sports and Recreation for the Disabled: A Resource Manual. Indianapolis, Benchmark Press, 1989.

letics, focusing on the enlightenment of rehabilitation providers as possible advocates in a variety of capacities. Most importantly, knowledgeable rehabilitation professionals can identify future disabled athletes and educate other professionals about the world of disabled athletics and the benefits for those who choose to get involved.

ORGANIZATIONAL STRUCTURE OF DISABLED ATHLETICS

The organizational structure appears complex to newcomers to disabled athletics. In most instances, the basic structure follows the same format used for able-bodied amateur athletics, with one exception. Because most disabled sports organizations (DSOs) arose to meet the needs of athletes with similar disabilities, disabled athletics has historically been governed by "disability-specific" organizations as opposed to "sport-specific" organizations as in able-bodied sports. For example, each of the eight DSOs offers track and field to its athletes; therefore, eight governing bodies exist for rules, competitions, and medal criteria (Table 42–1).[1] In contrast, in able-bodied sports in the United States, all track and field is governed

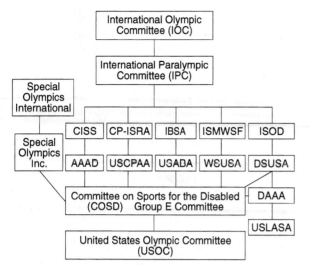

FIGURE 42–1. Organizational Chart for the International Sports Organizations. IOC, International Olympic Committee; IPC, International Paralympic Committee; CISS, Comité International des Sports des Soudes; CP-ISRA, Cerebral Palsy International Sports and Recreational Association; IBSA, International Blind Sport Association; ISMWSF, International Stoke-Mandeville Wheelchair Sports Federation; ISOD, International Sports Organization for the Disabled; AAAD, American Athletic Association for the Deaf; USCPAA, United States Cerebral Palsy Athletic Association; USABA, United States Association for Blind Athletes; WSUSA, Wheelchair Sports USA; DSUSA, Disabled Sports USA; DAAA, Dwarf Athletic Association of America; USLASA, United States Les Autres Sports Association. (Adapted from Paciorek MJ, Jones JA: Sports and Recreation for the Disabled: A Resource Manual. Indianapolis, Benchmark Press, 1989.)

by the National Governing Body (NGB), Track and Field USA.

Currently, many philosophical and structural changes are occurring at all levels of disabled athletics. Some sports are moving toward becoming entirely sport-specific with regard to organizational structure, whereas other more complex sports are weighing the advantages and disadvantages of such a change. The evolution of disabled sports has been rapid and appears to be gaining momentum. The organizational structure presented in this text will change to some degree in the future, as will some of the organizations' names, but the basic format will probably remain the same.

The International Olympic Committee (IOC) presides over all international Olympic-sanctioned sporting events and governing bodies. The parallel organization for the disabled is the International Paralympic Committee (IPC). The IPC's primary responsibility is to sanction disabled sporting events and act as a coordinating committee among the host city of the Paralympic Games and the five international disabled sports organizations (IDSOs), which are the Comite International des Sports des Soudes (CISS), Cerebral Palsy International Sports and Recreational Association (CP-ISRA), International Blind Sport Association (IBSA), International Stoke-Mandeville Wheelchair Sports Federation (ISMWSF), International Sports Organization for the Disabled (ISOD), and International Sport Federation for Persons with Mental Handicaps (INAS-FMH). Representation to the IDSOs is granted to DSOs from all countries that meet the criteria for membership. The IDSOs process information from participating countries and communicate directly to the IPC or the hosting Paralympic Games city. Policy and international rules for competition are governed by the IDSOs (Fig. 42–1). The IOC works with member countries, which are represented by their individual National Organizing Committees (NOCs) and international sports federations. The United States Olympic Committee (USOC) is the NOC for the United States and is the coordinating body for amateur sports, with the primary purpose of preparing Olympic and Pan American Games' teams. The five membership categories within the USOC are group A, Olympic/Pan American sports organizations, which includes the 42 national governing bodies (NGBs) for each sport; group B, community-based multisport organizations, armed forces, and education-based multisport organizations; group C, affiliated sport organizations; group D, state Olympic organizations; and group E, organizations of sport for the disabled (Fig. 42–2).

The Committee on Sports for the Disabled currently recognizes six DSOs: American Athletic Association for the Deaf (AAAD), Dwarf Athletic Association of America (DAAA), United States Cerebral Palsy Athletic Association (USCPAA), United States Association for Blind Athletes (USABA), Wheelchair Sports USA (WSUSA),

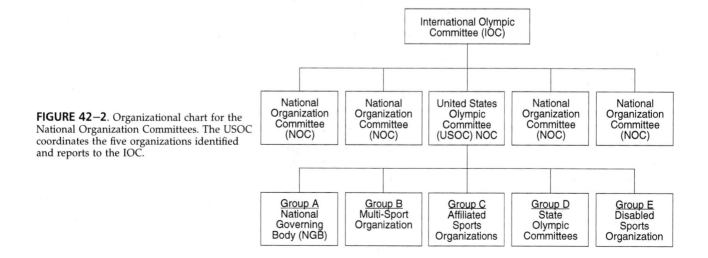

FIGURE 42–2. Organizational chart for the National Organization Committees. The USOC coordinates the five organizations identified and reports to the IOC.

TABLE 42–2
Classification Systems for Athletes with Disabilities

Organization	Sport	Classification System
2,3,4,5,6,7	Alpine skiing	10 classifications, based on type of ski equipment used
3,4,7	Basketball (wheelchair)	3-class U.S. system based on neurologic function; 4-class international system based on functional trunk movement in wheelchair; combined classification points of players on court limited by rules
3	Cycling	3-class system, based on limb involvement
2,3,4,5,7	Powerlifting	Competition by weight classes
2,3,4,7	Swimming	10-class integrated system, with different classifications for breaststroke, backstroke, and freestyle
3,7	Table tennis (standing)	5-class system for standing athletes
3,4,7	Table tennis (wheelchair)	5 seated classes based on upper extremity and trunk function
3	Track and field (amputees, standing)*	9-class system based on upper vs. lower extremity involvement and level of amputation
3,4,7	Track and field (wheelchair)	4 classes for track events; 7 seated classes for field events; 1 standing class for field events
3,7	Volleyball (sitting)	All players must sit
3	Volleyball (standing)	8-class system; uses combined classification points of players on court
1	All sports for AAAD	Must have hearing loss greater than 55 db in best ear
2	All sports for DAAA	Eligibility based on height less than 5'0"
5	All sports for USABA†	3-class system, based on visual field and acuity
6	All sports for USCPAA‡	8-class system, based on level of function of extremities and ambulatory status
7	All sports for USLASA§	6-class system, based on extremity and trunk function in sitting and standing competition
8	All	Participants compete in classes by age, gender, and ability level

Key:
1. AAAD: American Athletic Association of the Deaf
2. DAAA: Dwarf Athletic Association of America
3. DSUSA: Disabled Sports USA (amputees)
4. WSUSA: Wheelchair Sports USA
5. USABA: United States Association of Blind Athletes
6. USCPAA: United States Cerebral Palsy Athletic Association
7. USLASA: United States Les Autres Sports Association (other disabilities)
8. SOI: Special Olympics International (developmentally disabled)
*Bilateral above-knee amputees can compete in a wheelchair or standing.
†In cycling, athletes ride tandem.
‡In international swimming competition, an integrated system is used.
§Most athletes compete under specific functional classifications for wheelchair or ambulatory athletes.

and Disabled Sports USA (DSUSA). The United States Les Autres Sports Association (USLASA) is currently not recognized by the USOC, but the organization contributes significantly to the disabled sports movement. Each of the U.S. DSOs has representation to its respective international DSO as a voting member.

CLASSIFICATION OF ATHLETES WITH DISABILITIES

Classification systems have existed almost as long as sports for persons with disabilities. The systems are intended to provide a means to ensure equitable competition, where ability and skills, not degree of physical disability, are the variables among competitors. Accordingly, athletes of similar levels of disability are grouped together in a "class" designated for competition. Individuals in the same class compete against each other in individual sports, such as track and field or swimming. In team sports, athletes in various classes are allowed to compete as a team only in prescribed combinations, which serve to ensure that the most severely disabled players will not be excluded from the sport.

Traditionally, athlete classification was primarily a medical decision, based on the results of a physical examination of such criteria as neurologic function, degree of visual deficit, or length of residual limbs. There were inherent problems in both the intent and the implementation of such systems. These systems classified athletes within a disability group for all sports in which they competed, regardless of the relative advantage of having certain functions for a particular sport. For example, a sport such as wheelchair racing requires considerably less trunk rotation for performance than a sport such as wheelchair basketball. In addition, the divisions between classes were arbitrary and did not reflect parallel increments in performance across all sports. Further, it became apparent that as disabled sports organizations such as Wheelchair Sports USA (WSUSA) tried to mix athletes with different disabilities in a classification system designed for spinal cord–injured athletes, the system clearly favored certain athletes. Weiss and Curtis[2] studied the distribution of disabilities across finalists in each class of competition at a national (WSUSA) multisport championship. They found that the finalists comprised a disproportionate number of athletes with postpolio paralysis and athletes with amputations compared with the number of athletes with paraplegia and spina bifida in the organization. Athletes with cerebral palsy were also underrepresented in the finalist groups.

For some of these reasons, athletes within a DSO were prevented from competing against athletes from other DSOs, as each DSO developed separate meets for its national championships. At the world championship events, where multiple DSOs represented various countries, amputees competing in wheelchairs had a different competition from paraplegics in wheelchairs for each distance of a track meet. In the 1988 Seoul Paralympics, this division by classification and by disability group resulted in over 40 different 100-meter races being run. This was confusing and nonproductive for meet organizers, athletes, and spectators.

Dissatisfaction with classification systems has been the norm, rather than the exception, throughout the history of sports for the disabled. In the mid-1980s, Horst Strohkendl developed the first classification system that was based on observation of an athlete's function during actual wheelchair basketball competition rather than the athlete's neurologic level.[3] Other sports have followed, in an effort to consolidate athletes by classification in their sports rather than by their disabilities. Sport-specific functional classification systems have now been developed for track and field,

swimming, table tennis, and shooting.[4] For example, between the 1988 and 1992 Paralympics, a 10-class function classification system for swimming was implemented. This system combines cerebral palsy, amputee, and wheelchair athletes who would have competed in 25 classes in the 1992 Paralympic Games. The 10-class system is intended to reduce the time and organizational effort required to hold the competition. Classification systems in winter sports focus on the type of adaptive ski equipment used.

Despite the benefits of simplifying an athletic event, Richter et al.[5] argue that this system lacks reliability and validity by integrating disability groups and applying arbitrary criteria that disadvantage certain disability groups. Classification systems are currently in flux and are expected to evolve further as a result of the experiences in sport-specific functional classification. Performance and degree of disability do not always show a direct relationship. To describe each classification system currently used goes beyond the scope of this chapter. Table 42–2 summarizes the various systems used in some competitive sports.

Rehabilitation professionals and physicians have traditionally been involved as classifiers in most DSOs, since traditional classification involved physical examination and disability assessment. These traditional observations still play a part in some functional classification systems, but more important now is the observation of athletic performance in the sport. Thus the role of the classifier in the era of functional classification is to observe performance in sports competition. Classification is frequently carried out by a team of classifiers, including medical personnel, sports technical experts, athletes, and coaches. Physical therapists are particularly well suited for this role due to their strengths in the observation of normal and abnormal movement. An ability to observe movement carefully during functional performance is critical to the classification process.

TECHNICAL ASSESSMENT

Traditionally, a coach is responsible for the training of an athlete, and the medical team plays a supportive role, responding to injuries or implementing injury prevention programs. Disabled athletes present a unique situation in which a growing number of therapists and other medical professionals have become involved in the training process. One reason for their involvement is that the coaching process of a disabled athlete must include some knowledge in the following areas: sport performance (the actual biomechanics of the event), pathology, kinesiology, pathokinesiology, adaptive physiology, prosthetics or orthotics, and motivational psychology. The criteria for coaching the disabled athlete go well beyond those required to coach an able-bodied athlete, in terms of assessing physical and technical methods for performance enhancement.

Two approaches to the analysis of biomechanical events may be employed to study human movement. The first is the quantitative approach, which applies numerical values to describe all movements. This

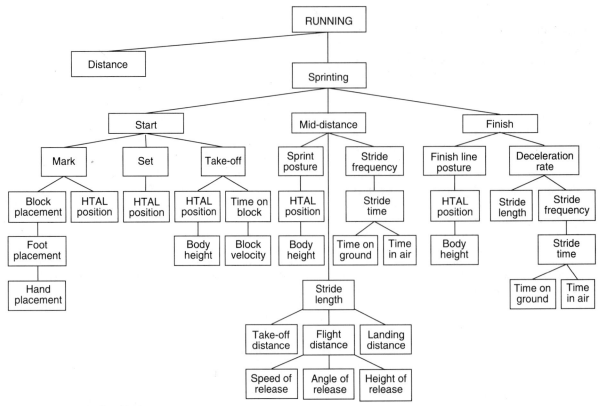

FIGURE 42–3. A model of the components of sprinting, divided into three phases: start, mid-distance, and finish. HTAL: Head, trunk, arm, and leg. (Courtesy of Advanced Rehabilitation Therapy, Inc., Miami, FL.)

method is the most explicit, but it is complex, expensive, time consuming, and, for the average athlete, unnecessary. In contrast, the qualitative approach describes movement in non-numerical terms utilizing observation, qualitative data, and applied physical principles as the foundation for interpretations made by the observer. Qualitative analysis is more easily employed than quantitative analysis. Qualitative analysis can be performed simply by general observation, memory of a performance, or use of videotape. Obviously, videotaped recordings provide a more accurate account of the movement being analyzed and can be reviewed to verify the impressions of the observer.[6]

The disability of the athlete adds another factor to the equation when attempting to enhance athletic performance and prevent injury. Each athlete presents with some form of biomechanical restriction: either a physical limitation, such as increased tone, weakened muscles, loss of range of motion, or vision loss, or the need for an additional mechanical device such as a wheelchair or prosthesis. A systematic assessment of each component of the athlete's sport must be made, as with able-bodied athletes, yet the therapist or coach must now take into consideration how each component of the skill being learned can be mastered by either physical or mechanical compensation. This is the challenge put before all those who work with disabled athletes, and that is what makes this work so exciting and gratifying.

Regardless of the approach—quantitative, qualitative, or a combination of the two—movement analysis must be performed in a systematic manner. The following is provided to give some insight into the performance enhancement process and the role that the medical professional can play.

DEFINE THE MOVEMENT OR SKILL TO BE ANALYZED. Before any analysis of movement can begin, the specific movement or skill to be analyzed must be defined. The more specifically the movement is defined, the greater the chance of success. For example, if a track sprinter is being analyzed, the first question that would have to be asked is what part of the sprint requires analysis? The start, mid-distance, or finish? Once the phase of the sprint has been determined, a host of splinter components would have to be identified and assessed for that phase (Fig. 42–3).

IDENTIFY THE BIOMECHANICAL PRINCIPLES THAT GOVERN THE DESIRED MOVEMENT OR SKILL. Once the component parts of the sprint have been identified, the mechanical effects throughout the kinetic chain of the sprinter's body must be examined in order to determine the effect one body segment has on another. The mechanical effects can be the result of either internal or external influence. This process can be either complex or general. In many cases, an educated coach can visually observe the majority of biomechanical constraints that may hinder an athlete's performance. Often an in-depth quantitative analysis only confirms what the coach has observed.

The following is a brief outline suggesting the major topic areas that should be considered when performing a movement analysis.

The Physiologic Laws That Relate to the Neuromuscular and Musculoskeletal Systems. The athlete's body size and weight, strength, range of motion, muscular tone, limb length, sensation, balance, coordination, agility, vision, hearing, endurance, and other physiologic considerations that may be inherent to the type of disability or to the athlete's current physical condition must be analyzed. For example, athletes with quadriplegia or paraplegia are able to maximize their performance using different wheelchair strokes and trunk position as a result of the level of disability and the motor function available. Likewise, many swimmers with various disabilities find the backstroke to be faster for them than the crawl stroke and therefore choose the backstroke when competing in freestyle events.

The Mechanical Laws Based on Newton's Laws of Motion. The effects of physical laws such as gravity, friction, inertia, and momentum should be examined, especially as they relate to any physical compensation by an athlete. Likewise, mechanical advantages and disadvantages with regard to adaptive devices should be explored to determine the best modification for a particular athlete participating in a specific sport. Disabled athletics has been the catalyst for numerous technical advances as a result of modifications developed by athletes.

The Physical Environment and External Conditions. The playing surface (e.g., concrete, grass, wood, or synthetic surface) can have a tremendous impact on an athlete's performance. For example, a wheelchair racer may vary tire pressure with different track surfaces such as asphalt or a synthetic material. Every athlete must make important decisions based on environmental and external conditions. Another example would be a blind sprinter having the option of a sighted guide or a caller who provides auditory instruction to keep the athlete on line. In a noisy stadium, a caller may not be possible or too confusing, and a sighted guide would be mandatory.

The Movements Immediately Preceding or Following the Desired Skill. As with any movement skill, all the components of that skill build on each other and have a direct cause and effect. For example, all throwing performances depend on the windup, acceleration, release, and deceleration or follow-through phases. No one phase acts independently of the others. Therefore, if a cerebral palsy athlete has increased tone in the throwing arm (or anywhere throughout the body), one if not all of the throwing phases may be affected to some degree. As a result, alternative solutions that promote motion away from the limitations may enhance a throwing performance. Throwing the implement backwards over the shoulder or sideways over the head may help increase the arc of motion during the acceleration or deceleration phase.

The Mechanical Efficiency of Adaptive Equipment. Once all the aspects of movement analysis have been completed, the evaluation team must ask how an adaptive device can provide a mechanical advantage to overcome a given limitation. Historically, the majority of innovative adaptive devices for disabled athletics have arisen through the efforts of disabled athletes themselves. One of the most significant advances in recent years has benefited lower extremity amputees. Prosthetic designs have been developed to maximize athletic performance rather than just to facilitate walking. Contemporary socket designs take muscular efficiency into account, prosthetic knees meet the superior cadence demands placed on them, and newer foot materials and configurations optimize athletic performance. The same can be said about wheelchairs, orthotic devices, and other adaptive innovations that have been introduced in recent years. Despite these achievements, there is still considerable room for improvement in this area.

IDENTIFY PERFORMANCE ENHANCEMENT METHODS. Finally, after each of the component skills has been identified and the athlete's current level of performance has been evaluated, a program designed to improve the performance must be outlined. For a disabled athlete, training, equipment, and motivation are paramount when designing a strategy to prepare for competition. Performance enhancement in itself is a major topic of discussion. The following is a brief overview of some considerations for planning a training program for a disabled athlete.

Training Methods. Today there are as many different training programs for athletes as there are successful athletes who would like to share their secret to success. Many of these training methods are sound and well worth taking under advisement. Coaches and medical professionals must consider the nature of the athlete's disability and what, if any, limitations must be placed on the athlete to prevent injury or unnecessary medical complications. Although few disabled athletes have activity restrictions, there are many athletes who will benefit from the following preventive measures when participating in sports or training. Major considerations are outlined in Table 42–3.

Once any precautions are identified, the disabled athlete must begin a physical training program comparable to that of any able-bodied athlete. Similar training principles apply when selecting a strengthening, endurance, agility, speed, or any other type of program. Often a brief biomechanical analysis must be performed when creating a training program. If the athlete cannot use a traditional weight training apparatus because of physical limitations, such as inability to use the hands to grip, alternative methods, such as securing the hand to the handle, may have to be employed. If environmental conditions such as poor weather prohibit a wheelchair athlete from performing the necessary road work for cardiovascular endurance, a roller trainer may be used. In short, the problem-solving process must continue with training as it does with competition, placing as few limitations on the athlete as possible.

Equipment Enhancement. As previously discussed, sport- and disability-specific adaptive equipment can enhance an athlete's performance in a number of ways. The selection and development of adaptive equipment for an individual athlete should be a collective decision, including the athlete, coach, therapist, orthotist, prosthetist, or equipment manufacturer.

TABLE 42–3
Injuries and Disability-Specific Medical Conditions of Athletes with Disabilities

Problem	Prevention	Treatment
Chronic overuse syndromes (shoulder impingement, tendinitis, bursitis, carpal tunnel syndrome)	Taping, splinting, protective padding, proper wheelchair positioning, good technique	Rest; apply injury-specific principles of care; selective strengthening, muscle balancing, flexibility; analysis of technique
Overexertion (muscle strains)	Warm-up and stretching; proper conditioning and equipment	Rest; gradual progression of exercise program
Falls, physical contact (sprains, contusions)	Equipment safety; appropriate padding for sport; appropriate sport-specific spotting; qualified assistance/guides for athletes	Apply injury-specific principles of care; check for signs of fracture in athletes without movement or sensation
Blisters	Encourage callus formation; protective taping, gloves, padding, cushioning; adequate clothing	Apply injury-specific principles of care; be aware of areas that lack sensation; make prosthetic adjustments
Abrasions/lacerations	Check equipment for sharp or abrasive surfaces; wear protective clothing; use cushions or towels in all transfers; use mats on hard surfaces; camber wheelchair wheels	Apply injury-specific principles of care; be aware of areas that lack sensation
Decubitus ulcers and burns	Adequate cushioning; proper weight shifting; dry clothing; special precautions for areas wthout sensation; skin inspection; good nutrition and hygiene	Bed rest if necessary to remove all pressure from a weight-bearing surface; open wound care as necessary; check equipment
Hyperthermia	Minimize exposure to direct sun; provide shade; wear adequate clothing for insulation and maintain hydration; spray externally with water; avoid hot and humid conditions	Remove from ambient conditions; cool immediately; seek medical assistance
Hypothermia	Minimize exposure; wear adequate clothing, keeping head covered; maintain hydration; avoid exposure to cold and wet conditions	Cover and seek medical assistance
Autonomic dysreflexia	Encourage regular bowel and bladder habits in competitive situations	Lift to sitting position; search for source of stimulus, usually full bladder or bowel; attempt to relieve condition; this is a medical emergency
Orthostatic hypotension	Wear elastic stockings or corset supports; avoid heat	Recline in wheelchair or on ground/bed; encourage deep breathing
Seizures	Avoid stress, dehydration, extremes of temperatures, and fatigue	Protect head and keep airway open by jaw thrust; avoid putting objects in the mouth
Unexplained fever (often urinary tract infections)	Drink fluids; practice good hygiene for self-catheterization	Seek medical treatment
Allergies (bee sting, drug)	Notify medical personnel at competition site of potential problem; be prepared	Seek medical treatment
Eye injuries	Protective eyewear, goggles, safety glasses	Apply injury-specific principles of care

Motivation. The motivation of a disabled athlete is no different from the motivation of an able-bodied athlete. As with all athletes, the intrinsic desires that compel an individual to succeed may vary, but the positive methods of motivation available to coaches remain the same. A discussion of the various motivational techniques that may be employed is beyond the scope of this chapter. Supportive personnel must develop a working relationship, and each must learn how to maintain the quest to strive for mutual goals and continued success.

It is important to keep in mind that success is not always defined by winning.

PSYCHOSOCIAL CONSIDERATIONS

Sports involvement has been reported to have positive effects on the physical conditioning and self-image of adults with disabilities.[7] In fact, elite wheelchair athletes have psychologic profiles that are similar to those of elite able-bodied athletes.[8] An athlete with a disability is likely to present similar challenges to medical professionals as an able-bodied athlete, with a few exceptions.

Depending on the age at the onset of the disability and the time since its onset, an athlete with a disability may still be actively engaged in the various stages of the coping process, such as denial, anger, or depression. Frustrations encountered in athletic competition or following an athletic injury may compound already existing feelings of loss or anger. An individual's ability to cope with outside stresses may vary widely, depending on the nature of the disability and the person's internal resources and social support system. However, there is considerable evidence in the literature to support the premise that sports involvement among adults with disabilities promotes improved self-concepts and psychologic well-being.[9]

Additionally, it is important to remember that disabled individuals may have different experiences with the health care system than their able-bodied counterparts. Their access to the health care system has traditionally been through rehabilitation medicine rather than sports medicine. If injured disabled athletes are viewed as disabled persons with injuries, their treatment may be quite different than if they are seen as athletes with injuries who also happen to have permanent disabilities. The goals of the health professionals who treat these patients may vary from merely returning these individuals to an everyday level of performance to returning them to an elite athletic level. It is very important, therefore, to assess the individual athlete's goals and preinjury performance level and design realistic programs accordingly.

Some athletes with disabilities self-treat serious injuries rather than seeking medical assistance.[10,11] This may result in reinjury and the progression to chronic disability. Their training programs may also lack sufficient attention to flexibility and conditioning.[12] The sports rehabilitation team's ability to intervene and prevent chronic soft tissue changes, which increase further risk of injury, is of critical importance.

The active socialization and actual physical activity involved with sports participation may provide benefits for an individual with a disability. Active individuals with disabilities have been reported to have fewer problems with body image, a higher degree of physical function, and fewer medical complications than members of the inactive disabled population.[7,13,14]

It is also important to look at the skills developed through athletic participation. Athletics is an acceptable way to reintegrate with the community. Through athletic participation, there is a de-emphasis on the disability and a focus on goal-oriented objectives and resources. Athletic participation encourages the development of networking skills and interpersonal relationships that may be useful in work settings as well. An individual who participates in athletics becomes less dependent on society and makes more contributions to society. Athletes are motivated to raise funds for equipment and travel and are responsible for themselves during travel. This discipline often carries over to educational and employment endeavors.[15]

Like their able-bodied counterparts, some individuals with disabilities who participate in sports have substance abuse problems with alcohol or drugs. Many athletes with spinal cord injuries were initially injured in an alcohol- or drug-related incident.[16] Sports medicine professionals who work with athletes with disabilities need to be aware of the signs and symptoms of substance abuse and know the appropriate referrals to make.

Another segment of the population of athletes with disabilities has various cognitive and sensory disorders. Athletes who have sustained brain injuries sometimes exhibit behavior that is difficult to understand. Any athlete who becomes combative, abusive, or a danger to himself or herself or to other athletes should be removed to an area where he or she can refocus and calm down, away from any overstimulation that might add to the problem. Athletes who are unable to communicate verbally may use sign language or communication boards. Although not all athletes with disabilities are able to understand instructions, health professionals should not address a companion or coach instead of the athlete.

COMMON INJURIES AND DISABILITY-SPECIFIC MEDICAL PROBLEMS OF ATHLETES WITH DISABILITIES

Preventive practices for disabled athletes are becoming a growing concern among coaches and medical staff alike. Coaches and athletes must be educated in proper warm-up techniques, including stretching, elevating core body temperature, and sport-specific drills. Moreover, all athletes should be required to wear or use the recommended safety gear for every sport. Coaches and event organizers should also be obligated to provide certified or skilled spotters, sighted guides, or assistive personnel to ensure every athlete's safety during competition.

The health professional providing care to athletes with disabilities needs to be aware of common injuries and conditions that are inherent to certain disability groups. Table 42–3 provides information concerning prevention and treatment of common injuries and medical problems of athletes with disabilities. Table 42–4 presents the type and frequency of commonly reported injuries sustained by wheelchair athletes.

INJURIES OF ATHLETES WHO COMPETE IN WHEELCHAIRS

Athletes with disabilities experience athletic injuries related to the specific risks and demands of their sport. Track, road racing, and wheelchair basketball are among the highest-risk sports for athletes who compete in wheelchairs.[10,17] Athletes who train more hours per week and over a longer period of time generally report

TABLE 42–4
Common Injuries of Wheelchair Athletes

	128 Adult Athletes, All Sports[10] (% of 291 Reported Injuries)	90 Adult Athletes, All Sports[17] (% of 346 Reported Injuries)	69 Pediatric Track Athletes[28] (% of Athletes Reporting)	19 Elite Adult Athletes[11] (% of 50 Reported Injuries)
Soft tissue injuries	33	32	34	52
Blisters	18	25	77	6
Lacerations/abrasions	17	27	38	24
Decubitus/pressure areas	7	3	14	Not reported
Arthritis/joint inflammation	5	1.5	Not reported	Not reported
Fractures	5	2	6	6
Hand weakness/numbness	5	Not reported	Not reported	Not reported
Bruises/contusions	Not reported	8	41	10
Temperature regulation disorders	3	Not reported	49	Not reported
Head injury/concussion	2	2	Not reported	Not reported
Dental injury	1	1	Not reported	Not reported
Dislocation	Not reported	<1	Not reported	Not reported
Eye injury	Not reported	<1	Not reported	Not reported
Wheel burns	Included with lacerations	Not reported	71	Not reported
Other illness	Not reported	Not reported	Not reported	2

more injuries than those who have a shorter duration and less intense training history.[10]

The most common injuries to athletes competing in wheelchairs are soft tissue injuries of the shoulder, elbow, and wrist; abrasions and contusions of the arms and hands; and blisters of the hands.[10,11] In addition, the spinal cord–injured population may experience some unique problems, including skin ulceration, temperature regulation disorders, and delayed recognition of injuries in areas that lack sensation.

SOFT TISSUE INJURIES OF UPPER EXTREMITIES

Both novice and veteran wheelchair athletes experience chronic soft tissue problems of the upper extremities. Wheelchair basketball players often practice and play in excess of 15 to 20 hours per week during the basketball season. Elite road racers frequently have training schedules that entail total distances in excess of 100 miles per week. Propelling a wheelchair such distances requires specific repetitive upper extremity motion and therefore stresses the shoulder, elbow, and wrist joints. Rotator cuff injuries, bicipital tendinitis, shoulder impingement syndromes, lateral epicondylitis (tennis elbow), radial extensor muscle tendinitis, and carpal tunnel syndrome are common problems in wheelchair users.[10,18–22] The excessive forces imposed by weight bearing and continuous shoulder use are implicated in the development of chronic shoulder problems. Bayley et al.[23] reported shoulder intra-articular pressures to be 2½ times greater than arterial pressure during wheelchair transfers. Impingement positioning is also frequent in this population, which must frequently engage in overhead activity, even to carry out daily activities.[24] Surgical decompression via

acromioplasty has been reported to be effective in relieving chronic shoulder pain.[25,26] In addition to chronic soft tissue problems, osteonecrosis of the shoulder has been reported in wheelchair users.[27]

Poor flexibility may be a predisposing factor to the development of chronic shoulder problems. Wheelchair pushing stresses development of the chest, anterior shoulder, triceps, and biceps muscles. Specific stretching must be done before and after activity to emphasize flexibility in shoulder flexion, extension, horizontal abduction, and external rotation and to achieve full length of the triceps and biceps muscles, since they are two-joint muscles.

Strength training should emphasize achieving balance at the shoulder, specifically, strengthening of the posterior shoulder, including the posterior deltoid, latissimus dorsi, external rotators, rhomboids, and middle and lower trapezius muscles. Many chronic soft tissue injuries can be prevented and managed by achieving such balance.

Athletes with chronic soft tissue problems of the shoulders or elbows may benefit from preventive use of ice after training. Preventive taping may also be useful with hand, wrist, and elbow problems. The well-known principles of RICE (rest, ice, compression, and elevation) apply to injuries sustained by athletes who compete in wheelchairs. The use of anti-inflammatory medications is also of value in assisting athletes with acute or chronic soft tissue problems. Stretching and strengthening are essential to prevent reinjury.

ABRASIONS AND CONTUSIONS

When athletes use equipment such as wheelchairs, they are also at risk for accidental injury from incidental

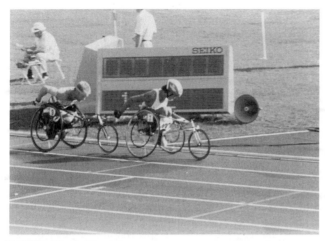

FIGURE 42–4. Wheelchair racers wear protection on the upper arms and use gloves.

contact with the wheelchair parts.[10,28] For example, athletes frequently report friction burns of the inner arms from accidental contact with the large tires during the downstroke in pushing a racing wheelchair. Beginning athletes who are not using equipment that is specific for sports may attempt to train in wheelchairs with wheelchair brakes that are placed dangerously close to the wheelchair push rim. Traumatic injuries of the thumb can easily result from a slip forward during high-intensity pushing.

Simple preventive measures include protecting the upper arm from accidental contact with wheelchair tires, wearing gloves, and wearing a bicycle-type helmet to prevent head injury in the event of collision. Many athletes find it useful to protect the upper arm with the elasticized top of an athletic sock (Fig. 42–4). All wheelchair parts or sharp surfaces that could accidentally result in a contact injury should be removed or covered with protective foam.

BLISTERS

Blisters are a frequent problem for most wheelchair athletes. Because the hands are used continuously for propulsion, athletes may experience frequent problems with blisters of the fingers and thumb from contact with the wheelchair push rim. Thick calluses may develop on the palm of the hand; they can crack and result in painful fissures, open to infection.

Hands should be cleaned frequently and calluses filed with a pumice stone. Open cracks or fissures, blisters, and other abrasions should be managed with antibiotic creams and covered with Band-Aids or dressings, as appropriate. Wheelchair athletes often develop symptoms of carpal tunnel syndrome from the repetitive trauma of wheelchair propulsion, causing compression in the carpal tunnel area.[10,29] Gloves are recommended for training and competition, but recent evidence questions their efficacy in preventing carpal tunnel syndrome.[29] Any athlete with symptoms of hand tingling or numbness should be referred for evaluation for carpal tunnel syndrome.

Leather batting gloves or handball gloves are most easily adapted and reinforced for wheelchair pushing, with layers of tape applied to the areas of highest pressure. Custom-designed leather mitts with reinforced neoprene use Velcro to keep the hand in a closed position, creating a fist, and are widely used in road racing. This innovative glove design incorporates high-friction materials and maximizes the force generated during contact with the push rim. Because of the enhanced power available to the athlete, stroke dynamics have changed, and wrist and elbow injuries may decrease in frequency.

LACK OF PROTECTIVE SENSATION

Spinal cord injury, multiple sclerosis, and other neurologic disorders interfere with the normal protection that pressure, temperature, and pain sensation provide. Pressure points, especially under sitting areas, may lead to skin breakdown, ulceration, and infection. Insensitive skin must be inspected frequently.

Any time there is persistent redness of the skin, that area should have all pressure from sitting, clothes, or equipment relieved until the redness resolves and normal skin color returns. Otherwise, these areas may go on to ulcerate and may progress to serious infections. Athletes with open pressure sores should not participate in competition. Training should cease, and the athlete should avoid sitting or any position that may place him or her at risk for additional pressure damage, until the area is completely healed.

Athletes with chronic pressure sore problems may need customized seating systems that alleviate areas of pressure. Wheelchair cushions can be modified to accommodate an athlete's individual needs. If an athlete has chronic problems due to positioning in the sports wheelchair, he or she should be referred to a physical or occupational therapist for evaluation and recommendations for possible adaptations.

Fractures account for less than 5 percent of all injuries sustained by wheelchair athletes.[10] However, osteoporosis is frequently associated with lower extremity paralysis. As a result, athletes may be susceptible to lower extremity fractures from relatively minor injuries. These fractures may go unnoticed because of the lack of sensation that would normally accompany a bony fracture. Therefore, following any injury, one must be aware of signs and symptoms such as abnormal body position, bruising, edema, or grinding sensations with movement. The athlete should be evaluated by x-ray to rule out a fracture, as movement of bony fragments may interfere with healing and cause further damage to muscles and blood vessels.

By using such simple preventive techniques, athletes who compete in wheelchairs can have safe and productive competitive careers.

INJURIES OF ATHLETES WHO COMPETE STANDING

Athletes with disabilities who compete while standing represent a variety of physical disabilities and sports interests. They often compete with disabilities such as upper and lower extremity amputations, visual deficits, and cerebral palsy. These athletes do not appear to be at greater risk for the common musculoskeletal problems associated with sports participation in the general population.[12] Although musculoskeletal problems may be no more frequent for athletes with disabilities, disability-related problems are seen among athletes who wear prostheses for running and athletes who sustain falls and other accidental injuries secondary to their disabilities or the use of assistive devices.

ABRASIONS AND BLISTERS TO BONY PROMINENCES WITHIN PROSTHETIC SOCKET

Many lower extremity amputees run wearing prostheses. Common problems are skin breakdown, bruising, abrasion, blistering, skin rashes, and swelling on the residual limb, within the prosthetic socket, after or during exercise. These problems can sometimes be prevented by proper adjustment of prosthetic fit and alignment and prompt management of developing skin lesions.

Common sites for these problems in below-knee amputees are the fibula head, distal anterior end of the tibia, distal end of the fibula, medial and lateral femoral condyles, over the patella, and over scar tissue and poorly healed skin. Above-knee amputees may experience similar problems over the pubic or ischial rami, over the ischial tuberosities, at the distal lateral femur, over the greater trochanter, or over sites of scar tissue or poor healing.

Depending on the nature of the injury or trauma sustained, it may be appropriate to use a number of different management strategies. For bruising and blisters, the athlete can relieve friction by wearing additional (dry) stump socks or foam pads, or by applying abrasion protection products (Second Skin, Spenco; Bioclusive, Johnson & Johnson; DuoDerm, E. R. Squibb; Tegaderm, 3M Canada, Inc.; Ampu-Balm, Southern Prosthetic Supply) over soft tissue areas that commonly break down as a result of continual friction. Unfortunately, in most cases the application of foam or leather padding may cause total-contact suction sockets to lose suction, and pistoning may result.

Ideally, the pads are used prophylactically prior to the event. However, often they are applied after a blister has formed to permit continued participation. Use of these protective pads must be monitored regularly, especially during long-distance events, because once the inner silicone gel dries out, the outer covering material can become a source of irritation.

It may be appropriate to use rest, ice, and compression and to decrease additional trauma to the limb through supported ambulation with crutches or a cane.

COMPRESSION INJURIES

The absorption of ground reaction forces generated during support limb impact in able-bodied athletes is accomplished by the mechanics of the foot-ankle complex, rotation of long bones, flexion of all lower extremity joints, and insulation of muscle. Amputee runners lack many, if not all, of these shock-absorbing mechanisms and thus are prone to many "impact" or "compression" injuries. All these injuries are the result of the ground forces being transmitted to the socket via the prosthetic pylon. Above- and below-knee amputees often experience bruising over the bony prominences listed above. In addition, above-knee amputees with ischial containment socket designs often complain of excessive pressure from the medial wall.

Recurrent skin problems, bruising, or recurrent tendinitis should lead to suspicion of prosthetic malalignment or a misfitting socket. The prosthetist, coach, and athlete should be able to work together to evaluate the athlete's needs and adjust or redesign an appropriate prosthesis. Modification of the patella tendon bar for below-knee amputees or modification of the height of the anterior or medial socket wall for above-knee amputees may provide some relief from compressive forces.

FALLS

Accidental falls are likely to occur in runners with disabilities, as a result of uneven ground surfaces and environmental conditions. Falling is the most common cause of hand abrasions. Ambulatory athletes with disabilities may use special equipment such as prostheses, crutches, and canes, which are subject to fatigue and sudden breakdown, especially in the face of the uncommon stress associated with athletics. Blind runners present an obvious problem in that they lack the visual acuity to detect environmental hazards in their path. Sighted guides are critical to their optimal and safe performance.

Some athletes with disabilities wear bicycle helmets when running to provide an extra measure of safety, if they have problems with footing or balance. Athletes who use assistive devices such as crutches or canes should check for cracks or fissures in metal shafts or rubber tips prior to use.

All athletes with disabilities should take the same precautions recommended to athletes in the general population to help prevent accidents. Wearing reflective clothing at night, running defensively when there are cars or bicycles present, carrying identification that includes pertinent medical information, and dressing appropriately for a workout will help improve safety margins.

It is strongly recommended that athletes with disabilities train with other athletes or groups who can provide companionship, support, and an extra measure of safety. Volunteers who run with blind athletes especially must be able to concentrate on obstacles and sudden environmental changes, as well as individual athletic needs and performance.

LOW BACK PAIN

Some athletes with disabilities also experience chronic low back pain. Athletes with tightness of the hip flexor muscles often compensate with increased mobil-

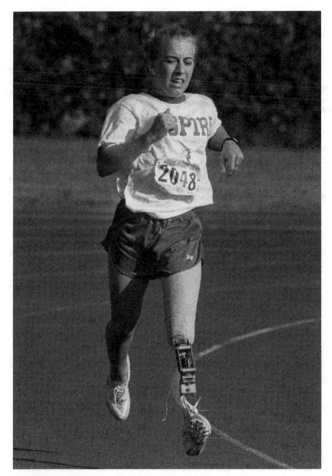

FIGURE 42–5. Above-knee amputee sprinter.

ity in the lumbar spine. Amputees often overuse the lumbar spine as a compensatory mechanism. Because of the forces transmitted through a rigid, unforgiving prosthesis, amputees, especially above-knee amputees, must compensate for the lack of lower extremity joint flexion with excessive lumbar spine lateral flexion and extension (Fig. 42–5). Greater lateral lumbar flexion is observed during early support, and increased lumbar extension is observed during late support as the maximal hip extension is being achieved. As a result of daily ambulation and running, an imbalance in back musculature, as well as a functional scoliosis, may be observed in many amputees.

Muscle balancing, stretching, and traditional prophylactic low back pain measures may be employed to assist an athlete experiencing low back pain as the result of excessive lumbar movement or hip flexor tightness.

BURSITIS

Rarely, amputees complain of bursa pain from socket irritation. On these occasions, below-knee amputees most frequently experience prepatellar, infrapatellar, or pretibial bursa pain. Above-knee amputees complain of ischial and trochanteric bursitis. Bursitis, when it occurs in amputees, is often the result of poor prosthetic fit. Necessary prosthetic modifications should be made.

KNEE INJURIES

Athletes with cerebral palsy often show genu valgum and mechanical instability at the knee. In addition, quadriceps muscles may be spastic and tight. Even though knee instability and muscle imbalance may be present, it is not clear that these predispose such athletes to a higher risk of injury.

Below-knee and Syme's amputees may be considered vulnerable to many more knee injuries than actually occur because of the rigid lever constituted by the prosthesis. Most socket designs bring the medial and lateral wall well above the knee joint line, reducing the chance of collateral ligament injury. In most cases, the residual limb pulls away from the socket rather than being fixed within the socket.

Jumping events such as the long jump put amputees at the greatest risk of knee injury. Occasionally, hyperextension injuries occur as a result of the body's forward momentum over a fixed prosthesis and residual limb.

INJURIES TO THE SOUND LIMB

In amputee athletes, the sound limb often sustains injuries as a result of the stresses endured by compensating for the prosthetic limb. Frequently, chronic hamstring problems arise as a result of the altered hip flexion of both lower extremities.

The sound limb foot also must adapt to the additional weight bearing that is often associated with amputees who hop on and utilize the sound limb more than the prosthetic limb. Some individuals develop plantar fasciitis, stretched plantar ligaments, or foot imbalances such as pronation because of the additional abnormal forces.

Treatment of injuries to runners with disabilities should follow the same principles and guidelines that apply to able-bodied and sighted runners. Rest, ice, compression, and elevation (RICE), sport orthotics, athletic taping, and sports rehabilitation are all effective techniques for treating the musculoskeletal problems of runners with disabilities.

INJURIES TO THE UPPER EXTREMITIES IN CRUTCH USERS

Some lower extremity amputees prefer to compete without a prosthesis, using crutches to assist in their mobility. As with all crutch users, care must be taken to avoid hand and wrist injuries such as carpal tunnel problems at the wrist and neurovascular compression at the axilla. Athletes who use crutches should be encouraged to use and frequently replace rubber padding on hand grips and under axillae.

ENERGY REQUIREMENTS FOR AMPUTEE RUNNERS

The metabolic cost of ambulation has been well documented as being 15 to 30 percent higher for transtibial amputees while walking at a pace 10 to 40 percent slower than nonamputees[30–37] and 40 to 65 percent higher for transfemoral amputees who ambulate at a pace 15 to 50 percent slower than nonamputees.[37–40] The discrepancy in metabolic cost of ambulation is directly related to age, cause of amputation, length of residual limb, and prosthetic design.[37,41,42] To date, no studies have been published examining the metabolic cost of amputee running, but it appears that a considerable physiologic demand is placed on amputee runners for several reasons. In addition to the reasons previously stated, alteration of the normal kinematics of the running gait, such as a transfemoral amputee's inability to flex the prosthetic knee during stance or the lack of normal foot-ankle motions, increases the physiologic demands.[43–47] There are also kinetic and musculoskeletal disadvantages, such as the fact that an amputee's knee musculature absorbs only 1.4 times as much energy as it generates, compared with 3.6 times as much for a nonamputee jogger.[43,45] Increased demands are placed on the sound limb as well; for example, the sound limb is responsible for approximately 90 percent of the total energy generated during running.[43] The loss of the amputated limb also decreases the total body surface area available for physiologic thermoregulation for cooling the body.

Collectively, all these influences can increase the physiologic demands placed on an amputee runner and result in greater fatigue, potential hyperthermia, and injuries related to musculoskeletal imbalances. Hyperthermia is rarely a problem in running events, since 1500 meters is the longest distance permitted in international amputee track competition. However, there are a few amputee marathon runners and a great number of cyclists who could be at risk for developing hyperthermia.

REHABILITATION OF SPORTS INJURIES

The rehabilitative management of disabled athletes is similar to that of any other athlete. The rehabilitation must be a comprehensive program designed to return the disabled athlete to his or her sport with the greatest degree of function and in the shortest time possible. Just as an able-bodied athlete's program must be progressive and functional, so must a disabled athlete's rehabilitation program. Therefore, a general rehabilitation program should include warm-up, strengthening, flexibility, coordination, proprioception, balance, speed, agility, and muscular and cardiovascular endurance and conclude with a cool-down period. Some exercises may have to be adapted to meet the needs of the individual athlete.

One such adaptation is for cardiorespiratory endurance training. Athletes with sympathetic nervous system involvement, such as individuals with neurologic lesions above T4, have diminished heart rate and blood pressure responses to exercise. This diminished sympathetic response limits the use of heart rate and blood pressure as effective indicators of exercise intensity. Age-adjusted formulas for calculating target heart rates cannot be used easily with this population. Therefore, exercise prescriptions for these athletes may include parameters of speed, duration, frequency, or mechanical resistance rather than using a target heart rate to vary intensity.

It is also important to note that an athlete with a disability is often unable to rest an injury completely due to the demands for continued daily function. For example, a wheelchair athlete who sustains a shoulder injury is unable to rest because demands of everyday mobility require the use of the shoulder joint. An amputee who injures the sound limb will have increased difficulty with ambulation if the prosthetic limb becomes the dominant limb. In order to regain the ability to perform everyday tasks, the temptation to increase the use of the injured extremity prematurely may increase recovery time and the risk of injury. Alternatives to daily activities, rehabilitation, and training methods designed to reduce the risk of insult to the injured limb should be explored by the physical therapist and athlete.

EDUCATION AND INJURY PREVENTION

Educating athletes as to the most effective means of prevention is an important task for both coaching and sports medicine staff. Commonsense coaching and sports medicine techniques; familiarization with the disability by the athlete, coach, and volunteers; planned workouts; and a thought toward safety can help prevent injuries, minimize risks, and ensure success.

DISABILITY-SPECIFIC MEDICAL PROBLEMS

In addition to injuries, pre-existing medical conditions, the requirements of sport participation, and environmental conditions expose athletes with disabilities to the risk of specific medical problems.

TEMPERATURE REGULATION DISORDERS

Thermal injuries are common problems in all athletes with disabilities. Exposure to heat and cold often provides unique challenges to an athlete with a disability.[48] The athlete may be intolerant to conditions that would not particularly trouble an able-bodied athlete, due to sensory impairments, sympathetic nervous system dysfunction, and inadequate body mechanisms for cooling or warming. Additionally, specific medications (tranquilizers, diuretics, sedative-hypnotics, alcohol, sympathomimetics, anticholinergics, and thyroid replacement drugs) predispose an athlete to problems with temperature regulation.

Equipment and surfaces such as asphalt or metal may heat up in the sun and cause burns to a person without sensation. Similarly, individuals with paralyzed limbs often have impaired circulation, with a tendency to develop swelling of their feet, since their muscles do not assist in venous return. Along with this is a relatively lower blood flow to the skin and deep tissues. This makes the limb more susceptible to sunburn or frostbite, and even lesser degrees of heat or cold may cause serious deep tissue damage.

In addition, in spinal cord injury and in multiple sclerosis, there are problems with regulation of core body temperature due to a loss of normal blood flow regulation via the central nervous system. Athletes with quadriplegia often report heat and cold intolerance.[10] This is compounded by an inability to sweat below the level of a spinal cord injury. Many medications used for pain, depression, allergy, bladder dysfunction, high blood pressure, and other problems also interfere with normal sweating.

HYPOTHERMIA

Tolerance to cold is affected by an athlete's level of physical fitness, percentage of body fat, wind, and water immersion. There are adverse effects on athletic performance if the body's core temperature drops. Early symptoms of hypothermia include weakness, fatigue, clumsy movements, slurring speech, and a decreased shivering response. Later symptoms are collapse and unconsciousness. Hypothermia is potentially serious, or even fatal, because it may result in cardiac arrhythmias and dysfunction of other body systems.[49] The risk of hypothermia is greatly increased by exercising in extremely cold weather, especially if there is a high windchill factor or the athlete does not pay attention to skin and clothes wetness.

An athlete who has had a spinal cord injury (usually competing in a wheelchair or sit-ski) may not have sensation below the level of the neurologic lesion to feel cold extremities. In addition, normal mechanisms of piloerection (goose bumps), shivering, and circulatory shunting for warming may not take place. This is especially a problem when it is both cold and wet. Even temperatures around 50° F may be a problem for an athlete with a spinal cord injury above the midthoracic level.[48]

The following general principles apply to prevent hypothermia in an athlete with a disability. Protective clothing should be worn whenever possible, and the clothing should keep the athlete comfortable during the activity. Multiple layers of clothes should be used to take advantage of air trapped between the layers. The innermost layer should carry moisture away from the body, as cooling occurs more rapidly if the skin surface is wet. Polypropylene and cotton are recommended materials. Additionally, the head should be covered to prevent heat loss, since as much as 25 percent of heat loss occurs from the head. Wearing hats and helmets when training or competing in cold weather is essential to maintain body temperature.

Athletes should be encouraged to drink adequate fluids. Thirst is an unreliable indicator of the state of hydration, and athletes may become as quickly dehydrated in cold, dry climates as in hot climates. Water is lost with hard breathing and perspiration under cold conditions as well as hot conditions.

Those athletes who are predisposed to cold intolerance should take special precautions during training and competition. Athletes with a past history of cold injury (frostbite) may suffer further trauma. Older athletes may have poorer circulation to the extremities and may be subject to greater intolerance to cold. In addition, an athlete who has a communication or cognitive disorder may not be able to communicate symptoms of cold intolerance readily. Special attention must be given to making sure that these athletes are well supervised to recognize potential problems.

Special attention should be given to awareness of environmental conditions (windchill factor, wet conditions), wearing appropriate clothing and head covering, hydration, and training intensity and duration. After training or competition, the athlete should go to a warm, dry environment and remove cold or wet garments and dress in warm, dry garments so that there is no postexercise lowering of the body temperature. Superficial frostbite can be treated by placing the affected area under a warmer body part or by blowing warm air onto the body part.[49] The most effective treatment for an athlete with hypothermia is medically supervised rewarming by using thermal blankets, intravenous fluid replacement, and warm baths. Hypothermia can be a life-threatening condition, requiring prompt medical attention.[50] The principles of treating a hypothermic athlete with a disability are essentially the same as for treating athletes without disabilities, with added awareness of the possibility of pre-existing sensory and autonomic nervous system dysfunction.

HYPERTHERMIA

Intolerance to heat is exacerbated by the environmental temperature and humidity. Mild symptoms of heat illness are characterized by muscle cramps after exercising in the heat. More severe heat illness results in heat exhaustion, and the athlete may complain of headache, nausea, vomiting, lightheadedness, weakness, cramps, and general malaise. Most severe is heatstroke, where the athlete's body temperature may rise dangerously high. The athlete's performance will deteriorate, and he or she may become confused and disoriented and may faint. He or she may not sweat normally and may experience personality changes. This athlete is at risk for multiple organ damage, which can be prevented with quick treatment.

Athletes with disabilities should exercise extreme caution when high temperatures are accompanied by high humidity. High humidity prevents cooling of the body by normal sweating. High ambient temperatures do not allow for heat dissipation from the body to the environment. In warm climates, under these conditions, athletes and coaches should plan training and competitions in the early morning or evening hours to prevent exposure to peak heat conditions.

Clothing should be worn to provide shade and hold moisture for heat loss. Light clothing, in light colors, with "breathable" fibers are the best attire for exercise in very hot conditions. Disabled athletes should be encouraged to wear shirts, instead of removing them in hot conditions, because of the added protection. Clothing can provide protection from the sun's rays as well as assist with cooling by holding moisture close to the skin.

Sunscreens should be used whenever athletes will be exposed to the sun. An athlete with a spinal cord injury may have a particularly increased risk of sunburn in areas without sensation due to circulatory changes. Although sunscreens are helpful in protecting against sunburn, water-resistant sunscreens can also make the athlete more susceptible to heat intolerance by impeding perspiration. Thus, care should be taken to cover only those areas exposed to the sun, especially in athletes who may not perspire normally.

Athletes with disabilities sometimes lack physiologic mechanisms for cooling. Athletes with spinal cord injuries (especially quadriplegia) and others with neurologic dysfunction above the level of the first thoracic segment (T1) are particularly susceptible to heat intolerance. These athletes do not sweat below the level of the neurologic lesion and therefore cannot lower their body temperature by this form of heat exchange.

Close monitoring and preventive measures, such as spraying the surface of the face, neck, upper trunk, and arms with water from a spray bottle, should be routine. Although there is no evidence that spraying with water lowers the core temperature of normal athletes, the experience of spinal cord–injured athletes seems to support that this is a useful practice. Even more important, however, is staying out of the sun and wearing protective clothing.

Special attention should be paid during field event competition, which may involve hours of waiting in hot, sunny conditions. Athletes should be encouraged to rest in shaded, cooler, well-ventilated areas prior to and following competition.

Athletes who have medical conditions that predispose them to heat intolerance should be closely monitored. Older athletes and young children may also experience more severe problems. In addition, athletes with heart disease, diabetes, high blood pressure, and sweat gland dysfunction may have a higher incidence of heat illness. Of course, any athlete who has an acute problem such as an infection, nausea, vomiting, fever, diarrhea, fatigue, or pre-existing dehydration may be particularly intolerant to the heat. These individuals should refrain from training and competition until the acute condition improves. Close monitoring of clothing, fluid intake, and body temperature is essential to the safe participation of high-risk athletes in extreme environmental conditions.

Any athlete showing signs of heat intolerance should be removed to a shaded, cool, well-ventilated area and treated for heat illness. Any athlete displaying headache, lightheadedness, or general malaise in the heat should discontinue exercise and be taken to a shaded, well-ventilated area. Medical attention is essential to cool the athlete as quickly as possible. Fluid replacement and cooling at the neck, groin, and armpits are often adequate to reverse symptoms, although more extensive treatment may be indicated.

Athletes who have communication or cognitive disorders may not communicate symptoms of heat intolerance readily. Special attention must be given to making sure that these athletes are well supervised to recognize potential problems. Fluid replacement should be offered frequently by coaches or staff to all cognitively impaired athletes to prevent heat illness.

HYDRATION

Thirst is an unreliable indicator of the state of hydration. Athletes should be encouraged to drink water continually, regardless of thirst, and to avoid salt tablets and undiluted electrolyte solutions. Athletes should drink at least 1 liter (about a quart) of water 1 to 2 hours before competition or training and half a liter (16 oz) of water 15 to 30 minutes before the event. Fluid replacement should continue at a rate of at least 400 to 500 cc (13 to 16 oz) every 15 to 30 minutes during training or competition. Following practice or competition, the athlete should continue with 1 to 2 liters of fluid.[50]

Cool (45 to 55° F) water is the best form of fluid replacement for events lasting less than 1 hour, as they tend to be more rapidly absorbed than warm water.[50] Glucose and electrolyte solutions and carbohydrate polymer solutions may be beneficial in events lasting over 1 hour, as they delay the onset of fatigue. Solutions should be of a concentration of less than 10 percent; a concentration of 6 to 8 percent is ideal. If an athlete drinks electrolyte solutions or sweetened drinks, he or she should be sure that the drink is well diluted or should drink an equal amount of water. Alcoholic beverages and caffeine-containing beverages should be avoided because they cause further dehydration.

Certain athletes with developmental disabilities may not be able to reliably monitor their own fluid intake. Coaches should be especially cognizant of the fluid needs of this population or cognitively impaired athletes. It may be helpful to monitor the athlete's weight daily in hot conditions and increase fluid replacement accordingly. Any change in weight greater than 2 percent daily may indicate dehydration and should be treated accordingly.

Some athletes with disabilities restrict water intake because of bladder incontinence. Coaches need to assure that athletes have access to adequate bathroom facilities rather than risk heatstroke due to poor fluid intake in hot weather.

BLADDER DYSFUNCTION

Athletes with neurologic disorders such as spinal cord injury or multiple sclerosis often have a neurogenic bladder. Because the bladder does not always empty properly or completely, bladder infections, bladder stones, and bladder obstruction are common to wheelchair athletes with neurogenic bladder.

Those who have indwelling catheters to drain the bladder and, to a lesser degree, those who use catheters to drain the bladder on an intermittent schedule usually have frequent, if not constant, bacteria in their urine. When bacteria invade the bladder wall, the infection can spread into the kidneys and blood stream, causing severe illness and death. Therefore, any infection needs prompt treatment with antibiotics. Athletes should refrain from competition and training for at least 8 hours after the initiation of antibiotic treatment and should be without a fever for at least 24 hours before resuming participation.

To prevent recurrent bladder infection, athletes should ensure adequate fluid intake to flush the bladder regularly. They must also have access to clean areas to allow good technique to avoid contamination during the handling and use of catheters and connecting tubing and bags.

If catheter tubing becomes blocked, the athlete may develop a bladder obstruction and be unable to urinate. Bladder obstruction can obstruct blood flow back to the heart by pressure on the inferior vena cava, or cause abnormally high blood pressure by stimulation of reflex activity. If bladder obstruction precipitates autonomic dysreflexia, blood pressure can rise dangerously high and even cause a cerebral hemorrhage. Also, rapid relief of an obstruction may cause a precipitous drop in blood pressure and result in shock damage to the heart or kidneys. Exercise may exacerbate these problems.

HYPOTENSION

Wheelchair athletes with multiple sclerosis and spinal cord injury may experience hypotension with rapid position changes, due to the inability of the sympathetic nervous system to accommodate for a rapidly shifting blood volume. Infections from pressure sores may also cause pressure drop. Pain, antispasticity, antiseizure, and bladder and bowel medications may all affect blood pressure regulation. This may cause problems in endurance activities and even lead to lightheadedness or fainting.

If an athlete in a wheelchair experiences lightheadedness due to hypotension, help the individual to a recumbent position or tip the wheelchair back. These maneuvers will help increase venous return. Gentle pressure on the abdomen with deep breathing may also be helpful. If problems with lightheadedness continue, the athlete should be referred to a physician for evaluation of the problem.

HYPERTENSION

Autonomic dysreflexia is a serious problem of spinal cord–injured athletes whose lesions are above the midthoracic level. This reflexive process, causing massive sympathetic outflow, often begins from an obstruction of bowel or bladder. Any spinal cord–injured athlete with sudden hypertension or pounding headache should be suspected of having autonomic dysreflexia.

This is a medical emergency. The individual should assume or remain in a sitting position if possible to minimize blood pressure. The bladder should be emptied and the bowel evacuated; the condition should then be re-evaluated. Immediate medical intervention should follow if the hypertension has not resolved.

Recent studies have revealed that many elite wheelchair athletes with quadriplegia routinely self-induce autonomic dysreflexia to increase sympathetic outflow and improve performance during competition.[51,52] With autonomic dysreflexia, the athlete experiences uncontrollably high hypertension, which may lead to cerebral hemorrhage and death. "Boosting" via clamping a catheter or inducing a painful stimulus is a dangerous and foolhardy practice and should be discouraged among all athletes.

BLOOD FLOW

Some muscle and joint diseases have associated problems with spasm of the arteries of the hands and feet that may be induced by cold. Edema or swelling in paralyzed limbs may be increased by generalized increased blood flow with exercise or prolonged sitting with straps around the legs or trunk. If blood flow is obstructed, there may be problems with venous return and development of thrombophlebitis. Persistent swelling in a leg that does not get better with elevation may indicate thrombophlebitis, although symptoms usually occur without warning. Fragments of the thrombus may break off, resulting in pulmonary embolus, often a life-threatening complication.

Edema should resolve with elevation of the extremities. Redness or heat in the area can signify a serious problem. Edema of the lower extremities should be treated by removing obstructive straps and reclining and elevating the limbs above the heart. Individuals with persistent edema with signs of inflammation should be properly evaluated for infectious processes or thrombophlebitis and treated appropriately.

DYSPHAGIA

Athletes with cerebral palsy sometimes present with dysphagia or difficulty swallowing. An athlete with dysphagia may drool saliva from the mouth, which can cause a great deal of fluid loss. In addition, an athlete who has difficulty swallowing may choke on water or soft drinks.

Since an athlete with dysphagia is at risk for losing fluids by drooling, coaches and supportive personnel should ensure that the athlete has access to fluids that are easy to swallow and that straws are available. Generally, athletes with dysphagia are able to swallow frequent small amounts of thicker liquids, such as juices, more easily than water. Since dehydration may be a problem, avoiding exposure to the sun is also important.

DYSARTHRIA

Dysarthria, or difficulty controlling the oral and vocal musculature to speak, may be seen in the cerebral palsy and brain-injured populations. Although many athletes have both dysphagia and dysarthria, the two conditions are not always present together. An athlete with dysarthria may not be able to express his or her needs quickly or in a way that is easy to understand. Health professionals should be careful not to assume, however, that expressive problems also mean that the athlete does not understand. They should take the time to communicate simply and directly. It may help to speak clearly and slowly, using simple, direct instructions.

APHASIA

Brain-injured athletes and a small percentage of cerebral palsy athletes may present with aphasia. This is a problem either in receiving and processing the verbal information presented (usually fluent aphasia) or in formulating a verbal message to be expressed (usually nonfluent aphasia).

It may be helpful to use writing or gestures to communicate if there is a language problem. Those with significant communication problems may need to communicate through a coach. Always use direct communication with the athlete first, before communicating through another person. Athletes with pre-existing medical problems should carry written instructions or wear Medic-Alert bracelets at all times in the event that a coach or team member is not present and an emergency arises.

BEHAVIORAL PROBLEMS

With the overstimulation of athletic competition, some brain-injured athletes may become agitated, excited, or occasionally hostile or abusive. Specific intervention techniques to remove the athlete from the situation and redirect his or her attention may help reduce distress. It may be helpful to isolate the athlete from the stimulus in a medical tent or other quiet area. Attempting to reason, argue, or debate may only make the situation worse and provoke a more agitated response. It is usually helpful to redirect the athlete's attention.

SEIZURE DISORDERS

Some cerebral palsy athletes have a history of seizure disorders. Seizures do not often occur during sports competition because the state of metabolic acidosis that frequently accompanies hypoxia stabilizes neuronal membranes. The most likely time for a seizure to occur is during travel and other times of stress, dehydration, and extremes of temperature. Seizure activity should be suspected following a syncopal episode in which there is no other explanation.

Routine safety measures apply during seizure activity to protect the head and airway. Following the seizure or in the postictal period, it is important to do a neurologic examination to look for deficits, signs of head injury, contusions, or neck pain. The athlete may be confused and should be encouraged to rest. Hos-

pitalization is required only if the seizure activity is new or different from that experienced previously. A coach or other responsible party should, however, check the athlete's responsiveness every 2 hours for the first 24 hours.

A medication history and schedule should be reviewed, as athletes often forget to take seizure medications such as phenytoin (Dilantin), carbamazepine (Tegretol), or phenobarbital in the excitement of travel and competition. Fatigue and dehydration may also precipitate the onset of seizure activity and may need to be addressed.

CRITERIA FOR TRAVEL

There are numerous areas in which sports medicine applies to athletes and teams that are traveling for competition. A medical staff member with a group of athletes with disabilities has many significant roles in the pretrip planning, as well as providing services during the competition.

PRETRIP HEALTH SCREENING AND EMERGENCY CONTACT INFORMATION

Athletes should complete forms that include current name and address, physician's name and address, emergency contacts, insurance coverage, past medical history, a list of current medications, and current medical problems. Some organizations and teams require that athletes have a physical examination within 3 to 6 months of departure. It is also important to have a mechanism to ensure that other medical problems have not developed in the interim between sending in the medical information and the departure date. Infections, pressure sores, traumatic injuries, seizures, or hospitalizations that have occurred in this interim period require attention by the medical staff to determine the current stability of the athlete's condition and his or her fitness for travel and competition.

EDUCATION ON DOPING FOR INTERNATIONAL COMPETITIONS

Athletes with disabilities are subject to the same antidoping regulations as able-bodied athletes, regardless of their medical problems. Athletes need to be educated about banned over-the-counter and prescription medications. If an athlete is taking a medication that is banned, he or she needs to call the USOC Drug Hotline (1-800-233-0393) in Colorado Springs, Colorado, or the Sport Medicine and Science Council of Canada in Ottawa, Ontario (613-748-5671), to discuss alternatives. The athlete then needs to consult with his or her physician to determine which nonbanned medications could be substituted. Athletes with disabilities must be especially careful, because even traces of prescription medications such as sympathomimetics, antihypertensives, diuretics, corticosteroids, or pain medications routinely prescribed in the management of their chronic medical conditions may result in a positive drug test. It is critical that alternative nonbanned medications be prescribed well in advance of the competition, as some banned medications can be detected in the urine as long as several months after the last dose was taken. It is also important to remember that all over-the-counter medications and prescription medications that the medical team brings should meet the USOC or SMSCC guidelines as well.

PRETRIP INFORMATION AND PLANNING

Athletes who are traveling must bring sufficient medications and supplies, such as catheters and gloves, for their care for the duration of the trip. This needs to be emphasized in writing to all athletes, as medications, services, and supplies are often difficult to find in other countries. State Department and Centers for Disease Control advisories for pretrip immunizations should be followed. Athletes and staff must receive this information several months prior to departure, in many cases, to achieve desired immunity.

JET LAG EDUCATION

Athletes traveling over several time zones often experience problems with eating and sleep cycles due to the abrupt time change. These changes can impact performance dramatically. To minimize changes, athletes are encouraged to change watches to the destination time zone immediately on departure. They are encouraged to sleep and wake at a time appropriate for the destination. Meals should also be adjusted accordingly. Athletes are encouraged to stay well hydrated and to use natural light, rather than stimulants such as caffeine, to assist in staying awake during the day in the new time zone. Sleep cycles should remain at 6 to 8 hours, and athletes should avoid the temptation to take long naps during midday. Alcohol should be avoided during the trip due to its depressant and diuretic effects.

ATTENTION TO HYDRATION AND NUTRITION OUTSIDE NORTH AMERICA

Athletes may not tolerate all food and water in other countries, and water and food may not meet standards of sanitation. Unlabeled water sources, in particular, may not be safe for consumption. It is important to provide a clean water source for the athletes' hydration needs, which may mean that the team must immediately purchase cases of bottled water to be kept in the housing area and brought to the competition site. Athletes should be aware of when it is essential to drink bottled water and to be cautious about food choices. Food from street vendors in any country should be avoided. Ice made from contaminated water is often overlooked and may cause serious gastrointestinal problems when added to bottled water.

Athlete nutrition may suffer from changes in diet. With decreased protein intake, immune system function may be compromised.[53] It is a good idea to advise athletes to bring a supply of high-protein food sources from home for emergencies and for supplementation of the local diet. Choices such as nuts, trail mix, peanut butter, cans of tuna fish, and small packages of cereal may provide protein to supplement the diet at the competition site.

EQUIPMENT FOR TRAVEL

Medical staff who are traveling with groups of athletes with disabilities should bring a well-stocked trainer's bag, including first-aid supplies and emergency equipment (Table 42–5). It is helpful to have

TABLE 42–5
Suggested Items for First-Aid Kit for Travel with Disabled Athletic Teams

Scissors: 7-in. tape scissors, small suture scissors
Tape cutter
Fingernail cutter
Penlight
Tongue forceps
Tweezers
1-in. adhesive tape (2–3)
1½-in adhesive tape (6–8)
½-in adhesive tape (2)
2-in Elastikon tape (2–3)
1-in dermal tape (1–2)
Ace wraps 2-in., 4-in, 6-in (2 each)
Contact lens solution
Eye wash
Taping base (Tuf Skin spray)
Tape underwrap (4–6)
Gauze pads (4 × 4, 3 × 3, large) (4–6 each)
Telfa pads (nonadherent, various sizes) (2–3 each)
Finger splints
Petroleum jelly
Antiseptic soap
Aspirin, Tylenol, ibuprofen
Antacid (liquid or tablets)
Band-Aids (various sizes)
Steri-strips (butterfly bandages are second choice)
Cotton-tipped applicators
Padding: cotton; sponge (miscellaneous) ¼ and ½ in.; only felt (miscellaneous) ¼ and ½ in.
Fungicide ointment
Alcohol and/or Betadine swabs
Antibacterial cream
Plastic bags for ice or instant cold paks
Moleskin
Second Skin Blister Pak
Peroxide, 6 oz.
Ampu Balm
Sterile catheters
Sterile and nonsterile rubber gloves
Mirror (small)
Thermometer (oral)
Sunscreen lotion (seasonal/location)
Small spray bottle
Triangular bandage or sling
Pocket CPR mask or shield
Portable, battery-operated ultrasound and electrical stimulation units

TABLE 42–6
Typical Committees for a Competition for Athletes with Disabilities

- Sponsorship
- Medical
- Classification
- Technical/event/officiating
- Manpower
- Accommodations
- Meals/refreshments
- Transportation
- Registration/packets
- Command post (on-site information center)
- Awards
- Computer operations
- Correspondence
- Entertainment
- Equipment
- Outfitters
- Athlete assistance
- Public relations and marketing

TABLE 42–7
Typical Responsibilities of Medical Committee Members

- Medical history forms (athletes, coaches, staff, and volunteers)
- Command post directives/hot lines
- Medical information flyers (athletes, coaches, staff, and volunteers)
- Local hospital notification and coordination
- Community medical staff alert (emergency medical staff, doctors, nurses, etc.)
- Event medical coverage
- Practice field medical coverage
- Medical tent for events
- Adaptive equipment repair tent (wheelchair, prosthesis, etc.)
- Injury report forms
- Disability emergent care information sheets for staff (a memory jogger for medical staff who don't often work with disabled athletes)
- First-aid kit checklist
- Appropriate personal coverage

electrical stimulation and ultrasound units that are battery operated, can be recharged, or run on local current. Since voltages (and wall plugs) often vary, staff should be prepared with a variety of adapters and converters. It is often easier to use a battery-operated unit and bring a supply of batteries.

FOREIGN FACILITIES

It is important to remember that the facilities for treating athletes or acquiring ice in other countries may be quite different from those at home. A treatment room may not be available, and a medical staff person must sometimes improvise by providing treatment on the team bus, in the athlete's room, or on a bench at a sport venue. Ice is frequently not as available as it is in North America.

The medical staff must be aware of the mechanism for managing a serious injury or problem. Emergency services and contacts should be established, and the local hospital identified. Local organizers should provide emergency systems access at competition sites and a mechanism for doing so at the housing site as well. In cases of severe injury or illness, the U.S. or Canadian consulate may be able to assist with information on local resources to provide appropriate care to injured or ill athletes.

INJURY MANAGEMENT PRINCIPLES

SERIOUS INJURIES

Serious injuries or illnesses may require hospitalization. It is important to remember that medical personnel are not usually licensed to practice in other countries. Plans for transport of injured or ill athletes should be established early. An athlete who is seriously ill in a

foreign country is often hospitalized in an environment where he or she may not speak the same language and the standards for treatment may differ markedly. It has been our experience that it is beneficial to evacuate a seriously injured athlete as soon as it is medically advisable.

MINOR INJURIES

Even minor injuries and illnesses that occur at the competition site may impact athlete participation in competition. It is inadvisable for an athlete with a fever to compete under any circumstances. Injuries that may become worse with continued physical activity should be identified. Athletes and coaching staff should be educated about the serious sequelae of continued activity. Medical staff members should enforce precautions and activity restrictions as needed and look to the team administrative leaders for support of those recommendations.

TABLE 42–8
Typical Responsibilities of Classification Committee Members

- Notification of certified classifiers
- Current classification manuals
- Current classification cards
- Appropriate medical information on athletes for classifiers
- Necessary evaluation equipment as outlined by classifiers
- Appropriate space for classifiers to classify athletes
- Processing table and staff to direct athletes
- Instruction sheet describing the classification process for coaches and athletes
- Arrangements for protest submission and hearings

ORGANIZATION OF DISABLED ATHLETIC EVENTS

The logistics of hosting and organizing an event for disabled athletes is an enormous task. The process of organizing an event is not a topic specific to this chapter, but therapists and other medical personnel are frequently asked to assume many roles when they become involved with event organizing committees. Most commonly, they are asked to provide medical coverage or, if certified as a classifier, to classify athletes or assume the role of a technical consultant. Tables 42–6, 42–7, and 42–8 list the specific needs of organizing, medical, and classification committees, respectively.

CONCLUSION

Sports medicine team members involved in disabled athletics have the ability to serve in many roles. The traditional role of providing emergency and rehabilitative medical care is only a fraction of the contribution that may be offered. Classifying, coaching, consulting with coaches, officiating, organizing, and administering are some of the many functions that medical personnel have the professional training and expertise to perform in order to enhance the overall performance of disabled athletes. Another integral responsibility that must be assumed by medical professionals is the education and recruitment of athletes through hospitals, rehabilitation centers, and other medical facilities where potential disabled athletes can be educated as to the availability of various sports organizations and quality training programs.

As the disabled athletics movement continues to flourish, and athletes continue to achieve physical feats once only imagined, the general public is beginning to recognize that the sporting events of physically challenged athletes are in fact demonstrations of true athleticism. With the support of health professionals, these athletes will be able to continue to maximize their performance with minimized injury risk.

REFERENCES

1. Paciorek MJ, Jones JA: Sports and Recreation for the Disabled: A Resource Manual. Indianapolis, Benchmark Press, 1989.
2. Weiss M, Curtis KA: Controversies in medical classification of wheelchair athletes. *In* Sherrill C. (ed): Sport and Disabled Athletes. Champaign, IL, Human Kinetics, 1986.
3. Strohkendl H: The new classification system for wheelchair basketball. *In* Sherrill C (ed): Sport and Disabled Athletes. Champaign, IL, Human Kinetics, 1986.
4. Curtis KA: Sport-specific functional classification for wheelchair athletes. Sports 'n' Spokes 1991; 17:45–48.
5. Richter KJ, Adams-Mushett C, Ferrara MS, McCann BC: Integrated swimming classification: a faulted system. APAQ 1992; 9:5–13.
6. Hay JG: The Biomechanics of Sports Techniques. Englewood Cliffs, NJ, Prentice-Hall, 1985.
7. Goldberg G, Shephard RJ: Personality profiles of disabled individuals in relation to physical activity patterns. J Sports Med 1982; 22:477–484.
8. Horvat M, French R, Henschen K: A comparison of the psychological characteristics of male and female able-bodied and wheelchair athletes. Paraplegia 1986; 24:115–122.
9. Sherrill C, Silliman L, Gench B, Hinson M: Self-actualisation of elite wheelchair athletes. Paraplegia 1990; 28:252–260.
10. Curtis KA, Dillon DA: Survey of wheelchair athletic injuries: common patterns and prevention. Paraplegia 1985; 23:170–175.
11. Ferrara MS, Davis RW: Injuries to elite wheelchair athletes. Paraplegia 1990; 28:335–341.
12. Ferrara MS, Buckley WE, McCann BC, et al: The injury experience of the competitive athlete with a disability: prevention implications. Med Sci Sports Exerc 1992; 24:184–188.
13. Curtis KA, McClanahan S, Hall KM, et al: Health, vocational, and functional status in spinal cord injured athletes and nonathletes. Arch Phys Med Rehabil 1986; 67:862–865.
14. Stotts KM: Health maintenance: paraplegic athletes and nonathletes. Arch Phys Med Rehabil 1986; 67:109–114.
15. Shephard RJ: Benefits of sport and physical activity for the disabled: implications for the individual and for society. Scand J Rehabil Med 1991; 23:51–59.
16. Sweeney FF, Foote JE: Treatment of drug and alcohol abuse in spinal cord injured veterans. Int J Addict 1982; 17:897–904.
17. McCormack DAR, Reid DC, Steadward RD, Syrotuik DG: Injury profiles in wheelchair athletes: results of a retrospective survey. Clin J Sport Med 1991; 1:35–40.
18. Aljure J, Eltorai I, Bradley WE, et al: Carpal tunnel syndrome in paraplegic patients. Paraplegia 1985; 23:182–186.
19. Gellman H, Sie I, Waters RL: Late complications of the weight-bearing upper extremity in the paraplegic patient. Clin Orthop Rel Res 1988; 233:132–135.
20. Burnham R, Newell E, Steadward R: Sports medicine for the physically disabled: the Canadian team experience at the 1988 Seoul Paralympic Games. Clin J Sport Med 1991; 1:193–196.
21. Sie I, Waters RL, Adkins RH, Gellman H: Upper extremity pain in the post rehabilitation spinal cord injured patient. Arch Phys Med Rehabil 1992; 73:44–48.
22. Burnham RS, Steadward RD: Upper extremity peripheral nerve entrapments among wheelchair athletes: prevalence, location and risk factors. Arch Phys Med Rehabil 1994; 75:519–524.
23. Bayley JC, Cochran TP, Sledge CB: The weightbearing shoulder-impingement syndrome in paraplegics. J Bone Joint Surg 1987; 69A:676–678.
24. Burnham RS, May L, Nelson E, Steadward R: Shoulder pain in wheelchair athletes—the role of muscle imbalance. Am J Sports Med 1993; 21:238–242.
25. Robinson MD, Hussey RW, Ha CY: Surgical decompression of impingement syndrome in the weight-bearing shoulder. Arch Phys Med Rehabil 1993; 74:324–332.
26. Neer CS: Anterior acromioplasty for the chronic impingement syndrome in the shoulder. J Bone Joint Surg 1972; 54A:41–50.
27. Barber DB, Gall NG: Osteonecrosis: an overuse injury of the shoulder in paraplegia: case report. Paraplegia 1991; 29:423–426.
28. Wilson PE, Washington RL: Pediatric wheelchair athletics: sports injuries and prevention. Paraplegia 1993; 31:330–337.
29. Burnham RS, Chan M, Hazlett C, et al: Acute median nerve dysfunction from wheelchair propulsion: the development of a model and study of the effect of hand protection. Arch Phys Med Rehabil 1994; 75:513–518.
30. Ganguli S, Datta SR, Chatterjee BB: Metabolic cost of walking at different speeds with patellar tendon bearing prosthesis. J Appl Physiol 1974; 36:440–443.
31. Gonzalez EG, Corcoran PJ, Reyes RL: Energy expenditure in below-knee amputees: correlation with stump length. Arch Phys Med Rehabil 1974; 55:111–119.
32. Molen NH: Energy/speed relation of below-knee amputees walking on motor-driven treadmill. Int Z Angew Physiol 1973; 31:173–185.
33. Pagliarulo MA, Waters R, Hislop HJ: Energy cost of walking of below-knee amputees having no vascular disease. Phys Ther 1979; 59:538–542.
34. Torburn L, Perry J, Ayyappa E, Shanfield SL: Below-knee amputee gait with dynamic elastic response prosthetic feet: a pilot study. J Rehabil Res Dev 1990; 27:369–384.

35. Waters RL, Perry J, Antonelli EE, et al: Energy cost of walking of amputees: the influence of level of amputation. J Bone Joint Surg 1976; 58A:42–46.

36. Waters RL, Yakura JS: The energy expenditure of normal and pathological gait. Crit Rev Phys Med 1989; 1:183.

37. Fisher SV, Gullickson G: Energy cost of ambulation in health and disability: a literature review. Arch Phys Med Rehabil 1978; 59:121–132.

38. Huang CT, Jackson JR, Moore NB, et al: Amputation: energy cost of ambulation. Arch Phys Med Rehabil 1979; 60:18–24.

39. James U: Oxygen uptake and heart rate during prosthetic walking in healthy male unilateral above-knee amputees. Scand J Rehabil Med 1973; 5:71–80.

40. Traugh GH, Corcoran PJ, Rudolpho LR: Energy expenditure of ambulation in patients with above-knee amputations. Arch Phys Med Rehabil 1975; 56:67–71.

41. Flandry E, Beskin J, Chambers R, et al: The effects of the CAT-CAM above-knee prosthesis on functional rehabilitation. Clin Orthop 1989; 239:249–262.

42. Gailey RS, Lawrence D, Burditt C, et al: The CAT-CAM socket and quadrilateral socket: a comparison of energy cost during ambulation. Prosthet Orthot Int 1993; 17:95–100.

43. DiAngelo DJ, Winter DA, Dhanjoo N, Newcombe WR: Performance assessment of the Terry Fox jogging prosthesis for above-knee amputees. J Biomech 1989; 22:543–558.

44. Enoka RM, Miller DI, Burgess EM: Below-knee amputee running gait. Am J Phys Med 1982; 61:68–84.

45. Winter DA, Sienko SE: Biomechanics of below-knee amputee gait. J Biomech 1988; 21:361–367.

46. Smith AW: A biomechanical analysis of amputee athlete gait. Int J Sports Biomech 1990; 6:262–282.

47. Czerniecki JM, Gitter A, Munro C: Joint moment and muscle power output characteristics of below knee amputees during running: the influence of energy storing prosthetic feet. J Biomech 1991; 24:63–75.

48. Corcoran PJ: Sports medicine and the physiology of wheelchair marathon racing. Orthop Clin North Am 1980; 11:697–716.

49. Arnheim DD: Modern Principles of Athletic Training, 6th ed. St. Louis, Times Mirror/Mosby College Publishing, 1985.

50. Roy S, Irvin R: Sports Medicine: Prevention, Evaluation, Management and Rehabilitation. Englewood Cliffs, NJ, Prentice-Hall, 1983.

51. Burnham R: Boosting self-induced autonomic dysreflexia in wheelchair athletes. Paper presented at Vista '93 Conference, Jasper, Alberta, Canada, May 19, 1993.

52. Raymond S: Using dysreflexia to enhance athletic performance: an athlete's opinion. Paper presented at Vista '93 Conference, Jasper, Alberta, Canada, May 19, 1993.

53. Good RA, Lorenz BA: Nutrition, immunity, aging, and cancer. Nutr Rev 1988; 46:62–67.

CHAPTER 43

Pharmacology and Drugs in Sports: Common Use, Abuse, and Testing

RON COURSON *PT, ATC, NREMT*
BILL McDONALD *MA, ATC*
JAMES B. ROBINSON *MD*
KEN WRIGHT *DA, ATC*

Humans have been using alcohol and plant-derived drugs for thousands of years, as far as is known, ever since *Homo sapiens* first appeared on the planet. Recorded history indicates that some of these drugs were used not just for their presumed therapeutic effects but also for recreational purposes. In some of the highly developed ancient cultures, psychoactive plants played important economic and religious roles. There is evidence that people have always overused, misused, or abused these substances. Although drugs appear to have always coexisted with humans, they certainly play a much different role in modern society than they did even 100 years ago. Major events have occurred in pharmacology and medicine that have produced revolutionary changes in the way drugs are viewed. In addition, recent cultural revolutions have influenced our attitudes and behavior regarding drugs and drug use.[1]

Drug use by athletes has been an unfortunate aspect of sports probably since the beginning of organized competition. It has been documented that the ancient Greeks used herbs and mushrooms in an attempt to improve athletic performance. Cyclists used stimulants in the nineteenth century to improve endurance, and anabolic and androgenic aids were first used during World War II to make German troops more aggressive.[2]

"There is no argument that drugs pose at least as serious a health problem in major league sports as they do in most high schools. By the time athletes have made the pros, most have been given so many pills, salves, injections, and potions by amateur and pro coaches, doctors, and trainers to pick them up, cool them down, kill pain, enhance performance, reduce inflammation, and erase anxiety that there isn't much they won't sniff, spread, stick in, or swallow to get bigger or smaller, or to feel good."[3] Athletes are at least as vulnerable to drug abuse as other members of society.[1,3,4] How did this happen? How do athletes become so involved in the use and abuse of drugs?

Society has become drug obsessed. Have a pain, take a pill. Want to lose weight, take a pill. Can't sleep, take a pill. Without a doubt, escalating medical and pharmaceutical advances, coupled with media sensationalism, have divided society into groups of pill poppers. Individuals are constantly told to say no. Yet society is confronted with the conflicting message, "If you've got an ill, take a pill."

As a result, it takes minimal knowledge to figure out where an athlete without proper guidance will go when seeking answers to questions such as how to become bigger, how to get stronger, and how to become fitter. Many are and will be looking to find their solutions in a pill. It is the "pill for every ill" mentality that has laid the foundation for global epidemic drug abuse and is the great lie of the present era. This deception promises solutions to problems when it in fact trades one problem for another one. It creates in individuals a dependency and an insecurity, a belief that one is inadequate. Individuals learn to rely on external potions rather than self-reliance on internal potential.

The "win at all costs" mentality often profanes athletics and promotes the message that winning isn't everything—it's the only thing. The influence of this mentality has been so profound as to shape the way athletes perceive themselves. Athletes often see their worth as human beings as being conditional on the outcome of their performance, creating tremendous stress and pressure to constantly improve and compete successfully. Put simply, one's value as a human being seems to be determined solely by what one does rather than who one is. The stress of success may prove risky for athletes, who by their nature are competitive and compulsive.

Coupled with the consent of self-serving coaches and agents, careless parents, and unscrupulous racketeers in a sports-crazed society, sports often promise escalating financial fortune and elevated social fame. It is no wonder that overly ambitious athletes are quick to embrace anything that promises the gaining of a competitive edge. In addition, it is important to remember that athletes did not make all their decisions on their own. Behind many successful athletes are small armies of supporters, family members, neighbors, and friends, all of them urging, cheering, cajoling, threatening, begging, supporting, criticizing, and pushing the athlete onward. Even though this is intended in the best interest of the competitor, it may push him or her toward dangerous activities. Some of these friends are quite willing for the athlete to do whatever is necessary to gain the edge that will enhance their own as well as the athlete's future.

In a survey conducted at the 1984 Summer Olympic Games in Los Angeles, 100 elite world-class athletes were asked, if there were a magic pill that would ensure them a gold medal, but it would mean losing their lives within the year, how many would take it. Fifty responded affirmatively.[5] In other words, winning was chosen over living.

The desire to win can be so great that athletes sometimes lose the concept of right and wrong as a result of being such single-minded, driven individuals. Sometimes it is difficult to view life as a whole, and sports goals may be the only true tangible goals perceived by an obsessed individual. These goals may totally dominate the obsessed athlete's life and effectively shut out any vision of a world beyond. In some athletes' minds, the present is a stairway of relatively minor competitions leading up to the moment when they have the opportunity to be the best in their designated sport.

TYPES OF DRUGS

Athletic performance can be influenced by several factors, including genetic composition, fitness level, skill level, diet, quality of the opponent, environment, health, coaching, location of competition, sleep, motivation, psychology, and luck. Also influencing performance are various drugs. Drug use by athletes can be divided into three categories: therapeutic drugs, recreational drugs, and performance enhancing drugs. Therapeutic drugs are any medication used by an athlete, either over-the-counter (OTC) or prescribed by a physician, to treat some injury or illness. Recreational drugs, or drugs of abuse, are chemicals that are used to alter the mental status of the user. These include alcohol, cocaine, marijuana, narcotics, and other "street drugs." Performance, or "ergogenic," drugs are those compounds that are used by athletes to gain a competitive edge over other athletes. These drugs are discussed in Chapter 15.

THERAPEUTIC DRUGS

The use of various oils, liniments, salves, and pills to treat ill or injured athletes is an extremely important aspect of the day-to-day care of these athletes. Often proper diagnosis and treatment can make a significant difference in the performance of an athlete, such that the outcome of an event may be influenced. Therapeutic medications can be divided into OTC medications and prescription medications. OTC medications include any compound that can be purchased by an individual without having been dispensed by a physician and used at the discretion of the purchaser. Although these drugs are generally considered safe, inappropriate use can cause severe adverse effects and even death. In the United States, drugs are approved by the Food and Drug Administration (FDA) and have strict dosing instructions and clearly labeled warnings. Unfortunately, even OTC medications can cause problems for athletes. For example, indiscriminate use of ibuprofen can cause gastric bleeding or kidney damage. Allergic reactions can occur, including anaphylaxis, if a preparation containing aspirin is ingested by someone who is sensitive to it. Another problem encountered by athletes taking OTC medications is the possibility of that drug being on a banned substance list and showing up in a drug screening. Unfortunately, this has happened to Olympic athletes on more than one occasion, resulting in disqualification or loss of a medal. As will be discussed later, the dispensing of OTC medications by athletic trainers, physical therapists, or individuals other than physicians is controversial, especially to minors. Even giving aspirin or acetaminophen (Tylenol) to a minor without a parent's consent could have legal ramifications. The best policy to observe is not to dispense any medications to minors and to be careful about distributing medications in any athletic setting.

Prescription medications are compounds that can be dispensed only by a person licensed to do so, such as a physician or dentist. In the United States, each state has its own regulations on the control of these medications, with ultimate guidelines provided by the Drug Enforcement Agency (DEA). The DEA has also developed a controlled drug system for the classification of prescription drugs that have the potential for abuse.[6] These range from Schedule I drugs that have a high potential for abuse and no accepted medical use, such as heroin and LSD, to Schedule V drugs that have a low potential for abuse and currently have accepted medical uses, such as codeine. All other medications in this classification (such as anti-inflammatory drugs and antibiotics) that are not scheduled need a prescription for dispensation. The following is a brief discussion of some of the therapeutic drugs used by sports medicine teams.

ANALGESICS

No sport is devoid of injury. The high demands of training and competition often lead to myriad injuries, ranging from acute traumatic injuries to chronic overuse injuries. Most of these injuries cause pain and are treated with various analgesics.

ACETAMINOPHEN (TYLENOL). Acetaminophen is by far the most common medication used to relieve pain, due to the fact that it is well tolerated, without many of the adverse effects associated with aspirin, and is available without a prescription. Acetaminophen is a major metabolite of one of the first antipyretic medications, phenacetin, first introduced in 1893.[7] It has analgesic and antipyretic effects similar to those of aspirin, but no anti-inflammatory effects. Once absorbed from the gastrointestinal tract, it has a peak onset of action in 30 to 60 minutes. It is available in tablets, capsules, suppositories, liquids, and combined with other medications. Dosage should not exceed 4000 mg per day. Adverse effects are rare. However, due to its metabolism by the liver, severe liver damage and even death can be caused by overingestion, whether accidental or intentional. The drug has no effect on physical performance other than to decrease pain, which may then permit activity.

OPIOID ANALGESICS

Opioids are a group of compounds that have morphine-like actions. Some of the more familiar opioid drugs are listed in Table 43–1. These medications are used to relieve moderate to severe pain not relieved by milder analgesics. Opium is derived from the seeds of the poppy plant *(Papaver somniferum)* and has been used since the third century B.C.[7] These compounds work at the central nervous system level by attaching to specific receptors for the body's own natural pain killers, enkephalins and endorphins. Opioids may have many effects, including analgesia, drowsiness, changes in

TABLE 43–1
Common Opioid Analgesics

Generic Name	Brand Name
Codeine	–
Morphine	–
Meperidine	Demerol
Hydrocodone	Lortab, Vicodin
Oxycodone	Percodan, Tylox
Propoxyphene	Darvocet
Pentazocine	Talwin
Heroin	–
Methadone	–

mood, respiratory depression, nausea, and a decrease in gastric mobility, which is useful to treat diarrhea but may also cause constipation. Opioids may also cause constriction of the pupils (pinpoint pupils), which is a telltale sign of their use and abuse. These compounds are all addictive. Tolerance may develop to prolonged use and produce physical dependence, characterized by withdrawal symptoms. They all can have an adverse impact on athletic performance due to their effects on the central nervous system.

Opioids must be administered only by a licensed physician and should never be given out by athletic trainers or physical therapists. They must be kept in a locked cabinet at all times. All opioids are on the banned drug lists except codeine, and they are often tested for in routine random drug screenings associated with amateur athletic events. Care must be taken with testing, however, as positive drug tests have been caused by the ingestion of foods with poppy seeds in them, such as bagels.

ANTI-INFLAMMATORY MEDICATIONS[8,9]

Nonsteroidal anti-inflammatory drugs (NSAIDs) are fast becoming the most popular medications used in the training room (Table 43–2). They have analgesic, antipyretic (fever reducing), and anti-inflammatory properties; therefore, they are often used to treat injuries and inflammatory conditions in athletes. All NSAIDs are chemically related to aspirin and work by inhibiting prostaglandin synthesis.

When tissue damage occurs either by macrotraumatic or microtraumatic means, the arachidonic cascade that produces prostaglandins is initiated (Fig. 43–1). These prostaglandins are responsible for the cardinal signs of inflammation—pain, swelling, erythema (redness), and warmth—by their action on the surrounding blood vessels and various inflammatory cells. When tissue is damaged, phospholipids in the cell membranes are exposed to surrounding enzymes, particularly phospholipase, which forms arachidonic acid. Arachidonic acid can then be converted either into leukotrienes, which have various effects on white blood cells, by the enzyme lipooxygenase, or into the various prostaglandins by the action of the enzyme cyclooxygenase.

TABLE 43–2
Common NSAIDs

Generic name	Brand Name
Acetylsalicylic acid	Aspirin
Choline salicylate	Arthropan
Diflunisal	Dolobid
Choline magnesium trisalicylate	Trilisate
Salsalate	Disalcid
Ibuprofen	Motrin, Rufen
Fenoprofen	Nalfon
Ketoprofen	Orudis, Oruvail
Naproxen	Naprosyn, Anaprox
Flurbiprofen	Ansaid
Indomethacin	Indocin
Sulindac	Clinoril
Tolmetin	Tolectin
Diclofenac	Voltaren
Meclofenamate	Meclomen
Nabumetone	Relafen
Oxaprozin	Daypro
Piroxicam	Feldene
Phenylbutazone	Butzolodin

Aspirin and NSAIDs inhibit the function of cyclooxygenase, thus prohibiting the formation of the various prostaglandins.

The prostaglandins PGD_2, PGE_2, and PGF_2 cause dilation of blood vessels and leakage of fluid into the surrounding tissues and work with other chemicals, such as histamine and bradykinin, to cause pain. Thromboxane A_2 causes constriction of blood vessels and platelet aggregation (clot formation). Prostacyclin (PGI_2) causes relaxation of blood vessels and bronchial tubes. Inhibition of these prostaglandins can help modify the inflammatory response and thus enhance the healing process and the return to normal activity.

The adverse effects of NSAIDs can all be linked to their inhibition of prostaglandins in all areas of the body. The action of NSAIDs is local, but the inhibition is indiscriminate. The most common adverse reaction is gastric upset, including nausea, vomiting, and bleeding ulcers. These reactions are due to the inhibition of the prostaglandins that produce a protective mucus coating of the stomach and intestinal lining but may also cause an increase in acid production. Other adverse effects include those on pregnancy and labor and kidney damage. NSAIDs can also inhibit platelet function similar to aspirin and thus prolong bleeding times. However, this effect is reversible with cessation of the drug, unlike aspirin. Injudicious use of OTC NSAIDs, aspirin, and acetaminophen can lead to severe adverse effects in some individuals. Therefore, the practice of athletic trainers and physical therapists suggesting their use should be discouraged.

ASPIRIN (ACETYLSALICYLIC ACID, OR ASA). Aspirin is derived from willow bark and has been used to reduce fever since the early 1800s. It belongs to a group of compounds called salicylates and was first developed by a chemist employed by Bayer and introduced in 1899.[7] Aspirin is a nonprescription medication and is the standard to which all other anti-inflammatories are compared. It is well tolerated by most people, but it can upset the stomach and thus tends to be coated (Empirin) or combined with an antacid (Ascriptin). It should be used with caution in children due to its role in the development of Reye syndrome (an acute disease of the brain occurring as a complication of viral infections that can cause seizures and death). Aspirin may also inhibit platelet cyclooxygenase, which prevents platelets from aggregating and thus thins the blood, which may prolong bleeding times. This effect lasts the lifetime of the platelet, which is generally 4 to 7 days. For this reason, aspirin should not be used in athletes who are at risk for hematoma formation or head injuries. The dose should not exceed 3600 mg per day. Toxic effects include salicylism, manifested by headache, nausea, tinnitus (ringing in ears), and even death. Aspirin has no effects on performance and is not a banned substance.

IBUPROFEN. Ibuprofen has been made available in a nonprescription form (Advil, Nuprin, Motrin) containing 200 mg per tablet. It is an analgesic at low doses (up to 1600 mg per day) and an anti-inflammatory at high doses (1800 to 3200 mg per day). It has adverse effects similar to those of all the NSAIDs, including stomach upset or bleeding stomach ulcers. It should not be dispensed or its use suggested by athletic trainers or physical therapists in doses equivalent to the prescription dosage (by increasing the number of pills taken) due to legal ramifications. It should not be used by athletes who are allergic to aspirin or other NSAIDs, by pregnant athletes, or by individuals with kidney damage. Prolonged indiscriminate use without a physician's knowledge should be discouraged. Ibuprofen has no adverse effect on athletic performance and is not a banned substance.

NAPROXEN. Naproxen sodium (Aleve) is the newest anti-inflammatory available over the counter. It is the same medication as prescription-strength Naprosyn

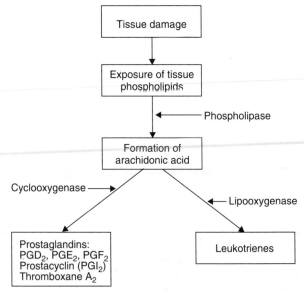

FIGURE 43–1. The arachidonic cascade.

and Anaprox but contains only 220 mg per tablet. The maximal suggested dose for analgesia is 660 mg per day, which is far lower than the anti-inflammatory dose of 1000 to 1500 mg per day. It has similar adverse effects and precautions as ibuprofen.

PRESCRIPTION NSAIDS. There are numerous prescription NSAIDs available today to be used in the armamentarium of the sports medicine physician. Each compound has its own set of advantages and uses, with the choice usually dependent on the physician's personal experience. NSAIDs are usually divided by chemical groups, but there is no uniform acceptance of the classification. Each manufacturer usually claims to be in a different chemical group, often confusing the issue. In general, an NSAID is chosen based on its effectiveness, ease of administration, cost, and adverse effects. Although drugs given once daily are easier to take and usually have a higher compliance rate, they are generally more expensive. The adverse effect profile is the same for each of the NSAIDs, as was discussed previously. If one NSAID does not appear to work or stops working after a period of use, switching to another chemical class or compound is often successful. None of these substances has an adverse effect on physical performance, and none is a banned substance.

CORTICOSTEROIDS. Corticosteroids are the most potent anti-inflammatories available for use in the athletic setting. This is due to their ability to inhibit the formation of both prostaglandins and leukotrienes by the inhibition of phospholipase (see Fig. 43–1). These chemicals are related to the steroids secreted by the adrenal cortex and are different from the anabolic-androgenic steroids used as ergogenic aids. Cortisone and its related compounds are classified as glucocorticoids. The effects of corticosteroids are numerous and widespread, affecting carbohydrate, protein, and lipid metabolism; electrolyte and water balance; and the immune system. Therefore, these drugs should be used with caution and for only short periods of time. Adverse effects include systemic reactions such as suppression of the pituitary gland, diabetes, osteoporosis, avascular necrosis of bone, high blood pressure, growth inhibition in children, and overwhelming infections. Injection of these preparations in joints can cause inhibition of articular cartilage formation, severe local reactions, and pain and may mask symptoms, leading to worsening of the effects of repetitive trauma to damaged tissue. Injection of these agents in soft tissue can lead to delayed wound healing, tendon rupture, loss of protective fat coverings, and loss of pigment in the skin.[10,11] The indiscriminate use of corticosteroids on the skin during phonophoresis and iontophoresis can cause the systemic effects discussed previously as well as severe, irreversible skin damage by loss of subcutaneous fat, loss of pigmentation, and thinning of the skin. Corticosteroid use should be strictly limited and under the direct supervision of a physician. The use of corticosteroids is banned by the International Olympic Committee (IOC) except for topical use, inhalation therapy, or local or intra-articular injection; however, any injection or oral use requires written notification to the IOC.[12]

DIMETHYL SULFOXIDE (DMSO). DMSO is a chemical solvent derived from wood processing that has little FDA-approved medical use. It is a very water- and fat-soluble chemical and is thus rapidly absorbed through the skin, which makes it useful to transport other chemicals such as local anesthetics and corticosteroids. However, DMSO can also transport impurities through the skin. It has its own unique effects by providing analgesia (through nerve blockade), vasodilation, muscle relaxation, anti-inflammatory action, and inhibition of bacterial growth.[13] DMSO is available in several preparations. A 50 percent solution is approved in the United States for treatment of interstitial cystitis, a 70 percent solution is approved for medicinal purposes by some states within the United States and Canada, a 90 percent solution is approved for veterinary use only, and a 99 percent solution is used as an industrial degreaser but contains too many impurities to be used by athletes. Studies show that at least a 70 percent solution must be used to achieve an anti-inflammatory effect.[14] Adverse effects include local redness and itching at the site of application, a garlic taste in the mouth, nausea, headache, and the transportation of impurities across the skin. The use of DMSO has also been demonstrated to cause clouding of the lens in the eyes of experimental rabbits, but this has not been demonstrated in humans.[14] Use of an unapproved form by athletic trainers, physical therapists, or physicians could have legal ramifications.

OTHER MEDICATIONS

Numerous other therapeutic medications—both OTC and prescription—are used by sports medicine personnel to help take care of the day-to-day injuries and illnesses of athletes. Each drug has its own set of clinical uses and specific adverse effects. Some of these may affect physical performance and thus should be used with caution. Many are banned substances that could disqualify an athlete. The following is a brief description of some of the more common classes of medications used.

ANTIBIOTICS. Antibiotics are medications available by prescription only and are used to fight infections, ranging from local skin infections to severe systemic infections such as pneumonia and kidney infections. There are numerous antibiotics available, and the choice by a physician usually depends on the site of the infection, the most likely pathogen involved, age of the patient, drug allergies, physician experience with the drug, concurrent medical illnesses, cost, dosing interval, results of cultures and sensitivity tests, and local resistant patterns to antibiotics by bacteria.

The most common group of antibiotics used are the penicillins and related compounds such as amoxicillin, ampicillin, and the cephalosporins (such as Keflex, Ceclor, and Suprax). For individuals allergic to penicillin, antibiotics such as erythromycin or tetracycline are used. Some of the newer antibiotics have the advantage of requiring only one dose per day but are usually considered overkill and are often cost prohibitive.

All antibiotics have adverse reactions, ranging from nausea, diarrhea, and skin rash to severe systemic anaphylactic shock. They should be used with caution in athletes taking birth control pills because of the decreased effectiveness of the oral contraceptives when combined with antibiotics. Antibiotics have no effect on physical performance, although the condition that is being treated may. They are not banned by any organization.

ANTIHYPERTENSIVE MEDICATIONS. Drugs used to treat high blood pressure are often taken by athletes with this condition. There are several different classes of antihypertensives, each with its own unique mode of action.[15] Beta blockers such as Inderal are common first-line drugs for the treatment of hypertension. However, their use by athletes should be limited due to a possible adverse effect on performance as a result of decreased maximum heart rate, decreased cardiac output, increased severity of exercise-induced bronchospasm, and development of muscle fatigue caused by decreased stores of metabolic substrates. Beta blockers are banned by the IOC owing to their calming effects and the consequent steadiness that can be achieved by athletes in shooting sports such as riflery, biathlon, and archery.

Diuretics should be avoided because they may cause dehydration and place an athlete at risk for heat illness. They are banned substances due to their ability to alter the integrity and validity of urine samples used in drug testing by diluting the concentration of the urine and producing a more rapid excretion of drugs. Diuretics also produce a fluid loss, which could assist athletes who want to deliberately lose weight in order to compete in a lower weight class. Such use is banned.

There are several classes of antihypertensive medications that are used by athletes because they have little or no effect on physical performance and are not banned. These include calcium channel blockers (Procardia, verapamil), angiotensin converting enzyme (ACE) inhibitors (Vasotec, Capoten), and vasodilators such as terazosin (Hytrin) and prazosin (Minipress).

COUGH AND COLD PREPARATIONS. There are multitudes of drugs available for the treatment of coughs, colds, and upper respiratory infections. Most of these are OTC preparations. Decongestants are medications that decrease the swelling of the mucous membranes by constriction of the blood vessels. They are generally classified as sympathomimetic and are thus banned by the IOC because of their stimulant effects. They are used for the treatment of nasal congestion associated with cold and flu symptoms. However, one must be careful in advising athletes who are subjected to drug screening, because even most nasal sprays are prohibited because of the medications they contain.

Antihistamines are a class of drug used to treat the symptoms associated with common seasonal allergies such as sneezing, watery eyes, and nasal drainage. They do this by their inhibition of histamine, which is responsible for these symptoms. All antihistamines except the newer prescription antihistamines—terfenadine (Seldane), loratadine (Claritin), and astemizole (Hismanal)—are sedating and must be used with caution in active athletes. Because of their sedating effect, some antihistamines may be useful as a sleep aid for some athletes with insomnia. The pure antihistamines are not banned, but combination products with decongestants are not allowed.

Cough preparations contain several different medications to prevent cough. The OTC medications that contain only dextromethorphan, which is not a banned substance, may be used. Caution must be observed, however, because many cough preparations also contain banned decongestants. Prescription cough preparations usually contain codeine or a synthetic codeine such as hydrocodone. Although codeine is not banned, hydrocodone is. These medications are also usually sedating. One cough preparation available by prescription only, benzonatate (Tessalon Perles), is useful in athletes due to its nonsedating activity and is not a banned substance.

GASTROINTESTINAL MEDICATIONS. Most of the medications used to treat various gastrointestinal problems such as nausea, vomiting, and diarrhea are not banned substances. Most antinausea medications such as promethazine hydrochloride (Phenergan) are classified as antihistamines and are thus allowed, but they may cause sedation. Antidiarrheal medications except paregoric are allowed, but the combination of diphenoxylate hydrochloride and atropine sulfate (Lomotil) is chemically related to meperidine (Demerol) and may cause severe drowsiness, so it must be used with caution in athletes. Although once banned, it is now approved by the IOC. All medications used to treat gastritis and peptic ulcer disease, such as antacids, are approved.

ASTHMA MEDICATIONS. In 1984, 11 percent of the athletes competing in the Summer Olympic Games in Los Angeles had asthma or exercise-induced bronchospasm, and a total of 41 medals were won by these athletes. Medications used to treat asthma can be divided into several categories. Specific β agonists are the most common medications used to treat asthma in athletes. Only albuterol (Ventolin, Proventil) and terbutaline (Brethaire) are approved in the inhalant or nasal form and must have prior written approval by the IOC. All other β agonists are now banned. Sympathomimetic medications such as ephedrine are classified as stimulants and are banned by the IOC. The inhaled corticosteroids beclomethasone, dexamethasone, triamcinolone, and flunisolide, as well as cromolyn (Intal) and nedocromil (Tilade), are approved and are useful as adjunct therapy. Theophylline is also approved for the treatment of asthma in athletes.

THERAPEUTIC MEDICATION DISPENSATION

LEGAL CONSIDERATIONS

In the United States, federal and state laws and codes govern the storage, handling, dispensation, and documentation of the use of therapeutic medications. Only qualified personnel are permitted to prescribe or dispense medications.[16–27] Questions often arise regarding the role of nonphysicians and pharmacists in medication prescription and dispensation. Legal proceedings have questioned the involvement of athletic trainers in dispensing both OTC and prescription drugs.[6,19,20,23,28]

Hawkins[19] states that athletic trainers should perform only those acts that are consistent with their professional qualifications and existing legal regulations. The same holds true for other sports medicine clinicians such as physical therapists. Among the most legally compromising situations is that in which an athletic trainer or physical therapist performs a function for which he or she is not qualified or is not permitted by law to perform. It is every athletic trainer's and physical therapist's responsibility to know his or her professional limitations and restrictions as specified by existing sports medicine legislation, and to perform only those acts that are consistent with personal professional qualifications and legal regulations. For example, prescription medications should not be dispensed by an athletic trainer, since such an act would be inconsistent with the professional qualifications and the legal regulations governing the provision of sports medicine services.[19]

In addition to federal and state laws regarding medication dispensation, athletic trainers and physical therapists must be aware of state laws that regulate their professions. Thirty states in the United States currently have some type of athletic training practice regulation, ranging from licensure to certification to registration to exemption. All 50 states have physical therapy practice regulations. There are variances in practice acts from state to state. Therefore, it is paramount that practicing athletic trainers and physical therapists be familiar with state laws. In those states without specific athletic training credentialing, the athletic trainer should obtain a copy of the state's medical practice act to determine the scope and setting of practice permitted to athletic trainers and other health care providers.[29]

All athletic trainers and physical therapists should be concerned with pharmaceutical regulations, but athletic trainers and physical therapists working within collegiate and professional sports may have more requirements regarding dispensation practices. Typically, athletic trainers and physical therapists who treat athletes in the sports medicine clinical setting are following patients under the care of private physicians and are generally out of the pharmaceutical loop. Due to legal considerations in dealing with minors, many high school sports medicine providers are restricted from dispensing even OTC medications.[23]

Research sponsored by the National Collegiate Athletic Association (NCAA) in 1985 revealed that prescription medications were being provided to student-athletes by persons other than legally authorized physicians.[30] A 1991 study sponsored by the NCAA on drug distribution in athletics programs revealed that this practice has not changed.[21–23,31,32] Seventy percent of the Division I institutions studied dispensed prescription medications from the training room. Forty-seven percent of the athletic trainers questioned dispensed prescription medications from the training room, and 23 percent dispensed them while traveling without a

physician. The research also showed that state and federal regulations regarding packaging, labeling, record keeping, and storage of medications are being overlooked or disregarded when medications are dispensed from the training room. Many states have recently adopted more restrictive regulations regarding packaging, labeling, record keeping, and storage of prescription and nonprescription medications. Athletic departments must be concerned about the risks to student-athletes when these regulations are not followed.[21,22,31,32] In the preface to the 1991 NCAA study, the investigators stated, "It should be made clear that the investigators believe that athletics personnel involved in this study truly tried to act in the best interest of the athlete and did not knowingly violate any laws."[31,32] However, the old adage "ignorance of the law is no excuse" is applicable in this situation. Sports medicine personnel must be aware of both federal and state statutes and how they may impact their professional practice.

The NCAA *Sports Medicine Handbook*'s guideline for dispensing prescription medication states: "Physicians cannot delegate the authority for dispensing prescription medications to athletic trainers under current medication dispensing laws, since athletic trainers are not authorized by law to dispense under any circumstances. The improper delegation of authority by the physician or the dispensing of prescription medications by the athletic trainer (even with permission of the physician) places both parties at risk for legal liability."[25,26,31,32]

Drug dispensation practices are subject to, and should be in compliance with, all state, federal, and DEA regulations. Federal laws include the Federal Food, Drug, Cosmetic Act; Federal Controlled Drug Act; Fair Packaging and Labeling Act; USP official standards; and Federal Anti-Tampering Act. State laws include controlled substances acts, pharmacy acts, and professional practice acts. State laws and codes should be consulted, as there are variations from state to state.[22] When there are variations between federal and state laws, an acceptable practice is to comply with the more stringent law.[24]

POLICIES AND PROCEDURES

In the collegiate and professional sports setting, the sports medicine team may maintain inventories of both OTC and prescription medications for dispensation. Many team physicians maintain a medical kit stocked for travel. A commercially prepared emergency kit, such as the Banyan Stat Kit, may be utilized by the physician. These emergency kits contain various drugs, many of which are in prefilled syringes for quick preparation and administration. This enables the physician to initiate treatment in many emergencies, including cardiac and allergic reactions. The sports medicine team may also maintain small amounts of medications in a secured storage area in the athletic training facility or physician examination room so that initial starter doses may be dispensed to the athlete in the interim period before the physician's prescription can be filled.

In the event that medications are dispensed in the practice of sports medicine, the sports medicine team should develop written policies and procedures to ensure that dispensation is carried out safely, appropriately, and within legal guidelines. The following concerns should be addressed:

1. LEGAL COMPLIANCE. The sports medicine team should be cognizant of state regulations regarding the dispensation of medications and ensure compliance with the law. Investigations and legal cases have arisen in recent years involving procedures for dispensing medications in the athletic training room.[6,23]

2. APPROPRIATE PERSONNEL AND STATE LICENSURE. Medication should be dispensed by the appropriate personnel who are licensed by the state to perform such a task. The 1991 NCAA study found that unqualified personnel in the athletic department were often dispensing prescription and nonprescription medication to athletes. Responsibilities that should have been handled by a team physician or a pharmacist were routinely being performed by athletic trainers, assistants, and student trainers.[21–23] This activity may be construed as practicing medicine and/or pharmacy without a license.

3. PROPER PACKAGING AND LABELING. In the past, many sports medicine providers dispensed medicine to athletes in small white pill envelopes or medicine tins. However, this practice does not follow packaging and labeling regulations. In the United States, the FDA requires the following information as a minimum to be included on the labels of medicines: the name of the patient, the date the substance was dispensed, the name and quantity of the substance, instruction for administration, the name of the physician prescribing the medication, and a statement explaining what the drug is intended to be used for. State laws may require the name and address of the pharmacy, the address of the patient, the name of the manufacturer or distributor, and the strength and name of the drug. On repackaged medication, some state and federal laws require the lot number, manufacturer, and expiration date. In addition, containers must often be child and light resistant.[22,23]

4. DRUG DISTRIBUTION RECORDS. Extensive and accurate medication dispensation records should be kept. The following information should be recorded as a minimum: patient name, date, medication, strength, dosage, injury or illness, allergies, pertinent history, and signature of the individual dispensing the medication.[2,20,23,25] It should be noted that all medications, whether purchased from a licensed distributor or received in the form of sample packages, must be documented in the same fashion.[2] Accountability remains constant in the issuance of all pharmacologic substances.[16,18] The sports medicine team should have a policy for record retention and be aware that some states have regulations for maintaining files for athletic departments within state-funded organizations.

5. STORAGE CONSIDERATIONS AND SECURITY. Medications should be housed in a secure and protective environment. It must be realized that medications are chemical compounds and will degrade if stored in a less than optimal environment. Most medications should be housed in an environment between 59° and 86°F (15° to 30°C); however, some medications must be refrigerated. Light may affect a medication, as may movement.[22] For example, carrying drugs in a travel kit may cause rapid breakdown due to excessive movement. If prescription medications are kept in the sports medicine facility, they should be stored in a minimum double-lock facility, with only the physician and/or pharmacist having a key to the medication cabinet. Prescriptive treatment medications, such as iontophoresis medications and Fluoro-Methan, should also be stored under lock and key. Travel kits containing medications should be locked or kept in a locked storage area. OTC medications should also be secured.

6. INVENTORY. Medications should be inventoried on a regular basis, checking expiration dates and properly disposing of expired medications.

7. TRAVEL KIT GUIDELINES. Emergency and travel kits should be routinely inspected for drug quality and security, especially to make sure that movement from travel has not caused medication breakdown or damage. Prescription drugs should not be carried in the travel kit unless authorized by a state pharmacy board and by a physician's authorizing letter. However, it is appropriate for the athletic trainer to carry specific medications that have been prescribed for an individual athlete, such as allergy medication or a bronchodilator for an athlete with exercise-induced asthma. Care must be taken to carefully document medications dispensed from the travel kit, just as medications are documented when dispensed from the pharmacy, physician office, or sports medicine facility. The travel kit should be kept locked and stored in a locked area when not in use.

8. PATIENT EDUCATION. In the United States, federal and state regulations have placed an increased emphasis on patient education regarding the use of medications. When dispensed a medication, an athlete should be instructed in the type and purpose of the medication, proper dosage and administration, precautions, and possible adverse effects. A medication history should be obtained to ensure that the athlete has no allergy to the medication and is not currently taking any other medications that could possibly react with the prescribed medication. The sports medicine staff may utilize commercially prepared medication information cards or devise their own. With the increased health awareness today, the sports medicine staff may regularly encounter questions regarding medications and should be prepared to provide up-to-date factual information in an understandable form. Updated medication reference guides should be maintained to provide information.

9. BANNED MEDICATIONS. Before dispensing any medications, the sports medicine team must ensure that the specific medication is not a banned substance. A number of OTC and prescription medications are banned by certain athletic organizations and/or sports governing bodies. Additionally, some vitamin, herbal, and nutritional supplements may contain banned substances. Failure to check these reference lists may inadvertently cause an athlete to test positive for a banned substance on a drug test, such as those conducted by the NCAA, the USOC, or the IOC. Reference guides detailing banned substances are available. Additionally, the USOC maintains a drug hot line (1-800-233-0393) to provide further information or clarification. When in doubt, the sports medicine team should not dispense a medication until checking with the appropriate resource. Additionally, the athlete should be advised to declare any OTC or prescription medication usage prior to taking a drug test.

10. FOLLOW-UP. With the administration of any OTC or prescription medication, the sports medicine team should closely follow the athlete to ensure that the medication has the desired effects and that no drug interactions or complications arise.

RECOMMENDATIONS

The dispensation of medications is a complex issue that is governed by a wide range of federal and state regulations. The sports medicine team should ensure that strict compliance with these measures is maintained at all times. The dispensing of prescription medications should be performed by individuals licensed to perform such duties—the physician and the pharmacist. Patient education should accompany the dispensation of any medication, and strict documentation should be maintained.

RECREATIONAL DRUG USE

Unfortunately, recreational drug use is a part of sports, just as it is for society as a whole. Athletes find themselves associating with social groups and friends and frequenting clubs in which alcohol is served, just as nonathletes do. They succumb to the same pressures that other young people face in society today regarding experimentation with and use of alcohol and drugs. Contrary to popular belief, athletes do not use alcohol or drugs more frequently than their nonathlete counterparts; however, often due to their newsworthy status, more is heard of athletes with drug problems. The following is a brief description of some of the common recreational drugs used by athletes.

ALCOHOL. Alcohol has been a part of society since the beginning of recorded history. It has been used as a drug, food, medicine, solvent, and religious ritual. The problems associated with excessive alcohol use are well publicized. Approximately 13.3 million individuals in the United States have alcohol-related problems.[2] Half of motor vehicle fatalities each year are alcohol related, and alcohol is responsible for 98,000 deaths per year.[2] However, alcohol remains a legal substance and is the number one substance of abuse in teenagers.

Recent studies have indicated that there is no difference in alcohol use, attitudes toward alcohol, or problems associated with alcohol between athletes and nonathletes.[33] However, one study indicated that college athletes had a higher proportion of risk-taking behavior than nonathletes, including consuming larger quantities of alcohol per sitting and driving more

frequently while intoxicated, as well as a greater family history of alcohol or drug abuse.[34]

Alcohol functions as a central nervous system depressant by interfering with the reticular activating system and cerebral cortex. These effects are directly related to the blood concentration and alcohol tolerance. Dependency can develop. Alcohol has an adverse effect on performance by impairing balance and steadiness, reaction time, fine and complex motor coordination, visual tracking, and information processing. It has no effect on endurance and may have a calming effect on athletes in whom tension and tremors may affect performance, such as marksmen. Alcohol is thus banned by the IOC.

MARIJUANA. Marijuana is derived from the plant *Cannabis sativa.* The principal active compound is δ-9-tetrahydrocannabinol (THC). Although marijuana is the most common illegal drug used by adolescents, a recent study indicates a slight decline in usage among college athletes from 36 to 28 percent.[30] Effects from inhalation or ingestion include decreased attention span and concentrating ability, decreased memory, relaxation, and euphoria, but it can cause excitement or anxiety. Its adverse effects on athletes can be attributable to its distortion of visual perception, decrement in psychomotor performance, and distortion of time. Marijuana has also been associated with the so-called antimotivational syndrome, characterized by apathy, impaired judgment, and loss of ambition. Adverse effects with long-term use include chronic respiratory problems, impaired immunity, decreased sperm production, gynecomastia, and tachycardia. It may produce tolerance as well as physical and psychological dependence. It is banned by the IOC.

COCAINE. The use of cocaine by athletes has drawn widespread media attention, especially with the deaths of such athletes as Len Bias and Don Rogers in 1986. Almost daily one is bombarded with information about athletes and nonathletes who use and abuse cocaine and crack. The 1989 study by Anderson et al.,[30] however, showed a decrease in cocaine usage from 17 to 5 percent in collegiate athletes.

Cocaine is derived from the coca plant and is classified as a stimulant. It was first used as a local anesthetic in the 1800s but rapidly became a drug of abuse. Cocaine works by potentiating the action of catecholamines in the central nervous system, thus elevating mood, decreasing fatigue, increasing activity, and producing euphoria. It can be used orally, nasally, intravenously, or by inhalation.

Cocaine's effects on performance are debatable. Some experts believe that cocaine may be ergogenic by increasing muscle strength and reaction time, like amphetamines. However, most think that cocaine's effects are detrimental to athletic performance, and it is thus not classified as an ergogenic drug.

More disturbing are the adverse effects associated with cocaine use. The most widely recognized are its effects on the cardiovascular system, such as arrhythmias, myocardial infarction, and even sudden death. Other adverse effects include stroke, seizures, psychosis, anorexia, increased risk of heatstroke, and addiction.

Cocaine is an illegal substance and is banned by the IOC.

DRUG TESTING

Drug testing began with the 1968 Olympic games. Since that time, each Olympic Committee has spent considerable amounts of money to equip a drug testing laboratory. In January 1986, the member institutions of the NCAA voted overwhelmingly to expand the NCAA drug education program to include mandatory drug testing during and after NCAA championship events. The major goals of both organizations are to protect the health of athletes and to help ensure that competition is fair and equitable. It is not, however, the intent of this text to provide a detailed description of how to set up a drug testing program. The *U.S. Olympic Committee Drug Education Handbook*[35] and L. E. Bolling's *NCAA Drug Testing/Education Programs*[36] are excellent resources that detail how to set up a drug testing program. These publications are available through the USOC and the NCAA.

Drug testing is a controversial issue in contemporary athletics. Although most of the discussion about drug testing has centered on its legal ramifications, drug testing is now standard practice in national and international competitions. Reviewing the legal ramifications of drug testing is beyond the scope of this chapter, so discussion is limited to specific components of a drug testing program that must be in place before an athlete is tested for a banned substance. The NCAA has established the following guidelines for colleges and universities that are considering implementing a drug testing program:

1. The college's or university's legal counsel must be kept informed at every stage, particularly in regard to right-to-privacy statutes.
2. Before initiating drug testing, a specific written policy on drug testing should be developed, distributed, and publicized. The policy should include such information as (a) a clear explanation of the purposes of the program; (b) the drugs to be tested for, how often, and under what conditions; and (c) actions to be taken, if any, against an athlete who tests positive.
3. An appropriate waiver form should be developed wherein the athlete agrees to submit to drug testing.
4. The types of drugs to be tested for must be determined. The NCAA provides schools with a list of its banned substances. The NCAA and IOC have similar banned substance lists and update their lists annually. It is advisable that all athletes be made aware of these lists so that they, along with their physicians and athletic trainers, can make sure that any medications they are presently using are not banned.

Logistical aspects of a drug testing program must also be in place before any athlete is tested. These administrative components include:

1. When, from whom, and how will urine samples be collected, secured, and transported to the laboratory?
2. Who will select the laboratory that will analyze the urine samples? Questions concerning the laboratory staff's qualifications and experience with drug testing need to be addressed. Does the laboratory have the necessary equipment to test the types of drugs to be analyzed?
3. How will urine samples be stored, and how soon will analysis be initiated?
4. What type of analytic procedures will be conducted? Radioimmunologic assay or gas chromatography? Is the laboratory capable of performing mass spectrometry analysis as well?
5. What are the laboratory's false-positive and false-negative rates?
6. How will false-positives be identified and processed?
7. Who will receive the test results, and how will the results be used?

It is important throughout the entire process to protect the athlete's right to privacy and to make available to the athlete materials and resources on drug education and related topics.

During a drug test, a urine specimen is analyzed for any substances on the list of banned drugs. A careful procedure is followed to ensure that no cheating on the part of the athlete is taking place and to ensure as much accuracy as possible. The anonymity of the athlete is maintained at all times. For routine screening, the more economical thin-layer chromatography (TLC) or gas-liquid chromatography (GLC) is used. When either one is positive, to obtain positive drug identification, gas chromatography–mass spectrometry is used. This method is extremely sensitive and is able to confirm selective drugs with almost 100 percent certainty, and it provides legally admissible data. Drug testing programs should be random to ensure success and to avoid being financially prohibitive. It must be realized that no system or device is completely failproof. False-positives can occur. Great care must be taken that an athlete's personal rights are not violated.

The question of who should perform the routine collection and testing of urine arises when considering drug testing. In many programs, the athletic trainer is given this responsibility. This, however, undermines what the athletic trainer stands for—an impartial, unbiased health professional who, in many cases, is a confidant to the athlete. Whenever possible, an outside organization should run the drug testing program. If the athletic trainer must be involved with the program, he or she should be removed as far as possible from the actual testing phase. Any drug testing program must stay within state legal guidelines and at all times must be confidential and concerned with the well-being of the athlete.

One of the most important aspects of any drug testing program is how a positive test result is handled. Before a drug testing program is initiated, there must be specific

TABLE 43–3
Doping Classes

A. Stimulants
Amphetamines
Cocaine
Caffeine (>12 mcg/ml)
Ephedrine

B. Narcotics
Codeine
Morphine
Pethidine and related compounds

C. Anabolic Agents
Nandrolone
Stanozolol
Testosterone and related compounds

D. Diuretics
Furosemide
Triamterene
Hydrochlorothiazide and related compounds

E. Peptide Hormones and Analogues
Growth hormone
Human chorionic gonadotropin
Adrenocorticotropic hormone
EPO (Erythropoietin)

policies that clearly state what the treatment plan and course of action will be if an athlete's drug test is positive. Only the team physician should be aware of the results of the drug tests. This eliminates any potential invasion of privacy and prevents harmful gossip. The team physician is responsible for implementing the treatment plan to ensure that an athlete receives proper medical care and counseling for any potential abuse pattern. Specific steps in the initiation of treatment, counseling, and further testing must be clearly delineated. Punitive action must be withheld until these appropriate steps have been completed. In the event of repeated offenses, the athlete will lose his or her right to privacy, and coaches, athletic director, and parents will be notified so that proper communication and punitive action can be initiated. Each institution must decide what punitive action will be taken in each case and how to handle repeat offenders. It is imperative that athletes be given every possible chance to "clean up their acts" so that they do not fall into the same abuse patterns once they leave the institution.

GUIDE TO BANNED MEDICATIONS

Most associations that govern athletic competition classify "doping" as the administration of or use by a competing athlete of any substance foreign to that body or any physiological substance, taken in abnormal quantity or taken by an abnormal route of entry into the body with the sole intention of increasing in an artificial and unfair manner his/her performance in competition.

As a result of this problem, banned medications have been outlined (Table 43–3). An athlete's misuse of drugs threatens the health of the athlete, the dignity of amateur sport, and public support. Before taking any medication prior to competition, the athlete should have it verified by the head physician or some other knowledgeable member of the sports medicine staff for that specific event. In addition, prior to drug testing athletes should always declare every drug or substance that they are taking.

REFERENCES

1. Ray O, Dsir C: Drugs, Society, and Human Behavior. St. Louis, Times-Mirror/Mosby, 1990.
2. Wadler GI, Hainline B: Drugs and the Athlete. Philadelphia, FA Davis, 1989, pp 234–237.
3. Lipsyte R: Baseball and drugs. The Nation, May 23, 1988, p 613.
4. Ryen AJ: Causes and remedies of drug misuse and abuse by athletes. JAMA 1984; 252:517.
5. Goldman B: Death in The Locker Room. Chicago, Elite Sports Medicine Publications, 1992.
6. Whitehill WR, Wright KE, Robinson JB: Guidelines for dispensing medications. J Athletic Training 1992; 27:20–22.
7. Goodman A, Gillman A: The Pharmacological Basis of Therapeutics, 8th ed. Elmsford, CT, Pergamon Press, 1990.
8. Clyman B: Role of NSAIDs in sports medicine. Sports Med 1986; 3:242–246.
9. Simon LE, Mills JA: Nonsteroidal anti-inflammatory drugs: Parts 1 and 2. N Engl J Med 1980; 302:1179–1185, 1237–1243.
10. Karpman RR, McComb JE, Voltz RG: Tendon rupture following local steroid injection: report of four cases. Postgrad Med 1980; 68:169–174.
11. Noyes FR, Grood E, Nussbaum N: Effect of intraarticular corticosteroids on ligament properties. Clin Orthop Rel Res 1977; 123:197–209.
12. United States Olympic Committee Drug Education and Doping Control Program. Colorado Springs, United States Olympic Committee, May 27, 1993.
13. Jacob SW, Herschler R: Biological actions of dimethylsulfoxide. Ann NY Acad Sci 1975; 243:1–508.
14. Percy EC, Carsen JD: The use of DMSO in tennis elbow and rotator cuff tendinitis: a double blind study. Med Sci Sports Exerc 1981, 13:215–219.
15. Lund-Johnson PER: Exercise and antihypertensive therapy. Am J Cardiol 1987; 59:98A–107A.
16. Administrative functions, practices and procedures. In Code of Federal Regulations, title 21, part 1316. Washington, DC, Drug Enforcement Administration, Department of Justice, 1990; pp 222–225.
17. Arnheim DD, Prentice WE: Drugs and sports. In Arnheim DD, Prentice WE (eds): Principles of Athletic Training, 8th ed. St. Louis, Mosby–Year Book, 1993, pp 385–417.
18. General enforcement regulation. In Code of Federal Regulations, title 21, part 1. Washington, DC, Food and Drug Administration, Health and Human Services, 1990, pp 5–7.
19. Hawkins JD: Legal aspects of sports medicine services. In Hawkins JD (ed): The Practical Delivery of Sports Medicine Services: A Conceptual Approach. Canton, OH, PRC Publishing, 1993, pp 31–48.
20. Herbert DL: Dispensing prescription medications to athletes. In Herbert, DL (ed): The Legal Aspects of Sports Medicine. Canton, OH, Professional Sports Publications, 1991, pp 215–224.
21. Laster-Bradley M, Berger BA: Evaluation of drug distribution systems in university athletics programs: Development of a model or optimal drug distribution system for athletics programs. Unpublished report, 1991.
22. Laster-Bradley M: Drug distribution in college athletics. Presentation at NATA Annual Clinical Symposium, Denver, 1992.
23. Pharmaceuticals in the training room. Dallas, TX, National Athletic Trainers Association, February 1994; pp 4–5, 27.

24. Pharmacy Law Digest. St. Louis, JB Lippincott, 1987, pp CS-4, DC16–19.

25. Prentice WE: Pharmacological considerations in a rehabilitation program. *In* Prentice WE (ed): Rehabilitation Techniques in Sports Medicine. St. Louis, Times Mirror/Mosby, 1990, pp 140–150.

26. Ray R: Management Strategies in Athletic Training. Champaign, IL, Human Kinetics, 1994.

27. Tucker AM: Prescription and over-the-counter medications. Presentation at American Sports Medicine Institute—Injuries in Football. Birmingham, AL, 1992.

28. Drugs in sports. *In* Athletic Training and Sports Medicine, 2nd ed. Park Ridge, IL, American Academy of Orthopaedic Surgeons, 1991.

29. Ray R: Management Strategies in Athletic Training. Champaign, IL, Human Kinetics, 1994.

30. Anderson WA, McDeag DB, McGrew CA: A national survey of alcohol and drug use by college athletes. Phys Sports Med 1991; 19:91–104.

31. NCAA Sports Medicine Handbook, 5th ed. Overland Park, KS, National Collegiate Athletic Association, 1992.

32. NCAA Sports Medicine Handbook, 7th ed. Overland Park, KS, National Collegiate Athletic Association, 1994.

33. Overman SJ, Terry T: Alcohol use and attitudes: A comparison of college athletes and non-athletes. J Drug Educ 1991; 21:107–117.

34. Nattiv A, Puffer JC: Lifestyles and health risks of college athletes. J Fam Pract 1991; 33:585–590.

35. United States Olympic Committee Drug Education Program. United States Olympic Committee, Colorado Springs, 1994.

36. Benton MT: 1993–94 NCAA Drug-Testing Education Program. Overland Park, KS, National Collegiate Athletic Association, 1994.

INDEX